HANDBUCH DER HAUT- UND GESCHLECHTSKRANKHEITEN

J. JADASSOHN
ERGÄNZUNGSWERK

BEARBEITET VON

G. ACHTEN · J. ALKIEWICZ · R. ANDRADE · R. D. AZULAY · H.-J. BANDMANN · L. M. BECHELLI
M. BETETTO · H. H. BIBERSTEIN † · R. M. BOHNSTEDT · G. BONSE · S. BORELLI · W. BORN
O. BRAUN-FALCO · I. BRODY · S. R. BRUNAUER · W. BURCKHARDT · J. CABRÉ · F.T. CALLOMON†
C. CARRIÉ · H. CHIARI · G. B. COTTINI · H. J. CRAMER · R. DOEPFMER † · G. DOTZAUER · CHR.
EBERHARTINGER · H. EBNER · G. EHLERS · G. EHRMANN · R. A. ELLIS · A. ENGELHARDT · F.
FEGELER · E. FISCHER · H. FISCHER · H. FLEISCHHACKER · H. FRITZ-NIGGLI · H. GÄRTNER
O. GANS · M. GARZA TOBA · P. E. GEHRELS · H. GÖTZ · L. GOLDMAN · H. GOLDSCHMIDT
A. GREITHER · H. GRIMMER · P. GROSS · TH. GRÜNEBERG · J. HÄMEL · E. HAGEN · D.
HARDER · W. HAUSER · E. HEERD · E. HEINKE · H.-J. HEITE · S. HELLERSTRÖM · A. HENSCHLER-GREIFELT · J. J. HERZBERG · J. HEWITT · G. VON DER HEYDT · G. E. HEYDT · H. HILMER
H. HOBITZ · H. HOFF · K. HOLUBAR · G. HOPF · O. HORNSTEIN · L. ILLIG · W. JADASSOHN
M. JÄNNER · E. G. JUNG · R. KADEN · K. H. KÄRCHER · FR. KAIL · K. W. KALKOFF · W. D.
KEIDEL · PH. KELLER · J. KIMMIG · G. KLINGMÜLLER · N. KLÜKEN · W. KLUNKER · A. G.
KOCHS† · H. U. KOECKE · FR. KOGOJ · G. W. KORTING · E. KRÜGER-THIEMER · H. KUSKE
F. LATAPI · H. LAUSECKER † · P. LAVALLE · A. LEINBROCK · K. LENNERT · G. LEONHARDI
W. F. LEVER · W. LINDEMAYR · K. LINSER · H. LÖHE † · L. LÖHNER · L. J. A. LOEWENTHAL
A. LUGER · E. MACHER · F. D. MALKINSON · C. MARCH · J. T. McCARTHY · R. T. McCLUSKEY
K. MEINICKE · W. MEISTERERNST · N. MELCZER · A. M. MEMMESHEIMER · J. MEYER-ROHN
A. MIESCHER · G. MIESCHER† · P. A. MIESCHER · G. MORETTI · E. MÜLLER · A. MUSGER
TH. NASEMANN · FR. NEUWALD · G. NIEBAUER · H. NIERMANN · W. NIKOLOWSKI · F. NÖDL
H. OLLENDORFF-CURTH · F. PASCHER · R. PFISTER · K. PHILIPP · A. PILLAT · H. PINKUS
P. POCHI · W. POHLIT · H. PORTUGAL · M. I. QUIROGA · W. RAAB · R. V. RAJAM · B. RAJEWSKY · J. RAMOS E SILVA · H. REICH · R. RICHTER · G. RIEHL · H. RIETH · H. RÖCKL · N. F.
ROTHFIELD · ST. ROTHMAN† · M. RUPEC · S. RUST · T. ŠALAMON · S. A. P. SAMPAIO · R.
SANTLER · K. F. SCHALLER · E. SCHEICHER-GOTTRON · A. SCHIMPF · C. SCHIRREN · C.
G. SCHIRREN · H. SCHLIACK · W. SCHMIDT, MANNHEIM · W. SCHMIDT, MÜNCHEN · R.
SCHMITZ · W. SCHNEIDER · U. W. SCHNYDER · H. E. SCHREINER · H. SCHUERMANN† · K.-H.
SCHULZ · R. SCHUPPLI · E. SCHWARZ · J. SCHWARZ · M. SCHWARZ-SPECK · H.-P.-R. SEELIGER
R. D. G. PH. SIMONS† · J. SÖLTZ'-SZÖTS · E. SOHAR · C. E. SONCK · H.W. SPIER · R. SPITZER
D. STARCK · Z. STARY · G. K. STEIGLEDER · H. STORCK · J. S. STRAUSS · G. STÜTTGEN · M.
SULZBERGER · A. SZAKALL† · L. TAMÁSKA · A. TANAY · J. TAPPEINER · J. THEUNE · W.THIES
W. UNDEUTSCH · G. VELTMAN · J. VONKENNEL† · F.WACHSMANN · G. WAGNER · W. H. WAGNER · E. WALCH · G. WEBER · R. WEHRMANN · K. WEINGARTEN · G. G. WENDT · A. WIEDMANN
H. WILDE · A. WINKLER · D. WISE · A. WISKEMANN · P. WODNIANSKY · KH. WOEBER · H. WÜST
K. WULF · L. ZALA · H. ZAUN · J. ZEITLHOFER · J. ZELGER · M. ZINGSHEIM · L. ZIPRKOWSKI

HERAUSGEGEBEN GEMEINSAM MIT

R. DOEPFMER† · O. GANS · H. GÖTZ · H. A. GOTTRON · J. KIMMIG · A. LEINBROCK · G. MIESCHER† · TH. NASEMANN · H. RÖCKL · C. G. SCHIRREN · U.W.
SCHNYDER · H. SCHUERMANN† · H. W. SPIER · G. K. STEIGLEDER · H. STORCK
A. WIEDMANN

VON

A. MARCHIONINI†

SCHRIFTLEITUNG: C. G. SCHIRREN

ERSTER BAND · ERSTER TEIL

SPRINGER-VERLAG BERLIN HEIDELBERG GMBH
1968

NORMALE UND PATHOLOGISCHE ANATOMIE DER HAUT I

BEARBEITET VON

G. ACHTEN · I. BRODY · O. BRAUN-FALCO · H. J. CRAMER
G. DOTZAUER · CHR. EBERHARTINGER · H. EBNER
G. EHLERS · R. A. ELLIS · E. HAGEN · H. U. KOECKE · G. MORETTI
G. NIEBAUER · H. PINKUS · P. E. POCHI · M. RUPEC
W. SCHMIDT · J. S. STRAUSS · L. TAMÁSKA · A. TANAY · H. ZAUN

HERAUSGEGEBEN VON

O. GANS UND G. K. STEIGLEDER

MIT 535 TEILS FARBIGEN ABBILDUNGEN

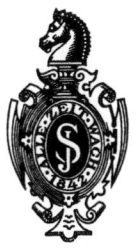

SPRINGER-VERLAG BERLIN HEIDELBERG GMBH
1968

Alle Rechte vorbehalten. Kein Teil dieses Buches darf ohne schriftliche Genehmigung des Springer-Verlages übersetzt oder in irgendeiner Form vervielfältigt werden.

© by Springer-Verlag Berlin Heidelberg 1968
Ursprünglich erschienen bei Springer-Verlag Berlin Heidelberg New York 1968
Softcover reprint of the hardcover 1st edition 1968

Library of Congress Catalog Card Number 28-17078

ISBN 978-3-662-30269-9   ISBN 978-3-662-30268-2(eBook)
DOI 10.1007/978-3-662-30268-2

Die Wiedergabe von Gebrauchsnamen, Handelsnamen, Warenbezeichnungen usw. in diesem Werk berechtigen auch ohne besondere Kennzeichnung nicht zu der Annahme, daß solche Namen im Sinn der Warenzeichen- oder Markenschutz-Gesetzgebung als frei zu betrachten wären und daher von jedermann benutzt werden dürften

Druck der Universitätsdruckerei H. Stürtz AG, Würzburg

Titel-Nr. 5518

Vorwort

Dieser Ergänzungsband über die normale Anatomie der Haut erscheint gerade ein Jahrhundert nach dem Geburtstage von FELIX PINKUS (geb. am 4. April 1868), der — abgesehen von dem Beitrag über die Blutgefäße der Haut von W. SPALTEHOLZ und dem über das Pigment der Haut von B. BLOCH — den ersten Band des Jadassohnschen Handbuches der Haut- und Geschlechtskrankheiten geschrieben und die normale Anatomie der Haut mit einmaliger Gründlichkeit, Weitsicht und Kritik behandelt hat. Ein wesentlicher Teil der Fakten mußte von FELIX PINKUS selbst erarbeitet werden. Wenn man sich dieser Tatsache bewußt ist, kann man erst die Leistung des Autors voll würdigen.

Wir möchten den vorliegenden Band dem Gedächtnis von FELIX PINKUS widmen.

Dem Buch wünschen wir, daß die Leser nach vier Jahrzehnten ebenso wie nach dem Studium des ursprünglichen Beitrages über die Anatomie der Haut sagen werden, daß er nichts von seiner Bedeutung verloren hat und ein Meilenstein der wissenschaftlichen Entwicklung geblieben ist.

O. GANS und G. K. STEIGLEDER

Inhaltsverzeichnis

A. Histologie der normalen Haut

The Epidermis. By Ass. Professor Isser Brody, M. D., Stockholm. (With 54 Figures) . 1
Introduction 1

A. Dermo-Epidermal Junction 2
    I. The Attachment of the Epidermis to the Dermis 2
    II. The Dermo-Epidermal Interface 4

B. Epidermal Sub-Layers 8
    I. Stratum Basale 8
    II. Transitional Cells between the Strata basale and spinosum 10
    III. Stratum spinosum 10
    IV. Stratum intermedium 11
    V. Transitional Cells or T-Cells 12
    VI. Stratum lucidum 13
        1. Plantar and Palmar Skin 13
        2. Non-Plantar and -Palmar Skin 14
    VII. Stratum corneum 14
        1. Plantar and Palmar Skin 15
        2. Non-Plantar and -Palmar Skin 15
    VIII. Transitional Zone 17

C. The Morphology of the Keratinocytes 18
    I. Cell Surface 18
        1. Cell Relief 18
        2. Plasma Membrane 20
            a) The "Horny Membrane" of Unna 20
            b) The Plasma Membrane as Revealed by Electron Microscopy 21
    II. Intercellular Space 23
    III. Attachment Zones 31
        1. Desmosomes 31
            a) The Regular Desmosome 32
            b) The Simple Desmosome 34
        2. Nexus 34
        3. The Junctional Desmosomes 35
    IV. Epidermal Fibrils 36
        1. Definitions 36
        2. General Features 37
        3. The Development of the Fibrils into Keratin Fibrils 42
            a) The Speckled Pattern 42
            b) The Keratohyalin 43
            c) The Keratin 49
    V. Mitochondria 55
    VI. The Golgi Apparatus 57
    VII. Ribosomes and alpha-Cytomembranes 57
    VIII. Other Cytoplasmic Constituents 58
    IX. Nucleus 60
    X. Cell Regeneration 61

D. The Histochemistry of the Keratinocytes 66
    I. Inorganic Substances 66

II. Amino Acids, Proteins, Nucleic Acids and Protein-bound Sulfhydryl and Disulfide Groups 67
   1. Amino Acids and Proteins 67
   2. Nucleic Acids 68
      a) Deoxyribonucleic Acid (DNA) 68
      b) Ribonucleic Acid (RNA) 69
   3. Sulfhydryl and Disulfide Groups 70
III. Carbohydrates 76
   1. Glycogen 76
   2. PAS-Reactive, Diastase-Resistant Polysaccharides 78
IV. Lipids 81
V. Enzymes 85
   1. Cytochrome Oxidase 85
   2. Monoamine Oxidase 87
   3. Succinic Dehydrogenase 87
   4. NADH- and NADPH-Tetrazolium Reductases 89
   5. Specific Coenzyme-Linked Dehydrogenases 90
   6. Phosphorylase and Amylo-1,4 → 1,6-transglucosidase 91
   7. Esterases 92
      a) Aliesterases 92
         α) Alpha-Naphtol or Non-Specific Esterases 92
         β) Indoxyl Acetate Esterases 95
         γ) Tween 60 Esterases 95
         δ) AS Esterases 95
      b) Cholinesterases 96
   8. Phosphomonoesterases 96
      a) Acid Phosphatase 96
      b) Alkaline Phosphatase 99
   9. Adenosine Triphosphatase (ATPase) 99
   10. Phosphamidase 100
   11. Nucleases 100
      a) Ribonuclease (RNase) 100
      b) Deoxyribonuclease (DNAse) 100
   12. Beta-Glucuronidase 100
   13. Proteolytic Enzymes 101
   14. Carbonic Anhydrase 102
   15. Ubiquinone 102
   16. Desulfhydrase 103

E. Dendritic Cells 103
  I. The Melanocyte 103
   1. Origin 103
   2. Demonstration, Distribution and Frequency 106
   3. Morphology 107
   4. The Transfer Process of Melanin Granules 113
   5. Enzymatic Activity 114
      a) Phenol-Oxydase 114
      b) Adenosintriphosphatase 115
  II. Langerhans Cells 116
   1. Origin 116
   2. Morphology 117
   3. Enzymatic Activity 119

References 120

Histologie, Histochemie und Wachstumsdynamik des Haarfollikels. Von Priv.-Doz. Dr. med. Hansotto Zaun, Homburg a. d. Saar. (Mit 20 Abbildungen, davon 2 farbige)

Einleitung 143
  I. Die Struktur des aktiven Haarfollikels 143
   1. Die Haarzwiebel (Bulbus) 145
   2. Das Haar 147
      a) Die Haarrinde (Cortex) 148
      b) Das Haarmark (Medulla) 148
      c) Das Oberhäutchen (Epidermicula) 149

3. Die epithelialen Wurzelscheiden 150
   a) Innere Wurzelscheide 150
   b) Äußere Wurzelscheide 152
4. Die dermale Papille 153
5. Die bindegewebigen Follikelhüllen 153
   a) Glashaut 153
   b) Haarbalg 154
6. Differenzierung der Matrixzellen und Verhornung im elektronenoptischen Bild . 154
7. Der Haarfollikel in funktioneller Sicht 157
II. Die Strukturveränderungen des Follikels während des Haarcyclus 157
III. Altersveränderung des Follikels und der Kopfhaut (einschließlich sog. „Alopecia praematura") 165
IV. Histochemie des Haarfollikels 169
  1. Histotopographie anorganischer Substanzen 170
  2. Histotopographie von Kohlenhydraten 170
    a) Glykogen 170
    b) Saure Mucopolysaccharide 171
  3. Lipoide 171
  4. Histotopographie von Aminosäuren 172
  5. Sulfhydryl-(SH-) und Disulfid-(SS-)Gruppen 173
  6. Nucleinsäuren 174
  7. Histotopographie von Enzymen 175
V. Autoradiographische Befunde am Haarfollikel 175
Schluß 178
Literatur 178

Histology, Histochemistry and Electron Microscopy of Sebaceous Glands in Man. By Prof. Dr. JOHN S. STRAUSS and Dr. PETER E. POCHI, Boston. (With 22 Figures) 184

A. Distribution, Regional Variation and Gross Anatomy 184
B. Histology 192
C. Histochemistry 195
  I. Lipids 196
  II. Other Specific Substances 201
  III. Enzymes 201
D. Ultrastructure of the Human Sebaceous Gland 204
  I. Peripheral Cells 205
  II. Partially Differentiated Cells 210
  III. Fully Differentiated Cells 216
E. Sebaceous Glands in Mucous Membranes and Ectopic Sites 216
  I. Lip and Oval Mucosae 217
  II. External Genitalia 218
    1. Female 218
    2. Male 218
  III. Nipple 218
  IV. Eyelids 218
  V. Salivary Glands 218
  VI. Miscellaneous Sites 219
F. Growth and Proliferation of the Glands 219
References 220

Eccrine Sweat Glands: Elektron Microscopy; Cytochemistry and Anatomy. By Prof. Dr. RICHARD A. ELLIS, Providence. (With 23 Figures) 224

Introduction 224
I. Development of the Eccrine Sweat Glands 225
II. The Secretory Tubule 230
  1. Myoepithelial Cells 230
    a) Electron Microscopy 231
    b) Cytochemistry 235
    c) Function 236

2. Clear Cells 237
   a) Electron Microscopy 237
   b) Cytochemistry 241
   c) Function 243
3. Dark Cells 244
   a) Electron Microscopy 245
   b) Cytochemistry 247
   c) Function 248
III. The Intradermal Sweat Duct 249
   1. Basal Cells 250
      a) Electron Microscopy 250
      b) Cytochemistry 252
      c) Function 253
   2. Superficial Cells 254
      a) Electron Microscopy 254
      b) Cytochemistry 256
      c) Function 257
IV. The Epidermal Sweat Duct 258
   a) Electron Microscopy 258
   b) Cytochemistry 260
V. Vascularization of the Eccrine Sweat Glands 261
VI. Innervation of Eccrine Sweat Glands 262
References 263

Apokrine Schweißdrüsen. Von Prof. Dr. Otto Braun-Falco, München, und Dr. M. Rupec, Marburg. (Mit 46 Abbildungen, davon 1 farbig) 267

A. Historischer Überblick und Embryonalentwicklung 267
   I. Historischer Überblick 267
   II. Die Embryonalentwicklung 268
B. Die Struktur der apokrinen Schweißdrüsen 271
   I. Lokalisation und makroskopische Anatomie 271
   II. Mikroskopische Anatomie 275
      1. Der sekretorische Abschnitt 275
         a) Drüsenzellen 275
         b) Die Zellen des sog. hellen intermediären Abschnittes 279
         c) Die Myoepithelzellen 279
         d) Die Basalmembran 280
         e) Lumeninhalt 281
         f) Altersbedingte Veränderungen 282
         g) Die Innervation 284
      2. Der Ausführungsgang 284
      3. Postmortale Veränderungen 285
   III. Elektronenmikroskopische Anatomie 287
      1. Die apokrinen Drüsenzellen 287
      2. Die Myoepithelzellen 301
      3. Die Zellen des sog. hellen intermediären Abschnittes 304
      4. Ausführungsgang 304
C. Die Histochemie der apokrinen Schweißdrüsen 305
   I. Nucleinsäuren 305
   II. Proteine 305
   III. Lipide 306
   IV. Kohlenhydrate 307
   V. Eisen 309
   VI. Enzyme des energieliefernden Stoffwechsels 311
      1. Enzyme der Glykolyse 312
      2. Glycerin-1-Phosphat-Dehydrogenase (GDH) und Glycerin-1-Phosphat-Oxydase (GPOX) 314
      3. Malic Enzym (ME) 315
      4. Enzyme des Pentosephosphat-Cyclus 315

     5. Enzyme des Citronensäure-Cyclus 316
     6. Enzyme der Atmungskette 318
  VII. Weitere Dehydrogenasen 320
 VIII. Monoaminooxydase (MOA) 321
  IX. Hydrolytische Enzyme 321
     1. Esterasen 321
        a) Cholinesterasen 321
        b) Aliesterasen 322
     2. Phosphomonoesterasen 322
     3. Adenosintriphosphatase 324
     4. Thiaminpyrophosphatase 324
     5. β-Glucuronidase 325
     6. Leucinaminopeptidase 325
     7. Chondrosulphatase 325
D. Über den Sekretionsmodus der apokrinen Schweißdrüsen 325
E. Über hormonelle Einflüsse auf apokrine Schweißdrüsen 328
Literatur 330

Normale Histologie und Histochemie des Nagels. Von Prof. Dr. med. GEORGES ACHTEN, Brüssel. (Mit 34 Abbildungen) 339
Einleitung 339
A. Anatomie des Nagels 340
   I. Die Nageleinheit 340
      1. Nagelmatrix 341
      2. Nagelplatte 342
      3. Periunguiale Gewebe 342
         a) Die Nagelfurchen 342
         b) Das Eponychium 342
         c) Das Hyponychium 342
         d) Die Fingerkuppe 342
  II. Der Altersnagel 342
B. Embryologie 342
   I. Makroskopische Untersuchung 343
  II. Mikroskopische Untersuchung 344
      1. Der Nagel und seine Matrix 345
      2. Das Nagelbett (Hyponychium) 346
      3. Das Periunguiale Gewebe 346
         a) Das Eponychium 346
         b) Das Hyponychium 347
         c) Die Fingerbeere 347
         d) Lederhaut und Subcutis 348
      4. Die drei Nagelschichten 348
C. Histologie 349
   I. Der Nagel und seine Matrix 349
  II. Das Nagelbett (Hyponychium) 351
 III. Das Periunguiale Gewebe 352
      1. Eponychium 352
      2. Hyponychium 353
      3. Fingerbeere 353
      4. Lederhaut 354
      5. Gefäßversorgung 354
      6. Innervation 357
  IV. Der Altersnagel 360
D. Histochemie 361
   I. Nagelmatrix 361
      Nagelbett (Hyponychium) 361
      Periunguiale Gewebe 361
      1. Das Glykogen 361

2. Die Mucopolysaccharide 362
a) Basalmembran und Corium 363
b) Intercellularräume der Epidermis 363
3. Ribonucleinsäure 364
4. Die Enzyme 365
a) Saure Phosphatasen 365
b) Alkalische Phosphatasen 366
c) Cholinesterasen 366
d) Amylo-Phosphorylase 367
Schlußfolgerungen 368
II. Der eigentliche Nagel 369
1. PAS-positive Substanzen 369
2. Basophilie 370
3. Proteine mit Sulfhydrylgruppen 370
Schlußfolgerungen 371
4. Elektronische Mikroskopie 373
Literatur 374

Zur Innervation der Haut. Von Frau Prof. Dr. E. Hagen, Bonn. (Mit 47 Abbildungen) . 377
Einleitung 377
Methoden 377
1. Epidermale Nerven 378
2. Das subepidermale Nervengeflecht 389
3. Gefäßnerven 398
4. Spezifisch gebaute, sensible Nervenformationen 400
a) Der Nervenapparat des Haares 400
b) Sensible Endkörperchen 411
Literatur 423

Die normale Histologie von Corium und Subcutis. Von Prof. Dr. W. Schmidt, München.
(Mit 22 Abbildungen) 430
A. Die Bauelemente des Bindegewebes von Corium und Subcutis 430
I. Die zelligen Bestandteile des Bindegewebes 430
1. Fibrocyten und Fibroblasten 431
2. Histiocyten 434
3. Gewebsmastzellen 436
4. Plasmazellen 438
5. Die Reticulumzelle und Fettzelle 439
II. Die Fasern des Bindegewebes 439
Entstehung des Kollagens und Bildung der kollagenen Fibrille 440
1. Die argyrophile Faser 443
2. Die kollagene Faser 445
3. Die elastische Faser 447
III. Die Grundsubstanz 450
B. Aggregationsweise der Bauteile und Gewebebildung 453
Fettgewebe und Fettorgane 455
1. Die Primitivorgane 455
2. Das Gewebe univacuolärer Fettzellen 455
3. Das Gewebe plurivacuolärer Fettzellen 456
4. Cyto- und histochemische Unterschiede von weißem und braunem Fett . . . 456
5. Fettgewebe oder Fettorgane 458
6. Die funktionelle Bedeutung des subcutanen Fettgewebes 458
7. Vorgänge bei der Speicherung und Entspeicherung 459
C. Mikroskopische und submikroskopische Anatomie von Corium und Subcutis 461
I. Die Basalmembran 461
II. Das Corium 465
1. Das Stratum papillare 465
2. Das Stratum reticulare 470
3. Das Corium als Ganzes 471

III. Die Subcutis 474
    Der Einbau der Gefäße in Subcutis und Corium 478
IV. Die Muskulatur der Haut 479
    1. Glatte Muskulatur 479
    2. Skeletmuskulatur 482
    3. Die myoepithelialen Zellen 482
Literatur 482

The Blood Vessels of the Skin. By Prof. Dr. GUISEPPE MORETTI, Genova. (With 165 Figures, of which are 10 in Colour) 491

A. Introduction 491
  I. General Considerations 491
  II. Historical Considerations 493
  III. Technical Considerations 495
    1. Capillaroscopic Methods 496
    2. Injection Methods 497
    3. Histological Methods 498
    4. Histochemical Methods 498
    5. Physical Methods 498
B. Notes on Comparative Anatomy, Embryology, and Prenatal and Postnatal Development of Cutaneous Blood Vessels 499
  I. General Observations 499
  II. Indications From Comparative Embryology and Comparative Anatomy in Mammals (Excluding Man) 500
    1. The Order Chioptera 503
    2. The Order Primates 505
    3. The Order Lagomorpha 506
    4. The Order Rodentia 507
    5. The Order Carnivora 507
    6. The Order Cetacea 508
    7. The Order Perissodactyla 508
    8. The Order Artiodactyla 510
  III. Embryology, Prenatal, and Postnatal Development of the Vessel Network in Man 511
C. Building Stones for the Cutaneous Blood Vessel Network 517
  I. Introductory Observations 517
  II. Arteries and Arterioles 517
    1. Artery types 517
    2. Arterioles: Types and Distributive Characteristics 519
    3. The Structure of the Arteries and Arterioles 523
    4. The Transition of the Arteries into Arterioles and of these into Capillaries . . 524
    5. The Histochemistry and Electron Microscopy of the Arterioles 525
  III. The Capillaries 529
    1. Definition and General Characteristics 529
    2. Papillary Loops 533
    3. Structure of the Capillaries 534
    4. Histochemistry of the Capillaries 536
    5. Electron Microscopy of the Capillaries 539
  IV. The Venules and Veins of the Skin 546
    1. Types of Venules and Veins 546
    2. The structure of the Venules and Veins 547
    3. Histochemistry and Electron Microscopy of Venules 550
  V. Arteriovenous Anastomosis (AVA) 551
    1. Types of Anastomoses 551
    2. Number and Size of Anastomoses 552
    3. Structure of the Arteriovenous Anastomoses 553
    4. Histochemistry of the Arteriovenous Anastomoses 556
  VI. Notes on the Biological Modifications of the Blood Vessels in the Skin . . 558
    1. Indications on the Periodic or Permanent Regeneration of Cutaneous Vessels 558
    2. Notes on the Histochemistry and Electron Microscopy of Neoformed Vessels 559
    3. Indications of Degenerative Phenomena in the Cutaneous Blood Network . . 563

VII. The Nerves of the Cutaneous Blood Vessels 564
   1. General Principles 564
   2. The Nerves of the Arteries and Arterioles, Veins and Venules and Arteriovenous
      Anastomoses 565
   3. The Problem of Capillary Innervation 566
D. The Architecture of the Cutaneous Blood Network 567
   I. General Observations 567
   II. The Distribution of the Arterial Vessels in the Subcutaneous and in the Dermis
       (apart from the Appendages) 567
       1. Networks Formed in the Subcutaneous 567
       2. Regional Aspects of the "Cutaneous" and "Fascial" Network 568
       3. Networks Formed in the Dermis 572
       4. Regional Aspects of the Dermal Networks 575
   III. The Distribution of Arterioles and Capillaries Around the Appendages 580
       1. Periglandular Networks 581
       2. Perifollicular Networks, their Static and Dynamic Aspects 583
       3. The Vascular Unit 590
       4. Smooth Muscles 594
       5. Nerve Structures 594
   IV. The Distribution of the Venous Vessels in the Dermis and Subcutaneous (Appendages Included) 595
       1. Networks Formed in the Dermis and Subcutaneous Tissue 595
       2. The Veins and Venules of the Appendages 597
       3. Regional Aspects and Factors which May Influence the Appearance of the
          Veins and Cutaneous Venules 598
       4. Smooth Muscles 598
       5. Nerve Structures 598
   V. Arteriovenous Anastomosis of the Dermis 598
E. An Outline of the Blood Cutaneous Network Design 599
   I. Preliminary Remarks 599
   II. How the Blood Vessel Cutaneous Network was Envisaged before Spalteholz . . 599
   III. Spalteholz's View of the Blood Network 600
   IV. The Modern Conception of the Cutaneous Blood Network 602
F. Conclusions 607
References 609

Embryologie der Haut. Von Prof. Dr. med. HERMANN PINKUS, Detroit, und Dr. med. ANTOINETTE TANAY, Detroit. (Mit 37 Abbildungen) 624
Einleitung 624
A. Entwicklung der Epidermis 625
   1. Allgemeines 625
   2. Ultrastruktur 628
   3. Histochemie 631
   4. Topographische Unterschiede 633
   5. Epidermis der Neugeborenen 636
B. Entwicklung des Coriums und des Fettgewebes 636
   1. Allgemeines 636
   2. Fasern und Zellen 638
   3. Basalmembran 639
   4. Blut- und Lymphgefäße 639
   5. Subcutanes Fettgewebe 640
   6. Histochemie 641
C. Entwicklungsmechanik der menschlichen Haut 641
D. Der Haarkomplex 644
   I. Morphologische Entwicklung 644
      1. Frühe Stadien 644
      2. Entwicklung der verschiedenen Teile 650
         a) Der Bulbus 650
         b) Unterer Follikelabschnitt 652

c) Wulst 653
d) Isthmus 653
e) Talgdrüse 653
f) Infundibulum 653
g) Haarkanal 653
h) Haar und innere Wurzelscheide 655
i) Arrector-Muskel 656
k) Apokrine Drüse 657
II. Topographische Entwicklung der Haare 658
III. Histochemie 659
IV. Quantitative Daten über fetale Haarkomplexe 660
V. Spezialisierte Drüsen 661
1. Freie und spezialisierte Talgdrüsen 661
2. Mammaregion 661
3. Gehörgang und Nasenvorhof 663
E. Ekkrine Drüsen 663
1. Allgemeines 663
2. Ultrastruktur 665
3. Histochemie 665
4. Quantitative Daten und Drüsen des Neugeborenen 668
F. Nagel 669
1. Allgemeines 669
2. Histochemie 673
3. Ultrastruktur 673
G. Nerven und andere Neuralleisten-Abkömmlinge 673
1. Frühstadium 673
2. Nerven der Finger- und Zehenbeeren 674
3. Melanocyten und Langerhanssche Zellen 676
H. Schlußbemerkungen 677
Literatur 677

Die Altersveränderungen der Haut. Von Dozent Dr. med. H. J. Cramer, Erfurt. (Mit
7 Abbildungen) 683
Einleitung 683
1. Über Unterschiede der Altersveränderungen an bedeckter und unbedeckter Haut . 684
2. Dicke der Haut 686
3. Epidermis 686
4. Pigmentierung 691
5. Corium 691
6. Glatte Muskulatur 695
7. Talgdrüsen 695
8. Ekkrine Schweißdrüsen 696
9. Apokrine Schweißdrüsen 696
10. Die Brustdrüse 698
11. Haar und Haarfollikel 698
12. Nägel 699
13. Blutgefäße 700
14. Lymphgefäße 702
15. Nerven 702
16. Fettgewebe 703
17. Unterschiede durch Geschlecht, Konstitution und Rasse 703
Literatur 705

Hautveränderungen an Leichen. Von Prof. Dr. med. G. Dotzauer, Köln, und Dr. L. Tamáska, Köln. (Mit 22 Abbildungen, davon 5 farbig) 708
Einleitung und Problemstellung 708
I. Die Haut der frühen Leichenzeit 708
1. Algor 708
2. Palor 710

3. Livores 710
  a) Differentialdiagnose zwischen Cyanose und Totenflecken 714
  b) Postmortale Reoxydation der Livores 714
  c) Differentialdiagnose vitaler und postmortaler Blutungen 715
4. Postmortale Gewebswasserverschiebung 718
5. pH-Wasserstoffionenkonzentration 718
6. Autolyse 718
7. Rigor 722
8. Fettstarre 724
9. Vertrocknung der Haut 724
  a) Regulation des Wassergehaltes der intakten Haut, der sichtbaren Schleimhäute 724
    α) Vertrocknungen der intakten Haut und der sichtbaren Schleimhäute in der Agone 724
    β) Vertrocknung der intakten Haut und der Schleimhäute post mortem . . 725
  b) Vertrocknung der versehrten Haut 727
    α) Vertrocknung der Epidermis nach vitalen Verletzungen 727
    β) Vertrocknungen der Haut nach agonalen Verletzungen 727
    γ) Vertrocknungen nach postmortalen Verletzungen 728
  c) Vertrocknungen der Haut nach Einwirkung von Nekrophagen 728
10. Indentitätfeststellung über die Haut in der frühen Leichenzeit 728
II. Die Haut und Anhangsgebilde in der späteren Leichenzeit 730
  1. Putrifikation 730
  2. Dekomposition 733
  3. Nekrophagen 733
    a) Fauna 734
    b) Flora 735
  4. Mumifikation 739
  5. Saponifikation (Fettwachsbildung) 741
    a) Die Haut in feuchtem Milieu 741
    b) Die Haut in feuchtem Milieu nach dem Tode 742
    c) Wasserleiche: Direkte Einwirkung des Wassers 742
  6. Moormumifikation 749
  7. Indentitätsfeststellung über die Haut in der späteren Leichenzeit 751
III. Gewalteinwirkungen auf die Haut einer Leiche 752
  1. Abgrenzung gegenüber agonalen wie vitalen Prozessen 752
  2. Stumpfe Gewalt 755
    a) Druckanämie 756
    b) Hautblutungen 756
    c) Hautabschürfungen 757
  3. Stich-, Schnitt- und Hiebverletzungen an der Leichenhaut 760
  4. Schußverletzung 764
    a) Fernschuß 764
    b) Nahschuß (relativer Nahschuß) 765
    c) Einschuß bei aufgesetzter Waffe (absoluter Nahschuß) 766
    d) Ausschußverletzungen 767
  5. Verbrennung 768
  6. Verbrühung 772
  7. Verätzung der Leichenhaut 773
  8. Strom- und stromähnliche Veränderungen der Leichenhaut 774
  9. Die postmortale percutane Resorption von Gasen 778
Literatur 780

B. Allgemeine Pathologie

Allgemeine Pathologie des Fettgewebes. Von Priv.-Doz. Dr. GÜNTER EHLERS, Gießen. (Mit 15 Abbildungen) 787
  I. Vorbemerkungen 787
  II. Anatomie des Fettgewebes 788
  III. Atrophien der Haut unter besonderer Berücksichtigung des Fettgewebes . . . 789
    Definition und Einteilung 789
    1. Primäre, physiologisch bedingte Atrophien, Atrophia cutis senilis 790

2. Sekundäre, degenerativ bedingte Atrophien 790
   a) Inanitionsatrophie 790
   b) Inaktivitätsatrophie 791
   c) Mechanisch bedingte Atrophie (Druckatrophie) 791
   d) Neurotrophisch bedingte Atrophie 792
3. Sekundäre, entzündlich bedingte Atrophien 793
   a) Atrophien nach allergischen, toxischen oder infektiösen Prozessen 793
   b) Umschriebene, entzündlich bedingte Atrophien 794
IV. Entzündliche und vorwiegend gefäßbedingte Erkrankungen des Fettgewebes . . 795
  1. Patho-Histologie der Erkrankungen des subcutanen Fettgewebes 795
    a) Erythema nodosum 796
    b) Erythema induratum Bazin 798
    c) Nodular Vasculitis 799
    d) Sarcoid Darier-Roussy 800
    e) Spontanpanniculitis Typ Pfeifer-Weber-Christian 800
    f) Spontanpanniculitis Typ Rothmann-Makai 802
    g) Panniculitis subacuta nodosa migrans 803
    h) Spontan auftretende Fettgewebsnekrosen und Fettgranulome 803
    i) Traumatogene Fettgewebsnekrose 803
    j) Fettgewebsnekrose der Brustdrüse 803
    k) Medikamentöse Lipodystrophie 804
    l) Sclerema neonatorum 805
    m) Adiponecrosis subcutanea neonatorum 806
    n) Necrosis progressiva subcutanea neonatorum 808
  2. Patho-Histologie vorwiegend gefäßbedingter Erkrankungen des subcutanen Fettgewebes 808
    a) Periarteriitis nodosa-Gruppe 809
    b) Necrobiosis lipoidica 814
    c) Necrobiosis maculosa 815
    d) Granulomatosis disciformis chronica et progressiva 815
    e) Lipogranulomatosis subcutanea hypertonica Gottron 816
    f) Pingranliquose 817
V. Tumoren des subcutanen Fettgewebes 818
  1. Gutartige Tumoren 820
    a) Lipoblastoma cutis 820
    b) Fibrolipom — Angiolipom 820
    c) Hämangioblastom 821
    d) Hibernom 821
    e) Naevus lipomatosus cutaneus superficialis Hoffmann-Zurhelle 823
  2. Bösartige Tumoren 823
    a) Liposarkom 823
    b) Hibernoma malignum 824
  3. Reticulo-histiocytäre Tumoren, systemische Erkrankungen und Metastasen des subcutanen Fettgewebes 824
VI. Experimentelle Pathologie des Fettgewebes 826
VII. Ätiologie und Pathogenese der Fettgewebserkrankungen 832
VIII. Zusammenfassende Besprechung 839
Literatur 843

Ablagerung und Speicherung in der Cutis. Von Doz. Dr. Christoph Eberhartinger, Wien, Dr. Herwig Ebner, Wien, und Dr. Gustav Niebauer, Wien 862
Einleitung 862
  I. Amyloide 862
  II. Hyalin 868
  III. Mucin 874
    1. Hyalinosis cutis et mucosae Urbach-Wiethe (Lipoidproteinose) 870
    2. Pseudomilium colloidale (Pellizari) 872
  IV. Lipide 880
    1. Intracellulär 881
      a) Xanthom 881
      b) Histiocytose (Lichtenstein, Lever). Xanthogranulomatose 882
      c) Angiokeratoma corporis diffusum Fabry 884

2. Extracellulär 884
   a) Necrobiosis lipoidica 884
   b) Extracelluläre Cholesterinose Kerl-Urbach 885
V. Glykogen 885
VI. Kalk 887
VII. Urate 888
VIII. Melanin 889
IX. Porphyrine 892
X. Ablagerungen von Eisen (Hämosiderin) 895
XI. Carotinoide 897
XII. Silber 898
XIII. Gold 900
XIV. Fremdkörper 900
Literatur 901

Vergleichende Histologie der Haut. Von Prof. Dr. H. U. KOECKE, Köln. (Mit 21 Abbildungen, davon 1 farbig) 920
Einleitung 920
   Die Feinstruktur des Integumentes bei den Chordata 921
I. Grundzüge des Aufbaues der Chordatenhaut 921
II. Die Haut der Acrania 922
III. Die Haut der Craniota (Vertebrata) 927
   1. Cyclostomata (Rundmäuler) 927
      a) Neunaugen (Petromyzonidae) 927
      b) Schleimaale (Myxinidae) 936
   2. Chondrichthyes (Knorpelfische) 941
      a) Der Bau der Haut 941
      b) Der physiologische Farbwechsel 946
      c) Das Seitenlinien-System, Funktion und Bedeutung als Fern-Tastsinnesorgan 951
   3. Teleostei (Knochenfische) 956
   4. Amphibia (Lurche) 969
      a) Der Bau der Haut und die Bildung der Basalmembran 969
      b) Die Veränderungen während der Metamorphose 986
   5. Reptilia (Kriechtiere) 987
   6. Vögel 997
Literatur 1015
   Anhang 1029
      Die Haut der Säugetiere; ausgewählte Literatur 1029

Namenverzeichnis 1034
Sachverzeichnis 1085

A. Histologie der normalen Haut

The Epidermis

By

Isser Brody, Stockholm

With 54 Figures

Introduction

Since the presentation, in the first edition of JADASSOHN's "Handbuch der Haut- und Geschlechtskrankheiten", of the histology and histochemistry of the normal epidermis (PINKUS, 1927) and of different aspects of the melanin pigment (BLOCH, 1927), research activities in these two fields have been much intensified. Our knowledge of both the structure and function of the epidermis has been considerably extended, and this advance has been rendered possible chiefly by the development and application of electron-microscopic, histochemical, autoradiographic, X-ray diffraction and biochemical methods.

In view of the explosive development and the constantly changing front-line of research it is on the whole impossible to do justice even to the most essential advances in a short introduction. Research on the epidermis has been concentrated on attempts to elucidate the structural and functional connection between epidermis and dermis. With electron microscopy it has been possible to show the finer structural connection between these two layers. With the same technique it has also been possible to show that the epidermis is built up of cells in part separated by an intercellular space and nowhere forming a syncytium. Numerous morphological and histochemical studies have been devoted to research on the investigation of one of the most important epidermal functions, *viz.* the formation of a horny layer, and to the elucidation of the "barrier"-function of the epidermis between the organism and its surroundings. It has been electron microscopically demonstrated that the process of "keratinization" or "cornification" starts in the stratum basale. With the displacement of the Malpighian cells or the so-called keratinocytes towards the skin-surface the ultrastructure of the cells and the intercellular space is changed at distinct levels of the epidermis.

The histochemical technique offers a method of ascertaining the histotopography of chemical substances, more especially the enzymes. In this way it is possible to get a certain insight into the metabolism of the cells in the different epidermal sub-layers, and the histochemical results may then be related to the structural variations of the different epidermal functions. It does in fact emerge from the results of numerous histochemical investigations that during the transitional phase of the cell displacement towards the skin-surface, the metabolism of the undifferentiated basal keratinocytes is the subject, with increasing differentiation and therewith increasing remoteness from the O_2-supply, to considerable readaptations.

For the study of the synthesis of nucleic and amino acids and proteins the histochemical methods are as yet all too crude. Here, however, autoradiography has contributed essential information.

Especially the last 20 years have yielded fruitful results as regards the research on melanin pigment. The formation of this pigment has in normal epidermis been found to be restricted to certain definite cells, the melanocytes. Combined biochemical and morphological studies, first with histological technique and later and above all with electron microscopy, have made essential contributions to the investigation of the formation of melanin pigment. The melanocytes and cells of Langerhans show a roughly similar appearance, consisting of a cell body with dendritic processes. They are here jointly presented under the heading "Dendritic Cells". The charting of the morphology of the melanocytes and the cells of Langerhans has been rendered possible by above all electron microscopy.

A. Dermo-Epidermal Junction
I. The Attachment of the Epidermis to the Dermis

The junction between the epidermis and dermis has been the subject of numerous morphological studies. Among the points particularly discussed by the histologists has been whether the two layers are connected through a membrane. HERXHEIMER (1916), reviewing the earlier concepts, assumed the presence of a translucent membrane. He, however, considered this membrane morphologically as well as tinctorially to be analogous to the connective tissue fibers in the dermis. SCHAFFER (1933) has suggested the hypothesis that between the epidermis and dermis there is a real cuticular cement substance. DICK (1947) has described the occurrence of a reticular layer consisting of intercellular colloids and fibers. FRIBOES (1920, 1922), KOGOJ (1923), PINKUS (1927) and SZODORAY (1931), on the other hand, have denied the occurrence of a real membrane. They think that on the dermal side there is a dense network of argyrophilic reticulum fibers which are in direct contact with the "spiral fibers" of HERXHEIMER (1889). The latter were assumed to constitute the so-called "Wurzelfüßchen" at the basal surface of the keratinocytes.

Gradually the conception has been accepted according to which the junction is formed of a dermal membrane, the "basement membrane" or "basal membrane" of DUHRING, consisting of a network of fibrils embedded in a structureless matrix that embraces the cytoplasmic protrusions of the basal surface of the cells in the stratum basale, *i.e.*, the "Wurzelfüßchen" in German literature (HOEPKE, 1927; PLENK, 1927; PAUTRIER and WORINGER, 1930; SZODORAY, 1931; DICK, 1947; ODLAND, 1950; BRAUN-FALCO, 1954, 1957a, b, 1964; BRAUN-FALCO and RATHJENS, 1954a; GRAUMANN, 1954; MONTAGNA, 1956; HORSTMANN, 1957, 1961; LEVER, 1961; RITZENFELD, 1962).

In electron-microscopic investigations the presence of a membrane in the extracellular space at the transition between the dermis and epidermis has been definitely established (Figs. 1 and 19). This membrane was for the first time described by OTTOSON, SJÖSTRAND, STENSTRÖM and SVAETICHIN (1953) in frog skin. This submicroscopic membrane, about 150 to 700 Å in thickness, has constantly been demonstrated in subsequent electron-microscopical studies of the dermoepidermal junction in frog skin (PORTER, 1954, 1956; WEISS and FERRIS, 1954a, b; FARQUHAR and PALADE, 1965; PALADE and FARQUHAR, 1965), and in mammalian skin, such as that from man (SELBY, 1955, 1956; ODLAND, 1958, 1964; BRODY, 1960b, 1964b; PEARSON and SPARGO, 1961; HU and CARDELL, 1962; WILGRAM, CAULFIELD and LEVER, 1962; RHODIN, 1965), from rat (SELBY, 1955; MERCER, 1958a, 1961; FARQUHAR and PALADE, 1965), from mouse (SELBY, 1955; SETÄLÄ, MERENMIES, STJERNVALL and NYHOLM, 1960; RHODIN, 1963; ROTH and CLARK, 1964), from rabbit (v. BARGEN, 1959) and from guinea pig (SNELL, 1965a).

OTTOSON, SJÖSTRAND, STENSTRÖM and SVAETICHIN (1953) have proposed the name "basement membrane" for this submicroscopic membrane because of its structural similarity to the basement membranes of capillary endothelial cells, renal tubular cells and pancreatic excretory cells. The authors stress that this membrane should be distinctly separated from the structure that in the histological literature has been named the "basement or basal membrane". The latter is a zone where the connective tissue fibrils of the dermis form a dense layer facing the basal surface of the epidermis. OTTOSON, SJÖSTRAND, STENSTRÖM and SVAETICHIN suggest the term "subepithelial reticulum" as a more adequate expression for this dense connective-tissue zone and reserve the name "basement membrane" for the structure which is discerned only in the electron microscope. WEISS and FERRIS (1954a, b) describe the latter structure as "a continuous sharp interface" above the "basement lamellae". SELBY (1955, 1956) has called it the "dermal membrane" in order to distinguish it from the "thicker, typical basement membranes found in other tissues". The name "basement membrane" as proposed by OTTOSON, SJÖSTRAND, STENSTRÖM and SVAETICHIN (1953) has been generally accepted, but the expression "basal membrane" is also used for this submicroscopic membrane (MERCER, 1958a, 1961; v. BARGEN, 1959; BRAUN-FALCO, 1963b; HORSTMANN, 1963b; BREATNACH, 1964a; RITZENFELD, 1964; BRAUN-FALCO and PETRY, 1965).

How this membrane is formed is unknown. It is questionable whether, as is assumed by v. BARGEN (1959), it has only a connective tissue origin. MERCER (1961) has pointed out that "membranes of this special character appear to form wherever two populations of cells which have followed sufficiently different embryonic pathways, and become differently differentiated, are brought again into physical contiguity. Thus they are found, wherever mesodermal tissues contact ecto- or endothelial tissues".

What electron microscopically corresponds to the "basement membrane" of the histologists has not yet been elucidated. Below the submicroscopic basement membrane different types of dermal fibrils occur. Associated with the basement membrane is a network of fine filaments (Figs. 1 and 19) described in the adult skin of man (BRODY, 1960b) and of frog and rat (PALADE and FARQUHAR, 1965), and in embryonal mouse skin (MENEFEE, 1957). These differ from the collagen filaments both with respect to the diameter and the cross-banding pattern (BRODY, 1960b; PALADE and FARQUHAR, 1965). They vary in diameter from 200 to 750 Å (PALADE and FARQUHAR, 1965). PALADE and FARQUHAR (1965) have given detailed data of their cross-banding pattern and pointed out that this is characteristic and unique for these filaments. Their length is difficult to determine because they branch and fuse frequently. The filaments separate the basement membrane from the collagen filaments, with which they do not show any continuity (BRODY, 1960b, PALADE and FARQUHAR, 1965). Their chemistry and function are unknown. They may in part be followed into the basement membrane (BRODY, in press), which seems to consist of a filamentous component embedded in a homogeneous matrix. In the electron micrographs there is no continuity between the dermal and epidermal fibrils, a hypothesis earlier maintained by some histologists (FRIBOES, 1920, 1922; KOGOJ, 1923; PINKUS, 1927; SZODORAY, 1931).

The basement membrane closely follows the basal surface of the epidermis and is partly separated from it by a space which is about 300 Å in width (OTTOSON, SJÖSTRAND, STENSTRÖM and SVAETICHIN, 1953; PORTER, 1954, 1956; WEISS and FERRIS, 1954a, b; SELBY, 1955; MERCER, 1958a, 1961; ODLAND, 1958, 1964; v. BARGEN, 1959; BRODY, 1960b; SETÄLÄ, MERENMIES, STJERNVALL and NYHOLM, 1960; PEARSON and SPARGO, 1961; HU and CARDELL, 1962; WILGRAM, CAUL-

FIELD and LEVER, 1962; ROTH and CLARK, 1964; FARQUHAR and PALADE, 1965; PALADE and FARQUHAR, 1965; RHODIN, 1965). The basement membrane is in continuity with the keratinocytes at the so-called "junctional desmosomes" (BRODY, 1960, 1962a, in press; CAULFIELD and WILGRAM, 1962; Figs. 1 and 19). The junction between the dermis and epidermis is thus formed by the junctional desmosomes, the submicroscopic basement membrane and the fine dermal filaments associated with this membrane. The junctional desmosomes are rather frequent along the whole basal surface of the keratinocytes.

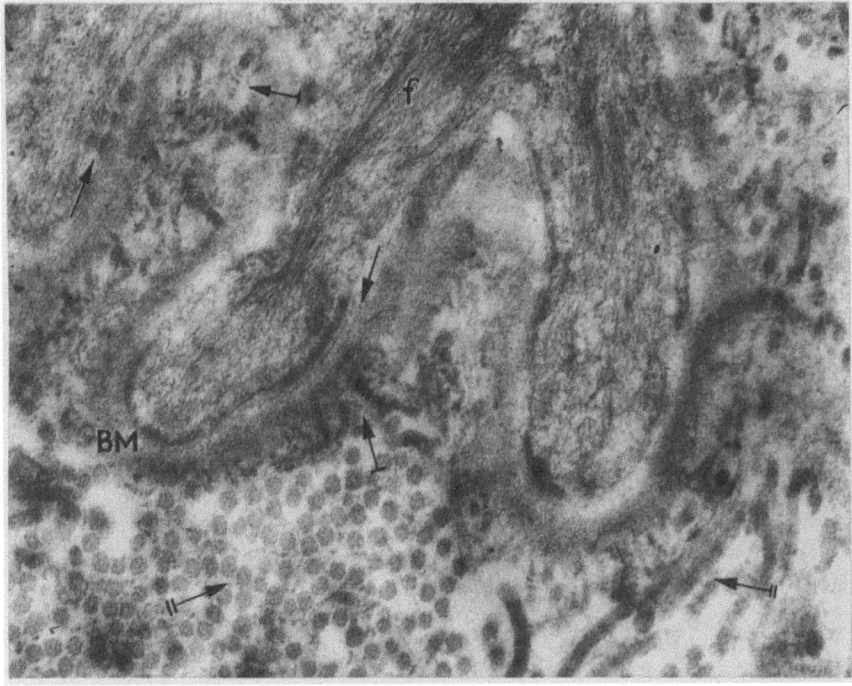

Fig. 1. Junction between dermis and epidermis in skin from the upper arm showing distinct cytoplasmic protrusions. *f* bundles of epidermal filaments, *BM* basement membrane in contact with the extracellular component of the junctional desmosomes (→). A special type of filament (↦) associated with the basement membrane at its dermal surface. The filaments differ in thickness and cross-banding pattern from the collagen filaments (⊢→). × 47,000. (From BRODY, 1960b. Courtesy of J. Ultrastruct. Res., Academic Press Inc., New York-London)

II. The Dermo-Epidermal Interface

In the light microscope, the transition between the epidermis and dermis in cross-sections of the skin appears as an irregularly undulating borderline. This undulating shape is due to an irregular projection into the dermis of parts of the non-cornified epidermis in the shape of so-called rete pegs or epidermal ridges which enclose the vascularized dermal papillae (LEVER, 1956, 1961; MONTAGNA, 1956, 1962). The irregularity of the borderline is furthermore accentuated by the occurrence of the cytoplasmic protrusions along the basal surface of each keratinocyte in the stratum basale (Fig. 1).

This borderline may vary conspicuously in shape in one and the same area of the skin and it also displays pronounced variations in the skin from different sites. The morphological investigations of the dermo-epidermal interface are of great importance for our understanding of the functional interaction of the dermis and the epidermis. This interface has been studied in detail after the separation, fixation and staining of the epidermis and the dermis.

Different methods have been used for the separation. The skin has been treated with weak acetic acid solution (BLASCHKO, 1884; PERNKOPF and PATZELT, 1933; FELSHER, 1946; COWDRY, 1950; FLEISCHAUER, 1952; HORSTMANN, 1952a, b, 1957, 1961, 1963a), weak ammonia solution (BAUMBERGER, SUNTZEFF and COWDRY, 1942), or 2 N sodium bromide solution (STARICCO and PINKUS, 1957). The skin has been exposed to enzymatic activity such as that of crude trypsin solutions (MEDAWAR, 1941; BILLINGHAM and MEDAWAR, 1948; SZABÓ, 1955), hyaluronidase (OBERSTE-LEHN, 1952, 1962; ROSS, 1965), or pancreatin (BECKER, FITZPATRICK and MONTGOMERY, 1952). Finally, the skin has been heated to 50° C (BAUMBERGER, SUNTZEFF and COWDRY, 1942) or stretched (VAN SCOTT, 1952). According to BILLINGHAM and SILVERS (1960), the enzymatic method with crude trypsin solutions is preferable to other methods. The cells remain alive, so that apart investigations of the relief of the undersurface of the epidermis, sheets of the epidermis so prepared can be grafted, stained supravitally or be used for enzymatic studies (BILLINGHAM and REYNOLDS, 1952; BILLINGHAM and MEDAWAR, 1953; BILLINGHAM and SILVERS, 1960). The method of VAN SCOTT (1952), involving stretching of the skin, has also been used for biochemical studies of the epidermis on mucopolysaccharides (BRAUN-FALCO and WEBER, 1958) and on enzymes (RASSNER, 1966).

The architecture of the basal surface of the epidermis displays a complicated relief of a network of epidermal ridges, mounds and depressions of varying size which structurally constitute a negative counterpart to the dermal valleys, craters, hills and papillae (BLASCHKO, 1884, 1887; PERNKOPF and PATZELT, 1933; GREB, 1939; HORSTMANN, 1952a, b, 1957, 1961, 1963a; MEDAWAR, 1953; SZABÓ, 1959a, 1962; BILLINGHAM and SILVERS, 1960; MONTAGNA, 1962). Roughly, the relief of the undersurface of the epidermis becomes bolder with increasing thickness of the epidermis. Thus the epidermal ridges and craters display a greater depth, breadth and complexity in the skin of the palms and soles than in that from the abdomen or the medial side of the thigh (MONTAGNA, 1956, 1962; BILLINGHAM and SILVERS, 1960).

Of greater importance than only a comparison of the relief of the interface of the epidermis and dermis in the skin from the palm and sole on the one hand and that from other sites on the other hand are the detailed comparative studies of this interface from the main areas of the body (BLASCHKO, 1887; GREB, 1939; HORSTMANN, 1952a, b, 1957, 1961, 1963a; SZABÓ, 1959a, 1962; ROSS, 1965). BLASCHKO (1887) has investigated the epidermal undersurface in skin mainly from embryos, new-born and young children and, though only to a small extent from adults. He divides the skin into two main groups, hair-covered and non-hair-covered skin, and then into further subgroups. GREB (1939) has studied the dermal papillae and subdivided the whole skin into five groups according to the shape and size of the papillae.

We are indebted to HORSTMANN (1952a, b, 1957, 1961, 1963a) for much of our knowledge of the intricate architecture of the interface of the epidermis and dermis. Thanks to HORSTMANN's method (1952a, b) in preserving the material in such a way that fine details can be inspected and photographed in incident light, the evaluation of macerated specimens has become of diagnostic value in various dermatoses (OBERSTE-LEHN, 1962). On the grounds of division upon which BLASCHKO (1887) and GREB (1939) have based their descriptions, they have not sufficiently taken into consideration the age of the individual or the arrangement and development of the appendages of the skin. With respect to these factors HORSTMANN (1952a, b, 1957, 1961, 1963a) made very detailed studies of the interface of the epidermis and dermis in skin from the main sites of the body.

HORSTMANN (1952b) has observed that the epidermal ridges, dermal papillae and skin appendages usually appear in a certain arrangement, and he discerns three motifs or patterns: a) a "clock-dial"-motif: a concentric arrangement of the sweat-glands around the hair follicles; b) a "rosette"-motif: a radial course of the epidermal ridges that surround and separate the papillae; c) a "cockade"-motif: a concentric arrangement of the epidermal ridges around the hair follicles and the sweat glands. Because these motifs are observed in most sites HORSTMANN (1952b) has assumed that these regular formations have arisen through particular fixed processes in the course of their development.

With regard to the development and number of the dermal papillae, their arrangement in relation to the skin appendages and the reciprocal arrangement of the hairs, HORSTMANN (1952a, b, 1957, 1961, 1963a) subdivides the skin into five groups:

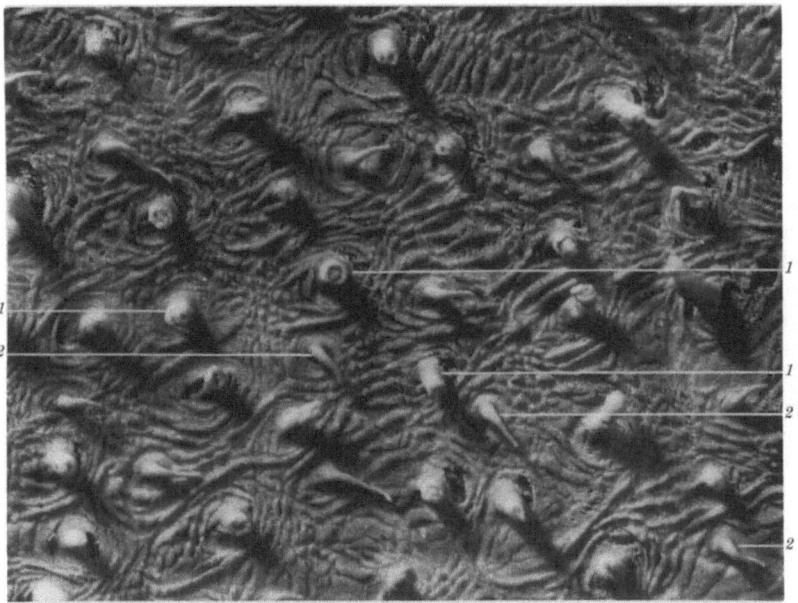

Fig. 2. Broken hairroots (*1*) and ducts of sweat glands (*2*) are to be seen in the epidermis from the lower eyelid of a 58 years old man. × 20. (From HORSTMANN, 1963a. Courtesy of Excerpta Med. Found.)

Group 1: the skin is here characterized by the totally absent, infrequently or poorly developed papillae (face; Fig. 2);

Group 2: the skin shows a uniform distribution of the papillae as well as of the arrangement of the hairs and sweat glands (dorsum of the foot, ear, back and mamma; Fig. 3);

Group 3: in this type of skin the hairs are distinctly arranged in rows (the region over the patella and os ischii, and the abdomen);

Group 4: includes all skin areas where the epidermal ridges appear very distinctly *e.g.* rima ani, scrotum, mammilla, lips, labiae majorae et minorae, palma, planta and the hair-free region of the outer auditory canal.

This picture is also found to a moderate extent in the skin of the palpebra (group 1), mamma (group 2) and abdomen (group 3).

Group 5: In the skin of the palma, planta and the hair-free region of the outer auditory canal the epidermal ridges are not only very distinct, but their regular arrangement is so prominent (Fig. 4) that HORSTMANN (1952b) considered it justified to classify the skin from these areas in a separate group.

Skin from different areas can thus be distinctly divided into groups, but transitional types and also subgroups are discerned. Of very great importance from both the physiological and pathophysiological points of view are HORSTMANN's (1952b) observations to the effect that even normally there are differences between the folds almost completely free of papillae and the adjacent epidermal ridges very strongly indented by papillae.

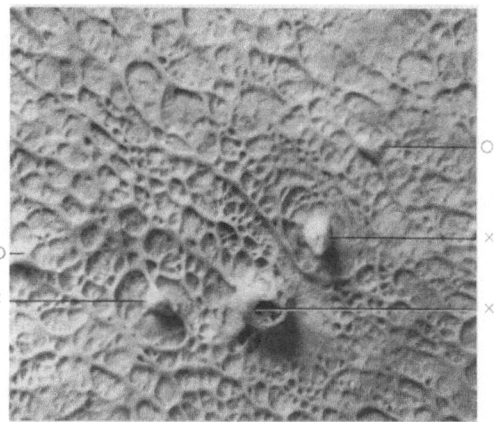

Fig. 3. The epidermis of the pectoral skin of a 55 years old man. ×,× = root of the hair, partially with cockades. ○,○ = sweat glands. × 20. (From HORSTMANN, 1963a. Courtesy of Excerpta Med. Found.)

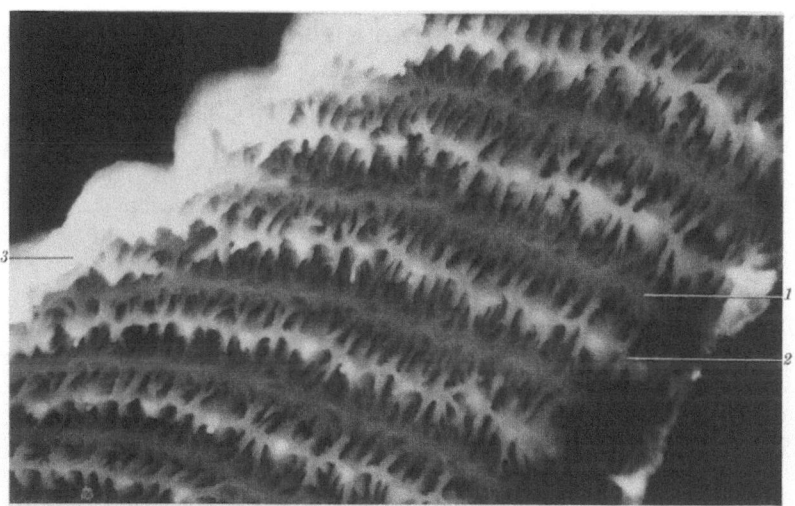

Fig. 4. The epidermis of the fingertip equipped by adhering groin (1) and glandular groin (2) as seen upside down in the side-light. (3) border of the section. × 20. (From HORSTMANN, 1963a. Courtesy of Excerpta Med. Found.)

The profound influence of the hair follicles upon the structure of the epidermal ridges and other skin appendages in normal and pathological conditions has been furthermore stressed by SZABÓ (1959a) and Ross (1965).

A close correlation seems to exist between the boldness of the relief of the dermo-epidermal interface and the wealth of capillary loops and blood vessels (ELLIS, 1958, 1961, 1964; MORETTI, ELLIS and MESCON, 1959; HORSTMANN, 1964).

No apparent relationship has been observed between the network of epidermal ridges and the skin-texture lines (Ross, 1965).

B. Epidermal Sub-Layers

Adult human epidermis varies conspicuously in thickness in skin from the different areas of the body. The order of magnitude of the given numerical data diverges, however, considerably. According to ELLIS (1964), the epidermis over the medial surface of the leg is about 27, over the sacral region 32, over the scapular region 35 and over the knee 42 μ. From a report by DROSDOFF, PERNKOPF and PATZELT (1933) have culled the following figures: the epidermis of the cheek is about 90 to 120, of the extremities 70 to 100, of the palm 500 to 650, of the finger tip 800 to 900 and of the plantar surface of the third phalanx on the second toe 1,000 to 1,400 μ in thickness. In a more detailed table DROSDOFF has reported the thickness of the epidermis when measuring between two dermal papillae or above one papilla. Both data are important to know, because in some areas the rete pegs and dermal papillae are very pronounced, and the thickness of the epidermis in these areas may therefore vary conspicuously, whereas in other sites the epidermis has throughout a rather even thickness.

The regeneration of the cells occurs in the proximal part of the epidermis. As the cells move towards the skin surface pronounced morphological and histochemical alterations of the cells and the intercellular space appear at distinct levels, which permit of a division of the epidermis into sub-layers (Figs. 5 and 7).

I. Stratum basale

The sub-layer close to the basement membrane is called stratum basale (Fig. 5). It forms a continuous layer in all areas of the human body (HORSTMANN, 1957). The cells have a more deeply basophilic cytoplasm and a more dark-staining nucleus than in the cell-layers above (LEVER, 1954, 1961; LEBLOND, GREULICH and PEREIRA, 1964). It is also possible with electron microscopy to distinguish the cells of the stratum basale from those of the stratum spinosum with respect to the stainability and ultrastructure of the epidermal fibrils (BRODY, 1959a, 1960b, 1962e, 1964b; Fig. 5).

HOEPKE (1927) considers that the cells of the stratum basale differ from those of the stratum spinosum only with respect to their shape. However, as HORSTMANN (1957) very rightly points out, the cell configuration is not a constant feature of the stratum basale. In thin epidermis containing only few cell layers the cells of the stratum basale may be flattened or more or less round, with their longitudinal axis oriented more or less parallelly to the dermo-epidermal interface. Stratum basale has also been named "stratum cylindricum" (cf. PERNKOPF and PATZELT, 1933) because in many sites of the body the cells are predominantly cylindrical in shape and are arranged in the form of a palisade with the longitudinal axis perpendicular to the dermo-epidermal interface. This picture is particularly distinct in the palmar and plantar skin.

HOEPKE (1927) assumes that the cylindrical shape and palisade arrangement of the cells is a result of increased pressure from the side. But with such close packing of the cells more cells per unit area will come in contact with the dermis and its vascular bed. ELLIS (1958, 1961, 1964), MORETTI, ELLIS and MESCON (1959) and HORSTMANN (1964) have observed a close correlation between the thickness of the epidermis and the boldness of relief of the dermo-epidermal interface on the one hand and the vascular pattern and richness of the blood supply on the other hand.

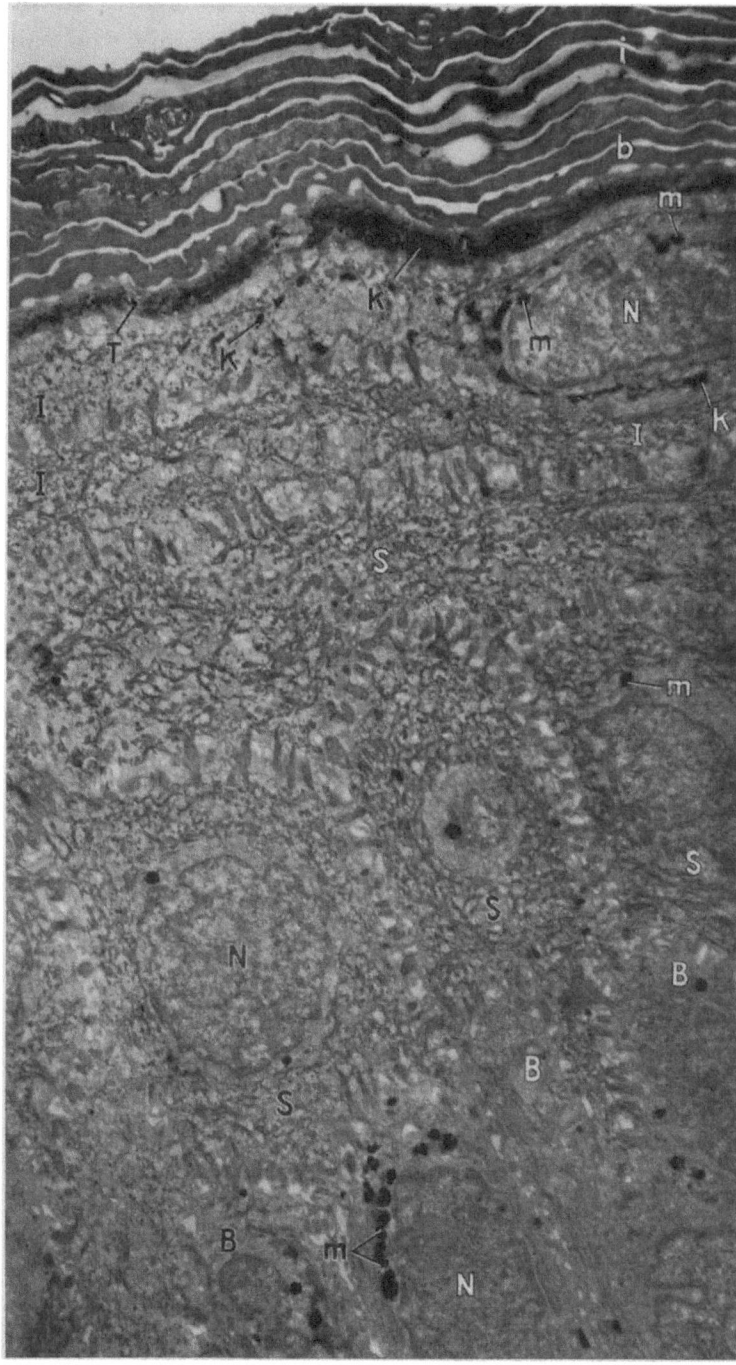

Fig. 5. Survey of the epidermis in skin from the upper arm. *B* stratum basale, *S* stratum spinosum, *I* stratum intermedium, *T* T-cell, *b* basal layer of the stratum corneum, *i* intermediate layer of the stratum corneum, *N* nucleus, *m* melanin granule, *k* keratohyalin. The epidermal fibrils are less opaque in the basal cells than in the spinous cells. × 7,000. (From BRODY, 1960b. Courtesy of J. Ultrastruct. Res., Academic Press Inc., New York-London)

According to Pinkus (1958), the average diameter of a basal cell is about 6 μ.

In human skin the basal layer has been described as only one cell thick (Hoepke, 1927; Pernkopf and Patzelt, 1933; Horstmann, 1957, 1963a; Montagna, 1962). While in thicker epidermis the sub-layers above the stratum basale are considered to contain more cell layers than in thinner epidermis, the cells in the basal layer have been thought to change only with respect to the orientation of their longitudinal axis towards the dermo-epidermal interface, with an increased number of cylindrical, palisade-arranged cells (Hoepke, 1927; Pinkus, 1927; Horstmann, 1957). In the plantar epidermis from the rat Leblond, Greulich and Pereira (1964), however, have shown that the stratum basale comprises two to three cell layers. Although such investigations on normal human plantar epidermis have not yet been published, the findings are probably also applicable here. Such an assumption is favored by studies on pathologically thickened epidermis from other sites than the palm or sole. Thus in the psoriatic epidermis an increase in the number of cell layers has been observed in the stratum basale. This consists of one to three cell layers (Brody, 1962a; van Scott and Ekel, 1963).

II. Transitional Cells between the Strata basale and spinosum

In the plantar epidermis of the rat cells displaying features intermediate between those in the strata basale and spinosum have in light microscope been observed across the hypothetical line separating the two sub-layers; these have been referred to as "transitional cells" (Leblond, Greulich and Pereira, 1964). These cells make it difficult to establish the upper limit of the stratum basale in the plantar epidermis.

III. Stratum spinosum

In 1883 Unna introduced the name "stratum spinosum or spinous layer" for the sub-layer located distally to the stratum basale (Fig. 5).

In the light microscope the "desmosomes" (Schaffer, 1927) appear most distinctly between the cells in this stratum of the epidermis. A cursory glance in the light microscope shows the desmosomes as spines on the cell surface, "spina" or "acantha", from which the terms "stratum spinosum" and "stratum acanthoticum" are derived (Siemens, 1952). Another name for this layer is "stratum or rete Malpighii" (Goldblum, Piper and Campbell, 1954; Lever, 1956, 1961; Goltz, Fusaro and Jarvis, 1958). The expression "rete Malpighii" often also refers jointly to strata basale and spinosum (Siemens, 1952; Brody, 1962a, c; Montagna, 1962; Ellis, 1964). In 1956 Montagna had included strata basale, spinosum as well as granulosum in the expressions "rete or mucus Malpighii", "rete mucosum", "stratum Malphigii". According to Lever (1956, 1961) the spinous cells are also called "squamous" cells.

Pinkus (1927) considered stratum spinosum as "der eigentliche Körper der Epidermis der Vorbereiter der Hauptfunktion der Epidermis (der Hornschicht)". It is composed of polygonal cells forming a mosaic (Lever, 1961). The cells usually become flattened as they move towards the skin surface. The height of the cell and the degree of flattening are related to the thickness of the epidermis and to the distance to the skin surface (Pinkus, 1927; Horstmann, 1957). The number of cell layers is also correlated to the thickness of the epidermis (Horstmann, 1957). There is no doubt but that the stratum spinosum comprises more cell layers in thicker than in thinner epidermis. However, in the light of the observations by Leblond, Greulich and Pereira (1964) on the normal epidermis of the rat foot and by Brody (1962a) and van Scott and Ekel (1963) on psoriatic epidermis, further studies are necessary in order to elucidate whether in thicker normal human epidermis the increase of cells in the proximal part of the epidermis is due exclusively to spinous cells, or whether there is also an increase of basal and/or transitional cells. Electron-microscopic investigations have, moreover, revealed that some of the distal cells previously included in the stratum spinosum, do indeed belong to the upper third layer of the non-cornified epidermis (Fig. 5). In these cells the keratohyalin is so weakly developed that it is not discernible in the light microscope, though it is seen in the electron microscope (BRODY, 1960b, 1964b).

IV. Stratum intermedium

Stratum spinosum is according to UNNA (1883) succeeded by the most interesting sub-layer of the epidermis (Fig. 5). The cells here contain a basophil component referred to by WALDEYER (1882) as "keratohyalin granules". Since the keratohyalin is a constant constituent of normal cornifying epidermis, UNNA (1883) gave this sub-layer the name "stratum granulosum or granular layer". In 1921 UNNA wrote: "Herewith a new epidermal layer was established, a transitional layer between the spinous and horny cells, the stratum granulosum, the granular layer of the skin which was later to play an important role in the pathology, as its easily demonstrable disappearance is used to characterize certain epidermal conditions, the parakeratoses."

Parakeratosis is often interpreted as equivalent to the psoriasiform parakeratosis, because in its classical form parakeratosis occurs precisely in psoriasis (STEIGLEDER, 1960a). The histopathological picture of psoriasis is characterized of a mixing of para- and hyperkeratosis (UNNA, 1894; GANS, 1932; STEIGLEDER, 1960a). The electron-microscopic investigations of the psoriatic epidermis in macroscopically changed skin have revealed the occurrence of three types of disturbance in the keratinization process, *i.e.*, parakeratosis without keratohyalin, parakeratosis with keratohyalin and hyperkeratosis, where keratohyalin is always present (BRODY, 1962a, b, c, d, e, f, g, 1963a, b, c, d, 1964c). The lack of keratohyalin in the epidermis of the psoriasiform parakeratosis has by histologists been misinterpreted as an expression for the absence of an intermediate layer between the spinous and horny cells; the keratinization process has here been presumed to occur directly from the stratum spinosum to the stratum corneum (UNNA, 1894, 1921; SIEMENS, 1952; BRAUN-FALCO, 1957c; HELWIG, 1958; JARRETT, SPEARMAN and HARDY, 1959; LEVER, 1961; JARRETT and SPEARMAN, 1964; MONTAGNA, 1964; SZODORAY and NAGY-VEZEKÉNYI, 1965). However, with electron microscopy BRODY (1962a, c, d, e, 1963a, b) has definitely demonstrated the presence of an upper, third layer of the non-cornified epidermis in all three types of disturbance in the keratinization process in psoriatic epidermis, *i.e.*, also in parakeratosis without keratohyalin. It comprises four to five cell layers.

The observations that in certain pathological conditions keratohyalin is not formed at all (BRODY, 1962a, c, d, e), or that in normal epidermis it may be so weakly developed that it is not discernible in the light microscope (HORSTMANN, 1957b; BRODY, 1960, 1964b) seemed to justify the introduction of the expression "stratum intermedium" (BRODY, 1962a, c, e), instead of "stratum granulosum" (UNNA, 1883), for the upper third layer in normal and pathologic non-cornified epidermis in order to define this sub-layer with respect to its topography and not to a particular cellular component. This layer forms, irrespectively of the presence or absence of keratohyalin, an intermediate stage in the evolution of the spinous cells into horny cells. In normal epidermis the stratum intermedium is distinguished from the subjacent spinous layer also with respect to the ultrastructure of the cell surface and the intercellular space (BRODY, 1959b, 1960a, b, 1964b; FREI and SHELDON, 1961; BRODY and LARSSON, 1965; MATOLTSY and PARAKKAL, 1965; RUPEC and BRAUN-FALCO, 1965; BREATHNACH and WYLLIE, 1966; Figs. 8 and 26).

On the basis of histological investigations it has been pointed out that a continuous stratum intermedium is only formed in a multi-layered epidermis, whereas in thin epidermis this layer may be incomplete (HORSTMANN, 1957). Whether this observation will also hold in the electron microscope is not yet clear. The thickness of the stratum intermedium has been correlated to the thickness of the other epidermal strata (OLIN, 1943) and also to the development of the dermal papillae and epidermal ridges (PINKUS, 1927). In histological sections of skin from the hair-covered scalp and from the cheek the dermal papillae are few and poorly developed and a one-layered stratum intermedium is observed. In skin of the chest, where the papillae are denser, the stratum intermedium consists of two layers. In the skin on the back of the hand, the forehead, elbow, the gluteal and patellae regions the dermal papillae are distinct and the stratum intermedium here comprises two to three cell layers. In the palmar skin this stratum is two to six cells thick.

The cells are more or less flattened with their longitudinal axis oriented parallely to the skin surface (Figs. 5, 6 and 23). FERREIRA-MARQUES and PARRA (1960) have reported that the diameter of one cell in the stratum intermedium may cover 6 spinous and 8 basal cells respectively.

V. Transitional Cells or T-Cells

At the transition between the strata intermedium and lucidum in plantar skin and between the strata intermedium and corneum in skin from other sites BRODY (1959a, b, 1960a, b, 1963c, 1964b) has with electron microscopy demonstrated the occurrence of cells which he names "transitional cells or T-cells" (Figs. 5, 6 and 26).

In the skin from the sole of guinea-pig and man the T-cells form a 1- to 2-cell thick continuous layer (BRODY, 1959b, 1963c).

In the skin from other sites of the body (abdomen, breast, back, upper arm, thigh and gluteal region) the T-cells seem not to form a continuous layer (BRODY, 1959b, 1960a, b, 1964b; ROTH and CLARK, 1964; RUPEC and BRAUN-FALCO, 1965). In human epidermis regional variations occur, however, with respect to their frequency (BRODY, 1960b). They are observed either at the same level as the superficial cells of the stratum intermedium or as the basal cells of the stratum corneum. They are more flattened than the cells in the stratum intermedium. Their height is on an average 0.7 μ (BRODY, 1960b).

A characteristic feature of the T-cells is the very opaque plasma membrane (Figs. 6 and 26) which with respect to its ultrastructure is identical with that of the horny cells (BRODY, 1959b, 1960b, 1966; Fig. 17). The T-cells are similar to the basal horny cells and to the cells of the stratum lucidum also with respect to the dense and opaque cytoplasm (BRODY, 1959b, 1960a, b, 1963c, 1964b; ROTH and CLARK, 1964; Fig. 6). They show resemblances to the cells of the stratum intermedium with regard to the stainability, arrangement and ultrastructure of the fibrillar substance, and the occurrence of nuclei and ribosomes (BRODY, 1959b, 1960b, 1963c, 1964b; ROTH and CLARK, 1964; RUPEC and BRAUN-FALCO, 1965; Fig. 6).

On the basis of the ultrastructure of the fibrils the T-cells can be subdivided into different types. This for instance is very distinct in psoriatic epidermis (BRODY, 1963c). In the normal human plantar skin, where the T-cells form a continuous layer, two types of T-cells are discerned, *i.e.*, types A and B (BRODY, 1963c), whereas in other areas of the body only T-cells of type A have been observed (BRODY, 1959b, 1960a, b, 1964b; ROTH and CLARK, 1964; RUPEC and BRAUN-FALCO, 1965). BRODY (1963c) suggests that the cells in the stratum intermedium pass *via* the T-cells of type A and B in this order of progression in those skin areas where these types occur, and *via* the T-cell of type A in those skin areas where only this cell type appears.

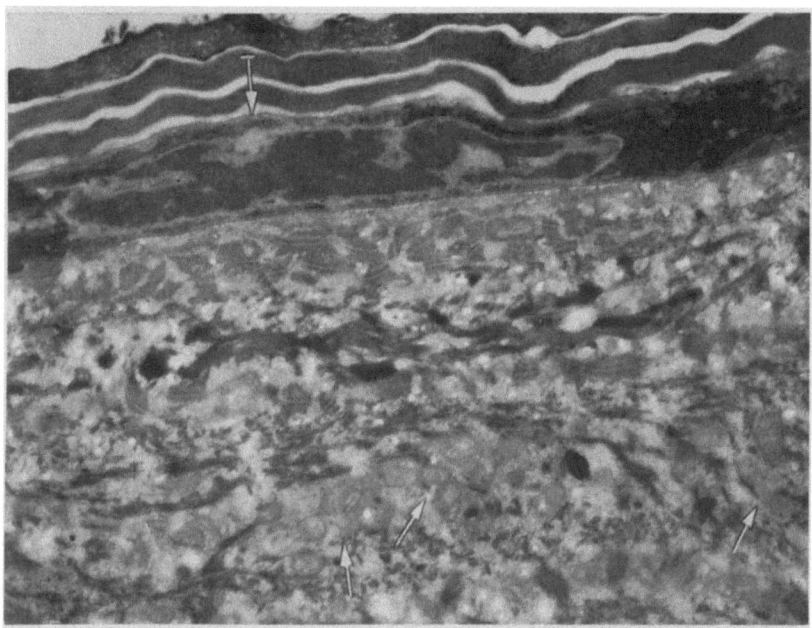

Fig. 6. Skin from the upper arm. In the stratum intermedium the keratohyalin is rather poorly developed. In the proximal cell, groups with numerous mitochondria (→). In the T-cell a flattened nucleus with condensed, opaque karyoplasm. The fibrils are in the main changed into a keratohyalin-like substance. They surround the nucleus but leave free a perinuclear zone. The modified plasma membrane of the T-cell appears very opaque (↦). × 13,000.
(From BRODY, 1960b. Courtesy of J. Ultrastruct. Res., Academic Press Inc., New York-London)

VI. Stratum lucidum

In the light microscope the sub-layer immediately above stratum intermedium is the so-called stratum lucidum of OEHL (1857). Opinion varies, however, as to whether a stratum lucidum is present only in the plantar and palmar skin and corresponding areas of the toes and fingers (HOEPKE, 1927; PINKUS, 1927; ROTHMAN, 1929, 1932, 1954; PERNKOPF and PATZELT, 1933; LEVER, 1954; HORSTMANN, 1961) or whether it also appears in skin from other sites of the body (GRÜNEBERG and SZAKALL, 1955; SZAKALL, 1955, 1959, 1963; MONTAGNA, 1956, 1962; KIMMIG and WEHRMAN, 1961; ZELICKSON and HARTMANN, 1961b; KLIGMAN, 1964).

1. Plantar and Palmar Skin

UNNA (1883) subdivided the stratum corneum of the foot skin into four sublayers (looking from the stratum intermedium towards the skin surface): a basal, superbasal, intermediate and superficial layer. He considered the basal layer to correspond to the stratum lucidum of OEHL (1857). In the usual histological stains the stratum lucidum is seldom colored (MONTAGNA, 1956). By using osmic acid UNNA (1883, 1921) was able to discern two sub-layers in what he called the basal layer (*i.e.*, OEHL's stratum lucidum). The proximal layer close to the stratum intermedium he named "stratum infrabasale". This layer was 1—2 cells thick, did not contain any keratohyalin and was not blackened by osmic acid.

The distal layer of the basal layer comprised 3—5 cell layers and was blackened by osmic acid.

Brody (1959b, 1963c) assumes that the T-cell layer in plantar skin demonstrated with electron microscopy probably corresponds to the "infrabasal layer" of Unna. Both are 1—2 cell layers in thickness and show the same topography. This hypothesis is further supported by the observation of Hoepke (1927) that keratohyalin, contrary to the findings of Unna (1921), appears in the stratum lucidum.

As has been mentioned earlier, the T-cells in human plantar skin are of two types: types A and B (Brody, 1963c). Only type A contains keratohyalin, whereas in type B so-called "heterogeneous areas" of the fibrillar substance have been observed. In some parts of these areas a "keratin pattern" has been discerned (Brody, 1963c).

From an electron-microscopic viewpoint it seemed justifiable to consider the T-cells as a particular stage in the development of the keratinocytes (Brody, 1959b, 1960b, 1962e, 1964b). The character of a developmental stage as represented by the T-cells is particularly well seen in psoriatic epidermis characterized by hyperkeratosis (Brody, 1963c). In accordance with this argument the T-cell layer in the foot skin may be considered as a separate stratum and only the upper layer of the basal layer of Unna (1883) may represent a "stratum lucidum proper" (Brody, 1963f).

2. Non-Plantar and -Palmar Skin

According to Montagna (1956, 1962), Zelickson and Hartmann (1961b) and Kligman (1964) a stratum lucidum is also present in other sites than in the skin of the palms and soles. It comprises 1—2 cell layers. According to Montagna it appears in transverse sections in the light microscope as a hyaline layer. According to Kligman it is distinctly revealed by the hematoxylin staining of isolated sheets of horny layer, but can barely be made out in transverse sections. The cells are nucleated and contain basophilic cytoplasm. On the basis of electron micrographs Zelickson and Hartmann (1961b) described these cells as having a moth-eaten appearance.

In the type of skin here considered there are no electron microscopic criteria for the occurrence of a stratum lucidum proper as it appears in the epidermis of the plantar skin (Brody, 1963f). Between the strata intermedium and corneum there are only a varying number of T-cells, which here do not form a continuous layer (Brody, 1960b, 1962e, 1964b; Roth and Clark, 1964; Rupec and Braun-Falco, 1965). Microradiographic studies by Steigleder, McCarthy and Nurnberg (1964) also favor the opinion of Hoepke (1927), Pinkus (1927), Rothman (1929, 1932, 1954), Pernkopf and Patzelt (1933) and Lever (1954) that a stratum lucidum occurs only in the plantar and palmar skin.

From the electron-microscopic viewpoint, moreover, it seems unjustifiable to consider the "stratum corneum compactum" of Rothman (1954) as equivalent to the stratum lucidum of the foot skin, as has been suggested by Grüneberg and Szakall (1955), Szakall (1955, 1959, 1963) and Kimmig and Wehrmann (1961).

VII. Stratum corneum

The horny layer exhibits conspicuous variations in thickness in one and the same area, as well as between different areas of the body. Thus in abdominal skin the stratum corneum varies between 6 and 32 μ. In the plantar skin it attains a thickness of 80 μ (STÜTTGEN, 1965). MARZULLI (1962) mentions an average thickness of 37 μ (33.7—40.0 μ) for the stratum corneum of the skin covering the anterior forearm. The relation in thickness between the horny layer and the non-cornified epidermis varies in the palmo-plantar surfaces between 4—20:1 and more, and in other sites between 1:1.5 and 1:4 (SPIER, 1964).

The stratum corneum displays pronounced variations also with regard to its structure.

1. Plantar and Palmar Skin

UNNA (1883) demonstrated that in plantar skin the stratum corneum comprises three sub-layers above the stratum basale (*i.e.*, stratum lucidum of OEHL): (a) a superbasal layer containing a dense cytoplasm (like the upper layer of UNNA's basal layer, the superbasal layer was blackened by osmic acid, though the two layers could be separated because they showed different colors with picro-carmine and iodide-violet stains); (b) an intermediate layer with a loose cytoplasm; and (c) a superficial layer, where the cells again displayed a dense cytoplasm.

In microradiographic studies of the skin of the flexor surface of the toe only two layers were discerned above OEHL's stratum lucidum (STEIGLEDER, MCCARTHY and NURNBERN, 1964). The upper layer allowed a minimal passage of roentgen rays. The stratum lucidum transmitted somewhat more, whereas the layer between the two allowed a maximal passage of X-rays. STEIGLEDER, MCCARTHY and NURNBERG (1964) thus show that the outermost sub-layer of the stratum corneum in the foot skin has the greatest physical density and not the stratum lucidum as suggested by ZEIGER (1936 a, b).

2. Non-Plantar and -Palmar Skin

In the light microscope two sub-layers of the stratum corneum have been discerned in this type of skin: a proximal stratum compactum, where the fibrils were assumed to be closely packed, and a superficial stratum disjunctum, where they appeared looser (ROTHMAN, 1954). In contradistinction to the stratum corneum disjunctum, the stratum compactum has a hyaline appearance because of its high light refraction. It is further characterized by high anisotropy, and shows an intense reaction to Gram- and amido-black-staining as well as a strong pyrinophilia and secondary fluorescence (BRAUN-FALCO, 1965a).

Also in microradiographic studies of the skin of the abdomen, face, upper lip and calf of the leg two layers were observed (STEIGLEDER, MCCARTHY and NURNBERG, 1964). The outer looser layer allowed very free passage of roentgen rays, whereas the deeper region of the stratum corneum in the main prevented the passage of X-rays. Just above the stratum intermedium a thin cornified layer showing a very high density was often discerned. This layer was not considered as identical with the stratum lucidum of the plantar skin. It showed a positive PAS-reaction, even after preincubation with diastase.

The stratum corneum of the skin covering the elbow and knee shows different microradiograms than those of the face, abdomen etc. It is thicker and is on the whole more obstructive to roentgen rays. Unlike the other regions of the body, the whole stratum corneum was here red-stained in the PAS-reaction (STEIGLEDER, MCCARTHY and NURNBERG, 1964).

With electron microscopy it has been decisively demonstrated that the stratum corneum does not form a syncytium, as had been earlier suggested (WEIDENREICH, 1900; HOEPKE, 1927; LEVER, 1954; ROTHMAN, 1954). The horny cells are

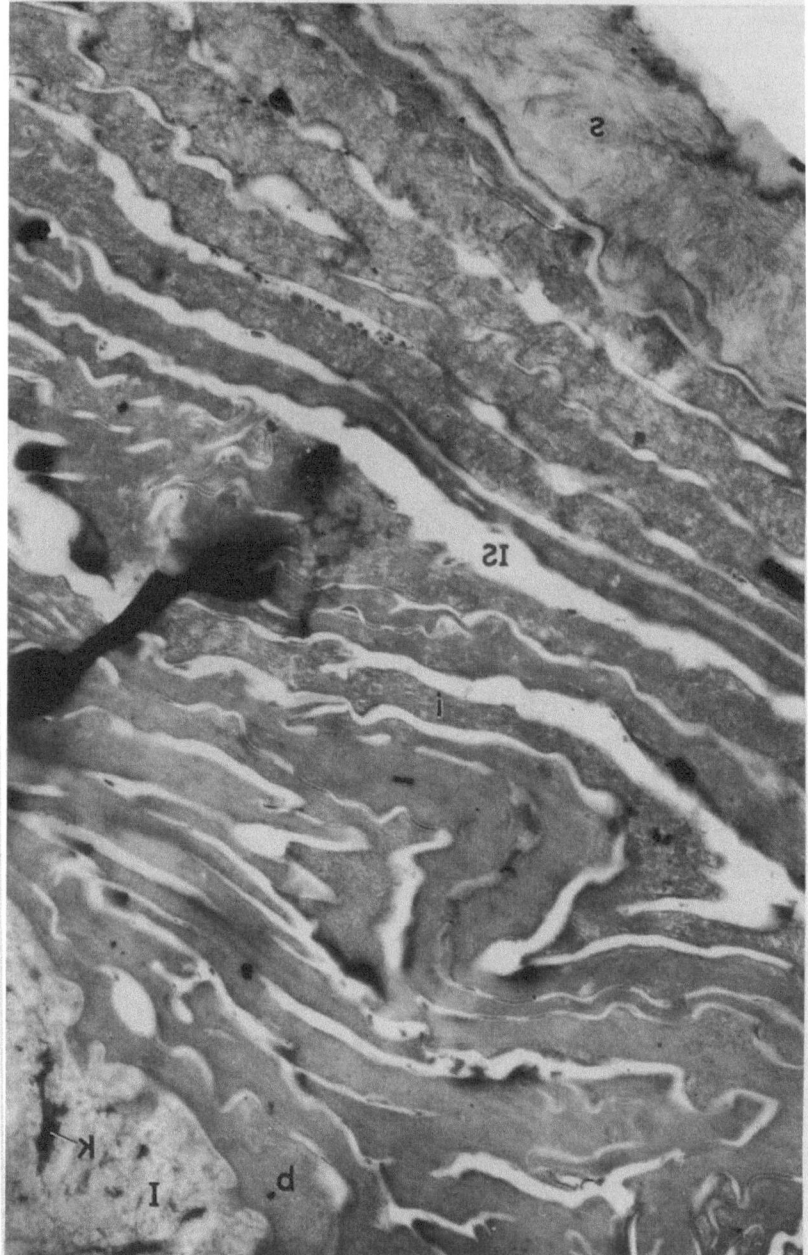

Fig. 7. Survey of the stratum corneum of the epidermis in skin from the upper arm. Three sub-layers are distinguished with respect to the stainability of the fibrils with uranyl acetate: basal (*b*), intermediate (*i*) and superficial (*s*) layer. The fibrils are best stained in the intermediate and least stained in the superficial layer. *IS* intercellular space, *I* stratum intermedium, *k* keratohyalin. × 12,000. (From BRODY, 1962g. Courtesy of J. invest. Derm., The Williams and Wilkins Co., Baltimore)

bounded by a distinct plasma membrane and are separated by an intercellular space (Figs. 7, 9, 10, 27 and 28).

From an electron-microscopic point of view the stratum corneum of guinea-pig and human epidermis can be divided into three sub-layers: a basal, an intermediate and a superficial layer (BRODY, 1959a, 1962g; Fig. 7). This division into three sub-layers is based on the different stainability of the keratin fibrils for uranyl acetate at the various levels of the stratum corneum and not upon the density of the fibrils.

The basal layer comprises 4—10, the intermediate 8—12 and the superficial layer 2—3 cell layers in skin from the regions of the upper arm, sacrum and abdomen (Brody, 1962g).

The long diameter of a horny cell is about 30 μ (Pinkus, 1959). The height of a cell may vary distinctly, as does also the height between different cells. The widest range of height is between 0.12 and 2.34 μ. However, in the basal and intermediate layers the cell height usually varies between 0.12 and 0.90 μ, whereas in the superficial layer it is between 0.12 and 2 μ (Brody, 1962g, 1966). Horstmann (Fig. 13 in 1960) mentions a great variation in the height also of the horny cells in rat hair.

The horny cells are constituted of fibrils, of a non-fibrillar substance and to a lesser extent of mitochondria and different types of granules (Brody, 1959a, b, 1960a, b, 1962g, 1964a, b). In principle two types of cells are seen (Figs. 27 and 28). In one type practically the whole cytoplasm is filled with closely packed fibrils. These cells may appear single, form a layer or occur in consecutive layers at all levels of the stratum corneum. The second type of cell seems to predominate. Between the fibrils and along the plasma membrane a varying amount of non-fibrillar substance is here observed. This substance is usually distinctly seen in the basal layer, whereas in the intermediate and superficial layers it is more or less dissolved, owing to the technique for tissue preparation (Brody, 1959a, b, 1960a, b, 1962g, 1964a, b, 1966; Odland, 1964). By decreasing the time period for fixation and dehydratation the non-fibrillar substance is dissolved to a lesser extent and is distinctly found also in the intermediate and superficial layers (Brody, 1966).

In this text the expressions "non-cornified" and "cornified" epidermis are also used. Non-cornified epidermis comprises the strata basale, spinosum and intermedium. The cornified epidermis includes the strata lucidum proper and corneum in plantar and palmar skin, and only the horny layer in skin from other sites. The T-cells will be particularly referred to.

VIII. Transitional Zone

Histologists and histochemists have considered that the actual keratinization process takes place in the stratum intermedium and in a zone located between this layer and the stratum corneum. Within this narrow area the most conspicuous alterations occur. These have been believed to result in the formation of keratin. This region has been named "Übergangs-Epithelien" (Unna, 1894; Gans, 1932), "Übergangsschichten" (Rothman, 1929), "Grenzzone" (Zeiger, 1936a), "transitional layers" (Rothman, 1954), "transitional region" (Ward and Lundgren, 1954), "keratogenous zone" (Montagna, 1956), "Intermediärzone" (Braun-Falco, 1957c), and "transitional layer" (Montagna, 1964). The expression "transitional zone" will be used here.

Steigleder and Gans (1964) and Braun-Falco (1965a) point out that it is difficult to define more precisely the topography of the transitional zone. Mescon and Flesch (1952), Eisen, Montagna and Chase (1953), Montagna, Eisen, Rademacher and Chase (1954) and Braun-Falco (1957c) have described a narrow layer located between the strata intermedium and corneum. They believed it to consist of partly cornified cells containing a still discernible nucleus. Montagna (1964) considers the transitional zone equivalent to the stratum corneum compactum. Steigleder and Gans (1964) and Braun-Falco (1965a) included at least the upper layers of the stratum intermedium, the T-cells and parts of or the whole of stratum corneum compactum.

The transitional zone is easier to define with respect to its histochemistry (MONTAGNA, 1956, 1962; STEIGLEDER, 1957, 1958c, 1959a; BRAUN-FALCO, 1958, 1959, 1965a; STEIGLEDER and GANS, 1964; SZODORAY and NAGY-VEZEKÉNYI, 1965). Enzymes such as acid phosphatases (Figs. 45—47), non-specific esterases (Fig. 42), nucleases, proteolytic enzymes, lipases and beta-glucuronidase display a high activity in this zone. Furthermore, there are here histochemically demonstrable lipids (Fig. s. 37a—c and 38), probably also phospholipids, numerous free sulfhydryl groups (Fig. 33) and PAS-positive substances.

The assumption that the keratinization starts in the stratum intermedium (JARRETT, 1964; JARRETT and SPEARMAN, 1964) is to a great extent based on the investigations by UNNA (1883, 1913), RABL (1901), UNNA and GOLODETZ (1907a, b, 1909) and SZODORAY (1930), who restricted the "true keratin" to the cell membrane (cf. chapters C I and C II). As pointed out by BRODY (1966), the cell membrane of the horny cell is, however, not equivalent to UNNA's (1883, 1913) "horny membrane" or "keratin A".

With roentgen-diffraction technique it has been shown that an alpha-keratin diffraction pattern characteristic for hair keratin, myosin and fibrin (ASTBURY and STREET, 1931; ASTBURY and WOODS, 1933; ASTBURY and DICKINSON, 1935a, b; BAILEY, ASTBURY and RUDALL, 1943) is also discerned in the non-cornified as well as the cornified epidermis (DERKSEN and HERINGA, 1938; GIROUD and CHAMPETIER, 1938; DERKSEN, HERINGA and WEIDINGER, 1937; CHAMPETIER and LITVAC, 1940; RUDALL, 1946, 1947, 1952). On the basis of these observations it has been suggested that the keratinization process starts in the basal region of the epidermis and is associated with the so-called tonofibrils (DERKSEN and HERINGA, 1936; GIROUD and CHAMPETIER, 1936; DERKSEN, HERINGA and WEIDINGER, 1937; CHAMPETIER and LITVAC, 1940; KÜNTZEL, 1944a, b; GRASSMAN and TRUPKE, 1944, 1951; RUDALL, 1946, 1947, 1952).

The electron-microscopic investigations, on the other hand, have revealed that the differentiation of the epidermis in terms of the formation of a functionally mature stratum corneum involves a complete transformation of the whole keratinocyte. Equally essential seems to be the occurrence of what appears to be a normal distribution of non-fibrillar and fibrillar substances, the development of a characteristic plasma membrane and attachment zones as well as the formation of intercellular components. The various steps in the transformation appear at different levels of the epidermis during the displacement of the keratinocyte from the stratum basale to the outermost layer of the stratum corneum.

C. The Morphology of the Keratinocytes
I. Cell Surface
1. Cell Relief

In the light and electron microscope cytoplasmic protrusions at the basal surface of the keratinocytes facing the dermis have been distinctly observed in normal human epidermis (cf. MONTAGNA, 1962; Fig. 1). The number and size of the protrusions may vary conspicuously in adjacent cells in the same skin area of the body, but in normal human epidermis they seem on the whole to increase in number and size with increasing thickness of the epidermis (MONTAGNA, 1956, 1962). They are particularly distinctly seen in the palm and sole.

In adult mouse (SETÄLÄ, MERENMIES, STJERNVALL and NYHOLM, 1960) and guinea-pig epidermis (SNELL, 1965a) the protrusions are on the whole smaller than in normal human epidermis. In frog skin the protrusions are well developed (FARQUHAR and PALADE, 1965).

At the lateral and distal surfaces of the basal cells and at the entire surface of the spinous cells finger-like protrusions have been observed with light (UNNA, 1883) and electron microscopy (ODLAND, 1958; V. BARGEN, 1959; HIBBS and CLARK, 1959; BRODY, 1960b; EDWARDS and MAKK, 1960; HU and CARDELL, 1962; SNELL, 1965a).

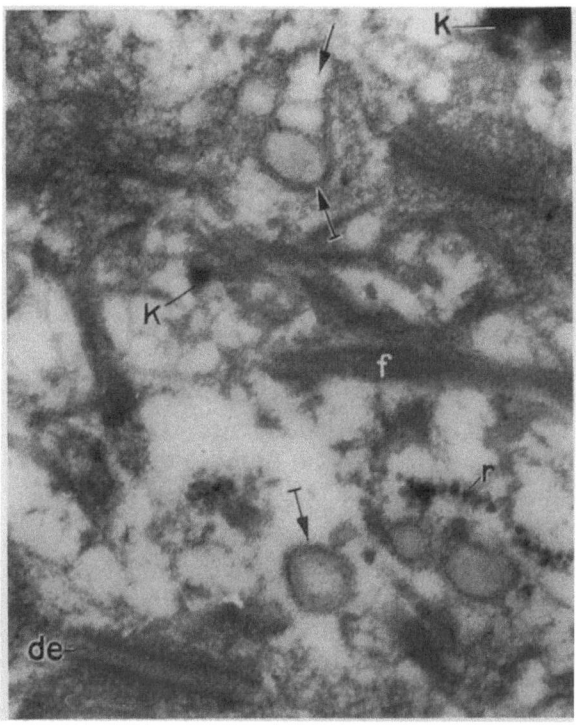

Fig. 8. Parts of cells in the stratum intermedium of the epidermis in human skin from the sacral region. Intracellularly and intercellularly in the invagination (→) are seen bodies (↦) — the so-called lamellated bodies. *de* regular desmosome, *k* keratohyalin, *f* epidermal fibril, *r* ribosomes. × 66,000

The protrusions project more or less far into the intercellular space. Where the latter is narrow the protrusions of the adjacent cells may fit into each other like cog-wheels.

The lateral surface of the basal cells is usually more even than the distal one or the cell surfaces of the spinous cells. The surfaces of the cells in both the strata basale and spinosum are even where they face a melanocyte or a Langerhans cell (Figs. 49, 51 and 53).

At the surfaces of the cells facing each other at the transition between the strata spinosum and intermedium, protrusions are still observed, but they are smaller in size and number than those at the other cell surfaces in the stratum spinosum. In the stratum intermedium the cell surfaces change their relief. At the cell surfaces facing the T- and horny cells deep invaginations have been described by BRODY (1959a, 1960a, b) in guinea-pig and human epidermis (Fig.26). This finding has been confirmed in mouse epidermis by FREI and SHELDON (1961), in human epidermis by Matoltsy and Parakkal (1965) and Rupec and Braun-Falco (1965), who extended the observations of invaginations also to the lateral surfaces of the cell layer close to the stratum corneum. In normal human epidermis Rupec and Braun-Falco (1965) and in hyperplastic mouse epidermis Frei and Sheldon (1961) have furthermore shown that invaginations also occur at the surfaces of the deeper located cells in a multi-layered stratum intermedium (Fig. 8).

These observations thus imply that invaginations are present at all cell surfaces in the stratum intermedium except at those facing the spinous cells. In human epidermis the frequency of invaginations may vary conspicuously in adjacent cells within the same area of the body, and it also shows distinct variations in the skin from different sites. Between the invaginations and the cell junctions the cell surface is mainly even.

In embryonal mouse epidermis the appearance of the invaginations shows a close correlation to the degree of differentiation of the epidermis (Brody and Larsson, 1965).

The surfaces of the T- and horny cells in human epidermis from the abdomen, mamma, forearm, upper arm, back and thigh are strikingly even (Brody, 1960b; Figs. 5, 6, 7 and 9). The surfaces of the T- and horny cells of guinea-pig epidermis from the back display a more or less pronounced wavy course (Brody, 1959a, b; cf. also electron micrographs in Snell, 1965a). In plantar skin from rat the relief of the horny cell is strongly undulated (Horstmann and Knoop, 1958; Horstmann, 1960).

2. Plasma Membrane

a) The "Horny Membrane" of Unna

Friboes (1920, 1922) considered the entire epidermis as a syncytium. Patzelt (1926) stresses that throughout the epidermis, *i.e.*, also in the stratum corneum, the isolable cells constitute the biological unit of the epidermis. In spite of this suggestion, however, Patzelt shares the general histological notion that the cell junctions are made up of cytoplasmic processes, "intercellular bridges", through which the fibrils run from cell to cell (for survey and references see Patzelt, 1926; Hoepke, 1927; Pinkus, 1927; Pernkopf and Patzelt, 1933; Braun-Falco, 1954; Montagna, 1956).

As regards the boundary of the epidermal cells, Unna (1903, 1921, 1928) and Unna and Golodetz (1907a, b, 1909) held the view that a cell membrane exists from the stratum spinosum and upwards. Unna assumed that a particular ectoplasm constitutes the cell membrane of the stratum spinosum. This ectoplasm consists of what has by other authors been interpreted as the intercellular space. In an electron-microscopic study of human skin Pease (1951) supports this view of Unna. In the stratum intermedium the cell membrane appears, according to the latter (1883), as a light border clearly distinguishable from the remaining cytoplasm.

On the basis of the degree of solubility Unna (1883, 1913) and Unna and Golodetz (1907a, b, 1909) were able to distinguish three horny substances. When they treated the stratum corneum with nitric acid or alkaline solutions a membrane-like component insoluble in these solutions was all that remained of the stratum corneum. This, the most resistant substance of the horny layer, was called "keratin A" by Unna. From the light-microscopic picture of the arrangement of the membrane-component Unna (1883) assumed that only the border layer of the protoplasm was completely cornified, and he therefore suggested that the keratin A constitutes the cell border layer which he called the "horny membrane". The horny membrane has later also been referred to as the "horny cell membrane". Keratin B has been considered to represent the fibrillar component of the cytoplasm. It occurs in various amounts and is like keratin A insoluble in pepsin-hydrochloric acid but soluble in nitric acid and in cold alkaline solution. A larger or smaller content of the cytoplasm was considered by UNNA to be constituted by the horn albumoses which, unlike the keratins, is soluble also in pepsin-hydrochloric acid.

RABL (1901), SZODORAY (1930), MATOLTSY and BALSAMO (1955a, b) and MATOLTSY and MATOLTSY (1962a) assume that the cell membrane is first discernible in the stratum intermedium. In the stratum corneum it is transformed into UNNA's horny membrane.

HOEPKE (1924, 1927), PATZELT (1926), PINKUS (1927) and PERNKOPF and PATZELT (1933), again, stress that the cells in the non-cornified epidermis lack a cell membrane but exhibit a fine border layer. With the exception of PINKUS (1927) these authors assume that in the stratum corneum the border layer is transformed into the horny membrane of UNNA. According to PINKUS, however, a cell membrane is not even discernible in the stratum corneum.

UNNA's assumption (1883, 1913) that "true" keratin (keratin A) is only limited to the cell membranes of the horny cells and is distinctly discernible in the light microscope has gained many supporters (WEIDENREICH, 1900; HOEPKE, 1927; SZODORAY, 1930; PERNKOPF and PATZELT, 1933; CHAMPETIER and LITVAC, 1939; MATOLTSY and BALSAMO, 1955a, b; MATOLTSY and HERBST, 1956; SPIER and CANEGHEM, 1957; MATOLTSY, 1962a; MATOLTSY and MATOLTSY, 1962a; CHRISTOPHERS and KLIGMAN, 1964; JARRETT, 1964; JARRETT and SPEARMAN, 1964; KLIGMAN, 1964; PASCHER, 1964; MATOLTSY and PARAKKAL, 1965; MATOLTSY and MATOLTSY, 1966).

b) The Plasma Membrane as Revealed by Electron Microscopy

In an electron-microscopic investigation of the dorsal skin of the frog OTTOSON, SJÖSTRAND, STENSTRÖM and SVAETICHIN (1953) have for the first time demonstrated that the cells in the non-cornified epidermis are delimited by a complete cell membrane, or "plasma membrane", as it also often is called. They found the plasma membrane to be particularly well marked at the cell junctions. On the basis of this observation the authors have suggested that the epidermis does not represent a syncytium. PORTER (1954, 1956) has also observed that there is no evident continuity of filaments or cytoplasm at the cell junctions. With few exceptions these observations have been repeatedly confirmed both in the non-cornified and cornified epidermis (SELBY, 1955, 1956, 1957; HORSTMANN and KNOOP, 1958; ODLAND, 1958, 1960, 1964; BRODY, 1959a, b, 1960a, b, 1962e, g, 1963a, 1964a, b, 1966; v. BARGEN, 1959; HORSTMANN, 1960, 1961; LEVER, 1961; ZELICKSON and HARTMANN, 1961b; RHODIN and REITH, 1962; HU and CARDELL, 1962; WILGRAM, CAULFIELD and LEVER, 1962; ROTH and CLARK, 1964; BRAUN-FALCO, 1965a; WILGRAM, CAULFIELD and MADGIC, 1965; FARQUHAR and PALADE, 1965; RHODIN, 1965; RUPEC and BRAUN-FALCO, 1965; MATOLTSY and PARAKKAL, 1965; SNELL, 1965a, b).

In the entire non-cornified normal human (BRODY, 1964a) and frog epidermis (FARQUHAR and PALADE, 1965) the plasma membrane appears as an asymmetrical triple-layered pattern with a total thickness of about 70 to 90 Å (Fig. 18). It consists of a more opaque layer facing the cytoplasm, a somewhat less opaque peripheral layer and a light intermediate layer. The plasma membrane displays the same ultrastructure and thickness as that in non-cornified psoriatic epidermis

(BRODY, 1962b, e), oral epithelium (MATOLTSY and PARAKKAL, 1965) and various other tissues (SJÖSTRAND, 1960, 1963a, b, 1964).

The plasma membrane and most other membrane systems of the cell (mitochondrial and nuclear membranes, alpha-cytomembranes etc.) are thought to consist of a lipid-protein system (DANIELLI, 1958; ROBERTSON, 1959, 1960; SJÖSTRAND, 1960, 1963a, b, 1964; BROWN and DANIELLI, 1964; NICOLAIDES, 1964). The hypothesis has been advanced that the light, intermediate layer of the plasma membrane represents a double layer of oriented lipid molecules, and that the opaque layers correspond to the location of the polar groups of the phospholipids and a thin layer of protein or glycoprotein. The more strongly stained cytoplasmic leaflet of the plasma membrane which accounts for the asymmetry of the cell membrane may consist of an additional layer of globular protein molecules (SJÖSTRAND, 1960, 1964).

With paper chromatography RIEMERSMA (1963) has investigated the possible reaction mechanisms involved in osmium tetroxide fixation as used in electron microscopy. His observations may lend support to the hypothesis that osmium is deposited in the polar strata and not in the hydrophobic interior of the lipid micelles.

In the T- and horny cells a modified plasma membrane appears (Figs. 17 and 26). BRODY (1959a, b, 1960b) observed two layers, *viz.* an outer approx. 40 Å thick, opaque layer, and immediately adjacent to this a broader, somewhat less opaque inner zone facing the cytoplasm. Since it was impossible to judge whether both these layers belong to the plasma membrane or whether the broad zone represents a condensation of the cytoplasm at the cell surface, BRODY (1959a) introduced the expression " cell boundary".

According to FARQUHAR and PALADE (1965), a distinct, symmetrical, triple-layered cell membrane about 100 Å thick is observed in the horny cells of frog skin. All around the cell surface the cell membrane is backed by a continuous (200 to 300 Å thick) shell of dense material located in the cytoplasm immediately adjacent to the inner layer of the plasma membrane. The "cell boundary" earlier described by BRODY (1959a) corresponds to the inner leaflet of the cell membrane and the shell of dense material. In a subsequent study of normal human stratum corneum BRODY (1966) has verified the observation by FARQUHAR and PALADE (1965) of a triple-layered cell membrane, but he finds it to be asymmetrical like that of the non-cornified epidermis (Figs. 11a and 26). A retrospective analysis of my earlier electron micrographs of the horny layer (BRODY, 1960b, 1964a) confirms this picture (Fig. 17). The plasma membrane of the keratinized tongue epithelial cell of the rat displays a similar ultrastructure (FARBMAN, 1966).

It may be questioned whether the "broad zone" (BRODY, 1959a) or the "shell of dense material" (FARQUHAR and PALADE, 1965) is not to be considered as part of the plasma membrane. The "broad zone" is distinctly delimited from the cytoplasm by a narrow opaque layer (BRODY, 1964a; Figs. 17 and 27). In the expression "broad, cytoplasmic zone" of the modified plasma membrane BRODY (1966) has included the outer, narrow, opaque layer corresponding to the cytoplasmic layer of the plasma membrane in the non-cornified epidermis, the above-mentioned "broad zone" (BRODY, 1959a) and the narrow, opaque layer facing the cytoplasm (BRODY, 1964a). The intermediate layer constitutes the main part of the "broad cytoplasmic zone" and is here referred to as the "inner broad intermediate layer" in order to distinguish it from the "outer intermediate layer" located between the peripheral opaque layer facing the intercellular space and the broad cytoplasmic zone (Figs. 17, 26 and 27). In normal human epidermis the total thickness of the modified plasma membrane is about 200 Å (BRODY,

1966). The modified plasma membranes of the T- and horny cells in psoriatic and guinea-pig epidermis exhibits the same ultrastructural pattern as that of normal human epidermis but differ in thickness. A characteristic feature of the T-cell is the very high opacity of its plasma membrane, in contradistinction to the lesser opacity of the plasma membrane of the horny cells (BRODY, 1959a, b, 1960a, b, 1964a, b). The inner broad intermediate layer of the modified plasma membrane of the T-cells is responsible for this high opacity (Fig. 26).

MATOLTSY and PARAKKAL (1965) describe the plasma membrane of the stratum corneum in human plantar epidermis as a thickened membrane and an outer amorphous coat. They have interpreted this coat as intercellular substance. Their electron micrographs, however, indicate rather that the "outer amorphous coat" constitutes a part of the modified plasma membrane.

The electron-microscopic investigations of normal human epidermis have thus revealed that the plasma membrane of the non-cornified epidermis is about 70 to 90 Å thick. In the T- and horny cells it is transformed into a modified plasma membrane with an average thickness of 200 Å. BRODY (1966) points out that the electron microscopic results are entirely incompatible with the assumption by histologists that the membrane-like component, the only structure that remains after the horny layer has been treated with nitric acid or alkaline solution, corresponds to the two adjacent horny membranes, as suggested by UNNA (1883), or to the fused horny cell membrane as suggested by WEIDENREICH (1900), HOEPKE (1927) and others. No peripherally located intracellular component which as a consequence of the preparation technique might fuse with the plasma membrane to form a membrane-structure corresponding in thickness to that observable in the light microscope is discernible in the electron microscope. The inference is therefore that the structure considered by histologists to be the cell membranes in fact constitute components located in the intercellular space (BRODY, 1966).

II. Intercellular Space

Contrary to the view advanced by UNNA (1903, 1921, 1928), HOEPKE (1927), PINKUS (1927), PERNKOPF und PATZELT (1933) and MELCZER and CSEPLÁK (1957) consider that an intercellular space is present in the stratum spinosum. Most histologists have assumed that the space becomes narrower in the stratum intermedium and that it is absent in the stratum corneum. WEIDENREICH (1900) and HOEPKE (1927) have suggested that the cell membranes of the adjacent horny cells fuse.

In his work of 1883 UNNA mentions the presence of a narrow intercellular space in the stratum corneum which is filled with lipids. PERNKOPF and PATZELT (1933) also note the existence of an intercellular space in the horny layer, containing a substance that stains black with silver nitrate.

In histochemical studies mucopolysaccharides have been localized to the intercellular space throughout the epidermis (WISLOCKI, FAWCETT and DEMPSEY, 1951; DUPRÉ, 1952, 1953; BRAUN-FALCO, 1954, 1958, 1961a; BRAUN-FALCO and WEBER, 1958; STEIGLEDER and WEAKLEY, 1961). Lipids have been demonstrated in the intercellular space of the stratum spinosum or stratum intermedium and in the transitional zone (BRAUN-FALCO and WEBER, 1958). If an esterase activity is present in the stratum corneum this is slight and appears only in the intercellular space (STEIGLEDER and LÖFFLER, 1956; STEIGLEDER, 1957, 1959a, 1964; STEIGLEDER and ELSCHNER, 1959).

In spite of these repeated light-microscopic observations of substances in the intercellular space in the stratum corneum it has still been maintained that if there is an intercellular space in the stratum corneum this is only of a submicroscopic order of magnitude (LEVER, 1956, 1961; SELBY, 1957; KLIGMAN, 1964).

With electron microscopy a distinct extracellular space is discerned throughout the epidermis. It forms a continuous system from the basement membrane to the

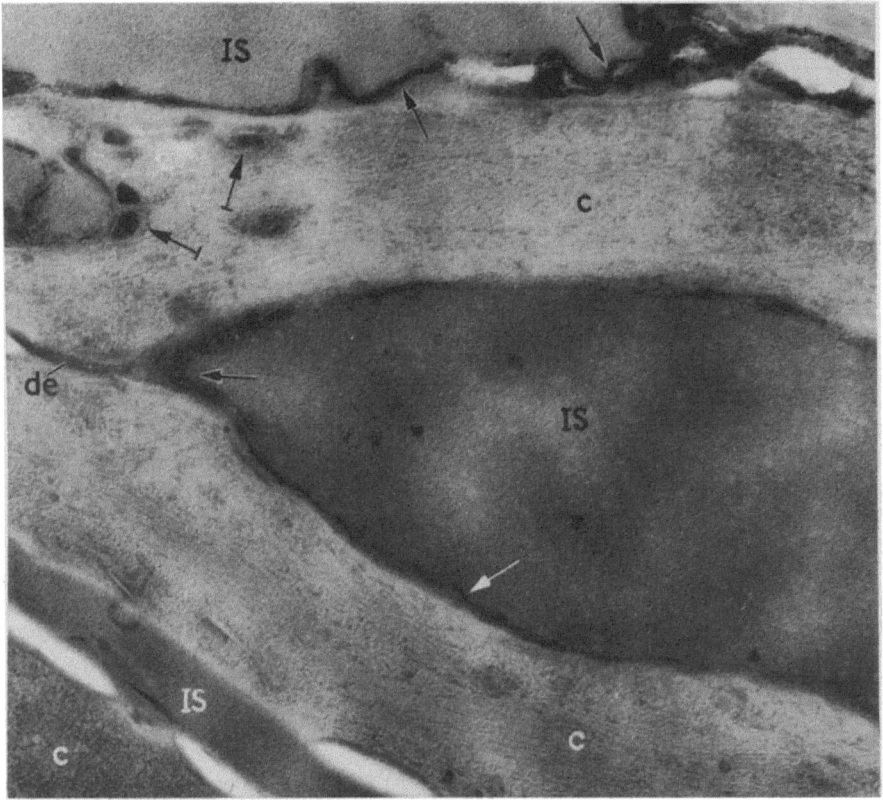

Fig. 9. Part of the basal layer of the stratum corneum in abdominal skin. The intercellular space (*IS*) varies conspicuously in width and in some areas exceeds the height of the cells (*c*). The *IS* is filled with non-homogeneous substance. A highly opaque membrane-component (→) appears mainly at the periphery of the *IS*. *de* regular desmosome. The fibrils in the cells show a distinct keratin pattern. Granules of unknown nature (↦). × 61,000.
[From BRODY, 1966. Courtesy of Nature, Macmillan (Journals) Limited, London]

skin surface. The extracellular space between the basement membrane and the basal surface of the cells in the stratum basale has a width of about 300 Å (for references see chapter A:I) and it is in direct continuity with the intercellular space in the stratum basale (MERCER, 1961).

In the non-cornified epidermis the intercellular space appears most distinctly in the stratum spinosum (Fig. 20). HIBBS and CLARK (1959) state that they have found only a narrow space in this layer. Sections of the epidermis from different sites, however, show variations in the width of the intercellular space in the stratum spinosum, and variations probably also occur within the same area.

In the stratum intermedium the cells may lie close to each other and the width of the intercellular space is then no more than 200 to 300 Å, or it may here become widened through the occurrence of the invaginations of the cell surfaces (Fig. 8). The intercellular space may also have about the same width as that in the stratum spinosum.

In the stratum corneum the intercellular space may have a width of 200 to 300 Å or it may vary conspicuously and attain a maximal width of about 2 μ (BRODY, 1966). This means that in some parts its width may exceed the height of the horny cells, whereas in other parts it is only of submicroscopic order of magnitude (Figs. 9, 14a and 14b).

In the normal guinea-pig and human epidermis BRODY (1959b, 1960a, b, 1964b) has demonstrated that the intercellular space between the stratum intermedium and the T- and horny cells is filled with an opaque, amorphous material in which round or oval vesicles of low opacity are dispersed. The vesicles were mainly found in the invaginations. BRODY (1959b) has suggested that the intercellular substance may be derived from the cells on their transformation to T- and horny cells and may perhaps be reabsorbed by the cells of the stratum intermedium. In a study of normal and hyperplastic mouse epidermis FREI and SHELDON (1961) confirm and extend the findings of BRODY. They have observed substances in the whole intercellular space of the stratum intermedium. They have shown, moreover, the occurrence of opaque granules both in the invaginations and in the cells of the stratum intermedium (Fig. 8). They call these granules "corpuscula". The corpuscula are similar in appearance to the intracellular bodies earlier described by SELBY (1957) and ODLAND (1960). Some of the corpuscula were homogeneously dense and structureless, whereas others displayed an internal structure. FREI and SHELDON (1961) assume that the content of the corpuscula is extruded into the intercellular space and there forms the amorphous substance. Later electron-microscopic investigations of normal epidermis (MATOLTSY and PARAKKAL, 1965; BREATHNACH and WYLLIE, 1966) and of normal and pathologic mucous membranes (MATOLTSY and PARAKKAL, 1965; FRITHIOF and WERSÄLL,

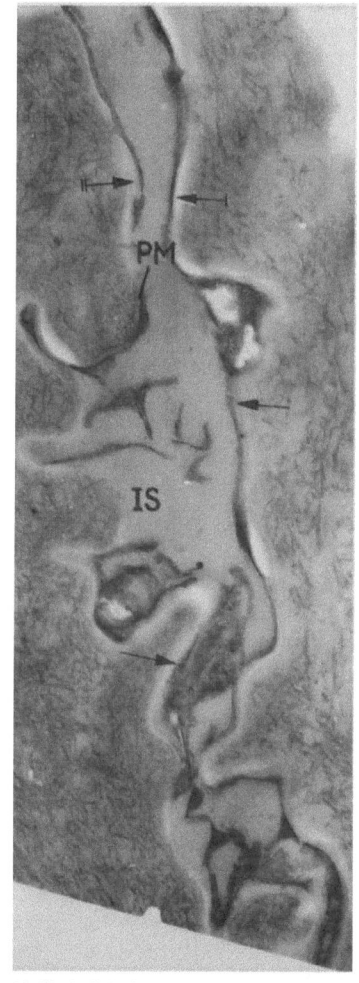

Fig. 10. Part of the intermediate layer of the stratum corneum in abdominal skin. The intercellular space (*IS*) is filled with a non-homogeneous substance. A highly opaque membrane-component (→) and bodies incorporated in it (→) are observed mainly along the periphery of the *IS*. The membrane may show a triple-layered pattern (⊢→) or appear blurred (⊢→). *PM* plasma membrane. × 30,000. [From BRODY, 1966. Courtesy of Nature, Macmillan (Journals) Limited, London]

1965; OLÁH and RÖHLICH, 1966) in man and laboratory animals support the findings by FREI and SHELDON (1961) that one type of granule occurs both intracellularly and intercellularly in the invaginations. These granules contain a system of densely packed membranes and are bounded by an asymmetrical triple-layered membrane (ODLAND, 1964; FRITHIOF and WERSÄLL, 1965; MATOLTSY and PARAKKAL, 1965; WILGRAM, 1965; BREATHNACH and WYLLIE, 1966; OLÁH and RÖHLICH, 1966; WILGRAM and WEINSTOCK, 1966). The size of these organelles has been given as

1000 to 5000 Å (MATOLTSY and PARAKKAL, 1965), and as 1000 to 2000 Å (FRITHIOF and WERSÄLL, 1965). According to BREATHNACH and WYLLIE (1966) the length of the granule is 1300 to 2400 Å and the breadth 1200 to 2000 Å. The granules have been called "Odland's bodies" (JARRETT and SPEARMAN, 1964), "Selby-Odland's bodies" (WILGRAM, 1965), "lamellated bodies" (FRITHIOF and WERSÄLL, 1965), "membrane-coating granules" (MATOLTSY and PARAKKAL, 1965) and "keratinosomes" (WILGRAM, 1965; WILGRAM and WEINSTOCK, 1966). The expression "lamellated bodies" will be used here. FRITHIOF and WERSÄLL (1965), MATOLTSY and PARAKKAL (1965), BREATHNACH and WYLLIE (1966) and OLÁH and RÖHLICH (1966)

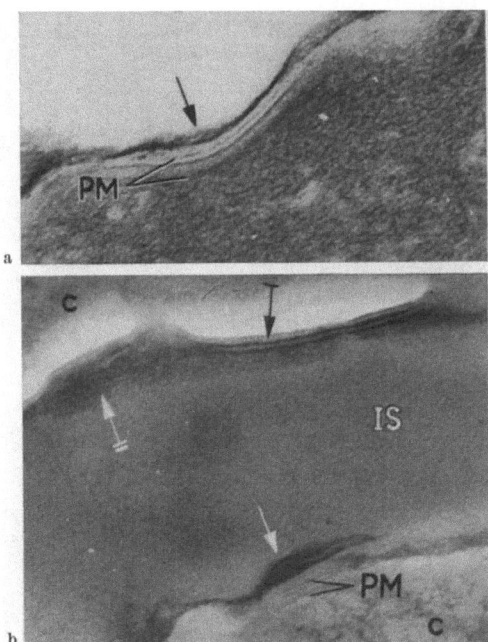

Fig. 11. a Part of a cell in the superficial layer of the stratum corneum. The membrane-component (→) located at the periphery of the intercellular space is distinctly separated from the plasma membrane (PM) of the cell. × 146,000. [From BRODY, 1966. Courtesy of Nature, Macmillan (Journals) Limited, London.] b Part of the intermediate layer of the stratum corneum. A body (→) incorporated in the membrane-component is located at the periphery of the intercellular space (IS) and is also distinctly separated from the plasma membrane (PM). The membrane-component shows a triple-layered pattern (⊢→). The non-homogeneous substance in the IS displays indications of fine filaments (⊢→). c cell. × 76,000

assume that the granules are excreted into the intercellular space in the stratum intermedium. RUPEC and BRAUN-FALCO (1965) have made the same observations, but they think that the invaginations are constricted and thus become intracytoplasmic organelles which are ultrastructurally identical with the intracellular lamellated bodies.

With FREI and SHELDON (1961) MATOLTSY and PARAKKAL (1965) also believe that the lamellated bodies empty their content into the intercellular space, but only after first having become attached to the plasma membrane. At a later stage the content of the bodies was thought to form the thickened plasma membrane of the horny cells (MATOLTSY and PARAKKAL, 1965). There is, however, no evidence that the modified plasma membranes of the T- and horny cells are formed in this way.

Nor is there any evidence that the amorphous substance in the intercellular space derives from the lamellated bodies, as FREI and SHELDON (1961) and MATOLTSY and PARAKKAL (1965) suggest. This substance is also seen in those parts of the intercellular space in which no bodies appear and it also fills the entire intercellular space of the stratum corneum in human skin from the abdominal and sacral regions (BRODY, 1966; Figs. 9—12). Higher magnifications have revealed that this intercellular substance is not amorphous but displays a pattern with indications of fine opaque filaments (BRODY, 1966; Figs. 9 and 11b). Dispersed in this substance are found lamellated bodies and other types of granule and vesicle of different shape, size and ultrastructure which occur at all levels of the stratum corneum and also close to the skin surface (BRODY, 1966; Figs. 12—14). In some parts of the intercellular space they are frequently observed and in other regions they are sparser.

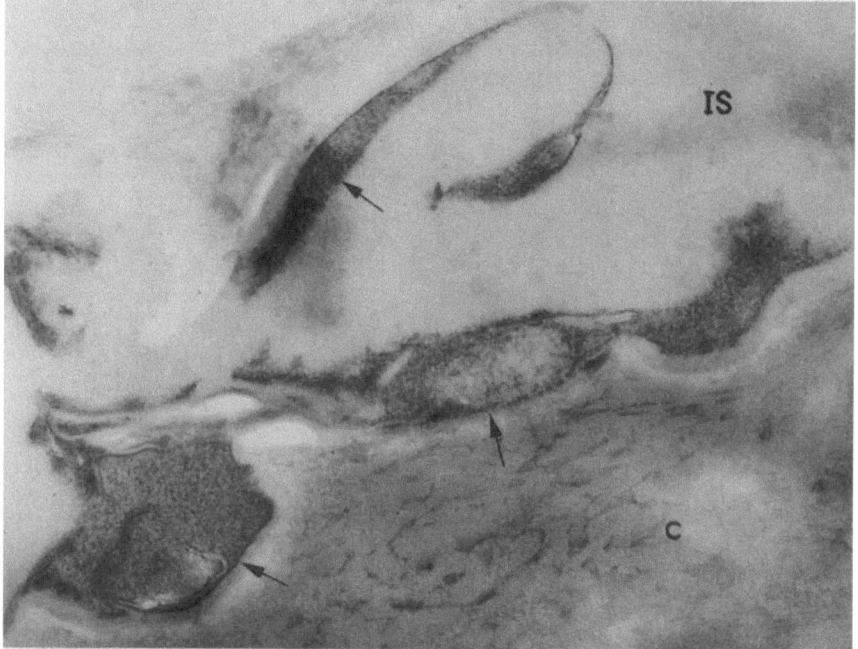

Fig. 12. Part of the superficial layer of the stratum corneum. Lamellated bodies (→) incorporated in the membrane-component. *IS* intercellular space, *c* cell. × 50,000. [From BRODY, 1966. Courtesy of Nature, Macmillan (Journals) Limited, London]

In the stratum corneum the lamellated bodies seem to be incorporated in a membrane-like component (BRODY, 1966). This structure has not yet been distinguished either intercellularly or intracellularly in the stratum intermedium. The membrane-like component is very opaque (Figs. 9—12). It appears mainly at the periphery of the intercellular space close to the cell surface, but like the lamellated bodies is distinctly separated from the plasma membrane (Figs. 11a and b). It may be observed along the length of the cells or may occur only fragmentarily. In some areas it exhibits a triple-layered pattern and in others it appears as a multi-layered structure or as a single, blurred layer (Figs. 9, 11a and b). The membrane varies here between 100 and 400 Å in thickness. The incorporated lamellated bodies have a length of 2400 to 7300 Å and a breadth of 450 to 5100 Å (Fig. 12).

Granules containing triple-layered membranes are often observed. It is, however, not yet clear whether the outer, bounding membrane is single- or triple-layered. The granules have a length of 2700 to 5200 Å and a breadth of 1500 to 2200 Å (Fig. 13a). Another larger organelle seems to be at least partly constituted of a system of triple- and multi-layered membranes (Fig. 13d). A frequently seen granule displays a diffuse ultrastructure. It seems to be bounded by an opaque, single layer. It has a rather low opacity, but some parts appear to be more, and others less, opaque. It is about 3600 Å in length and about 1300 Å in breadth. Close to this granule, smaller, dense, opaque bodies are often observed (Fig. 13b).

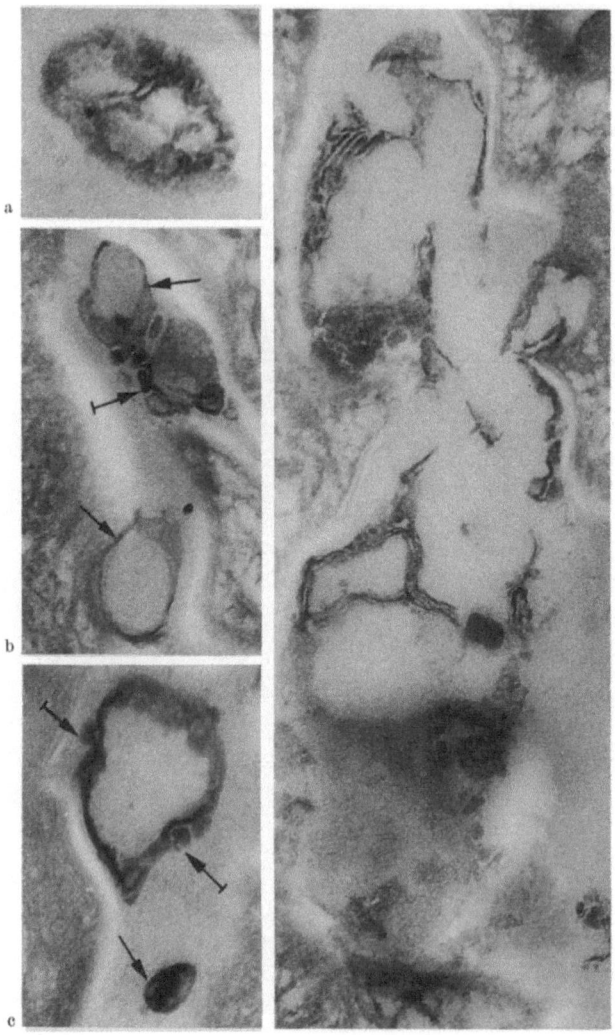

Figs. 13a—d showing different types of structures appearing in the intercellular space of the stratum corneum in human skin from the abdominal and sacral regions. [From BRODY, 1966. Courtesy of Nature, Macmillan (Journals) Limited, London.] a Granule displaying a triple-layered inner membrane. The outer limiting membrane is indistinct. × 100,000. b The granules (→) seem to be partly bounded by an opaque, single-layered membrane. Some parts of the granules are more, and others less, opaque. Small, opaque corpuscles (⊢→) appear close to the longitudinally sectioned granule. × 68,000. c At the bottom a small oval granule with uneven opacity (→). In the upper part of the picture a granule or vesicle bounded by a rather broad, opaque membrane. Small corpuscles (⊢→) close to the membrane. × 80,000. d Disrupted granules which consist partly of triple- and multiple-layered membranes. × 68,000

Another type of granules appears as mainly dense corpuscles with a round or oval shape. These vary in size and opacity. They have a length of 170 to 1300 Å and a breadth of 170 to 900 Å (Fig. 29). A granule or vesicle bounded by a rather broad, opaque membrane, adjacent to which appear smaller granules, can also be seen. It has a length of about 3,200 Å and a breadth of about 2,300 Å (Fig.13c).

Several of the lamellated bodies incorporated in the membrane-like component and several of the other granules are of such an order of magnitude that they may be seen in the light microscope, and may there give the impression of a diffuse membranous component if they occur closely enough. Granules and bodies of a size which is close to the lower limit of the resolution of the light microscope should also be discernible with optical microscopy if they are numerous and occur densely in the intercellular space (BRODY, 1966).

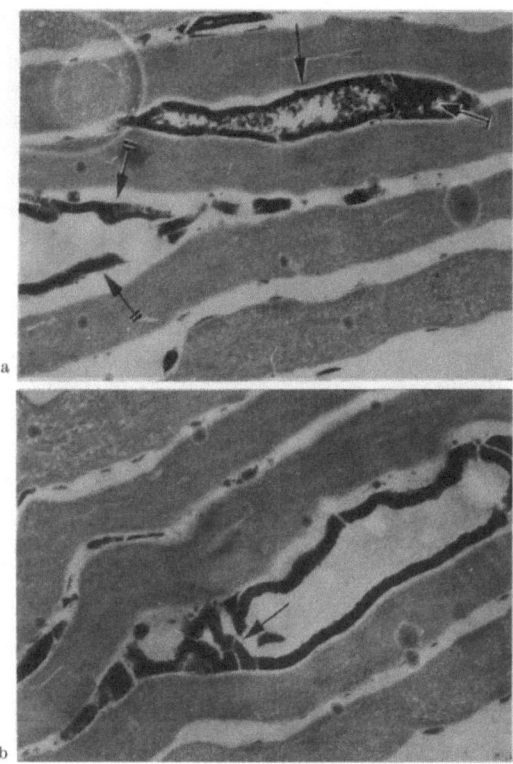

Fig. 14. a Part of the intermediate layer of the stratum corneum in human skin from the upper arm. In the intercellular space a granule (→) displaying a broad, very opaque outer membrane. At one end the content is very opaque and shows indications of an inner membrane (↦) with thickness and opacity similar to those of the outer membrane. In the adjacent part of the intercellular space remains of a similar granule showing only fragments of the outer membrane (↦). × 20,000. b A granule similar to that shown in Fig. 14a. The outer membrane is thick and opaque. At one end (→) inner membranes of thickness and opacity similar to those of the outer membrane. The breadth of the granule exceeds the height of the cells. In other parts the intercellular space is rather narrow. × 20,000

MATOLTSY and PARAKKAL (1965) treated human skin and bovine oral epithelium with 0.1 N sodium hydroxyde, and after centrifugation obtained a membrane-like structure which they examined in the electron microscope. They assume that this structure represents isolated envelopes of the horny cells, in accordance with the view earlier suggested by histologists (UNNA, 1883, 1913; WEIDENREICH, 1900; HOEPKE, 1927; PERNKOPF and PATZELT, 1933; MATOLTSY and BALSAMO, 1955; CHRISTOPHERS and KLIGMAN, 1964; KLIGMAN, 1964). The membranous component obtained by MATOLTSY and PARAKKAL (1965), however, is similar in arrangement, ultrastructure and thickness to the membrane-like component with the incorporated lamellated bodies which BRODY (1966) has distinctly demonstrated in the intercellular space of the stratum corneum. These components and the different types of granule are the only organelles of a size recognizable in the light microscope, whereas the plasma membrane itself is only of a submicroscopic order of magnitude. On the basis of these different observations Brody (1966) advances the hypothesis that the diffuse membranous structure observed in the light microscope and retained in the horny layer after skin has been treated with cold alkaline solution or nitric acid (*i.e.*, the most resistant material of the stratum corneum or what Unna has called "keratin A") does not represent the cell membranes but is constituted by a complex of structures located in the intercellular space.

This assumption is further strongly supported by different data respecting the "horny membrane" of Unna or the "horny cell membrane" that have been presented. Unna (1883) himself gave the following description of it: "Very thin sections of the horny layer therefore show, after digestion, a coarse-meshed network of horny substance without any content, whose trabeculae are formed from two adjacent horny fibres which are joined by rather short horny bridges. These horny fibres, the cross-sections of the horny membranes, have everywhere the same thickness, of about 1 μ, even through the whole thickness of the stratum corneum of the heel."

By means of polarization-optical and X-ray diffraction methods Champetier and Litvac (1939) have investigated untreated sections of the stratum corneum and sections of the horny layer treated with cold alkaline solution. In the untreated sections the anisotropic fibril keratin (Keratin B of Unna) showed an alpha-diffraction pattern which under pressure or in autoclave could be transformed into a beta-pattern. The membrane-component remaining after the treatment with the alkaline solution did not show any diffraction pattern, and Champetier and Litvac therefore consider this isotropic membrane-keratin as an entirely different substance from the keratin B.

In histochemical studies Spier and Caneghem (1957), and Jarrett and Spearman (1964) propose that the disulfide groups in the stratum corneum are mainly concentrated to the "cell membrane".

According to Pascher (1964) only the keratin A of Unna, identical to the "horny cell membrane component", fulfils the claims which the definition of keratins implies, *viz.* that the keratins should be insoluble in water, in diluted acids and alkalis and be resistant to proteolytic enzymes (Flaschenträger and Lehnartz, 1951).

Matoltsy and Matoltsy (1966) have investigated the biochemistry of the membranous component isolated from the stratum corneum of the plantar epidermis with centrifugation after extraction in 0.1 N sodium hydroxide. They found a high proline and cystine content. The large quantities of proline may according to the authors imply that the membrane-protein is not a fibrous protein. This observation lends support to the view advanced by Champetier and Litvac (1939). The high cystine content also accords well with the histochemical results obtained by Spier and Caneghem (1957) and Jarrett and Spearman (1964).

It is, moreover, of great interest to note the remarkable differences in the amounts of "cell membranes" which Pascher (1964), in a biochemical study, obtained from the normal human stratum corneum of the back and from callus (which means a further thickening of the already normally very thick horny layers of the plantar or palmar skin). The native total stratum corneum of the back contains 24.5 per cent "cell membrane" (stratum corneum compactum 11.0 per cent and stratum corneum disjunctum 13.5 per cent), whereas that of the callus contains only 3.5 per cent "cell membrane". From homogenized abdominal epidermis Matoltsy and Balsamo (1955a, b) and Matoltsy and Herbst (1956) obtained 5 to 10 per cent insoluble residues, which consist of "cell membrane", granules and some cellular debris. Human plantar and palmar skin contains 5 per cent resistant "cell-membrane" material (MATOLTSY, 1962a).

III. Attachment Zones

1. Desmosomes

Among histologists the view has been held that the epidermal cells are connected through "intercellular bridges" (cf. surveys by PATZELT, 1926; SCHAFFER, 1927; BRAUN-FALCO, 1954). The cytoplasmic processes of the adjacent cells were assumed to form these bridges. At the point where the processes were thought to meet, a thickening is observed in the light microscope. This has been called "bridge nodule", the "nodule of Bizzozero", the "nodule of Ranvier" or the "desmosome" of SCHAFFER (1927).

In an electron-microscopic investigation of adult frog skin OTTOSON, SJÖSTRAND, STENSTRÖM and SVAETICHIN (1953) point out that where the adjacent cells connect, the cell membrane is particularly well marked. In embryonic frog skin PORTER (1954a, b) was also able to show that there is no continuity of fibrous elements or cytoplasm across the cell membrane at the cell junctions.

The subsequent investigations on the normal epidermis of man (ODLAND, 1958; HIBBS and CLARK, 1959; BRODY, 1960b, 1964a, b, in press; ZELICKSON, 1961; ZELICKSON and HARTMANN, 1961b; RHODIN, 1965; WILGRAM, CAULFIELD and MADGIC, 1965; RUPEC, 1966; cf. also review by MERCER, 1961), of rat (HORSTMANN and KNOOP, 1958; MERCER, 1958a; BIRBECK, 1961), of guinea-pig (BRODY, 1959a, 1960b; SNELL, 1965a, b), of mouse (VOGEL, 1960; ROTH and CLARK, 1964), of frog (FARQUHAR and PALADE, 1964, 1965), of the embryonic epidermis of different laboratory animals (OVERTON, 1962; BRODY and LARSSON, 1965; KELLY, 1965) and of pathologic human epidermis (WILGRAM, CAULFIELD and LEVER, 1961; BRODY, 1962a, b, c, d, 1963a, b, c; WILGRAM, CAULFIELD and MADGIC, 1964a, b, 1965; BRAUN-FALCO and PETRY, 1965, 1966; BRAUN-FALCO and VOGELL, 1965, 1966) have greatly increased our knowledge of the ultrastructure of the cell junctions occurring at the points where the light microscopists have assumed the presence of cytoplasmic "intercellular bridges". Among the electron microscopists the expression "desmosome", coined by SCHAFFER (1927), is generally used for these cell junctions. FARQUHAR and PALADE (1963, 1964, 1965) have also introduced the name "macula adhaerens" for this type of cell junction.

Desmosomes are present not only in the epidermis, but also in mucous membranes (FASSKE and THEMANN, 1959b; KARRER, 1960; VOGEL, 1960; MERKER, 1961), and in other tissues (SJÖSTRAND, ANDERSSON-CEDERGREN and DEWEY, 1958; WOOD, 1959; GRIMLEY and EDWARDS, 1960; HAMA, 1960; FARQUHAR and PALADE, 1963; TAMARIN and SREEBNY, 1963; LOCKE, 1965; ROSS and GREENLEE, 1966).

In frog epidermis, FARQUHAR and PALADE (1965) distinguish three types of desmosomes, viz. "regular", "composite" and "modified" desmosomes. In human epidermis RUPEC (1956) has described two types: a desmosomal structure that probably corresponds to the regular desmosome in frog epidermis, and a "simple" desmosome. The latter is by FARQUHAR and PALADE (1963) named "zonula adhaerens". The desmosomes of the normal human epidermis will here be referred to as "regular" and "simple" desmosomes.

The desmosomes display a symmetric ultrastructure and consist of a cellular component contributed by each cell and of an intercellular component. The two types of desmosomes differ, however, with respect to both the cellular and intercellular components (Figs. 15).

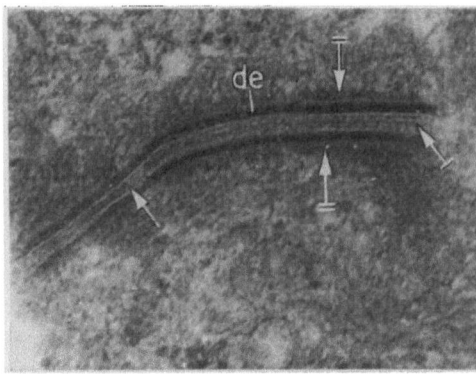

Fig. 15 shows a regular (*de*) and simple (→) desmosome. The simple desmosome lacks the central layer (↦) of the intercellular component of the regular desmosome. The filaments insert into a filamentous striation (⊢→) running parallel to the plaques but separated from them by a less opaque layer. × 98,000

a) The Regular Desmosome

In a study of normal human epidermis ODLAND (1958) observed that the intercellular component of the regular desmosomes consists of seven layers and that the so-called attachment plaques (here referred to as "plaques") form thickenings of the single-layered plasma membrane. This electron-microscopic picture of the regular desmosome suggested by ODLAND has been supported in some later investigations on the epidermis and mucous membranes (HIBBS and CLARK, 1959; BRODY, 1960b; TAMARIN and SREEBNY, 1963; PUCCINELLI, 1964; ROTH and CLARK, 1964; WILGRAM, CAULFIELD and MADGIC, 1964a).

VOGEL (1960), investigating the epidermis and cervical epithelium of the mouse, and KARRER (1960), investigating the human cervical epithelium, showed independently, however, that the plasma membrane in the non-cornified epidermis is triple-layered and that the intercellular component of the regular desmosomes consists only of two light layers and a central, opaque, single layer. The "intermediate dense layers" and "proximal light layers" which ODLAND (1958) referred to as belonging to the intercellular component are thus by VOGEL (1960) and KARRER (1960) considered to represent the outer leaflets and intermediate light layers of the adjacent plasma membranes respectively. These findings have since been confirmed (PETRY, 1962; FARQUHAR and PALADE, 1965; RUPEC, 1966; BRODY, in press; Figs. 15 and 16).

In a study of normal human epidermis HIBBS and CLARK (1959) show that the central, opaque layer of the intercellular component — the so-called "intercellular contact layer" of ODLAND (1958), "stratum x" of KARRER (1960) or the "M-layer" of RUPEC (1966) — is triple-layered. In a recent investigation BRODY (in press) supports this finding (see also Fig. 25). The latter author has, moreover, demonstrated that the layer earlier considered as the outer leaflet of the plasma membrane within the desmosomal area also appears as triple-layered. The intercellular component thus consists here of nine layers, *i.e.*, two plates separated centrally from each other and laterally from the outer leaflets of the plasma membranes by a narrow, light layer. Each plate consists of a broad, intermediate, light layer limited by narrow, opaque layers (BRODY, in press).

Within the desmosomal area ODLAND (1958) assumed that the cell membrane is thickened. He called this part of the cell membrane "attachment plaque", since he believed that the epidermal filaments insert into this plaque. According to KARRER (1960) and FARQUHAR and PALADE (1965), the plaque is formed by "condensed" cytoplasm along the inner leaflet of the plasma membrane. VOGEL (1960) suggests that it represents a thickening of the cytoplasmic leaflet of the plasma membrane. RUPEC (1966) and BRODY (in press; see also Fig. 16) have demonstrated that the plaque, together with the cytoplasmic leaflet of the plasma membrane, forms a five-layered, very opaque structure. The plaque and the intercellular component have each a width of about 150 Å (RUPEC, 1966).

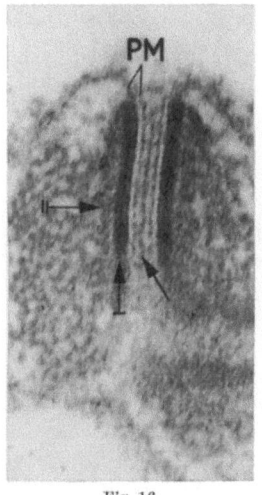
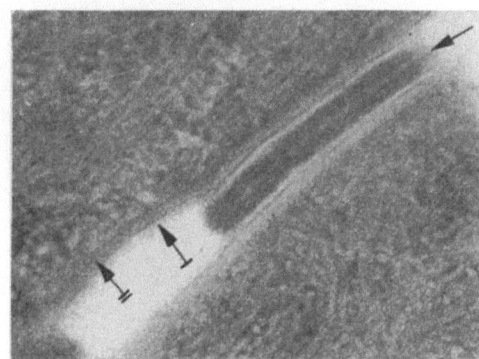

Fig. 16. Fig. 17

Fig. 16. Higher magnification of a regular desmosome in the stratum basale. The intercellular component consists of three layers: a central, opaque layer (→) and two less opaque layers on each side. *PM* triple-layered plasma membrane. The plaques (↦) with the cytoplasmic leaflet of the plasma membrane included consist of three opaque and two less opaque layers. The filamentous striation (↦) into which the filaments insert is separated from the plaques by a less opaque layer. × 173,000

Fig. 17. Higher magnification of a regular desmosome in the stratum corneum. The intercellular component (→) is on the whole more opaque than that of the desmosomes in the non-cornified epidermis (cf. Fig. 16). The layering is still distinguishable. The modified plasma membrane consists of a peripheral, faintly opaque layer (↦), a broad cytoplasmic zone and an outer intermediate light layer in between. The main part of the broad cytoplasmic zone is constituted by the inner broad intermediate layer (↦), which is bounded on either side by narrow opaque layers. The outer of these opaque layers represents the cytoplasmic leaflet of the plasma membrane in the non-cornified epidermis. In the cells the fibrils show a keratin pattern. × 133,000. (From BRODY, 1960b. Courtesy of J. Ultrastruct. Res., Academic Press Inc., New York-London)

In accordance with the hypothesis by ODLAND (1958), it is generally held that the epidermal filaments terminate at the plaques (MERCER, 1961; WILGRAM CAULFIELD and LEVER, 1961; FARQUHAR and PALADE, 1965; KELLY, 1966; WILGRAM and WEINSTOCK, 1966). This finding is at variance with the observations of BRODY (1960b, 1964b, in press). According to the latter author, the filaments do not insert into the plaques, but terminate at an opaque, filamentous striation which runs parallel to the plaques (Figs. 15 and 16). This is separated from the latter by a less opaque, about 40 Å thick layer (BRODY, 1960b). RUPEC (1966) has observed that the probably obliquely sectioned filament bundles are separated from the plaques by a narrow, light layer. He thus partly supports the findings by BRODY (1960b, 1964b, in press).

In the normal human stratum corneum the regular desmosomes display an altered ultrastructure as compared to those in the non-cornified epidermis (BRODY, 1960b, 1964b, in press). A similar layering of the intercellular component is observed (Fig. 17), but the altered appearance seems to be due to an increase in the opacity of the broad, intermediate layers of the plates of the intercellular component (BRODY, in press). The plaques are no longer distinguishable, since they form parts of the modified plasma membrane. The filamentous striation is only faintly indicated.

b) The Simple Desmosome

In an electron-microscopic investigation of the epidermis in rat-foot skin HORSTMANN and KNOOP (1958) found different appearances of the desmosomes in the various strata. In the upper layer of the stratum intermedium and in the stratum corneum they observed that the intercellular component of the desmosomes consists of two opaque and three less opaque layers. This ultrastructure differs from that of the intercellular component of the regular desmosomes. This type of desmosome probably corresponds to that described by RUPEC (1966) as a simple desmosome. It is characterized by the occurrence of a relatively thin intercellular component (Fig. 15) which lacks the opaque "M-layer" (RUPEC, 1966) or "intercellular contact layer" (ODLAND, 1958) of the regular desmosomes. The triple-layered pattern of the plasma membrane is distinctly discernible also in the simple desmosomes. Associated with the cytoplasmic leaflet of the plasma membrane, a condensed cytoplasmic, about 50 Å thick zone is observed. Within this zone a somewhat less opaque layer is seen (RUPEC, 1966).

2. Nexus

Besides the two types of desmosomes a third type of cell junction is found between the keratinocytes in the non-cornified human epidermis. It has been

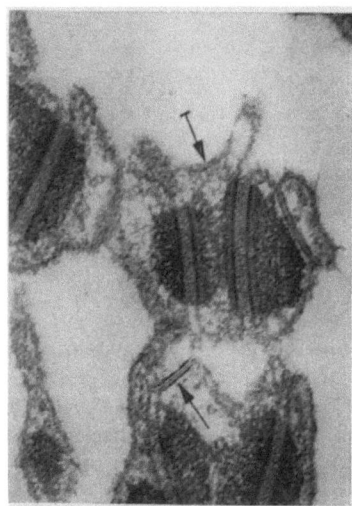

Fig. 18 shows regular desmosomes and a nexus (→). The plasma membrane is triple-layered (⊢→). ×48,000

described in normal human epidermis (RUPEC, 1966) and in psoriatic epidermis (BRODY, 1962a). It is also observed in frog epidermis (DEWEY and BARR, 1964; FARQUHAR and PALADE, 1964, 1965), in normal human cervical epithelium (KARRER, 1960) and in other tissues (for references see DEWEY and BARR, 1964). It appears as a five-layered structure formed by the fusion of two adjacent triple-layered cell membranes (Fig. 18). DEWEY and BARR (1964) have introduced the term "nexus" for this contact zone, which expression is used here. Other expressions have been suggested, such as "longitudinal connecting surface" (SJÖSTRAND, ANDERSSON-CEDERGREN and DEWEY, 1958), "quintuple-layered cell interconnection" (KARRER, 1960), "external compound membrane" (ROBERTSON, 1960), "tight junction" (FARQUHAR and PALADE, 1961), "zonula and macula occludens" (FARQUHAR and PALADE, 1963, 1965).

With electron microscopy BRODY and LARSSON (1965) have investigated the development of sub-layers in embryonic mouse epidermis. They found that the nexuses are more numerous in earlier than in later stages, whereas the number of desmosomes increases with the increasing differentiation of the epidermis. In adult normal human epidermis the nexuses are few. In psoriatic epidermis characterized by parakeratosis without keratohyalin the nexuses are often observed, whereas the desmosomes occur in smaller numbers than in normal tissue (BRODY, 1962a, b, c, d). In psoriatic epidermis with hyperkeratosis there are, again, numerous desmosomes but only few nexuses (BRODY, 1963b, c, d). These observations may indicate that in the epidermis the number of nexuses and desmosomes is related to the stage of differentiation (BRODY and LARSSON, 1965). Further support for this assumption is afforded by the observations of human epidermis with chronic nummular eczema (BRAUN-FALCO and PETRY, 1965, 1966) and of normal frog epidermis (FARQUHAR and PALADE, 1965). The latter type of epidermis differs greatly from the normal human epidermis. Although FARQUHAR and PALADE (1965) use the term "stratum granulosum", no keratohyalin is discernible in this type of epidermis. The horny cells contain nuclei, and the epidermal fibrils do not undergo a differentiation with the development of a "keratin pattern" (BRODY, 1959a, 1960b, 1964b). The epidermis of the frog skin is thus in some respects similar to the parakeratotic psoriatic epidermis without keratohyalin as described by BRODY (1962a, b, c, d, e), and like this it contains numerous well-developed nexuses.

According to FARQUHAR and PALADE (1963, 1965) the nexuses (zonula and macula occludens) are impermeable by macromolecules, water, ions and small water-soluble molecules. They may also represent areas of low resistance coupling and may offer pathways for electric current between the cell interiors (DEWEY and BARR, 1964).

3. The Junctional Desmosomes

Along the dermo-epidermal junction a special type of attachment zone occurs (Figs. 1 and 19). It is generally known as "half- or hemi-desmosome" (PORTER, 1956; CHARLES and SMIDDY, 1957; MERCER, 1961; KELLY, 1966; WILGRAM and WEINSTOCK, 1966). The expressions "bobbin" (WEISS and FERRIS, 1954a; FARQUHAR and PALADE, 1965), "basal plate" (FARQUHAR and PALADE, 1965) and "junctional granule" (WILGRAM and WEINSTOCK, 1966) have also been used. This type of attachment zone is considered to differ from the regular desmosomes only inasmuch it does not form a contact between two cells. From an ultrastructural point of view it is believed to represent a half of a regular desmosome. BRODY (in press) has, however, demonstrated that the attachment zones along the dermo-epidermal junction differ also ultrastructurally from the regular desmosomes as well as from the other types of attachment zone described in the epidermis. He terms them "junctional desmosomes". They do not contain any plaques as they were earlier assumed to do (WEISS and FERRIS, 1954a; PORTER, 1956; SELBY, 1956; CHARLES and SMIDDY, 1957; ODLAND, 1958; FARQUHAR and PALADE, 1965; KELLY, 1966). The filaments terminate at a filamentous striation which is separated from the plasma membrane by a narrow, light layer (BRODY, in press).

The junctional desmosomes are numerous and occur fairly regularly along the entire plasma membrane of the keratinocytes (SELBY, 1955; MERCER, 1958a, 1961; ODLAND, 1958; BRODY, 1960b; WILGRAM, CAULFIELD and MADGIC, 1964a, b, 1965). The extracellular component is in close contact with the basement membrane (BRODY, 1962a, in press; CAULFIELD and WILGRAM, 1962; ROTH and CLARK, 1964; Figs. 1 and 19).

PETRY, OVERBECK and VOGELL (1961a, b) and PETRY (1962) state that the displacement of the individual cells from the basal layer towards the surface of the vaginal epithelium must imply that the regular desmosomes represent temporary and variable structures: they become dissolved and new desmosomes are formed according to the situation. The observations of the different types of attachment zone in the epidermis (FARQUHAR and PALADE, 1965; RUPEC, 1966; BRODY, in press) strongly support this view.

The desmosomal structures are considered to be involved primarily in the attachment of the cells (MERCER, 1961; FARQUHAR and PALADE, 1965), or in the case of the junctional desmosomes in the attachment of the keratinocytes to the basement membrane (BRODY, 1962a, in press; CAULFIELD and WILGRAM, 1962; ROTH and CLARK, 1964). It has also been assumed that they serve to anchor and orient the epidermal fibrils (MERCER, 1961; WILGRAM, CAULFIELD

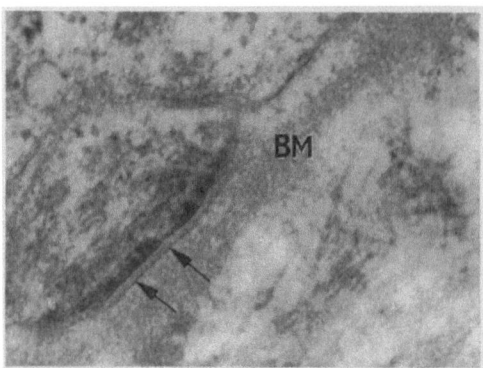

Fig. 19 shows a junctional desmosome along the dermo-epidermal junction. The peripheral leaflet of the plasma membrane is faintly indicated within the junctional desmosome. Extracellular component of the junctional desmosome (→). *BM* basement membrane. × 81,000

and LEVER, 1961; WILGRAM, CAULFIELD and MADGIC, 1964a; FARQUHAR and PALADE, 1965) and to provide suitable sites for initiating fibrinogenesis (MERCER, 1961; ROTH and CLARK, 1964; WILGRAM, CAULFIELD and MADGIC, 1964a).

IV. Epidermal Fibrils

1. Definitions

RANVIER (1879, 1882) was the first to describe the occurrence of epithelial fibers in the epidermis. On the basis of the general histological conception that the fibers run *via* the "intercellular bridges" from cell to cell throughout the epidermis and that they are responsible for the tonus of the epidermis, HEIDENHAIN (1907) introduced the name "tonofibrils" for these structures.

Whether the fibrils exist *in vivo* or represent artefacts resulting from postmortal changes or brought about by the fixing agents is a question that is decisive for studies of the morphology, chemistry, and function of the fibrils, and one which has long been debated. The most widely varying histological statements have been made as to what the true facts concerning the tonofibrils may be. PATZELT (1926) gives a collocation of the relevant literature, *i.e.*, that relating to the point on which a consensus of opinion has by no means been arrived at: whether in the process of cornification the fibrils persist, whether in this connection they are disintegrated or what otherwise may be the facts regarding them.

The discussion of the question whether the fibrils are artefacts or not was, however, first brought seriously to the fore by the investigations of living epidermal cells by DE MOULIN (1923) and CHAMBERS and RÉNYI (1925), of living epidermal cells in tissue culture by PARSHLEY and SIMMS (1950) and by electron-microscopic investigations of osmium-fixed epidermis by GESSLER, GREY, SCHUSTER, KELSCH and RICHTER (1948) and PEASE (1951). These investigations did not show any evidence for the existence of the intracellular fibrils so frequently observed in histological, fixed material.

However, a wide range of studies in which a variety of techniques are used, has clearly brought direct and indirect evidence for the existence of fibrils in the epidermis. This has been done by phase-contrast microscopic (v. ALBERTINI, 1946; MELCZER and CZEPLÁK, 1957) and polarization-optical (HORSTMANN, 1957; MELCZER and CCEPLÁK, 1957) investigations of living epidermis; with phase-contrast microscopy on living cells (LEWIS, POMERAT and EZELL, 1949) and on fixed and embedded epidermal cells (PINKUS, 1932, 1939) in tissue culture; by X-ray diffraction studies of sectioned epidermis (DERKSEN and HERINGA, 1936; GIROUD and CHAMPETIER, 1936; DERKSEN, HERINGA and WEIDINGER, 1937; CHAMPETIER and LITVAC, 1939) and of chemically extracted epidermal fibrous protein (RUDALL, 1946, 1947, 1952; ROE, 1956; MATOLTSY, 1964, 1965); and, finally, by electron-microscopic investigations of fixed and embedded epidermis of man and laboratory animals (PORTER, 1954, 1956; WEISS and FERRIS, 1954; SELBY, 1955, 1956, 1957; CHARLES and SMIDDY, 1957; HORSTMANN, 1957b, 1960; HORSTMANN and KNOOP, 1958; MERCER, 1958a, b, 1961; ODLAND, 1958, 1964; v. BARGEN, 1959; BRODY, 1959a, b, 1960a, b, 1962e, g, 1963a, 1964a, b; CHARLES, 1959; HIBBS and CLARK, 1959; EDWARDS and MAKK, 1960; SETÄLÄ, MERENMIES, STJERNVALL and NYHOLM, 1960; FREI and SHELDON, 1961; ZELICKSON, 1961; ZELICKSON and HARTMANN, 1961; HU and CARDELL, 1962; MATOLTSY and MATOLTSY, 1962a; RHODIN and REITH, 1962; WILGRAM, CAUFIELD and LEVER, 1962; FARQUHAR and PALADE, 1963, 1964, 1965; RHODIN, 1963, 1965; ROTH and CLARK, 1964; WILGRAM, CAULFIELD and MADGIC, 1964a, b, 1965; BRAUN-FALCO, 1965a; SNELL, 1965a, b; RUPEC, 1966).

These congruent results afford strong support for the assumption that the fibrils represent true cytoplasmic differentiations and are not due to the action of fixatives or to postmortal changes. The earlier held electron-microscopic view that the cytoplasm is granular, and not fibrillar (GESSLER, GREY, SCHUSTER and KELSCH, 1948; PEASE, 1951; ADOLPH, BAKER and LEIBY, 1951; LADEN, ERICKSON and ARMEN, 1952), has in subsequent studies been completely disproved (for references see above).

Although elastic properties are ascribed to the epidermal fibrous protein (RUDALL, 1952, 1953), MERCER, MUNGER, ROGERS and ROTH (1963) consider that there is no conclusive evidence that all fibrils are simultaneously in a state of tension. The electron-microscopic studies by PORTER (1954, 1956), WEISS and FERRIS (1954), SELBY (1955, 1956, 1957) and subsequent investigators have, moreover, shown unequivocally that the tonofibrils do not pass from cell to cell, but constitute exclusively intracellular components. MERCER, MUNGER, ROGERS and ROTH (1963) therefore suggest that the prefix "tono" be dropped. In order to arrive at a simplified and consistent nomenclature of similar components in keratinizing epithelia and related non-keratinizing epithelia they also propose a change of the terminology.

They define "keratins" as proteins produced by epithelial cells and usually retained within the cell. They are insoluble in the usual protein solvents, owing to the presence of numerous disulfide bonds between the peptide chains. The keratins are predominantly filamentous, predominantly amorphous, or mixtures of filamentous and amorphous elements.

A "fiber" ("fibre") is that portion of the hair protruding above the epidermis, including the cuticle of the cortex, the cortex and the medulla.

A "fibril" consists of a group of filaments. It may or may not contain a matrix.

A "filament" represents a long thread-like unit. It is usually 50—100 Å in diameter but may, e.g. in feather keratin, have a diameter of 30 Å. The filament is present in many keratins, in prekeratinized cells and in the cells of non-keratinizing epithelia.

"Protofilaments" are thread-like units associated with each other to form a filament.

"Intrafibrillar matrix" constitutes an opaque layer between the filaments (it corresponds to the term "interfilamentous substance", which is used here).

"Intrafilamentous matrix" forms the opaque layer that is found between the protofilaments.

In order to distinguish the fibrils in different tissues MERCER, MUNGER, ROGERS and ROTH further suggest the use of modifying adjectives such as "basal cell filaments", "epidermal fibrils", "mucous membrane fibrils" etc.

2. General Features

The fibrils are composed of bundles of filaments, first described in the non-cornified epidermis of embryonic frog skin by PORTER (1954, 1956) and WEISS and FERRIS (1954) and of embryonic and adult human and adult rat skin by SELBY (1955, 1956, 1957), and in the stratum corneum of adult guinea-pig and human skin by BRODY (1959a, b, 1960a, b). In the non-cornified as well as in the cornified epidermis the filaments seem to have a smaller diameter in the human skin than those in the skin of hair-covered mammalian laboratory animals. In the non-cornified human epidermis they have a diameter of about 50 Å (Selby, 1955, 1956, 1957; Brody, 1960b, 1964b; Zelickson, 1961). In the horny layer of human epidermis they attain a diameter of about 74 Å (Brody, 1960b, 1964b). The corresponding data for the filaments in guinea-pig skin are 70 to 80 Å (Brody, unpublished) and 100 Å (Brody, 1959a) respectively. The diameter of the filaments in the non-cornified epidermis of rat (Horstmann and Knoop, 1958) and of rabbit (v. Bargen, 1959) is about 80 Å.

In which sub-layer or sub-layers the increase of the diameter occurs has not yet been shown. In, for instance, psoriatic epidermis — irrespectively of whether there is a parakeratosis without keratohyalin, parakeratosis with keratohyalin or hyperkeratosis — the filaments in the entire epidermis, including the horny layer, have the same diameter of about 50 Å (Brody, 1962a, b, c, d, e, 1963a, b, c, 1964c).

In the strata spinosum and intermedium the filaments have generally been considered to be arranged in bundles, fibrils. There are, however, divergent opinions as to their arrangement in the stratum basale. In studies of adult epidermis Brody (1960b, 1964b; Figs. 20 and 21), Farquhar and Palade (1964), Roth and Clark (1964), Wilgram, Caulfield and Madgic (1965), and of embryonic epidermis Brody and Larsson (1965) and Breathnach and Wyllie (1965a) have clearly demonstrated that the filaments throughout the cytoplasm of the basal cells are aggregated into fibrils. The same aggregation of the filaments into fibrils has been repeatedly observed in pathologic epidermis (Wilgram, Caulfield and Lever, 1961; Brody, 1962a, 1963a; Braun-Falco and Petry, 1965; Braun-Falco and Vogell, 1965; Wilgram, Caulfield and Madgic, 1964a, b, 1965). In the stratum basale of adult epidermis Zelickson and Hartmann (1961) and Snell (1965a) have noted that the filaments are either arranged in fibrils or occur randomly. Finally, in other studies both of adult epidermis (Selby, 1955, 1956; Hibbs and Clark, 1959; Rhodin and Reith, 1962) and of embryonic epidermis (Selby, 1955; Hashimoto, Gross and Lever, 1965) it has been stated that the filaments appear loosely scattered throughout the cytoplasm without any aggregation into fibrils.

On the basis of electron micrographs Birbeck (1964) and Roth and Clark (1964) point out that the fibrils increase in number in the stratum spinosum. Mercer (1958a, 1961) and Horstmann (1960) suggest that the fibrils increase in number in the stratum intermedium. Hibbs and Clark (1959), on the other hand, think that the fibrils partly disappear in the stratum intermedium, a view that has had many advocates among histologists (cf. Patzelt's survey, 1926). The investigations by Selby (1956) and later by Brody (1960b, 1964b) do not support any of these suggestions. There is no electron-microscopic evidence for an increase or decrease in the numbers of fibrils in the non-cornified epidermis above the stratum basale. A distinct feature in the electron micrographs of the normal epidermis is the variation in the numbers of fibrils in adjacent cells in all strata throughout the epidermis (Brody, 1959a, b, 1960a, b, 1962g, 1963a, 1964a, b; Fig. 20).

The fibrils anastomose and form a network, the main direction of which is oriented parallel to the longitudinal axis of the cells (Horstmann, 1960; Brody, 1960b, 1964b; Figs. 6, 20—24, 31 and 32). This picture is similar to that obtained with polarization microscopy of the birefringent fibrils (Matoltsy and Balsamo, 1955; Montagna, 1956, 1962; Mercer, 1961; Matoltsy, 1962b). The magnitude of birefringence in the epidermis, however, is low as compared to that in wool or hair (MERCER, 1949; MATOLTSY, 1962b). According to MERCER (1961), there is a rise of the birefringence in the stratum intermedium that may be due to the appearance of the keratohyalin substance. According to SELBY (1955, 1956), there is a close association between the filaments and the nuclear membrane.

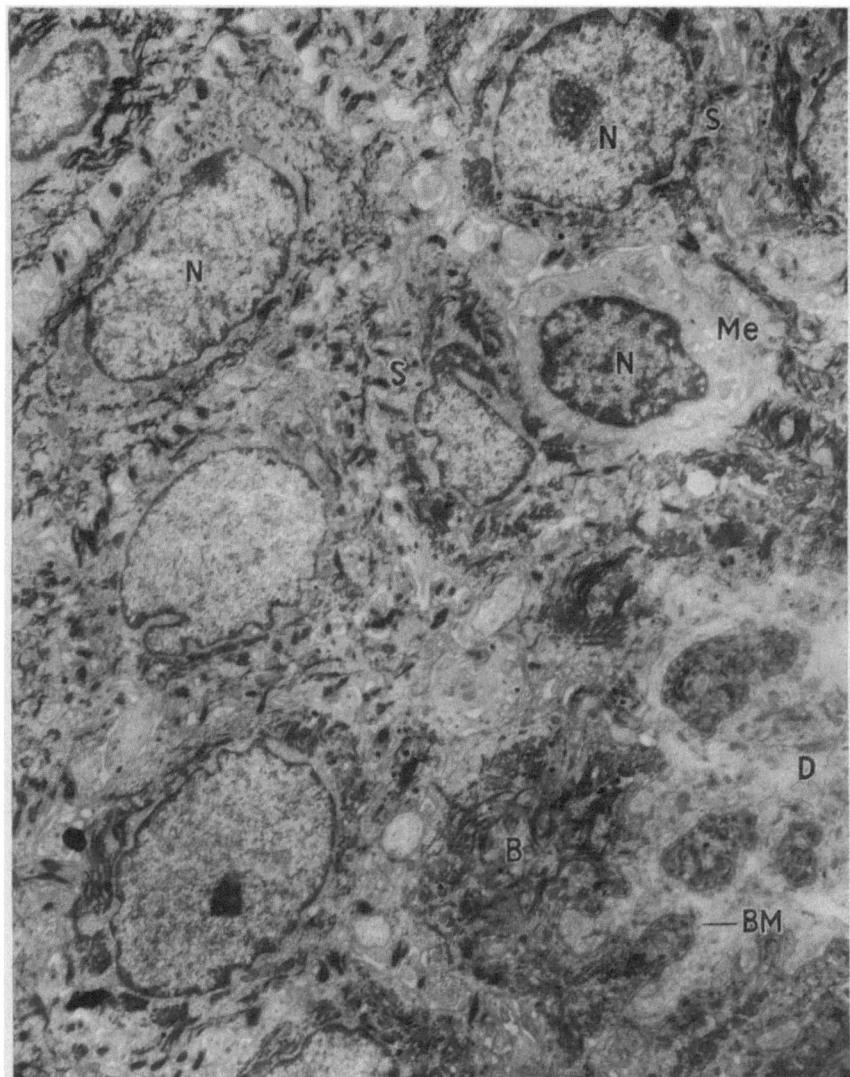

Fig. 20. Survey of the dermo-epidermal junction in human epidermis from the upper arm. *D* dermis, *BM* basement membrane, *B* stratum basale, *S* stratum spinosum, *Me* melanocytes displaying a "clear" cytoplasm and containing fairly numerous mitochondria. The epidermal fibrils surround the nuclei (*N*) but leave everywhere a distinct fibril-free perinuclear zone. The adjacent cells in the strata basale and spinosum show distinct variations with respect to the fibrillar content and the arrangement of fibrils in bundles. × 6,000

This notion has not, however, been verified. In the cells containing nuclei the fibrils often show a concentric arrangement around the nuclei, and always leave a distinct perinuclear zone free (BRODY, 1960b). The fibrils bounding this zone are usually parallel to the contour of the nuclei (Figs. 5, 6, 20, 31 and 32).

SMIDDY and CLARK (1957) have advanced the hypothesis that the fibrils are attached at both their ends to the desmosomes. MERCER (1961) and ROTH and

CLARK (1964) have not been able to confirm this observation, but consider that every fibril is at least at one end attached to the desmosomes. In order to express the assumed close association between the epidermal fibrils and the "attachment plaques" (ODLAND, 1958) of the desmosomes WILGRAM, CAULFIELD and LEVER (1961) have introduced the expression "tonofilament-desmosome complex". Among their various functions the desmosomes are assumed to anchor and orient the fibrilar system in the cells (MERCER, 1961; WILGRAM, CAULFIELD and LEVER, 1961, 1962, 1963; WILGRAM, CAULFIELD and MADGIC, 1964a, b, 1965; ROTH and CLARK, 1964; FARQUHAR and PALADE, 1965).

Thus WILGRAM and his co-workers assume that in pemphigus the alteration in the orientation and arrangement of the fibrils is due to a disintegration of the tonofilament-desmosome complex with a retraction of the fibrils. In electron-microscopic investigations of chronic nummular eczema and of pemphigus vulgaris BRAUN-FALCO and PETRY (1965, 1966) and BRAUN-FALCO and VOGELL (1965, 1966) discuss in detail the relationship between fibrils and desmosomes. They suggest that the formation of desmosomes and the development and orientation of the fibrils in the cells are subject to tensions within and between the cells in the cell unions. Following this view they do not think that the acantholysis and the disorder in the fibrillar system in pemphigus are primarily due to a separation of fibrils and desmosomes. They assume that the changes are due rather to a defective ability of the cells to develop desmosomal structures, a disability which results in alterations of the tensions between and within the cells. The latter changes may result in a disorganization of the fibrils (BRAUN-FALCO and PETRY, 1965, 1966; BRAUN-FALCO and VOGELL, 1965, 1966).

The suggestion by MENEFEE (1957), with respect to normal embryonic mouse epidermis, that the fibrils are associated with the mitochondrial membranes has not been verified in subsequent studies of the same tissue (BRODY and LARSSON, 1965) or of pathologic human epidermis (BRODY, 1962a; BRAUN-FALCO and PETRY, 1965).

As regards their thickness and aggregation into bundles the fibrils show the same variations in the stratum basale and stratum spinosum (BRODY, 1960b, 1964b; Fig. 20). The increased aggregation into bundles in the stratum spinosum suggested by WILGRAM, CAULFIELD and MADGIC (1965) has not been observed by the present writer. In the stratum intermedium either the fibrils may show the same arrangement as in the subjacent sub-layers (Figs. 5, 6, 24 and 25) or an increase packing of the fibrils into bundles is observed (BRODY, 1960b, 1964b). Occasionally, almost all the fibrils in the cells are packed together (Fig. 23). In the T- and horny cells these structures show an arrangement similar to that in the stratum intermedium. Here, however, more cells in which the fibrils are packed into larger bundles are usually found (BRODY, 1959a, b, 1960a, b, 1962g, 1964a, b; Figs. 5, 6, 26—29).

In sections which have not been "stained" or which have been stained with different metal salt solutions in room temperature according to GIBSON and BRADFIELD (1957), WATSON (1958), KARNOVSKY (1961), MILLONIG (1961) and REYNOLDS (1963) the individual opaque filaments appear distinctly in all strata of the non-cornified epidermis (SELBY, 1955, 1956, 1957; HORSTMANN, 1957b, 1960; HORSTMANN and KNOOP, 1958; MERCER, 1958a, b, 1961; ROTH and CLARK, 1964; WILGRAM, CAULFIELD and MADGIC, 1965). According to ROTH and CLARK (1964) and WILGRAM, CAULFIELD and MADGIC (1965) the filaments within the fibrils are more packed in the stratum spinosum than in the stratum basale.

BRODY (1959a) has introduced a section-staining with saturated aqueous solution of uranyl acetate at 40 to 70° C for 20 to 120 minutes. This staining technique has been shown to be particularly suitable for studies of the epidermal fibrils in normal and pathologic epidermis (BRODY, 1959a, b, 1960a, b, 1962a, b, c, d, e, g, h, 1963a, b, c, d, 1964a, b, c; BRODY and LARSSON, 1965). In the entire epidermis the fibrillar structure appears distinctly, and nowhere are observed isolated, scattered filaments. On the strength of this observation BRODY (1964b) suggests that the fibrils represent the fibrous unit in fixed and embedded epidermis.

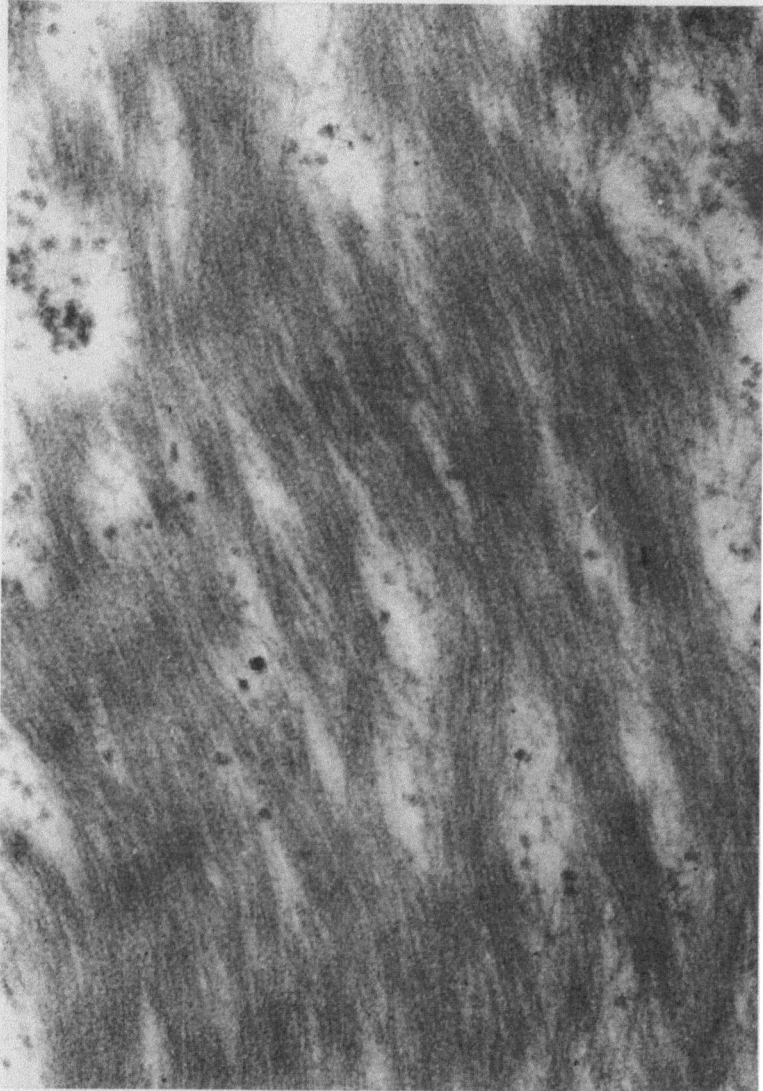

Fig. 21 shows the characteristic picture of the fibrils in the stratum basale. They anastomose and aggregate into bundles of varying size. The individual filaments are distinctly seen. × 85,000. (From BRODY, 1960b. Courtesy of J. Ultrastruct. Res., Academic Press Inc., New York-London)

This staining technique has further revealed that the epidermal fibrils undergo characteristic changes in their ultrastructure and stainability during the displacement of the keratinocytes from the stratum basale to the superficial layer of the stratum corneum. The process of transformation is geared through a successive series of characteristic ultrastructural patterns occurring in a well-defined fashion in the various epidermal sub-layers (BRODY, 1959a, 1960b, 1962g, 1964b).

3. The Development of the Fibrils into Keratin Fibrils

In the non-cornified epidermis the outlines of the individual filaments in the fibrils are, when the sections are stained with uranyl acetate according to BRODY (1959a), only distinguishable in the stratum basale (BRODY, 1960b, 1962e, 1964b). The fibrils are here constituted by approximately 50 Å thick, opaque filaments embedded in a less opaque, interfilamentous substance (BRODY, 1964b; Fig. 21). They show a fairly low opacity (1960b; Fig. 5).

In hyperkeratotic psoriatic epidermis, where on analogy with the conditions in normal skin a development of a "keratin pattern" (for definition see BRODY, 1959a) is observed, individual filaments in the fibrils in the non-cornified strata are also seen exclusively in the stratum basale (BRODY, 1963a, b, c).

a) The Speckled Pattern

In the stratum spinosum the fibrils are more opaque than those in the stratum basale (BRODY, 1960b, 1964b; Fig. 5). They appear here as compact structures in which the individual filaments cannot be distinguished (Fig. 22). A distinct "speckled

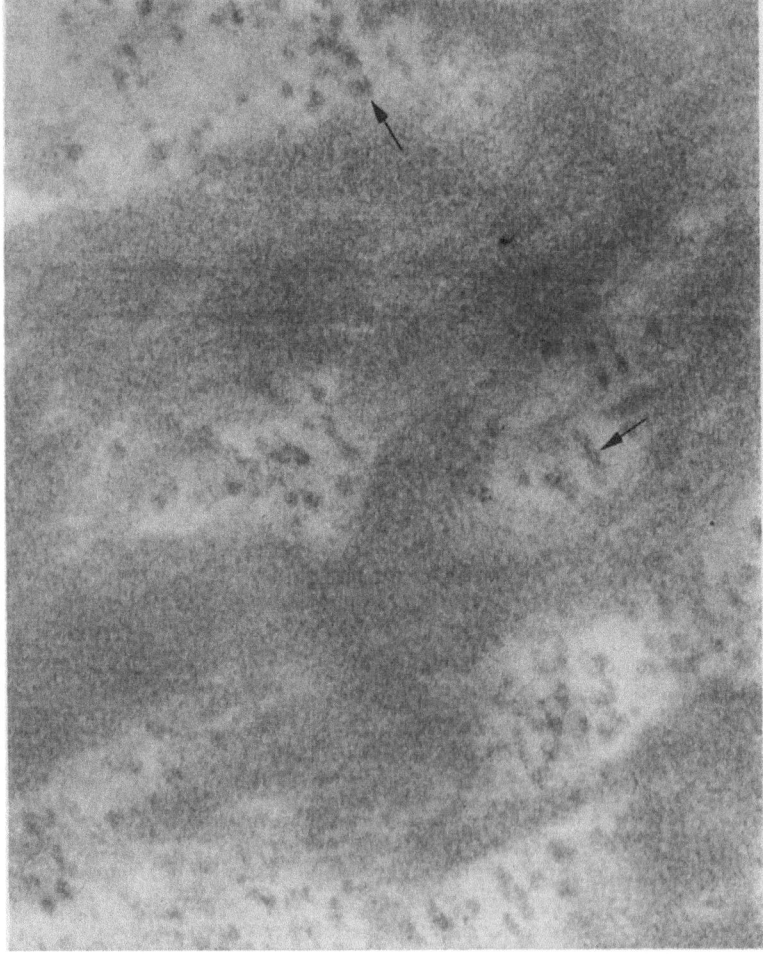

Fig. 22. In the stratum spinosum the fibrils exhibit the same arrangement as in the stratum basale, but display a different ultrastructure. The individual filaments are no longer discernible, but a speckled pattern appear distinctly. The ribosomes show indications of an internal pattern (→). × 131,000. (From BRODY, 1960b. Courtesy of J. Ultrastruct. Res., Academic Press Inc., New York-London)

pattern" is observable in the fibrils owing to differences in affinity to the stain of rather regularly disposed regions (BRODY, 1960b, 1964b). WEIBEL and SCHNYDER (1966) have noted that the fibrils show an intersected periodicity of 120 Å which is inclined 45° in relation to the filamentous direction.

These changes in fibrillar morphology do not occur abruptly with the transition of the basal cell to the stratum spinosum, but are already indicated in the apical parts of the cells in the stratum basale and reflect different stages in the differentiation of the fibrils (BRODY, 1960b). It seems likely that the alterations in question are an expression for chemical changes in the fibrillar substance. It is also possible that a change in the medium in which the filaments are suspended may contribute to the characteristic aggregation of the filaments observed in the stratum spinosum.

b) The Keratohyalin

Since the demonstration of keratohyalin in the epidermis (AUFHAMMER), this cellular component has been the subject of strongly controversial theories with regard to its origin, morphology, histochemistry, and, not least, its role in the keratinization process.

MERTSCHNIGG (1889), KREIBICH (1915) and LUDFORD (1925) assume that the keratohyalin derives from the nuclear substance since they are similarly stained with basic stains such as hematoxylin. RABL (1887) and MARTINOTTI (1915) have suggested that both the nucleus and the cytoplasm take part in the formation of the keratohyalin. As further support for the assumption of a correlation between the disappearance of nuclear material and the appearance of the keratohyalin STEIGLEDER and GANS (1964) have advanced the following histological observations. In the stratum intermedium of normal human epidermis the nucleoli appear close to the nuclear membrane. In the dyskeratotic cell the nucleus seems to be poorer in substance at the appearance of the keratohyalin. And, finally, in parakeratosis the occurrence of nuclei in the horny layer is associated with a simultaneous absence of keratohyalin. On the strength of electron-microscopic studies SOGNNAES and ALBRIGHT (1956) and v. BARGEN (1959) also suggest that the nucleus is involved in the formation of keratohyalin. According to v. BARGEN the nuclear membrane is no longer to be seen in the stratum intermedium of the epidermis in rabbit skin, and the karyoplasm is condensed at the periphery. In the cytoplasm around the nuclei irregular, homogeneous structures appear which can with certainty be identified as keratohyalin only after the larger part of the cell is filled with this substance (v. BARGEN, 1959).

However, the electron micrographs hitherto published seem not to permit any conclusions bearing out the possible relationship between nuclear function and the formation of keratohyalin (SELBY, 1956; HORSTMANN and KNOOP, 1957, 1958; BRODY, 1960b). In adult human and rat epidermis the nuclei in the stratum intermedium usually have the same appearance as those in the stratum spinosum and they display a distinct nuclear membrane (Figs. 5 and 31). Only in exceptional cases are in normal human epidermis nuclei seen with a condensed karyoplasm at the periphery (Fig. 32), which v. BARGEN (1959) suggests is a normal feature in rabbit epidermis. The condensed karyoplasm is less opaque than the keratohyalin material (Fig. 32). The nuclei of the T-cells are flattened and dark, and the karyoplasm appears mainly compact. It is also here less opaque than the keratohyalin-like substance (Fig. 6). In contradistinction to v. BARGEN (1959), BRODY (1960b, 1964b) has never found keratohyalin close to the nuclei in normal human epidermis. Like the fibrils, it always leaves a distinct perinuclear zone free (Figs. 31 and 32). Further, the electron-microscopic studies of psoriatic epidermis (BRODY, 1962a, e, 1964c) do not lend any support to the findings by STEIGLEDER and GANS (1964). On the contrary, parakeratosis is often associated with the presence of keratohyalin in the stratum intermedium.

KROMAYER (1897) and PATZELT (1926) have proposed that the keratohyalin is formed by the disintegration of the intraprotoplasmic plexus of fibrils. PATZELT (1954) believes that the keratohyalin stands in a certain relation to the fibrils but does not consider that it is a precursor to the keratin or constitutes a regular concomitant in the formation of the keratin. ROTHMAN (1954) and DE BERSAQUES and ROTHMAN (1962) have advanced the view that cellular proteins are hydrolysed to free amino acids with subsequent *de novo* formation of keratin in the transitional zone.

BLASCHKO (1889a, b) has advanced the hypothesis that the keratohyalin is formed in the fibrils as "drops or lumps of a soft firm mass arranged in rows". These then fuse and in the stratum lucidum and stratum corneum are reconstituted as intracellular fibrils once again. He called the keratohyalin in the stratum intermedium "prokeratin I", and the "eleidin" in the stratum lucidum "prokeratin II".

HUECK (1937) believed that the keratohyalin represents a degeneration product in a cell layer constituting "an intermediary zone between life and death". In the fifties this view gained many supporters, since with histochemical methods no protein-bound sulfhydryl or disulfide groups were demonstrated in the keratohyalin (MESCON and FLESCH, 1952; BARRNETT, 1953; MONTAGNA, EISEN, RADEMACHER and CHASE, 1954; BERN, ELLIAS, POWERS and HARKNESS, 1955; MONTAGNA, 1956; MATOLTSY, 1958b). SELBY (1956, 1957) has investigated human epidermis and epidermis of the rat skin with electron microscopy, and she points out that the morphology of the keratohyalin is consistent with the wide-spread belief that it represents a particular type of debris or side-product in keratinization.

On the basis of electron-microscopic investigations a close correlation between the fibrils and keratohyalin has been assumed by several authors (HORSTMANN, 1957b, 1960; HORSTMANN and KNOOP, 1958; MERCER, 1958a, 1961; v. BARGEN, 1959; BRODY, 1959a, b, 1960a, b, 1962e, 1964b; CHARLES, 1959; ZELICKSON, 1961; MATOLTSY, 1962b; MATOLTSY and MATOLTSY, 1962a; BIRBECK, 1964; ODLAND, 1964; ROTH and CLARK, 1964). Different theories concerning this relationship have, however, been proposed.

According to MERCER (1958a, 1961) the fibrillar substance formed in the basal cells is insufficient in amount to constitute the fibrous keratin in the stratum corneum. He has therefore suggested that the keratohyalin represents centres for the formation of a new type of fibril which forms the main part of the fibrous keratin. If this interpretation of the function of the keratohyalin were correct, one would expect to find a decrease of the keratohyalin material towards the surface of the stratum intermedium. The opposite, however, is the case (BRODY, 1962e).

HORSTMANN (1957b, 1960), HORSTMANN and KNOOP (1958), v. BARGEN (1959), BRODY (1959a, b), CHARLES (1959), ZELICKSON (1961), ROTH and CLARK (1964) and ODLAND (1964) describe the keratohyalin as being deposited on and around the fibrils and between the filaments, but as appearing also beyond the fibrils. HORSTMANN and KNOOP (1958) mention that when the keratohyalin substance is deposited on the filament bundles it is also pressed between the filaments, which according to these authors are still discerned within keratohyalin substance. BRODY (1959a, b) has interpreted his pictures as showing an incorporation of the filaments by keratohyalin diffusing along the filament bundles. He assumes that the keratohyalin later forms the interfilamentous substance in the "keratin pattern" of the keratin fibrils. ODLAND (1964) suggests that the keratohyalin appears at the interstices of the fibril and filament network.

In more recent studies it has been distinctly shown that the keratohyalin is entirely restricted to the fibrillar substance (BRODY, 1960b, 1964b). It appears as intensely stained regions and BRODY assumes that it represents chemically altered fibrillar substance. When it comprises larger parts of the fibrillar substance, it appears as the fibrillar network itself (Figs. 23, 24 and 31). No keratohyalin is observed in the interfibrillar cytoplasm or in the perinuclear fibril-free zone. The keratohyalin does not show any preference regarding its location in the cell and is not found in particularly large amounts around the nucleus (Fig. 31), as has often been suggested by histologists (for references see PATZELT, 1926). The hypothesis that the keratohyalin is restricted to the fibrils is also supported by the findings of MATOLTSY (1962b) and MATOLTSY and MATOLTSY (1962a). These authors however, assert that the ultimate fate of the keratohyalin is a "dissociation and mixing with constituents of epithelial cells during a late stage of maturation".

In ultrathin, uranyl-acetate stained sections the fibrils in the stratum intermedium appear compact. The speckled pattern so characteristic of the fibrils in the stratum spinosum is here less pronounced or absent. In the less stained parts of the fibrillar substance, where this change is distinguishable, the fibrils show at the same time less opacity than that of those in the subjacent stratum (BRODY, 1960b). Where the keratohyalin first appears it forms small, round or elongated, intensely stained regions with a breadth of 100 to 300 Å or less (HORSTMANN, 1957b; BRODY, 1960b, 1964b; ODLAND, 1964; Figs. 24 and 25). Usually, the keratohyalin regions increase in size towards the surface of the stratum intermedium. Occasionally it may comprise practically the whole fibrillar substance (Fig. 23). It is, however, of importance to point out that small stained areas are observed throughout the stratum intermedium (BRODY, 1960b, 1964b), indicating that keratohyalin is formed in all cells. It may further be mentioned that

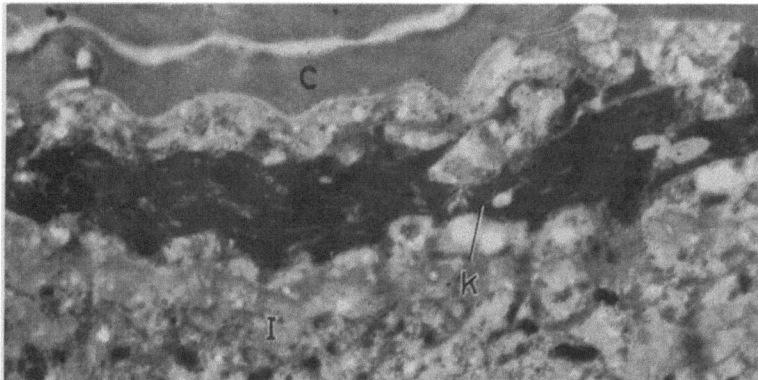

Fig. 23 shows that the main part of the fibrillar substance in the upper cell in the stratum intermedium (*I*) appears as keratohyalin (*k*). *C* stratum corneum. × 16,000. (From BRODY, 1960b. Courtesy of J. Ultrastruct. Res., Academic Press Inc., New York-London)

the intensely stained regions appear irrespective of whether the fibrils are thin or aggregated into smaller or larger bundles (HORSTMANN and KNOOP, 1958; BRODY, 1960b, 1964b; Fig. 24).

When the embedded epidermis is irradiated with ultraviolet light before the sections are stained with uranyl acetate (BRODY, 1962f) a change in the ultrastructure of the fibrillar substance in the stratum intermedium is observed (BRODY, 1964b). In the less stained parts of the fibrils a pattern similar to the speckled pattern characteristic of the fibrils in the stratum spinosum becomes visible. Where the keratohyalin appears first it seems to accentuate this pattern, or it appears as an opaque, linear component (Fig. 25). Where the keratohyalin comprises larger regions of the fibrils an indication of a two-component system is seen, *viz.*, a more opaque component surrounding less opaque areas (Fig. 25). This two-component system is similar to the "keratin pattern" (BRODY, 1959a) in the stratum corneum. A similar appearance of the keratohyalin is described by ODLAND (1964). In agreement with the finding by HORSTMANN and KNOOP, (1958) he observed that the more opaque keratohyalin material surrounds the less opaque filaments. ODLAND considers this image to be analogous to the "keratin pattern" in the stratum corneum.

In the T-cell the fibrils display the same ultrastructure and arrangement as those in the stratum intermedium, with the exception that the keratohyalin-like substance is here less opaque than the keratohyalin (BRODY, 1959b, 1960b, 1964b; Figs. 5, 6 and 26). In the stratum corneum, finally, the keratin fibrils exhibit a so-called "keratin pattern" (BRODY, 1959a; Figs. 27—29). This has subsequently been repeatedly confirmed (BRODY, 1959b, 1960a, b, 1964a, b; ODLAND, 1964; BRAUN-FALCO, 1965).

The electron-microscopic results here presented thus favour the idea, first proposed by BLASCHKO (1889a, b), of a direct development of the keratin fibrils from the fibrillar material in the stratum basale without any disintegration of the fibrils in the stratum intermedium or in the T-cells (BRODY, 1959a, b, 1960b,

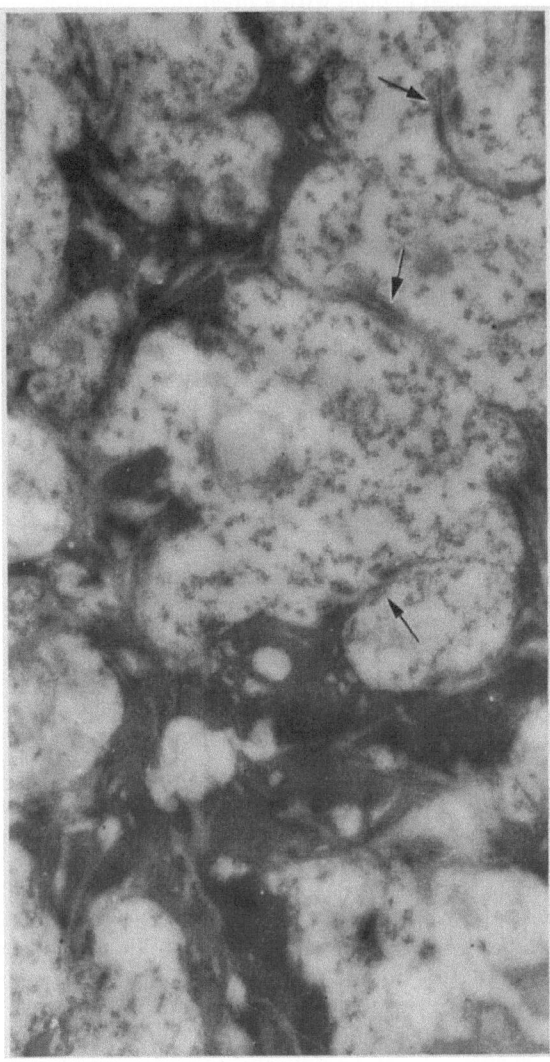

Fig. 24. Skin from sacrum. In an upper cell of the stratum intermedium smaller (→) and larger areas of the fibrillar substance are changed into keratohyalin. Like the fibrils the keratohyalin therefore appears as a network. × 26,000. (From BRODY, 1964b. Courtesy of Academic Press Inc., New York-London)

1962e, 1964b; ODLAND, 1964). However, when the filaments and interfilamentous substance in the stratum basale are compared with those in the stratum corneum these components show a reversed affinity to the stains used, *i.e.*, in the stratum basale the filaments appear more opaque, whereas in the stratum corneum the interfilamentous substance is more intensely stained. It is likely that the fibrils in the intensely stained regions of the fibrils in the stratum intermedium are infiltrated with an interfilamentous material which has a strong affinity to the stains used, and which also affects the affinity of the filaments to these stains by chemical interaction (BRODY, 1960b). A change of the staining properties of the filamentous and interfilamentous components therefore occurs at this level in keratinization. In the light of both its ultrastructure and its stainability the keratohyalin seems to form the immediate precursor of the keratin pattern (BRODY, 1960b, 1964b; ODLAND, 1964).

The ribosomes show an obvious topographical relationship to the fibrillar substance (BRODY, 1959a, b, 1960b, 1964b; RHODIN and REITH, 1962; ODLAND, 1964; ROTH and CLARK, 1964). These particles are considered to be the site for protein synthesis in the cells (LOFTFIELD, 1957; SIEKEVITZ and PALADE, 1960a, b).

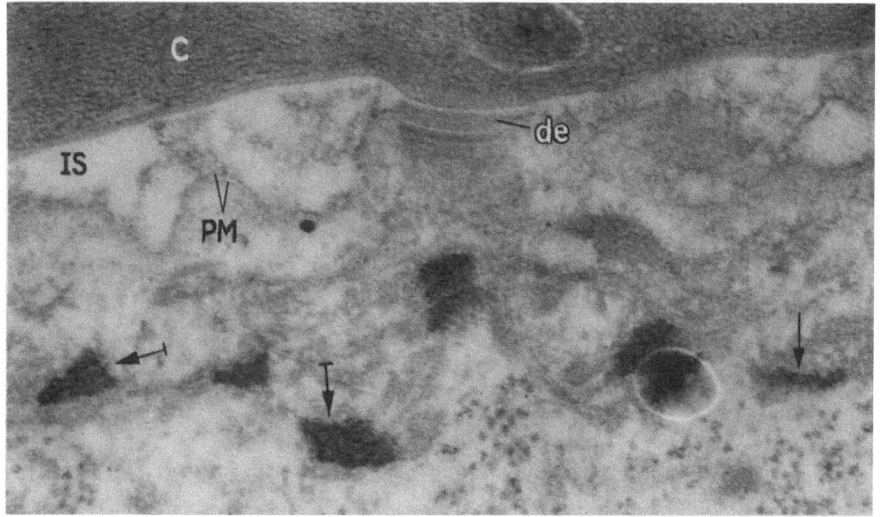

Fig. 25. Skin from the upper arm. The keratohyalin may first appear as a thin linear opaque component (→). When the keratohyalin constitutes actual areas of the fibrillar substance these areas are on the whole more opaque than the fibrillar substance that is not changed. In the keratohyalin is discerned a pattern of less opaque regions surrounded by more opaque material (↦). This pattern is similar to the keratin pattern in the horny cell (C). *de* regular desmosome. The intercellular space (*IS*) is rather wide, owing to the presence of invaginations of the surface of the cell in the stratum intermedium, whereas the horny-cell surface is even. *PM* triple-layered plasma membrane. × 72,000. (From BRODY, 1964b. Courtesy of Academic Press Inc., New York-London)

The very opaque keratohyalin material might be derived from the ribosomes in the cells of the stratum intermedium (BRODY, 1959a, b, 1960b, 1964b). There may be a synthesis of a particular protein in the cells of the stratum intermedium which may be incorporated into the preformed fibrils (BRODY, 1960b, 1964b). This view is strongly supported by earlier and more recent investigations with other techniques. Histochemically, ribonucleic acid has been demonstrated in the keratohyalin (LEUCHTENBERGER and LUND, 1951; SPIER and CANEGHEM, 1957). With the method of ultraviolet absorption CASPERSSON (1950) has demonstrated an accumulation of ribosenucleotides during the process of keratinization. Also autoradiographic investigations indicate the synthesis of ribonucleic acid in the stratum intermedium (FUKUYAMA and BERNSTEIN, 1963; BERNSTEIN, 1964). LEUCHTENBERGER and LUND (1951) have suggested that the keratohyalin is synthesized in the stratum intermedium and does not form a degeneration product. When histidine-H^3 is administered to newborn rats it is particularly concentrated in the stratum intermedium (BERNSTEIN, 1964). According to REAVEN and COX (1965) there is a close relationship between histidine and keratohyalin. Histidine is histochemically also distinguishable in the stratum corneum, and it may perhaps reflect the participation of material from keratohyalin in the final keratin product (REAVEN and COX, 1965).

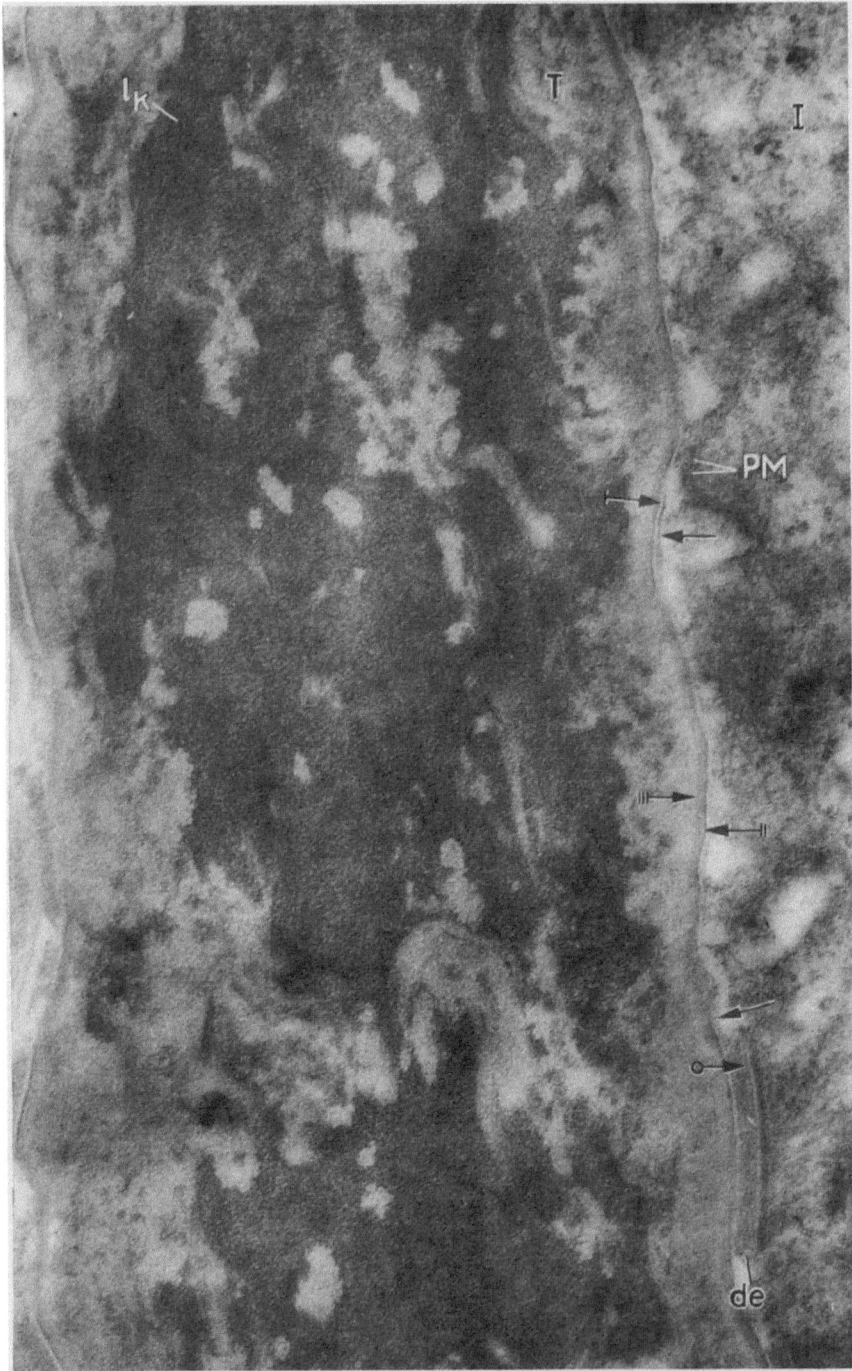

Fig. 26. Human skin from sacral region. Higher magnification of a T-cell (*T*). *I* stratum intermedium, *k* keratohyalin-like substance. The modified plasma membrane is more opaque than that of the horny cell but displays the same ultrastructure. The peripheral opaque leaflet appears distinct (→) as does also the outer intermediate light layer (⊢→). The outer opaque layer (⊢⊢→) of the broad cytoplasmic zone (⊢⊢⊢→) corresponding to the cytoplasmic leaflet of the triple layered plasma membrane (*PM*) in the non-cornified epidermis is here distinctly seen. *de* regular desmosome. Indication of a triple-layered pattern of the central layer of the intercellular component (o→). × 87,000

In the strata basale and spinosum the ribosomes also appear to be topographically related to the fibrils (BRODY, 1960b). There is no evidence that the fibrils increase in numbers in the normal stratum spinosum. Whether the ultrastructural change of the fibrils with the appearance of a speckled pattern is associated with protein synthesis is not known. From a morphological viewpoint, however, the development of a speckled pattern seems to be a prerequisite condition for the appearance of keratohyalin in the stratum intermedium. Thus in psoriatic epidermis without keratohyalin the fibrils throughout the epidermis mainly show the same ultrastructure as the fibrils in the stratum basale (BRODY, 1962a, b, c, d, e). This is also the case with the epidermis in frog skin, which is characterized by a horny layer containing nuclei, by a stratum intermedium where keratohyalin is absent and by the same ultrastructure of the fibrils throughout the epidermis (cf. electron micrographs by FARQUHAR and PALADE, 1965). In psoriatic epidermis characterized by hyperkeratosis a distinct speckled pattern is found both in the stratum spinosum and stratum intermedium, in which latter layer distinct intensely stained regions of the fibrils occur (BRODY, 1963a, b, c). In the early stages in the differentiation of embryonic mouse epidermis the fibrils display the same ultrastructure throughout, but when keratohyalin appears a speckled pattern is simultaneously found in the fibrils in the stratum spinosum (BRODY and LARSSON, 1965).

On the strength of electron-microscopic studies other theories have, however, also been advanced with regard to the role of the fibrils and the keratohyalin in the keratinization process. SNELL (1965a) points out that the involvement of the filaments in the keratohyalin is entirely coincidental. According to this author proteins and other substances are synthesized in the stratum basale, accumulate in the cytoplasm of the cells and are deposited in the stratum intermedium as keratohyalin. The ribosomes also take part in the formation of the latter substance. The keratohyalin "granules" increase in size and fuse with one another. In this connection they come to absorb an ever greater part of the cytoplasm of the cell, and only as a consequence of this do they incorporate the fibrils. When the keratohyalin finally reaches the stratum corneum it undergoes certain chemical changes and is now called keratin.

Thus while SNELL does not ascribe to the fibrils any role in the formation of keratin BRAUN-FALCO, KINT and VOGELL (1963) question whether the keratohyalin in its well-known shape is of any importance in this process. According to these authors a "basaloid cell type" in Verruca seborrhoica may be transformed into a normal horny cell without having passed the keratohyalin-stage. CHARLES (1959), too, believes the keratohyalin to be of no importance in the keratinization process, but considers it as "being merely the first precipitation from the cytoplasm".

c) The Keratin

The keratins may be classified with respect to various properties, and functional and structural aspects (cf. survey by LUNDGREN and WARD, 1963). Owing to the sulfur-content the keratins are grouped into "soft" keratin, such as that in the epidermal horny layer, with a low sulfur-content, and "hard" keratin, comprising hair, horn, hoof and feathers, with a high concentration of sulfur. Another classification is based on the extensive wide-angle X-ray diffraction studies by ASTBURY and co-workers (ASTBURY and STREET, 1931; ASTBURY and WOODS, 1934; ASTBURY and DICKINSON, 1935a, b; BAILEY, ASTBURY and RUDALL, 1943; ASTBURY, 1945, 1947, 1953a, b; RUDALL, 1946, 1947, 1952, 1953).

Astbury and Woods (1934) have suggested that the polypeptide chains in mammalian hairs occur in a "folded" configuration. This configuration was designated as an alpha-keratin structure in order to distinguish it from the "extended" configuration of the beta-keratin. The X-ray diffraction pattern of alpha-keratin is characterized by meridional spacings of 1.5 and 5.1 Å and by a longitudinal period of 198 Å. The beta-keratin type exhibits a meridional spacing at 3.3 Å and two equatorial spacings at 4.65 and 9.7 Å. By a stretching of the mammalian hairs more than 50 per cent the alpha-keratin structure is transformed into a beta-pattern. This phenomenon is reversible (Astbury and Woods, 1934).

In later studies Pauling, Corey and Branson (1951) and Pauling (1953, 1954) suggest that the alpha-polypeptide chains are not "folded" but "spiral-shaped". They have therefore designated the alpha-polypeptide chains as alpha-helices. Crick (1953) and Pauling and Corey (1953a, b) have independently advanced the theory that the axis of the alpha-helices themselves form a helix, so that the structure is constituted of coiled coils. The alpha-helix gives meridional spacings of 1.5 Å and 5.4 Å instead of the 5.1-Å spacing for the "folded" alpha-keratin. The helices have a diameter of 11 Å (Pauling and Corey, 1953b). For more detailed studies the reader is referred to the exhaustive reviews by Mercer (1961), Lundgren and Ward (1962, 1963) and Cohen (1966).

The alpha-keratin configuration is common to several fibrous proteins of divers properties such as keratin, muscle, epidermis, fibrinogen and fibrin. These proteins have therefore been grouped together as the "KMEF"-group (Bailey, Astbury and Rudall, 1943; Rudall, 1952). All the fibrous proteins here show the phenomenon of alpha $\rightleftharpoons$ beta transformation. By denaturation they also display a shortened or "supercontracted" form (Astbury, 1945).

X-ray diffraction studies of the epidermis have revealed an alpha-keratin structure in the non-cornified as well as in the cornified layers (Derksen and Heringa, 1936; Giroud and Champetier, 1936; Derksen, Heringa and Weidinger, 1937; Champetier and Litvac, 1939). The epidermal fibrils were considered to give this configuration. Through the stretching of the epidermis the alpha-pattern was transformed into a beta-configuration (Derksen and Heringa, 1936; Champetier and Litvac, 1939).

Definite evidence that the epidermal fibrils are responsible for the alpha-keratin structure has been presented by Rudall (1952) and Matoltsy (1964, 1965) in biochemical, X-ray diffraction and electron-microscopic investigations on the epidermis from the cow's nose. From the whole epidermis, including the stratum corneum, Rudall has isolated two protein fractions. The major fraction is constituted by the fibrous protein, which he called "epidermin". It displays a characteristic alpha-type diffraction pattern which by stretching is transformed into a beta-configuration. The smaller fraction represents a non-fibrous protein which does not show any orientation with reference to the plane of the film. In later studies Matoltsy (1964, 1965) has isolated a prekeratin molecule from the non-cornified layers of the epidermis from the cow's nose. This prekeratin molecule has a molecular weight of 640,000. It has a diameter of about 34 Å and a length of about 1,050 Å. The prekeratin molecule has a characteristic alpha-keratin configuration with a meridional spacing of 5.4 Å and an equatorial spacing of 9.7 Å. Measurements have given a helix-content of about 40 per cent. The prekeratin molecules aggregate readily to form long filaments. They contain protein, lipids and carbohydrates. Only small amounts of proline and sulfur-containing amino acids were found.

Biochemical investigations have revealed a heterogeneous composition of the stratum corneum (Unna, 1883, 1913; Grüneberg and Szakall, 1955; Matoltsy and BALSAMO, 1955a, b; SPIER and PASCHER, 1959; MATOLTSY, 1962a). UNNA obtained three fractions all of which he assumed to be constituents of the cell, viz. the keratin A or the "horny membrane", keratin B or the fibrous keratin and the horn albumoses. In later studies two main fractions were discerned, viz. the fibrous keratin and a non-keratinous fraction. The "cell membrane", nuclear remnants and various cytoplasmic constituents are included in the latter (GRÜNE-BERG and SZAKALL, 1955; SPIER and PASCHER, 1959; MATOLTSY, 1962a). The keratin:non-keratin ratio has been reported to be 7:3 to 5:5 (MATOLTSY, 1962a).

In the interpretations of the biochemical results only the horny cells seem to have been taken into consideration, since the stratum corneum has been considered to consist only of cells. However, electronmicroscopic investigations have distinctly revealed that the intercellular space constitutes a substantial part of the horny layer and is filled throughout with different structures (BRODY, 1966; cf. also chapter C II). On the strength of this observation it seems reasonable to assume that the fibrous keratin forms a larger part of the cellular constituents than is indicated in the keratin: non-keratin ratio mentioned above.

The electron-microscopic investigations of the stratum corneum in normal human epidermis show that the fibrils usually constitute the main component (BRODY, 1960b, 1962g, 1964a, b; Figs. 27—29). Certain variations are seen, reflecting the variations in the number of fibrils already distinguished in the non-cornified layers. The cells also contain to a varying extent a non-fibrous substance appearing between the fibrils. This substance is distinct in the basal horny layer. In the intermediate and superficial layers of the human stratum corneum small electron-optically empty spaces usually appear which seem to replace the non-fibrous substance in the basal layer. The appearance of these empty spaces seems to be partly due to a dissolving of the non-fibrous substance during the tissue preparation (BRODY, 1966). Whether the empty spaces are merely due to a dissolving of the non-fibrous substance, or whether also the fibrillar substance is dissolved is not known. In the superficial horny cells of the guinea-pig epidermis large electron-optically empty spaces often dominate the picture (BRODY, 1959a; SNELL, 1965a). Large spaces are occasionally also observed in human stratum corneum (Fig. 29).

In the staining of the sections with uranyl acetate at 40 to 70° C (BRODY, 1959a) the fibrils in the intermediate layer are best stained and those in the superficial layer of the human stratum corneum are least stained (BRODY, 1962g; Fig. 7).

In higher magnification the fibrils display a keratin pattern. This consists of bundles of less opaque filaments embedded in an opaque interfilamentous substance (BRODY, 1959a, b, 1960a, b, 1964a, b; ODLAND, 1964; BRAUN-FALCO, 1965; Figs. 27—29). In human epidermis the filaments have a diameter of 74 Å (BRODY, 1960b). In guinea-pig epidermis their diameter is about 100 Å and the interfilamentous substance is estimated as 30 Å at its thinnest points. The ratio of filament:interfilamentous substance was estimated as approximately 2:3 (BRODY, 1959a). According to FILSHIE and ROGERS (1961), the filaments in the fully keratinized hair has a diameter of 80 Å. The ratio of filament:interfilamentous substance in hair is reported as 1:1 (BIRBECK and MERCER, 1957a, b; ROGERS, 1959c).

According to LUNDGREN and WARD (1963), a group of about 30 to 60 alpha-helices with associated, perhaps non-protein substance are required to make up a filament. How the helices are packed within the filaments has not yet been elucidated but several models for the packing have been suggested (cf. LUND

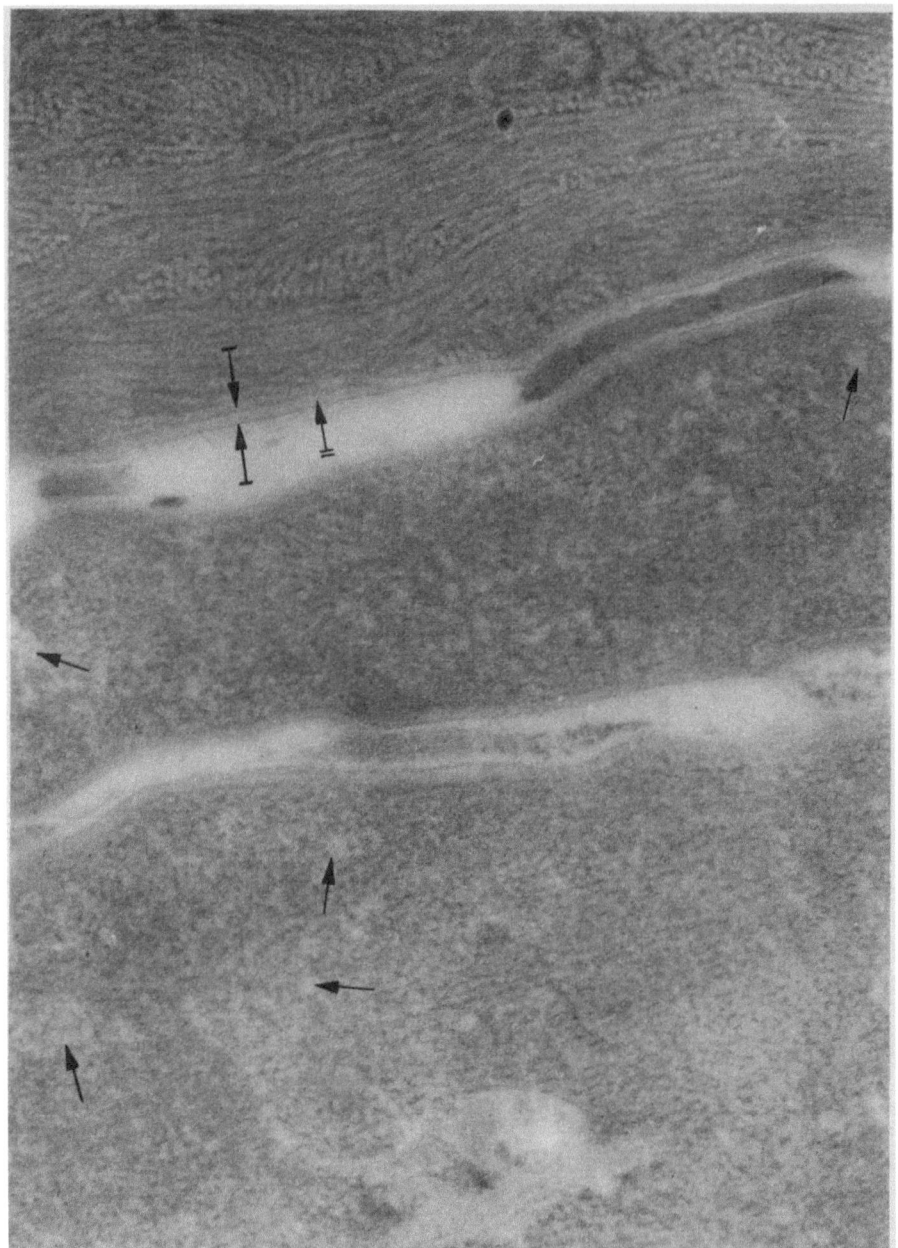

Fig. 27. Human skin from shoulder. Parts of cells in the basal layer of the stratum corneum displaying varying distinctness of the keratin pattern. In the upper cell the keratin pattern is distinctly visible. The keratin fibrils are closely packed throughout the cell. In the lower cells a keratin pattern is discerned but is less distinct. Areas of less opaque, non-fibrillar substance (→) are irregularly scattered between the keratin fibrils. The broad cytoplasmic zone of the modified plasma membrane is distinctly seen with two opaque narrow layers (↦) bounding the inner, broad intermediate layer (⊢→). × 131,000. (From BRODY, 1964a. Courtesy of J. invest. Derm., The Williams and Wilkins Co., Baltimore)

GREN and WARD, 1963). In an electron-microscopic study of Australian fine merino wool, human hair and porcupine quill tip ROGERS and FILSHIE (1961) have demonstrated that the filaments are constituted of protofilaments with a diameter of 20 Å. They have shown that these protofilaments exhibit a "9+2" arrangement.

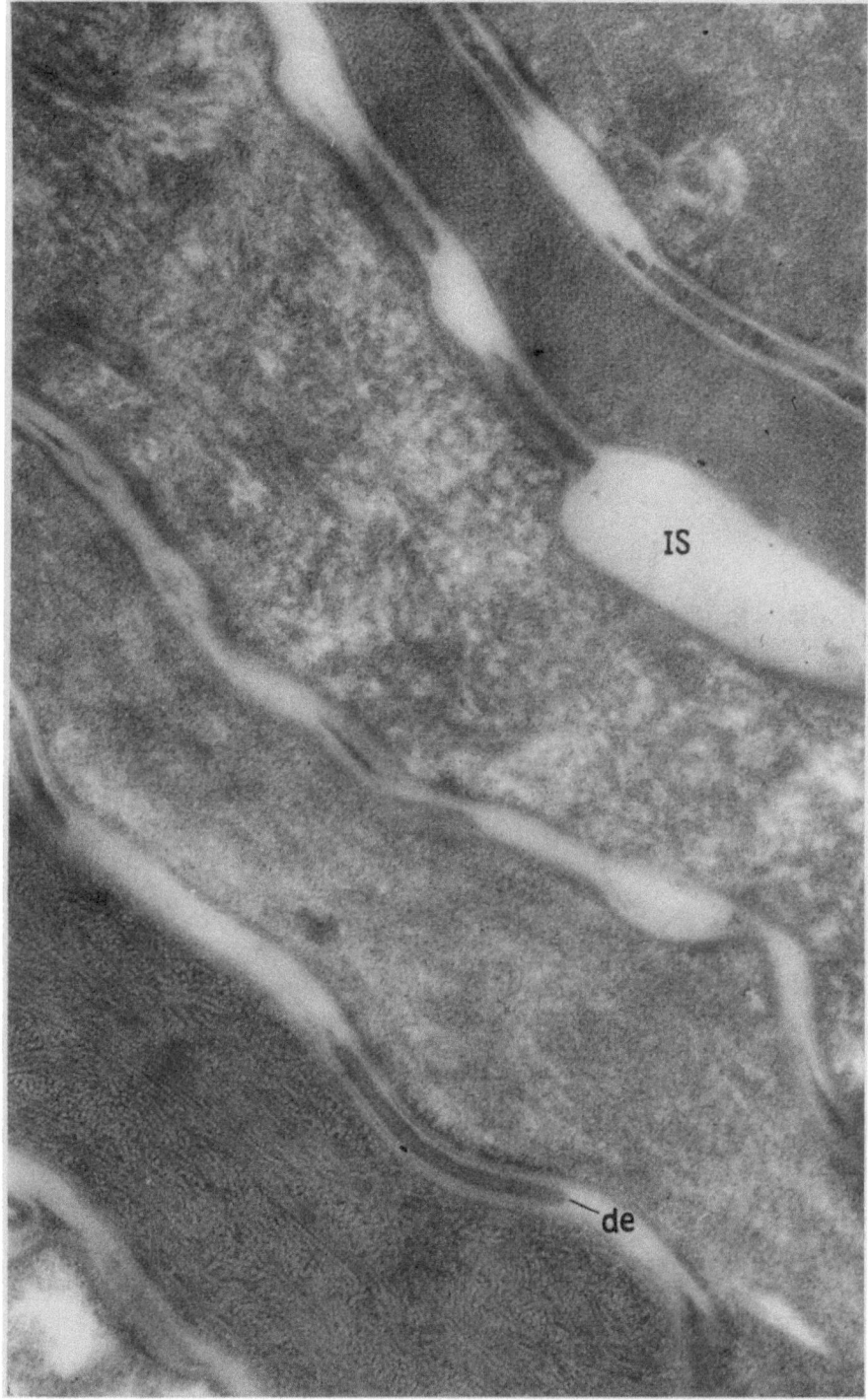

Fig. 28. Skin from the shoulder. Part of the intermediate layer of the stratum corneum with varying ultrastructure of the fibrils in adjacent horny cells. *IS* intercellular space, *de* regular desmosome. × 89,000.
(From BRODY, 1964a. Courtesy of J. invest. Derm., The Williams and Wilkins Co., Baltimore)

On the strength of electron-microscopic and X-ray diffraction results FRASER, MACRAE and ROGERS (1962) have further suggested that each protofilament consists of a 3-strand rope of alpha-helices, and each strand is regularly divided into a repeating sequence of three distinct proportions of similar length. Whether this pattern is also valid for the epidermal keratin filament is not yet known.

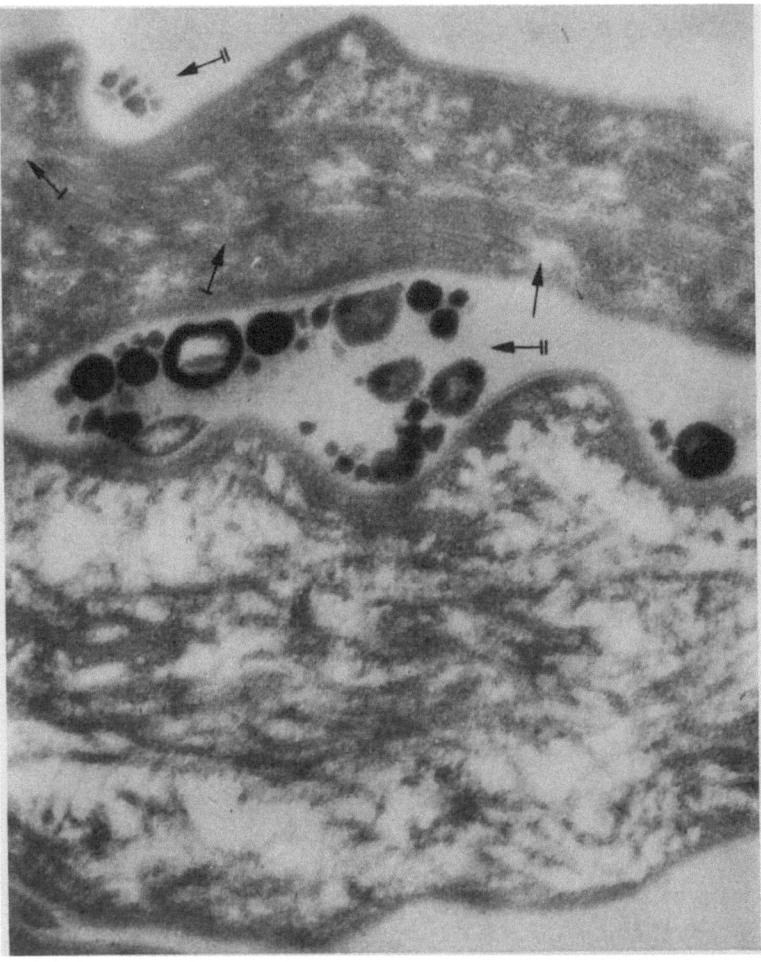

Fig. 29. Skin from the shoulder. Two horny cells showing distinctly varying numbers of fibrils. In the lower cell electron-optically empty spaces dominate the picture. In the upper cell the main part of the cytoplasm consists of fibrils. Between the fibrils small electron-optically empty spaces (→) and small areas with less opaque non-fibrillar substance (↦). In the intercellular space, components (↦) of various shape and opacity. × 85,000.
(From BRODY, 1964a. Courtesy of J. invest. Derm., The Williams and Wilkins Co., Baltimore)

No protofilaments have yet been shown in the cross-sections of filaments in ultra thin sections of the epidermis. The prekeratin molecule isolated by MATOLTSY (1964, 1965) from the non-cornified epidermis of the cow's nose has a diameter of 34 Å. Further studies are needed to ascertain whether the diameter of protofilaments agrees in normal epidermis and hair, and in other types of epidermis such as the parakeratosis occurring under normal conditions e.g. in the epidermis from the cow's nose (DERKSEN and HERINGA, 1936) and frog skin, and under pathological conditions.

V. Mitochondria

By mitochondria are histologically understood the cytoplasmic organelles which in living cells appear in a dark-field or phase-contrast microscope as motile filaments, rods or granules. They are stained selectively with Janus green, and are also stained with Regaud's and Heidenhain's hematoxylin or with Altmann's technique (MONTAGNA, 1962; BOURNE and TEWARI, 1964).

When studied with histological methods the mitochondria in the epidermis have often been mixed up with epidermal fibrils and desmosomes (for survey and references see MONTAGNA, 1956, 1962; HORSTMANN, 1957, 1960; RITZENFELD, 1965).

Electron microscopy opened up new ways of studying the morphology of the mitochondria and their relationship to other cytoplasmic constituents. The fine structure of the mitochondria was first described by PALADE (1952a, b, 1953), SJÖSTRAND (1953a, b, c, 1955, 1956a, b) and SJÖSTRAND and RHODIN (1953). The mitochondria (Fig. 30) appear as rounded or oval organelles bounded by an outer membrane and containing a system of inner membranes (SJÖSTRAND) or cristae mitochondriales (PALADE). The inner membranes are immersed in a ground substance which appears finely granular. The arrangement and number of inner membranes vary considerably in the mitochondria of different tissues (SJÖSTRAND, 1955). Subsequent studies have revealed that the outer and inner mitochondrial membranes show a five-layered pattern, with three opaque layers separated by two light layers (for survey and references see SJÖSTRAND, 1960). In a study of mouse kidney and pancreas SJÖSTRAND (1963c, d, e) has further demonstrated that the mitochondrial outer and inner membranes display a globular pattern. This observation has since been confirmed by ROSA and TSOU (1965) and WALKER and SCHRODT (1965).

In the normal human epidermis the mitochondria have a length of 2,500 to 10,000 Å and a breadth of 1,500 to 2,500 Å (ZELICKSON and HARTMANN, 1961b). In electron-microscopic studies of epidermis from man (SELBY, 1955, 1957; ZELICKSON and HARTMANN, 1961b; BRAUN-FALCO, 1965), from rat (HORSTMANN and KNOOP, 1958; HORSTMANN, 1960), from rabbit (V. BARGEN, 1959) and from guinea-pig (SNELL, 1965a) it has been constantly pointed out that the mitochondria are numerous in the stratum basale, show the same number or are less numerous in the stratum spinosum, are few or absent in the stratum intermedium and are absent in the strata lucidum and corneum. BRODY (1960b), on the other hand, reports that the mitochondria in the stratum intermedium of human epidermis may be seen as distinctly as in the subjacent strata and also show the same pattern of distribution. Mitochondria displaying a distinct structure were also found in the stratum corneum, in accordance with earlier studies on the guinea-pig epidermis (BRODY, 1959a). On the whole, there is a decrease in the number of mitochondria from the stratum basale to the skin-surface. This decrease is most striking at the transition between the stratum intermedium and the T-cells and horny cells. If one studies survey-pictures of epidermis one finds that the number of mitochondria varies considerably in adjacent cells in the strata basale, spinosum and intermedium. In the stratum intermedium are seen cells which seem to contain as many mitochondria as cells in the stratum basale (Fig. 6). Throughout the non-cornified epidermis the mitochondria are scattered over the whole cytoplasm. They do not show an increased tendency to a perinuclear arrangement in the strata spinosum and intermedium as compared to those in the stratum basale. They occur in groups or singly.

The occurrence of the enzyme succinic dehydrogenase in the mitochondria (for references see SCHNEIDER and KUFF, 1964) has been used to demonstrate histologically the distribution of the mitochondria in the epidermis (ZELICKSON, 1960; RITZENFELD, 1965; RITZENFELD and KOCH, 1966). The occurrence of the enzymes NADH- and NADPH-tetrazolium reductases in the mitochondria (PEARSE, 1960; BRAUN-FALCO and PETZOLDT, 1964) has in a similar way been used to show the distribution pattern of the mitochondria in normal and pathological epidermis (RITZENFELD and KOCH, 1966). The results arrived at by ZELICKSON (1960) and RITZENFELD and KOCH (1966) are similar to BRODY's (1960b), whereas those of RITZENFELD (1965) agree rather with the electron-microscopic observations made by SELBY (1955, 1957), ZELICKSON and HARTMANN (1961b) and BRAUN-FALCO (1965a).

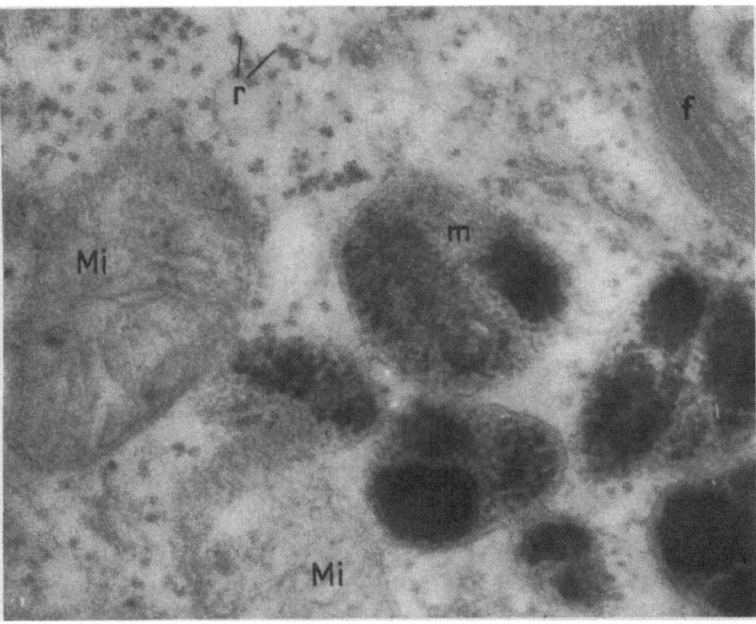

Fig. 30. Mitochondrion (*Mi*) and melanin granules (*m*) in a cell of the stratum basale. The mitochondrion is bounded by an outer triple-layered membrane and contains inner membranes. The melanin granules are also bounded by a triple-layered membrane and show areas of different ultrastructure and opacity. *f* fibril, *r* ribosomes. × 79,000. (From BRODY, 1964b. Courtesy of Academic Press Inc., New York-London)

FASSKE and THEMANN (1959b), investigating pathological oral epithelium, have stated that with a decreasing number of mitochondria the fibrils increase. This correlation has not been observed in normal human epidermis or in parakeratotic or hyperkeratotic psoriatic epidermis (BRODY, 1960b, 1962a, b, c, d, 1963b, c, d). There is no evidence in the electron micrographs that the fibrils in normal human epidermis increase in number above the stratum basale (SELBY, 1956; BRODY, 1960b, 1964b). In parakeratotic psoriatic epidermis the mitochondria occur in greater numbers in the strata basale, spinosum, intermedium and corneum than those in normal human epidermis (BRODY, 1962a, b, c, d, e, f). The fibrils in this type of epidermis are relatively few. A decrease in the number of mitochondria from the stratum basale towards the skin-surface is also observed here, but a corresponding increase in the fibrils is not seen.

In an electron-microscopic study of the corneal epithelium in mice with A-vitamin deficiency SHELDON and ZETTERQVIST (1956) have suggested that the keratohyalin material is formed from the mitochondria. This observation has not been verified in human epidermis (BRODY, 1960b, 1964b) or in rat epidermis (HORSTMANN and KNOOP, 1958).

VI. The Golgi Apparatus

After the prolonged immersion of sections of neural tissue in a solution of osmium tetroxide and rubidium bichromate, GOLGI (1898) discovered a cellular constituent that he called the "internal reticular apparatus". This is generally known as the *Golgi apparatus*. Apart from the mitochondria, no cellular component has aroused more controversy than the Golgi apparatus (for survey and references see BOURNE and TEWARI, 1964). HORSTMANN (1957) and MONTAGNA (1962) have comprehensively surveyed the pertinent literature with regard to the epidermis.

With phase-contrast microscopy DALTON and FELIX (1952, 1953) succeeded in demonstrating the occurrence of this apparatus in living cells of different tissues.

The fine structure of the Golgi apparatus as revealed by electron microscopy was first described by DALTON and FELIX (1954), RHODIN (1954) and SJÖSTRAND and HANZON (1954a, b).

SJÖSTRAND and HANZON (1954a, b), investigating the exocrine pancreatic cells in mouse, have shown that the Golgi apparatus is constituted of three different elements: the Golgi membranes, the Golgi ground substance and the Golgi granules. The Golgi membranes are arranged in pairs. They occur in groups of mostly two to five tightly packed pairs of membranes. The average thickness of a pair of membranes is 180 Å. The distance between the centres of the constituent membranes has been estimated as 130 Å. The single membrane has a thickness of 60 Å. The width of the space in between the two membranes of a pair is 60 Å. The pairs of membranes may be arranged roughly parallel. A characteristic feature is the occurrence of empty vacuoles, or what FAWCETT (1966) calls cisternae, in between the split membrane-pairs (SJÖSTRAND and HANSSON, 1954b). Here the pairs of membranes are embedded in the homogeneous, granulated or reticulated Golgi ground substance. In the pancreas the Golgi granules range from a diameter of 40 Å to the varying size of the zymogen granules. In various cell types secretion granules of different kinds occur (cf. chapter on "Melanocytes"; FAWCETT, 1966).

In the normal human epidermis the Golgi apparatus seems to be poorly developed. In the majority of electron-microscopic investigations it is not mentioned at all. It is usually located supranuclearly. In rabbit skin v. BARGEN (1959) observed Golgi apparatus in the stratum basale and lower stratum spinosum. In the latter layer they occurred within a larger area than in the stratum basale. In the upper stratum spinosum the apparatus was no longer distinguished. In an electron-microscopic study of normal human epidermis ZELICKSON and HARTMANN (1961b) have noted a Golgi apparatus only in the stratum basale. According to light-microscopic investigations it is also found in the stratum intermedium (cf. review by HORSTMANN, 1957).

VII. Ribosomes and alpha-Cytomembranes

In the non-cornified epidermis of man and of different laboratory animals the free ribosomes or microsomal particles (cf. SJÖSTRAND, 1962) dominate the picture, whereas alpha-cytomembranes (for definition see SJÖSTRAND, 1956a, b) are few (MERCER, 1958a, 1961; HORSTMANN and KNOOP, 1958; HORSTMANN, 1960; BRODY, 1960b, 1964b; ODLAND, 1964; ROTH and CLARK, 1964). The ribosomes have an approximate diameter of 150 Å. In small magnifications they appear with even opacity, but in higher magnifications each particle shows indications of a less intensely stained spot contrasting with more intensely stained regions surrounding it (BRODY, 1960b; Fig. 22). They occur singly, in groups, or in short, straight, or somewhat wavy chains. Throughout the non-cornified epidermis they are numerous in the perinuclear, fibril-free zone. In the strata basale and spinosum they occur in large numbers, usually in groups or singly in the meshes of the fibrillar network. In the stratum intermedium they are often collected in groups occurring close to the fibrils. Also in the T-cells groups of ribosomes are seen (BRODY, 1959b, 1960b; ROTH and CLARK, 1964). No ribosomes have been found in the strata lucidum or corneum.

In electron-microscopic studies PORTER and KALLMANN (1952) and PALADE and PORTER (1952) introduced the term endoplasmic reticulum for the system of tubules and vesicles observed in the cells. SJÖSTRAND (1953b) demonstrated that the endoplasmic reticulum is constituted of various types of membranous components. He introduced the term alpha-cytomembranes for one type of cytoplasmic membranes (SJÖSTRAND, 1956a, b; see also survey, 1964). These measure about 50 Å in thickness and are arranged in pairs or as single membranes associated with the nuclear membrane and with adherent ribosomes. The expression rough cisternae of the endoplasmic reticulum is also used for this type of cytoplasmic membranes (for survey and references see PORTER, 1963; FAWCETT, 1966).

The alpha-cytomembranes are few in the normal human keratinocytes. ZELICKSON and HARTMANN (1961b) have only observed them in the strata basale and spinosum, whereas ODLAND (1964) has also found them in the perinuclear, fibril-free zone in the stratum intermedium (Fig. 31).

Cytochemical and electron-microscopic studies of exocrine pancreatic cells have revealed that the ribosomes contain a high concentration of ribonucleic acid (SIEKEVITZ and PALADE, 1958a, b). The free and attached ribosomes are considered to be the site of protein synthesis in the cells (LOFTFIELD, 1957; SIEKEVITZ and PALADE, 1960a, b).

In the epidermis the ribosomes are responsible for a part of the basophilia. MONTAGNA (1962) has given a detailed account of the different chemical substances responsible for the basophilia in epidermis.

VIII. Other Cytoplasmic Constituents

Throughout the normal human epidermis have with electron microscopy been observed a small number of so-called lipid droplets (BRODY, 1963e; HANUŠOVÁ, 1965; BRAUN-FALCO, 1965b) whose histochemical nature has been studied by STEIGLEDER (1958c, 1960b) and HANUŠOVÁ (1960, 1961, 1965) (cf. chapter on "Lipids").

In the cells of the upper stratum spinosum and of the stratum intermedium in normal human epidermis so-called *lamellated bodies* (FRITHIOF and WERSÄLL, 1965; cf. chapter C II) occur in varying numbers (CHARLES and SMIDDY, 1957; SELBY, 1957; ODLAND, 1960, 1964; MATOLTSY and PARAKKAL, 1965; RUPEC and BRAUN-FALCO, 1965; WILGRAM, 1965; Fig. 8). They have a diameter of between 1000 and 5000 Å. ODLAND (1960) indicates the presence of membranes within the bodies. In a study of normal and hyperplastic mouse epidermis FREI and SHELDON (1961) also distinguished indications of an internal structure. In a later study on normal human epidermis ODLAND (1964) clearly showed that the bodies contain a system of parallel membranes. In subsequent studies of normal epidermis from man and laboratory animals (MATOLTSY and PARAKKAL, 1965; WILGRAM, 1965; BREATHNACH and WYLLIE, 1966) and of normal and pathological mucous membranes (MATOLTSY and

PARAKKAL, 1965; FRITHIOF and WERSÄLL, 1965; OLÁH and RÖHLICH, 1966) this observation has been confirmed and further extended. Thus FRITHIOF and WERSÄLL (1965) have been able to demonstrate that the bodies in human mucous membrane present a highly ordered structural organization. The bodies may contain a system of densely packed layers or their interior is subdivided into two or three sectors exhibiting different main orientations of the layers. The layers are opaque, have a thickness of 25 Å and are separated by a light zone. The latter has a width of 35 Å. In the middle of the light zone a narrow dense layer appears.

According to MATOLTSY and PARAKKAL (1965) the lamellated bodies are first observed in the vicinity of the Golgi apparatus. They seem to be most numerous in the upper cells of the stratum spinosum and decrease in numbers in the cells of the stratum intermedium. However, simultaneously with this intracellular decrease they increase in number in the intercellular space of the stratum intermedium in the epidermis (FREI and SHELDON, 1961; MATOLTSY and PARAKKAL, 1965; RUPEC and BRAUN-FALCO, 1965), and in the mucous membranes (MATOLTSY and PARAKKAL, 1965; FRITHIOF and WERSÄLL, 1965; OLÁH and RÖHLICH, 1966). BRODY (1966) has also demonstrated their occurrence in the intercellular space of the stratum corneum in normal human epidermis (Fig. 12).

Their function is as yet unknown. A suggested relationship between the lamellated bodies and mitochondria, according to which they are attenuated mitochondria (SELBY, 1957; ODLAND, 1960; ZELICKSON and HARTMANN, 1961, 1962), has not been confirmed in subsequent studies (MATOLTSY and PARAKKAL, 1965; RUPEC and BRAUN-FALCO, 1965; FRITHIOF and WERSÄLL, 1965; OLÁH and RÖHLICH, 1966). These bodies and other types of organelles occur in larger numbers in pathological epidermis such as that occurring in psoriatic skin (BRODY, 1962a, b, c, d, f), in mucinosis follicularis (ORFANOS and GAHLEN, 1964), in dermatoses characterized by acantholysis, and in ichthyosis (WILGRAM, 1965), and in epidermolytic hyperkeratosis (WILGRAM and CAULFIELD, 1966). ORGANOS and GAHLEN (1964) point out that the presence of the bodies in normal human epidermis speaks against a virus hypothesis. They discuss the possibility that the bodies may perhaps represent an electron-microscopic equivalent to the light-microscopic, diastase-resistant PAS-granules observed in the epidermis. WILGRAM (1965) indicates that the laminated ultrastructure of the bodies may indicate a lysosome character. MATOLTSY and PARAKKAL (1965) and HASHIMOTO, GROSS, NELSON and LEVER (1966) suggest that the lamellated bodies contain mucopolysaccharides, whereas FRITHIOF and WERSÄLL (1965) and OLÁH and RÖHLICH (1966) consider them to be phospholipid in nature.

Electron-microscopic investigations have shown that the *melanin* granules are most numerous in the basal cells, where they occur scattered throughout the cytoplasm or in the perinuclear, fibril-free zone (BRODY, 1960b; ZELICKSON and HARTMANN, 1961b; Figs. 5 and 30). In higher strata they are found mainly in the perinuclear zone. In a light-microscopic study KEDDIE and SAKAI (1965) have shown their occurrence also in the horny cells.

In normal human epidermis ZELICKSON and HARTMANN (1961b) observed a centriole close to the Golgi apparatus in the cells of the stratum basale. No centriole was distinguished in stratum spinosum.

According to STOECKENIUS (1957) there may be a spatial relationship between the centriole and the Golgi apparatus. The centriole is a self-replicating component located in the juxtanuclear area of living cells (cf. FAWCETT, 1966). It appears as a hollow cylinder with a length of 3000—5000 Å and a diameter of 1500 Å. Nine evenly spaced tubulus embedded in a dense amorphous substance form the wall. This seems to be closed at one end and open at the other.

IX. The Nucleus

Nuclei are present in all non-cornified cells as well as in the T-cells (BRODY, 1960b; ROTH and CLARK, 1964). They have an oval shape with the longitudinal axis oriented parallelly to that of the cells. In the T-cells the nuclei have a long, flattened shape (Fig. 6).

The nuclei are everywhere bounded by a distinct membrane consisting of two opaque layers separated by a 200 to 700 Å wide space. The inner layer is about 300 Å thick (ZELICKSON and HARTMANN, 1961b; SNELL, 1965a). Through pores in the outer layer the light interspace is in direct continuity with the spaces delimited by alpha-cytomembranes. Ribosomes may also adhere to the cytoplasmic face of the outer layer of the nuclear membrane. At the site corresponding to the pore in the outer layer the inner leaflet of the nuclear membrane is replaced by a thin septum (Fig. 31). In normal human epidermis a distinct membrane has been observed around all nuclei in the stratum intermedium and T-cells (BRODY, 1960b). In the cells of the stratum intermedium in rat-foot epidermis a distinct nuclear membrane has also been found (HORSTMANN and KNOOP, 1957, 1958). In other electron-microscopic studies of rabbit (v. BARGEN, 1959) and guinea-pig epidermis (SNELL, 1965a) it has been pointed out that the nuclear membrane is less distinctly seen than that in the subjacent strata or may even be degenerated.

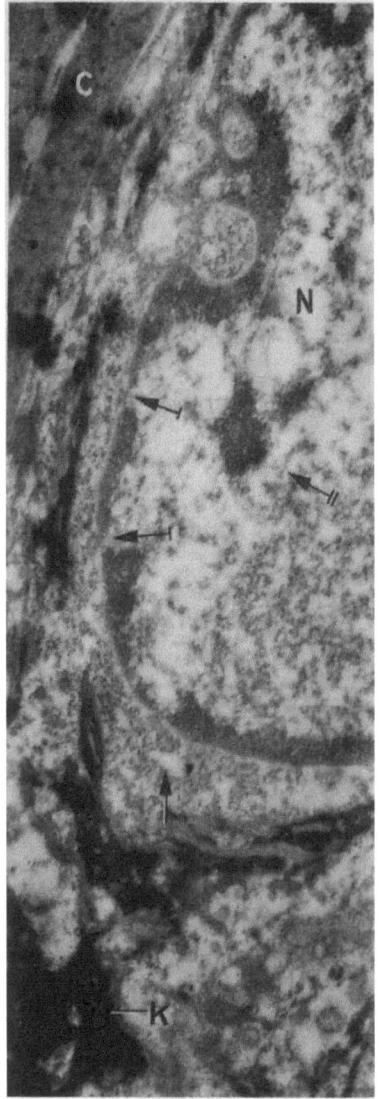

Fig. 31. Nucleus (*N*) of an upper cell of the stratum intermedium in abdominal epidermis, bounded by a nuclear membrane. Through pores in the outer leaflet of the membrane the light interspace of the nuclear membrane is in continuity with alpha-cytomembranes (→). The inner leaflet is in some areas replaced by a thin septum (↦). The karyoplasm appears as fine opaque, more or less densely occurring particles associated with less opaque, fine filaments (↦). A large number of ribosomes in the fibril-free perinuclear zone. The keratohyalin (*k*) is not found in larger amounts around the nucleus than in other parts of the cell. *C* stratum corneum. × 22,000

The karyoplasm appears as fine opaque, more or less densely occurring particles associated with less opaque filaments (HORSTMANN, 1960; Fig. 31). The nuclei contain one or several nucleoli. The latter appear as opaque, rounded bodies mainly eccentrically placed in the nucleus. No membrane separates them from the rest of the karyoplasm (HORSTMANN, 1960; ZELICKSON and HARTMANN, 1961b).

In the normal human epidermis the nuclei in the stratum intermedium usually have the same appearance as those in the subjacent strata (Figs. 5 and 31). Occasionally, nuclei occur where the karyoplasm is condensed at the periphery

(Fig. 32). In the stratum intermedium of rabbit epidermis only the latter type has been described (v. BARGEN, 1959). In the T-cells of human epidermis, however, the nuclei always display a condensed karyoplasm. The condensed karyoplasm in the nuclei in the T-cells is less opaque than that in the nuclei in the stratum intermedium (Fig. 6).

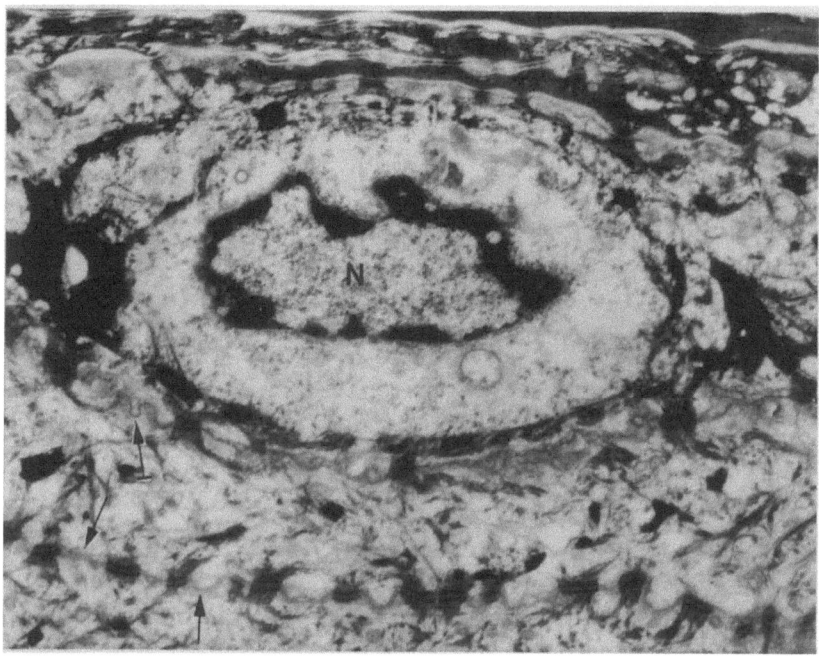

Fig. 32. Nucleus (*N*) of an upper cell of the stratum intermedium in abdominal epidermis showing a condensed opaque karyoplasm at the periphery. The condensed karyoplasm is less opaque than the keratohyalin. The nucleus is bounded by a nuclear membrane. A distinct fibril-free perinuclear zone is seen. The keratohyalin does not predominate around the nucleus. The cell surfaces between the regular desmosomes are rather even (→) or show invaginations (↦). × 7,000

X. Cell Regeneration

The physiologic regeneration replaces the horny cells which shed off successively at the skin surface. The renewal time of the epidermis has been studied with different techniques. v. VOLKMANN (1954) injected Indian ink in the epidermis and followed its disappearance from the skin surface. It disappeared from the surface of the palmar epidermis after 32 to 36 days, of the arm after about 17 days, and of the leg after about 30 days. ROTHBERG, CROUNSE and LEE (1961) injected glycine-2-C^{14} intravenously in two patients with chronic myelogenous leukemia and measured the appearance of radioactivity in scraped stratum corneum from the back. The renewal time was found to be 26 to 28 days. With vital microscopy EHRING (1962) investigated the renewal time of the human epidermis at the side of the finger-nail. It varied between 15 and 38 days. EPSTEIN and MAIBACH (1966) injected thymidine-H^3 intradermally at several sites on normally appearing human skin of the upper arm and the thigh. The renewal time for the non-cornified epidermis was estimated at 13 to 18 days.

The number of mitoses in the fixed and embedded epidermis is low. According to THURINGER (1928, 1939), the small number is partly due to the effect of postmortal changes, and the number of mitotic figures decreases in relation to the time elapsing between the removal of the tissue and its fixation. FULAR (1955) observed very few mitoses in normal epidermis, whereas psoriatic epidermis and squamous epithelium carcinoma displayed numerous mitoses on fixation undertaken immediately after the removal of the tissues. On the strength of these observations FULAR (1955) concludes that in normal epidermis the number of mitoses is, simply, small.

THURINGER (1928) observed great regional variations of the mitosis-index, *i.e.*, the number of cells showing mitosis in relation to the whole cell population. This index is in the epidermis of the scalp 1:2414, of the ear 1:268,275 and of the leg 1:378,325. MESSIER and LEBLOND (1960), however, point out that the mitotic index is only a rough indication of the rate of cell proliferation.

ANDREW (1949, 1951) and ANDREW and ANDREW (1949, 1954) considered the number of mitoses of the keratinocytes to be insufficient to replace the successive shedding of the epidermal cells. They therefore suggested that the keratinocytes are partly replaced by lymphocytes deriving from the dermis. They assumed that the lymphocytes in the epidermis are transformed into keratinocytes *via* "clear cells" and "intermediate cells". ANDREASEN (1952) also observed lymphocytes in the normal epidermis, but was unable to verify the observations of a transformation of these cells into keratinocytes. MEDAWAR (1953) points out that the lymphocytes presumed to occur in the epidermis in fact correspond to the perikaryon of the melanocytes, the so-called "clear cells" of MASSON (1948a, b).

Another hypothesis has been advanced, *viz.* that besides mitosis an amitotic cell division also occurs in the epidermis. The latter has been presumed to take place in the upper layer of the stratum spinosum (PATZELT, 1926, 1929; HOEPKE, 1927) and in the stratum intermedium (FERREIRA-MARQUES and PARRA, 1960), where two nuclei are often observed. According to PINKUS (1927), no evidence has been presented to show the presence of an amitotic fission in the epidermis. HORSTMANN (1957) also doubts that all binuclear cells originate from amitotic cell division.

In a schematic drawing PINKUS (1958, 1966) explains the small number of mitoses and the long life span of the normal epidermal cells (cf. also Fig. 49 in PINKUS, 1964). As the diagram shows, the basal cells give rise to clones of maturing keratinocytes. In the drawing two clones are depicted. These have the forms of inverted cones, owing to increasing traverse diameter of the maturing cells towards the skin surface. In the upper layers the cells per unit area are sparser, as may be seen from the diagram (with surface area = 4 cells, base = 100 cells).

A question that has long been debated and is not yet resolved is in which stratum or strata mitosis normally occurs. It has been hypothetically suggested that the germinative layer is constituted by both strata basale and spinosum (cf. MASSHOFF, 1955; HORSTMANN, 1957, 1961 and VERNE, 1960). According to THURINGER (1924, 1928, 1939), MILLER and MACMANUS (1940), COWDRY and THOMPSON (1944) and THURINGER and COOPER (1949, 1950) most mitoses occur in the lower and middle third of the stratum spinosum. ZANDER (1888), RABL (1901), ORITZ PICON (1933), MEDAWAR (1953) and MERCER (1961), on the other hand, consider that nearly all dividing cells are found in the stratum basale, and only a few occur in the lower third of the stratum spinosum. A third theory, first suggested by PINKUS (1927), *viz.* that the germinative layer is restricted to the stratum basale, is now gaining an increasing number of adherents (HANSON, 1947; LEBLOND, 1951; MESSIER and LEBLOND, 1960; MONTAGNA, 1962; LEBLOND, GREULICH and PEREIRA, 1964; VAN SCOTT, 1964). In order to explain the observations by THURINGER (1924, 1928, 1939), HANSON (1947) and LEBLOND (1951) suggest that in obliquely sectioned epidermis the mitoses may give the impression of occuring in the suprabasal layers. Another explanation is given by VAN SCOTT (1964), viz. that the mitoses assumed to occur in higher strata are in fact juxtaposed to the dermal papillae, as may be shown by serial sectioning of the tissue. In view of the changes of the fibrillar ultrastructure at the transition of the cells from the stratum basale to the stratum spinosum (BRODY, 1960b, 1964b), it seems reasonable also from an electron-microscopic viewpoint, to assume that cell regeneration is restricted to the basal layer.

In order to ascertain more definitely in which layer mitosis occurs, autoradiographic studies have been carried out after the administration of thymidine-H^3. Thymidine or thymine deoxyriboside is considered to be the most suitable labelled precursor for the study of the deoxyribose nucleic acid (DNA) synthesis which takes place prior to mitosis (SWIFT, 1950; REICHARD and ESTBORN, 1951; LEBLOND and WALKER, 1956; CRONKITE, BOND, FLIEDNER and RUBIN, 1959; LEBLOND, MESSIER and KOPRIWA, 1959; MESSIER and LEBLOND, 1960; BERNSTEIN, 1964; LEBLOND, GREULICH and PEREIRA, 1964). In the epithelium of the tongue of young adult mice LEBLOND, MESSIER and KOPRIWA (1959) observed that only the basal cells were labelled 8 hours after the administration of thymidine-H^3. In similar studies of the epidermis and oesophageal epithelium of young adult mice and rats SCHULTZE and OEHLERT (1960) found that $1^1/_2$ hours after the administration the labelled nuclei occurred only in the basal layer. In a more extensive study of the oesophageal epithelium in rat and mouse LEBLOND, GREULICH and PEREIRA (1964) have demonstrated that initially (15 minutes and one hour after the administration of thymidine-H^3) practically all labelled nuclei appear in the basal layer (99 per cent in rat and 97 per cent in mouse). The authors state that the few labelled cells that seemed to be just above the stratum basale histologically still exhibit the characteristic features of basal cells. No distinct labelled nuclei were observed in the transitional cells between the strata basale and spinosum or in the spinous cells. Similar results have been obtained in autoradiographic studies of the plantar epidermis of the rat (LEBLOND, GREULICH and PEREIRA, 1964). Here, too, the initially labelled cells were throughout only of the basal cell type. In plantar epidermis, however, the stratum basale is constituted by three rows of cell layers. From their observations the authors conclude that all cells in the stratum basale are able to synthesize DNA and to divide.

In a similar autoradiographic study of the skin from young rats FUKUYAMA and BERNSTEIN (1961) obtained labelled nuclei in the basal and spinous cells of the epidermis 15 minutes after administration. According to BERNSTEIN (1964), most of the label was restricted to the basal cells even 12 hours after the administration of thymidine-H^3. These results suggest that most, if not all, of the DNA synthesis and mitotic activity is restricted to the stratum basale. In a subsequent autoradiographic study of human skin *in vitro* FUKUYAMA, NAKAMURA and BERNSTEIN (1965) state, however, that DNA synthesis occurs both in the basal layer and in the layer just above the stratum basale.

THURINGER (1928) noted that the mitotic axis in the stratum basale of the human epidermis is parallel to the dermo-epidermal interface. In the stratum spinosum it is oblique to this interface (THURINGER and COOPER, 1949). PINKUS and HUNTER (1966) have found that the mitotic axis may be vertical, oblique or horizontal to the skin surface.

Statistically, the maintenance of the "steady state" of the stratified squamous epithelium (LEBLOND and WALKER, 1956) through the division of a basal cell implies that one daughter cell migrates, undergoes differentiation, and is finally eliminated at the surface, whereas the other remains in the stratum basale and may undergo further fission. In an autoradiographic study of the oesophageal epithelium in adult mouse Greulich (1964) has investigated the proliferative and differentiative behaviour of the individual basal cells in greater detail. First, the basal cell may divide, thus giving rise to one daughter cell which immediately migrates and differentiates, and to another daughter cell that remains in the basal layer. Second, a basal cell may divide and both daughter cells may immediately move outwards. In order to maintain the structural integrity of the tissue this alternative means that in some other part another basal cell undergoes fission and the two daughter cells must remain in the stratum basale. Third, all basal cells may divide, the division in this case resulting only in the production of more basal cells. In normal human epidermis Pinkus and Hunter (1966) have observed the same alternatives in the behaviour of the individual daughter cells. In addition, they also suggest a fourth alternative, *viz.* a mitotic division of suprabasal cells. This finding is at variance with the observations by Greulich (1964) and Leblond, Greulich and Pereira (1964), who consider that all mitosis is restricted to the basal layer, and that if a cell is squeezed out from this layer it still displays the characteristic features of a basal cell type. Pinkus and Hunter (1966), however, point out that their data do not permit any definite conclusion as to whether in the fourth alternative the division of the cell has already started in the basal layer, or whether the migrated daughter cell is able to undergo mitosis.

According to Greulich (1964), the migration of the single cells from the stratum basale towards the mucous membrane surface occurs randomly. This takes place for the most part independently of the mitosis from which the migrating cell took its origin (Greulich, 1964).

Various factors influence the frequency of mitosis, and the literature pertinent to this aspect of cell regeneration has been fully reviewed by Bullough (1952a, 1955a, b), Swann (1957), Montagna (1962) and Bullough and Rytömaa (1965). These factors have been mainly studied in *in vitro* and *in vivo* investigations of mouse epidermis.

In vitro studies of mouse epidermis have shown that if glucose, fructose, pyruvate or lactate are added to the substrate the number of mitoses will increase (Bullough and Johnson, 1951; Bullough, 1952a; Gelfant, 1959, 1960a, b). A high oxygen-tension also results in a increase of mitoses (Bullough and Johnson, 1951). The energy that a cell needs for fission must be mobilized and stored before division starts (Bullough, 1952a, b). Anaerobic conditions or respiratory inhibitors prevent the onset of mitosis but are without effect on a cell undergoing division.

The mitotic frequency is subject to a diurnal cycle, with the highest mitotic rate during sleep and the lowest during active muscular exercise (Bullough, 1948a, b). Further investigations have revealed that in well-fed adult mammals the epidermis is continuously furnished with an adequate supply of glucose and oxygen. The supply of these raw materials is, however, influenced by variations in the hormone-content in the blood (for survey and references see Montagna, 1962). The estrogens, androgens and possibly insulin are the only hormones which in physiological concentration *in vivo* have an obviously stimulating effect on mitosis. Adrenalin has a distinct antimitotic effect, and this is shown both in *in vivo* and *in vitro* studies (Bullough, 1952a, b, 1955b).

In *in vitro* studies of mouse epidermis Evensen and Heldaas (1964) have found that the immediate effect of adrenalin is promotion of the mitosis. The increased cell proliferation cannot, however, be followed for more than one hour. Colcemid in the concentrations used by the authors does not arrest the immediate effect of adrenalin for more than an hour. Evensen and Heldaas conclude that the effect of adrenalin is to give the epidermal cells in the "premitotic resting phase" an impulse to start mitosis.

BULLOUGH and LAURENCE (1959/60) have shown that if the epidermis is totally removed from one side of the mouse ear this will result in a high mitotic activity in the intact epidermis on the opposite side of the ear. The authors assumed the presence of a diffusible inhibitor that in normal epidermis controls the mitosis. BULLOUGH (1962) has given this inhibitor the name "chalone". There are probably at least three distinct chalones produced in mouse skin (BULLOUGH and LAURENCE, 1960), and each chalone is assumed to be produced by the tissue on which it specifically acts (BULLOUGH and LAURENCE, 1964a). An epidermal chalone is isolated from the back of adult mouse (BULLOUGH, HEWETT and LAURENCE, 1964). This substance is water-soluble and non-dialyzable and is precipitated by alcohol and destroyed by boiling. It does not survive in water solution but survives for at least a year when lyophilized. On the strength of its chemistry BULLOUGH, HEWETT and LAURENCE (1964) assume that the epidermal chalone is a protein. It is only active in the presence of adrenalin, with which it forms an unstable compound which is the actual inhibitor (BULLOUGH and LAURENCE, 1964a). The effect of the chalone is to reduce the number of cells preparing for mitosis (BULLOUGH and LAURENCE, 1964b). Loss of chalone accelerates the DNA synthesis and results in increased fission. If chalone were absent in the tissue the cells would tend to grow and to divide indefinitely.

BULLOUGH and RYTÖMAA (1965) have devoted a detailed discussion to the homeostatic mechanisms of mitosis. The finding that the actual mitotic inhibitor may be an unstable chalone-adrenalin complex (BULLOUGH and LAURENCE, 1964a) affords an explanation for the diurnal mitotic rhythm. When the mouse is sleeping the output of adrenalin is low, the chalone-adrenalin complex breaks down and the mitotic rate rises. During muscular activity the output of adrenalin rises, the complex re-forms and the mitotic rate falls.

BULLOUGH (1963) suggested the division of the cycle through which a cell passes from one mitosis to the next into four phases. "Dichophase" is the phase when a cell "decides" whether to prepare for another mitosis or to prepare for function within the tissue. "Prophase" is characterized by the period of preparation for mitosis and includes the phase of DNA synthesis and the antephase. Prophase is followed by mitosis. Finally, there is an "apophase" where each daughter cell re-establishes its normal synthetic mechanisms and grows to full size. The effect of a chalone is to reduce the number of cells preparing for mitosis. Chalone will therefore probably act in the dichophase, prior to the prophase. The cell is most sensitive to chalone during the dichophase and the antephase, both of which may be blocked by excess of chalone. The cell is least sensitive during prophase and mitosis, which may both be slowed down but not stopped. In the presence of sufficient chalone the cell will "decide" to synthesize those enzymes which are needed for tissue function. In the absence of chalone the DNA synthesis starts and the cell enters into mitosis. BULLOUGH and RYTÖMAA consider that any such "decision" relating to synthetic activities most likely involves gene action. This action may be under the control of two groups of genes, i.e., "mitosis operon" and "tissue operon". The tissue operon, which is probably tissue-specific, controls the synthesis for the activity within the tissue. The mitosis operon controls the DNA synthesis. The operon theory of chalone action may also be used to explain the duration of the mitotic cycles. The concentration of chalone affects the speed of these cycles. In the normal epidermis the mitotic rate is low and the speed at which cells pass through the antephase is moderate. In any typical tissue the specialization for mitosis and the specialization for function are merely opposite expressions of the same homeostatic mechanism. A typical tissue is composed of at least four distinct cell-types: the "progenitor" cells (P), which are involved in the mitotic cycle; the immature cells (I), which are preparing for tissue function; the mature cells (M), which are specialized for tissue function but which, if the effective chalone concentration falls, are capable of reversion to mitosis; and the mature cells called D, which are also specialized for tissue function but are unable to revert to mitosis. According to BULLOUGH and RYTÖMAA only the cells in the stratum intermedium of the mouse epidermis represent the D-cells, and the chalone is considered to be chiefly produced by the D-cells.

D. The Histochemistry of the Keratinocytes
I. Inorganic Substances

Histochemical methods for the demonstration of inorganic substances are not yet sufficiently advanced to give reliable results (BRAUN-FALCO, 1961a).

With histochemical methods GANS (1924), GANS and PARKHEISER (1924) and DÄHN (1926) studied the distribution of calcium and potassium in human skin. They noted that normal human epidermis contains a high concentration of potassium and a low concentration of calcium, whereas in the dermis the concentrations were reversed.

Zinc is of importance for the effect of many enzymes and forms a constituent in the enzyme carbonic anhydrase (BRAUN-FALCO, 1961a). Using the dithizone reagent (MAGER, MCNARY and LIONETTI, 1953), BRAUN-FALCO and RATHJENS (1956) investigated the histotopography of zinc in normal human epidermis. The stratum basale and lower stratum spinosum reacted strongly. The upper stratum spinosum and the stratum intermedium appeared light pinky, indicating a moderate concentration of zinc. The stratum corneum exhibited a varying reaction. Some areas showed a light positive reaction. In other areas a more intense reaction appeared. BRAUN-FALCO and RATHJENS assumed the latter to be of artificial nature and due to an external inhibition by zinc-containing substances. REAVEN and COX (1962) obtained the same distribution pattern when they stained the sections with dithizone immediately after sectioning. However, when the sections were kept in room air for a day or more before staining with dithizone a quite different distribution pattern of the zinc was observed. The transitional zone appeared intensely stained. The authors interpreted this to mean that the transitional zone has the capacity *in vitro* to bind and concentrate zinc when the ion is supplied in very dilute solutions.

Another way of studying the histotopography of the inorganic substances was opened up with the elaboration of the microincineration method. HINTZSCHE (1956) and recently KRUSZYNSKI (1966) have presented comprehensive surveys of the microincineration technique and its results.

Sections of tissue are simply reduced to ash by heating at high temperature on a glass slide. Proteins, lipids and carbohydrates are calcined and a pattern of inorganic substances is left. According to KOOYMAN (1935) and MONTAGNA (1956) also this method is of limited value. MONTAGNA (1956) points out that it is likely that the original topographic relationship of the inorganic material is disturbed after the microincineration. Iron, silica and uranium are practically the only elements which can be recognized with any degree of certainty (SCOTT, 1933; KOOYMAN, 1935). However, caution is probably to be recommended as regards conclusions concerning the occurrence of iron, as the nuclei can absorb iron from the ambience (WIENER, 1916). Minerals such as sodium, potassium, calcium and magnesium, which are most abundant in the tissue, are not easy to distinguish (KOOYMAN, 1935). Calcium and magnesium leave white ash, whereas the bluish ash is assumed to be due to sodium and potassium (GANS, 1930; KOOYMAN, 1935; ENGMAN and MACCARDLE, 1940; MACCARDLE, ENGMAN and ENGMAN, 1943).

With microincineration of the epidermis a high amount of ash is obtained in the strata corneum and basale (GANS, 1930; HERRMANN, 1932, 1935; HORNING, 1934; KOOYMAN, 1935; MACCARDLY, ENGMAN and ENGMAN, 1943). The total amount of ash shows regional variations, variations with respect to age, and sex differences (RIVELLONI, 1938).

GANS (1930) suggests that the main part of the compact white ash consists of calcium salts, and their distribution corresponds to that of the total ash. A similar distribution pattern was obtained by KRUSE (1958). HERRMANN (1932, 1935) has reported the occurrence of calcium, magnesium, phosphate and sulphate ash. He observed that phosphate occurs in the strata basale, spinosum and corneum. Calcium and magnesium usually appear as phosphate salts. Sulphate occurs in the strata corneum and basale.

HERRMANN (1935) and MACCARDLE, ENGMAN and ENGMAN (1943) have shown that calcium and magnesium display regional variations with respect to age. With increasing age there is an increase in the calcium and magnesium concentrations, but there is no corresponding increase in the concentration of the total ash.

II. Amino Acids, Proteins, Nucleic Acids and Protein-bound Sulfhydryl and Disulfide Groups

1. Amino Acids and Proteins

That there are so few histochemical investigations on the occurrence of amino acids and proteins in the epidermis is according to BRAUN-FALCO (1961a) due to the circumstance that most of the methods hitherto available have been relatively crude and injurious to tissue. In their surveys SPIER and CANEGHEM (1957), STEIGLEDER (1957) and BRAUN-FALCO (1961a) have discussed in detail the available methods and the results.

However, the autoradiographic technique should be able to offer new possibilities of following amino-acid incorporation and enable researchers to determine the location in the epidermis of protein synthesis *de novo*, i.e., the synthesis of protein from individual amino acids (BERNSTEIN, 1964).

Using the alloxan- and ninhydrin-Schiff-techniques (YASUMA and ICHIKAWA, 1953) for the demonstration of free amino acids, BRAUN-FALCO (1955, 1961a) has shown that normal human non-cornified epidermis reacts strongly. The horny layer gives a fainter reaction.

With ultraviolet microspectrographic methods SANDRITTER (1953) found that the intracellular content of proteins of the type serum globulin and albumin as well as aliphatic amino acids increase in amount towards the skin surface.

In a histochemical study REAVEN and COX (1963) have shown that certain components in the transitional zone of normal human epidermis react strongly to the Pauly reaction with diazotized sulfanilic acid. They suggest that this reaction is due to histidine. In a subsequent study REAVEN and COX (1965) have confirmed and extended these observations. In normal human abdominal epidermis the keratohyalin substance and the deep layers of the stratum corneum react strongly, whereas the upper layers of the horny layer generally give a less intense reaction to histidine. In the thick plantar and palmar epidermis, on the other hand, a strong reaction by Pauly-positive material was obtained throughout the stratum corneum. The amount of histidine in diseased skin is directly related to the amount of keratohyalin substance. In regions where keratohyalin is absent the overlying stratum corneum was not stained by the Pauly reagent. In other areas of the epidermis, where keratohyalin appeared in the stratum intermedium, the overlying horny layer reacted positively. These observations may lend support to the view, based upon electron-microscopic investigations of normal epidermis (MERCER, 1958a, 1961; BRODY, 1959a, b, 1960b, 1964b; ODLAND, 1964; ROTH and CLARK, 1964) and of psoriatic epidermis (BRODY, 1962a, b, c, d, e, 1963b, c, d, 1964b), that the keratohyalin material may contribute to the structure of keratin (REAVEN and COX, 1965).

In *in vitro* studies REAVEN and COX (1965) have further demonstrated that the histidine in most specimens is converted into urocanic acid. This observation is in accordance with the results arrived at by SCHWARZ (1961). In biochemical investigations the presence of urocanic acid in the normal human stratum corneum has also been shown (SPIER and PASCHER, 1959; SCHWARZ and SPIER, 1965). TABACHNIK (1957) found urocanic acid throughout the epidermis of the guinea-pig.

Autoradiographic studies of normal human epidermis indicate a glycine (ROTHBERG, CROUNSE and LEE, 1961) and leucine (KAKU, IGARASHI, MASU and FUJITA, 1964) incorporation in the stratum basale.

With histidine-H^3 FEGELER and RAHMANN-ESSER (1966b) have investigated the non-affected and affected skin of patients with Psoriasis vulgaris. In the non-affected skin they have found a maximal incorporation of tritiated histidine in the stratum intermedium, less in the strata basale and spinosum and none in the stratum corneum. These results agree with those arrived at by FUKUYAMA, NAKAMURA and BERNSTEIN (1965) on the epidermis of newborn rats. In the affected psoriatic skin there is increased incorporation in the strata basale and spinosum as compared to corresponding layers in the non-affected skin. No activity has, however, been observed in the strata intermedium or corneum. These results may support the observations by REAVEN and COX (1963, 1965).

With autoradiography BERNSTEIN (1964) and FUKUYAMA, NAKAMURA and BERNSTEIN (1965b) studied the incorporation of tritiated methionine, phenylalanine, leucine, glycine and histidine in protein in the epidermis of newborn rats. Thirty minutes after injection, labelling from methionine, phenylalanine and leucine was detected in the nuclei and the cytoplasm of the cells in the strata basale, spinosum and intermedium, with a maximum over the stratum basale and lower stratum spinosum. Labelling from glycine and histidine was also detected 30 minutes after injection in each strata, but here with a maximum over the stratum intermedium and the upper stratum spinosum. If these results indicate a protein synthesis *de novo*, the major sites of protein synthesis in the epidermis of newborn rats would then be in the stratum basale and lower stratum spinosum and in the stratum intermedium and upper stratum spinosum.

2. Nucleic Acids

a) Deoxyribonucleic Acid (DNA)

DNA is found only in the nucleus. The DNA-content and the metabolism of the nucleus have in recent years been the subject of intensive investigation (for review see MOSES, 1964).

LEUCHTENBERGER and LUND (1951) have reported that the DNA-content in the nuclei in the stratum intermedium is approximately the same as that in the nuclei in the subjacent layers. In subsequent studies it has, however, been shown that the DNA-content is high in the nuclei in the stratum basale and lower stratum spinosum, whereas in the outer layers of the non-cornified epidermis the DNA-content is relatively low (HARDY, 1952; SANDRITTER, 1953; WASHBURN and BLOCKER, 1954; BERN, ALFERT and BLAIR, 1957).

In order to ascertain where in the epidermis the DNA-synthesis occurs, autoradiographic studies have been carried out after the administration of thymidine-H^3. In an *in vitro* study of human skin FUKUYAMA, NAKAMURA and BERNSTEIN (1965a) report that DNA-synthesis occurs in the nuclei in the stratum basale as well as in the cells above this layer.

In an autoradiographic study on the epidermis from young rats FUKUYAMA and BERNSTEIN (1961) obtained labelled nuclei in the basal and spinous cells 15 minutes after administration. BERNSTEIN (1964) points out that most of the label is restricted to the nuclei in the basal cells even 12 hours after injection with tritiated thymidine, and he therefore suggests that most, if not all, of the DNA-synthesis is restricted to the stratum basale. In similar studies of the epidermis from rat (SCHULTZE and OEHLERT, 1960; LEBLOND, GREULICH and PEREIRA, 1964), from mouse (SCHULTZE and OEHLERT, 1960) and from pig (WEINSTEIN, 1965) labelled nuclei occurred only in the stratum basale from 15 minutes to 6 hours after the injection of thymidine-H^3, indicating that all DNA-synthesis in the laboratory animals is restricted to the nuclei in the stratum basale.

b) Ribonucleic Acid (RNA)

Independently, CASPERSSON and SCHULTZ (1939, 1940) and BRACHET (1940) demonstrated RNA in the cytoplasm and in the nuclei. They assumed a correlation between RNA- and protein-synthesis. The high RNA-content in the ribosomes (SIEKEWITZ and PALADE, 1958a, b, 1960b) in the cytoplasm, make the ribosomes responsible for the cytoplasmic basophilia. For as yet unexplained reasons the cytoplasmatic ribonucleoproteins are consumed during the protein synthesis. The replacement is made for the most part from the RNA-depot of the nucleolus in the cell nucleus (BRAUN-FALCO, 1961a). The role of the RNA and the nucleocytoplasmic relationships have during the last decades been the subject of intensive research (for review see GOLDSTEIN, 1964).

SANDRITTER (1953), using ultraviolet microspectrographic methods, has demonstrated that the RNA-concentration decreases from the stratum basale to the stratum spinosum and is approximately the same in the strata spinosum and intermedium. In conformity with these observations STEIGLEDER (1957) found with histochemical technique that the RNA-content is greatest in the basal layers, comprising the stratum basale and the lower layers of stratum spinosum (STEIGLEDER, 1955), and decreases towards the stratum corneum. MOBERGER and DE (1955) point out that the stratum intermedium does not contain more RNA than the subjacent strata and they consider, furthermore, that the keratohyalin does not contain any RNA. The latter finding is at variance with the observations by LEUCHTENBERGER and LUND (1951), SPIER and CANEGHEM (1957) and RUST and STEIGLEDER (1965), according to which the keratohyalin substance contains RNA. Histochemically RUST and STEIGLEDER (1965) show that the RNA is diffusely scattered in the strata basale and spinosum. In the upper stratum spinosum the RNA appears as fine granules which in the stratum intermedium become larger and, with respect to localization, size and staining properties, correspond to the RNA-containing keratohyalin "granules".

In autoradiographic studies no labelled precursor is available for localizing RNA-synthesis with the same degree of specificity as is the case for DNA (BERN-

STEIN, 1964). According to KAKU, IGARASHI, MASU and FUJITA (1964) the highest RNA-synthesis occurs in the stratum spinosum of normal human epidermis. FEGLER and RAHMANN-ESSER (1965), on the other hand, have found a decrease in the RNA-synthesis from the stratum basale towards stratum corneum.

RAHMANN-ESSER and FEGELER (1966b) have investigated with uridine-H^3 the non-affected and affected skin of patients with Psoriasis vulgaris. Here, too, in accordance with their earlier results on normal human epidermis (FEGELER and RAHMANN-ESSER, 1965) they obtained a maximal RNA-synthesis in the stratum basale and a decrease in the synthesis towards the stratum corneum. The latter layer did not show any activity. On the strength of their observations RAHMANN-ESSER and FEGELER (1966b) conclude that the stratum intermedium is characterized by a minimal RNA-synthesis and a maximal protein-synthesis.

The site of RNA-synthesis in the epidermis of young rats has been investigated with autoradiographic technique after the administration of cytidine-H^3 (FUKUYAMA and BERNSTEIN, 1963; BERNSTEIN, 1964). The first labelling appeared after 15 minutes. This experiment showed that most of the early labelling was concentrated over the nucleoli in the nuclei throughout the strata basale, spinosum and intermedium. Two hours after administration radioactivity was seen to be extensive over the remainder of the nucleus, and not until 6 hours after the injection with cytidine-H^3 did the label appear extensively also over the cytoplasm. At 24 hours after injection the labelling was greater in the cytoplasm than in the nuclei.

In an autoradiographic study of normal human epidermis FEGELER and RAHMANN-ESSER (1966a) investigated the effect of vitamin C and folic acid on the protein- and RNA-metabolism. They found that vitamin C has a depressing effect, whereas folic acid leaves the protein and RNA-metabolism unaffected.

3. Sulfhydryl and Disulfide Groups

With the nitroprusside test (GIROUD and BULLIARD, 1930, 1933, 1935; GIROUD and LEBLOND, 1951; LEBLOND, 1951; for further references see also RAUSCH and GLODNY, 1956) and with the Prussian blue method with ferricyanide (CHÈVREMONT and FRÉDERIC, 1943) the sulfhydryl groups in the entire non-cornified epidermis react intensely. When a modification of BENNETT's (1951) method with 1-(4-chloromercuriphenylazo)-naphthol-2 reagent is used the stratum basale reacts more strongly than the stratum spinosum (MESCON and FLESCH, 1952). The more intense reaction in the former layer was in part ascribed to the larger numbers of melanin granules occurring there. With this technique the nuclei and nucleoli in the stratum spinosum reacted more strongly than the cytoplasm, and the desmosomes stained better in this layer than those in the subjacent layer. With the 2,2'-dihydroxy-6,6'-dinaphthyl disulfide reagent introduced by BARRNETT and SELIGMAN (1952a, b), BARRNETT (1953) obtained a homogenous staining for sulfhydryl groups in the strata basale and spinosum; the nuclei did not react, and the desmosomes, particularly those in the stratum basale, were well stained. GOLDBLUM, PIPER and CAMPBELL (1954) modified the methods by CHÈVREMONT and FRÉDERIC (1943), BENNETT (1951) and BARRNETT and SELIGMAN (1952a) and in principle obtained consistent results with the three methods. This observation was subsequently confirmed by STEIGLEDER (1960b) in studies on the psoriatic epidermis. With all three modifications GOLDBLUM, PIPER and CAMPBELL have shown that in the strata basale and spinosum the nuclei stain lightly except in the periphery. In these layers also the cytoplasm stained lightly, except at the periphery, where particularly the desmosomes reacted strongly. The melanin granules were especially clearly seen with the modification of BARRNETT and SELIGMAN's method.

CHÈVREMONT and FRÉDÉRIC (1943) showed that the keratohyalin in the stratum intermedium reacts particularly intensely with the Prussian blue method. On the strength of this finding the authors advanced the hypothesis that the keratohyalin represents the immediate precursor to the keratin. According to GOLDBLUM, PIPER and CAMPBELL (1954), the keratohyalin shows a positive reaction with all three modifications, but the reaction is best seen with the modification of the Prussian blue method. In other studies no reaction was observed, either for sulfhydryl or disulfide groups. In the fifties, the prevailing view among histochemists was therefore that the keratohyalin is only a degeneration product without any importance for the formation of keratin (MESCON and FLESCH, 1952; BARRNETT, 1953; EISEN, MONTAGNA and CHASE, 1953; MONTAGNA, EISEN, RADEMACHER and CHASE, 1954; MONTAGNA, 1956; BERN, ELLIS, PICKETT, POWERS and HARKNESS, 1955; MATOLTSY, 1958b).

CHÈVREMONT and FRÉDÉRIC (1943), MESCON and FLESCH (1952), BARRNETT (1953), EISEN, MONTAGNA and CHASE (1953), MONTAGNA, EISEN, RADEMACHER and CHASE (1954) and MONTAGNA (1956, 1962) have observed a strong reaction for -SH groups in the transitional zone (Fig. 33), which reaction was not demonstrable with the nitroprusside method (GIROUD and BULLIARD, 1930, 1933, 1935; GIROUD and LEBLOND, 1951). This zone corresponds to the "phanerogenous zone" (GIROUD and BULLIARD, 1930) in the skin appendages such as the nails, hair etc., where the sulfhydryl groups react strongly. The observation of this zone also in the epidermis implies that a clear distinction between "soft" and "hard" keratinization is not possible in view of the histotopography of the sulfhydryl groups.

None of the methods hitherto used is, however, specific for sulfhydryl groups, which may in part explain the somewhat various results obtained with the different reagents (MESCON and FLESCH, 1952; RUDALL, 1952; BARRNETT, 1953; GOLDBLUM, PIPER and CAMPBELL, 1954; JOHNSON, HOFFMANN and ROLLE, 1957). Another important point is that the different reagents react with the different types of -SH groups occurring in the native protein, *i.e.*, freely reacting, sluggishly reacting and masked sulfhydryls (BARRON, 1951). Moreover, there are certain proteins which have only one or two of the three types of the sulfhydryls (OGURA, KNOX and GRIFFIN, 1961).

The freely reacting sulfhydryl groups react easily with nitroprusside and ferricyanide. The sluggishly reacting type does not give any reaction with nitroprusside but reacts with stronger reagents such as iodine and mercaptic-forming compounds. As a rule, all heavy metals which form mercaptans with thiols react in a similar manner with the —SH groups. The masked sulfhydryls, finally, remain in the native protein so well protected that the known —SH reagents do not attack them until the geometric configuration of the molecules is altered through rupture of the hydrogen bonds as this occurs e.g. in denaturation (BARRON, 1951). According to BARRNETT (1953), the results of the method by BARRNETT and SELIGMAN (1952a, b) may be due to the reaction of both "free" and "bound" sulfhydryls, since denaturation of the proteins occurs during fixation. SPIER and CANEGHEM (1957) suggest that a denaturation occurs in connection with all the methods, including the nitroprusside and Prussian blue methods.

OGURA, KNOX and GRIFFIN (1960a, b, 1961) and OGURA, KNOX, GRIFFIN and KUSUHARA (1962) have measured the sulfhydryl and disulfide concentrations in normal human epidermis with the amperometric titration technique. In biopsy specimens from living skin the sulfhydryls and disulfides occur in significantly higher concentrations than in skin from autopsy material. In infant skin there is a high sulfhydryl concentration but low disulfide concentrations. With advance in age the cysteine-cystine-sulfur and methionine-sulfur decrease in quantity.

The highest value for sulfhydryls is found in Caucasian skin, the lowest in Negro and in intermediate value in Latin American skin. In Caucasian and Negro skin the disulfide values are of the same order of magnitude. In the skin of the palms and soles the concentrations of sulfhydryl and disulfide are unexpectedly low (OGURA, KNOX, GRIFFIN and KUSUHARA, 1962).

The sulfhydryl groups are of great importance for numerous biological reactions (see surveys by BARRON, 1951; ROTHMAN, 1954; RAUSCH and GLODNY, 1956). They are essential for cellular respiration and for the activity of a large number of enzymes. In the epidermis they show a close correlation to the distribution of succinic dehydrogenase (EISEN, MONTAGNA and CHASE, 1953; ROGERS, 1953; FORAKER and WINGO, 1955, 1956). The protein-bound sulfhydryls are probably a constituent part of the active centre of the succinic dehydrogenase protein (HOFFMANN-OSTENHOF, 1954). The thiols are particularly numerous in the transitional zone, which is also characterized by its high enzymatic activity (cf. chapter on "Transitional zone"). Soluble as well as fixed sulfhydryl groups are essential for cell division and growth (RAPKINE, 1937; HAMMETT and WALP, 1939; BRACHET, 1950). It has also been claimed that they are concerned with cell permeability (LE FEVRE, 1948), the synthesis and activity of hormones (BARRON, 1951) and with melanogenesis (for survery and references see RAUSCH and GLODNY, 1956).

In a large number of investigations particular attention has been given to the histotopography of the sulfur (-SH and -S-S-) groups in the epidermis with a view to elucidating their function in the formation of keratin (cf. reviews by GIROUD and LEBLOND, 1951; MONTAGNA, 1952, 1956, 1962; RAUSCH and GLODNY, 1956; HORSTMANN, 1957; FLESCH, 1958; MATOLTSY, 1958a, b).

With the nitroprusside test (for references see RAUSCH and GLODNY, 1956) and the Prussian blue method (CHÈVREMONT and FRÉDERIC, 1943) the non-cornified epidermis stained intensely, while the strata lucidum and corneum remained unstained. On the strength of these observations it has long been held that during the keratinization process all sulfhydryl-containing amino-acid residues facing each other on neighbouring polypeptide chains close, to form disulfide cross-linkages (GIROUD and BULLIARD, 1930, 1933, 1935; GIROUD and LEBLOND, 1951; LEBLOND, 1951; MONTAGNA, 1952, 1956, 1962; ROTHMAN, 1954; HORSTMANN, 1957).

These observations by GIROUD and his co-workers have, however, not been verified in subsequent investigations in which the modification of BENNETT'S (1951) method and the method of BARRNETT and SELIGMAN (1952a, b) have been used (MESCON and FLESCH, 1952; BARRNETT, 1953; EISEN, MONTAGNA and CHASE, 1953; MONTAGNA, EISEN, RADEMACHER and CHASE, 1954; MONTAGNA, 1956, 1962; STEIGLEDER, 1956, 1957; MATOLTSY, 1958b). Thus a positive staining for sulfhydryl groups has also been obtained in the stratum corneum (Fig. 33). This reaction is less intense than that for the non-cornified epidermis (BARRNETT, 1953). GOLDBLUM, PIPER and CAMPBELL (1954) also demonstrated that the epidermal horny layer stained quite intensely for sulfhydryls with the modifications of the methods of CHÈVREMONT and FRÉDERIC (1943), BENNETT (1951) and BARRNETT and SELIGMAN (1952a).

Also in biochemical (VAN SCOTT and FLESCH, 1954; FLESCH and SATANOVE, 1955) and spectromicrophotometric (STEINER, 1960) investigations the occurrence of sulfhydryl groups in the stratum corneum has been shown. FLESCH and SATANOVE report that the -SH values in the non-cornified and cornified layers are 14 and 8 per cent of the "total" sulfur-content (-SH + -S-S-) respectively. VAN SCOTT and FLESCH point out that if during the epidermal keratinization process there is an oxidation of sulfhydryl to disulfide groups this conversion of sulfhydryls is incomplete and occurs in the proximal strata of the non-cornified epidermis.

BARRNETT (1953) questions whether the keratinization process in the epidermis really does involve an oxidation of -SH to -S-S- groups at all. According to him, no direct evidence of the occurrence in human epidermis of an oxidizing substance, a metallic catalyst or an enzyme system capable of oxidizing cysteine to cystine has been presented. RONY, SCHEFF, COHEN and RENNAGEL (1958) have succeeded

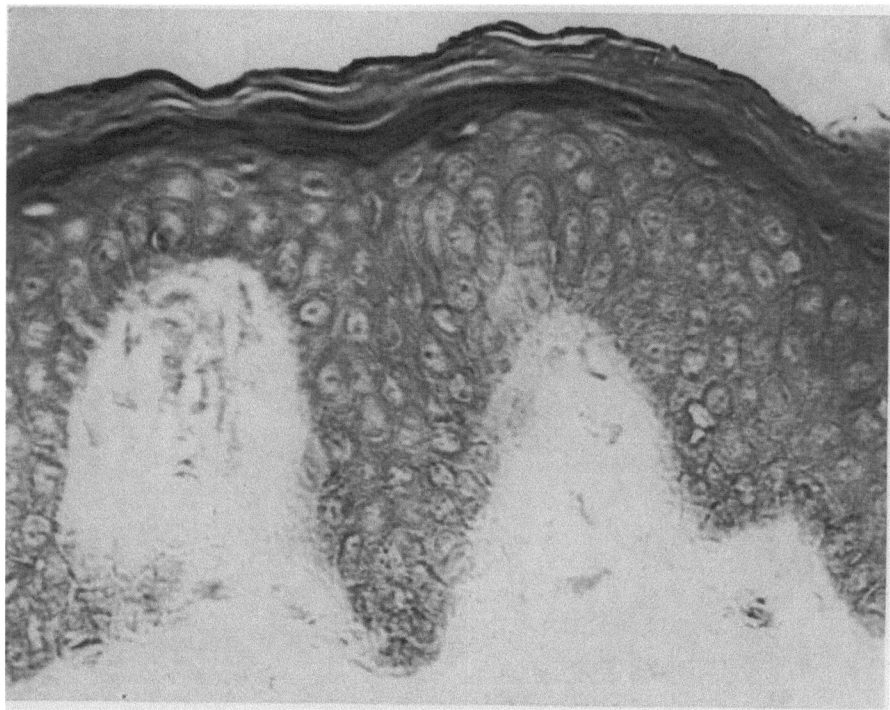

Fig. 33. The normal epidermis of the scalp showing the histotopy of -SH groups. The non-cornified epidermis displays a homogeneous distribution. The keratohyalin is negative. The transitional zone is strongly reactive, whereas the stratum corneum is mildly reactive. (From MONTAGNA, 1962. Courtesy of Academic Press Inc., New York-London)

in demonstrating the presence of a sulfhydryl-oxidase system in rabbit skin homogenates. They assume that this enzyme is involved in the keratinization process but can not entirely exclude the possibility that it is also associated with other factors than those related to this process.

According to ROTHMAN (1954), a high cystine content has been regarded as probably the only constant chemical feature of the hydrolytic products of the keratins in contrast to the cell proteins from which the keratins derive. Histochemical (BARRNETT, 1954; BARRNETT and SELIGMAN, 1954; MONTAGNA, 1956, 1962; STEIGLEDER, 1956b, 1957), biochemical (VAN SCOTT and FLESCH, 1954; FLESCH and SATANOVE, 1955) and spectromicrophotometric (STEINER, 1960) investigations on the distribution of disulfide groups in the epidermis do not seem to support the notion that this view holds also for epidermis. VAN SCOTT and FLESCH (1954) and FLESCH and SATANOVE (1955) show that the main part of the "total" sulfur (-SH + -S-S-) in the non-cornified epidermis is present as disulfide groups, and that the disulfide concentration is practically identical with that of the stratum corneum. On the strength of these results VAN SCOTT and FLESCH assume the occurrence of an -S-S- containing keratin precursor in the non-cornified epidermis which forms the main part of the disulfide-content in the stratum corneum. Disulfide groups have been histochemically demonstrated in the entire non-cornified epidermis (BARRNETT, 1954; MONTAGNA, 1956, 1962; STEIGLEDER, 1956b, 1957). According to MONTAGNA and his co-workers (MONTAGNA, EISEN, RADEMACHER and CHASE, 1954; MONTAGNA, 1956, 1962) the basal cytoplasmic protrusions, the desmosomes and the fibrils show a strong sulfhydryl and disulfide reaction. The stratum corneum reacts stronger to -S-S- groups than

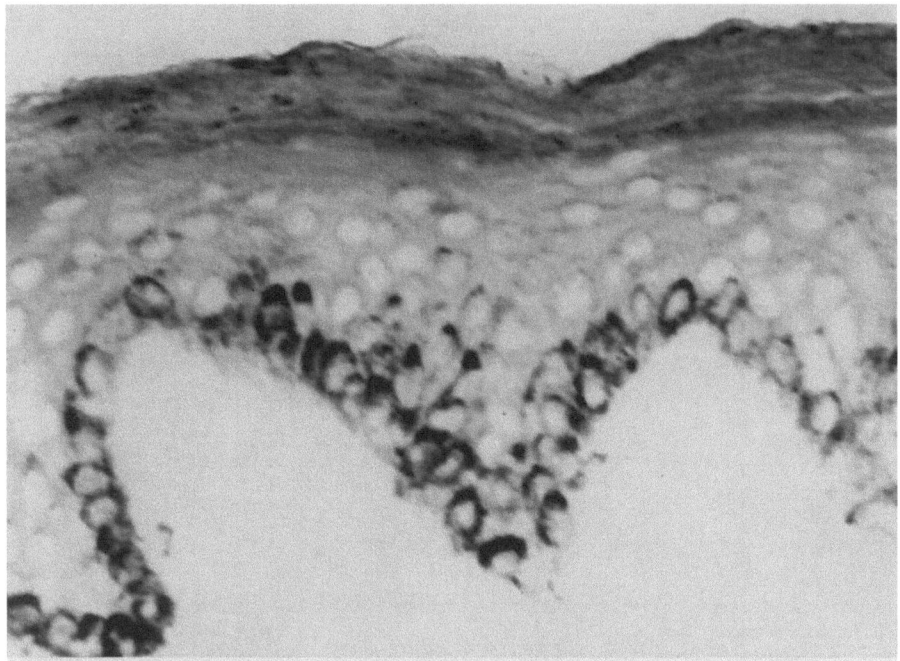

Fig. 34. The normal epidermis of the scalp showing the histotopy of -S-S- groups. The entire stratum corneum stains darker than the non-cornified epidermis. The basal cytoplasmic protrusions, desmosomes and fibrils show also a strong reaction. (From MONTAGNA, 1962. Courtesy of Academic Press Inc., New York-London)

to -SH groups (Fig. 33 and 34). Under the phase-contrast microscope most of the -SH and -S-S- groups in the cells seemed to be localized on the fibrils (MONTAGNA, 1962). These observations by MONTAGNA and his co-workers are not, however, supported by the biochemical investigations in which the epidermal fibrous protein has been extracted and isolated. In the fibrous protein of the non-cornified human epidermis ROE (1956) was not able to demonstrate any sulfur; and the fibrous protein in the non-cornified (RUDALL, 1952; MATOLTSY, 1964, 1965) and the cornified layers (RUDALL, 1952) of the parakeratotic epidermis from the cow's nose were found to contain only small quantities of sulfur-containing amino acids.

The epidermal horny layer differs from other keratinized tissues also with respect to the cystine-content. The stratum corneum contains only 3.8 per cent cystine (ECKSTEIN, 1935), while the cystine-content in human hair and in fingernail amounts to 15.5 and 12.0 per cent (BLOCH, 1939) respectively.

X-ray diffraction studies (ASTBURY and WOODS, 1934; FRASER, MACRAE and ROGERS, 1959; ROGERS, FINCH and YOUATT, 1963) and biochemical investigations (ALEXANDER and HUDSON, 1954; CORFIELD, ROBSON and SKINNER, 1958; ROGERS, 1959a, 1964; GILLESPIE, O'DONELL, THOMPSON and WOODS, 1960; GILLESPIE,

1962, 1965) have shown that the alpha-keratins in hair, hooves, fur, nails, quills and baleen can be separated into two fractions: an alpha-keratose fraction consisting of sulfur-poor proteins displaying an alpha-type X-ray diffraction pattern, and a gamma-keratose fraction containing sulfur-rich proteins exhibiting a poorly oriented cross-beta-diffraction pattern. The "filament + matrix" complex predicted by X-ray and chemical studies has also been demonstrated with electron microscopy (JEFFREY, SIKORSKI and WOODS, 1956; BIRBECK and MERCER, 1957a, b; MERCER, 1957, 1958a, b, 1961; ROGERS, 1959b, c, 1964; FRASER, MACRAE and ROGERS, 1959; FILSHIE and ROGERS, 1961). The less opaque component in this two-phase system is assumed to represent the cystine-poor filaments and corresponds to the alpha-keratose fraction, while the opaque interfilamentous substance is thought to form the cystine-rich matrix and represents the gamma-keratose fraction.

In contradistinction to the content of the alpha-keratins in the appendages of the skin, a biochemical investigation has shown that the epidermal alpha-keratin does not contain a high-sulfur protein (CROUNSE, 1963). Electron-microscopic investigations of guinea-pig's and human epidermis (BRODY, 1959a, b, 1960a, b, 1962e, g, 1963a, 1964a, b; ODLAND, 1964; BRAUN-FALCO, 1965) have, however, distinctly shown the presence of a "filament + matrix" system which BRODY (1959a) has called the "keratin pattern". On the basis of the electron micrographs BRODY (1959a, b, 1960b, 1964b) assumes that the keratohyalin represents the immediate percursor to the keratin pattern. On the strength of the histochemical observations by FRÉDERIC and CHÈVREMONT (1943) and GOLDBLUM, PIPER and CAMPBELL (1954), BRODY (1959a) has further suggested that in accordance with the assumptions respecting hair (BIRBECK and MERCER, 1957a, b; ROGERS, 1959b, c), the interfilamentous substance in the keratin pattern contains sulfur, whereas the less opaque filaments are poor on sulfur. This view is in agreement with that of MONTAGNA (1962) and MATOLTSY (1966) that the epidermal keratin may be stabilized by disulfide bonds. We do not yet know the finer biochemical and morphological differences between the filaments and the interfilamentous substance in the keratin pattern in the stratum corneum and hair (MILLARD and RUDALL, 1960). But from a morphological viewpoint there seem to be striking differences in the respective occurrences of a distinct keratin pattern in the epidermal horny layer and in hair. In the keratogenous zone (BIRBECK and MERCER, 1957a, b; MERCER, 1958, 1961) as well as in the fully keratinized hair (ROGERS, 1964b, c; FILSHIE and ROGERS, 1961; PATRIZI and MUNGER, 1966) a distinct keratin pattern is everywhere observed in the cells in the published micrographs. On the other hand, in all three sub-layers of the human stratum corneum the fibrils in the adjacent cells may show conspicious differences with respect to the distinctness of the keratin pattern or no pattern at all (BRODY, 1962g, 1964a; Figs. 27—29). These variations in the morphology of the fibrils may perhaps reflect differences in their chemical composition.

SPIER and CANEGHEM (1957) have raised further objections to the hypothesis of a conversion of -SH to -S-S- groups during the keratinization process. Like JARRETT and SPEARMAN (1964), these authors have assumed that the amino-acid sulfur is mainly concentrated to the cell periphery which encloses the sulfur-poor or sulfur-free scleroproteins like a protective sheath. With this suggestion the authors have fallen in line with the conception that the "horny membrane" or UNNA's (1883, 1913) keratin A constitutes the most resistant substance of the horny layer and represents the "true" keratin of the stratum corneum (cf. chapters on "Cell surface" and "Intercellular space"). Recent electron-microscopic studies on the intercellular space in the stratum corneum indicate that the membrane-structure considered by histologists and biochemists to form the horny cell membrane in fact seems to represent an intercellular membrane-component (BRODY, 1966). If this is the case the structure has a high cystine-content (MATOLTSY and MATOLTSY, 1966). BARRON (1951) mentions that the rigidity of the keratin molecule containing -S-S- groups may also be found in the intercellular frame. The membrane-component observed in the intercellular space in the stratum corneum (BRODY, 1966) is not observed in the non-cornified epidermis. Whether the so-called lamellated bodies incorporated in the membrane also participate in the formation of this membrane-structure is not yet known. With a histochemical method with nitro blue tetrazolium for the detection of sulfhydryl and disulfide groups DEGUCHI (1964) has obtained distinct formazan precipitation due to sulfhydryl groups in the intercellular substances in the strata intermedium and corneum in plantar skin.

III. Carbohydrates

The metabolism of carbohydrates in the skin has been the subject of numerous biochemical, histochemical and quantitative histochemical investigations (cf. reviews by ROTHMAN, 1954; LEONHARDI, 1959; KIMMIG and WEHRMAN, 1961; FREINKEL, 1964; HERSHEY, 1964; WEBER, 1964).

Among the carbohydrates, glycogen and PAS-reactive, diastase-resistant polysaccharides have been histochemically demonstrated in the epidermis. Detailed accounts of methods, results of investigation and function have been presented by PEARSE (1953, 1960), BRAUN-FALCO (1954, 1961a), MONTAGNA (1956, 1962), HORSTMANN (1957), STEIGLEDER (1957) and FALIN (1961).

1. Glycogen

BERNARD (1859), BRUNNER (1906), SASAKAWA (1921) and PATZELT (1954) were unable to demonstrate any glycogen in the adult epidermis, whereas BRADFIELD (1951), MONTAGNA and his co-workers (MONTAGNA, NOBACK and ZAK, 1948; MONTAGNA, CHASE and HAMILTON, 1951; MONTAGNA, CHASE and LOBITZ, 1952; MONTAGNA, 1952, 1956, 1962), BRAUN-FALCO (1953, 1954, 1961a), STEIGLEDER (1957) and FERREIRA-MARQUES and PARRA (1960) observed a dotty occurrence of small amounts of glycogen. The glycogen-content exhibits certain topographical variations, and slightly more glycogen is found in the epidermis of the scrotum and the scalp than in other sites (MONTAGNA, CHASE and LOBITZ, 1952; MONTAGNA, 1962).

When glycogen occurs in the tissue it is usually found in the upper layers of the stratum spinosum, whereas the proximal spinous and the basal cells are free from glycogen (Fig. 35). The cells of the stratum intermedium are also usually free from this substance (MONTAGNA, CHASE and LOBITZ, 1952; BRAUN-FALCO, 1954). If, nevertheless, glycogen appears in the last-mentioned stratum, BRAUN-FALCO (1954) considers that it is only demonstrable in the lateral cell processes, whereas SMITH and PARKHURST (1949) and STEIGLEDER (1957) have also observed it between the keratohyalin "granules".

UNNA and GOLODETZ (1910a, b) have found a substance in the so-called "infrabasal horny layer" (UNNA, 1883) which they assume to be glycogen and to be formed through a transformation of the keratohyalin. HANAWA (1913) carried out detailed investigations of this substance and observed that some of its properties were similar to those of glycogen. In accordance with the view of UNNA and GOLODETZ (1910a, b), HANAWA thought that the substance in question was of importance for the formation of "eleidin". Small glycogen granules have been demonstrated in the stratum corneum of the lining epithelium of the external auditory meatus (MONTAGNA, NOBACK and ZAK, 1948). WASHBURN and BLOCKER (1954) also observed glycogen in the stratum lucidum. In other studies, however, no glycogen has been found either in the keratohyalin in the stratum intermedium or in any part of the stratum corneum (SMITH and PARKHURST, 1949; MONTAGNA, CHASE and HAMILTON, 1951; MONTAGNA, CHASE and LOBITZ, 1952; MONTAGNA, 1956, 1962; BRAUN-FALCO, 1954; STEIGLEDER, 1957). The PAS-positive granules

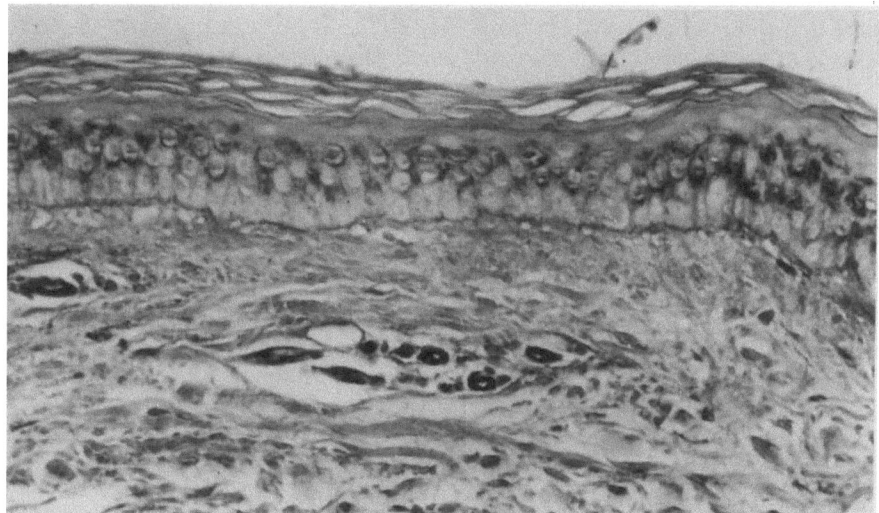

Fig. 35. Histotopy of glycogen in normal epidermis. Basal cells free of glycogen. Glycogen in cytoplasmic distribution within the spinous cells. Stratum intermedium practically free of glycogen. PAS-reaction.
(From BRAUN-FALCO 1965a. Courtesy of Acta Facultatis Medicae Universitatis Brunensis)

which LANSING and OPDYKE (1950) assumed to represent glycogen-containing keratohyalin are probably glycogen granules located between the keratohyalin (SMITH and PARKHURST, 1949; STEIGLEDER, 1957).

With electron microscopy of normal human epidermis small quantities of glycogen have also been demonstrated in the stratum spinosum (MEIRELES PINTO, FALCÃO, CRUZ-SOBRAL and MORATO, 1963). The glycogen appears in the cytoplasm as 150- to 250-Å large, randomly scattered, opaque particles.

All non-cornified epidermal cells display a more or less strong phosphorylase and amylo-1,4 → 1,6-transglucosidase activity (BRAUN-FALCO, 1956a, 1961a; SPIER and CANEGHEM, 1957; ELLIS and MONTAGNA, 1958; MONTAGNA, 1962; ELLIS, 1963, 1964). The demonstration of these enzymes implies that in principle all living epidermal cells are capable of glycogenesis. This finding speaks against the view that so-called sessile glycogen is present in the skin as a fixed cytoplasmic constituent (BRAUN-FALCO, 1961a). BRAUN-FALCO (1961a) suggests that the glycogen-content in the epidermis at a certain moment rather characterizes the metabolic situation at this moment and in this situation it may change fast. BRAUN-FALCO (1956a) stressed as particularly noteworthy the positive reaction to phosphorylase in the basal layer. This observation may imply either that the paucity of glycogen or its absence in the cells of the stratum basale is due to an increased breaking down of the glycogen (BRAUN-FALCO, 1956a), or that after a successful glycogenesis the cells have already been transferred into the stratum spinosum (STEIGLEDER, 1959a).

In a comprehensive survey of the research on the glycogen in the skin and mucous membranes Falin (1961) points out that as a source of energy or plastic material glycogen is related to several important cellular processes such as regeneration, differentiation and growth. Braun-Falco (1961a) has also taken up for detailed examination the different interpretations that have been advanced, and particularly those advanced on the basis of morphologic observations of the accumulation of glycogen in the skin in pathologic conditions. With Lobitz and Holyoke (1954), Braun-Falco (1961a) considered that the observations made to date do not permit of any definite conclusion as to the function of the glycogen. There is thus no unequivocal evidence that an increase of the glycogen-content is connected with the proliferating capacity or with a retarded keratinization process. Many findings also cast doubt upon the correctness of the interpretation that the type of cornification is a determining factor for the occurrence of glycogen or that the breaking down of glycogen in case of insufficient oxygen supply is a source of cell energy.

However, on the strength of new results concerning the histotopography of succinic dehydrogenase in normal epidermis (Zelickson, 1960) and of cytochrome oxidase in normal and pathologic epidermis (Braun-Falco, 1961b) on the one hand, and the histological observations of the distribution of the mitochondria in normal epidermis (Montagna, 1952, 1956; Zelickson, 1960) and the electron-microscopic finds regarding the distribution of the mitochondria in pathologically changed mucous membrane (Fasske and Themann, 1959a) on the other hand, Braun-Falco (1961b) once more took up for discussion the possibility of anerobic glycolysis as a source of energy, in accordance with earlier view (Bradfield, 1951; Firket, 1951; Ferreira-Marques and Parra, 1960). Ferreira-Marques and Parra (1960) have suggested the subdivision of the epidermis into two regions. The proximal region, the "stratum oxybioticum", comprises the strata basale and spinosum. This layer is said to get its energy through the oxidative cell respiration. The distal "stratum anoxybioticum", comprising the strata intermedium, lucidum and corneum, is presumed to get its energy through the breaking down of glycogen to lactic acid through anaerobic glycolysis with the participation of nuclearly bound glycolytic processes (Bradfield, 1951; Firket, 1951; Fasske and Themann, 1959a; Ferreira-Marques and Parra, 1960; Ferreira-Marques, 1961; Braun-Falco, 1961b). Braun-Falco (1965a), however, asserts that it is not possible to make a distinct delimitation of the two regions from each other without the occurrence of gradual transitions. The correctness of this last-mentioned view is supported by Brody's (1960b) electron-microscopic observations of the distribution of the mitochondria in normal human epidermis. (Fig. 6).

2. PAS-Reactive, Diastase-Resistent Polysaccharides

Besides the histochemically demonstrable glycogen, normal epidermis also contains non-glycogen, PAS-positive substances that are not hydrolized by saliva or diastase. They presumably consist of neutral and acid mucopolysaccharides and glycoproteins (Wislocki, Fawcett and Dempsey, 1951; Dupré, 1952, 1953; Braun-Falco, 1954, 1958, 1961a; Braun-Falco and Weber, 1958; Montagna, 1956, 1962; Steigleder, 1958; Flesch, 1959; Flesch, Roe and Esoda, 1960; Flesch and Esoda, 1960; Roe, Flesch and Esoda, 1961; Steigleder and Weakley, 1961; Flesch and Esoda, 1962, 1963).

In the intercellular space and on the cell surfaces of the strata spinosum and corneum Wislocki, Fawcett and Dempsey (1951), Braun-Falco (1954), and

STEIGLEDER and WEAKLEY (1961) have observed a PAS-reactive, diastase-resistant material. This material was less distinctly demonstrable in the intercellular space of the stratum intermedium. WISLOCKI, FAWCETT and DEMPSEY (1951) described its appearance as a homogeneous substance filling the intercellular spaces and as granules located on, or possibly in, the "cell membranes", whereas BRAUN-FALCO (1954) assumed that it was disposed as a layer on the cell surface. A similar material has also been found on the desmosomes in the strata basale and spinosum and in the proximal layers of the stratum intermedium (DUPRÉ, 1952, 1953; BRAUN-FALCO, 1954; STEIGLEDER and WEAKLEY, 1961). In man and monkey the skin contains conspicuously less amounts of this PAS-positive substance than the mucous membranes (WISLOCKI, FAWCETT and DEMPSEY, 1951). These writers observed distinct topographical variations in the skin. The largest amounts appeared in the skin of man and monkey sole; barely recognizable traces were found in that of the monkey thigh, lips and vulva; and no PAS-reactive substances were demonstrated in the skin of the monkey abdomen and ear (WISLOCKI, FAWCETT and DEMPSEY, 1951).

WISLOCKI, FAWCETT and DEMPSEY (1951) have suggested that the PAS-reactive, diastase-resistant material may be a local metabolic product of the epidermal cells formed in or on their surfaces and discharged or secreted into the intercellular spaces. However, they also mentioned the possibility that this material may reach its destination through the diffusion of an unstained precursor from the underlying lamina propria. BRAUN-FALCO (1954) stressed the striking sameness in the histochemical character of the PAS-reactivity of the "basement membrane" and the intercellular substances, which according to BRAUN-FALCO may speak strongly in favour of a mesenchymal origin of the intercellular "cementing ground substance". This substance has been generally considered as a mucopolysaccharide or glycoprotein. However, whereas DUPRÉ (1952, 1953) suggested that it consists of acid chondroitin sulfate B, BRAUN-FALCO (1954) came to the conclusion that the only groups of substances that may come into the question are neutral mucopolysaccharides and glycoproteins.

Further histochemical investigations have revealed the presence of a Hale-PAS-reactive material disposed on the desmosomes and the cell surfaces in the intercellular space of the strata basale and spinosum (BRAUN-FALCO and WEBER, 1958; STEIGLEDER and WEAKLEY, 1961). This substance increases in amount towards the stratum spinosum (Fig. 36), disappears in the stratum intermedium, and is no longer detectable in the stratum corneum.

With Alcian-blue staining, which is presumed at least partly to reveal acid mucopolysaccharides, GOLTZ, FUSARO and JARVIS (1958) obtained a small accumulation of Alcian-blue-positive material on the desmosomes and close to the cell surface in the stratum spinosum. The cell-outlines of the stratum corneum were not stained.

BRAUN-FALCO and WEBER (1958) and STEIGLEDER and WEAKLEY (1961) assumed that the Hale-PAS-reactive material probably consists of an acid mucopolysaccharide and is derived largely from the epidermal cells and not from the corium. Strong support for this hypothesis has been presented by BRAUN-FALCO, LANGNER and CHRISTOPHERS (1966). In autoradiographic studies on the uptake of S^{35}-labelled sodium sulphate BOSTRÖM, ODEBLAD and FRIBERG (1953) and MONTAGNA and HILL (1957) observed moderate amounts of S^{35} in the basal and spinous cells. BRAUN-FALCO, LANGNER and CHRISTOPHERS (1966) obtained a high concentration of S^{35}-containing silver granules in the strata basale and spinosum. Only few granules appeared in the stratum intermedium, and the stratum corneum was always negative. The authors drew the conclusion that especially the proximal epidermal cells are capable of synthesizing sulfate-containing acid mucopolysaccharides.

Using his adhesive celluloid-strip method, Wolf (1939) investigated with Gram-stain the stratum corneum desquamans (*i.e.*, stratum corneum disjunctum) of the epidermis from different sites. The Gram-positive material appeared as granules showing regional variations with respect to size and number. The nature of these granules is unknown.

In later studies it was demonstrated that in cross-sections of the normal epidermis with a thin stratum corneum Gram-positive material appears in a narrow band corresponding to the transitional zone (Steigleder, 1958; Flesch, Roe and Esoda, 1960; Szodoray and Nagy-Vezekényi, 1965). In the epidermis

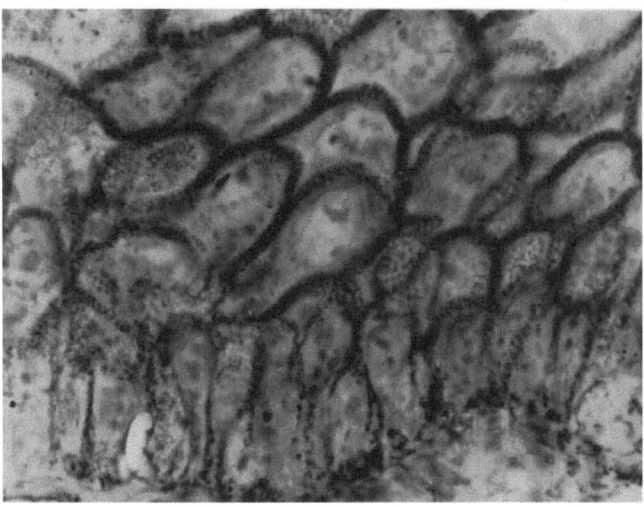

Fig. 36. Normal skin. Hale-reactive substances of mucopolysaccharide character within the intercellular spaces of the epidermis, between basal cells in granular distribution and between spinous cells more homogeneous. (From Braun-Falco and Weber, 1958. Courtesy of Arch. klin. exp. Derm., Springer, Berlin-Göttingen-Heidelberg)

of the sole this material is more widely distributed, and a positive Gram-staining is obtained of the keratohyalin, the transitional zone and also in scattered areas of the more superficial layers of the stratum corneum. Flesch, Roe and Esoda (1960) and Szodoray and Nagy-Vezekényi (1965) ascribe the Gram-positive staining to the presence in the tissue of acid mucopolysaccharides. With earlier and later investigators (Wislocki, Fawcett and Dempsey, 1951; Braun-Falco and Weber, 1958; Steigleder and Weakley, 1961; Braun-Falco, Langner and Christophers, 1966) Flesch, Roe and Esoda (1960) suggested that the epidermal cells are capable of synthesizing a highly resistant, glucosamine-containing material, probably a mucopolysaccharide. Flesch and his co-workers (Flesch, Roe and Esoda, 1960; Flesch and Esoda, 1960; Roe, Flesch and Esoda, 1961; Flesch and Esoda, 1963) furthermore postulated that during normal keratinization the acid mucopolysaccharide, forming a constituent of the keratohyalin, is largely decomposed in the fully developed horny layer.

With Fischer (1953), Steigleder (1956), on the other hand, assumed that the Gram-positivity of the tissue was due to the presence of -SH groups. He observed a correlation between the localization of the Gram-staining material and the distribution of the -SH groups as revealed by the method of Barrnett and Seligman (1952a).

Horstmann (1957) points out that mucopolysaccharides like keratin contain sulfur as sulfhydryl or disulfide groups. Steigleder and Weakley (1961) have observed that the acid mucopolysaccharides disposed on and between the desmosomes are very resistant to extraction by lithium bromide. This finding, according to the authors, may suggest that the mucopolysaccharides are fixed to the desmosomes by other forces than hydrogen bonds. Besides mucopolysaccharides, also protein-bound sulfhydryl groups have been demonstrated on the desmosomes (MESCON and FLESCH, 1952; BARRNETT, 1953; GOLDBLUM, PIPER and CAMPBELL, 1954; MONTAGNA, 1956, 1962). STEIGLEDER and WEAKLEY (1961) have discussed the controversial interpretation (cf. FLESCH, ROE and ESODA, 1960; ROE, FLESCH and ESODA, 1961; FISCHER, 1953; STEIGLEDER, 1956) of the substances responsible for the Gram-staining. They questioned whether the observed reactions were due to the presence of several chemical compounds or whether only one substance contained all of the molecules necessary for the observed Gram-positive staining.

In a histochemical investigation on the autolysis of the skin BRAUN-FALCO and WINTER (1964) observed that the Hale-PAS-positive material of the keratohyalin remained for a longer time than the Hale-PAS positive substances in the intercellular space of the epidermis and in the dermis. While the latter substances have been considered as acid mucopolysaccharides (BRAUN-FALCO and WEBER, 1958; STEIGLEDER and WEAKLEY, 1961), the biochemical nature of the PAS-Hale reactive material in the keratohyalin is unknown (BRAUN-FALCO and WINTER, 1964).

IV. Lipids

In their reviews on the histotopography of lipids in the epidermis STEIGLEDER (1957) and BRAUN-FALCO (1961a) mention that our knowledge in the field of the histochemistry of lipids has not greatly increased since the investigations by NICOLAU (1911). The difficulties in demonstrating cellular lipids with histochemical techniques have been largely ascribed to the association of the lipids to proteins, by which association the lipids were thought to be masked. The stainability of a substance is due not only to its chemical nature, but also to its physico-chemical characteristics (LISON, 1953).

In the human epidermis (NICOLAU, 1911; MONTAGNA, CHASE and HAMILTON, 1951) and in the epidermis of laboratory mammals (MONTAGNA, 1950) discrete sudanophil lipid granules have been discerned in all strata except in the horny layer. These writers found a mainly perinuclear arrangement. Many of the granules are of a small size, usually just within the resolving power of the light microscope, whereas others are coarser, contain a sudanophobic center and are often linked together to form short chains (MONTAGNA, 1950; MONTAGNA, CHASE and HAMILTON, 1951). NICOLAU has observed certain topographical variations with a larger number of granules in the skin of the axilla, the hair-covered scalp, the face and the lobe of the ear. MONTAGNA (1950) suggests that the granules may represent the Golgi complex or parts of it.

RANVIER (1898) reported the presence of lipids in the stratum corneum. UNNA (1928) has described the occurrence of cholesterol esters in the keratinized layers, but only free cholesterol in the non-cornified strata. In frozen sections of the surface epithelium of the auditory tube stained with Nile blue sulfate MONTAGNA, NOBACK and ZAK (1948) have demonstrated a bright pink color of the stratum corneum which they think may indicate the presence of neutral lipids.

At the staining of the epidermis for lipids the transitional zone reacted more strongly than any other region of the epidermis (BRAUN-FALCO, 1958, 1965a). The following fatty substances were observed here: phospholipids by BAKER's acid hematein test (BRAUN-FALCO, 1958; JARRETT, 1960; JARRETT and SPEARMAN, 1964; SZODORAY and NAGY-VEZEKÉNYI, 1965; Fig. 37a), fatty acid by FISCHLER's

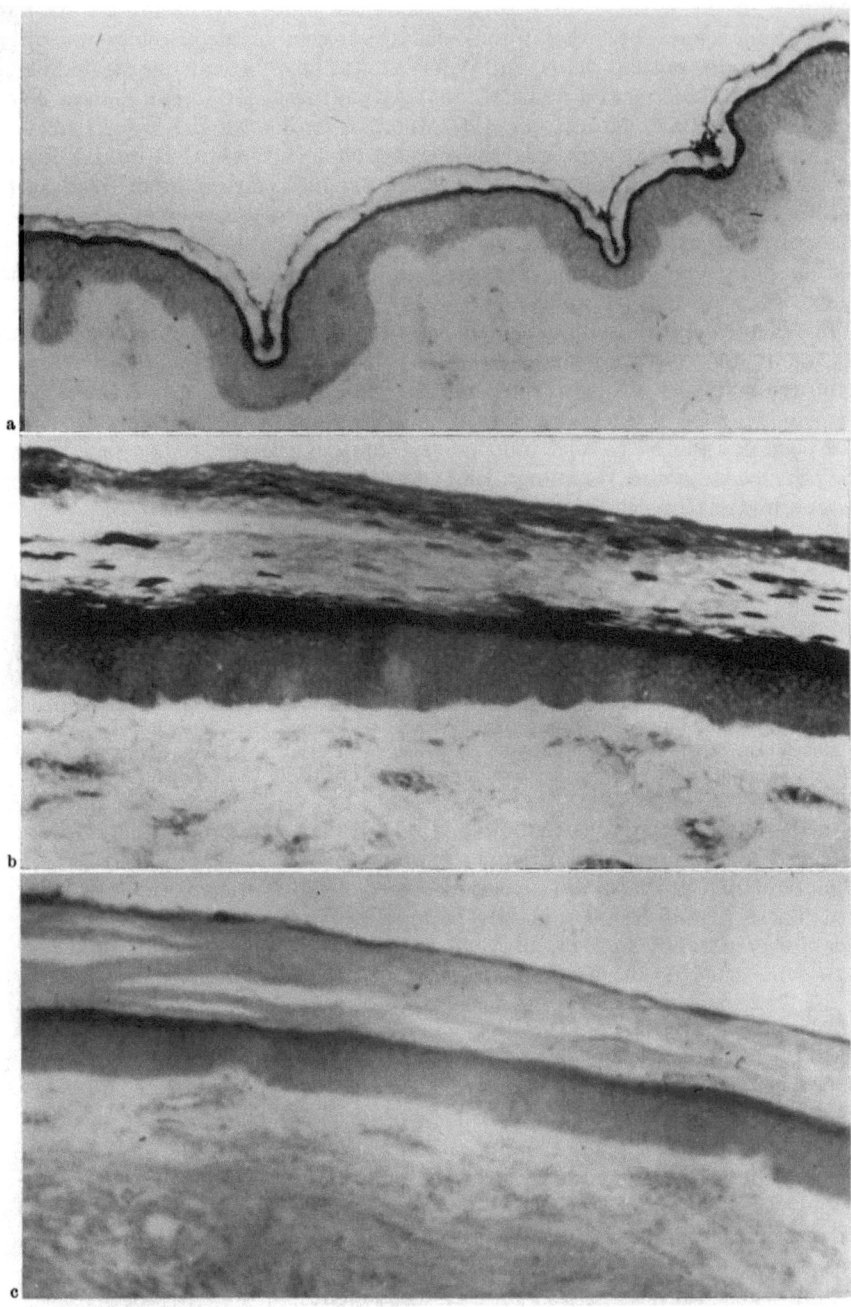

Fig. 37a—c. Normal skin. a) Baker's acid hematein for localizing phospholipids. Intensive positive reaction in the subcorneal transitional zone, horny layer negative. Weakly positive reaction on the skin surface, due to surface phospholipids. b) Fischler's reaction for staining fatty acids. Intensive positive reaction in the subcorneal transitional zone. Horny layer with exception of a few cells negative. Positive reaction on the skin surface. c) UV-Schiff reaction for staining unsaturated fatty acids and lipids. Intensive positive reaction in the subcorneal transitional zone. Horny layer negative. Skin surface positive. (From BRAUN-Falco, 1958. Courtesy of Ann. N.Y. Acad. Sci., The New York Academy of Sciences)

reagent (BRAUN-FALCO, 1958; Fig. 37b) and unsaturated lipids by the LILLIE's performic acid-Schiff and the UV-Schiff reactions (BRAUN-FALCO, 1958; Fig. 37c). With these four methods the skin surface also stained positively, whereas the intermediate area of the stratum corneum (with the exception of a few cells in FISCHLER's reagent) appeared negatively.

In electron-microscopic studies a few intracellular so-called lipid droplets or granules have been observed throughout normal human epidermis (BRODY, 1963e; HANUŠOVÁ, 1965; BRAUN-FALCO, 1965b) and have also been reported in normal nail plate (HANUŠOVÁ, 1965). These droplets were for the first time described in the epidermis by STEIGLEDER (1958c, 1960b) in a histochemical investigation of parakeratosis as PAS-positive granules which are partly stained with Sudan black B. HANUŠOVÁ (1960, 1961, 1965) has made a detailed study of their histochemical and ultrastructural nature. She investigated different types of epidermis, such as parakeratosis in Psoriasis vulgaris and squamous eczema, hyperkeratosis in Lichen ruber planus and Pityriasis rubra pilaris, alternating para- and hyperkeratosis in Verruca vulgaris and, finally, the orthokeratotic epidermis in the clinical normal skin of psoriatics. She observed the granules in all the studied material.

The granules are light-refractive in a dark field, non-birefringent in polarized light and stain gray-blue with Sudan black B (HANUŠOVÁ, 1960, 1961). They are also stained according to PAPPENHEIM, GIEMSA and GRAM and with PAS and touluidine blue (HANUŠOVÁ, 1965). On the strength of the stainability of the granules with these different stains HANUŠOVÁ (1965) assumes that they consist of a complex of lipoglycoproteins, and perhaps also contain enzymes.

HANUŠOVÁ (1960, 1961, 1965) found the granules particularly numerous in the parakeratotic horny layers, whereas in the hyperkeratotic horny layers and in the orthokeratotic horny layer in patients with psoriasis they appeared only sparsely. HANUŠOVÁ (1961, 1965) therefore suggests that the granules form a characteristic feature of parakeratosis and calls them "parakeratotic lipid granules". With HANUŠOVÁ (1960, 1961, 1965), BRODY (1962c, d, f, 1964c) and SWANBECK and THYRESSON (1962) also observed them in particularly large numbers in parakeratotic psoriatic epidermis. But a distinct increase in numbers as compared to normal human epidermis (BRODY, 1963e) is also observed in hyperkeratotic psoriatic epidermis (BRODY, 1963c, d, 1964). They seem to be fairly numerous also in toe-nail infected by T. rubra (MATOLTSY and MATOLTSY, 1962b). These latter observations indicate rather that an increase in the number of lipid droplets occurs in diseased skin and nail, irrespective of the type of keratinization disturbance, even if the largest increase is found in parakeratosis.

In the stratum corneum the granules are usually oval or round with a fairly even surface (HANUŠOVÁ, 1960, 1961, 1965; BRODY, 1962c, d, f, 1963c, d, e, 1964c; MATOLTSY and MATOLTSY, 1962b). They are delimited by an opaque membrane (BRODY, 1962c, d, 1963e, 1964c). HANUŠOVÁ (1960, 1961) has given their size as 0.1 to 0.5 μ. BRODY (1962c, d) has observed a length of 0.38 to 0.57 μ and a width of 0.20 to 0.40 μ. Occasionally they exhibit a more irregular shape with a wrinkled outer membrane and are then similar to the lipid droplets in the non-cornified layers of the epidermis (BRODY, 1962b, c, d, 1963e, 1964c). The granules vary in number from cell to cell and are scattered all over the cytoplasm, single of close together. In the electron-microscopic picture, in sections irradiated with ultraviolet light, the granules show a fairly low, uniform opacity (BRODY, 1962f, 1963c, d, e), whereas in non-irradiated sections they often show a more uneven opacity with less opacity along the outer opaque membrane (HANUŠOVÁ, 1960, 1961, 1965; BRODY, 1962c, d, 1963e, 1964c).

Centrifugal isolation of subcellular components has made it possible to analyze their chemical composition (cf. review by SCHNEIDER and KUFF, 1964). In different tissues the various types of membrane (*e.g.* mitochondrial, microsomal, Golgi complex, nuclear and plasma membrane) show a high content of lipids, and particularly of phospholipids.

In the non-cornified epidermis are present cell membranes and nuclei and to a varying extent mitochondria, Golgi apparatus, alpha-cytomembranes, and granules and vesicles of different appearance. The lipid layer of the modified plasma membrane of the T- and horny cells seems to be ultrastructurally like the corresponding layer of the plasma membrane in the non-cornified epidermis (FAR-

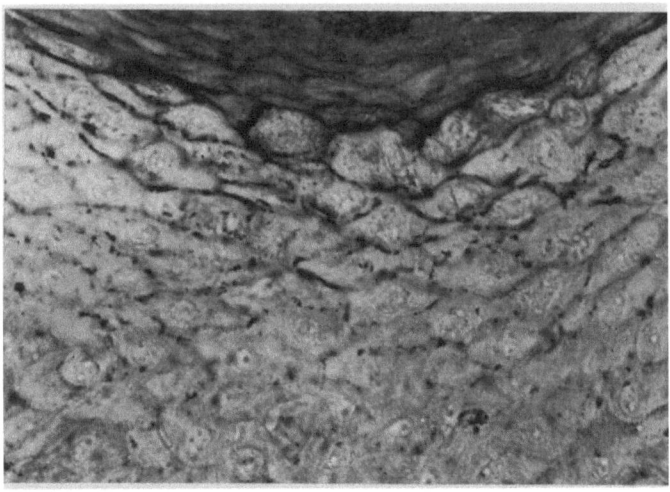

Fig. 38. Normal skin. Sudanophilic lipid material within the intercellular spaces, especially in the higher layers of stratum spinosum and in the keratogeneous zone. (From BRAUN-FALCO and WEBER, 1958. Courtesy of Arch. klin. exp. Derm., Springer, Berlin-Göttingen-Heidelberg)

QUHAR and PALADE, 1965; BRODY, 1966; FARBMAN, 1966). The nuclei, Golgi apparatus and alpha-cytomembranes are reduced in number in the upper spinous cells and in the stratum intermedium. Golgi apparatus and the alpha-cytomembranes are not found above the stratum intermedium; nuclei are still seen in the T-cells (BRODY, 1960b; ROTH and CLARK, 1964), and a small number of mitochondria are present in the T-cells and the stratum corneum (BRODY, 1959a, 1960b; RHODIN, 1963). The "lamellated bodies" (FRITHIOF and WERSÄLL, 1965) increase in number towards the stratum intermedium, where they occur both intra- and intercellularly (for further references cf. chapters C II and C VIII). They are also present in the intercellular space of the stratum corneum, where, however, also other types of granule are observable (BRODY, 1966; Figs. 10—14). FRITHIOF and WERSÄLL (1965) and OLÁH and RÖHLICH (1966) have suggested that the "lamellated bodies" are phospholipid in nature.

FEULGEN and VOIT (1924) and FEULGEN, IMHÄUSER and BEHRENS (1929) discovered the plasmalogens. These are phosphoglycerides which liberate higher fatty aldehydes on hydrolysis under acidic conditions (RAPPAPORT and FRANZL, 1957). With differential centrifugation technique SCHNEIDER and KUFF (1954) isolated Golgi-material from epididymides. They obtained a substance that gave an intense reaction to the periodic acid Schiff (PAS) reagent. This substance could be extracted with lipid solvents. The nature of this PAS-reactive lipid is unknown. There was no evidence for the presence of PAS-reactive mucopolysaccharides or mucoproteins (SCHNEIDER and KUFF, 1954) but plasmalogens or acetalphosphatides might qualify (SCHNEIDER and KUFF, 1964).

Voss (1941) investigated the normal human skin for plasmalogens. The whole non-cornified epidermis was stained, with a stronger reaction for the stratum basale.

Dupré (1953) has described the presence of a glycolipoprotein complex in the intercellular space of the whole epidermis in the skin of the sole. In the human epidermis (Montagna, 1952; Dupré, 1953; Prunieras, 1957) and in the oral and vaginal epithelium (Wislocki, Bunting and Dempsey, 1950; Wislocki, 1951) the desmosomes reacted positively to the Sudan black B and the Baker's acid hematein test, indicating the presence of phospholipids. These observations were later confirmed by Steigleder (1957), Braun-Falco and Weber (1958) and Montagna (1962).

Already in 1952 Montagna noted lipid granules in the intercellular space. Because they seemed to increase in number in poorly fixed tissues or in tissues kept in fixative for longer than one month he commented the finding with the words: "One is cautioned against too literal an interpretation of these intercellular lipids." Braun-Falco and Weber (1958) distinctly demonstrated that not only the desmosomes give a phospholipid reaction, but sudanophilic (Sudan black B) substances also occur in the intercellular space between the desmosomes. These substances increase in amount in the upper layer of the stratum spinosum or in the stratum intermedium and in the transitional zone (Fig. 38).

V. Enzymes

1. Cytochrome Oxidase

All living cells of mammalian origin contain cytochrome-cytochrome-oxidase systems (Lerner, 1954). These systems act as electron-transferring mechanisms in the oxidative reactions of the Krebs cycle as well as in many other oxidative reactions, and probably also in the phosphate metabolism related to glycolysis. Electrons removed from the substrate molecules are oxidatively transferred ultimately to molecular oxygen through a series of reversibly oxidized and reduced intermediary carriers. The final step of the reactions takes place through the cytochrome-cytochrome-oxidase system, in the order cytochrome b, c, a and cytochrome oxidase to oxygen. Cytochrome oxidase or Warburg's yellow ferment is thus of fundamental importance for the cell respiration (Schuemmelfeder, 1948; Green, 1954; Hoffmann-Ostenhof, 1954; Lerner, 1954).

The Nadi reaction for the demonstration of cytochrome oxidase devised for histological use by Gräff (1916, 1922) has not been widely adopted (Dempsey and Wislocki, 1944; Schuemmelfeeder, 1948; Steigleder, 1952, 1957, 1959a; Braun-Falco, 1961a). This method has not proved quite reliable, and it has often been difficult to repeat the results (Braun-Falco, 1961b; Montagna and Yun, 1961; Montagna, 1962). These disadvantages have been ascribed to the instability and lipid solubility of the final dye stuff and the therewith connected diffusion artefacts (Gomori, 1952; Pearse, 1953; Burstone, 1959; Braun-Falco, 1961b).

It is only through the methods introduced by Burstone (1959, 1960, 1961) that reliable histochemical investigations of cytochrome oxidase have become possible. These methods permit of a detailed study of the histotopography of this enzyme in the skin (Braun-Falco, 1961b; Montagna and Yun, 1961; Montagna, 1962).

The cytochrome oxidase activity is restricted to the living epidermal layers, while the "Intermediärzone" of Braun-Falco (1957c) and the stratum corneum always react negatively (Braun-Falco, 1961b; Montagna and Yun, 1961; Montagna, 1962). With shorter periods of incubation the proximal epidermal layers react more strongly than the distal layers which are in process of transformation into the cell layers of the stratum intermedium. With longer periods of incubation the entire non-cornified epidermis reacts intensely (Braun-Falco, 1961b).

A more detailed study (Fig. 39) reveals that the distribution of the cytochrome-oxidase positive granules is dense and uniform throughout the cytoplasm in the cells of the stratum basale. In the stratum spinosum the reactive particles decrease in number, and arrange themselves more around the nuclei, particularly close to the poles of the latter. In the cells of the stratum intermedium they are only found in smaller numbers, and here the perinuclear arrangement dominates (BRAUN-FALCO, 1961 b; MONTAGNA and YUN, 1961; MONTAGNA, 1962).

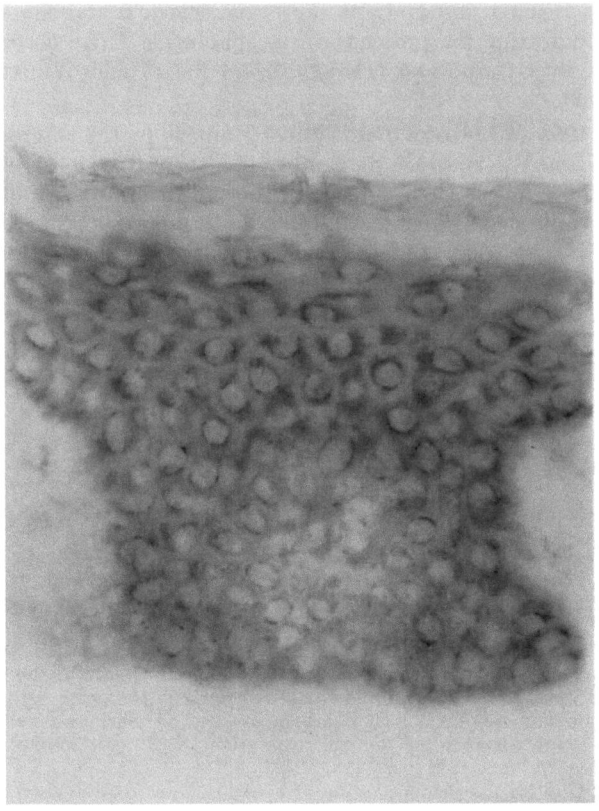

Fig. 39. Histotopy of cytochrome oxidase in normal skin. Granular distribution of enzyme activity indicating precipitates. In the higher layers of the stratum spinosum more perinuclear distribution of the precipitates. Decrease of the reaction in the stratum intermedium, horny layer negative. (From BRAUN-Falco, 1961 b. Courtesy of Arch. klin. exp. Derm., Springer, Berlin-Göttingen-Heidelberg)

BRAUN-FALCO (1961 b) and MONTAGNA (MONTAGNA and YUN, 1961; MONTAGNA, 1962) consider that the distinct granular structures showing cytochrome oxidase activity completely correspond to the distribution of the mitochondria in the epidermis, as these organelles have been demonstrated with histological staining methods (MONTAGNA, 1952, 1956, 1962; HORSTMANN, 1957) and shown in some electron-microscopic investigations of the epidermis (SELBY, 1957; HORSTMANN and KNOOP, 1958; BRAUN-FALCO, 1965 a) and of mucous membrane (FASSKE and THEMANN, 1959).

On the strength of the well-known fact that the cytochrome-oxidase activity is restricted to the mitochondria (STAFFORD, 1951; GREEN, 1954; LINDBERG and ERNSTER, 1954; SIEBERT, 1955; PEARSE and SCARPELLI, 1959; LEONHARDI, 1959; for further references see BOURNE and TEWARI, 1964) BRAUN-FALCO (1961 b) takes up for more detailed discussion the possibility of using the histochemical methods employed for the detection of cytochrome oxidase (and also of succinic dehydrogenase) for the demonstration of the mitochondria in tissue. This technique, *i.e.*, to locate succinic dehydrogenase and thus the mitochondria, has been used by ZELICKSON (1960), RITZENFELD (1965) and RITZENFELD and KOCH (1966).

2. Monoamine Oxidase

Monoamine oxidase is widely distributed in the animal world and is present in different tissues (EDER, 1957). In cellular metabolism its role seems to vary with the function of the organ. Through oxidative deamination it degrades alkylamine, and indol-, phenyl- and oxyphenylalkylamine.

HELLMANN (1955) has only been able to demonstrate monoamine oxidase activity in the sweat and sebaceous glands of the horse and cat skin but the skin of dog, rat, guinea pig, monkey or man did not show any reaction. SHELLEY, COHEN and KOELLE (1955) have observed a faint diffuse staining of the human non-cornified epidermis. Using the method of GLENNER, BURTNER and BROWN (1957) with tetrazolium salts, MONTAGNA (1962) has obtained a fairly intense reaction of monoamine oxidase in the non-cornified layers of the epidermis in different mammals. The strongest reaction appeared in the cells of the stratum basale and the lower cells of the stratum spinosum. The enzymatic activity faded gradually upwards and disappeared in the stratum intermedium.

In a study of liver cells HAWKINS (1952) demonstrated that about two-thirds of the amine oxidase activity is present in the mitochondrial fraction and the remainder is found in the microsomes. The distribution of this enzyme is therefore to a great extent similar to that of cytochrome oxidase and succinic dehydrogenase. However, by adding potassium cyanide to the incubation mixture it is histochemically possible to separate monoamine oxidase from cytochrome oxidase and succinic dehydrogenase (MONTAGNA, 1962). The latter enzymes are inhibited by potassium cyanide which is not the case with monoamine oxidase.

3. Succinic Dehydrogenase

The biological significance of succinic dehydrogenase resides mainly in its function as a link in the chain of reactions of Krebs citric acid cycle. Since these reactions are concerned with the oxidation of lipids, carbohydrates and proteins, it is likely that this enzyme is present in all living cells (SUMNER and SOMERS, 1947; THUNBERG, 1951).

According to MONTAGNA (1962) and ELLIS (1964), there are several modifications of the original method of SELIGMAN and RUTENBURG (1951) available for the demonstration of succinic dehydrogenase, but none is more satisfying than that of FARBER and LOUVIERE (1956). Attention may also be drawn to the fact that BURSTONE (1964) has given an account of the history, methods and applied histochemistry of dehydrogenases. BRAUN-FALCO and PETZOLD (1965) have studied the optimal reaction conditions for the histochemical demonstration of dehydrogenases in guinea-pig epidermis.

Repeated investigations on the histotopography of the succinic dehydrogenase activity in the epidermis have shown a distribution similar to that in man (ROGERS, 1953; BRAUN-FALCO and RATHJENS, 1954b; FORAKER and WINGO, 1955; MONTAGNA and FORMISANO, 1955a; MONTAGNA, 1956, 1962; STEIGLEDER, 1957, 1959a; BRAUN-FALCO, 1958, 1963a, 1965a; MORETTI, ADACHI, MESCON and POCHI, 1963; ELLIS, 1964) and in laboratory animals (PADYKULA, 1952; ROGERS, 1953; FORMISANO and MONTAGNA, 1954; BRAUN-FALCO and PETZOLD, 1965). The succinic dehydrogenase activity (formazan crystal deposits) is most intense in the stratum basale and fades gradually towards the transitional zone. BRAUN-FALCO and RATHJENS (1954b) have pointed out that while the stratum basale always displays a high enzymatic activity, this may vary conspicuously in the stratum spinosum. In the stratum intermedium discrete granules are only occasionally discerned. Stratum corneum always appeared negative. The reactive granules are located only intracellularly and show a mainly perinuclear distribution.

According to STEIGLEDER (1959a) the histochemically demonstrable intensity of the enzyme reaction seemed to be related to the thickness of the sections. Thus the differences between the succinic dehydrogenase acitivities in the cells of the stratum basale and those of the stratum spinosum are less distinct in 5 μ thick cryostat sections than they are in thicker sections.

The epidermis of the palm reacted somewhat more strongly than the thinner epidermis of the scalp, axilla, back and chest (MONTAGNA and FORMISANO, 1955a). Further, regional differences have been revealed by visual and photometric determinations of the succinic dehydrogenase activity (MORETTI, ADACHI, MESCON and POCHI, 1963). The strongest activity was found in the epidermis of the skin covering the sole, knee and sacral regions, while that of the arm, chest and scapular areas displayed the least. Although the degree of enzymatic reactivity in many sites of the body seemed to be related to the thickness of the epidermis, there were many exceptions to this rule.

ELLIS (1964) has furthermore observed good correlation between the wealth of the vascular bed and the enzymatic activity in the epidermis. Thus the skin of the thigh has a poorly developed capillary pattern and the epidermis displays a low succinic dehydrogenase activity, while the skin of the sacral region, on the other hand, shows a rich vascular bed and a high succinic dehydrogenase activity in the epidermis. ELLIS stresses that although the pattern of cause and effect is not clear in this instance, it seemed reasonable to assume that substrates reaching the epidermis from the circulation may be of importance for the inducement of the enzyme synthesis. A close relationship between the thickness of the epidermis and the wealth of the blood supply has also been reported (ELLIS, 1958, 1961, 1964; MORETTI, ELLIS and MESCON, 1959; HORSTMANN, 1964).

In hypertensive kidneys a good correlativity between the oxygen consumption, as measured with the Warburg technique, and the intensity of the formazan crystal deposits has also been observed by ZWEIFACH, BLACK and SCHORR (1950). Most of the succinic dehydrogenase and cytochrome oxidase activity in a cell is found in the mitochondria (see survey by BOURNE and TEWARI, 1964). The distribution of these enzymes in the epidermis is thought to correspond closely to the distribution of these organelles (BRAUN-FALCO and RATHJENS, 1954b; FORMISANO and MONTAGNA, 1954; MONTAGNA and FORMISANO, 1955a; BRAUN-FALCO, 1961a, 1965a; BRAUN-FALCO and PETZOLD, 1964; ELLIS, 1964). The distribution of the formazan-reactive granules thus shows that the enzymatic activity is greatest where the cellular metabolism is most intense and where particular cell achievements such as mitosis are required. The regional variations in the succinic dehydrogenase activity may reflect differences in the epidermal mitotic rate over the surface of the body and variations in the rates of growth and differentiation (ELLIS, 1964).

SERRI and RABIOSI (1956) have investigated with semiquantitative methods the succinic dehydrogenase activity of the human epidermis in different age-groups (8 to 44, 53 to 70 and 71 to 82 years of age). They found that the enzymatic activity decreased with increasing age. The reaction of succinic dehydrogenase fluctuates also in the epidermis throughout the hair-growth cycle of the mouse (ARGYRIS, 1956; HERSHEY, 1964). HERSHEY has compared the succinic dehydrogenase concentration measured with quantitative histochemical methods and the oxygen consumption of full thickness mouse skin at various stages of the hair cycle. He finds a close relationship between the oxygen consumption and the succinic dehydrogenase content at all phases of the hair cycle.

Good correlation between the distribution of succinic dehydrogenase and of sulfhydryl groups has been repeatedly observed (EISEN, MONTAGNA and CHASE,

1953; ROGERS, 1953; FORAKER and WINGO, 1955, 1956). BRAUN-FALCO and RATHJENS (1954b) considered this observation understandable in the light of the fact that the presence of sulfhydryl groups is necessary for the enzymatic activity. All reagents for the demonstration of -SH groups are strong inhibitors of the succinic dehydrogenase reaction (BARRON and KALNITZKY, 1947; BARRON, 1951). The thiol groups probably constitute a part in the active centre of the enzyme protein (HOFFMANN-OSTENHOF, 1954).

4. NADH- and NADPH-Tetrazolium Reductases

BRAUN-FALCO and PETZOLD (1964) have given a detailed review of earlier biochemical and histochemical data on the NADH- and NADPH-tetrazolium reductases, in connection with which they have reported their own observations on the histotopography of these enzymes in normal human epidermis.

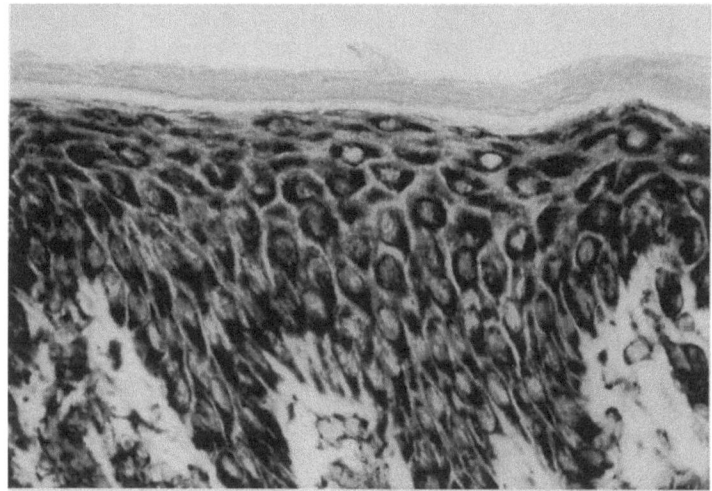

Fig. 40. Histotopy of NADH-tetrazolium salt reductase in normal epidermis. Strong positive reaction in all living epidermal cells within the cytoplasm. Nuclei and intercellular spaces negative. In some cells enzyme activity indicating perinuclear distribution of formazane precipitates. (From BRAUN-FALCO and PETZOLDT, 1964). Courtesy of Arch. klin. exp. Derm., Springer, Berlin-Göttingen-Heidelberg)

For the histochemical demonstration of dehydrogenases tetrazolium salts are used. These salts are reduced to visible formazan granules only in the presence of a substrate-specific dehydrogenase (i.e. specific coenzyme-linked dehydrogenases) and the so-called tetrazolium reductases (BRODIE and GOTS, 1953; FARBER, STERNBERG and DUNLAP, 1961). NOVIKOFF (1963) has introduced the term "tetrazolium reductases" for the enzymes that reduce the tetrazolium salts, instead of the earlier used expression "diaphorases" (ADLER, EULER and GÜNTHER, 1938). The reduction of the tetrazolium salts with the formation of visible formazan takes place in two stages. In the first stage there is a transfer of hydrogen ions from the substrate (malate, lactate etc.) to the coenzyme NAD or NADP through the action of the substrate-specific or coenzyme-linked dehydrogenases. During the second stage the hydrogen ions are transferred from the reduced coenzyme to the tetrazolium salt through the action of the NADH- or NADPH-tetrazolium reductase. The absence of tetrazolium reductases would therefore imply that visible formazan fails to appear and the possible occurrence of dehydrogenase activity in the tissue would then remain unknown (BRAUN-FALCO and PETZOLD, 1964). The dehydrogenase activity here in question is, however, brought about by other substrate-specific dehydrogenases than succinic dehydrogenase. The latter is a flavoprotein and transfers the hydrogen ions directly to the tetrazolium salt (PEARSE and SCARPELLI, 1959; BRAUN-FALCO and PETZOLD, 1964).

The NADH- (Fig. 40) and NADPH-tetrazolium reductase activity is entirely restricted to the non-cornified epidermis (BRAUN-FALCO and PETZOLD, 1964). It is distinctly visible all the way up to the upper cell layers of the stratum intermedium. The layers above, *i.e.*, the "Intermediärzone" of BRAUN-FALCO (1957c) and the stratum corneum, always stain negatively. Occasionally the enzymatic activity seems to be higher in the stratum basale than in the strata located above this.

In the epidermis the NADH-tetrazolium reductase reacts on the whole more strongly than the NADPH-tetrazolium reductase. Both enzymes appear in the form of dense formazan granules with a distinct intracytoplasmic, often perinuclear arrangement.

BRAUN-FALCO and PETZOLD (1964) have devoted a more detailed discussion to the question whether the distribution of NADH- and NADPH-tetrazolium reductase-positive formazan granules corresponds to that of the mitochondria. It has earlier been assumed that the two enzymes are bound to the mitochondria (for survey and references see PEARSE and SCARPELLI, 1959) and that the NADPH-tetrazolium reductase is also present in the microsomes (WILLIAMS, GIBBS and KAMIN, 1959; ERNSTER, LJUNGGREN and DANIELSON, 1960). In the epidermis the two enzymes do not show the same histotopographic distribution as succinic dehydrogenase (BRAUN-FALCO and RATHJENS, 1954b; MONTAGNA and FORMISANO, 1955a) and cytochrome oxidase (BRAUN-FALCO, 1961b; MONTAGNA and YUN, 1961). The two last-mentioned enzymes correspond in their decreasing activity towards the upper non-cornified epidermal layers to the distribution pattern shown for the mitochondria by MONTAGNA (1952, 1956, 1962), BRAUN-FALCO (1965a) and RITZENFELD (1965). The NADH- and NADPH-tetrazolium reductases, on the other hand, show about the same high activity throughout the non-cornified epidermis. These histochemical observations may suggest caution in localizing the tetrazolium reductase to the mitochondria in the epidermis, and also permit the assumption that the two enzymes may at least partly appear in the non-mitochondrial cytoplasm (BRAUN-FALCO and PETZOLD, 1964).

5. Specific Coenzyme-Linked Dehydrogenases

To the specific coenzyme-linked dehydrogenases belong (1) diphosphopyridine nucleotide (DPN)-linked dehydrogenases which catalyze the oxidation of lactic, malic, isocitric, alpha-glycero-phosphate, glutamic and beta-hydroxybutyric acids, and (2) triphosphopyridine nucleotide (TPN)-linked dehydrogenases which catalyze the oxidation of isocitric acid, glucose 6-phosphate and 6-phosphogluconate (IM 1965). PEARSE (1960) and BURSTONE (1964) have given detailed accounts of the history, methods and applied histochemistry of these enzymes. As appears from the foregoing chapter, the coenzymes NAD and NADP are here necessary in order to transfer the colourless, soluble forerunner of the tetrazolium salt to the coloured, insoluble formazan granules.

CORMANE and CLAESSENS (1963) have investigated the distribution of beta-hydroxybutyric dehydrogenase in normal human skin. The enzymatic activity was restricted to the non-cornified layers of the epidermis, but the strata basale and intermedium displayed a stronger reaction than the stratum spinosum (Fig. 41).

In the epidermis of the Rhesus monkey only the non-cornified epidermis reacted, whereas the stratum corneum appeared negatively (IM, 1965). The enzymes differ with respect to intensity in the various layers. The DPN-linked enzymes such as malic, lactic and beta-hydroxybutyric dehydrogenases showed a strong reaction throughout the non-cornified epidermis. The glutamic and alpha-glycerophosphate (DPN-linked) dehydrogenases reacted strongly in the stratum basale and decreased in intensity towards the stratum intermedium. The TPN-linked dehydrogenases stained weakly in the stratum basale and increased to a moderate reaction in the stratum intermedium.

The observations of the distribution of DPN- and TPN-linked dehydrogenases in the non-cornified epidermis (IM, 1965) support the findings of BRAUN-FALCO and PETZOLD (1964) as regards the distribution of NADH- and NADPH-tetrazolium reductases and their suggestion that these enzymes are linked to both the mitochondrial and the non-mitochondrial fractions of the cytoplasm.

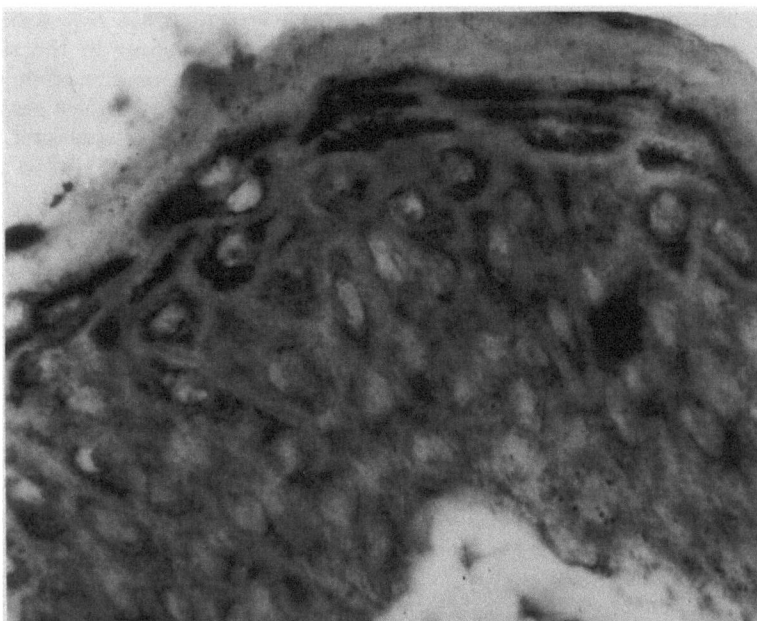

Fig. 41. Histotopy of beta-hydroxy butyryl dehydrogenase activity in normal skin of the back. The epidermis shows a positive reaction in all layers except stratum corneum. The amount of the reaction product in the stratum intermedium and basale is larger than the intensity in the stratum spinosum. Localization is mainly perinuclear.
(From CORMANE and CLAESSENS, 1963. Courtesy of Dermatologica, Karger, Basel-New York)

6. Phosphorylase and Amylo-1,4 → 1,6-transglucosidase

Phosphorylase (amylo-phosphorylase) and amylo-1,4 → 1,6-transglucosidase (branching factor of CORI and CORI, 1943 or Q-enzyme of potato of HAWORTH, PEAT and BOURNE, 1943) are enzymes involved in the process of glycogenesis (TAKEUCHI, HIGASHI and WATAMUKI, 1955; BRAUN-FALCO, 1956a, 1961a; SPIER and CANEGHEM, 1957; ELLIS and MONTAGNA, 1958; TAKEUCHI, 1958; MONTAGNA, 1962; ELLIS, 1963, 1964). Indirect evidence of the presence of phosphorylase and amylo-1,4 → 1,6-transglucosidase is the histochemical demonstration of glycogen in the tissue. These enzymes are thus present in tissues that normally store glycogen or utilize glycogen or amylose (ELLIS and MONTAGNA, 1958). They catalyze the last step in the glycogen synthesis, i.e., the reversible glucose-1-phosphate ⇌ glycogen and phosphate.

Phosphorylase alone catalyzes the synthesis of alpha-1,4-glucosidic bonds at the non-reducing ends of polysaccharide chains, making the 1,4-linked chains longer by the addition of glucose units from glucose-1-phosphate and producing straight chain polymers of the amylose type. When the straight chain polymers reach a certain critical length the amylo-1,4 → 1,6-transglucosidase presumably acts in such a manner that a 1,6 link is formed from a 1,4 link. Together the two enzymes synthesize the large branched polysaccharide molecule of glycogen (ELLIS and MONTAGNA, 1958; TAKEUCHI, 1958).

TAKEUCHI, HIGASHI and WATAMUKI (1955) found phosphorylase only in the stratum basale of the human epidermis. BRAUN-FALCO (1956a, 1961a) and SPIER and CANEGHEM (1957) observed a more or less strong enzymatic activity in the whole non-cornified epidermis. However, whereas in some areas the cells of the stratum intermedium did not show any reaction, in other areas the cells reacted strongly, indicating a synthesis of polysaccharide also in this layer of the epidermis (BRAUN-FALCO, 1956a).

ELLIS and MONTAGNA (1958) and MONTAGNA (1962) succeeded in demonstrating the presence of amylo-1,4 → 1,6-transglucosidase in the skin, and observed that this enzyme was usually found in the same sites in the skin of man as phosphorylase. In the normal adult epidermis the two enzymes mostly show moderate concentrations, but both may vary with respect to the site and the age of the subject. Thus in very thin epidermis the enzymes are either absent or cannot be detected. In thick epidermis some phosphorylase may appear in the stratum basale; the stratum spinosum is rich in both enzymes, and a weak reaction may be seen in the stratum intermedium. The palms and soles show the highest enzymatic activity, with both enzymes present in the strata basale and spinosum. Some enzymatic reaction may occasionally also be seen in the stratum lucidum (ELLIS and MONTAGNA, 1958; MONTAGNA, 1962). According to ELLIS (1964), however, no enzymes are present either in the stratum intermedium or in the transitional zone.

The stratum corneum does not respond with any activity to either phosphorylase or amylo-1,4 → 1,6-transglucosidase in any region of the body (BRAUN-FALCO, 1956a, 1961; SPIER and CANEGHEM, 1957; ELLIS and MONTAGNA, 1958; MONTAGNA, 1962; ELLIS, 1964).

There seems to be a direct relationship between the amount and distribution of the two enzymes in the epidermis and the height of the stratum corneum (ELLIS and MONTAGNA, 1958). A very high concentration of phosphorylase and amylo-1,4 → 1,6-transglucosidase is found in the epidermis of children, while there is a virtual absence of these enzymes in the skin of the aged (ELLIS and MONTAGNA, 1958; MONTAGNA, 1962).

7. Esterases

Under the name esterases are assorted all enzymes that hydrolyze esters of carboxylic acids (GOMORI, 1952a, b). A division of the esterases into groups based in principle on the ground of division proposed by GOMORI (1952a, b) has been followed in a number of histochemical investigations of esterases in the skin (FINDLAY, 1955; HELLMANN, 1955; MONTAGNA, 1955, 1956, 1962; MONTAGNA and FORMISANO, 1955b; ARGYRIS, 1956; BRAUN-FALCO, 1956b, 1958, 1961a; STEIGLEDER, 1956a, 1957, 1958a, b, c, 1959a, b, 1960c, 1964; STEIGLEDER and LÖFFLER, 1956; STEIGLEDER and SCHULTIS, 1957; MONTAGNA and BECKETT, 1958; MONTAGNA and ELLIS, 1958; STEIGLEDER and ELSCHNER, 1958; MORETTI, ADACHI and ELLIS, 1960; WELLS, 1960; STEIGLEDER and WEAKLEY, 1961; ELLIS, 1964).

Two main groups are distinguished: aliesterases and cholinesterases. Most investigators have subdivided the aliesterases into non-specific esterases and lipases. The former are defined as those aliesterases that hydrolyze short-chain aliphatic esters, while lipases act on fatty acid esters with a long carbon chain.

Although the enzymatic activity obtained with various substrates and techniques may not be indicative of different enzymes, MONTAGNA (1962), still in accordance with the principle of GOMORI (1952a, b) has suggested that the aliesterases may be subdivided into groups identified with the name of the substrate that they split. *Alpha-naphthol* or *non-specific esterases* split alpha-naphthyl acetate. According to BRAUN-FALCO (1956b) not only the non-specific esterases, but also acetyl cholinesterases, non-specific cholinesterases and lipases are able to hydrolyze alpha-naphthyl acetate. *Indoxyl acetate esterases* convert indoxyl to indigo blue (BARRNETT, 1952). Indoxyl acetate is hydrolyzed by lipases, non-specific esterases and cholinesterases (BARRNETT and SELIGMAN, 1951). *Tween 60 esterases* split Tween 60 and are probably similar to pancreatic lipases (GOMORI, 1952; STEIGLEDER and SCHULTIS, 1957). According to ELLIS (1964) both lipases and esterases are demonstrated with the Tween esterase technique. *AS esterases* split naphthol AS acetate (GOMORI, 1952a, b).

In the same way it is possible to subdivide the cholinesterases into *specific* or *acetylcholinesterases* that split either acetyl or butyrylthiocholine iodide and non-specific or pseudocholinesterases that split either acetyl- or buturylthiocholine iodide.

The different groups of esterases may furthermore be characterized with respect to their susceptibility to different activators and inhibitors (NACHLAS and SELIGMAN, 1949; BRAUN-FALCO, 1956b; STEIGLEDER and SCHULTIS, 1957; MARGHESCU and BRAUN-FALCO, 1966; for further references see the survey by BURSTONE, 1964).

a) Aliesterases
α) Alpha-Naphthol or Non-Specific Esterases

Non-Palmar and -Plantar Skin. A diffuse, moderate esterase activity has been observed in the cell layers below the transitional zone (FINDLAY, 1955; MONTAGNA,

1955, 1956, 1962; BRAUN-FALCO, 1956b). According to STEIGLEDER and LÖFFLER (1956) the cells of the stratum basale exhibit a somewhat higher reaction than those of the stratum spinosum. The authors thought that this increased reaction was perhaps not completely ascribable to the melanin.

An intense band of non-specific esterases activity (Fig. 42) has been repeatedly demonstrated in an area of the epidermis corresponding to the transitional zone (FINDLAY, 1955; MONTAGNA, 1955, 1956, 1962; BRAUN-FALCO, 1956b, 1958, 1963a, 1965a; STEIGLEDER, 1957, 1958a, c, 1959a, b, 1960c, 1964; STEIGLEDER and LÖFFLER, 1956; MONTAGNA and ELLIS, 1958; WELLS, 1960; KNOTH, RUBACH and EHLERS 1965).

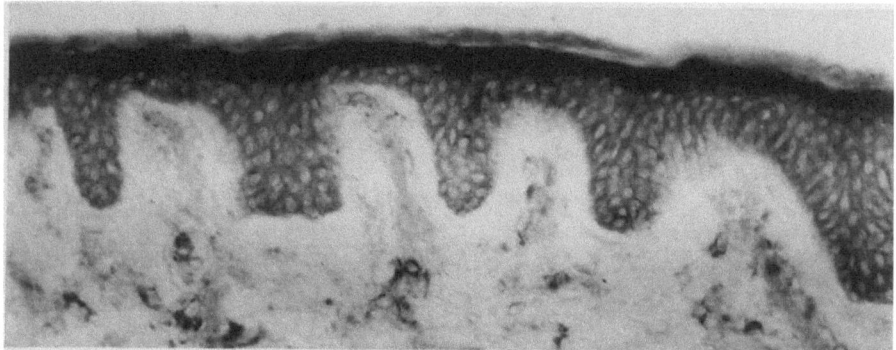

Fig. 42. Histotopy of nonspecific esterases in normal epidermis. Non-cornified epidermis weakly positive. Band-like strong positive reaction in the transitional zone. Horny layer practically negative. Azo-dye coupling technique. (Courtesy of Prof. Dr. O. BRAUN-FALCO, Marburg a. d. Lahn, Germany)

The histochemical demonstration of this esterase-rich band of cells is partly due to the type of incubation substrate that is used. Thus WELLS (1960) did not obtain any reaction with naphthol AS acetate or 5-bromoindoxyl acetate. The results are also dependent on the fixation and embedding methods used (STEIGLEDER, 1960). Regional variations of the band also occur (FINDLAY, 1955; BRAUN-FALCO, 1956b; STEIGLEDER and LÖFFLER, 1956). It is mainly absent in the epidermis of the palm and sole (see below). STEIGLEDER and LÖFFLER (1956) have observed that the esterase-rich area is very distinct in those types of epidermis in which the horny layer is not particularly thick, as for instance in the skin of the upper arm and the back. It seemed to be fainter in the epidermis of the face, the hair-covered scalp, the mons pubis and in the epithelium of the mucous membrane folds at the anus.

Within the cells of the transitional zone STEIGLEDER (1958c, 1959a, 1960c) has observed round granules exhibiting a strong non-specific esterase activity. These were located close to the nuclear membrane, at the nuclear poles, and close to the "cell membranes". They did not stain with Nile blue, but the granules close to the "cell membranes" appeared with Sudan black B-staining.

The area of the horny layer located between the transitional zone and the skin surface shows no or only slight esterase activity (STEIGLEDER, 1964). Where a reaction appeared it was mainly found close to the "cell membranes" and between the cell layers (STEIGLEDER and LÖFFLER, 1956; STEIGLEDER, 1957, 1959a, 1964; STEIGLEDER and ELSCHNER, 1959). The non-specific esterases are thus here so-called exoenzymes, i.e., enzymes with extracellular activity (THUNBERG, 1951).

A strong non-specific esterase activity has, finally, been observed also at the skin surface (STEIGLEDER and LÖFFLER, 1956; STEIGLEDER, 1958a, 1959b, 1964;

STEIGLEDER and ELSCHNER, 1959). STEIGLEDER and his co-worker (STEIGLEDER, 1958a, 1959a, b; STEIGLEDER and ELSCHNER, 1959) have further been able to confirm this observation by modifying the histochemical technique and applying

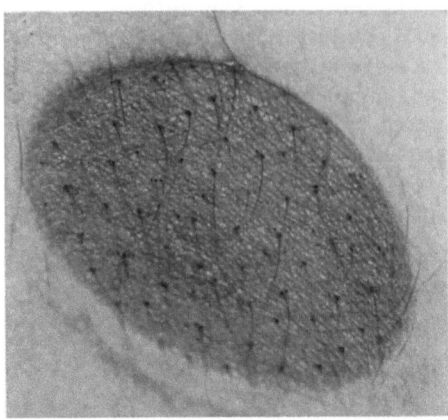

Fig. 43. Demonstration of an activity of non-specific esterases on the skin surface. Test on the flexor-surface of the lower part of the arm. The entire surface of the incubated skin reacts, but the openings of the hair follicles are more intensively stained. (From STEIGLEDER and ELSCHNER, 1959. Courtesy of Arch. klin. exp. Derm., Springer, Berlin-Göttingen-Heidelberg)

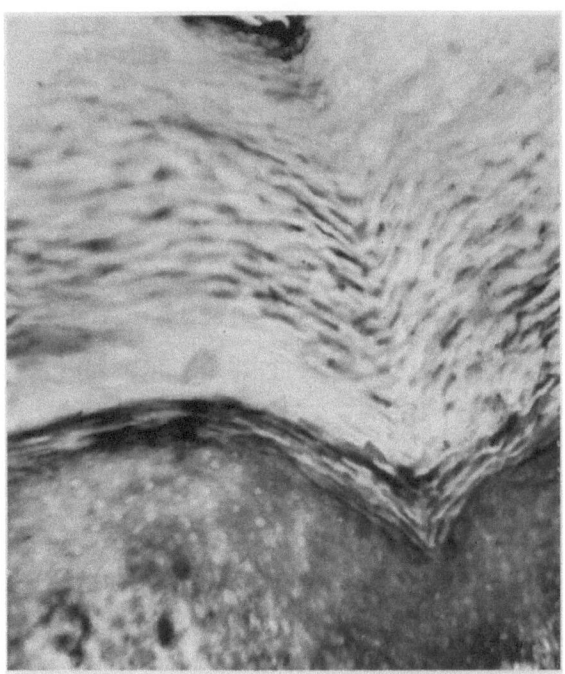

Fig. 44. Skin from the volar side of the finger. Histochemical demonstration of an activity of non-specific esterases. The subcorneal esterase-positive area less pronounced than in other parts of the skin; Stratum lucidum negative, but the higher layers of the stratum corneum in contrast to other areas of the skin partially positive. Positive material on the horny layer near the opening of a sweat duct. (From STEIGLEDER and LÖFFLER, 1956. Courtesy of Arch. klin. exp. Derm., Springer, Berlin-Göttingen-Heidelberg)

it direct to the surface of the living skin, thus permitting a macroscopical reading of the results (Fig. 43). The enzymes on the skin surface may derive from four sources, *i.e.*, the epidermis, the sweat, the sebaceous glands and parasites on the skin surface (STEIGLEDER, 1958a). The histochemical reaction in the horny layer to non-specific esterases was not parallel to the staining with Sudan black B, but in the outer layers of the stratum corneum it better corresponded to the staining with Nile blue. According to LENNERT and WEITZEL (1952/53) the latter stain reacts with more lipid substances than does Sudan black B.

Plantar and Palmar Skin. The non-specific esterases are here particularly rich in the stratum basale (FINDLAY, 1955; STEIGLEDER and LÖFFLER, 1956; MONTAGNA and ELLIS, 1958; WELLS, 1960; MONTAGNA, 1962; ELLIS, 1964). Stratum spinosum always stained weaker than the stratum basale (STEIGLEDER and LÖFFLER, 1956). The epidermis of the palm and sole differed from that from other sites, particularly with respect to the absence of an esterase-rich band corresponding to the transitional zone (FINDLAY, 1955; STEIGLEDER and LÖFFLER, 1956; MONTAGNA and ELLIS, 1958; MONTAGNA, 1962; ELLIS, 1964). The stratum lucidum stained negatively, except for an occasional reaction in its upper cells (FINDLAY, 1955; STEIGLEDER and LÖFFLER, 1956). Esterase-containing material was here also present between the cell layers (STEIGLEDER and LÖFFLER, 1956; Fig. 44) and at the surface of the stratum corneum (FINDLAY, 1955; STEIGLEDER and LÖFFLER, 1956).

β) Indoxyl Acetate Esterases

With indoxyl acetate as substrate BRAUN-FALCO (1956b) and MONTAGNA and ELLIS (1958) have obtained a distinct enzyme activity in the strata basale, spinosum and intermedium. According to MONTAGNA and ELLIS the esterase activity appeared evenly distributed in the stratum intermedium and was found both intra- and intercellularly. In the zone corresponding to the basal horny layer BRAUN-FALCO (1956b) has observed larger indigo crystals than in the subjacent layers. Whereas according to BRAUN-FALCO the upper part of the stratum corneum stained negatively, MONTAGNA and ELLIS found a sparse occurrence of small, curving sticks displaying an esterase activity.

From the results of the effect of inhibitors on the indoxyl-acetate esterase activity BRAUN-FALCO (1956b) concluded that cholinesterases did not play any role for the reaction, which was due, instead, to the presence of non-specific esterases and lipases. The lipases, he believed, formed a minor part and were located mainly in the area below the transitional zone.

γ) Tween 60 Esterases

Tween 60 esterases have been demonstrated in the epidermis of man, chimpanzee and macaque (MORETTI, ADACHI and ELLIS, 1960; MORETTI, ADACHI, MESCON and POCHI, 1963). The basal and spinous layers show the strongest reaction. Semiquantitative methods reveal great regional variations in the epidermis of the chimpanzee and macaque (MORETTI, ADACHI and ELLIS, 1960). A correlation between the esterase activity and the hair growth, as observed by ARGYRIS (1956) in the skin of mouse, is probably unlikely in the skin of primates because the cyclic activity of the hair follicles does not sweep through the epidermis of the primates in predictable waves as it does in the mouse (ELLIS, 1964).

δ) AS Esterases

According to MONTAGNA and ELLIS (1958) all cells in the strata basale and spinosum contain an AS esterase. Stratum intermedium lacks reactivity, whereas the stratum corneum stains strongly, particularly in its proximal part.

In the palm and sole the esterase granules are evenly distributed in the basal and spinous layers. They are absent in the strata intermedium and corneum, whereas the stratum lucidum exhibits a weak reaction.

b) Cholinesterases

In a biochemical study of human skin MAGNUS and THOMPSON (1954) have observed small amounts of non-specific cholinesterases. HURLEY, SHELLEY and KOELLE (1953), AAVIK (1955), BRAUN-FALCO (1956b) and YAMAZAKI (1964) have not been able to confirm this finding in their histochemical investigations of the skin. HELLMANN (1955), on the other hand, has obtained a diffuse reaction for cholinesterase throughout the epidermis of the rat and occasionally a cholinesterase activity in the strata basale and lucidum of the human epidermis. The epidermis of the cat, dog, guinea pig and monkey does not show any reaction. According to MONTAGNA and ELLIS (1958) an activity appears in the strata basale and intermedium. According to MAGNUS and THOMPSON (1954), HELLMANN (1955) and MONTAGNA and ELLIS (1958) assume that the reaction is due to non-specific cholinesterases. Investigating inhibitors and activators of esterase activity in skin STEIGLEDER and SCHULTIS (1957) recommend caution in the interpretation of histochemical observations. Their results, however, indicate the presence of both specific and non-specific cholinesterases in the human epidermis. MONTAGNA and BECKETT (1958) have investigated the lip of rat and observed a diffuse reaction throughout the epidermis. They conclude that this reaction may be due to either both specific and non-specific cholinesterases, or non-specific cholinesterases and a third type of cholinesterases.

8. Phosphomonoesterases

Three types of hydrolytic enzymes responsible for the breakdown of phosphate esters have been demonstrated, viz. mono-, di-, and triphosphatases (PEARSE, 1960). For histochemical purposes it is in the main only the monophosphatases, or, as they are also called, the phosphomonoesterases or phosphatases that come into the question. On the basis of optimum pH levels in vitro "alkaline" and "acid" phosphatases are distinguished.

BRAUN-FALCO (1958, 1961a) has pointed out that since the original works of GOMORI (1939, 1949) innumerable studies have been published on the distribution of phosphatases in all kinds of tissue, but that our knowledge of the natural substrates of the phosphatases is still very limited. The enzymes probably play an important role in the carbohydrate, protein, and possibly also in the lipid metabolism (for survey and references see KOPF, 1957; BRAUN-FALCO, 1961a; BURSTONE, 1964). In fracture callus in rat ROSIN (1952) has observed a close correlation between the amount of ribonucleic acid and alkaline phosphatases. This finding has, however, not been confirmed in skin (BRAUN-FALCO, 1961a).

a) Acid Phosphatase

Acid phosphatase is present in the entire epidermis but is most distinctly evident in the transitional zone (MORETTI and MESCON, 1956; SPIER and MARTIN, 1956; BRAUN-FALCO, 1958, 1961a, 1963a, 1965a; STEIGLEDER, 1959a, b, 1960c, 1964; BRADSHAW, WACHSTEIN, SPENCE and ELIAS, 1963; JARRETT and SPEARMAN, 1964; ELSEN, ARNDT and CLARK, 1964; KNOTH, RUBACH and EHLERS, 1965; Fig. 45). This enzyme exhibits a distribution pattern similar to that of the nonspecific esterases, beta-glucuronidase, deoxyribonuclease and ribonuclease (for references see the respective chapters). BRAUN-FALCO (1958) has suggested that the concentration of hydrolytic enzymes in the transitional zone may be related to the decomposition of cytoplasm and nuclei taking place in this region of the epidermis.

In a histochemical and biochemical study acid phosphatase has also been demonstrated in the stratum corneum disjunctum (SPIER, PASCHER and MARTIN,

1955). The presence of the enzyme in this region of the stratum corneum has been assumed to be connected with the disintegration of the nuclei in the transitional zone.

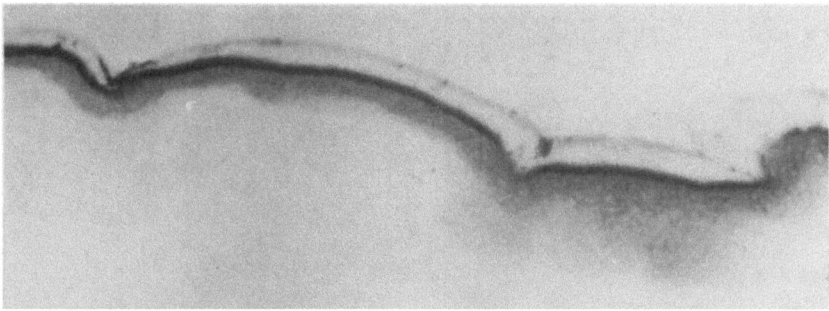

Fig. 45. Histotopy of acid phosphatase in normal epidermis. Weakly positive reaction in the non-cornified epidermis; strong positive reaction in the transitional zone and negative reaction in the horny layer. (From BRAUN-FALCO, 1958. Courtesy of Ann. N.Y. Acad. Sci., The New York Academy of Sciences)

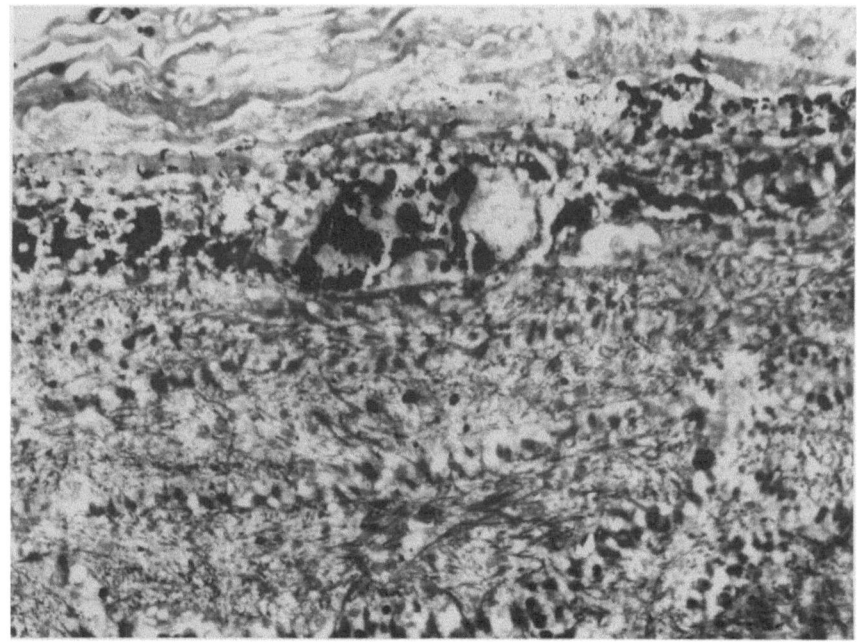

Fig. 46. Electron microscopy reveals acid phosphatase activity by electron opaque accumulation of lead sulfide as intense nuclear and keratohyalin granular localization in the granular layer and as some diffuse distribution in the keratin layer of human epidermis. No distinct lysosomes are seen. Modified Gomori's reaction. Prefixed with phosphate buffered formalin and postfixed with $KMNO_4$ after Gomori's reaction and stained with phosphotungstic acid and uranyl acetate. × 6,200. (From MISHIMA, 1966a. Courtesy of J. invest. Derm., The Williams and Wilkins Co., Baltimore)

In studies on rat liver homogenates APPELMANS, WATTIAUX and DE DUVE (1955) and DE DUVE, PRESSMAN, GIANETTO, WATTIAUX and APPELMANS (1955) have demonstrated that acid phosphatase is present in a fraction intermediate between the mitochondria and the microsomes. This fraction also contains ribonuclease, deoxyribonuclease, cathepsin and beta-glucuronidase. Electron-microscopic studies have revealed the occurrence of a dense, 0.25 to 0.5 µ large granule in this fraction (NOVIKOFF, BEAUFAY and DE DUVE, 1956). DE DUVE and his group have called this granule "lysosome". The enzymatic activities of the lysosomes could not, however, be measured unless the granules were damaged by various methods, indicating a delimiting membrane around the granules (BERTHET and DE DUVE, 1951; DE DUVE, PRESSMAN, GIANETTO, WATTIAUX and APPELMANS, 1955; WATTIAUX and DE DUVE,

1956). SCARPELLI and PEARSE (1958) have localized acid phosphatase in short rods and ovoid structures measuring 0.5 to 1.2 μ. These components were considered to represent the lysosomes. According to BURNE and TEWARI (1964) lysosomes do not have any characteristic ultrastructural appearance, but vary conspicuously in size and shape. They can therefore only be identified through the demonstration of their content of acid phosphatase. DE DUVE and WATTIAUX (1966) have given a detailed review on the lysosome concept.

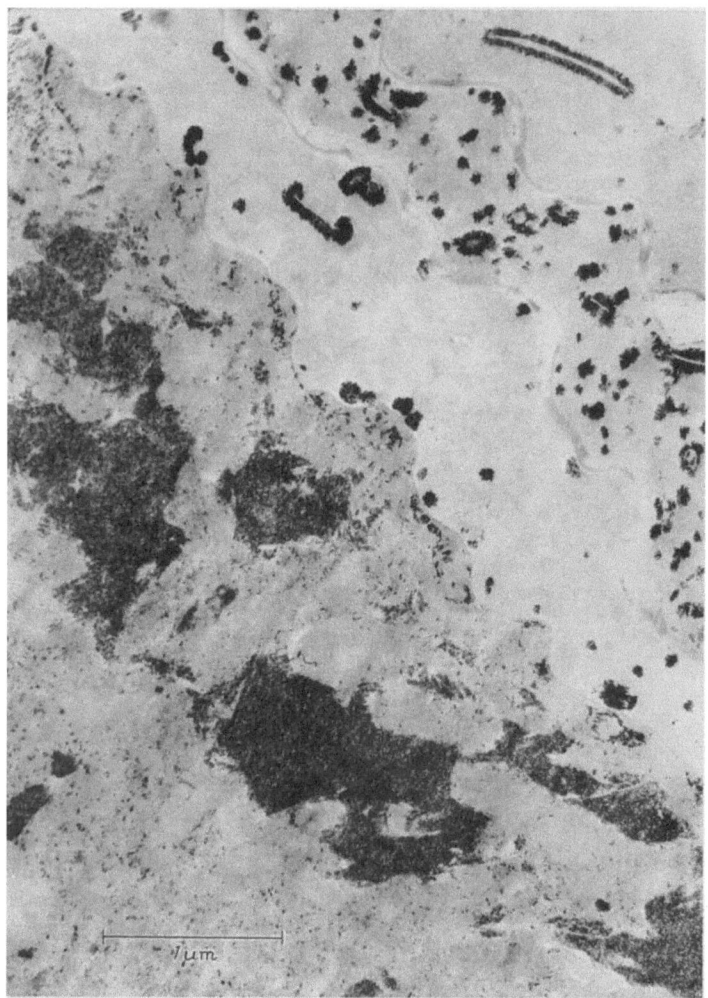

Fig. 47. Electron-histochemical demonstration of acid phosphatase in normal human epidermis. Acid phosphatase indicating lead precipitates within keratohyalin granules and in the basal portions of the horny layer. Incubation time 35 min. Noncontrasted. × 23,000. (From BRAUN-FALCO and RUPEC, 1965. Courtesy of Naturwissenschaften, Springer, Berlin-Göttingen-Heidelberg)

With electron microscopy OLSON and NORDQUIST (1966) have investigated normal human epidermis and demonstrated acid phosphatase activity in membrane-bound granules in the basal and spinous cells. These granules occurred randomly scattered throughout the cytoplasm and were assumed to be lysosomes.

In the transitional zone, where a high acid-phosphatase activity has been histochemically demonstrated, this enzyme seems to occur only in a non-lysosomal form (EISEN, ARNDT and CLARK, 1964; MISHIMA, 1964, 1966; BRAUN-FALCO and RUPEC, 1965). In the stratum intermedium acid phosphatase occurs in the nuclei (EISEN, ARNDT and CLARK, 1964; MISHIMA, 1964, 1966a; Fig. 46) and is particularly evident at the periphery close to the nuclear membrane (EISEN, ARNDT and CLARK, 1964). In the cytoplasm it is found diffusely distributed (EISEN, ARNDT and CLARK, 1964; BRAUN-FALCO and RUPEC, 1965), and the keratohyalin, moreover, displays an intense reaction to it (BRAUN-FALCO and RUPEC, 1965; MISHIMA, 1966a; Figs. 46 and 47).

In the stratum corneum a rather diffuse reaction to acid phosphatase has been observed (EISEN, ARNDT and CLARK, 1964; MISHIMA, 1964, 1966a; BRAUN-FALCO and RUPEC, 1965), but in the basal part of the horny layer intensely stained cells occur alternately with cells displaying no reaction (BRAUN-FALCO and RUPEC, 1965; Figs. 46 and 47). Occasionally acid phosphatase is also distinctly shown in the desmosomes (EISEN, ARNDT and CLARK, 1964).

b) Alkaline Phosphatase

Biochemically, SPIER, PASCHER and MARTIN (1955) have obtained small amounts (1/50 or less of the acid phosphatase content) in the stratum corneum disjunctum. According to KOPF (1957) and MONTAGNA (1962) no enzymatic activity is histochemically demonstrable in the epidermis, whereas PIRILÄ and ERÄNKÖ (1950) and SPIER and MARTIN (1956) have observed a faint reaction of the keratohyalin. JARRETT, SPEARMAN, RILEY and CANE (1965), again, have demonstrated a distinct reaction to alkaline phosphatase in the stratum intermedium.

9. Adenosine Triphosphatase (ATPase)

The enzyme adenosine triphosphatase plays a fundamental role in the release of energy in living systems effected by the breakdown of adenosine triphosphate to adenosine diphosphate (PEARSE, 1960).

ATPase is localized to the mitochondria and the cell membranes of the keratinocytes (MUSTAKALLIO, 1962; JARRETT and RILEY, 1963; BRADSHAW, WACHSTEIN, SPENCE and ELIAS, 1963; CORMANE and KALSBEEK, 1963; FARQUHAR and PALADE, 1966).

The mitochondria are observed as small rod-shaped structures in the perinuclear zone (BRADSHAW, WACHSTEIN, SPENCE and ELIAS, 1963; CORMANE and KALSBEEK, 1963). In accordance with the histological distribution of the mitochondria the ATPase activity is greatest in the stratum basale, decreases progressively in the cells of the stratum spinosum until, in the stratum intermedium, no activity is histochemically distinguishable (BRADSHAW, WACHSTEIN, SPENCE and ELIAS, 1963).

WOLFF (1964a) has obtained a diffuse yellow-brown colour of the epidermis with maximal staining of the stratum intermedium. Occasionally, the keratohyalin appeared very distinctly. WOLFF referred this reaction to enzymatic activity. BRADSHAW, WACHSTEIN, SPENCE and ELIAS (1963) also obtained a staining of the keratohyalin and, further, of the melanin granules. These authors, however, consider this reaction to be non-specific. Whereas WOLFF (1963a) could not observe the nuclei, CORMANE and KALSBEEK (1963) observed a faintly coloured nucleolus.

In a beautiful light- and electron-microscopic study of the localization of ATPase activity in the epidermis of *Rana pipiens*, *Rana catesbiana* and *Bufo marinus*, FARQUHAR and PALADE (1966) have shown that the reaction product is found in contact with the outer leaflet of all plasma membranes facing the intercellular space. It was absent from the membrane areas involved in cell junctions (desmosomes, zonulae and maculae occludentes), and from the cell membranes facing the external medium and the dermis. Most intracellular deposits were found in the mitochondria.

On the basis of their observations FARQUHAR and PALADE (1966) suggest that the Na⁺ pump is localized along all plasma membranes facing the intercellular space of the epidermis in frog and toad skin.

10. Phosphamidase

Phosphamidase belongs to the phosphatases (PEARSE, 1960; BURSTONE, 1964). This enzyme has not yet been demonstrated in either normal or pathological human epidermis (STEIGLEDER, 1959; BRAUN-FALCO, 1961a; MONTAGNA, 1962). In the epidermal epithelium of the cheek and the lip of the rat, MEYER and WEIMANN (1957) have observed an intense reaction in the stratum intermedium and a fainter activity of phosphamidase in the distal spinous cells. The subjacent cell layers of the non-cornified epidermis and the stratum corneum did not stain. In the stratum intermedium the enzymatic activity was restricted to the keratohyalin and to the nucleoli. MEYER and WEIMANN (1957) suggest that the phosphamidase may play a role in condensing processes, such as the withdrawal of water and of cellular constituents, and in the formation of disulfide bonds.

11. Nucleases

The breakdown of nucleic acids is considered to occur through the effect of a succession of enzymes such as nucleases or nucleodepolymerases, nucleotidases (nucleophosphatases) and nucleosidases (PEARSE, 1960). The histochemistry is mainly concerned with the first-mentioned group, the nucleases or nucleodepolymerases, whether the substrate is ribonucleic acid (RNA) or deoxyribonucleic acid (DNA).

a) Ribonuclease (RNase)

In the transitional zone and at the surface of the stratum corneum a high RNAse-activity has been observed (STEIGLEDER and RAAB, 1962; STEIGLEDER and FISCHER, 1963). The intermediate region of the stratum corneum and the epidermis below the transitional zone stained negatively. The enzymatic activity in the transitional zone was related to the keratinization process, whereas that in the upper layers of the stratum corneum was considered to be due to the presence of sebum (STEIGLEDER and RAAB, 1962; STEIGLEDER, 1964).

b) Deoxyribonuclease (DNAse)

The physiological disintegration of the nuclei during normal keratinization may possibly be initiated by DNAse (SPIER and CANEGHEM, 1957; SANTOIANNI and ROTHMAN, 1961). The disappearance of the second step of nuclear disintegration effected by the splitting of mono- and oligo-nucleotides through acid phosphatases is more or less simultaneously observable in the transitional zone (SPIER and CANEGHEM, 1957).

SPIER and CANEGHEM (1957) have demonstrated the occurrence of DNAse in an area corresponding to the stratum intermedium. This enzyme displays a moderate activity as compared to that of acid phosphatase. In further studies STEIGLEDER and RAAB (1962) have noticed that DNAse is less active in human skin than RNAse. A moderately active band of DNAse has been observed in the lowest layers of the stratum corneum immediately above the stratum intermedium (STEIGLEDER and RAAB, 1962; STEIGLEDER and FISCHER, 1963). In the palm and sole a DNAse activity has also been shown in the stratum corneum above the stratum lucidum (STEIGLEDER and RAAB, 1962).

12. Beta-Glucuronidase

Beta-glucuronidase belongs to the glucosidases, which hydrolyze glycosidic linkages. The latter consists of a bond between the aldehyde group of a sugar (glycone) and the hydroxyl group of aglycone (for survey and references see BURSTONE, 1964).

The biological function of beta-glucuronidase has not yet been elucidated, but a mutual relationship has been observed between the activity of this enzyme and the growth of cancerous tissue (FISHMAN and BAKER, 1956; FISHMAN, BAKER and BORGES, 1959), as well as between the activities of this enzyme and of ovarian hormones (FISHMAN and BAKER, 1956; HAYASHI and FISHMAN, 1961, 1962). MONIS, BANKS and RUTENBURG (1960) have confirmed the observations of FISHMAN and his group with respect to the intense reaction of beta-glucuronidase in human malignant tumors of epithelial origin. Mesenchymal tumors, on the other hand, showed only little or no reaction (MONIS and RUTENBURG, 1958; MONIS, BANKS and RUTENBURG, 1960).

In 1954 SELIGMAN, TSOU, RUTENBURG and COHEN demonstrated for the first time the presence of beta-glucuronidase in the epidermis. This finding has later been confirmed in histochemical (BRAUN-FALCO, 1956c, 1958, 1961a, 1965a; MONTAGNA, 1957, 1962; STEIGLEDER, 1958d, 1959a, 1964; JARRETT and SPEARMAN, 1964), and biochemical (MESIROW and STOUGHTON, 1954) investigations.

The whole epidermis reacts distinctly but the various layers show a clear difference with respect to the amount of enzymatic activity (BRAUN-FALCO, 1956c). The strata basale and spinosum stain moderately with a somewhat higher reaction for the stratum basale. An intense activity has been observed in the transitional zone. The keratohyalin did not stain. STEIGLEDER (1958), who has investigated the skin surface in this respect, has observed there a strong reaction to this enzyme. Unlike the non-specific esterases, the "cell membranes" of the horny cells were not stained.

The intense reaction of beta-glucuronidase in the transitional zone in normal epidermis, and in a region below the horny layer and in the upper dermis in pathological skin may according to BRAUN-FALCO (1961a) indicate a correlation between this enzyme and the mechanism of cornification. He discussed a possible role of beta-glucuronidase in the decomposition of the epithelial acid mucopolysaccharides in the intercellular space. JARRETT and SPEARMAN (1964) have suggested that the so-called ODLAND's bodies (cf. chapters CII and CVIII) are lysosomes, and that the increased activity of beta-glucuronidase in the stratum intermedium may be due to the release of this enzyme from the cellular lysosomes (DE DUVE and BEAUFAY, 1959). This enzyme is to a significant extent also present in the microsomes (DE DUVE and BEAUFAY, 1959).

13. Proteolytic Enzymes

Proteolytic enzymes are subdivided into exo- and endopeptidases (KARLSON, 1966). The exopeptidases split the polypeptide chains of the protein molecules by breaking the peptide bonds of the alpha-amino groups. The endopeptidases split the proteins at certain places within the polypeptide chains. Aminopeptidase belongs to the exopeptidases, whereas chymotrypsin is an endopeptidase.

Normal skin has been investigated with respect to the aminopeptidase activity (BRAUN-FALCO, 1956d, 1961a; STEIGLEDER, 1959a, 1962; ADACHI and MONTAGNA, 1961; MONTAGNA, 1962; STEIGLEDER, KUDICKE and KAMEI, 1962; WOLFF, 1963b). According to STEIGLEDER, KAMEI and KUDICKE (1963) the substrate that they had earlier used in order to show aminopeptidase-activity in the skin (STEIGLEDER, 1962; STEIGLEDER, KUDICKE and KAMEI, 1962) can also be split by chymotrypsin (HASEGAWA and SIEGEL, 1962; SYLVÉN and BOIS, 1962). As it is not yet possible other than theoretically to separate the two types of enzymes, STEIGLEDER, KAMEI and KUDICKE (1963) and STEIGLEDER (1964) propose that instead of "aminopeptidase-activity" the expression "proteolytic activity" should be used in accordance with the definition (KARLSON, 1966).

Epidermis displays a moderate proteolytic activity (BRAUN-FALCO, 1956d, 1961a; STEIGLEDER, 1959a; ADACHI and MONTAGNA, 1961; MONTAGNA, 1962; STEIGLEDER, KUDICKE and KAMEI, 1962; WOLFF, 1963b). The reaction is strongest in the stratum basale and decreases towards the skin surface. In the skin of the palm and sole the strata basale and intermedium show a higher activity than the stratum spinosum (ADACHI and MONTAGNA, 1961; MONTAGNA, 1962; STEIGLEDER, KUDICKE and KAMEI, 1962). The stratum lucidum stained occasionally (ADACHI and MONTAGNA, 1961). A reaction by the stratum corneum of the scalp and face was sometimes obtained (STEIGLEDER, KUDICKE and KAMEI, 1962). According to STEIGLEDER (1962, 1964) and STEIGLEDER, KUDICKE and KAMEI (1962) a proteolytic activity at the skin surface is observed macroscopically as well as histologically in transverse sections of the skin. The enzymes may here originate partly from the epidermis itself and partly from microbes (STEIGLEDER, 1962).

WOLFF (1963b) has investigated the occurrence of proteolytic enzymes (aminopeptidases) in the skin with l-leucyl-beta-naphthylamide (LNA) and l-leucyl-4-methoxy-beta-naphthylamide (LMNA) substrates. In LNA-incubated sections a moderate activity of the epidermis was obtained with maximum staining in the stratum basale, with decreased reactivity towards the skin surface. The entire stratum corneum stained negatively. With the LNA substrate WOLFF thus got the same results as BRAUN-FALCO (1956d, 1961a), ADACHI and MONTAGNA (1961) and MONTAGNA (1962) in non-palmar and non-plantar skin. His results, however, differed from those of STEIGLEDER, KUDICKE and KAMEI (1962) with respect to the positive reaction of the stratum corneum and the skin surface demonstrated by the latter authors.

In LMNA-incubated sections the whole epidermis appeared completely negative. On the basis of this negative result WOLFF (1963b) interpreted the positive reaction obtained with LNA-substrate as a diffusion artefact with the primary reaction products localized to the intensely stained subepidermal connective tissue.

Although this interpretation seemed most attractive to WOLFF, he could not rule out the possibility that the different results obtained with the LNA- and LMNA-substrates might be due to two different enzymes in the tissue.

14. Carbonic Anhydrase

Through the action of carbonic anhydrase carbonic acid is split to give CO_2 and H_2O and, in the reverse direction CO_2 is hydrated to carbonic acid (PEARSE, 1960).

According to BRAUN-FALCO and RATHJENS (1955) the cells of the stratum basale show the highest activity. However, the distribution of the cobalt sulfide precipitases showing the enzymatic activity is by no means even in the stratum basale cells. Within the rete pegs several layers of the spinous cells exhibit a reaction, whereas suprapapillarly the reaction soon disappears above the stratum basale. In the upper stratum spinosum and in the stratum corneum no precipitates were distinguished. The horny layer exhibited an even dark-brown staining, but this was considered as an artefact due to the fixation.

15. Ubiquinone

Ubiquinone or coenzyme Q belongs chemically to the group benzoquinone (KARLSON, 1966). It is widely distributed and occurs in plants as well as animals (for references see BRAUN-FALCO and PETZOLD, 1966). Ubiquinone is found in rather high concentrations as a constituent of the lipoprotein membranes of the mitochondria (KARLSON, 1966). Histochemical studies have revealed that it is also present as a non-mitochondrial cytoplasmic component (TRANZER and PEARSE, 1963). Ubiquinone acts as an oxidation and reduction catalyzer, respectively, in the transfer of hydrogen ions between the flavoproteins and the cytochromes in the respiration chain (GREEN, ZIEGLER and DOEG, 1959; HATEFI, LESTER, CRANE and WIDMER, 1959; DOEG, KRUEGER and ZIEGLER, 1960; REDFEARN and PUMPHREY, 1960). It is considered as a coenzyme for the flavoproteins.

In the non-cornified epidermis ubiquinone shows the same intense reaction in the strata basale, spinosum and intermedium (BRAUN-FALCO and PETZOLD, 1966). Stratum corneum stains negatively (Fig. 48). In the plantar skin the transitional zone is not more reactive than the subjacent layers of the stratum intermedium. The formazan granules are densely packed in the cytoplasm, whereas the nuclei and intercellular space are always free of granules.

The histotopography of the ubiquinone-reactive formazan granules corresponds entirely to that of the NADH- and NADPH-tetrazolium reductases (BRAUN-FALCO and PETZOLD, 1964). On the basis of the studies on the distribution of the mitochondria by RITZENFELD (1965) and ZELICKSON and HARTMANN (1961b), BRAUN-FALCO and PETZOLD (1966) have suggested, in accordance with the observations by TRANZER and PEARSE (1963) that ubiquinone in the epidermis is bound to the mitochondria as well as to a non-mitochondrial cytoplasmic component.

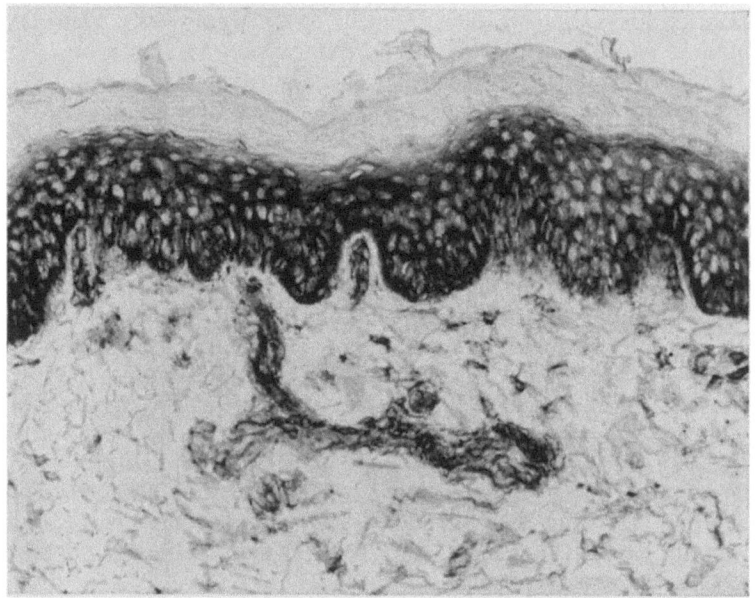

Fig. 48. Histotopy of ubiquinone in normal skin. All living epidermal cells and mesenchymal cells contain ubiquinone. (From BRAUN-FALCO and PETZOLDT, 1966. Courtesy of Arch. klin. exp. Derm., Springer, Berlin-Göttingen-Heidelberg)

16. Desulfhydrase

The enzyme desulfhydrase (cysteine desulfhurase) removes the sulfhydryl groups from the cysteine molecule and forms pyruvic acid and hydrogen sulfide (JARRETT, 1962; JARRETT and SPEARMAN, 1964; KARLSON, 1966).

JARRETT (1962) has demonstrated the occurrence of desulfhydrase in the stratum intermedium. There is a reduction of sulfhydryl groups above the stratum intermedium. Some of the excess of the sulfhydryl groups in the stratum intermedium may perhaps be removed by desulfhydrase (JARRETT and SPEARMAN, 1964).

E. Dendritic Cells
I. The Melanocyte
1. Origin

In 1884 RIEHL described for the first time the presence of dendritic cells in human skin (in leukoderma syphiliticum and in normal hair matrix). In 1885 EHRMANN also succeeded in demonstrating them in normal human epidermis.

The origin, shape and mode of division of the dentritic cell and its role in the formation of pigment have been the subject of controversy (cf. reviews by HOEPKE, 1927; BLOCH, 1927, 1929; PERCIVAL and STEWART, 1930; LATERJET,

1938; Meirowsky, 1940; Masson, 1948a; Montagna, 1956, 1962; Horstmann, 1957, 1961; Billingham and Silvers, 1960).

According to Becker (1927), three main theories as to the nature of the dendritic cell have been advanced. According to one theory, every cell in the stratum basale is dendritic, but only a few are identified as such by their content of pigment. The view proposed by Bloch (1917, 1927, 1929) that all epidermal cells are under appropriate stimuli able to produce the pigment that they contain in their cytoplasm was the prevalent theory during the thirties and forties (Peck, 1930; Danneel and Lubnow, 1936; Lubnow, 1939; Meirowsky, 1940; Danneel, 1941; Ormsby and Montgomery, 1948; Meirowsky, Freeman and Wiseman, 1951). Allen (1949, 1953) considers that the dendritic cell does not differ in any essential respect from the keratinocytes. He assumes that the cells have "intercellular bridges" and questions whether they possess true dendritic processes.

The third theory, put forward by Masson (1926), implies that the mammalian epidermis is composed of two distinct varieties of cell, viz. keratinocytes and pigment-forming dendritic cells. This view has been generally accepted, thanks to histological works on skin (Masson, 1948a, b; Billingham, 1948, 1949; Billingham and Medawar, 1948, 1953; Becker, Fitzpatrick and Montgomery, 1952; Szabó, 1954, 1959b; Breathnach, 1957; Staricco and Pinkus, 1957; Hu, Staricco, Pinkus and Fosnaugh, 1957; Hu, 1959), and to electron-microscopic works on skin (Barnicot and Birbeck, 1958; Clark and Hibbs, 1958; Odland, 1958; Charles and Ingram, 1959; Drochmans, 1960a; Zelickson and Hartmann, 1961a; Rappaport, Makai and Swift, 1963; Breatnach and Wyllie, 1964; Breathnach, Goodwin and Wyllie, 1965), and on hair (Barnicot, Birbeck and Cuckow, 1955; Birbeck, Mercer and Barnicot, 1956; Barnicot and Birbeck, 1958; Birbeck and Barnicot, 1959; cf. also surveys by Medawar, 1953; Lerner, 1955; Horstmann, 1957, 1961; Billingham and Silvers, 1960; Mercer, 1961; Montagna, 1962).

No indications of a transformation of keratinocytes into dendritic cells have been observed in adult human skin (Masson, 1948a; Staricco, 1957; Staricco and Pinkus, 1957; Szabó, 1959b) or in embryonic human skin (Zimmermann and Becker, 1959).

Bloch (1929) and Masson (1948a) called the melanin-forming cells "melanoblasts". The cells containing phagocytized pigment were referred to by Bloch as "chromatophores" and by Masson as "chromatophores" or "melanophores". Since in modern usage the suffix "blast" has been given to the immature cells which differentiate into mature cells, Becker, Fitzpatrick and Montgomery (1952) have suggested the expressions "melanodendrocyte" or "melanogenocyte" as more appropriate designations for the mature, melanin-forming dendritic cell.

At the third Conference on the Biology of the Normal and Atypical Pigment Cell in New York in 1951 Fitzpatrick and Lerner (1953) introduced a revised terminology of the pigment cells which has become generally accepted.

Table. *Terminology of pigment cells*

	Earlier terminology		Terminology according to Fitzpatrick and Lerner (1953)
	Biology	Medicine	
Mature melanin-forming cell	melanophore	melanoblast	melanocyte
Immature melanin-forming cell	melanoblast	—	melanoblast
Cell with phagocytized melanin	macrophage	melanophore	macrophage or melanophage
"Contractile" cell	melanophore	melanophore	melanophore

Compare the above table with the recently proposed terminology of the pigment cells presented at the sixth International Pigment Cell Conference in Sofia 1965 (DELLA PORTA and MÜHLBOCK, 1966).

BLOCH (1927, 1929) believed that the melanin-forming epidermal cells are of ectodermal origin, and that only the dermal pigmented cells occurring close to the dermo-epidermal junction are macrophages. HARRISON (1910a, b, 1938), on the other hand, advanced the hypothesis that the melanocyte system is of neural crest origin. This view has been repeatedly confirmed in amphibia (DU SHANE, 1934, 1935; TWITTY, 1936), in birds (DORRIS, 1939; EASTLICK, 1939; HAMILTON, 1941) and in mice (RAWLES, 1947, 1953), and is considered to be valid also for mammals in general (cf. the review by ZIMMERMANN and BECKER, 1959a). HORSTMANN (1957) and STARCK (1964) have thoroughly reviewed the literature pertinent to the latter theory.

ZIMMERMANN and CORNBLEET (1948), ZIMMERMANN (1954), and ZIMMERMANN and BECKER (1959a, b) have investigated the melanoblasts and melanocytes in fetal negro skin. They define the melanoblast as an embryonic cell existing exclusively in the dermis and potentially capable of producing melanin, but not containing the fully elaborated pigment (ZIMMERMANN and BECKER, 1959a, b). The melanoblasts differentiate in the dermis into immature melanocytes. A few melanocytes appear in the epidermis in the eleventh embryonic week. Between the twelfth and fourteenth weeks a sharp increase in the numbers of epidermal melanocytes occurs, indicating a period of rapid influx. The number of epidermal melanocytes remains fairly stabilized after the fifth fetal month. By the time of birth there are approximately 1035 epidermal melanocytes per mm^2. In later fetal life, *i.e.*, between the sixth month and birth, the "dermal" melanocytes are identifiable only in certain skin areas (ZIMMERMANN and BECKER, 1959a, b).

Postnatally the epidermal melanocytes have been considered to form a self-reproducing system without any further recruitment from the dermis (MASSON, 1948a; BILLINGHAM and MEDAWAR, 1953; MEDAWAR, 1953; BILLINGHAM and SILVERS, 1960; BREATHNACH, 1964, 1965). Although mitotic figures are far from easy to see (MEDAWAR, 1953), such have been reported by BILLINGHAM (1948), MASSON (1948a), PINKUS (1949), and BECKER, FITZPATRICK and MONTGOMERY (1952). During cell division the "cytochrine" activity (MASSON, 1948a) of the melanocyte ceases, but the latter does not lose its pigment (MEDAWAR, 1953). Thus MEDAWAR (1953) did not find any evidence for the supposition that the generative cell is a non-pigmented melanoblast which differentiates into a pigmentary melanocyte that is no longer capable of fission. According to PINKUS (1949), the dendritic cells do not retract their processes during cell division, as is considered to be the case by BILLINGHAM and SILVERS (1960).

In an electron-microscopic investigation of adult human epidermis CHARLES and INGRAM (1959) observed cells in the dermis, close to the dermo-epidermal junction. They described the cells as having the appearance of melanocytes and being in a position to enter or leave the epidermis. These cells observed by CHARLES and INGRAM may perhaps represent the so-called "dermal" melanocytes of ZIMMERMANN and BECKER (1959a, b).

According to an earlier proposed view there is a histogenetic relationship between the melanin-pigment granules and the mast-cell granules (MICHELS, 1938). NAY (1956) has advanced the hypothesis that the mast cells are precursors of the melanocytes in mouse hair. OKUN (1965) has studied the histogenesis of melanocytes in man and laboratory animals. On the basis of morphologic, histochemical, ultrastructural and embryologic parallels between melanocytes and mast cells he suggests that these two cell types have a common tissue stem cell.

OKUN further assumes that under certain circumstances the mast cells may represent a transitional phase in the development of melanocytes.

On the basis of his observations OKUN (1965) discusses the validity of the evidences for the currently accepted theory that the epidermal melanocytes in adult animals form a closed and self-reproducing system of cells. Contrary to this view he assumes that the precursors of the epidermal melanocytes are present in the subepidermal bed of loose connective tissue.

2. Demonstration, Distribution and Frequency

With dihydroxyphenylalanine (Dopa) BLOCH (1917, 1927, 1929) had obtained a staining of the dendritic cells as well as of the keratinocytes, and he therefore drew the incorrect conclusion that all epidermal cells are able to produce melanin pigment.

With the modified Dopa reactions according to LAIDLAW and BLACKBERG (1932) and BECKER (1935), MASSON (1948a) and BILLINGHAM (1948) were able to show clearly that only the dendritic cells are stained with Dopa.

BILLINGHAM (1948) distinguished two types of dendritic cells, *viz.* "pigmented" and "white" dendritic cells. The former are present in the heavily pigmented areas of the skin in black and white guinea-pigs. The white dendritic cells occur in "non-pigmented epidermis" as in *e.g.* the "non-pigmented skin of spotted guinea-pigs, of rabbits and of man".

The pigmented dendritic cells show a positive Dopa reaction, whereas the white dendritic cell is revealed with the gold impregnation technique of GAIRNS (1930), with methylene blue and azan staining. The white dendritic cells are assumed by BILLINGHAM to lack the melanogenic properties characteristic of the pigmented dendritic cells. In all other respects they closely resemble the latter: with regard to their size, shape, position, number, mode of branching, the number and length of their processes, the disposition and mode of termination of the latter, the relation which may exist between two such dendritic cells and, finally, their nucleate nature (BILLINGHAM, 1948).

In further studies it has been shown that the pigmented dendritic cell and the white dendritic cell, *i.e.*, the "clear cell" of MASSON (1948a, b), are merely different preparation images of the same cell, the melanocyte, the different appearance being due to differences in the rate of melanogenesis (MASSON, 1948a, b; ZIMMERMANN and CORNBLEET, 1948; BILLINGHAM, 1949; BECKER, FITZPATRICK and MONTGOMERY, 1952; BILLINGHAM and MEDAWAR, 1953). BILLINGHAM (1949) points out that the pigmented dendritic cell of the epidermis in Indian and Negro skin and the white dendritic cell of the epidermis in Caucasian skin only differ with respect to the rate of melanogenesis. BECKER, FITZPATRICK and MONTGOMERY (1952) confirm the presence of the so-called white dendritic cells of BILLINGHAM (1948). Unlike BILLINGHAM (1948), however, they succeeded in staining this type of melanocyte with gold and methylene blue as well as with Dopa. This cell does not, on the other hand, show any tyrosinase activity (BECKER, FITZPATRICK and MONTGOMERY, 1952).

As "true" melanocytes have been considered only the dendritic cells occurring in the stratum basale of the epidermis close to the dermo-epidermal junction (MASSON, 1948a, b; BILLINGHAM, 1948, 1949; PINKUS, 1949; BECKER, FITZPATRICK and MONTGOMERY, 1952; BILLINGHAM and MEDAWAR, 1953; SZABÓ, 1954, 1959b; PINKUS and STARICCO, 1957; BILLINGHAM and SILVERS, 1960).

SZABÓ (1954, 1959b) has made a thorough study of the distribution and frequency of the melanocytes in skin. Melanocytes are present in all areas irrespective of whether the skin is exposed to sunlight or covered by clothing. There are on an average 1560 melanocytes per square millimeter of the skin surface. There are, however, great regional variations. For instance, the epidermis of the face and the forehead is about twice as densely populated by melanocytes as is the epidermis of other regions. Szabó has further shown that the melanocytes are symmetrically distributed throughout the body. No significant sexual or racial differences are observed with respect to their frequency distribution, and the Caucasian epidermis is anatomically as well provided with melanocytes as is the epidermis of coloured skin.

Pinkus, Staricco, Kropp and Fan (1959) confirm Szabó's figures with respect to the regional variations in the number of melanocytes, and also the observation that there are no significant differences in their number as between white and coloured skin.

Becker, Fitzpatrick and Montgomery (1952) have demonstrated that the darkness of the skin is directly correlated to the number of melanin granules in the melanocytes.

3. Morphology

The melanocyte consists of a body called the "perikaryon", from which processes (branches or dendrites) arise and travel outwards to pass between the surrounding basal cells (Billingham, 1948; Masson, 1948a; Billingham and Medawar, 1953; Medawar, 1953). The cells may have between two and ten branches, but on an average these number about five. In cells having only few processes, the base diameter of the dendrites is usually greater than that in cells furnished with many branches. Some processes exceed 70 μ in length, although the majority of branches vary between 30 and 40 μ (Billingham, 1948).

The surface of the whole melanocyte (*i.e.*, the perikaryon and the dendrites) does not show the typical finger-like processes of the keratinocytes, but is smooth (Clark and Hibbs, 1958; Zelickson and Hartmann, 1961a). The button-shaped bodies at the terminations of the dendrites referred to by the histologists (Billingham, 1948; Masson, 1948a) are not distinguished in the electron micrographs. The surface of the keratinocytes facing the melanocytes are also smooth. The intercellular space between the two cell types is along their whole surface mainly very narrow (Figs. 49 and 51).

The electron-microscopic studies carried out have distinctly shown that the melanocytes are not attached to the adjacent keratinocytes or to the basement membrane by desmosomes or junctional desmosomes (Clark and Hibbs, 1958; Odland, 1958; Charles and Ingram, 1959; Birbeck, Breathnach and Everall, 1961; Zelickson and Hartmann, 1961a; Birbeck, 1962; Figs. 49 and 51). Birbeck (1962) points out that in spite of the absence of junctional desmosomes the melanocytes are firmly attached to the basement membrane, so that a special mechanism must be involved. In the retinal melanocytes desmosomes have been demonstrated (Moyer, 1961). Birbeck (1962) interprets the differences in the skin and the eye as being due to differences in the embryological development of the melanocytes in these two tissues.

The melanocytes are bounded by a plasma membrane (Clark and Hibbs, 1958; Odland, 1958; Charles and Ingram, 1959; Drochmans, 1960a; Birbeck, Breathnach and Everall, 1961; Zelickson and Hartmann, 1961a; Birbeck, 1962). This displays the same ultrastructure as that of the keratinocytes, with an asymmetric triple-layered pattern and a thickness of 80 to 90 Å.

In histological stains such as hematoxylin and eosin the nuclei of the melanocytes appear basophilic and darker than those of the keratinocytes, whereas the cytoplasm has a clear appearance (MASSON, 1948a, b; LEVER, 1961; SHUKLA, 1965). Also in electron micrographs the nuclei of the melanocytes are often more opaque than those in the adjacent basal cells (Fig. 51; cf. also electron micrographs by ODLAND, 1958; BREATHNACH, GOODWIN and WYLLIE, 1964). A nuclear mem-

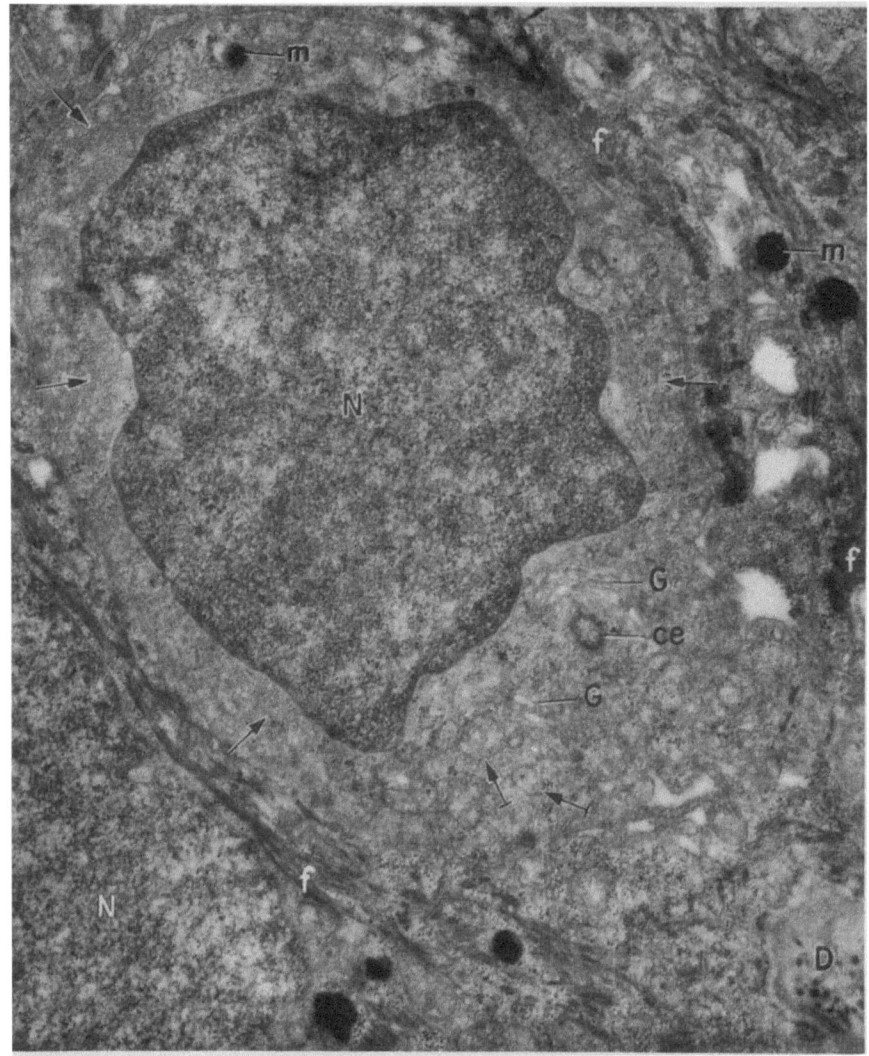

Fig. 49. Human abdominal epidermis. Survey of a melanocyte with rather light-stained cytoplasm. Large number of longitudinally and cross-sectioned bundles of filaments (→). The filament bundles are on the whole less opaque than the epidermal fibrils (f). ce centriole, mitochondria (↦), G Golgi apparatus, m melanin granule, N nucleus. The cell surface of the melanocyte is even, as are also the adjacent surfaces of the keratinocytes. No desmosomes are here visible. D dermis. × 20,000

brane of smooth regular outline is usually seen (ODLAND, 1958; BIRBECK, BREATHNACH and EVERALL, 1961; ZELICKSON and HARTMANN, 1961a). The nuclear membrane is triple-layered (ZELICKSON and HARTMANN, 1961a).

The content of the various cellular components may vary conspicuously in the different melanocytes. In the electron-microscopic studies it has repeatedly been pointed out that the melanocytes lack the type of filaments that characterize the keratinocytes (BARNICOT and BIRBECK, 1958; CLARK and HIBBS, 1958;

ODLAND, 1958; CHARLES and INGRAM, 1959; DROCHMANS, 1960a; BIRBECK, BREATHNACH and EVERALL, 1961; ZELICKSON and HARTMANN, 1961; BIRBECK, 1962). In a few investigations, however, filaments are distinguished also in the melanocytes (DROCHMANS, 1960a; BREATHNACH, 1963; Figs. 49 and 50). The filaments have a diameter of about 70 Å, and occur in the perikaryon as well as in the dendrites. They do not show any relationship to other cellular components (DROCHMANS, 1960a). DROCHMANS considers that they are not epidermal filaments because they do not show any tendency to approach the plasma membrane or to aggregate into bundles. In my own studies the filaments seem not to occur

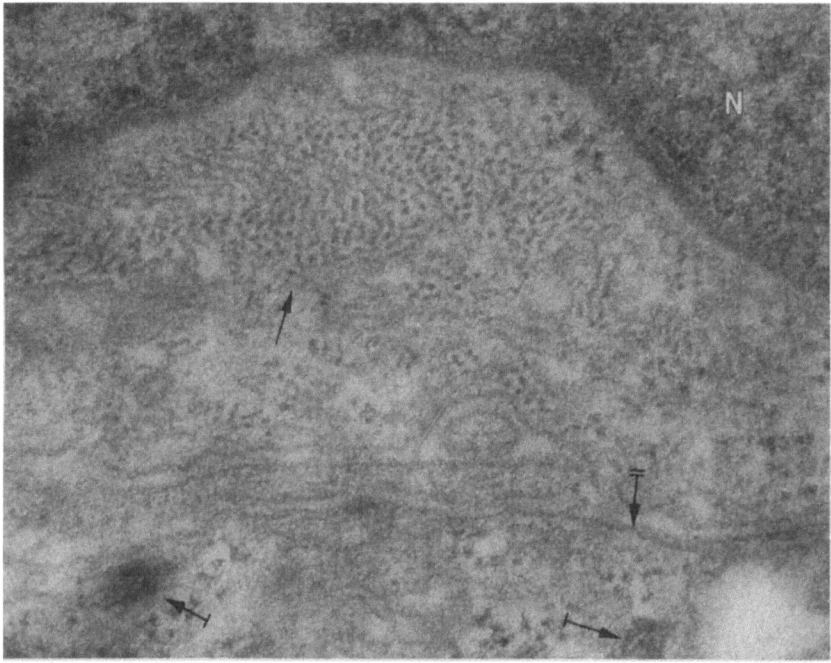

Fig. 50. Part of a melanocyte showing bundles of longitudinally and cross-sectioned filaments (→). The bundles are less opaque than the epidermal fibrils (⊢→) but the individual filaments are rather well stained. N nucleus, narrow intercellular space (⊢→). × 103,000

isolated, but are everywhere arranged in fibrils (Figs. 49 and 50) in a way similar to that of the filaments in the keratinocytes of the stratum basale. Rather do the two types of fibrils differ with respect to their stainability by the metal salts used for the fixation and staining of the tissue, to the varying occurrence of the fibrils in the melanocytes, and to the different filament diameter.

Mitochondria may be so abundant that they almost entirely fill the cytoplasm (CLARK and HIBBS, 1958; ZELICKSON and HARTMANN, 1961a), or, again they are not very numerous (BIRBECK, BREATHNACH and EVERALL, 1961). While CLARK and HIBBS (1958) point out that they are larger than the mitochondria in adjacent keratinocytes, BIRBECK, BREATHNACH and EVERALL (1961) mention that they are small, but no numerical data are given.

The Golgi apparatus is well developed (BARNICOT and BIRBECK, 1958; CLARK and HIBBS, 1958; CHARLES and INGRAM, 1959; DROCHMANS, 1960a; BIRBECK, BREATHNACH and EVERALL, 1961; ZELICKSON and HARTMANN, 1961a; BIRBECK, 1962). It consists of large, flattened, smooth-walled vesicles (4100 Å × 900 Å) which are in their turn surrounded by numerous small, round (500 Å), smooth-walled vesicles (ZELICKSON and HARTMANN, 1961a). The Golgi apparatus seems usually to occur on the far side of the nucleus from the basement both in the epidermis (BARNICOT and BIRBECK, 1958) and in the hair-bulb (BIRBECK, 1963), but in the epidermis it may also be observed in other areas of the cell.

Alpha-cytomembranes (for definition see SJÖSTRAND, 1956a, b; cf. also SJÖSTRAND, 1964), or the so-called rough cisternae of the endoplasmic reticulum (cf. PORTER, 1963; FAWCETT, 1966), are usually well developed in the melanocytes (CLARK and HIBBS, 1958; BIRBECK, 1962, 1963).

MASSON (1948a, b), ZIMMERMANN and CORNBLEET (1948) and BILLINGHAM and MEDAWAR (1953) have suggested that in the "white dendritic cell" or "clear cell", the melanin pigment is restricted to the dendrites, whereas in the heavily pigmented melanocytes the melanin granules are densely distributed throughout the perikaryon and its branches.

MASSON (1948a), using ammonium silver nitrate, has found that the melanin pigment of the keratinocytes and of the branches of the melanocytes darkens before that of the perikaryon. The melanocytes of the palm and sole contain reducing melanin mainly in the dendrites. But with reduced silver nitrate the melanocytes appear filled with granules (MASSON, 1948a). MASSON assumes that these granules represent an early primitive form of melanin granules and he has used the term "premelanin" introduced by HORTEGA for this primitive form of melanin granule. He further believes that premelanin granules are also present in the melanocytes rich in melanin-pigment, and that they appear first in the perikaryon and come to maturity during their migration into the dendrites of the melanocytes.

The site of melanogenesis has for a long time been a controversial question, and different theories have been advanced. MEIROWSKY (1908) and MEIROWSKY and FREEMAN (1951) have suggested that the melanin granules consist of extruded nuclear substance. This hypothesis has not been verified with electron microscopy (BARNICOT and BIRBECK, 1958). According to GODA (1928/1931), DU BUY, WOODS, BURK and LACKEY (1949), and WOODS (1959), the granules are of mitochondrial origin. Electron-microscopic studies of normal and pathologic melanocytes in the epidermis, in the hair and the eye have, however, clearly shown that the melanin granules and the mitochondria are two distinctly separated organelles (BARNICOT and BIRBECK, 1958; BIRBECK and BARNICOT, 1959; DALTON, 1959; MOYER, 1961). These observations have been further strongly supported by combined biochemical and electron-microscopic investigations on mouse melanoma (BAKER, BIRBECK, BLASCHKO, FITZPATRICK and SEIJI, 1960; SEIJI, FITZPATRICK and BIRBECK, 1961; SEIJI, SHIMAO, BIRBECK and FITZPATRICK, 1963). In a high — resolution autoradiographic study of mouse melanoma the mitochondria seemed not to be of any importance for the melanogenesis (ZELICKSON, HIRSCH and HARTMANN, 1965).

A third theory has been proposed by DANNEEL and LUBNOW (1936), LUBNOW (1939), and GÜTTES (1953), according to whom the Golgi apparatus plays a role in the formation of the melanin granules. BOWEN (1929) localized the synthesis of the granules to the Golgi apparatus. KIRKMAN and SEVERINGHAUS (1938), on the other hand, assumed that the Golgi apparatus concentrated a protein synthesized elsewhere into visible granules. On the basis of electron-microscopic studies of melanocytes in normal human epidermis, and in normal and albino hair (BARNICOT and BIRBECK, 1958; BIRBECK and BARNICOT, 1959; BIRBECK, 1962, 1963) and of melanocytes in mouse melanoma (WELLING and SIEGEL, 1959, 1960, 1963; HU and CARDELL, 1964) it has been postulated that the early stages of the melanin granules occur in the Golgi apparatus.

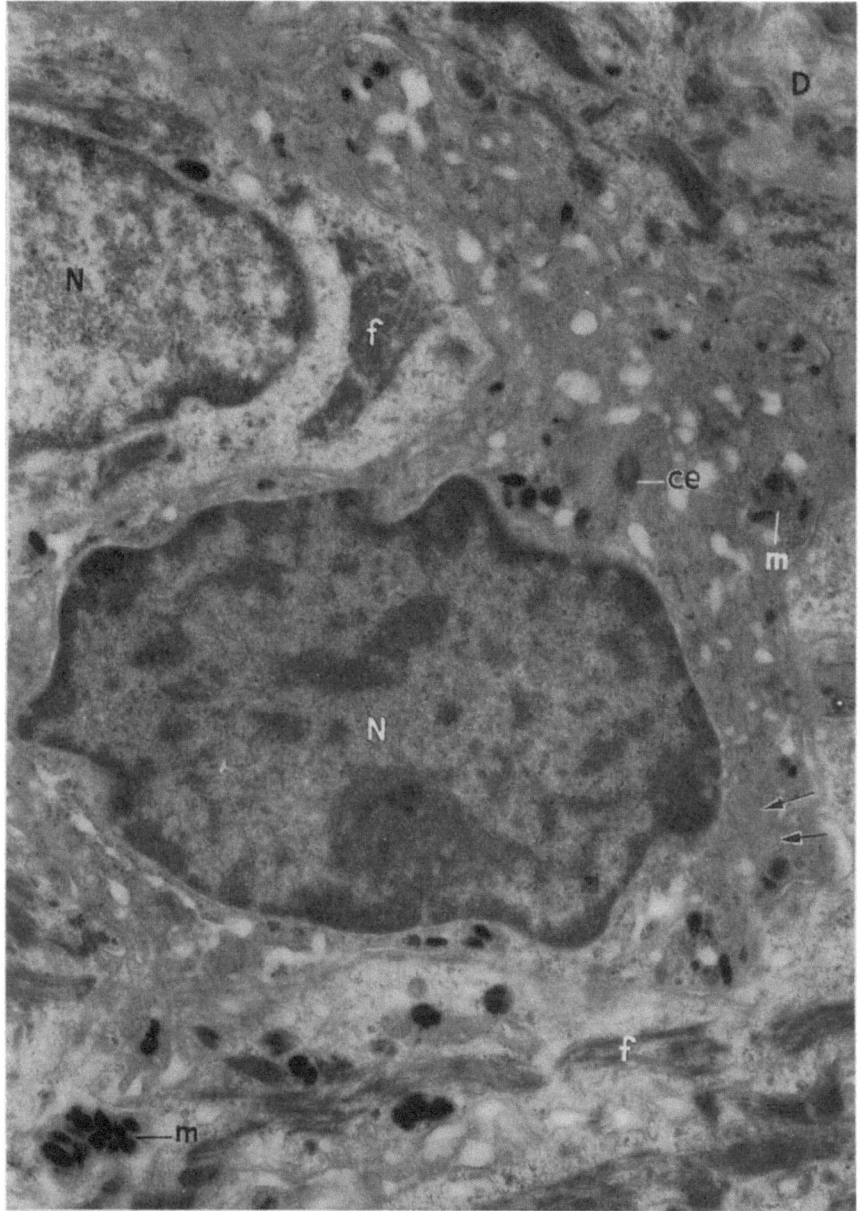

Fig. 51. Survey of a melanocyte showing a rather opaque cytoplasm as compared with that of the adjacent keratinocytes. Also the nucleus (N) is more darkly stained. The cell surface of the melanocyte and the adjacent surfaces of the circumambient keratinocytes are rather even and the intercellular space is narrow. A fairly large number of melanin granules (m) occur. Mitochondria (→), f epidermal fibrils, ce centriole, D dermis. × 16,000.
(From BRODY, 1964b. Courtesy of Academic Press Inc., New York-London)

In an electron-microscopic study of the melanocytes in human hair hollow, ellipsoidal bodies, 0.25 to 0.5 μ in size, and bounded by a thin moderately opaque wall, as well as distinct, large, melanin granules, were observed (BARNICOT, BIRBECK and CUCKOW, 1955). The authors consider the ellipsoidal bodies as formative stages to the large melanin granules. In further electron-microscopic investigations of the melanocytes in the epidermis (BARNICOT and BIRBECK, 1958; CLARK and

HIBBS, 1958) and in the hair (BARNICOT and BIRBECK, 1958; BIRBECK and BARNICOT, 1958) small, dense granules were found besides the melanin granules. According to CLARK and HIBBS these dense granules are neither melanin granules nor mitochondria. BARNICOT and BIRBECK (1958) and BIRBECK and BARNICOT (1959) point to their similarity to the ellipsoidal bodies earlier described by

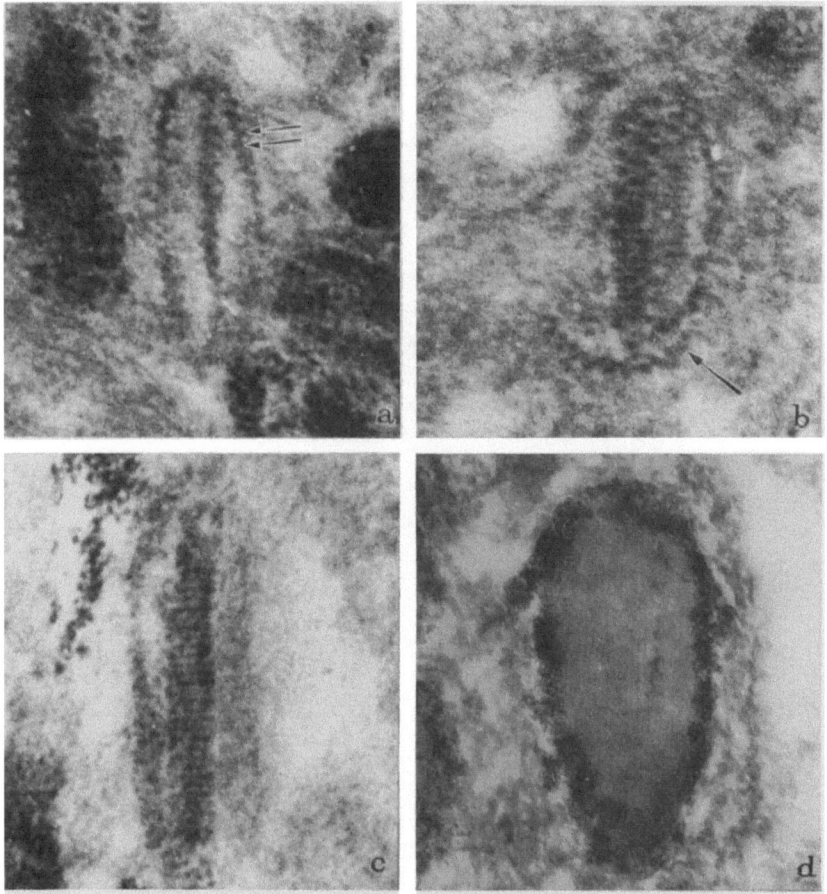

Fig. 52 shows different developmental stages of the melanosomes in human skin. a) a primary fibrillar melanosome which shows 3 coiled fibrils with a pitch (arrows) of about 110 Å. b) and c) striated melanosomes: a condensation of the fibrils seems to occur along the axis of the melanosomes. Some coiled peripheral fibrils remain free and present a spiral configuration (b, arrow). d) dense melanosome with a central core and an osmiophilic shell. Stain on blocks: phosphotungstic acid, embedded in methacrylate. × 150,000. (From DROCHMANS, 1966.
Courtesy of Springer, Berlin-Göttingen-Heidelberg)

BARNICOT, BIRBECK and CUCKOW (1955). In the hair and in the epidermis they are stated to appear in the Golgi region, where no mature melanin granules are found. BARNICOT and BIRBECK (1958) and BIRBECK and BARNICOT (1959) therefore postulate that the Golgi apparatus may be regarded as a zone of melanin formation in accordance with the light-microscopic view by BOWEN (1929), DANEEL and LUBNOW (1936), KIRKMAN and SEVERINGHAUS (1938), LUBNOW (1939) and GÜTTES (1953). Between the Golgi region and the peripherally located mature melanin granules intermediate granular stages have been seen in the dark hair melanocyte (BIRBECK and BARNICOT, 1959).

In normal human epidermis and more distinctly in hyperplastic epidermis, such as that found in condyloma, DROCHMANS (1960a) describes two stages of the melanin granules: an earlier stage, the "light" melanin granule, and a later stage, the "dense" melanin granule. He suggests that the material constituting the light melanin granule represents the main structural component. The granule is formed of a basic framework in which a striated pattern appears with a line spacing of about 70 Å. In the dense granule a similar pattern is present. In the basic framework a diffuse greyish substance is embedded which is responsible for the compact dense appearance of the granule. The dense granule is further surrounded by a shell of a coarse, non-organized granular material (cf. also text to Figs. 52 a—d).

For the melanocytes of human hair a more detailed description of the melanogenesis has been presented by BIRBECK and BARNICOT (1959) and BIRBECK (1962, 1963). In the Golgi region the earliest morphological structures are small vesicles with a diameter of about 0.05 μ. These vesicles are transformed into large vesicles by fusion or by growth. Initially the large vesicles are round to oval. Later, they become elongated until they are approximately the size of a mature melanin granule. At the same time a system of inner membranes appear. The outer limiting membrane displays a triple-layered pattern, where the intermediate light layer is about 70 Å thick. The inner membranes do not show this ultrastructure. They display either a concentric cylindrical arrangement or appear as a single membrane wrapped in a spiral. A fine structure is imprinted upon the inner membrane and this structure is similar to the striated pattern described by DROCHMANS (1960a). The structure appears in the hair melanin as an orthogonal array of particles (BIRBECK, 1963). The spacing of the particles is about 80 Å in the direction along the length of the inner membrane. BIRBECK (1963) suggests that the inner membranes are made up of units with the dimensions 80 Å $\times$ 30 Å. Each unit contains one site of melanin synthesis. At a later stage in the development the internal membranes show an increase in thickness and opacity (BIRBECK and BARNICOT, 1959). The spaces between the membranes become filled and the mature melanin granule appears highly opaque and structureless.

A similar development of the melanin granules has also been shown by WELLINGS and SIEGEL (1963) and by HU and CARDELL (1964) in human, mouse and Syrian hamster melanomas.

4. The Transfer Process of Melanin Granules

MASSON (1948a) considers the melanocyte as a glandular cell. Its secretion product, the mature melanin granule, is not secreted directly externally like that of the exocrine glands or in vessels like that of the endocrine glands but in other cells. MASSON has therefore coined the expression "cytochrine" for the dispersion of the melanin granules to the keratinocytes (BILLINGHAM, 1948; MASSON, 1948a; cf. also survey of BILLINGHAM and SILVERS, 1960).

MAGNIN and ROTHMAN (1957) were the first to demonstrate that the keratinocytes may influence the production and transfer of the melanin granules. From a physiological viewpoint FINDLAY (1961) has discussed the reciprocal relation between the epidermis and its degree of pigmentation. FITZPATRICK and BREATHNACH (1963) consider that the melanocytes and keratinocytes structurally and functionally constitute a unit, which they call the "epidermal melanin unit". This unit is defined as a "melanocyte in a functional association with a group of keratinocytes, which latter may vary in numbers". The relative ratio of melanocytes to keratinocytes shows certain regional variations (SZABÓ, 1959b). In the epidermis of the cheek there are four to five keratinocytes to each melanocyte, whereas in that of the arm and thigh about ten to twelve keratinocytes. In the latter two sites the number of keratinocytes to each melanocyte may, however, vary.

The actual mechanism of the transfer process of the melanin granules is not yet known. The granules may reach the keratinocytes through active ingestion by the keratinocytes and/or by an active inoculation or penetration by the dendritic processes of the melanocytes.

In vitro studies have shown an active uptake of melanin granules by the keratinocytes (MATSUMOTO, 1918; SMITH, 1921; LEWIS, POMERAT and EZELL, 1949; CRUICKSHANK and HARCOURT, 1964).

In the electron microscopic study of hair BARNICOT and BIRBECK (1958) sometimes observed that the ends of the dendrites containing aggregates of granules were lying in the cytoplasm of the cortical cell. Occasionally the clump of granules was surrounded by a distinct cell membrane. BARNICOT and BIRBECK suggest that together with the melanin granules other cellular constituents of the melanocytes may be transferred to the keratinocytes. DROCHMANS (1960b, c), who has performed an electron-microscopic study on human epidermis, assumes that the transfer of melanin granules occurs through the penetration or invagination of the keratinocyte by the dendrites of the melanocyte. The dendrites then become detached. SWIFT (1964) believes that the granules are excreted from the end of the dendrites into the intercellular space and are subsequently phagocytized by the cortical cell. Neither the *in vitro* nor the electron-microscopic studies, however, reveal to what extent the penetration of the dendritic processes is of importance for the mechanism of transfer.

STRAILE (1964) has demonstrated that a dispersion of melanin granules may also occur when the melanocytes of the hair follicle have lost their dendrites, as is the case after exposing the skin to X-rays. The dendrites thus seem not to be essential for the cytochrine process as such. The occurrence of dendrites may at least mean that a larger surface for the process of transfer is available.

5. Enzymatic Activity

a) Phenol-Oxydase

FITZPATRICK, BECKER, LERNER and MONTGOMERY (1950) were the first to demonstrate the presence of phenol-oxydase (earlier tyrosinase, phenolase) in human epidermis, thus providing the decisive proof that an enzymatic process forms the basis for the melanin formation in the melanocytes.

The enzyme phenol-oxydase is alone responsible for the conversion of tyrosine into melanin (PEARSE, 1960; KARLSON, 1966). Phenol-oxydase transfers tyrosine into Dopa (=dihydroxyphenylalanine) and oxidizes this diphenol into quinone. Through a number of sequential reactions which take place in part spontaneously, without enzyme catalysis, there finally arises the black or brown-black melanin (cf. KARLSON, 1966). Several physico-chemical factors are of importance for the reaction, such as copper as activator, sulfhydryl groups as inhibitors, the temperature, the pH-value, the electrolyte concentration (see survey by HORSTMANN, 1957), as well as hormonal influence (LERNER, 1955, 1960, 1964; SNELL, 1964). For the biochemistry of the melanogenesis the reader must be referred to summarizing presentations (LERNER and FITZPATRICK, 1950; BECKER, FITZPATRICK and MONTGOMERY, 1952; FITZPATRICK and LERNER, 1954; VOLLAND, 1954; HORSTMANN, 1957; FITZPATRICK, 1958, 1959; MASON, 1959; YASUNOBU, 1959; THOMSON, 1962; SWAN, 1963).

For the histochemical visualization of the melanocytes in human epidermis the phenol-oxydase- and the Dopa-reactions have been used (SZABÓ, 1954, 1959b;

Staricco and Pinkus, 1957; Pinkus, Staricco, Kropp and Fan, 1959). Mishima (1960) has elaborated a combined method with the Dopa-reaction and Masson's (1948a) ammoniated silver nitrate method for the demonstration of melanin, premelanin and phenol-oxydase sites.

In combined biochemical and electron-microscopic investigations of mouse melanoma Seiji, Fitzpatrick and Birbeck (1961), Seiji, Shimao, Fitzpatrick and Birbeck (1961), Seiji, Shimao, Birbeck and Fitzpatrick (1963), and Seiji and Iwashita (1965) have demonstrated phenol-oxydase activity in the ribosomes, the rough surface membranes (alpha-cytomembranes), the smooth surface membranes (Golgi apparatus) and in the melanosomes. On the basis of these findings the authors suggest that phenol-oxydase is synthesized in the ribosomes associated with the rough cisternae of the endoplasmic reticulum (alpha-cytomembranes) and subsequently transferred to the Golgi apparatus. Electron microscopy (Wellings and Siegel, 1963; Hu and Cardell, 1964) and electron-microscopic autoradiography (Zelickson, Hirsch and Hartmann, 1965) on mouse melanoma and electron microscopy on duck embryo melanocytes (Koecke, 1966) also lend support to the hypothesis that the alpha-cytomembranes and the Golgi apparatus are involved in the process of melanization.

On the basis of combined biochemical and electron-microscopic studies three intermediate stages have been recognized in the formation of the melanin granules in the mouse melanoma (Seiji, Shimao, Birbeck and Fitzpatrick, 1963). Stage 1 is characterized by the synthesis and condensation of polypeptides into secondary and tertiary structures ("protyrosinase") of the enzymic protein molecules ("intermediate vesicle"). In stage 2 the "protyrosinase" molecules are arranged in an ordered structure ("premelanosome"). Melanin is here not yet synthesized. During this stage the arrangement, shape and size of the premelanosomes are believed to be both species- and site-dependent. In stage 3 the synthesis of melanin starts, and melanin accumulates inside the premelanosome which develops into the "melanosome". Finally with the formation of the melanin granules the melanization process is completed. No phenol-oxydase activity is found in the end product.

Investigations of neoplastic melanocytes (Nakai and Shubik, 1964) and of melanoma (Seiji and Iwashita, 1965) with radioactive dihydroxyphenylalanine have shown that Dopa-C^{14} is only incorporated into the melanosomes, indicating that in malignant melanocytes the melanosomes are the specific site of melanin formation.

In the electron-microscopic studies of the melanocytes in the normal human hair bulb (Birbeck, 1963), in human, mouse and Syrian hamster melanomas (Wellings and Siegel, 1963; Hu and Cardell, 1964) and in the normal duck embryo (Koecke, 1966) premelanosomes, melanosomes and melanin granules have been distinguished. In an electron-microscopic study of the melanocytes in human epidermis Drochmans (1966) has introduced the expressions "primary fibrillar melanosomes", "striated melanosomes" and "dense melanosomes" for the different stages of development (Fig. 52a—d).

b) Adenosintriphosphatase

According to Bradshaw, Wachstein, Spence and Elias (1963) the basal melanocytes and the suprabasal Langerhans cells show the same strong ATPase activity. The authors localize the enzymatic reaction to the mitochondria and the cell membranes. Wolff (1963a, 1964a, b) has also obtained an ATPase reaction in the dendritic cells of the stratum basale, but the ATPase-positive dendritic cells are here fewer in number than those in the suprabasal layers. A comparison between "ATPase"- and "Dopa"-sections shows no agreement in the localization of the ATPase and the Dopa-oxydase reactions. WOLFF (1964b) interprets these observations to mean that either there are only some basal melanocytes which are ATPase positive, or there are no ATPase-active, Dopa-positive melanocytes, but that the cells that give this reaction are basally located Langerhans cells (BREATHNACH, 1963).

In their light- and electron-microscopic investigations of the localization of ATPase in the epidermis of frog and toad skin FARQUHAR and PALADE (1966) demonstrate that the reaction is much heavier along the cell membranes of the basal and suprabasal dendritic cells than along the keratinocytes. The reaction product appears in the intercellular space in close association with the outer leaflet of the plasma membrane. Intracellularly the mitochondria show the strongest reaction.

II. Langerhans Cells
1. Origin

In 1868 LANGERHANS demonstrated a branched cell type in the suprabasal strata of the epidermis which has become known as "Langerhans cell". With respect to the nature and significance of this cell there have been many diverging views. The different theories have been exhaustively reviewed by FERREIRA-MARQUES (1951), BREATHNACH (1965) and WOLFF (1967a, b). According to BREATHNACH (1965) there are two current main theories. One view is that the Langerhans cells represent functional neural elements. According to the other notion they form a stage in the life-cycle of the melanocytes.

The Langerhans cell has been considered as a Schwann cell (FERREIRA-MARQUES, 1951), as a specialized intraepidermal component of the peripheral autonomic neurovegetative system (RICHTER, 1956), and as part of the "neurohormonal" system of the skin (NIEBAUER, 1956; WIEDMANN, 1960, 1963a, b). BREATHNACH (1965) discusses in detail these different theories and comes to the conclusion that there is no substantial evidence for the view that the Langerhans cell represents a neural element in the epidermis.

The resemblance in shape between the Langerhans cells and the melanocytes has led several authors to assume a close relationship between these two types of cell (MASSON, 1948a, 1951; MEDAWAR, 1953; BILLINGHAM and MEDAWAR, 1953; cf. also reviews by FERREIRA-MARQUES, 1951; BILLINGHAM and SILVERS, 1960; BREATHNACH, 1965). MASSON (1951) and MEDAWAR and BILLINGHAM (1953) have suggested that the Langerhans cell is an effete or dead melanocyte.

In vitiliginous human epidermis, cells appearing in the stratum basale seem to replace the basal melanocytes occurring in the normal epidermis (BIRBECK, BREATHNACH and EVERALL, 1961). These cells are indistinguishable from the suprabasal Langerhans cells. On the basis of these observations BREATNACH (1963) has advanced the hypothesis that the basal melanocytes divide into two daughter cells which have the appearance of Langerhans cells. In the normal epidermis one daughter cell is equipped with melanogenic attributes, whereas the other is not, but immediately ascends to the suprabasal strata and is eventually exfoliated. In vitiligo, on the other hand, no daughter cell becomes melanogenic, and this would explain the great frequency of Langerhans cells in the stratum basale of vitiliginous epidermis. BREATHNACH (1964, 1965) has clearly shown that the Langerhans cell is not an effete cell but is engaged in active protein synthesis.

Analogously with the observations in the vitiliginous human epidermis, a basal Langerhans cell-type is also found in the basal layer of the epidermis in the skin of the black-and-white spotted guinea-pig (BREATHNACH, GOODWIN and WYLLIE, 1965).

An important contribution to the discussion of the nature of the Langerhans cells has recently been presented by WOLFF (1967a, b) and WOLFF, WINKELMANN and HOLUBAR (1967). According to these authors the Langerhans cells and the melanocytes form two autochthonous and independent cell systems. This assumption is based on the observations that the Langerhans cells differ from the melanocytes with respect to their ultrastructure, their enzymatic reactions, their quantitative behaviour and their failure to be affected by stimuli which induce considerable changes in the number of melanocytes. Further, the Langerhans cells lack the capacity for pigment production.

The Langerhans cells possess enzymes characteristic for connective tissue (WOLFF, 1967a, b) and are capable of phagocytosis (BREATHNACH and WYLLIE, 1966; MISHIMA, 1966). WOLFF (1967a, b) and WOLFF, WINKELMANN and HOLUBAR (1967) also point to the fact that the cells show an ultrastructure identical to that of the histiocytes in Histiocytosis X (BASSET, MALLET and TURIAF, 1965; BASSET and TURIAF, 1965; TURIAF and BASSET, 1965; BASSET and NEZELOF, 1966; TURIAF and BASSET, 1966). These different data may imply a probable mesenchymal nature of the Langerhans cells (WOLFF, 1967a, b; WOLFF, WINKELMANN and HOLUBAR, 1967).

According to WOLFF (1967a, b), different findings also favor the assumption of a direct functional correlation between the Langerhans cells and the keratinocytes. To express this functional correlation WOLFF and WINKELMANN (in press) have suggested the term "epidermal-Langerhans-cell-unit", on analogy with the expression "epidermal-melanin-unit" coined by FITZPATRICK and BREATHNACH (1963) for the close relationship between the melanocytes and the keratinocytes. JARRETT and SPEARMAN (1964) have advanced the hypothesis that the Langerhans cells may be intimately associated with the cells of the stratum intermedium, and may add their enzymatic activity to that already produced by the keratinocytes themselves.

2. Morphology

The Langerhans cells are equipped with dendrites of the same number and appearance as the basal melanocytes (MEDAWAR, 1953). No dendrites have been observed above the stratum intermedium. With respect to the ultrastructure and thickness of the plasma membrane the two cells agree. Although the Langerhans cells are not attached to the surrounding keratinocytes, the intercellular space is usually very narrow (Fig. 53).

One of the characteristic features of the Langerhans cell is the marked indentations of the nuclei (BARNICOT and BIRBECK, 1958; BREATHNACH, 1965; Fig. 53). The intranuclear material is finely granulated and a nucleolus is present. The nuclear membrane is distinct.

Filaments typical for the keratinocytes are absent (BARNICOT and BIRBECK, 1958; CLARK and HIBBS, 1958; ZELICKSON and HARTMANN, 1961; BREATHNACH, 1964, 1965), but fine filaments of unknown nature similar to those in the basal melanocytes (DROCHMANS, 1960a; Figs. 49 and 50) do also occur in the Langerhans cells (BREATHNACH, 1965). Golgi apparatus, centriolar bodies, mitochondria and endoplasmic reticulum are present to varying extents.

In the Langerhans cells rod-shaped organelles with curved ends and a line exhibiting 90 Å striation running down the centre have been shown (BIRBECK, BREATHNACH and EVERALL, 1961; BREATHNACH, 1965; Fig. 54). BIRBECK, BREATH-

NACH and EVERALL (1961) consider the rod-shaped structures as sectional profiles of disc-shaped granules which in a plane cut at right angles to their surface show a two-dimensional array of particles with a spacing of 90 Å in both directions.

A system of vesicles and vacuoles similar to those in the basal melanocytes is seen in the cells (Fig. 54). They have a diameter of 0.1 to 0.2 μ and are bounded

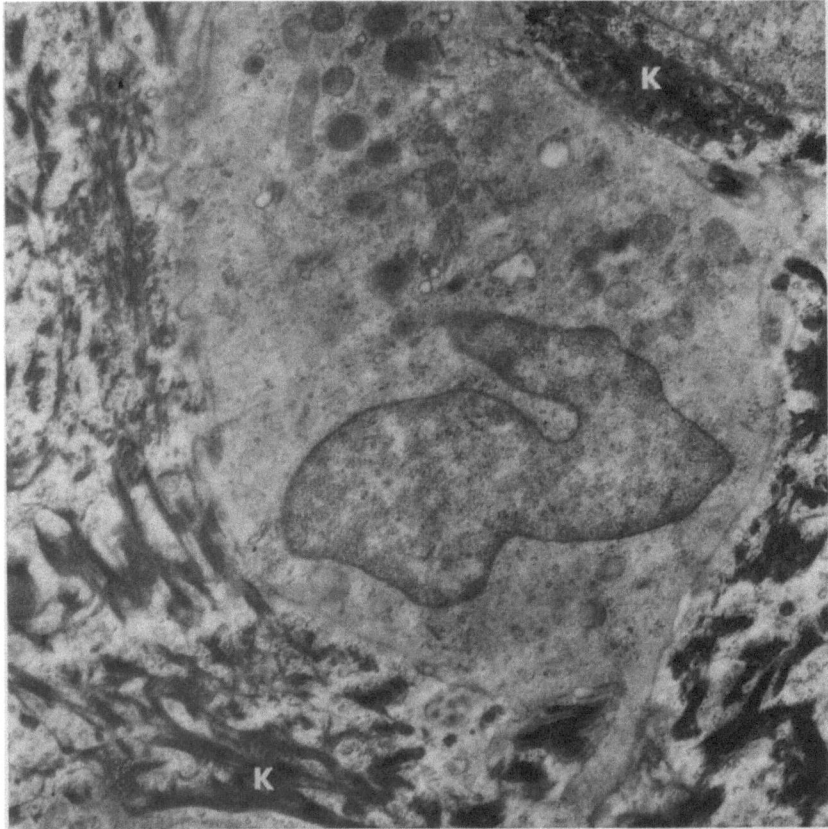

Fig. 53. Langerhans cell from stratum spinosum of human epidermis. Note indented nucleus, "clear" cytoplasm due to the absence of epidermal fibrils which are abundantly present in adjacent keratinocytes (K), and cytoplasmic organelles of various character. × 12,000. (From BREATHNACH, 1965. Courtesy of Int. Rev. Cyt., Academic Press Inc., New York-London)

by a 150 Å thick membrane. The disc-shaped granules are closely associated with these structures and seem to be formed by a transformation of the vesicles. A similar close association is also found between the disc-shaped organelles and the plasma membrane (BREATHNACH, 1965). According to BIRBECK, BREATHNACH and EVERALL (1961) and BREATHNACH (1965), the disc-shaped granules may perhaps represent a modified type of pre-melanosomes.

ZELICKSON (1963) and BREATHNACH (1965) have also demonstrated a rounded or oval granule containing uniformly dispersed fine particles. Their diameter is approximately 0.3 μ.

In the Langerhans cells are also found sacs of varying size with ill-defined inclusions, small, round bodies with lamellated or whorled internal membranes, and small vesicles (BREATHNACH, 1964, 1965). BREATHNACH (1965) points out that these structures are similar in appearance to the lysosomes. In some of them rod-shaped profiles have been distinguished (BREATHNACH, 1965).

According to ZELICKSON (1963), the Langerhans cells also contain melanin granules, though this finding has not been confirmed (BIRBECK, BREATHNACH and EVERALL, 1961; BREATHNACH, 1965).

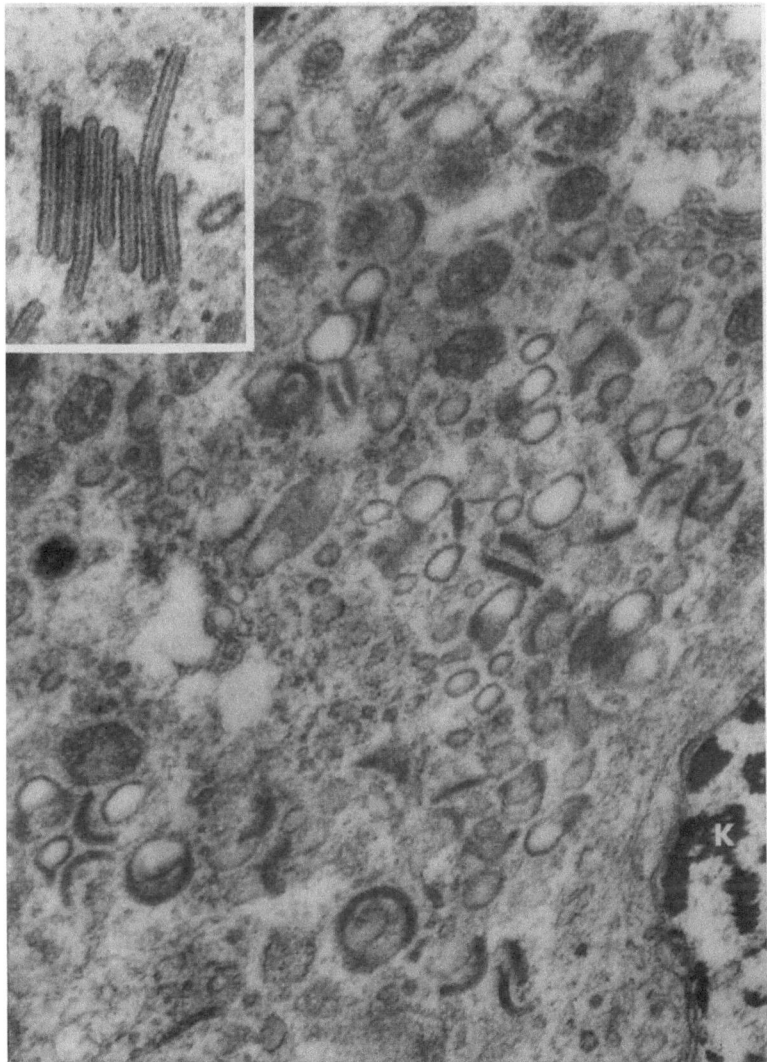

Fig. 54. Cytoplasm of Langerhans cell. Vesicles and rod-shaped profiles are present. K portion of adjacent keratinocyte. × 32,000. Inset: a cluster of rod-shaped profiles from the cytoplasm of another Langerhans cell. × 66,000. (From BREATHNACH, 1965. Courtesy of Int. Rev. Cyt., Academic Press Inc., New York-London)

3. Enzymatic Activity

With histochemistry the enzymes adenosine triphosphatase (ATPase) (MUSTAKALLIO, 1962; JARRETT and RILEY, 1963; WOLFF, 1963a, 1964a, b; BRADSHAW, WACHSTEIN, SPENCE and ELIAS, 1963; CORMANE and KALSBEEK, 1963), nonspecific esterases (JARRETT and RILEY, 1963), adenosine diphosphatase (ADPase) and inosine triphosphatase (CORMANE and KALSBEEK, 1963; WOLFF, 1964a, b), aminopeptidase (WOLFF, 1963b, 1964b), and acetylcholinesterase (LYNE and CHASE, 1966) have been demonstrated in the Langerhans cells.

According to WOLFF (1963b, 1964b), these cells show a more intense aminopeptidase activity than do the keratinocytes, and the "aminopeptidase-method" may therefore be used for the histochemical visualization of the Langerhans cells.

MUSTAKALLIO (1962), WOLFF (1963a, 1964a, b) and JARRETT and RILEY (1963) hold the view that the ATPase reaction is particularly high in the Langerhans cells. BRADSHAW, WACHSTEIN, SPENCE and ELIAS (1963), on the other hand, have demonstrated that the basal melanocytes and the suprabasal Langerhans cells exhibit the same strong reaction. These results agree with those arrived at by FARQUHAR and PALADE (1966) on frog epidermis. In all histochemical investigations, moreover, it has been shown that the dendritic cells react more strongly than do the keratinocytes. The "ATPase-method" seems therefore to be useful for a histochemical visualization of the dendritic cells in the epidermis, irrespective of whether these are melanocytes or Langerhans cells. Concerning further data on the morphology and histochemistry of the Langerhans cells the reader is referred to the comprehensive survey recently presented by WOLFF (1967a, b).

References

AAVIK, O. R.: Cholinesterases in human skin. J. invest. Derm. 24, 103—106 (1955). — ADACHI, K., and W. MONTAGNA: Histology and cytochemistry of human skin. XXII. Sites of leucine aminopeptidase. J. invest. Derm. 37, 145—152 (1961). — ADLER, E., H. v. EULER, and G. GÜNTHER: Enzymatische Aldehyd-Dismutation und Alkohol-Dehydrierung. Sv. Vet. Akad. Arkiv Kemi 12, Nr 54, 1—7 (1938). — ADOLPH, W. E., R. F. BAKER, and G. M. LEIBY: Electron microscope study of epidermal fibers. Science 113, 685—686 (1951). — ALBERTINI, A. v.: Pflasterepithelzellen im Phasenkontrastbild. Acta anat. (Basel) 1, 463—468 (1946). — ALEXANDER, P., and R. F. HUDSON: Wool: Its chemistry and physics. London: Chapman & Hall Ltd. 1954. — ALLEN, A. C.: A reorientation on the histogenesis and clinical significance of cutaneous nevi and melanomas. Cancer (Philad.) 2, 28—56 (1949). — Malignant melanoma. A clinicopathological analysis of the criteria for diagnosis and prognosis. Cancer (Philad.) 6, 1—45 (1953). — ANDREASEN, E.: On the occurrence of the lymphocytes in the normal epidermis. Acta derm.-venereol. (Stockh.) 32, Suppl. 29, 17—21 (1952). — ANDREW, W.: The role of lymphocytes in the normal epidermis. Anat. Rec. 103, 419 (1949). — Age changes in the skin of Wistar institute rats with particular reference to the epidermis. Amer. J. Anat. 89, 283—319 (1951). — ANDREW, W., and N. V. ANDREW: Lymphocytes in the normal epidermis of the rat and of man. Anat. Rec. 104, 217—241 (1949). — Lymphocytes in normal epidermis of young, older, middleaged and senile rats. J. Geront. 9, 412—420 (1954). — APPELMANS, F., R. WATTIAUX, and C. DE DUVE: Tissue fractionation studies. 5. The association of acid phosphatase with a special class of cytoplasmic granules in rat liver. Biochem. J. 59, 438—445 (1955). — ARGYRIS, F. S.: The distribution of succinic dehydrogenase and non-specific esterase in mouse skin throughout the hair cycle. Anat. Rec. 125, 105—114 (1956). — ASTBURY, W. T.: Artificial protein fibres: their conception and preparation. Nature (Lond.) 155, 501—503 (1945). — Introduction to A discussion on the structure of proteins. Proc. roy. Soc. B 141, 1—9 (1953a). — The forms of biological molecules. In: Essays on growth and form, presented to D'Arcy Wentworth Thompson (W. E. LE GROS CLARK, and P. B. MEDAWAR, eds.), p. 309—354 (1953b). — ASTBURY, W. T., and S. DICKINSON: α—β-intramolecular transformation of myosin. Nature (Lond.) 135, 95 (1935a). — α—β transformation of muscle protein in situ. Nature (Lond.) 135, 765 (1935b). — ASTBURY, W. T., and A. STREET: X-ray studies of the structure of hair, wool, and related fibers. I. General. Phil. Trans. A 230, 75—101 (1931). — ASTBURY, W. T., and H. J. WOODS: X-ray studies of the structure of hair, wool, and related fibers. II. The molecular structure and elastic properties of hair keratin. Phil. Trans. A 232, 333—394 (1934). — AUFHAMMER: Quoted from P. G. UNNA: In: Handbuch der speziellen Pathologie und Therapie (H. v. ZIEMSSEN, Hrsg.), Bd. XIV, Teil 1, S. 1—114. Leipzig F. C. W. Vogel 1883.

BAILEY, K., W. T. ASTBURY, and K. M. RUDALL: Fibrinogen and fibrin as members of the keratin-myosin group. Nature (Lond.) 151, 716—717 (1943). — BAKER, R. V., M. S. C. BIRBECK, H. BLASCHKO, T. B. FITZPATRICK, and M. SEIJI: Melanin granules and mitochondria. Nature (Lond.) 187, 392—394 (1960). — BARGEN, G. v.: Elektronenmikroskopische Untersuchung der Kaninchenhaut (Epidermis). Z. Zellforsch. 50, 459—471 (1959). — BARNICOT, N. A., and M. S. C. BIRBECK: The electron microscopy of human melanocytes and melanin granules. In: The biology of hair growth (W. MONTAGNA and R. A. ELLIS, eds.), p. 239—253. New York: Academic Press 1958. — BARNICOT, N. A., M. S. C. BIRBECK, and

F. W. Cuckow: The electron microscopy of human hair pigments. Ann. hum. Genet. 19, 231—249 (1955). — Barrnett, R. J.: The distribution of esterolytic activity in the tissues of the albino rat as demonstrated with indoxyl acetate. Anat. Rec. 114, 577—599 (1952). — The histochemical distribution of protein-bound sulfhydryl groups. J. nat. Cancer Inst. 13, 905—925 (1953). — Lecture given at 3rd Symp. on the biology of the skin, Brown University, 1954, quoted from P. Flesch and A. Satanove. Brit. J. Derm. 67, 343—347 (1955). — Barrnett, R. J., and A. M. Seligman: Histochemical demonstration of esterases by production of indigo. Science 114, 579—582 (1951). — Histochemical demonstration of protein-bound sulfhydryl groups. Science 116, 323—327 (1952a). — Demonstration of protein-bound sulfhydryl and disulfide groups by two new histochemical methods. J. nat. Cancer Inst. (Abstract) 13, 215—216 (1952b). — Histochemical demonstration of sulfhydryl and disulfide groups of protein. J. nat. Cancer Inst. 14, 769—803 (1954). — Barron, E. S. G.: Thiol groups of biological importance. Advanc. Enzymol. 11, 201—266 (1951). — Barron, E. S. G., and G. Kalnitzky: The inhibition of succinoxidase by heavy metals and its reactivations with dithiols. Biochem. J. 41, 346—351 (1947). — Basset, F., R. Mallet et J. Turiaf: Nouvelle mise en évidence, par la microscopie électronique, de particules d'allure virale dans une seconde forme clinique de l'histiocytose X, le granulome éosinophile des l'os. C.R. Acad. Sci (Paris) 261, 5719—5720 (1965). — Basset, F., et C. Nézelof: Présence en microscopie électronique de structures filamenteuses originales dans les lésions pulmonaires et osseuses de l'histiocytose X. Etat actuel de la question. Bull. Soc. méd. Hop. Paris 117, 413—426 (1966). — Basset, F., et J. Turiaf: Identification par la microscopie électronique de particules de nature probablement virale dans liaisons granulomateuses d'une histiocytose "X" pulmonaire. C.R. Acad. Sci. (Paris) 261, 3701 et 3703 (1965). — Baumberger, J.P., V. Suntzeff, and E. V. Cowdry: Methods for the separation of epidermis from dermis and some physiologic and chemical properties of isolated epidermis. J. nat. Cancer Inst. 2, 413—423 (1942). — Becker, S. W.: Melanin pigmentation. A systematic study of the pigment of the human skin and upper mucous membranes, with special consideration of pigmented dendritic cells. Arch. Derm. Syph. (Chic.) 16, 259—290 (1927). — An improved (paraffin section) method for the Dopa reaction. Arch. Derm. Syph. (Chic.) 31, 190—195 (1935). — Becker jr., S. W., T. B. Fitzpatrick, and H. Montgomery: Human melanogenesis: cytology and histology of pigment cells (melanodendrocytes). Arch. Derm. Syph. (Chic.) 65, 511—523 (1952). — Bennett, H. S.: The demonstration of thiol groups in certain tissues by means of a new colored sulfhydryl reagent. Anat. Rec. 110, 231—246 (1951). — Bern, H. A., M. Alfert, and S. M. Blair: Cytochemical studies of keratin formation and of epithelial metaplasia in the rodent vagina and prostate. J. Histochem. Cytochem. 5, 105—119 (1957). — Bern, H. A., J. J. Ellias, P. B. Pickett, T. R. Powers, and M. N. Harkness: The influence of vitamin A on the epidermis. Amer. J. Anat. 96, 419—447 (1955). — Bernard, C.: De la matière glycogène considérés comme condition de développement de certains tissus chez le foetus. J. Physiol. (Paris) 2, 326—337 (1859). — Bernstein, I. A.: Relation of the nucleic acid to protein synthesis in the mammalian epidermis. In: The epidermis (W. Montagna and W. C. Lobitz jr., eds.), p. 471—483. New York and London: Academic Press 1964. — Bersaques, J. de., and S. Rothman: Mechanism of keratin formation. Nature (Lond.) 193, 147—148 (1962). — Berthet, J., and C. de Duve: The existence of a mitochondria-linked, enzymatically inactive form of acid phosphatase in rat-liver tissue. Biochem. J. 50, 174—181 (1951). — Billingham, R. E.: Dendritic cells. J. Anat. (Lond.) 82, 93—109 (1948). — Dendritic cells in pigmented human skin. J. Anat. (Lond.) 83, 109—115 (1949). — Billingham, R. E., and P. B. Medawar: Pigment spread and cell heredity in guinea-pig's skin. Heredity 2, 29—47 (1948). — A study of the branched cells of the mammalian epidermis with special reference to the fate of their division products. Phil. Trans. B 237, 151—171 (1953). — Billingham, R. E., and J. Reynolds: Transplantation studies on sheets of pure epidermal epithelium and on epidermal cell suspensions. Brit. J. plast. Surg. 5, 25—36 (1952). — Billingham, R. E., and W. K. Silvers: The melanocytes of mammals. Quart. Rev. Biol. 35, 1—40 (1960). — Birbeck, M. S. C.: Quoted from E. H.Mercer: Keratin and keratinization. An essay in molecular biology. New York: Pergamon Press 1961. — Electron microscopy of melanocytes. Brit. med. Bull. 18, 220—229 (1962). — Electron microscopy of melanocytes: the fine structure of hair-bulb premelanosomes. In: The pigment cell. Molecular, biological and clinical aspects (V. Riley and J. G. Fortner, eds.). Ann. N.Y. Acad. Sci. 100, 540—547 (1963). — Birbeck, M. S. C., and N. A. Barnicot: Electron microscope studies on pigment formation in human hair follicles. In: Pigment cell biology (M. Gordon, ed.), p. 549—561. New York: Academic Press 1959. — Birbeck, M. S. C., A. S. Breathnach, and J. D. Everall: An electron microscope study of basal melanocytes and high-level clear cells (Langerhans cells) in Vitiligo. J. invest. Derm. 37, 51—64 (1961). — Birbeck, M. S. C., and E. H. Mercer: Electron microscopic, X-ray and birefringence studies on the proteins of the hair follicle. In: Proc. Stockholm Conf. Electron Microscopy 1956 (F. S. Sjöstrand and J. Rhodin, eds.), p.158—160. Stockholm: Almqvist & Wiksell and New York: Academic Press 1957a. — Electron microscopy of the human hair follicle. Part I, Introduction and the hair cortex. J. Biophys. biochem. Cytol. **3**, 203—213 (1957b). — BIRBECK, M. S. C., E. H. MERCER, and N. A. BARNICOT: The structure and formation of pigment granules in human hair. Exp. Cell Res. **10**, 505—514 (1956). — BLASCHKO, A.: Zur Anatomie und Entwicklungsgeschichte der Oberhaut. Arch. Anat. Physiol., Physiol. Abt. (Leipzig), 173—175 (1884). — Beiträge zur Anatomie der Oberhaut. Arch. mikr. Anat. **30**, 495—528 (1887). — Über den Verhornungsprocess (I). Arch. Anat. Physiol., Physiol. Abt. (Leipzig), 366—367 (1889a). — Über den Verhornungsprocess (II). Arch. Anat. Physiol., Physiol. Abt. (Leipzig), 539—540 (1889b). — BLOCH, BR.: Das Problem der Pigmentbildung in der Haut. Arch. Derm. Syph. (Chic.) **124**, 129—208 (1917). — Das Problem der Pigmentbildung in der Haut. In: J. JADASSOHN, Handbuch der Haut- und Geschlechtskrankheiten, Bd. I/1, S. 434—541. Berlin: Springer 1927. — The problem of pigment formation. Amer. J. med. Sci. **177**, 609—618 (1929). — BLOCK, R. J.: The composition of keratins; the amino acid composition of hair, wool, horn and other eukeratins. J. biol. Chem. **128**, 181—186 (1939). — BOSTRÖM, H., E. ODEBLAD, and U. FRIBERG: A qualitative and quantitative autoradiographic study on the uptake of S^{35}-labelled sodium sulphate in the skin of the adult rat. Acta path. microbiol. scand. **32**, 516—521 (1953). — BOURNE, G. H., and H. B. TEWARI: Mitochondria and Golgi apparatus. In: Cytology and cell physiology (G. H. BOURNE, ed.), 3rd ed., p. 377—421. New York and London: Academic Press 1964. — BOWEN, R. H.: Cytology of glandular secretion. Quart. Rev. Biol. **4**, 484—519 (1929). — BRACHET, J.: La detection histochimique des acides pentosenucleiques. Compt. R. Soc. Biol. (Paris) **133**, 88—90 (1940). — Chemical embryology (Transl. by L. G. BARTH). New York: Interscience Publ. 1950. — BRADFIELD, J. R. G.: Glycogen of vertebrate epidermis. Nature (Lond.) **167**, 40—41 (1951). — BRADSHAW, M., M. WACHSTEIN, J. SPENCE, and J. M. ELIAS: Adenosine triphosphatase activity in melanocytes and epidermal cells of human skin. J. Histochem. Cytochem. **11**, 465—473 (1963). — BRAUN-FALCO, O.: Über die Verteilung von Polysacchariden in der Epidermis bei Dermatosen, die mit Akanthose einhergehen. Derm. Wschr. **128**, 1021—1029 (1953). — Histochemische und morphologische Studien an normaler und pathologisch veränderter Haut. Arch. Derm. **198**, 111—198 (1954). — Weitere histochemische Untersuchungen am homogenen Anteil des subepidermalen Grenzstreifens normaler menschlicher Haut. Arch. klin. exp. Derm. **201**, 521—530 (1955). — Über die Fähigkeit der menschlichen Haut zur Polysaccharidsynthese, ein Beitrag zur Histotopochemie der Phosphorylase. Arch. klin. exp. Derm. **202**, 163—170 (1956a). — Beitrag zum histochemischen Nachweis von Esterasen in normaler und psoriatischer Haut. Arch. klin. exp. Derm. **202**, 153—162 (1956b). — Zur Histotopographie der β-Glucuronidase in normaler menschlicher Haut. Arch. klin. exp. Derm. **203**, 61—67 (1956c). — Histochemische Aminopeptidase-Darstellung in normaler Haut, bei Psoriasis, Dermatitis, Basaliom, spinozellulärem Karzinom und Molluscum sebaceum. Derm. Wschr. **134**, 1341—1349 (1956d). — Histochemie des Bindegewebes. Arch. klin. exp. Derm. **206**, 319—363 (1957a). — Über Untersuchungen des Hautbindegewebes mit der Hale-PAS-Reaktion (Ritter und Oleson) unter normalen Bedingungen und bei Erkrankungen des Hautbindegewebes. Acta histochem (Jena) **5**, 10—24 (1957b). — Das Wesen des parakeratotischen Verhornungsmodus aus histochemischer Sicht. Klin. Wschr. **35**, 1182—1184 (1957c). — The histochemistry of Psoriasis. Ann. N.Y. Acad. Sci. **73**, 936—976 (1958). — Die Histochemie der Haut. In: Dermatologie und Venereologie (H. A. GOTTRON u. W. SCHÖNFELD, Hrsg.), Bd. I/1, S. 366—472. Stuttgart: Georg Thieme 1961a. — Zur Histotopographie der Cytochromoxydase in normaler und pathologisch veränderter Haut sowie in Hauttumoren. Arch. klin. exp. Derm. **214**, 176—224 (1961b). — Histochemische Morphologie der abnormalen Verhornung. In: Proc. XII. Intern. Congr. Derm., Washington D.C., 1962 (D. M. PILLSBURY and C. S. LIVINGOOD, eds.), vol. I, p. 416—422. Intern. Congr. Ser. No. 55 Exc. Med. Found. 1963a. — (1963b) quoted from P. RITZENFELD, Arch. klin. exp. Derm. **220**, 261—265 (1964). — Pathologische Veränderungen an Grundsubstanz, Kollagen und Elastica. In: J. JADASSOHN, Ergänzungswerk Handbuch der Haut- und Geschlechtskrankheiten (A. MARCHIONINI, Hrsg.), Bd. I/2, S. 519—651. Berlin-Göttingen-Heidelberg-New York: Springer 1964. — Die Histochemie der Barriere. In: De structura et functione stratorum epidermidis s. d. barrierrae. Proc. 2nd intern. sympos. Brno 1964 (G. LEJHANEC and P. HYBÁŠEK, eds.). Acta Fac. Med. Univ. Brunensis (Lékařska fakulta, Universita J.E. Purkyně, Brno) **16**, 49—64 (1965a). — Diskussion. In: De structura et functione stratorum epidermidis s. d. barrierrae. Proc. 2nd intern. Sympos. Brno 1964 (G. LEJHANEC and P. HYBÁŠEK, eds.). Acta Fac. Med. Univ. Brunensis **16**, 133—134 (1965b). — BRAUN-FALCO, O., A. KINT u. W. VOGELL: Zur Histogenese der Verruca seborrhoica. II. Elektronenmikroskopische Befunde. Arch. klin. exp. Derm. **217**, 627—651 (1963). — BRAUN-FALCO, O., A. LANGNER u. E. CHRISTOPHERS: Über den Einbau von ^{35}S-markiertem Sulfat in die Haut bei Psoriasis (in vitro). Gleichzeitig ein Beitrag zur Frage epidermaler saurer Mucopolysaccharide. Arch. klin. exp. Derm. **224**, 310—317 (1966). — BRAUN-FALCO, O., u. G. PETRY: Zur Feinstruktur der Epidermis bei chronischem nummulärem Ekzem. I. Stratum basale. Arch. klin. exp. Derm. **222**, 219—241 (1965). — Zur Feinstruktur der Epidermis bei chronischem nummulärem Ekzem. II. Stratum spinosum. Arch. klin. exp. Derm. **224**, 63—80 (1966). — BRAUN-FALCO, O., and D. PETZOLD: Über die Histotopie von NADH- und NADPH-Tetrazoliumreduktase in menschlicher Haut. I. Normale Haut. Arch. klin. exp. Derm. **220**, 455—473 (1964). — Zur Frage optimaler Reaktionsbedingungen bei der histochemischen Darstellung von Enzymen des Energie-liefernden Stoffwechsels in der Epidermis. I. Dehydrogenasen. Arch. klin. exp. Derm. **223**, 620—633 (1965). — Über die Histotopie von Ubichinon in menschlicher Haut. I. Normale Haut. Arch. klin. exp. Derm. **224**, 362—372 (1966). — BRAUN-FALCO, O., u. B. RATHJENS: Beitrag zum Studium histochemischer Reaktionen an Keratinen und anderen cutanen Gewebeanteilen. Acta histochem. (Jena) **1**, 82—94 (1954a). — Histochemische Darstellung der Bernsteinsäuredehydrogenase in der menschlichen Haut. Derm. Wschr. **130**, 1271—1276 (1954b). — Über die histochemische Darstellung der Kohlensäureanhydratase in normaler Haut (gleichzeitig ein Beitrag zur Technik ihres Nachweises). Arch. klin. exp. Derm. **201**, 73—82 (1955). — Histochemische Darstellung von Zink in normaler menschlicher Haut. Arch. klin. exp. Derm. **203**, 130—136 (1956). — BRAUN-FALCO, O., u. M. RUPEC: Über das Vorkommen von saurer Phosphatase in Keratohyalin-Granula normaler menschlicher Epidermis. Naturwissenschaften **109**, 1—2 (1965). — BRAUN-FALCO, O,. u. W. VOGELL: Elektronenmikroskopische Untersuchungen zur Dynamik der Acantholyse bei Pemphigus vulgaris. I. Die klinisch normal aussehende Haut in der Umgebung von Blasen mit positivem Nikolski-Phänomen. Arch. klin. exp. Derm. **223**, 328—346 (1965). — Elektronenmikroskopische Untersuchungen zur Dynamik der Acantholyse bei Pemphigus vulgaris. II. Die acantholytische Blase. Arch. klin. exp. Derm. **223**, 533—550 (1966). — BRAUN-FALCO, O., u. G. WEBER: Zur Histo- und Biochemie des epidermalen Intercellularraumes unter normalen und pathologischen Verhältnissen. Arch. klin. exp. Derm. **207**, 459—471 (1958). — BRAUN-FALCO, O., u. W. WINTER: Untersuchungen über die Autolyse der Haut. Arch. klin. exp. Derm. **220**, 417—442 (1964). — BREATHNACH, A. S.: Melanocyte distribution in forearm epidermis of freckled human subjects. J. invest. Derm. **29**, 253—261 (1957). — A new concept of the relation between the Langerhans cell and the melanocyte. J. invest. Derm. **40**, 279—281 (1963). — The dermo-epidermal junction. In: Progress in the biological sciences in relation to dermatology — 2 (A. ROOK and R. H. CHAMPION, eds.), p. 415—425. Cambridge: Cambridge University Press 1964. — The cell of Langerhans. Int. Rev. Cytol. **18**, 1—28 (1965). — BREATHNACH, A. S., D. GOODWIN, and L. M.-A. WYLLIE: "Clear cells" in the basal layer of white epidermis of the black and white spotted guinea-pig. J. Anat. (Lond.) **99**, 163 (1965). — BREATHNACH, A. S., and L. M.-A. WYLLIE: Electron microscopy of melanocytes and melanosomes in freckled human epidermis. J. invest. Derm. **42**, 389—394 (1964). — Fine structure of cells forming the surface layer of the epidermis in human fetuses at fourteen and twelve weeks. J. invest. Derm. **45**, 179—189 (1965a). — Melanin in Langerhans cells. J. invest. Derm. **45**, 401—403 (1965b). — Osmium iodide positive granules in spinous and granular layer of guinea pig epidermis. J. invest. Derm. **47**, 58—60 (1966). — BRODIE, A. F., and J. S. GOTS: Effects of an isolated dehydrogenase enzyme and flavoprotein on the reduction of triphenyltetrazoliumchloride. Science **114**, 40—41 (1953). — BRODY, I.: The keratinization of epidermal cells of normal guinea pig skin as revealed by electron microscopy. J. Ultrastruct. Res. **2**, 482—511 (1959a). — An ultrastructural study on the role of the keratohyalin granules in the keratinization process. J. Ultrastruct. Res. **3**, 84—104 (1959b). — An electron microscopic investigation of the keratinization process in the epidermis. In Proc. 15th Meet. Northern Derm. Soc., Oslo, 1959. Acta derm.-venereol. (Stockh.) **40**, 74—84 (1960a). — The ultrastructure of the tonofibrils in the keratinization process of normal human epidermis. J. Ultrastruct. Res. **4**, 264—297 (1960b). — The ultrastructure of the epidermis in Psoriasis vulgaris as revealed by electron microscopy. 1. The dermo-epidermal junction and the stratum basale in parakeratosis without keratohyalin. J. Ultrastruct. Res. **6**, 304—323 (1962a). — The ultrastructure of the epidermis in Psoriasis vulgaris as revealed by electron microscopy. 2. The stratum spinosum in parakeratosis without keratohyalin. J. Ultrastruct. Res. **6**, 324—340 (1962b). — The ultrastructure of the epidermis in Psoriasis vulgaris as revealed by electron microscopy. 3. The stratum intermedium in parakeratosis without keratohyalin. J. Ultrastruct. Res. **6**, 341—353 (1962c). — The ultrastructure of the epidermis in Psoriasis vulgaris as revealed by electron microscopy. 4. The stratum corneum in parakeratosis without keratohyalin. J. Ultrastruct. Res. **6**, 354—367 (1962d). — Electron microscopic observations on the keratinization process in normal and psoriatic epidermis. Thesis. Uppsala: Almqvist & Wiksells 1962e. — Electron microscopic demonstration of mitochondria and α-cytomembranes with negative contrast in the horny layer of parakeratotic psoriatic epidermis. J. Ultrastruct. Res. **7**, 346—358 (1962f). — The ultrastructure of the horny layer in normal and psoriatic epidermis as revealed by electron microscopy. J. invest. Derm. **39**, 519—527 (1962g). — Ultrastructural aspects on the keratinization process in normal human epidermis and in psoriatic epidermis as revealed by electron microscopy. In: Proc. XII. Intern. Congr. Derm. Washington D.C. 1962 (D. M. PILLSBURY and C. S. LIVINGOOD, eds.), vol. II, p. 1283—1288. Intern. Congr. Ser. No. 55. Exc. Med. Found. 1963a. — The ultrastructure of the epidermis in Psoriasis vulgaris as revealed by electron microscopy. 5. The non-cornified layers in hyperkeratosis. J. Ultrastruct. Res. 8, 566—579 (1963b). — The ultrastructure of the epidermis in Psoriasis vulgaris as revealed by electron microscopy. 6. The transition cells in hyperkeratosis. J. Ultrastruct. Res. 8, 580—594 (1963c). — The ultrastructure of the epidermis in Psoriasis vulgaris as revealed by electron microscopy. 7. The stratum corneum in hyperkeratosis. J. Ultrastruct. Res. 8, 595—606 (1963d). — Unpublished data 1963e. Quoted from I. BRODY. In: The epidermis (W. MONTAGNA and W. C. LOBITZ jr., eds.), p. 551—572. New York and London: Academic Press 1964c. — Unpublished data 1963f. — Observations on the fine structure of the horny layer in the normal human epidermis. J. invest. Derm. **42**, 27—31 (1964a). — Different staining methods for the electronmicroscopic elucidation of the tonofibrillar differentiation in normal epidermis. In: The epidermis (W. MONTAGNA and W. C. LOBITZ jr., eds.), p. 251—273. New York and London: Academic Press 1964b. — Cytoplasmic components in the psoriatic horny layers with special reference to electron-microscopic findings. In: The epidermis (W. MONTAGNA and W. C. LOBITZ jr., eds.), p. 551—572. New York and London: Academic Press 1964c. — The intercellular space in normal human stratum corneum. Nature (Lond.) **209**, 472—476 (1966). — An electron-microscopic study of the junctional and regular desmosomes in normal human epidermis. Acta derm.-venereol. (Stockh.) (in press). — BRODY, I., and K. S. LARSSON: Morphology of mammalian skin: Embryonic development of the epidermal sub-layers. In: Biology of the skin and hair growth. Proc. Sympos. Canberra 1964 (A. G. LYNE and B. F. SHORT, eds.), p. 267—290. Sydney and London: Angus & Robertson LTD 1965. — BRUNNER, H.: Über Glykogen in der gesunden und kranken Haut. Verh. dtsch. derm. Ges. **9**, 521—535 (1906). — BULLOUGH, W. S.: Mitotic activity in the adult male mouse, Mus musculus L. The diurnal cycles and their relation to waking and sleeping. Proc. roy. Soc. B **135**, 212—233 (1948a). — The effects of experimentally induced rest and excercise on the epidermal mitotic activity of the adult male mouse, Mus musculus L. Proc. roy. Soc. B **135**, 233—242 (1948b). — The energy relations of mitotic activity. Biol. Rev. **27**, 133—168 (1952a). — Stress and epidermal mitotic activity. I. The effects of the adrenal hormones. J. Endocr. **8**, 265—274 (1952b). — Hormones and mitotic activity. Vitam. and Horm. **13**, 261—292 (1955a). — A study of the hormonal relations of epidermal mitotic activity in vitro. III. Adrenalin. Exp. Cell Res. **9**, 108—115 (1955b). — The control of mitotic activity in adult mammalian tissues. Biol. Rev. **37**, 307—342 (1962). — Analysis of the life-cycle in mammalian cells. Nature (Lond.) **199**, 859—862 (1963). — BULLOUGH, W. S., C. L. HEWETT, and E. B. LAURENCE: The epidermal chalone: a preliminary attempt at isolation. Exp. Cell Res. **36**, 192—200 (1964). — BULLOUGH, W. S., and M. JOHNSON: The energy relations of mitotic activity in adult mouse epidermis. Proc. roy. Soc. B **138**, 562—575 (1951). — BULLOUGH, W. S., and E. B. LAURENCE: The control of epidermal mitotic activity in the mouse. Proc. roy. Soc. B **151**, 517—536 (1959/60). — The control of mitotic activity in mouse skin. Exp. Cell Res. **21**, 394—405 (1960). — The study of mammalian epidermal mitosis in vitro. A critical analysis of technique. Exp. Cell Res. **24**, 289—297 (1961). — Mitotic control by internal secretion: the role of the chalone-adrenalin complex. Exp. Cell Res. **33**, 176—194 (1964a). — Duration of epidermal mitosis in vitro. Effect of the chalone-adrenalin complex and of energy production. Exp. Cell Res. **35**, 629—641 (1964b). — BULLOUGH, W. S., and T. RYTÖMAA: Mitotic homeostasis. Nature (Lond.) **205**, 573—578 (1965). — BURSTONE, M. S.: New histochemical technique for the demonstration of tissue oxidase (cytochrom oxidase). J. Histochem. Cytochem. **7**, 112—122 (1959). — Histochemical demonstration of cytochrom oxidase with new amine reagents. J. Histochem. Cytochem. **8**, 63—70 (1960). — Modifications of histochemical techniques for the demonstration of cytochrom oxidase. J. Histochem. Cytochem. **9**, 59—65 (1961). — Enzyme histochemistry and cytochemistry. In: Cytology and cell physiology (G. H. BOURNE, ed.), p. 182—237. New York and London: Academic Press 1964.

CASPERSSON, T. O.: Cell growth and cell function. New York: W. Norton Co. 1950. — CASPERSSON, T., and J. SCHULTZ: Pentose nucleotides in the cytoplasm of growing tissue. Nature (Lond.) **143**, 602—603 (1939). — Ribonucleic acids in both nucleus and cytoplasm, and the function of the nucleolus. Proc. nat. Acad. Sci. (Wash.) **26**, 507—515 (1940). — CAULFIELD, J. B., and G. F. WILGRAM: An electron microscopic study of blister formation in erythema multiforme. J. invest. Derm. **39**, 307—316 (1962). — CHAMBERS, R., and G. S. RÉNYI: The structure of the cells in tissues as revealed by microdissection. I. The physical relationships of the cells in epithelia. Amer. J. Anat. **34**, 385—402 (1925). — CHAMPETIER, G., et A. LITVAC: Structures histologiques et structures moleculaires au cours de la kératinisation épidermique. Arch. Anat. micr. Morph. exp. **35**, 65—76 (1939). — CHARLES, A.: An electron microscope study of cornification in the human skin. J. invest. Derm. **33**, 65—74 (1959). — CHARLES, A., and J. T. INGRAM: Electron microscope observations of the melanocyte of the human epidermis. J. Biophys. biochem. Cytol. **6**, 41—44 (1959). — CHARLES, A., and F. G. SMIDDY: The tonofibrils of the human epidermis. J. invest. Derm. **29**, 327—338 (1957). — CHÈVREMONT, M., et J. FRÉDERIC: Une nouvelle methode histochimique de mise en évidence des substances à fraction sulfhydrile. Application à l'epiderme, au poil et à la levure. Arch.

Biol. (Liège) **54**, 589—605 (1943). — CHRISTOPHERS, E., and A. M. KLIGMAN: Visualization of the cell layers of the stratum corneum. J. invest. Derm. **42**, 407—409 (1964). — CLARK jr., W. H., and R. G. HIBBS: Electron microscope studies of the human epidermis. The clear cell of Masson (dendritic cell or melanocyte). J. Biophys. biochem. Cytol. **4**, 679—683 (1958). — COHEN, C.: Architecture of the α-class of fibrous proteins. In: Molecular architecture in cell physiology (T. HAYASHI and A. G. SZENT-GYÖRGYI, eds.), p. 169—190. New Jersey: Prentice-Hall, Inc. Englewoods Cliffs 1966. — COREY, R. B., and L. PAULING: Fundamental dimensions of polypeptide chains. Proc. roy. Soc. B **141**, 10—20 (1953). — CORFIELD, M. C., A. ROBSON, and B. SKINNER: The amino acid composition of three fractions from oxidized wool. Biochem. J. **68**, 348—352 (1958). — CORI, G. T., and C. F. CORI: Crystalline muscle phosphorylase. IV. Formation of glycogen. J. biol. Chem. **151**, 57—63 (1943). — CORMANE, R. H., and F. L. E. CLAESSENS: Some aspects of beta-hydroxy-buturyl dehydrogenase activity in the human skin (normal — abnormal). Dermatologica (Basel-New York) **126**, 369—379 (1963). — CORMANE, R. H., G. and L. KALSBEEK: ATP-hydrolyzing enzymes in normal human skin. Dermatologica (Basel) **127**, 381—397 (1963). — COWDRY, E. V.: Laboratory technique in biology and medicine, 2nd. ed. Baltimore: Williams & Wilkins Co. 1948. — Skin. In: Text book of histology. Philadelphia: Lea & Febiger 1950. — COWDRY, E. V., and H. C. THOMPSON jr.: Localization of maximum cell division in epidermis. Anat. Rec. **88**, 403—409 (1944). — CRICK, F. H. C.: The packing of α-helices: simple coiled-coils. Acta crystallogr. London **6**, 689—697 (1953). — CRONKITE, E. P., V. P. BOND, T. M. FLIEDNER, and J. R. RUBIN: The use of tritiated thymidine in the study of deoxyribonucleic acid synthesis and cell turnover in hemopoietic tissues. Lab. Invest. **8**, 263—275 (1959). — CROUNSE, R. G.: Epidermal keratin: a re-evaluation. Nature (Lond.) **200**, 539—542 (1963). — CRUICKSHANK, C. N. D., and S. A. HARCOURT: Pigment donation *in vitro*. J. invest. Derm. **42**, 183—184 (1964).

DÄHN, W.: Über die Kalzium- und Kaliumverteilung in der normalen Haut. Derm. Wschr. **82**, 425—433 (1926). — DALTON, A. J.: Organization in benign and malignant cells. Lab. Invest. **8**, 510—537 (1959). — DALTON, A. J., and M. D. FELIX: "Lipochondria" and the Golgi substance in epithelial cells of the epididymis. Nature (Lond.) **170**, 541 (1952). — Studies on the Golgi substance of the epithelial cells of the epididymis and duodenum of the mouse. Amer. J. Anat. **92**, 277—305 (1953). — Cytologic and cytochemical characteristics of the Golgi substance of epithelial cells of the epididymis — *in situ*, in homogenates and after isolation. Amer. J. Anat. **94**, 171—208 (1954). — DANNEEL, R.: Phänogenetik der Kaninchenfärbung. Ergebn. Biol. **18**, 55—87 (1941). — DANNEEL, R., u. E. LUBNOW: Zur Physiologie der Kälteschwärzung beim Russenkaninchen. II. Der Einfluß von Röntgenstrahlen auf die Pigmentbildung. Biol. Zbl. **56**, 572—584 (1936). — DEGUCHI, Y.: A histochemical method for demonstrating protein-bound sulfhydryl and disulfide groups with nitro blue tetrazolium. J. Histochem. Cytochem. **12**, 261—265 (1964). — DELLA PORTA, G., and O. MÜLHBOCK: Structure and control of the melanocyte. Berlin-Heidelberg-New York: Springer 1966. — DEMPSEY, E. W., and G. B. WISLOCKI: Observations on some histochemical reactions in the human placenta, with special reference to the significance of the lipoids, glycogen and iron. Endocrinol. **35**, 409—429 (1944). — DERKSEN, J., u. G. C. HERINGA: Verhornung und Tonofibrillen der Epidermis. Festschrift für Prof. SZYMONOWICZ, Lwów. Pol. Gaz. lek. **15**, 592—594 (1936). — DERKSEN, J. C., G. C. HERINGA, and A. WEIDINGER: On keratin and cornification. Acta neerl. Morph. **1**, 31—37 (1937). — DEWEY, M. M., and L. BARR: A study of the structure and distribution of the nexus. J. Cell Biol. **23**, 553—585 (1964). — DICK, J. C.: Observations on the elastic tissue of the skin with a note on the reticular layer at the junction of the dermis and epidermis. J. Anat. (Lond.) **81**, 201—211 (1947). — DOEG, K. A., S. KRUEGER, and D. M. ZIEGLER: Studies on the electron transfer system. XXIX. The isolation and properties of a succinic dehydrogenase-cytochrome b complex from beef heart mitochondria. Biochim. biophys. Acta (Amst.) **41**, 491—497 (1960). — DORRIS, F.: The production of pigment by chick neural crest in grafts to the 3-day limb bud. J. exp. Zool. **80**, 315—345 (1939). — DROCHMANS, P.: Electron microscope studies of epidermal melanocytes, and the fine structure of melanin granules. J. biophys. biochem. Cytol. **8**, 165—180 (1960a). — Étude au microscope électronique du mechanisme de la pigmentation melanique. Arch. belges Derm. **16**, 155—163 (1960b). — Étude au microscope électronique du mécanisme de la pigmentation mélanique: la distribution des grains de mélanine aux cellules malpighiennes. Path. et Biol. **9**, 947—954 (1960c). — The fine structure of melanin granules (the early, mature and compound forms). In: Structure and control of the melanocyte (G. DELLA PORTA and O. MÜHLBOCK, eds.), p. 90—95. Berlin-Heidelberg-New York: Springer 1966. — DROSDOFF: Zit. von E. PERNKOPF u. V. PATZELT. In: Die Haut- und Geschlechtskrankheiten (L. ARZT and K. ZIELER, Hrsg.), Bd. I, S. 1—140. Berlin u. Wien: Urban & Schwarzenberg 1934. — DU BUY, H. G., M. W. WOODS, D. BURK, and M. D. LACKEY: Enzymatic activities of isolated amelanotic and melanotic granules of mouse melanomas and a suggested relationship to mitochondria. J. nat. Cancer Inst. **9**, 325—336 (1949). — DUHRING: Quoted from K. HERXHEIMER. Derm. Z. **23**, 129—134 (1916). — DUPRÉ, A.: Étude histochimique des glucide de la peau humaine (glycogène et polysaccharides acides) par la reaction d'Hotchkiss-MacManus. Thèse. Toulouse 1952. — Études histochimiques de la peau humaine. II. Les espaces intercellulaires. Filaments d'union. Nodules de Bizzozero. Substance "cimentante". Substance intercellulaire. Ann. Derm. Syph. (Paris) **80**, 490—500 (1953). — DU SHANE, G. P.: The origin of pigment cells in Amphibia. Science **80**, 620—621 (1934). — An experimental study of the origin of pigment cells in Amphibia. J. exp. Zool. **72**, 1—31 (1935). — DUVE, C. DE, and H. BEAUFAY: Tissue fraction studies. 10. Influence of ischemia on the state of some bound enzymes in rat liver. Biochem. J. **73**, 610—616 (1959). — DUVE, C. DE, B. C. PRESSMAN, R. GIANETTO, R. WATTIAUX, and F. APPELMANS: Tissue fraction studies. 6. Intracellular distribution patterns of enzymes in rat-liver tissues. Biochem. J. **60**, 604—617 (1955). — DUVE, C. DE, and R. WATTIAUX: Functions of lysosomes. Ann. Rev. Physiol. **28**, 435—492 (1966).

EASTLICK, H. L.: The point of origin of the melanophores in chick embryos as shown by means of limb bud transplants. J. exp. Zool. **83**, 131—157 (1939). — ECKSTEIN, H. C.: Amino acids in human skin. Proc. Soc. exp. Biol. (N.Y.) **32**, 1573—1574 (1935). — EDER, M.: Der histochemische Nachweis des Fermentes Monoaminoxydase. Beitr. path. Anat. **117**, 343—396 (1957). — EDWARDS, G. A., and L. MAKK: A comparative micromorphologic study of normal human epidermis and a human squamous cell carcinoma transplant. Amer. J. Path. **37**, 101—120 (1960). — EHRING, F.: Die Regenerationszeit der menschlichen Epidermis. Hautarzt **13**, 499—502 (1962). — EHRMANN, S.: Untersuchungen über die Physiologie und Pathologie des Hautpigmentes. Arch. Derm. Syph. (Wien) **12**, 507—532 (1885). — EISEN, A. Z., K. A. ARNDT, and W. H. CLARK: The ultrastructural localization of acid phosphatase in human epidermis. J. invest. Derm. **43**, 319—326 (1964). — EISEN, A. Z., W. MONTAGNA, and H. B. CHASE: Sulfhydryl groups in the skin of the mouse and guinea pig. J. nat. Cancer Inst. **14**, 341—353 (1953). — ELLIS, R. A.: Aging of the human male scalp. In: The biology of hair growth (W. MONTAGNA and R. A. ELLIS, eds.), p. 469—485. New York: Academic Press 1958. — Vascular patterns of the skin. In: Advances in biology of skin (W. MONTAGNA and R. A. ELLIS, eds.), vol. 2, p. 20—37. New York: Pergamon Press 1961. — Histochemistry of the epidermis. In: Proc. XII. Intern. Congr. Derm. Washington D.C. 1962 (D. M. PILLSBURY and C. S. LIVINGOOD, eds.), vol. I, p. 373—375. Intern. Congr. Ser. No. 55. Excerpta Med. Found. Amsterdam-New York-London-Milan-Tokyo 1963. — Enzymes of the epidermis. In: The epidermis (W. MONTAGNA and W. C. LOBITZ jr., eds.), p. 135—144. New York and London: Academic Press 1964. — ELLIS, R. A., and W. MONTAGNA: Histology and cytochemistry of human skin. XV. Sites of phosphorylase and amylo-1,6-glucosidase activity. J. Histochem. Cytochem. **6**, 201—207 (1958). — ENGMAN, M. F., and R. C. MACCARDLE: Histochemical study of neurodermatitis; microincineration and spectrographic analysis. Arch. Derm. **42**, 109—111 (1940). — EPSTEIN, W. L., and H. I. MAIBACH: Cell renewal in human epidermis. Arch. Derm. **92**, 462—468 (1966). — ERNSTER, L., M. LJUNGGREEN, and L. DANIELSON: Purification and some properties of highly dicumarol-sensitive liver diaphorase. Biochem. biophys. Res. Commun. **2**, 88—92 (1960). — EVENSEN, A., and O. HELDAAS: The effect of adrenalin on the mitotic rate in the epidermis of hairless mice in *vitro*. Acta path. microbiol. scand. **62**, 24—28 (1964).

FALIN, L. I.: Glycogen in the epithelium of mucous membranes and skin and its significance. Acta anat. (Basel) **46**, 244—276 (1961). — FARBER, E., and C. D. LOUVIERE: Histochemical localization of specific oxidative enzymes. IV. Soluble oxidation-reduction dyes as aids in the histochemical localization of oxidative enzymes with tetrazolium salts. J. Histochem. Cytochem. **4**, 347—356 (1956). — FARBER, E., W. H. STERNBERG, and C. E. DUNLAP: Histochemical localization of specific oxidative enzymes. I. Tetrazolium stains for DPN- and TPN-diaphorase. J. Histochem. Cytochem. **4**, 254—265 (1961). — FARBMAN, A. I.: Plasma membrane changes during keratinization. Anat. Rec. **156**, 269—282 (1966). — FARQUHAR, M. G., and G. E. PALADE: Tight intercellular junctions. First Ann. Meet. Amer. Soc. Cell Biol. 1961. Quoted from M. M. DEWEY and L. BARR: A study of the structure and distribution of the nexus. J. Cell Biol. **23**, 553—585 (1964). — Junction complexes in various epithelia. J. Cell Biol. **17**, 375—412 (1963). — Functional organization of amphibian skin. Proc. nat. Acad. Sci. (Wash.) **51**, 569—577 (1964). — Cell junctions in amphibian skin. J. Cell Biol. **26**, 263—291 (1965). — Adenosine triphosphatase localization in amphibian epidermis. J. Cell Biol. **30**, 359—379 (1966). — FASSKE, E., u. H. THEMANN: Die pathologische Schleimhautverhornung und ihre Beziehung zur Glykogensynthese. Beitr. path. Anat. **121**, 442—469 (1959a). — Über das Deckepithel der menschlichen Mundschleimhaut. Z. Zellforsch. **49**, 447—463 (1959b). — FAWCETT, D. W.: An atlas of fine structure. The cell, its organelles and inclusions. Philadelphia and London: W. B. Saunders Co. 1966. — FEGELER, F., u. M. RAHMANN-ESSER: Autoradiographische Untersuchungen zum Protein- und RNS-Stoffwechsel der normalen menschlichen Haut. Arch. klin. exp. Derm. **223**, 255—262 (1965). — Einfluß von Vitamin C und Folsäure auf den Eiweiß- und Ribonucleinsäure-Stoffwechsel normaler und psoriasiskranker Haut. Autoradiographische Untersuchungen. Arch. klin. exp. Derm. **224**, 424—436 (1966a). — Autoradiographische Untersuchungen zum Proteinstoffwechsel der Epidermis gesunder und durch Psoriasis vulgaris veränderter Haut. Arch. klin. exp. Derm. **227**, 847—851 (1966b). — FELSHER, Z.: Studies on the adherence of the epidermis to the corium. Proc. Soc. exp. Biol. (N.Y.) **62**, 213—215 (1946). — FERREIRA-MARQUES, J.: Systema sensitivum intraepidermicum. Die Langerhansschen Zellen als Rezeptoren des hellen Schmerzes: Doloriceptores. Arch. Derm. Syph. (Berl.) **193**, 191—250 (1951). — A contribution to the biology of the epidermis: stratum oxybioticum and stratum anoxybioticum. J. invest. Derm. **36**, 63—64 (1961). — FERREIRA-MARQUES, J., and C. A. PARRA: Contribution to the study of stratum granulosum and the epidermis biology: stratum oxybioticum and stratum anoxybioticum. Acta derm.-venereol. (Stockh.) **40**, 241—255 (1960). — FEULGEN, R., K. IMHÄUSER u. M. BEHRENS: Zur Kenntnis des Plasmalogens. I. Eigenschaften des Plasmalogens, Darstellung und Natur des Plasmals. Hoppe-Seylers Z. physiol. Chem. **180**, 161—179 (1929). — FEULGEN, R., u. K. VOIT: Über einen weitverbreiteten festen Aldehyd. Seine Entstehung aus einer Vorstufe, sein mikrochemischer und mikroskopisch-chemischer Nachweis und die Wege zu seiner präparativen Darstellung. Pflügers Arch. ges. Physiol. **206**, 389—410 (1924). — FILSHIE, B. K., and G. E. ROGERS: The fine structure of α-keratin. J. molec. Biol. **3**, 784—786 (1961). — FINDLAY, G. H.: The simple esterases of human skin. Brit. J. Derm. **67**, 83—91 (1955). — The influence of the human epidermis on melanin synthesis. South Afr. J. Lab. clin. Med. **7**, 26—30 (1961). — FIRKET, H.: Recherches sur la régénération de la peau de mammifères. II. Etude histochimique. Arch .Biol. (Liège) **62**, 335—350 (1951). — FISCHER, R.: The selectivity of the Gram-stain for keratins. Experientia (Basel) **9**, 20—21 (1953). — FISHMAN, W. H., and J. R. BAKER: Cellular localization of β-glucuronidase in rat tissue. J. Histochem. Cytochem. **4**, 570—587 (1956). — FISHMAN, W. H., J. R. BAKER, and P. R. F. BORGES: Localization of β-glucuronidase in some human tumors. Cancer (Philad.) **12**, 240—245 (1959). — FITZPATRICK, T. B.: Zur Rolle der Tyrosinase bei der Säugetier-Melanogenese. Hautarzt **10**, 520—525 (1959). — FITZPATRICK, T. B., S. W. BECKER jr., A. B. LERNER, and H. MONTGOMERY: Tyrosinase in human skin: demonstration of its presence and its role in human melanin formation. Science **112**, 223—225 (1950). — FITZPATRICK, T. B., and A. S. BREATHNACH: Das epidermale Melanin-EinheitSystem. Derm. Wschr. **147**, 481—489 (1963). — FITZPATRICK, T. B., P. BRUNET, and A. KUKITA: The nature of hair pigment. In: The biology of hair growth (W. MONTAGNA and R. A. ELLIS, eds.), p. 255—303. New York: Academic Press 1958. — FITZPATRICK, T. B., and A. B. LERNER: Terminology of pigment cells. Science **117**, 640 (1953). — Biochemical basis of human melanin pigmentation. Arch. Derm. Syph. (Chic.) **69**, 133—149 (1954). — FLASCHENTRÄGER, B., u. E. LEHNARTZ: Physiologische Chemie. Berlin-Göttingen-Heidelberg: Springer 1951. — FLEISCHAUER, K.: Über die Morphogenese des Haarstrichs und der Papillenleisten. Z. Zellforsch. **38**, 50—68 (1952). — FLESCH, P.: Chemical data on human epidermal keratinization and differentiation. J. invest. Derm. **31**, 63—73 (1958). — Mucopolysaccharides in human epidermis. J. Soc. cosmet. Chem. **10**, 154—159 (1959). — FLESCH, P., and E. C. J. ESODA: Mucopolysaccharides in human epidermis. J. invest. Derm. **35**, 43—46 (1960). — Isolation of a glycoproteolipid from human horny layers. J. invest. Derm. **39**, 409—415 (1962). — Further studies of epidermal mucopolysaccharides. Arch. Derm. **88**, 706—708 (1963). — FLESCH, P., D. A. ROE, and E. C. J. ESODA: The Gram-staining material of human epidermis. J. invest. Derm. **34**, 17—28 (1960). — FLESCH, P., and A. SATANOVE: Sulphydryl groups and disulphide linkage in human epidermal components. Brit. J. Derm. **67**, 343—347 (1955). — FORAKER, A. G., and W. J. WINGO: Histochemical studies of skin. Localization of dehydrogenase activity. Protein-bound sulfhydryl and disulfide groups. Arch. Derm. **72**, 1—6 (1955). — Protein-bound sulfhydryl and disulfide groups and succinic dehydrogenase activity in basal cell carcinoma of the skin. Exp. Med. Surg. **14**, 122—129 (1956). — FORMISANO, V. R., and W. MONTAGNA: Succinic dehydrogenase activity in the skin of the guinea pig. Anat. Rec. **120**, 893—905 (1954). — FRASER, R. D. B., and T. P. MACRAE: Quoted from G. E. ROGERS. Ann. N.Y. Acad. Sci. **83**, 378—399 (1959b). — FRASER, R. D. B., T. P. MACRAE, and G. E. ROGERS: Structure of the α-keratin. Nature (Lond.) **183**, 592—594 (1959). — Molecular organization in alpha-keratin. Nature (Lond.) **193**, 1052—1055 (1962). — FREI, J. V., and H. SHELDON: A small granular component of the cytoplasm of keratinizing epithelia. J. biophys. biochem. Cytol. **11**, 719—724 (1961). — FREINKEL, R. K.: Carbohydrate metabolism in the skin. In: The epidermis (W. MONTAGNA and W. C. LOBITZ jr., eds.), p. 485—492. New York and London: Academic Press 1964. — FRIBOES, W.: Basalmembran. Bau des Deckepithels (I). Physiologische und pathologische Ausblicke. Derm. Z. **31**, 57—83 (1920). — Beiträge zur Anatomie und Biologie der Haut. IX. Nochmals epidermale Basalmembran. Eine Entgegnung gegen HERXHEIMER und SOPHIE BORN. Arch. Derm. Syph. (Berl.) **140**, 201—207 (1922). — FRITHIOF, L., and J. WERSÄLL: A highly ordered structure in keratinizing oral epithelium. J. Ultrastruct. Res. **12**, 371—379 (1965). — FUKUYAMA, K., and I. A. BERNSTEIN: Autoradiographic studies of the incorporation of thymidine-H^3 into deoxyribonucleic acid in the skin of young rats. J. invest. Derm. **36**, 321—326 (1961). — Site of synthesis of ribonucleic acid in mammalian epidermis. J. invest. Derm. **41**, 47—52 (1963). — FUKUYAMA, K., T. NAKAMURA, and I. A. BERNSTEIN: DNA synthesis in human skin studied in *vitro* by autoradiography. J. invest. Derm. **44**, 29—32 (1965a). — Differentially localized incorporation of amino acids in relation to epidermal keratinization in the newborn rat. Anat. Rec. **152**, 525—535 (1965b). — FULAR, W.: Der Zellersatz in der menschlichen Epidermis. Morph. Jb. **96**, 1—13 (1955).

GAIRNS, F. W.: A modified gold chloride method for demonstration of nerve endings. Quart. J. micr. Sci. **74**, 151—154 (1930). — GANS, O.: Über den Calciumgehalt der gesunden und kranken Haut. Arch. Derm. Syph. (Berl.) **145**, 135—137 (1924). — Zur Histotopochemie der gesunden und kranken Haut. Untersuchung des anorganischen Aufbaues mittels der Schnittveraschung. Arch. Derm. **161**, 607—646 (1930). — Die allgemeine pathologische Anatomie der Haut. In: J. JADASSOHN, Handbuch der Haut- und Geschlechtskrankheiten, Bd. IV/3, S. 1—175. Berlin: Springer 1932. — GANS, O., u. T. PARKHEISER: Über den Kalziumgehalt der gesunden und kranken Haut. Derm. Wschr. **78**, 249—260 (1924). — GELFANT, S.: A study of mitosis in mouse ear epidermis *in vitro*. II. Effects of oxygen tension and glucose concentration. Exp. Cell Res. **18**, 494—503 (1959). — A study of mitosis in mouse ear epidermis *in vitro*. III. Effects of glucolytic and Krebs cycle intermediates. Exp. Cell Res. **19**, 65—72 (1960a). — A study of mitosis in mouse ear epidermis *in vitro*. IV. Effects of metabolic inhibitors. Exp. Cell Res. **19**, 72—82 (1960b). — GESSLER, A. E., C. E. GREY, M. C. SCHUSTER, J. J. KELSCH, and M. N. RICHTER: Notes on electron microscopy of tissue section. 1. Normal tissue. Cancer Res. **8**, 534—547 (1948). — GIBBONS, I. R., and J. R. G. BRADFIELD: Experiments on staining thin-sections for electron microscopy. In: Proc. Stockh. Conf. on Electron Microsc. 1956 (F. S. SJÖSTRAND and J. RHODIN, eds.), p. 121—124. Stockholm: Almqvist & Wiksell 1957. — GILLESPIE, J. M.: The isolation and properties of some soluble proteins from wool. VII. The heterogeneity of the high-sulphur proteins $SCMKB1$. Aust. J. biol. Sci. **15**, 572—588 (1962). — The high-sulphur proteins of normal and aberrant keratins. In: Biology of the skin and hair growth (A. G. LYNE and B. F. SHORT, eds.), p. 377—398. Sydney: Angus & Robertson 1965. — GILLESPIE, J. M., I. J. O'DONELL, E. O. P. THOMPSON, and E. F. WOODS: Preparation and properties of wool proteins. J. Textile Inst. **51**, T 703—T 716 (1960). — GIROUD, A., et H. BULLIARD: La keratinisation de l'epiderme et des phanerès. Paris: Gaston Doin 1930. — Reactions des substances a fonction sulfhydryle. Protoplasma (Berl.) **19**, 381—384 (1933). — Les substances a fonction sulfhydryle dans l'épiderme. Arch. anat. micr. Morph. exp. **31**, 271—290 (1935). — GIROUD, A., H. BULLIARD et C. P. LEBLOND: Les deux types fondamentaux de kératinisation. Bull. Histol. appl. **11**, 129—144 (1934). — GIROUD, A., et G. CHAMPETIER: Recherches sur les roentgénogrammes des keratines. Bull. Soc. Chim. biol. (Paris) **18**, 656-664 (1936). — GIROUD, A., and C. P. LEBLOND: The keratinization of epidermis and its derivatives, especially the hair, as shown by X-ray diffraction and histochemical studies. Ann. N.Y. Acad. Sci. **53**, 613—626 (1951). — GLENNER, G. G., H. J. BURTNER, and G. W. BROWN: The histochemical demonstration of monoamine oxidase activity by tetrazolium salts. J. Histochem. Cytochem. **5**, 591—600 (1957). — GODA, T.: Quoted from E. HORSTMANN. In: Dermatologie and venerologie (H. A. GOTTRON and W. SCHÖNFELD, eds.), vol. I/1, p. 62. Stuttgart: Georg Thieme 1961. — GOLDBLUM, R. W., W. N. PIPER, and A. W. CAMPBELL: A comparison of three histochemical stains for the demonstration of protein-bound sulfhydryl groups in normal human skin. J. invest. Derm. **23**, 375—383 (1954). — GOLDSTEIN, L.: Nucleocytoplasmic relationships. In: Cytology and cell physiology (G. H. BOURNE, ed.), 3rd ed., p. 559—635. New York and London: Academic Press 1964. — GOLTZ, R. W., R. M. FUSARO, and J. JARVIS: The demonstration of acid substances in normal skin by alcian blue. J. invest. Derm. **31**, 183—194 (1958). — GOMORI, G.: Microtechnical demonstration of phosphatase in the tissue sections. Proc. Soc. exp. Biol. (N.Y.) **42**, 23—26 (1939). — Further studies on the histochemical specificity of phosphates. Proc. Soc. exp. Biol. (N.Y.) **72**, 449—450 (1949). — The histochemistry of esterases. Int. Cytol. Rev. **1**, 323—335 (1952a). — Microscopic histochemistry. Principles and practice. Chicago: University of Chicago Press 1952b. — GRÄFF, S.: Eine Anweisung zur Herstellung von Dauerpräparaten bei Anwendung der Naphtholblau-Oxydasereaktion mit einigen Bemerkungen zur Theorie und Technik der Reaktion. Zbl. allg. Path. path. Anat. **27**, 313—318 (1916). — Intracelluläre Oxydation und Nadireaktion (Indophenolblausynthese). Beitr. path. Anat. **70**, 1—19 (1922). — GRASSMANN, W., u. I. TRUPKE: Chemie der Haut unter besonderer Berücksichtigung der Proteine. In: Handbuch der Gerbereichemie und Lederfabrikation (W. GRASSMANN, Hrsg.), Bd. I/1, S. 359—510. Wien: Springer 1944. — Aminosäuren und Peptide. In: Physiologische Chemie (B. FLASCHENTRÄGER, Hrsg.), Bd. I, S. 489—584. Berlin-Göttingen-Heidelberg: Springer 1951. — GRAUMANN, W.: Die histochemische Perjodatreaktion der Reticulin- und Kollagenfasern. Acta histochem. (Jena) **1**, 116—126 (1954). — GREB, W.: Untersuchungen über die Gestalt des Papillarkörpers der menschlichen Haut. Z. Anat. Entwickl.-Gesch. **110**, 247—263 (1939). — GREEN, D. E.: Enzymes in metabolic sequences. In: Chemical pathways of metabolism (D. M. GREENBERG, ed.), vol. 1, p. 27—65. New York: Academic Press 1954. — GREEN, D. E., D. M. ZIEGLER, and K. A. DOEG: Sequence of components in the succinic chain of the mitochondrial electron transport system. Arch. Biochem. **85**, 280—282 (1959). —

GREULICH, R. C.: Aspects of cell individuality in the renewal of stratified squamous epithelia. In: The epidermis (W. MONTAGNA and W. C. LOBITZ jr., eds.), p. 117—133. New York and London: Academic Press 1964. — GRIMLEY, PH. M., and G. A. EDWARDS: The ultrastructure of cardiac desmosomes in the toad and their relationship to the intercalated discs. J. biophys. biochem. Cytol. 8, 305—318 (1960). — GRÜNEBERG, TH., u. A. SZAKALL: Über den Gehalt an Schwefel und wasserlöslichen Bestandteilen in der verhornten Epidermis bei normaler und pathologischer Verhornung (Psoriasis). Arch. klin. exp. Derm. 201, 361—377 (1955). — GÜTTES, E.: Die Herkunft des Augenpigmentes beim Kaninchenembryo. Z. Zellforsch. 39, 168—202 (1953a). — Über die Beeinflussung der Pigmentgenese im Auge des Hühnerembryos durch Röntgenstrahlen und über die Herkunft der Pigmentgranula. Z. Zellforsch. 39, 260-275 (1953b). HAMA, K.: The fine structure of the desmosomes in frog mesothelium. J. biophys. biochem. Cytol. 7, 575—577 (1960). — HAMILTON, H. L.: Influence of adrenal and sex hormones on the differentiation of melanophores in the chick. J. exp. Zool. 88, 275—305 (1941). — HAMMETT, F. S., and L. WALP: The influence of SH on cell proliferation of blue-green algae. Growth 3, 427—433 (1939). — HANAWA, S.: Zur Kenntnis des Glykogens und des Eleidins in der Oberhaut. Arch. Derm. Syph. (Wien) 118, 357—385 (1913). — HANSON, J.: The histogenesis of the epidermis in the rat and mouse. J. Anat. (Lond.) 81, 174—197 (1947). — HANUŠOVÁ, S.: Psoriasis im Flächenbild. Arch. klin. exp. Derm. 210, 227—251 (1960). — Parakeratotische Lipoidgranula. Arch. klin. exp. Derm. 214, 6—20 (1961). — Parakeratotische Lipoidgranula. In: De structura et functione stratorum epidermidis s. d. barrierrae. Proc. 2nd intern. sympos. Brno 1964 (G. LEJHANEC and P. HYBÁŠEK, eds.). Acta Fac. Med. Univ. Brunensis 16, 123—134 (1965). — HARDY, M. H.: The histochemistry of hair follicle in the mouse. Amer. J. Anat. 90, 285—338 (1952). — HARRISON, R. G.: The outgrowth of the peripheral nerve fibers in altered surroundings. Wilhelm Roux' Arch. Entwickl.-Mech. Org. 30, 15—33 (1910a). — Heteroplastic graftings in embryology. J. exp. Zool. 9, 787—848 (1910b). — Die Neuralliste. Anat. Anz., Erg.-H. 85, 4—30 (1938). — HASEGAWA, J., and A. SIEGEL: Hydrolysis of 1-leucyl-β-naphthyl amide by chymotrypsin. J. Histochem. Cytochem. 10, 766—767 (1962). — HASHIMOTO, K., B. G. GROSS, and W. F. LEVER: The ultrastructure of the skin of human embryos. I. Intraepidermal eccrine sweat duct. J. invest. Derm. 45, 139—151 (1965). — HASHIMOTO, K., B. G. GROSS, R. NELSON, and W. F. LEVER: The ultrastructure of the skin of human embryos. III. The formation of the nail in 16—18 weeks old embryos. J. invest. Derm. 47, 205—217 (1966). — HATEFI, Y., R. L. LESTER, F. L. CRANE, and C. WIDMER: Studies on the electron transport system. XVI. Enzymic oxidoreduction reactions of coenzyme Q. Biochim biophys. Acta (Amst.) 31, 490—501 (1959). — HAWKINS, J.: The localization of amine oxidase in the liver cell. Biochem. J. 50, 577—581 (1952). — HAWORTH, W. N., S. PEAT, and E. J. BOURNE: Synthesis of amylopectin. Nature (Lond.) 154, 236—238 (1944). — HAYASHI, M., and W. H. FISHMAN: Enzymorphologic observations in the uterus and vagina of castrate rats receiving ovarian hormones. Acta endocr. (Kbh.) 38, 107—120 (1961). — Enzymorphology of rat vagina during the oestrus cycle; β-glucuronidase. Acta endocr. (Kbh.) 39, 154—162 (1962). — HEIDENHAIN, M.: Plasma und Zelle. I. In: v. BARDELEBEN, Handbuch der Anatomie des Menschen, Bd. VIII/1. Jena 1907. — HELLMANN, K.: Cholinesterase and amine oxidase in the skin: a histochemical investigation. J. Physiol. (Lond.) 129, 454—463 (1955). — HELWIG, E. B.: Pathology of psoriasis. Ann. N.Y. Acad. Sci. 73, 924—935 (1958). — HERRMANN, F.: Zur Methode der Veraschung von Gewebsschnitten und Aschendifferenzierung (Darstellung von Magnesiumsalzen und Phosphaten). Z. wiss. Mikrosk. 49, 313—330 (1932). — Erweiterung des Verfahrens der Schnittveraschung. Differenzierung der anorganischen Struktur gesunder und kranker Haut. Z. wiss. Mikr. 52, 257—275 (1935). — HERSHEY, F. B.: Quantitative histochemistry of skin. In: The Epidermis (W. MONTAGNA and W. C. LOBITZ jr., eds.), p. 145—160. New York and London: Academic Press 1964. — HERXHEIMER, K.: Über eigentümliche Fasern in der Epidermis und im Epithel gewisser Schleimhäute beim Menschen. Arch. Derm. Syph. (Wien) 21, 645—657 (1889). — Über die epidermale Basalmembran. Derm. Z. 23, 129—134 (1916). — HIBBS, R. G., and W. H. CLARK: Electron microscope studies of the human epidermis. The cell boundaries and topography of the stratum Malpighii. J. biophys. biochem. Cytol. 6, 71—76 (1959). — HINTZSCHE, E.: Das Aschenbild tierischer Gewebe und Organe. Methodik, Ergebnisse und Bibliographie. Berlin-Göttingen-Heidelberg: Springer 1956. — HOEPKE, H.: Epithelfasern und Basalmembran. Anat. Anz. Erg.-H. 58, 147—156 (1924b). — Die Haut. In: W. v. MÖLLENDORFF, Handbuch der mikroskopischen Anatomie des Menschen, Bd. III/1, S. 1—116. Berlin: Springer 1927. — HOFFMANN-OSTENHOF, O.: Enzymologie. Wien: Springer 1954. — HORSTMANN, E.: Zur Morphologie der gesunden und kranken Haut. Arch. Derm. Syph. (Berl.) 194, 164—173 (1952a). — Über den Papillarkörper der menschlichen Haut und seine regionalen Unterschiede. Acta anat. (Basel) 14, 23—42 (1952b). — Die Haut. In: W. v. MÖLLENDORFF, Handbuch der mikroskopischen Anatomie des Menschen, Erg.-Bd. (W. BARGMANN, Hrsg.), Bd. III/3, S. 1—276. Berlin-Göttingen-Heidelberg: Springer 1957a. — Zur Elektronenmikroskopie der Epidermis. In: W. v. MÖLLENDORFF, Handbuch der mikroskopischen Anatomie des Menschen, Erg.-Bd. (W. BARGMANN, Hrsg.), Bd. III/3, S. 486—488. Berlin-Göttingen-Heidelberg: Springer 1957b. — Elektronenoptische Struktur der Haut. Arch. klin. exp. Derm. **211**, 18—35 (1960). — Anatomie der Haut und ihrer Anhangsorgane. In: Dermatologie und Venereologie (H. A. GOTTRON and W. SCHÖNFELD, Hrsg.), Bd. I/1, S. 42—103. Stuttgart: Georg Thieme 1961. — Die Morphologie der Epidermis. In: Proc. XII. Intern. Congr. Derm., Washington D.C. 1962 (D. M. PILLSBURY and C. S. LIVINGOOD, eds.), vol. I, p. 362—372. Intern. Congr. Ser. No. 55. Excerpta Med. Found. Amsterdam-New York-London-Milan-Tokyo 1963a. — Unpublished data 1963b. Quoted from P. RITZENFELD. Arch. klin. exp. Derm. **220**, 261—265 (1964). — Das Muster der Blutgefäße. In: Probleme der Haut- und Muskeldurchblutung. Bad Oeynhausener Gespräche VI, 1962 (L. DELIUS u. E. WITZLEB, Hrsg.), S. 1—10. Berlin-Göttingen-Heidelberg: Springer 1964. — HORSTMANN, E., u. A. KNOOP: Zur Struktur des Nucleolus und des Kernes. Z. Zellforsch. **46**, 100—107 (1957). — Elektronenmikroskopische Studien an der Epidermis. I. Rattenpfote. Z. Zellforsch. **47**, 348—362 (1958). — HU, F.: Cytological studies of human pigment cells in tissue culture. In: Pigment cell biology (M. GORDON, ed.), p. 147—158. New York: Academic Press 1959. — HU, F., and R. R. CARDELL jr.: Observations on the ultrastructure of human skin. Henry Ford Hosp. Bull. **10**, 63—87 (1962). — HU, F., R. J. STARRICO, H. PINKUS, and R. P. FOSNAUGH: Human melanocytes in tissue culture. J. invest. Derm. **28**, 15—32 (1957). — HUECK, W.: Morphologische Pathologie. Leipzig: Georg Thieme 1937. — HURLEY, H. J., W. B. SHELLEY, and G. B. KOELLE: The distribution of cholinesterases in human skin, with special reference to eccrine and apocrine sweat glands. J. invest. Derm. **21**, 139—147 (1953).

IM, M. J. C.: Distribution of dehydrogenases in the skin of the rhesus monkey (Maccaca mulatta). J. Histochem. Cytochem. **13**, 668—676 (1965).

JARRETT, A.: Some problems of keratinization as studied by fluorescence microscopy. In: Proc. 11th Intern. Congr. Derm. Stockholm 1957 (S. HELLERSTRÖM, K. WIKSTRÖM and A.-M. HELLERSTRÖM, eds.). Acta derm.-venereol. (Stockh.) **3**, 430—432 (1960). — The histochemistry of keratinization. In: Progress in the biological sciences in relation to dermatology (A. ROOK, ed.), p. 135—140. Cambridge: Cambridge University Press 1960. — A histological method for the demonstration of cysteine desulphurase. J. Histochem. Cytochem. **10**, 400—401 (1962). — Chairman's introduction to the discussion. In: Progress in the biological sciences in relation to dermatology — 2 (A. ROOK and R. H. CHAMPION, eds.), p. 241—242. Cambridge: Cambridge University Press 1964. — JARRETT, A., and P. A. RILEY: Esterase activity in dendritic cells. Brit. J. Derm. **75**, 79—81 (1963). — JARRETT, A., and R. I. C. SPEARMAN: Histochemistry of the skin Psoriasis. London: English Universities Press LTD 1964. — JARRETT, A., R. I. SPEARMAN, and J. A. HARDY: The histochemistry of keratinization. Brit. J. Derm. **71**, 277—295 (1959). — JEFFREY, G. M., J. SIKORSKI, and H. J. WOODS: The micro-fibrillar structure of keratin fibers. Proc. Int. Wool Text. Res. Conf. Aust. 1955, vol. F: 130—141 (1956). — JOHNSON, P. L., H. HOFFMANN, and G. K. ROLLE: The gram staining mechanisms of cat tongue keratin. J. Histochem. Cytochem. **5**, 84—90 (1957).

KAKU, H., Y. IGARASHI, S. MASU, and S. FUJITA: Autoradiographic studies on RNA and protein synthesis of human skin in vivo in normal and pathologic conditions by H-3-uridine and H-3-leucine. Arch. histol. jap. **24**, 515—523 (1964). — KARLSON, P.: Kurzes Lehrbuch der Biochemie. Stuttgart: Georg Thieme 1966. — KARNOVSKY, M. J.: Simple methods for "staining with lead" at high pH in electron microscopy. J. biochem. biophys. Cytol. **11**, 729—732 (1961). — KARRER, H. E.: Interconnections in normal human cervical epithelium. J. biophys. biochem. Cytol. **7**, 181—184 (1960). — KEDDIE, F., and D. SAKAI: Morphology of the horny cells of the superficial stratum corneum: cell membranes and melanin granules. J. invest. Derm. **44**, 135—138 (1965). — KELLY, D. E.: Fine structure of desmosomes, hemidesmosomes, and an adepidermal globular layer in developing newt epidermis. J. Cell Biol. **28**, 51—72 (1966). — KIMMIG, J., u. R. WEHRMANN: Biochemie der Haut. In: Dermatologie und Venerologie (H. A. GOTTRON and W. SCHÖNFELD, Hrsg.), Bd. I/2, S. 1178—1238. Stuttgart: Georg Thieme 1961. — KIRKMAN, H., and A. E. SEVERINGHAUS: A review of the Golgi apparatus. III. Anat. Rec. **71**, 79—103 (1938). — KLIGMAN, A. M.: The biology of the stratum corneum. In: The epidermis (W. MONTAGNA and W. C. LOBITZ jr., eds.), p. 387—433. New York and London: Academic Press 1964. — KNOTH, W., M. RUHBACH u. G. EHLERS: Vergleichende ferment-histochemische Untersuchungen nach Anwendung vier verschiedener Schnittherstellungsverfahren. I. Nachweis der sauren Phosphatasen und unspezifische Esterase in Meerschweinchenniere, -zunge und -haut. Arch. klin. exp. Derm. **222**, 403—422 (1965). — KOECKE, H. U.: Die Anwendung des Elektronmikroskopes bei der Untersuchung entwicklungsphysiologischer Probleme. Zeiss Informationen **60**, 47—51 (1966). — KOGOJ, F.: Über die Art der Verbindung zwischen Epidermis und Kutis. Derm. Z. **39**, 203—212 (1923). — KOOYMAN, D. J.: State and localization of inorganic salts in the skin as revealed by extraction and microincineration. Arch. Derm. Syph. (Chic.) **132**, 394—403 (1935). — KOPF, A. W.: The distribution of alkaline phosphatase in normal and pathologic human skin. Arch. Derm. (Chic.) **75**, 1—37 (1957). — KREIBICH, C.: Keratohyalin. Arch. Derm. Syph. (Berl.)

121, 313—318 (1916). — Kromayer, F.: Einige epitheliale Gebilde in neuer Auffassung. Beiträge zur Pigmentfrage. Derm. Z. 4, 335—400 (1897). — Kruse, M.: Aschenbilder von normaler, psoriatischer und neurodermitischer Haut mit besonderer Berücksichtigung des Magnesiumbildes. Z. Haut- u. Geschl.-Kr. 24, 127—131 (1958). — Kruszynski, J.: The microincineration technique and its results. In: Handbuch der Histochemie (W. Graumann u. K. Neumann, Hrsg.), Bd. I/2, S. 96—187. Stuttgart: Gustav Fischer 1966. — Küntzel, A.: Histologie der tierischen Haut. In: Handbuch der Gerbereichemie und Lederfabrikation (E. Grassmann, Hrsg.), Bd. I/1, S. 183—358. Wien: Springer 1944a. — Physikalische Chemie und Kolloidchemie der Eiweißkörper unter besonderer Berücksichtigung des Kollagens. In: Handbuch der Gerbereichemie und Lederfabrikation (E. Grassmann, Hrsg.), Bd. I/1, S. 511—619. Wien: Springer 1944b.

Laden, E. L., J. O. Erickson, and D. Armen: Electron microscopic study of epidermal prickle cells. J. invest. Derm. 19, 211—215 (1952). — Laidlaw, G. F., and S. N. Blackberg: Melanoma studies. A simple technique for the Dopa reaction. Amer. J. Path. 8, 491—498 (1932). — Langerhans, P.: Über die Nerven der menschlichen Haut. Virchows Arch. path. Anat. 44, 325—337 (1868). — Lansing, A. I., and D. I. Opdyke: Histological and histochemical studies of the nipples of estrogen treated guinea pigs with special reference to keratohyalin granules. Anat. Rec. 107, 379—397 (1950). — Laterjet, R.: La physiologie normale du pigment mélanique cutané chez l'homme. Biol. méd. (Nikrói) 28, 1—40 (1938). — Leblond, C. P.: Histological structure of hair, with a brief comparison to other epidermal appendages and the epidermis itself. Ann. N.Y. Acad. Sci. 53, 464—475 (1951). — Leblond, C. P., R. C. Greulich, and J. P. M. Pereira: Relationship of cell formation and cell migration in the renewal of stratified squamous epithelia. In: Advances in biology of skin (W. Montagna and R. E. Billingham, eds.), vol. V, p. 39—67. Oxford-London-Edinburgh-New York-Paris-Frankfurt: Pergamon Press 1964. — Leblond, C. P., B. Messier, and B. Kopriwa: Thymide-H^3 as a tool for the investigation of the renewal of cell populations. Lab. Invest. 8, 296—308 (1959). — Leblond, C. P., and B. E. Walker: Renewal of cell populations. Physiol. Rev. 36, 255—275 (1956). — Le Fevre, P. G.: Evidence of active transfer of certain non-electrolytes across the human red cell membrane. J. gen. Physiol. 31, 505—527 (1948). — Lennert, K., u. G. Weitzel: Zur Spezifität der histologischen Fettfärbungsmethoden. Z. wiss. Mikr. 61, 20—29 (1952/53). — Leonhardi, G.: Die physiologische und pathologische Chemie der Enzyme in der Haut. Akt. Probl. Derm. I, 47—106 (1959). — Stand der Fermentforschung auf dem Gebiete der Dermatologie. Arch. klin. exp. Derm. 211, 75—104 (1960). — Lerner, A. B.: Enzymes. In: S. Rothman, Physiology and biochemistry of the skin, p. 564—579. Chicago: University Chicago Press 1954. — Melanin pigmentation. Amer. J. Med. 19, 902—924 (1955). — Hormonal control of pigmentation. Ann. Rev. Med. 11, 187—194 (1960). — Lerner, A. B., and T. B. Fitzpatrick: Biochemistry of melanin formation. Physiol. Rev. 30, 91—126 (1950). — Lerner, A. B., and J. S. McGuire: Melanocyte-stimulating hormone and adenocorticotrophic hormone. Their relation to pigmentation. New Engl. J. Med. 270, 539—546 (1964). — Leuchtenberger, C., and H. Z. Lund: The chemical nature of the so-called keratohyalin granules of the stratum granulosum of the skin. Exp. Cell Res. 2, 150—152 (1951). — Lever, W. F.: Histopathology of the skin. Philadelphia and Montreal: J. B. Lippincott Co. 1954. — Histopathology of the skin, 3rd ed. Philadelphia and Montreal: J. B. Lippincott Co. 1961. — Lewis, S. R., C. M. Pomerat, and D. Ezell: Human epidermal cells observed in tissue culture with phase contrast microscopy. Anat. Rec. 104, 487—503 (1949). — Lindberg, O., and L. Ernster: Chemistry and physiology of mitochondria and microsomes. In: Protoplasmatologia, Handbuch Protoplasmaforschung, Bd. III, A 4. Wien: Springer 1954. — Lison, L.: Histochimie et Cytochimie Animale. Paris: Gauthiers-Villars 1953. — Lobitz jr., W. C., and J. B. Holyoke: The histochemical response of the human epidermis to controlled injury; glycogen. J. invest. Derm. 22, 189—198 (1954). — Locke, M.: The structure of septate desmosomes. J. Cell Biol. 25, 166—169 (1965). — Loftfield, R. B.: The biosynthesis of protein. Progr. Biophys. 8, 347—386 (1957). — Lubnow, E.: Die Wirkung der Röntgenstrahlen auf die Pigmentbildung im Kaninchenhaar. Z. indukt. Abstamm. u. Vererb.-L. 77, 516—532 (1939). — Ludford, R. J.: Cell organs during keratinization in normal and malignant growth. Quart. J. micr. Sci. 69, 27—57 (1925). — Lundgren, H. P., and W. H. Ward: Levels of molecular organization in α-keratins. Arch. Biochem., Suppl. 1, 78—111 (1962). — The keratins. In: Ultrastructure of protein fibers (R. Borasky, ed.), p. 39—122. New York: Academic Press 1963. — Lyne, A. G., and H. B. Chase: Branched cells in the epidermis of the sheep. Nature (Lond.) 209, 1357—1358 (1966).

MacCardle, R. C., M. F. Engman jr., and M. F. Engman sen.: Mineral changes in neurodermatitis revealed by microincineration. Arch. Derm. Syph. (Chic.) 47, 335—372 (1943). — Mager, M., W. McNary jr., and F. Lionetti: The histochemical detection of zinc. J. Histochem. Cytochem. 1, 493—504 (1953). — Magnin, P. H., and S. Rothman: Inhibition of melanin formation by human epidermis. Dermatologica (Basel) 115, 315—320 (1957). — Magnus, I. A., and R. H. S. Thompson: Cholinesterase activity of human skin. Brit. J. Derm.

66, 163—173 (1954). — MARGHESCU, S., u. O. BRAUN-FALCO: Über Esterasen-Isozyme in der Hornschicht bei Hautgesunden sowie bei Psoriasis, Ekzem und Ichtyosis. Enzymelektrophoretische Untersuchungen an Schuppenextrakten. Arch. klin. exp. Derm. 224, 42—47 (1966). — MARTINOTTI, L.: Richerche sulla fine struttura dell'epidermide humana normale in rapporto alla sua funzione eleidochekeratinica. Nota II. Lo strato granuloso e la funzione cheratojalinica. Arch. Zellforsch. 13, 446—458 (1915). — MARZULLI, F. N.: Barriers to skin penetration. J. invest. Derm. 39, 387—393 (1962). — MASON, H. S.: Structure of melanins. In: Pigment cell biology (M. GORDON, ed.), p. 563—582. New York: Academic Press 1959. — MASSHOFF, W.: Die physiologische Regeneration. In: Handbuch der allgemeinen Pathologie (F. BÜCKNER, E. LETTERER u. F. ROULET, Hrsg.), Bd. VI/1, S. 441—514. Berlin-Göttingen-Heidelberg: Springer 1955. — MASSON, P.: Les naevi pigmentaires, tumeurs nerveuses. Ann. Anat. path. méd.-chir. 3, 417—453 (1926). — Pigment cells in man. In: The biology of melanocytes (M. GORDON, ed.). Spec. publ. N.Y. Acad Sci. 4, 15—51 (1948a). — La "cellule claire" de l'epiderme normal. Mikroskopie 3, 129—135 (1948b). — My conception of cellular nevi. Cancer (Philad.) 4, 9—38 (1951). — MATOLTSY, A. G.: Keratinization of embryonic skin. J. invest. Derm. 31, 343—346 (1958a). — The chemistry of keratinization. In: The biology of hair growth (W. MONTAGNA and R. A. ELLIS, eds.), p. 135—165. New York: Academic Press 1958b. — Structural and chemical properties of keratin-forming tissues. In: Comparative biochemistry. A comprehensive treatise (M. FLORKIN and H. S. MASON, eds.), vol. IV/B, p. 343—369. New York and London: Academic Press 1962a. — Mechanism of keratinization. In: Fundamentals of keratinization (E. O. BUTCHER and R. F. SOGNNAES, eds.), p. 1—25. AAAS, Publ. No 70. Washington, D.C. 1962b. — Prekeratin. Nature (Lond.) 201, 1130—1131 (1964). — Soluble prekeratin. In: Biology of the skin and hair growth (A. G. LYNE and B. F. SHORT, eds.), p. 291—305. Sydney: Angus & Robertson 1965. — Membrane-coating granules of the epidermis. J. Ultrastruct. Res. 15, 510—515 (1966). — MATOLTSY, A. G., and C. A. BALSAMO: A study of the components of the cornified epithelium of human skin. J. biophys. biochem. Cytol. 1, 339—360 (1955a). — The components of the cornified epithelium of the human skin. J. invest. Derm. 25, 71—74 (1955b). — MATOLTSY, A. G., and F. S. M. HERBST: A study of human epidermal proteins. J. invest. Derm. 26, 339—342 (1956). — MATOLTSY, A. G., and M. MATOLTSY: A study of morphological and chemical properties of keratohyalin granules. J. invest. Derm. 38, 237—247 (1962a). — Cytoplasmic droplets of pathologic horny cells. J. invest. Derm. 38, 323—325 (1962b). — The membrane protein of horny cells. J. invest. Derm. 46, 127—129 (1966). — MATOLTSY, A. G., and P. F. PARAKKAL: Membrane-coating granules of keratinizing epithelia. J. Cell Biol. 24, 297—307 (1965). — MATSUMOTO, S.: Demonstration of epithelial movements by the use of vital staining with observations on phagocytosis in the corneal epithelium. J. exp. Zool. 27, 37—47 (1918). — MEDAWAR, P. B.: Sheets of pure epidermal epithelium from human skin. Nature (Lond.) 148, 783 (1941). — The micro-anatomy of the mammalian epidermis. Quart. J. micr. Sci. 94, 481—506 (1953). — MEIRELES PINTO, M. I., L. FALCAO, F. CRUZ-SOBRAL et M. J. X. MORATO: Étude sur glycogène de l'epiderme normal et psoriatique. Ann. Derm. Syph. (Paris) 90, 497—508 (1963). — MEIROWSKY, E.: Origin of melanotic pigment of skin and eye. Leipzig: W. Klinkhardt 1908. — A critical review of pigment research in the last hundred years. Brit. J. Derm. 52, 205—217 (1940). — MEIROWSKY, E., and L. W. FREEMAN: Chromatin-melanin relationships in malignant melanoma. J. invest. Derm. 16, 257—260 (1951). — MEIROWSKY, E., L. W. FREEMAN, and A. WISEMAN: Observation on melanization in isolated hair cells. Acta derm.-venereol. (Stockh.) 31, 723—728 (1951). — MELCZER, N., and G. CSEPLÁK: Epithelfasern und Intercellularspalten der normalen und pathologisch veränderten menschlichen Epidermis in überlebendem Zustande. Arch. klin. exp. Derm. 205, 219—227 (1957). — MENEFEE, M. G.: Some fine structure changes occurring in the epidermis of embryo mice during differentiation. J. Ultrastruct. Res. 1, 49—61 (1957). — MERCER, E. H.: Some experiments on the orientation and hardening of keratin in the hair follicle. Biochim. biophys. Acta (Amst.) 3, 161—169 (1949). — The fine structure of keratin. Textile Res. J. 27, 860—866 (1957). — The electron microscopy of keratinized tissues. In: The biology of hair growth (W. MONTAGNA and R. A. ELLIS, eds.), p. 91—111. New York: Academic Press 1958a. — Electron microscopy and the biosynthesis of fibers. In: The biology of hair growth (W. MONTAGNA and R. A. ELLIS, eds.), p. 113—133. New York: Academic Press 1958b. — Keratin and keratinization. An essay in molecular biology. New York: Pergamon Press 1961. — Protein synthesis and epidermal differentiation. In: The epidermis (W. MONTAGNA and W. C. LOBITZ jr., eds.), p. 161—178. New York and London: Academic Press 1964. — MERCER, E. H., B. L. MUNGER, G. E. ROGERS, and S. I. ROTH: A suggested nomenclature for fine-structural components of keratin and keratin-like products of cells. Nature (Lond.) 201, 367—368 (1963). — MERKER, H. J.: Das elektronenmikroskopische Bild der Haftstellen (Desmosomen) im Vaginalepithel der Ratte. Berl. Med. 12, 555—558 (1961). — MERTSCHNIGG: Histologische Studien über Keratohyalin und Pigment. Virchows Arch. path. Anat. 116, 484—516 (1889). — MESCON, H., and P. FLESCH: Modification of Bennett's method for the histochemical demonstration of free sulfhydryl groups in skin. J. invest. Derm. 18, 261—266 (1952). — MESIROW, S. M., and R. B. STOUGHTON: Demonstration of beta-glucuronidase in human skin. J. invest. Derm. 23, 315—316 (1954). — MESSIER, B., and C. P. LEBLOND: Cell proliferation and migration as revealed by autoradiography after injection of thymidine-H^3 into male rats and mice. Amer. J. Anat. 106, 247—265 (1960). — MEYER, J., and J. P. WEINMANN: Occurrence of phosphamidase in keratinizing epithelia. J. invest. Derm. 29, 393—405 (1957). — MICHELS, N. A.: The mast cells. In: Handbook of haematology (H. DOWNEY, ed.), vol. I/4, p. 318. New York: P. B. Hoeber 1938. — MILLARD, A., and K. M. RUDALL: Light and electron microscope studies of fibres. J. roy. micr. Soc. 79, 227—231 (1960). — MILLER, J., and J. F. A. MACMANUS: The part played by the basal and prickle layers of the epidermis in regeneration and neoplasia. Trans. roy. Soc. Can., Sect. V 34, 81—86 (1940). — MILLONIG, G.: A modified procedure for lead staining of thin sections. J. biochem. biophys. Cytol. 11, 736—739 (1961). — MISHIMA, Y.: New technic for comprehensive demonstration of melanin, premelanin, and tyrosinase sites. Combined Dopa-premelanin reaction. J. invest. Derm. 34, 355—360 (1960). — Lysosomal and non-lysosomal acid phosphatase activity of the human skin. J. Cell Biol. 23, 122 A (1964). — Cellular and subcellular differentiation of melanin phagocytosis and synthesis by lysosomal and melanosomal activity. J. invest. Derm. 46, 70—75 (1966a). — Melanosomes in phagocytic vacuoles in Langerhans cells. J. Cell Biol. 30, 417—423 (1966b). — MOBERGER, G., and P. DE: A cytochemical study of the cellular granules in the stratum granulosum of the epidermis. Exp. Cell Res. 8, 578—582 (1955). — MONIS, B., B. M. BANKS, and A. M. RUTENBURG: β-D-glucuronidase activity in malignant neoplasms of man. Cancer (Philad.) 13, 386—393 (1960). — MONIS, B., and A. M. RUTENBURG: Histochemical distribution of β-D-glucuronidase activity in malignant tumors. J. Histochem. Cytochem. 6, 89—90 (1958). — MONTAGNA, W.: Perinuclear sudanophil bodies in mammalian epidermis. Quart. J. micr. Sci. 91, 205—208 (1950). — The cytology of mammalian epidermis and sebaceous glands. Int. Rev. Cytol. 1, 265—304 (1952). — Histology and cytochemistry of human skin. IX. The distribution of non-specific esterases. J. biophys. biochem. Cytol. 1, 13—16 (1955). — The structure and function of skin. New York: Academic Press 1956. — Histology and cytochemistry of human skin. XI. The distribution of β-glucuronidase. J. biophys. biochem. Cytol. 3, 343—347 (1957). — Skin, integument and pigment cells. In: The Cell (J. BRACHET and A. E. MIRSKY, eds.), vol. V, p. 267—322. New York: Academic Press 1961. — The structure and function of skin, 2nd. ed. New York and London: Academic Press 1962. — The anatomy and histology of normal skin. In: The evaluation of therapeutic agents and cosmetics (T. H. STERNBERG and V. D. NEWCOMER, eds.), p. 1—24. New York-Toronto-London: McGraw-Hill Book Co. 1964. — MONTAGNA, W., and E. B. BECKETT: Cholinesterases and alpha esterases in the lip of the rat. Acta anat. (Basel) 32, 256—261 (1958). — MONTAGNA, W., H. B. CHASE, and J. B. HAMILTON: The distribution of the glycogen and lipids in human skin. J. invest. Derm. 17, 147—157 (1951). — MONTAGNA, W., H. B. CHASE, and W. C. LOBITZ jr.: Histology and cytochemistry of human skin. II. The distribution of glycogen in the epidermis, hair follicles, sebaceous glands and eccrine sweat glands. Anat. Rec. 114, 231—247 (1952). — MONTAGNA, W., A. Z. EISEN, A. H. RADEMACHER, and H. B. CHASE: Histology and cytochemistry of human skin. VI. The distribution of sulfhydryl and disulfide groups. J. invest. Derm. 23, 23—32 (1954). — MONTAGNA, W., et R. A. ELLIS: L'histologie et la cytologie de la peau humaine. XVI. Répartition et concentration des estérases carboxyliques. Ann. Histochim. 3, 1—17 (1958). — MONTAGNA, W., and V. FORMISANO: Histology and cytochemistry of human skin. VII. The distribution of succinic dehydrogenase activity. Anat. Rec. 122, 65—77 (1955a). — Esterase activity in the skin of mammals. J. Anat. (Lond.) 89, 425-429 (1955b). — MONTAGNA, W., and C. R. HILL: The localization of S^{35} in the skin of the rat. Anat. Rec. 127, 163—171 (1957). — MONTAGNA, W., C. R. NOBACK, and F. G. ZAK: Pigment, lipids and other substances in the glands of the external auditory meatus of man. Amer. J. Anat. 83, 409—435 (1948). — MONTAGNA, W., and J. S. YUN: Histology and cytochemistry of human skin. XXIII. The distribution of cytochrome oxidase. J. Histochem. Cytochem. 9, 694—698 (1961). — MORETTI, G., N. K. ADACHI, and R. A. ELLIS: Regional differences in acid phosphatase and tween esterase activity in the chimpanzee and the macaque. J. Histochem. Cytochem. 8, 237—241 (1960). — MORETTI, G., N. K. ADACHI, H. MESCON, and P. POCHI: Regional variations of enzymes in human skin. Unpubl. data 1963. Quoted from R. A. ELLIS. In: The epidermis (W. MONTAGNA and W. C. LOBITZ jr., eds.), p. 135—144. New York and London: Academic Press 1964. — MORETTI, G., R. A. ELLIS, and H. MESCON: Vascular patterns in the skin of the face. J. invest. Derm. 33, 103—112 (1959). — MORETTI, G., and H. MESCON: Histochemical distribution of acid phosphatases in normal human skin. J. invest. Derm. 26, 347—360 (1956). — MOSES, M. J.: The nucleus and chromosomes: a cytological perspective. In: Cytology and cell physiology (G. H. BOURNE, ed.), 3rd. ed., p. 423—558. New York and London: Academic Press 1964. — MOULIN, F. DE: Der Verhornungsprozeß der Haut und der Hautderivate. Anat. Anz. 56, 461—468 (1923). — MOYER, F.: Electron microscope observations on the origin, development and genetic control of melanin granules in the mouse eye. In: The structure of the eye (G. K. SMELSER, ed.), p. 469—489. New York: Academic Press 1961. — MUSTAKALLIO, K.: Adenosine triphosphatase activity in neural elements of human epidermis. Exp. Cell Res. **28**, 449—451 (1962).

NACHLAS, M. M., and A. M. SELIGMAN: Evidence for the specificity of esterase and lipase by the use of three chromogenic substrates. J. biol. Chem. **181**, 343—355 (1949). — NAKAI, T., and P. SHUBIK: Electronmicroscopic autoradiography: the melanosomes as a site of melanogenesis in neoplastic melanocytes. J. invest. Derm. **43**, 267—269 (1964). — NAY, T.: Mast cells and hair growth in the mouse (1956). Quoted from M. R. OKUN. J. invest. Derm. **44**, 285—299 (1965). — NICOLAU, S.: Recherches histologiques sur la graisse cutanée. Ann. Derm. Syph. (Paris) Ser. 5, **2**, 641—658 (1911). — NOVIKOFF, A. B.: Electron transport enzymes: biochemical and tetrazolium staining studies. In: Histochemistry and cytochemistry. Proc. 1st Intern. Congr., p. 465—481. London: Pergamon Press 1963. — NOVIKOFF, A. B., H. BEAUFAY, and C. DE DUVE: Electron microscopy of lysosome-rich fractions from rat liver. J. biophys. biochem. Cytol. **2**, 179—184 (1956). — NIEBAUER, G.: Über die interstitiellen Zellen der Haut. Hautarzt **7**, 123—126 (1956).

OBERSTE-LEHN, H.: Characteristica der epidermalen Formelemente bei einigen Dermatosen im epidermo-cutanen Grenzflächenbild. Hautarzt **3**, 351—355 (1952). — Dermoepidermal interface. Arch. Derm. **86**, 770—778 (1962). — ODLAND, G. F.: The morphology of the attachment between the dermis and the epidermis. Anat. Rec. **108**, 399—413 (1950). — The fine structure of the interrelationship of cells in the human epidermis. J. biophys. biochem. Cytol. **4**, 529—538 (1958). — A submicroscopic granular component in human epidermis. J. invest. Derm. **34**, 11—15 (1960). — Tonofilaments and keratohyalin. In: The epidermis (W. MONTAGNA and W. C. LOBITZ jr., eds.), p. 237—249. New York and London: Academic Press 1964. — OEHL (1857): Quoted from H. HOEPKE. In: W. v. MÖLLENDORFF, Handbuch der mikroskopischen Anatomie des Menschen, Bd. III/1, S. 1—116. Berlin: Springer 1927. — OGURA, R., J. M. KNOX, and A. C. GRIFFIN: An evaluation of methods for the sulfhydryl and disulfide concentration in the stratum corneum. J. invest. Derm. **35**, 125—129 (1960a). — The application of an ultramicromethod for determining sulfhydryl compounds in the epidermis. J. invest. Derm. **35**, 319—321 (1960b). — Quantitative studies of epidermal sulfhydryl. J. invest. Derm. **36**, 29—35 (1961). — The concentration of sulfhydryl and disulfide in human epidermis, hair and nail. J. invest. Derm. **38**, 69—75 (1962). — OKUN, M. R.: Histogenesis of melanocytes. J. invest. Derm. **44**, 285—299 (1965). — OLÁH, I., u. P. RÖHLICH: Phospholipidgranula im verhornenden Oesophagusepithel. Z. Zellforsch. **73**, 205—219 (1966). — OLIN, T. E. (1942): Zit. von E. HORSTMANN. In: W. v. MÖLLENDORFF, Handbuch der mikroskopischen Anatomie des Menschen. Erg.-Werk, Bd. III/3, S. 1—276. Berlin: Springer 1957a. — OLSON, R. L., and R. E. NORDQUIST: Ultramicroscopic localization of acid phosphatase in human epidermis. J. invest. Derm. **46**, 431—435 (1966). — ORMSBY, O. S., and H. MONTGOMERY: Diseases of the skin. 7th ed., p. 32. Philadelphia 1948. — ORTIZ PICON, J. M.: Über Zellteilungsfrequenz und Zellteilungsrhythmus in der Epidermis der Maus. Z. Zellforsch. **19**, 408—509 (1933). — OTTOSON, D., F. SJÖSTRAND, S. STENSTRÖM, and G. SVAETICHIN: Microelectrode studies on the E.M.F. of the frog skin related to electron microscopy of the dermo-epidermal junction. Acta physiol. scand. **29**, Suppl. 106, 611—624 (1953). — OVERTON, J.: Desmosome development in normal and reassociation cells in the early chick blastoderm. Develop. Biol. **4**, 532—548 (1962).

PADYKULA, H. A.: The localization of succinic dehydrogenase in tissue sections of the rat. Amer. J. Anat. **91**, 107—146 (1952). — PALADE, G. E.: The fine structure of mitochondria. Anat. Rec. **114**, 427—451 (1952a). — Study of fixation for electron microscopy. J. exp. Med. **95**, 285—298 (1952b). — Electron microscope study of mitochondrial structure. J. Histochem. Cytochem. **1**, 188—211 (1953). — PALADE, G. E., and M. G. FARQUHAR: A special fibril of the dermis. J. Cell Biol. **27**, 215—222 (1965). — PALADE, G. E., and K. R. PORTER: The endoplasmic reticulum. Anat. Rec. (Abstract) **112**, 370 (1952). — PARSHLEY, M. S., and H. S. SIMMS: Cultivation of adult skin epithelial cells (chicken and human) in vitro. Amer. J. Anat. **86**, 163—190 (1950). — PASCHER, G.: Bestandteile der menschlichen Hornschicht. Quantitative Skleroprotein-Bausteinanalysen. Arch. klin. exp. Derm. **218**, 111—125 (1964). — PATRIZI, G., and B. L. MUNGER: The maturation of cortical keratin in filiform hairs of the rat penis. J. Ultrastruct. Res. **14**, 329—344 (1966). — PATZELT, V.: Zum Bau der menschlichen Epidermis. Z. mikr.-anat. Forsch. **5**, 371—462 (1926). — Histologische und biologische Probleme der Haut. Z. mikr.-anat. Forsch. **17**, 253—302 (1929). — Über Tonofibrillen, Keratohyalin, Glykogen und Verhornung in der Epidermis. Acta anat. (Basel) **21**, 349—356 (1954). — PAULING, L.: General chemistry, 2nd ed. San Francisco 1953. — The nature of the chemical bond, 2nd ed. Cornell University Press 1948. Ninth Printing 1954. — PAULING, L., and R. B. COREY: Stable configurations of polypeptide chains. Proc. roy. Soc. B **141**, 21—33 (1953a). — Compound helical configurations of polypeptide chains: structure of proteins of the α-keratin type. Nature (Lond.) **171**, 59—61 (1953b). — PAULING, L., R. B. COREY, and H. R. BRANSON: α-helix in the keratin-myosin-fibrinogen group. Proc. nat. Acad. Sci. (Wash.) **37**, 205—211

(1951). — PAUTRIER, L.-M., et FR. WORINGER: Contribution à l'étude de l'histo-physiologie cutanée. III. Les rapports morphologiques entre l'epiderme et le derme. Ann. Derm. Syph. (Paris) **1**, 985—1005 (1930). — PARSE, A. G. E.: Histochemistry. Theoretical and applied. London: J. & A. Churchill Ltd. 1953. — Histochemistry. Theoretical and applied, 2nd ed. London: J. & A. Churchill 1960. — PEARSE, A. G. E., and D. G. SCARPELLI: Intramitochondrial localization of oxidative enzyme systems. Exp. Cell Res., Suppl. **7**, 50—64 (1959). — PEARSON, R. W.: Studies on the pathogenesis of epidermolysis bullosa. J. invest. Derm. **39**, 551—575 (1962). — PEARSON, R. W., and B. SPARGO: Electron microscope studies of dermal-epidermal separation in human skin. J. invest. Derm. **36**, 213—224 (1961). — PEASE, D. C.: Electron microscopy of human skin. Amer. J. Anat. **89**, 469—497 (1951). — PECK, S. M.: Pigment studies of the human skin after application of thorium X. With special reference of origin and function of dendritic cells. Arch. Derm. **21**, 916—956 (1930). — PERCIVAL G. H., and C. P. STEWART: Melanogenesis: a review. Edinb. med. J. **37**, 497—523, (1930). — PERNKOPF, E., u. V. PATZELT: Anatomie und Histologie der Haut. In: Die Haut- und Geschlechtskrankheiten (L. ARZT and K. ZIELER, Hrsg.), Bd. I, S. 1—140. Berlin u. Wien: Urban & Schwarzenberg 1933. — PETRY, G.: Desmosomen. Dtsch. med. Wschr. **87**, 1012—1014 (1962). — PETRY, G., L. OVERBECK u. W. VOGELL: Sind Desmosomen statische oder temporäre Zellverbindungen? Naturwissenschaften **48**, 166—167 (1961a). — Vergleichende elektronen- und lichtmikroskopische Untersuchungen am Vaginalepithel in der Schwangerschaft. Z. Zellforsch. **54**, 382—401 (1961b). — PINKUS, F.: Die normale Anatomie der Haut. In: J. JADASSOHN, Handbuch der Haut- und Geschlechtskrankheiten, Bd. I/1, S. 1—378. Berlin: Springer 1927. — PINKUS, H.: Über Gewebekulturen menschlicher Epidermis. Ein Beitrag zur Anatomie der Haut. Arch. Derm. **165**, 53—85 (1932). — Notes on structure and biological properties of human epidermis and sweat gland cells in tissue culture and in the organism. Arch. exp. Zellforsch. **22**, 47—52 (1939). — Mitotic division of human dendritic melanoblasts. J. invest. Derm. **13**, 309—311 (1949). — Keratosis senilis; a biological concept of its pathogenesis and diagnosis based on the study of normal epidermis and 1730 seborrheic and senile keratoses. Amer. J. clin. Path. **29**, 193—207 (1958). — Die makroskopische Anatomie der Haut. In: J. JADASSOHN, Handbuch der Haut- und Geschlechtskrankheiten, Erg.-Werk (A. MARCHIONINI, Hrsg.), Bd. I/2, S. 1—138. Berlin-Göttingen-Heidelberg-New York: Springer 1964. — Malignant transformation of epithelium. In: Modern trends in dermatology — 3 (R. M. B. MACKENNA, ed.), p. 275—293. London: Butterworths & Co. 1966. — PINKUS, H., and R. HUNTER: The direction of the mitotic axis in human epidermis. Arch. Derm. **94**, 351—354 (1966). — PINKUS, H., R. J. STARRICO, P. J. KROPP, and J. FAN: The symbiosis of melanocytes and human epidermis under normal and abnormal conditions. In: Pigment cell biology (M. GORDON, ed.), p. 127—138. New York: Academic Press 1959. — PIRILÄ, V., and O. ERÄNKÖ: Distribution of histochemically demonstrable alkaline phosphatase in normal and pathological human skin. Acta path. microbiol. scand. **27**, 650—661 (1950). — PLENK, H.: Über argyrophile Fasern (Gitterfasern) und ihre Bildungszellen. Ergebn. Anat. Entwickl.-Gesch. **27**, 302—412 (1927). — PORTER, K. R.: Observations on the submicroscopic structure of animal epidermis. Anat. Rec. (Abstract) **118**, 433 (1954). — Observations on the fine structure of animal epidermis. In: Proc. 3rd Intern. Conf. E.M. 1954 (R. ROSS, ed.), p. 539—546. London: Roy. Microsc. Soc. 1956. — Diversity of the subcellular level and its significance. In: The nature of biological diversity (J. M. ALLEN, ed.), p. 121—163. New York: McGraw-Hill Book Co. 1963. — PORTER, K. R., and F. L. KALLMANN: Significance of cell particulates as seen by electron microscopy. Ann. N.Y. Acad. Sci. **54**, 882—891 (1952). — PRUNIERAS, M. (1957): Quoted from O. BRAUN-FALCO and G. WEBER. Arch. klin. exp. Derm. **207**, 459—471 (1958). — PUCCINELLI, V.: Il desmosoma nell' epithelio cutaneo. G. ital. Derm. **105**, 281—294 (1964).

RABL, H.: Untersuchungen über die menschliche Oberhaut und ihre Anhangsgebilde mit besonderer Rücksicht auf die Verhornung. Arch. mikr. Anat. **48**, 430—495 (1896). — Bleiben die Protoplasmafasern in der Körnerschichte der Oberhaut erhalten? Arch. Derm. Syph. (Wien) **41**, 1—12 (1897a). — Haut. Ergebn. Anat. Entw.-Gesch. **7**, 339—402 (1897b). — Histologie der normalen Haut des Menschen. In: F. MRAČEK, Handbuch der Hautkrankheiten, Bd. I, S. 1—163. Wien: Alfred Hölder 1901. — RAHMANN-ESSER, M., u. F. FEGELER: Autoradiographische Untersuchungen zum RNS-Stoffwechsel der Epidermis gesunder und durch Psoriasis vulgaris veränderter Haut. Arch. klin. exp. Derm. **227**, 852—855 (1966). — RANVIER, M. L.: Nouvelles recherches sur le mode d'union des cellules du corps muqueux de Malpighi. C. R. Acad. Sci. (Paris) **89**, 667—669 (1879). — Sur la structure des cellules du corps muqueux de Malpighi. C. R. Acad. Sci. (Paris) 1374—1377 (1882). — Histologie de la peau. I. La matière grasse de la couche cornée de l'epiderme chez l'homme et les mammifères. Arch. Anat. micr. Morph. exp. **2**, 510—517 (1898). — RAPKINE, L.: Sur les processus chimiques au cours de la division cellulaire. III. Inhibition et rétablissment de la division cellulaire. J. chem. Physics **34**, 416—427 (1937). — RAPPAPORT, M. M., and R. E. FRANZL: The structure of plasmalogens. III. The nature and significance of the aldehydogenic linkage. J. Neurochem. **1**,

303—310 (1957). — RAPPAPORT, H., T. MAKAI, and H. SWIFT: The fine structure of normal and neoplastic melanocytes in the Syrian hamster with particular reference to carcinogen-induced melanotic tumors. J. Cell Biol. **16**, 171—186 (1963). — RASSNER, G.: Aktivitätsmuster von Enzymen des energieliefernden Stoffwechsels in normaler menschlicher Epidermis und bei Psoriasis vulgaris. I. Enzymaktivitätsbestimmungen in normaler menschlicher Epidermis und klinisch nicht veränderter Epidermis bei Psoriasis vulgaris. Arch. klin. exp. Derm. **225**, 398—407 (1966). — RAUSCH, L., u. H. GLODNY: Entwicklungen und Ergebnisse der Thiolforschung in dermatologischer Sicht. Zbl. Haut- u. Geschl.-Kr. **94**, 1—23 (1956). — RAWLES, M. E.: Origin of pigment cells from the neural crest in the mouse embryo. Physiol. Zool. **20**, 248—266 (1947). — Origin of the mammalian pigment cell and its role in the pigmentation of hair. In: Pigment cell growth (M. GORDON, ed.), p. 1—13. New York: Academic Press 1953. — REAVEN, E. P., and A. J. COX jr.: Binding of zinc by the transitional layer of the epidermis. J. invest. Derm. **39**, 133—137 (1962). — The histochemical localization of histidine in the human epidermis, and its relationship to zinc binding. J. Histochem. Cytochem. **11**, 782—790 (1963). — Histidine and keratinization. J. invest. Derm. **45**, 422—431 (1965). — REDFEARN, E. R., and A. M. PUMPHREY: Oxidation-reduction levels of ubiquinone (coenzyme Q) in different metabolic states of rat liver mitochondria. Biochem. biophys. Res. Commun. **3**, 650—653 (1960). — REICHARD, P., and B. ESTBORN: Utilization of desoxyribosides in the synthesis of polynucleotides. J. biol. Chem. **188**, 839—846 (1951). — REYNOLDS, E. S.: The use of lead citrate at high pH as an electron-opaque stain in electron microscopy. J. Cell Biol. **17**, 208—212 (1963). — RHODIN, J.: Correlation of ultrastructural organization and function in normal and experimentally changed proximal convoluted tubule cells of the mouse. Thesis. Karolinska Institutet, Stockholm, p. 1—76, 1954. — An atlas of ultrastructure, p. 132—133. Philadelphia and London: W. B. Saunders Co. 1963. — Ultrastructure of human skin. J. Pediat. **66**, 171—177 (1965). — RHODIN, J. A. G., and E. J. REITH: Ultrastructure of keratin in oral mucosa, skin, oesophagus, claw, and hair. In: Fundamentals of keratinization (E. O. BUTCHER, and R. F. SOGNNAES, eds.), No 70, p. 61—94. AAAS Washington D.C. 1962. — RICHTER, R.: Studien zur Neurohistologie der nervösen vegetativen Peripherie der Haut bei verschiedenen chronischen infektiösen Granulomen mit besonderer Berücksichtigung der Langerhansschen Zellen. Arch. klin. exp. Derm. **202**, 466—495 (1956). — RIEHL, G.: Zur Kenntnis des Pigmentes im menschlichen Haar. Arch. Derm. Syph. (Wien) **11**, 33—39 (1884). — RIEMERSMA, J. C.: Osmium tetroxide fixation of lipids: Nature of the reaction products. J. Histochem. Cytochem. **11**, 436—442 (1963). — RITZENFELD, P.: Über die Dermis-Epidermis-Verbindung. Arch. klin. exp. Derm. **215**, 362—368 (1962). — Über die Basalmembran. Arch. klin. exp. Derm. **220**, 261—265 (1964). — Die Mitochondrien der menschlichen Epidermis unter besonderer Berücksichtigung des fibrillären Apparates. Arch. klin. exp. Derm. **222**, 500—526 (1965). — RITZENFELD, P., u. R. KOCK: Die Mitochondrien und ihre Transformation in der menschlichen Epidermis. Arch. klin. exp. Derm. **225**, 269—285 (1966). — RIVELLONI, G.: Richerche spodografiche in cute umana normale. G. ital. Derm. Sif. **79**, 31—73 (1938). — ROBERTSON, J. D.: The structure and function of subcellular components. Biochem. Soc. Symp. **16**, 3—43 (1959). — The molecular structure and contact relationships of cell membranes. Progr. Biophys. **10**, 343—418 (1960). — ROE, D. A.: A fibrous keratin precursor from the human epidermis. J. invest. Derm. **27**, 1—8 (1956). — ROE, D. A., P. FLESCH, and E. C. J. ESODA: Present status of epidermal mucopolysaccharides. Arch. Derm. **84**, 213—218 (1961). — ROGERS, G. E.: The localization of dehydrogenase activity and sulphydryl groups in wool and hair follicles by the use of tetrazolium salts. Quart. J. micr. Sci. **94**, 253—268 (1953). — Electron microscope studies of hair and wool. Ann. N.Y. Acad. Sci. **83**, 378—399 (1959a). — Newer findings on the enzymes and proteins of hair follicles. Ann. N.Y. Acad. Sci. **83**, 408—428 (1959b). — Electron microscopy of wool. J. Ultrastruct. Res. **2**, 309—330 (1959c). — Structural and biochemical features of the hair follicle. In: The epidermis (W. MONTAGNA and W. C. LOBITZ jr., eds.), p. 179—236. New York and London: Academic Press 1964. — ROGERS, G. E., L. FINCH, and G. YOUATT: Quoted from G. E. ROGERS. In: The epidermis (W. MONTAGNA and W. C. LOBITZ jr., eds.), p. 179—236. New York and London: Academic Press 1964. — RONY, H. R., G. J. SCHEFF, D. M. COHEN, and W. R. RENNAGEL: Sulfhydryl oxidase activity in skin homogenates. J. invest. Derm. **30**, 43—50 (1958). — ROSA, C. G., and K. C. TSOU: Demonstration of the Sjöstrand membrane particles by the electron cytochemical method. Nature (Lond.) **206**, 103—105 (1965). — ROSIN, A.: Über das Verhalten der alkalischen Phosphatase im Frakturkallus der Ratte. Acta anat. (Basel) **16**, 29—44 (1952). — Ross, J. B.: The dermo-epidermal interface in health and disease. Brit. J. Derm. **77**, 77—87 (1965). — Ross, R., and T. K. GREENLEE jr.: Electron microscopy: attachment sites between connective tissue cells. Science **153**, 997—999 (1966). — ROTH, S. I., and W. H. CLARK: Ultrastructural evidence related to the mechanism of keratin synthesis. In: The epidermis (W. MONTAGNA and W. C. LOBITZ jr., eds.), p. 303—337. New York and London: Academic Press 1964. — ROTHBERG, S., R. G. CROUNSE, and J. L. LEE: Glycine-C^{14} incorporation into the proteins of normal stratum corneum and the abnormal stratum corneum of psoriasis.

J. invest. Derm. **37**, 497—505 (1961). — ROTHMAN, S.: Resorption durch die Haut. In: A. BERTHE, Handbuch der normalen und pathologischen Physiologie, Bd. IV, S. 107—151. Berlin: Springer 1929. — Physiology and biochemistry of the skin. Chicago: University of Chicago Press 1954. — ROTHMAN, S., u. FR. SCHAAF: Chemie der Haut. In: J. JADASSOHN, Handbuch der Haut- und Geschlechtskrankheiten, Bd. I/2, S. 161—377. Berlin: Springer 1929. — RUDALL, K. M.: The structure of epidermal protein. In: Symposium on fibrous proteins (Soc. Dyers and Colourists), p. 15—23 (1946). — X-ray studies of the distribution of protein chain types in the vertebrate epidermis. Biochim. biophys. Acta (Amst.) **1**, 549—562 (1947). — The proteins of the mammalian epidermis. Advanc. Protein Chem. **7**, 253—290 (1952). — Elastic properties and α-β-transformation of fibrous proteins. Proc. roy. Soc. B **141**, 39—45 (1953). — The biomolecular structure of hair keratin. In: Progr. in the biological sciences in relation to dermatology — 2 (A. ROOK and R. H. CHAMPION, eds.), p. 355—368. Cambridge: Cambridge University Press 1964. — RUPEC, M.: Über intercelluläre Verbindungen in normaler menschlicher Epidermis. Arch. klin. exp. Derm. **224**, 32—41 (1966). — RUPEC, M., u. O. BRAUN-FALCO: Zur Ultrastruktur und Genese der intracytoplasmatischen Körperchen in normaler menschlicher Epidermis. Arch. klin. exp. Derm. **221**, 184—193 (1965). — RUST, S., u. G. K. STEIGLEDER: Über die Verteilung der Ribonucleinsäure in der gesunden und psoriatisch veränderten Epidermis. Arch. klin. exp. Derm. **221**, 194—202 (1965).

SANDRITTER, W.: Ultraviolettmikroskopische Untersuchungen an Plattenepithel. Frankfurt. Z. Path. **64**, 520—530 (1953). — SANTOIANNI, P., and S. ROTHMAN: Nucleic acid-splitting enzymes in human epidermis and their possible role in keratinization. J. invest. Derm. **37**, 489—495 (1961). — SASAKAWA, M.: Beiträge zur Glykogenverteilung in der Haut unter normalen und pathologischen Zuständen. Arch. Derm. Syph. (Berl.) **134**, 418—443 (1921). — SCARPELLI, D. G., and A. G. E. PEARSE: Physical and chemical protection of cell constituents and the precise localization of enzymes. J. Histochem. Cytochem. **6**, 369—376 (1958). — SCHAFFER, J.: Das Epithelgewebe. In: W. v. MÖLLENDORFF, Handbuch der mikroskopischen Anatomie des Menschen, Bd. II/1, S. 1—231. Berlin: Springer 1927. — Lehrbuch der Histologie und Histogenese, 3. Aufl. Leipzig: Wilhelm Engelmann 1933. — SCHMIDT, W. J.: Die Bausteine des Tierkörpers im polarisierten Lichte. Bonn 1924. — SCHNEIDER, W. C., and E. L. KUFF: On the isolation and some biochemical properties of the Golgi substance. Amer. J. Anat. **94**, 209—224 (1954). — Centrifugal isolation of subcellular components. In: Cytology and cell physiology (G. H. BOURNE, ed.), 3rd ed., p. 19—89. New York and London: Academic Press 1964. — SCHULTZE, B., and W. OEHLERT: Autoradiographic investigation of incorporation of H^3-thymidine into cells of the rat and mouse. Science **131**, 737—738 (1960). — SCHUEMMELFEDER, N.: Histochemie der Zellatmung. Verh. Dtsch. Ges. Path. (G. B. GRUBER, Hrsg.), 32, Tagg, S. 117—125 (1948). — SCHWARZ, E.: Abbau von Histidin zu Urocainsäure in der Epidermis. Biochem. Z. **334**, 415—424 (1961). — SCHWARZ, E., and H. W. SPIER: About the proof of urocanic acid in callus and in normal human horny layer. J. invest. Derm. **45**, 319—323 (1965). — SCOTT, E. J. VAN: Mechanical separation of the epidermis from the corium. J. invest. Derm. **18**, 377—379 (1952). — Definition of epidermal cancer. In: The epidermis (W. MONTAGNA and W. C. LOBITZ jr., eds.), p. 573—586. New York and London: Academic Press 1964. — SCOTT, E. J. VAN, and T. M. EKEL: Kinetics of hyperplasia in psoriasis. Arch. Derm. **88**, 337—381 (1963). — SCOTT, E. J. VAN, and P. FLESCH: Sulfhydryl groups and disulfide linkages in normal and pathological keratinization. Arch. Derm. Syph. (Chic.) **70**, 141—154 (1954). — SCOTT, G. H.: The localization of mineral salts in cells of some mammalian tissues by microincineration. Amer. J. Anat. **53**, 243—288 (1933). — SEIJI, M., T. B. FITZPATRICK, and M. S. C. BIRBECK: The melanosome: a distinctive subcellular particle of mammalian melanocytes and the site of melanogenesis. J. invest. Derm. **36**, 243—252 (1961). — SEIJI, M., and S. IWASHITA: Intracellular localization of tyrosinase and the site of melanin formation in melanocyte. J. invest. Derm. **45**, 305—314 (1965). — SEIJI, M., K. SHIMAO, M. S. C. BIRBECK, and T. B. FITZPATRICK: Subcellular localization of melanin biosynthesis. Ann. N.Y. Acad. Sci. **100**, 497—533 (1963). — SEIJI, M., K. SHIMAO, T. B. FITZPATRICK, and M. S. C. BIRBECK: The site of biosynthesis of mammalian tyrosinase. J. invest. Derm. **37**, 359—368 (1961). — SELBY, C. C.: An electron microscope study of the epidermis of mammalian skin in thin sections. I. Dermo-epidermal junction and basal cell layer. J. biophys. biochem. Cytol. **1**, 429—444 (1955). — The fine structure of human epidermis as revealed by the electron microscope. J. soc. cosmet. Chemists **7**, 584—599 (1956). — An electron microscope study of thin sections of human skin. II. Superficial cell layers of footpad epidermis. J. invest. Derm. **29**, 131—150 (1957). — SELIGMAN, A. M., and S. H. RUTENBURG: The histochemical demonstration of succinic dehydrogenase. Science **113**, 317—320 (1951). — SELIGMAN, A. M., K.-C. TSOU, S. H. RUTENBURG, and R. B. COHEN: Histochemical demonstration of β-D-glucuronidase with a synthetic substrate. J. Histochem. Cytochem. **2**, 209—229 (1954). — SERRI, F.: La succinodeidrasi nella cute umana normale e pathologica. Minerva derm. **30**, Suppl. 12, 636—646 (1955). — SERRI, F., e G. RABBIOSI: Indagini sull'attività enzimatica cutanea della deidrasi succinia nelle differenti età della vita. Minerva med. **47**, 1515—1516

(1956). — SETÄLÄ, K., L. MERENMIES, L. STJERNVALL, and M. NYHOLM: Mechanism of experimental tumorigenesis. IV. Ultrastructure of interfollicular epidermis of normal adult mouse. J. nat. Cancer Inst. 24, 329—353 (1960). — SHELLEY, W. B., S. B. COHEN, and G. B. KOELLE: Histochemical demonstration of monoamine oxidase in human skin. J. invest. Derm. 24, 561—565 (1955). — SHELDON, H., and H. ZETTERQVIST: Experimentally induced changes in mitochondrial morphology: Vitamin A deficiency. Exp. Cell Res. 10, 225—228 (1956). — SHUKLA, R. C.: Visualization of the nuclei of the basal melanocytes of the black guinea-pig and of human skin under the bright field microscope. Nature (Lond.) 207, 1102—1103 (1965). — SIEBERT, G.: Biochemie der Enzyme. Acta histochem. (Jena) 2, 122—134 (1955). — SIEKEVITZ, P., and G. E. PALADE: A cytochemical study on the pancreas of the guinea pig. I. Isolation and enzymatic activities of cell fractions. J. biophys. biochem. Cytol. 4, 203—218 (1958a). — A cytochemical study on the pancreas of the guinea pig. II. Functional variations in the enzymatic activity of microsomes. J. biophys. biochem. Cytol. 4, 309—318 (1958b). — A cytochemical study on the pancreas of the guinea pig. V. *In vivo* incorporation of leucine-1-C^{14} into the chymotrypsinogen of various cell fractions. J. biophys. biochem. Cytol. 7, 619—630 (1960a). — A cytochemical study on the pancreas of the guinea pig. VI. Release of enzymes and ribonucleic acid from ribonucleoprotein particles. J. biophys. biochem. Cytol. 7, 631—644 (1960b). — SIEMENS, H. W.: Allgemeine Diagnostik und Therapie der Hautkrankheiten. Berlin-Göttingen-Heidelberg: Springer 1952. — SJÖSTRAND, F.S.: Electron microscopy of mitochondria and cytoplasmic double membrane. Nature (Lond.) 171, 30—32 (1953a). — The organization of the cytoplasm of the excretory cells of the mouse pancreas. J. appl. Phys. (Abstract) 24, 116 (1953b). — The ultrastructure of the inner segment of the retinal rods of the guinea pig eye as revealed by electron microscopy J. cell. comp. Physiol. 42, 45—70 (1953c). — The ultrastructure of the mitochondria. In: Fine structure of cells. Leiden 1954. Intern. Union Biol. Sci. Ser. B, No 21, p. 16—30. Groningen: P. Noordhoff 1955. — The ultrastructure of cells as revealed by electron microscope. Int. Rev.Cytol. 5, 455—533 (1956a). — Electron microscopy of cells and tissues. In: Physical techniques in biological research (G. OSTER and A. W.POLLISTER, eds.), vol. 3, p. 241—298. NewYork: Academic Press 1956b. — Morphology of ordered biological structures. Radiat. Res., Suppl. 2, 349—386 (1960). — The fine structure of the exocrine pancreas cell. Ciba Found. Symp. Exocrine Pancreas (A. V. S. DE RUECK and M. P. CAMERON, eds.), p. 1—19. London: J. & A. Churchill 1962. — The ultrastructure of the plasma membrane of columnar epithelium cells of the mouse intestine. J. Ultrastruct. Res. 8, 517—541 (1963a). — The fine structure of the columnar epithelium of the mouse intestine with special reference to fat absorption. In: Biochemical problems of lipids (A. C. FRAZER, ed.), B. B. A. library, vol. 1, p. 91—115. Amsterdam: Elsevier Publ. Co. 1963b. — A new repeat structural element of mitochondrial and certain cytoplasmic membranes. Nature (Lond.) 199, 1262—1264 (1963c) — A new ultrastructural element of the membranes in mitochondria and of some cytoplasmic membranes. J. Ultrastruct. Res. 9, 340—361 (1963d). — A comparison of plasma membrane, cytomembranes, and mitochondrial elements with respect to ultrastructural features. J. Ultrastruct. Res. 9, 561—580 (1963e). — The endoplasmic reticulum. In: Cytology and cell physiology (G. H. BOURNE, ed.), p. 311—375. New York and London: Academic Press 1964. — SJÖSTRAND, F. S., E. ANDERSSON-CEDERGREN, and M. M. DEWEY: The ultrastructure of the intercalated discs of frog, mouse and guinea pig cardiac muscle. J. Ultrastruct. Res. 1, 271—287 (1958). — SJÖSTRAND, F. S., and V. HANZON: Electron microscopy of the Golgi apparatus of the exocrine pancreas cell. Experientia (Basel) 10, 367—368 (1954a). — Ultrastructure of Golgi apparatus of exocrine cells of mouse pancreas . Exp. Cell Res. 7, 415—429 (1954b). — SJÖSTRAND, F. S., and J. RHODIN: The ultrastructure of the proximal convoluted tubules of the mouse kidney as revealed by high resolution electron microscopy. Exp. Cell Res. 4, 426—456 (1953). — SMITH, C., and H. T. PARKHURST: Studies on the thymus of the mammal. II. A comparison of the staining properties of Hassal's corpuscles and of thick skin of the guinea pig. Anat. Rec. 103, 649—673 (1949). — SMITH, D. T.: The ingestion of melanin pigment granules by tissue cultures. Johns Hopk. Hosp. Bull. 32, 240—244 (1921). — SNELL, R. S.: Effect of the alpha melanocyte stimulating hormone of the pituitary on mammalian epidermal melanocytes. J. invest. Derm. 42, 337—347 (1964). — An electron microscopic study of keratinization in the epidermal cells of the guinea-pig. Z. Zellforsch. 65, 829—846 (1965a). — The fate of epidermal desmosomes in mammalian skin. Z. Zellforsch. 66, 471—487 (1965b). — SOGNNAES, R. F., and J. T. ALBRIGHT: Preliminary observations on the fine structure of oral mucosa. Anat. Rec. 126, 225—240 (1956). — SPIER, H. W.: Biochemische Grundprobleme der epidermalen Verhornung. Arch. klin. exp. Derm. 219, 568—571 (1964). — SPIER, H. W., u. P. v. CANEGHEM: Zur Histochemie der Verhornung. Arch. klin. exp. Derm. 206, 344—363 (1957). — SPIER, H. W., u. K. MARTIN: Histochemische Untersuchungen über Phosphomonoesterasen der gesunden Haut mit Hinweis auf Befunde bei Hauterkrankungen. Arch. klin. exp. Derm. 202, 120—152 (1956). — SPIER, H. W., u. G. PASCHER: Zur analytischen und funktionellen Physiologie der Hautoberfläche. Hautarzt 7, 55—60 (1956). —

Die wasserlöslichen Bestandteile der peripheren Hornschicht (Hautoberfläche). Quantitative Analysen. VI. Das Substrat der UV-Absorption des wasserlöslichen Urocaninsäure-Gehalt der Hornschicht. Arch. klin. exp. Derm. **209**, 181—193 (1959). — SPIER, H. W., G. PASCHER u. K. MARTIN: Phosphomonoesterasen an der Hautoberfläche. Dermatologica (Basel) **111**, 9—13 (1955). — STAFFORD, H. A.: Intracellular localization of enzymes in pea seedlings. Physiol. Plant. (København) **4**, 696—741 (1951). — STARCK, D.: Herkunft und Entwicklung der Pigmentzellen. In: J. JADASSOHN, Handbuch der Haut- und Geschlechtskrankheiten, Erg.-Werk (A. MARCHIONINI, Hrsg.), Bd. I/2, S. 139—175. Berlin-Göttingen-Heidelberg-New York: Springer 1964. — STARRICO, R. J.: Qualitative and quantitative data on melanocytes in human epidermis treated with thorium X. J. invest. Derm. **29**, 185—195 (1957). — STARRICO, R. J., and H. PINKUS: Quantitative and qualitative data on the pigment cells of adult human epidermis. J. invest. Derm. **28**, 33—44 (1957). — STEIGLEDER, G. K.: Histochemische Untersuchungen im psoriatischen Herd über Oxydation, Reduktion und Lipoidstoffwechsel. Arch. Derm. Syph. (Berl.) **194**, 296—307 (1952). — Zur Funktion der Acanthose. Arch. Derm. Syph. (Berl.) **200**, 377—395 (1955). — Zum histochemischen Nachweis von Lipase in der normalen Haut und Leber und der normalen und pathologisch veränderten Haut des Menschen. Z. Haut- u. Geschl.-Kr. **20**, 270—272 (1956a). — Zum histochemischen Nachweis SH- und S-S-gruppenhaltiger Substanzen in der normalen und pathologisch veränderten Haut des Menschen. Klin. Wschr. **34**, 495—496 (1956b). — Die Histochemie der Epidermis und ihrer Anhangsgebilde. Arch. klin. exp. Derm. **206**, 276—317 (1957). — Zum Verhalten des esterspaltenden Fermentes in der Haut des behaarten Kopfes. Hautarzt **9**, 67—71 (1958a). — Histochemistry of plantar hyperkeratosis. A contribution to the physiology of the skin surface. J. invest. Derm. **31**, 29—34 (1958b). — Morphologische und histochemische Befunde in pathologischer Hornschicht, insbesondere bei Parakeratose. Ein Beitrag zur Biologie der Hautoberfläche. Arch. klin. exp. Derm. **207**, 209—229 (1958c). — Über den Nachweis der β-glucuronidase auf der Hautoberfläche. Klin. Wschr. **36**, 984—985 (1958d). — Die Histotopochemie der Enzyme in der Haut. In: Aktuelle Probleme der Dermatologie I (R. SCHUPPLI, Hrsg.), S. 84—106. Basel and New York: S. Karger 1959a. — Die Fähigkeit der Hautoberfläche zur Esterspaltung und Esterbildung. III. Das Verhalten der esterspaltenden Enzyme (unspez. Esterasen und Phosphatasen) auf der Hautoberfläche und unter der Hornschicht unter normalen und pathologischen Bedingungen, mit besonderen Hinweisen auf die Acne vulgaris und die Psoriasis. Arch. klin. exp. Derm. **209**, 313—326 (1959b). — Die Struktur der Haut als Grundlage ihrer Leistung und Erkrankung. In: Handbuch der allgemeinen Pathologie, Bd. III/2, S. 539—665. Berlin-Göttingen-Heidelberg: Springer 1960a. — Kritische Analyse der Histochemie der parakeratotischen Hornschicht und der zugehörigen Epidermis mit besonderer Berücksichtigung der Perjodsäure-positiven (PAS-pos.) Substanzen. In: Proc. 11th Intern. Congr. Derm. Stockholm 1957 (S. HELLERSTRÖM, K. WIKSTRÖM, and A.-M. HELLERSTRÖM, eds.). Acta derm.-venereol. (Stockh.) **3**, 383—390 (1960b). — Bemerkungen über das Vorkommen von Enzymen auf, unter und in normaler und pathologisch veränderter Hornschicht. Arch. klin. exp. Derm. **211**, 203—207 (1960c). — Aminopeptidasen-Aktivität auf der Hautoberfläche. Klin. Wschr. **40**, 1154—1156 (1962). — An der Hautoberfläche nachweisbare Enzyme. Zur Frage ihrer Bedeutung bei der epidermalen Verhornung. Arch. klin. exp. Derm. **219**, 585—593 (1964). — STEIGLEDER, G. K., u. H. ELSCHNER: Die Fähigkeit der Hautoberfläche zur Esterspaltung. Arch. klin. exp. Derm. **208**, 489—501 (1959). — STEIGLEDER, G. K., u. I. FISCHER: Über die Lokalisation von Ribonuclease- (RNAse) und Deoxyribonuclease (DNAse)- Aktivität in normaler, in entzündlich veränderter Haut und bei Hauttumoren. Arch. klin. exp. Derm. **217**, 553—562 (1963). — STEIGLEDER, G. K., u. O. GANS: Pathologische Reaktionen in der Epidermis. In: J. JADASSOHN, Handbuch der Haut- und Geschlechtskrankheiten, Erg.-Werk (A. MARCHIONINI, Hrsg.), Bd. I/2, S. 178—298. Berlin-Göttingen-Heidelberg: Springer 1964. — STEIGLEDER, G. K., Y. KAMEI u. KUDICKE: Lokalisation von proteolytischer Aktivität in entzündlich veränderter Haut. Arch. klin. exp. Derm. **217**, 417—437 (1963). — STEIGLEDER, G. K., R. KUDICKE u. Y. KAMEI: Die Lokalisation der Aminopeptidasen-Aktivität in normaler Haut. Arch. klin. exp. Derm. **215**, 307—325 (1962). — STEIGLEDER, G. K., u. H. LÖFFLER: Zum histochemischen Nachweis unspezifischer Esterasen und Lipasen. Arch. klin. exp. Derm. **203**, 41—60 (1956). — STEIGLEDER, G. K., J. T. MCCARTHY u. M. NURNBERG: Strukturanalytische Untersuchungen an gesunder und kranker Haut unter besonderer Berücksichtigung der Hornschicht. Arch. klin. exp. Derm. **220**, 8—18 (1964). — STEIGLEDER, G. K., and W. P. RAAB: The localization of ribonuclease and deoxyribonuclease activities in normal and psoriatic epidermis. J. invest. Derm. **38**, 209—214 (1962). — STEIGLEDER, G. K., u. K. SCHULTIS: Zur Histochemie der Esterasen der Haut. Arch. klin. exp. Derm. **205**, 196—211 (1957). — STEIGLEDER, G. K., and D. R. WEAKLEY: Mucopolysaccharides in human epidermis. Brit. J. Derm. **73**, 171—179 (1961). — STEINER, K.: Sulfur levels in normal and pathologic epidermis. J. invest. Derm. **34**, 189—196 (1960). — STOECKENIUS, W.: Golgi-Apparat und Centriol menschlicher Plasmazellen. Frankfurt. Z. Path. **68**, 404—409 (1957). — STRAILE, W. E.: A study of the hair follicle and its melanocytes. Develop. Biol. **10**, 45—70 (1964). — STÜTTGEN, G.: Die normale und pathologische Physiologie der Haut. Stuttgart: Gustav Fischer 1965. — SUMNER, J. B., and G. F. SOMERS: Chemistry and methods of enzymes, 2nd. ed. New York: Academic Press 1947. — SWAN, G. A.: Chemical structure of melanins. Ann. N.Y. Acad. Sci. **100**, 1005—1019 (1963). — SWANBECK, G., and N. THYRESSON: A study of the state of aggregation of the lipids in normal and psoriatic horny layer. Acta derm.-venereol. (Stockh.) **42**, 445—457 (1962). — SWANN, M. M.: The control of cell division: A review. I. General mechanisms. Cancer Res. **17**, 727—757 (1957). — SWIFT, H. H.: The desoxyribose nucleic acid content of animal nuclei. Physiol. Zool. **23**, 169—200 (1950). — SWIFT, J. A.: Transfer of melanin granules from melanocytes to the cortical cells of human hair. Nature (Lond.) **203**, 976—977 (1964). — SYLVÉN, B., and I. BOIS: Studies on the histochemical "leucine aminopeptidase" reaction. I. Identity of the enzymes possibly involved. Histochemie **3**, 65—78 (1962). — SZABÓ, G.: The number of melanocytes in human epidermis. Brit. med. J. **1**, 1016—1017 (1954). — A modification of the technique of "skin splitting" with trypsin. J. Path. Bact. **70**, 545 (1955). — The regional anatomy of the human skin and the frequency of hair follicles and sweat ducts. In: Proc. 11th Intern. Congr. Derm. Stockholm 1957 (S. HELLERSTRÖM, K. WIKSTRÖM, and A.-M. HELLERSTRÖM, eds.). Acta derm.-venereol. (Stockh.) **2**, 150 (1959a). — Quantitative histological investigations on the melanocyte system of the human epidermis. In: Pigment cell biology (M. GORDON, ed.), p. 99—125. New York: Academic Press 1959b. — Quoted from W. MONTAGNA: The structure and function of skin, 2nd ed., p. 22. New York and London: Academic Press 1962. — SZAKALL, A.: Über die Eigenschaften, Herkunft und physiologischen Funktionen der die H-Ionen-Konzentration bestimmenden Wirkstoffe in der verhornten Epidermis. Arch. klin. exp. Derm. **201**, 331—360 (1955). — Biologie der Hautoberfläche. In: Proc. 11th. Intern. Congr. Derm. Stockholm 1957 (S. HELLERSTRÖM, K. WIKSTRÖM, and A.-M. HELLERSTRÖM, eds.). Acta derm.-venereol. (Stockh.) **2**, 23—26 (1959). — The epidermal barrier layer. In: Proc. XII. Intern. Congr. Derm. Washington, D. C. 1962 (D. M. PILLSBURY, and C. S. LIVINGOOD, eds.), vol. I, p. 404—406. Intern. Congr. Ser. No. 55. Excerpta Med. Found. Amsterdam-New York-London-Milan-Tokyo 1963. — SZODORAY, L.: Beiträge zur Eiweißstruktur des Hautepithels. Arch. Derm. Syph. (Berl.) **159**, 605—610 (1930). — The structure of the junction of the epidermis and the corium. Arch. Derm. Syph. (Chic.) **23**, 920—925 (1931). — SZODORAY, L., u. K. NAGY-VEZEKÉNYI: Entwicklung und Keratinisation der menschlichen Epidermis mit besonderer Berücksichtigung der Barriere. In: De structura et functione stratorum epidermidis s. d. barrierrae. Proc. 2nd. intern. sympos. Brno 1964 (G. LEJHANEC and P. HYBÁŠEK, eds.). Acta Fac. Med. Univ. Brunensis **16**, 93—97 (1965).

TABACHNIK, J.: Urocanic acid, the major acid-soluble, ultra-violet-absorbing compound in guinea-pig epidermis. Arch. Biochem. **70**, 295—298 (1957). — TAKEUCHI, T.: Histochemical demonstration of branching enzyme (amylo-1,4 → 1,6-transglucosidase) in animal tissue. J. Histochem. Cytochem. **6**, 208—216 (1958). — TAKEUCHI, T., K. HIGASHI, and S. WATAMUKI: Distribution of amylophosphorylase in various tissues of human and mammalian organs. J. Histochem. Cytochem. **3**, 485—491 (1955). — TAMARIN, A., and L. M. SREEBNY: An analysis of the desmosome shape, size, and orientation by the use of histometric and densitometric methods with electron microscopy. J. Cell Biol. **18**, 125—134 (1963). — THOMSON, R. H.: Melanins. In: Comparative biochemistry. A comprehensive treatise (M. FLORKIN, and H. S. MASON, eds.), vol. III, part A, p. 727—753. New York and London: Academic Press 1962. — THUNBERG, T.: Die Enzyme der elementaren Atmung. In: Physiologische Chemie (B. FLASCHENTRÄGER und E. LEHNARTZ, Hrsg.), S. 1171—1245. Berlin-Göttingen-Heidelberg: Springer 1951. — THURINGER, J. M.: Regeneration of stratified squamous epithelium. Anat. Rec. **28**, 31—43 (1924). — Studies on cell division in the human epidermis. Anat. Rec. **40**, 1—13 (1928). — The mitotic index of the palmar and plantar epidermis in response to stimulation. J. invest. Derm. **2**, 313—326 (1939). — THURINGER, J. M., and Z. K. COOPER: Age changes in the human epidermis. Rep. Progr. Res. Proj. Amer. Canc. Soc. C.P. **22**, 1—6 (1949). — The mitotic index of the human epidermis, the site of maximum cell proliferation, and the development of the epidermal pattern. Anat. Rec. **106**, 255 (1950). — TRANZER, J. P., and A. G. E. PEARSE: Cytochemical demonstration of ubiquinones in animal tissues. Nature (Lond.) **199**, 1063—1066 (1963). — TURIAF, J., et F. BASSET: Une case, d'histiocytose X pulmonaire avec présence de particule de nature probablement virale dans les lésions granulomateuses, pulmonaires examinées au microscope électronique. Bull. Soc. méd. Hôp. Paris **116**, 1197—1208 (1965). — Deux nouveaux cas d'histiocytose X à localisations pulmonaires et osseuses avec présence dans les lésions granulomateuses de particules tubulaires intracytoplasmiques suggérant une structure virale. Bull. Soc. méd. Hôp. Paris **117**, 373—383 (1966). — TWITTY, V. C.: Correlated genetic and embryological experiments on Triturus. J. J. exp. Zool. **74**, 239—302 (1936).

UNNA, P. G.: Entwicklungsgeschichte und Anatomie. In: H. v. ZIEMSSEN, Handbuch der speziellen Pathologie und Therapie, Bd. XIV/1, S. 1—114. Leipzig: F. C. W. Vogel 1883. — Histopathologie der Hautkrankheiten. In: J. ORTH, Lehrbuch der speziellen pathologischen

Anatomie, Erg.-Bd., Teil 2, S. 265—272. Berlin: August Hirschwald 1894. — Eine neue Darstellung der Epithelfasern und die Membran der Stachelzellen. Mh. prakt. Derm. **37**, 289—301 (1903a). — Eine neue Darstellung der Epithelfasern und die Membran der Stachelzellen. Mh. prakt. Derm. **37**, 337—342 (1903b). — Biochemie der Haut. Jena: Gustav Fischer 1913. — Zur feineren Anatomie der Haut. III. Von der Stachelschicht zur Hornschicht. Berl. klin. Wschr. **58**, 447—449 (1921). — (1928). Quoted from D. J. KOOYMAN: Lipids of the skin. Arch. Derm. Syph. (Chic.) **25**, 444—450 (1932). — UNNA, P. G., u. L. GOLODETZ: Neue Studien über die Hornsubstanz. Mh. prakt. Derm. **44**, 397—422 (1907a). — Neue Studien über die Hornsubstanz. Mh. prakt. Derm. **44**, 459—468 (1907b). — Die Hautfette. Biochem. Z. **20**, 469—502 (1909). — Zur Chemie der Haut. Das Eigenfett der Hornschicht. Mh. prakt. Derm. **50**, 95—115 (1910a). — Die Hautfette. Mh. prakt. Derm. **51**, 42—44 (1910b).

VERNE, J.: Précis d'Histologie. La Cellule — les Tissus — les Organes, 5th. ed. Paris: Masson & Cie. 1960. — VOGEL, A.: Zum Feinbau der Intercellularbrücken nach Kontrastierung mit Phosphorwolframsäure. In: 4th Intern. Conf. EM, vol. II, p. 286—289. Berlin-Göttingen-Heidelberg: Springer 1960. — VOLKMANN, R. v.: Versuche zur Feststellung der Erneuerungsdauer geschichteter Plattenepithelien. Anat. Nachr. **1**, 86—88 (1950). — VOLLAND, W.: Aktuelle Melaninprobleme. Med. Mschr. **8**, 652—660 (1954). — VOSS, H.: Histochemische Untersuchungen über das Verhalten der menschlichen Haut zur Plasmalreaktion. Dtsch. med. Wschr. **67**, 127—128 (1941).

WALDEYER, W.: Untersuchungen über die Histogenese der Horngebilde, insbesondere der Haare und Federn. Beitr. Anat. Embryol. als Festgabe JACOB HENLE, S. 141—163. Bonn: Max Cohen & Sohn 1882. — WALKER, S. M., and G. R. SCHRODT: Membrane-like structures within sarcoplasmic reticulum. Nature (Lond.) **206**, 150—154 (1965). — WARD, W. H., and H. P. LUNDGREN: The formation, composition, and properties of the keratins. Advanc. Protein Chem. **9**, 243—297 (1954). — WASHBURN jr., W. W., and T. G. BLOCKER jr.: The histochemistry of burned human skin. I. Glycogen, ribonucleic acid and deoxyribonucleic acid. Plast. reconstr. Surg. **14**, 393—402 (1954). — WATSON, M. L.: Staining of tissue sections for electron microscopy with heavy salts. J. biochem. biophys. Cytol. **4**, 475—478 (1958). — WATTIAUX, R., and C. DE DUVE: Tissue fractionation studies. 7. Release of bound hydrolases by means of triton X-100. Biochem. J. **63**, 606—608 (1956). — WEBER, G.: Some aspects of the carbohydrate metabolism enzymes in the human epidermis under normal and pathological conditions. In: The epidermis (W. MONTAGNA and W. C. LOBITZ jr., eds.), p. 453—470. New York and London: Academic Press 1964. — WEIBEL, E. R., u. U. W. SCHNYDER: Zur Ultrastruktur und Histochemie der granulösen Degeneration bei bullöser Erythrodermie congénitale ichtyosiforme. Arch. klin. exp. Derm. **225**, 286—298 (1966). — WEIDENREICH, F.: Über Bau und Verhornung der menschlichen Oberhaut. Arch. mikr. Anat. **56**, 169—229 (1900). — WEINSTEIN, G. D.: Autoradiographic studies of turnover time and protein synthesis in pig epidermis. J. invest. Derm. **44**, 413—419 (1965). — WEISS, P., and W. FERRIS: Electron micrograms of larval amphibian epidermis. Exp. Cell Res. **6**, 546—549 (1954a). — Electronmicroscopic study of the texture of the basement membrane of larval amphibian skin. Proc. nat. Acad. Sci. U.S. **40**, 528—540 (1954b). — WELLINGS, S. R., and V. SIEGEL: Role of Golgi apparatus in the formation of melanin granules in human malignant melanoma. J. Ultrastruct. Res. **3**, 147—154 (1959). — Electron microscopy of human malignant melanoma. J. nat. Cancer Inst. **24**, 437—461 (1960). — WELLS, G. C.: Esterases in normal human skin and in chronic granulomata. In: Progress in the biological sciences in relation to dermatology (A. ROOK, ed.), p. 120—134. Cambridge: Cambridge University Press 1960. — WIEDMANN, A.: Das Verhalten des neurohormonalen Systems der Haut beim Ekzem. Z. Haut- u. Geschl.-Kr. **24**, 34—37 (1960). — Über das neurohormonale System der Haut. Hautarzt **14**, 60—64 (1963a). — Das neurohormonale System der Haut in seinen Beziehungen zu den Gefäßen bei allergischen Prozessen. Derm. Wschr. **147**, 129—133 (1963b). — WIENER, A.: Beitrag zum mikrochemischen Nachweis des Eisens in der Pflanze, insbesondere des „maskierten". Biochem. Z. **77**, 27—50 (1916). — WILGRAM, G.: Das Keratinosom: ein Faktor im Verhornungsprozeß der Haut. Hautarzt **16**, 377—379 (1965). — WILGRAM, G. F., J. B. CAULFIELD, and W. F. LEVER: An electron microscopic study of acantholysis in Pemphigus vulgaris. J. invest. Derm. **36**, 373—382 (1961). — An electron microscopic study of acantholysis and dyskeratosis in Hailey and Hailey's disease. J. invest. Derm. **39**, 373—381 (1962). — Elektronenmikroskopische Untersuchungen bei Hauterkrankungen mit Akantholyse (Pemphigus vulgaris, Pemphigus familiaris benignus chronicus, Morbus Darier). Derm. Wschr. **147**, 281—293 (1963). — WILGRAM, G. F., J. B. CAULFIELD and E. B. MADGIC: A possible role of the desmosome in the process of keratinization. An electron microscopic study of acantholysis and dyskeratosis. In: The epidermis (W. MONTAGNA and W. C. LOBITZ jr., eds.), p. 275—301. New York and London 1964a. — An electron microscopic study of acantholysis and dyskeratosis in Pemphigus foliaceus with a special note on peculiar intracytoplasmic bodies. J. invest. Derm. **43**, 287—299 (1964b). — An electron microscopic study of genetic errors in keratinization of man. In: Biology of the skin and hair growth. Proc. Sympos. Canberra 1964 (A. G. LYNE and B. F. SHORT, eds.), p. 251—266. Sydney: Angus & Robertson 1965. — WILGRAM, G. E., and A. WEINSTOCK:

Advances in genetic dermatology. Arch. Derm. **94**, 456—479 (1966). — WILLIAMS jr., CH. H., R. H. GIBBS, and H. KAMIN: A microsomal TPNH-neotetrazolium diaphorase. Biochim. biophys. Acta (Amst.) **32**, 568—569 (1959). — WISLOCKI, G. B.: The staining of the intercellular bridges of the stratified squamous epithelium of the oral and vaginal mucosa by Sudan black B and Baker's hematein method. Anat. Rec. (Abstract) **109**, 128—129 (1951). — WISLOCKI, G. B., H. BUNTING, and E. W. DEMPSEY: The chemical histology of the human uterine cervix with supplementary notes on the endometrium. In: Menstruation and its disorders (E. T. ENGLE, ed.), p. 23—50. Springfield (Ill.): Ch. C. Thomas 1950. — WISLOCKI, G. B., D. W. FAWCETT, and E. W. DEMPSEY: Staining of stratified squamous epithelium of mucous membranes and skin of man and monkey by the periodic acid-Schiff method. Anat. Rec. **110**, 359—375 (1951). — WOLF, J.: Die innere Struktur der Zellen des Stratum desquamans der menschlichen Epidermis. Z. mikr.-anat. Forsch. **46**, 170—202 (1939). — WOLFF, K.: Histologische Beobachtungen an der normalen menschlichen Haut bei der Durchführung ferment-histochemischer Untersuchungen mit Adenosintriphosphat als Substrat. Arch. klin. exp. Derm. **216**, 1—17 (1963a). — Zur Orthotopie der histochemisch erfaßbaren Aminopeptidasenaktivität der menschlichen Haut. Arch. klin. exp. Derm. **217**, 534—552 (1963b). — Über die Adenosintriphosphataseaktivität der menschlichen Haut. Arch. klin. exp. Derm. **218**, 254—273 (1964a). — Zur Enzymaktivität in den Langerhansschen Zellen. Arch. klin. exp. Derm. **218**, 446—460 (1964b). — Die Langerhans-Zelle. Ergebnisse neuer experimenteller Untersuchungen. I. Mitteilung. Arch. klin. exp. Derm. **229**, 54—75 (1967a). — Die Langerhans-Zelle. Ergebnisse neuer experimenteller Untersuchungen. II. Mitteilung. Arch. klin. exp. Derm. **229**, 76—101 (1967b). — WOLFF, K., and R. K. WINKELMANN: Quantitative studies on the Langerhans cell population of guinea-pig epidermis. J. invest. Derm. (in press). — WOLFF, K., R. K. WINKELMANN, and K. HOLUBAR: Recent observations on Langerhans cells. Exhibition at the XIII. Intern. Congr. Derm. in Munich, 1967. — WOOD, R. L.: Intercellular attachment in the epithelium of hydra as revealed by electron microscopy. J. biophys. biochem. Cytol. **6**, 343—351 (1959). — WOODS, M. W.: Discussion. In: Pigment cell biology (M. GORDON, ed.), p. 560. New York: Academic Press 1959.

YASUMA, A., and T. ICHIKAWA: Ninhydrine-Schiff and alloxan-Schiff staining. A new histochemical staining method for protein. J. Lab. clin. Med. **41**, 296—299 (1953). — YASUNOBU, K. T.: Mode of action of tyrosinase. In: Pigment cell biology (M. GORDON, ed.), p. 583—608. New York: Academic Press 1959.

ZANDER, R.: Der Bau der menschlichen Epidermis. Arch. Anat. Entwickl.-Gesch., 51—96 (1888). — ZEIGER, K.: Das Ladungsmosaik der Epidermis. Z. Zellforsch. **23**, 431—441 (1936a). — Kolloidhistologische Untersuchungen an Epithelien. Z. Zellforsch. **24**, 10—41 (1936b). — ZELICKSON, A. S.: Histochemical localization of mitochondria in human skin. J. invest. Derm. **35**, 265—268 (1960). — Normal human keratinization process as demonstrated by electron microscopy. J. invest. Derm. **37**, 369—379 (1961). — Electron microscopy of skin and mucous membrane. Springfield (Ill.): Ch. C. Thomas 1963. — ZELICKSON, A. S., and J. F. HARTMANN: The fine structure of the melanocyte and melanin granule. J. invest. Derm. **36**, 23—27 (1961a). — An electron microscopic study of human epidermis. J. invest. Derm. **36**, 65—72 (1961b). — ZELICKSON, A. S., H. M. HIRSCH, and J. F. HARTMANN: Localization of melanin synthesis. J. invest. Derm. **45**, 458—463 (1965). — ZIMMERMANN, A. A.: Die Entwicklung der Hautfarbe beim Neger vor der Geburt. Mitt. naturforsch. Ges. Bern **37**, 33—71 (1954). — ZIMMERMANN, A. A., and S. W. BECKER jr.: Precursors of epidermal melanocytes in the negro fetus. In: Pigment cell biology (M. GORDON, ed.), p. 159—170. New York: Academic Press 1959a. — Melanoblasts and melanocytes in fetal negro skin. Ill. Monogr. med. sci. **6**, 1—59 (1959b). — ZIMMERMANN, A. A., and TH. CORNBLEET: The development of epidermal pigmentation in the negro fetus. J. invest. Derm. **11**, 382—392 (1948). — ZWEIFACH, B. W., M. M. BLACK, and E. SCHORR: Histochemical alterations revealed by tetrazolium chloride in hypertensive kidneys in relation to renal VEM mechanisms. Proc. Soc. exp. Biol. (N.Y.) **74**, 848—854 (1950).

Histologie, Histochemie und Wachstumsdynamik des Haarfollikels

Von

Hansotto Zaun, Homburg/Saar

Mit 20 Abbildungen, davon 2 farbige

Einleitung

Der vorliegende Beitrag befaßt sich mit den durch Anwendung mikromorphologischer Untersuchungsverfahren gewonnenen Kenntnissen über die Struktur des normalen Haarfollikels, über seine Strukturwandlungen im Ablauf des cyclischen Haarwachstums und über Topographie und Schicksal einiger seiner Gewebsbausteine. Auch der Altersformwandel der Kopfhaut und die Morphologie epilierter Haarwurzeln werden in ihm besprochen. Gefäß- und Nervenversorgung und die Entwicklung des Haars bleiben ebenso wie die drüsigen Anhangsorgane des Haarfollikels — die Talgdrüsen — unberücksichtigt bzw. sind nur erwähnt, wo es die Geschlossenheit der Darstellung erfordert. Im übrigen muß dazu auf die entsprechenden Kapitel dieses Bandes verwiesen werden. Soweit im Rahmen unseres Themas abzuhandelnde Fakten bereits an anderer Stelle in diesem Ergänzungswerk ausführlicher erörtert sind, wird hier — unter Hinweis auf den betreffenden Beitrag — auf eine erneute Besprechung verzichtet.

In den vier Jahrzehnten nach der Bearbeitung der Histologie des Haarfollikels durch F. PINKUS im Originalwerk dieses Handbuchs ist unser Wissen vom Haar in vieler Hinsicht erweitert und ergänzt worden. Die Tatsache, daß der Haarfollikel als relativ einfaches biologisches System für das Studium von Wachstums- und Differenzierungsvorgängen ein besonders geeignetes Objekt ist (MONTAGNA, 1962), gab Anlaß zu immer genauerem Studium der Morphologie und Wachstumsdynamik des Follikels, wobei eine Reihe neuer Untersuchungsverfahren der Haarforschung dienstbar gemacht wurden. Da im Folgenden auf manche Einzelheit nur andeutungsweise eingegangen werden kann, sei hier auf die monographischen Berichte über die drei in den letzten 15 Jahren abgehaltenen großen Haarsymposien hingewiesen (HAMILTON und LIGHT; MONTAGNA und ELLIS, 1958; LUBOWE), die eine Fülle detaillierten neuen Befundmaterials enthalten.

I. Die Struktur des aktiven Haarfollikels

Ein aktiver (haarproduzierender) Follikel besteht aus dem Haar mit seiner in die Haut eingesenkten Wurzel, den Haarbildungsstätten an der Basis der Wurzel und den epithelialen und bindegewebigen Hüllen der Haarwurzel. Haarfollikel liegen schräg in der Haut. Sie sind in charakteristischen Gruppen angeordnet. Die Basis längerer Follikel erstreckt sich unter die Ebene der Cutis ins subcutane Fettgewebe. Eine gute Orientierung über den Einbau der Follikel in Cutis und

Subcutis und über ihre Dichte und Stellung zueinander erlaubt die Methode des dicken Schnitts (SANDERSON und THIEDE; MARON). Die Gruppenstellung der Follikel kann man an Macerationspräparaten erkennen (OBERSTE-LEHN und NOBIS, 1963; s.a. Abb. 13). Aufgrund von Serienschnitten gefertigte maßstabgetreue Modelle zeigen eindrucksvoll die äußeren Strukturen der Follikel und ihre Größenverhältnisse zueinander und zu den Talgdrüsen (MONTAGNA und VAN SCOTT). Angaben über Zahl und Gruppenstellung von Haarfollikeln in verschiedenen Körperregionen sowie Meßergebnisse von Bestimmungen des Haut-Haarwurzelwinkels und des Tiefstands der Follikel finden sich im Beitrag von H. PINKUS (Bd. I/2).

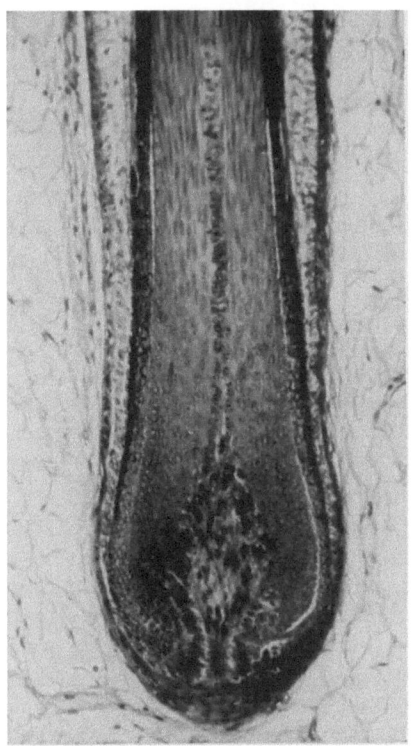

Abb. 1. Sagittalschnitt median durch den unteren Teil der Haarwurzel. Azan-Färbung. Num. Apert. 0,32 Planapochromat. [Aus: H.-J. BANDMANN u. K. BOSSE: Arch. klin. exp. Derm. 227, 390—409 (1966)]

Lichtmikroskopisch stellt sich der Aufbau des Follikels wie folgt dar:

Im Zentrum befindet sich das Haar, dessen aus zwei oder drei verschiedenartigen Zellschichten (s.u.) aufgebauter Schaft aus der Haut herausragt. Die Wurzel des Haars (Abb. 1) endet mit einer zwiebelförmigen Verdickung, dem Bulbus, der vom radialen Ende her eiförmig ausgehöhlt ist. Der Hohlraum wird vom lockeren Bindegewebe der dermalen Papille — des ernährenden Organs — vollständig ausgefüllt. Im Bereich des Bulbus hat der Follikel seinen größten Durchmesser. Die Haarwurzel wird umgeben von zwei röhrenförmigen epithelialen Wurzelscheiden, deren innere aus drei Zellschichten gebildet ist. Äußere und innere Wurzelscheide laufen im unteren und mittleren Drittel des Follikels parallel. Die innere Wurzelscheide, deren Differenzierung in drei Lagen mit zunehmender Verhornung verlorengeht, zerbröckelt — nachdem sie vollständig verhornt ist — etwas unterhalb der Grenze zum oberen Drittel. Die abgebröckelten Fragmente gelangen mit dem sezernierten Talg nach außen. Die äußere Wurzelscheide geht etwa an der Grenze zwischen mittlerem und distalem Follikeldrittel in Höhe der Mündung des Talgdrüsenausführungsgangs ohne scharfe Grenze in das dem Oberflächenepithel entsprechende Epithel des Haarkanals über.

Eine hyaline Membran, die Glashaut, trennt die äußere Wurzelscheide von dem besonders deutlich in der Subcutis hervortretenden bindegewebigen Haarbalg. Der Haarbalg, der den Follikel wie ein Fingerling überzieht, geht oben in den Papillarkörper der Haut über und ist unten mit der dermalen Papille verbunden. An der Seite des Follikels, die mit der Hautoberfläche einen stumpfen Winkel bildet, zieht der Musculus arrector pili schräg aus dem subepidermalen Bindegewebe zum Haarbalg. Oberhalb des Muskels liegen die Talgdrüsen, deren unterschiedlich langer Ausführungsgang in den Haarkanal einmündet. Jenseits dieser Einmündung ist der Haarkanal gleichzeitig Ausführungsgang für die Talgdrüsensekrete (Ductus pilo-sebaceus).

1. Die Haarzwiebel (Bulbus)

Nach Ansicht der meisten Autoren (AUBER; CHASE, 1954; MONTAGNA und VAN SCOTT; MONTAGNA, 1962; BRAUN-FALCO, 1962; ROTH und HELWIG, 1964a), die sich mit der Struktur des Bulbus befaßt haben, besteht die Haarzwiebel aus zwei funktionell unterschiedlichen Regionen, die durch eine durch den weitesten Teil der Papille gelegte imaginäre Ebene getrennt sind. Unterhalb dieser „kritischen Ebene" (AUBER) liegt die eigentliche Haarmatrix, die

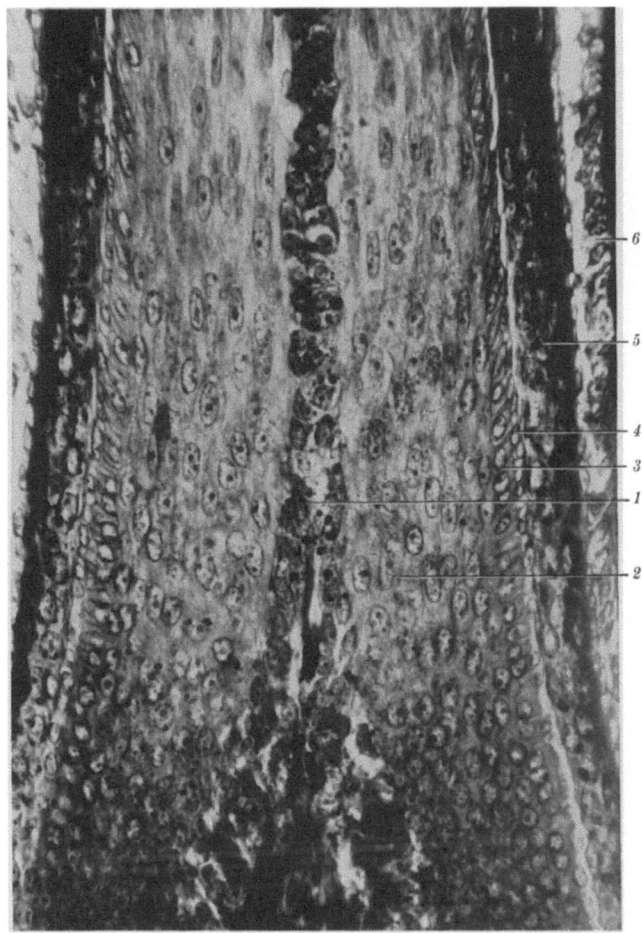

Abb. 2. Zellschichten des oberen Bulbus. Azan-Färbung. Num. Apert. 0,63 Planapochromat. *1* Markzellen, *2* Rindenzellen, *3* Epidermicula, *4* Scheidencuticula, *5* innere Wurzelscheide, *6* äußere Wurzelscheide. [Aus: H.-J. BANDMANN u. K. BOSSE: Arch. klin. exp. Derm. **227**, 390—409 (1966)]

Region der Zellproliferation, oberhalb liegt die Region der Zelldifferenzierung. Im Gegensatz dazu steht die Auffassung KLIGMANs (1959), daß der Bulbus in seiner Gesamtheit Haarmatrix ist, und daß der Auberschen Ebene eine funktionelle Bedeutung als Matrixgrenze nicht zukommt. KLIGMAN stützt sich dabei auf die Tatsache, daß auch im oberen Bulbusbereich (bis zur Höhe der Papillenspitze, BRAUN-FALCO, 1962) noch mitotische Zellaktivität nachgewiesen werden kann. Nach MONTAGNA und VAN SCOTT ist aber die Zahl der mitotisch aktiven Zellen oberhalb der kritischen Ebene zu gering, als daß ihnen für das Haarwachstum eine wesentliche Bedeutung beigemessen werden könnte. Die Ergebnisse zahlenmäßiger Bestimmungen der Mitosen in verschiedenen Bulbusabschnitten (BRAUN-FALCO, 1962; BULLOUGH und LAURENCE; VAN SCOTT und EKEL; VAN SCOTT, EKEL und AUERBACH) stützen diese Anschauung (s. auch unter II und V).

Der unterhalb der kritischen Ebene gelegene Bulbusanteil besteht aus undifferenzierten Zellen und ist völlig melaninfrei. Die papillennahen Matrixzellen sind zylindrisch, die weiter peripher liegenden Zellen ellipsoid. Die Längsachsen papillennaher Zellen stehen senkrecht zum Haarschaft. Mit zunehmender Entfernung von der Papille wird die Richtung der Zellachsen der Richtung der Follikelachse immer mehr angenähert. Matrixzellen zeigen deutliche Nucleoli in großen Kernen und ein mäßig elektronendichtes homogenes Cytoplasma, das die gewöhnlichen cytoplasmatischen Organellen enthält (ROTH und HELWIG, 1964a). Die durch Desmosomen verbundenen Zellmembranen sind glatt und laufen parallel. Zwischen ihnen liegen enge gewundene Kanäle (0,3—0,5 µ Durchmesser), die wahrscheinlich den lichtmikroskopisch sichtbaren „Fusi" (s.u.) entsprechen. Von

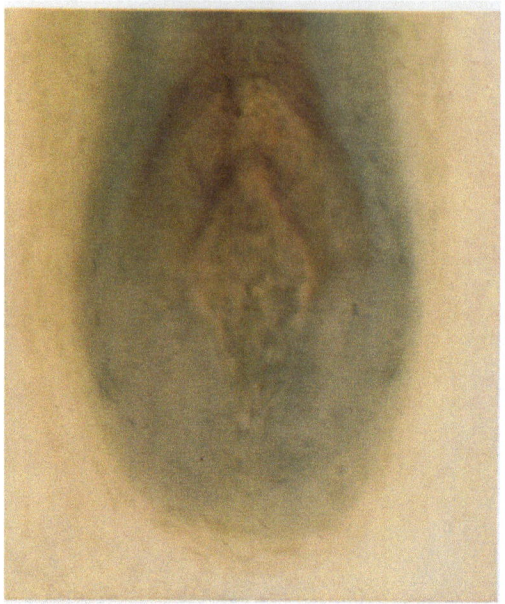

Abb. 3. Pigmenthaube über der Papillenkuppel. Dicker Schnitt. Gallocyaninfärbung. Num. Apert. 0,20 Neofluar
(Präparat und Photo: Prof. H.-J. BANDMANN und Doz. K. BOSSE)

der Matrix steigen die Zellen zum oberen Bulbus auf und formieren sich hier zu 6 elektronenoptisch schon unmittelbar über der Auberschen Ebene unterscheidbaren konzentrischen Zellröhren (BIRBECK und MERCER, 1957), aus denen die je 3 Schichten des Haars und der inneren Wurzelscheide (Abb. 2) hervorgehen. Die Zellen ähneln elektronenmikroskopisch denen der Matrix, sind aber etwas cytoplasmareicher (ROTH und HELWIG, 1964a). Die schon in der Matrix sichtbaren intercellulären Kanäle sind im oberen Bulbus, vor allem in den zentralen Follikelregionen nahe der Papillenspitze, besonders deutlich zu erkennen.

Eine Haube säulenförmiger dentritischer Melanocyten liegt der Basalmembran im Bereich der Papillenkuppel an (Abb. 3). Durch ihre Größe sowie die große Zahl reifer Melaningranula und das Fehlen von Keratinfibrillen im Cytoplasma sind sie von keratinisierenden Zellen leicht zu unterscheiden (BIRBECK). Sie entsprechen in ihren Eigenschaften völlig den Melanocyten der oberflächlichen Epidermis (MEDAWAR). Ihre pigmentreichen Dentriten erstrecken sich zwischen die undifferenzierten Zellen der Rinde und des Marks. Wahrscheinlich werden die Pigmentgranula in die Zellzwischenräume exsudiert und von dort durch Phagocytose in die Haarzellen aufgenommen (SWIFT). Genauere elektronenoptische Untersuchungen über Melanocyten und Melaninbildung im Haar wurden von

BIRBECK, MERCER und BARNICOT sowie BIRBECK durchgeführt. Hinsichtlich näherer Einzelheiten muß hier auf die aufschlußreichen Originalarbeiten verwiesen werden.

Nach dem Grad der Differenzierung der präsumtiven Rindenzellen unterteilen MONTAGNA und VAN SCOTT den Bereich zwischen Matrix und verhorntem Haarschaft in 4 Zonen. In der Zone unmittelbar über der kritischen Ebene („*pre-elongation region*") richten sich die Zellen unter mäßiger Vergrößerung vertikal aus (AUBER). Oberhalb, im engeren Bulbusanteil („*cellular elongation region*"), werden die Zellen beträchtlich verlängert. Es folgt die Verhornungs-Vorzone („*cortical preceratinization region*"), in der zahlreiche basophile Fibrillen in den lang ausgezogenen Rindenzellen sichtbar werden. In der „*keratogenen Zone*" (GIROUD und BULLIARD) werden die Rindenzellen hyalinisiert und verlieren ihren cellulären Charakter.

MERCER (1949) hat den gleichen Bezirk im Hinblick auf Ausrichtung und Stabilität der Haarrindenstrukturen in drei Zonen unterteilt. Er unterscheidet aufgrund polarisationsoptischer und röntgenographischer Untersuchungen 1. isotropen Bulbus, 2. Zone des faserigen, nicht konsolidierten Präkeratins, 3. Zone der fortschreitenden Härtung. Die 2. und 3. Zone von MERCER zeichnen sich durch das Vorliegen doppelbrechender Substanzen aus. Eine Anisotropie ist am Follikel überall dort festzustellen, wo fibrilläre Strukturen vorhanden sind (Abb. 4). In der Haarzwiebel ist das zunächst in der Henleschen Schicht, etwa in der Höhe der Einschnürung des Bulbus in der Huxleyschen Schicht der Fall (SCHMIDT, 1925/26,

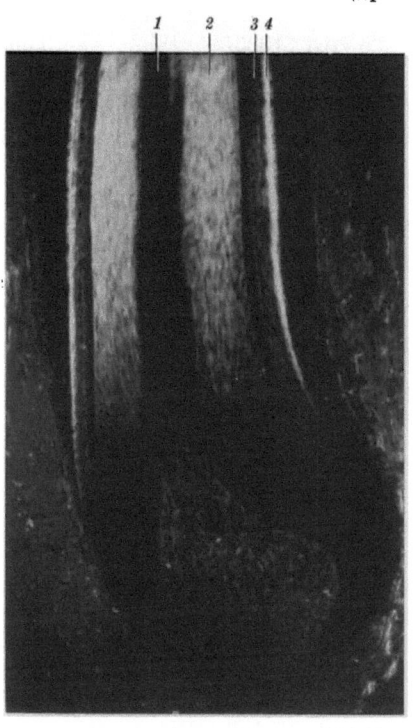

Abb. 4. Unterer Abschnitt einer Haarwurzel aus der Lippe in polarisiertem Licht. *1* Haarmark, *2* Rinde, *3* Huxleysche Schicht, *4* Henlesche Schicht. Die Schwingungsebene des Mikroskops in 45°-Stellung. (Aus: E. HORSTMANN: Handbuch der mikroskopischen Anatomie des Menschen, Bd. III/3, S. 159. Berlin-Göttingen-Heidelberg: Springer 1957)

1932). In der Rindenzone des Bulbus sieht man eine zunehmende Doppelbrechung von der Höhe des oberen Papillenpols an aufwärts (ODLAND).

2. Das Haar

Das Haar ist zusammengesetzt aus der Rinde, dem Oberhäutchen und dem nicht immer vorhandenen Haarmark. Form, Durchmesser und Markausbildung der Haare zeigen in verschiedenen Lebensaltern, bei verschiedenen Rassen und bei beiden Geschlechtern deutliche Unterschiede (DUGGINS und TROTTER; LOCHTE 1951; vgl. auch H. PINKUS, Bd. I/2). Die Schaftbreite der Haare schwankt beträchtlich, auch beim gleichen Individuum und in der gleichen Region. Haardickenmessungen stammen meist aus der Zeit vor Abfassung des Originalwerks (s. dort). Neuere Messungen — tabellarisch zusammengestellt bei HIRSCH — zeigten keine wesentlichen Abweichungen. Für das Kopfhaar werden Breiten von 25—125 μ (Europäer) bzw. bis 150 μ (Asiaten) angegeben.

a) Die Haarrinde (Cortex)

Die Rinde bildet die Hauptmasse des Haars. Sie besteht aus fest miteinander verbundenen faden- bzw. spindelförmigen völlig verhornten Zellen, die 90—120 μ lang und 3—7 μ dick sind (HIRSCH). In diesen Zellen sind Tonofibrillen sehr dicht und parallel zur Längsachse gelagert. Auf der Ausrichtung der Tonofibrillen beruht die starke und bei Dehnung des Haars zunehmende Anisotropie der Rinde (SCHMIDT, 1925/26, 1932). Die Tonofibrillen verleihen dem Haar seine mechanische Festigkeit.

In pigmentierten Haaren sind Melaningranula zwischen den Tonofibrillen in Längsreihen eingelagert (CHARLES). Die Zahl der Pigmentgranula in der Rindensubstanz, die neben dem Luftgehalt des Haars und der Rauhigkeit seiner Oberfläche die Haarfarbe bestimmt, nimmt von außen nach innen ab (VERNALL). Zahl und Verteilung der Granula in der Rinde zeigen bei verschiedenen Rassen deutliche Unterschiede (VERNALL).

Zwischen den Rindenzellen finden sich die Fusi (HAUSMAN, 1932, 1944), zarte Spalträume in unterschiedlicher Zahl, die in der noch lebenden Haarwurzel mit Flüssigkeit gefüllt waren und beim Hochwachsen infolge Austrocknung des Haars Luft aufgenommen haben.

b) Das Haarmark (Medulla)

Das Mark ist der variabelste Teil des Haarschafts. Es kann vollkommen fehlen, unzusammenhängend, zusammenhängend oder fragmental vorhanden sein (HAUSMAN, 1930). Gelegentlich sind in einem Haar nur einzelne wenige Markinseln sichtbar (LOCHTE, 1938a). In seltenen Fällen ist das Mark auch — in ganzer Länge des Haars oder stellenweise — paarig angelegt (CHOWDHURI und BHATTACHARYYA). Gewöhnlich kann man beim gleichen Individuum verschiedene Marktypen beobachten, zuweilen sogar am gleichen Haar. Meist haben dünne Haare keine oder eine unzusammenhängende, dicke Haare eine fragmentale oder zusammenhängende Medulla (WYNKOOP).

Beim Menschen sind zum Zeitpunkt der Geburt in der Regel nur wenige Haare medulliert. Der Anteil markhaltiger Haare zeigt eine Abhängigkeit von Alter, Geschlecht und Rasse (MONTAGNA, 1962). Mit Ausnahme sehr dünner Haare haben beim Erwachsenen fast alle Haare eine Medulla, die aber oft einen so geringen Durchmesser hat, daß sie lichtmikroskopisch nicht zu erkennen ist. Bei polarisationsoptischer Untersuchung tritt sie deutlich hervor, da das Mark im Gegensatz zur Rinde kaum doppelbrechende Strukturen enthält, so daß es als isotroper Einschluß in der anisotropen Rindensubstanz erscheint (GARN). Nach LUELL und ARCHER nimmt der Markdurchmesser im Laufe des Lebens ständig zu. Diese Autoren konnten bei Untersuchung einer großen Zahl epilierter Haarbüschel von Probanden verschiedener Altersklassen und verschiedener Rasse eine eindeutige Beziehung zwischen der maximalen meßbaren Markbreite und dem Lebensalter feststellen. Rassenunterschiede waren nicht zu erkennen. LOCHTE (1938a) gibt an, daß die Medulla beim Menschen bis zu $1/3$ der Schaftbreite des Haars einnehmen kann.

Die locker gebauten Zellen des Marks sind in Papillennähe kubisch und flachen sich ab, wenn sie aufsteigen. Sie zeigen dann geldrollenartige Lagerung (BARGMANN). Da sie später als die Rindenzellen und nur unvollständig verhornen, sind ihre Kerne weiter spitzenwärts anfärbbar als die der Rindenzellen. Markzellen sind nur schwach pigmentiert. Im polarisierten Licht erscheinen die Pigmentgranula aufgrund ihrer spezifischen Absorption als dunkle Körner in den hellen Markzellen (GARN). Häufig sind in den Zellen des Marks basophile Tröpfchen (HORSTMANN, 1957) bzw. acidophile lichtbrechende Granula (BARGMANN) sichtbar, auf deren Natur bei der Besprechung der Verhornungsvorgänge (I/6) näher eingegangen wird. Inter- und intracellulär enthält das Mark mit Luft gefüllte Hohlräume. Elektronenmikroskopisch zeigen papillennahe Markzellen die üblichen Zellorganellen. Mit Ausnahme des Kerns verschwinden diese beim Hochwachsen der Zellen sehr plötzlich, und das Cytoplasma zwischen den Vacuolen wird von einem granulären elektronendichten Material ausgefüllt (ROTH und HELWIG, 1964b). Die Zahl der Vacuolen nimmt nach distal hin zu (ROGERS, 1964). Eine detaillierte Beschreibung der Ultrastruktur der Markzellen in verschiedenen Höhen des Follikels geben ROTH und HELWIG (1964b).

c) Das Oberhäutchen (Epidermicula)

Die Zellen der Epidermicula, die einen festen Schuppenmantel um das Haar bilden, steigen in einer Zellage von der Matrix auf. Ihre Differenzierung ist elektronenmikroskopisch schon am Übergang vom unteren zum mittleren Bulbusdrittel an einer auffälligen Glättung der aneinandergrenzenden Membranen über-

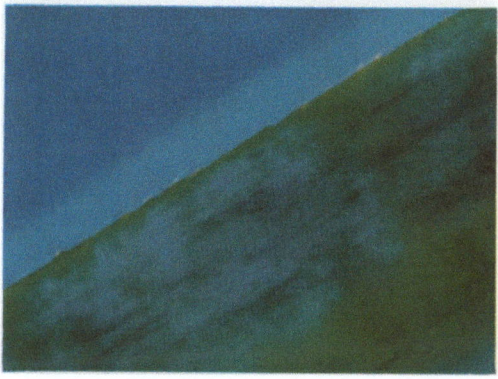

Abb. 5. Dachziegelartige Staffelung der Epidermiculaschuppen. Fluorchromierung mit Chlor-Tetracyclin. Num. Apert. 0,32 Planapochromat. (Präparat und Photo: Prof. H.-J. BANDMANN und Doz. K. BOSSE)

einanderliegender Zellen zu erkennen (BIRBECK und MERCER, 1957b). Die in Bulbusmitte kuboiden Zellen, die die üblichen Zellorganellen enthalten und durch ein elektronendichtes Zementmaterial fest miteinander verbunden sind, werden im oberen Bulbus säulenförmig, wobei ihre Längsachse radial ausgerichtet ist. Aufgrund der lückenlosen Verbindung der Epidermiculazellen können Melanocytenfortsätze nicht zwischen sie eindringen. Die Epidermicula bleibt daher unpigmentiert.

Etwas oberhalb des Bulbus legen sich die Zellen des Oberhäutchens infolge stärkeren Hochrückens ihrer Außenkanten schindelförmig übereinander und werden flacher, wobei ihr Kern an die rindennahe Zellseite rückt und in Scheibenform gepreßt wird. Bis zur Mitte des Follikels flachen sich die Zellen zunehmend ab und gewinnen Schuppenform. In der oberen Follikelhälfte werden die Schuppen hyalinisiert und verlieren ihre Kernreste. In diesem Bereich ist die Epidermicula doppelbrechend.

Am freien Haarschaft liegen 2—7 Schuppen (LOCHTE, 1938a) dachziegelartig übereinander, wobei nur $1/4$ (F. PINKUS) bis $1/6$ (HIRSCH) einer Schuppe freiliegt, der Rest von proximalen Zellen bedeckt ist. Die dachziegelartige Staffelung ist fluorescenzmikroskopisch besonders schön darzustellen (BANDMANN und BOSSE; Abb. 5). Die Schuppen sind beim Menschen durchschnittlich 0,33 µ dick und 30 µ lang (APPLEYARD und GREVILLE).

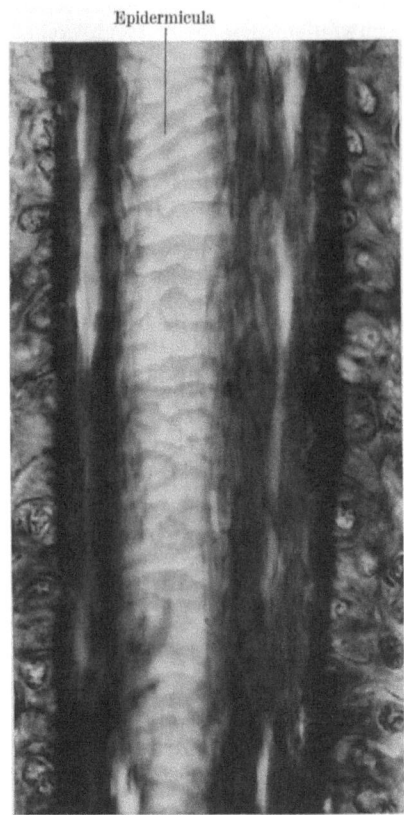

Die Form der Epidermiculaschuppen und die durch ihre freiliegenden Ränder bestimmte Oberflächenzeichnungen des Haars wurde bereits im Originalwerk von F. PINKUS ausführlich besprochen. Durch in der Zwischenzeit vorgelegte weitere Untersuchungsergebnisse von HAUSMAN (1930), MÜLLER sowie LOCHTE (1938a, 1954) konnte erhärtet werden, daß die Zeichnung des Haaroberhäutchens artspezifisch ist. MÜLLER hat darauf hingewiesen, daß es sich bei den von HAUSMAN als „coronal" klassifizierten, das Haar rings umgreifenden Schuppen nicht — wie HAUSMAN vermutete — um geschlossene Ringe handelt, sondern um Verwachsungsprodukte ein und derselben oder (häufiger) verschiedener nebeneinander liegender Schuppen. Zwischen diesen sind Verwachsungsnähte deutlich darstellbar. LOCHTE stellte bei seinen besonders eingehenden Studien über die Oberflächenstruktur des Haars (1938a, b, 1954) fest, daß „traumatische" Einwirkungen die Gestalt der Schuppensäume beeinflussen. Beim Menschen sind die freien Schuppenränder in Wurzelnähe glatt oder leicht gewellt (Abb. 6) und werden zur Haarspitze hin zunehmend eingekerbt. Solche Kerbungen fehlen beim Neugeborenen (LOCHTE, 1938b).

Abb. 6. Epidermicula. Azan-Färbung. Num. Apert. 0,63 Planapochromat. [Aus: H.-J. BANDMANN und K. BOSSE: Arch. klin. exp. Derm. **227**, 390—409 (1966)]

3. Die epithelialen Wurzelscheiden

a) Innere Wurzelscheide

Drei konzentrische Zellschichten, die von der Peripherie der Matrix aufsteigen, bilden die innere Wurzelscheide (Abb. 7). Von außen nach innen unterscheidet man Henlesche Schicht, Huxleysche Schicht und Cuticula. Die funktionelle Bedeutung der mehrschichtigen Gliederung ist unbekannt (BARGMANN). Die Schichten sind bei den meisten Säugern je eine Zellage breit. Beim Menschen kann die Huxleysche Schicht auch zwei Zellen dick sein. In den Zellen der inneren Wurzelscheide findet sich als charakteristisches Intracellularprodukt das Trichohyalin (BIRBECK und MERCER, 1957c), eine lichtmikroskopisch sichtbare Keratinvorstufe (s. I/6). Wie die Zellen der Epidermicula sind auch die Zellen der drei Schichten der inneren Wurzelscheide durch eine etwa in Bulbusmitte auftretende Zementsubstanz fest miteinander verbunden (BIRBECK und MERCER, 1957c). Sie sind frei von Melanin.

In der Henleschen Schicht sind kleine Trichohyalingranula schon in Bulbusmitte in den hier kuboiden Zellen sichtbar. Wenn diese Zellen zum oberen Bulbus hochsteigen, werden sie vertikal verlängert, und ihre Trichohyalingranula vereinigen sich zu homogenen Tropfen und parallel angeordneten Stäbchen. Gleichzeitig setzt die Hyalinisierung der Zellen ein. Ihre Kerne werden unscharf und verschwinden bald.

Bis vor kurzem wurde angenommen, daß die äußere Seite der verhornten Henleschen Schicht völlig glatt ist und bei ihrem Hochwachsen mit dem Haar über die glatte Grenzfläche der teilweise verhornten äußeren Wurzelscheide hinweggleitet (vgl. MONTAGNA und VAN SCOTT;

MONTAGNA, 1962). Nach den elektronenmikroskopischen Befunden von HAPPEY und JOHNSON sowie ROTH und HELWIG (1964a) bestehen aber zwischen Henlescher Schicht und äußerer Wurzelscheide Reihen von Desmosomen oder intercellulären Verbindungspunkten, so daß man — zumindest für den unteren Follikelanteil — annehmen muß, daß Henlesche Schicht und äußere Wurzelscheide miteinander verhaftet sind. In diesem Sinne spricht auch die Tatsache, daß bei Epilation wachsender Haare oft die äußere Wurzelscheide mit extrahiert wird und daß Haar und innere Wurzelscheide nicht etwa aus der äußeren Wurzelscheide herausgleiten.

Erst am Gipfel des Bulbus, wo die Henlesche Schicht schon vollständig hyalinisiert ist, treten in den Zellen der Huxleyschen Schicht Trichohyalingranula

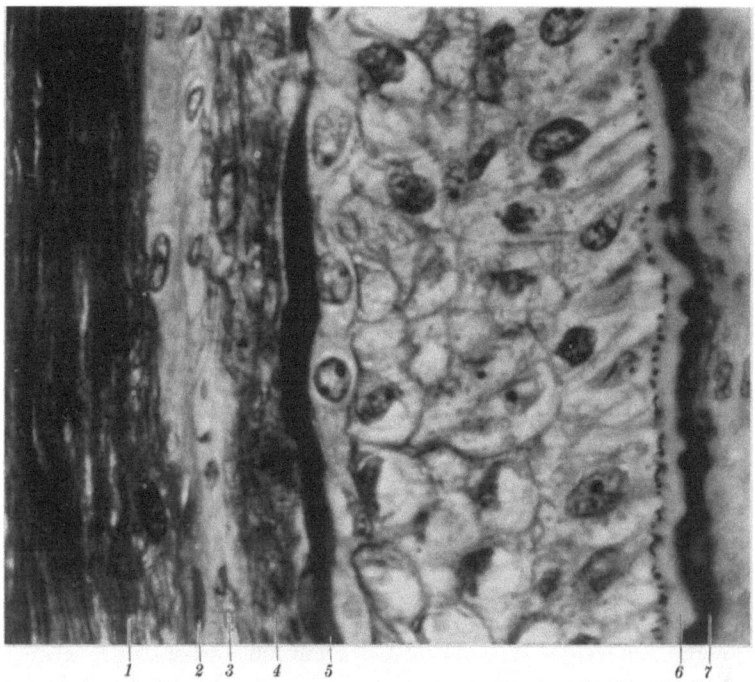

Abb. 7. Haarwurzel. Längsschnitt unterhalb des Haarwulstes. *1* Rinde, *2* Haarcuticula, *3* Scheidencuticula *4* Huxleysche Schicht, *5* Henlesche Schicht, *6* Glashaut, die gegen die äußere Wurzelscheide in feinen Leisten (dunkle Punktreihe) vorspringt, *7* Haarbalg. Vergr. 780fach (Eisen-Hämatoxylin nach HEIDENHAIN). (Aus: E. HORSTMANN: Handbuch der mikroskopischen Anatomie des Menschen, Bd. III/3, S. 157. Berlin-Göttingen-Heidelberg: Springer 1957)

auf. Man sieht hier einige Zellen, aus denen sich cytoplasmatische Ausläufer durch die Henlesche Schicht bis an die äußere Wurzelscheide erstrecken. In diesen „*Flügelzellen*" (HOEPKE) sind lichtmikroskopisch Trichohyalingranula nicht zu erkennen (MONTAGNA, 1962). Sie sollen aber beträchtliche Mengen elektronenmikroskopisch sichtbaren Trichohyalins enthalten (HAPPEY und JOHNSON). Die Ausläufer der Flügelzellen stellen lebende Brücken durch die tote Henlesche Schicht dar und dienen wahrscheinlich der Stoffwechselversorgung der noch lebenden Huxleyschen Schicht, die erst bis zur Follikelmitte hyalinisiert wird.

Die zunächst kuboiden Cuticulazellen, die kleinsten Zellen des Follikels, sind schon im unteren Bulbus zu erkennen. Oberhalb des Bulbus werden diese Zellen und ihre Kerne vertikal elongiert. Die proximalen Enden der abgeflachten Zellen werden etwa in halber Follikelhöhe zum Follikelzentrum hin verschoben, wobei sie die distalen Enden der nachfolgenden Zellen dachziegelartig überlagern. Sie verzahnen sich mit den apikalwärts gerichteten Rändern der Epidermiculazellen (DE GROODT und DE GROODT) und tragen so zur festen Verankerung des wachsenden Haars im Follikel bei. In Follikelmitte treten regelmäßig verteilte Trichohyalingranula in den Zellen auf und kurz danach wird die Cuticula hyalinisiert und die Zellkerne verschwinden.

Die drei vollständig verhornten Schichten der inneren Wurzelscheide verschmelzen etwas oberhalb der Mitte des Follikels zu einer soliden hyalinen Röhre, die sich weiter aufwärts auflockert und in den Haarkanal abbröckelt. Vermutlich erfolgt dieser Abbau durch enzymatische Keratinolyse (MONTAGNA und VAN SCOTT).

Das polarisationsoptische Verhalten der inneren Wurzelscheide läßt den Ablauf der Verhornungsgänge erkennen. In den einzelnen Schichten tritt Anisotropie fortlaufend mit dem Auftreten der Trichohyalingranula, die selbst zunächst isotrop sind (BIRBECK und MERCER, 1957c), in Erscheinung. Eine ausführliche moderne Darstellung polarisationsmikroskopischer Befunde an den Wurzelscheiden gibt HORSTMANN (1957).

b) Äußere Wurzelscheide

Die äußere Wurzelscheide erstreckt sich von den Matrixzellen am unteren Ende der Haarzwiebel aufwärts und geht im Ductus pilosebaceus unmerklich in das den obersten Teil des Haarkanals auskleidende Oberflächenepithel über. Der dem Bulbus anliegende Teil ist dünn (vgl. Abb. 1) und besteht aus 1—3 (meist 2) Lagen abgeflachter Zellen, die einen ellipsoiden Kern und elektronenmikroskopisch die gewöhnlichen cytoplasmatischen Organellen aufweisen (ROTH und HELWIG, 1964a). Von den peripheren Zellen im unteren Follikelbereich gehen zarte cytoplasmatische Fortsätze aus, die seitwärts durch die dicke Glasmembran stoßen. Unmittelbar oberhalb des Bulbus sind diese Ausläufer am deutlichsten entwickelt. Wo sich der Bulbus verjüngt, nimmt die Zahl der Zellschichten zu und die Wurzelscheide verdickt sich zunehmend (s. Abb. 7). Diese Verdickung, der *Haarwulst*, erreicht ihr Maximum am Übergang vom unteren zum mittleren Follikeldrittel. Die Zellen sind hier groß und — abgesehen von der zentralen Zellschicht — von Vacuolen durchsetzt. Der Haarwulst ist meist gleichmäßig ausgebildet, kann aber auch zum Ansatz des Musculus arrector pili hin stärker aufgetrieben sein. Er ist nicht bei allen Säugern vorhanden (MONTAGNA und YUN). Oberhalb des Haarwulstes flachen sich alle Zellagen stark ab, so daß bei gleichbleibender Zahl der Zellschichten die Dicke der Scheide deutlich abnimmt. Die Zahl der Vacuolen vermindert sich.

Distal vom Ende der inneren Wurzelscheide ist der Haarkanal zunächst noch eine kurze Strecke von unverhornten Zellen der äußeren Wurzelscheide ausgekleidet (HORSTMANN, 1957). Nach der Oberfläche zu wird die Wurzelscheide hyalinisiert und verhornt unvollständig. Oberhalb der Talgdrüseneinmündung bildet die äußere Wurzelscheide eine keratinisierte oberflächliche Lage, die in den Haarkanal abgeworfen wird. Die Zellen sind hier weder lichtmikroskopisch noch elektronenmikroskopisch (ROTH und HELWIG, 1964a) von Oberflächenepithelzellen zu unterscheiden. Mitosen, die auch an anderen Stellen der äußeren Wurzelscheide gelegentlich sichtbar sind, finden sich in diesem Bereich besonders häufig. In Höhe der Talgdrüseneinmündung hat ZIMMERMANN eigenartige ringförmige Ausziehungen der äußeren Wurzelscheide, sog. „Kragen", beschrieben, deren peripherer Anteil gegen die Subcutis („Hängekragen") oder gegen die Epidermis („Stehkragen") abgebogen sein kann. Die Bedeutung dieser Bildungen, die vorwiegend an Follikeln des mittleren Gesichtsbereichs beobachtet werden, ist unbekannt.

Im unteren und mittleren Anteil des menschlichen Follikels — unterhalb des Haarkanals — konnte STARICCO (1959, 1960, 1963) zwischen den basalen Anteilen der Zellen, die die periphere Schicht der äußeren Wurzelscheide bilden, unregelmäßig verteilte, von einem hellen Hof umgebene runde Zellen mit dunklem Kern nachweisen. Es handelt sich dabei um amelanotische Melanocyten, die sich in die pigmentierten dentritischen Melanocyten des Haarkanals umwandeln, wenn sie beim Hochwachsen mit der Wurzelscheide die „melanogenetische Ebene" (STARICCO, 1960) in Höhe der unteren Grenze des Haarkanals erreichen. Bei verschiedenen Säugern werden dentritische Melanocyten in der ganzen äußeren Wurzelscheide gefunden (MONTAGNA und HARRISON; MONTAGNA und YUN).

Die äußere Wurzelscheide ist reich an doppelbrechenden Tonofibrillen, die in kompliziert verflochtenen gegenläufigen spiraligen Zügen einen Aufhängeapparat bilden, durch den am Haar wirkende Zug- und Stauchungskräfte auf die äußere Wurzelscheide übertragen und von der empfindlichen Haarwurzel ferngehalten werden sollen (HORSTMANN, 1957).

4. Die dermale Papille

Die bindegewebigen Elemente, die während der Funktionsphase des Follikels von der Haarzwiebel umschlossen sind, bilden die dermale Papille (vgl. Abb. 1 und 3). Ihre Gestalt ist abhängig von der Gestalt des Bulbus. Durch einen basalen Stengel ist die dermale Papille mit der Bindegewebsscheide verbunden. Papillen großer Follikel sind reich vascularisiert, Papillen sehr kleiner Follikel überhaupt nicht. Die Zellen der dermalen Papille zeigen große ovale Kerne und ein vacuolisiertes Cytoplasma. Sie liegen locker verteilt in einer hyalinen Grundsubstanz, in der sich ein zartes argyrophiles Netzwerk darstellen läßt. Nach den elektronenmikroskopischen Befunden von ROTH und HELWIG (1964a) zeigen bei der Maus die mit den üblichen cytoplasmatischen Organellen ausgestatteten Papillenzellen zahlreiche kurze cytoplasmatische Fortsätze. Diese greifen an der Spitze der Papille zwischen die von der Basalmembran des Bulbus umgebenen Fortsätze der Haarzellen. Von einigen Bindegewebszellen an der Basis der Papille, die durch Grundsubstanz deutlich von den anderen Papillenzellen separiert sind, erstrecken sich lange cytoplasmatische Ausläufer an der Außenseite der Basalmembran entlang. Diese Ausläufer sind durch Desmosomen miteinander verbunden und trennen die Basalmembran vom Capillarnetz ab. Gelegentlich finden sich in der Grundsubstanz kollagene Fasern. VAN SCOTT und EKEL haben zeigen können, daß bei normalen menschlichen Haaren konstante Beziehungen zwischen dem Volumen der Papille und dem der Matrix (1:10) sowie zwischen der Zahl der Papillenzellen und der Zahl der mitotisch aktiven Matrixzellen (9:1) bestehen.

5. Die bindegewebigen Follikelhüllen

a) Glashaut

Die Glashaut ist eine homogene zylindrische Membran zwischen der äußeren Wurzelscheide und der Bindegewebsscheide. Sie ist die Basalmembran des Follikelepithels und hängt mit der Basalmembran der Epidermis zusammen. Um den oberen Teil des Follikels herum ist die Glashaut einschichtig und sehr dünn. Im mittleren und unteren Follikelbereich wird sie dicker und erreicht ihre maximale Breite in Höhe des größten Bulbusdurchmessers. Hier sind zwei Schichten deutlich zu unterscheiden. In Matrixhöhe ist die Basalmembran dünn, in der Papille kaum sichtbar.

Die äußere, im ganzen Follikelbereich sichtbare Schicht besteht aus zarten kollagenen Fasern, die ein vom normalen Kollagen etwas abweichendes färberisches Verhalten zeigen (MONTAGNA, 1962). Die innere Schicht, die in Form schmaler Ringblenden zwischen die Basalzellen der äußeren Wurzelscheide eindringt (s. Abb. 7) und in die die basalen cytoplasmatischen Fortsätze der Wurzelscheidenzellen hineinragen, erscheint im histologischen Schnitt als verflochtener Fibrillenfilz. Das lichtmikroskopische Bild ergänzen die elektronenmikroskopischen Befunde von ROGERS (1957). Seine an Follikeln von Meerschweinchen und Mäusen durchgeführten Untersuchungen zeigten, daß die zwei Lagen der Glashaut aus langen kollagenen Fibrillen mit einem Durchmesser von 500 Å bestehen. Diese Fibrillen verlaufen in der inneren Schicht parallel zur Längsachse des Follikels, in der äußeren Schicht senkrecht dazu.

Die Glashaut leitet sich von den Fibroblasten der Bindegewebsscheide her. Ob es an ihr eine innere Lamelle epithelialer Abkunft gibt (F. PINKUS; COOPER), ist Gegenstand der Diskussion (HORSTMANN, 1957; MONTAGNA, 1962).

Anisotropie findet sich in der Glasmembran nur im mittleren Teil der äußeren Schicht — von oberhalb des Bulbus bis zum Beginn des Haarkanals — und nur im Längsschnitt.

b) Haarbalg

Der Haarbalg besteht aus einer inneren Schicht vorwiegend zirkulär verlaufender und einer äußeren — dickeren — Schicht längsverlaufender kollagener Fasern. Im histologischen Schnitt sind in beiden Schichten, jedoch bevorzugt in der äußeren, einige Fibroblasten sichtbar. Auch die zwischen den kollagenen Fasern spärlich anzutreffenden zarten elastischen Fasern liegen großenteils in der peripheren Schicht. Der Faserrichtung entsprechend ist die innere Schicht in Längsschnitten isotrop, in Querschnitten anisotrop, die äußere Schicht in Längsschnitten anisotrop und in Querschnitten isotrop.

Unterhalb des Ansatzes des M. arrector pili finden sich im Haarbalg häufiger zirkulär verlaufende Muskelfasern, die manchmal so zahlreich sind, daß am Querschnitt ein kräftiger Ringmuskel in Erscheinung tritt (ZIMMERMANN). Die Funktion dieses Muskels ist nicht bekannt.

6. Differenzierung der Matrixzellen und Verhornung im elektronenoptischen Bild

Nach der Definition von MERCER, MUNGER, ROGERS und ROTH sind Keratine von epithelialen Zellen produzierte Proteine, die gewöhnlich in den Zellen verbleiben und aufgrund der Gegenwart zahlreicher Disulfidbrücken zwischen den Peptidketten mit üblichen Eiweißlösungsmitteln nicht löslich sind. Sie können vorwiegend faserig, vorwiegend amorph oder Mischungen faseriger und amorpher Elemente sein.

Ziel der Differenzierungsvorgänge in den epithelialen Zellen des Haarfollikels ist die Keratinisation. Im elektronenmikroskopischen Bild kann das Auftreten früher Keratinvorstufen in den Zellen und das Schicksal dieser Differenzierungsprodukte bis zur vollständigen Verhornung sichtbar gemacht werden. Dabei zeigt sich, daß in den verschiedenen von der Matrix aufsteigenden Zellstrukturen unterschiedliche Verhornungsvorgänge zu unterschiedlichen Endprodukten führen (Abb. 8). Die Matrixzellen enthalten noch keine elektronenoptisch darstellbaren Differenzierungsprodukte (PARAKKAL und MATOLTSY; BIRBECK und MERCER, 1957a—c). Über ihre Zellorganellen s. Abschnitt I/1.

In den von der Matrix aufsteigenden Rindenzellen werden im mittleren Bulbus viele zarte Filamente[1] sichtbar (BIRBECK und MERCER, 1957a; MERCER, 1958),

---

[1] Filamente: 50—100 Å dicke fadenförmige Einheiten; Protofilamente: 20 Å dicke fadenförmige Einheiten, die miteinander verbunden sind und Filamente bilden; Fibrillen: lichtmikroskopisch sichtbare Gruppe von Filamenten (vgl. MERCER, MUNGER, ROGERS und ROTH).

die einen Durchmesser von 80 Å haben und aus 20 Å dicken Protofilamenten zusammengesetzt sind (FILSHIE und ROGERS). Diese Filamente lagern sich aneinander und bilden parallel zur Längsachse des Follikels orientierte Bündel. Von der Höhe der Bulbusverengung an wird zwischen die Filamente eine amorphe Zementsubstanz eingelagert und verbindet die Filamentbündel zu Fibrillen. Filamente und Zementsubstanz nehmen mit dem Aufsteigen der Zellen zu, bis der

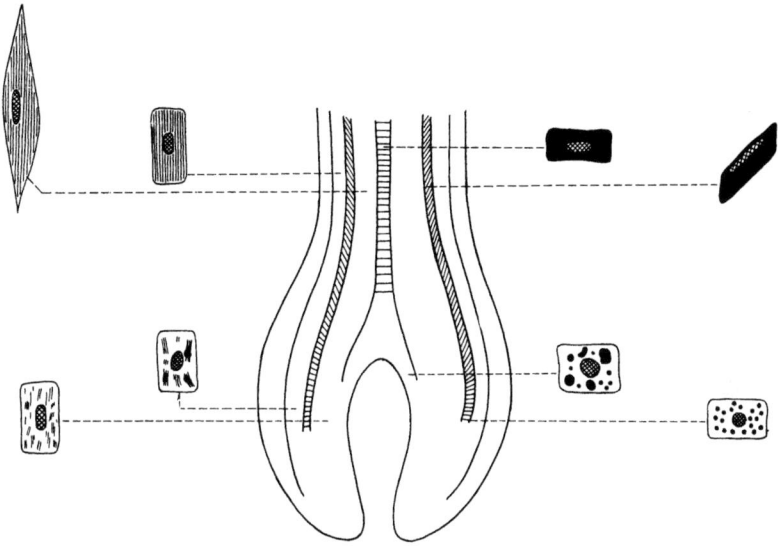

Abb. 8. Schematische Darstellung der elektronenoptisch sichtbaren, in den verschiedenen Zellschichten des Follikels unterschiedlich ablaufenden Verhornungsvorgänge

Cytoplasmaraum mit Fibrillen vollgepackt ist, die schließlich zu Keratinblöcken kondensieren. Das Keratin der Rindenzellen ist dementsprechend ein Komplex aus faserigen Elementen, die in eine amorphe Substanz eingebettet sind (BIRBECK und MERCER, 1957a; ROTH und HELWIG, 1964b). In den verhornten Rindenzellen liegt der von längsausgerichteten Fibrillen eingemauerte Kernrest in der Mitte (ROGERS, 1959).

In den Markzellen treten kurz oberhalb der Papille amorphe runde Granula auf, die zunächst etwa 300 Å dick sind, sich durch fortgesetzte Anlagerung eines amorphen Materials vergrößern und, während die Zellen höher steigen, auch zahlenmäßig zunehmen (PARAKKAL und MATOLTSY). Sie können einen Durchmesser von 1—2 μ erreichen, sind nicht mit Fibrillen vergesellschaftet und lassen keine nur mit Hilfe des Elektronenmikroskopes erfaßbare Feinstruktur erkennen (ROTH und HELWIG, 1964b). Während des weiteren Differenzierungsvorgangs verschwinden die Zellorganellen (s. I/2c) mit Ausnahme des Kerns und der Vacuolen, und das Cytoplasma zwischen den Vacuolen wird mit amorphen Granula vollständig ausgefüllt. Wenn der Zellkern degeneriert, fließen die Granula zu einer homogenen strukturlosen Masse an der Zellperipherie zusammen (PARAKKAL und MATOLTSY).

In den Cuticulazellen treten zwischen Bulbusmitte und Höhe der Follikelconstriction runde amorphe Granula auf (BIRBECK und MERCER, 1957b; ROGERS, 1959) mit einem Durchmesser von etwa 300 Å. Daneben finden sich auch wenige Filamente (HAPPEY und JOHNSON; CHARLES). Während der Zellreifung nehmen die amorphen Granula an Zahl und — durch Anlagerung amorpher Substanz an ihrer Außenfläche — an Größe zu. Sie haben keine Beziehung zu den Filamenten (CHARLES). Die Granula aggregieren sich in der Nähe der lateralen Zellmembran und füllen allmählich die Zelle aus, wobei flachgedrückter Kern und cytoplasmatische Organellen (s. I/2a) an die mediale Zellwand gedrückt werden (ROTH und HELWIG, 1964b). Die Verhornung erfolgt durch Zusammenfließen der Granula zu einer amorphen Masse, in die fibrilläres Material nicht eingeschlossen ist (CHARLES). Diese homogene Masse nimmt die lateralen $2/3$ der Zelle ein. Das mediale Zelldrittel besteht aus einer in keratinolytischen Lösungsmitteln unlöslichen Schicht aus verdichtetem cytoplasmatischen Material (BIRBECK und MERCER, 1957b). Nach HAPPEY und JOHNSON liegt zwischen diesen beiden Schichten eine dünne dritte Schicht aus parallel zur Haarachse angeordneten Fibrillenbündeln, die sich von den schon sehr früh in den Zellen sichtbaren Filamenten herleitet.

Über die Differenzierung der Zellen der inneren Wurzelscheide wurden einander widersprechende Beobachtungen mitgeteilt. Nach BIRBECK und MERCER (1957c) sowie MERCER (1958) enthalten die Zellen in frühen Stadien der Differenzierung keine Filamente, sondern nur amorphes Trichohyalin, das später einer fibrösen Umwandlung unterliegen soll. CHARLES stellte demgegenüber fest, daß Filamente als erste Differenzierungsprodukte erkennbar werden. PARAKKAL und MATOLTSY sowie ROTH und HELWIG (1964a) bestätigten diesen Befund. Nach diesen Autoren erscheinen in der Ebene, in der die verschiedenen Schichten des Haars unterscheidbar werden, 60—80 Å dicke Filamente in den Wurzelscheidenzellen, die sich zu Bündeln (Fibrillen) zusammenlegen. Dicht oberhalb der Region, wo gut umschriebene Filamentbündel sichtbar werden, erscheinen elektronendichte Anlagerungen einer amorphen Substanz an bzw. zwischen den Filamenten. In filamentfreien Bezirken des Cytoplasmas wird diese Substanz nicht beobachtet. Die lichtmikroskopisch sichtbaren Trichohyalingranula sind komplexe Strukturen aus Filamenten und amorpher Substanz (PARAKKAL und MATOLTSY). Sie vergrößern sich durch fortgesetzte Anlagerung der amorphen Substanz an Filamente und gewinnen sehr unterschiedliche Form und Größe. Gleichzeitig nimmt überall in den Zellen die Zahl der Filamente zu. Im Endstadium der Differenzierung verschwindet die amorphe Substanz der Trichohyalingranula. Diese Transformation betrifft zunächst die Henlesche Schicht, dann die Cuticula und zuletzt die Huxleysche Schicht (ROTH und HELWIG, 1964a). Die verhornten Zellen, deren Kerne degeneriert sind und in denen Zellorganellen nicht mehr zu identifizieren sind, sind fast vollständig von 70—80 Å dicken Filamenten ausgefüllt. Zwischen ihnen ist zunächst noch stellenweise amorphes Material — wahrscheinlich Trichohyalinreste — sichtbar, das mit weiterem Aufsteigen der Zellen verschwindet.

Zusammenfassend ergibt sich, daß in Mark und Epidermicula ein amorphes Keratin, in Rinde und Wurzelscheide ein faseriges Keratin entsteht. PARAKKAL und MATOLTSY haben darauf hingewiesen, daß die morphologisch ähnlichen Keratine von Mark und Epidermicula ebenso wie die von Rinde und Wurzelscheide sich ihrer chemischen Natur nach deutlich unterscheiden. Auf diesbezügliche Einzelheiten kann hier nicht eingegangen werden. Chemie und Klassifikation der Keratine sind im Beitrag von RICHTER (Bd. I/3) besprochen.

Aus den Untersuchungen von PARAKKAL und MATOLTSY ergibt sich auch, daß die lichtmikroskopisch ähnlichen granulären Substanzen in innerer Wurzelscheide und Markzellen elektronenmikroskopisch unterschiedlich sind und somit nicht beide als Trichohyalin angesprochen werden können. Die Autoren haben daher vorgeschlagen, die Differenzierungsprodukte der Markzellen als amorphe Granula, die der Wurzelscheidenzellen als Trichohyalingranula zu bezeichnen.

7. Der Haarfollikel in funktioneller Sicht

Die Strukturen des Haarfollikels bilden eine funktionelle Einheit, deren Aufgabe die Haarproduktion ist. Wie MONTAGNA und VAN SCOTT (vgl. auch MONTAGNA, 1962) dargelegt haben, lassen sich aus der Architektur des Follikels einige interessante Rückschlüsse hinsichtlich der mutmaßlichen Bedeutung bestimmter Follikelstrukturen bei der Erfüllung dieser Aufgabe ziehen. So kann die Anschwellung des Bulbus nicht nur durch den Einschluß der dermalen Papille erklärt werden, sondern eine zweckgerichtete Struktur sein, die einen ständigen Anstrom der für ein gleichmäßiges Haarwachstum erforderlichen Zellmengen garantieren soll. Dadurch, daß die Masse der auf breiter Ebene von der Matrix aufsteigenden Zellen im oberen Bulbus durch einen engen „Flaschenhals" getrichtert wird, kann die Wachstumsrate leichter gleichmäßig aufrechterhalten werden, als wenn Matrix und Bulbus den gleichen Durchmesser wie das Haar hätten. Die schon unmittelbar oberhalb der Auberschen Ebene verhornende Henlesche Schicht der inneren Wurzelscheide könnte das Skelet des Trichters bilden, in den die hochsteigenden Zellen hineingedrückt werden. Die mit Glykogen vollgestopften Zellen der äußeren Wurzelscheide und die bindegewebigen Follikelhüllen geben dem Trichter Elastizität und Festigkeit und könnten — gemeinsam mit der inneren Scheide — für das sich bildende Haar formbestimmend sein.

II. Die Strukturveränderungen des Follikels während des Haarcyclus

Die Produktion eines Haars ist kein kontinuierlicher Prozeß, sondern in jedem Follikel wiederholen sich in rhythmischer Folge Phasen der Entwicklung, der Funktion, der Involution und der Ruhe. Jede derartige Phasenfolge bildet einen Haarcyclus, in dessen Ablauf der Follikel tiefgreifenden strukturellen Um-

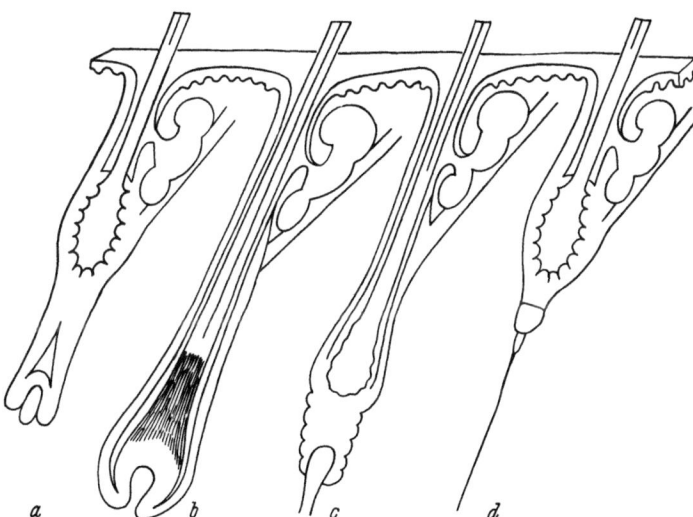

Abb. 9a—d. Die Phasen des Haarcyclus (schematisch). a Entwicklungsphase (wiedergegeben ist das Anagen III), b Funktionsphase (Anagen VI), c Involutionsphase (Katagen), d Ruhephase (Telogen)

wandlungen unterliegt (Abb. 9). Im Prinzip sind die Vorgänge des cyclischen Wachstums im Haarfollikel schon seit langem bekannt, und die Umwandlung des „Papillenhaars" in ein hochsteigendes Kolbenhaar wurde bereits im Originalwerk dieses Handbuchs von F. PINKUS dargestellt. Genauere Untersuchungen über das charakteristische morphologische Substrat der einzelnen Stadien des Haarcyclus wurden aber erst in den letzten Jahrzehnten durchgeführt.

Die gebräuchliche Benennung der Hauptphasen des Haarcyclus geht zurück auf DRY, der aufgrund seiner Untersuchungen an Mäusen vorschlug, die Entwicklungs- und die Funktionsphase als Anagen, die Involutionsphase als Katagen und die Ruhephase als Telogen zu bezeichnen. CHASE, RAUCH und SMITH unterteilten die Anagenphase in sechs morphologisch einwandfrei abgrenzbare Teilphasen (Anagen I—VI)[1]. Die Dynamik der Katagenphase wurde von KLIGMAN (1959) sowie BRAUN-FALCO und KINT genauer studiert, wobei letztere Autoren zeigten, daß drei Teilphasen des Katagen unterschieden werden können.

Ausgehend von dem im vorhergehenden Abschnitt beschriebenen mikromorphologischen Bild des Follikels in der Funktionsphase (Anagen VI) stellen sich die Strukturveränderungen im Ablauf des Haarcyclus bis zur erneuten Bildung eines Follikels mit voll wachsendem Haar im einzelnen wie folgt dar:

Katagen I (Dedifferenzierungsphase). Das erste morphologisch wahrnehmbare Kennzeichen für die Beendigung der Anagenphase ist eine Verkleinerung des Haarbulbus infolge drastischer Reduktion der mitotischen Aktivität. Mit dieser Bulbusverkleinerung kommt es zum Sistieren der Differenzierungsvorgänge. Die Bildung der inneren Wurzelscheide hört völlig auf, und die zentralen Matrixzellen treten nur noch verzögert hoch, wodurch sich die keratogene Zone verlängert (Abb. 10a). Haar und Medulla verschmälern sich zunehmend und auch die Dicke der äußeren Wurzelscheide nimmt beträchtlich ab. Mit der völligen Einstellung der Markbildung — schon von älteren Autoren (DRY, LOCHTE, 1938c) als frühes Zeichen der Beendigung des Haarwachstums erkannt — findet die Dedifferenzierungsphase ihren Abschluß.

Im *Katagen II (Phase der präsumtiven Kolbenhaarbildung)* kommt es im noch nicht wesentlich verkürzten Follikel zu kolbenartiger Anschwellung der untersten Partien der keratogenen Zone (Abb. 10b). Der vorwiegend von nicht definitiv verhornten Matrixzellen gebildete präsumtive Kolben wird seitlich umgeben von einer einlagigen Schicht von Zellen der äußeren Wurzelscheide, an die sich — den Haarkanal nach unten abschließend — ein Strang aus wenig differenzierten Zellen anschließt. Die dermale Papille wird sehr klein.

Im *Katagen III (Expulsionsphase)* wird der parakeratotisch verhornte präsumtive Haarkolben kontinuierlich aufwärts befördert (Abb. 10c—e), bis er die definitive Lage der Telogenphase unterhalb der Einmündung des Talgdrüsenausführungsgangs erreicht hat. Während dieser Zeit verlängert sich der dedifferenzierte Zellstrang in dem Maße, in dem der präsumtive Kolben hochrückt.

Welche Mechanismen das Hochsteigen des Haars im sich verkürzenden Follikel bewirken, ist Gegenstand der Diskussion. Die Annahme von SCHWANITZ, daß der proximale Haaranteil bis zur Höhe der Telogenstellung mit dem Follikel atrophiert, kann aufgrund neuerer Untersuchungen (BRAUN-FALCO und KINT) als widerlegt gelten. WOLBACH glaubt, daß durch massive Verdickung von Haarbalg und Glasmembran und gleichzeitige Verkürzung der äußeren Wurzelscheide das Haar passiv aufwärts geschoben bzw. gezogen wird. KLIGMAN (1959) sowie SAVILL und WARREN sehen in dem Druck, der durch den infolge zahlenmäßiger Zunahme undifferenzierter Zellen sich verlängernden Zellstrang auf den präsumtiven Kolben ausgeübt wird, die treibende Kraft für die Katagenbewegung des Haars. Gegen diese Auffassungen haben BRAUN-FALCO und KINT aufgrund ihrer sorgfältigen Beobachtungen bei Ratten eingewandt, daß sie bei ihren Versuchstieren eine Verdickung von Bindegewebsscheide und Glasmembran nicht feststellen konnten und daß der sich verlängernde dedifferenzierte Zellstrang oft so dünn und unregelmäßig ausgebildet ist, daß man ihm eine aktive Funktion in obigem Sinne kaum

---

[1] Der terminologischen Anregung von DAVIS, das Stadium der Haarbildung — beginnend mit dem Einsetzen der Keratinisation und endend mit dem Abschluß der Haarproduktion — als *Metagen* zu bezeichnen und damit von der Entwicklungs-(Anagen-)phase abzugrenzen, wurde bislang im Schrifttum nicht gefolgt, obwohl das unter physiologischen Gesichtspunkten begrüßenswert wäre.

Die Strukturveränderungen des Follikels während des Haarcyclus 159

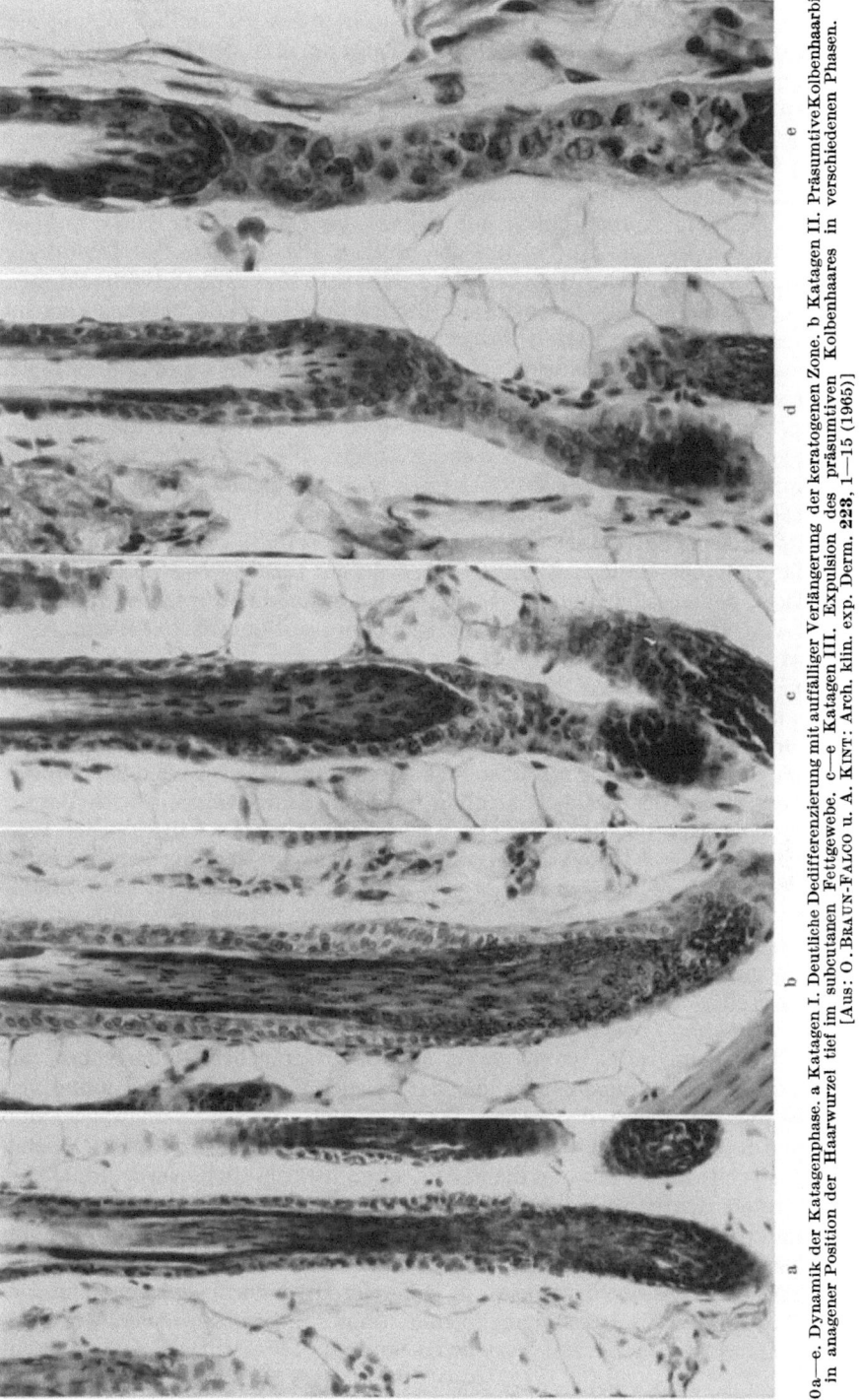

Abb. 10a—e. Dynamik der Katagenphase. a Katagen I. Deutliche Dedifferenzierung mit auffälliger Verlängerung der keratogenen Zone. b Katagen II. Präsumtive Kolbenhaarbildung in anagener Position der Haarwurzel tief im subcutanen Fettgewebe. c—e Katagen III. Expulsion des präsumtiven Kolbenhaares in verschiedenen Phasen.
[Aus: O. BRAUN-FALCO u. A. KINT: Arch. klin. exp. Derm. **223**, 1—15 (1965)]

beimessen kann. Nach Meinung letzterer Autoren ist die katagene Aufwärtsbewegung eine Funktion der äußeren Wurzelscheide, deren Zellen den mit seiner Umgebung nicht verhafteten Haarkolben nach unten zu umfließen, um sich unterhalb des sukzessiv höher steigenden Kolbens zum dedifferenzierten Zellstrang zu formieren.

Wenn der präsumtive Kolben seine definitive Lage erreicht hat, verkleinert er sich und verhornt total. Der definitive Haarkolben wird von einem mehrere Zellagen dicken Sack epidermaler Zellen umgeben, der sich von der äußeren Wurzelscheide herleitet und an seiner Basis in den dedifferenzierten Zellstrang übergeht. Die dem Kolben anliegende Zellage des epidermalen Sacks verhornt teilweise und bildet eine Kapsel um den Kolben, die in Höhe des Talgdrüsengangs mit dem Epithel des Haarkanals verschmilzt (MONTAGNA, 1962). Bürstenartig vom Haarkolben in den epidermalen Sack ausstrahlende schwach keratinisierte Fasern verankern den Kolben. Nach völliger Verhornung des Kolbens kommt es infolge Zelldegeneration vom proximalen Ende her zu einer drastischen Verkürzung des dedifferenzierten Zellstrangs, wobei die zu einer kleinen kugelförmigen Zellgruppe kondensierte dermale Papille — von WOLBACH als ,,Papillenrest" bezeichnet — dem sich verkürzenden Zellstrang aufwärts folgt. Schließlich bleibt unterhalb des epidermalen Sacks nur noch ein kleiner Strang undifferenzierter Zellen erhalten, der sekundäre Haarkeim, dem die Papille proximal anliegt. Vom unteren Ende des Follikels, der jetzt nur noch etwa $1/3$ seiner ursprünglichen Länge hat und vollständig im Corium liegt, zieht der zurückgelassene Haarstengel in die Tiefe, der aus den fibrösen Strukturen des kollabierten leeren Haarbalgs gebildet wird. Die Glasmembran zerfällt, wenn der dedifferenzierte Zellstrang sich verkürzt, und wird resorbiert[1].

Wenn die beschriebenen Strukturänderungen abgeschlossen sind, beginnt das Telogen, die Phase völliger Ruhe.

Bei der Beschreibung der Neubildung eines Follikels aus dem sekundären Haarkeim können wir uns kürzer fassen, da dieser Prozeß weitgehend der embryonalen Entwicklung des Follikels aus dem primären Haarkeim entspricht, die in einem anderen Kapitel dieses Bandes besprochen wird (s.a. H. PINKUS, 1958, 1959). Die wesentlichen Unterschiede zur embryonalen Haarbildung bestehen darin, daß jetzt der Keim nicht mehr primär von der Epidermis herabwachsen muß, daß ein Kanal von der Talgdrüsenmündung zur Oberfläche bereits ausgebildet ist und daß im Haarstengel eine Schiene für den herabwachsenden Follikel vorliegt.

Den Beginn der Entwicklungsphase *(Anagen I)* kennzeichnet das Einsetzen reger mitotischer Zellteilung in den undifferenzierten Zellen des sekundären Haarkeims. Im *Anagen II* wächst der Haarkeim abwärts, wobei er die hochstehende dermale Papille umgreift. Damit deutet sich der Beginn der Bulbusbildung an. Gleichzeitig entsteht unmittelbar über der basalen Zellschicht eine dünne verhornte Kuppel als Beginn der inneren Wurzelscheide. Diese Keratinkuppel spitzt sich zu und beginnt im *Anagen III* durch den Haarkanal hochzuwachsen. Der Bulbus ist jetzt voll ausgebildet und die Matrixregion tritt deutlich hervor. Im oberen Bulbus treten dentritische Pigmentzellen auf. Infolge fortgesetzten Längenwachstums der äußeren Wurzelscheide dringt der untere Pol des Haarbulbus weiter in die Tiefe vor. Im *Anagen IV* wird ein in Rinde und Mark differenzierter Haarschaft erkennbar, dessen Spitze etwa in Höhe der Basis der Talgdrüse steht. Der untere Pol des Bulbus hat seinen tiefsten Stand — tief im subcutanen Fettgewebe — erreicht. Die dermale Papille ist lang und schmal. Im *Anagen V* steht

---

[1] An der Auflösung der Glasmembran kann morphologisch erkannt werden, daß es sich um einen sich verkürzenden katagenen und nicht um einen im frühen Anagen befindlichen Zellstrang handelt (KLIGMAN 1959).

die Haarspitze in Höhe der Epidermisoberfläche, die innere Wurzelscheide in ihrer definitiven Höhe. Der Bulbus gewinnt seinen maximalen Durchmesser, und die Papille wird noch schmaler. Damit ist die Entwicklung des neuen Follikels abgeschlossen, und im *Anagen VI* wächst das Haar für die Dauer der Funktionsphase ohne weitere sichtbare Formveränderungen des Bulbus.

Im Zusammenhang mit der regen Zellvermehrung bei der Entwicklung des aktiven Follikels und beim Wachstum des Haars sind Untersuchungen über Zahl und Lokalisation von Mitosen während verschiedener Cyclusphasen von besonderem Interesse. BULLOUGH und LAURENCE bestimmten die Mitosen im Haarfollikel der Maus bei unbehandelten Tieren und nach subcutaner Colcemid-

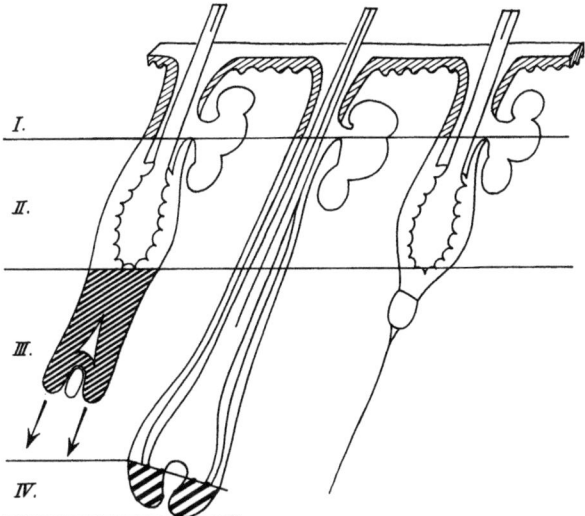

Abb. 11. Schemata des herabwachsenden, tiefstehenden und ruhenden Follikels, zur Verdeutlichung der von BULLOUGH und LAURENCE unterschiedenen Zonen mitotischer Aktivität. I: Zone, in der die mitotische Aktivität der der Basalschicht der Epidermis entspricht. II: Mitosenfreie Zone. III: Zone intensiver mitotischer Aktivität während der Entwicklungsphase. IV: Haarmatrix

Injektion. Durch letzteres Verfahren werden die Mitosen nach Duplikation der Chromosomen in der Metaphase arretiert. Es zeigte sich, daß am Follikel verschiedene Zonen unterschieden werden können, die sich hinsichtlich des Vorkommens mitotischer Aktivität im Ablauf des Cyclus unterschiedlich verhalten. In den basalen Zellagen des oberen Follikelanteils von der Talgdrüsenmündung aufwärts entspricht die mitotische Aktivität der der Basalschicht der Epidermis. Sie ändert sich während des Haarcyclus nur geringfügig, wobei im Anagen II und III eine gesteigerte, im Anagen IV—VI eine verminderte Aktivität — auch in der Epidermis — festzustellen ist. Zwischen der Talgdrüsenmündung und der Ebene, in der der untere Pol des ruhenden Haarkolbens steht, liegt eine in allen Phasen des Cyclus mitosenfreie Zone. Unter dieser Ebene liegt eine Zone, in der zeitweilig, und zwar während der Verlängerung des aktiven Follikels, rege mitotische Aktivität vorhanden ist. In den Zellen, die sich während des Herabwachsens des Follikels bereits in Haar und innere Wurzelscheide differenzieren, sind Mitosen nicht mehr nachweisbar. Wenn der Bulbus seinen tiefsten Stand in der Subcutis erreicht hat, beschränkt sich die mitotische Aktivität fast ausschließlich auf die Matrix (vgl. Abb. 11).

Genauere Angaben über die Zahl der Mitosen und die Mitosenrate[1] in der Haarmatrix während eines künstlich induzierten Haarcyclus verdanken wir

---
[1] Prozentsatz der Mitosen an der Gesamtzahl der Matrixzellen.

Tabelle 1. *Durchschnittliche Mitosenzahl in 50 Haarmatrices pro Maus im Verlauf eines Haarcyclus und prozentualer Anteil der Mitosen unbehandelter Tiere (d, e) an der Mitosenzahl Colchicin-vorbehandelter Tiere (a, b, c).* (Aus: BRAUN-FALCO, 1962)

Wachstumsphase	Tag nach Epilation	Versuchsgruppe	Durchschnittliche Mitosenzahl in 50 Haarbulbi pro Maus der Tiere a, b, c	Durchschnittliche Mitosenzahl in 50 Haarbulbi pro Maus der Tiere d, e	Prozentualer Anteil der Mitosen der unvorbehandelten Tiere (d, e) an der Mitosenzahl der Colchicinvorbehandelten Tiere (a, b, c) %
A I—II	2.	1	96,3	11,0	11,7
A III	4.	2	192,0	21,0	10,9
A IV	6.	3	392,0	43,0	10,9
A V	8.	4	468,7	54,0	11,5
A VI	10.	5	710,0	73,5	10,3
A VI	12.	6	849,0	87,5	10,1
A VI	14.	7	744,7	74,5	10,0
A VI	16.	8	653,7	62,0	9,4
A VI	18.	9	592,3	54,5	9,2
Cat.	20.	10	51,3	6,0	11,4
Tel.	22.	11	6,3	1,0	15,8
Tel.	24.	12	3,3	1,5	45,4
Tel.	26.	13	5,6	0	0
A I—II	28.	14	90,3	9,0	9,9

BRAUN-FALCO (1962). Die von ihm registrierten Mitosenzahlen sind in Tabelle 1 wiedergegeben. Hervorzuheben ist, daß Mitosenzahl und Mitosenrate im Anagen VI nicht gleichbleiben, sondern bereits lange vor Beendigung der Funktionsphase allmählich wieder absinken.

Ohne auf nähere Einzelheiten einzugehen, soll hier noch kurz erwähnt werden, daß BRAUN-FALCO anhand seiner Ergebnisse berechnen konnte, daß jede Matrixzelle etwa alle 22 Std in eine Zellteilung eintritt und daß jede Mitose in etwa 25 min beendet sein muß. BULLOUGH und LAURENCE berechneten für den von ihnen untersuchten Mäusestamm eine Teilung aller Matrixzellen innerhalb 13 Std und eine Dauer der einzelnen Zellteilung von 15—30 min.

Die rhythmischen Entwicklungs- und Wachstumsvorgänge im Haarfollikel laufen im Prinzip bei allen Säugern gleich ab. Hinsichtlich der Dauer des gesamten Haarcyclus und der einzelnen Cyclusphasen bestehen aber zwischen verschiedenen Säugern und — oft — auch zwischen verschiedenen Hautgebieten des gleichen Tiers Differenzen (MORETTI, 1965). Auch beim Menschen haben die Haare verschiedener Körperregionen Cyclen unterschiedlicher Länge (BUTCHER, 1951). Für das menschliche Kopfhaar gibt KLIGMAN (1959) an, daß die Anagenphase Jahre, die Katagenphase 2—3 Wochen und die Telogenphase mehrere Monate dauert.

Bei vielen Tieren (z. B. Ratte, Maus, Kaninchen) verläuft das Haarwachstum wellenförmig, d. h. es treten in einer bestimmten Körperregion die Follikel synchron ins Anagenstadium ein, und von dieser Region wird in zeitlich und räumlich geordneter Folge der Beginn der Wachstumsphase in den Follikeln peripherer Hautregionen induziert (CHASE und EATON). Auch simultaner Beginn des Anagen in allen Follikeln kann beobachtet werden. Andere Tiere (z. B. Meerschweinchen) und der Mensch zeigen demgegenüber kein synchronisiertes Haarwachstum, sondern der Haarcyclus läuft in jedem Follikel individuell und zeitlich von den Cyclen der umgebenden Follikel völlig unabhängig ab („mosaic pattern"; FLESCH, CHASE, 1954).

Anhand von Haarwurzeluntersuchungen (s. u.) wurde festgestellt, daß sich beim Menschen unter physiologischen Bedingungen etwa 80—85% der Kopfhaare im Anagen, etwa 1% im Katagen und etwa 15—20% im Telogen befinden (BARMAN, ASTORE und PECORARO; BARMAN, PECORARO und ASTORE; CROUNSE und VAN SCOTT; KLIGMAN, 1961; LYNFIELD; VAN SCOTT, 1958; VAN SCOTT, REINERTSON und STEINMULLER; WITZEL und BRAUN-FALCO), wobei gewisse Alters- und Geschlechtsunterschiede bei Untersuchung größerer Kollektive deutlich werden (WITZEL und BRAUN-FALCO). Bei noch unveröffentlichten vergleichenden Bestimmungen der prozentualen Häufigkeit von Haaren der verschiedenen Cyclusphasen im Haarwurzelstatus und in aufgehellten dicken Schnitten fand ich mit letzterer Methode durchweg um etwa 5% weniger Telogenhaare.

Auf die strukturellen und funktionellen Veränderungen, die in den Geweben, die den Haarfollikel umgeben, während des Haarcyclus in Erscheinung treten, kann hier leider im einzelnen nicht eingegangen werden. Sie können deutlich nur bei Tieren mit synchronisiertem bzw. wellenförmigem Haarwachstum beobachtet werden. Eine kurze Übersicht findet sich bei MORETTI. Hier sei nur darauf hingewiesen, daß während bestimmter Cyclusphasen Veränderungen in der Dicke der Haut (ANDREASEN; BORODACH und MONTAGNA; BUTCHER, 1934; CHASE, 1954; CHASE, MONTAGNA und MALLONE; GIBBS), ihrem Flüssigkeitsgehalt (BRAUN-FALCO und FRENZ, 1960; BUTCHER und GROKOEST; THYRESSON), ihrem Fettgehalt (BRAUN-FALCO und FRENZ, 1961), ihrem Gehalt an Histamin und Serotonin (MORETTI, GIACOMETTI, BOIDO und REBORA) sowie in der Dicke der Kollagenfasern und der Menge und Struktur interfibrillärer mesenchymaler Substanzen (BRAUN-FALCO und THEISEN, 1959) beobachtet wurden.

Anhang: Morphologie epilierter Haarwurzeln. Der Haarwurzelstatus.

Untersucht man aus der Haut ausgezogene ungefärbte Haare[1] bei Lupenvergrößerung, dann kann man feststellen, daß ihre Wurzeln sehr unterschiedlich gestaltet sein können und daß die Form der Haarwurzeln von der Histologie her bekannte Bilder bestimmter Cyclusphasen deutlich wiedererkennen läßt. Die folgende Beschreibung stützt sich auf Angaben von VAN SCOTT, REINERTSON und STEINMULLER, VAN SCOTT (1958) sowie BRAUN-FALCO und ZAUN (1962a, b).

Normale epilierte Anagenhaare (Abb. 12a, b) sind — meist relativ scharf — etwa im Bereich des mittleren Bulbus abgerissen. In den untersten vorhandenen Bulbusanteilen findet sich oft Melanin. Besonders charakteristisch ist die durch einen helleren Abschnitt von den pigmenthaltigen Bulbusanteilen getrennte dunkle keratogene Zone oberhalb des Bulbus. Zwei deutlich zu unterscheidende Wurzelscheiden können den unteren Haarabschnitt umgeben. Oft sind die Wurzelscheiden nur teilweise vorhanden oder fehlen (scheinbar; s. u.) gänzlich.

Dysplastische Anagenhaare (Abb. 12c, d) haben die grundsätzlichen Charakteristika normaler Anagenhaare, sind jedoch viel dünner und haben einen schmaleren, oft deformierten Bulbus. Die Wurzelscheiden fehlen meist. Derartige Haare findet man bei bestimmten Krankheitszuständen. Vereinzeltes Vorkommen bei Gesunden könnte evtl. damit erklärt werden, daß die Haarwurzeln im Katagen I in ihrer Struktur dysplastischen Haaren entsprechen (BRAUN-FALCO und KINT). Größere prozentuale Anteile von dysplastischen Haaren bei Gesunden sind auf zu langsamen Epilationszug zurückzuführen.

Epilierte Katagenhaare zeigen am proximalen Ende des Haarschafts eine kolbenartige Auftreibung. Dem Haarschaft liegen die Wurzelscheiden deutlich erkennbar an. In frühen Stadien des Katagen (der Phase der präsumtiven Kolbenhaarbildung entsprechend) erscheint der unvollständig verhornte Haarkolben — wie die keratogene Zone anagener Haare — dunkel (Abb. 12e, f), im Katagen III zunehmend heller (Abb. 12g) (unveröffentlichte eigene Beobachtung).

Telogenhaare zeigen einen hellen (vollständig verhornten) Kolben mit etwas dunklerer Kapsel. Wurzelscheiden fehlen. Der Kolben epilierter Telogenhaare ist meist von einem transparenten Sack umgeben (Abb. 12h). An beim physiologischen Haarwechsel spontan ausgefallenen Haaren fehlt dieser Sack oft (Abb. 12i).

Das Vorkommen dystrophischer, d.h. während des Anagenstadiums infolge zunehmender Verdünnung des Haarschafts im Wurzelbereich abgebrochener Haare (Abb. 12j) bei Gesunden ist umstritten. Gelegentliche derartige Beobachtungen sollen auf fehlerhafter Epilation beruhen. Für bestimmte Krankheiten ist ein großer Anteil dystrophischer Haare typisch (Übersicht: ZAUN).

---

[1] Die Epilation muß rasch erfolgen, da durch langsamen Epilationszug anagene Haarwurzeln artifiziell verändert und pathologische Wurzelformen vorgetäuscht werden können (BRAUN-FALCO und RASSNER, 1965; MAGUIRE und KLIGMAN).

Durch Färbung mit Gallocyanin oder durch Fluorochromierung wird es möglich, weitere Struktureinzelheiten an epilierten Haaren zur Darstellung zu bringen (BANDMANN und BOSSE). Mit derartigen Verfahren konnten BANDMANN und BOSSE eine innere Wurzelscheide an epilierten Anagenhaaren stets darstellen.

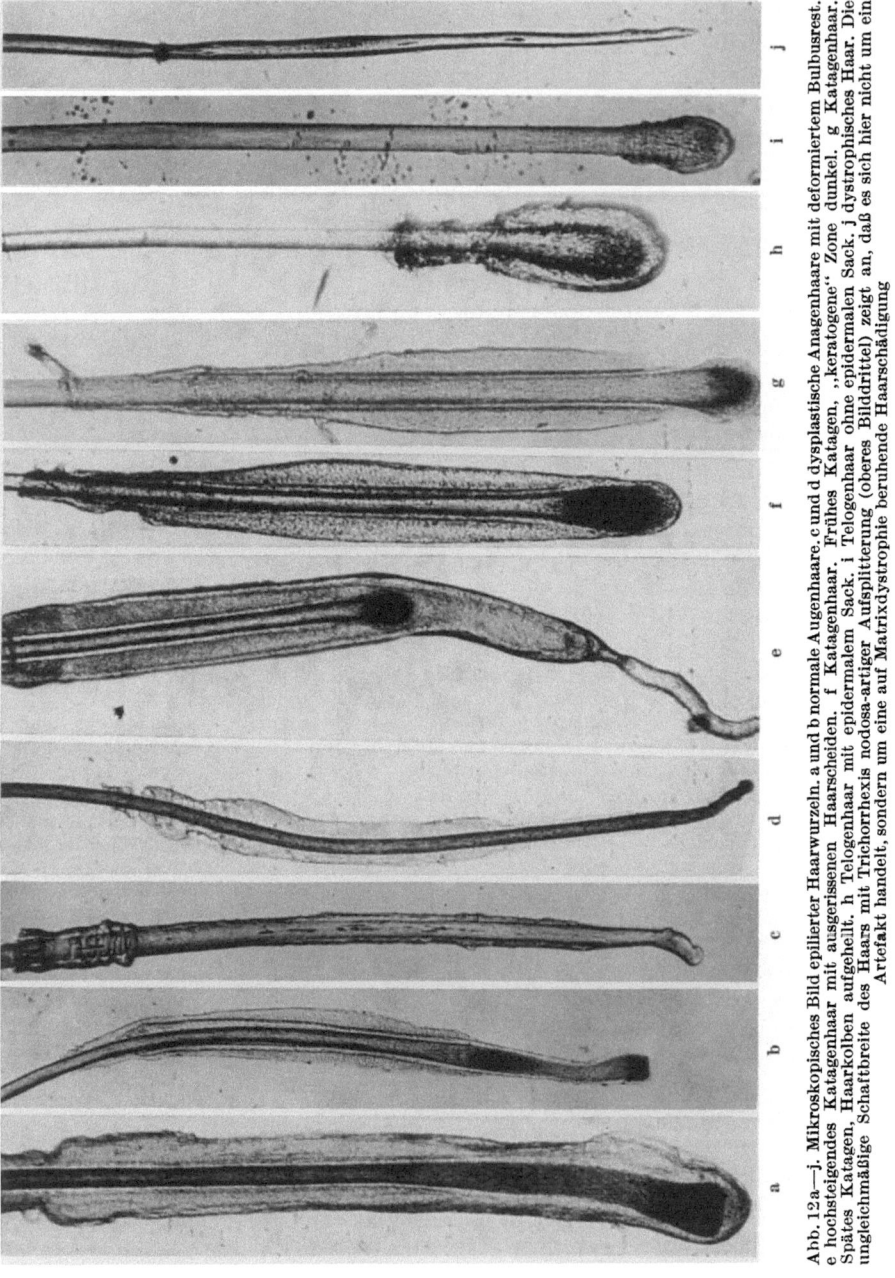

Abb. 12a—j. Mikroskopisches Bild epilierter Haarwurzeln. a und b normale Augenhaare. c und d dysplastische Anagenhaare mit deformiertem Bulbusrest. e hochsteigendes Katagenhaar mit ausgerissenen Haarscheiden. f Katagenhaar, Frühes Katagen, „keratogene" Zone dunkel. g Katagenhaar. Spätes Katagen, Haarkolben aufgehellt. h Telogenhaar mit epidermalem Sack. i Telogenhaar ohne epidermalen Sack. j dystrophisches Haar. Die ungleichmäßige Schaftbreite des Haars mit Trichorrhexis nodosa-artiger Aufsplitterung (oberes Bilddrittel) zeigt an, daß es sich hier nicht um ein Artefakt handelt, sondern um eine auf Matrixdystrophie beruhende Haarschädigung

Die Tatsache, daß es möglich ist, aus der Gestalt epilierter Haarwurzeln die jeweilige Cyclusphase ihrer Ursprungsfollikel zu erschließen, macht man sich bei der Bestimmung des *Haarwurzelstatus* (VAN SCOTT, REINERTSON und STEINMULLER) zunutze. Dabei differenziert man die Wurzeln eines rasch und einzeitig epilierten genügend großen Haarbüschels (60—100 Haare). Das festgestellte prozentuale Verhältnis normaler und gegebenenfalls pathologischer Wurzelformen (Haarverteilungsmuster) läßt weitgehende Rückschlüsse hinsichtlich der Wachstumssituation im Epilationsbereich zu. Die mit der Methode gefundenen Normwerte wurden bereits bei der Besprechung des Haarcyclus (S. 162) angegeben. Daß Kolbenhaare auch aus im frühen Anagen befindlichen Follikeln epiliert werden können, muß bei der Beurteilung eines Haarstatus berücksichtigt werden, schränkt aber den praktischen Wert der Methode nicht ein.

III. Altersveränderungen des Follikels und der Kopfhaut (einschließlich sog. „Alopecia praematura")

Kopfhaut und Haarfollikel zeigen nicht nur im Ablauf des Haarcyclus strukturelle Veränderungen, sondern auch einen altersbedingten Formwandel. Obwohl kaum zu übersehen ist, daß die Haare des Kopfes bei den meisten Menschen mit zunehmendem Alter dünner und in ihrer Gesamtzahl vermindert werden, sind Ergebnisse systematischer Untersuchungen über Altersveränderungen der Kopfhaut in der Literatur nur vereinzelt mitgeteilt worden.

Nach ELLIS, der das histologische Bild der Haut im Scheitelbereich männlicher Individuen vom Geburtsalter bis zum 88. Lebensjahr studierte, erfährt die Epidermis im Alter eine deutliche Verdünnung, und die bei jungen Männern tief ins Corium hineinragenden Reteleisten werden zu dünnen Rippen reduziert oder schwinden völlig. Diese Veränderungen sieht ELLIS als direkte Folge der verminderten Zirkulation im subepidermalen Plexus an, dessen Gefäßschlingen — wie auch CORMIA zeigte — mit zunehmendem Alter verkürzt und zahlenmäßig reduziert werden. Dabei bleibt die Gefäßversorgung der Talg- und Schweißdrüsen bis ins hohe Alter erhalten (ELLIS, CORMIA).

Die in der Kindheit kleinen Talgdrüsen vergrößern sich in der Pubertät. Mit fortschreitendem Alter können sie sich durchaus unterschiedlich verhalten, was die widersprüchlichen Angaben in der Literatur erklärt. Während EJIRI keine altersabhängigen Talgdrüsenveränderungen feststellen konnte, nehmen die Talgdrüsen nach ELLIS mit zunehmendem Alter — und bei der Glatzenbildung oft besonders deutlich — an Größe zu. CORMIA fand demgegenüber die Talgdrüsen bei jungen Glatzenträgern unverändert, bei älteren Glatzenträgern häufig verkleinert. Schweißdrüsen zeigen keine deutlichen altersbedingten Strukturänderungen.

Von KOSUGI und KIM wurde herausgestellt, daß die elastischen Fasern im Bereich des Capillitiums mit zunehmendem Alter reduziert werden. SINGH und McKENZIE fanden in den subepidermalen Lagen der Kopfhaut alter Menschen — und besonders bei Glatzenbildung — vermehrt sulfatierte Mucopolysaccharide und eine Verdickung der kollagenen Fasern. ATKINSON, CORMIA und UNRAU bestimmten Wachstumsphasen und maximale Durchmesser der Haare des Scheitelbereichs im histologischen Schnitt und stellten mit zunehmendem Alter eine Verminderung des mittleren Haardurchmessers und — erstaunlicherweise — eine Verminderung der Zahl der Telogenhaare fest. Sie glauben, letzteren Befund damit erklären zu können, daß Ruhehaare bei älteren Menschen rascher ausfallen.

Die Häufigkeitsverteilung der Haaranordnungsmuster (Follikelgruppen, Follikelbündel und Einzelfollikel — vgl. H. PINKUS, Bd. I/2) untersuchten OBERSTE-LEHN und NOBIS (1959) an Grenzflächenpräparaten. Sie stellten fest, daß es während des Alterungsvorgangs zu einer Abnahme gruppiert stehender Follikel kommt.

Eine Reihe neuartiger und die bekannten Einzelbefunde in vieler Hinsicht ergänzender Einblicke in die strukturellen Veränderungen, denen die Kopfhaut im Laufe des Lebens unterliegt, vermitteln die kürzlich von GOERTTLER mitgeteilten Befunde. GOERTTLER untersuchte gemeinsam mit GÖRDEL vergleichend histologische Präparate und epidermocutane Grenzflächenpräparate von Kopfhautstücken, die bei einem größeren Sektionsgut an drei normierten Stellen entnommen waren. Fassen wir seine Ergebnisse — unter Vernachlässigung der regionalen Unterschiede — zusammen, dann stellt sich der postnatale Formwandel der Kopfhaut wie folgt dar: Bei Säuglingen sind Epidermisunterfläche und Corium noch nicht verzahnt. Histologisch läßt die Grenzfläche eine sanfte Wellung erkennen. Die Talgdrüsen variieren an Zahl und Größe erheblich und auch die Dicke der Subcutis variiert. Das Grenzflächenbild wird beherrscht von Haarfollikeln, die meist in einigem Abstand rings von Schweißdrüsen umgeben sind (Abb. 13a). Erst im zweiten Lebenshalbjahr sind Andeutungen eines Leistenmusters zu erkennen. Ihre charakteristische Gestalt gewinnt die epidermocutane Grenzfläche bei Kindern und Jugendlichen (1—15 Jahre). In dieser Altersgruppe senkt die Epidermisunterseite ein kompliziertes bogen- und säulenförmiges Maschensystem ins Corium ein, das zunächst die Follikel nicht mit einbezieht. Diese stehen in napfartigen Ausbuchtungen mit erhabenem Rand („Burggraben"). Histologisch erscheint die Epidermis verdickt und springt mit tiefen Leisten ins Corium vor. Die Talgdrüsen sind meist klein. Bei älteren Jugendlichen und jungen Erwachsenen (16—30 Jahre) erreicht die Entwicklung der Kopfhaut ihren Höhepunkt. Die tief ins Corium ragenden Epidermisleisten greifen jetzt auch auf die vorher durch den „Burggraben" abgegrenzten Follikel über. Sie bilden engmaschig unregelmäßige oder mehr weitmaschig-regelmäßige und weniger tief gestaffelte Netzstrukturen, worin sich die Differenzierung in ein „männliches" und ein „weibliches" Reliefmuster andeutet. Die Haarfollikel ragen hoch aus der Grenzfläche hervor (Abb. 13b). Die Größe der Talgdrüsen variiert im histologischen Schnitt sehr stark. Das Subcutangewebe enthält nur einzelne Bindegewebszüge, die sich um die Follikel verdichten.

In der Altersgruppe der 31—45jährigen werden diskrete bis deutliche regressive Veränderungen der Kopfhaut bei beiden Geschlechtern sichtbar. Die Tiefe des Maschennetzes nimmt ab. Geschlechtsgebundene Besonderheiten im Aufbau der epidermocutanen Grenzfläche werden in der Mehrzahl der Fälle deutlich erkennbar. Frauen zeigen weitmaschig-regelmäßige Netze mit schmaleren Leisten, Männer ein variables Maschenwerk aus meist engmaschigen Netzen, dessen Muster arealweise oder abrupt wechseln. Ein Zusammenhang zwischen Haarwachstum und Ausbildung der Epidermisleisten besteht offensichtlich nicht. Vielmehr kann bei starkem Haarbesatz das Subepidermalrelief stark reduziert und andererseits bei spärlichem Haarwuchs das Grenzflächenbild völlig erhalten sein. Der Reduktion der Reliefleisten entsprechend zeigt sich auch im histologischen Schnitt eine Abflachung der Epidermiszapfen. Die Zahl der Epidermislagen kann vermindert oder — im Sinne einer Pachydermie — leicht vermehrt sein. Die Haarfollikel lassen deutliche regressive Umwandlungen erkennen und der Ductus pilosebaceus wird trichterförmig ausgeweitet. Die Talgdrüsen sind meist unverändert. Die hohe Subcutis wird nur von einzelnen Bindegewebssepten durchzogen.

In der Gruppe der 46—60jährigen tritt die Alterung der Haut immer deutlicher hervor. Bei Männern sind die Maschenformationen im Grenzflächenbild meist weitgehend reduziert, und Maschenmuster und Maschenweite wechseln ganz abrupt. Bei Frauen ist die Reduktion nicht so stark, und auch in Feldern stärkerer Reduktion bleibt das ursprüngliche Maschenmuster noch erkennbar. Auch im histologischen Schnitt wird die Abnahme der Verzahnung von Epidermis und

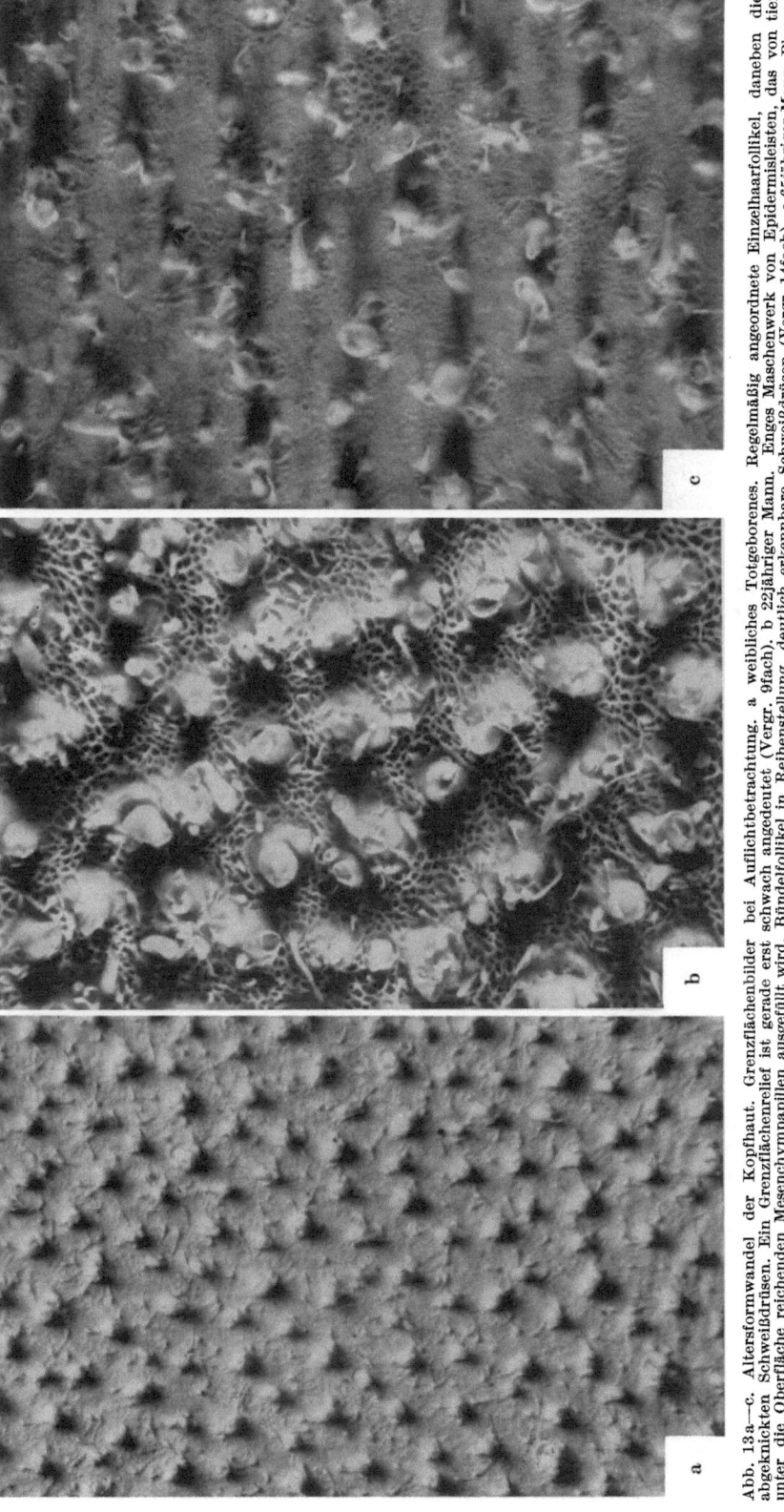

Abb. 13a—c. Altersformwandel der Kopfhaut. Grenzflächenbilder bei Auflichtbetrachtung. a weibliches Totgeborenes. Regelmäßig angeordnete Einzelhaarfollikel, daneben die abgeknickten Schweißdrüsen. Ein Grenzflächenrelief ist gerade erst schwach angedeutet (Vergr. 9fach). b 22jähriger Mann. Enges Maschenwerk von Epidermisleisten, das von tief unter die Oberfläche reichenden Mesenchymrpapillen ausgefüllt wird. Bündelfollikel in Reihenstellung, deutlich erkennbare Schweißdrüsen (Vergr. 14fach). c 65jähriger Mann. Plumpe Follikel, Atrophie des Subepidermalreliefs. Mitte rechts: Mosaik mit erhaltenem Maschenmuster (Vergr. 14fach). (Aus: K. GOERTTLER: Die menschliche Glatze im Altersformwandel der behaarten Kopfhaut. Stuttgart: Georg Thieme 1965)

Corium deutlich. Die Haarfollikel werden kleiner. Dünnere Haare mit kleinem Bulbus haben oft sehr dicke äußere Wurzelscheiden. Die Talgdrüsengröße variiert beträchtlich. Das subcutane Fettpolster wird vermehrt von Bindegewebssepten durchzogen, und die Stärke der die Anhangsorgane umgebenden Bindegewebsscheiden hat zugenommen.

In höherem Alter entsprechen die Befunde prinzipiell den für die letzte Altersgruppe geschilderten, jedoch treten Differenzen in der Ausbildung des Grenz-

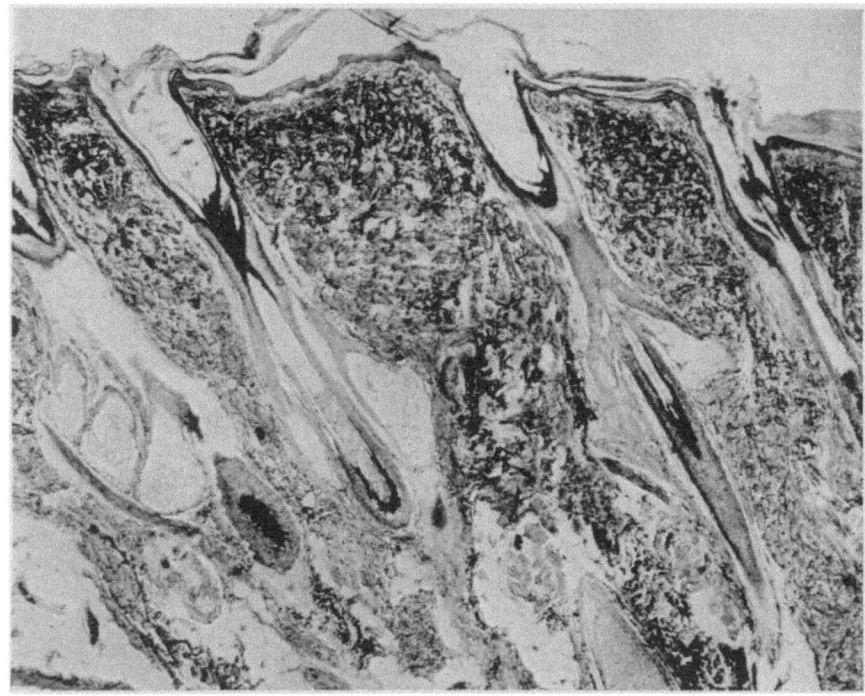

Abb. 14. Histologisches Bild der Glatzenhaut. 75jähriger Mann. Miniaturfollikel. Zwischen den erweiterten Haarkanälen und — in geringerem Umfang — in der Tiefe elasticapositives Material. Färbung: Goldner Elastica; Vergr. 75fach. (Aus: K. GOERTTLER: Die menschliche Glatze im Altersformwandel der behaarten Kopfhaut. Stuttgart: Georg Thieme 1965)

reliefs noch stärker in Erscheinung (Abb. 13c). Die Haarfollikel reichen weniger tief in die Cutis. Die schon geschilderten Geschlechtsunterschiede werden besonders deutlich. Im histologischen Bild sieht man verkürzte Follikel mit kleinen dermalen Papillen und verdünnten Haaren. Der Anteil katagener oder telogener Haare ist auffällig vermehrt. Auch die Talgdrüsen zeigen im hohen Alter Rückbildungserscheinungen, während sich die Schweißdrüsen über alle Altersstufen hinweg als stabiles Element erweisen. Das subcutane Bindegewebe ist bei beiden Geschlechtern verdickt.

Im Zusammenhang mit den physiologischen Altersveränderungen der Kopfhaut soll auch kurz auf das histologische Substrat der sog. Alopecia praematura[1] und der Alopecia senilis eingegangen werden (Abb. 14). Bei der Glatzenbildung unterliegen die Haarfollikel einer retrograden Metamorphose (MONTAGNA, 1959) und werden in Miniaturfollikel umgewandelt, die nur noch ein dünnes lanugoartiges Haar zu produzieren vermögen. Diese Reduktion der Haare zu Lanugohaaren ist der einzige konstante histologisch erfaßbare Befund, der als typisch für die

---
[1] Die von ORENTREICH vorgeschlagene Bezeichnung „androgenetische Alopecie" ist besser und sollte allgemein übernommen werden.

Alopecia praematura angesehen werden kann (GOERTTLER). Alle Veränderungen, die darüber hinaus in der Glatzenhaut beobachtet wurden (CORMIA; GALEWSKY; GOERTTLER; KNOCHE; LIGHT; SINGH und McKENCIE), entsprechen den oben beschriebenen normalen Altersveränderungen der Kopfhaut, wobei die Abbauvorgänge zuweilen akzentuiert erscheinen. Der Grad der Ausprägung dieser Altersveränderungen variiert bei Glatzenträgern beträchtlich und stärker als bei Personen mit vollem Haupthaar. Das gilt auch für das Grenzflächenbild (Abb. 15), das von völlig normalen Musterbildern mit typischem Hochrelief und regelmäßigen Follikeln (die aber nur Lanugohaare enthalten) bis zu hochgradig reduzierten Mustern mit atypischen Follikeln und teilweisem Follikelverlust alle Übergänge zeigen kann (GOERTTLER).

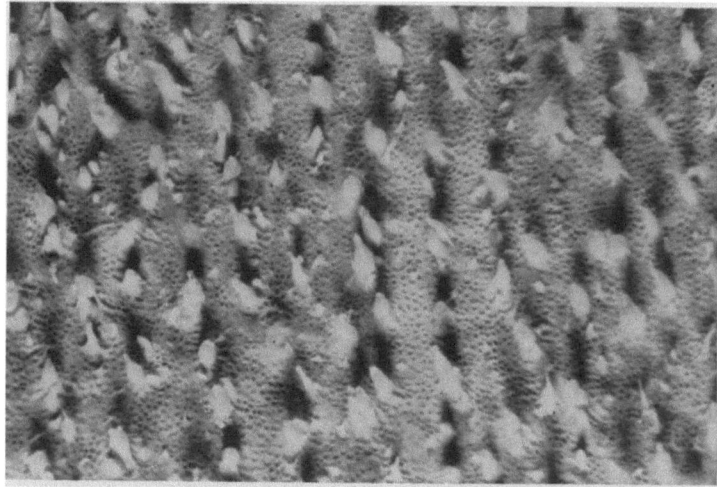

Abb. 15. Grenzflächenbild der Kopfhaut bei 71jährigem Mann mit Glatzenbildung im Entnahmebereich. Regelmäßiges Rete Malpighi, wohlerhaltene Follikel, die ausschließlich mit Lanugohaaren gefüllt sind. (Aus: K. GOERTTLER: Die menschliche Glatze im Altersformwandel der behaarten Kopfhaut. Stuttgart: Georg Thieme 1965)

Geht man vom morphologischen Substrat aus, dann kann man die Alopecia praematura zwanglos den Altersveränderungen der Kopfhaut zuordnen. Mit den wenigen gesicherten Kenntnissen, die wir über die Ursache der Glatzenentstehung haben (HAMILTON; LUDWIG; RASSNER, ZAUN und BRAUN-FALCO; SANTLER), ist diese Auffassung vom Wesen der Alopecia praematura gut in Einklang zu bringen. In diesem Zusammenhang ist auch die Feststellung erwähnenswert, daß bei der Alopecia praematura in den sich verkleinernden Follikeln die normalen Größenbeziehungen zwischen dermaler Papille und Haarmatrix erhalten bleiben und Haar und Haarwurzel somit — abgesehen von ihrer Größe — normal sind (VAN SCOTT und EKEL, VAN SCOTT, 1959).

IV. Histochemie des Haarfollikels

Zur Zeit der Abfassung des Originalwerks dieses Handbuchs steckte die Histochemie noch in den Anfängen. Die rapide Entwicklung dieses Forschungszweiges in den letzten Jahrzehnten hat dazu geführt, daß wir heute über Vorkommen und Lokalisation zahlreicher Zell- und Gewebsbestandteile im Haarfollikel gesicherte Kenntnisse haben. Eine besonders ausführliche Besprechung der histochemischen Befunde am Haarfollikel verdanken wir BRAUN-FALCO (1958). Eine Reihe ergänzender Einzelheiten finden sich bei MONTAGNA (1962). Die folgende Übersicht lehnt sich — unter Berücksichtigung neuerer Befunde — weitgehend an die Darstellungen der genannten Autoren an.

1. Histotopographie anorganischer Substanzen

Von den zahlreichen anorganischen Substanzen, die im Haarfollikel chemisch nachweisbar sind, konnte bisher nur Zink histochemisch dargestellt werden (BRAUN-FALCO und RATHJENS, 1956). Zink ist in großen Mengen in der äußeren Wurzelscheide lokalisiert. Im Haarschaft, der nach analytischen Untersuchungen zinkhaltig ist, gelang der histochemische Nachweis nicht.

2. Histotopographie von Kohlenhydraten

a) Glykogen

Aktive Haarfollikel sind sehr glykogenreich (Abb. 16a). Im Haarbalg findet sich Glykogen im Cytoplasma der Fibroblasten und extracellulär entlang der Fasern

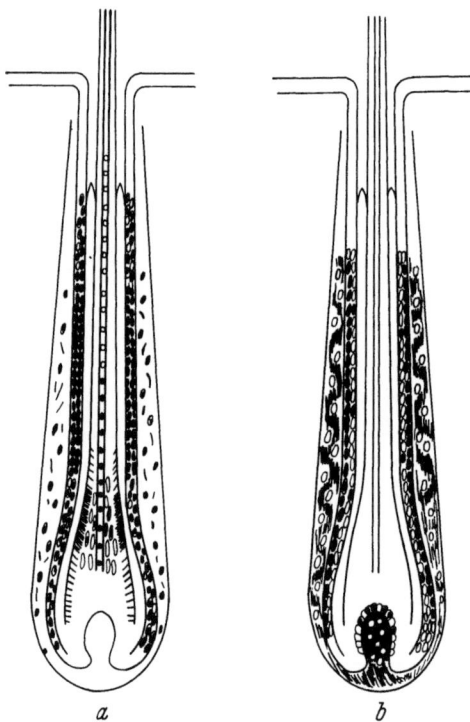

Abb. 16a u. b. Histotopographie von Kohlenhydraten (schematisch). a Verteilung von Glykogen (dunkel) im wachsenden Haarfollikel. b Lokalisation metachromatischer Substanzen (saure Mucopolysaccharide) im wachsenden Haarfollikel

(MONTAGNA, CHASE und HAMILTON). Besonders viel Glykogen enthält die äußere Wurzelscheide. Ihre Zellen sind im mittleren Follikeldrittel so mit Glykogen beladen, daß nur ein schmales cytoplasmatisches Netzwerk dazwischen übrig bleibt (SASAKAWA; MONTAGNA, CHASE und HAMILTON). Unteres und oberes Drittel der äußeren Wurzelscheide enthalten weniger Glykogen. Die Zellen der inneren Wurzelscheide sind glykogenfrei. Die Epidermicula enthält unmittelbar oberhalb des Bulbus viel Glykogen. In gleicher Höhe finden sich in manchen Rindenzellen Glykogenspuren. In beiden Schichten verschwindet das Glykogen abrupt, wenn die Zellen in den Verhornungsvorgang eintreten. Die Markzellen enthalten Glykogen bis etwa zur Follikelmitte. Haarmatrix und dermale Papille sind glykogenfrei.

Während des Haarcyclus ändert sich der Glykogengehalt des Follikels (MONTAGNA und CHASE; SHIPMAN, CHASE und MONTAGNA). Im Katagen verschwindet das Glykogen plötzlich. Bei der Maus enthält der Ruhefollikel kein Glykogen. Bei Primaten finden sich beträchtliche Glykogenmengen in den Zellen des epidermalen Sacks (LOMBARDO; MONTAGNA und ELLIS, 1959). Im Anagen I und II bleibt der Follikel glykogenfrei, im Anagen III erscheinen Glykogengranula an der Peripherie der äußeren Wurzelscheide. Im Anagen IV findet sich Glykogen in den unteren Zellen von Mark und Epidermicula und reichlich im mittleren Segment der äußeren Wurzelscheide. Die Speicherung von Glykogen im Haarfollikel zeigt eine inverse Beziehung zur mitotischen Aktivität und zur Keratinisation (MONTAGNA, 1962). Verhornende und mitotisch aktive Zellen enthalten kein Glykogen. Übereinstimmend mit den histochemischen Befunden sind Glykogengranula auch elektronenmikroskopisch in den verschiedenen Schichten des Follikels nachweisbar (ROTH und HELWIG, 1964a, b).

b) Saure Mucopolysaccharide

Das Vorhandensein saurer Mucopolysaccharide im Follikel gibt sich zu erkennen durch Metachromasie und PAS-Reaktivität. Im aktiven Haarfollikel finden sich metachromatische Substanzen an zahlreichen Stellen. In der dermalen Papille färbt sich die Grundsubstanz intensiv metachromatisch, das Cytoplasma der Papillenzellen orthochromatisch (MONTAGNA, CHASE und MELARAGNO). Am Haarbalg zeigt sich im unteren Follikeldrittel schwache, im mittleren Follikeldrittel stärkere, vorwiegend an die Grundsubstanz gebundene Metachromasie. Die äußere Wurzelscheide zeigt Metachromasie vorwiegend in den peripheren Zellschichten, die auch besonders glykogenreich sind. Schwache, oft durch die Basophilie der Zellen maskierte Metachromasie zeigt sich in den Bulbuszellen, die an die Papille angrenzen (Abb. 16b).

Fast alle metachromatischen Gewebselemente des Follikels sind auch PAS-reaktiv. Die Glasmembran ist stark PAS-reaktiv, zeigt aber keine Metachromasie (vgl. MONTAGNA, 1962). Da das metachromatische Material in der dermalen Papille und der äußeren Wurzelscheide durch Hyaluronidase nicht verdaut wird (MONTAGNA, CHASE und MELARAGNO; MONTAGNA, CHASE und LOBITZ), glauben MONTAGNA u. Mitarb., daß es sich um Chondroitinsulfat B (das neben Hyaluronsäure in größeren Mengen in der Haut vorkommende saure Polysaccharid) handelt.

Das Verhalten von Metachromasie und PAS-Reaktivität während der Phasen des Haarcyclus untersuchten MONTAGNA, CHASE, MALONE und MELARAGNO. Metachromatische und PAS-reaktive Substanzen sind in der Papille vom Anagen III, unmittelbar vor Einsetzen der Haarproduktion, an bis zum Ende des Anagen VI, festzustellen und verschwinden im Katagen abrupt. Der ruhende Follikel färbt sich orthochromatisch.

3. Lipoide

Sudanophile Lipoidkörper in Form diskreter Granula finden sich perinucleär in fast allen unverhornten Zellen des Follikels. In Größe, Form und Anordnung entsprechen sie den Golgi-Elementen (MONTAGNA, CHASE und HAMILTON). Die Matrixzellen zeigen an ihren Polen zwei oder mehr große Lipoidkörper mit jeweils einer exzentrischen sudanophoben Vacuole und diffus im Cytoplasma eine schwache, staubförmige sudanophile Tüpfelung. Im oberen Bulbus sind die Lipoidkörper durch Pigmentgranula verdeckt. Die äußere Wurzelscheide weist im Bereich des unteren Bulbus sehr viele Lipoidkörper auf. Weiter aufwärts enthalten nur die peripheren, der Glashaut anliegenden Zellen deutlich sichtbare sudanophile Elemente. Die sudanophilen Bestandteile der Zellen des Haarkanals entsprechen denen der Epidermiszellen (MONTAGNA, 1950). Die Zellen der präsumtiven inneren Wurzelscheide zeigen in Höhe des oberen Bulbus diskrete Lipoidgranula, die verschwinden, sobald in den Zellen Trichohyalin auftritt (MONTAGNA, 1950). Die aufbröckelnde innere Wurzelscheide im Haarkanal ist stark sudanophil. Das Haar ist relativ frei von sudanophilen Körpern. Zarte aber deutliche sichtbare Granula sieht man in den Zellen der dermalen Papille.

Phospholipoide lassen sich mit dem sauren Hämateintest nach BAKER in großer Menge in den Matrixzellen und der inneren Wurzelscheide nachweisen (BRAUN-FALCO, 1958). Mit dem Einsetzen der Verhornung nimmt ihre Menge ab, jedoch zeigt die keratogene Zone noch eine starke Reaktion (CRAMER; s. Abb. 17).

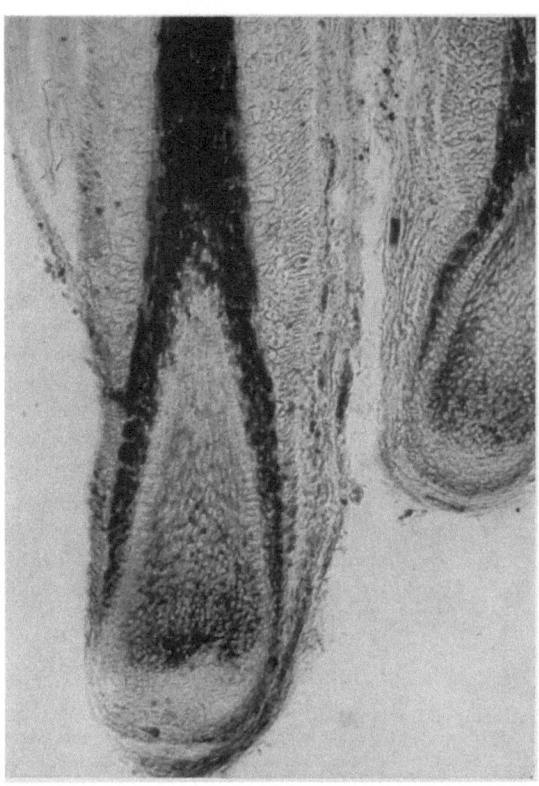

Abb. 17. Anfärbung der „keratogenen Zone" des Haarfollikels mit dem sauren Hämatein-Test nach BAKER. Vergr. 150fach. [Aus: H. J. CRAMER: Arch. klin. exp. Derm. **218**, 191—202 (1964)]

Während des Katagen enthalten Follikelzellen und dermale Papille vermehrt Lipoide. Im Ruhefollikel sind in fast allen Zellen des epidermalen Sacks Lipoidgranula sichtbar, während der restliche Follikel frei ist (MONTAGNA, 1962).

4. Histotopographie von Aminosäuren

Hier liegen nur spärliche Ergebnisse vor. Arginin findet sich in der inneren Wurzelscheide (STEIGLEDER, 1957; Abb. 18). Es ist dort in den Trichohyalin-Tröpfchen lokalisiert und verschwindet bei der Verhornung (ROGERS, 1963). Auch die amorphen Granula des Marks enthalten Arginin. In den verhornten Anteilen der inneren Wurzelscheide und des Marks ist reichlich Citrullin nachweisbar (ROGERS, 1963, 1964). Größere Mengen von Tyrosin finden sich in der Medulla (GIROUD, BULLIARD und LEBLOND; STOVES). Das Haarkeratin enthält Tryptophan. Freie Aminosäuren werden in hoher Konzentration in der keratogenen Zone und in der zentralen Zellschicht der äußeren Wurzelscheide gefunden (BRAUN-FALCO, 1958).

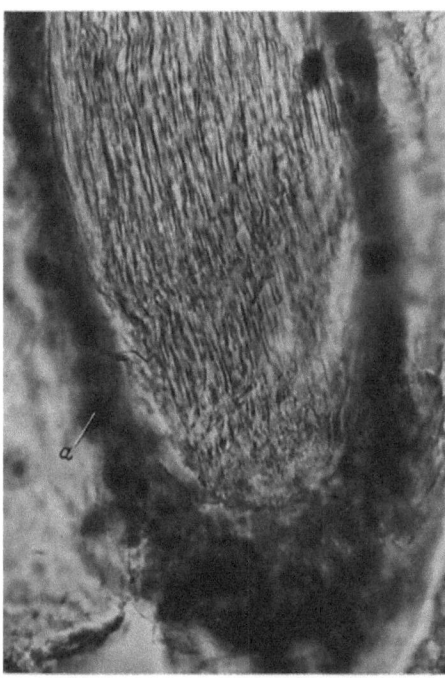

Abb. 18. Tiefer Abschnitt eines Haarfollikels. Die innere Wurzelscheide gibt eine intensive Anfärbung in der Reaktion auf Arginin (a). Nachweis nach SAKAGUCHI, modifiziert nach WARREN und MCMANUS. Vergr. 320fach. [Aus: G. K. STEIGLEDER: Arch. klin. exp. Derm. **206**, 276—317 (1957)]

5. Sulfhydryl-(SH-) und Disulfid-(SS-) Gruppen

Die Bedeutung proteingebundener SH-Gruppen bei der Keratinisation ist im Beitrag von RICHTER (Bd. I/3) besprochen. Untersuchungen über die Histotopochemie von Sulfhydryl-Gruppen wurden vorgelegt von BARRNETT und SELIGMAN; HARDY; EISEN, MONTAGNA und CHASE; ODLAND; MONTAGNA, EISEN, RADEMACHER und CHASE; GOLDBLUM, PIPER und CAMPBELL sowie FORACER und WINGO. In der äußeren Wurzelscheide gelingt gleichmäßiger Nachweis von SH-Gruppen vom Bulbus bis zum Ausgang des Haarkanals. Die Henlesche Schicht der inneren Wurzelscheide ist reicher an SH-Gruppen als die Huxleysche Schicht. Die Scheidencuticula enthält nur wenige, die Epidermicula viele SH-Gruppen. Reich an Sulfhydryl-Gruppen ist der obere Bulbus und besonders die keratogene Zone, wohingegen im Haarschaft ein Nachweis nicht gelingt.

In der Katagenphase enthält die äußere Wurzelscheide mehr Sulfhydryl-Gruppen als im Anagen, und in der Umgebung des sich entwickelnden Kolbenhaars sind sehr reichlich SH-Gruppen nachweisbar (EISEN, MONTAGNA und CHASE). Im Ruhefollikel finden sich SH-Gruppen in mäßiger Menge im epithelialen Sack, reichlich in der Kapsel des Haarkolbens (MONTAGNA, EISEN, RADEMACHER und CHASE). Die Lokalisation von SH-Gruppen im menschlichen Follikel stimmt mit den experimentell gewonnenen Ergebnissen bei Maus und Meerschweinchen überein (FORAKER und WINGO).

Die Verteilung von Disulfid-Gruppen entspricht im wesentlichen der Verteilung der SH-Gruppen, jedoch sind in der Sulfhydryl-freien verhornten Haarrinde die meisten SS-Gruppen nachweisbar (MONTAGNA, EISEN, RADEMACHER und CHASE). Im Ruhefollikel zeigt der verhornte Haarkolben die für SS-Gruppen charakteristische Färbung nur schwach.

6. Nucleinsäuren

Desoxyribonucleinsäure (DNS), die histochemisch mit der Feulgen-Methode nachgewiesen wird, kommt nur in Zellkernen vor. Sie wird ausschließlich in den unverhornten Anteilen des Haarfollikels gefunden (HARDY). In aktiven Follikeln färben sich die Kerne in der Matrix am stärksten, im oberen Bulbus zunehmend schwächer an. Die Kerne der äußeren Wurzelscheide sind in Bulbushöhe nur schwach, oberhalb des Haarwulstes stark Feulgen-reaktiv. Die Zellkerne in der Henleschen Schicht verlieren ihre Feulgen-Reaktivität mit dem Auftreten der Trichohyalingranula in den Zellen. Die Kerne der Zellen von Huxleyscher Schicht, Cuticula und Epidermicula sind etwa bis zur halben Follikelhöhe Feulgen-reaktiv. Im Bereich der Haarrinde verliert sich die Feulgen-Färbbarkeit in der keratogenen Zone, in den Markzellen oberhalb der Follikelmitte (MONTAGNA, 1962).

Ribonucleinsäure (RNS) findet sich in größeren Mengen in Kern und Cytoplasma von Zellen, in denen Syntheseleistungen erfolgen. In aktiven Follikeln enthalten die undifferenzierten Zellen der Matrix sehr viel RNS. Bis zur keratogenen Zone nimmt der RNS-Gehalt langsam ab. Mit der Beendigung der Protein-

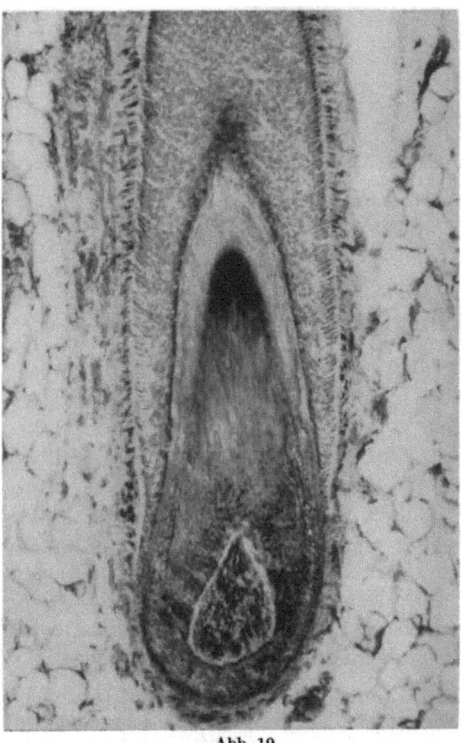
Abb. 19

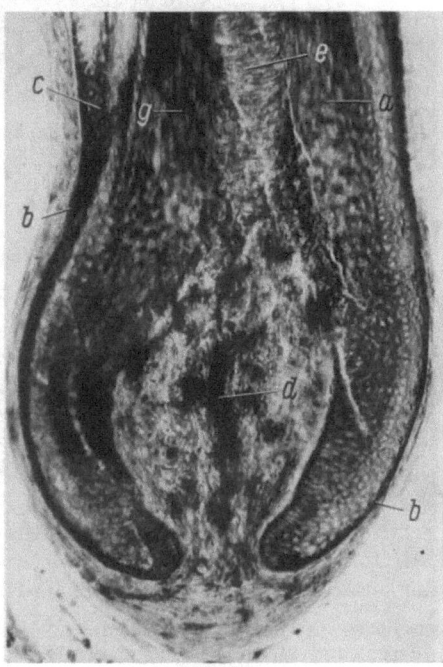
Abb. 20

Abb. 19. Anagene Haarfollikel NADH-Tetrazoliumreductase-Reaktion nach Acetonfixierung. Haarmatrixzellen mäßig positiv. Keratogene Zone diffus unspezifisch positiv auf NADH-Tetrazoliumreductase. Hyalinisierte innere Wurzelscheide negativ. Die äußere Wurzelscheide zeigt mäßige Enzymaktivität. In der dermalen Haarpapille fleckige Formazanniederschläge als Zeichen von NADH-Tetrazoliumreductase-Aktivität. Mikroskopische Vergr. 25fach. [Aus: O. BRAUN-FALCO u. D. PETZOLDT: Arch. klin. exp. Derm. **220**, 455—473 (1964)]

Abb. 20. Reaktion auf unspezifische Esterasen (Azofarbstoff-Kupplungsreaktion). Tiefer Abschnitt eines Haarfollikels im Bartbereich. Man erkennt die starke Reaktion der äußersten Epithellage (b). Am linken oberen Rand beginnt sich die Zone der starken Reaktion in der äußeren Wurzelschicht zu teilen und sich dem verhornenden Haar zu nähern (c). Deutliche Reaktion der inneren Wurzelscheide, die dann in das verhornende Haar übergeht. Dessen dunkle Anfärbung (a, g) ist nur auf den Pigmentgehalt, aber nicht auf eine echte Reaktion zurückzuführen. Man beachte ferner die Reaktion in der Papille. Die intensiv angefärbten Zellen sind wahrscheinlich Melaninbildner (d). Ferner kann man in der Mitte über der Papille die Reaktion des Haarmarks (e) verfolgen. Hier erscheinen die Zellgrenzen angefärbt. [Aus: G. K. STEIGLEDER: Hautarzt **9**, 67—71 (1958)]

synthese in den Zellen ist die Ribonucleinsäure in der Haarrinde nicht mehr nachweisbar. In der inneren Wurzelscheide nimmt der RNS-Gehalt mit dem Einsetzen der Hyalinisierung gleichfalls stark ab, jedoch findet man auch in der völlig hyalinisierten Wurzelscheide noch RNS (BRAUN-FALCO, 1958).

7. Histotopographie von Enzymen

Mitteilungen über den histochemischen Nachweis von Enzymaktivitäten im Bereich des Haarfollikels wurden in den letzten Jahren in so großer Zahl publiziert, daß eine ausführlichere Besprechung einzelner Arbeiten und insbesondere ein näheres Eingehen auf die angewandten Methoden und ihre Spezifität den Rahmen dieses Beitrags sprengen würde. Es soll daher, unter Hinweis auf die ausführlichen Übersichten von BRAUN-FALCO (1958), LEONHARDI und STEIGLEDER sowie STEIGLEDER (1957), hier nur eine tabellarische Übersicht gegeben werden, in der nach Angaben der jeweils zitierten Autoren aufgezeigt ist, welche Enzyme bislang in welchen Gewebspartien des Follikels histochemisch dargestellt werden konnten. Auf detaillierte Angaben über unterschiedliche Aktivitätsstärken in verschiedenen Bereichen wurde dabei verzichtet, da einerseits die von verschiedenen Autoren gewonnenen Ergebnisse diesbezüglich nicht immer ganz übereinstimmen und da andererseits ein stärkerer oder schwächerer Aktivitätsnachweis keinen Rückschluß auf die aktuelle Stoffwechselgröße erlaubt. Der histochemische Fermentnachweis zeigt nämlich lediglich potentielle Stoffwechselleistungen an (BRAUN-FALCO, 1961b). Die in lebenden Geweben vorliegenden Enzymkonzentrationen übersteigen die zum Normalumsatz erforderlichen Konzentrationen um das 50—600fache (SIEBERT, 1956), so daß selbst eine Aktivitätshemmung von etwa 99% eine Einschränkung der normalen Stoffwechselleistungen nicht bedingen muß (BRAUN-FALCO, 1958). Die Abb. 19 und 20 verdeutlichen einige der tabellarisch wiedergegebenen Befunde.

V. Autoradiographische Befunde am Haarfollikel

Bei der Autoradiographie wird die Verteilung ins Gewebe eingebauter radioaktiver Substanzen durch Schwärzung eines auf einen histologischen Schnitt aufgebrachten photographischen Films dargestellt. Die Methode erlaubt, das Schicksal von markierten Substanzen, die dem Organismus parenteral, percutan oder auf anderem Wege zugeführt wurden, genauer zu verfolgen und vermittelt damit wichtige Einblicke in örtliche Stoffwechselprozesse. Sie kann histochemische Verfahren in vieler Hinsicht ergänzen. Autoradiographische Untersuchungen haben uns besonders bezüglich des Einbaus von Aminosäuren in die Haarwurzel und des Eiweißumsatzes im Follikel eine Reihe neuer und wichtiger Erkenntnisse gebracht.

Daß Haarwurzeln einen im Vergleich mit den meisten anderen Geweben recht beträchtlichen Eiweißumsatz haben, zeigten Untersuchungen von NIKLAS und OEHLERT. Diese Autoren bestimmten den Einbau von Thioaminosäuren in verschiedene Gewebe nach Gabe eines Hydrolysats von S-35-markiertem Hefeeiweiß und fanden in den Zellen der Haarwurzel auffallend starke Radioaktivität. Da bei der Schnittbearbeitung freie Aminosäuren aus dem Gewebe herausgelöst werden, kann die Radioaktivität nur darauf beruhen, daß markierte Substanzen in Gewebseiweiße fest eingebaut wurden[1] und daß somit an diesen Stellen Eiweißumsatz erfolgt. Interessanterweise ist das Ausmaß des so autoradiographisch festgestellten Proteinumsatzes dem Gehalt der Zellen an Ribonucleinsäure direkt proportional.

Der Einbau S^{35}-markierten Cystins in den Follikel ist wiederholt studiert worden. Dabei hat sich gezeigt, daß Cystin direkt in der keratogenen Zone aufgenommen und — wahrscheinlich als Cystein — eingebaut wird. Bereits 1 Std nach intraperitonealer Injektion von S^{35}-Cystin ist dessen Inkorporation in der keratogenen Zone aktiver Follikel nachweisbar (NAKAI). 6—8 Std nach der Applikation zeigt die keratogene Zone hohe Radioaktivität, der Bulbus nur mäßig starke Aktivität (BERN; HARKNESS und BERN; NAKAI). Entsprechende Befunde

---
[1] Das gilt in gleicher Weise für alle nachfolgend besprochenen Versuchsergebnisse mit markierten Aminosäuren.

Tabelle 2. *Histotopochemie von Enzymen im Bereich des Haarfollikels.* Übersicht
+ = Enzymaktivität histochemisch nachweisbar; — = Enzymaktivität histochemisch nicht nachweisba

Lokalisation der Aktivitäten / Enzym	äußere Wurzelscheide	innere Wurzelscheide	Aktiver Follikel – dermale Papille	Matrix	oberer Bulbus	keratogene Zone	Haarschaft	Ruhefollikel – epithelialer Sack	Haarstengel	M. arrect. pilorum	bindegewebiger Haarbalg	Autoren
Phosphorylase	+	+		+	+	—	+	+	+	—		BRAUN-FALCO (1956b); ELLI u. MONTAGNA; NAKAMURA
Cytochromoxydase	+	+[a]	+	+	—	—	+	—	+	—		ROGERS (1953); BRAUN-FALCO (1961a); MONTAGNA (1962)
Bernsteinsäuredehydrogenase	+		+	+	+	—	—	+	—	+	—	FORMISANO u. MONTAGNA; BRAUN-FALCO u. RATHJENS (1954); MONTAGNA u. FORMISANO; FORAKER u. WINGO; ZELICKSON (1960)
NADH- und NADPH-Tetrazoliumreductase	+	+[a]	+	+	+	+	—	+	+	+	—	BRAUN-FALCO u. PETZOLD
β-Glucuronidase	+	+[a]		+	+	+	—	—	+	+		BRAUN-FALCO (1956c); MONTAGNA (1957)
Aminopeptidasen	+			+	+	—	+	+	+	+	+	BRAUN-FALCO (1956e); ADACHI u. MONTAGNA; STEIGLEDER, KUDICKE u. KAMEI; WOLFF (1963b)[b]
Unspezifische Esterasen	+	+	—	+	+	+		+	—	+		FINDLAY; MONTAGNA (1955); BRAUN-FALCO (1956a); STEIGLEDER u. LÖFFLER; STEIGLEDER (1958); KNOTH, RUHBACH u. EHLERS
Alkalische Phosphatase	—	—	+	+	—	—	—				+	JOHNSON, BUTCHER u. BEVELANDER; SPIER u. MARTIN KOPF
Saure Phosphatase	+	+	—[c]	+	+	+	—[d]			+	—	SPIER u. MARTIN; SPIER u. v. CANEGHEM; WOLFF (1963a) KNOTH, RUHBACH u. EHLERS
Glucose-6-Phosphatase			+	+								BRAUN-FALCO (1956d, 1958)
5-Nucleotidase			+	+						+	+	SPIER u. MARTIN; WOLFF (1963a)
Ribonuclease						+						SPIER u. v. CANEGHEM; STEIGLEDER u. RAAB; STEIGLEDER u. FISCHER
Adenosintriphosphatase	+	+	+	+		+				+	+	CORMANE u. KALSBEEK; WOLFF (1963a)
Monoaminooxydase	+			+	+	+		+	+	+		SHELLEY, COHEN u. KOELLE (1955); YASUDA u. MONTAGN
β-hydroxy-Butyryl-Dehydrogenase	+	+		+	+	+	—			+		CORMANE u. CLAESSENS
Kohlensäureanhydratase	+	+										BRAUN-FALCO u. RATHJENS (1955)

[a] Hyalinisierte Anteile: —.
[b] WOLFF erhob — abhängig von dem bei der Inkubation angewandten Substrat — teilweise von de dargestellten Ergebnissen stark abweichende Befunde.
[c] In den Untersuchungen von WOLFF: +.
[d] Proximale Anteile des Haarschafts: +.

erhob BÉLANGER nach subcutaner Radiocystin-Injektion. Demgegenüber werden C^{14}-enthaltende Proteinhydrolysate von Bulbus und keratogener Zone gleichmäßig aufgenommen, was auf eine relativ selektive Aufnahme des Cystins in der keratogenen Zone schließen läßt (HARKNESS und BERN). Auch im Katagen nimmt der Follikel Radiocystin auf, während das Telogenhaar keine radioautographische Aktivität zeigt (HARKNESS und BERN). Die Frage nach der Art des Einbaus des Cystins suchten BERN, HARKNESS und BLAIR durch Behandlung der autoradiographischen Schnitte mit verschiedenartigen Lösungsmitteln zu klären. Nach diesen Untersuchungen ist es wahrscheinlich, daß das Cystin durch Peptid-Bindung in die Hauptkette der Keratinmoleküle eingebaut ist. NAKAI bestimmte nach S^{35}-Cystinapplikation mittels elektronenmikroskopischer Autoradiographie die Korndichte über den cellulären Strukturen der keratogenen Zone und stellte fest, daß etwa 64% der Körner über den Tonofibrillen der Rinde lagen. Die Tonofibrillen sind also der Ort, an dem die markierte Aminosäure in hoher Konzentration vorliegt. Andere celluläre Elemente zeigen demgegenüber keine durch Zählung der geschwärzten Körner erfaßbare stärkere Radioaktivität. Aus diesen Beobachtungen ergibt sich, daß das Cystin nicht in freier Form in den Zellen angereichert, sondern direkt in Tonofibrillen eingebaut wird.

Wie rasch das Cystin vom Blutstrom in die Haarwurzel diffundiert, zeigt ein Versuch von RYDER. Dieser Autor tötete eine Maus 30 sec nach intravenöser Applikation von S^{35}-Cystin und konnte bereits nach dieser kurzen Zeit schwache Radioaktivität in Anagenfollikeln nachweisen.

Auch der Einbau von S^{35}-Methionin ist autoradiographisch vorwiegend in der keratogenen Zone nachweisbar (BÉLANGER; NAKAI), wobei nach LEBLOND, EVERETT und SIMMONS die proximalen Anteile dieser Zone auffällig bevorzugt sind. EDWARDS konnte durch chromatographische Untersuchungen zeigen, daß das markierte Schwefelatom von S^{35}-Methionin im Cystein eingebaut wird.

Intraperitoneale Injektion von Tritium-markiertem Tyrosin führt bei Ratten innerhalb kurzer Zeit (10 min) zu autoradiographisch erfaßbarer Aktivität in Matrix, oberem Bulbus und keratogener Zone bis zur Höhe, in der der Haarschaft voll verhornt ist (SIMS). Es ist dies ein eindeutiges Zeichen dafür, daß in den Rindenzellen erst unmittelbar vor der völligen Verhornung die Proteinsynthese beendet wird.

Interessante Ergebnisse zur Lokalisation der DNS-Synthese im Haarfollikel lieferten Untersuchungen von ALLEGRA und MARCHESELLI. Diese Autoren injizierten eine Lösung von H^3-Thymidin zu verschiedenen Zeiten des durch mechanische Epilation synchron angeregten Haarcyclus in die Haut von Ratten. Während der ersten Phase der Follikelentwicklung wird der markierte DNS-Baustein in den peripheren Zellen des nach unten wachsenden Haarkeims angereichert, im Stadium vollen Haarwachstums nur im Bulbus, und zwar ganz überwiegend unterhalb einer Ebene, die der „kritischen Ebene" von AUBER entspricht. Diese Befunde können als weiterer Beweis dafür herangezogen werden, daß die mitotische Aktivität im Follikel auf die unteren Bulbusanteile beschränkt ist und daß die Aubersche Ebene als funktionelle Grenze zwischen Zellbildungs- und Zelldifferenzierungszone tatsächlich existiert.

MONTAGNA und HILL bestimmten in Haaren verschiedener Cyclusphasen den Einbau des Schwefels nach Gabe von S^{35}-markiertem Na_2SO_4. Sie fanden Radioaktivität an Stellen und zu Zeiten, wo histochemisch saure Mucopolysaccharide nachweisbar sind. Auf die autoradiographisch darstellbaren Verteilungsmuster weiterer markierter Substanzen im Haarfollikel kann hier nicht eingegangen werden. Mitgeteilt wurden Beobachtungen über die Ansammlung von Jod-131, Selen-75, Vanadium-48, Strontium-90, Zink-65 (STRAIN, LANKAU und PORIES), ferner Kohlenstoff-14 (LEBLOND; HARKNESS und BERN), C^{14}-markierter Glucose (RYDER) und Phosphor-32 (HARKNESS und BERN). Verschiedene markierte Carcinogene wie Benzpyren und Methylcholantren werden ebenfalls in wachsende Haare eingebaut (OEHLERT und GRIMM).

Außer für das Studium von Einbauprozessen kann die Autoradiographie auch zur Bestimmung der Wachstumsgeschwindigkeit des Haares herangezogen werden und ist hier anderen Verfahren deutlich überlegen. ASHMORE und UTTLEY lieferten Wachstumskurven für die Haare von Mäusen, denen sie während eines durch Epilation synchron angeregten Haarcyclus in 24stündigen Abständen S^{35}-markiertes Cystin intraperitoneal injizierten. Auf den autoradiographischen Aufnahmen der nach Beendigung des Cyclus epilierten Haare konnten die Abstände der Zonen der täglichen Einlagerung exakt bestimmt werden. MUNRO führte entsprechende Messungen bei drei Versuchspersonen durch, denen er S^{35}-Cystin intradermal injizierte. Die dabei erforderlichen Dosen von 0,05 µc S^{35} pro Injektion sind so gering, daß auch bei mehrfacher Applikation die Gefahr einer Strahlenschädigung nicht besteht. In den Haaren sind die oberen Grenzen der Aktivitätszonen sehr scharf zu erkennen. Durch Ausmessung der Abstände dieser Grenzen konnte MUNRO für das Kopfhaar ein mittleres tägliches Wachstum von 0,37 mm bestimmen.

Schluß

In der vorstehenden Übersicht über den derzeitigen Stand des Wissens vom Haarfollikel konnte bei den uns hinsichtlich des Umfangs gesetzten Grenzen manches Problem nur in sehr geraffter Form dargestellt, manche für die Bearbeitung spezieller Fragen wichtige Einzeltatsache nur am Rande erwähnt werden. Die von subjektiven Wertungen nicht freie Auswahl der Schwerpunkte unserer Darstellung erfolgte in Hinblick darauf, daß es zweckmäßig sei, über eine bloße Bestandsaufnahme hinaus für die Erforschung der noch ungelösten Probleme der Biologie des Haares und für das Verständnis pathologischer Reaktionen des Follikels grundlegende Fakten ausführlicher darzustellen und damit den am Haar Interessierten eine Arbeits- und Orientierungshilfe für die weitergehende Forschung zu geben.

Literatur

(Einige bei der Abfassung herangezogene Übersichtsarbeiten und Monographien, die im Text nicht zitiert sind, sind mit einem * vor dem Autorennamen gekennzeichnet.)

ADACHI, K., and W. MONTAGNA: Histology and cytochemistry of human skin. XXII. Sites of leucine aminopeptidase (LAP). J. invest. Derm. **37**, 145—151 (1961). — ALLEGRA, F., and W. MARCHESELLI: The regrowing hair follicle of the guinea pig. Arch. Derm. Syph. (Chic.) **90**, 310—313 (1964). — ANDREASEN, E.: Cyclic changes in the skin of the mouse. Acta path. microbiol. scand. **32**, 157—163 (1953). — APPLEYARD, H. M., and C. M. GREVILLE: The cuticle of mammalian hair. Nature (Lond.) **166**, 1031 (1950). — ASHMORE, H., and M. UTTLEY: Measurement of rate of growth of rodent hair using cystine labelled with sulphur-35. Nature (Lond.) **206**, 108—109 (1965). — ATKINSON, S., F. CORMIA, and S. A. UNRAU: The diameter and growth phase of hair in relation to age. Brit. J. Derm. **71**, 309—311 (1959). — AUBER, L.: The anatomy of follicles producing wool-fibres, with special reference to keratinization. Trans. roy. Soc. Edinb. **62**, 191—254 (1952).

BANDMANN, H.-J., u. K. BOSSE: Histologie und mikroskopische Anatomie des Haarfollikels im Verlauf des Haarcyclus. Arch. klin. exp. Derm. **227**, 390—409 (1966). — BARGMANN, W.: Histologie und mikroskopische Anatomie des Menschen, 5. Aufl. Stuttgart: Georg Thieme 1964. — BARMAN, J. M., I. ASTORE, and V. PECORARO: The normal trichogram of the adult. J. invest. Derm. **44**, 233—236 (1965). — BARMAN, J. M., V. PECORARO, and I. ASTORE: Method, technic and computations in the study of the trophic state of the human scalp hair. J. invest. Derm. **42**, 421—425 (1964). — BARRNETT, R. J., and A. M. SELIGMAN: Histochemical demonstration of protein-bound sulfhydryl groups. Science **116**, 323—327 (1952).— *BEHRMAN, H. T.: The scalp in health and disease. St. Louis: C. V. Mosby Co. 1952. —

Bélanger, L. F.: Autoradiographic visualization of the entry and transit of S 35 methionine and cystine in the soft an hard tissues of the growing rat. Anat. Rec. **124**, 555—579 (1956). — Bern, H. A.: Histology and chemistry of keratin formation. Nature (Lond.) **174**, 509—511 (1954). — Bern, H. A., D. R. Harkness, and S. M. Blair: Radioautographic studies of keratin formation. Proc. nat. Acad. Sci. (Wash.) **41**, 55—60 (1955). — Birbeck, M. S. C.: Electron microscopy of melanocytes: The fine structure of hair-bulb premelanosomes. Ann. N.Y. Acad. Sci. **100**, 540—547 (1963). — Birbeck, M. S. C., and E. H. Mercer: The electron microscopy of the human hair follicle. 1. Introduction and the hair cortex. J. biophys. biochem. Cytol. **3**, 203—214 (1957a). — The electron microscopy of the human hair follicle. 2. The hair cuticle. J. biophys. biochem. Cytol. **3**, 215—222 (1957b). — The electron microscopy of the human hair follicle. 3. The inner root sheath and trichohyaline. J. biophys. biochem. Cytol. **3**, 223—230 (1957c). — Birbeck, M. S. C., E. H. Mercer, and N. A. Barnicot: The structure and formation of pigment granules in human hair. Exp. Cell Res. **10**, 505—514 (1956). — Borodach, G. N., and W. Montagna: Fat in the skin of the mouse during cycles of hair growth. J. invest. Derm. **26**, 229—232 (1956). — Braun-Falco, O.: Beitrag zum histochemischen Nachweis von Esterasen in normaler und psoriatischer Haut. Arch. klin. exp. Derm. **202**, 153—162 (1956a). — Über die Fähigkeit der menschlichen Haut zur Polysaccharidsynthese, ein Beitrag zur Histotopochemie der Phosphorylase. Arch. klin. exp. Derm. **202**, 163—170 (1956b). — Zur Histotopographie der β-Glucuronidase in normaler menschlicher Haut. Arch. klin. exp. Derm. **203**, 61—67 (1956c). — Zur histochemischen Darstellung von Glucose-6-Phosphatase in normaler Haut. Derm. Wschr. **134**, 1252—1257 (1956d). — Histochemische Aminopeptidase-Darstellung in normaler Haut, bei Psoriasis, Dermatitis, Basaliom, spinozellulärem Karzinom und Molluscum sebaceum. Derm. Wschr. **134**, 1341—1349 (1956e). — The histochemistry of the hair follicle. In: The biology of hair growth (W. Montagna and R. A. Ellis, eds.), p. 65—90. New York: Academic Press 1958. — Zur Histotopographie der Cytochromoxydase in normaler und pathologisch veränderter Haut sowie in Hauttumoren. Arch. klin. exp. Derm. **214**, 176—224 (1961a). — Die Histochemie der Haut. In: Dermatologie und Venerologie (H. A. Gottron u. W. Schönfeld, Hrsg.), Bd. I/1, S. 366—472. Stuttgart: Georg Thieme 1961b. — Über die mitotische Aktivität in der Haarmatrix bei der Albinomaus während eines künstlich induzierten Haarcyclus. Arch. klin. exp. Derm. **215**, 63—78 (1962). — Braun-Falco, O., u. O. Frenz: Über Veränderungen des Wassergehaltes der Haut während des Haarwachstumscyclus bei der Ratte. Arch. klin. exp. Derm. **212**, 64—68 (1960). — Über Veränderungen im Fettgehalt der Rattenhaut während des Haarcyclus. Arch. klin. exp. Derm. **212**, 173—179 (1961). — Braun-Falco, O., u. A. Kint: Zur Dynamik der Katagenphase. Arch. klin. exp. Derm. **223**, 1—15 (1965). — Braun-Falco, O., u. D. Petzold: Über die Histotopie von NADH- und NADPH-Tetrazoliumreduktase in menschlicher Haut. I. Normale Haut. Arch. klin. exp. Derm. **220**, 455—473 (1964). — Braun-Falco, O., u. B. Rassner: Über den Einfluß der Epilationstechnik auf normale und pathologische Haarwurzelmuster. Arch. klin. exp. Derm. **223**, 501—508 (1965). — Braun-Falco, O., u. B. Rathjens: Histochemische Darstellung der Bernsteinsäuredehydrogenase in der menschlichen Haut. Derm. Wschr. **130**, 1271—1276 (1954). — Über die histochemische Darstellung der Kohlensäureanhydratase in normaler Haut. Arch. klin. exp. Derm. **201**, 73—82 (1955). — Histochemische Darstellung von Zink in normaler menschlicher Haut. Arch. klin. exp. Derm. **203**, 130—136 (1956). — Braun-Falco, O., u. H. Theisen: Über Veränderungen im Hautbindegewebe während des Haarwachstumscyclus bei der Maus. Arch. klin. exp. Derm. **209**, 426—434 (1959). — Braun-Falco, O., u. H. Zaun: Über die Beteiligung des gesamten Capillitiums bei Alopecia areata. Hautarzt **13**, 342—348 (1962a). — Zum Wesen der chronischen diffusen Alopecie bei Frauen. Arch. klin. exp. Derm. **215**, 165—180 (1962b). — Bullough, W. S., and E. B. Laurence: The mitotic activity of the follicle. In: The biology of hair growth (W. Montagna and R. A. Ellis, eds.), p. 171—187. New York: Academic Press 1958. — Butcher, E. O.: The hair cycles in the albino rat. Anat. Rec. **61**, 5—19 (1934). — Development of the pilary system and the replacement of hair in Mammals. Ann. N.Y. Acad. Sci. **53**, 508—516 (1951). — Butcher, E. O., and A. W. Grokoest: The influence of tissue fluid on hair growth. Growth **5**, 175—181 (1941).

Charles, A.: Electron microscope observations on hardening in the hair follicle. Exp. Cell Res. **18**, 138—149 (1959). — Chase, H. B.: Growth of the hair. Physiol. Rev. **34**, 113—126 (1954). — * The behavior of pigment cells and epithelial cells in the hair follicle. In: The biology of hair growth (W. Montagna and R. A. Ellis, eds.), p. 229—237. New York: Academic Press 1958. — Chase, H. B., and G. J. Eaton: The growth of hair follicles in waves. Ann. N.Y. Acad. Sci. **83**, 365—368 (1959). — Chase, H. B., W. Montagna, and J. D. Malone: Changes in the skin in relation to the hair growth cycle. Anat. Rec. **116**, 75—82 (1953). — Chase, H. B., H. Rauch, and V. W. Smith: Critical stages of hair development and pigmentation in the mouse. Physiol. Zool. **24**, 1—8 (1951). — Chowdhuri, S., and B. Bhattacharyya: Paired medulla in human hair. Curr. Sci. **33**, 748—749 (1964). — Cooper, Z. K.: A histological study of the integument of the armadillo. Amer. J. Anat. **45**, 1—37

(1930). — CORMANE, R. H., and F. L. E. CLAESSENS: Some aspects of beta-hydroxy butyryl dehydrogenase activity in the human skin (normal-abnormal). Dermatologica (Basel) **126**, 369—379 (1963). — CORMANE, R. H., and G. L. KALSBEEK: ATP-hydrolyzing enzymes in normal human skin. Dermatologica (Basel) **127**, 381—397 (1963). — CORMIA, F. E.: Vasculature of the normal scalp. Arch. Derm. Syph. (Chic.) **88**, 692—701 (1963). — CRAMER, H. J.: Histochemische Untersuchungen mit dem sauren Hämateintest nach Baker an normaler und pathologisch veränderter Haut. I. Normale Haut. Arch. klin. exp. Derm. **218**, 191—202 (1964). — CROUNSE, R. G., and E. J. VAN SCOTT: Changes in scalp hair roots as a measure of toxicity from cancer chemotherapeutic drugs. J. invest. Derm. **35**, 83—90 (1960).

DAVIS, B. K.: Phases of the hair-growth cycle. Nature (Lond.) **194**, 694 (1962). — DRY, F. W.: The coat of the mouse (Mus musculus). J. Genet. **16**, 287—340 (1926). — DUGGINS, O. H., and M. TROTTER: Changes in morphology of hair during childhood. Ann. N.Y. Acad. Sci. **53**, 569—575 (1951).

EDWARDS, L. J.: The absorption of methionine by the skin of the guinea pig. Biochem. J. **57**, 542—547 (1954). — EISEN, A. Z., W. MONTAGNA, and H. B. CHASE: Sulfhydryl groups in the skin of mouse and guinea pig. J. nat. Cancer Inst. **14**, 341—353 (1953). — EJIRI, I.: Studien über die Histologie der menschlichen Haut: über die regionären und Altersunterschiede der verschiedenen Hautelemente mit besonderer Berücksichtigung der Altersveränderung der elastischen Fasern. Jap. J. Derm. Urol. **41**, 8—12 (1937). — Zit. nach ELLIS. — ELLIS, R. A.: Ageing of the human male scalp. In: The biology of hair growth (W. MONTAGNA and R. A. ELLIS, eds.), p. 469—485. New York: Academic Press 1958. — ELLIS, R. A., and W. MONTAGNA: Histology and cytochemistry of human skin. XV. Sites of phosphorylase and amylo-1,6-glucosidase activity. J. Histochem. Cytochem. **6**, 201—207 (1958).

FILSHIE, B. K., and G. E. ROGERS: The fine structure of α-keratin. J. molec. Biol. **3**, 784—786 (1961). — FINDLAY, G. H.: The simple esterases of human skin. Brit. J. Derm. **67**, 83—91 (1955). — *FLECK, F., u. M. FLECK: Die Haarkrankheiten des Menschen. Berlin: VEB Verlag Volk und Gesundheit 1962. — FLESCH, P.: Hair growth. In: S. ROTHMAN, Physiology and biochemistry of the skin, p. 601—661. Chicago: University of Chicago Press 1954. — FORAKER, A. E., and W. J. WINGO: Histochemical studies of skin. Arch. Derm. (Chic.) **72**, 1—6 (1955). — FORMISANO, V. R., and W. MONTAGNA: Succinic dehydrogenase activity in the skin of the guinea pig. Anat. Rec. **120**, 893—905 (1954).

GALEWSKY, E.: Erkrankungen der Haare und des Haarbodens. In: Handbuch der Haut- und Geschlechtskrankheiten (J. JADASSOHN, Hrsg.), Bd. XIII/1, S. 129—437. Berlin: Springer 1932. — GARN, S. M.: The examination of hair under the polarizing microscope. Ann. N.Y. Acad. Sci. **53**, 649—652 (1951). — GIBBS, H. F.: A study of the post-natal development of skin and hair of the mouse. Anat. Rec. **80**, 61—81 (1941). — GIROUD, A., et H. BULLIARD: La kératinisation de l'épiderme et des phaneres. Genèse des substances soufrées de la kératine. Arch. Morph. gén. exp. **29**, 7—83 (1930). — GIROUD, A., H. BULLIARD, and C. P. LEBLOND: (1934) zit. nach BRAUN-FALCO (1958). — *GIROUD, A., and C. P. LEBLOND: The keratinization of epidermis and its derivates, especially the hair, as shown by X-ray diffraction and histochemical studies. Ann. N.Y. Acad. Sci. **53**, 613—626 (1951). — GOERTTLER, K. (unter Mitarb. v. P. GÖRDEL): Die menschliche Glatze im Altersformwandel der behaarten Kopfhaut. In: Zwanglose Abhandlungen aus dem Gebiet der normalen und pathologischen Anatomie (W. BARGMANN u. W. DOERR, Hrsg.), H. 17. Stuttgart: Georg Thieme 1965. — GOLDBLUM, R. W., W. N. PIPER, and A. W. CAMPBELL: A comparision of three histochemical stains for the demonstration of protein-bound sulfhydryl groups in normal human skin. J. invest. Derm. **23**, 375—383 (1954). — GROODT, A. DE, u. FR. DE GROODT: Stand, Lage und Anordnung einer Gruppe von Haarcuticulazellen mit Hilfe von darstellender Geometrie. Z. mikr.-anat. Forsch. **36**, 637—644 (1934).

HAMILTON, H. B.: Patterned loss of hair in man: Types and incidence. Ann. N.Y. Acad. Sci. **53**, 708—728 (1951). — HAMILTON, J. B., and A. E. LIGHT (eds.): The growth, replacement and types of hair. Ann. N.Y. Acad. Sci. **53**, 461—752 (1951). — HAPPEY, F., and A. G. JOHNSON: Some electron microscope observations on hardening in the human hair follicle. J. Ultrastruct. Res. **7**, 316—327 (1962). — HARDY, M. H.: The histochemistry of hair follicles in the mouse. Amer. J. Anat. **90**, 285—337 (1952). — HARKNESS, D. R., and H. A. BERN: Radioautographic studies of hair growth in the mouse. Acta anat. (Basel) **31**, 35—45 (1957). — HAUSMAN, L. A.: Recent studies of hair structure relationships. Sci. Mounthly **30**, 258—277 (1930). — The cortical fusi of mammalian hair shafts. Amer. Naturalist **66**, 461—470 (1932). — Applied microscopy of hair. Sci. Monthly **59**, 195—202 (1944). — HIRSCH, F.: Das Haar des Menschen. Ulm: Haug 1956. — HOEPKE, H.: Die Haare. In: Handbuch der mikroskopischen Anatomie des Menschen (Hrsg. W. v. MÖLLENDORFF), Bd. III/1, S. 1—116. Berlin: Springer 1927. — HORSTMANN, E.: Die Haut. In: Handbuch der mikroskopischen Anatomie des Menschen (W. BARGMANN, Hrsg.), Bd. III/3, S. 1—276. Berlin-Göttingen-Heidelberg: Springer 1957. — * Die elektronenmikroskopische Struktur der Haut. Arch. klin. exp. Derm. **211**, 18—35 (1960).

JOHNSON, P. L., E. O. BUTCHER, and G. BEVELANDER: The distribution of alkaline phosphatase in the cyclic growth of the rat hair follicle. Anat. Rec. **93**, 355—361 (1945). KLIGMAN, A. M.: The human hair cycle. J. invest. Derm. **33**, 307—316 (1959). — Pathologic dynamics of human hair loss. I. Telogen effluvium. Arch. Derm. (Chic.) **83**, 175—198 (1961). — KNOCHE, H.: Degenerative Veränderungen des vegetativen Nervensystems in der Glatzenhaut. Arch. Derm. Syph. (Berl.) **197**, 505—512 (1954). — KNOTH, W., M. RUHBACH u. G. EHLERS: Vergleichende ferment-histochemische Untersuchungen nach Anwendung vier verschiedener Schnittherstellungsverfahren. Arch. klin. exp. Derm. **222**, 403—422 (1965). — KOPF, A. W.: The distribution of alkaline phosphatase in normal and pathologic human skin. Arch. Derm. (Chic.) **75**, 1—37 (1957). — KOSUGI, T., u. Y. S. KIM: Zur Pathohistologie der Glatze der Kopfhaut und des Ergrauens der Kopfhaare. Trans. Soc. path. jap. **27**, 651—653 (1937). Ref. Zbl. Haut- u. Geschl.-Kr. **59**, 663 (1938).

LEBLOND, C. P.: Histological structure of hair, with brief comparision to other epidermal appendages and epidermis itself. Ann. N.Y. Acad. Sci. **53**, 464—475 (1951). — LEBLOND, C. P., N. B. EVERETT, and B. SIMMONS: Sites of protein synthesis as shown by radioautography after administration of S 35-labelled methionine. Amer. J. Anat. **101**, 225—271 (1957). — LEONHARDI, G., u. G. K. STEIGLEDER: Biochemie und Histochemie der Enzyme in der Haut. In: Aktuelle Probleme der Dermatologie (R. SCHUPPLI, Hrsg.), Bd. I, S. 47—106. Basel u. New York: Karger 1959. — LIGHT, A. E.: Histological study of human scalps exhibiting various degrees of nonspecific baldness. J. invest. Derm. **13**, 53—59 (1949). — LOCHTE, T.: Atlas der menschlichen und tierischen Haare. Leipzig: Schöps 1938. — Cuticulastudien am menschlichen Haar. Zbl. Kleintierk.- u. Pelztierk. **14**, 1—26 (1938b). — Über die Kopfhaarlänge beim Säugling und Kleinkinde und über den Haarwechsel des Kopfhaares des Neugeborenen. Zbl. Kleintierk.- u. Pelztierk. **14**, 27—48 (1938c). — Grundriß der Entwicklung des menschlichen Haares. Frankfurt a. Main: Schöps 1951. — Tafeln zur Haarkunde. Leipzig: Geest & Portig/Schöps 1954. — LOMBARDO, C.: Il glicogeno in alcuni derivati epidermici della cute umana. G. ital. Derm. Sif. **75**, 185—186 (1934). Zit. nach MONTAGNA 1962. — LUBOWE, I. I. (ed.): Hair growth and hair regeneration. Ann. N.Y. Acad. Sci. **83**, 359—512 (1959). — LUDWIG, E.: Der heutige Stand unseres Wissens über die Glatze. Hautarzt **13**, 337—339 (1962). — LUELL, E., and V. E. ARCHER: Hair medulla variation with age in human males. Amer. J. phys. Anthropol. **22**, 107—109 (1964). — LYNFIELD, Y. L.: Effect of pregnancy on the human hair cycle. J. invest. Derm. **35**, 323—327 (1960).

MAGUIRE, H. C., and A. M. KLIGMAN: Hair plucking as a diagnostic tool. J. invest. Derm. **43**, 77—79 (1964). — MARON, H.: Die Tiefe der Haarzwiebeln in der menschlichen Kopfhaut. Derm. Wschr. **143**, 8—19 (1961). — MEDAWAR, P. B.: The micro-anatomy of the mammaliau epidermis. Quart. J. micr. Sci. **94**, 481—506 (1953). — MERCER, E. H.: Some experiments on the orientation and hardening of keratin in the hair follicle. Biochim. biophys. Acta (Amst.) **3**, 161—169 (1949). — The electron microscopy of keratinized tissues. In: The biology of hair growth (W. MONTAGNA and R. A. ELLIS, eds.), p. 91—111. New York: Academic Press 1958.— MERCER, E. H., B. L. MUNGER, G. E. ROGERS, and S. I. ROTH: A suggested nomenclature for fine-structural components of keratin and keratin-like products of cells. Nature (Lond.) **201**, 367—368 (1964). — MONTAGNA, W.: Perinuclear sudanophil bodies in mammalian epidermis. Quart. J. micr. Sci. **91**, 205—208 (1950). — Histology and cytochemistry of human skin. IX. The distribution of non-specific esterases. J. biophys. biochem. Cytol. **1**, 13—16 (1955). — Histology and cytochemistry of human skin. XI. The distribution of β-glucuronidase. J. biophys. biochem. Cytol. **3**, 343—348 (1957). — Hair growth and hair regeneration. Introduction. Ann. N.Y. Acad. Sci. **83**, 362—364 (1959). — The structure and function of skin, 2nd ed. New York and London: Academic Press 1962. — MONTAGNA, W., and H. B. CHASE: Histology and cytochemistry of human skin X. X-irradiation of the scalp. Amer. J. Anat. **99**, 415—446 (1956). — MONTAGNA, W., H. B. CHASE, and J. B. HAMILTON: The distribution of glycogen and lipids in human skin. J. invest. Derm. **17**, 147—157 (1951). — MONTAGNA, W., H. B. CHASE, and W. C. LOBITZ jr.: Histology and cytochemistry of human skin II. The distribution of glycogen in the epidermis, hair pollicles, sebaceous glands and eccrine sweat glands. Anat. Rec. **114**, 231—247 (1952). — MONTAGNA, W., H. B. CHASE, J. D. MALONE, and H. P. MELARAGNO: Cyclic changes in polysaccharides of the papilla of the hair follicle. Quart. J. micr. Sci. **93**, 241—245 (1952). — MONTAGNA, W., H. B. CHASE, and H. P. MELARAGNO: Histology and cytochemistry of human skin I. Metachromasia in the mons pubis. J. nat. Cancer Inst. **12**, 591—597 (1951). — MONTAGNA, W., A. Z. EISEN, A. H. RADEMACHER, and H. B. CHASE: Histology and cytochemistry of human skin VI. The distribution of sulfhydryl and disulfide groups. J. invest. Derm. **23**, 23—32 (1954). — MONTAGNA, W., and R. A. ELLIS (eds.): The biology of hair growth. New York: Academic Press 1958. — The skin of the potto (Perodicticus potto). Amer. J. phys. Anthropol. **17**, 137—162 (1959). — MONTAGNA, W., and V. R. FORMISANO: Histology and cytochemistry of human skin. VII. The distribution of succinic dehydrogenase activity. Anat. Rec. **122**, 65—77 (1955). — MONTAGNA, W., and R. J. HARRISON: Specialization in the skin of the seal (Phoca vitulina). Amer. J. Anat. **100**, 81—114

(1957). — MONTAGNA, W., and C. R. HILL: The localization of S 35 in the skin of the rat. Anat. Rec. **127**, 163—172 (1957). — MONTAGNA, W., and E. J. VAN SCOTT: The anatomy of the hair follicle. In: The biology of hair growth (W. MONTAGNA and R. A. ELLIS, eds.), p. 39—64. New York: Academic Press 1958. — MONTAGNA, W., and J. S. YUN: The skin of the domestic pig. J. invest. Derm. **43**, 11—21 (1964). — MORETTI, G.: Das Haar. In: STÜTTGEN, G., Die normale und pathologische Physiologie der Haut, S. 506—553. Stuttgart: Gustav Fischer 1965. — MORETTI, G., C. GIACOMETTI, V. BOIDO, and R. REBORA: Histamine, serotonin and mast cells in the skin of the rat during the hair cycle. J. invest. Derm. **40**, 205—212 (1963). — MÜLLER, C.: Über den Bau der koronalen Schüppchen des Säugetierhaares. Zool. Anz. **126**, 97—107 (1939). — MUNRO, D. D.: Hair growth measurement using intradermal sulfur 35 cystine. Arch. Derm. Syph. (Chic.) **93**, 119—122 (1966).

NAKAMURA, J.: Studies on phosphorylase activity in the skin. Jap. J. Derm. **73**, 71—75 (1963). Ref. Zbl. Haut- u. Geschl.-Kr. **115**, 205 (1964). — NAKAI, T.: A study of the ultrastructural localization of hair keratin synthesis utilizing electron microscope autoradiography in a magnetic field. J. Cell Biol. **21**, 63—74 (1964). — NIKLAS, A., u. W. OEHLERT: Autoradiographische Untersuchungen der Größe des Eiweißstoffwechsels verschiedener Organe, Gewebe und Zellarten. Beitr. path. Anat. **116**, 92—123 (1956). — *NOBACK, C. R.: Morphology und phylogeny of hair. Ann. N.Y. Acad. Sci. **53**, 476—491 (1951).

OBERSTE-LEHN, H., u. A. NOBIS: Beobachtungen am Papillarkörper und an den Haarfollikeln während der Alterung des Menschen. Med. Kosmetik **8**, 176—181 (1959). — OBERSTE-LEHN, H., u. A. NOBIS: Die Haaranordnung beim Menschen und bei einigen Säugetieren. Z. Anat. Entwickl.-Gesch. **123**, 589—642 (1963). — ODLAND, G. F.: Some microscopic studies of the keratinization of human hair. J. invest. Derm. **21**, 305—312 (1953). — OEHLERT, W., u. D. GRIMM: Das Verteilungs- und Einbaumuster radioaktiv markierter Carcinogene in der Mäuseepidermis nach lokaler Applikation. Z. Krebsforschung (im Druck). — ORENTREICH, N.: J. Soc. cosm. Chem. **11**, 479 (1960). Zit. nach LUDWIG.

PARAKKAL, P. F., and A. G. MATOLTSY: A study of the differentiation products of the hair follicle cells with the electron miscroscope. J. invest. Derm. **43**, 23—34 (1964). — PINKUS, F.: Die normale Anatomie der Haut. In: Handbuch der Haut- und Geschlechtskrankheiten (J. JADASSOHN, Hrsg.), Bd. I/1, S. 1—378. Berlin: Springer 1927. — PINKUS, H.: Embryology of hair. In: The biology of hair growth (W. MONTAGNA and R. A. ELLIS, eds.), p. 1—32. New York: Academic Press 1958. — Zur Entwicklung des Haarfollikels beim Menschen, insbesondere des Infundibulums und des bindegewebigen Anteils. Hautarzt **10**, 164—170 (1959). — Die makroskopische Anatomie der Haut. In: Handbuch der Haut- und Geschlechtskrankheiten, Erg.-Werk (A. MARCHIONINI, Hrsg.), Bd. I/2, S. 1—138. Berlin-Göttingen-Heidelberg-New York: Springer 1964.

RASSNER, B., H. ZAUN u. O. BRAUN-FALCO: Zum Pathomechanismus der männlichen Glatzenbildung. Arch. klin. exp. Derm. **216**, 307—318 (1963). — RICHTER, R.: Die Haare. In: Handbuch der Haut- und Geschlechtskrankheiten, Erg.-Werk (A. MARCHIONINI, Hrsg.), Bd. I/3, S. 282—576. Berlin-Göttingen-Heidelberg: Springer 1963. — ROGERS, G. E.: The localization of dehydrogenase activity and sulphydryl groups in wool and hair follicles by the use of tetrazolium salts. Quart. J. micr. Sci. **94**, 253—268 (1953). — Electron microscope observations on the glassy layer of the hair follicle. Expt. Cell Res. **13**, 521—528 (1957). — Electron microscope studies of hair and wool. Ann. N.Y. Acad. Sci. **83**, 378—399 (1959). — The localization and significance of arginine and citrulline in proteins of the hair follicle. J. Histochem. Cytochem. **11**, 700—705 (1963). — Isolation and properties of inner sheath cells of hair follicles. Exp. Cell Res. **33**, 264—276 (1964). — *ROOK, A.: Some chemical influences on hair growth and pigmentation. Brit. J. Derm. **77**, 115—129 (1965). — ROTH, S. I., and E. B. HELWIG: The cytology of the dermal papilla, the bulb, and the root sheaths of the mouse hair. J. Ultrastruct. Res. **11**, 33—51 (1964a). — The cytology of the cuticle of the cortex, the cortex and the medulla of the mouse hair. J. Ultrastruct. Res. **11**, 52—67 (1964b). — RYDER, M. L.: Nutritional factors influencing hair and wool growth. In: The biology of hair growth (W. MONTAGNA and R. A. ELLIS, eds.), p. 305—334. New York: Academic Press 1958.

SANDERSON, K. V., and H. THIEDE: The micro-anatomy of normal skin as seen in thick sections. Brit. J. Derm. **73**, 43—56 (1961). — SANTLER, R.: Gesichtspunkte zur „sogenannten Glatzenoperation". Hautarzt **12**, 516—520 (1961). — SASAKAWA, M.: Beiträge zur Glykogenverteilung in der Haut unter normalen und pathologischen Zuständen. Arch. Derm. Syph. (Berl.) **134**, 418—443 (1921). — SAVILL, A., and C. WARREN: The hair and scalp, 5. Aufl. London: Edward Arnold 1962. — SCHMIDT, W. J.: Menschliches Haar im polarisierten Lichte. Mikrokosmos **19**, 65—69, 89—93 (1925/26). — Beiträge zur Doppelbrechung des menschlichen Kopfhaares. Z. Zellforsch. **15**, 188—206 (1932). — SCHWANITZ, J.: Untersuchungen zur Morphologie und Physiologie des Haarwechsels beim Hauskaninchen. Z. Morph. Ökol. Tiere **33**, 496—526 (1938). Zit. nach BRAUN-FALCO u. KINT. — SCOTT, E. J. VAN: Response of hair roots to chemical and physical influence. In: The biology of hair growth (W. MONTAGNA and

R. A. ELLIS, eds.), p. 441—449. New York: Academic Press 1958. — Evaluation of disturbed hair growth in alopecia areata and other alopecias. Ann. N.Y. Acad. Sci. 83, 480—490 (1959). — SCOTT, E. J. VAN, and T. M. EKEL: Geometric relationships between the matrix of the hair bulb an its dermal papilla in normal and alopecic scalp. J. invest. Derm. 31, 281—287 (1958). — SCOTT, E. J. VAN, T. M. EKEL, and R. AUERBACH: Determinants of rate and kinetics of cell division in scalp hair. J. invest. Derm. 41, 269—273 (1963). — SCOTT, E. J. VAN, R. P. REINERTSON, and R. STEINMULLER: The growing hair roots of the human scalp and morphologic changes therein following amethopterin therapy. J. invest. Derm. 29, 197—204 (1957). — SHELLEY, W. B., S. B. COHEN, and G. B. KOELLE: Histochemical demonstration of monoamine oxidase in human skin. J. invest. Derm. 24, 561—565 (1955). — SHIPMAN, M., H. B. CHASE, and W. MONTAGNA: Glycogen in skin of the mouse during cycles of hair growth. Proc. Soc. exp. Biol. (N.Y.) 88, 449—451 (1955). — SIEBERT, G.: Biochemie der Enzyme. Acta histochem. (Jena) 2, 122—134 (1956). — SIMS, R. T.: The incorporation and fate of H3-tyrosine in the hair cortex of rats observed by radioautography. J. Cell Biol. 22, 403—412 (1964). — SINGH, M., and J. MCKENZIE: The histology and histochemistry of the dermis in hairy and non-hairy parts of the human skin with special reference to baldness. J. Anat. (Lond.) 95, 569—574 (1961). — SPIER, H. W., u. P. v. CANEGHEM: Zur Histochemie der Verhornung. Arch. klin. exp. Derm. 206, 344—363 (1957). — SPIER, H. W., u. K. MARTIN: Histochemische Untersuchungen über die Phosphomonoesterasen der gesunden Haut mit Hinweis auf Befunde bei Hauterkrankungen. Arch. klin. exp. Derm. 202, 120—152 (1956). — STARICCO, R. G.: Amelanotic melanocytes in the outer sheath of the human hair follicle. J. invest. Derm. 33, 295—297 (1959). — The melanocytes and the hair follicle. J. invest. Derm. 35, 185—194 (1960). — Amelanotic melanocytes in the outer sheath of the human hair follicle and their role in the repigmentation of regenerated epidermis. Ann. N.Y. Acad. Sci. 100, 239—254 (1963). — STEIGLEDER, G. K.: Histochemie der Epidermis und ihrer Anhangsgebilde. Arch. klin. exp. Derm. 206, 276—317 (1957). — Zum Verhalten der esterspaltenden Fermente in der Haut des behaarten Kopfes. Hautarzt 9, 67—71 (1958). — STEIGLEDER, G. K., u. I. FISCHER: Über die Lokalisation von Ribonuclease (RNAse)- und Deoxyribonuclease (DNAse)-Aktivität in normaler, in entzündlich veränderter Haut und bei Hauttumoren. Arch. klin. exp. Derm. 217, 553—562 (1963). — STEIGLEDER, G. K., R. KUDICKE u. Y. KAMEI: Die Lokalisation der Aminopeptidasenaktivität in normaler Haut. Arch. klin. exp. Derm. 215, 307—325 (1962). — STEIGLEDER, G. K., u. H. LÖFFLER: Zum histochemischen Nachweis unspezifischer Esterasen und Lipasen. Arch. klin. exp. Derm. 203, 41—60 (1956). — STEIGLEDER, G. K., and W. P. RAAB: The localisation of ribonuclease and deoxyribonuclease activities in normal an psoriatic epidermis. J. invest. Derm. 38, 209—214 (1962). — STOVES, J. L.: Structure of keratin fibres. Nature (Lond.) 151, 304 (1943). Zit. nach BRAUN-FALCO 1958. — STRAIN, W. H., C. A. LANKAU jr., and W. J. PORIES: Zink-65 in human hair. Nature (Lond.) 204, 490—491 (1964). — SWIFT, J. A.: Transfer of melanin granules from melanocytes to the cortical cells of human hair. Nature (Lond.) 203, 976—977 (1964). — *SZABÓ, G.: The regional frequency and distribution of hair follicles in human skin. In: The biology of hair growth (W. MONTAGNA and R. A. ELLIS, eds.), p. 33—38. New York: Academic Press 1958.
THYRESSON, N.: Experimental investigation on thallium poisoning in the rat. Acta derm.-venereol. (Stockh.) 31, 3—27 (1951).
VERNALL, D. G.: A study of the density of pigment granules in hair from four races of men. Amer. J. phys. Anthropol. 21, 489—496 (1963).
WITZEL, M., u. O. BRAUN-FALCO: Über den Haarwurzelstatus am menschlichen Capillitium unter physiologischen Bedingungen. Arch. klin. exp. Derm. 216, 221—230 (1963). — WOLBACH, S. B.: The hair cycle of the mouse and its importance in the study of sequences of experimental carcinogenesis. Ann. N.Y. Acad. Sci. 53, 517—536 (1951). — WOLFF, K.: Histologische Beobachtungen an der normalen menschlichen Haut bei der Durchführung fermenthistochemischer Untersuchungen mit Adenosintriphosphat als Substrat. Arch. klin. exp. Derm. 216, 1—17 (1963a). — Zur Orthotopie der histochemisch erfaßbaren Aminopeptidaseaktivität der menschlichen Haut. Arch. klin. exp. Derm. 217, 534—552 (1963b). — WYNKOOP, E. M.: A study of the age correlation of the cuticular scales, medullas, an shaft diameters of human head hair. Amer. J. phys. Anthropol. 13, 177—188 (1929).
YASUDA, K., and W. MONTAGNA: Histology and cytochemistry of human skin. XX. The distribution of monoamine oxidase. J. Histochem. Cytochem. 8, 356—366 (1960).
ZAUN, H.: Pathophysiologische Grundlagen des nicht-narbigen Haarausfalls. Med. Welt 17 (N.F.) 1401—1403 (1966). — ZELICKSON, A. S.: Histochemical localization of mitochondria in human skin. J. invest. Derm. 35, 265—268 (1960). — *Electron microscopy of skin and mucous membrane. Springfield (Ill.): Ch. C. Thomas 1963. — ZIMMERMANN, K. W.: Über einige Formverhältnisse der Haarfollikel des Menschen. Z. mikr.-anat. Forsch. 38, 503—553 (1935).

Histology, Histochemistry, and Electron Microscopy of Sebaceous Glands in Man

By

John S. Strauss and **Peter E. Pochi**, Boston/Mass.

With 22 Figures

A. Distribution, Regional Variation and Gross Anatomy

The sebaceous glands of man are distributed in the skin throughout all areas of the body except the palm, soles and the dorsum of the feet. Sebaceous glands are also found in the ear canal where they should not be confused with the ceruminal glands which are of apocrine origin. The sebaceous glands are associated with hair follicles, although in mucous membranes, as will be subsequently mentioned, they open directly to the surface. Wherever they are found, a great variation is observed in the number of the sebaceous glands per unit area of the skin surface. Detailed studies on the density of gland distribution are at best incomplete. A series of papers from Okajima's laboratory have described the distribution and size of the various appendages, including the sebaceous glands, of human skin. Unfortunately, while meticulous calculations have been made, it is difficult to interpret the data since each report considers the appendages of single individuals, and there is a wide variation evident with respect to age and race. Included in the reports are results of the examination of an 8-month Japanese fetus (KOSAKA, 1932), a Japanese newborn infant (TANIGUCHI, 1931), a 2 year-old Korean child (TANIGUCHI, KOSAKA and NAKANO, 1933), a 6 year-old Japanese child (KOIBUCHI, 1932), and a 45 year-old German man (YAMADA, 1932). The volume of the sebaceous glands was greatest in the only adult subject studied in this series (YAMADA, 1932). As will be indicated later in this chapter, the sebaceous glands would be expected to be larger in adults than in children. Thus, it is erroneous to consider that the above findings indicate that large glands are a racial characteristic as has been interpreted by KALLAPRAVIT (1963). The average values for sebaceous gland volume in the areas studied in the adult man (YAMADA, 1932) are shown in Table 1. The gland volumes, in descending order of size, were found on the forehead, scalp, back, forearm, upper arm, stomach, thigh and calf. The table also shows that individual gland volume decreases in a similar fashion.

BENFENATI and BRILLANTI (1939) have also studied the distribution of human sebaceous glands. They counted the number of glands and hairs in biopsies from as many as 26 separate areas in 4 males and 3 females, ranging in age from 11 to 73 years. Based upon the number of glands found, the areas of the body could be grouped into two broad categories, viz. 1) face and scalp, and 2) other areas. The face, including the chin, cheeks and forehead, together with the scalp, had the

Table 1. *Sebaceous gland volume in a middle-aged adult man* (adapted from YAMADA, 1932)

Site	Total gland volume (mm^3/cm^2 of skin)	Individual gland volume (mm^3)
Forehead	9.29	.065
Scalp	9.25	.070
Back	0.46	.019
Forearm	0.40	.017
Upper arm	0.17	.007
Stomach	0.16	.006
Thigh	0.09	.004
Calf	0.04	.002

greatest number of sebaceous glands — 367 to 876 sebaceous glands per square centimeter of skin surface. In their specimens, the highest gland density was found on the chin with an average of 821 glands per square centimeter, whereas the cheeks and forehead showed a mean value of 537 glands per square centimeter. It should be pointed out that no biopsies were taken from the nose, an area where one might also expect to find a high gland density. The scalp, cheek and forehead contained approximately the same number of glands. In agreement with the earlier Japanese study, these authors found that in all other areas of the body there were fewer than 100 glands per square centimeter, although the scrotum, another area with large glands, was not examined. In fact, with few exceptions there were fewer than 50 glands per square centimeter. On the trunk the greatest number of glands were found, in general, in the median dorsal, gluteal, scapular and sternal regions. BENFENATI and BRILLANTI (1939) also reported that more glands were seen in the mid-line of the trunk than in the lateral regions. A striking example of this difference is illustrated in Fig. 1. The data of BENFENATI and BRILLANTI (1939), as with the earlier quoted studies from Okajima's laboratory, suffer from certain deficiencies such as the fact that the age span of their subjects was very great. In addition, in the regions examined less than 50% of the hairs had associated sebaceous glands. Although MONTAGNA and VAN SCOTT (1958) have reported the occurrence of hairs without sebaceous glands, this is not a common finding. Careful examination of serial sections will almost invariably show sebaceous glands to be associated with hair follicles.

BENFENATI and BRILLANTI (1939) reported a wide variation in the number of glands in any given area from subject to subject. A similar variation was noted by JOHNSEN and KIRK (1952) who restricted their observations to the distribution of the sebaceous glands on the dorsum of the hands. In their study of five males, age 64—76 years, they found zero to 50 glands per square centimeter. Since the sebaceous glands are holocrine glands, measurements of their functional capacity (sebum production) can be correlated with gland size (MIESCHER and SCHÖNBERG, 1944; KLIGMAN and SHELLEY, 1958; STRAUSS and POCHI, 1961). It is noteworthy that POCHI and STRAUSS (1964, 1965) have also shown a wide variation in sebum production from individual to individual.

The size of the sebaceous glands tends to be correlated with the distribution of the glands; i.e., the largest glands are generally found in areas where the glands are most numerous. This is well illustrated in the data of YAMADA (1932) as summarized in Table 1. This correlation has also been shown by BENFENATI and BRILLANTI (1939) and by JOHNSEN and KIRK (1952). The latter authors made very careful measurements of gland volume. On the forehead, gland volume averaged 0.07 mm^3 while for the dorsum of the hand the average volume was 0.00044 mm^3.

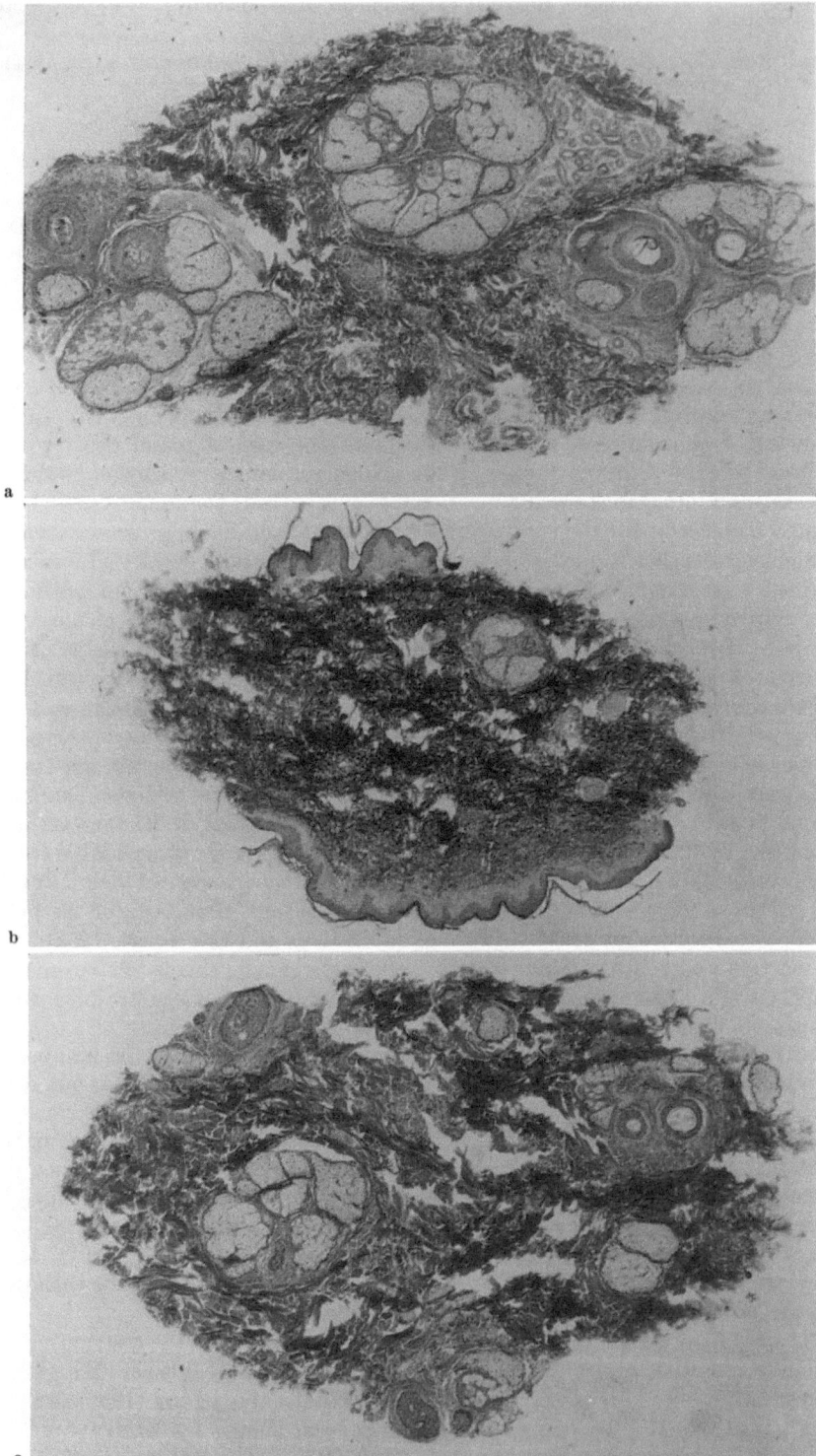

Fig. 1a—c. Cross sections of skin of the trunk region to illustrate regional variation in size and number of sebaceous glands. a: mid-line of chest. b: midaxillary line. c: mid-line of back. These cross sections clearly illustrate the abundance of sebaceous glands in the mid-line of the chest and back and the relative paucity of glands in the midaxillary line. All hematoxylin and eosin. (All × 32)

Another factor that must be taken into consideration in evaluating gland size is the age of the patient. The sebaceous glands are under endocrine control, and as a result, cannot be expected to be uniform in size throughout an individual's life. Furthermore, there are differences in sebaceous gland size between the sexes. In recent years considerable data have been gathered on the hormonal control of the sebaceous glands and have primarily concerned the large glands of the face. Whether the same relationship applies to the glands of the rest of the skin is not known. It should be noted that most of this new information on gland size has been gathered from studies of sebum production. Since sebaceous secretion is a holocrine process in which the individual cells comprise the secretory product, sebum production, as already indicated, can be correlated with gland size.

The sebaceous glands are well developed during fetal life and at the time of birth (SERRI and HUBER, 1963). The stimulus for this development has not been clearly established. However, it is most likely due to the effect of maternal hormones but also may be, in part, the result of endogenous production of steroids by the fetus. At some indeterminate time after birth the sebaceous glands undergo considerable atrophy. During the first few years of life, the glands are represented for the most part by tiny lateral outpocketings of undifferentiated cells from the follicular wall (STRAUSS, KLIGMAN and POCHI, 1962; STRAUSS and POCHI, 1963a, 1963b) (Fig. 2a). Areas of sebaceous differentiation may be present, but these tend to be small and infrequent and certainly do not approach the size seen in the adult (Fig. 2b).

Many investigators have shown that the human sebaceous glands are highly androgen-sensitive (HAMILTON, 1941; RONY and ZAKON, 1943; STRAUSS, KLIGMAN and POCHI, 1962; STRAUSS and POCHI, 1963a, 1963b). Furthermore, to date, androgens are the only hormones clearly shown to have a direct tropic effect on the sebaceous glands of man (STRAUSS, KLIGMAN and POCHI, 1962; STRAUSS and POCHI, 1963a, 1963b). Therefore, as a result of increased androgen output at puberty, the sebaceous glands undergo great enlargement, and the tiny outpocketings of undifferentiated epithelial cells develop into large multiacinar glands. Endocrinologists have shown that in addition to the testis, the ovary and the adrenal gland are sources of androgen production, and POCHI, STRAUSS and MESCON (1963) have reported that the principal adrenal androgen, dehydroepiandrosterone, can stimulate the sebaceous gland in man.

However, it is necessary to consider factors other than merely the difference between the prepuberal and post-puberal subject, since there are differences in gland size between males and females, and in the two sexes with advancing age. These factors have been studied by several investigators (KIRK, 1948; KVORNING, 1949; BRUN, ENDERLIN and DE WECK, 1955; GRASSET and BRUN, 1959; SMITH, 1959; POCHI and STRAUSS, 1963). KIRK (1948) was the first to report that sebaceous gland activity decreases in elderly women. Values for sebum production at various ages are given in Table 2. It can be seen that sebum production, and, by

Table 2. *Sebum production in normal males and females* (adapted from POCHI and STRAUSS, 1965)

Age	Males		Females	
	No.	Sebum production (mg. lipid/10 cm^2/3 hrs.)	No.	Sebum production (mg. lipid/10 cm^2/3 hrs.)
20—29	61	2.45	56	1.88
30—39	50	2.49	26	1.84
40—49	29	2.21	30	1.83
50—69	22	2.39	17	0.96
70—90	13	1.69	11	0.89

inference gland size, decreases in the female after the age of 50, a change postulated to be the result of a decrease in ovarian androgen production. That it is not due to a decrease in progesterone is evidenced by studies in which it has been shown that physiologic amounts of progesterone do not influence the functional status of the sebaceous glands (STRAUSS and KLIGMAN, 1961). It should be noted, however, that SMITH (1959) and ZELIGMAN and HUBENER (1957) have presented

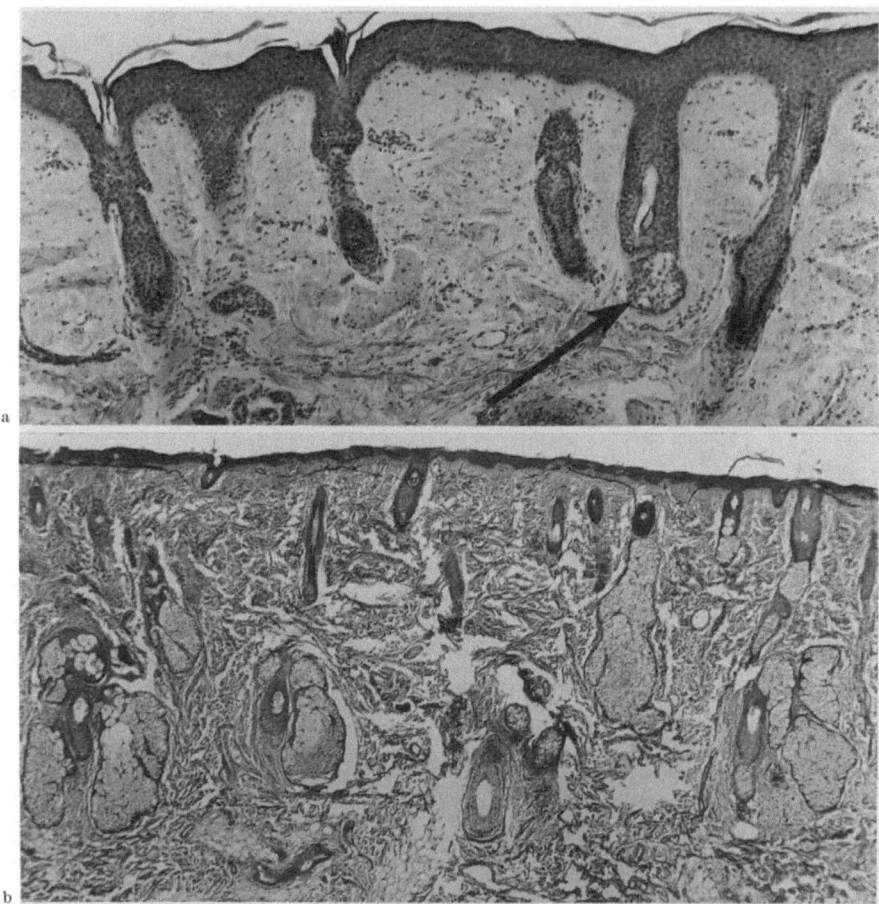

Fig. 2a and b. Comparison of sebaceous glands of the cheek in the child and the adult. a: Biopsy from a prepuberal child. The sebaceous gland anlagen are represented by small, lateral outpocketings of undifferentiated epithelial cells. The arrow indicates a small group of cells which have undergone some sebaceous differentiation. b: Biopsy from a young adult. Multiacinar glands of varying size and degree of complexity are present. Both hematoxylin and eosin. (a: × 72; b: × 28)

data which would indicate that progesterone increases the size of human sebaceous glands. Their data are not based on controlled quantitative studies. POCHI and STRAUSS (1963) have also noted a slight decrease in sebum production in the elderly male. BRUN, ENDERLIN and DE WECK (1955) and GRASSET and BRUN (1959) also observed a decrease in sebaceous gland activity, whereas KIRK (1948) did not. The maintenance of the sebaceous glands at a high level of activity until old age is clearly dependent on testicular androgen since castration of elderly males results in a prompt decrease in the activity of the sebaceous glands (POCHI and STRAUSS, 1963).

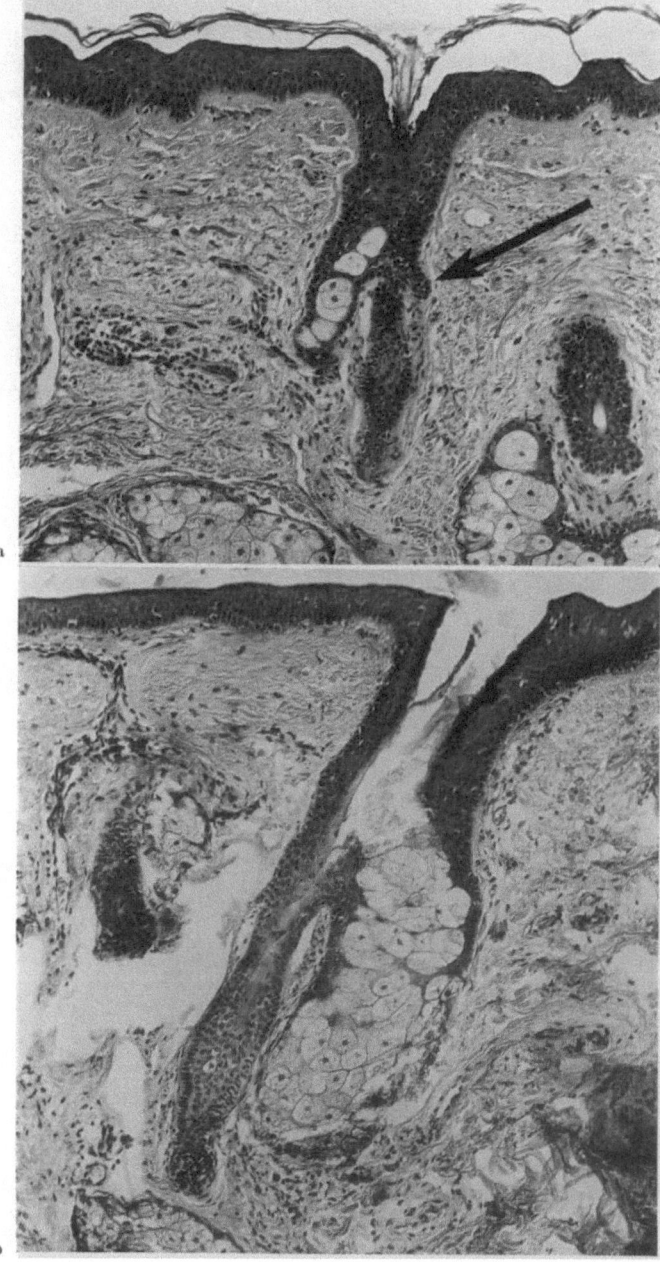

Fig. 3a and b. Two vellus follicles from the adult cheek. a: Small follicle with a partially differentiated sebaceous acinus on the left and a small sebaceous anlage of undifferentiated epithelial cells on the right (indicated by arrow). b: Medium-sized vellus follicle. Both hematoxylin and eosin. (Both × 109)

Evidence that the adrenal gland is a source for the maintenance of sebaceous gland activity in the absence of the gonads is available from studies of castrated males. Orchiectomy in elderly men causes a rapid decrease in sebum production (POCHI and STRAUSS, 1963). However, in these individuals as well as in those castrated at an earlier age, sebum production does not fall to prepuberal levels

(POCHI, STRAUSS and MESCON, 1962). Furthermore, sebum production in adults castrated prior to puberty is higher than that of the prepuberal subject (POCHI, STRAUSS and MESCON, 1962).

Estrogens have been shown to decrease sebaceous gland size and sebum production in man (JARRETT, 1955; STRAUSS, KLIGMAN and POCHI, 1962; STRAUSS

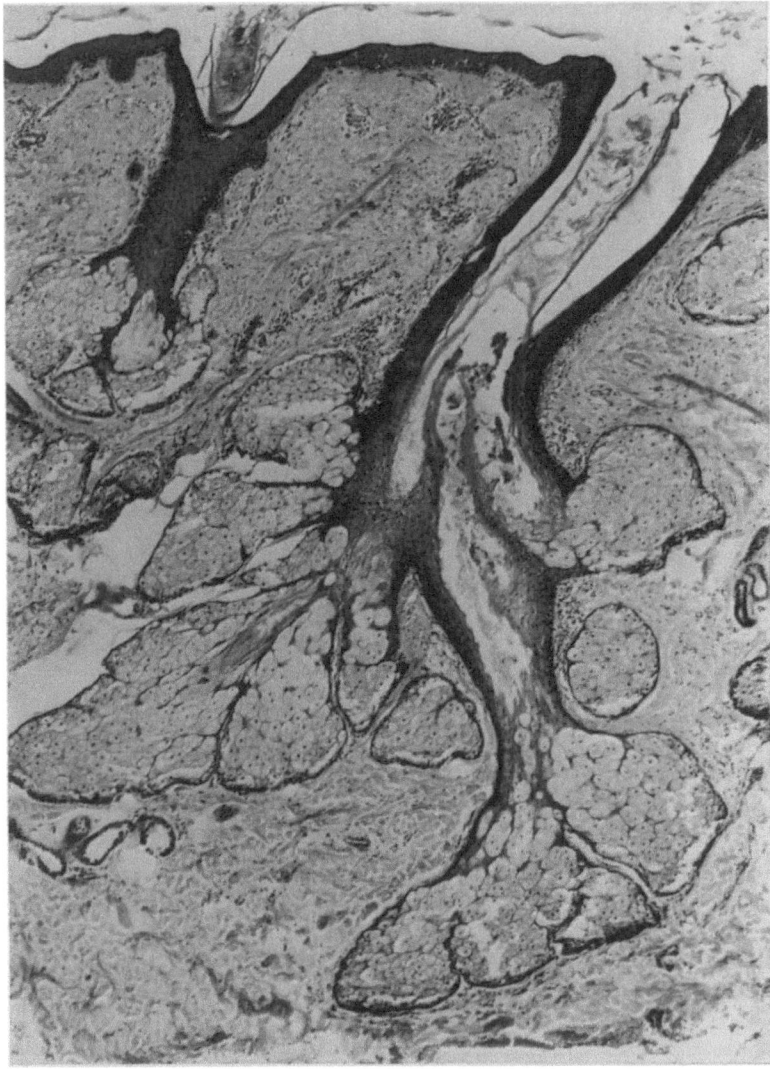

Fig. 4a and b. Large sebaceous follicles of the cheek. Both sections show a large, dilated follicular canal lined by a stratified squamous epithelium. The canal contains keratinous debris, sebum and microorganisms (primarily *Corynebacterium acnes* and *Pityrosporon ovale*). The sebaceous glands vary in size and shape. The hair is present in b (see arrow) but is not evident in the section shown in a. Both hematoxylin and eosin. (a: × 55; b: × 68)

and POCHI, 1963a, 1963b). In the male, at least, the effect appears to be primarily a central one involving pituitary-gonadal suppression (FORCHIELLI, RAO, SARDA, GIBREE, POCHI, STRAUSS and DORFMAN, 1965) rather than inhibition of androgens at the peripheral sebaceous gland level.

The individual's racial origin is another factor which may influence sebaceous gland size, but studies on racial differences are far from conclusive. KALLAPRAVIT

(1963) found greater glandular development in Caucasians and American Negroes than in Siamese Orientals. However, he studied only 4 to 5 subjects in each group, and the age span was very great — stillborn to 73 years. Actually, in his series there were only two young adult subjects. Therefore, it is difficult to attach significance to his results.

Sebaceous gland size is related not only to the density of glands per unit volume but also to the structural configuration of the glands. Thus, the large

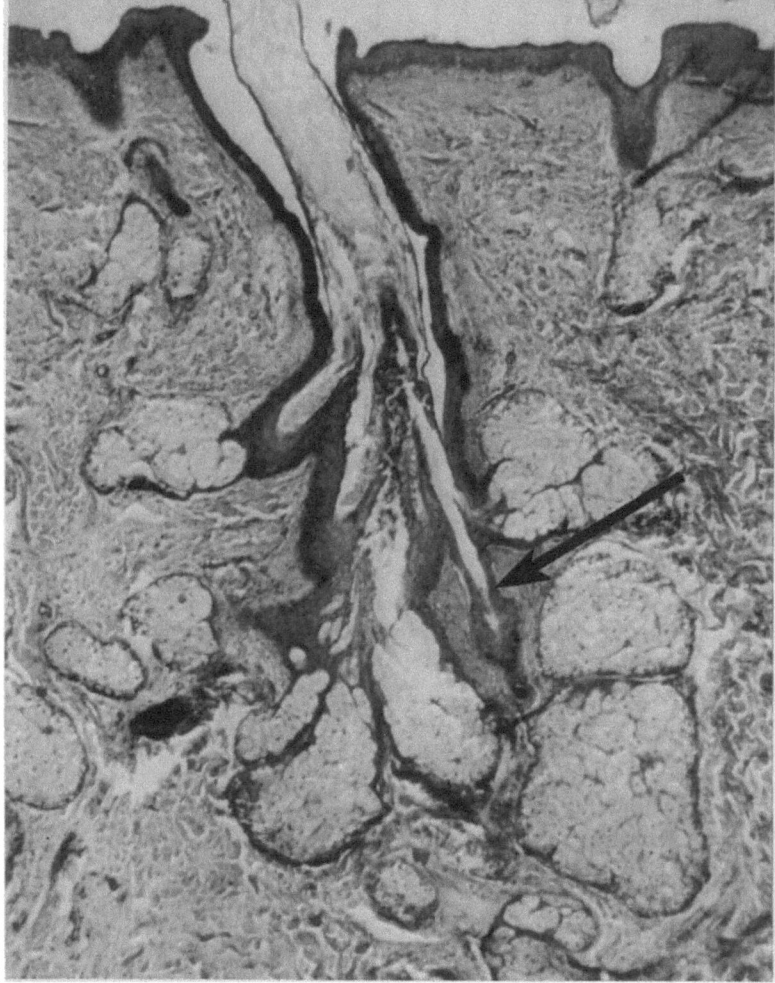

Fig. 4b

glands on the face and scalp and in the mid-line of the trunk are multilobular, but the smaller glands in other areas are usually unilobular (BENFENATI and BRILLANTI, 1939; STRAUSS and POCHI, 1966). It is not surprising, therefore, that the glands of the back of the hands are unilobular (JOHNSEN and KIRK, 1952). CLARA (1929) attributed this difference to the type of connective tissue surrounding the sebaceous glands but did not present any evidence to support this viewpoint.

In addition to the variation in number, size and structural complexity of the sebaceous glands that occurs from area to area, considerable variation occurs from gland unit to gland unit within the same area. This is most evident in sites such as the face where there is a high gland density. Furthermore, both vellus and terminal hairs can be associated with large sebaceous glands, and there is no direct relationship between gland size and hair size. One has only to view the three-dimensional balsa-wood models of hair follicles constructed by VAN SCOTT and co-workers (VAN SCOTT and MACCARDLE, 1956; MONTAGNA and VAN SCOTT, 1958) to appreciate the complexities of these interrelationships. A good example of the heterogeneity of sebaceous glandular organization is afforded by examination of the skin of the face. Many small vellus follicles with varying degrees of sebaceous gland development are present (Fig. 3). In addition, there are very large multi-acinar sebaceous glands attached to very large follicles (Fig. 4). These are the sebaceous follicles, a term originally used by HORNER in 1846. These follicles are still pilosebaceous follicles, for even if a hair is not readily evident on histologic examination, serial sections will always disclose the presence of a small vellus hair. The hair, however, is a minor appendage, and the widely dilated follicular canal connects directly with the ducts of the many acini of each unit structure. The follicular canal is filled with keratinous material, sebum, bacteria (*Corynebacterium acnes*) and fungi (*Pityrosporon ovale*). The enormous variation in sebaceous gland size in an area such as the cheek renders quantitative study of gland size a difficult task. On the extremities and most of the trunk the sebaceous glands are small, uniform in size and unilobular. Quantitation of these structures is considerably easier.

B. Histology

The cellular morphology of the sebaceous glands is uniform regardless of their shape or size. The individual acini are connected to the follicle by the sebaceous duct. This duct is a transitional zone between the lipid-producing cells of the sebaceous acinus and the stratified squamous epithelium of the follicular canal. The duct itself has a stratified squamous epithelium where it joins the follicular canal. A granular layer is present which disappears below. There is a rather abrupt transformation to lipid-forming cells as the duct wall becomes thinner and continuous with the single layer of peripheral undifferentiated cells of the sebaceous acinus (Fig. 5). The duct produces a stratum corneum although this is not readily apparent when the duct is narrow. However, in the large sebaceous follicles which have wide duct lumina, the desquamating material is readily evident. This is not a pathologic finding in the sebaceous duct, although thought to be so by VAN SCOTT and MACCARDLE (1956).

The cells in the outermost layer of the acinus are undifferentiated basal cells which rest on a basement membrane. This layer of cells is usually one cell in thickness but, as will be pointed out later, can be thicker under certain conditions. They are the germinative cells of the sebaceous gland and usually show no lipid differentiation. A few mitoses may be seen in this layer. The basal cells are small, flattened or cuboidal and are deeply basophilic. The nuclei are often flattened. Progressive lipid differentiation occurs in the acini in a centripetal direction. As lipids accumulate in the sebaceous cells, the cytoplasm appears foamy, and there is recognizable cellular enlargement (Figs. 6, 7). In routine histologic preparations, the fat is washed out so that the cells appear vacuolated, the walls of the vacuoles being formed by the cytoplasmic remnants which are progressively compressed into thin strands. The largest cells, located centrally, finally disrupt, and the lipid of the cells, together with cellular remnants, form the secretory product, sebum. Secretion of these glands is, therefore, holocrine. In the development of the

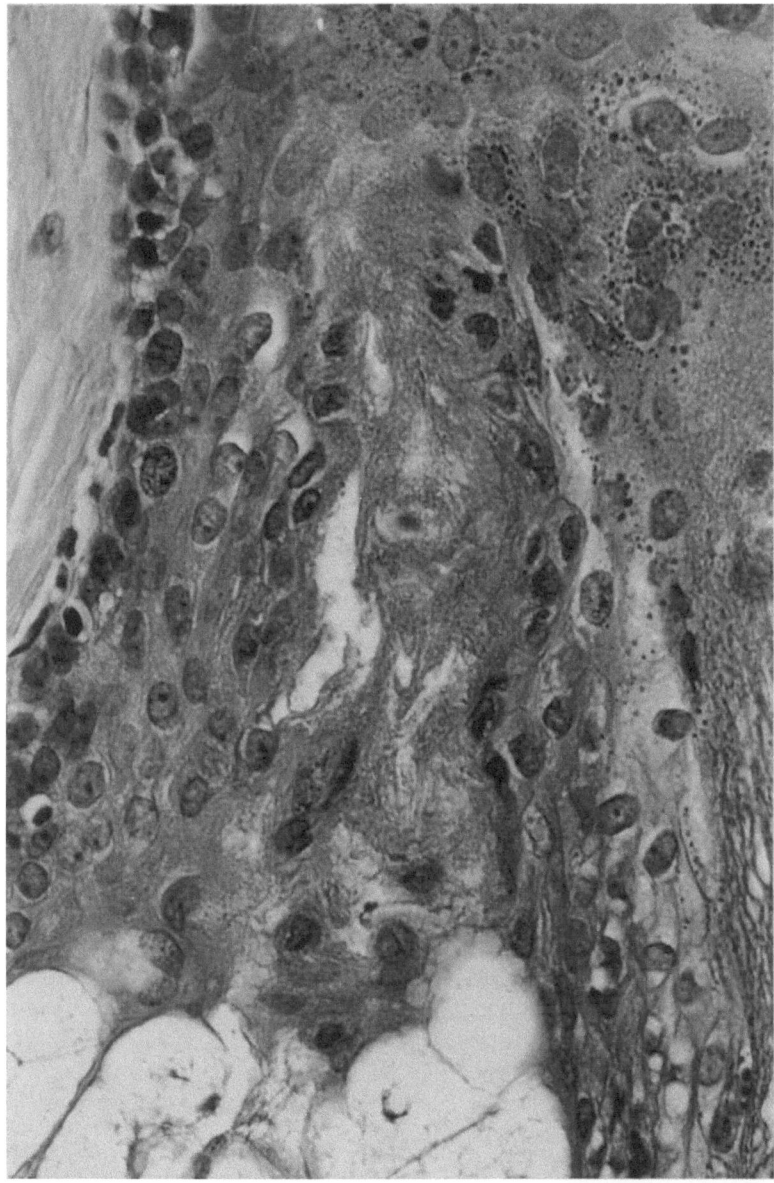

Fig. 5. High-power magnification of the sebaceous duct. A few sebaceous cells appear at the lower border. The dermis is shown in the upper left, adjacent to the wall of the duct. The follicular canal would be to the right of the photograph. A well-developed granular layer is evident at the upper right portion of the photograph. Hematoxylin and eosin. (× 740)

sebaceous acini, as will be discussed later, small fibrous trabeculae may become enclosed within the individual gland acini.

As mentioned above, the undifferentiated cells are strongly basophilic. This basophilia disappears when the sections are treated with ribonuclease (MONTAGNA, NOBACK and ZAK, 1948; MONTAGNA, 1962). Presumably, then, the basophilia is due to the presence of ribonucleoproteins. As the sebaceous cells differentiate, the basophilia disappears, and the spongy cytoplasm of lipid-laden cells becomes acidophilic.

Changes in the nuclei are seen as the cells undergo lipid differentiation. The nuclei of the basal layer are oval and resemble those of the basal layer of the epidermis. The nuclei do not enlarge as the cell becomes engorged with lipid. In

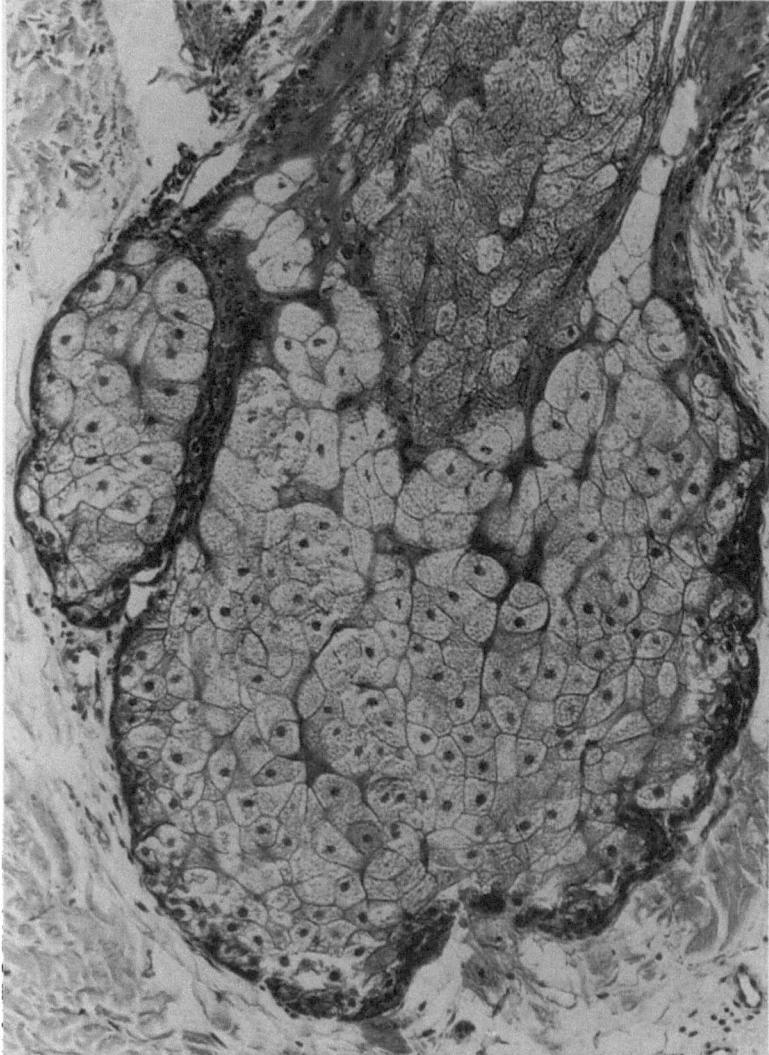

Fig. 6. Acinus of a sebaceous follicle. The basal cells appear as small, dark-staining peripheral cells. As lipid differentiation occurs, the cytoplasm becomes foamy. Cellular enlargement is also evident as the lipid accumulates. Ruptured cellular remnants appear in the secretory stream at the top of the photograph. Dark-staining areas in the center of the acinus are fibrous tissue trabeculae (see Fig. 7). Hematoxylin and eosin. ($\times$ 180)

fact, they become distorted as the lipid droplets encroach upon them and often are not visualized in the fully differentiated cells.

STEIGLEDER and MCCARTHY (1964) have studied the density of the cells of the skin utilizing microradiography. The amount of radiation absorbed is a measure of tissue density; i.e., the higher the tissue density the greater the absorption of soft x-rays used for this procedure. These workers have shown that the cytoplasm of the sebaceous cells absorbs relatively little of the incident beam, whereas the nucleus absorbs a considerable portion of the test radiation. This is the reverse of epidermal cells where the cytoplasm is denser than the nucleus.

Melanocytes have not been demonstrated in human sebaceous glands. However, BREATHNACH, BIRBECK and EVERALL (1963) have observed the presence of Langerhans cells in the sebaceous ducts and in the acinar tissue near the duct. Mitochondria (MONTAGNA, 1955a) and Golgi zones containing lipids (BOWEN, 1926, 1929; LUDFORD, 1925; MELCZER and DEME, 1942, 1943; MONTAGNA, NOBACK and ZAK, 1948) have been identified under the light microscope. However, these structures are so much more clearly resolved by the electron microscope that a discussion of these cellular organelles will be given in the section on ultrastructure.

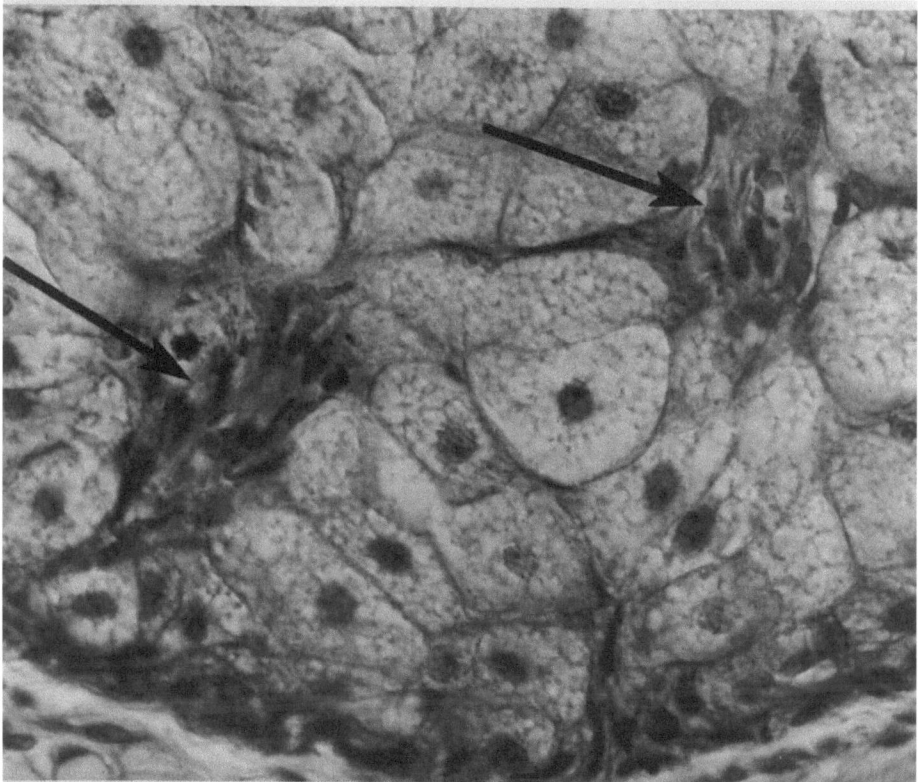

Fig. 7. High magnification of a portion of a sebaceous acinus. The dark-staining layer is the basal layer. Two fibrous tissue trabeculae with elongated fibroblasts are indicated by the arrows. A small blood vessel is present in the center of the group of cells on the right. Hematoxylin and eosin. ($\times$ 685)

C. Histochemistry

A considerable number of investigations have been done on the histochemistry of human and animal sebaceous glands. However, since the histochemical reactions often differ from species to species, the discussion herein will be restricted to studies of the sebaceous glands of man. For purposes of discussion, we shall describe separately the identification within human sebaceous glands of lipids, other specific substances, such as glycogen, and tissue enzymes. A summary of the histochemical reactions of the human sebaceous gland, as detailed below, is given in Table 3. The localization of these reactions, where specified, is summarized in Table 4.

Table 3. *Positive histochemical reactions demonstrated in sebaceous glands of man*

lipids	hydroxysteroid dehydrogenases
phospholipids	cytochrome oxidase
cholesterol esters	leucine aminopeptidase
glycogen	monoamine oxidase
sulfhydryl	succinic dehydrogenase
iron	acid phosphatase
phosphorylase	nonspecific esterases
amylo-1,6-glucosidase	lipases
β-glucuronidase	acetylcholinesterase

Table 4. *Localization of histochemical reactions in sebaceous glands of man*

1. Positive reactions in peripheral as well as differentiated sebaceous cells

lipids	β-glucuronidase
phospholipids	cytochrome oxidase

2. Positive reactions in peripheral cells with negative reaction in differentiated sebaceous cells

glycogen	succinic dehydrogenase
sulfhydryl	acid phosphatase
phosphorylase	nonspecific esterases
amylo-1,6-glucosidase	lipases
leucine aminopeptidase	acetylcholinesterase
monoamine oxidase	

3. Positive reactions in sebum

lipids	nonspecific esterases
phospholipids	lipases
cholesterol esters	

4. Positive reactions in sebaceous duct cells

glycogen	cytochrome oxidase
sulfhydryl	leucine aminopeptidase
phosphorylase	monoamine oxidase
amylo-1,6-glucosidase	succinic dehydrogenase
β-glucuronidase	acid phosphatase

1. Lipids

Sebum, which contains a high percentage of esterified fatty acids, is unique in its high content of squalene (NICOLAIDES, 1965; NICOLAIDES and RAY, 1965). Furthermore, odd-chain length fatty acids, as first isolated by WEITKAMP (1945) and WEITKAMP, SMILJANIC and ROTHMAN (1947), are found in greater concentration than in other body lipids. Unfortunately, in spite of these striking differences in the composition of sebum, histochemical studies of lipids have provided little help in delineating the mode of lipid synthesis. MELCZER and DEME (1942) proposed that there is a layering of the lipids in the sebaceous glands of man. They stated that the outermost cells in the acini contain mainly unsaturated fatty acids, the middle layer mainly long-chain alcohols and the inner layer of cells mainly neutral fats. However, the specificity of their stains is open to question, and subsequent investigations have been unable to confirm their findings (MONTAGNA, NOBACK and ZAK, 1948; SUSKIND, 1951).

The staining of lipid in the sebaceous glands has been investigated by MONTAGNA, NOBACK and ZAK (1948), SUSKIND (1951) and NASR (1965). The first mentioned authors studied the glands in the external auditory canal, while the latter investigators studied the glands in the scalp and the glabrous skin. Before presentation of their results, it should be pointed out that the uptake of lipid stains such as the various Sudans is based upon a preferential lipid solubility of the tissue to be stained. These stains are applied to the tissue sections, and excess dye is eluted with solvents such as alcohol. Because the stains are based solely on preferential solubility rather than irreversible tissue precipitation or fixation,

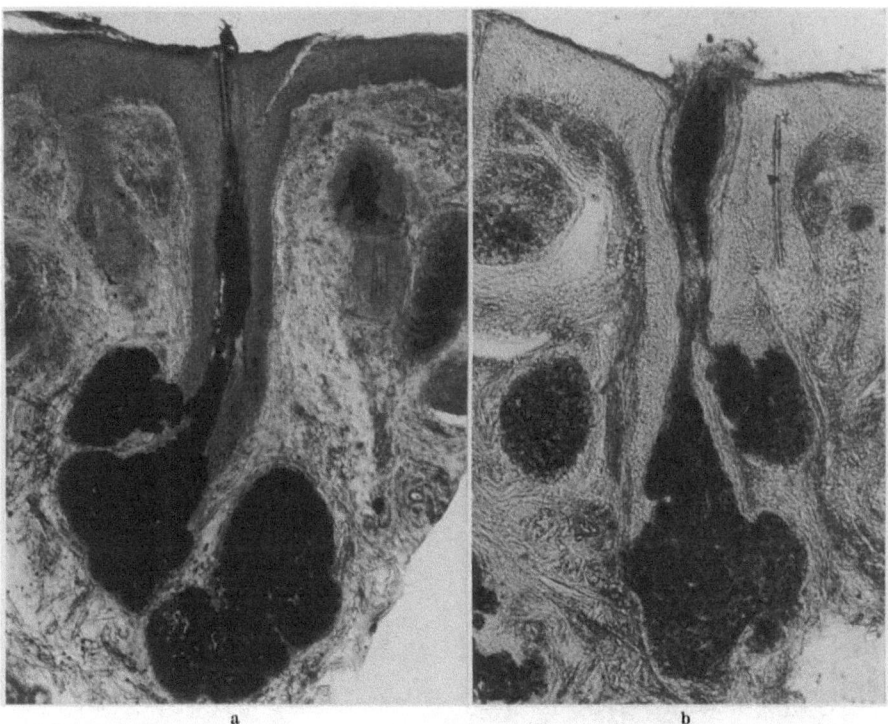

Fig. 8a and b. Medium-sized follicles of the face. a: Sudan Black B. b: Sudan IV (scarlet red). Greater cellular detail is present with this stain. (Both × 66)

exact localization of the dyes is difficult to define (Figs. 8, 9, 10). The peripheral cells usually contain little or no lipid. If lipid is present in these cells, the tiny lipid droplets may be scattered throughout the cytoplasm or clumped around the nucleus. The number of sudanophilic droplets increases progressively as the cells approach the center of the acinus. The size of the individual droplets also increases so that the central cells are several times their former size. By the time the cells are fully developed, they are completely filled with large fat globules. After the cells rupture, clumped sudanophilic material is found in the sebaceous duct and follicular canal. It has been alleged that, if the droplets within a given cell are uniform in size, the cells are healthy, and that, if the droplets are of different size, the cells are no longer normal (MONTAGNA, 1962, 1963).

Various other techniques have been used in an attempt to identify specific lipids. Nile blue sulfate has been used purporting to demonstrate the presence of free fatty acids in sebum. This stain was originally reported to be specific in that it would stain unsaturated triglycerides pink and fatty acids blue (SMITH, 1908, 1911). The use and significance of this dye have been critically reviewed by

CAIN (1947, 1948) who indicated that it is not altogether specific. A small amount of a pink dye, formed by oxidation, stains fatty substances indiscriminately as do the various Sudan stains. Also, the blue color is not specific for fatty acids; phospholipids are also stained blue by Nile blue sulfate. Therefore, the color changes

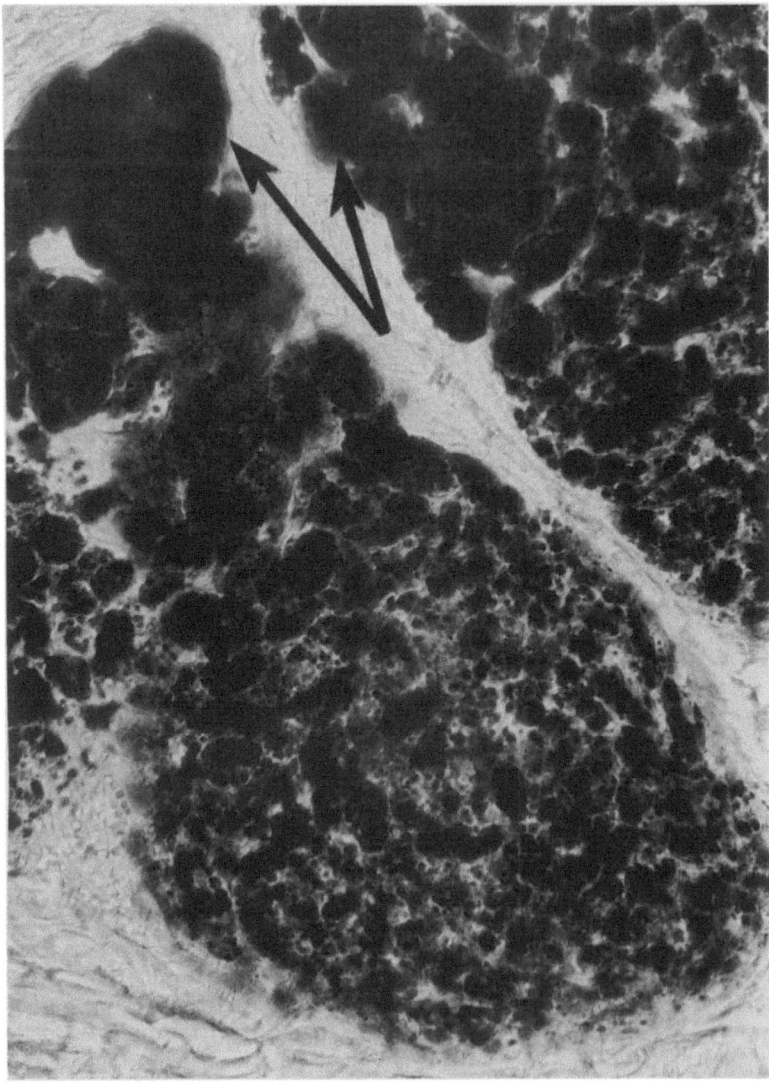

Fig. 9. High magnification of two sebaceous acini stained with Sudan IV. The region of the sebaceous ducts is indicated by the arrows. There is very little lipid in the peripheral cells. The lipid droplets enlarge as the cells approach the center of the gland. ($\times$ 295)

produced with this stain are difficult to interpret. The blue color in particular is now considered nonspecific. MONTAGNA, NOBACK and ZAK (1948) and SUSKIND (1951) have shown that most of the lipid in the maturing cells stains pink to red, probably indicating the presence of neutral lipids. After cell rupture the lipid stains pink to purple. Interpretation of these color changes presents formidable difficulties.

Another stain for fatty acids, which is probably more specific than Nile blue sulfate, is the Fischler stain, which has been studied by MONTAGNA, NOBACK and ZAK (1948). A small amount of particulate blue-black positive material is seen in the sebaceous cells, particularly at the edge of the lipid droplets. There is a

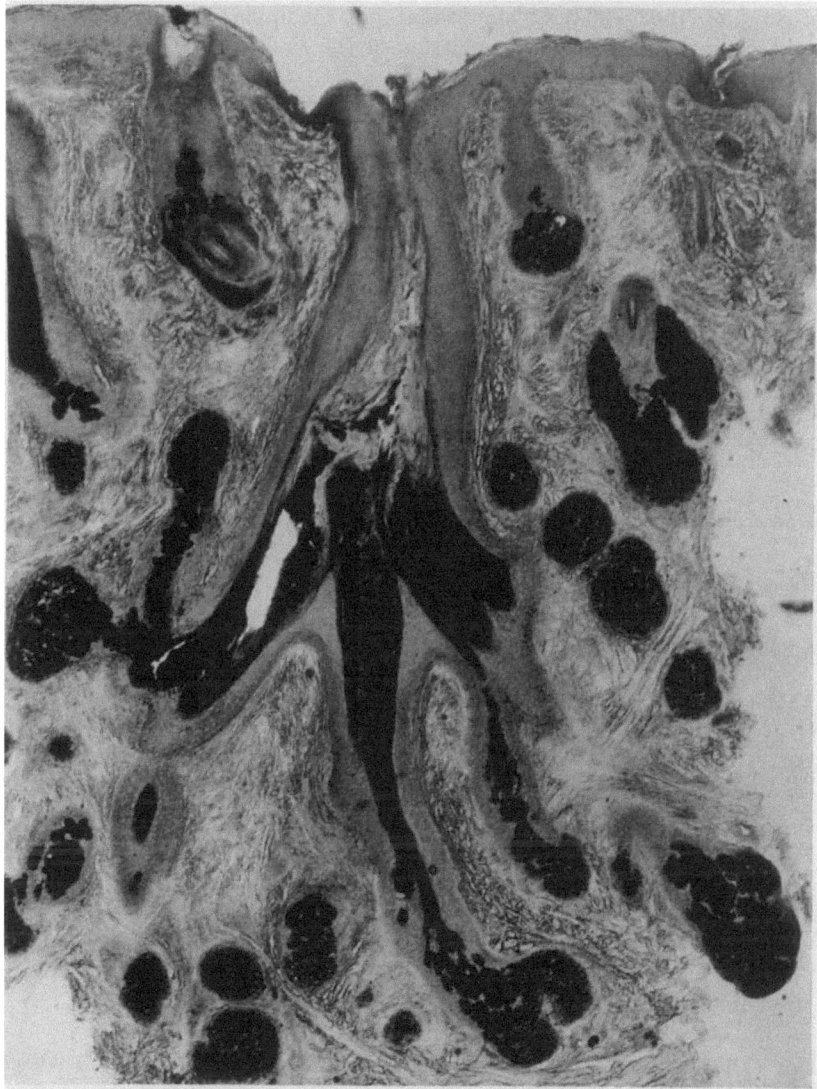

Fig. 10. Large sebaceous follicle of the cheek stained with Sudan Black B. There are many acini which are connected to the follicle by ducts of varying length. ($\times$ 51)

strong positive reaction in degenerating sebaceous cells and newly formed sebum, but old sebum does not stain. This finding that old sebum does not stain for fatty acids is not in agreement with the biochemical observations indicating that the content of free fatty acids is increased in older sebum (NICOLAIDES and WELLS, 1957). MONTAGNA, NOBACK and ZAK (1948) themselves question the validity of the stain and feel that their results are inconclusive.

Phospholipids have been demonstrated in sebaceous cells. They appear as small particles scattered throughout the cytoplasm and in the region believed to be the Golgi zone. Phospholipids apparently are structural components of the cell and not part of the lipid droplet. Some phospholipid is also found in sebum (MONTAGNA, 1962, 1963).

MONTAGNA (1962, 1963) has stated that only the lipids in the excretory ducts of the sebaceous glands stain on osmication of the tissue. We have stained frozen

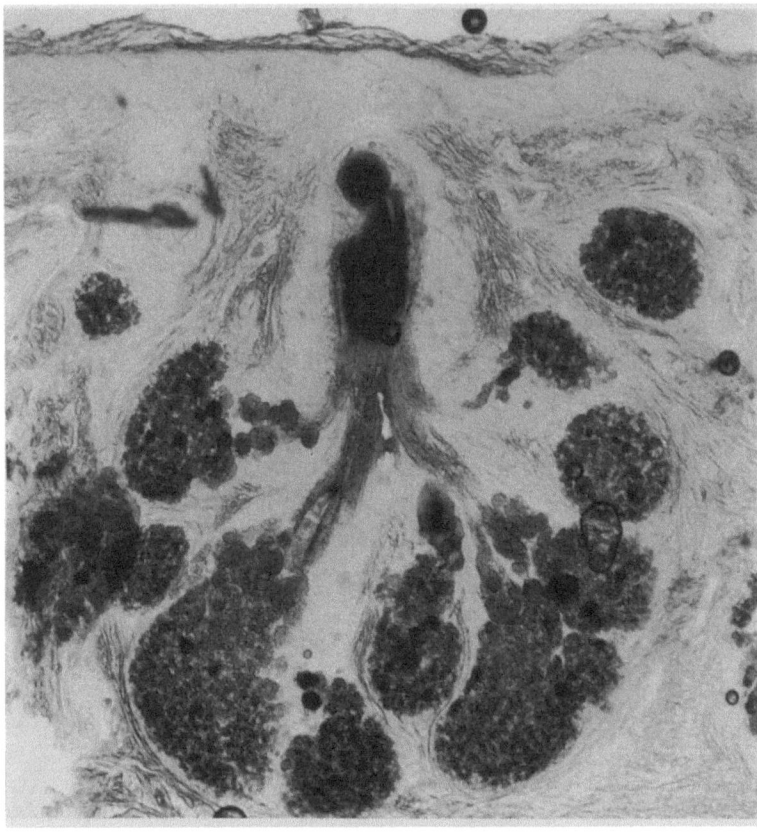

Fig. 11. Large sebaceous follicle of the cheek stained with osmium tetroxide. The most intense staining is in the follicular canal. However, a positive reaction, although less marked, also occurs throughout the sebaceous follicle. (× 86)

sections with osmium tetroxide. While it is true that a strong reaction is seen in the ducts, we have also seen stain uptake in the sebaceous acini although it is less intense (Fig. 11).

The Liebermann-Burchard reaction for cholesterol was positive in some of the specimens studied by both MONTAGNA, NOBACK and ZAK (1948) and SUSKIND (1951). This reaction was positive in the degenerating cells and in the sebum. The maturing cells and the peripheral cells did not show a positive reaction. Pretreatment of the specimens with digitonin eliminated the bluish-green color typical for this reaction. Since free cholesterol is digitonin-precipitable whereas cholesterol esters are soluble in digitonin, the authors have concluded that there is no free cholesterol in the degenerating cells or the excretory ducts.

A variable degree of birefringence has also been demonstrated in sebaceous glands (MONTAGNA, NOBACK and ZAK, 1948; SUSKIND, 1951). Both phospholipid and cholesterol have the property of anisotropy. Thus, since phospholipids are found in all sebaceous cells, the finding of birefringence cannot be interpreted as necessarily indicating the presence of cholesterol.

In summary, then, lipid stains have added very little to the knowledge of lipid synthesis other than the fact that the lipid accumulates as the cells progress in a centripetal direction. Current evidence also indicates that the phospholipid is a structural component of the cell and is not accumulated in the lipid droplets.

II. Other Specific Substances

Over the years, much attention has been focused on the presence of glycogen as a marker for metabolic activity of the epidermal cells (LOBITZ and HOLYOKE, 1954; LOBITZ, BROPHY, LARNER and DANIELS, 1962). Glycogen appears to be stored in such cells during periods of relative inactivity. The glycogen content decreases as the cells become metabolically active. It has been claimed that human sebaceous glands do not contain glycogen (SASAKAWA, 1921; LUDFORD, 1925). However, glycogen has been unequivocally demonstrated in human sebaceous glands (MONTAGNA, CHASE and HAMILTON, 1951; MONTAGNA, CHASE and LOBITZ, 1952). The cells of the ducts are very rich in glycogen, and many of the peripheral cells, too, contain it in abundance. As sebaceous differentiation occurs, the amount of glycogen decreases, and in the fully differentiated cells, glycogen cannot be detected. Thus, as lipid differentiation occurs, glycogen disappears.

Sulfhydryl stains are positive in the sebaceous glands (MONTAGNA, EISEN, RADEMACHER and CHASE, 1954). The duct cells and the undifferentiated peripheral cells show stippled cytoplasmic granules which also disappear as the cells show lipid differentiation.

Recently iron has been identified with the Perl stain in the sebaceous acinus in two biopsies by GROTS and TARGOVNIK (1966). Both biopsies were from women. One specimen was taken from the neck of a patient with pigmentation associated with lichen simplex chronicus. The other specimen was from the axilla in a patient with pseudoacanthosis nigricans. In an attempt to rule out the possibility of the iron being a contaminant, iron was added to the fixative solution of control biopsy specimens. This iron was not taken up by the sebaceous glands.

III. Enzymes

The sebaceous glands have been shown to contain a variety of enzymes. As was the case with glycogen, the characteristic pattern of many of the enzymes is one of abundant activity in the duct cells and the peripheral cells of the sebaceous glands with decreasing activity as the sebaceous cells mature and become filled with lipids (Table 4).

Since the sebaceous glands are rich in glycogen, they contain, as would be expected, phosphorylase and amylo-1,6-glucosidase activity (BRAUN-FALCO, 1956a; ELLIS and MONTAGNA, 1958; TAKEUCHI, 1958). Phosphorylase is necessary to form the 1, 4 linkages between glucose molecules forming straight-chain polymers. Amylo-1,6-glucosidase is necessary for the formation of the branched side chains of glycogen. Therefore, both enzymes are required for the reversible reaction between glucose-1-phosphate and glycogen. These enzymes are found in areas of glycogen utilization and storage. In fact, the presence of a positive stain for glycogen is considered evidence for the presence of these enzymes. Naturally, then, these enzymes are abundant in the duct cells and the peripheral cells. None are found in the mature cells of the sebaceous glands.

Another enzyme encountered in the sebaceous glands to which functional significance might be attached is β-glucuronidase. A great portion of the circulating testosterone is glucuronide-conjugated. The presence of the enzyme capable of disrupting the conjugated hormone could possibly play some role in the response of the androgen-sensitive sebaceous glands. Both BRAUN-FALCO (1956b) and MONTAGNA (1957) have found this enzyme in sebaceous glands. In fact, MONTAGNA (1957) has stated that of all the cutaneous appendages the sebaceous glands and the apocrine glands contain this enzyme in greatest abundance. The duct cells and the peripheral cells stain very strongly; however, activity is also present in the fully differentiated cells. The peripheral cells show a homogeneous reaction, whereas varying-sized reactive granules are seen in the differentiating and mature cells.

Recently, further evidence that the human sebaceous glands contain enzymes associated with steroid metabolism has been presented by BAILLIE, CALMAN and MILNE (1965). These authors have shown that there is hydroxysteroid dehydrogenase activity in the cytoplasm of sebaceous cells from the skin of the back. The cells demonstrated intense 3β- and 16β-hydroxysteroid dehydrogenase activity, moderate 3α-, 11β- and 17β-hydroxysteroid dehydrogenase activity, and trace 6β- und 20β-hydroxysteroid dehydrogenase activity.

Cytochrome oxidase is found throughout the cytoplasm of the sebaceous cells. MONTAGNA and YUN (1961) have stated that the sebaceous glands are "veritable wells of enzyme activity". All of the cells, even the fully mature lipid-laden cells, contain numerous enzyme-positive particles. The duct cells are also well endowed. Sebum, however, does not stain for this enzyme.

There is a good reaction for leucine aminopeptidase in the cells of the sebaceous ducts, a weak reaction in the peripheral cells, and none in the central cells (ADACHI and MONTAGNA, 1961). Since this enzyme is involved in protein and polypeptide cleavage, significance might be attached to the stronger reaction in the duct cells which are involved in protein metabolism. Its continued presence, albeit a weak reaction, in the peripheral cells may represent evidence for the pluripotential capability of these cells.

Monoamine oxidase is also found in the sebaceous glands (SHELLEY, COHEN and KOELLE, 1955; YASUDA and MONTAGNA, 1960). The reaction is most intense in the duct. In the peripheral cells many reactive coarse granules are found. The granules are less prominent in the more mature cells and are not found in the fully differentiated cells. This pattern of distribution, which is inversely proportional to the degree of lipid differentiation, is also found with respect to succinic dehydrogenase activity (MONTAGNA and FORMISANO, 1955). Acid phosphatase has also been identified (MORETTI and MESCON, 1956). Once again it is most prominent in the peripheral cells and is less evident in the differentiated cells.

Considerable attention has been directed to the esterases of the sebaceous glands (MONTAGNA, 1955b; FINDLAY, 1955; STEIGLEDER and LÖFFLER, 1956; NICOLAIDES and WELLS, 1957; MONTAGNA and ELLIS, 1958; STEIGLEDER, 1958). MONTAGNA (1955b) used alpha-naphthyl acetate as a substrate while FINDLAY (1955) used both the alpha-naphthyl acetate and butyrate as substrates. With these stains there was intense staining of the cells of the duct and the peripheral cells of the gland, but the mature cells were non-reactive, or, at most, slightly reactive.

NICOLAIDES and WELLS (1957) used alpha-naphthyl acetate, naphthol AS acetate, and 6-acetyl-5-bromo-indoxyl as substrates. It was their impression that there was inordinate false-positive staining with the alpha-naphthyl acetate and that the latter two esterases afforded more reliable results. With naphthol AS acetate and indoxyl acetate as substrates, there was no staining of the peripheral cells. However, MONTAGNA and ELLIS (1958) subsequently reported a strong reaction in the peripheral cells to both the indoxyl and naphthol AS esterase with only a slight reaction in differentiated cells. They also reported similar findings for Tween esterase using Tween 60 as a substrate.

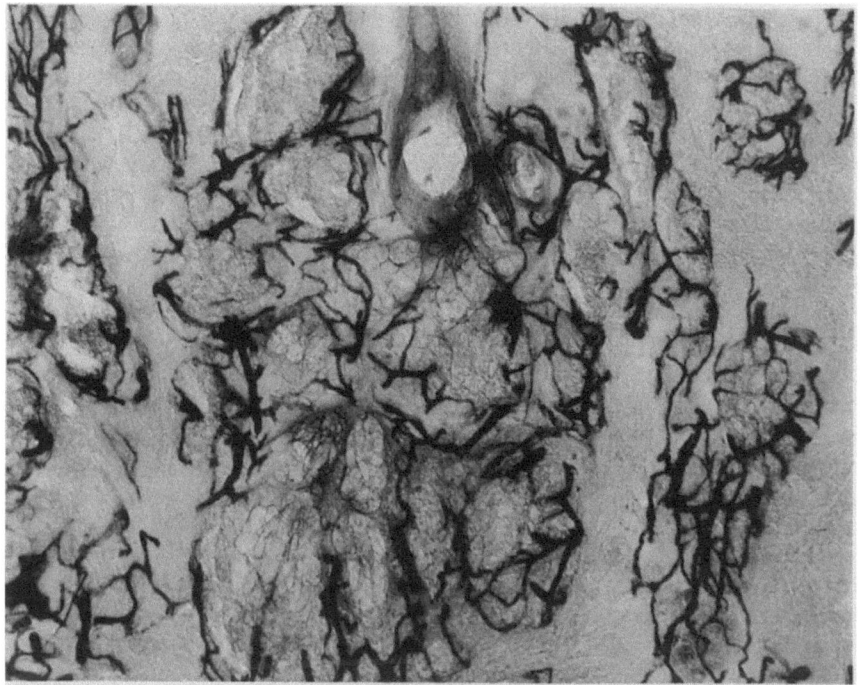

Fig. 12. Sebaceous glands of the face stained for alkaline phosphatase. There is no staining of the gland, but the extensive capillary network reacts positively. There are many vessels which penetrate into the trabeculae within the sebaceous glands. (× 142)

In addition to the studies on the sebaceous cells, attention has been focused on the esterase activity of the sebum in the ducts and follicles since biochemical evidence indicates that freshly secreted sebum has little or no free fatty acids and that enzymatic liberation of the free fatty acids from their esters occurs in the follicular canal (NICOLAIDES and WELLS, 1957). NICOLAIDES and WELLS (1957) found a strong reaction for naphthol AS acetate and the indoxyl acetate, extending from the point where sebum enters the follicular canal all the way to the skin surface. They did inhibitory studies to rule out the presence of cholinesterase or pseudocholinesterase and concluded that their findings indicated that there might be lipases in sebum. MONTAGNA and ELLIS (1958) arbitrarily divided the sebum into "recent" and "old". Recent sebum had a weak reaction for Tween esterase (Tween 60), alpha-naphthyl esterase, indoxyl esterase, and a strong reaction for naphthol AS esterase. However, old sebum had a strong reaction for Tween esterase and alpha-naphthyl esterase in addition to naphthol AS esterase. In contrast to the findings of NICOLAIDES and WELLS (1957), they did not observe any indoxyl esterase activity. STEIGLEDER and LÖFFLER (1956) and STEIGLEDER (1958) compared the Tween technique with Tween 60 as a substrate to the method using alpha-naphthyl acetate as a substrate. They found that the Tween esterase reaction was clearly positive in those follicular canals in human chin skin which contained appreciable amounts of sebum. With the alpha-naphthyl acetate reaction using True Blue BB as the coupling agent, they found that freshly formed sebum, as well as the centrally situated acinar cells gave a negative red stain. In contrast older sebum, especially near the skin surface, gave an intensely positive black reaction. The strongest reaction occurred in the region of the orifice of the pilosebaceous unit. A positive reaction was also observed at the periphery of the acini.

Human sebaceous glands do not contain alkaline phosphatase (SUSKIND, 1951; MONTAGNA, 1962, 1963). However, since the endothelium of small arterioles and capillaries is alkaline phosphatase-positive, this reaction has been useful for delineating the blood supply of the sebaceous glands (SUSKIND, 1951; MONTAGNA and ELLIS, 1957b; ELLIS, MONTAGNA and FANGER, 1958; MORETTI and MONTAGNA, 1959; MORETTI, ELLIS and MESCON, 1959; MONTAGNA, 1964). The sebaceous acini are surrounded by a rich plexus of small vessels (Fig. 12). Many of the large sebaceous lobules are complexes of fused small acini which may be separated by delicate connective-tissue trabeculae containing blood vessels. The vessels, which pass through these trabeculae, are easily demonstrated with the alkaline phosphatase stain and appear to lie freely within the gland.

A small amount of acetylcholinesterase has been observed in the peripheral cells of the sebaceous glands, and a stronger reaction for butyrylcholinesterase has been observed in the peripheral cells (MONTAGNA, 1964).

Motor innervation of the sebaceous glands in man has never been demonstrated. In this connection, it has been reported that there are no acetylcholinesterase-positive nerves in close proximity to the sebaceous acini (HURLEY, SHELLEY and KOELLE, 1953; HELLMANN, 1955; MONTAGNA and ELLIS, 1957a; THIES and GALANTE, 1957; MONTAGNA, 1964). However, cholinesterase-containing nerve fibers have been seen surrounding the meibomian gland (MONTAGNA and ELLIS, 1959), and recently MONTAGNA (1966) has observed other cholinesterase-containing nerves in human eyelid skin.

D. Ultrastructure of the Human Sebaceous Gland

CHARLES (1960), KUROSUMI, KITAMURA and KANO (1960), HIBBS (1962) and ELLIS and HENRIKSON (1963) have studied the ultrastructure of human sebaceous glands. The most comprehensive and detailed account of the processes concerned in the formation of sebum is found in the paper by ELLIS and HENRIKSON (1963). Dr. ELLIS kindly supplied the electron micrographs illustrated in this section and edited the material presented herein.

The exact site of lipogenesis in sebaceous cells has been a major point of disagreement among various workers. It was proposed by ROGERS (1957) originally, and then by PALAY (1958), that lipogenesis occurs on the smooth endoplasmic reticulum. ROGERS (1957) also theorized that mitochondria might contribute to lipogenesis in sebaceous cells as he observed opaque bodies within these particular cell organelles. Since his reported study, these granules have been observed in mitochondria of diverse cell types and have been correlated with calcium metabolism, not lipogenesis (PEACHEY, 1964). The studies by both ROGERS (1957) and PALAY (1958) were from animal skin (mouse and rat, respectively), whereas the reports to be detailed below have involved studies in man.

CHARLES (1960) studied sebaceous glands in three biopsy specimens taken from the scalp and forearm of men. Since he did not detect a system of smooth membranes limiting the lipid vacuoles, he concluded that the sebaceous material was not formed in endoplasmic reticulum.

HIBBS (1962) studied the sebaceous glands in axillary skin. He found many smooth-walled small vesicles scattered throughout the cytoplasm of the sebaceous cells. He did not ascribe any function of lipid formation to these, but he did allude to the fact that there might be some relationship of lipogenesis to the scattered ribonucleoprotein particles found in the cells in greater abundance at the time that lipid first appears in the cells. He also proposed that lipogenesis originates within the Golgi apparatus, although Golgi structures were rarely encountered in his preparations. His supposition for this statement was that in light microscopy the earliest visible fat droplets appear in the region of the Golgi apparatus. KUROSUMI, KITAMURA and KANO (1960) also studied the sebaceous glands of the axilla. They did not observe any Golgi structures in the sebaceous cells. They noted an inverse relationship between the number of cytoplasmic granules and vesicles and thereby concluded that the vesicles arose from granules. They were also of the opinion that lipogenesis occurred in mitochondria although no supporting evidence was given.

In contrast to these earlier publications, ELLIS and HENRIKSON (1963) have identified a prominent Golgi apparatus in sebaceous cells undergoing lipogenesis and have assigned a secretory function to this organelle, as well as to the smooth-walled membranous structures within the cytoplasm. They divide the cells of the sebaceous glands into three types depending on the stage of sebaceous transformation: the peripheral cells, the partially differentiated cells, and the fully differentiated cells. This classification will be followed in the description which follows. The electron micrographs of sebaceous cells which are presented herein were taken from specimens of the cheek of adult men.

I. Peripheral Cells
(Fig. 13, 14, 15)

The peripheral cells, which usually consist of only a single layer of cells, rest upon a basement membrane that is variable in its morphologic appearance. In some sections it is almost absent, while in other areas it is a well-organized structure composed of 2 to 5 electron-dense amorphous bands alternating with wider light-staining spaces. The cell border which rests on the basement membrane is quite regular. In contrast, the cell membrane between borders of adjacent sebaceous cells is somewhat irregular and is often thrown into multiple folds resembling microvilli (Fig. 13, 14, 15). There are spaces between the cells in the region of these microvilli suggesting that there may be nutrient canals between the cells. The oval nucleus of these peripheral cells occupies most of the cell (Fig. 13).

The thin band of cytoplasm which surrounds the nucleus contains many readily identifiable structures. As the sebaceous cells are derived from epidermal cells, they not unexpectedly contain tonofilaments, ranging in number from a few scattered strands to bundles of varying size (Fig. 13). They are most prominent in

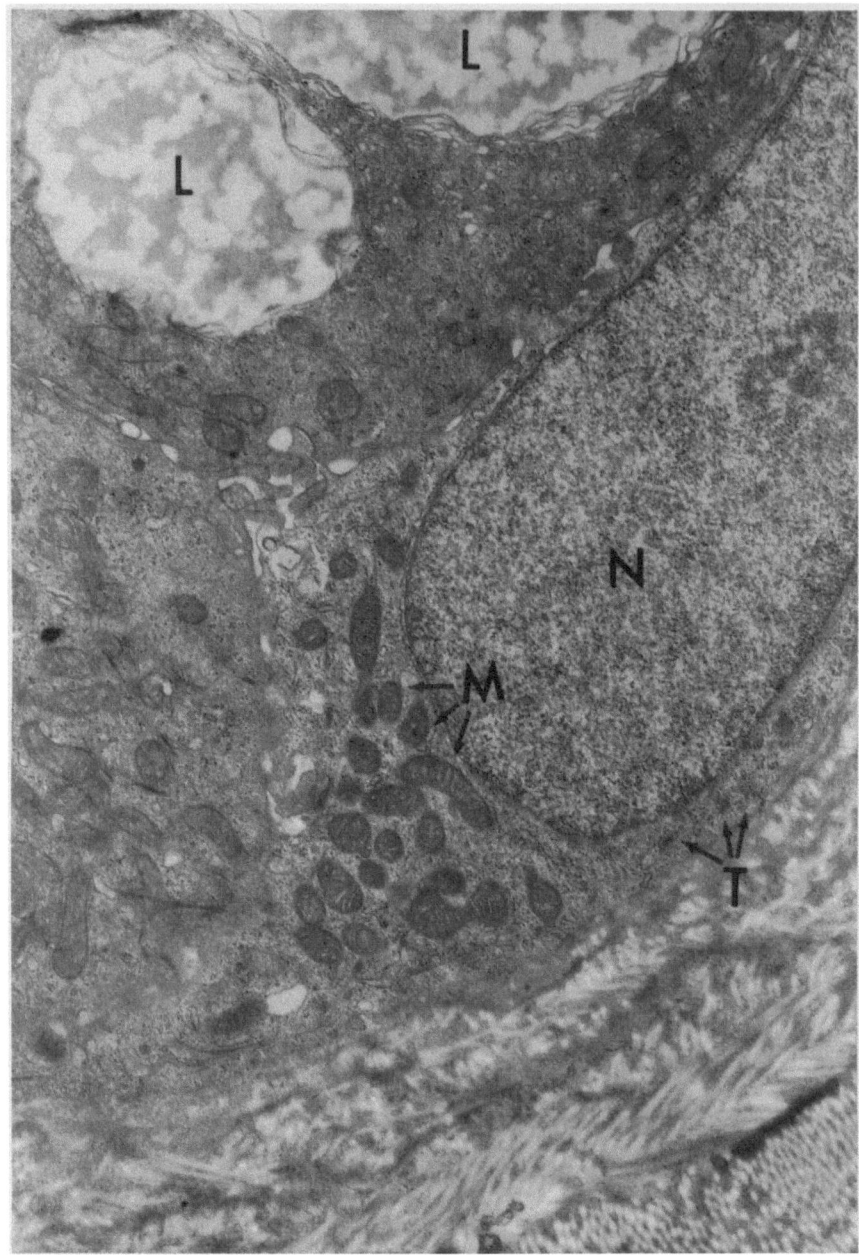

Fig. 13. Electron micrograph of portions of a peripheral cell (on the right) and two partially differentiated sebaceous cells (on the left and above). The dermis is at the lower portion of the photomicrograph. The basement membrane is not well delineated. There is relatively little cytoplasm in the peripheral cell with the nucleus (N) occupying most of the cell. Some tonofibrils (T) can be visualized. The mitochondria (M) with their cristae are prominent. The cytoplasm contains endoplasmic reticulum, ribonucleoprotein particles and glycogen granules. Microvilli are shown where the three cells join. The portion of the upper, partially differentiated cell contains two lipid vacuoles (L). These show the pallisading of the smooth membranes to form the limiting "husk". ($\times$ 10,600).
(Courtesy of Dr. R. A. Ellis, Brown University, Providence, R. I., U.S.A.)

the regions of the attachment zones. The tonofilaments, however, are not nearly as prominent in these cells as they are in the sebaceous duct cells (Fig. 16). The

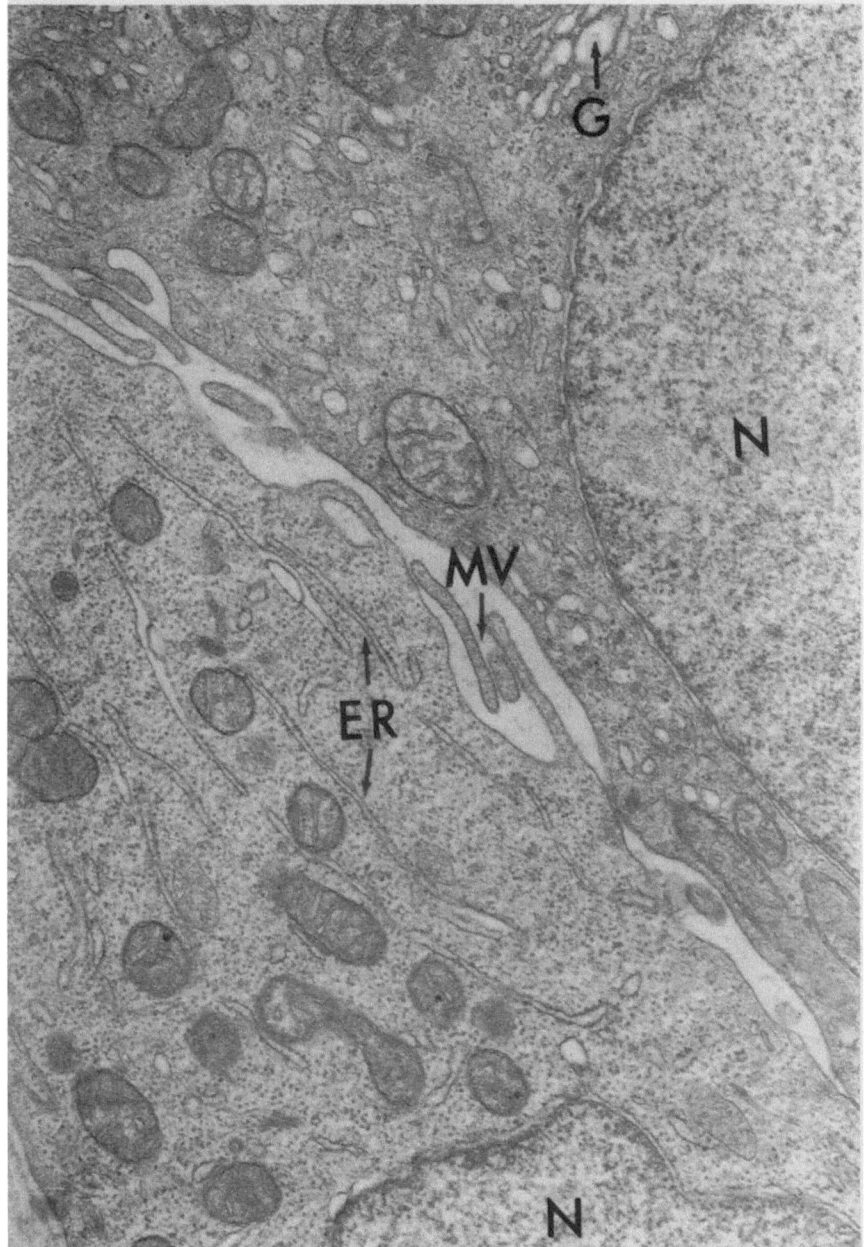

Fig. 14. Electron micrograph of portions of two adjacent peripheral cells. Parts of both nuclei (*N*) are shown. The microvilli (*MV*) are well developed. The lower cell contains rough endoplasmic reticulum (*ER*). A large number of free ribonucleoprotein granules (dark-staining particles) are also present. In the upper cell, the Golgi zone (*G*) is prominent. (× 28,500). (Courtesy of Dr .R. A. ELLIS, Brown University, Providence, R. I., U.S.A.)

latter cells, which become fully keratinized, undergo changes similar to those of the surface epidermis.

The peripheral cells contain abundant mitochondria which vary considerably in shape and show well-demarcated internal cristae (Fig. 13, 14, 15). A variable

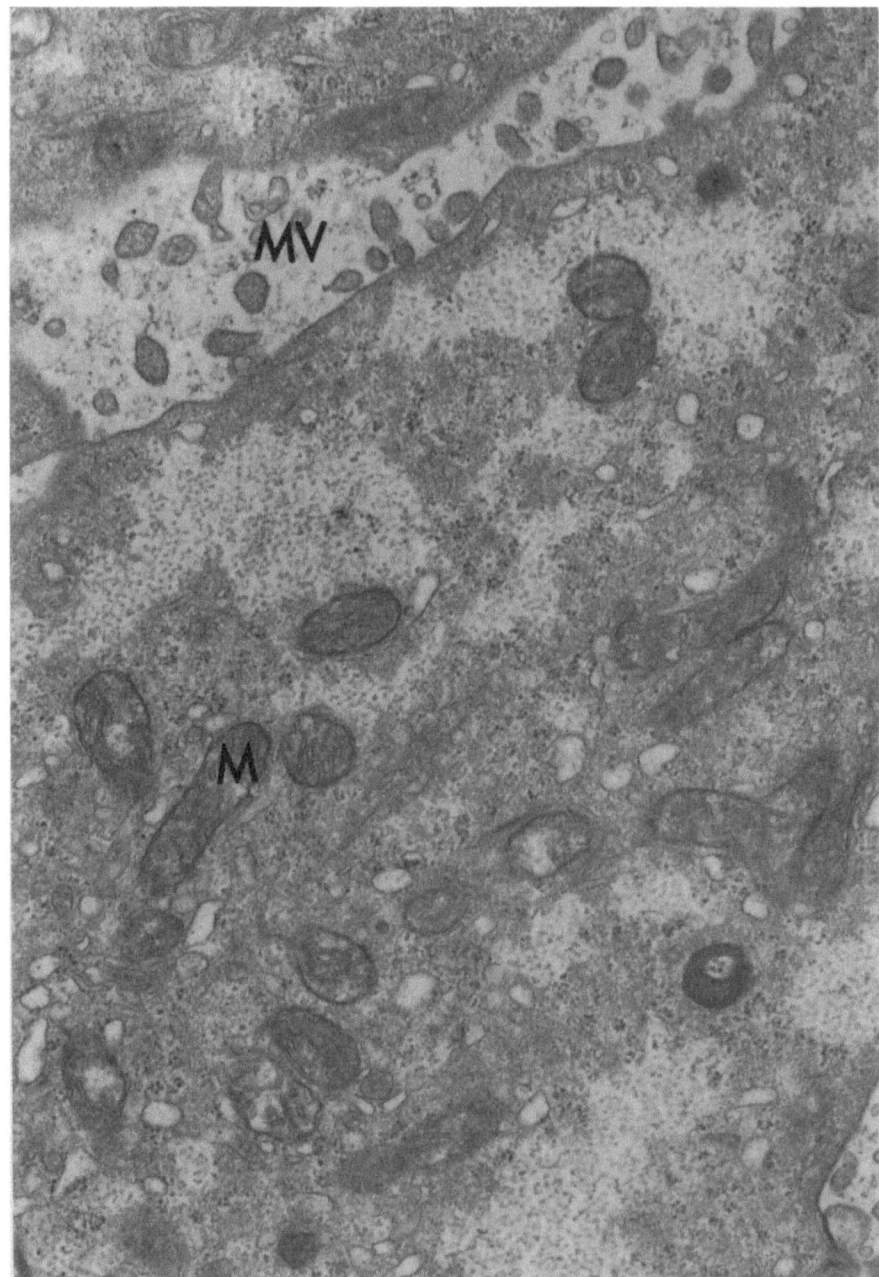

Fig. 15. Electron micrograph of a peripheral cell stained with lead citrate to demonstrate glycogen. The numerous, small light-staining particles are glycogen. The darker particles are free ribonucleoprotein granules. There are many mitochondria (*M*). In the space between the cells there are numerous cross sections of microvilli (*MV*). (× 22,000). (Courtesy of Dr. R. A. ELLIS, Brown University, Providence, R. I., U.S.A.)

amount of smooth and rough endoplasmic reticulum is found in the cytoplasm (Fig. 14, 15). In addition, there are free ribonucleoprotein particles scattered in the cytoplasm (Fig. 14). The cells often contain abundant glycogen granules (Fig. 15). The presence of glycogen and its association with sebaceous transformation have

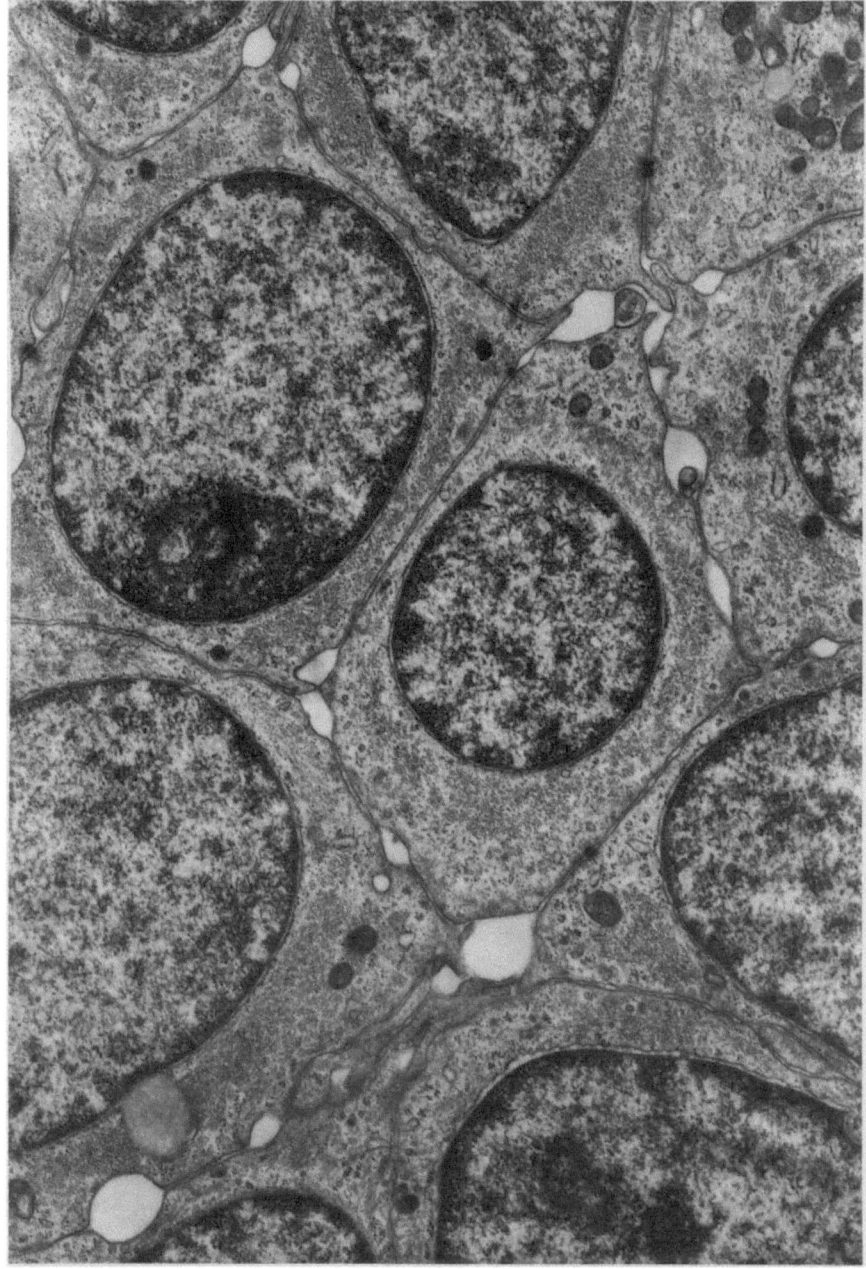

Fig. 16. Electron micrograph of sebaceous duct cells. Tonofilaments, ribonucleoprotein particles and glycogen granules are more prominent than in the peripheral cells. The mitochondria are less in evidence, and the cell walls are smoother. There are no lipid droplets. ($\times$ 14,100). (Courtesy of Dr. R. A. ELLIS, Brown University, Providence, R. I., U.S.A.)

been demonstrated by HENRIKSON (1965). The Golgi zone can be visualized in the peripheral cells (Fig. 14). Lipid vacuoles are usually not present although a few isolated droplets may appear in the peripheral cells.

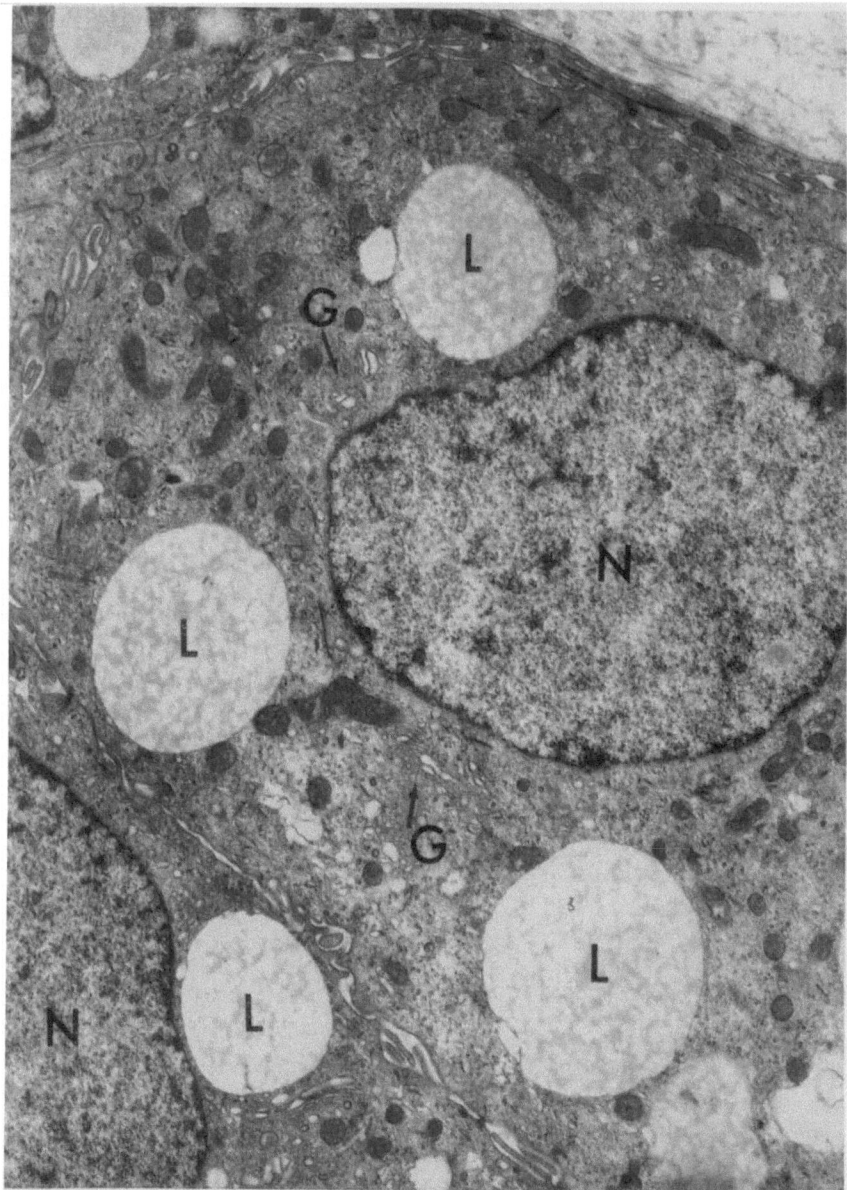

Fig. 17. Electron micrograph of partially differentiated sebaceous cells. The microvilli are quite prominent. The mitochondria are elongated. There are prominent perinuclear Golgi zones (G) in the central cell. There are large lipid vacuoles (L). The ribonucleoprotein particles are relatively scant. (× 9,100). (Courtesy of Dr. R. A. Ellis, Brown University, Providence, R. I., U.S.A.)

II. Partially Differentiated Cells
(Fig. 17, 18, 19, 20)

The nucleus of the partially differentiated cell frequently develops pale patches with concentric rings of fibrillar material surrounding a dark central core containing a few clumped ribonucleoprotein granules (Fig. 20). In addition, the differentiating cell shows many cytoplasmic differences. The cell membrane is

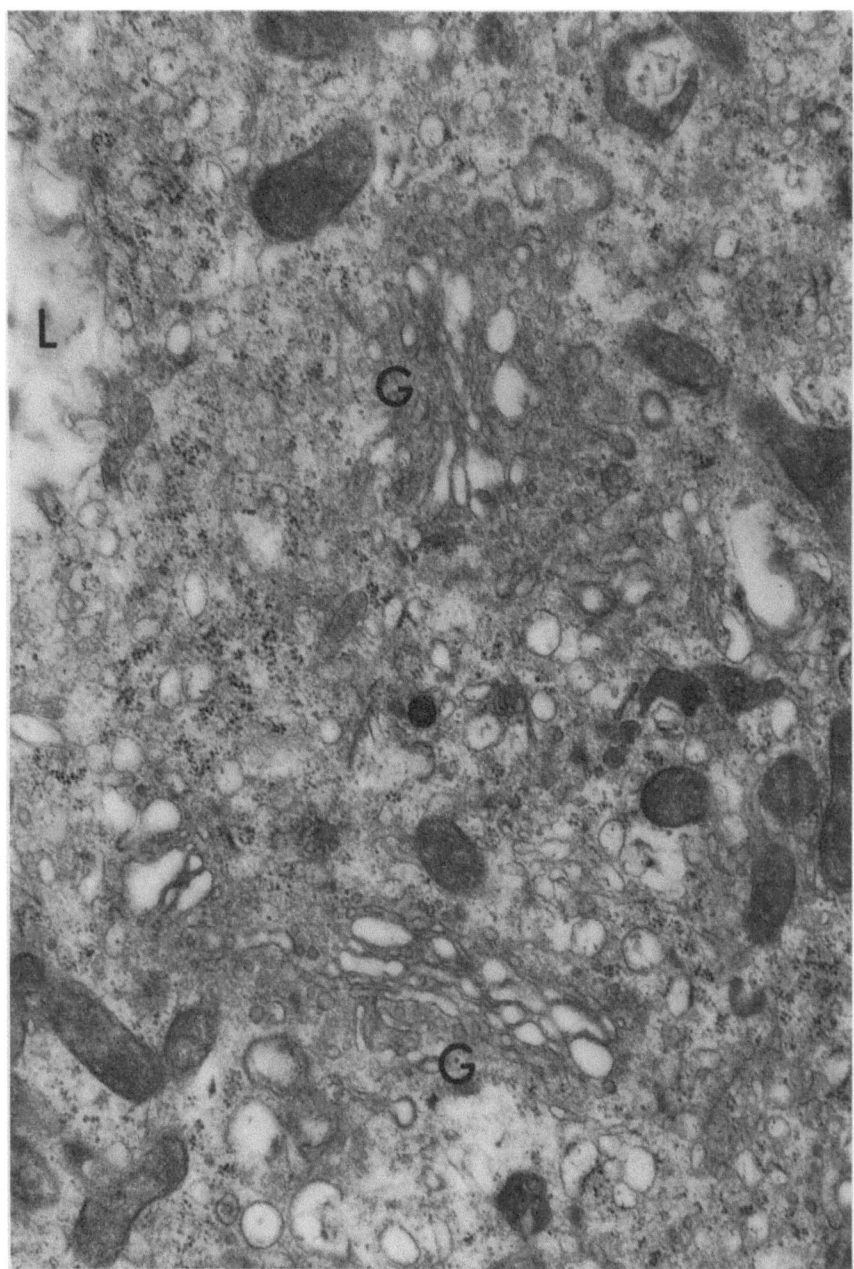

Fig. 18. Electron micrograph of partially differentiated sebaceous cells. The prominent Golgi apparatus (*G*) and the endoplasmic reticulum are illustrated in this high-magnification electron micrograph. A portion of a lipid vacuole (*L*) is shown on the left. There are few ribonucleoprotein particles. ($\times$ 18,100). (Courtesy Dr. R. A. ELLIS, Brown University, Providence, R. I., U.S.A.)

thrown up into more elaborate folding than is seen in peripheral cells (Fig. 17). The attachment plates have largely disappeared, and tonofilaments are rarely recognizable.

The cytoplasm is increased in absolute and relative amounts and contains more abundant endoplasmic reticulum (Fig. 18, 19, 20). This is predominantly of the

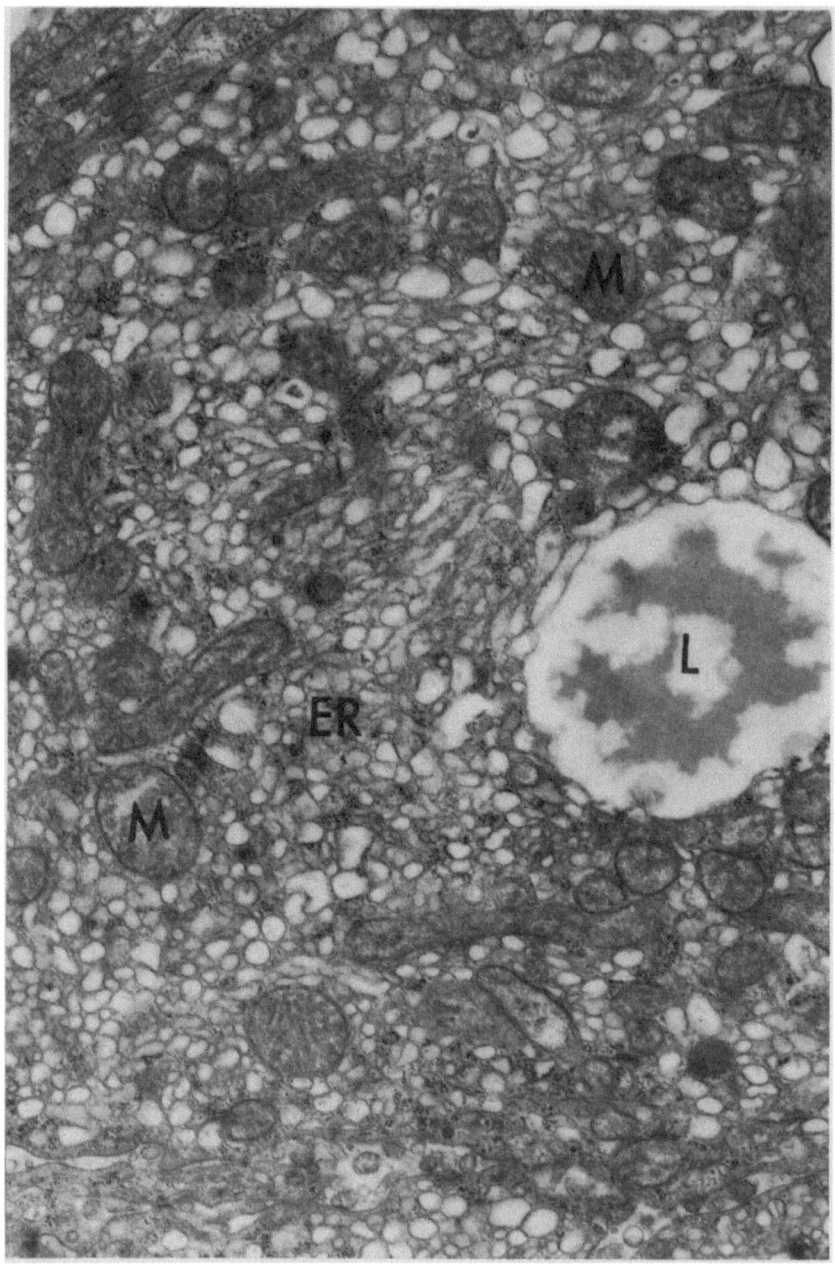

Fig. 19. Electron micrograph of partially differentiated sebaceous cell. In this cell the great abundance of the endoplasmic reticulum (*ER*) is illustrated. A portion of this endoplasmic reticulum is flattened around the large lipid vacuole (*L*). Openings of the endoplasmic reticulum into the lipid vacuole are shown. Some of the mitochondria (*M*) are elongated. Clumps of ribonucleoprotein particles are compressed among some of the small vesicles. (× 12,100). (Courtesy of Dr. R. A. ELLIS, Brown University, Providence, R. I., U.S.A.)

smooth type and exists in the earliest stages as small vesicles. The contents of the vesicles appear clear, and there are very few associated ribonucleoprotein particles. Glycogen granules are also sparse. The mitochondria are often elongated (Fig. 18, 19).

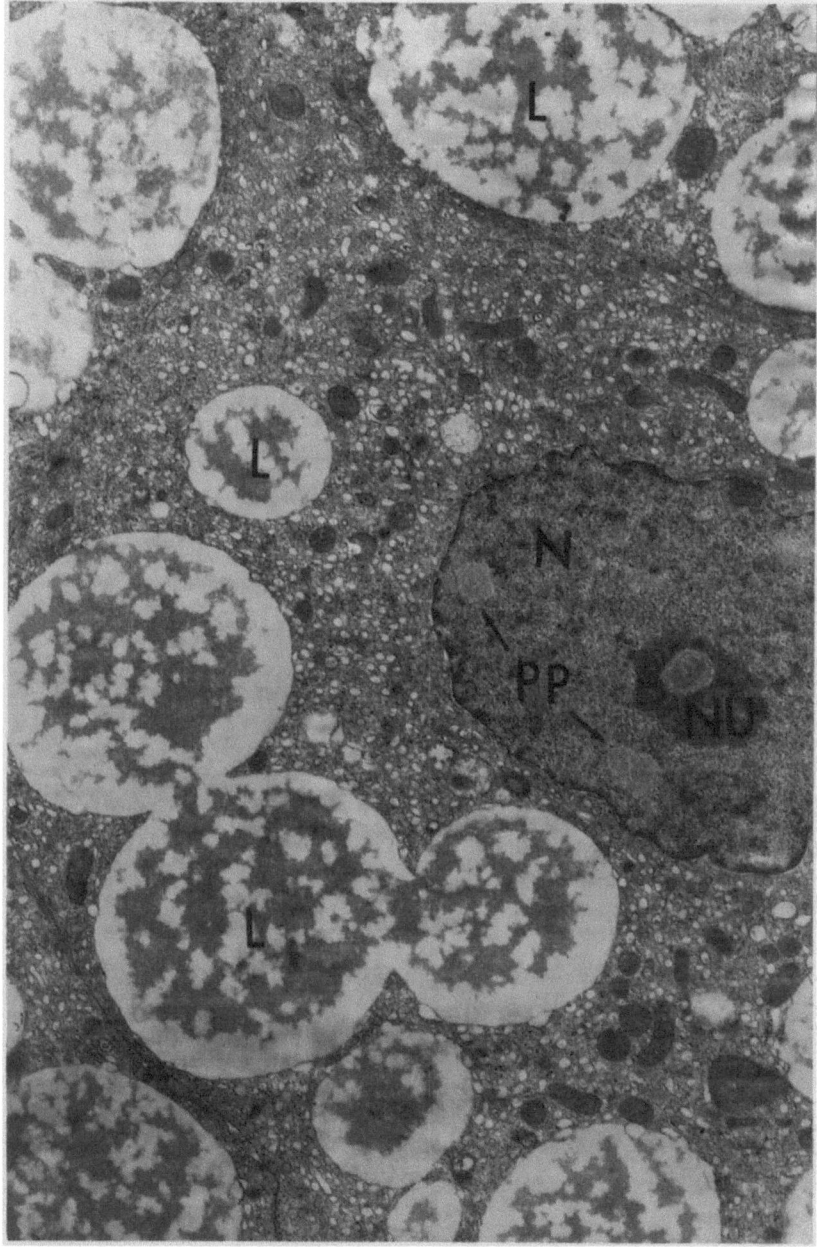

Fig. 20. Electron micrograph of partially differentiated sebaceous cell. Greater lipid differentiation is present. The lipid droplets are larger, and some fusion has occurred. The endoplasmic reticulum is well developed, and in some areas it is being incorporated into the lipid vacuoles. In the nucleus (N) there is a prominent nucleolus (NU). In addition, there are several pale patches (PP). (× 7,400). (Courtesy of Dr. R. A. Ellis, Brown University, Providence, R. I., U.S.A.)

Lipid droplets make their appearance in these cells (Fig. 17, 19, 20). The droplets are not uniform in size. A partial explanation for this may be that the lipid is formed at different times. With osmium fixation alone the contents of the smallest lipid droplets are almost uniformly osmiophilic. However, the larger

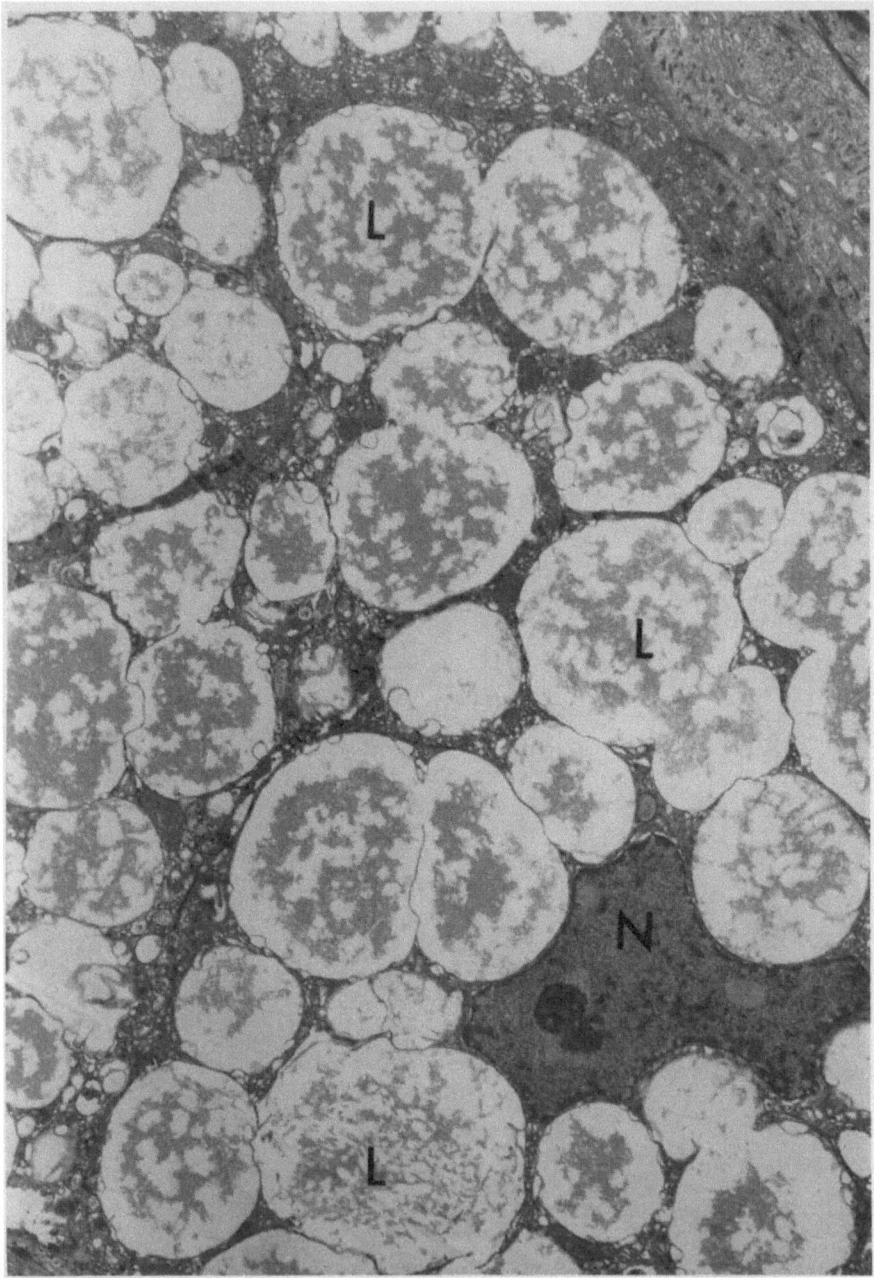

Fig. 21. Electron micrograph of nearly mature sebaceous cell. The nucleus (*N*) is deformed from encroachment of the lipid droplets. A nucleolus is seen. A few pale patches are present as well as some clumped RNP granules. The lipid droplets (*L*) are larger, and there is less cellular material between the droplets. Some fusion of the lipid droplets has occurred. ($\times$ 4,300). (Courtesy of Dr. R. A. ELLIS, Brown University, Providence, R. I., U.S.A.)

lipid vacuoles do not stain uniformly suggesting that the lipid is partially washed out during tissue processing. The lipid droplets have a limiting membrane which is made up of several compressed layers of smooth membranes (Fig. 13). This lamellar material is called the "husk", and its significance will be detailed below.

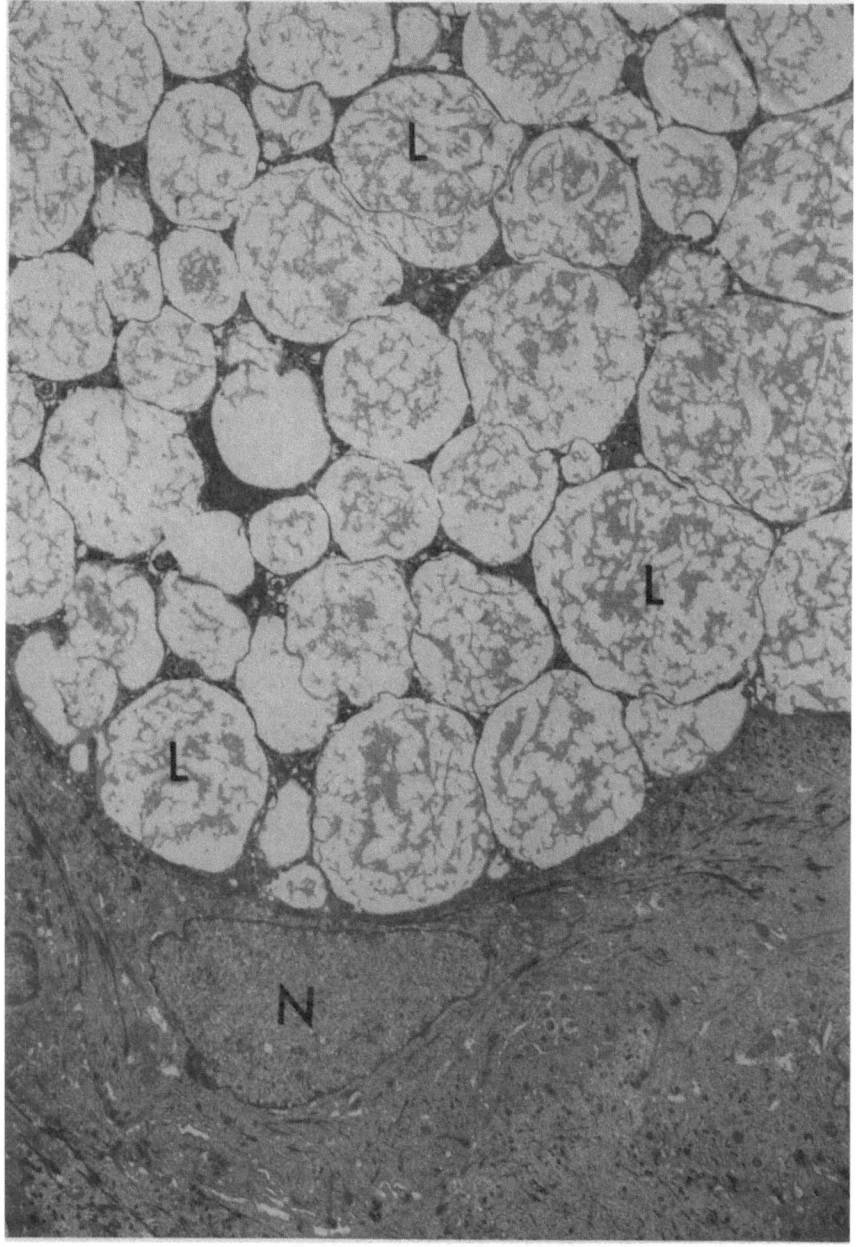

Fig. 22. Electron micrograph of fully differentiated sebaceous cell. The lipid droplets (L) now fill the cell completely. The dark staining cell with the prominent nucleus is a sebaceous duct cell. ($\times$ 3,400). (Courtesy of Dr. R. A. Ellis, Brown University, Providence, R. I., U.S.A.)

The "husk" is most obvious in osmium tetroxide-fixed tissue, but in glutaraldehyde-osmium tetroxide fixed material the "husk" is not well visualized.

In some of the partially differentiated cells a definite, well-developed Golgi apparatus is seen in the perinuclear zone (Fig. 18). Typically, the Golgi zone consists of parallel, smooth membranes, small vesicles and slightly dilated cisterns.

ELLIS and HENRIKSON (1963) have proposed that the Golgi zone and the abundant endoplasmic reticulum are both involved in the formation of lipid droplets in the sebaceous cells. According to their theory, the earliest lipid droplet originates as a dilated cistern in the Golgi apparatus. As lipid accumulates in this Golgi vesicle, the lipid droplet enlarges and the Golgi membranes and the adjacent endoplasmic reticulum are compressed in a lamellar fashion around the periphery of the droplet. As the droplet enlarges, the cisterns of the endoplasmic reticulum become continuous with the lipid vacuole at several points. Thus, with further enlargement of the vacuole, more and more of the endoplasmic reticulum becomes compressed, and the contents within the smooth membranes become incorporated into the lipid droplets. The smooth membranes themselves contribute to the formation of the "husk". Thus, their findings encompass much that has been proposed before, namely, that earliest lipid formation occurs in the Golgi apparatus, but that the endoplasmic reticulum also contributes to the formation of the droplets.

III. Fully Differentiated Cells
(Fig. 21, 22)

The fully differentiated sebaceous cells represent essentially an extension and elaboration of the changes described for partially differentiated cells. The nucleus remains relatively intact until sebaceous material comes to occupy almost the entire cell. Then, the nucleus becomes irregular in shape, there is clumping of the chromatin, and the nucleolar material becomes dispersed (Fig. 21). The amount of cytoplasm in these cells is greatly increased due to the accumulation of the lipid vacuoles. The cell membranes tend to be flatter with less prominent microvilli.

The predominant cytoplasmic organelles are the lipid vacuoles and the smooth endoplasmic reticulum (Fig. 21, 22). The lipid vacuoles are much larger and are more uniform in size. However, fusion between droplets may occur (Fig. 21, 22). It has been calculated that large sebaceous cells may contain more than 50 vacuoles. The endoplasmic reticulum is still prominent in these cells and is compressed around the edges of the lipid vacuoles giving rise to an increase in size of those droplets, as well as contributing to the "husk" of the lipid vacuoles.

Golgi zones may be present in these cells, but as full maturation occurs, the membrane systems become disorganized. Mitochondria persist, but they are widely dispersed in the cells due to the great increase in cell size.

E. Sebaceous Glands in Mucous Membranes and Ectopic Sites

Sebaceous glands are commonly encountered in areas other than the skin, particularly on the mucous membranes. Comprehensive reviews on this subject have appeared in recent years (MILES, 1958, 1963; GUIDUCCI and HYMAN, 1962; HYMAN and GUIDUCCI, 1963). In contrast to the sebaceous glands of the skin, these sebaceous glands, with rare exceptions, are not associated with hair follicles but open directly onto surface epithelia. In addition, when located in mucous membranes they are usually visible to the naked eye due to their superficial location and to the thinness of the overlying epithelium.

I. Lip and Oral Mucosa

Common locations for extra-cutaneous sebaceous glands are the vermilion or transition zone of the lip and the mucosa of the cheeks. These glands are designated as Fordyce spots in recognition of the description by FORDYCE (1896) of yellowish spots on the buccal mucosa and lips. In actuality, however, they had been described many years earlier and identified as sebaceous glands by KÖLLIKER (1862). Fordyce spots of the lips and oral mucosa are grossly visible and appear as well-circumscribed white to pale yellowish macules or papules varying in size from a pin-point to 1.5 mm. or more. On the lips, they are most numerous on the upper lip, being relatively sparse on the lower lip. Since few, if any, glands are seen on the border of the vermilion adjacent to the skin, the presence of these glands probably does not represent a mere extension of sebaceous structures from the skin to the mucosal surface.

In the oral mucosa the glands are most numerous in the occlusion plane of the teeth. The mucosa in this area differs from that above and below by being paler and more firmly attached to the underlying connective tissue (MILES, 1963). In addition, mucous glands are rare in this region, and in this respect it resembles the vermilion area of the lip. However, these anatomical differences cannot entirely explain the gland localization since sebaceous glands may also be found on other areas of the oral cavity such as the gingivae over the incisor, premolar and unerupted molar teeth, the anterior tonsillar pillars, the palate and the tongue. There is no direct relationship between the incidence or number of lip and oral mucosal glands — i.e. occasionally there are numerous lip glands with few or no oral glands, and vice versa.

The development of lip and oral mucosal sebaceous glands has been carefully studied, especially the latter (MILES, 1958, 1963). While small sebaceous glands are occasionally encountered in full-term fetuses, infancy and childhood, striking glandular development does not occur until puberty when there is a sudden increase in the size and total number of glands. Furthermore, there is evidence that neogenesis continues throughout adult life so that the total number of glandular units increases. This situation is different from that of sebaceous glands in the skin in which a decrease in sebaceous gland size occurs with aging, particularly in females (POCHI and STRAUSS, 1965). The increase in number of glands with age appears to occur through actual *de novo* formation from budding of new primordia in the basal cell layer of the epidermis (MILES, 1963). The process is a dynamic one of waxing and waning as one may observe atrophic, degenerating glands at the same time that new glands are forming.

Although HALTER (1937) found a lower incidence of sebaceous glands of the oral mucous membranes in females in certain age ranges, most investigators have felt that the incidence in males and females is equal (MARGOLIES and WEIDMAN, 1921; HALPERIN, KOLAS, JEFFERIS, HUDDLESTON and ROBINSON, 1953; MILES, 1958, 1963).

The sebaceous glands of the oral mucosa are similar to those encountered in most areas of the skin except that they are unassociated with hair follicles. They open directly onto the surface by a duct lined with stratified squamous epithelium. This duct is often quite wide and is filled with horny material. In the typical follicle, there are a number of globular acini arranged in a rosette around the duct. The microscopic structure and the histochemical reactions are essentially similar to those observed for cutaneous sebaceous glands (MILES, 1958, 1963).

There is no increase in the number and size of buccal sebaceous glands in acne vulgaris (SCHOBER, 1954), nor has any relationship been shown to exist between their occurrence and between alterations in serum cholesterol levels or the incidence of symptoms and signs of atherosclerosis (MARTIN and WALES, 1964).

II. External Genitalia

1. Female

Sebaceous glands are commonly encountered on the mucous membranes of the external genitalia. They are most numerous and invariably found on the medial surface of the labia minora. In newborns, the glands in this site are quite abundant and are often arranged around a vellus hair follicle which later disappears (MONTAGNA, 1962). While in the adult these glands open directly to the surface, one may on occasion observe them arranged around abortive hair follicles. The sebaceous glands are found less commonly on the labia majora and rarely on the hymen and the prepuce of the clitoris.

2. Male

Sebaceous glands, known as Tyson's glands, occur on the internal fold of the prepuce, and on the corona and glans. These glands are unilobulated or bilobulated. They are histologically similar to the glands of the oral mucosa and open directly onto the surface.

III. Nipple

The skin of the nipple and of the areola contains abundant sebaceous glands. In fact, PERKINS and MILLER (1926) found sebaceous glands in all of 40 nipple specimens examined from both males and females. They are not associated with either hair follicles or the mammary duct system and open to the surface through a short duct. These glands occur over the entire surface of the nipple and at the margin of the areolae peripheral to the alveolar glands of Montgomery which are not sebaceous glands.

IV. Eyelids

There are two types of special sebaceous glands in the eyelids. Small sebaceous glands are associated with the eyelashes and are known as the glands of Zeis. The larger glands of the eyelids are the meibomian glands which are embedded in the tarsal plates of the upper and lower eyelids. These glands are simple, elongated structures which are arranged parallel to one another in a single layer. Each gland empties into a long, straight, central duct which opens onto the inner free margin of the lid. There are no hairs associated with the meibomian glands. In contrast to sebaceous glands elsewhere, as already mentioned, the meibomian glands are surrounded by nerve networks rich in cholinesterase activity (MONTAGNA and ELLIS, 1959). However, since other sebaceous glands lack such innervation and since the formation of sebum is a holocrine process, it is likely that these nerves have a sensory rather than a secretory function.

V. Salivary Glands

Sebaceous glands have been noted frequently in parotid gland tissue since HARTZ (1946) first reported their presence here. MEZA-CHÁVEZ (1949) studied 100 normal parotid glands microscopically from 51 patients at autopsy and found sebaceous glands in 28% of the parotid glands, representing a patient incidence of 55%.

The submaxillary glands have also been reported to contain sebaceous glands (HAMPERL, 1931).

VI. Miscellaneous Sites

Sebaceous glands have been detected in the cervix (DONNELLY and NAVIDI, 1950), the esophagus (DE LA PAVA and PICKREN, 1962) and the larynx (GEIPEL, 1949).

F. Growth and Proliferation of the Glands

The embryology of sebaceous glands is discussed elsewhere in the Handbuch. However, the fact that the sebaceous gland takes origin as a small outpocketing of cells from the hair germ (SERRI and HUBER, 1963) is important in considering the subsequent changes that occur in the glands. Some of the cells of the glands maintain microscopic characteristics which are identical to those of the epithelial cells from which they are derived embryologically. Thus, the cells of the duct are identical to the epithelial cells of the follicle and constitute a similar stratified squamous epithelium. The peripheral cells of the acini have gross characteristics which are similar to the epithelial cells of the follicle. However, on electron microscopy, as already mentioned, they show evidence of protein synthesis (tonofilaments) plus lipid differentiation.

The peripheral cells normally differentiate with the formation of lipid as their end-product. However, under certain circumstances, the cells of the sebaceous acinus may differentiate to form a stratified squamous epithelium. This concept of "pluripotentiality" was proposed by PINKUS (1953). While injury to the epidermis, accompanied by only minimal follicular damage (e.g. contact dermatitis), does not produce any significant changes in the sebaceous glands, deeper injury, which of necessity involves the pilosebaceous unit (e.g. dermabrasion), produces profound changes in the sebaceous glands (EISEN, HOLYOKE and LOBITZ, 1955; STRAUSS and KLIGMAN, 1958; STRAUSS, 1959). Lipid differentiation ceases, and undifferentiated cells, which contribute to follicular repair, are formed. Furthermore, after removal of the epidermis, such as with dermabrasion, these undifferentiated cells, along with those from other epidermal appendages contribute a new epidermal mantle. Usually, the change from lipid differentiation proceeds only to the point of formation of undifferentiated cells. However, following certain types of injury, particularly experimentally induced severe inflammation, the pluripotentiality of the sebaceous cells is manifested by the actual formation of a stratified squamous epithelium. The types of change just discussed may be seen in various diseases of the skin (STRAUSS and KLIGMAN, 1960; MESCON and STRAUSS, 1960). It should be emphasized that the mature sebaceous cells do not participate in the reactive process. Once lipid differentiation occurs, the cells are irreversibly committed to this line of differentiation. They disappear as they are shed and are replaced by undifferentiated cells. Under experimental conditions the process of formation of undifferentiated cells is reversible, and sebaceous differentiation resumes following skin repair.

The mechanism of growth of individual acini and the replacement of sebaceous cells is a controversial and as yet unsettled subject. The classic view is that cell replacement is solely the result of mitotic division of the peripheral cells. However, while mitoses may be found in the peripheral cells, they are not numerous, and the question has been raised as to whether the number of mitoses is adequate to account for the replacement of cells lost in sebum secretion. Therefore, it has even been proposed that mitotic activity in the epithelium of the ducts is responsible for cell replacement in the sebaceous acinus with the cells from the duct migrating down into the acinus (BRINKMAN, 1912; CLARA, 1929).

Montagna (1962, 1963) has proposed a different theory to explain cell replacement. He does not feel that the peripheral cells are the germinative cells from which cell replacement for differentiation arises. Instead, new buds of undifferentiated epithelial cells arise from the excretory ducts and undergo sebaceous differentiation. According to his theory, lipid differentiation begins first in the most centrally located cells and proceeds towards the peripheral cells. As the new acini expand in size due to lipid accumulation in the cells, they may encroach upon and fuse with adjacent acini thus forming large sebaceous complexes. Evidence, cited by Montagna (1962, 1963), in favor of this process is the finding of connective-tissue stroma within the acini. This, however, does not prove his theory since these could be found without resorting to this explanation for gland replacement. In addition to the new buds arising from the ducts, Montagna (1962, 1963) feels that new acini may develop from areas of focal mitotic activity of the peripheral cells resulting in buds of undifferentiated cells which then undergo differentiation in the same fashion as the groups of cells which arise in the duct region. There can be little question that the sebaceous glands are subject to change in size and cellular structure as witnessed by their response to hormonal stimulation or suppression and to injury. However, Montagna's concepts have been challenged by Epstein and Epstein (1966), who studied cell turnover in human sebaceous glands by nuclear labeling with intracutaneous injection of thymidine-H^3. They found that the acini appear to maintain their anatomic integrity for a least one month. Furthermore, in serial studies, they were able to trace the migration of tagged material from the peripheral cells into the central regions of the acinus. They have interpreted their findings as indicating that cell replacement in the individual acinus is due to mitotic activity of the peripheral cells.

In preparing this chapter the authors have drawn extensively on material presented in the earlier chapter by the late Dr. Felix Pinkus (F. Pinkus, Die normale Anatomie der Haut. In: J. Jadassohn, Handb. Haut/Geschlechtskr., Bd. I/1. Berlin: Springer 1927), and on a more recent monograph on the sebaceous glands (Advances in biology of skin, vol. 4, The sebaceous glands (W. Montagna, R. A. Ellis and A. F. Silver, eds.). Oxford: Pergamon Press 1963).

This investigation was supported in part by research grants AM 07084 and AM 07388, and graduate training grant 2A-5295, National Institute of Arthritis and Metabolic Diseases, United States Public Health Service.

References

Adachi, K., and W. Montagna: Histology and cytochemistry of human skin. XXII. Sites of leucine aminopeptidase (LAP). J. invest. Derm. **37**, 145—152 (1961).
Baillie, A. H., K. C. Calman, and J. A. Milne: Histochemical distribution of hydroxysteroid dehydrogenases in human skin. Brit. J. Derm. **77**, 610—616 (1965). — Benfenati, A., and F. Brillanti: Sulla distribuzione delle ghiandole sebacee nella cute del corpo umano. Arch. ital. Derm. **15**, 33—42 (1939). — Bowen, R. H.: Studies on the Golgi apparatus in gland-cells. II. Glands producing lipoidal secretions — the so-called skin glands. Quart. J. micr. Sci. **70**, 193—215 (1926). — The cytology of glandular secretion. Quart. Rev. Biol. **4**, 484—519 (1929). — Braun-Falco, O.: Über die Fähigkeit der menschlichen Haut zur Polysaccharidsynthese, ein Beitrag zur Histotopochemie der Phosphorylase. Arch. klin. exp. Derm. **202**, 163—170 (1956a). — Zur Histotopographie der β-Glucuronidase in normaler menschlicher Haut. Arch. klin. exp. Derm. **203**, 61—67 (1956b). — Breathnach, A. S., M. S. Birbeck, and J. D. Everall: Observations bearing on the relationship between Langerhans cells and melanocytes. Ann. N.Y. Acad. Sci. **100**, 223—238 (1963). — Brinkman, A.: Die Hautdrüsen der Säugetiere (Bau und Secretionsverhältnisse). Ergebn. Anat. Entwickl.-Gesch. **20**, 1173—1231 (1912). — Brun, R., K. Enderlin et A. de Weck: Variations de la couche sébacée de l'avant-bras suivant l'age et le sexe. Acta derm.-venereol. (Stockh.) **35**, 311—317 (1955).
Cain, A. J.: The use of Nile blue in the examination of lipoids. Quart. J. micr. Sci. **88**, 383—392 (1947). — A further note on Nile blue. Quart. J. micr. Sci. **89**, 429 (1948). — Charles, A.: Electron microscopic observations of the human sebaceous gland. J. invest. Derm. **35**, 31—36 (1960). — Clara, M.: Morfologia e sviluppo delle ghiandole sebacee nell'uomo. Richerche Morfol. **9**, 121—182 (1929).

Donnelly, G. H., and S. Navidi: Sebaceous glands in the cervix uteri. J. Path. Bact. **62**, 453—454 (1950).
Eisen, A. Z., J. B. Holyoke, and W. C. Lobitz jr.: Responses of the superficial portion of the human pilosebaceous apparatus to controlled injury. J. invest. Derm. **25**, 145—156 (1955). — Ellis, R. A., and R. C. Henrikson: The ultrastructure of the sebaceous glands of man. In: Advances in biology of skin, vol. 4. The sebaceous glands (W. Montagna, R. A. Ellis and A. F. Silver, eds.). Oxford: Pergamon Press 1963. — Ellis, R. A., and W. Montagna: Histology and cytochemistry of human skin. XV. Sites of phosphorylase and amylo-1,6-glucosidase activity. J. Histochem. Cytochem. **6**, 201—207 (1958). — Ellis, R. A., W. Montagna, and H. Fanger: Histology and cytochemistry of human skin. XIV. The blood supply of the cutaneous glands. J. invest. Derm. **30**, 137—145 (1958). — Epstein jr., E. H., and W. L. Epstein: New cell formation in human sebaceous glands. J. invest. Derm. **46**, 453—458 (1966).
Findlay, G. H.: The simple esterases of human skin. Brit. J. Derm. **67**, 83—91 (1955). — Forchielli, E., G. S. Rao, I. R. Sarda, N. B. Gibree, P. E. Pochi, J. S. Strauss, and R. I. Dorfman: Effect of ethinyloestradiol on plasma testosterone levels and urinary testosterone excretion in man. Acta endocr. (Kbh.) **50**, 51—54 (1965). — Fordyce, J. A.: A peculiar affection of the mucous membrane of the lips and oral cavity. J. cutan. Dis. **14**, 413—419 (1896).
Geipel, P.: Talgdrüse im Kehlkopf. Zbl. allg. Path. path. Anat. **85**, 69—71 (1949). — Grasset, N., et R. Brun: Étude du film sebace de sujets sains et de patients atteints d'epilepsie ou de maladie de Parkinson. Dermatologica (Basel) **119**, 232—237 (1959). — Grots, I. A., and S. K. Targovnik: Personal communication 1966. — Guiducci, A. A., and A. B. Hyman: Ectopic sebaceous glands. Dermatologica (Basel) **125**, 44—63 (1962).
Halperin, V., S. Kolas, K. R. Jefferis, S. O. Huddleston, and H. B. G. Robinson: The occurrence of Fordyce spots, benign migratory glossitis, median rhomboid glossitis, and fissured tongue in 2,478 dental patients. Oral Surg. **6**, 1072—1077 (1953). — Halter, K.: Zur Kenntnis des Fordyceschen Zustandes und seiner Bedeutung für die Klärung der Lokalisationsfrage von Hautkrankheiten in der Mundhöhle. Arch. Derm. Syph. (Berl.) **176**, 201—213 (1937). — Hamilton, J. B.: Male hormone substance: a prime factor in acne. J. clin. Endocr. **1**, 570—592 (1941). — Hamperl, H.: Beiträge zur normalen und pathologischen Histologie menschlicher Speicheldrüsen. Z. mikr.-anat. Forsch. **27**, 1—55 (1931). — Hartz, P. H.: Development of sebaceous glands from intralobular ducts of the parotid gland. Arch. Path. **41**, 651—654 (1946). — Hellmann, K.: Cholinesterase and amine oxidase in the skin: a histochemical investigation. J. Physiol. (Lond.) **129**, 454—463 (1955). — Henrikson, R. C.: Glycogen and sebaceous transformation. J. invest. Derm. **44**, 435—437 (1965). — Hibbs, R. G.: Electron microscopy of human axillary sebaceous glands. J. invest. Derm. **38**, 329—336 (1962). — Horner, W. E.: On the odoriferous glands of the negro. Amer. J. med. Sci. **21**, 13—16 (1846). — Hurley jr., H. J., W. B. Shelley, and G. B. Koelle: The distribution of cholinesterases in human skin, with special reference to eccrine and apocrine sweat glands. J. invest. Derm. **21**, 139—147 (1953). — Hyman, A. B., and A. A. Guiducci: Ectopic sebaceous glands. In: Advances in biology of skin, vol. 4. The sebaceous glands (W. Montagna, R. A. Ellis and A. F. Silver, eds.). Oxford: Pergamon Press 1963.
Jarrett, A.: The effects of stilboestrol on the surface sebum and upon acne vulgaris. Brit. J. Derm. **67**, 165—179 (1955). — Johnsen, S. G., and J. E. Kirk: The number, distribution and size of the sebaceous glands in the dorsal region of the hand. Anat. Rec. **112**, 725—735 (1952).
Kallapravit, B.: Racial, age and regional differences in human sebaceous glands of the head and neck. Amer. J. phys. Anthropol. **21**, 121—133 (1963). — Kirk, E.: Quantitative determinations of the skin lipid secretion in middle-aged and old individuals. J. Geront. **3**, 251—266 (1948). — Kligman, A. M., and W. B. Shelley: An investigation of the biology of the human sebaceous gland. J. invest. Derm. **30**, 99—125 (1958). — Kölliker, A.: Über das Vorkommen von freien Talgdrüsen am Rothen Lippenrande des Menschen. Z. wiss. Zool. **11**, 341—343 (1862). — Koibuchi, S.: Quantitative Untersuchung der Anhangsorgane der Haut bei dem japanischen Kind. Folia anat. jap. **10**, 125—168 (1932). — Kosaka, Y.: Quantitative Untersuchung der Anhangsorgane der Haut bei einem japanischen Fetus. Folia anat. jap. **10**, 753—792 (1932). — Kurosumi, K., T. Kitamura, and K. Kano: Electron microscopy of the human sebaceous gland. Arch. histol. jap. **20**, 253—269 (1960). — Kvorning, S. A.: Investigations into the pharmacology of the skin fats and of ointments. II. On the occurrence and replenishment of fat on the skin in normal individuals. Acta pharmacol. (Kbh.) **5**, 262—269 (1949).
La Pava, S. de, and J. W. Pickren: Ectopic sebaceous glands in the esophagus. Arch. Path. **73**, 397—399 (1962). — Lobitz jr., W. C., D. Brophy, A. E. Larner, and F. Daniels jr.: Glycogen response in human epidermal basal cell. Arch. Derm. **86**, 207—211 (1962). Lobitz jr., W. C., and J. B. Holyoke: The histochemical response of the human epidermis

to controlled injury; glycogen. J. invest. Derm. 22, 189—195 (1954). — LUDFORD, R. J.: The cytology of tar tumors. Proc. roy. Soc. Med. B 98, 557—577 (1925).
MARGOLIES, A., and F. WEIDMAN: Statistical and histologic studies of Fordyce's disease. Arch. Derm. Syph. (Chic.) 3, 723—742 (1921). — MARTIN, E. A., and R. T. WALES: Sebaceous glands in the mouth. An investigation with particular reference to serum cholesterol and atherosclerosis. Irish J. med. Sci. 466, 481—486 (1964). — MELCZER, N., u. S. DEME: Beiträge zur Tätigkeit der menschlichen Talgdrüsen. I. Histologisch nachweisbare chemische Veränderungen während der Talgerzeugung. Dermatologica (Basel) 86, 24—36 (1942). — Beiträge zur Tätigkeit der menschlichen Talgdrüsen. I. Rolle und Formveränderungen des Golgi-Apparates während der Talgproduktion. Arch. Derm. Syph. (Berl.) 183, 388—395 (1943). — MESCON, H., and J. S. STRAUSS: Secondary histopathologic changes of the pilosebaceous unit. Arch. Derm. 81, 43—52 (1960). — MEZA-CHÁVEZ, L.: Sebaceous glands in normal and neoplastic parotid glands. Amer. J. Path. 25, 627—645 (1949). — MIESCHER, G., u. A. SCHÖNBERG: Untersuchungen über die Funktion der Talgdrüsen. Bull. schweiz. Akad. med. Wiss. 1, 101—114 (1944). — MILES, A. E. W.: Sebaceous glands in the lip and cheek mucosa of man. Brit. dent. J. 105, 235—248 (1958). — Sebaceous glands in oral and lip mucosa. In: Advances in biology of skin, vol. 4. The sebaceous glands (W. MONTAGNA, R. A. ELLIS and A. F. SILVER, eds.). Oxford: Pergamon Press 1963. — MONTAGNA, W.: Histology and cytochemistry of human skin. VIII. Mitochondria in the sebaceous glands. J. invest. Derm. 25, 117—121 (1955a). — Histology and cytochemistry of human skin. IX. The distribution of non-specific esterases. J. biophys. biochem. Cytol. 1, 13—16 (1955b). — Histology and cytochemistry of human skin. XI. The distribution of β-glucuronidase. J. biophys. biochem. Cytol. 3, 343—348 (1957). — The structure and function of skin, 2nd ed., p. 268—311. New York: Academic Press 1962. — The sebaceous glands in man. In: Advances in biology of skin, vol. 4. The sebaceous glands (W. MONTAGNA, R. A. ELLIS and A. F. SILVER, eds.). Oxford: Pergamon Press 1963. — Histology and cytochemistry of human skin. XXIV. Further observations on the axillary organ. J. invest. Derm. 42, 119—129 (1964). — Personal communication 1966. — MONTAGNA, W., H. B. CHASE, and J. B. HAMILTON: The distribution of glycogen and lipids in human skin. J. invest. Derm. 17, 147—157 (1951). — MONTAGNA, W., H. B. CHASE, and W. C. LOBITZ jr.: Histology and cytochemistry of human skin. II. The distribution of glycogen in the epidermis, hair follicles, sebaceous glands and eccrine sweat glands. Anat. Rec. 114, 231—248 (1952). — MONTAGNA, W., A. Z. EISEN, A. H. RADEMACHER, and H. B. CHASE: Histology and cytochemistry of human skin. VI. The distribution of sulfhydryl and disulfide groups. J. invest. Derm. 23, 23—32 (1954). — MONTAGNA, W., and R. A. ELLIS: Histology and cytochemistry of human skin. XII. Cholinesterases in the hair follicles of the scalp. J. invest. Derm. 29, 151—157 (1957a). — Histology and cytochemistry of human skin. XIII. The blood supply of the hair follicle. J. nat. Cancer Inst. 19, 451—463 (1957b). — L'histologie et la cytologie de la peau humaine. XVI. Répartition et concentration des estérases carboxyliques. Ann. Histochim. 3, 1—17 (1958). — Cholinergic innervation of the meibomian glands. Anat. Rec. 135, 121—128 (1959). — MONTAGNA, W., R. A. ELLIS, and A. F. SILVER: Advances in biology of skin, vol. 4. The sebaceous glands. Oxford: Pergamon Press 1963. — MONTAGNA, W., and V. FORMISANO: Histology and cytochemistry of human skin. VII. The distribution of succinic dehydrogenase activity. Anat. Rec. 122, 65—78 (1955). — MONTAGNA, W., C. R. NOBACK, and F. G. ZAK: Pigment, lipids, and other substances in the glands of the external auditory meatus of man. Amer. J. Anat. 83, 409—436 (1948). — MONTAGNA, W., and E. J. VAN SCOTT: The anatomy of the hair follicle. In: The biology of hair growth (W. MONTAGNA and R. A. ELLIS, eds.). New York: Academic Press 1958. — MONTAGNA, W., and J. S. YUN: Histology and cytochemistry of human skin. XXIII. The distribution of cytochrome oxidase. J. Histochem. Cytochem. 9, 694—698 (1961). — MORETTI, G., R. A. ELLIS, and H. MESCON: Vascular patterns in the skin of the face. J. invest. Derm. 33, 103—112 (1959). — MORETTI, G., and H. MESCON: Histochemical distribution of acid phosphatases in normal human skin. J. invest. Derm. 26, 347—360 (1956). — MORETTI, G., e W. MONTAGNA: Istologia e citochemica della cute umana. XVIII. Le unità vascolari. G. ital. Derm. 3, 243—254 (1959).
NASR, A. N.: Histochemical study of lipids in human sebaceous glands. J. Histochem. Cytochem. 13, 498—502 (1965). — NICOLAIDES, N.: Skin lipids. II. Lipid class composition of samples from various species and anatomical sites. J. amer. Oil Chem. Soc. 42, 691—702 (1965). — NICOLAIDES, N., and T. RAY: Skin lipids. III. Fatty chains in skin lipids. The use of *vernix caseosa* to differentiate between endogenous and exogenous components in human skin surface lipid. J. amer. Oil Chem. Soc. 42, 702—707 (1965). — NICOLAIDES, N., and G. C. WELLS: On the biogenesis of the free fatty acids in human skin surface fat. J. invest. Derm. 29, 423—433 (1957).
PALAY, S. L.: The morphology of secretion. In: Frontiers of cytology (S. L. PALAY, ed.), p. 322—325. New Haven: Yale University Press 1958. — PEACHEY, L. D.: Electron microscopic observations on the accumulation of divalent cations in intramitochondrial granules. J. Cell Biol. 20, 95—112 (1964). — PERKINS, O. C., and A. M. MILLER: Sebaceous glands in

the human nipple. Amer. J. Obstet. Gynec. 11, 789—794 (1926). — PINKUS, H.: Premalignant fibroepithelial tumors of skin. Arch. Derm. Syph. (Chic.) 67, 598—615 (1953). — POCHI, P. E., and J. S. STRAUSS: Sebaceous gland function before and after bilateral orchiectomy. Arch. Derm. 88, 729—731 (1963). — POCHI, P. E., and J. S. STRAUSS: Sebum production, casual sebum levels, titratable acidity of sebum, and urinary fractional 17-ketosteroid excretion in males with acne. J. invest. Derm. 43, 383—388 (1964). — POCHI, P. E., and J. S. STRAUSS: The effect of aging on the activity of the sebaceous gland in man. In: Advances in biology of skin, vol. 6. Aging (W. MONTAGNA, ed.). Oxford: Pergamon Press 1965. — POCHI, P. E., J. S. STRAUSS, and H. MESCON: Sebum secretion and urinary fractional 17-ketosteroid and total 17-hydroxycorticoid excretion in male castrates. J. invest. Derm. 39, 475—483 (1962). — The role of adrenocortical steroids in the control of human sebaceous gland activity. J. invest. Derm. 41, 391—399 (1963).

ROGERS, G. E.: Electron microscope observations on the structure of sebaceous glands. Exp. Cell Res. 13, 517—520 (1957). — RONY, H. R., and S. J. ZAKON: Effect of androgen on the sebaceous glands of human skin. Arch. Derm. Syph. (Chic.) 48, 601—604 (1943).

SASAKAWA, M.: Beiträge zur Glykogenverteilung in der Haut unter normalen und pathologischen Zuständen. Arch. Derm. Syph. (Berl.) 134, 418—443 (1921). — SCHOBER, B. (1954): Quoted by MILES 1963. — SCOTT, E. J. VAN, and R. C. MACCARDLE: Keratinization of the duct of the sebaceous gland and growth cycle of the hair follicle in the histogenesis of acne in human skin. J. invest. Derm. 27, 405—413 (1956). — SERRI, F., and W. H. HUBER: The development of sebaceous glands in man. In: Advances in biology of skin, vol. 4. The sebaceous glands (W. MONTAGNA, R. A. ELLIS and A. F. SILVER, eds.). Oxford: Pergamon Press 1963. — SHELLEY, W. B., S. B. COHEN, and G. B. KOELLE: Histochemical demonstration of monoamine oxidase in human skin. J. invest. Derm. 24, 561—565 (1955). — SMITH jr., J. G.: The aged human sebaceous gland. Arch. Derm. 80, 663—671 (1959). — SMITH, J. L.: The simultaneous staining of neutral fat and fatty acid by oxazine dyes. J. Path. Bact. 12, 1—4 (1908). — The staining of fat by Nile blue sulfate. J. Path. Bact. 15, 53—55 (1911). — STEIGLEDER, G. K.: Zum Verhalten der esterspaltenden Fermente in der Haut des behaarten Kopfes. Hautarzt 9, 67—71 (1958). — STEIGLEDER, G. K., u. H. LÖFFLER: Zum histochemischen Nachweis unspezifischer Esterasen und Lipasen. Arch. klin. exp. Derm. 203, 41—60 (1956). — STEIGLEDER, G. K., u. J. T. MCCARTHY: Strukturanalytische Untersuchungen an gesunder und kranker Haut unter besonderer Berücksichtigung der Hornschicht. Arch. klin. exp. Derm. 220, 8—18 (1964). — STRAUSS, J. S.: Response of the human sebaceous gland to experimental stress. J. Soc. cosmetic Chem. 10, 192—199 (1959). — STRAUSS, J. S., and A. M. KLIGMAN: Pathologic patterns of the sebaceous gland. J. invest. Derm. 30, 51—61 (1958). — The pathologic dynamics of acne vulgaris. Arch. Derm. 82, 779—790 (1960). — Effect of progesterone and progesterone-like compounds on the human sebaceous gland. J. invest. Derm. 36, 309—319 (1961). — STRAUSS, J. S., A. M. KLIGMAN, and P. E. POCHI: Effect of androgens and estrogens on human sebaceous glands. J. invest. Derm. 39, 139—155 (1962). — STRAUSS, J. S., and P. E. POCHI: The quantitative gravimetric determination of sebum production. J. invest. Derm. 36, 293—298 (1961). — The hormonal control of human sebaceous glands. In: Advances in biology of skin, vol. 4. The sebaceous glands (W. MONTAGNA, R. A. ELLIS and A. F. SILVER, eds.). Oxford: Pergamon Press 1963a. — The human sebaceous gland: its regulation by steroidal hormones and its use as an end organ for assaying androgenicity in vivo. Recent Progr. Hormone Res. 19, 385—444 (1963b). — Unpublished observations (1966). — SUSKIND, R. R.: The chemistry of the human sebaceous gland. I. Histochemical observations. J. invest. Derm. 17, 37—54 (1951).

TAKEUCHI, T.: Histochemical demonstration of branching enzyme (amylo-1,4-1,6 transglucosidase) in animal tissues. J. Histochem. Cytochem. 6, 208—216 (1958). — TANIGUCHI, T.: Quantitative Untersuchung der Anhangsorgane der Haut bei dem japanischen Neugeborenen. Folia anat. jap. 9, 215—265 (1931). — TANIGUCHI, T., Y. KOSAKA u. T. NAKANO: Quantitative Untersuchung der Anhangsorgane der Haut bei einem koreanischen Kind. Folia anat. jap. 11, 41—84 (1933). — THIES, W., u. L. F. GALENTE: Zur histochemischen Darstellung der Cholinesterasen im vegetativen Nervensystem der Haut. Hautarzt 8, 69—75 (1957).

WEITKAMP, A. W.: The acidic constituents of degras: a new method of structure elucidation. J. Amer. chem. Soc. 67, 447—454 (1945). — WEITKAMP, A. W., A. M. SMILJANIC, and S. ROTHMAN: The free fatty acids of human hair fat. J. Amer. chem. Soc. 69, 1936—1939 (1947).

YAMADA, K.: Quantitative Untersuchung der Anhangsorgane der Haut bei den Deutschen. Folia anat. jap. 10, 721—752 (1932). — YASUDA, K., and W. MONTAGNA: Histology and cytochemistry of human skin. XX. The distribution of monoamine oxidase. J. Histochem. Cytochem. 8, 356—366 (1960).

ZELIGMAN, I., and L. F. HUBENER: Experimental production of acne by progesterone. Arch. Derm. 76, 652—658 (1957).

Eccrine Sweat Glands: Electron Microscopy, Cytochemistry and Anatomy

By

Richard A. Ellis, Providence, Rhode Island, U.S.A.

With 23 Figures

Introduction

Although independent histological descriptions of the sweat glands were presented by PURKINJE and his pupil WENDT, in 1833, and by BRESCHET and ROUSSEL DE VAUZZENE, in 1834; it remained for SCHIEFFERDECHER (1917, 1922) to recognize that eccrine sweat glands were distinctly different from apocrine sweat glands. Now, when these structures are examined by modern cytological methods, the aptness of his designations is questionable since both types of sweat glands have a merocrine mode of secretion, but with some justification his terminology continues to be used (WEINER and HELLMAN, 1960). In man, the distinctions between eccrine and apocrine sweat glands are clear cut; they differ in their development, histology, fine structure, distribution, and in their function. The less versatile eccrine sweat glands serve principally in reducing body temperature by the production and surface evaporation of sweat; in moistening and lubricating the epidermis especially where it is greatly thickened; and in formation of sweat in response to emotional stimuli.

In man, sweat glands are particularly abundant in the plantar and volar surfaces of the hands and feet. Their tiny orifices dot the crests of the epidermal ridges that give dermatoglyphics their pattern. These sweat pores are scarcely visible to the naked eye, but they may be seen readily under low power magnification. It was MALPHIGI who first reported seeing clear watery droplets collecting at these orifices, and he concluded that these were the openings of sweat glands. In recent years, simple but elegant techniques have been developed for the visualization of sweat as it is secreted onto the surface of the skin, and these methods are extremely useful in revealing the numbers of active sweat glands in a given area of skin (WADA and TAKAGAKI, 1948; PAPA, 1963). The openings of the sweat glands at the skin surface (Fig. 1) may also be replicated and examined with the electron microscope (SARKANY and CARON, 1965).

Eccrine sweat glands are distributed over most of the body surface of man. Only the lips, the glans penis, the inner surface of the prepuce, the clitoris, and the labia minora are free of them (MONTAGNA, 1962a). In most of the remainder of the body skin eccrine sweat glands are admixed with apocrine sweat glands, although eccrine sweat glands predominate (PINKUS, 1927). Only eccrine sweat glands are present in the volar and plantar skin. Since sweat glands are not formed after birth, the original density of the sweat gland population is the same in all body regions. During the growth period of the body surface, they become spaced further apart in the fast growing regions of the trunk and the extremities than in the relatively slow expanding face (SZABO, 1962). From counts on twenty areas of skin on thirty-five adults KAWAHATA (1950) calculated that the skin of man contains 1.6 to 4.0 million sweat glands. KUNO (1956) estimates that human beings have from two to five million glands; while SZABO (1962) judges that there are approximately three million glands in the skin of a twenty-four year old man. Furthermore, SZABO finds that the eccrine sweat glands are the dominant skin

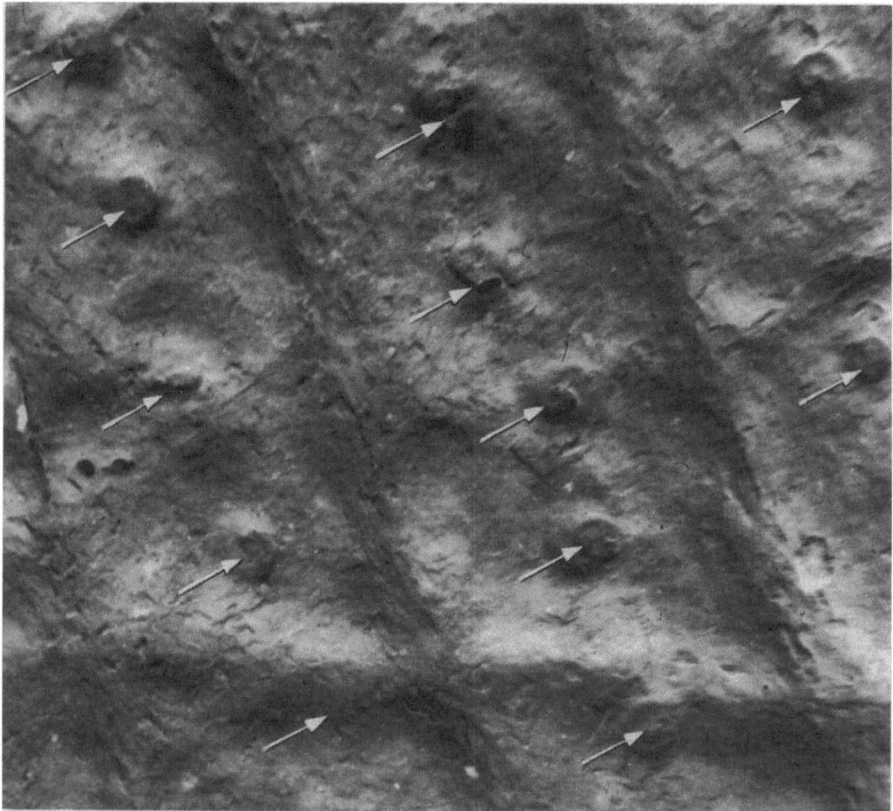

Fig. 1. In this electron micrograph of a shadowed replica of the skin surface, the spiraled openings of the epidermal sweat duct are demonstrated clearly along the crests of the epidermal ridges (arrows). This excellent preparation was kindly provided by I. SARKANY, M.R.C.P. (SARKANY and CARON, 1965). × 70

appendages, even outnumbering the hair follicles. In the adult, sweat glands are most numerous in the sole of the foot (620/cm^2) and the least abundant in the skin of the thigh 120/cm^2). The other regions of the body have population densities that fall between these two extremes.

I. Development of the Eccrine Sweat Glands

In man, the development of eccrine sweat glands is dyschronous in the body skin. Anlagen appear first, during the fourth month of fetal life, in the skin of the palms and soles. Early in the fifth fetal month anlagen of eccrine sweat glands make their appearance in the skin of the axilla; and later during the fifth fetal month they start developing in other regions of the skin (HORSTMANN, 1957). Thus, according to their developmental sequence the sweat glands fall into three broad groups: those in the glabrous skin of the palms and sole, those that together with large apocrine sweat glands constitute the axillary organ, and those that are distributed throughout the general body skin. In the general body skin the development of the eccrine sweat glands is also dyschronous, since the sweat glands are formed first in the forehead and scalp and appear later over the rest of the body. KUNO (1956) speculates that the eccrine sweat glands that form first

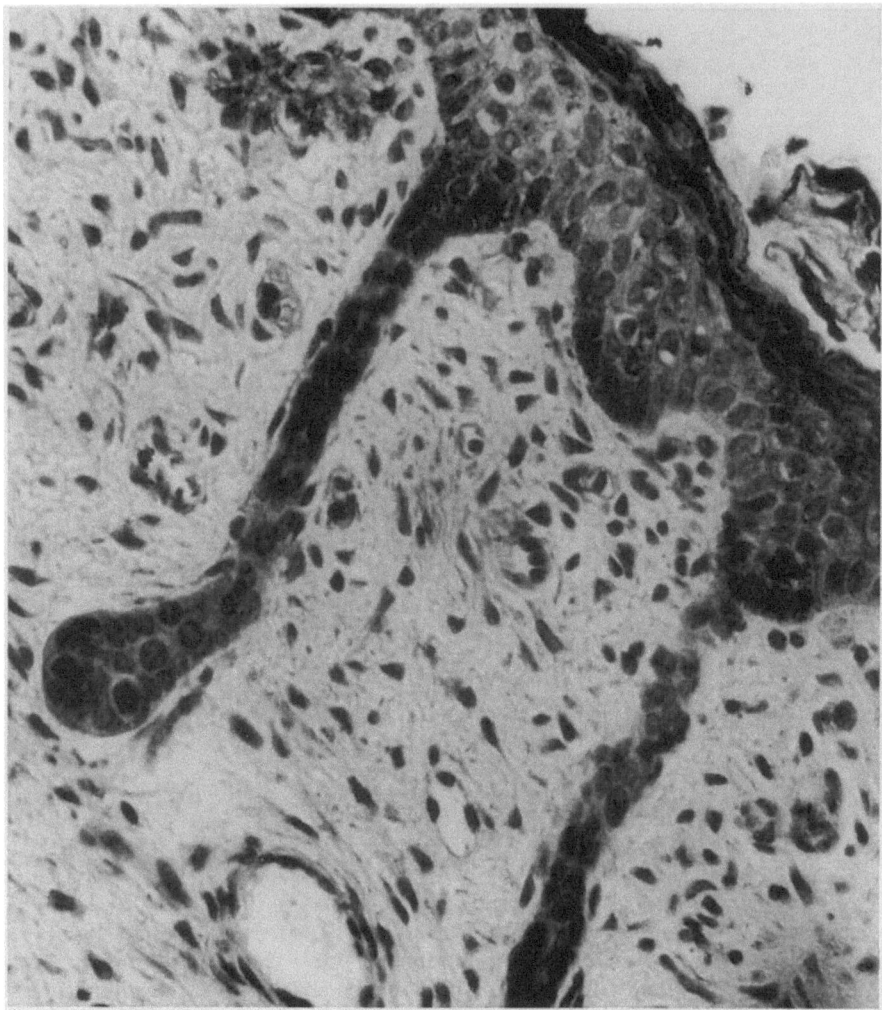

Fig. 2. The eccrine sweat glands in the finger of a 3 month old fetus consist of a cord of epithelial cells growing downward from the epidermis and a clavate end that will eventually develop into the coiled duct and the secretory coil. × 320

during fetal life may arise from a more primitive stem than those that develop later. There is some evidence that the development of the glands may be dependent upon their nerve supply, since in man as soon as the eccrine sweat glands are formed in the fetus they are associated with nerves rich in cholinesterase (BECKETT et al., 1956).

Between the thirteenth and nineteenth week of fetal life generative buds of cells appear and grow downward from the underside of the epidermal ridges on the hand and foot. The anlagen of the sweat glands are not restricted to the volar surfaces, but are also present at this time on the nail folds, the eponychium, and on the entire dorsal surface of the distal phalanx (MONTAGNA, 1962a). The anlagen for the eccrine sweat glands begin as small local condensations along the basal layer of epidermal cells (PINKUS, 1927): they are somewhat smaller and narrower

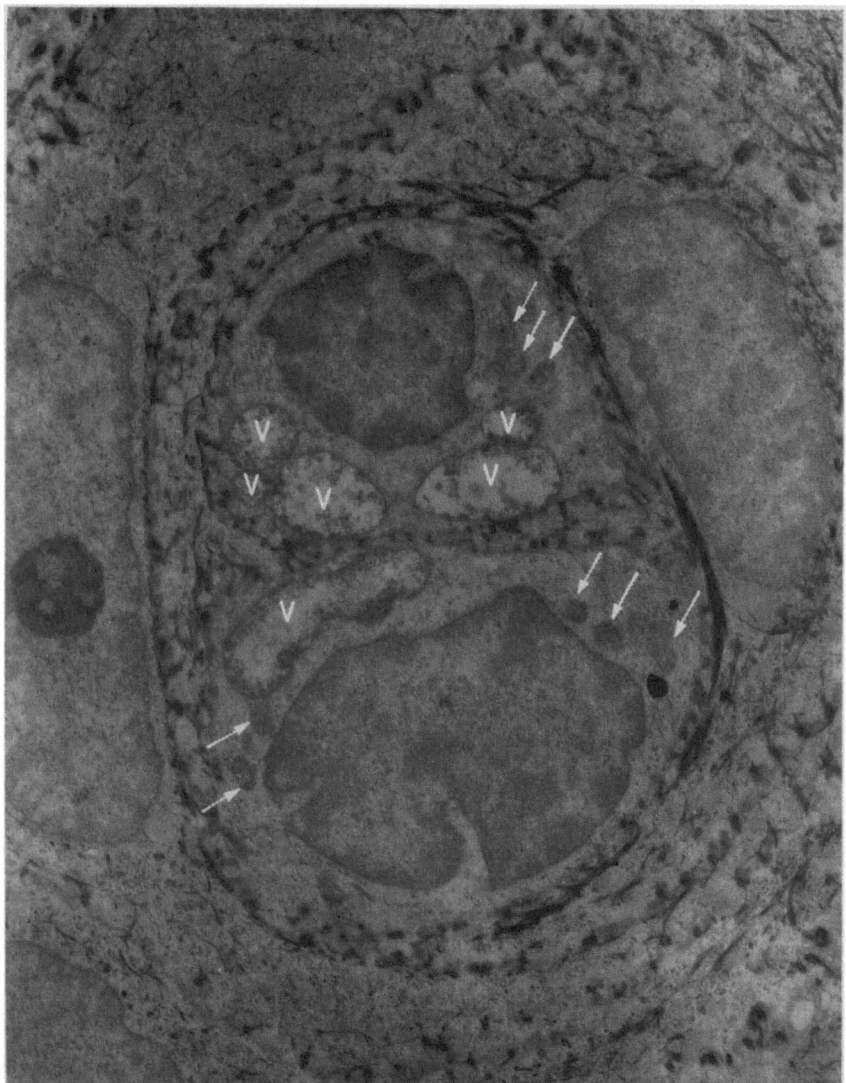

Fig. 3. Early stage (16 week old embryo) in development of lumen of epidermal sweat duct. Vacuoles (*V*) of different sizes have formed within the cytoplasm of two apposed luminal cells. The lysosomes (arrows) in the luminal cells contain small vesicles identical with those inside the large, coalescing vacuoles. × 8,500. This electron micrograph was kindly provided by K. HASHIMOTO, M.D. (HASHIMOTO et al., 1965)

than the anlagen of hair follicles and they do not have clumps of dermal papilla cells at their bases. The small club-shaped mass of mitotically active epithelial cells migrates quite rapidly toward the hypodermis leaving in its course a cord of cells that connect it to the overlying epidermis (Fig. 2). Glycogen is abundant in the cells that comprise the cord, but the cells at its swollen end contain almost none. At or near the level of the hypodermis the cells in the clavate stump of the anlagen continue to divide and form a column of epithelial cells that is tortuous, twisted and glomerate.

In embryos 14 to 15 weeks old the anlagen of the sweat glands have penetrated deep into the dermis and they have begun to form coils (HASHIMOTO et al., 1965).

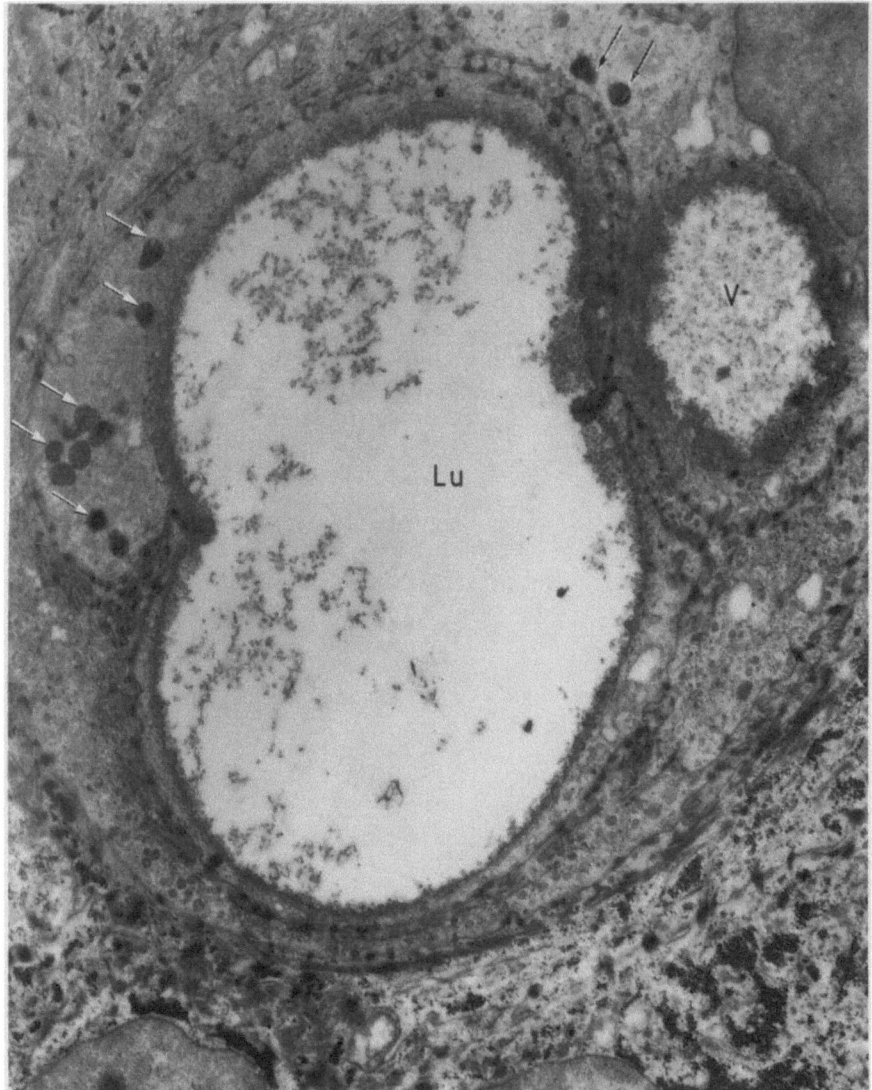

Fig. 4. Later stage (16 week old embryo) in the development of the lumen of the epidermal sweat duct. A large central cavity, the presumptive lumen (*Lu*), has formed through the fusion of vesicles in two apposed luminal cells. A large vacuole (*V*) within a third luminal cell has not yet fused with its neighbor. Lysosomes (arrows) are prominent in the cytoplasm of the luminal cells and clumps of glycogen are conspicuous in the surrounding squamous cells. × 8,500. This electron micrograph was kindly provided by K. HASHIMOTO, M.D. (HASHIMOTO et al., 1965)

At the base of the epidermis each sweat duct consists of a column of cells with two distinct layers. The innermost cells are readily identified by the numerous large dense vacuoles that contain small lucent vesicles surrounded by an amorphous osmiophilic substance. Since the anlagen contain an abundance of hydrolytic enzymes, both acid phosphatase and esterases, it seems likely that these dense vacuoles are lysosomal in nature. They appear within the central cells of the duct only during the period that the lumen of the duct is being established, but they are found in the luminal cells of the intraepidermal duct even in the adult. In the

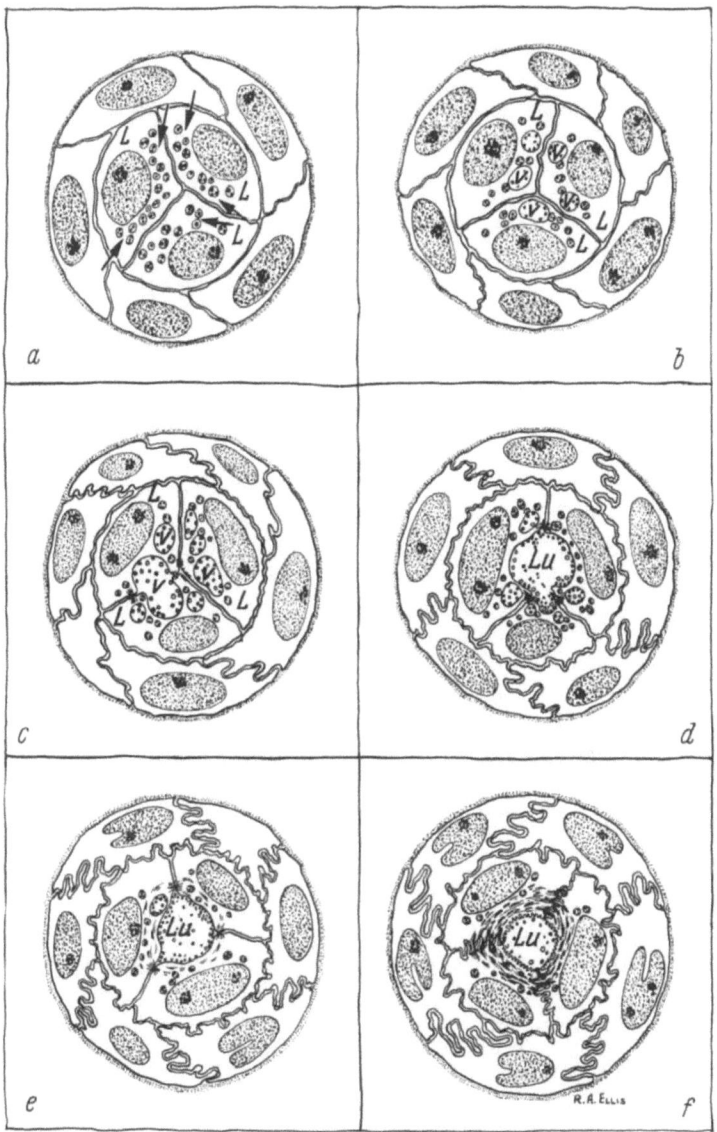

Fig. 5a—f. Diagram showing steps in the formation of the lumen of an epidermal sweat duct. a lysosomes (arrows) in unmodified luminal cells (*L*); b formation of vacuoles (*V*) within luminal cells through autolytic activity of lysosomes; c fusion of vacuoles within luminal cells and between apposed cells; d fusion of vacuoles of apposed cells and establishment of presumptive lumen (*Lu*); e completion of lumen and early formation of cuticular border; f final form of duct, lumen, and fibrous cuticular border with some lysosomes still evident in superficial cells. Diagrammatic interpretation of data presented by HASHIMOTO et al., 1965

early stages of lumen formation, intracytoplasmic cavities are formed within the central cells by local dissolution of the cytoplasm (HASHIMOTO et al., 1965). Since the same small vesicles that appear within dense vacuoles are also present in the smallest intracytoplasmic cavities, the large dense vacuoles are probably the foci

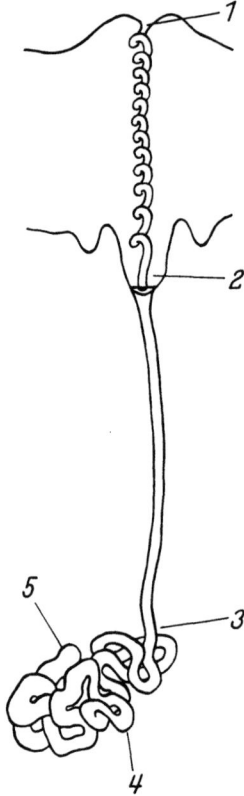

Fig. 6. Diagram of an eccrine sweat gland in the palm of man. Segment 1—2 is the intraepidermal sweat duct; segment 2—3 the straight duct; segment 3—4 the coiled duct and segment 4—5 the terminal secretory coil

for cytoplasmic dissolution (Fig. 3). The intracytoplasmic cavities enlarge through coalescence with one another and by fusion with adjacent dense vacuoles (Fig. 4). The intracytoplasmic cavities of adjoining cells then fuse, eventually forming a continuous lumen surrounded by an inner layer of superficial cells and an outer column of basal cells (Fig. 5). The lumen of the intraepidermal duct is thus established, and by the twenty-second week of fetal life it resembles closely that of the adult (HASHIMOTO et al., 1965).

By the end of the sixth fetal month, the coiled segment is fully formed and the club end of the anlagen is no longer apparent. Later, during the seventh and eighth fetal months, vacuoles appear within the cells lining the distal glomerate portion of the sweat gland. These vacuoles gradually coalesce to form a lumen that becomes continuous with that of the duct. Since not all of the glands develop synchronously these events do not proceed apace; but by the end of the eighth fetal month all of the eccrine sweat glands of the plantar and volar surfaces are hollow, having a continuous lumen along their entire length. The lumen broadens during the eighth month and the presumptive secretory cells take on some of the typical characteristics of the cells in adult glands (TSUCHIYA, 1954). In their final form the eccrine sweat glands of man are simple, coiled, tubular structures embedded in the dermis and opening onto the surface of the skin. The tubules are divisible into four distinct segments: the terminal secretory portion, the coiled duct, the straight duct and the intraepidermal duct (Fig. 6).

II. The Secretory Tubule

The secretory tubule is composed of three distinct cell types: peripheral myoepithelial cells, clear serous cells, and dark mucous cells (Fig. 7). Although these constituents of the secretory coil are described and discussed separately, they are closely integrated in both form and function.

1. Myoepithelial Cells

Within the secretory segment of the eccrine sweat glands of man, the myoepithelial cells form an incomplete pavement upon which the secretory cells rest (Fig. 7). The myoepithelial cells are elongate and sometimes branched; the thickest region of the cell is near the nucleus, with the cell tapering and flattening toward the poles of the long axis. The cells are aligned more or less parallel to the course of the secretory tubule (BUNTING et al., 1948) and they are loosely dovetailed with short gaps between most of the cells. At some sites myoepithelial cells adjoin one another. Binucleate myoepithelial cells are encountered occasionally even with the electron microscope, suggesting that this condition is not unusual (ELLIS, 1965). The nucleus is always displaced toward the apex of the cell and although somewhat ovate in shape, it is not obviously flattened or compressed by the underlying filamentous cytoplasm. In some cells, however, that have been sectioned longitudinally through the nucleus, the nuclear envelope may undulate, in a form

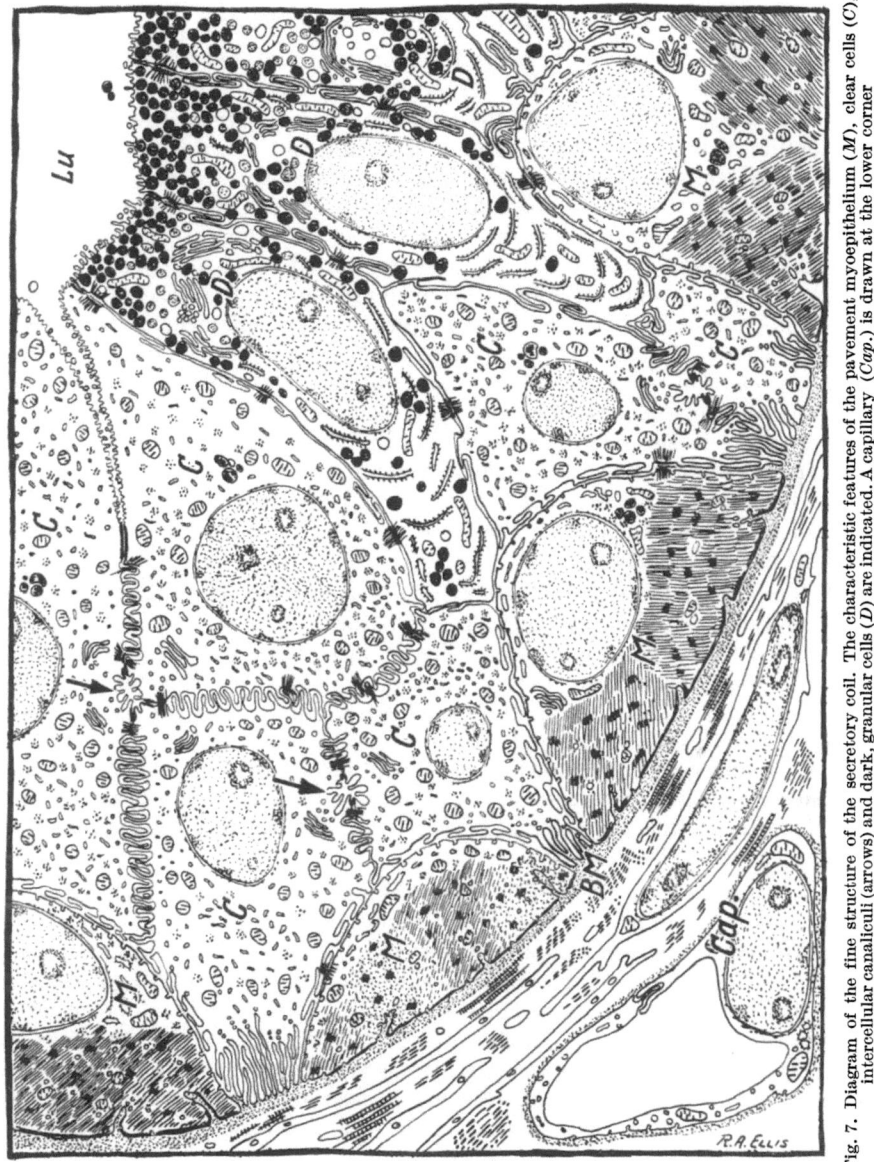

Fig. 7. Diagram of the fine structure of the secretory coil. The characteristic features of the pavement myoepithelium (*M*), clear cells (*C*), intercellular canaliculi (arrows) and dark, granular cells (*D*) are indicated. A capillary (*Cap.*) is drawn at the lower corner

similar to that observed in the nuclei of smooth muscle cells that have been fixed in a contractile state. This suggests that the form of the nucleus of the myoepithelial cells may be altered similarly during cell contraction.

a) Electron Microscopy

Dense masses of myofilaments fill most of the cytoplasm of the myoepithelial cell. The filaments are usually restricted to areas lateral and basal to the nucleus while the other cytoplasmic organelles are concentrated in the perinuclear cytoplasm and in a thin layer beneath the apical plasma membrane. Thin columns of unmodified cytoplasm also penetrate intermittently among the myofilaments and these may bear profiles of smooth surfaced endoplasmic reticulum, glycogen granules, and long, filamentous mitochondria (ELLIS, 1965).

The base of each myoepithelial cell is irregularly serrated (Fig. 8). Along the outer surface the basal invaginations are usually filled with the same dense amorphous substance that forms the adepithelial or basement membrane. The inner profile of the basement membrane that follows the basal contours of the myoepithelial cells is sculptured, but the outermost surface of the basement membrane is smooth. The amorphous substance thus forms a smoother outer sleeve of variable thickness around the secretory coil (Fig. 8). Loosely layered fibrocytes, masses of collagen fibers and unmyelinated nerve fibers lie external to the adepithelial membrane. Along the invaginations in the base of the myoepithelium, pits or caveoli are found frequently; the cell surface may also be closely associated with profiles of the endoplasmic reticulum suggesting continuity at these sites. The remainder of the basal surface of the plasma membrane is associated with cytoplasmic zones of high electron density (Fig. 8). The dense zones are more or less homogeneous and may serve as attachment sites for the myofilaments since many of the filaments seem to terminate in these regions. They are strikingly similar to the dense bands observed among the fibrillar masses. The dense zones are never found in the same regions where pits or caveoli appear along the plasma membrane.

The apical surface of the myoepithelial cell is nearly smooth, bears very few villous processes or folds, and seldom interdigitates with the elaborately folded surfaces of the adjacent secretory cells (Fig. 8). Pits, that are cup-shaped and have a central cavity nearly twice the diameter of the apical opening line the apical surface and seem identical with similar structures found along the plasma membranes of smooth muscle and endothelial cells. The pits or caveoli are all of the same size and shape and contain a substance of moderate electron density; these structures are entirely absent from the plasma membranes of the clear and dark secretory cells so this character alone serves to distinguish myoepithelial from secretory elements (ELLIS, 1965).

Myoepithelial cells contact each other infrequently, but where such contact is made the cell surfaces may be bonded by a tight junction or nexus, similar in form to that observed between smooth muscle cells. In these areas, too, occasional desmosomes may be seen joining adjacent myoepithelial cells. Gaps between neighboring myoepithelial cells are usually filled with the basal processes of interposed clear cells (Fig. 9). In these regions the surfaces of the clear cells are elaborately folded and intermeshed; here also originates a highly developed system of intercellular canaliculi (Fig. 9). A close relationship therefore exists between the basal, absorptive surfaces of the clear cells and the pavement myoepithelium.

In the perinuclear cytoplasm, in a thin rim of cytoplasm beneath the apical plasma membrane, and in the restricted cores of cytoplasm that penetrate the myofilaments are found the principal cytoplasmic organelles (Fig. 8). Coarse glycogen granules, variable in abundance, may appear separately or clumped in rosettes. Profiles of smooth endoplasmic reticulum (SER) appear both as irregular dilated cisternae and as small vesicles. The reticular structure of the SER is best visualized in the perinuclear cytoplasm, but individual components of this system also penetrate among the myofilaments (Fig. 10). Some myoepithelial cells have rough endoplasmic reticulum (RER) while others do not. When present, it is usually restricted to the perinuclear and apical zones and is not characteristic of the cytoplasmic cores penetrating the fibrillar areas. A Golgi apparatus with typical fine structure is not pervasive but occupies a supranuclear position. The mitochondria vary somewhat in size and shape according to their disposition

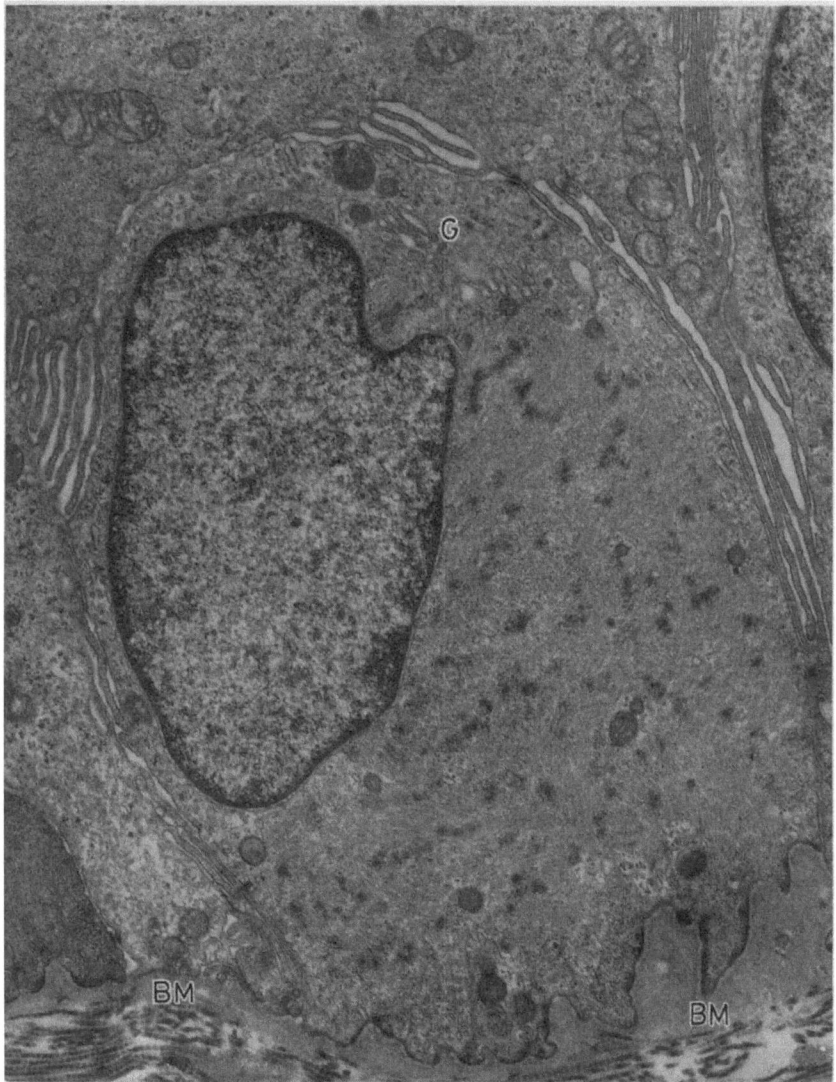

Fig. 8. A myoepithelial cell in cross-section bordered by the villous processes of clear cells. The serrated base of the cell rests on the basement membrane (*BM*). Myofilaments and dense zones fill most of the cytoplasm and a prominent Golgi zone (*G*) appears near the nucleus. × 16,200

within the cell, but they usually appear as long slender rods. They have a very dense matrix, the pseudomatrix of the cristae is frequently dilated and its contents are less electron dense than that of the true matrix. The cristae are oriented at right angles to the long axis of the mitochondrion and intramitochondrial granules are seldom present. Irregularly shaped particles of lipid and pigment, identified as lipofuchsin, are highly variable in their size and electron density, and they are not bounded by membranes. Small vesicles enclosing a dense granular substance are encountered occasionally and are presumed to be lysosomes.

The bulk of the cytoplasmic mass of the myoepithelial cell is filled with myofilaments that are oriented more or less parallel to the long axis of the secretory coil. Masses of myofilaments share a common orientation but various masses within a single cell may run in somewhat different directions. In cross-section the

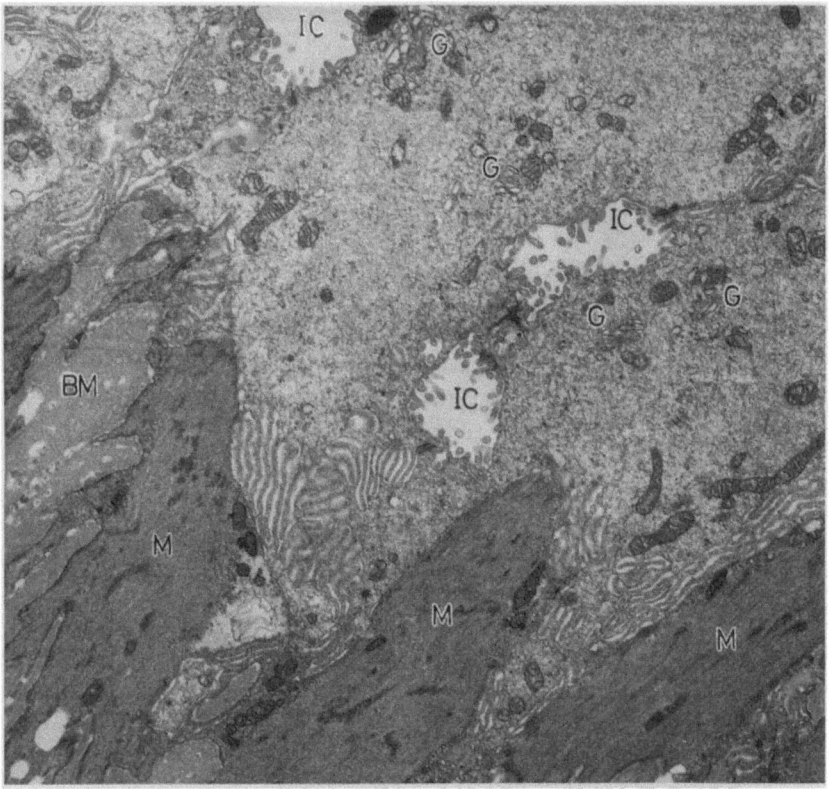

Fig. 9. In a section tangential to the secretory coil, the basal portions of several myoepithelial cells and clear cells are shown. Interdigitating folds at the bases of the clear cells fill the gaps in the myoepithelium. Three intercellular canaliculi (*IC*) and several Golgi zones (*G*) are distinguishing features of the clear cells. × 7,000

myofilaments appear as discrete spots approximately 50 Å in diameter; they are spaced irregularly and are mingled with a somewhat less dense amorphous substance that connects the dense filaments randomly. These components are all embedded in a matrix of low electron density. In the dense zones myofilaments and the amorphous substance predominate and the myofilaments are arranged more precisely in a pattern similar to that observed in the Z-band of striated skeletal muscle. In longitudinal section the myofilaments show parallel alignment, but individual filaments may be followed only for a short distance before they pass out of the plane of the section, suggesting that they are part of a meshwork (Fig. 9). Some myofilaments have a wavy appearance, and in some regions, especially where filament masses with different orientation converge on each other, they may criss-cross randomly. The myofilaments are of the same size as the F-actin filaments that have been identified in various types of smooth and striated muscle. The structure of the dense zones in the filamentous masses indicates that they are probably equivalent to the Z-bands of striated muscle (Fig. 8). The organization of the contractile apparatus of the myoepithelial cell seems, therefore, to be identical to the structure of the combined I and Z bands of striated muscle (FRANZINI-ARMSTRONG and PORTER, 1964).

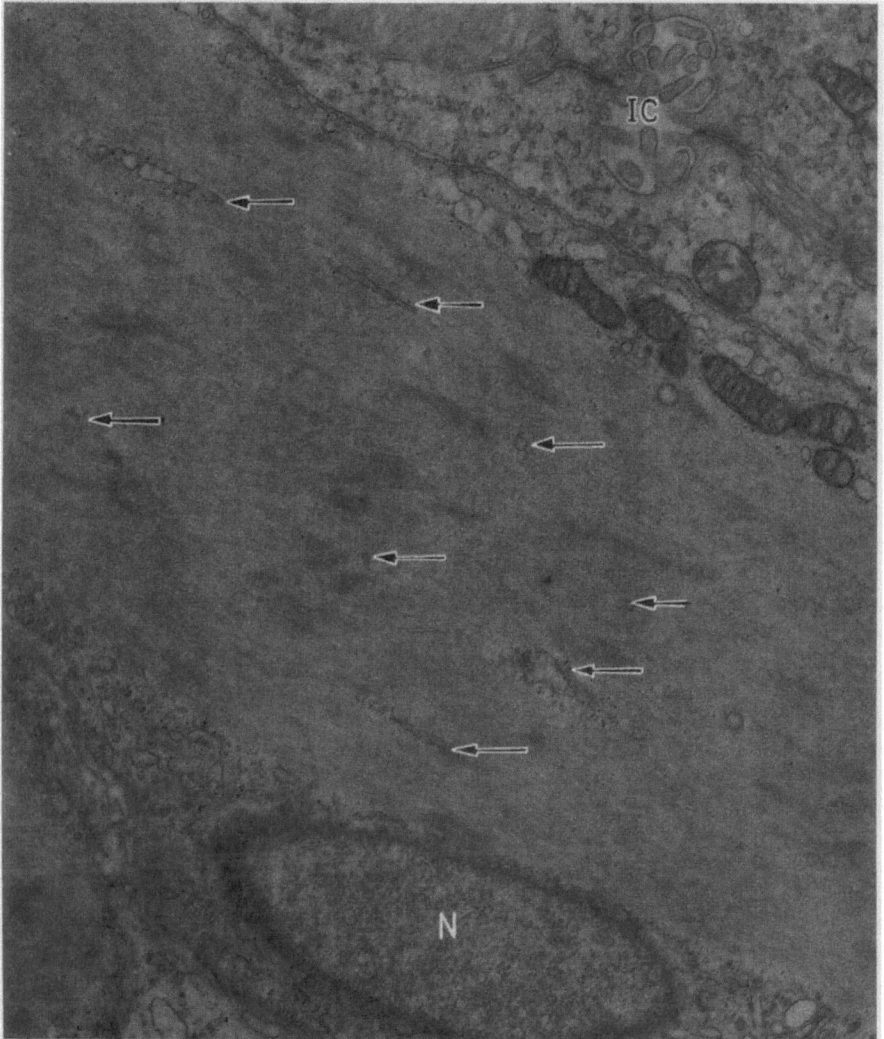

Fig. 10. In longitudinal section, smooth-membraned structures, dense glycogen granules and mitochondria (arrows) penetrate the masses of myofilaments. An intercellular canaliculus (*IC*) formed between two adjacent clear cells shows typical structure. Profiles of SER are obvious in the cytoplasm of the clear cells. × 18,000

b) Cytochemistry

The cytoplasm of myoepithelial cells is acidophilic. The oriented myofilaments that are anistropic under polarized light may be stained with phosphotungstic acid hematoxylin, with Regaud's hematoxylin and with Heidenhain's iron hematoxylin (MONTAGNA, 1962a).

The low reactivity of these cells for cytochrome oxidase (BRAUN-FALCO, 1961) and succinic dehydrogenase (BRAUN-FALCO and RATHJENS, 1954; MONTAGNA and

FORMISANO, 1955; SERRI, 1955) correlates well with the sparse numbers of mitochondria that populate them. The presence of delicate glycogen granules demonstrated within the cytoplasm by periodic acid Schiff staining is also confirmed with electron microscopy. Amylophosphorylase is consistently found in high concentration within the myoepithelium (BRAUN-FALCO, 1956a; ELLIS and MONTAGNA, 1958; YASUDA et al., 1958) and may be correlated with the glycogen and SER found in these cells. Esterase activity (MONTAGNA and ELLIS, 1958b) is probably associated with the lipid and lipofuchsin content of the cells as well as with the dense granules that are presumed to be lysosomes. Both sulfhydryl and disulfide groups are particularly concentrated in the myoepithelial cells (MONTAGNA et al., 1954). In the eccrine sweat glands of the rat foot pad, MATSUZAWA and KUROSUMI (1963) have reported that both alkaline phosphatase and adenosine triphosphatase are localized within the pits along the surface of the myoepithelial cell. These enzymes probably occupy similar sites in the eccrine sweat gland of man. In contrast to the secretory cells, the myoepithelium is only weakly reactive for monoamine oxidase (YASUDA and MONTAGNA, 1960).

c) Function

Both physiologists and morphologists consider the myoepithelial cells as contractile elements, and the same drugs that stimulate contraction in smooth muscle also induce myoepithelial contraction. The function of the myoepithelial cells in eccrine sweat glands is, however, not clear cut. HURLEY and WITKOWSKI (1961a, b) showed that after the intradermal injection of methylene blue, stimulation of the eccrine sweat glands with epinephrine resulted in the new formation of eccrine sweat and "not simply expulsion of preformed or pooled sweat by the myoepithelium". They concluded that in the eccrine sweat glands "the role of the myoepithelium as a primary or accessory force in the delivery of the sweat to the skin surface following its secretion is still not clear". Developmental studies show that eccrine sweat production in the rat parallels the cytodifferentiation of the secretory cell rather than the myoepithelial cell (MATSUZAWA and KUROSUMI, 1963). The close association between the clear cells and the myoepithelial cells in human eccrine sweat glands suggests that these two cell types may function in concert. Contraction of individual cells in the discontinuous myoepithelial pavement may serve to open wider the gaps between cells and expose a much broader surface of the highly folded base of the interposed clear cells to the extracellular fluid. In this way the myoepithelial cells could act as valves indirectly controlling the flow of sweat by regulating the area of the secretory cell exposed to the extracellular fluid (ELLIS, 1965).

In addition to their contractile function, the heterogeneity of structure observed among myoepithelial cells indicates a high number of cell activities. The pits lining the plasma membrane may be specialized receptor sites or they may be correlated with pinocytotic activity. Some cells have local concentrations of RER suggesting the synthesis of proteins for export. In other cells the Golgi zone is very conspicuous indicating that it is involved perhaps in synthetic or secretory processes. Some cells are binucleate others are interconnected by conjoined membranes. The cytoplasm of some cells is nearly filled with massed myofilaments while in others as much as one-half of the cytoplasmic space appears to be afilamentous. Such variability in the cell population shows that the myoepithelial cells are not engaged only in contraction but also in other diverse activities such as pinocytosis, cell division, the production of basement membrane or intercellular substances and impulse transmission (ELLIS, 1965).

2. Clear Cells

Observations from both light and electron microscopy indicate that under normal conditions there are approximately equal numbers of clear cells and dark cells within the secretory coil (MONTAGNA, 1962a). The clear cells are readily distinguished from myoepithelial cells and dark cells since they contain no myofilaments or secretory granules, they have elaborately folded basal membranes and they border on the intercellular canaliculi (HIBBS, 1958; KUROSUMI, 1958; CHARLES, 1960; MUNGER, 1961; ELLIS, 1962). The clear cells rest either directly upon the basement membrane that surrounds the secretory coil or upon the myoepithelial pavement. They are generally broader at the base than at the apex. The apical surface of the clear cell that borders the lumen of the secretory coil is often restricted by the overlying dark cells. The nucleus lies near the center of the cell, it is usually ovoid or round and shows no evidence of deformation during the secretory process.

Although mitotic activity is reported to be rare in the cells of the secretory tubules (BUNTING et al., 1948; HOLYOKE and LOBITZ, 1952) cell division is occasionally observed among the clear cells (MONTAGNA, 1962a). Apparently mitosis is not stimulated in the clear cells by repeated episodes of profuse sweating in either salt-loaded or salt-depleted subjects (DOBSON, 1962). Instead, in the salt-depleted subjects, fusion of some adjacent clear cells is reported to occur followed by a slow return to their normal cytology as the stress is continued.

a) Electron Microscopy

Along the base of the clear cell the plasma membrane is plicated, forming long villous folds (Figs. 9 and 11). The folds of adjacent clear cells interdigitate with each other in a regular pattern and the intercellular spaces between them are extremely irregular in width (MUNGER, 1961; ELLIS, 1962). This suggests true intercellular spaces may exist between the cells, and that extracellular coating substances may be sandwiched between them. Where the clear cells rest upon underlying myoepithelial cells the villous processes are flattened against the smooth surface of the myoepithelium. Where two clear cells abut intercellular canaliculi are often present between them (MUNGER, 1961; ELLIS, 1962). At these sites the interdigitating villous processes are interrupted by typical continuous junctional complexes that delimit the intercellular canaliculus (Figs. 9 and 11). The surfaces of two or sometimes three clear cells may border a single canaliculus. The microvilli lining the surface of each canaliculus are much stubbier than the folds that cover the base of the clear cell (Figs. 9, 11, and 12).

The typical junctional complex with the zonula occludens adjoining the lumen of the intercellular canaliculus, furnishes proof that the intercellular canaliculus represents the luminal surface of the cell. The villous folds at the basal and lateral surfaces of the cell form the absorptive surface of the cell. The canaliculi take their origin near the basement membrane and are already prominent only a few millimicrons within the secretory epithelium (Fig. 9). They are not necessarily straight and sometimes form a branching system.

In some biopsy specimens of eccrine sweat glands the secretory cells are reported by light microscopy to be riddled with evenly spaced "vacuoles" that contain neither lipid nor glycogen (HOLYOKE and LOBITZ, 1952). Under the electron microscope this configuration is present in glands that are actively secreting and the "vacuoles" are the dilated intracellular canaliculi whose contents are similar in structure and in electron density to the material found in the lumen of the secretory coil.

Intracellular canaliculi have been reported within the clear cells in both light (MONTAGNA et al., 1952, 1953; BUNTING et al., 1948) and electron microscopic (CHARLES, 1960; SCOTT, 1960) studies. Improved methods now indicate that such observations result from sectioning artifact, and that the canalicular profiles that appear within clear cells result from tangential cuts through the curved intercellular canaliculi (Fig. 12).

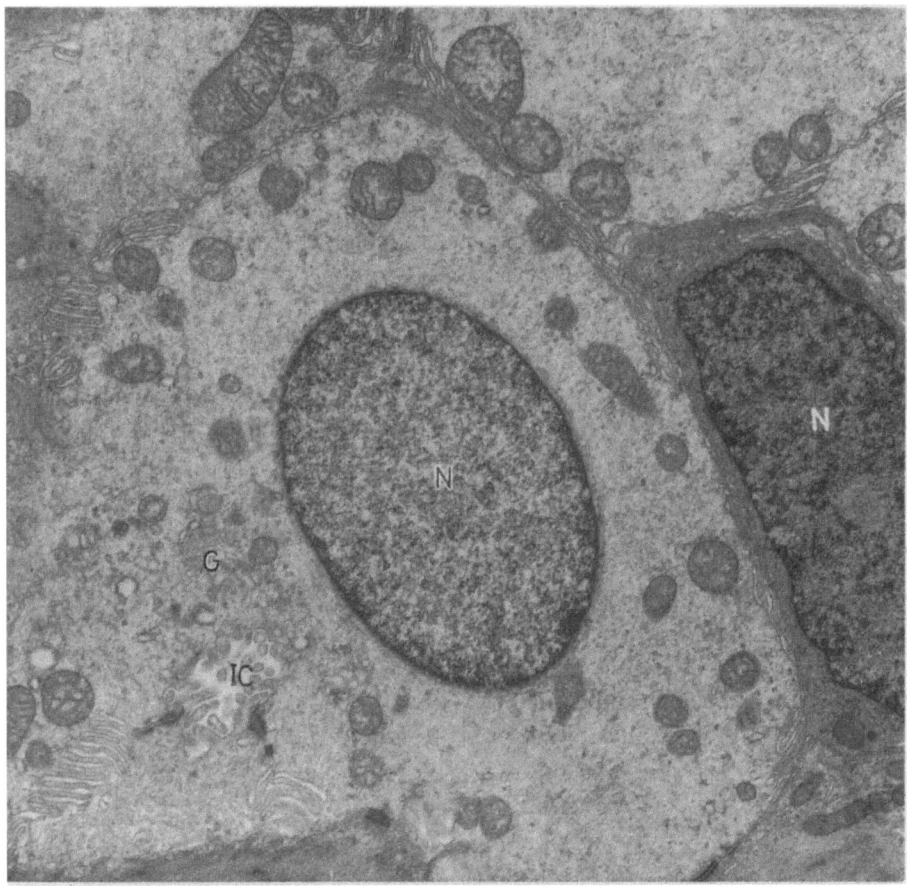

Fig. 11. Typical ultrastructural features of a clear cell are revealed in this electron micrograph. Variation in the character of the cell border is especially obvious. The nucleus and surrounding dense cytoplasm of a dark cell is shown at the lower center. Parts of two myoepithelial cells appear at the right. An intercellular canaliculus (*IC*), an adjacent Golgi zone (*G*), randomly distributed mitochondria and an ovate nucleus characterize the clear cell.
× 12,500

Wherever clear cells adjoin dark cells, the plasma membrane of the clear cell may be fashioned in a variety of patterns (Figs. 11 and 12). Rarely the surfaces of clear and dark cells are interfolded, more commonly the surface of the clear cell is thrown into villous folds and these are flattened against the smooth surface of the dark cells. At some sites the surfaces of both cells are smooth and the plasma membranes are apposed closely.

The apical surface of the clear cell may border the lumen of the secretory coil, but usually the exposed surface is restricted by overlying dark cells. Where the clear cell does extend inward to the lumen its surface membrane is smooth except for a few short, protruding microvilli. Specialization of the cell surface is least spectacular at this interface of the clear cell.

The cytoplasm of the clear cells is often permeated with glycogen in the form of coarse particles clustered in rosettes (Figs. 11, 12 and 13). The granules of

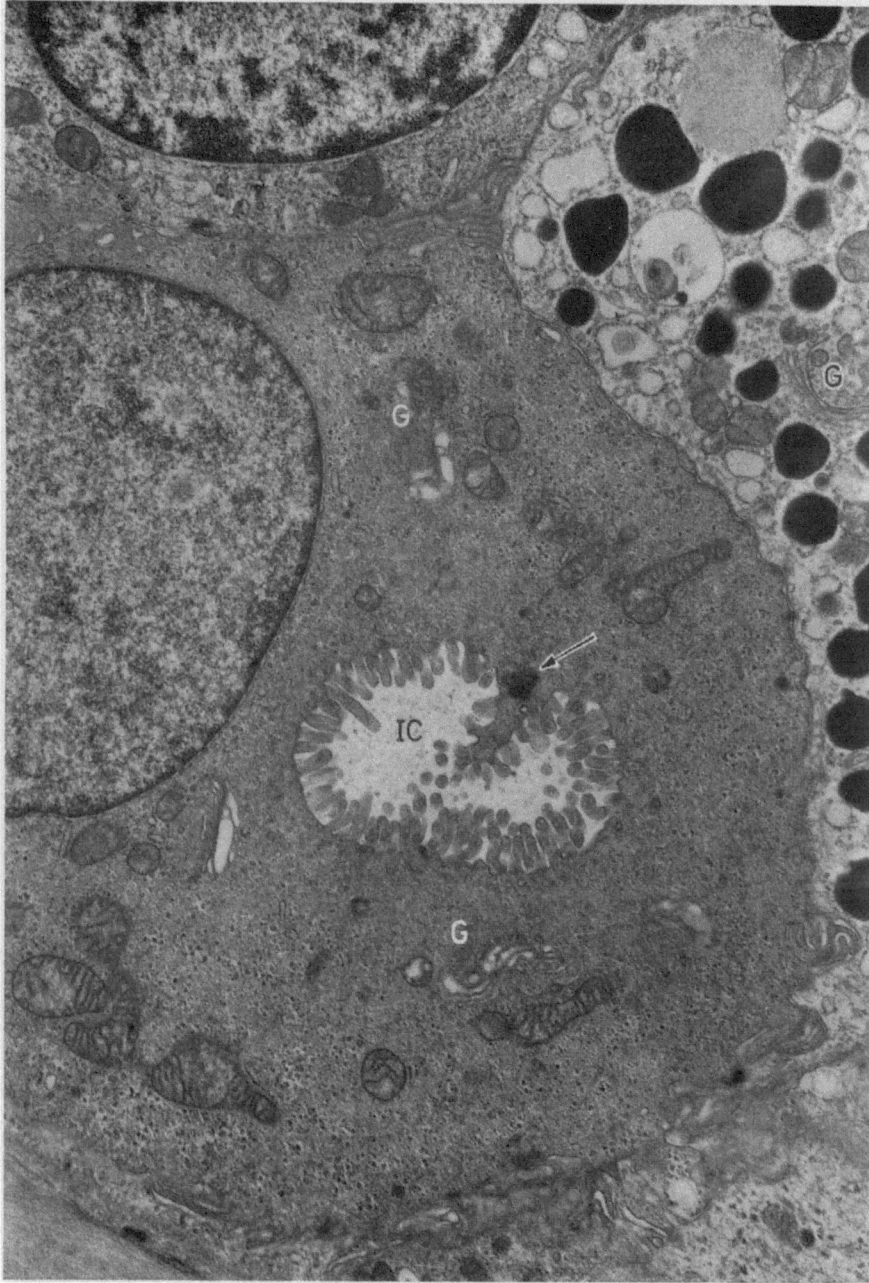

Fig. 12. The cytoplasm of adjacent clear and dark cells appear in sharp contrast in this electron micrograph. An intercellular canaliculus is sectioned tangentially and could be misinterpreted as an intracellular structure. The dense attachment plaque of a junctional complex, however, indicates that part of the wall of the intercellular canaliculus is formed by another clear cell that is not shown in this section. Dense rosettes of glycogen are scattered through the cytoplasm of the clear cell. The dark cell at the top is in an early stage of synthesis and the cytoplasm is dense with RNP particles. In the dark cell at the right, secretory granules in different stages of condensation and typical Golgi membranes appear in the cytoplasm. × 12,800

glycogen assume high electron density after staining with lead hydroxide. This feature is not always a reliable way to identify clear cells since the glycogen stores may be exhausted during prolonged activity of the gland (GUALDI and BALDINO, 1930; YUYAMA, 1935; SHELLY and MESCON, 1952; DOBSON, FORMISANO and LOBITZ, 1958). Other morphological criteria that are easily observed with the electron microscope such as the shape of the nucleus, the form and density of the

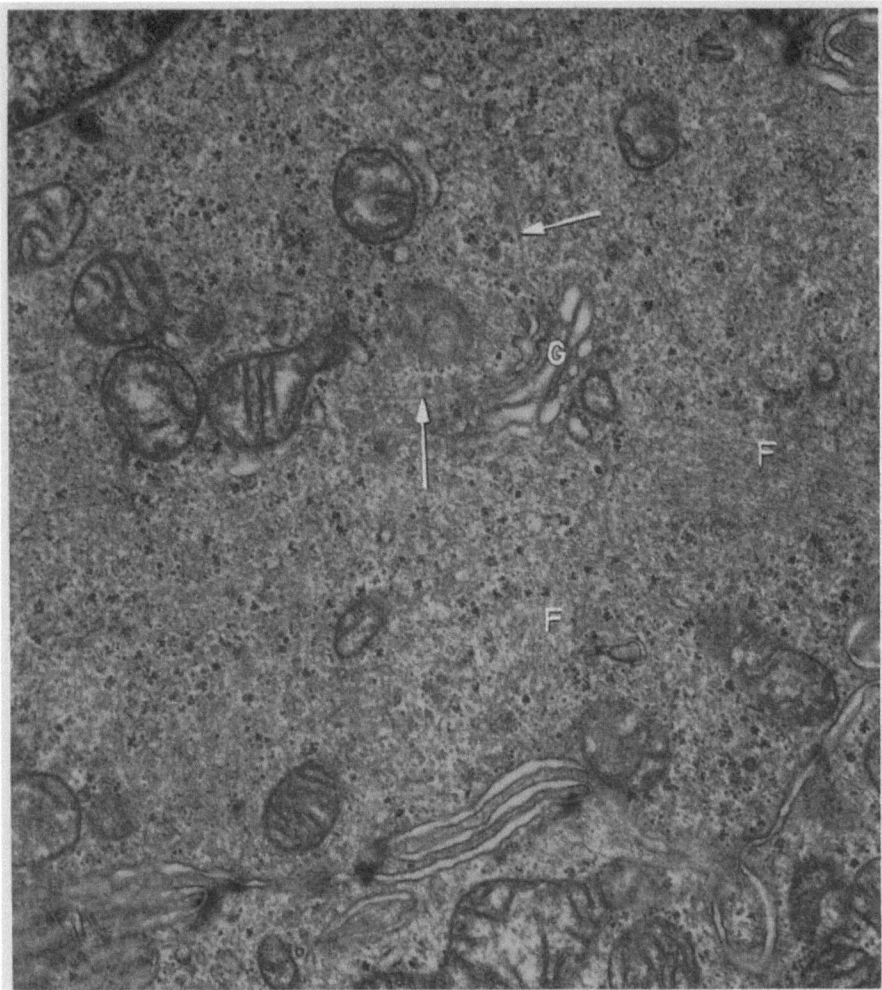

Fig. 13. At high magnification the cytoplasm of the clear cell contains fine filaments (*F*); a few microtubules (arrows) that are oriented toward the Golgi apparatus (*G*); dense rosettes of glycogen; mitochondria and profiles of smooth endoplasmic reticulum. × 23,400

mitochondria, the absence of secretory droplets or myofilaments, the folded plasma membranes and the intercellular canaliculi are more reliable.

The mitochondria of the clear cells are spherical or ovoid. They have a moderately dense matrix with several widely spaced cristae and occasional intramitochondrial granules. Since the mitochondria are scattered randomly throughout the cytoplasm, they apparently have no preferential orientation within the clear cells (Figs. 11, 12 and 13). Rarely, a mitochondrion may be closely applied to a lipid inclusion (ELLIS, 1962).

The endoplasmic reticulum of the clear cells is principally of the smooth type. Profiles of this system are distributed throughout the cytoplasm and seem to form a continuous pattern, and it is closely associated with the glycogen stores. A few profiles of rough endoplasmic reticulum are sometimes present in the clear cells. Usually this component is found only in scant amounts, but in some cells the rough endoplasmic reticulum may be more abundant and organized into stacked lamellae.

The Golgi apparatus of the clear cells is not pervasive. It is posed close to the intercellular canaliculi and consists of typical closely packed, parallel, smooth membranes and small peripheral vesicles (Figs. 11, 12 and 13). The large vacuoles that are a common component of the Golgi complex in other secretory cells are sparse or altogether lacking in the clear cells. Small clear vesicles, more or less uniform in size, are present in the cytoplasm between the Golgi membranes and the intercellular canaliculus, suggesting the transfer of a secretory product from the Golgi zone to the canaliculus. In addition, a few microtubules are oriented toward the Golgi zone (Fig. 13).

Lipid droplets of varying size as well as irregular complex pigment granules may also be present in the cytoplasm of the clear cells (HIBBS, 1958; KUROSUMI et al., 1960; CHARLES, 1960; MUNGER, 1961; ELLIS, 1962). Some of these inclusions are undoubtedly the lipofuchsin granules that have been observed within the clear cells with the light microscope. Others, especially the dense osmiophilic droplets are probably triglyceride. Some of the larger lipid droplets may have clear locules within them, suggesting that they have a complex composition of substances with different solubility. The clear holes may contain a non-osmiophilic saturated lipid or another substance that has been extracted by the solvents used in dehydrating and embedding the tissues. It is reported that lipid inclusions of this type (polyvesicular) are markedly increased in both number and size within the clear cells of eccrine sweat glands of aged persons (KUROSUMI et la., 1960).

b) Cytochemistry

Glycogen and lipid are common components of clear cells and with the appropriate methods they can be readily demonstrated. With light microscopic techniques, the glycogen is concentrated along the borders of the intercellular canaliculi (MONTAGNA et al., 1952); but this may be an artifact of fixation since a similar distribution is not seen with the improved fixation methods of electron microscopy (Fig. 14). The lipid droplets are composed of phospholipid (MONTAGNA et al., 1953), a Sudanophilic component that is extractable with acetone (BUNTING et al., 1948) and a florescent pigment that is partially preserved after extraction with lipid solvents (MONTAGNA et al., 1953). As indicated in electron microscopic observations there are two distinct types of lipid inclusions in the clear cells, triglyceride droplets and complex lipofuchsin granules.

Oxidative enzymes abound in the clear cells. There are moderate concentrations of succinic dehydrogenase within the clear cells (BRAUN-FALCO, 1954; MONTAGNA and FORMISANO, 1955; SERRI, 1955; LOEWENTHAL, 1961), and strong reactions are also elicited for cytochrome oxidase (BRAUN-FALCO, 1961; MONTAGNA, 1962b), and both NADH- and NADPH-tetrazolium reductase (BRAUN-FALCO and PETZOLDT, 1964). These enzymes are contained within the mitochondria, but the cytochemical reactions are somewhat stronger than the mitochondrial populations of these cells might indicate. This suggests that the mitochondria that are present in the clear cells are extremely active in oxidative respiration and in the synthesis of ATP.

Carbonic anhydrase has been demonstrated in high concentration within the clear cells (BRAUN-FALCO and RATHJENS, 1955), and may play an important role in maintaining the acid-base balance there. However, the method used to demonstrate the activity of the enzyme is not always reliable and the results may be questionable.

Monoamine oxidase can be demonstrated within the clear cells (YASUDA and MONTAGNA, 1960); the end product of the reaction takes the form of large granules that show a pattern of distribution similar to that of the mitochondria. This enzyme may attack adrenalin or other amines that affect the activity of the cell.

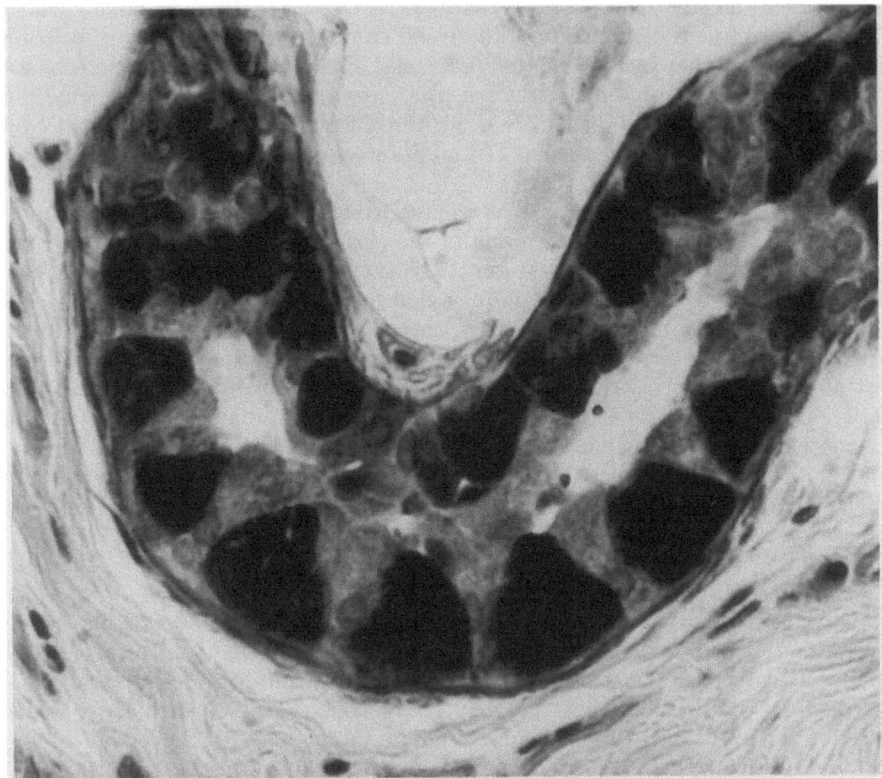

Fig. 14. With the light microscope, staining with periodic acid-Schiff reveals the high glycogen content of the clear cells in the secretory coil. The dark cells appear pale and do not contain glycogen. × 500

The secretory coil of the eccrine sweat glands is highly reactive for phosphorylase (BRAUN-FALCO, 1956a; ELLIS and MONTAGNA, 1958; YASUDA et al., 1958). Whereas epidermis and sebaceous glands may require 20—30 minutes in the substrate before detectable quantities of carbohydrate may be detected within the cells, the sweat glands give an intense iodine test for polysaccharide after only two minutes incubation. At first all of the cells are intensely colored but as the preparations age it is evident that the clear cells retain their color longest and are therefore the most reactive cells in the secretory coil. This correlates well with the normal distribution of glycogen within these cells.

Beta-glucuronidase (BRAUN-FALCO, 1956b; MONTAGNA, 1957) is reported to be present in high concentration within all the cells of the secretory coil including the clear cells; but acid phosphatase is not usually detectable. Esterases also are found in very modest concentration within the clear cells. These three enzymes are usually associated with lysosomes, and there are few structures in the clear cells that resemble lysosomes. Since some of the techniques used for demonstrating beta-glucuronidase in tissue sections have been challenged, the results obtained on eccrine sweat glands are certainly open to debate.

Alkaline phosphatase, demonstrated with the azo-dye method (GOMORI, 1952) is abundant around the intercellular canaliculi (MONTAGNA, 1962b) with the better resolution of electron microscopy, MATSUZAWA and KUROSUMI (1963) showed that in the eccrine sweat glands of the foot pads of the rat, alkaline phosphatase was concentrated along the folded basal membranes of the clear cells. They also demonstrated adenosine triphosphatase activity along the basal plasma membranes.

c) Function

The clear cells produce most of the watery secretion that emerges as sweat on the surface of the skin. This conclusion is supported by several observations. First, the eccrine sweat glands of some primates seem to contain only clear cells in the secretory coil (MONTAGNA et al., 1961; MONTAGNA and YUN, 1962). Second, after episodes of prolonged sweating, the clear cells are depleted of their glycogen and they undergo characteristic morphological alterations that are indicative of hyperactivity (DOBSON, 1962). Third, the clear cells resemble closely other types of serous secretory cells, e.g. those in lacrimal or salivary glands.

The cytological changes that occur in the sweat glands during periods of profuse sweating have been studied thoroughly (DOBSON et al., 1958; DOBSON, 1960; DOBSON, 1962). Profuse sweating causes virtually no changes in the secretory cells of the glands of salt-loaded subjects, but in salt-depleted subjects the clear cells become consistently atrophied, vacuolated and fused with one another. Six hours after the initiation of sweating the clear cells of the sweat glands contain no glycogen (YUYAMA, 1935; SHELLEY and MESCON, 1952). Approximately one hour after sweating commences small vacuoles appear at the base of the clear cells. The nuclei of the clear cells become progressively paler during periods of profuse sweating. Within twenty-four hours after the period of sweating, glycogen reappears in abundance within the clear cells. In subsequent periods of profuse sweating glycogen is not depleted from the clear cells, but they become progressively smaller, flatter and more vacuolated. After three periods of sweating the cytological changes in the clear cells are maximal, and subsequent periods do not evoke retrogressive changes in the clear cells. Instead adaptive mechanisms lead to the reestablishment of a secretory epithelium more or less normal in appearance. Since in subjects on a low salt intake, the rate of secretion of sodium in the sweat is consistently lower than in subjects on a high salt intake, this establishes an apparent association between diminished salt excretion and morphologic changes in the large clear cells (DOBSON, 1962).

Physiologic studies show that the secretion of the secretory coil is nearly isotonic with blood (DOBSON, 1962; SLEGERS, 1964; SCHULZ and ULLRICH, 1966). Thus the clear cells act essentially like a filter, permitting water and some specific ions to pass from its plasma to its luminal side, while effectively blocking the flow of other plasma components. The interstitial fluids are absorbed into the cell along the elaborately folded basal and lateral surfaces of the cell. The irregular intercellular spaces surrounding the basal folds are probably not artifacts (TERZAKIS, 1964) and may be very active areas of the cell surface involved either in membrane flow or in pinocytosis. The elaborate pleating of the cell surface is sufficient to enhance even the passive movement of water. Within the cell the smooth endoplasmic reticulum and the Golgi apparatus may assume active roles in selecting substances for secretion. The isotonic secretion is then released into the intercellular canaliculi which increase the surface area available for secretion without using the luminal surface of the cell (MUNGER, 1961) and are confluent with the lumen of the secretory coil. It is apparent from the electron micrographs that there are no direct passages between the connective tissue spaces that surround the glomus of the sweat gland and the intercellular canaliculi. Junctional complexes are continuous along the walls of the intercellular canaliculi (Fig. 10) and block any such pathway, and the only available route for substances passing into the lumen of the secretory coil is through the secretory cells. In this respect the eccrine sweat gland is entirely different from the nephron.

From a comparative point of view the clear cells resemble in fine structure other salt and water secreting epithelial cells (TERZAKIS, 1964); and it is reasonable to conclude that they play a major role in the transport of sodium for secretion in the sweat. This is especially evident in relation to the specializations of the cell surface that have been correlated with ion and water transport (FAWCETT, 1962). The population of mitochondria in the clear cells is sparse, however, when contrasted with that of cells found in the salt glands of marine reptiles (ELLIS and ABEL, 1964) and marine birds (DOYLE, 1960; KOMNICK, 1963) known to produce a hypertonic salt secretion. This is, perhaps, additional evidence that the secretory product of the clear cell is not hypertonic and that the energy requirements for its elaboration are not great.

3. Dark Cells

The dark cells have a narrow base and a broad apical surface that borders the lumen of the secretory coil (Fig. 15). It is the inverted pyramidal shape of these

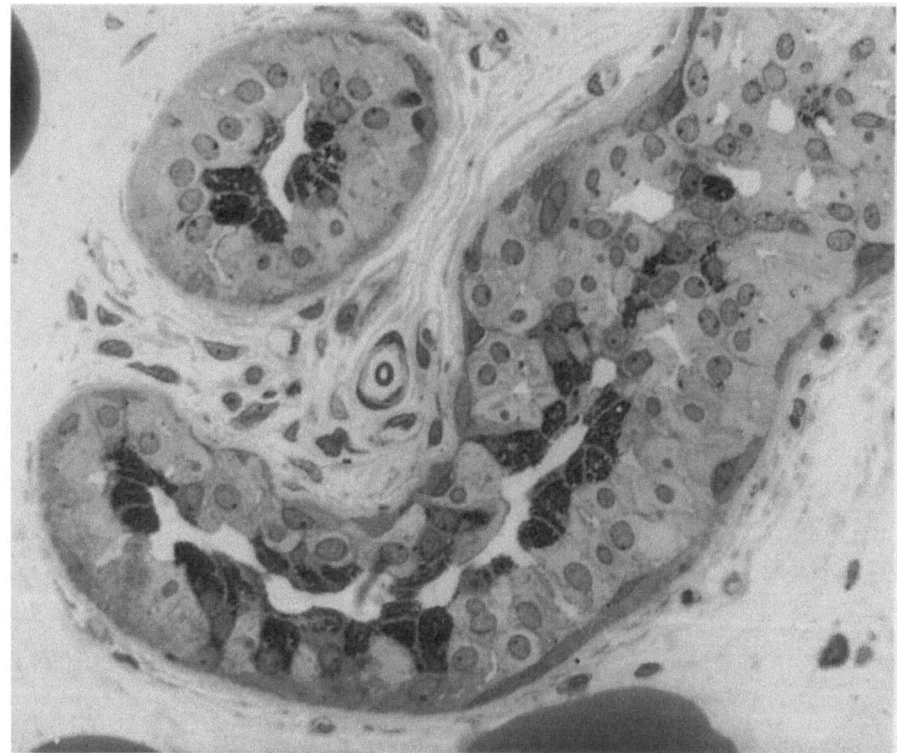

Fig. 15. Staining with borax-Toluidine blue, reveals the specific granulation of the dark cells under the light microscope. Clear cells, intercellular canaliculi and myoepithelial cells also appear clearly in this 0.5 μ Epon section. × 340

cells that give a pseudostratified appearance to the epithelium of the secretory coil. Since they are typical mucigenous cells (LEE, 1960), they may vary considerably in their shape, size, and internal organization during different periods in their secretory cycle. For example, some cells may be packed with small secretion granules but other cells may contain very few or none. In spite of this variability, however, the dark cells may be identified by the ribonucleoprotein that is always present in sufficient quantity to render them strongly basophilic when stained with basic dyes (MONTAGNA et al., 1953). A large and pervasive Golgi apparatus, filling much of the supranuclear cytoplasm, is also a striking feature of this cell type.

a) Electron Microscopy

The character of the surface of the dark cell changes at different interfaces; it has a border of short microvilli along the lumen of the secretory coil, it bears even villous folds where two dark cells are apposed and it is more or less flat and unmodified where it abuts clear cells (Figs. 12 and 16). The apical surface of the dark cells is irregular and has a ragged appearance in electron micrographs. Microvilli, of almost uniform diameter but unequal in length, and positioned haphazardly, line the lumen. Typical junctional complexes separate the luminal and lateral surfaces of the cell. In addition scattered desmosomes are spaced irregularly along the sides of the cells. The lateral surfaces of adjacent dark cells are closely adherent separated by a uniform gap of approximately 120 Å (Fig. 12). At intervals this margin of the cells is thrown into long, slender and even folds that are oriented parallel to the cell surface and intermesh in perfect alternating sequence with similar processes on the neighboring dark cell (ELLIS, 1962). These unions appear to be static configurations since the intercellular spaces are narrow and regular and the villous folds are smooth and flat. Their orientation to the long axis of the cell may not only block the flow of intercellular fluids toward the lumen but also lock the cells together. This pattern contrasts sharply with that seen between adjacent clear cells (Figs. 11 and 13). At the points where three or four dark cells join, these unions become more complex, but their design is similar in principle. The surface of the dark cell that borders on a clear cell or myoepithelial cell is usually smooth (Fig. 12) but it may have a few slender processes that interdigitate with its neighbor. Along these interfaces the gaps between the cells vary in width and the extensions of the cell surface may be sinuous. Here the dark cell is closest to the perimeter of the secretory coil and the cell metabolites must pass through this surface of the cell.

Profiles of rough and smooth endoplasmic reticulum pack the cytoplasm of the dark cell with the former predominating. In cells in the early stages of synthesis the rough endoplasmic reticulum is often arranged in closely stacked, flattened lamellae forming true ergastoplasm. Even cells that are well-filled with secretory granules, and in the terminal stage of the secretory cycle, have abundant particles of ribonucleoprotein (MUNGER, 1961), both associated with the endoplasmic reticulum and lying free in the cytoplasm (Fig. 12). Ribosomes are much more numerous in dark cells than in either the clear cells or myoepithelial cells, and their abundance must be primarily responsible for the strong basophilic staining that is characteristic of these cells.

Above the nucleus a pervasive Golgi apparatus extends through broad areas of the cytoplasm (ELLIS, 1962). The arched and closely-packed membranes form flattened lamellae that surround a few large central vacuoles; at their borders the lamellae are dilated and smaller vesicles frequently appear at their tips. Numerous other membrane-bounded vacuoles abound within the supranuclear cytoplasm. The relationships that these granules bear to one another is not entirely clear, but from their size and contents they seem to form a continuous series that can be correlated with the cycle of synthesis and secretion (Figs. 12 and 16).

The largest vacuoles contain a floculent substance that is electron lucid, and they are usually poised near the inner surface of the Golgi membranes. These vacuoles probably contain substances newly synthesized or recently conjugated within the Golgi apparatus. Other vesicles somewhat smaller in size and containing a moderately dense but still floculent material may lie beside the clearer vesicles

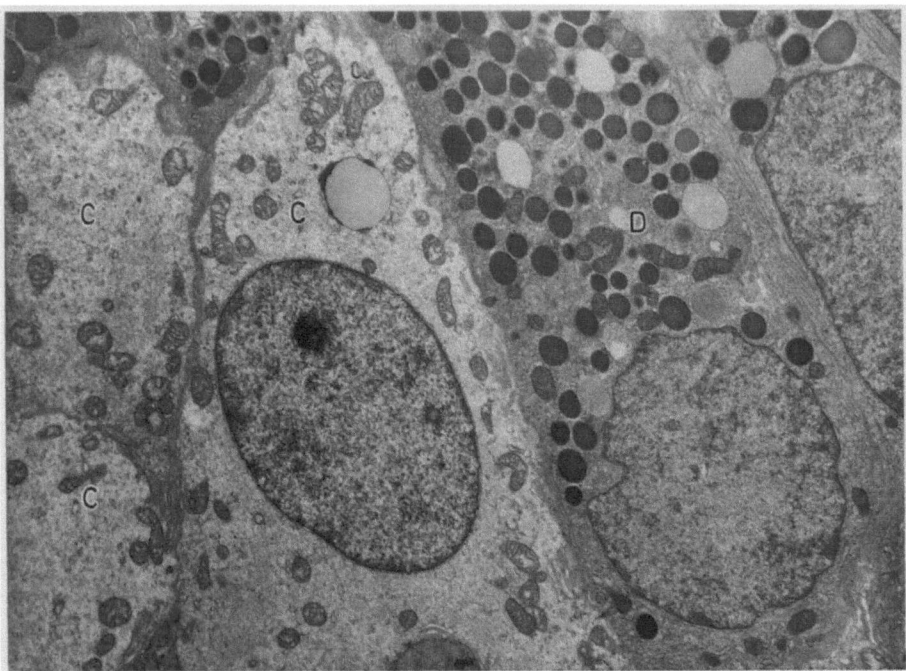

Fig. 16. The fine structure of dark cells and clear cells are contrasted strikingly in this electron micrograph. A lipid inclusion is shown in one of the clear cells (C) and secretion granules in different stages of condensation are evident in the dark cells (D). The nucleus of the clear cell is smooth and ovate, but the nuclei of the dark cells are irregular. The high RNP content of the cytoplasm of the dark cell renders it dense, but the paler cytoplasm of the clear cells contains many more mitochondria. (× 7,000)

but they also range widely through the supranuclear cytoplasm. The third class of vesicles, and usually the most numerous, contains a dense material that is perserved well with glutaraldehyde and stains more intensely with uranyl acetate than it does with lead citrate. These vesicles seem to have a uniformly dense interior, but upon close examination at high resolution it is finely granular. The three vesicular forms described above probably represent part of a continuum where the substances first compounded within the clear vesicles near the Golgi apparatus are concentrated and compressed into a smaller, more compact, and more electron dense form (Fig. 16). The floculent component observed within all of the vesicles supports this hypothesis. That the smaller dense vesicles contain the terminal secretory product is suggested by the occasional presence of dense spheres within the lumen of the secretory tubule. The secretory product is probably released by fusion of the membrane-bounded secretory vacuole with the plasma membrane at the surface of the dark cell, since the dense granules observed within the lumen have no membrane surrounding them.

In contrast to the spherical mitochondria in the clear cells, the dark cells contain sparse numbers of short rod-like or filamentous mitochondria (Fig. 16). Their matrix is dense and the cristae are most frequently oriented perpendicular to the long axis of the mitochondrion. Intramitochondrial granules are not observed in most specimens. The mitochondria are more abundant in the basal and perinuclear zones, but even in these areas they are seldom closely packed.

Lipid droplets of varying size may occur singly or clustered in groups within the cytoplasm (MUNGER, 1961; ELLIS, 1962). They usually lie among the secretory granules and are not different in appearance from the droplets observed in the clear cells. However, the amount of lipid is less and the droplets are usually of smaller size than within the clear cells. The lipid bodies seem to be surrounded by a membrane, but a substance with high electron density adheres closely to the rim of the vacuole and tends to obscure the envelope. The major portion of the vacuole is filled with a homogenous substance; a fine dense granular component delimits each vacuole and may subdivide it into two or more locules. This arrangement suggests that fusion may occur between smaller and larger lipid droplets.

A variety of other cell organelles are scattered through the cytoplasm of the dark cells. Microtubules, few in numbers, are usually aligned parallel to the long axis of the cells and are most frequent near the plasma membrane. Swirls of filaments, tentatively identified as tonofilaments, may be conspicuous in the supranuclear cytoplasm. Small membrane-bounded vesicles containing a dense granular substance are encountered occasionally in electron micrographs and resemble lysosomes. Paired centrioles are found consistently just beneath the plasma membrane at the secretory surface of the cell. Multivesicular bodies are rare components of the cytoplasm.

b) Cytochemistry

The dark cells contain fine lipid granules that may be stained with Sudan dyes. The amount of lipid found within the cells is highly variable and may differ even from gland to gland in the same individual. The lipid seems to be a stable component of the cell and is not secreted even when the glands are stimulated to sweat (SHELLY and MESCON, 1952; DOBSON and LOBITZ, 1958; DOBSON et al., 1958). A variable number of pigment granules that exhibit yellow or orange autoflorescence under near ultraviolet light are associated with the lipid droplets. These granules are not extracted with acetone, they contain no iron, they are not reactive for the periodic acid Schiff test and they increase both in size and number with advancing age. The pigment is probably the small dense component of the lipid droplets as they are seen with the electron microscope. Similar lipid complexes are more abundant in the clear cells (KUROSUMI et al., 1960) and occasionally they are seen in the myoepithelial cells (ELLIS, 1965). Traces of glycogen may sometimes be demonstrated in the dark cells with the periodic acid Schiff reaction.

The secretory vacuoles of the dark cells contain a substance that is moderately PAS-reactive but resistant to digestion with either saliva or diastase (FORMISANO and LOBITZ, 1957; FUSARO and GOLTZ, 1961). These vacuoles fill much of the apical cytoplasm of the cell. They stain deeply with basic dyes and often stain metachromatically with Toluidine blue. The basophilia is not affected by ribonuclease digestion. The apical vacuoles are also stained by Hale's colloidal iron method for mucopolysaccharide (MUNGER, 1961) and by Alcian blue (LEE, 1960). These various tests indicate that the secretion vacuoles contain an acid mucopolysaccharide (MUNGER, 1961; LEE, 1960). Since acid mucopolysaccharides are not stained by the PAS reaction the PAS staining must be due to carbohydrate-protein complexes that are also present within the secretion vacuoles (PEARSE, 1960, p. 235).

The dark cells are somewhat less reactive for both cytochrome oxidase (BRAUN-FALCO, 1961) and succinic dehydrogenase (BRAUN-FALCO and RATHJENS, 1954; SERRI, 1955; LOEWENTHAL, 1961) then are the clear cells. This observation correlates well with the mitochondrial population of these cells since there are fewer mitochondria in dark cells than in clear cells and these enzymes are reported to be localized within the mitochondria. The distribution of monoamine oxidase follows a similar pattern (YASUDA and MONTAGNA, 1960).

Phosphorylase is apparently present in dark cells even though typically they contain little glycogen (BRAUN-FALCO, 1956a; ELLIS and MONTAGNA, 1958; YASUDA et al., 1958). However, the reaction is so intense in the secretory coil that the exact disposition of the enzyme is difficult to determine.

The alpha-naphthol or AS esterase techniques are reliable methods of demonstrating specifically the dark cells within eccrine sweat glands (MONTAGNA and ELLIS, 1958). The secretory coil is moderately rich in esterase activity (STEIGLEDER and SCHULTIS, 1957) and the dark cells are much more reactive than the clear cells or myoepithelial cells for non-specific esterases. Acid phosphatase may be demonstrated in the dark cells, but it is present only in modest amount and is localized in small cytoplasmic granules. Alkaline phosphatase is not demonstrable within the dark cells, either with the azo-dye or the Gomori glycerophosphate techniques. Beta-glucuronidase may be demonstrated in high concentration within the secretory coil of the eccrine sweat glands but specific localization within the dark cells is uncertain (BRAUN-FALCO, 1956b; MONTAGNA, 1957).

c) Function

The function that the dark cells serve in the eccrine sweat glands is both obvious and obscure. They resemble other mucus-secreting cells in their fine struction and in the cytochemical reactivity, and they synthesize an epithelial mucin that is released into the lumen of the secretory coil (MUNGER, 1961). Comparative studies of other mammalian species indicate that mucus-secreting cells are not essential for the production of eccrine sweat and there is, even in man, great variability from one individual to another in the numbers of dark cells that are found within the secretory coil. The sweat glands of many of the lemurs (MONTAGNA et al., 1961; MONTAGNA and YUN, 1962) are devoid of dark cells but produce abundant sweat. These cells may then be considered as accessories, contributing to but not required for the production of eccrine sweat. The tonicity of the sweat produced by glands that lack dark cells may be quite different, however, from that of human sweat. The mucopolysaccharide that they produce may, in addition to the watery secretion of the clear cells, help lubricate and maintain the cornified cells of the skin surface in a supple state, and it may block the epidermal ducts of inactive sweat glands (LEE, 1960).

These dark cells undoubtedly provide or contribute to the PAS-reactive lining that coats the inner surface of the sweat duct (HASHIMOTO et al., 1966). The function that this coating serves is not yet clear, but it may act as a protective coating shielding the cells that line the duct from their own hydrolytic enzymes; or it may function directly in sodium reabsorption (MUNGER et al., 1961).

During periods of profuse sweating the PAS-positive diastase resistant material normally present in the dark cells is secreted and appears within the excretory duct or is deposited on the skin surface around the opening of the sweat pore (DOBSON and LOBITZ, 1958). This is substantiated by the demonstration of a glucoseamine component in human sweat when it is analyzed biochemically (JIRKA and KOTAS, 1957). Twenty-four hours after a period of profuse sweating small PAS-positive granules reappear in the dark cells, but they are smaller than those in normal cells and they do not stain metachromatically. During subsequent periods of profuse sweating the PAS-positive granules are not entirely depleted from the dark cells, but they may become fewer in number (DOBSON, 1960). Following periods of profuse sweating the PAS-positive non-glycogen material in the dark cells reappears at about the same rate that glycogen is restored in the clear cells (DOBSON, 1962).

These studies indicate that the constituents of the secretory vacuoles are synthesized at different rates. The PAS-positive diastase resistant substance, presumably a glycoprotein, is resynthesized rapidly, approximately at the same rate as glycogen after its release during periods of active sweating; but the acid mucopolysaccharide that stains metachromatically with Toluidine blue is either renewed at a much slower rate or secreted at the same rate that it is synthesized. Depletion and repletion of these substances is independent of salt intake (DOBSON et al., 1961). In repeated episodes of sweating, the rate of sodium excretion on the second day of sweating, when the small dark cells are free of secretory vacuoles, is essentially the same as on the first day when vacuoles are present (DOBSON, 1962). This suggests that the vacuoles are not directly involved in sodium excretion, but their contents, deposited along the wall of the duct, may still play an active role in sodium reabsorption.

III. The Intradermal Sweat Duct

The coiled duct of the eccrine sweat gland connects the secretory segment with the straight excretory duct. The secretory segment with its three cell types changes into a simple tube lined with two layers of cells. Neither of the two cell types that line the coiled duct bear any similarity to the cells in the secretory segment. Myoepithelial cells are completely lacking and there are no secretory cells of either serous or mucous types. Instead, the duct is formed by an outer ring of peripheral or basal cells and an inner ring of superficial, luminal or cuticular cells. The irregular ragged lumen of the secretory coil continues as the regular cylindrical cavity of the duct. At this point of juncture the lumen of the coiled duct has its maximum diameter, but it gradually diminishes to a narrow opening after a short distance. This short funnel-shaped portion of the coiled duct is not equivalent to either the "ampulla" or "sphincter" described by LOEWENTHAL (1960, 1961) and the overwhelming evidence from both light and electron microscopy shows that there are no such regional differentiations of either the secretory coil of the conjoined duct.

Although the cells of the duct do not divide frequently under normal conditions, they retain the ability to proliferate rapidly under conditions of stress. For example, LOBITZ et al. (1954b) described the remarkable regenerative behavior of the severed excretory ducts of eccrine sweat glands. Three days after a wound is inflicted the basal cells in the duct, near the wounded surface undergo a burst of mitotic activity. The cells produced through cell division radiate outward from the severed duct and form epithelial tongues under the granulation tissue. Continued proliferation of these cells results in the formation of a new epithelial covering under the granulation tissue that looks and behaves exactly like epidermis. Biologically, therefore the basal cells of the duct not only retain their capacity for cell division but also may revert to the epidermal cell type from which they took their origin. DOBSON (1962) reported that in salt-depleted subjects exposed to daily episodes of profuse sweating the basal cells in the ducts of the eccrine sweat glands show a striking burst of mitotic activity on the fourth day of the experiment, and a number of mitotic figures on subsequent days. Although no loss of luminal cells from the duct was reported in these experiments, MONTAGNA (1962a) has suggested that the loss of cells at the luminal side of the duct may provide the stimulus for mitosis in the basal cells. The evidence from DOBSON's (1962) study also indicates that low sodium intake under conditions of stress may induce mitotic activity in the basal cells. If the basal cells are active in sodium reabsorption this response would be highly adaptive.

Following periods of profuse sweating glycogen disappears from the cells of the duct. Recovery is slower in the luminal cells, where glycogen stores are not reestablished until seventy-two hours after the first episode of sweating, than it is in the basal cells where glycogen reappears 48 hours after profuse sweating. Once the cells of the duct regain their glycogen stores they do not loose it again during subsequent periods of sweating (DOBSON, 1962).

THOMPSON (1962) has found that parts of eccrine sweat glands may survive for years in dermal skin grafts even though they have no duct opening to the surface of the skin. The cells of the glands appear normal cytologically, except that intense acid phosphatase activity is found in the ductal cells of the graft and in the lumina of the excretory ducts. Lipid is also present within the ducts of the sweat glands of the graft. These observations suggest that the autolytic activity in the ducts of these glands is far greater than in normal sweat glands. THOMPSON (1962) concludes that "The survival in skin grafts of apparently functional sweat glands, when total obstruction of the excretory duct prevents the discharge of secretion, must be regarded as evidence supporting the existence of resorptive mechanisms in the sweat tubule; these probably reside chiefly in the remaining ductal elements." This study as well as evidence from other sources leaves little doubt that the duct cells play an active role in resorption.

Except for its convolutions the coiled duct is not especially different either histochemically or cytologically from the straight duct. The two cell types that form the duct change in character along the length of the duct but the differences are gradual, not dramatic.

1. Basal Cells

a) Electron Microscopy

The basal cells are distinctive in their morphology and are readily distinguished from other cells in the sweat glands by the fringe of short microvilli that covers all but the smooth basal surface of the cell, and by the abundant mitochondria that are packed into the cytoplasm (HIBBS, 1958; MUNGER, 1961). The plasma membrane along the base of each cell is slightly irregular with some small indentations; but for the most part it describes a regular arc (Fig. 17). Five or six basal cells form the outer perimeter of the secretory coil. At their periphery these cells are in turn invested with a thin amorphous adepithelial (basement) membrane and by a wrapping of collagenous fibers (Fig. 17). In addition, the processes of two or three circumferential layers of fibrocytes and a few unmyelinated nerve fibers are wrapped around the duct.

The villous borders of adjoining basal cells intermesh loosely in an irregular pattern (Fig. 17). The gaps between the basal cells are broken up by the microvilli into a tortuous system of uneven channels. At odd intervals the plasma membranes of adjacent basal cells are joined by desmosomes. The surfaces of the basal cells and the overlying superficial cells are intermeshed in a similar way, except that desmosomes link these cells more frequently.

Near the secretory segment the basal cells of the coiled duct seem to bear more villous processes and the intercellular channels are somewhat broader. A major portion of their cytoplasm is filled with spherical or ovoid mitochondria that are packed tightly side-by-side (HIBBS, 1958) (Fig. 17). The mitochondria differ strikingly from those in the other cells of the secretory coil and the duct (Fig. 18). They have the dilated cristae and the dense enlarged matrix characteristic of mitochondria primed with adenosine diphosphate and presumed to be actively synthesizing ATP (HACKENBROCK and BRANDT, 1965).

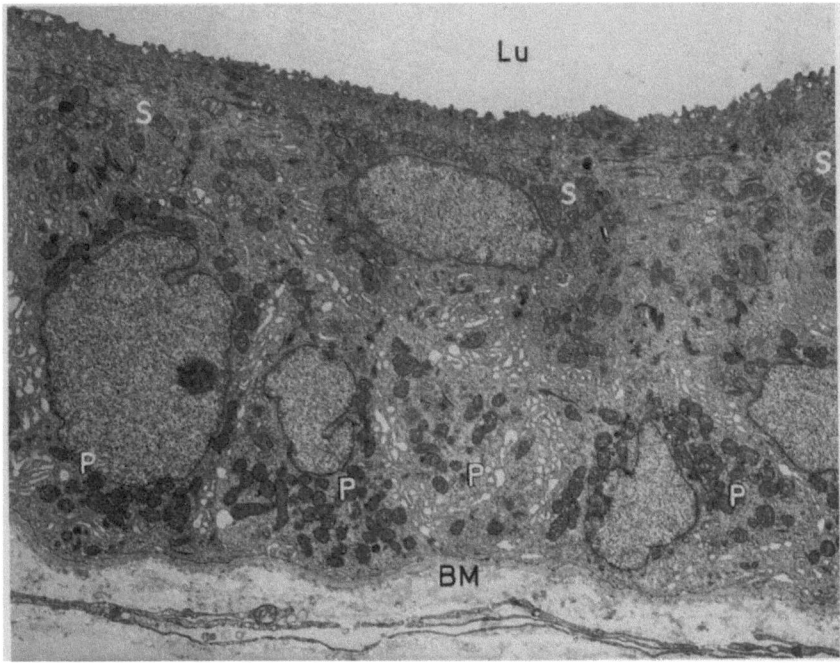

Fig. 17. A section through the coiled duct near its junction with the secretory coil shows the lumen, superficial cells (*S*), basal cells (*P*) and the basement membrane (*BM*). At this point the cuticular border in the superficial cells is narrow and poorly demarcated. The basal cells have irregular villous borders, they contain numerous mitochondria and a few tonofibrils. × 7,300

Glycogen granules are commonly found scattered throughout the cytoplasm of the basal cells. In addition, ribonucleoprotein particles are abundant, some are attached to profiles of the endoplasmic reticulum, but large numbers are loose in the cytoplasm. The endoplasmic reticulum of these cells is not highly developed consisting of some profiles of rough endoplasmic reticulum and scattered smooth membranes. Small vesicles are poised near the plasma membrane at all surfaces of the cell, but they do not seem to be part of a continuous membrane system (Fig. 18). Microtubules, few in number, run intermittently through the cytoplasm. The Golgi apparatus is small and inconspicuous. A few, small, membrane limited vesicles that contain a dense granular substance also seem to be constant components of the cytoplasm.

The nucleus of the basal cells is misshapen, usually it has numerous indentations and is deeply incised at one or more places (Fig. 17). It is usually kidney-shaped, curving slightly along the base of the cell to follow the contour of the tubule. One or two prominent nucleoli appear within the nucleoplasm.

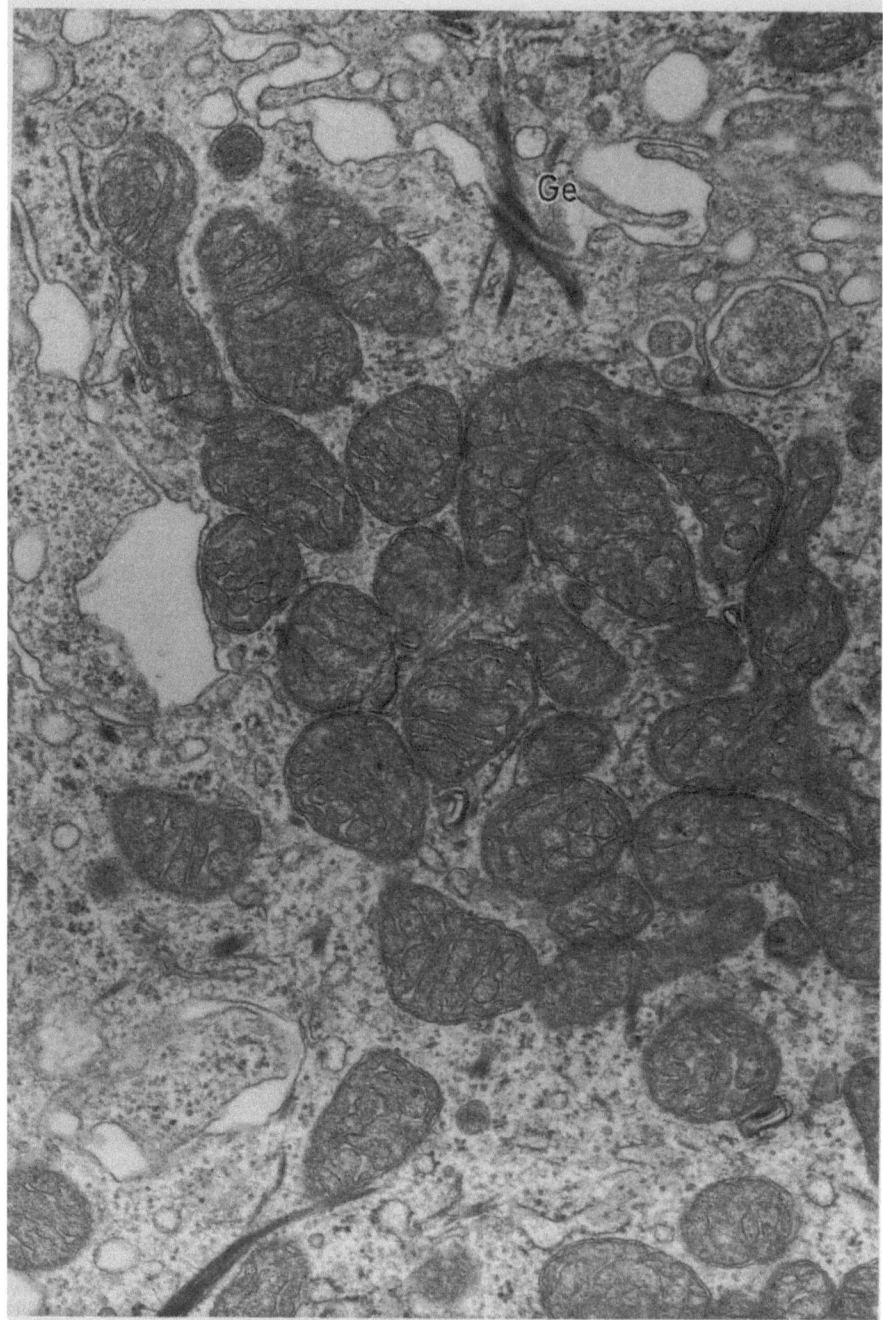

Fig. 18. The numerous mitochondria in the basal cells of the duct have dilated cristae and a dense matrix. Many villous processes cover the cell surface and smooth vesicles are common in the peripheral cytoplasm. Tonofilaments are restricted primarily to the sites of desmosomes ($De = Ge$ in the fig.). × 32,000

b) Cytochemistry

In consonance with the high numbers of mitochondria, the basal cells of the duct react strongly for succinic dehydrogenase (MONTAGNA and FORMISANO, 1955) and cytochrome oxidase (BRAUN-FALCO, 1961). The distribution of monoamine oxidase within the cells follows a similar pattern (YASUDA and MONTAGNA, 1960). Phosphorylase activity is intense in the basal cells, giving them a deep blue-black color with the iodine test after brief incubation in the substrate (ELLIS and MONTAGNA, 1958). Beta-glucuronidase is also reported to be in high concentration within the duct cells (BRAUN-FALCO, 1956b; MONTAGNA, 1957).

Little acid phosphatase or non-specific esterase can be detected histochemically within the basal cells. These tests reveal only a few scattered fine reactive granules within the cytoplasm (MONTAGNA, 1962a). Neither do the cells contain demonstrable amounts of alkaline phosphatase or cholinesterase. Aminopeptidase activity is reported to be somewhat more concentrated within the coiled duct than within the straight duct, but both segments have low reactivity. The precise cellular localization of this enzyme within the duct is uncertain (MONTAGNA, 1962b).

The basal cells do not contain stable lipid other than the phospholipids associated with the membranes of the cell, and both intrinsic and extrinsic pigment is lacking from the duct cells. The PAS reaction reveals glycogen in moderate concentration within the cytoplasm of the basal cells under normal conditions (FUSARO and GOLTZ, 1961). The glycogen content of the basal cells varies however under different conditions (DOBSON, 1962).

c) Function

Evidence from physiological studies shows conclusively that the duct of the eccrine sweat gland is engaged in the active reabsorption of sodium from the effluent elaborated by the secretory coil (ARAKI and ONDO, 1953; NITTA, 1953; SCHWARTZ et al., 1953; SCHWARTZ and THAYSEN, 1956; LOBITZ et al., 1955; LLOYD, 1962; DOBSON, 1962; SLEGERS, 1964). Direct sampling by microcanulation techniques also shows that sodium levels are higher in the effluent of the secretory tubule than in the duct (SCHULZ and ULLRICH, 1966). Other more circumstantial evidence also suggests that the duct plays an active role in sweat production (SCHIEFFERDECHER, 1922; ACKERMANN, 1939; LOBITZ and MASON, 1948; KUNO, 1956; MONTAGNA, 1956; THOMPSON, 1962). Comparative evidence from ultrastructural studies (MUNGER and BRUSILOW, 1961) also points logically to this conclusion, and gives the basal cells the principal responsibility for the extratubular transport of ions.

In their fine structure the basal cells are similar to many cells that are known to function in salt secretion (ELLIS, 1966). The loose fringe of microvilli that surround the cell are quite similar to the processes that characterize other typical ion secreting cells (FAWCETT, 1962). In the basal cell of the sweat duct however, the microvillous border of the cell is posed toward the lumen of the duct while the basal surface of the cell is nearly smooth. A comparison with other salt-secreting cells suggests that for these cells the absorptive surface is directed toward the lumen, while the secretory surface lies at the periphery of the duct. The basal cells of the duct contain more mitochondria than any of the other cells in the sweat glands. This fact is also consistent with their proposed role in sodium reabsorption, since all cells that are known to engage in ion transport or concentration have mitochondria in abundance (FAWCETT, 1962).

The gradual change in the fine structure of the basal cells that occurs from the junction with the secretory segment to the union with the intraepidermal duct are also consistent with their role in sodium transport. Near the secretory coil the basal cells contain more mitochondria and have an elaborate villous border, toward the junction of the coiled duct and straight duct the basal cells contain fewer mitochondria and increasing numbers of tonofilaments; they have shorter and probably fewer microvilli on their surface, along the length of the straight duct the basal cells show a continued reduction in the numbers of mitochondria, a conspicuous increase in tonofilaments (Fig. 19). This suggests that the basal cells are most active in sodium reabsorption near the secretory coil and that the capacity for reabsorption diminishes along the length of the duct as it approaches the epidermis.

2. Superficial Cells
a) Electron Microscopy

The superficial cells line the inner surface of the eccrine sweat duct. The apical cytoplasm of the cells is especially modified to form a cuticular border (ELLIS and

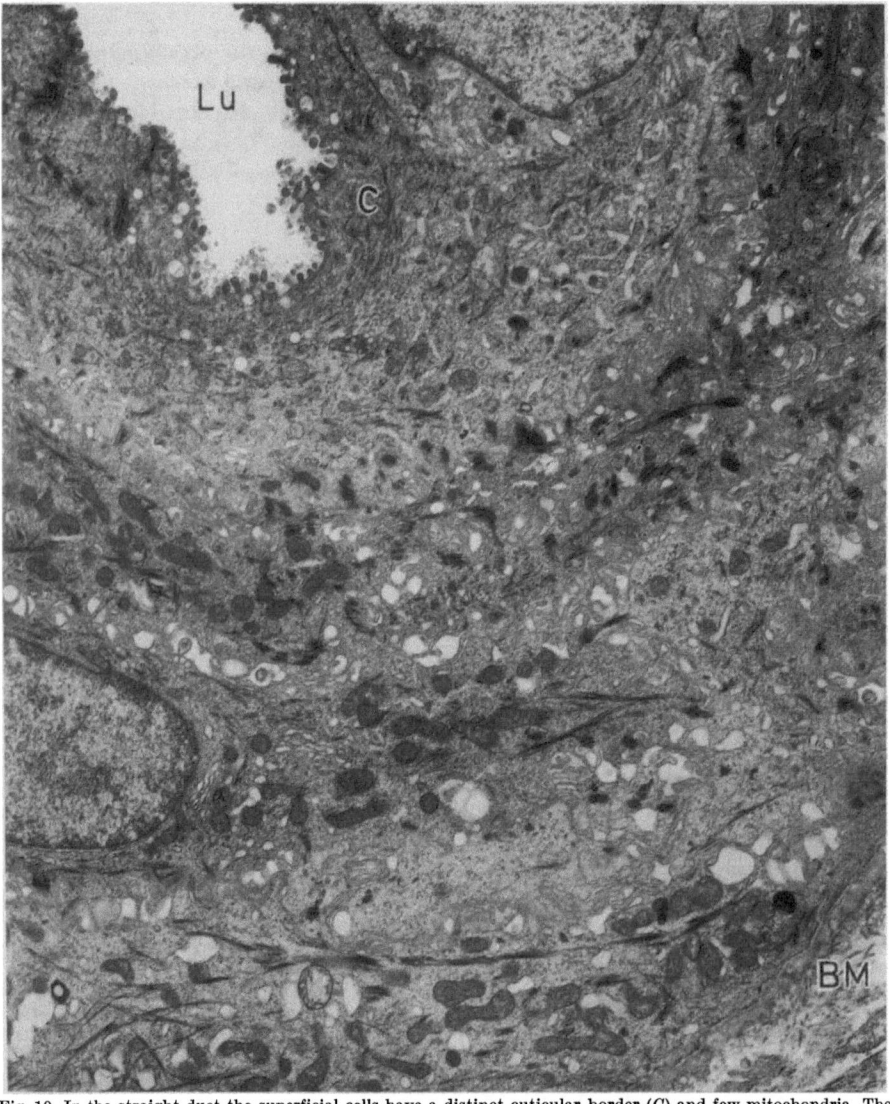

Fig. 19. In the straight duct the superficial cells have a distinct cuticular border (*C*) and few mitochondria. The basal cells have irregular borders, conspicuous tonofilaments, glycogen granules and dense mitochondria. The duct is surrounded by a definite basement membrane (*BM*) and layers of investing collagen fibers. × 8,400

MONTAGNA, 1961; MUNGER, 1961) and the cells are attached to each other laterally by a system of interdigitating plasma membranes and conspicuous desmosomes similar to those connecting the spinous cells of the Malphigian layer of the epidermis (Figs. 17, 19 and 20). The luminal border of the superficial cells bears low microvilli with plasma membranes that show typical unit membrane structure (Fig. 20).

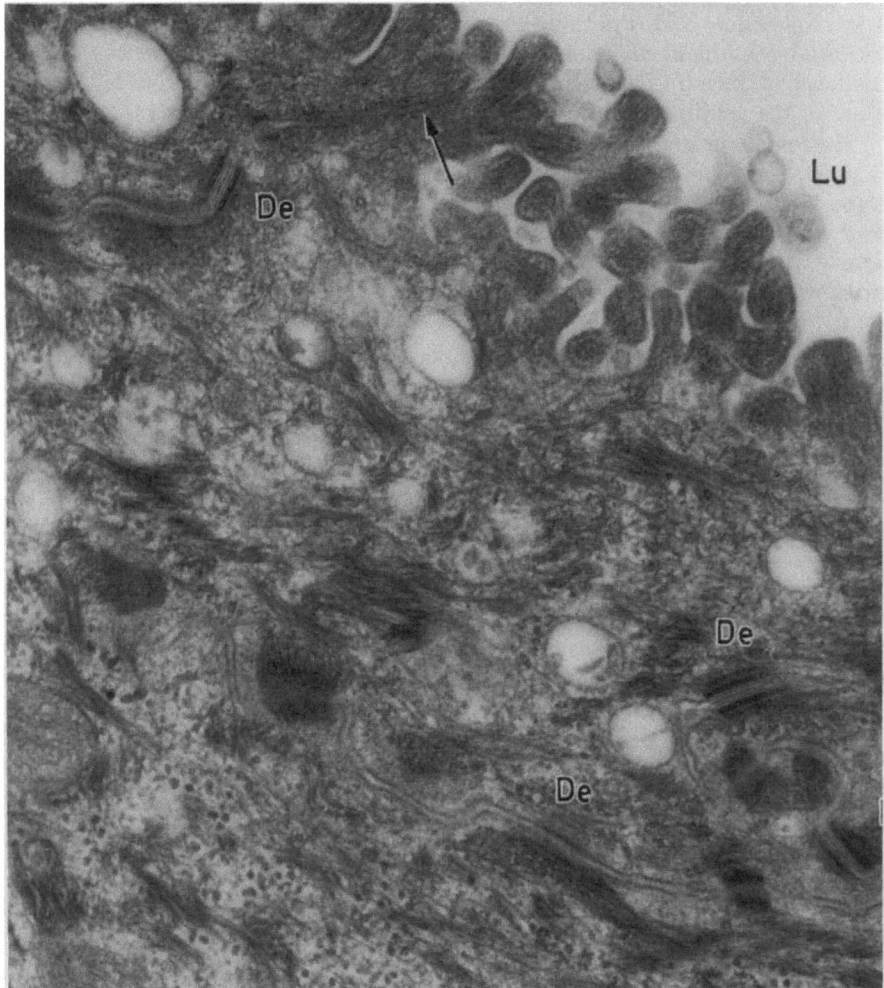

Fig. 20. At the upper level of the straight duct tonofilaments and tonofibrils form the cuticular border of the superficial cells. Short microvilli protrude into the lumen (*Lu*) of the duct and a typical junctional complex, consisting of zonula occludens (arrow) and a desmosome (*De*) join adjacent cells. Numerous desmosomes (*De*) connect the lateral borders of the cells. × 48,000

A few, small vesicles are present in the cytoplasm just beneath the microvilli, and some partially closed vesicles appear in the crypts between the short microvilli (Figs. 19 and 20). These vesicles may reflect either the pinocytotic or secretory activities at the cell surface. Just beneath the luminal surface of the cell, the cytoplasm is filled with moderately dense tonofilaments (Fig. 20).

It is this concentration of tonofilaments in the apical cytoplasm that forms the cuticular border of the duct. It is not a cuticle in the classical sense since it is an intracellular formation and not an extracellular secretion, but the term is well entrenched in the literature on sweat glands and so it is retained. A fibrous cuticular border is scarcely detectable in the superficial cells near the junction of the coiled duct and the secretory coil (HIBBS, 1958). At this point it consists of only a fine feltwork of tonofilaments loosely arranged within the cytoplasm (Fig. 17). Even here, however, mitochondria are excluded from the fibrous zone. The cuticular border becomes progressively broader and more prominent along the length of the coiled duct and it is fully developed in the straight duct, where a layer of thicker, dense tonofibrils underlies an apical zone of fine tonofilaments (Fig. 19). The layer of thick fibrils is sharp and distinct and separates the unmodified cytoplasm of the cell from the fibrous border (HASHIMOTO et al., 1966).

The tonofilaments that form the cuticular border are usually wavy and measure 35 to 70 Å in diameter. They are loosely organized, oriented more or less parallel to the luminal surface of the cell (Fig. 20). Some filaments seem to attach to the inner dense line of the plasma membrane producing zones of increased electron density. In its full expression the fibrous cuticular border, including both the more superficial layer of fine tonofilaments and the deeper band of coarse tonofibrils is about 1 μ wide comprising approximately one-fourth of the cell mass.

Below the cuticular border, in the perinuclear and infranuclear cytoplasm, there are mitochondria of various shapes, some profiles of both granular and agranular endoplasmic reticulum and glycogen granules all embedded in a homogeneous matrix. Occasionally these cells may contain organized ergastoplasm, but Golgi elements are characteristically lacking. Along the base of the superficial cell the plasma membrane is pressed into villous folds that complement those on the basal cells. On the lateral surface of the superficial cells the villous fringe changes in character as it approaches the lumen. At approximately one-third of the distance to the lumen, near the level of the nucleus, the villous processes gradually become shorter and broader and are transformed progressively into short sinuous stumps. In this zone of transition, desmosomes linking the surfaces of adjacent cells become both more conspicuous and more numerous (Fig. 20). Near the lumen each interlocking process of adjoining cells is marked by a prominent desmosome. The desmosomes become more noticeable because the tonofilaments that extend from the attachment plaques into the cytoplasm of the superficial cell increase both in numbers and apparent density. At the luminal interface the cell membranes of adjoining superficial cells are fused to form the typical zonula occludens or tight junction of the junctional complex (Fig. 20). HASHIMOTO et al. (1966) note that at the points where adjacent superficial cells meet in the intradermal duct, there are shallow clefts between the cells; but in the epidermal duct the cells are joined along raised ridges (Figs. 19 and 20).

b) Cytochemistry

Histochemically the superficial cells of the duct share much in common with the basal cells. It is the fibrous apical border of these cells that makes them unusual, and this distinguishing feature deserves special comment.

Although non-specific esterases are in low concentration within other sites of the duct, the luminal border of the superficial cells is strongly reactive (STEIGLEDER and SCHULTIS, 1957; MONTAGNA and ELLIS, 1958b). Only low levels of acid phosphatase activity are present in the superficial cells and there is no preferential localization of this enzyme at the luminal border. Enzymes that are linked to the mitochondria of the cell, such as cytochrome oxidase and succinic dehydrogenase are not demonstrable in the cuticular border. This is not surprising, since the electron microscope shows that mitochondria are excluded from that zone. Glycogen is frequently distributed along a fine line that marks the separation between the unmodified cytoplasm of the superficial cell and the fibrous border (LOBITZ et al., 1955), but it is never demonstrable within the cuticular zone.

Cytochemical tests show that the fibrous border of the superficial cells reacts strongly for both S-S and -SH groups (MONTAGNA et al., 1954), although studies by LEE (1960) indicate that S-S groups may be quantitatively insignificant. The positive identification of substances containing S-S and -SH linkages within the fibrous border supports the ultrastructural studies demonstrating that the cuticle consists of closely packed masses of tonofibrils and tonofiaments and is at least partially keratinized. Since the cuticular border is birefrigent under polarized light (SCHMIDT, 1959) the tonofilaments must be organized preferentially.

The luminal border of the superficial cells lining the duct gives a moderate reaction with the periodic acid Schiff method even after digestion of the sections with diastase or saliva (LOBITZ et al, 1954a, 1955; LEE, 1960; HASHIMOTO et al., 1966). LEE (1960) reported that the reaction is produced by the luminal contents but HASHIMOTO et al. (1966) suggested that this is an extracellular polysaccharide coat on the plasma membrane of the superficial cells. In any case, the cellular origin of this epithelial mucin is not clear. The superficial cells seem to have few of the intracellular organelles that in other cell types are ordinarily associated with polysaccharide synthesis and they may not themselves produce the surface coating. As an alternative source the dark cells within the secretory coil synthesize a polysaccharide and they could secrete the coating substance (LEE, 1960).

c) Function

The function that the superficial cells play in the elaboration of sweat is still a matter for debate. At least two possibilities exist: (1) that these are absorptive cells and that the cuticular border confers a capacity for selective reabsorption (or secretion) of material into the duct (MUNGER and BRUSILOW, 1961), (2) that the superficial cells function as supporting cells maintaining the shape and continuity of the lumen by their highly structured fibrous border (ELLIS and MONTAGNA, 1961).

The character of the cuticular border changes along the length of the duct. Near the secretory coil, the cuticular border is not well-developed and it consists primarily of a meshwork of tonofilaments (Fig. 17). In this same region the basal cells contain abundant mitochondria (MONTAGNA et al., 1953; HIBBS, 1958) and have an extensive surface area. In the remainder of the coiled duct and in the straight duct the fibrous border of the superficial cells is fully differentiated and the basal cells have fewer mitochondria, less surface area and increased numbers of tonofibrils. Thus the development of the cuticular border in the superficial cells may be inversely related to the specialization of the basal cells for sodium transport. This implies that a fully formed fibrous border may impede ion transport. On the other hand, small clear vesicles are as abundant in the fully developed fibrous border of the straight duct as they are within the partially developed cuticle of the coiled duct. If these vesicles reflect the pinocytotic activity at the luminal surface, then, the superficial cells seem to be equally active in this respect along the entire length of the duct. From electron micrographs the direction of movement of these vesicles cannot be ascertained, but the scant endoplasmic reticulum and the almost total absence of organized Golgi membranes suggests that these cells are not cells primarily engaged in secretion. Physiological studies of sweat secretion and reabsorption cannot distinguish between the function of the basal cells and the superficial cells, but from comparative ultrastructural evidence the superficial cells have no features in common with cells involved in ion secretion. It seems quite certain, therefore that although they may play some role in absorption, they do not play a role in active sodium transport. How the superficial cells may function in absorption is pure conjuncture. A specific surface coating of the plasma membrane, the organization of the tonofilaments or the nature of the proteins within the cuticular border could facilitate the selective reabsorption of ions from the lumen into these cells (MUNGER and BRUSILOW, 1961; ELLIS, 1966). As polyanions, mucopolysaccharides could assist the superficial cells in selectively absorbing sodium from the fluid within the lumen of the duct without disturbing the osmotic balance of the cell. Sodium absorbed in this manner could be released into the intercellular fluid where the basal cells could then actively transport it into the interstices of the dermis.

IV. The Epidermal Sweat Duct

From the point where the sweat gland opens onto the surface of the skin to the base of the rete ridges the sweat duct traverses the epidermis. In regions of the body where the epidermis is thin the length of this intraepidermal duct is short, but where the epidermis is thickened the duct follows a long and tortuous path (Fig. 6). This portion of the eccrine sweat gland that is distinct from the epidermis that surrounds it, was designated the "epidermal sweat duct unit" by LOBITZ et al. (1954a). Other authors have refered to it as the epidermal sweat duct (ZELICKSON, 1961) or the intraepidermal sweat duct (MONTAGNA, 1962a; HASHIMOTO et al., 1966). There is strong evidence supporting the epidermal sweat duct unit concept. For example, in some epidermal lesions such as senile keratosis, the epidermal sweat duct is relatively unaffected (LOBITZ et al., 1954a); the cells of the epidermal sweat duct contain no pigment, even in the skin of Negroes; and the cells of the intraepidermal sweat duct keratinize differently from the surrounding epidermal cells (LEE, 1960; HASHIMOTO et al., 1966). Biologically, however, the duct cells behave much like epidermal cells, in wound healing they contribute to the repair of denuded areas (LOBITZ et al., 1954b) and in normal skin the cells of the epidermal sweat duct are mitotically active only at the point where the straight duct joins with the epidermis, a site comparable to the basal germinative layer of the epidermis (LOBITZ et al., 1954b).

a) Electron Microscopy

The epidermal sweat duct shares many fine structural details with the straight duct. An inner ring of superficial or luminal cells lines the lumen, and two or three layers of peripheral ductal cells separate the luminal cells from typical epidermal cells (ZELICKSON, 1961).

In cross-sections through the epidermal sweat duct, two or three luminal cells form the inner rim of the canal. These cells are similar in most respects to the superficial cells that line the straight duct. The luminal surface of the cells is covered with short stumpy microvilli that are bent and twisted and have an inner fibrous core (Figs. 19 and 20). The fibrous cuticular border of the luminal cells is readily apparent, but not as highly developed as in the straight duct. Where two cells are joined at the luminal side, an evagination or tongue like papilla is formed (HASHIMOTO et al., 1966) and a typical junctional complex is observed (Figs. 19 and 20). Clear round vesicles lie just beneath villous surface of the luminal cells. Another feature that distinguishes these cells are the more numerous

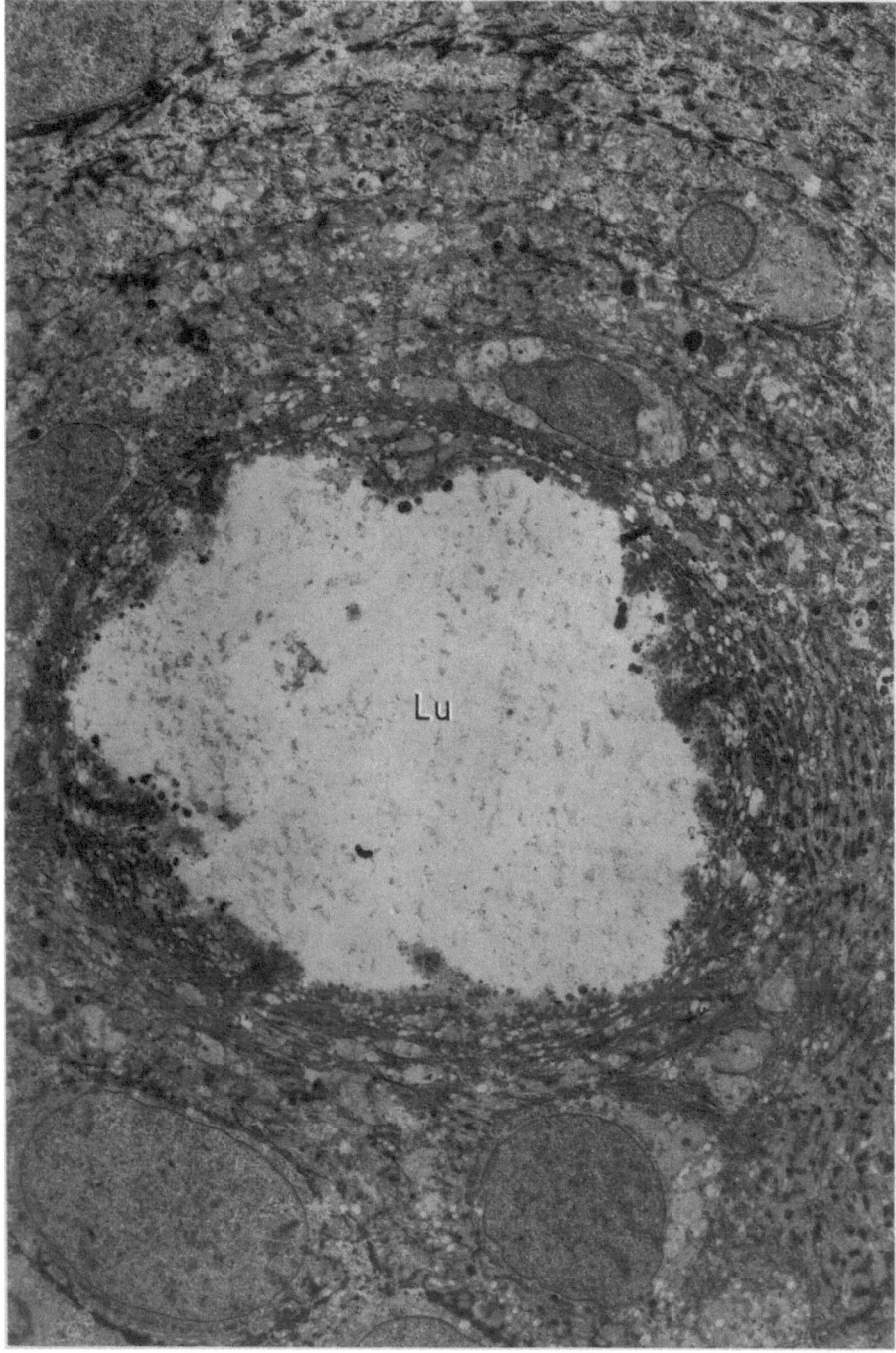

Fig. 21. In the fully-formed intraepidermal sweat duct of the fetus, the lumen (*Lu*) is broad and the cuticular border only partly developed. The superficial cells as well as the peripheral cells and the epidermal cells contain an abundance of dense glycogen granules in their cytoplasm. This electron micrograph was kindly provided by K. HASHIMOTO, M.D. (HASHIMOTO et al., 1965). × 4,200

lysosomes that are scattered through their cytoplasm. These are most abundant in the developing epidermal sweat ducts of embryonic skin (Figs. 3 and 4) (HASHIMOTO et al., 1965) but they persist in considerable numbers in the luminal cells of adults. These bodies may be responsible for the strong esterase activity that is associated with the epidermal sweat duct.

The relatively poor differentiation of the cuticular border in the luminal cells may be compensated for by the surrounding strong ductal walls that undergo keratinization much earlier than their epidermal neighbors (Table 1). The luminal

Table 1. *Degree of Keratinization of the Cells of the Intraepidermal Duct in Eccrine Sweat Glands from the Palm of the Hand.* (Adapted from LEE, 1960 and HASHIMOTO et al., 1966)

Epidermal Cells	Duct Cells	
	Outer Cells	Inner Cells
Sweat duct ridge	no KHG	no KHG
Basal layer	no KHG	no KHG
Lower spinous layer	few KHG	no KHG
Middle spinous layer	moderate KHG	few KHG
Upper spinous layer	abundant KHG	moderate KHG
Granular layer	keratinized	moderate KHG
Lower horny layer	keratinized	inc. keratinization
Middle horny layer	keratinized	inc. keratinization
Upper horny layer	keratinized	shed into lumen

KHG = keratohyalin granules.

cells do not contain membrane-coating granules (MATOLTSY and PARAKKAL, 1965) an observation consonant with their incomplete keratinization (HASHIMOTO et al., 1966).

The outer cells of the epidermal sweat duct resemble epidermal cells that are at comparable stages of differentiation. Since epidermal cells are discussed in detail in another chapter, detailed descriptions of these cells in the various stages of keratinization will not be repeated here.

Although some investigators have speculated that the epidermal sweat duct may function in the reabsorption or excretion of sweat (ZELICKSON, 1961) there is little physiological evidence to support such conclusions.

b) Cytochemistry

The histochemical reactions of the intraepidermal duct differ from the straight duct only in degree. In most respects the cells of the straight duct and the cells of the intraepidermal sweat duct may be equated. One striking feature, however, is the strong histochemical reactivity of the border of the luminal cells for non-specific esterases (STEIGLEDER and SCHULTIS, 1957; MONTAGNA and ELLIS, 1958b). The peripheral ductal cells are virtually indistinguishable in their histochemical reactivity from epidermal cells at comparable stages of differentiation. It will be seen from Table 1 that the peripheral ductal cells acquire keratohyalin granules and undergo keratinization before the epidermal cells that surround them (LEE, 1960; HASHIMOTO et al., 1966).

The coiled intraepidermal sweat duct is strongly reactive for amylophosphorylase up to the level of the stratum granulosum of the epidermis where reaction stops abruptly (ELLIS and MONTAGNA, 1958; YASUDA et al., 1958); but the surrounding epidermal cells are only lightly colored in the basal and lower Malpighian layers.

The esterase reaction is especially striking in the skin of the palms and soles where the spiral course of the intraepidermal duct is colored brightly in the otherwise unstained thick stratum corneum.

A PAS positive material coats the apical surface of the luminal cells (LEE, 1960; ZELICKSON, 1961; HASHIMOTO et al., 1966).

V. Vascularization of the Eccrine Sweat Glands

The precise relationship between the eccrine sweat glands and their blood supply has never been clearly delineated. The descriptions that appear in the literature outline the pattern of the blood supply, as it is observed in histological and histochemical preparations but they are not explicit in describing the specific relations between the blood vessels, the secretory segment of the eccrine sweat gland and the coiled and straight ducts.

Several approaches have been made to this problem. Most, like PETERSON (1935) have perfused the blood vessels of the skin with colored or opaque compounds. This technique is usually satisfactory, but it may fail to reveal many collapsed capillaries or constricted arterioles. EICHNER (1954) has used a silver impregnation method and iron hematoxylin staining, but this technique does not reveal the blood vessels specifically. Since red blood cells contain quantities of peroxidase, the G-Nadi reaction may be used to demonstrate the corpuscles within the blood vessels of the skin. The disadvantage of this method lies in the fact that in biopsy specimens most of the blood has drained from the vessels, and many, especially the smaller capillaries cannot be visualized. One of the most reliable methods for demonstrating the smaller vessels of the skin takes advantage of the alkaline phosphatase activity in their endothelium (BUNTING et al., 1948). Thick frozen sections of skin reacted for alkaline phosphatase show the paths of arterioles and capillaries, and have the added advantage of demonstrating both collapsed and constricted vessels as well as those that are distended.

The alkaline phosphatase preparations show that the entire glomerate portion of the gland is highly vascularized (Fig. 22). The blood vessels follow closely the contours of the gland and are intimately associated with both the coiled duct and the secretory segment (MONTAGNA and ELLIS, 1958a). In some glands all of the blood vessels seem to originate from one arteriole; but in others the blood supply may spring from several arterioles. In the scrotum, the glomerate portion of the eccrine sweat glands is loosely coiled and the capillaries around the different loops can be seen giving off branches and shunts which connect with the vessels around adjacent loops. In the tightly coiled tubular glands in the scalp, the axilla and the arm, the blood vessels form a dense plexus around the tubules.

The blood vessels supplying the straight duct may be somewhat variable in their origin. Some investigators assert that the deeper portion may be surrounded by capillaries that originate from the same arterioles that supply the glomerate portion of the gland, while the part of the duct nearer the epidermis is surrounded by capillaries stemming from the subepidermal plexus. Other studies indicate that two or more capillaries or arterioles, that connect to the hypodermal plexus, wind loosely around the straight portion of the excretory duct as it ascends toward the surface and that cross-shunts connect these roughly parallel vessels (MONTAGNA, 1962a). Near the base of the papillary body of the dermis the parallel vessels branch giving off capillary loops around the cone of the epidermis that contains the terminal coiled intraepidermal portion of the duct. Regional variations in the blood supply of the skin as well as in the architecture of the sweat glands may account for these different observations, and both may be accurate.

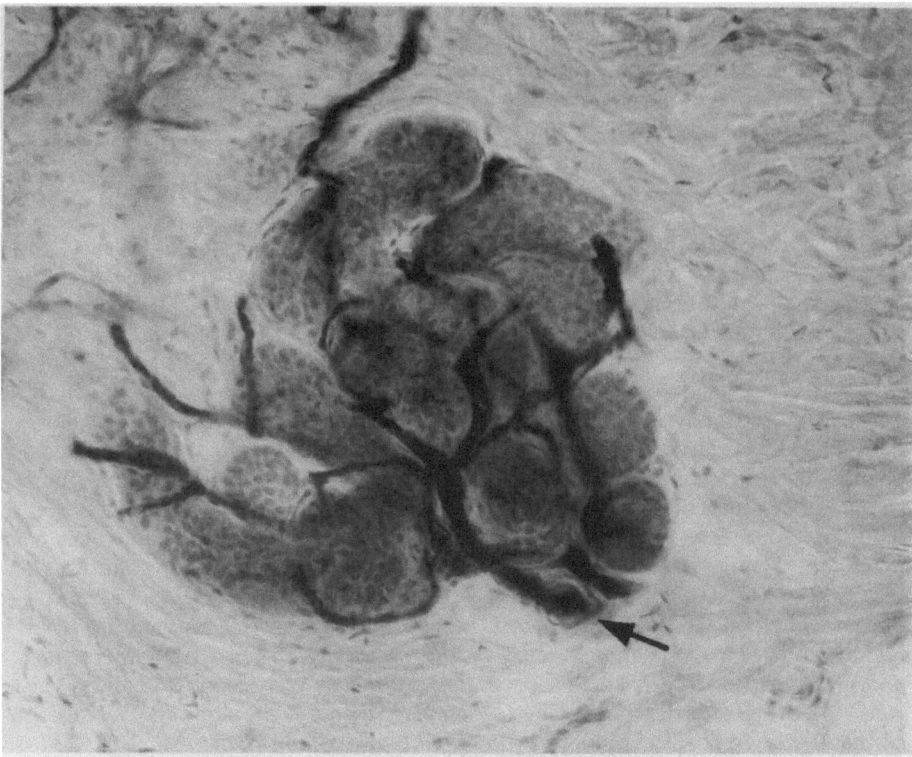

Fig. 22. Many of the capillaries that closely invest the coiled portion of this eccrine sweat gland seem to arise from a single arteriole (arrow). Alkaline phosphatase reaction. × 120

VI. Innervation of Eccrine Sweat Glands

Relationships between the nervous system and the eccrine sweat glands are established while the glands are still developing, and in the palms and soles such relationships may be demonstrated as early as the 18th week of fetal life (BECKETT et al., 1956). In man the delicate unmyelinated nerve fibers of the sympathetic nervous system, that surround the glomerate part of the eccrine sweat glands, are rich in specific cholinesterase (HELLMAN, 1955). The histochemical method for the demonstration of specific cholinesterase in tissue sections, is therefore, a far more reliable method of demonstrating the innervation of the sweat glands than any of the silver or gold impregnation techniques. The cholinesterase preparations show that the secretory coil is wrapped with strongly reactive nerve fibers that follow a more or less helical course relative to the axis of the tubule (Fig. 23). Some of the coils of the duct, but not the straight segments, are also surrounded by nerves that contain specific cholinesterases. The nerves that encircle the coiled duct are usually fewer in number than those around the secretory segment of the eccrine sweat glands (Fig. 23). There is no evidence that the eccrine sweat glands have a double innervation.

The nerves surrounding the coiled tubules of the eccrine sweat glands have the typical structure of unmyelinated nerve fibers of the peripheral nervous system and will not be described in detail here. The fine terminals, upon leaving the Schwann cell sheath adhere closely to the membrana propria of the epithelium.

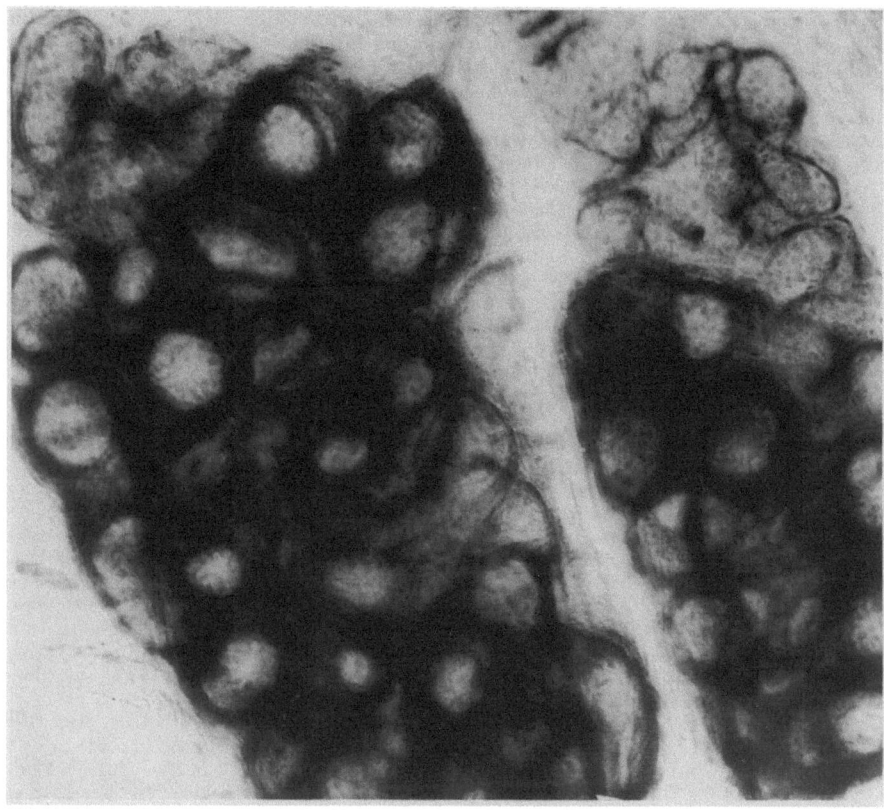

Fig. 23. Nerves strongly reactive for cholinesterase invest the coiled secretory tubules of two eccrine sweat glands in the scalp. The nerves wrapped about the coiled duct (upper right) are fewer in number and weaker in activity. Acetylthiocholine iodide substrate. Preparation courtesy of Dr. L. GIACOMETTI. × 120

None of the nerve processes penetrate the amorphous basement membrane however. Some investigators have suggested that the small circular profiles occasionally seen in the intercellular spaces may be the terminals of unmyelinated nerves. This interpretation seems untenable however, since these processes are of the same size and shape as cross-sections of the villous processes on the surfaces of the clear cells, and since nerve terminals are not observed penetrating the basement membrane. In a site where nerve fibers are present in such abundance the many electron microscopic studies of the eccrine glands would discover any direct innervation of the myoepithelial cells or the secretory cells, if there are such connections with the autonomic nervous system. This negative evidence seems to indicate that the sweat glands are stimulated to secrete by neurohumors released from nerves lying outside the basement membrane.

References

ACKERMANN, A.: Studien zur Physiologie der Schweißdrüsen, zur Pharmakologie und Funktionsweise der Schweißdrüsen. Dermatologica (Basel) 19, 151—174, 219—236 (1939). — ARAKI, Y., and S. ONDO: Urea, amino acid and ammonia in human sweat. Jap. J. Physiol. 3, 211—218 (1953).

BECKETT, E. B., G. H. BOURNE, and W. MONTAGNA: Histology and cytochemistry of human skin. The distribution of cholinesterase in the finger of the embryo and the adult. J. Physiol. (Lond.) 134, 202—206 (1956). — BRAUN-FALCO, O.: Histochemische und morphologische Studien an normaler und pathologisch veränderter Haut. Arch. Derm. Syph. **198**, 111—198 (1954). — Über die Fähigkeit der menschlichen Haut zur Polysaccharidsynthese, ein Beitrag zur Histotopochemie der Phosphorylase. Arch. klin. exp. Derm. **202**, 163—170 (1956a). — Zur Histotopographie der β-Glucuronidase in normaler menschlicher Haut. Arch. klin. exp. Derm. **203**, 61—67 (1956b). — Zur Histotopographie der Cytochromoxydase in normaler und pathologisch veränderter Haut sowie in Hauttumoren. Arch. klin. exp. Derm. **214**, 176—224 (1961). — BRAUN-FALCO, O., and D. PETZOLDT: Über die Histotopie von NADH- und NADPH-Tetrazoliumreduktase in menschlicher Haut. I. Normale Haut. Arch. klin. exp. Derm. **220**, 455—473 (1964). — BRAUN-FALCO, O., and B. RATHJENS: Histochemische Darstellung der Bernsteinsäuredehydrogenase in der menschlichen Haut. Derm. Wschr. **130**, 1271—1276 (1954). — Über die histochemische Darstellung der Kohlensäureanhydratase in normaler Haut. Arch. klin. exp. Derm. **201**, 73—82 (1955). — BRESCHET, G., et A. ROUSSEL DE VOUZEME: Recherches anatomiques et physiologiques sur les appareils tegumentaires des animaux. Ann. Sci. nat. (2) **2**, 167—238, 321—370 (1834). — BUNTING, H., G. B. WISLOCKI, and E. W. DEMPSEY: The chemical histology of human eccrine and apocrine sweat glands. Anat. Rec. **100**, 61—77 (1948).

CHARLES, A.: An electron microscope study of the eccrine sweat gland. J. invest. Derm. **34**, 81—88 (1960).

DOBSON, R. L.: The effect of repeated episodes of profuse sweating on the human eccrine sweat glands. J. invest. Derm. **35**, 195—198 (1960). — The correlation of structure and function in the human eccrine sweat gland. In: Advances in biology of skin (W. MONTAGNA, R. ELLIS and A. SILVER, eds.), vol. 3, p. 54—75. New York: Pergamon Press 1962. — DOBSON, R. L., D. C. ABELE, and D. M. HALE: The effect of high and low salt intake and repeated episodes of sweating on the human eccrine sweat gland. J. invest. Derm. **36**, 327—335 (1961). — DOBSON, R. L., V. FORMISANO, W. C. LOBITZ, and D. BROPHY: Some histochemical observations on the human eccrine sweat glands. III. The effects of profuse sweating. J. invest. Derm. **31**, 147—159 (1958). — DOBSON, R. L., and W. C. LOBITZ: Some histochemical observations on the human eccrine sweat glands. IV. The recovery from the effects of profuse sweating. J. invest. Derm. **31**, 207—213 (1958). — DOYLE, W. L.: The principal cells of the salt-gland of marine birds. Exp. Cell Res. **21**, 386—393 (1960).

EICHNER, F.: Zur Frage der Motivbildung in der menschlichen Haut. Anat. Anz. **100**, 303—310 (1954). — ELLIS, R. A.: The fine structure of eccrine sweat glands. In: Advances in biology of skin (W. MONTAGNA, R. ELLIS and A. SILVER, eds.), vol. 3, p. 30—53. New York: Pergamon Press 1962. — The fine structure of some salt-secreting epithelia. In: Research on pathogenesis of cystic fibrosis. Proc. IIIrd. Internat. Conf. p. 1—14. Maryland: N. I. H. Bethesda 1964. — Fine structure of the myoepithelium of the eccrine sweat glands of man. J. Cell Biol. **27**, 551—563 (1965). — ELLIS, R. A., and J. H. ABEL: Intercellular channels in the salt glands of marine turtles. Science **144**, 1340—1341 (1964). — ELLIS, R. A., and W. MONTAGNA: Histology and cytochemistry of human skin. XV. Sites of phosphorylase and amylo-1,6-glucosidase activity. J. Histochem. Cytochem. **6**, 201—207 (1958). — Electron microscopy of the duct, and especially the cuticular border of the eccrine sweat glands in *Macaca mulatta*. J. biophys. biochem. Cytol. **9**, 238—242 (1961).

FAWCETT, D. W.: Physiologically significant specializations of the cell surface. Circulation **26**, 1105—1125 (1962). — FORMISANO, V., and W. C. LOBITZ: The "Schiff-positive, nonglycogen material" in the human eccrine sweat glands. I. Histochemistry. Arch. Derm. **75**, 202—209 (1957). — FRANZINI-ARMSTRONG, C., and K. PORTER: Sarcolemmal invaginations constituting the T system in fish muscle fibers. J. Cell Biol. **22**, 675—696 (1964). — FUSARO, R. M., and R. W. GOLTZ: The normal human eccrine and apocrine glands. J. invest. Derm. **36**, 79—82 (1961).

GOMORI, G.: Microscopic histochemistry, principles and practice. Chicago: University of Chicago Press 1952. — GUALDI, A., e N. BALDINO: Ricerche sul metabolismo per variazioni della temperatura locale dei tessuti; il contenuto in glicogeno e in acido lattico della cute e dei muscoli raffreddati. Riv. Pat. clin. sper. **5**, 318—322 (1930).

HACKENBROCK, C. R., and P. W. BRANDT: Reversible ultrastructural changes in mitochondria in changes in functional state. J. Cell Biol. **27**, 40A (1965). — HASHIMOTO, K., B. G. GROSS, and W. F. LEVER: The ultrastructure of the skin of human embryos. I. The intraepidermal eccrine sweat duct. J. invest. Derm. **45**, 139—151 (1965). — Electron microscopic studies of the human adult eccrine gland. I. The duct. J. invest. Derm. **46**, 172—180 (1966). — HELLMANN, K.: Cholinesterase and amine oxidase in the skin: A histochemical investigation. J. Physiol. (Lond.) **129**, 454—463 (1955). — HIBBS, R. G.: The fine structure of human eccrine sweat glands. Amer. J. Anat. **103**, 201—218 (1958). — HOLYOKE, J. B., and W. C. LOBITZ: Histologie variations in the structure of human eccrine sweat glands. J. invest. Derm. **18**, 147—167 (1952). — HORSTMANN, E.: Die Haut. In: Handbuch der mikroskopischen Anatomie des Menschen (W. VON MÖLLENDORFF, ed.), Bd. 3, S. 1—488. Berlin: Springer 1957. — HURLEY, H. J., and J. WITKOWSKI: Dye clearance and eccrine sweat secretion in human skin.

J. invest. Derm. **36**, 259—272 (1961a). — Mechanism of epinephrine induced eccrine sweating in human skin. J. appl. Physiol. **16**, 652—654 (1961b).

JIRKA, M., and J. KOTAS: The occurrence of mucoprotein in human sweat. Clin. chim. Acta **2**, 292—296 (1957).

KAWAHATA, A.: Studies on the function of human sweat organs. Mie. med. J. **1**, 25—41 (1950). — KOMNICK, H.: Electronenmikroskopische Untersuchungen zur funktionellen Morphologie des Ionentransportes in der Solzdruse von *Larus argentatus*. III. Teil: Funktionelle Morphologie der Tubulusepithelzellen. Protoplasma (Wien) **56**, 605—636 (1963). — KUNO, Y.: In: Human perspiration. Springfield (Ill.): Ch. C. Thomas 1956. — KUROSUMI, K., T. KITAMURA, and K. KANO: Electron microscopy of the human eccrine sweat gland from an aged individual. Arch. histol. jap. **20**, 253—269 (1960).

LEE, M. C.: Histology and histochemistry of human eccrine sweat glands with special reference to their defense mechanisms. Anat. Rec. **136**, 97—105 (1960). — LLOYD, D. P. C.: Secretion and reabsorption in eccrine sweat glands. In: Advances in biology of skin (W. MONTAGNA, R. ELLIS and A. SILVER, eds.), vol. 3, p. 127—151. New York: Pergamon Press 1962. — LOBITZ, W. C., J. B. HOLYOKE, and D. BROPHY: Histochemical evidence for human eccrine sweat duct activity. Arch. Derm. **72**, 229—236 (1955). — LOBITZ, W. C., J. B. HOLYOKE, and W. MONTAGNA: The epidermal eccrine sweat duct unit. A morphologic and biologic entity. J. invest. Derm. **22**, 157—158 (1954a). — Responses of the human eccrine sweat duct to controlled injury. J. invest. Derm. **23**, 329—344 (1954b). — LOBITZ, W. C., and H. L. MASON: Chemistry of palmar sweat. VII. Discussion of studies on chloride urea, glucose, uric acid, ammonia-nitrogen and creatinine. Arch. Derm. Syph. **57**, 907—915 (1948). — LOEWENTHAL, L. J. A.: The human eccrine sweat gland ampulla. J. invest. Derm. **34**, 233—235 (1960). — The eccrine ampulla: morphology and function. J. invest. Derm. **36**, 171—182 (1961).

MATOLTSY, A. G., and P. PARAKKAL: Membrane-coating granules of keratinizing epithelia. J. Cell Biol. **24**, 297—307 (1965). — MATSUZAWA, T., and K. KUROSUMI: The ultrastructure, morphogenesis and histochemistry of the sweat glands in the rat foot pads as revealed by electron microscopy. J. Electronmic. **12**, 175—191 (1963). — MONTAGNA, W.: The structure and function of skin (1st ed.). New York: Academic Press 1956. — Histology and cytochemistry of human skin. XI. The distribution of β-glucuronidase. J. biophys. biochem. Cytol. **3**, 343—348 (1957). — The structure and function of skin (2nd ed.). New York: Academic Press 1962a. — Histological, histochemical and pharmacological properties. In: Advances in biology of skin (W. MONTAGNA, R. ELLIS and A. SILVER, eds.), vol. 3, p. 6—29. New York: Pergamon Press 1962b. — MONTAGNA, W., H. B. CHASE, and W. C. LOBITZ: Histology and cytochemistry of human skin. II. The distribution of glycogen in the epidermis, hair follicles, sebaceous glands and eccrine sweat glands. Anat. Rec. **114**, 231—237 (1952). — Histology and cytochemistry of human skin. IV. The eccrine sweat glands. J. invest. Derm. **20**, 415—423 (1953). — MONTAGNA, W., A. Z. EISEN, A. H. RADEMACHER, and H. B. CHASE: Histology and cytochemistry of human skin. VI. The distribution of sulfhydryl and disulfide groups. J. invest. Derm. **23**, 23—32 (1954). — MONTAGNA, W., and R. A. ELLIS: Histology and cytochemistry of human skin XIV. The blood supply of the cutaneous glands. J. invest. Derm. **30**, 135—145 (1958a). — L'histologie et la cytologie de le peau humaine. XVI. Repartition et concentration des esterases carboxyliques. Ann. Histochim. **3**, 1—17 (1958b). — MONTAGNA, W., and V. FORMISANO: Histology and cytochemistry of human skin. VII. The distribution of succinic dehydrogenase activity. Anat. Rec. **122**, 65—77 (1955). — MONTAGNA, W., K. YASUDA, and R. A. ELLIS: The skin of primates. III. The skin of the slow loris (*Nyctecebus coucang*). Amer. J. physic. Anthrop. **19**, 1—22 (1961). — MONTAGNA, W., and J. YUN: The skin of primates. VII. The skin of the great bushbaby (*Galgo crassicaudatus*). Amer. J. physic. Anthrop. **20**, 149—166 (1962). — MUNGER, B.: The ultrastructure and histophysiology of human eccrine sweat glands. J. biophys. biochem. Cytol. **11**, 385—402 (1961). — MUNGER, B. L., and S. W. BRUSILOW: An electron microscopic study of eccrine sweat glands of the cat foot and the toe pads — evidence for ductal reabsorption in the human. J. biophys. biochem. Cytol. **11**, 403—417 (1961). — MUNGER, B. L., S. W. BRUSILOW, and R. E. COOKE: An electron microscopic study of eccrine sweat glands in patients with cystic fibrosis of the pancreas. J. Pediat. **59**, 497—511 (1961).

NITTA, H.: On the possibility of a reabsorption in the excretory duct of the sweat gland: Experiments on the changes in sweat constituents resulting from application of collodion membrane on the skin. Nagoya med. J. **1**, 59 (1953).

PAPA, C. M.: A new technique to observe and record sweating. Arch. Derm. **88**, 732—733 (1963). — PEARSE, A. G.: Carbohydrates. In: Histochemistry, theoretical and applied, 2nd ed., p. 228—280. Boston: Little, Brown & Co. 1960. — PETERSON, H.: Histologie und mikroskopische Anatomie. München: J. F. Bergmann 1935. — PINKUS, F.: Die normale Anatomie der Haut. In: Handbuch der Haut- und Geschlechtskrankheiten (J. JADASSOHN, Hrsg.), Bd. 1, S. 1—378. Berlin: Springer 1927. — PURKINJE and WENDT: Quoted in GURLT, Vergleichende Untersuchungen über die Haut des Menschen und der Haussäugetiere, besonders in

Beziehung auf die Absonderungsorgane des Haut-Talges und des Schweißes. Arch. Anat. Physiol. (Lpz.) 399—418 (1835).
SARKANY, I., and G. A. CARON: Microtopography of the human skin. J. Anat. **99**, 359—364 (1965). — SCHIEFFERDECKER, P.: Die Hautdrusen des Menschen und der Säugetiere, ihre biologische und rassenanatomische Bedeutung, sowie die Muscularis sexualis. Biol. Zbl. **37**, 534—562 (1917). — Die Hautdrüsen des Menschen und der Säugetiere, ihre biologische und rassenanatomische Bedeutung, sowie die Muscularis sexualis. Zoologica **27**, 1—154 (1922). — SCHMIDT, W. J.: Doppelbrechung und Feinbau des Saumrohres (der sog. Cuticula) im Ausführgang der Schweißdrüsen des Menschen. Z. Zellforsch. **49**, 711—719 (1959). — SCHULZ, I., K. J. ULLRICH, E. FROMTER, H. M. EMRICH, A. FRICK, U. HEGEL, and H. HOLZGROVE: Micropuncture experiments on human sweat gland. In: Research on pathogenesis of cystic fibrosis. Proc. IIIrd Internat. Conf. p. 136—144. Maryland: N.I.H. Bethesda 1964. — SCHWARTZ, I. L., and J. H. THAYSEN: Excretion of sodium and potassium in human sweat. J. clin. Invest. **35**, 114—120 (1956). — SCHWARTZ, I. L., J. H. THAYSEN, and V. P. DOLE: Urea excretion in human sweat as a tracer for movement of water within the secreting gland. J. exp. Med. **97**, 429—437 (1953). — SCOTT, T. G.: Intracellular canals in human sweat glands. Nature (Lond.) **188**, 158—159 (1960). — SERRI, F.: Note de enzimologia cutana. II. Ricerche bio ed istochimiche sull'attivita succinodeidrasica della cute umana normale. Boll. soc. med.-chir. Pavia **69**, 3—19 (1955). — SHELLY, W. B., and H. MESCON: Histochemical demonstration of secretory activity in human eccrine sweat glands. J. invest. Derm. **18**, 289—301 (1952). — SLEGERS, J. F. G.: The mechanism of sweat-secretion. Pflügers Arch. ges. Physiol. **279**, 265—273 (1964). — STEIGLEDER, G. K., u. K. SCHULTIS: Zur Histochemie der Esterasen der Haut. Arch. klin. exp. Derm. **205**, 196—211 (1957). — SZABO, G.: The number of eccrine sweat glands in human skin. In: Advances in biology of skin (W. MONTAGNA, R. ELLIS and A. SILVER, eds.), vol. 3, p. 1—5. New York: Pergamon Press 1962.
TERZAKIS, J. A.: The ultrastructure of monkey eccrine sweat glands. Z. Zellforsch. **64**, 493—509 (1964). — THOMPSON, N.: Eccrine sweat glands in human skin grafts. In: Advances in biology of skin (W. MONTAGNA, R. ELLIS and A. SILVER, eds.), vol. 3, p. 76—96. New York: Pergamon Press 1962. — TSUCHIYA, K.: Über die ekkrine Schweißdrüse des menschlichen Embryo, mit besonderer Berücksichtigung ihrer Histo- und Cytogenese. Arch. histol. jap. **6**, 403—432 (1954).
WADA, M., and T. TAKAGAKI: A simple and accurate method for detecting the secretion of sweat. Tohoku J. exp. Med. **49**, 284 (1948). — WEINER, J. S., and K. HELLMAN: The sweat glands. Biol. Rev. **35**, 141—186 (1960).
YASUDA, K., H. FURUSAWA, and N. OGATA: Histochemical investigation on the phosphorylase in the sweat glands of axilla. Okajimas Folia anat. jap. **31**, 161—169 (1958). — YASUDA, K., and W. MONTAGNA: Histology and cytochemistry of human skin. XX. The distribution of monoamine oxidase. J. Histochem. Cytochem. **8**, 356—366 (1960).

Apokrine Schweißdrüsen*

Von

O. Braun-Falco und M. Rupec

Mit 46 Abbildungen (davon 1 vierfarbig)

A. Historischer Überblick und Embryonalentwicklung
I. Historischer Überblick

Bereits bevor SCHIEFFERDECKER (1917, 1922) die apokrinen Schweißdrüsen auf Grund ihrer Sekretart, ihres Sekretionsmodus und ihrer Formalgenese von den ekkrinen Schweißdrüsen abgetrennt hatte, waren diese — besonders im Achselbereich — als große Knäueldrüsen (Glandulae glomiformes) bekannt (KRAUSE, 1844; ROBIN, 1845; HORNER, 1846; KOELLIKER, 1850). So spricht beispielsweise HEYNOLD schon 1874 über zwei verschiedene Arten von Drüsen in der Achselhöhle, während RABL noch 1902 die Existenz zwei verschiedener Typen von Schweißdrüsen nicht für wahrscheinlich hielt. 1881 hat TARTUFERI Angaben von SCHAFFER (1940) zufolge die Ceruminaldrüsen, Achselhöhlendrüsen und Mollschen Drüsen als eine besondere Gruppe mit ‚dichtem Sekret' herausgestellt. Trotzdem bleibt es das unbestrittene Verdienst SCHIEFFERDECKERs, die Unterschiede zwischen ekkrinen und apokrinen Schweißdrüsen klar herausgearbeitet und die apokrinen Schweißdrüsen, welche auch phylogenetisch älter sein sollen, von den ekkrinen Drüsen abgetrennt zu haben. Die merokrinen Drüsen, d. h. große und kleine Schweißdrüsen, wurden in die *„merokrin-apokrinen Drüsen"* (Kuppel-, Schlauchdrüsen) und *„merokrin-ekkrinen Drüsen"* unterteilt (SCHIEFFERDECKER, 1917).

Später hat sich allerdings herausgestellt, daß beide Schweißdrüsenarten nicht nur morphologisch, sondern auch in bezug auf ihren Sekretionsmodus doch nicht so scharf voneinander abzutrennen sind. Was die Morphologie betrifft, so hat MINAMITANI (1941) als „atypische apokrine Drüsen ‚B'" eine *Zwischenform* zwischen apokrinen und ekkrinen Schweißdrüsen beschrieben. Er kommt mit dieser Feststellung früheren Vorstellungen LÜNEBURGs (1902) über die Umwandlung von kleinen in große Schweißdrüsen sehr nahe. Die Möglichkeit einer Umwandlung von ekkrinen in apokrine Schweißdrüsen ist neuerdings wieder von BORSETTO (1951) ventiliert worden. Auch BRINKMANN (1909) hat beide Schweißdrüsentypen für verwandt gehalten, eine Anschauung, die SCHAFFER (1926, 1940) ebenfalls für richtig hält. In diesem Zusammenhang ist erwähnenswert, daß auch die Drüsenzellen des antebrachialen Organs bei ,,Lemur catta" sich elektronenmikroskopisch teilweise als Strukturen mit ekkrinen, teilweise als solche mit apokrinen ultrastrukturellen Merkmalen erwiesen haben (KNEELAND, 1966). Als ein derartiger intermediärer Typ wären auch die Schweißdrüsen des Pferdes zu bezeichnen (KUROSUMI, MATSUZAWA und SAITO, 1963). Hier sind ebenfalls die lichtmikroskopischen Befunde O'BRIENS (1960) über die intermediären Schweiß-

---

* Unterstützt durch Mittel der Deutschen Forschungsgemeinschaft.

drüsen mit morphologischen Merkmalen ekkriner und apokriner Drüsen zu erwähnen.

Auch ein *apokriner Sekretionsmodus* wird neuerdings besonders von BARGMANN, FLEISCHHAUER und KNOOP (1961), HIBBS (1962), MUNGER (1965) sowie BIEMPICA und MONTES (1965) für nicht wahrscheinlich gehalten. Die Sekretion apokriner Schweißdrüsen soll nach diesen elektronenmikroskopischen Untersuchungen ohne eine „Dekapitation", also nicht apokrin erfolgen. (Näheres dazu s. S. 325.)

Das besondere Verdienst der Untersuchungen von SCHIEFFERDECKER ist nach F. PINKUS (1925) darin gelegen, als erster klar erkannt zu haben, daß die ekkrinen Schweißdrüsen keinen, die apokrinen Schweißdrüsen dagegen regelmäßig einen *Zusammenhang mit den Haarfollikeln* aufweisen. „Die ekkrine Drüse ... hat mit dem Haarbalg gar nichts zu tun" (SCHIEFFERDECKER, 1917). Auch diese Anschauung ist besonders in jüngster Zeit insoweit angezweifelt worden, als HORSTMANN (1952) auf enge räumliche Beziehungen zwischen beiden Strukturen anhand von Flächenpräparaten hingewiesen hat. Er konnte zeigen, daß die ekkrinen Schweißdrüsen eine Art „Zifferblatt" um den Haarfollikel bilden. Auf solche Beziehungen der ekkrinen Schweißdrüsen zum Haar in der Embryonalzeit hat auch FLEISCHHAUER (1953) aufmerksam gemacht. Außerdem sind sie schließlich auch nach BRINKMANN (1923/24) phylogenetisch nicht als „frei", sondern als einem Haarbezirk (F. PINKUS, 1927) zugehörige Organelle zu betrachten. Demgegenüber sind die direkten Beziehungen zwischen apokrinen Schweißdrüsen und Haarfollikeln allgemein anerkannt.

Die ersten Studien über die *Funktion der apokrinen Schweißdrüsen* wurden von OLIVET und NAUCK (1930) durchgeführt. Später haben sich vor allem HURLEY und SHELLEY (1954a, b, c, 1960), SHELLEY und HURLEY (1953, 1954, 1957) sowie SHELLEY (1951) mit dieser Fragestellung beschäftigt. In der letzten Zeit sind die apokrinen Schweißdrüsen besonders von japanischen (MINAMITANI, 1941; YASUDA, 1959, 1962, 1963; YASUDA et al., 1958, 1960a, b, 1962, 1963; KUROSUMI, 1961; KUROSUMI et al., 1959) und amerikanischen (MONTAGNA, 1956, 1959, 1962, 1963, 1964a, b; HURLEY und SHELLEY) Autoren bearbeitet worden. Zu ihrer *Phylogenese* haben besonders SCHIEFFERDECKER (1917, 1922, 1923), BRINKMANN (1909, 1923), KLAAR (1924, 1926), F. PINKUS (1910, 1925, 1926, 1927), SCHAFFER (1926, 1940), STRAUSS (1950), v. EGGELING (1923, 1940) und MONTAGNA (1962, 1963) Stellung genommen. Man glaubt, daß die apokrinen wie auch ekkrinen Schweißdrüsen von einem gemeinsamen Drüsentyp abstammen, welcher weder mit den heutigen ekkrinen noch den apokrinen Drüsen völlig übereinstimmt (MONTAGNA, 1963). Vielleicht sind als Bindeglied zwischen beiden Drüsentypen die Ballendrüsen (SCHAFFER, 1940) anzusehen.

II. Die Embryonalentwicklung

Die ersten apokrinen Schweißdrüsenanlagen sind im 4.—5. Monat (HURLEY und SHELLEY, 1960) bzw. im 5. Monat (MONTAGNA, 1962) zu beobachten. YANAGISAWA (1957) fand an der äußeren Nase erste Anlagen bei einem Embryo von 14,5 cm Länge[1]. ALVERDES (1934) sowie YANAGISAWA (1957) fanden Anlagen der Glandula vestibularis ebenfalls bei Embryonen von 14 cm, MOGI (1938) bei 11—14 cm Länge. Die Mollschen Drüsen sollen sich nach CONTINO (1907) schon bei einem 7,3 cm langen Embryo in der initialen Entwicklungsphase finden.

---

[1] Über die Fruchtlänge und den Zeitpunkt der Schwangerschaft siehe bei MARTIUS und HARTL (1959).

SIMONETTA und MAGNONI (1937) haben apokrine Drüsenanlagen im äußeren Gehörgang des Menschen im 3.—4. Monat feststellen können. STEINER (1925) fand erste Anlagen apokriner Schweißdrüsen beim weiblichen Fetus von 19,5 und beim männlichen von 22 cm und glaubt, daß sich die Drüsenanlagen bei männlichen Feten etwas später bilden. Diese Angaben stimmen mit der Auffassung von CAROSSINI (1912/13) überein. Es ist aber sicher mit gewissen individuellen

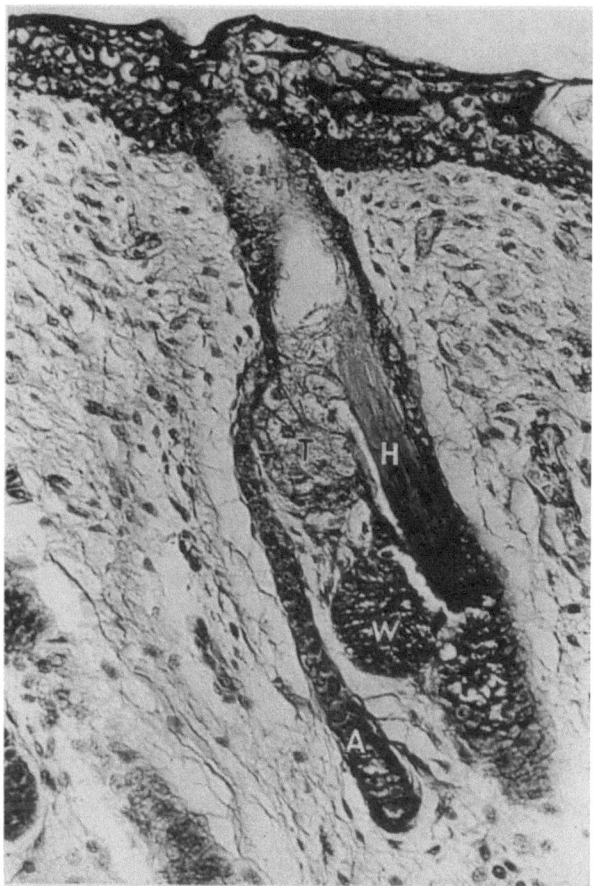

Abb. 1. Anlage einer apokrinen Schweißdrüse bei einem Fetus von 26 cm Länge. *A* apokrine Schweißdrüse, *T* Talgdrüse, *W* Wulst, *H* Haar. Reichlich Glykogen. PAS-Hämalaun. Vergr. 224 ×

Schwankungen zu rechnen. Wir haben die ersten Anlagen apokriner Schweißdrüsen in der Achsel zwischen 4. und 5. Monat des intrauterinen Lebens beobachtet (Abb. 1).

Die apokrinen Drüsen entwickeln sich von Haarfollikelanlagen als eine Epithelknospe an der hinteren Seite oberhalb der Talgdrüse. Daß der Ausführungsgang der apokrinen Schweißdrüsen an der Vorderseite des Haares liegt, ist nur selten beobachtet worden (STEINER, 1925). In relativ kurzer Zeit bildet sich zuerst ein solider Zellstrang, der im Corium etwa in der Haarpapillenhöhe endet. Im 6. Monat beginnt er sich zu knäueln (MONTAGNA, 1962). ALVERDES (1934) hat ebenfalls erste Windungen bei 30 cm langen Embryonen beobachten können. Bei Ceruminaldrüsen beginnt der Vorgang der Knäuelbildung nach SIMONETTA und MAGNONI (1937) bei 37 cm langen Embryonen. Bei Embryonen von 22 cm Länge läßt sich der Ausführungsgang bereits gut vom sekretorischen Abschnitt abgrenzen (MOGI, 1938). Eine Lichtung scheint sich zunächst im Ausführungsgang auszubilden (MONTAGNA, 1962). ALVERDES (1934) hat bei einem Embryo von 16,5 cm oft nur ein angedeutetes Lumen beobachtet, bei einem 25 cm langen Embryo war ein durchlaufendes Lumen vorhanden. Auch STEINER (1925) fand im 5. Monat, MORIOKA (1936) im 6. Monat eine Lichtung in apokrinen Schweißdrüsen. Dagegen sollen nach HERZENBERG (1926) die Drüsen der Neugeborenen nur selten ein Lumen besitzen. KYRLE (1925) bezeichnet in seinen „Vorlesungen" die apokrinen Drüsen des Neugeborenen als vorwiegend lumenlos und funktionsuntüchtig. Am Material von 44 Kindern fand HERZENBERG (1927), daß die apokrinen Drüsen erst ab 3.—5. Monat als solche sicher zu erkennen sind. Nur bei einem 3jährigen Knaben hat sie rudimentäre Sekretion feststellen können. Dagegen entsprachen bei einem 6jährigen Mädchen mit Pubertas praecox die apokrinen Drüsen morphologisch denjenigen bei Erwachsenen.

Die Anschauungen über den Zeitpunkt der Differenzierung der äußeren Zellreihe des sekretorischen Abschnittes in Myoepithelzellen stimmen nicht ganz überein. MONTAGNA (1962) hält es für möglich, daß sie bei Neugeborenen noch nicht abgeschlossen ist. Andererseits glauben ENDO (1934) sowie ALVERDES (1934), daß bisweilen diese zwei Zellarten doch gut zu unterscheiden sind. Die Drüsen des äußeren Gehörganges sollen demgegenüber schon intrauterin entwickelt sein (HURLEY und SHELLEY, 1960). Nach HORSTMANN (1957) ist die Histogenese der Ceruminaldrüsen erst extrauterin abgeschlossen.

Auf eine Beobachtung von SCHIEFFERDECKER (1922) stützend, die sich auf die Haut der Parotisgegend bezieht, ist man zu der Ansicht gekommen, daß die embryonalen Follikel regelmäßig solche rudimentäre apokrine Drüsenanlagen bilden, die sich später, abgesehen von Prädilektionsstellen, wieder zurückbilden. In diesem Sinne spricht auch die Beobachtung von CAROSSINI (1912/13) an der Haut in der Leistenbeuge. H. PINKUS (1958) hat bei 10 Feten diese Auffassung nicht ganz bestätigen können. Er war nämlich nicht imstande, sichtbar große Anlagen weder in der Rücken- noch in der Bauchhaut zu entdecken. Eine Ausnahme machte das Capillitium, wo sich aber sehr oft ektopische apokrine Schweißdrüsen finden können. Es hat schon WIMPFHEIMER (1907) auf Schweißdrüsen, die sich von Haaranlagen aus entwickeln, im Bereich der Kopfhaut menschlicher Feten hingewiesen. Wir haben die Achsel-, Rücken- und Bauchhaut bei 8 Feten (Länge 16—26 cm) systematisch untersucht und nur einmal mit Sicherheit eine apokrine Schweißdrüsenanlage in der Bauchhaut gefunden. Sonst konnten wir keine einwandfreien apokrinen Schweißdrüsenanlagen in den beiden letztgenannten Lokalisationen feststellen. In diesem Zusammenhang ist der Befund von SERRI (1962) bemerkenswert, der in der Brust-, Glutäal- und Gesichtshaut Anlagen der apokrinen Drüsen abgebildet hat.

Die Morphologie der apokrinen Drüsen im Kindesalter ist besonders von ENDO (1939) sowie MONTAGNA (1959) eingehend untersucht worden. Bei Neugeborenen fand ENDO im Knäuelbereich kubisches bzw. flachkubisches Epithel und gut differenzierte Myoepithelzellen. Bei Säuglingen war schon — obwohl selten — sog. kuppelförmige Sekretion vorhanden. Sie war in der nächsten Gruppe noch häufiger zu sehen. Im Lumen fanden sich homogene Massen. Im Schulalter unterscheiden sich die apokrinen Schweißdrüsen nicht viel von denen vom Spielalter. Sekretionsgranula in ihrer typischen Morphologie sind erst im 12. Lebensjahr zu erwarten (YASUI, 1960a). Wenn das Material vorher mit 1%iger Perjodsäure behandelt ist und anschließend mit Toluidinblau gefärbt wird, so ist nach YASUI (1960a) eine feingranuläre Substanz im Cytoplasma der apokrinen Drüsen beim ein- sowie auch beim 10monatigen Kind vorhanden. Nach MONTAGNA (1959) fängt die Sekretion im 8. Lebensjahr an. Lipide, Eisen und Pigment enthalten erst die Drüsen der Erwachsenen.

ENDO (1938) hat auch das Volumen der einzelnen apokrinen Drüsen bei Kindern von 3 Tagen bis 8,5 Jahren gemessen und fand ein durchschnittliches Volumen von 0,00737 cm³. Das größte bei einem 8,5jährigen Mädchen, das kleinste bei einem 5tägigen Kind. Dieses Volumen ist deutlich größer als das Volumen der ekkrinen Drüsen im Achselbereich. Da im Kindesalter die apokrinen Schweißdrüsen noch nicht voll entwickelt sind, ist eine Verwechslung mit ekkrinen Schweißdrüsen leicht möglich. Die Unterscheidung scheint bei Knaben leichter zu sein als bei Mädchen (ENDO, 1938). MONTAGNA (1962) gibt folgende Hinweise: nach dem ersten Jahr liegt das Knäuel der apokrinen Drüsen tiefer als das ekkriner Schweißdrüsen; nach ENDO liegen die apokrinen Schweißdrüsen bei japanischen Kindern nicht tiefer. Apokrine Drüsen haben ein weiteres Lumen, welches von kuboiden Zellen begrenzt ist, während die für ekkrine Schweißdrüsen typischen dunklen und hellen Zellen fehlen. Ferner ist die Basalmembran der apokrinen Drüsen bedeutend dichter als die ekkriner Schweißdrüsen. Über prinzipielle Unterscheidungsmerkmale der beiden Schweißdrüsengruppen hat sich schon SCHIEFFERDECKER (1917) geäußert: die apokrinen Drüsen besitzen makroskopisch eine ausgeprägte Variationsbreite, ihr Sekretionsschlauch ist weiter, ihr Knäuel lockerer, ihre Drüsenzellen mehr eosinophil, ihr Epithel wird kurz nach dem Tode ins Lumen abgestoßen, ihre Funktion fängt erst in der Pubertät an und ihr Ausführungsgang mündet in dem Haarbalg oder daneben, also in der Nähe eines Haarbalges.

Histochemische Untersuchungen apokriner Schweißdrüsen bei Feten stammen von SERRI, HUBER und MESCON (1962), SERRI, MONTAGNA und MESCON (1962), SERRI, MONTAGNA und HUBER (1963), bei Kindern von YASUI (1960b), YASUI und KAGEMOTO (1961) sowie YASUI und SUZUKI (1961).

B. Die Struktur der apokrinen Schweißdrüsen
I. Lokalisation und makroskopische Anatomie

Die apokrinen Schweißdrüsen sind beim Menschen auf ganz bestimmte Hautareale beschränkt. Die Anreicherung apokriner Schweißdrüsen in bestimmten Hautbezirken wurde auch bei Primaten beobachtet (MONTAGNA, 1963). Bei den Säugern kommen oft die sog. Duftorgane vor, die auch von apokrinen Drüsen gebildet sein können (ADAM, 1964). Apokrine Schweißdrüsen finden sich beim Menschen in folgenden Hautarealen: Axillen, Mons pubis, Labia majora, Circumanalregion, Scrotum, Areolae mammae, Mamillen, Vestibulum nasi, äußerer Gehörgang und Augenlid. Vielleicht ist auch das Gesicht hinzuzufügen (H. PINKUS, 1954). Nur in der Haut der Achselhöhlen stehen die apokrinen Schweißdrüsen dicht nebeneinander. Es sei außerdem betont, daß Glandulae uterinae wohl auch eine apokrine Sekretion aufweisen können, wie das WETZSTEIN und WAGNER (1960) elektronenmikroskopisch festgestellt haben und später auch ŠVAJGER (1963) lichtmikroskopisch bestätigt hat. Einen apokrinen (neben dem ekkrinen) Sekretionsmodus des Tubenepithels hat STEGNER (1962) postuliert.

Wir haben bei 29 (13 ♀ und 16 ♂) Leichen im Alter von 28—77 Jahren je ein Probestück aus der Axilla, Mons pubis und Scrotum bzw. Labia majora entnommen. Apokrine Schweißdrüsen waren in der Achselhaut reichlich und regelmäßig vorhanden, dagegen in der Regio pubis nur sechsmal (4 ♀ und 2 ♂), in Scrotalhaut dreimal und in der Labia majora viermal festzustellen. Das soll selbstverständlich nur ein Hinweis auf die Dichte und nicht auf das Vorhandensein bzw. Nichtvorhandensein apokriner Schweißdrüsen in den genannten Regionen sein.

Die Dicke des Drüsenlagers in der Axilla beträgt nach KLAAR (1926) bei der Frau 0,34—0,82 mm. Die knäuelförmigen sekretorischen Abschnitte der apokrinen Schweißdrüsen bilden nämlich eine gut sichtbare Schicht, das sog. Stratum glandulare (CAVAZZANA, 1947). Der größte Teil des Knäuels der axillaren apokrinen Schweißdrüsen liegt vorwiegend der Cutis an (PETER, 1935), so daß die Distanz von der Hautoberfläche bis zum tiefsten Punkt bis zu 5 mm beträgt (MONTAGNA, 1962). Zusammen mit den ekkrinen Schweißdrüsen sowie Talgdrüsen sind sie am Aufbau des sog. Axillarorgans beteiligt (SCHAFFER, 1940). SCHAFFER (1940) stimmt nicht mit KLAAR (1926) sowie F. PINKUS (1910) überein, welche unter dem Begriff des Axillarorgans nur die dort vorhandenen apokrinen Schweißdrüsen verstanden wissen möchten. Per analogiam spricht SCHIEFFERDECKER (1917) auch über das ,,Gehörgangsorgan", das ,,Circumanalorgan" (ähnlich WOOLLARD, 1930), das ,,Milchorgan". Die Ausbreitung apokriner Schweißdrüsen in der Achselhöhle entspricht praktisch der Ausbreitung der Haare (RICHTER, 1933; GLOOR-RUTISHAUSER, 1953). Am stärksten sind die Drüsen im Zentrum der Achselhöhle entwickelt (MONTAGNA, 1956). In Zusammenhang mit der Syntopie von Haaren und apokrinen Schweißdrüsen in der Achsel ist die Beobachtung von SHELLEY und BUTTERWORTH (1955) von Interesse. Diese Autoren fanden bei acht debilen Frauen mit normalem Menstruationscyclus, aber komplettem Fehlen der Axillarbehaarung nur eine sehr geringe Zahl von atropischen apokrinen Schweißdrüsen bzw. waren überhaupt keine apokrinen Schweißdrüsen nachzuweisen.

Heterotopie bzw. *Ektopie*, d.h. das Vorkommen von apokrinen Schweißdrüsen außerhalb der typischen Lokalisationsstellen ist seit den Untersuchungen von VOHWINKEL (1931) bekannt. H. PINKUS (1964) unterscheidet dagegen nur a-negative und potentiell a-positive Regionen (s. auch seine Abb. 11). VOHWINKEL (1931) hat zuerst bei einem Mulatten an der Stirn und an den Wangen und bei einem Weißen an der Bauchhaut apokrine Schweißdrüsen vorgefunden. Später sind heterotope apokrine Schweißdrüsen überwiegend in Verbindung mit Naevi und zwar besonders mit dem Naevus sebaceus von TAPPEINER (1939), SZODORAY (1948), HALTER (1956), WITTIG (1956), VAN CANEGHEM (1959), KOCH (1963) beschrieben worden (Abb. 2). Seltener ist die Syntopie mit Neurofibromen (TAPPEINER, 1939), Naevus syringocystadenomatosus (TAPPEINER, 1939), Naevus papillomatosus (ATUSI, 1940), mit mucinöser Umwandlung des Bindegewebes und Gefäßproliferation (ORMEA, 1952) beschrieben worden. OHNO und KINOSHITA (1927) haben apokrine Schweißdrüsen ebenfalls in Verbindung mit Naevus sebaceus, aber auch mit anderen Bildungen wie Naevus verruciformis, Fibrom, Papillom etc. beobachten können. Eisen konnten sie in den apokrinen Schweißdrüsen nicht nachweisen. Heterotope apokrine Schweißdrüsen sind — von seltenen Ausnahmen abgesehen (TAPPEINER, 1939; SZODORAY, 1948; ORMEA, 1952) — im Kopfbereich lokalisiert. HOMMA (1926) hat bei 6 von 10 Negern in der Brustregion apokrine Schweißdrüsen feststellen können, am Abdomen in 18,3% der Fälle. Die weißen Probanden seines Patientengutes wiesen keine ektopischen Schweißdrüsen in der erstgenannten Region und am Abdomen nur in 5% der Fälle auf. RICHTER und SCHMIDT (1934) haben bei 9 von 12 Fällen apokrine Schweißdrüsen in der Haut der Nasenflügel gefunden. In dieser Region hat bei den Japanern die apokrinen Schweißdrüsen KATO (1936) festgestellt und vorgeschlagen sie ,,Glandulae alae nasi" zu nennen. H. PINKUS (1954, 1964) hält das Gesicht und das Capillitium für den häufigsten Sitz ektopischer apokriner Schweißdrüsen. Vielleicht kommen apokrine Schweißdrüsen auch normalerweise im Gesicht vor (H. PINKUS, 1954), eine Vermutung, die von HALTER (1956) bestritten wird. Auch nach unserer Erfahrung ist der Kopfbereich die häufigste Lokalisation ektopischer apokriner Schweißdrüsen. Im

Gesicht — auch von VAN CANEGHEM (1959) mit Recht festgestellt — kommen sie nicht nur an Naevi gebunden vor. In diesem Zusammenhang ist eine Beobachtung von Chromhidrosis (SHELLEY und HURLEY, 1954) im Gesichtsbereich zu erwähnen, wo gefärbter Schweiß von ektopischen apokrinen Schweißdrüsen seinen Ausgang genommen hat. Auch die schwarzen Hidrocystome (Hydrocystome noir) sind mit ektopischen apokrinen Drüsen in Zusammenhang gebracht worden (MEHREGAN, 1964). In Basaliomen dagegen wurden nie Strukturen gefunden, die

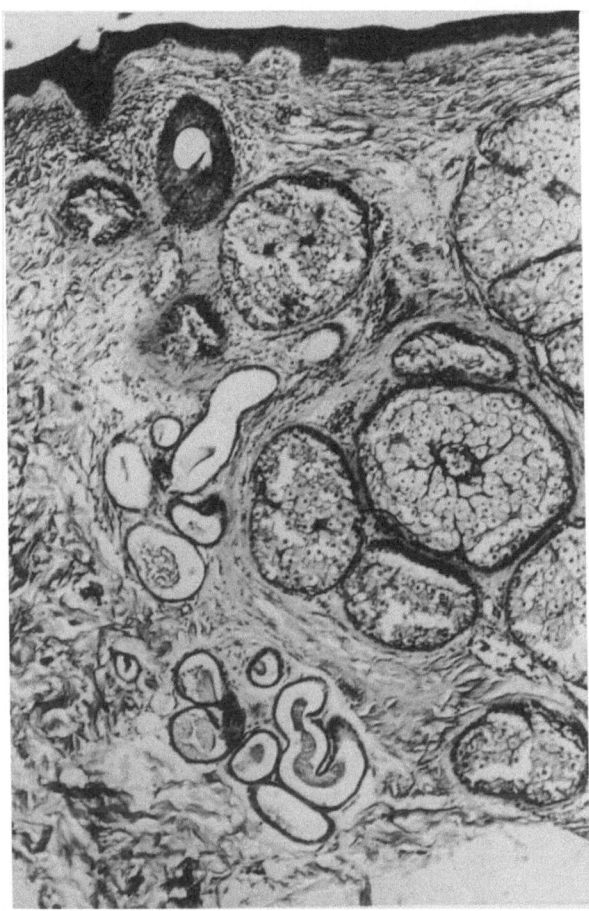

Abb. 2. Heterotope apokrine Schweißdrüsen innerhalb eines Naevus sebaceus (JADASSOHN). Hämatoxylin-Eosin. Vergr. 56 ×

apokrinen Schweißdrüsen entsprechen könnten (WOOD, PRANICH und BEERMAN, 1958).

VAN CANEGHEM (1959) hat zuerst auf ein unterschiedliches feingewebliches Aussehen heterotoper apokriner Schweißdrüsen hingewiesen. Er unterscheidet nämlich in Anlehnung an BRANCA (1927) sowie HOLMGREN (1922) auch bei den heterotopen Schweißdrüsen gemischte und intermediäre Drüsentypen.

Das *makroskopische Aussehen apokriner Schweißdrüsen* (Abb. 3) ist besonders an Wachsplattenmodellen untersucht worden (CONTINO, 1907; F. PINKUS, 1926; ALVERDES, 1932; PETER, 1935; SPERLING, 1935). ALVERDES (1934) hat auf den einfachen Bau des Drüsenkörpers der Glandulae vestibularis bei Neugeborenen, der einem unverzweigten Rohr ähnelt, hingewiesen. Die apokrinen

Schweißdrüsen Erwachsener sind in ihrer Form von der Lokalisation abhängig. Circumanaldrüsen, Mollsche Drüsen, Ceruminaldrüsen und die apokrinen Schweißdrüsen in den Axillen zeigen einen zunehmend komplizierteren Aufbau des sekretorischen Knäuels der Drüsen (SPERLING, 1935), wobei sich aber selbst bei den benachbarten Drüsen die Knäuel nicht durchdringen (PETER, 1935). Das Wachsplattenmodell der Ciliardrüse von CONTINO (1907), die als einfache Schlauchdrüse dargestellt ist, wurde von SPERLING (1935) als Ausnahme bezeichnet. Der ca.

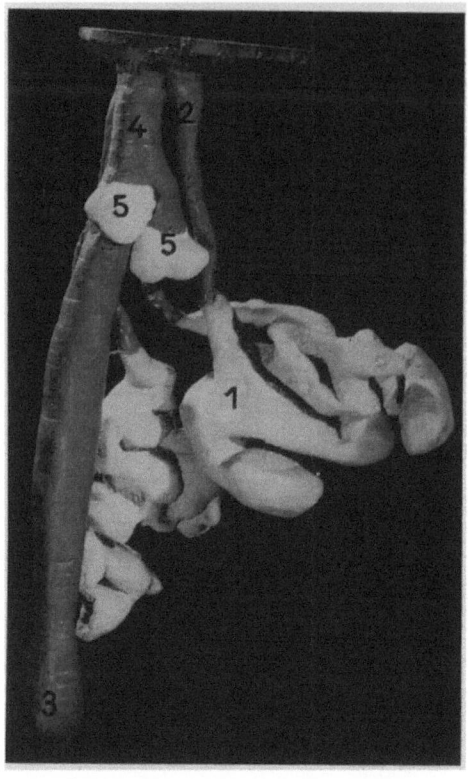

Abb. 3. Rekonstruktion einer apokrinen Schweißdrüse und Follikel-Talgdrüseneinheit. *1* Sekretorischer Abschnitt der apokrinen Schweißdrüse. *2* Ausführungsgang der apokrinen Schweißdrüse. *3* Anagenhaarwurzel. *4* Suprasebo-glanduläre Follikelportion. *5* Talgdrüse. Diese Abbildung verdanken wir der Freundlichkeit von Prof. Dr. med. EUGENE J. VAN SCOTT, National Institute of Health, Bethesda, Maryland (USA)

0,83—2,2 cm lange (PETER, 1935) sezernierende Abschnitt des Drüsenknäuels ist mit Auswüchsen, Seitensprossen, Nebenarmen (ALVERDES, 1934) bzw. Auszackungen und Ringbildungen (SPERLING, 1935) versehen, was GROTH (1935) sowie PETER (1935) allerdings nicht bestätigen konnten. Der Verlauf eines solchen Rohres soll einer rückläufigen Schlinge entsprechen (PETER, 1935). KATO und NAGATA (1938) konnten verzweigte Glandulae vestibulares nasi beobachten. SCHAFFER (1940) war nicht imstande, eine Verästelung apokriner Schweißdrüsen in der Achsel bei Menschen nachzuweisen. Die Größe des Modellknäuels apokriner Schweißdrüsen der Achselhöhle beträgt 1,2:0,8:0,6 mm und bei graphischer Rekonstruktion 1,9:1,8 mm bzw. 1,4:1,9 mm (PETER, 1935). MINE (1937) hat das Volumen der apokrinen Drüsen am Unterbauch bei den Japanerinnen gemessen und als Durchschnittsvolumen 0,04965 cm^3 angegeben. Nach dem 29. Lebensjahr vermindert sich langsam das Drüsenvolumen, ohne daß sich dabei die Form ändert.

II. Mikroskopische Anatomie

Bei apokrinen Schweißdrüsen kann man den sekretorischen Abschnitt und den Ausführungsgang unterscheiden.

1. Der sekretorische Abschnitt
a) Drüsenzellen

Innerhalb des sekretorischen Abschnittes, von BRANCA (1927) auch als glanduläres Segment bezeichnet, wären morphologisch (und funktionell?) wiederum zwei Teile zu differenzieren. ALVERDES (1934) spricht von einem proximalen trüben Teil mit typischem Drüsenepithel und einem hellen, dem Ausführungsgang benachbarten Teil. Nach demselben Autor hat bereits SCHIEFFERDECKER (1922) diese Abschnitte beschrieben. Auch HOLMGREN (1922) und BRANCA (1927) halten den „Anfangsteil" bzw. „segment à cellules claires" für einen besonderen Abschnitt des glandulären Teiles. Er besteht aus hellen Zellen ohne feingewebliche Merkmale einer apokrinen Sekretion und soll „einen wäßrigen Schweiß" produzieren (HOLMGREN, 1922). Das Charakteristische dieses Abschnittes sollen auch die epicellulären Canaliculi sein, die MONTAGNA, CHASE und LOBITZ (1953) allerdings nicht bestätigen konnten. Dieser Abschnitt ist wahrscheinlich mit dem sog. Zwischenteil von TEWFIK (1932) identisch. Heterotope apokrine Drüsen sollen manchmal ausschließlich aus diesen hellen Segmenten bestehen (VAN CANEGHEM, 1959). Im ganzen sind die Meinungen über diese Frage aber nicht einheitlich. Die Auffassung über zwei verschiedene Teile innerhalb des sekretorischen Abschnittes apokriner Schweißdrüsen sollte nur unter großem Vorbehalt angenommen werden (SCHAFFER, 1926; BRINKMANN, 1923/24).

Prinzipiell sind im sekretorischen Abschnitt zwei Zelltypen zu unterscheiden: Drüsenzellen und Myoepithelzellen. Das Drüsenepithel ist einschichtig. Dabei liegen die Drüsenzellen seitlich direkt nebeneinander und grenzen basal an die Myoepithelzellen bzw. direkt an die Basalmembran. Die Höhe des Drüsenepithels schwankt von 24—36 µ bis 18—24 µ (WAY und MEMMESHEIMER, 1938).

Die Gestalt der *Drüsenzellen* des sekretorischen Abschnittes scheint abhängig von dem jeweiligen Funktionszustand des betreffenden Teiles der apokrinen Schweißdrüse zu sein (HORSTMANN, 1957). Entweder sind die Drüsenzellen hochzylindrisch bzw. kubisch oder bei stark erweiterten Drüsentubuli abgeplattet. Wenn ein Tubulus exzessiv dilatiert ist, scheint er wie von einem Plattenepithel tapeziert zu sein (Abb. 9).

Der freie distale Rand einiger (MONTAGNA, 1962) hochzylindrischer Drüsenzellen ist bürstenförmig im Aussehen („brush border") und besitzt eine Reihe von dicht nebeneinander stehenden protoplasmatischen Ausläufern. Basalwärts folgt eine glasig imponierende (HEYNOLD, 1874), PAS-reaktive Schicht, die als *Cuticula* bezeichnet wurde (Abb. 4). Nach demselben Autor soll diese Cuticula zuerst von GAY (1871) in Drüsenzellen der Circumanaldrüsen abgebildet worden sein. Dieser Teil der Drüsenzellen wird auch heute in der Literatur „hyaline Plasmazone" (MINAMITANI, 1941) bzw. „crusta" (ITO, 1949) genannt und ist nach polarisationsoptischen Untersuchungen von TANAKA (1962) als doppelbrechend zu bezeichnen. Eine Cuticula ist nicht bei allen Drüsenzellen nachzuweisen, kann aber Angaben von MINAMITANI (1941) zufolge bei der Bildung der kuppelförmigen Ausbuchtungen (Abb. 5), die bei diesem Zelltyp lichtmikroskopisch so charakteristisch sind, erhalten bleiben. Es ist zu betonen, daß auf die kuppelförmig aussehenden Ausbuchtungen der Drüsenzellen („apocrine projection") unter anderem

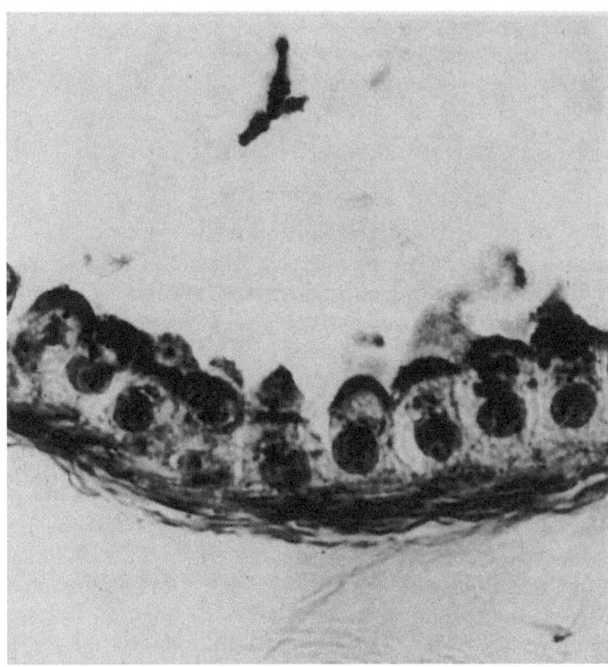

Abb. 4. Apokrine Schweißdrüse — sekretorischer Abschnitt. Cuticularsaum von intensiver PAS-Reaktivität an der apikalen Zellgrenze. Im lumennahen Zellabschnitt multiple PAS-reaktive Sekretgranula. Paraffinschnitt. PAS-Reaktion. Vergr. 740 ×

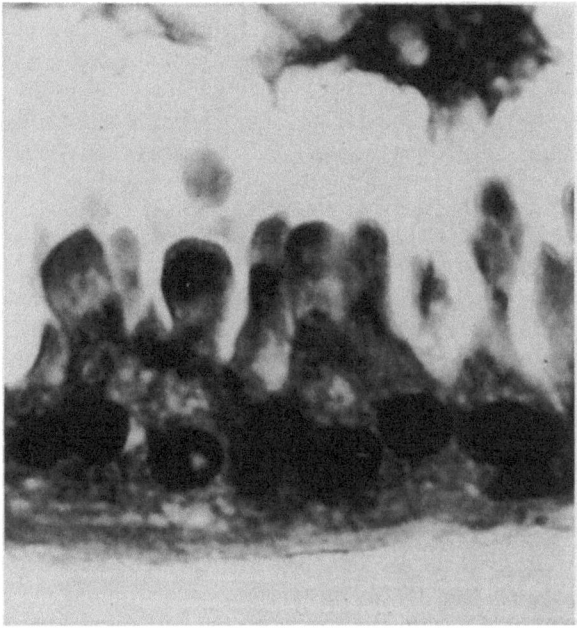

Abb. 5. Apokrine Schweißdrüse. Sog. sekretorische Ausbuchtungen der Drüsenzellen. Paraffinschnitt. Hämatoxylin-Eosin. Vergr. 890 ×

schon MISLAWSKY (1909) und BRINKMANN (1923/24) hingewiesen haben. BRINKMANN spricht direkt von ,,kuppelförmiger Sekretion".

Die Zellen sollen 1—2 (MONTAGNA, 1962), manchmal sogar drei (WAY und MEMMESHEIMER, 1938) *Zellkerne* besitzen, die wieder bis zu zwei RNS-haltige Nucleoli enthalten. Es soll eine direkte proportionelle Abhängigkeit zwischen der Intensität der cytoplasmatischen Basophilie und der Mitochondrienzahl und eine umgekehrte Proportion zwischen der cytoplasmatischen Basophilie und der Zahl der Sekretionsgranula bestehen (MONTAGNA, 1962). Basophilie ist in der Golgi-Zone nicht vorhanden. Da sie nach Ribonuclease-Bebrütung verschwindet (BUNTING, WISLOCKI und DEMPSEY 1958, MONTAGNA, 1962), ist sie im wesentlichen mit der cytoplasmatischen, ribosomal gebundenen RNS zu identifizieren und weist auf einen relativ hohen RNS-Gehalt der Zellen hin. (Zur Frage des RNS-Gehaltes der Mikrosomen und Ribosomen s. PALADE und SIEKEVITZ, 1956a und b, sowie MOULÉ, 1964).

Mitochondrien lassen sich lichtmikroskopisch durch verschiedene Techniken (Regauds Hämatoxylin, Heidenhainsches Hämatoxylin usw.) als große und pleomorphe Strukturen nachweisen oder zumindest markieren (MONTAGNA, 1962). Sie sind vor allem im basalen Abschnitt der Drüsenzellen anzutreffen, nicht dagegen im Bereich des Golgi-Apparates und im apikalen Zellbereich. In Zellen mit weniger Sekretionsgranula sollen sie zahlreicher vorkommen (OTA, 1950). Wie MONTAGNA (1962) mit Recht betonte, stehen die lichtmikroskopischen Befunde in gewisser Diskrepanz zu elektronenmikroskopischen Untersuchungsergebnissen, wonach die Zahl der Mitochondrien geringer zu sein scheint. Wahrscheinlich hat dies seinen Grund darin, daß bei Verwendung lichtmikroskopischer Färbeverfahren zur Darstellung von Mitochondrien vielleicht auch Lysosomen angefärbt werden (BOURNE und TEWARI, 1964). Da, wie noch zu zeigen sein wird, Lysosomen aber in den Drüsenzellen reichlich vorhanden sind, erklärt sich so die scheinbare Diskrepanz zwischen lichtmikroskopischen und elektronenmikroskopischen Untersuchungsergebnissen.

Die *Sekretgranula* sind ein sehr charakteristischer Bestandteil apokriner Drüsenzellen. Heute unterscheidet man lichtmikroskopisch: große Pigmentgranula, kleine gelbe Granula und eosinophile (acidophile) Granula (MONTAGNA, 1962). Man hält die Zone des Golgi-Apparates sowie auch den apikalen Zellbereich für granulafrei. Die sog. großen Sekretionsgranula sind wohl nur beim Menschen regelmäßig zu beobachten, da z.B. die Drüsenzellen der Circumanalregion der Katze (ATO, 1961) solche Granula nicht enthalten. Grundlegende Befunde über die chemische Zusammensetzung verdanken wir bereits den ersten Arbeiten über die sog. großen Schweißdrüsen. So hat beispielsweise HEYNOLD (1874) auf den Fettgehalt der Pigmentgranula der axillären apokrinen Schweißdrüsen nach Osmiumbehandlung hingewiesen, eine Beobachtung, die später wiederholt bestätigt wurde (WOOLLARD, 1930; MINAMITANI, 1941). HOMMA (1927) hat in Pigmentgranula Eisen nachgewiesen und kurze Zeit darauf betonte HERZENBERG (1927), daß sich die eosinophilen Granula der Eisenreaktion gegenüber refraktär verhalten. Die Gedanken, daß Eisen und Fett in ,,inniger Vermengung" vorkommen, hat schon RICHTER (1933) ausgesprochen. Außerdem hat er darauf hingewiesen, daß die Lagerung der ,,Fetttropfen" dem des Eisens entspricht.

Man hält es für sehr wahrscheinlich, daß die gelb-orange fluorescierenden großen Pigmentgranula einem Lipopigment entsprechen. Histochemische (SHELLEY und HURLEY, 1954; ROTHMAN, 1954; YASUDA und KAGEMOTO, 1960; YASUI, 1960a; PEARSE, 1961; KAWABATA, 1964; HASHIMOTO, GROSS und LEVER, 1966) und elektronenmikroskopisch-cytochemische (BIEMPICA und MONTES, 1965;

Rupec, 1966b) Arbeiten deuten heute eindeutig darauf hin, daß es sich um Lipofuscin handelt.

Es haben schon Montagna, Noback und Zak (1948) auf viele gemeinsame Eigenschaften des Pigmentes der apokrinen ceruminalen Drüsen mit dem Ceroid hingewiesen. Die Histogenese von Lipopigmenten ist besonders eingehend von Gedigk und Bontke (1956), Gedigk und Fischer (1959), Pearse (1961) sowie Gedigk (1964) bearbeitet worden. Auf einen Zusammenhang zwischen Pigmentgranula und Chromidrosis haben bereits Shelley und Hurley (1954) hingewiesen (zur Frage der Chromidrosis s. auch Greig, 1930). Es sei hier erwähnt, daß bereits Pissot (1899) unter anderem auch über eine Sekretion des Pigments von seiten der Ceruminaldrüsen geschrieben hat.

Die großen, überwiegend — aber nicht regelmäßig — sudanophilen Pigmentgranula sowie kleinere gelbe sudanophile Granula dürften einem „reifen" Stadium entsprechen. Diese Granula sind oft leicht basophil (Bunting et al., 1958). Die eosinophilen, nicht pigmentierten und nicht sudanophilen Granula sind wohl als unreife Granulaformen zu betrachten (Montagna, 1962). Pearse (1961) meint, daß eosinophile Granula kaum oxidierte Fettstoffe enthalten.

Was den Reichtum der Granula in vereinzelten Drüsenzellen betrifft, können wir im Grunde die Angaben von Montagna, Chase und Lobitz (1953) bestätigen. Er scheint nämlich nicht von der Höhe der Zellen abhängig zu sein; auch in flachen Zellen sind manchmal viele Pigmentgranula enthalten. Wir haben, obwohl selten, lichtmikroskopisch unterschiedlich große Aufhellung, d.h. optisch leere Zonen, innerhalb großer Pigmentgranula gesehen. Diese dürften elektronenmikroskopisch feststellbaren Desintegrationsbezirken dieser Granula (s. dort) entsprechen. Montagna (1962) glaubt, daß die nicht pigmentierten, bei Toluidinblau-Färbung „chromophoben", im übrigen eosinophilen, PAS-reaktiven Granula den elektronenmikroskopisch darstellbaren hellen Granula sehr wahrscheinlich entsprechen. Die Pigmentgranula sollen ultrastrukturell den dunklen Granula entsprechen. Mehr zur Ultrastruktur und Histochemie der sog. Sekretionsgranula der apokrinen Schweißdrüsen siehe in den entsprechenden Abschnitten.

Abschließend soll darauf hingewiesen werden, daß die Frage der lichtmikroskopisch sichtbaren verschiedenen Granulatypen infolge von Nomenklaturschwierigkeiten und dem so verschiedenartigen histochemischen Verhalten äußerst schwierig darzustellen ist. Es scheint so zu sein, daß die Granula in Abhängigkeit von ihrer Entwicklungsphase unterschiedliche färberische und histochemische Eigenschaften besitzen. Elektronenmikroskopische und elektronenmikroskopisch-cytochemische Befunde haben hier zu klareren Auffassungen geführt (s. S. 287).

Nach der ersten Beschreibung des *Golgi-Apparates* von v. Bergen (1904) ist er auch von anderen Autoren als ein supranuclear gelagertes System der Stäbchen und Körnchen dargestellt worden. (Über die anderen Befunde mit Licht- sowie Phasenkontrastmikroskop s. bei Bourne und Tewari, 1964.) Melczer (1935) hat nach Imprägnation mit OsO_4 sowie Silberimprägnation bei zylindrischen und kubischen Drüsenzellen ein „komplexes dreidimensionales Netz" gesehen. Ota (1950) behauptet, daß die apokrinen Schweißdrüsenzellen bei Osmidrosis über einen kleineren Golgi-Apparat verfügen sollen als das normalerweise der Fall ist. Brandes und Bourne (1954) haben eine hormonelle Kontrolle des Golgi-Apparates wahrscheinlich gemacht. Nach heutigen Auffassungen ist die Anschauung, daß via Golgi-Apparat die Sekretionsgranula Eisen, Pigment und Lipide erhalten (Minamitani, 1941) wohl nicht mehr haltbar. Auch Montagna (1962) hält diese Konzeption für nicht richtig.

Neben den typischen apokrinen Schweißdrüsen ist von Minamitani (1941) eine neue Gruppe der *sog. atypischen apokrinen Schweißdrüsen* herausgestellt worden. Er konnte diese Gruppe anhand seiner Untersuchungen an der Achselhaut bei Japanern in zwei Untergruppen „A" und „B" unterteilen. Die atypischen apokrinen Schweißdrüsen „A" sollen durch zylindrische, aber kleinere, schlank aussehende Drüsenzellen mit groben Sekretgranula und heftiger apokrinen Sekretion gekennzeichnet sein. Die atypischen apokrinen Schweißdrüsen „B" haben ein weites Lumen, welches mit unterschiedlich hohen zylindrischen Drüsenzellen tapeziert ist. Die Granula sind kleiner. Manche dieser Zellen enthalten keine Granula. Der Kern soll morphologisch dem Kern der ekkrinen Schweißdrüsen entsprechen (klein, rundlich bis oval). Man nimmt an, daß die erste Form unvollkommen entwickelten apokrinen Schweißdrüsen, die zweite vielleicht einer Zwischenform zwischen apokrinen und ekkrinen Drüsenzellen entspricht. MINAMITANI (1941) hat außerdem auch auf die gemischten Schweißdrüsen hingewiesen, d.h. solche Drüsen, wo zwischen apokrinen Drüsenzellen helle ekkrine Drüsenzellen bzw. zwischen ekkrinen Drüsenzellen apokrine Zellen liegen. YASUDA (1959) hat weitere atypische Zellen, die möglicherweise ihren Ausgang von Myoepithelzellen nehmen, beschrieben. Diese sind niedrige Zellen, die auf der Basalmembran zwischen zwei typischen apokrinen Drüsenzellen liegen und nicht immer das Lumen erreichen. Sie sollen eine gewisse Ähnlichkeit mit den hellen Zellen der ekkrinen Schweißdrüsen besitzen. Die zweite Form sind große rautenförmige Zellen, die auf der Basalmembran sitzen und keine Sekretionsgranula enthalten. Mit Eisenhämatoxylin färben sie sich dunkler als typische apokrine Drüsenzellen.

Mitosen im sekretorischen Abschnitt der apokrinen Schweißdrüsen werden nur selten beobachtet. So haben MONTAGNA, CHASE und LOBITZ (1953) apokrine Schweißdrüsen bei 52 Frauen und 2 Männern untersucht und nur bei 3 Frauen und einem Mann spontane Teilungsfiguren gefunden.

b) Die Zellen des sog. hellen intermediären Abschnittes

Diese sollen keine Zeichen einer apokrinen Sekretion aufweisen. Sie sind niedrig und besitzen ein helles Cytoplasma sowie einen Cuticula-ähnlichen Saum (HOLMGREN, 1922). Nach BRANCA (1927) soll ausnahmsweise nur eine Zellschicht vorkommen. Wir haben solche Zellen in den apokrinen Schweißdrüsen der Achselhöhle nicht mit Sicherheit feststellen können.

c) Die Myoepithelzellen

Zwischen der Basalmembran und dem Drüsenepithel sind die Myoepithelzellen (Abb. 6) zu finden. Auf ihre enge Verbindung mit den Drüsenzellen haben SARKAR und KALLENBACH (1966) hingewiesen. Diese Autoren haben zeigen können, daß auch Metastasen eines Mammacarcinoms Myoepithelzellen enthalten. Die kräftige Entwicklung dieser Zellen bei den apokrinen Schweißdrüsen soll sehr an primitive Muskelzellen bei Wirbellosen erinnern (SCHAFFER, 1940). Nach HORSTMANN (1957) sind die Myoepithelzellen der axillären apokrinen Schweißdrüsen zahlreicher und größer als die Myoepithelzellen der ekkrinen Schweißdrüsen. Es handelt sich dabei um spindelförmige Zellen, 5—10 μ breit, 50—100 μ lang (MONTAGNA, 1956), die im Querschnitt dreikantig bzw. stäbchenförmig aussehen (BARGMANN, 1959). Wie BUNTING et al. (1958) zeigen konnten, sind die Myofibrillen im Cytoplasma der Myoepithelzellen bei lichtmikroskopischer Betrachtung zahlreicher und gröber als in glatten Muskelzellen von Mm. arrectores pilorum oder Arteriolen. Lipidgranula finden sich parallel zur Zellachse angeordnet. GOLDSTEIN (1961) hat versucht, anhand seiner Studien an Ceruminaldrüsen einen Konnex zwischen den

Basalzellen des Ausführungsganges und der Myoepithelzellen auszumachen und glaubt, beim Menschen sowie beim Affen Cercopithecus aethiops eine intermediäre Myoepithelzellform gesehen zu haben. Diese Herausstellung der intermediären Myoepithelzellen gründet sich hauptsächlich auf die Kernform, welche zwischen dem runden Kern der Basalzelle des Ausführungsganges und dem abgeflachten stäbchenförmigen Kern einer typischen Myoepithelzelle liegen soll. Aber auch doppelbrechende Strukturen, wie sie für Myoepithelzellen typisch sind, können in diesen Zellen vorkommen. Nach Colchicinbehandlung hat GOLDSTEIN (1961)

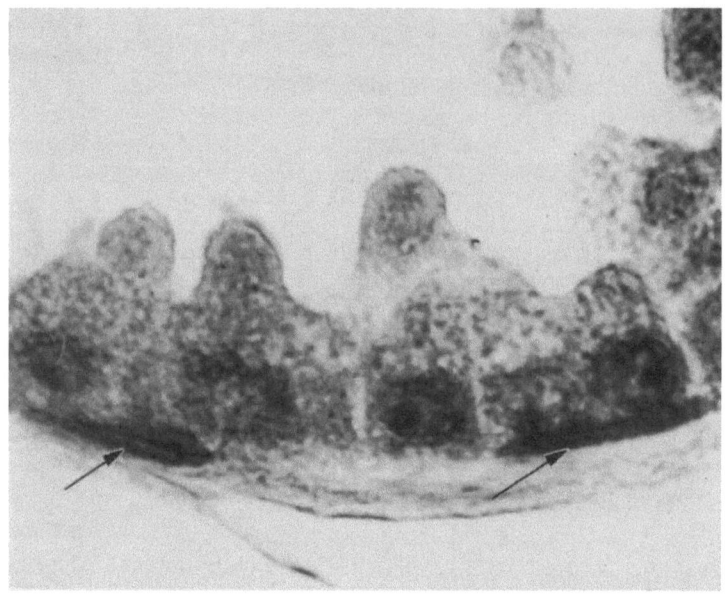

Abb. 6. Apokrine Schweißdrüse — sekretorischer Abschnitt. Typische Myoepithelzellen mit stäbchenförmigen Zellkernen an der Basis von Drüsenzellen (→). Paraffinschnitt. Toluidinblau. Vergr. 1300 ×

bei seinen Untersuchungen keine Mitosen in Myoepithelzellen, wohl aber 30 Teilungsfiguren im Ausführungsgang (bei 36 untersuchten Drüsen) gefunden. Auch dieser Befund könnte für eine Abstammung der Myoepithelzellen von den Basalzellen des Schweißdrüsenausführungsganges sprechen.

Was die Funktion der contractilen Myoepithelzellen betrifft, so haben HURLEY und SHELLEY (1954c, 1960) intra operationem nach Epinephrin bzw. Pitocin an apokrinen Schweißdrüsen peristaltische Wellen und Schweißausbruch beobachtet. In dilatierten, sekretorischen Abschnitten, z.B. bei alten Leuten, sind Myoepithelzellen nicht immer mit Sicherheit auszumachen. Allerdings haben MONTES u. Mitarb. (1960) in erweiterten sekretorischen Abschnitten mit flachen Drüsenzellen prominente myoepitheliale Zellen beschrieben. In Ceruminaldrüsen, Glandula vestibularis nasi und apokrinen Schweißdrüsen der Brust sind sie selten anzutreffen (HORSTMANN, 1957).

d) Die Basalmembran

Die lichtmikroskopische Basalmembran besteht nach MONTES u. Mitarb. (1960) aus einem intensiv PAS-reaktiven und einem schwach PAS-reaktiven Band (Abb. 33). Das erste soll aus Mucopolysacchariden bestehen. Häufig findet sich nur *eine* glasig wirkende, stark PAS-reaktive Basalmembran.

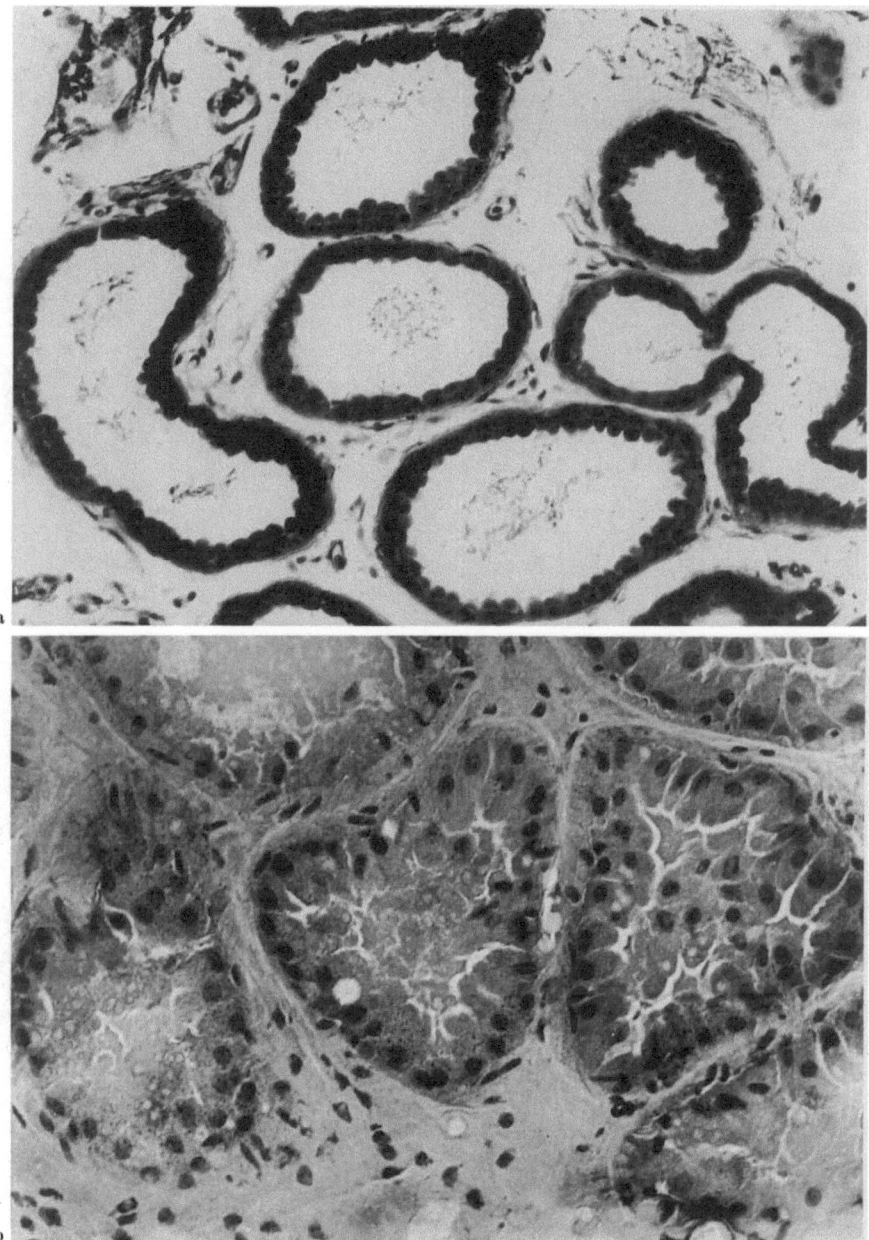

Abb. 7a u. b. Apokrine Schweißdrüse. a Paraffinschnitt. Hämatoxylin-Eosin. Vergr. 280 ×. b Im Kryostatschnitt sind die Drüsenlumina angefüllt mit einem homogenen Sekret und teilweise noch gut erhaltenen Zellkomplexen. Kryostatschnitt (System DITTES-DUSPIVA). Hämatoxylin-Eosin. Vergr. 300 ×

e) Lumeninhalt

Gewöhnlich ist das Lumen im sekretorischen Abschnitt apokriner Schweißdrüsen nicht leer (Abb. 7). Man findet entweder homogenes Material oder vereinzelte Zellen bzw. Zellkomplexe (Abb. 8), die sich histologisch und histochemisch als noch stoffwechselaktive Zellen erweisen können. In Kryostatschnitten fanden wir praktisch das ganze Lumen ausgefüllt (Abb. 7b).

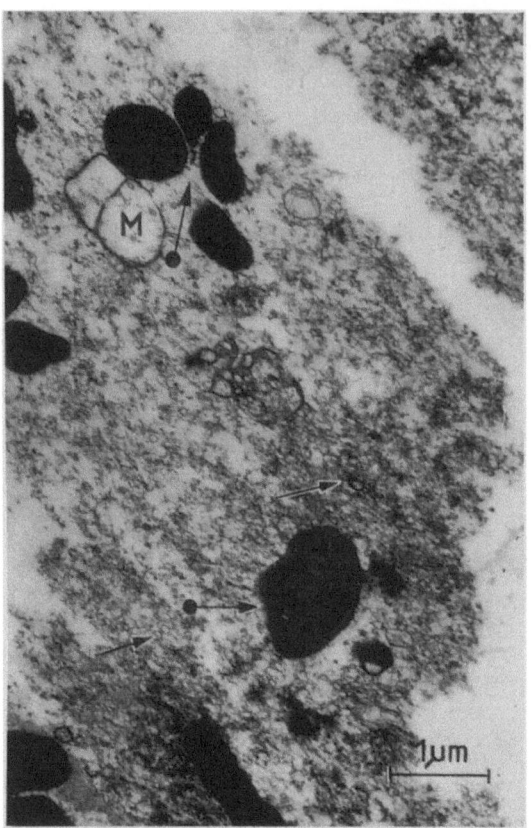

Abb. 8. Apokrine Schweißdrüse. Lumeninhalt: Granula, die wahrscheinlich den dunklen Granula (●→) entsprechen sowie Strukturen, die an untergegangene Mitochondrien (*M*) und vesiculös transformiertes endoplasmatisches Reticulum (→) erinnern

f) Altersbedingte Veränderungen

Die sekretorischen Abschnitte apokriner Schweißdrüsen neigen im Alter zu Dilatation (Abb. 9). Die Drüsenzellen werden immer flacher, manchmal bis zu einem Grade, daß sie Endothelzellen ähneln. Solche Veränderungen treten bei Frauen nach dem 30. Lebensjahr ein (MONTAGNA, 1959, 1964b). Auch der experimentelle Verschluß des Ausführungsganges durch einen Hornpfropf (z.B. nach Elektrodesikkation) kann zu cystischer Erweiterung mit Abflachung der Drüsenzellen führen (HURLEY und SHELLEY, 1954a, 1960). Daß solche Veränderungen auch spontan vorkommen können, wird aus Abb. 10 ersichtlich. Die flachen Zellen der blockierten Drüsen sind, wie das HURLEY und SHELLEY (1960) untersucht haben, leicht von ruhenden kubischen Drüsenzellen zu unterscheiden. Große cystische Erweiterungen in den apokrinen Schweißdrüsen betrachtet KLAAR (1926) als charakteristisch für das Postklimakterium. Seine Schlußfolgerungen beziehen sich auf 12 Frauen im Alter von 48—79 Jahren. Cystische Erweiterungen auch des Ausführungsganges sowie Mehrschichtigkeit und Sprossungsvorgänge hat schon BUSCHKE (1933) im höheren Alter beobachtet. Es ist hier zu erwähnen, daß durch Übereinanderschieben der Anschein eines geschichteten Epithels entstehen kann (SCHAFFER, 1926), wohl aber auch durch Schrägschnitte. Nach MONTES et al. (1960) sind die Zellen nach der Menopause kleiner, enthalten weniger PAS-reaktive Granula. Auch die cytoplasmatische RNS ist reduziert. Intraluminal sowie in Schweißdrüsenzellen und Myoepithelzellen kann auch Glykogen vorkommen. Mucinöse cystische Dilatation, die zuerst als pathologisches Geschehen bei Morbus Fox-Fordyce beschrieben wurde (WINKELMANN und MONTGOMERY, 1956), sich aber später als relativ regelmäßiger Befund herausgestellt hat (WINKELMANN und HULTIN, 1958), ist durch vacuolisiertes Epithel und intraluminale

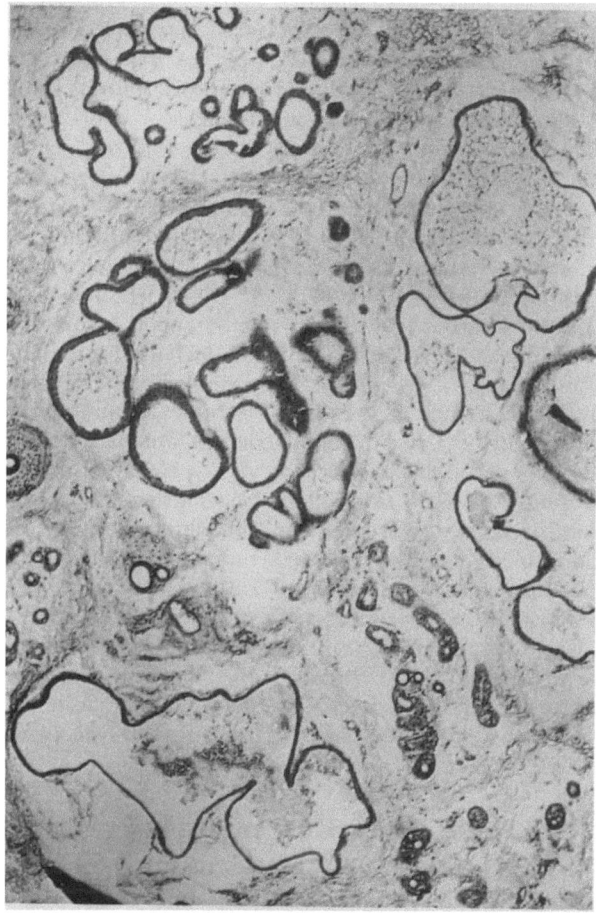

Abb. 9. Apokrine Schweißdrüse. Stark dilatierte apokrine Schweißdrüsen, teilweise mit Sekret im Lumen, bei einem 66jährigen Manne. Normale ekkrine Schweißdrüsen (rechts unten). Paraffinschnitt. Hämatoxylin-Eosin. Vergr. 35 ×

mucinöse Massen ausgezeichnet. Diese sind PAS-reaktiv, Diastase-resistent, Best-Carmin-positiv und bei Toluidinblau-Färbung orthochromatisch. Derartige Veränderungen sind vor allem im späteren Alter zu erwarten, obwohl sie auch schon bei einem 10jährigen Kind beobachtet wurden (WINKELMANN und HULTIN, 1958). Die mucinösen Einschlüsse sind auch in Drüsenzellen zu sehen (MONTAGNA, 1956). Eine Vermehrung des Bindegewebes, besonders aber der elastischen Fasern mit zunehmendem Alter hat RICHTER (1933) festgestellt. Man hat auch die Beobachtung gemacht, daß im späteren Alter die Talgdrüsen sowie ekkrinen und apokrinen Schweißdrüsen näher zusammenrücken (BECKER, 1964). MONTAGNA (1956) hat mit Recht vor zu weitgehenden Schlußfolgerungen in bezug auf mögliche Veränderungen von apokrinen Schweißdrüsen im späteren Alter gewarnt, da sie — im ganzen gesehen — als relativ resistent gegenüber Altersveränderungen zu bezeichnen sind.

g) Die Innervation

Die Innervation apokriner Schweißdrüsen ist bisher nur von wenigen Autoren bearbeitet worden. THIES (1958) hat mit der Jaboneroschen Silbercarbonatmethode ein syncytiales kernhaltiges Netz an vegetativen Plasmasträngen nachgewiesen. Es bestehen sehr wahrscheinlich keine Verbindungen zu Myoepithelzellen. Spezifische Cholinesterase ist nur selten nachzuweisen und leitet sich vielleicht von Synapsen her, was im Gegensatz zu den Befunden an ekkrinen Schweißdrüsen steht (HELLMANN, 1955; MONTAGNA, 1962 u. a.). Auch HURLEY und SHELLEY (1960) haben spezifische Cholinesterase — und zwar in Spuren — nach sehr langer Inkubationszeit (über 4 Std) festgestellt und glauben daher, daß es sich dabei um adrenergische Nerven handelt. Diese Untersuchungsergebnisse, die eindeutig für eine adrenergische Innervation der apokrinen Schweißdrüsen (HURLEY, SHELLEY und KOELLE, 1953; HURLEY und SHELLEY, 1960) sprechen sollen, stehen in einem gewissen Gegensatz zu den Befunden von MONTAGNA und ELLIS (1960) sowie MONTAGNA (1964), die Acetylcholinesterase-enthaltende Nerven um apokrine Drüsen bei Negern, seltener auch bei Weißen, festgestellt haben. Die Nerven um apokrine Schweißdrüsen enthalten nur Spuren der Butylcholinesterase (MONTAGNA, 1964). Diese Befunde decken sich auch mit den Angaben von AAVIK (1955) sowie ROTHMAN (1954) über Cholinesterase-enthaltende Nervenfasern um apokrine Drüsen, was wiederum mit den Befunden von AOKI (1955) über eine cholinergische Stimulation der apokrinen Drüsen gut übereinstimmt. Es ist interessant, daß Cholinesterase-enthaltende Nervenfasern auch bei den Primaten um apokrine Schweißdrüsen vorkommen (YASUDA, 1963). Intrauterin steigt die Zahl solcher Nervenfasern bis zum 10. Monat, später sinkt sie jedoch wieder ab. Es ist daher möglich, daß diese Fasern im Erwachsenenalter nur ein phylogenetisches Relikt bedeuten (YASUDA, 1963; YASUDA, MACHIDA und SUZUKI, 1963). Ein Netz autonomer Fibrillen um die Basalmembran des sekretorischen Teiles der apokrinen Schweißdrüsen haben CAHN und SHELLEY (1955) mit einer Hyaluronidase-Methylenblaumethode nachgewiesen. Ähnliche Befunde wie bei axillären apokrinen Drüsen sind auch bei Ceruminaldrüsen zu erheben (PERRY, HURLEY, GRAY und SHELLEY, 1955).

2. Der Ausführungsgang

Der Ausführungsgang (Abb. 10) mündet gewöhnlich im Trichter der supraseboglandulären Follikelportion („apopilosebaceous unit" — HURLEY und SHELLEY, 1960), manchmal aber auch frei an der Oberfläche, wobei man an eine Verschiebung der Mündung des Ausführungsganges beim Haarwechsel denken kann (SPERLING, 1935). Auch eine Einmündung in den Ductus der Talgdrüse, wie das auch bei den Ceruminaldrüsen möglich ist, wurde beobachtet. Besonders bei alten Personen ist der Ausführungsgang bei diesen Drüsen im Bereich des Orificiums in 1—2 mm breite Utriculi (MONTAGNA et al., 1948) erweitert. Solche Utriculi erinnern sehr an ähnliche Strukturen bei haarlosen Mäusen (s. auch DAVID, 1932). Beim Kamel münden die apokrinen Schweißdrüsen z.B. in die äußere Wurzelscheide der Grannenhaare (LEE und SCHMIDT-NIELSEN, 1962).

Der Ausführungsgang ist — obwohl nicht immer — im Vergleich mit dem sekretorischen Teil der Schweißdrüsen kürzer als der Ausführungsgang der ekkrinen Schweißdrüse im Vergleich mit ihrem sekretorischen Teil (HURLEY und SHELLEY, 1960), bei Neugeborenen soll aber das Verhältnis 1:1 sein (ALVERDES, 1934).

Das Epithel des Ausführungsganges ist ein zweischichtiges kubisches Epithel. Die luminale Zellschicht ist oft etwas abgeplattet, die Zellen besitzen eine Cuticula.

Die morphologische Ähnlichkeit mit dem Ausführungsgang ekkriner Schweißdrüsen ist sehr groß. Der apokrine Ausführungsgang soll etwas breiter sein und die Zellen sind etwas stärker eosinophil (HURLEY und SHELLEY, 1960).

Zur Frage eines möglichen Überganges von Zellen der Basalzellschicht des Ausführungsganges in Myoepithelzellen wurde bereits oben Stellung genommen.

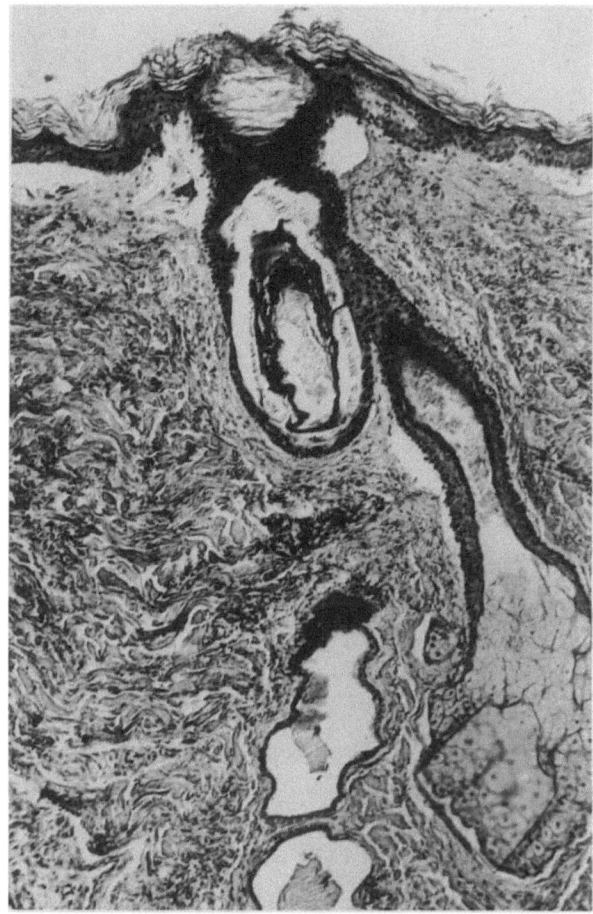

Abb. 10. Apokrine Schweißdrüsen. Der verschiedentlich getroffene erweiterte Ausführungsgang einer apokrinen Schweißdrüse mündet in den Follikelhals und zeigt keratotische Okklusion. Paraffinschnitt. Hämatoxylin-Eosin. Vergr. 99 ×

3. Postmortale Veränderungen

Die postmortalen Veränderungen des sekretorischen Teiles der apokrinen Schweißdrüsen sind schon seit KOELLIKER (1850) und VEIL (1911) bekannt. Das Nichtwissen über solche, bereits bald post mortem auftretenden Erscheinungen konnte zu Fehldeutungen, wie das wahrscheinlich im Falle von REBAUDI (1911) war, Anlaß geben. Die Neigung zur postmortalen Abschilferung ist unterschiedlich und hängt sehr wahrscheinlich von der Form, d.h. möglicherweise vom Sekretionszustand der Drüsenzellen ab. Nach RICHTER (1933) sowie MANCA (1934) sollen zylindrische Zellen sehr, kubische Zellen weniger, besonders wenig aber die flachen Zellen des sekretorischen Teiles zur postmortalen Abschilferung neigen. Bei den Ceruminaldrüsen treten die postmortalen Veränderungen später auf als bei axillären apokrinen Schweißdrüsen (MANCA, 1934). HOMMA (1925) glaubt, daß diese bald nach dem Tode auftretende Desquamation ein Unterscheidungsmerkmal gegenüber ekkrinen Schweißdrüsen ist, da sich das Drüsenepithel der ekkrinen Schweißdrüsen nicht so früh post mortem abschilfert. Auch KLAAR (1926) hat die starke Abschilferung des Drüsenepithels kurz nach dem Tode

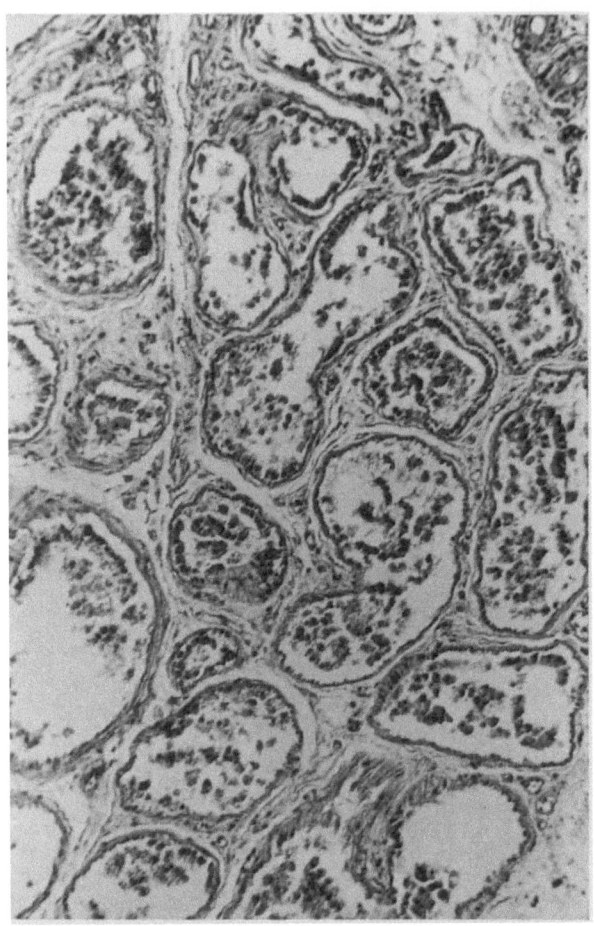

Abb. 11. Apokrine Schweißdrüsen. Typische postmortale Veränderungen in Form massiver Abschilferung der Drüsenepithelien. Paraffinschnitt. Hämatoxylin-Eosin. Vergr. 112 ×

unterstrichen. Die Epithelabstoßung als postmortales Ereignis (Abb. 11) ist sicher nicht mit dem Befund der cellulären Fragmente im Lumen der apokrinen Schweißdrüsen, die prompt nach der Entnahme fixiert bzw. gefroren waren (Abb. 7), gleichzustellen. Es ist sogar denkbar, daß es sich dabei noch um lebensfähige Zellen handelt (MONTAGNA, 1964). Dafür sprechen enzymatische Befunde.

Es ist weiter interessant, daß SPIELER (1964) von 100 Verstorbenen nur bei 4 eine Befundung wegen autolytischer Veränderungen nicht machen konnte, was im Gegensatz zur bedeutend rascheren Autolyse bei anderen drüsigen Organen stehen soll (BECKER und REITINGER, 1964). (Zur Frage der Autolyse ekkriner Schweißdrüsen s. BRAUN-FALCO und WINTER, 1965a und b sowie WINTER und BRAUN-FALCO, 1965.)

III. Elektronenmikroskopische Anatomie

Die Ultrastruktur der apokrinen Drüsenzellen (Allgemeines zur Ultrastruktur der Zelle s. bei SITTE, 1966) ist seit den ersten Arbeiten von CHARLES (1959) und KUROSUMI, KITAMURA und YIJIMA (1959) nur relativ wenig (HIBBS, 1962; YASUDA, ELLIS und MONTAGNA, 1962; KAWABATA, 1964; MUNGER, 1965; HASHIMOTO, GROSS und LEVER, 1966a und b) untersucht worden. SHIMIZU (1963) hat den Versuch unternommen, elektronenmikroskopisch den Einfluß verschiedener Pharmaka auf die apokrinen Schweißdrüsenzellen zu untersuchen.

Der bereits vom Lichtmikroskopischen her bekannte morphologische Aufbau der apokrinen Schweißdrüsen hat sich auch elektronenmikroskopisch grundsätzlich bestätigt.

1. Die apokrinen Drüsenzellen

Die *Zellmembran* (Plasmalemm) der apokrinen Drüsenzellen begrenzt den ganzen Zelleib, basal gegen myoepitheliale Zellen oder die Basalmembran, seitlich gegen benachbarte Drüsenzellen und apikal gegen das Lumen. Das Plasmalemm ist prinzipiell dreischichtig aufgebaut. Seine Dicke beträgt 80—95 Å (SJÖSTRAND, 1964), wobei erwähnenswert ist, daß die verschiedenartigen cellulären Membranen offensichtlich unterschiedlich dick sind (z.B. mitochondriale Membran 50—60 Å, Golgi-Membran 60—70 Å).

Im apikalen Bereich der Zelle finden sich viele ca. 1,0—1,5 μ [im Durchschnitt 1,0 μ (HIBBS, 1962)] lange, durch das Plasmalemm begrenzte Ausläufer des Cyto-

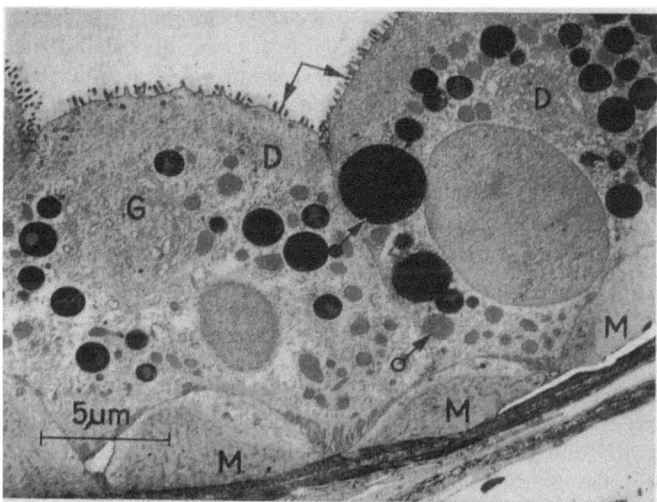

Abb. 12. Apokrine Schweißdrüse. Drüsenzellen (*D*), Myoepithelzellen (*M*), Mikrovilli (↙↘), Golgi-Apparat (*G*), helle Granula (o→), dunkle Granula (•→)

plasmas, die Mikrovilli (Abb. 12 und 13), welche an ihrer Basis fingerförmig verzweigt sein können. Die sekretorischen Ausbuchtungen („apocrine projections") sind regelmäßig frei von solchen Mikrovilli (KUROSUMI et al., 1959) und besitzen meistens einen klaren Inhalt mit nur wenigen Vesikeln. KUROSUMI (1961) hat sie mit den Pseudopodien von Leukocyten verglichen. Von einigen Autoren ist aber die Existenz solcher Ausbuchtungen in vivo angezweifelt worden (z.B. MUNGER, 1965; BIEMPICA und MONTES, 1965; HELANDER, 1965a und b). Wo die Drüsenzellen seitlich aneinander liegen, ist das Plasmalemm relativ geradlinig. Hier sind Drüsenzellen miteinander durch sog. „terminal bars" oder Schlußleisten verbunden. Diese Struktur soll nach FARQUHAR und PALADE (1963) einer zonula adhaerens, einer zonula occludens bzw. beiden entsprechen, was von dem untersuchten Material abhängt. Bei den von uns untersuchten apokrinen Schweißdrüsen der Achselhöhle entsprechen die Zwischenzellverbindungen hauptsächlich dem Typ der zonula adhaerens oder einfachen Desmosomen, wie wir gleichartige Strukturen in der Epidermis genannt haben (RUPEC, 1966a). Eine „Verdickung" des Plasmalemms in diesen Bereichen (KUROSUMI et al., 1959) ist wahrscheinlich auf die verdichtete cytoplasmatische Matrix zurückzuführen (Allgemeines zur Frage zwischencellulärer Verbindungen bzw. Membranenkontakte s. bei FARQUHAR und PALADE, 1963 sowie ROBERTSON, 1964.) Aber auch zwischen Myoepithelzellen und Drüsenzellen kommen Desmosomen stets vor.

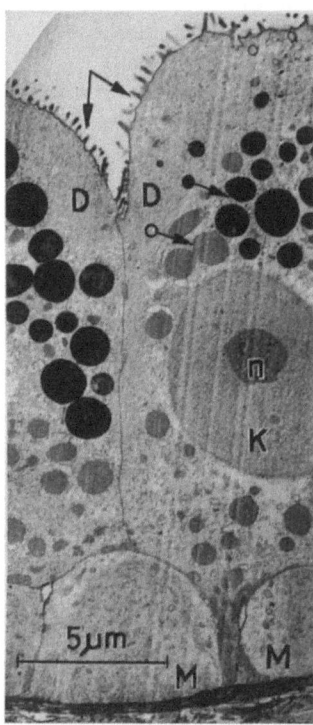

Abb. 13. Apokrine Schweißdrüse. Drüsenzellen (*D*), Myoepithelzellen (*M*), Mikrovilli (↙↘), Kern (*K*), Nucleolus (*n*), helle Granula (o→), dunkle Granula (•→)

Das basale Plasmalemm ist stark gefältelt (Abb. 14). Die Plasmalemmeinstülpungen zwischen zwei Myoepithelzellen, d. h. dort, wo die Drüsenzelle bis zur Basalmembran reicht, sind tief und verlaufen senkrecht zur Basalmembran. Dagegen sind die Falten oberhalb der Myoepithelzellen spärlicher und verlaufen mehr horizontal zur Oberfläche (KUROSUMI et al., 1959). Auf der Grundlage vergleichbarer Befunde an anderen Organen (PEASE, 1956) läßt sich vermuten, daß die reichliche Fältelung des basalen Plasmalemms funktionell eine Rolle bei der Absorption von Wasser sowie wasserlöslicher Substanzen spielt und damit von Wichtigkeit für die erste Sekretionsphase, nämlich Aufnahme des Ausgangsmaterials, sein dürfte (HELANDER, 1965a). Eine ähnliche Fältelung haben KUROSUMI und KITAMURA (1958) bei „pig's carpal organ" beschrieben (Näheres zur Struktur des Karpal-Organs beim Schwein s. bei SCHAFFER, 1940). Nach KAWABATA (1964) ist eine derartige Plasmalemm-Fältelung in dem basalen Anteil des Plasmalemms der Ceruminaldrüsen (Glandulae ceruminales) nicht vorhanden. Es bleibt fraglich, ob dadurch die unterschiedliche Konsistenz ihres Sekretes zu erklären ist.

Zwischen dem Bindegewebe und dem basalen Plasmalemm der Drüsenzelle ist eine extracelluläre ∼300 Å dicke elektronendichte *Basalmembran* vorhanden. Diese Membran ist von der Zellmembran durch eine etwa gleich breite helle Schicht getrennt. Auch an der Epidermis ist eine kontrastreiche ∼300—400 Å dicke Membran von der Basalzelle durch ein kontrastarmes ∼300 Å dickes Spatium getrennt (ZELICKSON, 1963). Sie entspricht wohl der adepidermalen Lamina von HAY (1964). Die Funktion der Basalmembran ist noch nicht definitiv geklärt. Vielleicht wirkt sie als eine Art Barriere (FREI, 1962). Die elektronenmikroskopische Basalmembran ist nicht mit dem PAS-reaktiven Grenzstreifen zu identifizieren (KOBAYASI, 1961). Letzterer umfaßt eine viel dickere Bindegewebszone. (Zur Frage der Basalmembran s. auch bei SWIFT und SAXTON, 1967).

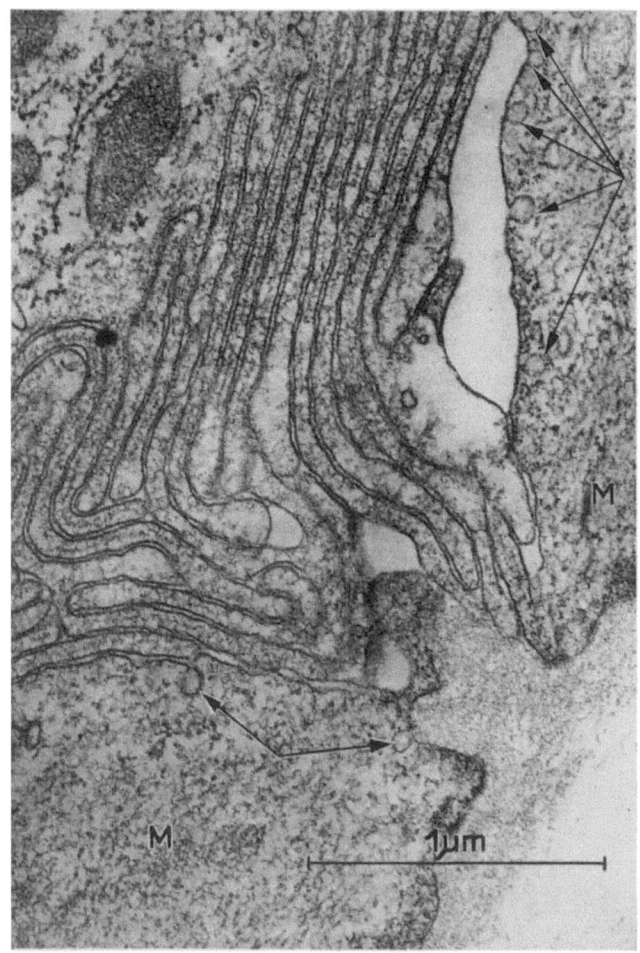

Abb. 14. Apokrine Schweißdrüse. Basale Fältelung des Plasmalemms. Vesikulation des Plasmalemms der Myoepithelzellen (*M*) ↖↑↗

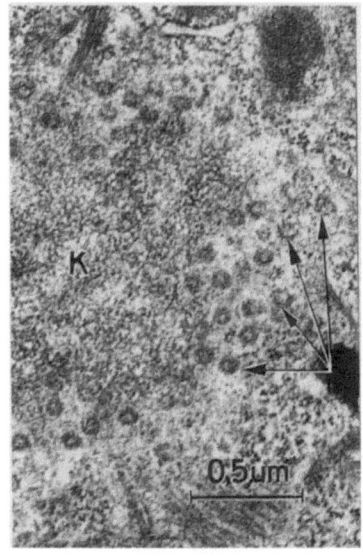

Abb. 15. Apokrine Schweißdrüse. Tangentialschnitt durch den Kern (*K*). Kernporen gut sichtbar (↖↑↗

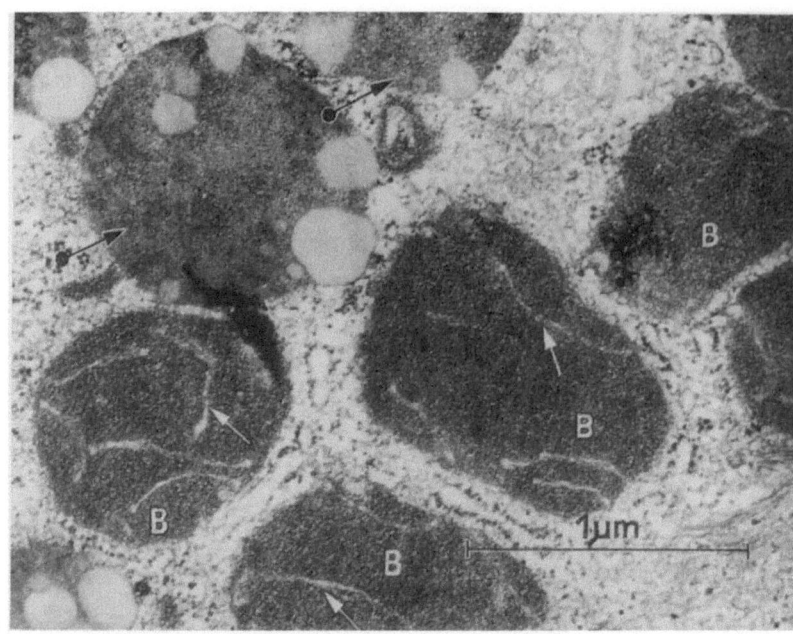

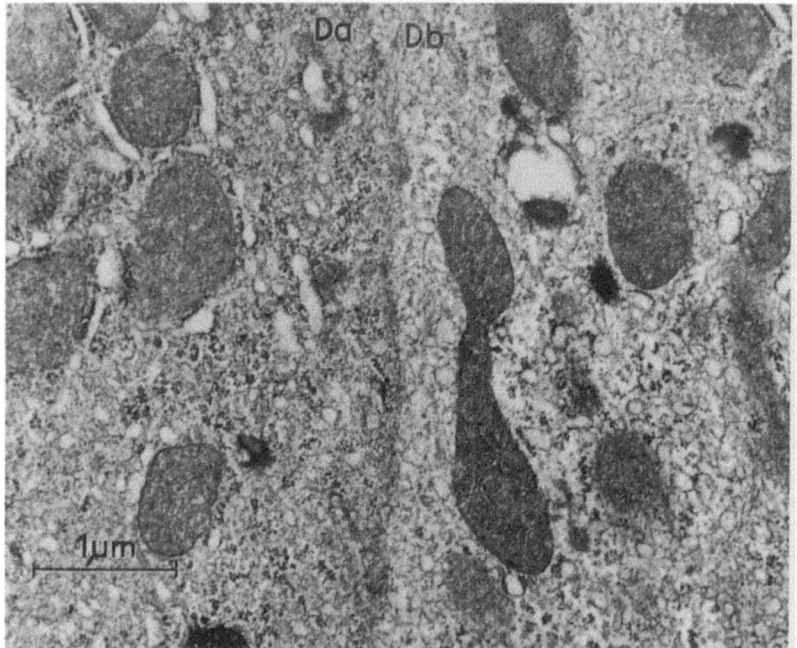

Abb. 16. Apokrine Schweißdrüse. Mitochondrien mit sehr elektronendichter Matrix (*B*). Cristae mitochondriales (→), Dunkle Granula (•→)

Abb. 17. Apokrine Schweißdrüse. Zwei benachbarte Drüsenzellen (*Da, Db*). Auffällig ist die unterschiedlich elektronendichte mitochondriale Matrix. Die Mitochondrien der etwas kontrastärmeren Zelle (*Db*) sind elektronendichter als die Mitochondrien der Zelle (*Da*)

Der *Zellkern* (Abb. 13) ist basal gelagert und als eine im basalen Anteil leicht abgeplattete Kugel zu interpretieren (KUROSUMI et al., 1959). Das Karyoplasma ist in von uns untersuchtem Material überwiegend gleichförmig. Manchmal sind randständige, der Membran anliegende Anlagerungen des Chromatins zu beobachten. (Zum normalen und pathologischen Aussehen der Kernstruktur s. bei DAVID, 1964.) Kernporen sind ein regelmäßiger Befund (KAWABATA, 1964). Wir haben sie besonders bei tangentialen Schnitten gesehen (Abb. 15). Nucleoli finden sich regelmäßig auch in von uns untersuchten Drüsenzellen meist in Einzahl (Abb. 13).

Die *Mitochondrien* als Sitz der für Oxydation des Substratwasserstoffes, Elektronentransport und oxydative Phosphorylierung (CAMERON, 1964) wichtige

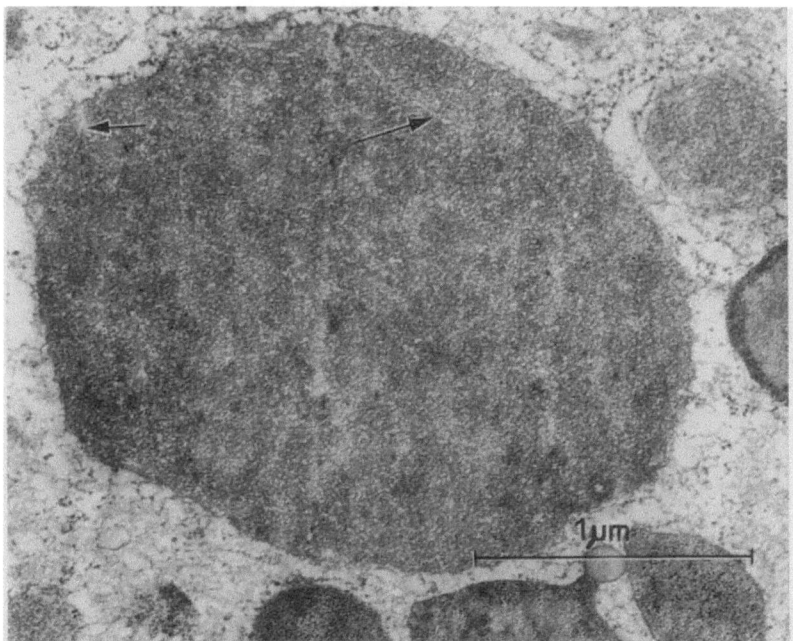

Abb. 18. Apokrine Schweißdrüse. Matrixreiches Riesenmitochondrium. Pfeile: wahrscheinlich Cristae mitochondriales

Enzymsysteme (dazu auch LEHNINGER, 1960) liegen hauptsächlich im basalen Abschnitt der Zelle, und zwar oberhalb der basalen Fältelung des Plasmalemms. Nach unserem Dafürhalten kommen sie einmal als ultrastrukturell unauffällige Mitochondrien vom Crista-Typ und zum anderen als modifizierte und schließlich auch als pathologisch alterierte Mitochondrien vor (Näheres zur Ultrastruktur der Mitochondrien s. bei VOGELL, 1963 und ANDRÉ, 1965). Bereits HIBBS (1962) sowie MUNGER (1965) haben darauf hingewiesen, daß die Mitochondrien über eine besonders elektronendichte Matrix verfügen können. Es ist die Frage, ob dieser „modifizierte" Mitochondrien-Typ einem besonderen Funktionszustand entspricht. Diese morphologischen Befunde können wir bestätigen (Abb. 16 und 17). Die Mitochondrien besitzen manchmal eine sehr dichte körnig faserige Matrix mit meistens gut erkennbarer Hüllmembran, aber wenig Cristae. Nach unserem Dafürhalten handelt es sich hierbei um Mitochondrien mit auffälliger Verschiebung der Matrix-Crista-Relation zugunsten der Matrix. Sie sind von der mit Ribosomen besetzten Seite der Ergastoplasmazisternen, wie dies sonst für Mitochondrien gilt, umgeben. Auch Riesenmitochondrien (5—10mal größer als normal) wurden in menschlichen Ceruminaldrüsen (KAWABATA, 1964) und in menschlichen apokrinen Schweißdrüsen (MUNGER, 1965) beschrieben (Abb. 18). Ähnliche Beobachtungen haben KUROSUMI, YAMAGISHI und SEKINE (1961) an den submandibularen Organen der Ratte machen können. (Zur Frage der Riesenmitochondrien und sog. hellen Granula s. unten). Andererseits können die Mitochondrien wohl beim Untergang einer Drüsenzelle vielleicht im Rahmen des Sekretionsvorganges auffällig geschwollen sein mit diesmal heller Matrix und reduzierten Cristae mitochondriales (Abb. 19 und 20). Diese pathologisch veränderten Mitochondrien sind

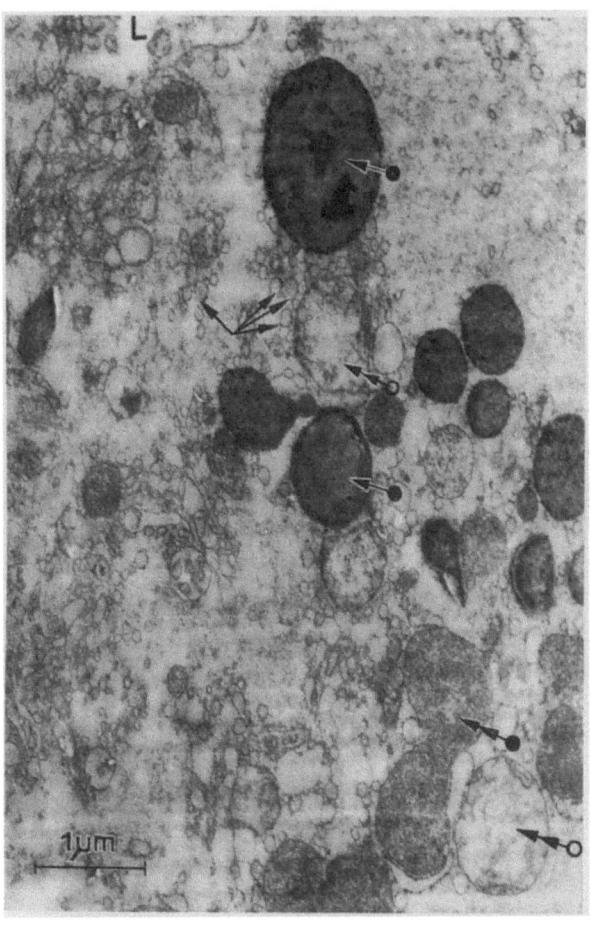

Abb. 19. Apokrine Schweißdrüse. Im Untergang begriffene Drüsenzelle. Dunkle Granula (•→). Geschwollene Mitochondrien (o→). Mitochondrien, die derartige Veränderungen noch nicht aufweisen (•→→), bläschenförmig transformiertes endoplasmatisches Reticulum (↖↑↗), Lumen (L)

bisher in apokrinen Schweißdrüsen nach unserem Wissen nicht beobachtet worden (Näheres zur Frage pathologisch veränderter Mitochondrien s. bei ROUILLER, 1960).

Schon in den ersten Abhandlungen über die Ultrastruktur der apokrinen Drüsenzellen sind *Sekretionsgranula* (Abb. 12 und 13) beobachtet und beschrieben worden. Dabei hat man zwei Typen herausgestellt: ,,smooth'' und ,,roogh'' (CHARLES, 1959) bzw. ,,light'' und ,,dark'' (KUROSUMI et al., 1959) Granula. Wir werden in Anlehnung an KUROSUMI et al. (1959) von hellen und dunklen Granula sprechen.

Helle Granula sind bis ~2 μ (KUROSUMI et al., 1959) bzw. 0,05—3 μ (YASUDA et al., 1962) groß und besitzen einen Inhalt, der gewöhnlich etwas kontrastärmer als der der mitochondrialen Matrix ist oder sich in dem Kontrast von mitochondrialer Matrix nicht wesentlich unterscheidet. Vereinzelte Granula enthalten im Innern pleomorphe Membranen, die an Cristae mitochondriales (YASUDA et al., 1962) erinnern. Sie sind von einer Doppelmembran umgeben. Selten wurden intragranulär auch Vesikel beobachtet, welche möglicherweise erweiterte Cristae mitochondriales darstellen können. Diese hellen Granula, deren mitochondriale Genese öfters diskutiert wurde (KUROSUMI et al., 1959; YASUDA et al., 1962; HASHIMOTO et al., 1966b), sind als modifizierte Mitochondrien zu betrachten (KAWABATA, 1964). Wir halten eine Identität mit den matrixreichen Riesenmitochondrien von THOENES (1966) für sehr wahrscheinlich. Es sind ultrastrukturelle Parallelen auch mit den vergrößerten Lebermitochondrien bei Delirium tremens (SZANTO, STEIG-

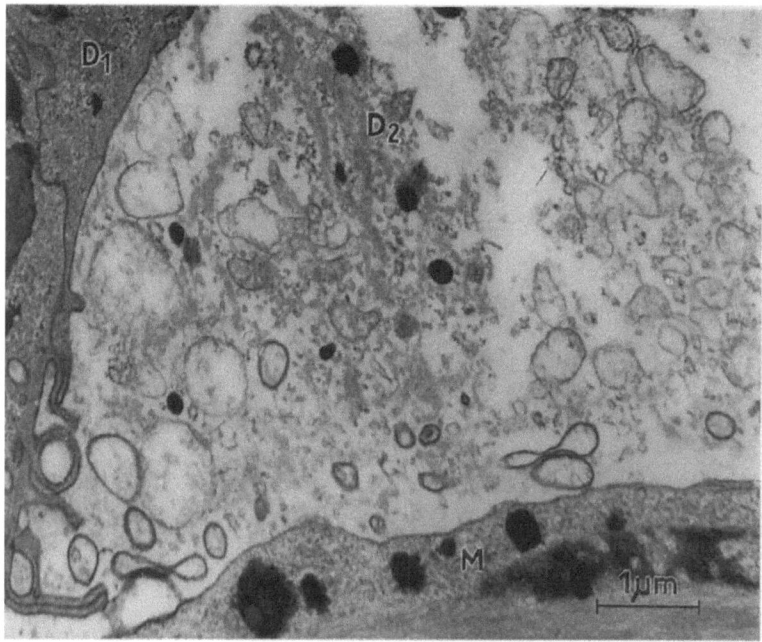

Abb. 20. Apokrine Schweißdrüse. Untergegangene apokrine Drüsenzelle (D_2). Geschwollene Mitochondrien sowie mehrere Vesikel gut erkennbar. Benachbarte Drüsenzelle (D_1) sowie Myoepithelzelle (M) ultrastrukturell unauffällig

MANN, PAMUKEN, FRIEDMAN und HADOK, 1965) zu ziehen. Aus diesem Grunde stimmen wir auch KAWABATA (1964) zu, wenn er dafür plädiert, den Begriff „light granules" überhaupt fallen zu lassen. Von diesem Blickwinkel aus ist es auch nicht angebracht, diese hellen Granula als Sekretionsgranula zu deuten, da die Theorie der mitochondrialen Genese der Sekretionsgranula nach dem heutigen Wissensstande nicht mehr haltbar ist (HIBBS, 1962; HELANDER, 1965a).

Die *dunklen Granula* sind größer als die hellen Granula (bis 7 μ groß) (KUROSUMI et al., 1959) und nach CHARLES (1959) durch eine periphere Anhäufung elektronendichter Partikel oder durch einen hellen Innenbereich und eine periphere Schicht aus elektronendichten Tropfen gekennzeichnet (Abb. 21—23). Eine sehr eingehende Beschreibung dieser Strukturen stammt von YASUDA et al. (1962). Diese Autoren haben innerhalb solcher nicht immer mit einer gut erkennbaren Membran umgebenen Granula 6 Komponenten beschrieben, und zwar: dunkle 300—1500 Å messende Spherula, weniger dunkle Globula, mäßig kontrastreiche ~200 Å große oder kleinere Vacuolen, die mit einem kontrastarmen Material angefüllt und von einer elektronendichten Substanz umgeben sind, sowie schließlich große und kleine blasse Areale. Auch Myelinfiguren wurden beobachtet. Diese Beschreibung steht in weitgehender Übereinstimmung mit der Ultrastruktur von

Lipofuscingranula, auch in bezug auf elektronenmikroskopisch-cytochemischen Nachweis der sauren Phosphatase (BIEMPICA und MONTES, 1965; RUPEC, 1966b). HASHIMOTO et al. (1966b) halten die dunklen Granula aufgrund ihrer Morphologie für Lysosomen (Näheres zur Frage der Lysosomen s. bei DE DUVE, 1963a und b; NOVIKOFF, 1961, 1963; MERKER, 1964; BERTHET, 1965; ERICSSON, TRUMP und WEIBEL, 1965; GORDIS und NITKOWSKY, 1965 u. a.). Auch die Autofluorescenz (KOENIG, 1963) scheint für den lysosomalen Charakter der Gebilde zu sprechen

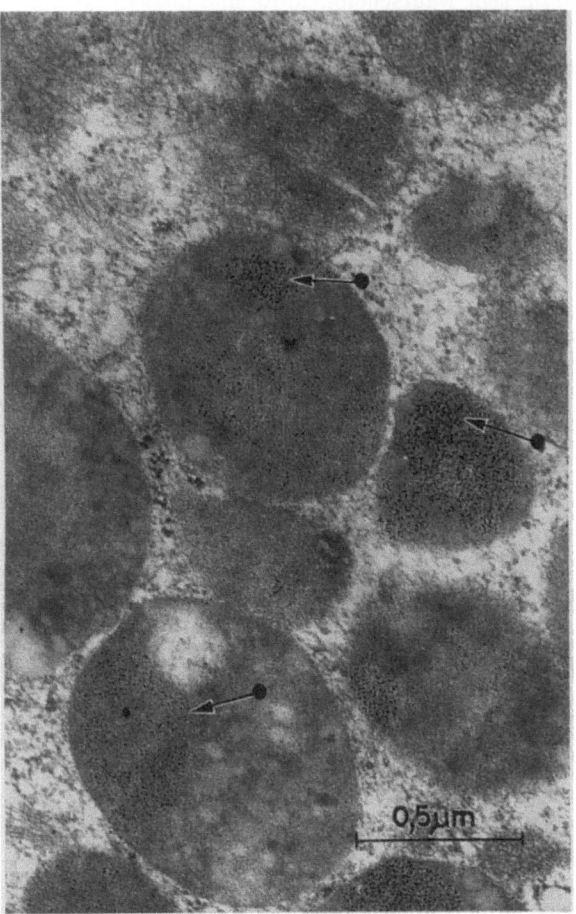

Abb. 21. Apokrine Schweißdrüse. Dunkle Granula, die größtenteils mit elektronendichten Partikeln (Ferritin-ähnliches Material) angefüllt sind (•→)

(BIEMPICA und MONTES, 1965). Es ist jedenfalls zu betonen, daß die Quantität des Lipopigmentes in umgekehrtem Verhältnis zu elektronenmikroskopisch-cytochemisch feststellbaren sauren Phosphataseaktivitäten dieser Gebilde steht. Schließlich können dunkle Granula wohl nur noch aus osmiophilem Pigment bestehen (RUPEC, 1966b) (Abb. 24 und 25). Es ist aber auch damit zu rechnen, daß Glutaraldehyd die hydrolytische Enzymaktivität hemmt und auf diese Weise Orte mit schwächerer Enzymaktivität nicht wahrgenommen werden können (DAEMS und PERSIJN, 1965; MAUNSBACH, 1966b). Nur MUNGER (1965b) hält aufgrund seiner lichtmikroskopisch-histochemischen sowie ultrastrukturellen Untersuchungen die dunklen Granula für ,,presumptive keratin granules".

Die apokrinen Drüsenzellen

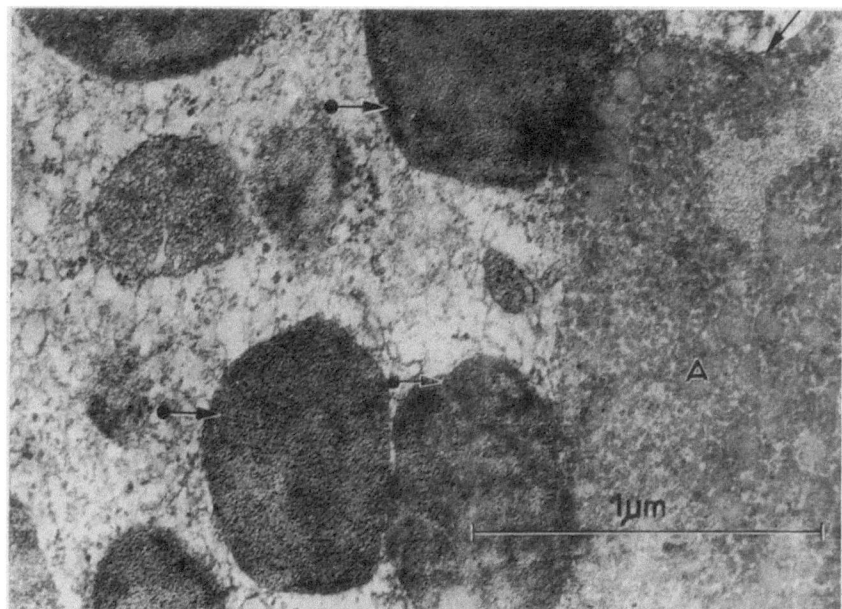

Abb. 22. Apokrine Schweißdrüse. Ein riesengroßes dunkles Granulum (*A*) mit unterschiedlich großen, kontrastreichen, kugelförmigen Gebilden, wenig elektronendichten Partikeln (Ferritin-ähnliches Material) und erkennbarer Membran (→). Die benachbarten dunklen Granula (•→) enthalten auch elektronendichte Partikel

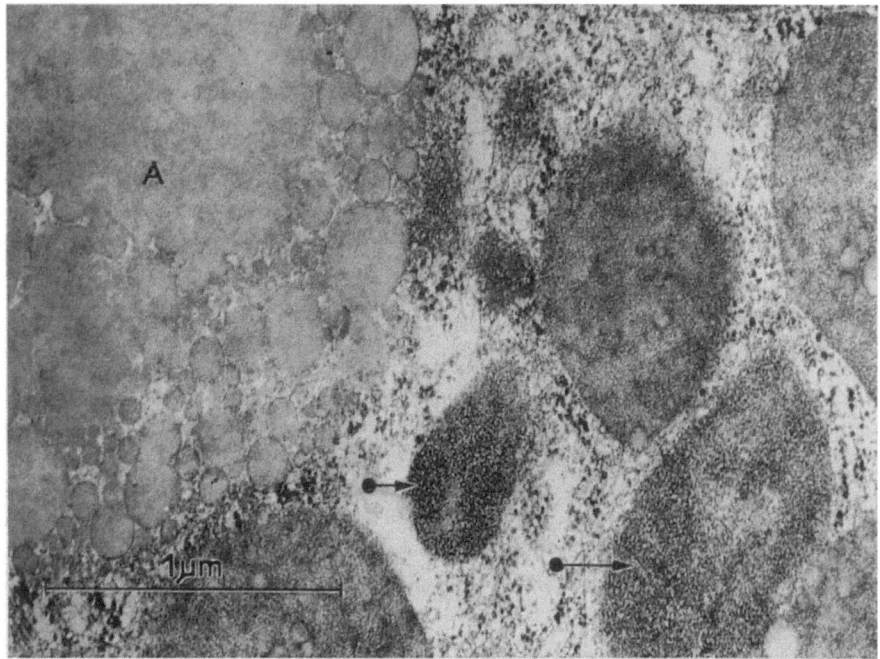

Abb. 23. Apokrine Schweißdrüse. Ein in Auflösung begriffenes dunkles Granulum (*A*). Das dunkle Granulum (•→) ist mit elektronendichten Partikeln (Ferritin-ähnliches Material) angefüllt

Eisenpartikel — wahrscheinlich ferritinähnliches Material — sind auch von YASUDA et al. (1962), MONTAGNA (1962), HIBBS (1962), RUPEC (1966b) u.a. in den dunklen Granula beobachtet worden (Abb. 21). Es wurde elektronenmikroskopisch gezeigt, daß es sich dabei vor allem um ein ferritinähnliches Material in saure Phosphatase enthaltenden Strukturen (wohl Lysosomen) handelt (Abb. 25) (RUPEC, 1966b). Eine solche Assoziation ist bisher in der Leber (ESSNER und NOVIKOFF, 1961; DAEMS, 1962) und der Rattenniere (ERICSSON, TRUMP und WEIBEL, 1965) beschrieben worden. Es wurde vermutet (BIEMPICA und MONTES,

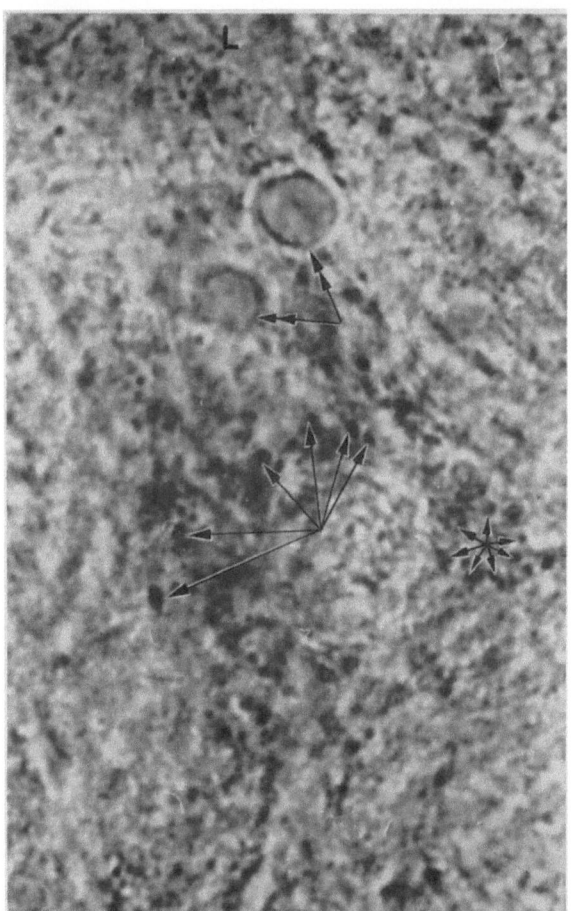

Abb. 24. Apokrine Schweißdrüse. Saure Phosphatasen. Im Cytoplasma einer Drüsenzelle feintropfige, intensiv positive Granula (Pfeile) und grobtropfige, schwach positive bzw. arreaktive Granula. Lumen (L). Kryostatschnitt. Saure Phosphatase nach GOMORI. Vergr. 2240 ×

1965), daß das Eisen von Mitochondrien abstammen könnte. Von historischem Interesse ist in diesem Zusammenhang, daß bereits RICHTER (1933) über eine „innige Vermengung" von Eisen und Fett sprach.

KUROSUMI et al. (1959) halten Granulationen und helle Areale innerhalb dunkler Granula für ein Zeichen beginnender Desintegration, wobei als Endzustand dieses Vorganges entweder nur noch eine Vacuole übrigbleibt oder wenn die Membran rupturiert wird, sich der ganze Inhalt intracytoplasmatisch verteilt (Abb. 23). Ein ähnliches Schicksal dieser Organelle hält auch HIBBS (1962) für wahrscheinlich. Nach HASHIMOTO et al. (1966b) besteht ein Sekretionstyp (s. dort), der durch Auflösung der Granula und das Übrigbleiben der Vacuolen (foamy vacuoles) gekennzeichnet sein soll. Eine intracelluläre Auflösung der dunklen Granula halten auch wir für bewiesen (Abb. 23).

Ob *Übergangsformen zwischen hellen und dunklen Granula* bestehen, ist noch nicht definitiv geklärt. Einige Autoren halten sie für möglich und für ultrastrukturell bewiesen (HIBBS, 1962). Wir haben Übergangsformen *nie* mit Sicherheit beobachten können. Wir halten nämlich die dunklen Granula für Lipopigment und eventuell auch Eisen enthaltende lysosomale Strukturen, während die hellen Granula, welche aller Wahrscheinlichkeit nach von Mitochondrien abstammen oder einer besonderen Form der Mitochondrien entsprechen, weder morphologisch noch sonst in irgendwelchem sicheren funktionellen Zusammenhang mit den dunklen Granula stehen. Nach KUROSUMI et al. (1959) sollen die hellen Granula

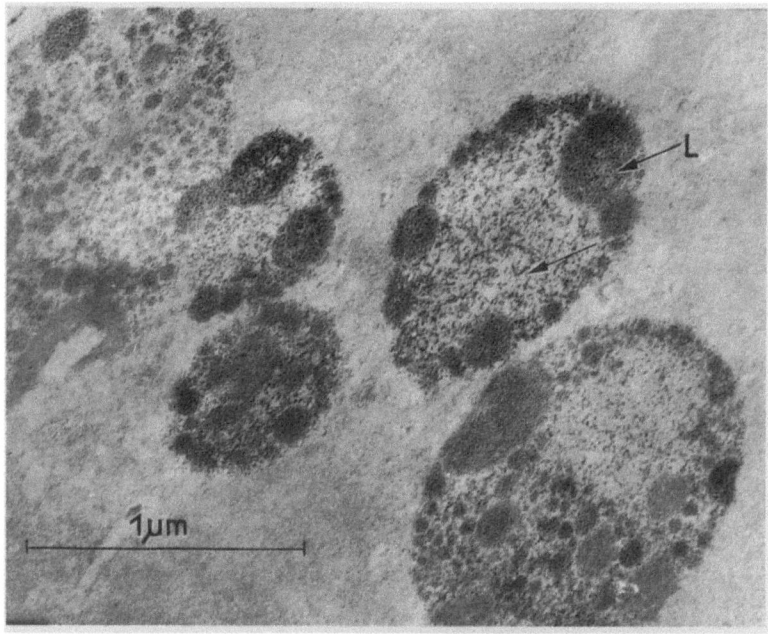

Abb. 25. Apokrine Schweißdrüse. Nachweis von saurer Phosphatase nach GOMORI in dunklen Granula einer apokrinen Drüsenzelle. Bleipräcipitate sind stäbchenförmig (→) und dadurch von anderen kontrastreichen Partikeln (Ferritin-ähnliches Material) zu unterscheiden (← L)

das Lipoidmaterial der apikal desintegrierten dunklen Granula absorbieren und auf diesem Wege in dunkle Granula übergehen können. Andererseits sind nach YASUDA et al. (1962) beide Granulatypen als eigenständige Strukturen aufzufassen. Ähnlicher Meinung ist auch YAMADA (1960).

Mit KAWABATA (1964) sind wir der Ansicht, daß die *Lipochondrien* wahrscheinlich den dunklen Granula entsprechen. Auch das graphisch dargestellte Schicksal von Lipochondrien (KUROSUMI, 1961) deckt sich weitgehend mit unseren heutigen Vorstellungen über das Schicksal der dunklen Granula. Außerdem haben wir auch in apokrinen Drüsenzellen polyvesiculäre Körperchen (Lipochondrien ?) gesehen (Abb. 26), die mit den in den ekkrinen Schweißdrüsen der Menschen (IIJIMA, 1959) morphologisch weitgehend übereinstimmen.

Die *irregulären Korpuskeln mit kristalliner Innenstruktur* (RUPEC, 1967a) kommen hauptsächlich als kantige, multianguläre bzw. längliche spindelförmige Korpuskeln in apokrinen Drüsenzellen vor (Abb. 27). Ihre Innenstruktur ist durch ein kristallines Muster gekennzeichnet. In der Form ähnliche Granula haben schon KUROSUMI et al. (1959) sowie HASHIMOTO et al. (1966b) beschrieben, ohne auf ihre Innenstruktur näher einzugehen. Das kristalline Muster dieser Korpuskeln ist mit

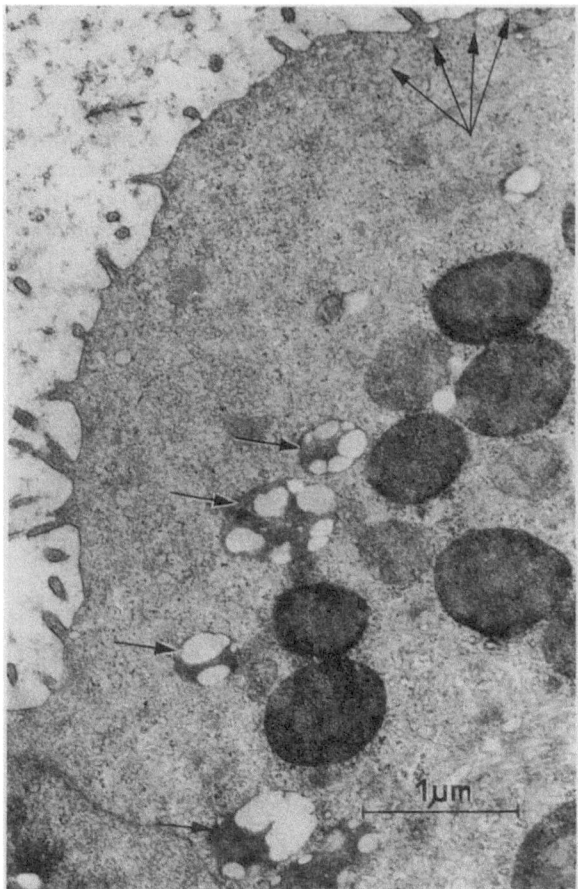

Abb. 26. Apokrine Schweißdrüse. Drüsenzelle mit dunklen Granula und Granula, die an sog. Lipochondrien erinnern (→). Vacuolen (↖ ↑ ↗)

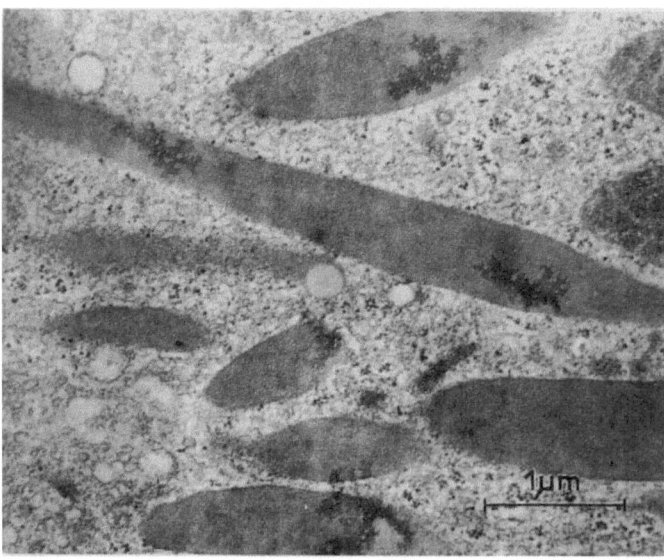

Abb. 27. Apokrine Schweißdrüse. Irreguläre Korpuskeln mit kristalliner Innenstruktur

dem in den Zellen der proximalen Tubuli der Rattenniere vorkommenden Proteinkristalle (MAUNSBACH, 1966a) zu vergleichen. In der Form ähnliche Korpuskeln sind auch z.B. in den Leydigschen Zellen (FAWCETT und BURGOS, 1960), Bindegewebszellen des Regenwurms (STAUBESAND, KUHLO und KERSTING, 1963), in den Zellen der Hühnchen-Thyreoidea (YOSHIMURA und IRIE, 1959) beobachtet worden. Wir glauben, daß sie den dunklen Granula zuzuordnen sind (Näheres bei RUPEC, 1967a). Einen Konnex der kristallinen Strukturen mit den Filamenten bzw. Filamentbündeln (s. unten), wie das beispielsweise NAGANO (1966) in Sertolischen Zellen beschrieben hat, konnten wir bisher nicht beobachten.

Nach YASUDA et al. (1962) soll noch eine dritte Form der *Vacuolen* neben den eben beschriebenen hellen bzw. dunklen Granula bestehen. Diese Vacuolen haben sie aufgrund morphologischer Kriterien mit Buchstaben A—D bezeichnet. Typ A besteht aus einer elektronendichten exzentrisch gelagerten Masse, die in ein helles Matrix eingebettet ist. Wahrscheinlich handelt es sich um die initiale Phase der dunklen Granula. Die beiden letztgenannten Gruppen (Typ C und Typ D) sind wohl als Lysosomen zu deuten. Typ C ist deshalb sehr interessant, weil er mit sehr elektronendichten Partikeln angefüllt ist, was ein Anlaß dazu war, diese Strukturen als „iron containing vesicles" zu bezeichnen. Die Vacuolen vom Typ B wurden auch als „multivesiculäre" Vesikeln beschrieben.

In ruhenden, besonders aber in sekretorisch aktiven Zellen sind vorwiegend im apikalen Bereich bis $\sim$500 Å breite Vacuolen vorhanden (Abb. 26), die sehr an pinocytotische Vesikel der Capillarendothelien erinnern (HIBBS, 1962). Wahrscheinlich hat CHARLES (1959) an diese Vesikel gedacht, als er von „apikalen Ansammlungen" sprach. Ihr Inhalt ist unterschiedlich kontrastreich. Solche Strukturen scheinen bei der „droplet secretion" (HIBBS, 1962) der apokrinen Schweißdrüsen aktiv beteiligt zu sein. Auch nach YASUDA et al. (1962) handelt es sich um sekretorische Vacuolen. Ähnlich glauben KAWABATA (1964), BIEMPICA und MONTES (1965) sowie HASHIMOTO et al. (1966b) in apikalen Vacuolen sekretorische Vacuolen zu sehen.

Wir haben fast regelmäßig in den apokrinen Drüsenzellen *Filamentenbündel* seltener vereinzelte Filamente, die manchmal parallel verlaufen, beobachten können, die in unserem Material nicht dazu neigen, im Bereich der Desmosomen zu enden. Die Filamentenbündel (Abb. 28) haben oft angedeutet ein „speckled pattern", ähnlich wie es z.B. BRODY (1960) in Stachelzellen der Epidermis beschrieben hat.

Der *Golgi-Apparat* besteht prinzipiell aus Golgi-Membranen und Golgi-Granula (SJÖSTRAND, 1964). In apokrinen Schweißdrüsenzellen ist er sehr voluminös (Abb. 12) und kann bis zu einem Drittel der Zelle einnehmen. Der Golgi-Apparat dieser Zellen besteht fast ausschließlich aus Vesikeln (KUROSUMI et al., 1959). Seine wichtigste Funktion soll in einer räumlichen Abtrennung von bestimmten Substanzen von Protein- sowie Polysaccharidcharakter vom Grundplasma beruhen (SIEVERS, 1965). Eine derartige Abtrennung erfolgt durch eine Membran. Vielleicht sind auch die Sekretionsprodukte in dieser Organelle einem Reifungsprozeß unterworfen (BOURNE und TEWARI, 1964). Ähnlich meint auch HELANDER (1965a), daß der Golgi-Apparat bei der Konzentration der Substanzen zu Sekretgranula eine entscheidende Rolle spielen kann. Wie bei den anderen Drüsen auch (KUROSUMI, 1965), ist der Golgi-Apparat der apokrinen Drüsenzellen bereits aufgrund licht- sowie elektronenmikroskopischer Untersuchungen mit der Bildung von Sekretionsgranula in Verbindung gebracht worden. In Übergangsepithelien ist auch seine Rolle bei der Plasmalemmbildung diskutiert worden (HICKS, 1966). (Näheres zur Frage des Golgi-Apparates s. bei DALTON und FELIX, 1956; KUFF und DALTON, 1959; CARASSO und FAVARD, 1961; MERCER, 1962 sowie SIEVERS, 1965).

Es besteht keine Übereinstimmung über den Entwicklungsgrad des *endoplasmatischen Reticulums*. So halten im Gegensatz zu KUROSUMI (1959) sowie HIBBS (1962), BIEMPICA und MONTES (1965) das Ergastoplasma (α-Cytomembran; SJÖSTRAND, 1964) für relativ gut entwickelt. Ein besonderer Konnex zwischen Ergastoplasmazisternen und dunklen Granula besteht offensichtlich nicht (YASUDA et al., 1962). Die Ergastoplasmamembranen sind überwiegend um die Mitochondrien (BIEMPICA und MONTES, 1965) und die sog. hellen Granula (HASHIMOTO et al., 1966b; eigene Befunde) zu finden. Als Ausdruck des Zelluntergangs ist eine bläschenförmige Transformation des Reticulums zu beobachten (Abb. 19). Solche

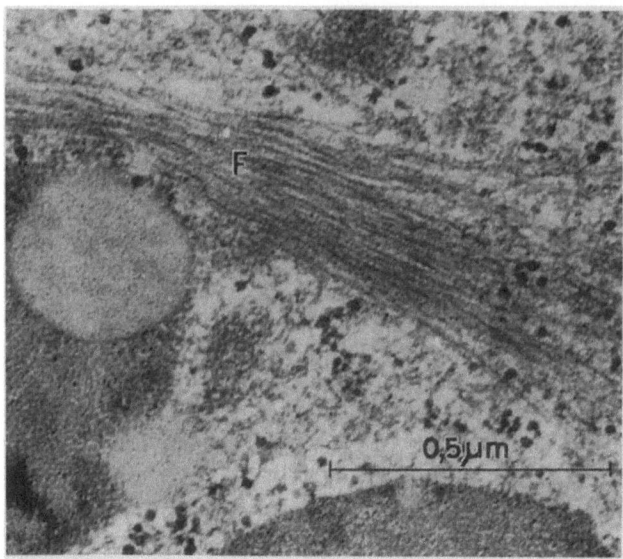

Abb. 28. Apokrine Schweißdrüse. Filamentenbündel (*F*) in einer Drüsenzelle

Veränderungen gehen in unserem Material regelmäßig mit der Mitochondrienschwellung und -abrundung einher. Sie erinnern sehr an von ITO (1962) beobachtete postmortale Veränderungen der Leberzellen.

Ribosomen [PALADE- (1955) Granula] sind oft frei im Cytoplasma, d.h. nicht membrangebunden, manchmal aber zu Gruppen aggregiert (Polysomen). Im übrigen sind sie der äußeren Fläche der ergastoplasmatischen Zisternen angelagert. Nach SJÖSTRAND (1964) sind diese nach OsO_4-Fixierung kontrastreichen Partikel durch ihre außerordentlich einheitliche Größe von 150 Å und die Anfärbbarkeit mit Uranylacetat bzw. Bleiverbindungen charakterisiert. Im „negative staining" zeigen sie eine unregelmäßige Form mit einem mittleren Durchmesser von 200 Å.

Vor kurzem hat GROSS (1966) die von AFZELIUS (1955) zuerst beschriebenen *„annulate lamellae"* auch in apokrinen Drüsenzellen sowie ebenfalls in den Zellen der apokrinen Hidrocystome (1965) dargestellt. An eigenem Material können wir diese Befunde bestätigen (Abb. 29). Das ist insoweit interessant, da solche, vielleicht von der Nuclearmembran abstammende Gebilde — die Annuli der Lamellen sind auch mit den Kernporen zu vergleichen — nur selten in somatischen Zellen gefunden wurden. Sie können mit Ribosomen verbunden sein (KESSEL, 1965) und sind auch zu Vesikelbildung fähig (SCHMIDT, 1965; HARRISON, 1966). Ihre Funktion ist bislang nicht sicher geklärt.

Außer den oben geschilderten typischen Drüsenzellen hat HIBBS (1962) *Zellen mit weniger dichtem Cytoplasma und weniger zahlreichen Sekretionsgranula* beschrieben. Diese Zellen sollen morphologisch den sog. dunklen Zellen der ekkrinen Schweißdrüsen weitgehend entsprechen. Wir haben öfter der Beschreibung nach ähnliche Drüsenzellen in unserem Material beobachten können. Dabei sind wir aber nicht geneigt, unbedingt eine Parallele mit den dunklen Zellen der ekkrinen Schweißdrüsen zu ziehen[1].

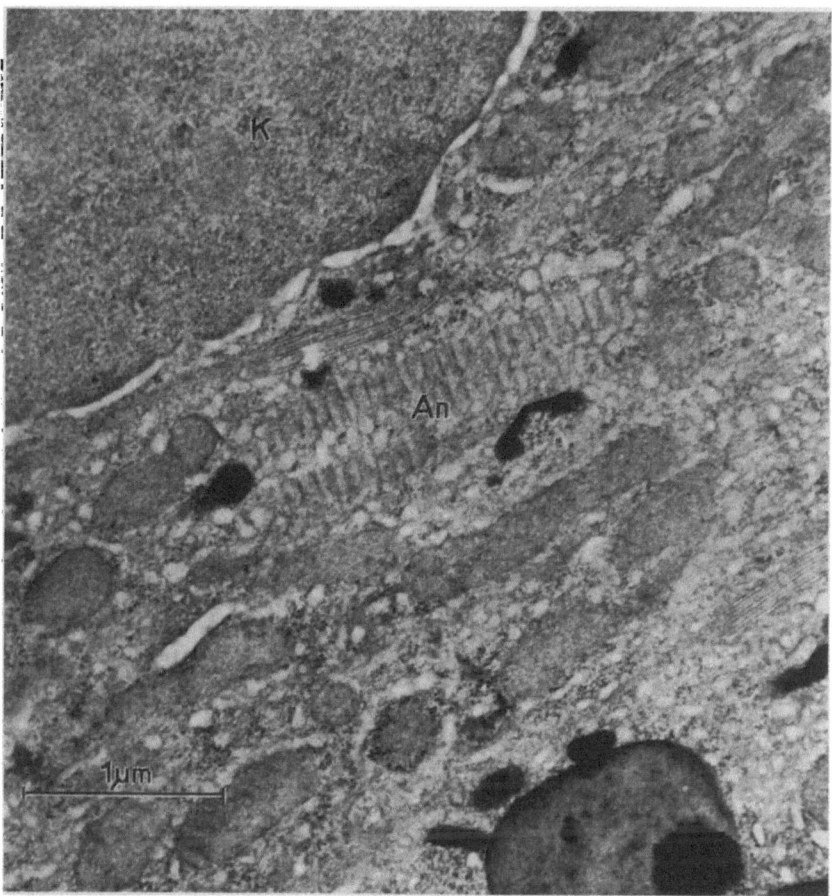

Abb. 29. Apokrine Schweißdrüse. In einer Drüsenzelle ‚annulate lamellae' (*An*). Kern (*K*)

Auch *die intercellulären Canaliculi*, wie sie z. B. bei ekkrinen Schweißdrüsen vorkommen, sind von CHARLES (1959) zwischen apokrinen Schweißdrüsenzellen beschrieben worden. Dieser Befund ist aber noch nicht bestätigt. In unserem Material konnten wir diese Strukturen nicht feststellen.

2. Die Myoepithelzellen

Untersuchungen an apokrinen Schweißdrüsen (KUROSUMI et al., 1959; CHARLES, 1959; HIBBS, 1962; KAWABATA, 1964; MUNGER, 1965a und b), ekkrinen Schweißdrüsen (HIBBS, 1958; TAKAHASHI, 1958a und b; MUNGER und BRUSILOW, 1961; MATSUZAWA und KUROSUMI, 1963; ELLIS, 1965), Schweißdrüsen des antebrachialen Organs bei Lemur catta (KNEELAND, 1966), Glandula mamma (RICHARDSON, 1949; TAKAHASHI, 1958; HAGUENAU, 1959; BARGMANN und KNOOP,

---

[1] Zur Ultrastruktur atypisch aussehender Zellen s. auch bei RUPEC (1967b).

1959; HOLLMANN, 1959 u.a.), der exorbitalen Drüse der Ratte (LEESON, 1960), und schließlich den submaxillären Drüsen beim Menschen (TANDLER, 1965) sowie der Ratte (SCOTT und PEASE, 1959; TAMARIN, 1966) haben erkennen lassen, daß die Feinstruktur von Myoepithelzellen in verschiedenen Arten von Drüsen ähnlich ist (Näheres dazu s. bei ELLIS, 1965). Morphologisch bestehen viele Übereinstimmungen zwischen Myoepithelzellen und glatten Muskelzellen (TAMARIN, 1966). Die Myoepithelzellen der apokrinen Schweißdrüsen sind spindelförmig und liegen zwischen der basalen Partie der Zellmembran der Drüsenzellen und der Basalmembran (Abb. 12 und 13), wobei auf oft vorhandene breite intercelluläre Spalt-

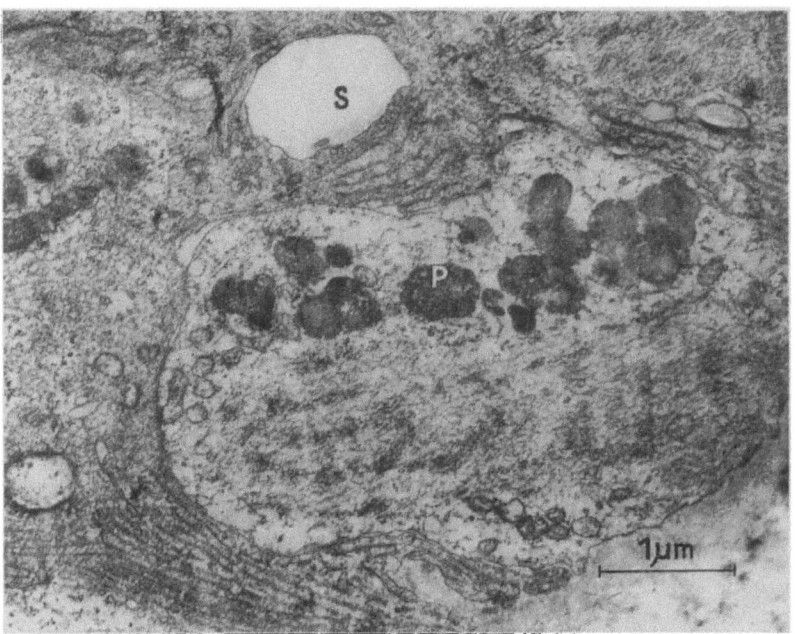

Abb. 30. Apokrine Schweißdrüse. Myoepithelzelle mit Pigmentgranula (*P*). Spaltraum (*S*)

räume (Abb. 30) zwischen einer Drüsenzelle und basalwärts liegender Myoepithelzelle hinzuweisen ist (CHARLES, 1959; HIBBS, 1962; eigene Untersuchungen). Die Myoepithelzellen der apokrinen Schweißdrüsen sind besonders eingehend von KUROSUMI et al. (1959) beschrieben worden. In der jüngsten Zeit haben vor allem ELLIS (1965), TANDLER (1965) sowie TAMARIN (1966) elektronenmikroskopisch das Myoepithelium der ekkrinen Schweißdrüsen bzw. Glandulae submandibularis bei Menschen und Ratten untersucht. Man unterscheidet auch bei den Myoepithelzellen der apokrinen Schweißdrüsen grundsätzlich einen filamentösen und einen nichtfilamentösen Anteil des Cytoplasmas.

Die *Myofilamente* sind 50—80 Å dick und entsprechen damit gut der Breite der Actinfilamente (NEEDHAM und SHOENBERG, 1964) wie kürzlich auch von TAMARIN (1966) betont wurde. Sie verlaufen parallel entsprechend der Längsachse der Zelle, wobei sie wohl ähnlich wie bei den ekkrinen Schweißdrüsen miteinander anastomosieren und so ein netzförmiges Aussehen bieten können. Es ist in diesem Zusammenhang interessant, daß die Anordnung der Myofilamente in den glatten Muskelzellen von Blutgefäßen in erschlafftem Zustand eine andere ist als in kontrahiertem Zustand. Die Myofilamente verlaufen nämlich im ersten Falle parallel zueinander, im zweiten aber bilden sie dichte Netzwerke (NEMETSCHEK, 1966). Entlang der Zellmembran und zwar dort, wo die Basalmembran an die

Zelle angrenzt, findet man elektronendichte plattenförmige Zonen, die Halbdesmosomen ähneln. In diesen Platten enden viele Myofilamente. Im Verlauf und parallel mit den Myofilamenten sind mehrere strichförmige elektronendichte Zonen zu finden (Abb. 31). Solche sog. ,,dark bodies" bestehen nach Untersuchungen von TANDLER (1965) sowie TAMARIN (1966) aus streckenweise dicht gepackten Filamenten. Sie sind vielleicht mit der Z-Linie der quergestreiften Muskelfasern zu vergleichen (HAGUENAU, 1959; ELLIS, 1965). Nach Ansicht von NEMETSCHEK (1966) sollen die vergleichbaren ,,spindelförmigen Verdichtungen" der glatten Muskelzellen Actomyosin entsprechen. Es sei erwähnt, daß derartige Strukturen in glatten Muskelzellen von Uteri trächtiger Ratten besonders zahlreich vorkommen, aber während der Austreibungsperiode weitgehend verschwinden (GANSLER, 1961). Man glaubt, daß Actin depolymerisiert wird.

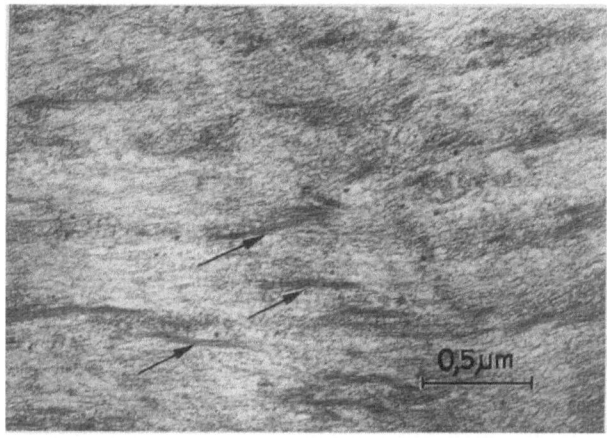

Abb. 31. Apokrine Schweißdrüsen. Myofilamente innerhalb einer Myoepithelzelle. Elektronendichte Zonen (→)

ELLIS hat perinucleär, aber auch im filamentösen Bereich in Glutaraldehydfixiertem Material *Mikrotubuli* beschrieben. Diese Strukturen sind sehr wahrscheinlich als eine ubiquitäre Komponente des Cytoplasmas zu interpretieren (DE-THÉ, 1964; BEHNKE, 1965). Ihre Funktion ist noch nicht definitiv geklärt. Es besteht die Möglichkeit, daß sie bei der Motilität der Zelle bzw. der Zellorganellen eine Rolle spielen (DE-THÉ, 1964; Näheres dazu s. auch bei TAYLOR, 1966).

Die längsausgezogen wirkenden *Zellkerne* der Myoepithelzellen sind apikal lokalisiert und ultrastrukturell grundsätzlich Drüsenzellkernen ähnlich (KUROSUMI et al., 1959). Die Kernporen waren im Material von TAMARIN (1966) in Myoepithelzellen nicht so oft anzutreffen wie in den sekretorischen Zellen.

Perinucleär sind oft elektronendichte, verschieden gestaltete *Granula* vorhanden, die als Pigment, vielleicht als Lipofuscin (ELLIS, 1965) zu deuten sind. Auch KAWABATA (1964) meint, daß diese Strukturen Lipofuscin entsprechen. Es würde also eine Beziehung zu Cytolysomen bzw. Lysosomen bestehen.

In der übrigen perinucleären, filamentfreien Zone finden sich regelmäßig auch andere Organellen: Golgi-Apparat, endoplasmatisches Reticulum, und zwar ohne und mit Ribosomenbesatz (Ergastoplasma), Mitochondrien und freie Ribosomen. Die Mitochondrien können sich auch zwischen Myofilamenten finden, wie es TAMARIN (1966), KNEELAND (1966) und auch wir beobachten konnten. Lumenwärts sind Myoepithelzellen durch relativ wenige *Desmosomen* mit den Drüsenzellen verbunden. Diese Tatsache, wie auch ihre Lage oberhalb der Basalmembran, wird als Argument für ihre epitheliale Herkunft gedeutet (TAMARIN, 1966).

Wo zwei Myoepithelzellen aneinanderstoßen, bilden sich Zwischenzellkontakte in Form von einfachen Desmosomen (tight junction) oder Nexus (ELLIS, 1965). TANDLER (1965) hat zwischen Myoepithelzellen und Drüsenzellen Nervenendigungen dargestellt. Die Situation, daß Nerven direkt an Myoepithelzellen oder Drüsenzellen enden, ist nach Untersuchungen von ELLIS (1965) unwahrscheinlich. In diesem Zusammenhang ist die vorwiegend entlang des basalen Plasmalemms vorhandene Vesikulation (Caveolae) zu erwähnen, die KUROSUMI et al. (1959) gerne als synaptischen Vesikeln ähnliche Strukturen deuten möchten. Solche Vesikel sind auch in anderen Myoepithelzellen (BARGMANN und KNOOP, 1959; TAMARIN, 1966 u.a.) sowie in anderen glatten Muskelzellen (SMITH, 1964) und in Zellen der Musculi arrectores pilorum (CHARLES, 1960) beschrieben worden. Außerdem hat man die Parallelen mit der Vesikulation des Capillarendothels (Näheres dazu bei WOLFF, 1966) gezogen (CHARLES, 1959). RHODIN (1962) hat für die glatten Muskelzellen zwei Möglichkeiten in bezug auf die Rolle einer solchen pinocytotischen Aktivität (Näheres zur Frage der Pinocytose s. bei HOLTER, 1965) angegeben, und zwar Transport der Metaboliten oder ihr Zusammenhang mit den enzymatischen Aktivitäten. Die alkalische Phosphataseaktivität in diesen Bläschen (MATSUZAWA und KUROSUMI, 1963) scheint für eine solche Anschauung zu sprechen. NEMETSCHEK (1966) sieht in dieser Membranvesikulation einen morphologischen Ausdruck für den Austausch von Flüssigkeit. Es ist von Interesse, daß SCOTT und PEASE (1959) in Myoepithelzellen der lacrimalen und salivaren Drüsen der Ratte überhaupt nicht bzw. nur selten solche Vesikel beobachtet haben, was ein Unterscheidungsmerkmal gegenüber den Zellen der glatten Muskulatur sein soll.

3. Die Zellen des sog. hellen intermediären Abschnittes

Es liegen bisher nach unserem Wissen keine ultrastrukturellen Beobachtungen über den sog. intermediären Abschnitt der apokrinen Schweißdrüsen (s. Histologie der apokrinen Schweißdrüsen) vor.

4. Ausführungsgang

Der Ausführungsgang ist zuerst von CHARLES (1959) eingehender untersucht worden. Dieser Autor hat einen relativen Reichtum an Mitochondrien und die Abwesenheit eines Golgi-Apparates in den Zellen der Ausführungsgänge beobachten können. Tonofilamentenbündel sind reichlich vorhanden. Im Cytoplasma sind Sekretionsgranula oder Vesikel nicht zu finden. HASHIMOTO, GROSS und LEVER (1966a) unterscheiden drei Zellschichten, und zwar die innere, die mittlere und die basale Zellschicht. Die Zellen der inneren Zellschicht besitzen an ihrer Oberfläche mehrere Mikrovilli. Basalwärts folgt sog. „terminal webb" mit Vesikeln, Tonofilamenten und Ribosomen und nach denselben Autoren die periluminale filamentöse Zone, die vor allem durch die Tonofilamentenbündel ausgezeichnet ist. Mitochondrien, Golgi-Apparat und das endoplasmatische Reticulum sind perinucleär angeordnet. Die Struktur der Zellen der mittleren Zellschicht entspricht der der inneren Zellschicht bis auf fehlende Mikrovilli und „terminal webb".

Die Zellen der basalen Zellschicht haben viel weniger Tonofilamente und reichlich Glykogengranula. Der Kern enthält viele Poren (HASHIMOTO et al., 1966a). Es ist bemerkenswert, daß HASHIMOTO et al. (1966a) glauben, die Ruptur des Plasmalemms sowie Abschnürungen der Mikrovilli als möglichen morphologischen Ausdruck einer Sekretion im Ausführungsgang gesehen zu haben. Diese Autoren (1966c) konnten einen ähnlichen Befund auch in dem Ausführungsgang der ekkrinen Schweißdrüsen erheben.

C. Die Histochemie der apokrinen Schweißdrüsen

An apokrinen Schweißdrüsen wurden auch zahlreiche histochemische Untersuchungen durchgeführt, vor allem, um einen Einblick in den Stoffwechsel und die Natur der verschiedenen intracytoplasmatischen Strukturen zu erhalten. Die Funktion der apokrinen Drüsenzellen läßt bereits vermuten, daß diese auch über intensive Stoffwechselleistungen verfügen müssen. Das dürfte sowohl für den Grundstoffwechsel wie auch für die Stoffwechselfunktionen gelten, welche mit der Sekretionstätigkeit dieser Drüsenzellen in Zusammenhang stehen. Im folgenden werden die Stoffe und Enzyme abgehandelt, soweit sie in apokrinen Schweißdrüsen bisher nachgewiesen wurden, wobei eigene Untersuchungen berücksichtigt werden.

I. Nucleinsäuren

Bereits in Hämalaun-Eosinschnitten, besonders aber bei Färbung mit Toluidinblau sind im sekretorischen Abschnitt die Drüsenzellen durch eine deutliche Basophilie charakterisiert, die auf den Reichtum basophiler Nucleinsäuren zurückzuführen ist. Neben den DNS-haltigen Zellkernen, welche mit der Feulgen-Reaktion darstellbar sind, ist auch bei Anfärbung mit Gallocyanin und Ribonuclease Verdauung der reichliche Gehalt dieser Zelle an Ribonucleinsäure im Cytoplasma und Nucleolus hervorzuheben (MONTAGNA, CHASE und LOBITZ, 1953; MONTES, BAKER und CURTIS, 1960). Die starke cytoplasmatische Basophilie steht in guter Übereinstimmung mit dem elektronenmikroskopisch feststellbaren Ribosomengehalt und deutet auch in Zusammenhang mit den großen Nucleolen darauf hin, daß diese Zellen über eine aktive Proteinsynthese verfügen. Dies gilt insbesondere für große Zellen mit starker Basophilie (MONTES et al., 1960).

In den Myoepithelzellen ist Ribonucleinsäure nicht in großen Mengen histochemisch nachweisbar (MONTES et al., 1960).

II. Proteine

Sulphydryl- und Disulfid-haltige Proteine. Wie in allen Epithelzellen sind auch die Reaktionen auf SH- und SS-Gruppen in den Zellen der apokrinen Schweißdrüsen positiv. In dem Drüsenepithel hat MUNGER (1965b) positive Reaktionsausfälle beobachtet und auch aufgrund vergleichender elektronenmikroskopischer Untersuchungen den Schluß gezogen, daß es sich dabei um sog. ,,presumptive keratin granules" handelt. Man kann dieser Interpretation nur schwer folgen, denn auch nicht verhornende Zellen, wie beispielsweise Leberzellen, können einen hohen Gehalt an SH- und SS-Gruppen-haltige Proteine besitzen, ohne daß dies etwas mit Verhornung zu tun hat.

Auffällig reichlich findet man SS- und SH-Gruppen-haltige Substanzen in den Myoepithelzellen (MONTAGNA et al., 1954). Hier scheinen sie an die Myofilamente gebunden zu sein.

Auch die alkalische Tetrazoliumreaktion wurde zur Identifizierung von Cystin und Cystin-haltigen Substanzen von YASUDA et al. (1960) herangezogen. Nach diesen Autoren sollen unreife Sekretionsgranula neben anderen Substanzen auch Cystin bzw. Cystin-haltige Stoffe enthalten, welche sich während des Reifungsvorganges dieser Granula offenbar verlieren.

Aminosäuren. Mit Reaktionen zum histochemischen Nachweis von Aminosäuren in Proteinen wie der Alloxan- bzw. Ninhydrin-Schifftechnik oder der gekuppelten Tetrazoliumreaktion zum Nachweis von Proteinen mit Phenolradikalen erhält man auch in den Epithelien der apokrinen Schweißdrüsen und den Myoepithelzellen wie in anderen epithelialen Strukturen der Haut positive Reaktionsausfälle. Wegen der Ubiquität der reagierenden Aminosäuren in Proteinen ist dies eigentlich auch nicht anders zu erwarten. YASUDA und KAGEMOTO (1960) haben besonders mit gekuppelter Tetrazoliumtechnik eingehende Untersuchungen durchgeführt und glauben in kleinen und großen Sekretionsgranula Histidin, nicht aber Tyrosin und Tryptophan, im Cytoplasma der Drüsenzellen neben eventuell nachgewiesenem Histidin regelmäßig Purin- und Pyrimidinbasen festgestellt zu haben. Auch mit der in ihrer Spezifität fraglichen (BARKA und ANDERSON, 1963) Bromphenolblaureaktion hat man eine Darstellung der cellulären Proteine in apokrinen Schweißdrüsen versucht (YASUI und SUZUKI, 1961). Das Cytoplasma der Drüsenzellen und die Epithelzellen fanden sich stets intensiv angefärbt. Die „cuticular border" im luminalen Randgebiet der Zelle fand sich erst nach dem 12. Lebensjahr intensiver reaktiv. Der Inhalt des Lumens war ebenfalls nur im Kindesalter durch eine stark positive Reaktion gekennzeichnet.

Zusammenfassend ist zu sagen, daß mit cytochemischen Reaktionen zum Nachweis von Aminosäuren und Proteinen, teils auch aufgrund geringer Spezifität der Methoden, im übrigen aber wegen des ubiquitären Vorkommens dieser Stoffe, streng spezifische Ergebnisse praktisch nicht gewonnen wurden.

III. Lipide

Lipide kommen in apokrinen Schweißdrüsen reichlich vor (Näheres s. bei MONTAGNA, 1962), im wesentlichen in sekretorischen Drüsenabschnitten (Abb. 32).

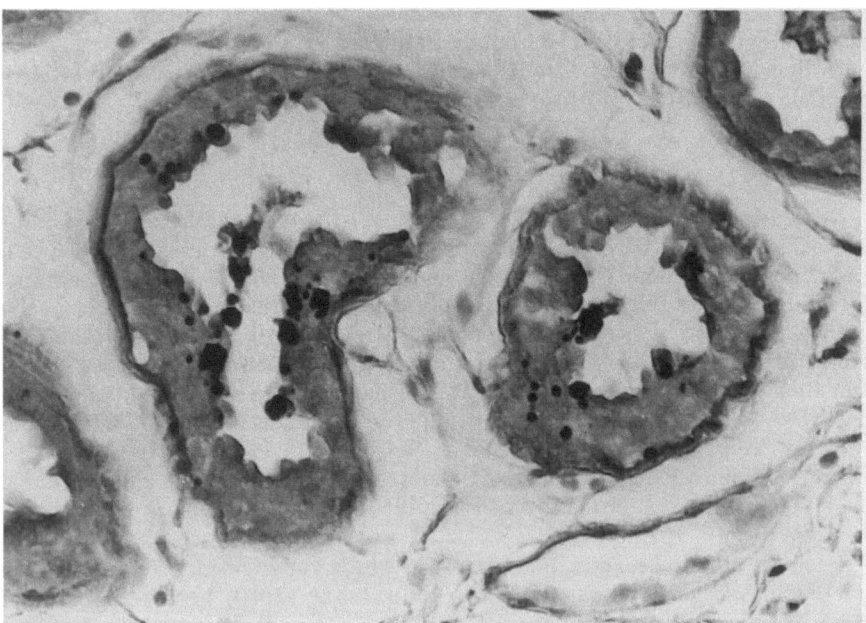

Abb. 32a u. b. Apkorine Schweißdrüse. a Reichlich sudanophile Granula in Drüsenepithelien. Kryostatschnitt. Sudanschwarz B. Vergr. 360 ×. b Lipopigmentgranula. Kryostatschnitt. Long-Ziehl-Neelsen. Vergr. 890 ×

In der Hauptsache handelt es sich dabei um Phospholipide, welche fluorescieren, Doppelbrechung aufweisen, sowie teilweise sudanophil oder sudanophob sind und andere für Lipopigmente typische Reaktionen zeigen (PEARSE, 1961). Es unterliegt wohl keinem Zweifel, daß es sich dabei um in ihrer chemischen Natur sich ändernde, aber bisher nicht definitiv aufgeklärte Fettstoffe handelt, die in gewisser Beziehung stehen zu dem sog. ,,Reifungsprozeß" der Sekretionsgranula. Es ist nämlich wahrscheinlich, daß verschiedene Reifungsstadien der Sekretionsgranula (z.B. gelbe, braune) verschiedenen Umwandlungs-(auch Oxydations-)Formen der sie integrierenden Lipopigmente entsprechen (Näheres ist im elektronenmikroskopischen Abschnitt über sekretorische Granula zu finden). Teilweise sind diese auch PAS-reaktiv (MONTES et al., 1960).

Neutralfette, Fettsäuren und Cholesterin scheinen in histochemisch einwandfrei nachweisbaren Mengen nicht vorzukommen (MONTAGNA, 1959, 1962).

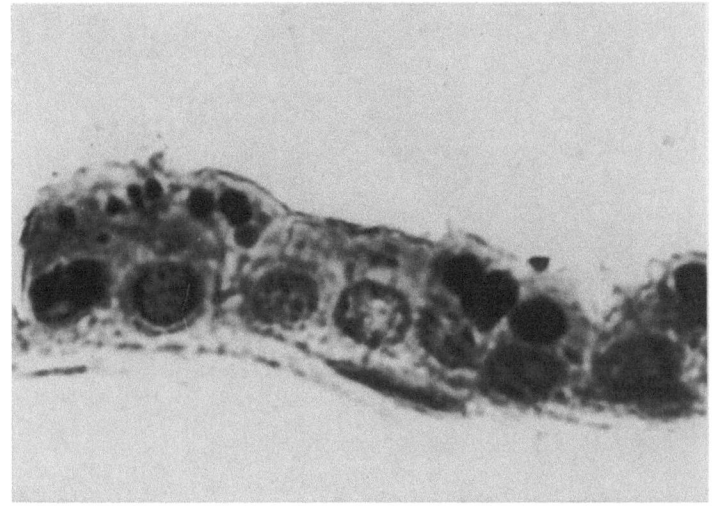

Abb. 32 b

IV. Kohlenhydrate

Unter den Kohlenhydraten wurden besonders mit der PAS-Reaktion unter Zuhilfenahme enzymatischer Identifizierungsmethoden Glykogen und Diastase-resistente PAS-reaktive Substanzen histochemisch in apokrinen Schweißdrüsen untersucht.

Glykogen. Im Gegensatz zu den ekkrinen Schweißdrüsen, welche durchweg — und besonders bei verminderter Sekretionsleistung — sehr reichlich Glykogen enthalten (Näheres s. bei BRAUN-FALCO, 1961), ist der geringe, oft fehlende Glykogengehalt in sekretorischen Abschnitten der apokrinen Schweißdrüsen bei Erwachsenen bemerkenswert.

Die Anlagen der apokrinen Schweißdrüsen beim Fetus von 4 Monaten enthalten nur geringe Mengen Glykogen. Später verschwindet das Glykogen, um zur Zeit der Bildung des sekretorischen Abschnittes wieder nachweisbar zu sein (Abb. 1) (SERRI, MONTAGNA und MESCON, 1962). Auch extrauterin ist Glykogen bis etwa zum 7. Lebensjahr weiter vorhanden (MONTAGNA, 1959). Später ist es — wie oben erwähnt — in axillären apokrinen Schweißdrüsen nicht nachzuweisen (MONTAGNA, CHASE und LOBITZ, 1953; MONTAGNA, 1959 sowie YASUI und KAGE-MOTO, 1961), wohl aber, abgesehen von axillären apokrinen Schweißdrüsen, bei den Negern (MONTAGNA, 1964a). Kleine Glykogenmengen sind ebenfalls in den Glandulae ceruminales nachgewiesen worden (MONTAGNA, NOBACK und ZAK, 1948 sowie KAGA, 1956). Die ceruminalen Drüsen des Hundes enthalten kein Glykogen (KAGA, 1956). Die Drüsenzellen der Regio pubis scheinen insoweit eine Ausnahme

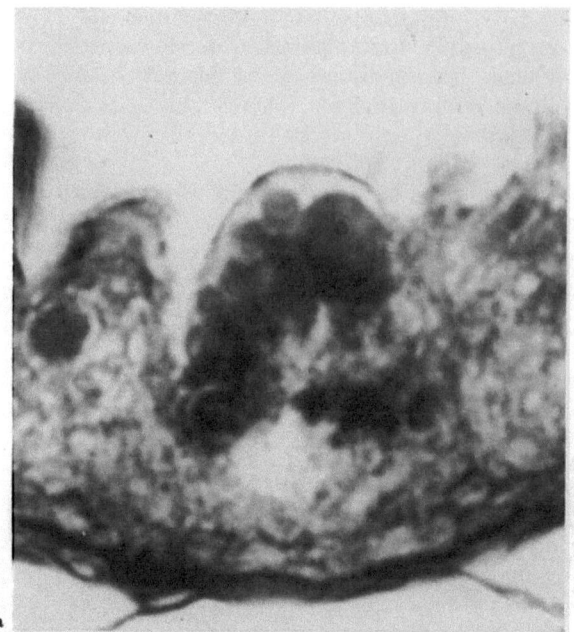

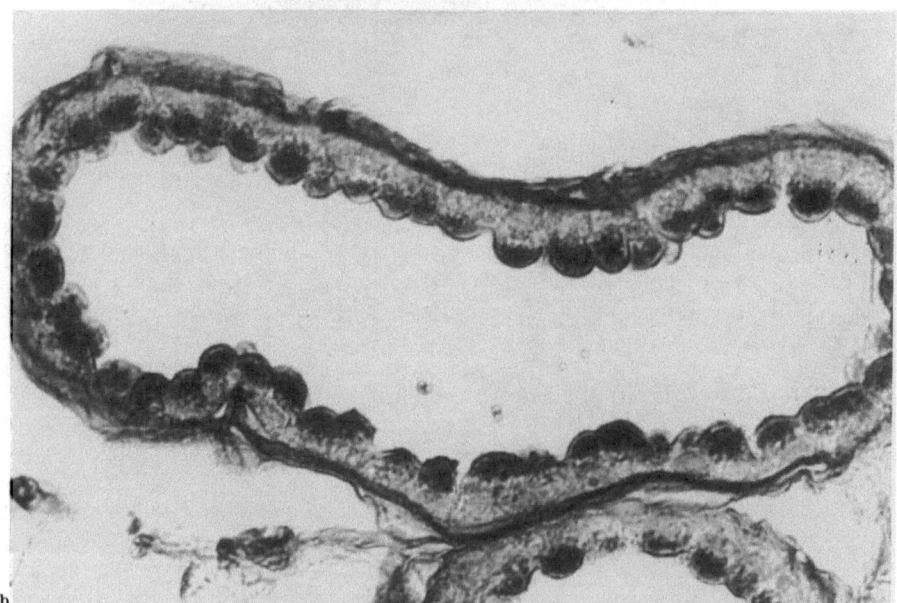

Abb. 33a u. b. Apokrine Schweißdrüsen. a Drüsenzelle mit PAS-reaktiven Granula. Deutliche Basalmembran. Paraffinschnitt. Hale-PAS-Reaktion. Vergr. 2300 ×. b PAS-reaktive Granula im apikalen Zellbereich. Paraffinschnitt. PAS-Reaktion

zu machen, als MONTAGNA, CHASE und HAMILTON (1951) in diesen basal wenige Glykogengranula gefunden haben. Nur in den Zellen der stark erweiterten sekretorischen Tubuli kann Glykogen in Spuren vorkommen (MONTAGNA, 1962; MONTAGNA und ELLIS, 1963). MONTES et al. (1960) berichten über die intracellulären Glykogengranula bei einem Fall nach der Menopause.

Luminaler Inhalt kann, obwohl selten, diskrete Glykogenkörnchen enthalten. Myoepithelzellen enthalten nur selten Glykogengranula.

Im Ausführungsgang sind die basalen, nicht dagegen die luminalen Zellen glykogenhaltig. Die Frage, weshalb im Gegensatz zu ekkrinen Schweißdrüsen apokrine Schweißdrüsen Glykogen als Reservestoff bei Erwachsenen im allgemeinen nicht enthalten, kann z.Z. nicht sicher beantwortet werden. Für die Bedeutung unterschiedlicher Funktionszustände könnte das Vorkommen von Glykogen bei Morbus Fox-Fordyce (auch verminderte Sekretionsleistung infolge Retention) sprechen (WINKELMANN und MONTGOMERY, 1956).

Diastase-resistente PAS-reaktive Substanzen. Sie können ebenfalls in apokrinen Schweißdrüsen in unterschiedlicher Form und Menge nachgewiesen werden. Nach MONTES et al. (1960) sind PAS-reaktive Diastase-resistente Granula oberhalb des Golgi-Apparates lokalisiert (Abb. 33), bei einer großen Anzahl auch basal und lateral von dem Kern. Die großen Pigmentgranula sind nach unseren Untersuchungen schwach reaktiv bzw. arreaktiv. Dieses PAS-reaktive, Diastase-resistente Material ist auch ein Anhaltspunkt für die Deutung dieser Gebilde als Lysosomen. Es ist nämlich bekannt, daß Leberlysosomen auch solche Substanzen enthalten (NOVIKOFF, 1961). MONTAGNA (1962) hat betont, daß die nicht pigmentierten Granula stark PAS-reaktiv und Diastase-resistent sind. Die Tatsache, daß der apikale Anteil des Cytoplasma, besonders aber die der Cuticula entsprechende Zone PAS-reaktiv ist — was mit unseren Untersuchungen übereinstimmt — aber keine Granula enthält, ist nach MONTAGNA (1962) so zu deuten, daß sich die Auflösung der reifen Granula in dem apikalen Cytoplasmaraum abspielt. Ausführliche Untersuchungen über Nicht-Glykogen-Polysaccharide haben auch FUSARO und GOLTZ (1961) durchgeführt, wie auch GOLTZ, FUSARO und JARVIS (1958) mit der Alcianblaureaktion *saure Mucopolysaccharide* in apokrinen Schweißdrüsen nachgewiesen haben.

Auch die Basalmembran der sekretorischen Abschnitte und die Cuticula in den Ausführungsgängen ist PAS-reaktiv und Diastase-resistent.

Über die chemische Natur des PAS-reaktiven Diastase-resistenten Materials kann eine nähere Aussage nicht gemacht werden. Wahrscheinlich handelt es sich um Polysaccharidproteinkomplexe (Näheres s. bei BRAUN-FALCO, 1961), teilweise wohl auch um PAS-reaktive Lipoproteide (MONTES et al., 1960).

V. Eisen

Eisen wird in den sekretorischen Epithelien apokriner Schweißdrüsen erst nach dem 11. (MONTAGNA, 1959) bzw. 12. Lebensjahr (YASUI und KAGEMOTO, 1961) nachweisbar (Abb. 34). HOMMA (1925) hat bei 13 von 16 untersuchten Fällen, d.h. in 81%, in gelben Granula eine positive Eisenreaktion nachgewiesen. HERZENBERG (1927) fand beim Manne in 40% der Fälle — und zwar auch in den gelben Granula — eine positive Eisenreaktion. Bei Frauen soll Eisen in Spuren, und zwar nur in der Schwangerschaft vorkommen. Zu ähnlichen Resultaten wie HOMMA (1925) kam auch RICHTER (1933), der die stärkste Reaktion zwischen dem 20. und 50. Lebensjahr fand. RICHTER (1933) meint, daß besonders in zylindrischen Drüsenzellen Eisen in großen Mengen vorkommt. Nach MANCA (1934) ist die Menge des Eisens in abgeplatteten Zellen klein, in zylindrischen aber wesentlich größer. Diese Resultate sind später auch von IWASHIGE (1951) bestätigt worden, der außerdem fand, daß Eisen intracellulär vor allem zwischen Golgi-Zone und sog. „cuticular border" im apikalen Zellbereich lokalisiert ist.

Auf eine Relation zwischen den sekretorischen Granula und Eisen hat bereits HOMMA (1925) hingewiesen, wobei er über Eisengehalt des Pigmentes schrieb,

Tabelle. *Histotopie von Enzymen des energieliefernden Stoffwechsels und angeschlossener*

Enzyme		PYASE	ALD	GAPDH	LDH	GDH	G-POX	ME	G-6-PDH
Apokrine Schweißdrüsen	Drüsenzellen apikal	0	2,5	3	4	2	2,5	2,5	3
	Drüsenzellen basal	0	2,5	3	4	2	2,5	2	3
	Myoepithelzellen	0—1	2,5	2—3	4	1,5—2	2	1,5	2
Ekkrine Schweißdrüsen	Schweißdrüsen-Endstücke	2,5	3	3	4	2,5	2—2,5	3	3

Intensität des Reaktionsausfalls: 0—4.

der von WAY und MEMMESHEIMER (1938) wohl für Hämosiderin gehalten wurde. BUNTING, WISLOCKI und DEMPSEY (1958) haben außer im Cytoplasma bei Anwendung der Berliner Blaureaktion Eisen in supranucleär liegenden Granula ge-

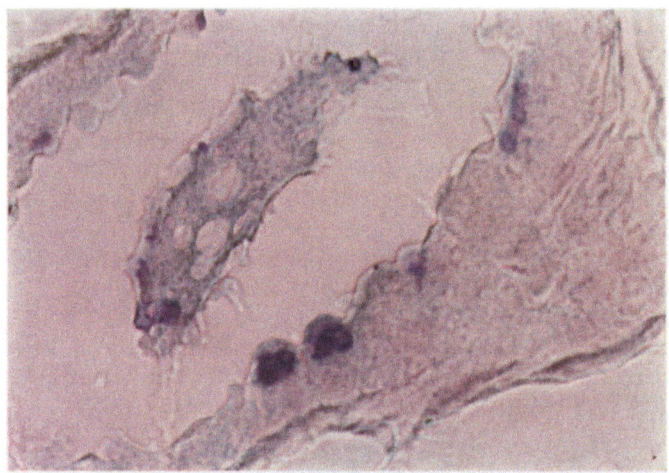

Abb. 34. Apokrine Schweißdrüse. Reichlich Eisen in Drüsenzellen. Berliner Blaureaktion. Mikroskopische Vergr. 256 ×

sehen. Diese Granula können manchmal auch die Größe eines Zellkernes einnehmen. Erst MONTAGNA, CHASE und LOBITZ (1953) sowie MONTAGNA (1962) haben eine genaue topische Zuordnung des anorganischen Eisens zu den Granula durchgeführt. Sie fanden, daß besonders die kleinen gelben Granula eisenhaltig sind. Die großen dunkelbraunen Granula enthalten es eventuell an der Peripherie. Diese Befunde stehen nicht in Einklang mit den Untersuchungen von ZORZOLI (1950), der keine registrierbare Relation zwischen Pigment und eisenhaltigen Granula nachweisen konnte.

Auch im Lumeninhalt ist von manchen Autoren Eisen nachgewiesen worden (MORIYAMA, 1927; NAGAMITSU, 1941; ZORZOLI, 1950; BUNTING et al., 1958; YASUI und KAGEMOTO, 1961; MUNGER, 1965b; eigene Befunde) (Abb. 34). Nach MONTAGNA (1962) ist im Lumen nur dann Eisen nachzuweisen, wenn Zellbestandteile vorhanden sind. Es ist bekannt, daß auch apokriner Schweiß Eisen enthalten kann (HURLEY und SHELLEY, 1960). Auch Achselhaare können Spuren von Eisen aufweisen (BUNTING et al., 1958). Außerdem hat sich schon RICHTER (1933) für

Stoffwechselwege im sekretorischen Abschnitt von apokrinen und ekkrinen Schweißdrüsen

6-PGDH	NAD-IDH	NADP-IDH	BDH	MDH	NADH-TR	NADPH-TR	CYASE	UBI	NAD-GLUDH	NADP-GLUDH	DHLDH
2,5	1,5	4	2,5	4	3	2	2,5	2,5	3	1,5	1
2,5	2	4	2,5	4	3	2,5	2,5	2,5	3	1,5	2,5
2,5	1,5	3—4	2	3—4	2,5	2	1	2	2	0—1	1
3	2	4	3	4	3	3—4	3	3	3	2	4

ein mindestens teilweises Übertreten des Eisens in das Sekret ausgesprochen. Es wurde behauptet, daß positive Eisenbefunde nur bei Personen mit Osmidrosis zu erhalten sind (IWASHIGE, 1951; YASUI und KAGEMOTO, 1961). Interessant ist die Feststellung (IWASHIGE, 1951), daß bei Japanern eine gewisse Parallelität zwischen der Intensität des Achselgeruches und Eisenreaktion bestehen soll. Mit hohem Alter werden nämlich der Achselgeruch sowie auch die Eisenreaktion schwächer. Die Drüsen in der Regio pubis und der Perianalregion sollen kein Eisen enthalten (MONTAGNA und ELLIS, 1959). Wir haben allerdings ebenfalls wie RICHTER (1933) anorganisches Eisen auch in apokrinen Schweißdrüsen in der Regio pubis finden können, allerdings nur in geringen Quantitäten.

Häufiger sind nicht alle, sondern nur vereinzelte Drüsenzellen, die das Lumen tapezieren, durch eine positive Eisenreaktion gekennzeichnet. RICHTER (1933) denkt dabei, daß Eisen vielleicht nur in bestimmten Phasen der Sekretbildung darstellbar ist. Elektronenmikroskopisch ist Eisen bzw. ein ferritinähnliches Material in unterschiedlichen Mengen in den dunklen Granula der apokrinen Schweißdrüsenzellen nachweisbar (MONTAGNA, 1962; RUPEC, 1966a u. b). Der Ausführungsgang ist frei von nachweisbaren Eisen.

Außer beim Menschen kann Eisen in kleinen Mengen auch bei erwachsenen Schimpansen vorkommen (MONTAGNA und ELLIS, 1963). Selten ist Eisen in den periglandulären Makrophagen beobachtet worden (MONTAGNA, 1964).

VI. Enzyme des energieliefernden Stoffwechsels

In diesem Abschnitt sollen die Enzyme des energieliefernden Stoffwechsels und der ihm angeschlossenen Stoffwechselwege besprochen werden. Unter dem Begriff „energieliefernder Stoffwechsel" werden Reaktionsfolgen zusammengefaßt, die durch schrittweise Oxydation der Substrate zu einem Gewinn chemischer Energie in Form energiereicher Phosphatverbindungen führen. Diese können direkt am Substrat (Substratphosphorylierung) oder nach Substratdehydrogenierung durch Oxydation des Wasserstoffes in der Atmungskette (Atmungskettenphosphorylierung) gewonnen werden. Glykolyse, Pentosephosphatcyclus, Citronensäurecyclus und Atmungskette stellen entsprechende Reaktionsfolgen dar, in welche der Katabolismus der Kohlenhydrate, Fette und Proteine einmündet (RASSNER, 1965)[1]. Über die histochemischen Reaktionsausfälle informiert die Tabelle.

---

[1] Der histochemische Nachweis der im folgenden besprochenen Enzyme erfolgte bei den eigenen Untersuchungen in der von BRAUN-FALCO und PETZOLDT (1965b) bzw. PETZOLDT und BRAUN-FALCO (1967) beschriebenen Technik.

1. Enzyme der Glykolyse

Phosphorylase (PYASE). Die Topie der histochemisch nachweisbaren Phosphorylaseaktivität beim Fetus stimmt weitgehend mit der des Glykogens überein (SERRI, MONTAGNA und MESCON, 1962). Auch später besteht gewisse Konkordanz zwischen histochemischem Nachweis des Glykogens und der Phosphorylase. Der sekretorische Teil ist nach Angaben der meisten Autoren areaktiv (Abb. 35) (ELLIS und MONTAGNA, 1958; YASUDA, FURUSAWA und OGATA, 1958; MONTAGNA, 1962). Bei Kindern, was wieder mit dem Glykogennachweis übereinstimmt, ist Phosphorylaseaktivität in den Drüsenzellen gefunden worden (MONTAGNA, 1959).

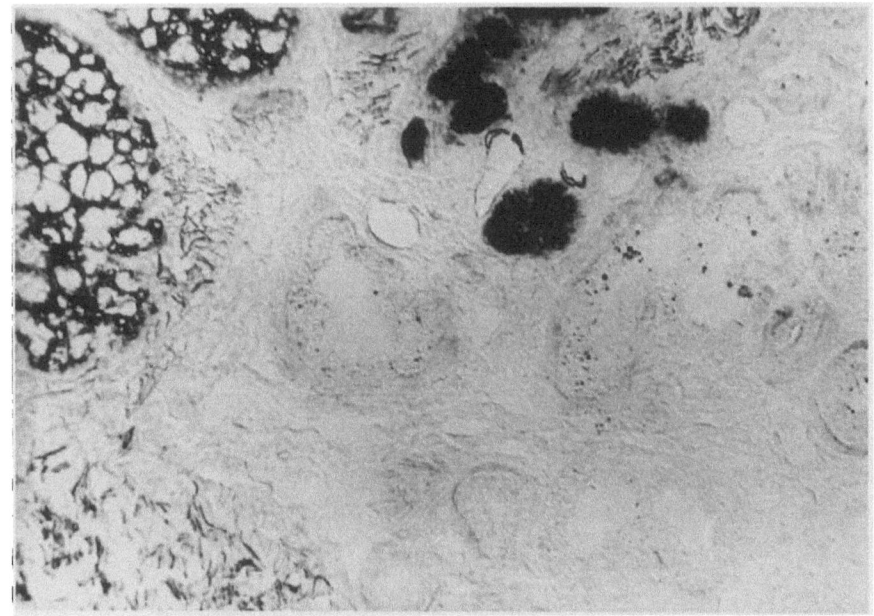

Abb. 35. Apokrine Schweißdrüse. Phosphorylaseaktivität ist in den Drüsenzellen (Mitte und rechts unten) nicht nachweisbar. Starke Phosphorylaseaktivität in ekkrinen Schweißdrüsen (rechts oben) und Talgdrüsen (links). Vergr. 112 ×

Interessant ist der Befund von YASUDA et al. (1963a), daß die Drüsen, die von Cholinesterase-enthaltenden Nervenfasern umgeben sind, auch über eine starke Phosphorylaseaktivität verfügen. Dieser Befund ist von phylogenetischem Interesse, da bei einigen Primaten (z.B. Nycticebus), wie MONTAGNA und ELLIS (1963) fanden, im sekretorischen Teil mäßige Phosphorylaseaktivitäten vorhanden waren. Andererseits sind Cholinesterase-haltige Nervenfasern bei Primaten oft gefunden worden (YASUDA, 1963). Man kann dabei mit einer gewissen Begründung an ein phylogenetisches Relikt denken (YASUDA et al., 1963a). Auch die sog. atypischen Zellen von YASUDA (1959) verfügen über Phosphorylaseaktivität. Die Zellen des Ausführungsganges sind ebenfalls im Gegensatz zu denjenigen des sekretorischen Abschnittes reaktiv (ELLIS und MONTAGNA, 1958; MONTAGNA 1962).

Die Myoepithelzellen verfügen über geringgradige Aktivität.

Vom Stoffwechsel her gesehen ist der Befund einer histochemisch praktisch fehlenden Phosphorylaseaktivität in den Zellen der sekretorischen Drüsenabschnitte — übrigens ebenfalls ein Fehlen des „branching enzyme" (ELLIS und MONTAGNA, 1958) — insofern von Interesse, als es die morphologische Grundlage für das Verständnis liefert, daß auch Glykogen in den Drüsenzellen des sekretorischen Abschnittes bei Erwachsenen praktisch nicht vorkommt. Aus beiden Befunden, die in einem deutlichen Gegensatz zu denjenigen bei ekkrinen Schweißdrüsen stehen und auf grundlegende Unterschiede zwischen diesen beiden Drüsen hinweisen, kann man auch vermuten, daß die apokrinen Schweißdrüsen zum einen eine mehr gleichmäßige sekretorische Tätigkeit aufweisen und zum andern so günstig mit Metaboliten versorgt werden, daß eine Energiespeicherung in Form von Glykogen offenbar nicht notwendig ist.

Aldolase (ALD). Die histochemisch nachweisbare, cytoplasmatisch lokalisierte Aldolaseaktivität (Abb. 36) ist nach eigenen Untersuchungen im ganzen als mäßig anzusprechen. Auffällig erscheint, daß in allen Zellen der apokrinen Schweiß-

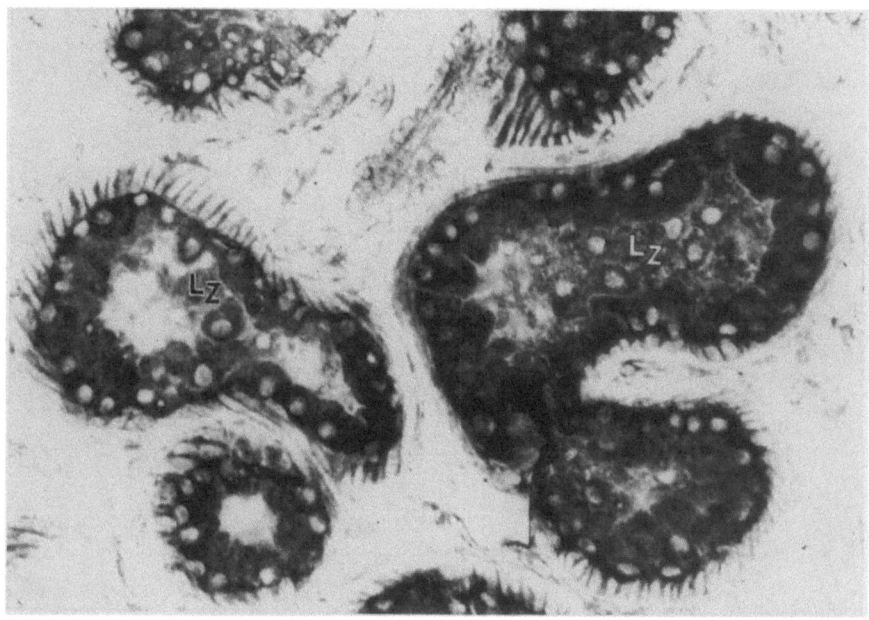

Abb. 36. Apokrine Schweißdrüse. Aldolase. Gut nachweisbare cytoplasmatische Aldolaseaktivität in den cytoplasmatischen Bereichen von Drüsenzellen und Myoepithelzellen. Deutliche Enzymaktivität auch des cellulären und nichtcellulären Lumeninhaltes (*Lz*). Kryostatschnitt. Vergr. 250 ×

drüsen, d.h. sowohl im sekretorischen Abschnitt wie auch im Ausführungsgang, dieses Enzym in etwas größerer Aktivität als in der Epidermis nachweisbar ist. Im sekretorischen Abschnitt fällt die Reaktion auf Aldolase im basalen Bereich der Drüsenzellen etwas stärker aus. Auch Myoepithelzellen scheinen über Aldolaseaktivität zu verfügen. Bemerkenswert ist schließlich, daß auch bereits im Lumen befindliche noch mehr oder wenig gut erhaltene Zellen histochemisch nachweisbare Enzymaktivitäten aufweisen.

Glycerinaldehyd-3-Phosphat-Dehydrogenase (GAPDH). Das für die Embden-Meyerhof-Kette repräsentative und wie die anderen Enzyme der Glykolyse extramitochondrial lokalisierte Enzym GAPDH kommt in apokrinen Schweißdrüsen histochemisch in etwa gleich hoher Aktivität vor wie in der Epidermis und in geringerer Aktivität als in ekkrinen Schweißdrüsen. In allen Drüsenzellen kann GAPDH stets in gleich starker Aktivität nachgewiesen werden (HASHIMOTO, 1961). In den Myoepithelzellen ist der histochemische Reaktionsausfall etwas geringer als in den Drüsenzellen. Da GAPDH in einer festliegenden Proportionskonstanz (PETTE und BÜCHER, 1963) mit anderen Enzymen der Embden-Meyerhof-Kette steht, darf man annehmen, daß der intensive histochemische Reaktionsausfall als

Zeichen einer ausgeprägten glykolytischen Aktivität gewertet werden kann, an deren Ende die Milchsäurebildung steht. In diesem Sinne spricht auch die histochemisch faßbare, viel stärkere Aktivität von Lactat-Dehydrogenase.

Lactat-Dehydrogenase (LDH). Dieses extramitochondriale Enzym, das für die Oxydierung der Milchsäure verantwortlich ist, kommt in den apokrinen Schweißdrüsenzellen in sehr hoher Aktivität vor (Abb. 37). Der intensive Reaktionsausfall ist vergleichsweise viel stärker als in Epidermiszellen und im Gegensatz zu Hashimoto (1961) selbst noch stärker als in den Zellen ekkriner Schweißdrüsenendstücke. Eine genaue intracelluläre Zuordnung ist, wie übrigens auch bei den

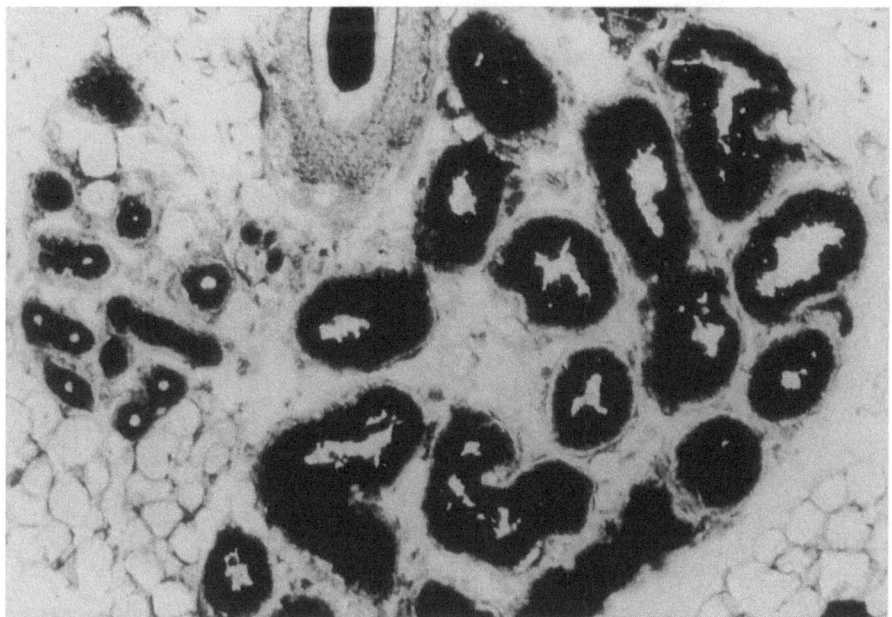

Abb. 37. Apokrine Schweißdrüse. Lactat-Dehydrogenase. Sehr starke LDH-Aktivität in apokrinen und ekkrinen (links) Schweißdrüsen. Kryostatschnitt. Vergr. 224 ×

anderen Dehydrogenasen, nicht möglich. Lediglich die Zellkerne erscheinen frei von Enzymaktivitäten. Die hohe LDH-Aktivität in den Drüsenzellen apokriner Schweißdrüsen ist ebenfalls als Zeichen einer hohen glykolytischen Aktivität dieser Zellen zu werten.

2. Glycerin-1-Phosphat-Dehydrogenase (GDH) und Glycerin-1-Phosphat-Oxydase (GPOX)

Die extramitochondriale **Glycerin-1-Phosphat-Dehydrogenase (GDH)** kann als ein Verbindungsenzym zwischen Glykolyse und Fettstoffwechsel angesehen werden. Auf histologischer Ebene ist ihre Aktivität in den apokrinen Schweißdrüsen im ganzen stärker als in der Epidermis, auf der anderen Seite etwas geringer als in ekkrinen Schweißdrüsen. Sowohl in den Drüsenzellen wie auch in den Zellen des Ausführungsganges findet sich ein deutlicher, mäßig starker cytoplasmatischer Reaktionsausfall. Die Myoepithelzellen besitzen anscheinend eine geringere Aktivität.

Bemerkenswerterweise finden wir im Lumen von apokrinen Schweißdrüsen keine histochemisch nachweisbare GDH-Aktivität. Man muß die GDH-Aktivität in apokrinen Schweißdrüsen als dahingehend interpretieren, daß diese Zellen auch zu aktiven Syntheseleistungen im Fettstoffwechsel fähig sind.

Die mitochondriale **Glycerin-1-Phosphat-Oxydase** (GPOX) (Meyerhof-Green-Enzym) (histochemischer Nachweis nach PETTE und BRANDAU, 1966) ist in apokrinen Schweißdrüsen etwa in gleich starker Aktivität wie die Glycerin-1-Phosphat-Dehydrogenase (GDH) nachweisbar. Die Drüsenzellen verhalten sich in gleicher Weise mäßig stark positiv, im ganzen etwa gleich stark wie die Zellen der ekkrinen Schweißdrüsenendstücke. Auffällig ist auch hier, daß die Myoepithelzellen etwas stärker positiv reagieren.

Als extramitochondriales Enzym steht die NAD-spezifische GDH in einer metabolischen mitochondrial-extramitochondrialen Wechselwirkung mit der mitochondrialen GPOX im sog. Glycerin-1-Phosphatcyclus (Näheres dazu s. bei BRANDAU und PETTE, 1966). Es ist interessant, daß beide Enzyme histochemisch in etwa gleich starker Aktivität in apokrinen Schweißdrüsen nachweisbar sind.

3. Malic Enzyme (ME)

Das NADP-spezifische extramitochondriale Malatenzym wird im allgemeinen einer Reaktionsfolge zugeordnet, welche eine Umgehung der energetisch ungünstigen Reaktion Pyruvat-Phosphoenolpyruvat darstellt, wobei über Oxalacetat auch Beziehungen zum Citratcyclus und dem Aminosäurestoffwechsel gegeben sind. So wurde die mögliche Bedeutung des ME als eines „extramitochondrialen Hilfsenzyms" des Citronensäurecyclus ventiliert (PETTE, 1965). Es ist bemerkenswert, daß dieses Enzym in apokrinen Schweißdrüsen in etwa gleich starker histochemisch feststellbarer Aktivität wie GAPDH vorkommt. Die cytoplasmatische Gesamtaktivität ist etwa gleich groß wie die der ekkrinen Schweißdrüsen (HASHIMOTO, 1961) und nach eigenen Untersuchungen geringfügig höher als in der Epidermis.

4. Enzyme des Pentosephosphatcyclus

Glucose-6-Phosphat-Dehydrogenase (G-6-PDH) und **6-Phosphat-Gluconat-Dehydrogenase** (6-PGDH).

Diese beiden Enzyme leiten den Pentosephosphatcyclus ein. Aus ihrem Vorkommen in apokrinen Schweißdrüsen kann mit großer Wahrscheinlichkeit auf den Ablauf dieses Cyclus geschlossen werden, auch wenn der Nachweis der übrigen Enzyme noch aussteht.

Die G-6-PDH liefert in apokrinen Schweißdrüsen eine stark positive Reaktion, etwa gleich stark wie in ekkrinen Schweißdrüsen, etwas stärker als in der Epidermis. Vergleichbare Resultate erhielt auch HASHIMOTO (1965). Alle Zellen apokriner Schweißdrüsen reagieren intensiv positiv in ihrem Cytoplasma. Der Reaktionsausfall in den Ausführungsgängen und Myoepithelzellen ist etwas schwächer als in den Drüsenzellen. G-6-PDH konnte innerhalb von im Lumen gelegener Zellanteile nicht sicher histochemisch nachgewiesen werden.

6-PGDH ist histochemisch ebenfalls in mäßig starker Aktivität nachweisbar. Im ganzen erscheint die Aktivität — in Übereinstimmung mit HASHIMOTO (1961) — etwas geringer als die der G-6-PDH.

Aus dem Vorkommen dieser Enzyme läßt sich entnehmen, daß in den Zellen der apokrinen Schweißdrüsen nicht nur Pentosen für andere Synthesen (z.B. Nucleinsäuren) bereitgestellt werden, sondern vor allen Dingen der hier gewonnene Wasserstoff von dem NADP-System übernommen wird und in dieser Form für

Synthesen (z. B. Lipidsynthese) zur Verfügung steht (s. dazu auch RASSNER, 1965). Die beachtlichen, histochemisch nachweisbaren Aktivitäten der beiden Enzyme sind ein indirekter Hinweis dafür, daß derartige synthetische Prozesse in den Zellen apokriner Schweißdrüsen eine wesentliche Rolle spielen. Dafür spricht übrigens auch die sehr hohe Aktivität der NADP-abhängigen Isocitronensäure-Dehydrogenase, welche ebenfalls z.T. cytoplasmatisch lokalisiert ist und Wasserstoff für das NADP-System liefert.

5. Enzyme des Citronensäurecyclus

Die Enzyme des Citronensäurecyclus sind zum größten Teil an Mitochondrien gebunden. Einige, wie MDH und NADP-IDH kommen auch cytoplasmatisch vor und haben als solche wahrscheinlich besondere Funktionen (s. auch bei PETTE und BRANDAU, BRANDAU und PETTE, 1966). Die Aktivität histochemisch nachweisbarer Enzyme des Citronensäurecyclus ist, soweit diese nur rein mitochondrial gebunden sind, etwas schwächer als in ekkrinen Schweißdrüsen, aber stärker als in der Epidermis.

NAD-Isocitrat-Dehydrogenase (NAD-IDH)

Sie kommt in apokrinen Schweißdrüsen histochemisch nur in mäßig starker Intensität vor. Eine sichere mitochondriale Zuordnung ist lichtmikroskopisch nicht möglich. Myoepithelzellen und Ausführungsgang reagieren schwächer (HASHIMOTO, 1961).

NADP-Isocitrat-Dehydrogenase (NADP-IDH)

Im Gegensatz zu der relativ schwachen NAD-IDH-Aktivität und im Gegensatz zu den Ergebnissen von HASHIMOTO (1961) steht nach eigenen Untersuchungen (Abb. 38) die sehr starke NADP-IDH-Aktivität in den apokrinen Schweißdrüsen. Diese ist vergleichsweise genauso stark wie in ekkrinen Schweißdrüsen und deutlich stärker als in der Epidermis. Es ist wahrscheinlich, daß zumindestens ein Teil dieses Enzyms nicht mitochondrial, sondern cytoplasmatisch lokalisiert ist und bei der Bereitstellung von Wasserstoff eine wichtige Rolle spielt.

Bernsteinsäure-Dehydrogenase (BDH)

BDH ist in apokrinen Schweißdrüsen nur relativ mäßig stark histochemisch nachweisbar. Die Myoepithelzellen sollen nach MONTAGNA (1962) stets areaktiv sein. Wir konnten indessen, ebenso wie HASHIMOTO (1961), auch in diesen Zellen deutlich mitochondriale BDH histochemisch nachweisen. Die Zellen der Ausführungsgänge sind oft stärker positiv als die Drüsenzellen.

Malat-Dehydrogenase (MDH)

MDH gehört ebenfalls zu den zweiörtigen Enzymen (PETTE und LUH, 1962), welche sowohl mitochondrial als auch cytoplasmatisch lokalisiert sind. Dieses Enzym gehört, wie auch die ebenfalls zweiörtige NADP-IDH zu denjenigen Enzymen, welche in apokrinen Schweißdrüsen durch eine sehr stark positive Reaktion charakterisiert sind (Abb. 39). Die Intensität des Reaktionsausfalles ist so groß, daß sich eine genaue intracelluläre Zuordnung nicht durchführen läßt. Lediglich die Zellkerne bleiben durch das negative Verhalten eindrucksvoll ausgespart.

Zusammenfassend ist zu sagen, daß die bisher vorliegenden histochemischen Untersuchungen über das Verhalten von Enzymen des Citronensäurecyclus dafür

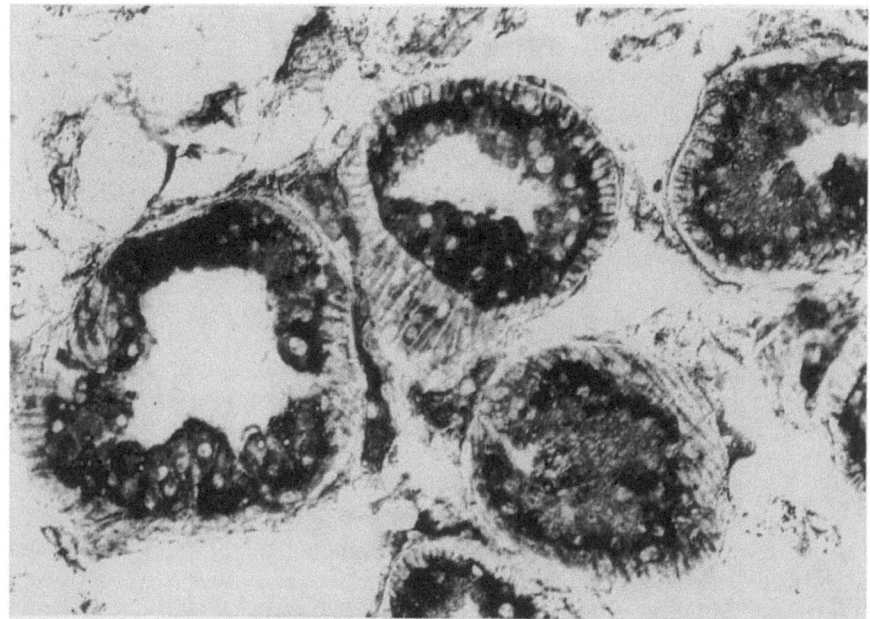

Abb. 38. Apokrine Schweißdrüse. NADP-abhängige Isocitrat-Dehydrogenase. Unterschiedlich starke Enzymaktivität in den Drüsenepithelien, besonders stark positive Reaktionen in den basalen Zellbereichen. Kerne reaktionslos. Myoepithelien mäßig positiv. Kryostatschnitt. Vergr. 224 ×

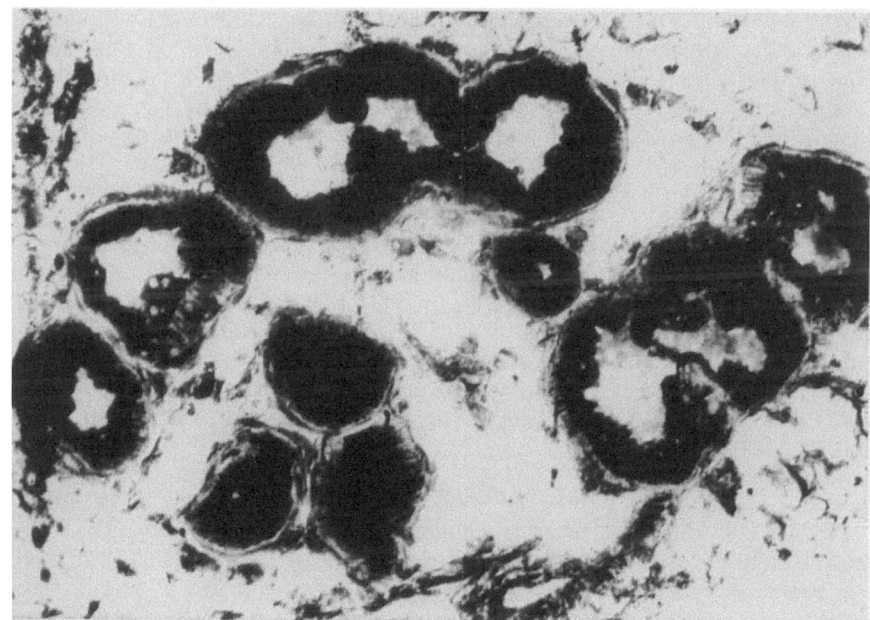

Abb. 39. Apokrine Schweißdrüse. Malat-Dehydrogenase. Sehr starker Reaktionsausfall in den sekretorischen Drüsenabschnitten und in den Myoepithelzellen. Kryostatschnitt. Vergr. 140 ×

sprechen, daß dieser auch in den Zellen, und vor allem in den Drüsenzellen apokriner Schweißdrüsen abläuft. Da die histochemisch faßbaren Aktivitäten von MDH und NADP-IDH wegen ihrer Zweiörtigkeit keine Rückschlüsse auf den mitochondrial auflaufenden Citronensäurecyclus zulassen, muß man auf der Basis der histochemischen Reaktionen für NADH-IDH und BDH annehmen, daß der Citratcyclus nicht sehr hoch dimensioniert ist.

Vielleicht spricht in diesem Sinne auch die Tatsache, daß ultrastrukturell normal aussehende Mitochondrien besonders in Drüsenzellen in recht unterschiedlicher Zahl vorkommen. Zumindest ergibt sich aus dem Vergleich der histochemisch faßbaren Aktivitäten der Enzyme des Citronensäurecyclus und der Glykolyse, daß die Drüsenzellen apokriner Schweißdrüsen den Energiebedarf für synthetisierende Zelleistungen offenbar mehr auf glykolytischem Wege zu gewinnen scheinen (s. auch RASSNER, 1965).

6. Enzyme der Atmungskette

Die Atmungskette ist bekanntlich der Hauptlieferant von energiereichem Adenosintriphosphat (ATP). Die verschiedenen mitochondrial gebundenen Enzyme sind histochemisch nur teilweise darstellbar.

NADH-Tetrazoliumsalzreductase (NADH-TR) und NADPH-Tetrazoliumsalzreductase (NADPH-TR)

Beide Enzyme (Näheres dazu s. BRAUN-FALCO und PETZOLDT, 1964 und 1965) sind in starker Aktivität histochemisch in apokrinen Schweißdrüsen nachweisbar (HASHIMOTO, 1961). Im ganzen ist der Reaktionsausfall auf NADH-TR intensiver als auf NADPH-TR (Abb. 40 und 41). Beide Enzyme entsprechen hinsichtlich ihrer histochemisch faßbaren Aktivitäten dem Verhalten ekkriner Schweißdrüsen. Nach BIEMPICA und MONTES (1965) sind besonders die basalen Partien der Drüsenzellen durch den histochemischen Reaktionsausfall charakterisiert, was auch mit der Topik der Mitochondrien weitgehend übereinstimmen würde. Wir fanden aber keine wesentlichen Unterschiede in der intracellulären Verteilung der Enzymanzeigenden Präcipitate, welche das Cytoplasma der Drüsenzellen massiv ausfüllen. Auch Myoepithelzellen und die Zellen der Ausführungsgänge reagieren relativ stark positiv.

Cytochromoxydase (CYASE)

Die Topie dieses mitochondrial lokalisierten Enzyms ist von MONTAGNA und YUN (1961) sowie MONTAGNA und ELLIS (1963) untersucht worden. Die Drüsenzellen sind regelmäßig sehr stark reaktiv, und zwar ist die Reaktivität gleichmäßig stark, abgesehen von der Drüsenzellenhöhe (MONTAGNA, 1962). Der Ausführungsgang ist mäßig reaktiv. Die Myoepithelzellen sind areaktiv (MONTAGNA und YUN, 1961). Wir konnten diese Befunde weitgehend bestätigen, allerdings auch in Myoepithelzellen CYASE nachweisen (zur Cytochromoxydase der Haut s. auch BRAUN-FALCO, 1961b).

Anhang: Ubichinon (UBI)

Obwohl Ubichinon kein Enzym, sondern ein ubiquitär vorkommendes Chinon darstellt, kommt diesem doch aller Wahrscheinlichkeit nach in der Atmungskette beim Elektronentransport eine wichtige Funktion zu (Näheres s. BRAUN-FALCO und PETZOLDT, 1966 und 1967). Es ist an Lipoproteine besonders der Mitochondrienmembran gebunden. Ubichinon läßt sich histochemisch in apokrinen Schweißdrüsen in mäßig starker Aktivität cytoplasmatisch nachweisen (Abb. 42). Eine genaue Zuordnung ist nicht möglich. Auch in Myoepithelzellen und den Zellen der Ausführungsgänge kommt es vor.

Zusammenfassend läßt sich sagen, daß auch Enzyme der Atmungskette in apokrinen Schweißdrüsen histochemisch nachgewiesen werden können. Ihre Akti-

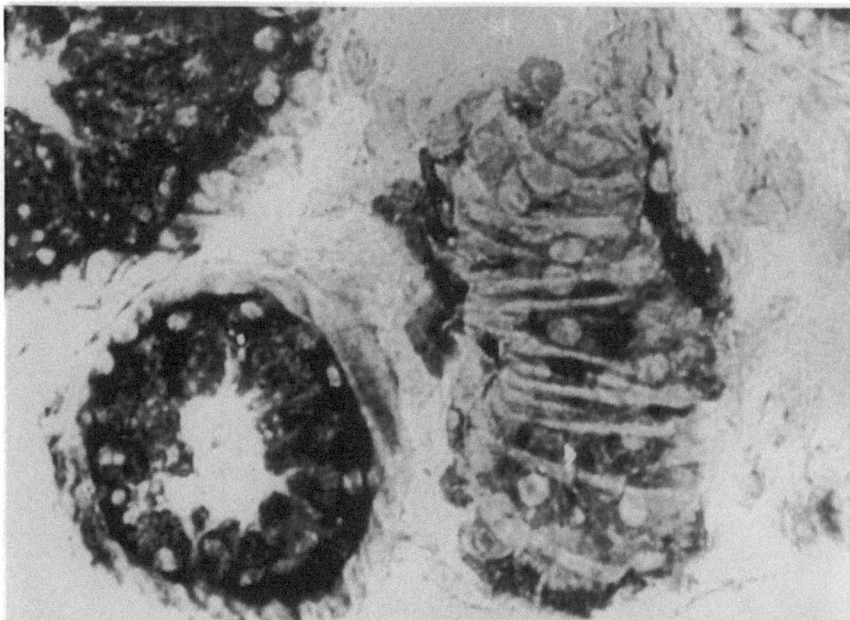

Abb. 40

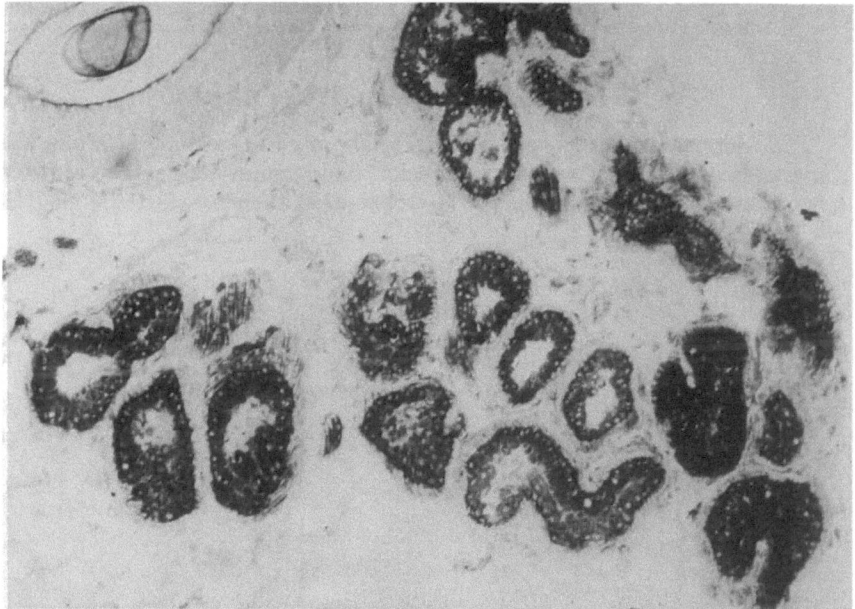

Abb. 41

Abb. 40. Apokrine Schweißdrüse. NADH-Tetrazoliumsalzreductase. Deutliche Enzymaktivität in den Drüsenzellen und den tangential getroffenen Myoepithelzellen (rechts). Kryostatschnitt. Vergr. 224 ×

Abb. 41. Apokrine Schweißdrüse. NADPH-Tetrazoliumsalzreductase. Deutliche, allerdings stellenweise unterschiedlich intensive Enzymaktivität in den Drüsenzellen und im Drüsenlumen. Kerne reaktionslos. Kryostatschnitt Vergr. 88 ×

vität ist histochemischen Befunden zufolge deutlich stärker als die von Enzymen des Citronensäurecyclus. Dies könnte darauf hindeuten, daß auch aus anderen Quellen der Atmungskette Wasserstoff zur Dehydrierung und damit zur Energiegewinnung zugeführt wird.

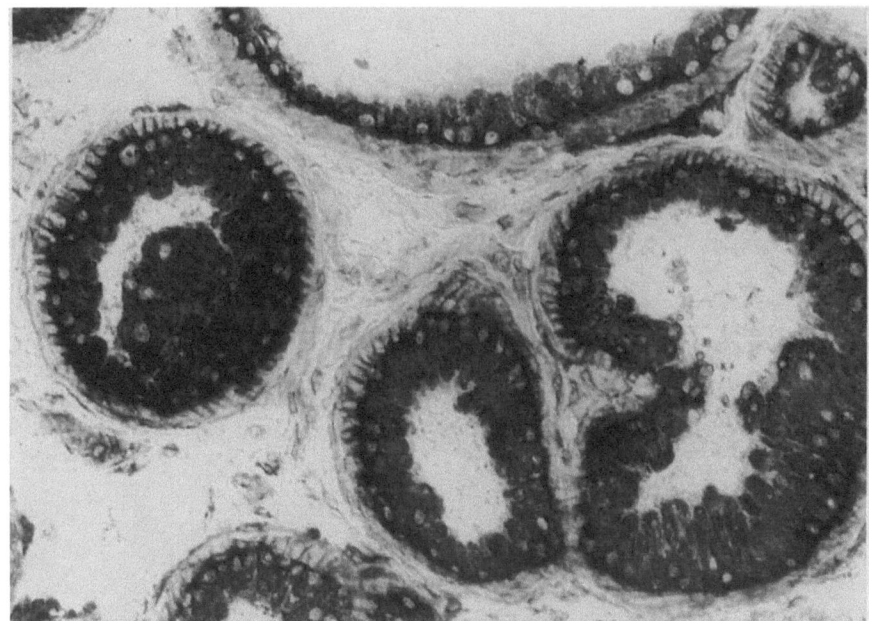

Abb. 42. Apokrine Schweißdrüse. Ubichinon. Relativ gleichmäßig starke cytoplasmatische Lokalisation von Ubichinon in den Drüsenzellen und in den Myoepithelzellen. Kryostatschnitt. Vergr. 250 ×

VII. Weitere Dehydrogenasen

Die **Glutamatdehydrogenase** (GluDH) kann als Enzym innerhalb des Verbindungsweges zwischen Citronensäurecyclus und Aminosäuremetabolismus angesehen werden. Dabei scheint der GluDH im wesentlichen eine Rolle im Rahmen

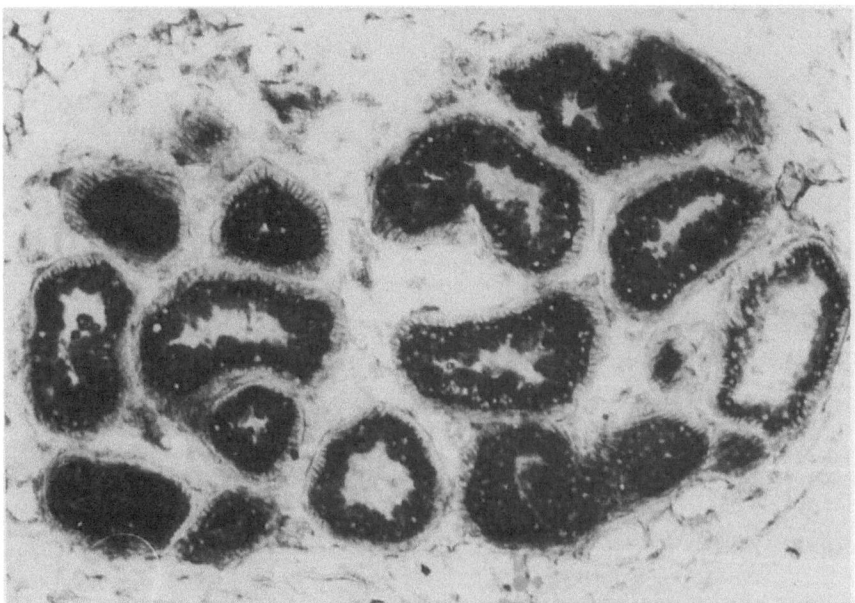

Abb. 43. Apokrine Schweißdrüse. NAD-abhängige Glutamat-Dehydrogenase. Intensive Enzymaktivität in den Drüsenepithelien auch innerhalb des Drüsenlumens. Kerne reaktionslos. Kryostatschnitt. Vergr. 110 ×

der oxydativen Desaminierung zuzukommen, was besagt, daß dieses Enzym mehr als abbauendes Enzym betrachtet werden kann, welches gleichzeitig Wasserstoff auf NAD oder NADP überträgt. Auffällig ist daher, daß die histochemischen Aktivitäten der NAD-GluDH wesentlich stärker sind als der relativ schwache Reaktionsausfall der NADP-GluDH (Abb. 43). Vergleichsweise zeichnen sich ekkrine Schweißdrüsen durch eine etwas stärkere Enzymaktivität aus. Eine nähere funktionelle Deutung lassen die histochemischen Untersuchungsergebnisse über dieses mitochondrial lokalisierte Enzym bisher nicht zu. Für Synthesevorgänge kann die Bereitstellung von NADPH bedeutsam sein.

Die Aktivität der **Dihydroliponsäure-Dehydrogenase** (DHLDH) kann im ganzen als sehr gering bezeichnet werden. In allen Zellen apokriner Schweißdrüsen läßt sich in etwa gleich starker Aktivität dieses Enzym nachweisen. In den Drüsenzellen findet man vor allem in den basalen Abschnitten stärkere Reaktionen.

VIII. Monoaminooxydase (MOA)

MOA ist ein Enzym, welches Noradrenalin bzw. Adrenalin zu oxydieren und damit zu inaktivieren vermag. Dies geschieht hauptsächlich innerhalb adrenergischer Nervenfasern (Näheres dazu s. auch bei STÜTTGEN, 1965). MOA kommt auch in apokrinen Schweißdrüsen vor. Bereits von SHELLEY, COHEN und KOELLE (1955) wurde MOA-Aktivität in den Drüsenzellen histochemisch festgestellt. Die exakte Histotopie wurde von YASUDA und MONTAGNA (1960) beschrieben. Die stärkste Reaktivität findet sich in den zylindrischen Drüsenzellen apikal sowie supra- und juxtanuclear, eine schwächere basal. In kubischen Zellen dagegen ist die Reaktivität in basalen Abschnitten der Zelle stärker als in apikalen. Golgi-Apparat, Kern und Granula sind frei von MOA-Aktivitäten.

Sehr schwache Enzymaktivität besteht in Myoepithelzellen. Die Zellen des Ausführungsganges sind stark reaktiv.

IX. Hydrolytische Enzyme

In apokrinen Schweißdrüsen wurden verschiedene hydrolytische Enzyme nachgewiesen.

1. Esterasen

Folgt man einem Einteilungsprinzip von GOMORI (1952), so kann man diese Enzymgruppe in die Cholinesterasen und Aliesterasen einteilen. Die Untergruppe der Cholinesterasen umfaßt die Acetylcholinesterase und die unspezifischen Cholinesterasen, die Untergruppe der Aliesterasen die unspezifischen Esterasen und die Lipasen.

a) Cholinesterasen

Acetylcholinesterase kommt in cholinergischen (aber auch in motorischen und sensorischen) Nervenfasern vor und ist auch in den Nerven um apokrine Schweißdrüsen histochemisch nachweisbar (YASUDA, SUZUKI und MACHIDA, 1963). Es ist allerdings beachtenswert, daß von einer Reihe von Autoren spezifische Cholinesterase nicht festgestellt werden konnte (HURLEY, SHELLEY und KOELLE, 1953; HELLMANN, 1955; MONTAGNA und ELLIS, 1959).

Auch der Nachweis von **unspezifischen Cholinesterasen** ist meistens nicht gelungen, auch wir selbst konnten Butyrylcholinesterase in Nerven um apokrine Schweißdrüsen nicht feststellen. Die Histotopie dieses Enzyms findet sich in dem Kapitel über die Innervation besprochen.

b) Aliesterasen

Unspezifische Esterasen, welche Ester kurzkettiger Fettsäuren (bis C_4) mit einfachen Alkoholen hydrolysieren, kommen in apokrinen Schweißdrüsen in starker Aktivität vor (MONTAGNA und ELLIS, 1963). In den Drüsenzellen ist die Aktivität intensiver als in den Zellen des Ausführungsganges. Gewöhnlich sind die Reaktionsausfälle in den Drüsenzellen so intensiv, daß eine nähere strukturelle Zuordnung nicht möglich ist, da die Zellen voll gefüllt sind mit Enzymaktivität anzeigenden Granula. Die Myoepithelzellen enthalten nach unseren Untersuchungen praktisch keine unspezifische Esterasenaktivität. Die funktionelle Bedeu-

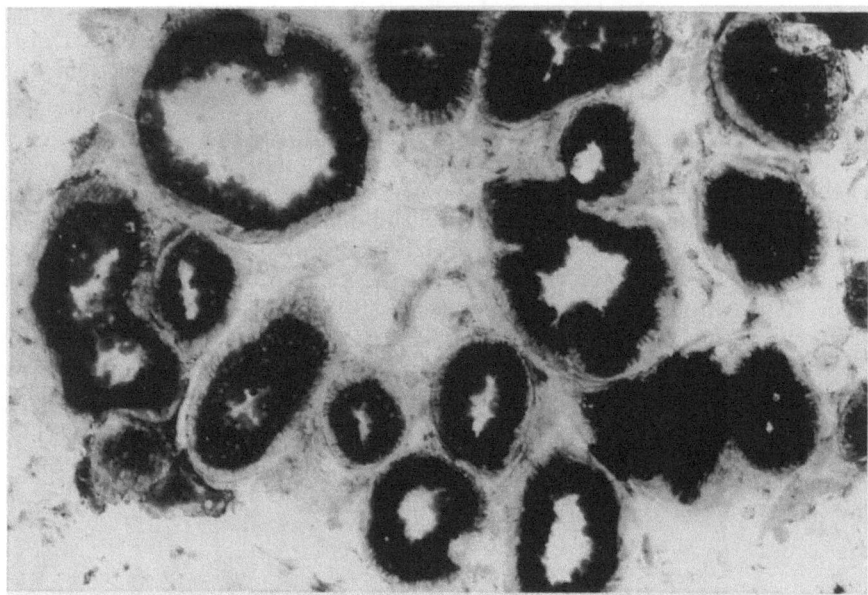

Abb. 44. Apokrine Schweißdrüsen. Unspezifische Esterasen. Intensiver cytoplasmatischer Reaktionsausfall in den Drüsenzellen und in den Myoepithelzellen. Kryostatschnitt. Vergr. 110 ×

tung dieser hohen Enzymaktivität ist bisher noch nicht klar. Man kann vermuten, daß sie im Zusammenhang mit den lysosomalen Aktivitäten steht.

Lipasen wurden von MONTAGNA (1962) in Form von Tweenesterasen in großer Aktivität innerhalb apokriner Schweißdrüsen nachgewiesen.

2. Phosphomonoesterasen

Bezüglich der Histochemie von Phosphomonoesterasen sei auf KOPF (1957) und BRAUN-FALCO (1961a) verwiesen. Im wesentlichen unterscheidet man unter den beiden klassischen Phosphomonoesterasen die alkalische Phosphatase (aPh) und die saure Phosphatase (sPh). Beide besitzen nur eine geringe Substratspezifität, wie besonders die Untersuchungen von SPIER und MARTIN (1956) gezeigt haben.

Saure Phosphatasen (sPh)

SERRI, HUBER und MESCON (1962) haben fetale apokrine Schweißdrüsen untersucht und in den Zellen des sekretorischen Abschnittes eine stärkere saure Phosphataseaktivität als in den Zellen des Ausführungsganges gefunden. Im Kindesalter sind die Drüsenzellen nur schwach reaktiv (YASUI, 1960b). Am stärksten scheinen die Aktivitäten im Pubertätsalter (15) Jahre) zu sein. Im Erwachsenenalter (25 Jahre) kommt es zu einer Verminderung der sPh.

Der Lumeninhalt ist stets frei von Enzymaktivität. MONTAGNA (1962) sowie MONTAGNA und ELLIS (1963) fanden in den Drüsenzellen apikal eine mäßige saure Phosphataseaktivität. Die Zellen des Ausführungsganges sind nur schwach reaktiv. Auf eine besonders starke Reaktion in den großen Granula der Drüsenzellen haben HASHIMOTO, GROSS und LEVER (1966b) hingewiesen. Eine positive Reaktion in dunklen Granula der Ceruminaldrüsen hat auch KAWABATA (1964) lichtmikroskopisch beobachten können. Dagegen ist es BUNTING, WISLOCKI und DEMPSEY (1948) nicht gelungen, sPh in apokrinen Schweißdrüsen nachzuweisen. Es wurden manchmal starke Enzymaktivitäten in Zellkernen beschrieben (z.B. TAKAMURA, 1958; YASUI, 1960b), die wohl als Artefakte zu interpretieren sind. KAGA (1956) fand keine nucleare Aktivität. (Zur Frage der sog. nucleären Aktivitäten der sPh s. auch PEARSE, 1961; sowie GOLDFISCHER, ESSNER und NOVIKOFF, 1964). In der jüngsten Zeit haben BIEMPICA und MONTES (1965) mit der Gomori-Methode lichtmikroskopisch (dazu Abb. 24) Lysosomen in der Golgi-Zone und apikal nachgewiesen. Diese Autoren sowie RUPEC (1966b) haben die Topik dieses Enzyms auch auf ultrastruktureller Ebene untersucht. Es ist sehr wahrscheinlich, daß die dunklen Granula elektronenmikroskopisch-cytochemisch Lipofuscin-enthaltende Lysosomen (alterierte Lysosomen) sind. Hier ist zu betonen, daß SHELLEY und HURLEY (1954) aufgrund ihrer Untersuchungen bei Chromidrosis sowie aufgrund ihrer Untersuchungen der normalen apokrinen Schweißdrüsen zu dem Schluß gekommen sind, daß die Pigmentgranula bei normalen, besonders aber bei chromidrotischen apokrinen Drüsen einem Lipopigment, und zwar dem Lipofuscin, entsprechen. Elektronenmikroskopisch-cytochemisch sind diese Befunde auch bestätigt worden (RUPEC, 1966b).

Alkalische Phosphatasen (aPh)

In den Anlagen apokriner Schweißdrüsen ist aPh histochemisch nicht nachweisbar. Erst wenn es zur Ausdifferenzierung des sekretorischen Abschnittes kommt, ist im Zentrum des entsprechenden Zellstranges eine sehr starke intracelluläre alkalische Phosphataseaktivtät festzustellen. Im Laufe der intrauterinen Entwicklung werden die Aktivitäten immer geringer. Bei einem 8 Monate alten Fetus hat YASUI (1960b) eine positive Reaktion nur noch in dem lumennahen Drüsenanteil der Drüsenzellen gefunden. Auch bei Erwachsenen (Abb. 45) haben mehrere Autoren nur noch positive Reaktionsausfälle in den lumennahen Abschnitten sekretorischer Zellen beobachten können (YASUI, 1960b; MONTAGNA, 1962; MONTAGNA und ELLIS, 1963). In ähnlicher Weise zeigen auch die ceruminalen Drüsen nur schwache apikale Aktivität, aber starke Aktivität des Inhaltes in der Drüsenlichtung (MONTAGNA, NOBACK und ZAK, 1948). Eine intensive alkalische Phosphataseaktivität des luminalen Teils des Cytoplasma fand KAGA (1956) beim Mann und anderen Mammifera, wobei sekretorische Ausbuchtungen (Kuppeln) besonders reaktiv sein sollen, sowie TAKAMURA (1958) bei Glandula vestibularis nasi der Katze. IHJIMA und OONO (1958) beobachteten nach Adrenalininjektion signifikante Erhöhungen der Enzymaktivität. Vielleicht ist die Reaktion nur an die Oberfläche der Mikrovilli gebunden, wie das z.B. CHASE (1963) für die Zellen des intestinalen Epithels zeigen konnte. KOPF (1957) sah Enzymaktivität anzeigende Präcipitate in den Drüsenzellen bipolar angeordnet, und zwar basal und luminal. Auch der Lumeninhalt war mäßig reaktiv. Auch nach Pilocarpininjektion scheinen die Aktivitäten zuzunehmen (WATANABE, 1961).

Schwächere Aktivitäten finden sich auch in Myoepithelzellen. Es scheint so zu sein, daß eher eine räumliche Beziehung zwischen alkalischer Phosphatase und Plasmamembran besteht als etwa eine solche zwischen diesem Enzym und dem kontraktilen Apparat der Myoepithelzellen (ELLIS, 1965). Zu solchen Überlegungen kommt man vor allem nach einer elektronenmikroskopisch-cytochemischen Untersuchung von MATSUZAWA und KUROSUMI (1963), die an Myoepithelzellen der Schweißdrüsen der Rattenpfote zeigen konnten, daß die Orte aPh-Aktivität im Bereich der Myoepithelzellen vor allem die pinocytotischen Bläschen sind und nicht die Myofilamente. Das stimmt auch mit den Befunden von GOLDSTEIN (1961) überein, der im polarisierten Licht zeigen konnte, daß Orte der Enzymlokalisation

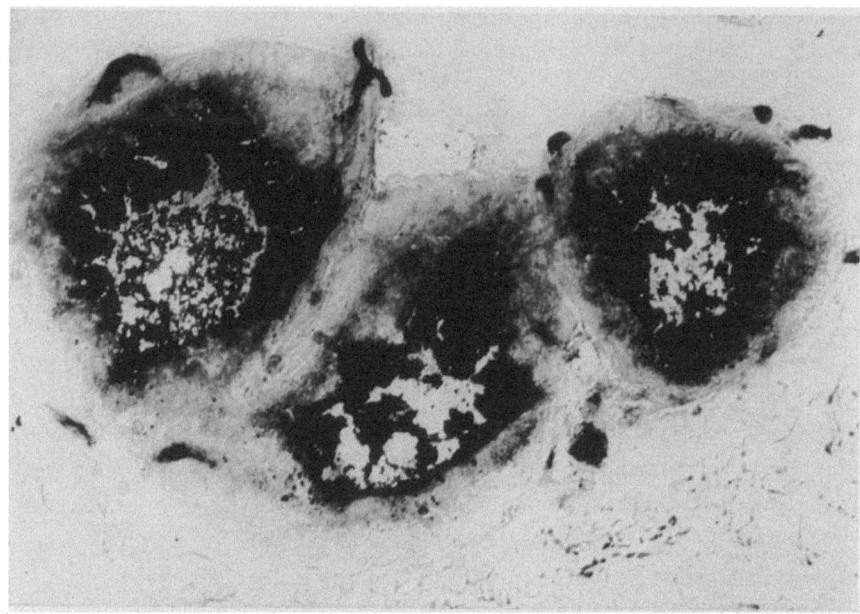

Abb. 45. Apokrine Schweißdrüsen. Alkalische Phosphatase. Intensiv positiver Reaktionsausfall in den Capillaren, um die Drüsenendstücke und in den apikalen Bereichen der Drüsenzellen sowie im Bereich des Lumeninhaltes. Kryostatschnitt. Vergr. 250 ×

die Zellwand und nicht die Myofilamente sind. Im Ausführungsgang sind die Epithelzellen frei von histochemisch nachweisbarer Enzymaktivität (KOPF, 1957; MONTAGNA, 1962).

Bereits bei Feten wird durch die starke aPh-Aktivität der Endothelzellen das *periglanduläre Capillarnetz* sehr gut markiert (SERRI, MONTAGNA und HUBER, 1963). Im Erwachsenenalter sind die Blutgefäße besonders von ELLIS, MONTAGNA und FANGER (1958) untersucht worden. Es scheint jeder Tubulus von einer gleichen Zahl von Capillaren versorgt zu sein. Ein Konnex zwischen dem Capillarplexus der apokrinen und ekkrinen Schweißdrüsen scheint nicht zu bestehen.

3. Adenosintriphosphatase

Starke Aktivität findet man im basalen Anteil der Zellmembran der sekretorischen Schweißdrüsen. Die gefaltete Partie der Membran kann auch andere Phosphate wie das Thiaminpyrophosphat spalten (BIEMPICA und MONTES, 1965). Zu ähnlichen Resultaten kamen auch MATSUZAWA und KUROSUMI (1963).

4. Thiaminpyrophosphatase

Wenn man Thiaminpyrophosphat als Substrat benutzt, läßt sich der Golgi-Apparat in seiner supranuclearen Lage gut darstellen (BIEMPICA und MONTES, 1965). Auf Enzymaktivitäten in der Golgi-Zone ist zuerst in der Epididymis der Maus von ALLEN und SLATER (1961) hingewiesen worden.

5. β-Glucuronidase

MONTAGNA (1962) fand starke β-Glucuronidaseaktivität in Zellen der sekretorischen Abschnitte der apokrinen Schweißdrüsen. Im Material von HASHIMOTO et al. (1966b) war der Reaktionsausfall besonders stark in den großen Granula, schwächer im Cytoplasma. Auch die Myoepithelzellen zeigten häufiger eine mäßig starke Reaktivität.

Die funktionelle Bedeutung der β-Glucuronidase in den apokrinen Schweißdrüsen ist nicht definitiv geklärt (Allgemeines dazu s. auch BRAUN-FALCO, 1961a). Es ist aber zu betonen, daß die β-Glucuronidase zu den lysosomalen Enzymen gehört (DE DUVE, 1963a und b).

6. Leucinaminopeptidase

Entsprechende Untersuchungen sind von ADACHI und MONTAGNA (1961) durchgeführt. Es fand sich eine mäßige bis starke Reaktivität in Drüsenzellen. Bei alten Individuen scheint der Reaktionsausfall etwas schwächer zu sein als bei jüngeren Menschen. Die Zellen des Ausführungsganges zeigen keinen positiven Reaktionsausfall.

In eigenen Untersuchungen konnten diese Untersuchungsergebnisse nicht bestätigt werden. Wir fanden auch in dem Ausführungsgang Leucinaminopeptidaseaktivität.

7. Chondrosulphatase

Diesbezügliche histochemische Untersuchungen haben nach unserem Wissen nur OHMURA und YASUDA (1961) durchgeführt und stärkere Aktivitäten im dem Lumen angrenzenden Teil der Drüsenzelle und Nucleolus gefunden. Das supranucleäre Cytoplasma verfügt über eine mäßige Aktivität.

Starke Aktivitäten sind auch in Myoepithelzellen festgestellt worden.

D. Über den Sekretionsmodus der apokrinen Schweißdrüsen

Lichtmikroskopische Beobachtungen waren dafür maßgebend, einen apokrinen Sekretionsmodus dieser Schweißdrüsen zu unterstellen und sie aufgrund dieser morphologischen Kriterien als apokrin herauszustellen (SCHIEFFERDECKER, 1917). Man nahm an, daß die sekretorisch aktive Drüsenzelle apikal eine ballonartige Auftreibung bildet, die nekrobiotisch abgestoßen werden soll oder daß die Kuppel durchbrochen wird und es dann zum Austritt von Cytoplasma und geformten Elementen („Kügelchen, Körnchen, Bläschen" SCHIEFFERDECKER, 1917) kommt. Durch einen solchen Sekretionsvorgang soll sich auch die Zelle insoweit in ihrem Aussehen ändern, daß sie niedriger, also nicht mehr zylindrisch, sondern kubisch wird. Es muß aber betont werden, daß bereits SCHIEFFERDECKER (1917) noch an einen zweiten, nämlich einen ekkrinen Sekretionsmodus der apokrinen Schweißdrüsen gedacht hat. Er spricht dabei von „einfacher Sekretion". Die von HURLEY und WITKOWSKI (1963) durchgeführten Untersuchungen scheinen einer solchen Auffassung nicht zu widersprechen.

Die Kuppel als wesentliches Merkmal einer apokrinen Drüsenzelle ist auch ultrastrukturell gesehen worden (KUROSUMI et al., 1959; KUROSUMI, 1961; KAWABATA, 1964; HASHIMOTO et al., 1966b), obwohl solche Befunde immer wieder mit der Begründung angezweifelt wurden (CHARLES, 1959; MONTAGNA, 1962; HIBBS,

1962; BIEMPICA und MONTES, 1965; MUNGER, 1965), daß die sog. ,,apocrine projection" vielleicht nur als Ausdruck von einer Anoxie absterbender Zellen, d.h. als ein Supravitalphänomen zu deuten wäre (HELANDER, 1965a und b; THOENES, 1965). Auch BARGMANN, FLEISCHHAUER und KNOOP (1961) möchten daher auf der Basis ihrer elektronenmikroskopischen Befunde den Begriff ,,apokrine Sekretion" fallen lassen. Von HOLMGREN (1922) wird eine holokrine Sekretion der apokrinen Schweißdrüsen für möglich gehalten.

Innerhalb der sekretorischen Aktivität der Drüsenzellen sind grundsätzlich drei Phasen zu unterscheiden (KUROSUMI, 1961; HELANDER, 1965a): 1. Die Aufnahme des Ausgangsmaterials, 2. die Synthese des Sekrets und 3. die Ausscheidung.

Bei der *Aufnahme* des Ausgangsmaterials (Metaboliten) spielt sehr wahrscheinlich das stark gefaltete basale Plasmalemm eine wesentliche Rolle (KUROSUMI et al., 1959; BIEMPICA und MONTES, 1965). So meint ELLIS (1965) aufgrund seiner Untersuchungen an ekkrinen Schweißdrüsen, daß durch die Kontraktion der Myoepithelzellen ein viel breiteres Areal des gefalteten Plasmalemms, d. h. eine größere Oberfläche der extracellulären Flüssigkeit exponiert wird. Dadurch ergibt sich bereits eine wichtige Rolle für die Myoepithelzellen in der ersten Phase der sekretorischen Aktivität. Diese interessante Auffassung trifft wohl auch für die apokrinen Schweißdrüsen zu. BIEMPICA und MONTES (1965) glauben, daß die in basalen Abschnitten der Drüsenzelle gelagerten Mitochondrien beim Absorptionsvorgang eine gewisse Rolle spielen können.

Die ersten *Synthesevorgänge* sind nach BIEMPICA und MONTES (1965) in den Zisternen des endoplasmatischen Reticulums zu suchen und weitere Bearbeitung erfolgt im Bereich des Golgi-Apparates. Es ist interessant zu betonen, daß die Caseinbildung bei lactierenden Mäusen, wie autoradiographisch von WELLINGS und PHILP (1964) mit DL-Leucin-4,5-H^3 gezeigt wurde, sich topisch über das Ergastoplasma und anschließend den Golgi-Apparat abspielt. Dieser Weg entspricht gut den allgemeinen Anschauungen, nach der die Synthese von Proteinen im Ergastoplasma erfolgt. Hier werden also die Vorstufen des Sekretes gebildet, die dann weiter zum Golgi-Apparat abtransportiert werden. HASHIMOTO et al. (1966) halten es für wahrscheinlich, daß sich die Bildung der dunklen Granula vom Golgi-Apparat ableitet. Auf die Rolle des voluminösen Golgi-Apparates in apokrinen Schweißdrüsen haben KUROSUMI et al. (1959), HIBBS (1962) sowie KAWABATA (1964) aufmerksam gemacht. In diesem Zusammenhang sei auf die funktionellen Beziehungen zwischen Lysosomen und Golgi-Apparat hingewiesen (NOVIKOFF, 1961, 1963). Es ist anzunehmen, daß die unreifen Sekretionsgranula (wohl Lysosomen) das in ihnen enthaltene Material verdauen, elektronendichter werden und schließlich ihren Inhalt in das apikale Cytoplasma entleeren. Eine Auflösung der Sekretionsgranula hat schon MONTAGNA (1956, 1962) für wahrscheinlich gehalten. Auch HASHIMOTO et al. (1966b) sind ähnlicher Auffassung und glauben, daß schließlich nur die noch schaumigen Vacuolen von den Sekretionsgranula übrigbleiben, die sich dann in das Drüsenlumen entleeren. Man diskutiert auch die Möglichkeit, daß sich Mitochondrien in Sekretionsgranula umwandeln können (Näheres bei KUROSUMI, 1961). Einen derartigen Entstehungsmodus der Granula hält HELANDER (1965) aber nach heutigen Auffassungen für unwahrscheinlich. Auch WATZKA (1966) bezweifelt, daß sich Mitochondrien in Zellsekret umwandeln können.

Nach BIEMPICA und MONTES (1965) soll die *Ausscheidung* des Sekretes durch den Vorgang der sog. Exocytose erfolgen. Eine apokrine Sekretion wird von diesen Autoren nicht für wahrscheinlich gehalten. Ebenso lehnt MUNGER (1965a) die apokrine Sekretion grundsätzlich ab. Für diesen Autor sind die apokrinen Drüsen nichts anderes als ekkrine Drüsen, denen die für ekkrine Drüsen typische Klarzellen fehlen. Die Sekretion soll durch die sekretorischen Vacuolen vor sich gehen. CHARLES (1959) hat schon früher über einen ekkrinen Sekretionsmodus der apokrinen Drüsen gesprochen. Dafür sollen die von ihm gefundenen intercellulären Canaliculi sprechen. Er erlaubt aber noch eine andere Sekretionsmöglichkeit, die durch einen nekrobiotischen Vorgang verwirklicht sein soll. Bereits SCHIEFFERDECKER (1917) hat einen Durchbruch der Kuppeln beschrieben. HASHIMOTO et al. (1966 b) haben versucht, entsprechende Kontinuitätsunterbrechungen des Plasmalemms auch elektronenmikroskopisch darzustellen. HIBBS (1962) spricht von sog. „droplet secretion", was wohl mit der Ausscheidung von Vacuolen zu vergleichen ist. Einen solchen Sekretionsmechanismus hält auch KAWABATA (1964) für wahrscheinlich, postuliert aber noch zwei weitere Sekretionstypen nach KUROSUMI (1961), und zwar Typ II, d. h. eine Abschnürung bzw. Dekapitation der apikalen Kuppeln der Drüsenzellen und Typ V, d. h. transmembranale Passage des Wassers und wasserlöslichen Materials ohne faßbare Veränderungen der Membran. ŠVAJGER (1965), der in Anlehnung an BARGMANN über eine apokrine Extrusion spricht, meint, daß diese mittels einer Vesikulation des Plasmalemms erfolgt. Die klassische, ultrastrukturell besonders von KUROSUMI et al. (1959) beschriebene apokrine Sekretion halten HASHIMOTO et al. (1966 b) für möglich. Dabei erwähnen sie auch noch andere Mechanismen, wie Abschnürung der Mikrovilli (mikroapokrine Sekretion — Typ III nach KUROSUMI, 1961), die schon erwähnte Sekretion durch Entleerung der Vacuolen ins Lumen und durch einen Membranendefekt. Andererseits meint MONTAGNA (1962), daß die apokrine Sekretion bei normalen apokrinen Schweißdrüsen überhaupt nicht vorkommt. Der ganze Sekretionsmechanismus erschöpft sich in der Abschnürung des terminalen Anteils der Mikrovilli, was nach KUROSUMI, MATSUZAWA und SAITO (1963) wohl als mikroapokrine Sekretion zu interpretieren wäre und in einer Exsudation durch diese Strukturen, was wieder dem Sekretionstyp V (KUROSUMI, 1961) entsprechen dürfte.

Zusammenfassend ist demnach festzustellen, daß bis heute noch keine einheitliche Auffassung über den Sekretionsmodus apokriner Schweißdrüsen existiert. Neben extremen Standpunkten, welche KUROSUMI et al. (1959), MUNGER (1965) sowie etwa auch BIEMPICA und MONTES (1965) vertreten, sind besonders in der jüngsten Zeit die Interpretationen von HASHIMOTO et al. (1966 b) zu erwähnen, welche sich prinzipiell nicht allzusehr von der bereits 1917 von SCHIEFFERDECKER vertretenen Auffassung unterscheiden.

Wir sind der Meinung, daß aller Wahrscheinlichkeit nach *mehrere Sekretionstypen* im Spiel sind, wobei wir die von KUROSUMI et al. (1959) abgebildete blasige, apikale Auftreibung in unserem Material mit Sicherheit nur sehr selten feststellen konnten. Vacuolen haben wir dagegen regelmäßig sehen können, auch die von HASHIMOTO et al. (1966 b) erwähnte Ruptur des Plasmalemms (Abb. 46), obwohl gerade hier auch mit Präparationsartefakten zu rechnen ist. Beachtenswert sind weiter die in unserem Material bisher an drei Zellen von ca. 100 untersuchten beobachteten Veränderungen, die mit Sicherheit auf ein Untergehen der ganzen Zelle hindeuten (Abb. 20). Die Beobachtung bezieht sich auf eine stark ausgeprägte Schwellung und Abrundung der Mitochondrien sowie eine vesiculöse Transformation des endoplasmatischen Reticulums. Das Plasmalemm ist in seiner Kontinuität oft unterbrochen, was wohl mit der erhöhten Fragilität zu erklären ist. Ob man derartige Befunde als Ausdruck einer holokrinen Sekretion interpretieren darf, bleibt noch fraglich. Es ist jedoch mit der Möglichkeit, daß die ganze apokrine Drüsenzelle schließlich einer Art Autolyse anheimfällt, bei der Diskussion des Sekretionsmechanismus zu rechnen. Dabei seien auch die Befunde von MESSIER und LEBLOND (1960) erwähnt, die radioautographisch zeigen konnten, daß eine anfänglich merokrine Zelle später „holocrin" (HELANDER, 1965a) abgestoßen werden kann. Auf jeden Fall liefern unsere ultrastrukturellen Untersuchungsergebnisse keinen sicheren Anhalt für die Annahme einer apokrinen Sekretion im klassischen Sinne, d. h. für eine Auftreibung und Abschnürung nur apikaler Zellabschnitte.

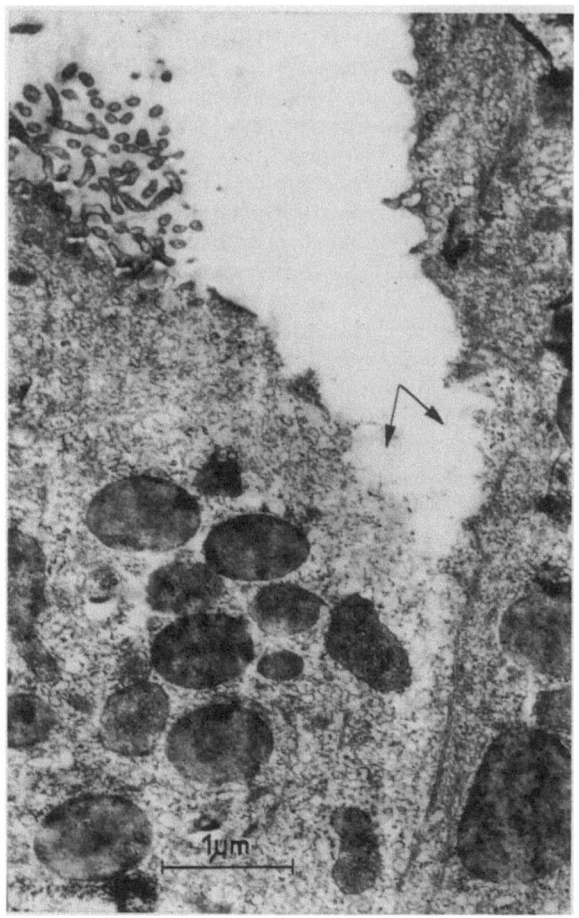

Abb. 46. Apokrine Schweißdrüse. Unterbrechung in der Kontinuität des Plasmalemms einer Drüsenzelle (↙↘) wahrscheinlich nicht als Artefakt zu deuten

E. Über hormonelle Einflüsse auf apokrine Schweißdrüsen

Seit LÜNEBURG (1902) auf die typische Morphologie der axillären apokrinen Schweißdrüsen erst in der Pubertätszeit hingewiesen hat, sind in der Literatur die Beziehungen zwischen diesen Drüsen und dem Zustand des Genitalapparates (Menses, Gravidität, Klimakterium, Senium) oft ventiliert worden. Da vom Morphologischen her vor etwa dem 12. Lebensjahr keine Anhaltspunkte für die aktive Sekretionsleistung apokriner Schweißdrüsen gegeben sind (YASUI, 1960a) — abgesehen von eventueller Pubertas praecox (HERZENBERG, 1927) — ist mit großer Wahrscheinlichkeit anzunehmen, daß die Sexualhormone dabei für die funktionelle Ingangsetzung und Kontrolle eine wichtige Rolle spielen (MONTAGNA,

1962). Die Entwicklung der apokrinen Schweißdrüsen ist offenbar fest an die Entwicklung der Haare in diesen Bereichen gebunden (SHELLEY und BUTTERWORTH, 1955). Es scheint so zu sein, daß die von mehreren Autoren registrierten Unterschiede in der Intensität der Entwicklung der axillären apokrinen Schweißdrüsen zwischen dem weiblichen und männlichen Geschlecht (WAELSCH, 1913; SCHIEFFERDECKER, 1917; LOESCHKE, 1925) nur auf die unterschiedliche Behaarungsstärke bezogen werden müssen (RICHTER, 1933; GLOOR-RUTISHAUSER, 1953). Auch HERZENBERG (1927) sowie WAY und MEMMESHEIMER (1938) haben einen geschlechtsabhängigen Entwicklungsgrad der apokrinen Schweißdrüsen nicht festgestellt.

Hormonelle Einflüsse der apokrinen Schweißdrüsen wurden beim Manne nur selten untersucht (PANÀ, 1934). Beim weiblichen Geschlecht interessierte besonders das Verhalten apokriner Schweißdrüsen während des Menstruationscyclus und der Gravidität.

Die Angaben über die Dicke des Drüsenlagers *im Verlauf des Menstruationscyclus* sind widersprechend. So haben LOESCHKE (1925) sowie HERZENBERG (1927) im Prämenstruum und im Menstruum eine Verdickung des Drüsenlagers in der Axilla beschrieben. Auch CAVAZZANA (1947) hat neben einer Hypertrophie hohe Drüsenzellen feststellen können. Auf der cytologischen Ebene haben MONTES et al. (1960) die Drüsen bei 23 Frauen untersucht und in den letzten Tagen der Menstruation bei 3 nur wenige PAS-reaktive Granula beobachtet, zwischen dem 5. und 10. Tag des Cyclusses dagegen bei 4 Frauen besonders viele Granula gefunden. Von KLAAR (1926) und MONTAGNA (1962) sind bei ein und denselben Individuen in verschiedenen Phasen des Cyclusses Biopsien in der Axilla vorgenommen worden. Es wurde keine Abhängigkeit des Axillarorgans von verschiedenen Phasen des Menstrualcyclus gesehen. Ähnliche Untersuchungen wurden auch von MONTES et al. (1960) bei 3 Frauen durchgeführt. Gleichzeitig wurden Gonadotropin und Oestrogene im Urin bestimmt, Vaginalabstriche und Temperaturmessungen durchgeführt. Irgendwelche signifikante Unterschiede in Abhängigkeit vom Menstrualcyclus bzw. der hormonellen Situation waren nicht zu registrieren. Es ist also wahrscheinlich gemacht, daß die apokrinen Schweißdrüsen weder strukturell noch funktionell vom Menstruationscyclus beeinflußt werden. PANÀ (1934) hält aufgrund experimenteller Untersuchungen eine Beeinflussung der Drüsen durch Ovarialhormone ebenfalls für wenig wahrscheinlich. So ist auch gut verständlich, daß die apokrinen Schweißdrüsen sogar 10 Jahre nach Ovariektomie noch immer in ihrem Aussehen normal sein können (MONTAGNA, 1962).

Während der *Gravidität* konnte MONTAGNA (1956) keine nennenswerten Veränderungen an apokrinen Schweißdrüsen feststellen. Seine Befunde stehen besonders im Gegensatz zu Arbeiten älterer Autoren, die über eine Hypertrophie bzw. Rückbildung und Hemmung der Drüsen während der Gravidität berichtet haben. Eine Hypertrophie der axillären Drüsen wurde von REBAUDI (1911) wie auch WAELSCH (1913), FRIEDRICH und SCHLOSSBERGER (1919) sowie HERZENBERG (1927) beobachtet. Der Fall von SEITZ (1906) mit angeblicher Drüsenschwellung im Achselbereich ist von KAYSER (1908) und WAELSCH (1913) als überzählige Brustdrüse gedeutet worden. In neuerer Zeit hat CAVAZZANA (1947) sehr hohe Drüsenzellen und hypertrophische Myoepithelzellen in der Gravidität beschrieben. Andererseits fand LOESCHKE (1925) die Dicke des Drüsenlagers beachtlich reduziert, was auf eine Hemmung im Wachstum hindeuten soll. Seine Befunde konnten auch KLAAR (1926) sowie RICHTER (1933), der Rückbildungserscheinungen mit Bindegewebsvermehrung festgestellt hat, bestätigen. Auch CORNBLEET (1952) ist der Meinung, daß die apokrinen Drüsen in der Gravidität weniger aktiv sind. Ein Beweis dafür soll aber in der Tatsache gelegen sein, daß Krankheiten apokriner

Schweißdrüsen, wie z. B. Morbus Fox-Fordyce, sich in der Schwangerschaft zurückbilden können. Auch Gestagene wirken bessernd bei Morbus Fox-Fordyce. MONTES et al. (1960) haben bei früher Gravidität eine Vermehrung der PAS-reaktiven Granula, dagegen eine Abnahme der Granula und Fülle des luminalen Inhaltes in den späteren Monaten der Gravidität sehen können.

Im Gegensatz dazu meint PANÀ (1934) ähnlich wie MONTAGNA (1962), daß die Gravidität keinen Einfluß auf die apokrinen Drüsen ausübt.

In bezug auf die hormonelle Beeinflussung der apokrinen Schweißdrüsen sind Untersuchungen über den direkten Einfluß von Hormonen von beachtlicher Bedeutung. So haben SHELLEY und CAHN (1955) nach lokaler sowie peroraler bzw. intramuskulärer Applikation von Hormonen mikroskopisch faßbare Veränderungen nicht feststellen können. Ähnlich sind nach subcutanen Implantationen von Testosteron und Oestradiol (SHELLEY und HURLEY, 1957) die apokrinen Schweißdrüsen morphologisch unverändert geblieben. Von HURLEY und SHELLEY (1960) wird eine hypophysäre Kontrolle der Drüsen postuliert.

Literatur

AAVIK, O. R.: Cholinesterases in human skin. J. invest. Derm. 24, 103—106 (1955). — ADACHI, K., and W. MONTAGNA: Histology and cytochemistry of human skin. XXII. Sites of leucine aminopeptidase (LAP). J. invest. Derm. 37, 145—151 (1961). — ADAM, H.: Die Haut der Säugetiere. Bau und Funktion. Studium Generale 17, 350—362 (1964). — AFZELIUS, B. A.: The ultrastructure of the nuclear envelope of the sea urchin oocytes studied with the electron microscope. Exp. Cell Res. 8, 147—158 (1955). — ALLEN, J. M., and J. J. SLATER: A cytochemical study of Golgi associated thiamine pyrophosphatase in the epididymis of the mouse. J. Histochem. Cytochem. 9, 418—423 (1961). — ALVERDES, K.: Die apokrinen Drüsen im Vestibulum nasi des Menschen. Z. mikr.-anat. Forsch. 28, 609—643 (1932). Ref. in: Ber. wiss. Biol. 22, 170—171 (1932). — Die Entwicklung der Glandulae vestibulares nasi des Menschen. Z. mikr.-anat. Forsch. 35, 119—145 (1934). — ANDRÉ, J.: Quelques données récentes sur la structure et la physiologie des mitochondries: glycogène, particules élémentaires, acides nucleiques. Arch. Biol. (Liège) 76, 277—304 (1965). — AOKI, T.: Stimulation of the sweat glands in the hairy skin of the dog by adrenaline, noradrenaline, acetylcholine, mecholyl and pilocarpine. J. invest. Derm. 24, 545—556 (1955). — ATO, N.: Histochemical study on the apocrine sweat gland in the circumanal region of cattle. Okajimas Folia anat. jap. 37, 19—27 (1961). Ref. in: Ber. wiss. Biol. 177, 123 (1962). — ATUSI, N.: Über das Vorkommen apokriner Drüsen im N. papillomatosus. Hiku-to-Hitunyo 8, 437—440 (1940). Ref. in: Zbl. Haut- u. Geschl.-Kr. 66, 607 (1961).

BARGMANN, W.: Histologie und mikroskopische Anatomie des Menschen. Stuttgart: Georg Thieme 1959. — BARGMANN, W., K. FLEISCHHAUER u. A. KNOOP: Über die Morphologie der Milchsekretion. II. Z. Zellforsch. 53, 545—568 (1961). — BARGMANN, W., u. A. KNOOP: Über die Morphologie der Milchsekretion. I. Z. Zellforsch. 49, 344—388 (1959). — BARKA, T., and J. P. ANDERSON: Histochemistry. New York-Evanston-London: Harper & Row Publ. Inc. 1963. — BECKER, V.: Funktionelle Morphologie der Schweißdrüsen. Fortschr. Med. 82, 901—906 (1964). — BECKER, V., u. J. REITINGER: Anatomische Untersuchungen an Schweiß- und Duftdrüsen. Verh. dtsch. Ges. Path. 48, 205—207 (1964). — BEHNKE, O.: Further studies on microtubules. A marginal bundle in human and rat thrombocytes. J. Ultrastruct. Res. 13, 469—477 (1965). — BERGEN, F. v.: Zur Kenntnis gewisser Strukturbilder („Netzapparate", „Saftkanälchen", „Trophospongium") im Protoplasma verschiedener Zellenarten. Arch. mikr. Anat. 64, 498—574 (1904). Zit. nach N. MELCZER 1935. — BERTHET, J.: La digestion intracellulaire et les lysosomes. Arch. Biol. (Liège) 76, 367—385 (1965). — BIEMPICA, L., and L. F. MONTES: Secretory epithelium of the large axillary sweat glands. Amer. J. Anat. 117, 47—72 (1965). — BORSETTO, P. L.: Osservazioni sullo sviluppo delle ghiandole sudoripare nelle diverse regioni della cute umana. Arch. ital. Anat. 66, 332—348 (1951). Zit. nach E. HORSTMANN 1957. — BOURNE, G. H., and H. B. TEWARI: Mitochondria and the Golgi complex. In: G. H. BOURNE, Cytology and cell physiology, p. 377—421. New York and London: Academic Press 1964. — BRANCA, P. A.: Sur la structure des glandes sudoripares. Ann. Derm. Syph. (Paris) 8, 1—2 (1927). — BRANDAU, H., u. D. PETTE: Topische Muster von Enzymen des energieliefernden Stoffwechsels im quergestreiften Muskel. Enzym. biol. clin. 6, 79—122 (1966). — BRANDES, D., and G. H. BOURNE: Brit. J. exp. Pathol. 35, 577 (1954). Zit. nach G. H. BOURNE u. H. B. TEWARI 1964. — BRAUN-FALCO, O.: Die Histochemie der Haut. In:

H. A. GOTTRON u. W. SCHÖNFELD, Dermatologie und Venerologie, Bd. I, Teil 1, S. 366—472. Stuttgart: Georg Thieme 1961a. — Zur Histotopographie der Cytochromoxydase in normaler und pathologisch veränderter Haut sowie in Hauttumoren. Arch. klin. exp. Derm. **214**, 176—224 (1961b). — BRAUN-FALCO, O., u. D. PETZOLDT: Über die Histotopie von NADH- und NADPH-Tetrazoliumreduktase in menschlicher Haut. Arch. klin. exp. Derm. **220**, 455—473 (1964). — Über die Histotopie von NADH- und NADPH-Tetrazoliumreduktase in menschlicher Haut. Arch. klin. exp. Derm. **221**, 410—432 (1965a). — Zur Frage optimaler Reaktionsbedingungen bei der histochemischen Darstellung von Enzymen des Energie-liefernden Stoffwechsels in der Epidermis. I. Dehydrogenasen. Arch. klin. exp. Derm. **223**, 620—633 (1965b). — Über die Histotopie von Ubichinon in menschlicher Haut. I. Normale Haut. Arch. klin. exp. Derm. **224**, 362—372 (1966). — Über die Histotopie von Ubichinon in menschlicher Haut. II. Pathologisch veränderte Haut und Hauttumoren. Arch. klin. exp. Derm. **228**, 290—306 (1967.) — BRAUN-FALCO, O., u. G. RASSNER: Zur morphologischen und funktionellen Organisation der menschlichen Epidermis. In: Medizinische Forschung in Marburg, Jahrbuch des Universitätsbundes 1966, S. 79—104. — BRAUN-FALCO, O., u. W. WINTER: Untersuchungen über die Autolyse der Haut. I. Mitt.: Morphologische Veränderungen. Arch. klin. exp. Derm. **220**, 344—361 (1964a). — Untersuchungen über die Autolyse der Haut. II. Mitt.: Histochemische Veränderungen. Arch. klin. exp. Derm. **220**, 417—442 (1964b). — BRINKMANN, A.: Über das Vorkommen von Hautdrüsenorganen bei den anthropomorphen Affen. Anat. Anz. **34**, 513—520 (1909). — Nachlese zu meinen Hautdrüsenuntersuchungen. In: BERGENS Museums Aarbok 1923/24, S. 3—36. — BRODY, I.: The ultrastructure of the tonofibrils in the keratinization process of normal human epidermis. J. Ultrastruct. Res. **4**, 264—297 (1960). — BUNTING, H., G. B. WISLOCKI, and E. W. DEMPSEY: The chemical histology of the human eccrine and apocrine sweat glands. Anat. Rec. **100**, 61—73 (1948). — BUSCHKE, W.: Cystenmamma und Axillarorgan. (Auf Grund von Untersuchungen an den apokrinen Achselschweißdrüsen im Klimakterium.) Arch. Gynäk. **152**, 431—446 (1933).

CAHN, M. M., and W. B. SHELLEY: Hyaluronidase-methylene blue staining of nerve fibers about the human axillary apocrine sweat gland. J. invest. Derm. **25**, 63—66 (1955). — CAMERON, R.: Pathological changes in cells. In: G. H. BOURNE, Cytology and cell physiology, p. 667—717. New York and London: Academic Press 1964. — CANEGHEM, P. VAN: Über die Struktur der heterotopen apokrinen Drüsen. Hautarzt **10**, 552—555 (1959). — CARASSO, N., et P. FAVARD: Les ultrastructures cytoplasmiques. In: C. MAGNAN, Traité de microscopie électronique, Teil II, p. 905—1117. Paris 1961. — CAROSSINI, G.: Lo sviluppo delle ghiandole sudoripare etc. Arch. ital. Anat. Embriol. (1912/13). Zit. nach K. STEINER 1925. — CAVAZZANA, P.: Indagini sul comportamento morfo-funzionale delle ghiandole glomerulari apocrine della pelle dell'ascella durante le fasi del ciclo mestruale e nella gravidanza. Riv. ital. Ginec. **30**, 114—134 (1947). — CHARLES, A.: An electron microscopic study of the human axillary apocrine gland. J. Anat. (Lond.) **93**, 226—232 (1959). — Electron microscopic observations of the arrector pili muscle of the human scalp. J. invest. Derm. **35**, 27—30 (1960). — CHASE, W. H.: The demonstration of alkaline phosphatase activity in frozen-dried mouse gut in the electron microscope. J. Histochem. Cytochem. **11**, 96—101 (1963). — CONTINO: Albrecht v. Graefes Arch. Ophthal. **66** (1907). Zit. nach G. SPERLING 1935. — CORNBLEET, T.: Pregnancy and apocrine gland diseases: hidradenitis, Fox-Fordyce disease. Arch. Derm. Syph. (Chic.) **65**, 12—19 (1952).

DAEMS, W. TH.: Mouse liver lysosomes and storage. A morphological and histochemical study. Thesis University of Leiden, Holland 1962. Zit. nach J. L. E. ERICSSON, B. F. TRUMP u. J. WEIBEL 1965. — DAEMS, W. TH., and J. P. PERSIJN: Enzyme histochemistry in electron microscopy. In: R. RUYSSEN and L. VANDENDRIESSCHE, Enzymes in clinical chemistry, p. 75—104. Amsterdam-New York-London: Elsevier Publ. Co. 1965. — DALTON, A. J., and D. M. FELIX: A comparative study of the Golgi complex. J. biophys. biochem. Cytol. **2**, 79—84 (1956). — DAVID, H.: Physiologische und pathologische Modifikationen der submikroskopischen Kernstruktur. Z. mikr.-anat. Forsch. **71**, 412—456 (1964). — DAVID, L. T.: The external expression and comparative dermal histology of hereditary hairlessness in mammals. Z. Zellforsch. **14**, 616—719 (1932). — DUVE, CH. DE: The lysosome concept. In: A. V. S. DE REUCK and M. P. CAMERON, Lysosomes, p. 1—31. London: J. & A. Churchill Ltd. 1963a. — The lysosome. Sci. Amer. **208**, 64—72 (1963b). — DE-THÉ, G.: Cytoplasmic microtubules in different animal cells. J. Cell Biol. **23**, 265—275 (1964).

EGGELING, H. v.: Über die phylogenetische Entstehung der Milchdrüsen und Haare. Anat. Anz. **56**, 65—71 (1923). — Über die Herkunft der Säugetierhautdrüsen. Anat. Anz. **90**, 149—157 (1940/41). — ELLIS, R. A.: Fine structure of the myoepithelium of the eccrine sweat glands of man. J. Cell Biol. **27**, 551—563 (1965). — ELLIS, R. A., and W. MONTAGNA: Histology and cytochemistry of human skin. XV. Sites of phosphorylase and amylo-1,6-glucosidase activity. J. Histochem. Cytochem. **6**, 201—207 (1958). — ELLIS, R. A., W. MONTAGNA, and H. FANGER: Histology and cytochemistry of human skin. XIV. The blood supply of the cutaneous glands. J. invest. Derm. **30**, 138—145 (1958). — ENDO, M.: Über die Größe der apokrinen Schweißdrüsen an der Achselhaut bei japanischen Kindern. Okajimas Folia anat. jap. **17**, 122—156 (1938). — Beiträge zur Kenntnis der apokrinen Schweißdrüsen an der Achselhaut bei japanischen Kindern. Okajimas Folia anat. jap. **17**, 607—617 (1939). — ERICSSON, J. L. E., B. F. TRUMP, and J. WEIBEL: Electron microscopic studies of the proximal tubule of the rat kidney. Lab. Invest. **14**, 1341—1365 (1965). — ESSNER, E., and A. B. NOVIKOFF: Localization of acid phosphatase activity in hepatic lysosomes by means of electron microscopy. J. biophys. biochem. Cytol. **9**, 773—784 (1961).

FARQUHAR, M. G., and G. E. PALADE: Functional complexes in various epithelia. J. Cell Biol. **17**, 375—412 (1963). — FAWCETT, D. W., and M. H. BURGOS: Studies on the fine structure of the mammalian testis. Amer. J. Anat. **107**, 245—269 (1960). — FLEISCHHAUER, K.: Über die Entstehung der Haaranordnung und das Zustandekommen räumlicher Beziehungen zwischen Haaren und Schweißdrüsen. Z. Zellforsch. **38**, 328—355 (1953). — FREI, J. V.: The fine structure of the basement membrane in epidermal tumors. J. Cell Biol. **15**, 335—342 (1962). — FRIEDRICH, u. SCHOSSBERGER: Zit. nach E. KROMPECHER 1919. — FUSARO, R. M., and R. W. GOLTZ: The normal human eccrine and apocrine glands. J. invest. Derm. **36**, 79—82 (1961).

GANSLER, H.: Struktur und Funktion der glatten Muskulatur, licht- und elektronenmikroskopische Befunde an Hohlorganen von Ratte, Meerschweinchen und Mensch. Z. Zellforsch. **55**, 724—762 (1961). — GAY: Die Circumanaldrüsen des Menschen. S.-B. Akad. Wiss. Wien **63**, 329 (1871). Zit. nach H. HEYNOLD 1874. — GEDIGK, P.: Über die Entstehung von Lipopigmenten. II. Internat. Kongr. für Histo- und Cytochemie Frankfurt a.M. 1964, S. 149—150. Berlin-Göttingen-Heidelberg: Springer 1964. — GEDIGK, P., u. E. BONTKE: Über den Nachweis von hydrolytischen Enzymen in Lipopigmenten. Z. Zellforsch. **44**, 495—518 (1956). — GEDIGK, P., u. R. FISCHER: Über die Entstehung von Lipopigmenten in Muskelfasern. Untersuchungen beim experimentellen Vitamin E-Mangel der Ratte und an Organen des Menschen. Virchows Arch. path. Anat. **332**, 431—468 (1959). — GLOOR-RUTISHAUSER, N.: Zur makroskopischen Anatomie der apokrinen Achseldrüsen. Acta anat. (Basel) **19**, 197—203 (1953). — GOLDFISCHER, S., E. ESSNER, and A. B. NOVIKOFF: The localization of phosphatase activities at the level of ultrastructure. J. Histochem. Cytochem. **12**, 72—95 (1964). — GOLDSTEIN, D. J.: On the origin and morphology of myoepithelial cells of apocrine sweat glands. J. invest. Derm. **37**, 301—309 (1961). — GOLTZ, R. W., R. M. FUSARO, and J. JARVIS: The demonstration of acid substances in normal skin by alcian blue. J. invest. Derm. **31**, 183—190 (1958). — GOMORI, G.: Int. Cytol. Rev. **1**, 323 (1952). Zit. nach O. BRAUN-FALCO 1961. — GORDIS, L., and H. M. NITKOWSKY: Lysosomes in human cell cultures. Exp. Cell Res. **38**, 556—569 (1965). — GREIG, D. M.: The analogy of black colostrum to melanhidrosis with some remarks on coloured milk and coloured sweat. Edinb. med. J. **37**, 524—544 (1930). — GROSS, B. G.: The fine structure of apocrine hidrocystoma. Arch. Derm. **92**, 706—712 (1965). — Annulate lamellae in the axillary apocrine glands of adult man. J. Ultrastruct. Res. **14**, 64—73 (1966). — GROTH, W.: Der Verlauf des Drüsenschlauchs in den a-Drüsen der Achselhaut des Menschen. Z. mikr.-anat. Forsch. **38**, 627—634 (1935). Ref. in: Ber. wiss. Biol. **38**, 128 (1936).

HAGUENAU, F.: Les myofilaments de la cellule myoépithéliale. Étude au microscope électronique. C.R. Acad. Sci. (Paris) **249**, 182—184 (1959). — HALTER, K.: Zur Frage der Heterotopie apokriner Drüsen. Z. Haut- u. Geschl.-Kr. **20**, 209—212 (1956). — HARRISON, G. A.: Some observations on the presence of annulate lamellae in alligator and sea gull adrenal cortical cells. J. Ultrastruct. Res. **14**, 158—166 (1966). — HASHIMOTO, K., B. G. GROSS, and W. F. LEVER: An electron microscopic study of the adult human apocrine duct. J. invest. Derm. **46**, 6—11 (1966a). — Electron microscopic study of apocrine secretion. J. invest. Derm. **46**, 378—390 (1966b). — Electron microscopic study of the human adult eccrine gland. I. The duct. J. invest. Derm. **46**, 172—185 (1966c). — HASHIMOTO, T.: Histochemical studies on various dehydrogenases related to glucose metabolism of the human skin. Skin. Res. **3**, 245—276 (1961). — HAY, E. D.: Secretion of connective tissue protein by developing epidermis. In: W. MONTAGNA and W. C. LOBITZ, The epidermis, p. 97—116. New York and London: Academic Press 1964. — HELANDER, H. F.: Morphology of animal secretory gland cells. In: K. E. WOHLFAHRT-BOTTERMANN, Sekretion und Exkretion, S. 2—26. Berlin-Heidelberg-New York: Springer 1965a. — Morphology of animal secretory gland cells. Diskussionsbemerkung. In: Sekretion und Exkretion. 2. wiss. Konf. d. Ges. Dtsch Naturf. und Ärzte Schloß Reinhardsbrunn 1964, S. 25. Berlin-Heidelberg-New York: Springer 1965b.— HELLMANN, K.: Cholinesterase and amine oxidase in the skin: a histochemical investigation. J. Physiol. (Lond.) **129**, 454—463 (1955). — HERZENBERG, H.: Neue Beiträge zur Lehre von den apokrinen Schweißdrüsen. Virchows Arch. path. Anat. **266**, 422—455 (1927). — HEYNOLD, H.: Über die Knäueldrüsen des Menschen. Virchows Arch. path. Anat. **61**, 77—90 (1874). — HIBBS, R. G.: The fine structure of human eccrine sweat glands. Amer. J. Anat. **103**, 201—217 (1958). — Electron microscopy of human apocrine sweat glands. J. invest. Derm. **38**, 77—84 (1962). — HICKS, R. M.: The function of the Golgi complex in transitional epithelium. J. Cell Biol. **30**, 623—643 (1966). — HOLLMANN, K.-H.: L'ultrastructure de la glande mammaire normale de la souris en lactation. J. Ultrastruct. Res. **2**, 423—443 (1959). — HOLMGREN, E.: Die Achseldrüsen des Menschen. Anat. Anz. **55**, 553—565 (1922). — HOLTER, H.: Physiologie der Pinocytose bei Amöben. In: K. E. WOHLFAHRT-BOTTERMANN, Sekretion und Exkretion, S. 119—146. Berlin-Heidelberg-New York: Springer 1965. — HOMMA, H.: Über positive Eisenbefunde in den Epithelien der apokrinen Schweißdrüsen menschlicher Axillarhaut. Arch. Derm. Syph. (Berl.) **148**, 464—469 (1925). — On apocrine sweat glands in white and negro man and woman. Bull. Johns Hopk. Hosp. **38**, 365—371 (1926). — HORNER, W. E.: Special anatomy and histology, vol. I, p. 378. Philadelphia: Lee & Blonehard 1846. Zit. nach ST. C. WAY u. A. MEMMESHEIMER 1938. — HORSTMANN, E.: Zur Morphologie der gesunden und kranken Haut. Arch. Derm. Syph. (Berl.) **194**, 164—173 (1952). — Die Haut. In: v. MÖLLENDORF-BARGMANN, Handbuch der mikroskopischen Anatomie des Menschen, Bd 3, Teil III, S. 1—276. Berlin-Göttingen-Heidelberg: Springer 1957. — HURLEY, H. J., and W. B. SHELLEY: Apocrine sweat retention in man. I. Experimental production of asymptomatic form. J. invest. Derm. **22**, 397—404 (1954a). — The human apocrine sweat gland: two secretions? Brit. J. Derm. **66**, 44—48 (1954b). — The role of the myoepithelium of the human apocrine sweat gland. J. invest. Derm. **22**, 143—156 (1954c). — The human apocrine sweat gland in health and disease. Springfield (Ill.): Ch. C. Thomas 1960. — HURLEY, H. J., W. B. SHELLEY, and G. B. KOELLE: The distribution of cholinesterases in human skin, with special reference to eccrine and apocrine sweat glands. J. invest. Derm. **21**, 139—147 (1953). — HURLEY, H. J., and J. A. WITKOWSKI: The merocrine component of apocrine secretion. Proc. Soc. exp. Biol. (N.Y.) **113**, 578—580 (1963).

IHJIMA, SH., and T. OONO: Cytochemical studies of gl. vestibulares nasi of the cat after adrenalin injection. Okajimas Folia anat. jap. **31**, 325—332 (1958). — IIJIMA, T.: Acta anat. Nippon (Tokyo) **34**, 649 (1959). Zit. nach K. KUROSUMI 1961. — ITO, S.: Histologie und Zytologie der Schweißdrüsen. Igaku no Shimpo **6**, 106—221 (1949). Zit. nach K. KUROSUMI, M. YAMAGISHI u. M. SEKINE 1961. — Light and electron microscopic study of membranous cytoplasmic organelles. In: R. J. C. HARRIS, The interpretation of ultrastructure, p. 129—147. New York and London: Academic Press 1962. — IWASHIGE, K.: Beiträge zur Kenntnis der Eisenreaktion bei den apokrinen Schweißdrüsen der Achselhaut von Japanern. Arch. histol. jap. **2**, 367—374 (1951).

KAGA, T.: Cytochemical studies of gl. ceruminosa in man and other mammals. Okajimas Folia anat. jap. **29**, 211—230 (1956). — KATO, S.: Über das Vorkommen apokriner Drüsen in der Außenhaut des Nasenflügels bei den Japanern. Okajimas Folia anat. jap. **14**, 97—100 (1936). — KATO, S., u. M. NAGATA: Kurze Mitteilung über die apokrinen Schweißdrüsen im Vestibulum nasi der Chinesen. Okajimas Folia anat. jap. **16**, 431—444 (1938). Zit. nach E. HORSTMANN 1957. — KAWABATA, I.: Electron microscope studies on the human ceruminous gland. Arch. histol. jap. **25**, 165—187 (1964). — KAYSER, F.: Achselhöhlenbrüste bei Wöchnerinnen. Arch. Gynäk. **85**, 458—482 (1908). — KESSEL, R. G.: Intranuclear and cytoplasmic annulate lamellae in tunicate oocytes. J. Cell Biol. **24**, 471—487 (1965). — KLAAR, J.: Über die axillaren Knäueldrüsen der Affen. Z. Anat. Entwickl.-Gesch. **72**, 609—627 (1924). — Zur Kenntnis des weiblichen Axillarorgans beim Menschen. Wien. klin. Wschr. **39**, 127—131 (1926). — KNEELAND, J. E.: Fine structure of the sweat glands of the antebrachial organ of "lemur catta". Z. Zellforsch. **73**, 521—533 (1966). — KOBAYASI, T.: An electron microscope study on the dermo-epidermal junction. Acta derm.-venereol. (Stockh.) **41**, 481—491 (1961). — KOCH, F.: Über das Vorkommen von apokrinen Drüsen in Talgdrüsennaevi. Arch. klin. exp. Derm. **174**, 126—131 (1963). — KOELLIKER, A.: Mikroskopische Anatomie, Bd 2, Teil 1. Leipzig 1850. — KOENIG, H.: The autofluorescence of lysosomes. Its value for the identification of lysosomal constituents. J. Histochem. Cytochem. **11**, 556—557 (1963). — KOPF, A. W.: The distribution of alkaline phosphatase in normal and pathologic human skin. Arch. Derm. **75**, 1—37 (1957). — KRAUSE, C.: Haut. In: WAGNERs Handbuch der Physiologie, Bd II, S. 126—131, 1844. Zit. nach J. SCHAFFER 1940. — KROMPECHER, E.: Zur Kenntnis der Geschwülste und Hypertrophien der Schweißdrüsen. Arch. Derm. Syph. (Berl.) **126**, 765—792 (1919). — KUFF, E. L., and A. J. DALTON: In: T. HAYASHI, Subcellular particles, p. 114. New York: Ronald 1959. Zit. nach F. S. SJÖSTRAND 1964. — KUROSUMI, K.: Electron microscopic analysis of the secretion mechanism. In: Int. Rev. Cytol. **11**, 1—117 (1961). — Golgi apparatus and its derivates with special reference to secretory granules. In: S. SENO and E. V. COWDRY, Intracellular membraneous structure. Japan Society for Cell Biology, Okayama 1965, p. 259—276. — KUROSUMI, K., and T. KITAMURA: Occurrence of foldings of plasma membrane (β-cyto-membrane) in cells of pig's carpal organ as revealed by electron microscopy. Nature (Lond.) **181**, 489 (1958). — KUROSUMI, K., T. KITAMURA, and T. IIJIMA: Electron microscope studies on the human axillary apocrine sweat glands. Arch. histol. jap. **16**, 523—566 (1959). — KUROSUMI, K., T. MATSUZAWA, and F. SAITO: Electron microscopic observations on the sweat glands of the horse. Arch. histol. jap. **23**, 295—310 (1963). — KUROSUMI, K., M. YAMAGISHI, and M. SEKINE: Mitochondrial deformation and apocrine secretory mechanism in the rabbit submandibular organ as revealed by electron microscopy.

Z. Zellforsch. **55**, 297—312 (1961). — KYRLE, J.: Vorlesungen über Histo-Biologie der menschlichen Haut und ihrer Erkrankungen, Bd I. Wien u. Berlin: Springer 1925.
LEE, D. G., and K. SCHMIDT-NIELSEN: The skin, sweat glands and hair follicles of the camel (camelus dromedarius). Anat. Rec. **143**, 71—77 (1962). Ref. in: Ber. wiss. Biol. **194**, 219 (1963). — LEESON, C. R.: The electron microscopy of the myoepithelium in the rat exorbital lacrimal gland. Anat. Rec. **137**, 45—55 (1960). — LEHNINGER, A. L.: The enzymic and morphologic organization of the mitochondria. Pediatrics **26**, 466—475 (1960). — LOESCHKE, H.: Über zyklische Vorgänge in den Drüsen des Achselhöhlenorgans und ihre Abhängigkeit vom Sexualzyklus des Weibes. Virchows Arch. path. Anat. **255**, 283—294 (1925). — LÜNEBURG: Beiträge zur Entwicklung und Histologie der Knäueldrüsen in der Achselhöhle des Menschen. Inaug.-Diss. Rostock 1902. Zit. nach J. KLAAR 1924.
MANCA, P. V.: Ricerche sulla struttura delle ghiandole apocrine. Studi sassaresi **11**, 883—890 (1933). — Ricerche sulla struttura delle ghiandole apocrine. G. ital. Derm. Sif. **75**, 187—193 (1934). — MARTIUS, H., u. H. HARTL: Lehrbuch der Geburtshilfe. Stuttgart: Georg Thieme 1959. — MATSUZAWA, T., and K. KUROSUMI: The ultrastructure morphogenesis and histochemistry of the sweat glands in the rat foot pads as revealed by electron microscopy. J. Electronmicroscopy **12**, 175—191 (1963). — MAUNSBACH, A. B.: Electron microscopic observations of cytoplasmic bodies with crystalline patterns in rat kidney proximal tubule cells. J. Ultrastruct. Res. **14**, 167—189 (1966a). — Observations on the ultrastructure and acid phosphatase activity of the cytoplasmic bodies in rat kidney proximal tubule cells. J. Ultrastruct. Res. **16**, 197—238 (1966b). — MEHREGAN, A. H.: Apocrine cystadenoma. Arch. Derm. **90**, 274—279 (1964). — MELCZER, N.: Über das Golgi-Kopsch'sche Binnennetz der menschlichen apokrinen Schweißdrüsenzellen. Derm. Wschr. **100**, 337—342 (1935). — MERCER, E. H.: The evolution of intracellular phospholipid membrane systems. In: R. J. C. HARRIS, The interpretation of ultrastructure, p. 369—384. New York and London: Academic Press 1962. — MERKER, H. J.: Die Lysosomen, eine neue Zellorganellengruppe. Berl. Med. **15**, 237—244 (1964). — MESSIER, B., and C. P. LEBLOND: Cell proliferation and migration as revealed by radioautography after injection of thymidine-H^3 into male rats and mice. Amer. J. Anat. **106**, 247—285 (1960). — MINAMITANI, K.: Zytologische und histologische Untersuchungen der Schweißdrüsen in menschlicher Achselhaut. Okajimas Folia anat. jap. **20**, 563—590 (1941). — MINE, T.: Über die Größe der apokrinen Schweißdrüsen an dem Unterbauch bei den Japanerinnen. Okajimas Folia anat. jap. **15**, 302—342 (1937). — MISLAWSKY, A. N.: Zur Lehre von der sogenannten blasenförmigen Sekretion. Arch. mikr.-anat. Forsch. **73** (1909). Zit. nach A. BRINKMANN 1909. — MOGI, E.: Beiträge zur Entwicklung der apokrinen Schweißdrüsen im Vestibulum nasi bei den japanischen Foeten. Okajimas Folia anat. jap. **16**, 147—182 (1938). — MONTAGNA, W.: Ageing of the axillary apocrine sweat glands in the human female. Ciba Foundation Colloquia on Ageing, vol. 2, p. 188—210. London: J. & A. Churchill Ltd. 1956. — Histology and cytochemistry of human skin. XIX. The development and fate of the axillary organ. J. invest. Derm. **33**, 151—162 (1959). — The structure and function of skin. New York and London: Academic Press 1962. — Phylogenetic significance of the skin of man. Arch. Derm. **88**, 1—19 (1963). — Histology and cytochemistry of human skin. XXIV. Further observations on the axillary organ. J. invest. Derm. **42**, 119—129 (1964a). — Morphology of the aging skin: the cutaneous appendages. In: W. MONTAGNA, Advances in biology of skin, vol. VI: Aging, p. 1—16. Oxford-London-Edinburgh-New York-Paris-Frankfurt: Pergamon Press 1964b. — MONTAGNA, W., H. B. CHASE, and J. B. HAMILTON: The distribution of glycogen and lipids in human skin. J. invest. Derm. **17**, 147—157 (1951). — MONTAGNA, W., H. B. CHASE and W. C. LOBITZ: Histology and cytochemistry of human skin. V. Axillary apocrine sweat glands. Amer. J. Anat. **92**, 451—470 (1953). — MONTAGNA, W., A. Z. EISEN, A. H. RADEMACHER, and H. B. CHASE: Histology and cytochemistry of human skin. VI. The distribution of sulfhydryl and disulfide groups. J. invest. Derm. **23**, 23—32 (1954). — MONTAGNA, W., e R. A. ELLIS: L'istochimica degli annessi cutanei. Minerva derm. **34**, 475—494 (1959). — Histology and cytochemistry of human skin. XXI. The nerves around the axillary apocrine glands. Amer. J. Phys. Anthrop. **18**, 69—70 (1960). — The histochemistry of skin and cutaneous glands. In: 1st Int. Congr. Histochem. Cytochem., p. 447—464. Oxford-London-New York-Paris: Pergamon Press 1963. — MONTAGNA, W., CH. R. NOBACK, and F. G. ZAK: Pigment, lipids and other substances in the glands of the external auditory meatus of man. Amer. J. Anat. **83**, 409—435 (1948). — MONTAGNA, W., and J. S. YUN: Histology and cytochemistry of human skin. XXIII. The distribution of cytochrome oxidase. J. Histochem. Cytochem. **9**, 694—698 (1961). — MONTES, L. F., B. L. BAKER, and A. C. CURTIS: The cytology of the large axillary sweat glands in man. J. invest. Derm. **35**, 273—291 (1960). — MORIOKA, Y.: Beiträge zur Entwicklungsgeschichte der menschlichen embryonalen Axillarschweißdrüsen. Okayama Igakkai Zasshi **48**, 1 (1936). Zit. nach M. ENDO 1938. — MORIYAMA, G.: Mikrochemische Untersuchung über die Achseldrüse, insbesondere Berücksichtigung der Osmidrosis axillae. Nagasaki Igakkai Zasshi **5**, 302 (1927). Zit. nach I. YASUI u. H. KAGEMOTO 1961. — MOULÉ, Y.: Endoplasmic reticulum and microsomes of rat liver. In: M. LOCKE, Cellular

membranes in development, p. 97—133. New York and London: Academic Press 1964. — MUNGER, B. L.: The cytology of apocrine sweat glands. I. Cat and monkey. Z. Zellforsch. 67, 373—389 (1965a). — The cytology of apocrine sweat glands. II. Human. Z. Zellforsch. 68, 837—851 (1965b). — MUNGER, B. L., and S. W. BRUSILOW: An electron microscope study of eccrine sweat glands of the cat foot and toe pads — evidence for ductal reabsorption in the human. J. biophys. biochem. Cytol. 11, 403—417 (1961).
NAGAMITSU, G.: Pathologisch-histologische Untersuchungen über die Osmidrosis axillae. Keio Igaku 21, 1011 (1941). Zit. nach I. YASUI u. H. KAGEMOTO 1961. — NAGANO, T.: Some observations on the fine structure of the Sertoli cells in the human testis. Z. Zellforsch. 73, 89—106 (1966). — NEEDHAM, D. M., and C. F. SHOENBERG: Proteins of the contractile mechanism of mammalian smooth muscle and their possible location in the cell. Proc. roy. Soc. B 160, 517—524 (1964). — NEMETSCHEK, H.: Elektronenmikroskopische Untersuchungen an der Gefäßmuskulatur unter Berücksichtigung definierter Funktionsstadien. Med. Klin. 61, 167—168 (1966). — NOVIKOFF, A. B.: Lysosomes and related particles. In: J. BRACHET and A. E. MIRSKY, The cell, p. 423—488. New York and London: Academic Press 1961. — Lysosomes in the physiology and pathology of cells: contributions of staining methods. In: A. V. S. DE REUCK and M. P. CAMERON, Lysosomes, p. 36—73. London: J. & A. Churchill Ltd. 1963.
O'BRIEN, J. P.: Persönliche Mitteilung an H. J. HURLEY u. W. B. SHELLEY 1960. — OHMURA, H., and T. YASUDA: Histochemical investigation on the chondrosulfatase in the sweat glands of the human axilla. In: K. SHIMAI and K. YASUDA, The skin, especially on the sweat glands, p. 153—167. Tokyo/Japan: Gakutjutsu-Tosho-Insatsu Co. Inc. 1961. — OHNO, T., u. H. KINOSHITA: Über die sogenannte apokrine Sekretionsveränderung bei verschiedenen pathologischen Zuständen. Jap. J. Derm. Urol. 27, 32 (1927). Ref. in: Zbl. Haut- u. Geschl.-Kr. 27, 358—359 (1928). — OLIVET, I., u. E. T. NAUCK: Z. ges. exp. Med. 71, 786 (1930). Zit. nach H. J. HURLEY u. W. B. SHELLEY 1960. — ORMEA, F.: Eterotopia nevica delle ghiandole apocrine con degenerazione mucosa del connettivo ed alterazioni vasali. Minerva der. 27, 69—72 (1952). Ref. in: Zbl. Haut- u. Geschl.-Kr. 84, 242 (1953). — OTA, R.: Zytologische und histologische Untersuchungen der apokrinen Schweißdrüsen in den normalen, keinen Achselgeruch (Osmidrosis axillae) gebenden Achselhäuten von Japanern. Arch. anat. Jap. 1, 285—308 (1950). Zit. nach W. MONTAGNA 1962.
PALADE, G. E.: A small particulate component of the cytoplasm. J. biophys. biochem. Cytol. 1, 59—68 (1955). — PALADE, G. E., and P. SIEKEVITZ: Liver microsomes. J. biophys. biochem. Cytol. 2, 171—200 (1956a). — Pancreatic microsomes. J. biophys. biochem. Cytol. 2, 671—690 (1956b). — PANÀ, C.: Ricerche sulle variazioni strutturali delle ghiandole apocrine ascellari in relazione allo stato delle ghiandole sessuali e della mammella. Sperimentale 88, 580—607 (1934). Ref. in: Zbl. Haut- u. Geschl.-Kr. 51, 165—166 (1935). — PEARSE, A. G. E.: Histochemistry, 3rd ed. London: J. & A. Churchill Ltd. 1961. — PEASE, D. C.: Infolded basal plasma membranes found in epithelia noted for their water transport. J. biophys. biochem. Cytol. 2, Suppl. 4, 203—208 (1956). — PERRY, E. T., H. J. HURLEY, M. B. GRAY, and W. B. SHELLEY: The adrenergic innervation of the apocrine (ceruminous) gland of the human ear canal. J. invest. Derm. 25, 219—221 (1955). — PETER, K.: Die Gestalt der Achselstoffdrüsen. Z. mikr.-anat. Forsch. 38, 330—340 (1935). — PETTE, D.: Plan und Muster im zellulären Stoffwechsel. Naturwissenschaften 52, 597—616 (1965). — PETTE, D., u. H. BRANDAU: Enzym-Histiogramme und Enzymaktivitätsmuster der Rattenleber. Enzym. biol. clin. 6, 79—122 (1966). — PETTE, D., u. TH. BÜCHER: Proportionskonstante Gruppen in Beziehung zur Differenzierung der Enzymaktivitätsmuster von Skelett-Muskeln des Kaninchens. Hoppe-Seylers Z. physiol. Chem. 331, 180—195 (1963). — PETTE, D., and W. LUH: Constant-proportion groups of multilocated enzymes. Biochem. biophys. Res. Commun. 8, 283—287 (1962). — PETZOLDT, D., u. O. BRAUN-FALCO: Zur Frage optimaler Reaktionsbedingungen bei der histochemischen Darstellung von Enzymen des Energie-liefernden Stoffwechsels in der Epidermis. II. Aldolase, Tetrazoliumreduktasen, Cytochromoxidase, Ubichinon. Arch. klin. exp. Derm. 227, 1005—1013 (1967). — PINKUS, F.: Die Entwicklungsgeschichte der Haut. In: KEIBEL u. MALL, Handbuch der Entwicklungsgeschichte des Menschen, Bd I, S. 249—295. 1910. Zit. nach J. SCHAFFER 1940. — Zur Kenntnis der menschlichen Schweißdrüsen. Derm. Z. 43, 253—259 (1925). — Zur Histologie der apokrinen Schweißdrüsen. Zbl. Haut- u. Geschl.-Kr. 19, 13 (1926). — Die normale Anatomie der Haut. In: J. JADASSOHN, Handbuch der Haut- und Geschlechtskrankheiten, Bd I, Teil 1, S. 1—378. Berlin: Springer 1927. — PINKUS, H.: Anatomy of the skin. Dermatologica (Basel) 108, 50—51 (1954). — Embryology of hair. In: W. MONTAGNA and R. A. ELLIS, The biology of hair growth, p. 1—32. New York and London: Academic Press 1958. — Die makroskopische Anatomie der Haut. In: O. GANS u. G. K. STEIGLEDER, Normale und pathologische Anatomie der Haut, Bd II. In: A. MARCHIONINI, Handbuch der Haut- und Geschlechtskrankheiten (Hrsg. J. JADASSOHN), S. 1—138. Berlin-Göttingen-Heidelberg-New York: Springer 1966. — PISSOT, L.: Essais sur les glandes du conduit auditive externe. Glandes dites cérumineuses. Thèse de Paris 1899, p. 44. Zit. nach J. SCHAFFER 1940.

Rabl, H.: Histologie der normalen Haut des Menschen. In: F. Mraček, Handbuch der Hautkrankheiten, Bd I, S. 1—163. Wien 1902. — Rassner, G.: Zur enzymatischen Organisation des energieliefernden Stoffwechsels des normalen Meerschweinchens. Arch. klin. exp. Derm. **222**, 391—402 (1965). — Rebaudi, St.: Der Schweißdrüsenapparat während der normalen und pathologischen Schwangerschaft. Hegars Beitr. z. Geburtsh. u. Gynäk. **17**, (1911). Zit. nach L. Waelsch 1913. — Rhodin, J. A. G.: Physiol. Rev. **42**, Suppl. 5, 48 (1962). Zit. nach D. S. Smith 1964. — Richardson, K. C.: Proc. roy. Soc. **136**, 30 (1949). Zit. nach A. Tamarin 1966. — Richter, W.: Beiträge zur normalen und pathologischen Anatomie der apokrinen Hautdrüsen des Menschen mit besonderer Berücksichtigung des Achselhöhlenorgans. Virchows Arch. path. Anat. **287**, 278—296 (1933). — Richter, W., u. W. Schmidt: Über das Vorkommen apokriner Drüsen in der Haut des Nasenflügels. Z. mikr.-anat. Forsch. **35**, 529—532 (1934). Ref. in: Ber. wiss. Biol. **30**, 505 (1934). — Robertson, J. D.: Unit membranes: A review with recent new studies of experimental alterations and a new subunit structure in synaptic membranes. In: M. Locke, Cellular membranes in development, p. 1—81. New York and London: Academic Press 1964. — Robin, Ch.: Note sur une espèce particulière de glandes de la peau de l'homme. Ann. Sc. nat. Sci. III, 380 (1845). Zit. nach J. Schaffer 1940. — Rothman, St.: Physiology and biochemistry of the skin. Chicago: University Press 1954. — Rouiller, Ch.: Physiological and pathological changes in mitochondrial morphology. Int. Rev. Cytol. **9**, 227—292 (1960). — Rupec, M.: Über intercelluläre Verbindungen in normaler menschlicher Epidermis. Arch. klin. exp. Derm. **224**, 32—41 (1966a). — Elektronenmikroskopischer Nachweis von saurer Phosphatase in Granula normaler menschlicher apokriner Schweißdrüsen. Arch. klin. exp. Derm. **225**, 472—479 (1966b). — Über irreguläre Korpuskeln mit kristalliner Innenstruktur in normalen menschlichen apokrinen Schweißdrüsen. Arch. klin. exp. Derm. **228**, 346—351 (1967a). — Zur Ultrastruktur atypisch aussehender Zellen in normalen menschlichen apokrinen Schweißdrüsen. Arch. klin. exp. Derm. **228**, 452—458 (1967b).

Sarkar, K., and E. Kallenbach: Myoepithelial cells in carcinoma of human breast. Amer. J. Path. **49**, 301—307 (1966). — Schaffer, J.: Über die Hautdrüsen. Wien. klin. Wschr. **39**, 1—5 (1926). — Die Hautdrüsenorgane der Säugetiere mit besonderer Berücksichtigung ihres histologischen Aufbaues und Bemerkungen über die Proktodäaldrüsen. Berlin u. Wien: Urban & Schwarzenberg 1940. — Schiefferdecker, P.: Die Hautdrüsen des Menschen und der Säugetiere, ihre biologische und rassenanatomische Bedeutung sowie die Muscularis sexualis. Biol. Zbl. **37**, 534—562 (1917). — Die Hautdrüsen des Menschen und des Säugetieres, ihre Bedeutung, sowie die Muscularis sexualis. Zoologica **72**, 1—154 (1922). — Die Bedeutung des Duftes für das Geschlechts- und Liebesleben des Menschen und der Tiere. Z. Sex.-Forsch. **10**, 137—140 (1923). Ref. in: Zbl. Haut- u. Geschl.-Kr. **13**, 411—412 (1924). — Schmidt, W.: Morphologische Aspekte der Stoffaufnahme und intrazellulären Stoffverarbeitung. In: K. F. Wohlfahrt-Bottermann, Sekretion und Ekretion, S. 147—160. Berlin-Heidelberg-New York: Springer 1965. — Scott, B. L., and D. C. Pease: Electron microscopy of the salivary and lacrimal glands of the rat. Amer. J. Anat. **104**, 115—161 (1959). — Seitz, L.: Über eine mit Schwellung einhergehende Hypersecretion der Schweiß- und Talgdrüsen in der Achselhöhle während des Wochenbettes, echte Milchsekretion vortäuschend. Arch. Gynäk. **80**, 517—531 (1906). — Serri, F.: Studi sulla cute del feto e del bambino. I. Peculiarità nello sviluppo e nella struttura della cute fetale. Boll. Soc. ital. Biol. sper. **36**, 1—6 (1962). — Serri, F., W. M. Huber e H. Mescon: Studi sulla cute del feto e del bambino. III. Attività della fosfatasi acida nella cute del feto. Boll. Soc. ital. Biol. sper. **38**, 1—5 (1962). — Serri, F., W. Montagna, and W. M. Huber: Studies of skin of fetus and the child. Arch. Derm. **87**, 234—245 (1963). — Serri, F., W. Montagna, and H. Mescon: Studies of the skin of the fetus and the child. J. invest. Derm. **39**, 199—217 (1962). — Shelley, W. B.: Apocrine sweat. J. invest. Derm. **17**, 255 (1951). — Shelley, W. B., and T. Butterworth: The absence of the apocrine glands and hair in the axilla in mongolism and idiocy. J. invest. Derm. **25**, 165—167 (1955). — Shelley, W. B., and M. M. Cahn: Experimental studies on the effect of hormones on the human skin with reference to the axillary apocrine sweat gland. J. invest. Derm. **25**, 127—158 (1955). — Shelley, W. B., S. B. Cohen, and G. B. Koelle: Histochemical demonstration of monoamine oxidase in human skin. J. invest. Derm. **24**, 561—565 (1955). — Shelley, W. B., and H. J. Hurley: The physiology of the human axillary apocrine sweat gland. J. invest. Derm. **20**, 285—297 (1953). — Localized chromidrosis. Arch. Derm. Syph. (Chic.) **69**, 449—471 (1954). — An experimental study of the effects of subcutaneous implantation of androgens and estrogens on human skin. J. invest. Derm. **28**, 155—158 (1957). — Shimizu, H.: Electron microscope observation of apocrine sweat gland from the viewpoint of clinical pharmacology. Bull. pharm. Res. Inst. **47**, 1—13 (1963). — Sievers, A.: Funktion des Golgi-Apparates in pflanzlichen und tierischen Zellen. In: K. F. Wohlfahrt-Bottermann, Sekretion und Exkretion, S. 89—111. Berlin-Heidelberg-New York: Springer 1965. — Simonetta, B., e A. Magnoni: Lo sviluppo delle ghiandole sebacee e ceruminose del condotto uditivo esterno nell'uomo. Arch. ital. Anat. Embriol. **39**, 245—261

(1937). Ref. in: Ber. wiss. Biol. **46**, 303 (1938). — SITTE, P.: Allgemeine Mikromorphologie der Zelle. In: H. METZNER, Die Zelle — Struktur und Funktion, S. 7—56. Stuttgart: Wissenschaftliche Verlagsgemeinschaft m.b.H. 1966. — SJÖSTRAND, F. S.: The endoplasmic reticulum. In: G. H. BOURNE, Cytology and cell physiology, p. 311—375. New York and London: Academic Press 1964. — SMITH, D. S.: Skeletal cardiac and smooth muscle. In: S. M. KURTZ, Electron microscopic anatomy, p. 267—293. New York and London: Academic Press 1964. — SPERLING, G.: Die Form der apokrinen Haardrüsen des Menschen. Z. mikr.-anat. Forsch. **38**, 241—252 (1935). — SPIELER, U.: Systematische anatomische Untersuchungen an Schweiß- und Duftdrüsen der Axilla des Menschen. Inaug.-Diss. Kiel 1964. — SPIER, H. W., u. K. MARTIN: Histochemische Untersuchungen über die Phosphomonoesterasen der gesunden Haut mit Hinweis auf Befunde bei Hauterkrankungen. Arch. klin. exp. Derm. **202**, 120—152 (1956). — STAUBESAND, G., B. KUHLO u. K. H. KERSTING: Licht- und elektronenmikroskopische Studien am Nervensystem des Regenwurmes. I. Mitt.: Die Hüllen des Bauchmarkes. Z. Zellforsch. **61**, 401—433 (1963). — STEGNER, H. E.: Elektronenmikroskopische Untersuchungen über die Sekretionsmorphologie des menschlichen Tubenepithels. Arch. Gynäk. **197**, 351—363 (1962). — STEINER, K.: Über die Entwicklung der großen Schweißdrüsen beim Menschen. Z. Anat. Entwickl.-Gesch. **78**, 83—97 (1925). — STRAUS jr., W. L.: The microscopic anatomy of the skin of the gorilla. In: The HENRY CUSHIER RAVEN Memorial volume (ed. W. K. GREGORY). New York: Columbia University Press 1950. — STÜTTGEN, G.: Die normale und pathologische Physiologie der Haut. Stuttgart: Gustav Fischer 1965. — ŠVAJGER, A.: Zur Sekretionsmorphologie menschlicher Endometriumdrüsen. Anat. Anz. **113**, 454—461 (1963). — Über den Begriff und die Definition der apokrinen Sekretion. VIII. Internat. Anatomen-Kongr. Wiesbaden 1965. — SWIFT, J. A., and C. A. SAXTON: The ultrastructural location of the periodate-Schiff-reactive basement membrane at the dermoepidermal junctions of human scalp and monkey gingiva. J. Ultrastruct. Res. **17**, 23—33 (1967). — SZANTO, P. B., F. STEIGMANN, F. PAMUKEN, I. FRIEDMAN, and R. HADOK: Alkoholic hepatitis in delirium tremens. Tijdschrift voor Gastro-enterologie 7b, 288—294 (1964). In: J. VANDENBROUCKE, G. DE GROOTE and L. O. STANDEERT, Advances in hepatology. Basel and New York: S. Karger 1965. — SZODORAY, L.: A heterotopiás apokrin mirigyekröl. Orv. Hetil. **4**, 360—364 (1948). TAKAHASHI, N.: Bull. Tokyo med. dent. Univ. **5**, 177 (1958a). Zit. nach A. TAMARIN 1966. — Bull. Tokyo med. dent. Univ. **4**, 259 (1958b). Zit. nach A. TAMARIN 1966. — TAKAMURA, K.: Cytochemical studies on glandulae vestibularis nasi of cat. Okajimas Folia anat. jap. **31**, 127—134 (1958). — TAMARIN, A.: Myoepithelium of the rat submaxillary gland. J. Ultrastruct. Res. **16**, 320—338 (1966). — TANAKA, K.: Polarisationsoptische Analyse der Axillarorgane des Menschen. Z. Zellforsch. **56**, 632—640 (1962). — TANDLER, B.: Ultrastructure of the human submaxillary gland. III. Myoepithelium. Z. Zellforsch. **68**, 852—863 (1965). — TAPPEINER, S.: Über das Vorkommen apokriner Drüsen in Naevusformationen. Arch. Derm. Syph. (Berl.) **179**, 144—150 (1939). — TARTUFERI, F.: Le glandule di Moll etc. Arch. per le Sc. med. **4**, 91 (1881). Zit. nach J. SCHAFFER 1940. — TAYLOR, A. C.: Microtubules in the microspikes and cortical cytoplasm of isolated cells. J. Cell Biol. **28**, 155—168 (1966). — TEWFIK, H.: Die apokrinen Drüsen der Achselhöhle. Prat. Dokt. (Istanbul) **5/6**, 228—229 (1932). Ref. in: Zbl. Haut- u. Geschl.-Kr. **43**, 619 (1933). — THIES, W.: Die Innervation der apokrinen Drüsen. Acta neuroveg. (Wien) **18**, 192—202 (1958). — THOENES, W.: Diskussionsbemerkung. In: K. E. WOHLFAHRT-BOTTERMANN, Sekretion und Exkretion, S. 25. Berlin-Heidelberg-New York: Springer 1965. — Über matrixreiche Riesenmitochondrien. Z. Zellforsch. **75**, 422—433 (1966).

VEIL, W.: Gibt es anatomische Veränderungen der Schweißdrüsen bei inneren Krankheiten? Dtsch. Arch. klin. Med. **103** (1911). Zit. nach L. WAELSCH 1913. — VOGELL, W.: Strukturelle und funktionelle Biochemie der Mitochondrien. I. Die Morphologie der Mitochondrien. In: P. KARLSON, Funktionelle und morphologische Organisation der Zelle. Berlin-Göttingen-Heidelberg: Springer 1963. — VOHWINKEL, K. H.: Über das Vorkommen von apokrinen Drüsen. Derm. Z. **60**, 314—321 (1931).

WAELSCH, L.: Über Veränderung der Achselschweißdrüsen während der Gravidität. Arch. Derm. Syph. (Berl.) **114**, 140—159 (1913). — WATANABE, H.: A cytochemical study of the human axillary apocrine sweat gland after pilocarpine injection. In: K. SHIMAI and K. YASUDA, The skin, especially on the sweat glands, p. 1—11. Tokyo/Japan: Gakujutsu-Tosho-Insatsu Co. Inc. 1961. — WATZKA, M.: Einige zu besonderen Leistungen differenzierte Zellen im Tierreich. In: H. METZNER, Die Zelle — Struktur und Funktion, S. 150—169. Stuttgart: Wissenschaftliche Verlagsgemeinschaft m.b.H. 1966. — WAY, ST. C., and A. MEMMESHEIMER: The sudoriparous glands. Arch. Derm. Syph. (Chic.) **38**, 373—382 (1938). — WELLINGS, S. R., and G. R. PHILP: The function of the Golgi apparatus in lactating cells of the Balb/c Crlg mouse. Z. Zellforsch. **61**, 871—882 (1964). — WETZSTEIN, R., u. H. WAGNER: Elektronenmikroskopische Untersuchungen am menschlichen Endometrium. Anat. Anz. **108**, 362—375 (1960). — WIMPFHEIMER, C.: Zur Entwicklung der Schweißdrüsen der behaarten Haut. Anat. Hefte **104** (1907). Zit. nach K. STEINER 1925. — WINKELMANN, R. K., and J. V.

HULTIN: Mucinous metaplasia in normal apocrine glands. Arch. Derm. 78, 309—313 (1958). — WINKELMANN, R. K., and H. MONTGOMERY: Fox-Fordyce disease. A histopathologic and histochemical investigation. Arch. Derm. Syph. (Chic.) 74, 63—68 (1956). — WINTER, W., u. O. BRAUN-FALCO: Untersuchungen über die Autolyse der Haut. III. Mitt.: Fluoreszenzmikroskopische Veränderungen. Arch. klin. exp. Derm. 222, 192—201 (1965). — WITTIG, R.: Die topographische Verteilung der Organ-Naevi am behaarten Kopf. Z. Haut- u. Geschl.-Kr. 20, 105—111 (1956). — WOLFF, J.: Elektronenmikroskopische Untersuchungen über die Vesikulation im Kapillarendothel. Z. Zellforsch. 73, 143—164 (1966). — WOOD, M. G., K. PRANICH, and H. BEERMAN: Investigation of possible apocrine gland component in basal cell epithelioma. J. invest. Derm. 30, 273—279 (1958). — WOOLLARD, H. H.: The cutaneous glands of man. J. Anat. (Lond.) 64, 415—421 (1930).

YAMADA, H.: Electron microscopic observations on the secretory processes of the axillary apocrine glands. Acta path. jap. 10, 173—187 (1960). Zit. nach K. YASUDA, R. A. ELLIS u. W. MONTAGNA 1962. — YANAGISAWA, N.: Die Entwicklung der Hautorgane im Nasenvorhof und in der Außenhaut der Nase, insbesondere unter Berücksichtigung der apokrinen-, ekkrinen- und Talgdrüse. Okajimas Folia anat. jap. 30, 129—138 (1957). Ref. in: Ber. wiss. Biol. 121, 140 (1958). — YASUDA, K.: On the non-typical cells in the axillary sweat gland. Okajimas Folia anat. jap. 33, 353—371 (1959). — The combined demonstration of monoamine oxidase and cholinesterase in the same section. Okajimas Folia anat. jap. 38, 139—147 (1962). — Considerations on the histochemical implication of phylogeny and ontogeny of the sweat glands. Riv. istochem. norm. pat. 10 (1963). Ber. del. V. Congr. naz. della Soc. ital. di istochem. Mailand 13.—14. Dez. 1963. — YASUDA, K., R. A. ELLIS, and W. MONTAGNA: The fine structural relationship between mitochondria and light granules in the human apocrine sweat glands. Okajimas Folia anat. jap. 38, 455—483 (1962). — YASUDA, K., H. FURUSAWA, and N. OGATA: Histochemical investigation on the phosphorylase in the sweat glands of axilla. Okajimas Folia anat. jap. 31, 162—169 (1958). — YASUDA, K., H. FURUSAWA, and O. SAEKI: A histochemical study of sweat glands in the axillary area particularly by using alkaline tetrazolium reaction. Okajimas Folia anat. jap. 35, 311—327 (1960). — YASUDA, K., and H. KAGEMOTO: A cytochemical study on the sweat gland of the human axilla (on the coupled tetrazolium reaction). Okajimas Folia anat. jap. 36, 185—193 (1960). — YASUDA, K., H. KAGEMOTO, and K. KOBAYASHI: A histochemical investigation on the sweat gland of human axilla, with special reference to the substances which increase basophilia after oxidation with periodic acid. Okajimas Folia anat. jap. 34, 587—597 (1960). — YASUDA, K., H. MACHIDA, and T. SUZUKI: Presence of cholinesterase-rich fibers around the apocrine sweat glands of japanese axilla. Okajimas Folia anat. jap. 39, 135—149 (1963a). — YASUDA, K., and W. MONTAGNA: Histology and cytochemistry of human skin. XX. The distribution of monoamine oxidase. J. Histochem. Cytochem. 8, 356—365 (1960). — YASUDA, K., T. SUZUKI, and H. MACHIDA: Distribution of phosphorylase in the human sweat glands. Okajimas Folia anat. jap. 39, 151—155 (1963b). — YASUI, I.: On the granules in the axillary apocrine sweat glands of the japanese children. Okajimas Folia anat. jap. 36, 309—328 (1960a). — Histochemical investigation on the axillary sweat glands (eccrine and apocrine glands) during childhood in Japanese, especially on the alkaline and acid phosphatase. Okajimas Folia anat. jap. 35, 275—309 (1960b). — YASUI, I., and H. KAGEMOTO: Histochemical investigation on the axillary sweat glands (eccrine and apocrine glands) during childhood in Japanese, especially on the PAS positive substance and iron. Okajimas Folia anat. jap. 37, 215—245 (1961). — YASUI, I., u. T. SUZUKI: Histochemische Untersuchung der Schweißdrüsen der Achselgegend bei japanischen Kindern mit besonderer Berücksichtigung der Eiweißkörper. Okajimas Folia anat. jap. 6, 123—128 (1961). Ref. in: Ber. wiss. Biol. 168, 243 (1963). — YOSHIMURA, F., and M. IRIE: Trans. 1st Asia and Oceania Regional Congr. Endocrinol. Kyoto 1959, p. 3. Zit. nach K. KUROSUMI 1961.

ZELICKSON, A. S.: Electron microscopy of skin and mucous membrane. Springfield (Ill.): Ch. C. Thomas 1963. — ZORZOLI, G.: Ricerche istochimiche sul pigmento intracellulare delle ghiandole ascellari dell'uomo. I. Boll. Soc. ital. Biol. sper. 26, 138—140 (1950).

Normale Histologie und Histochemie des Nagels

Von

Georges Achten, Brüssel

Mit 34 Abbildungen

Einleitung

Der Nagel ist ein verhorntes Anhangsgebilde der Finger- bzw. Zehenspitzenhaut. Dieses hochspezialisierte Anhängsel spielt im täglichen Leben eine wichtige Rolle:

es schützt vor mancherlei Verletzungen;

es erweist sich nützlich bei den kleinen Handreichungen des Alltags;

es kann als Waffe dienen, die in gewissen Situationen durchaus ihr Recht behauptet;

es hat auch eine ästhetische Funktion, deren Bedeutung nicht unterschätzt werden darf.

Bei den Tieren ist dieser verhornte Schild von noch wesentlich größerem Wert, wie dies die Kralle als Greif- und Scharrwerkzeug oder der Huf der Equiden beweist. Ein kurzer vergleichender Überblick soll die Hauptmerkmale des Aufbaus dieses Gebildes bei verschiedenen Tieren zeigen.

Der Huf, ein Hornfutteral, das einer oder mehreren Zehen eng aufsitzt, besteht, im Querschnitt sichtbar (Abb. 1), aus drei deutlich gesonderten Teilen:

aus der *Hufwand*, dem sichtbaren Teil des Hufs, wenn der Fuß auf dem Boden steht;

aus der *Hornsohle*, einer kreisförmigen Platte, die dem Boden aufliegt;

aus dem gegabelten sog. *Strahl*, welcher der Fingerbeere oder Fingerkuppe entspricht.

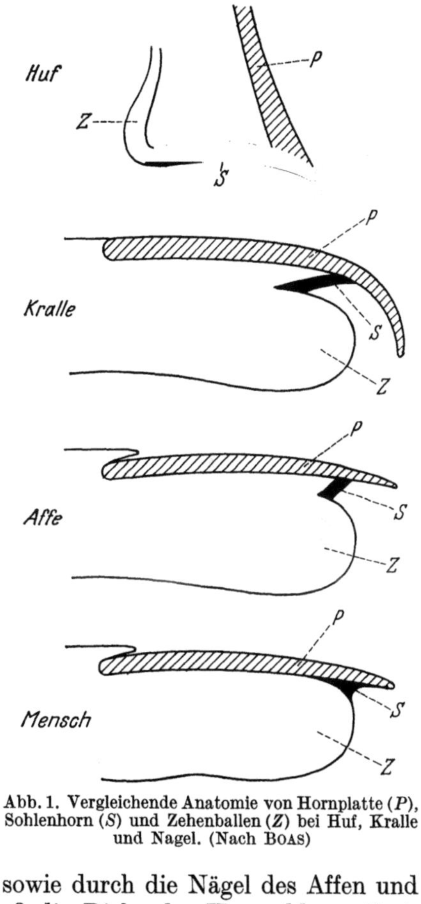

Abb. 1. Vergleichende Anatomie von Hornplatte (*P*), Sohlenhorn (*S*) und Zehenballen (*Z*) bei Huf, Kralle und Nagel. (Nach BOAS)

Schnitte durch die Krallen von Tieren sowie durch die Nägel des Affen und des Menschen (Abb. 1) lassen erkennen, daß die Dicke der Hornsohle variiert, die Nagelplatte aber überall gleichbleibt; bei den Primaten bildet letztere den oberen Teil der Kralle bzw. des Nagels, während hier die Hornsohle mit der Fingerkuppe verschmilzt (BOAS, 1884; BRUHAS, 1910; ZIEGLER, 1954).

A. Anatomie des Nagels
I. Die Nageleinheit

Gleich dem Haar ist der Nagel ein keratinisierter Anhang der Epidermis. Man kann daher zwischen diesen beiden Gebilden Parallelen ziehen. Ebenso wie man

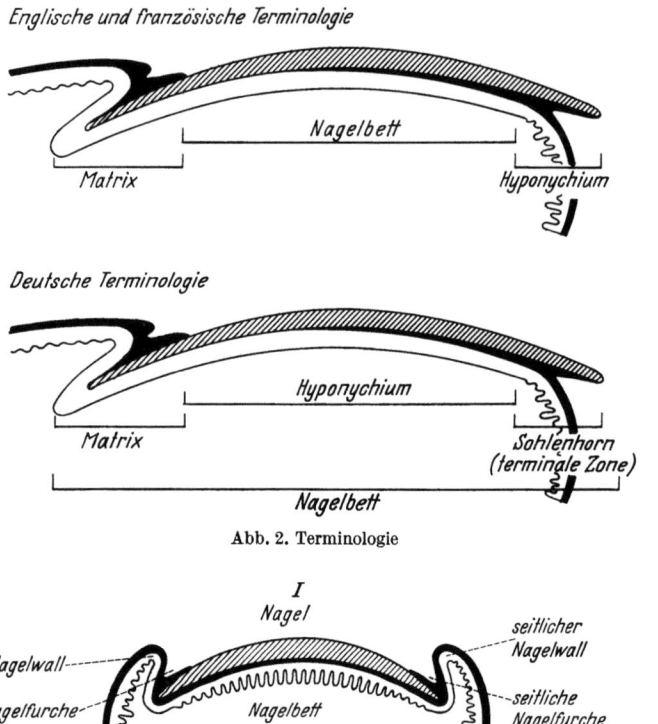

Abb. 2. Terminologie

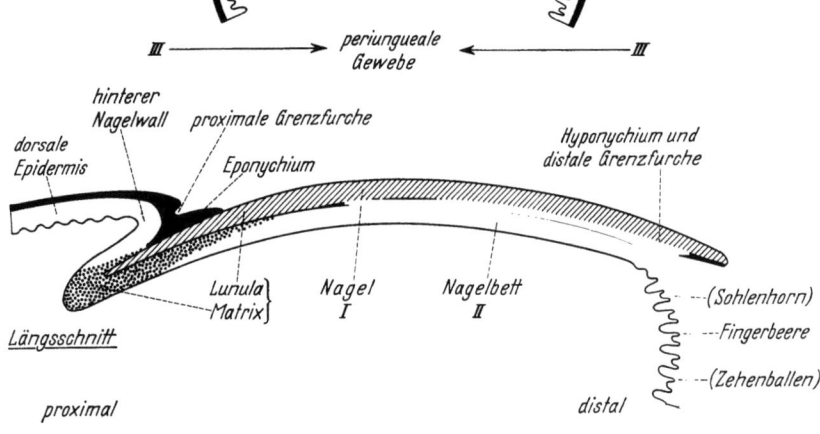

Abb. 3. Schema der Anatomie des Nagels im Querschnitt und Längsschnitt

von einer follikulären Einheit spricht, die aus dem eigentlichen Haar und seiner Matrix, der inneren und äußeren von der Epidermis gebildeten Wurzelscheide sowie aus dem perifollikulären Gewebe besteht, gibt es eine Einheit des Nagels.

Sie umfaßt die Nagelmatrix, die die Nagelplatte — den eigentlichen Nagel — hervorbringt, das Nagelbett, auf dem diese Platte ruht, und das periungueale Gewebe, das mit den beiden erstgenannten Regionen verwachsen ist.

Was die *Terminologie* betrifft (Abb. 2), unterscheiden die französisch- und englischsprachigen Autoren, von der proximalen Region bis zur distalen Region, Matrix, Nagelbett und Hyponychium.

Unter Hyponychium verstehen die deutschsprachigen Autoren die Zone, die bei dem distalen Teil der ungueaIen Matrix anfängt und am Sohlenhorn endigt, oftmals auch „Terminale Zone" genannt. Für diese Autoren besteht das Nagelbett aus Matrix, Hyponychium und Sohlenhorn.

In diesem Kapitel benützen wir die erst erwähnte Terminologie und, in Klammern, geben wir, sowohl im Text als auf den Bildern, den korrespondierenden deutschen Begriff.

Ein Längsschnitt durch die Fingerspitze (Abb. 3) erlaubt es, die Bestandteile der Nageleinheit voneinander zu unterscheiden.

1. Nagelmatrix

Aus der *Nagelmatrix*, einer Einstülpung der Epidermis des Fingerrückens, geht der eigentliche Nagel hervor, der von proximal nach distal wächst. Der Nagel selbst (Abb. 4) besteht aus einer harten, rechteckigen, dorsal-konvexen Platte, die

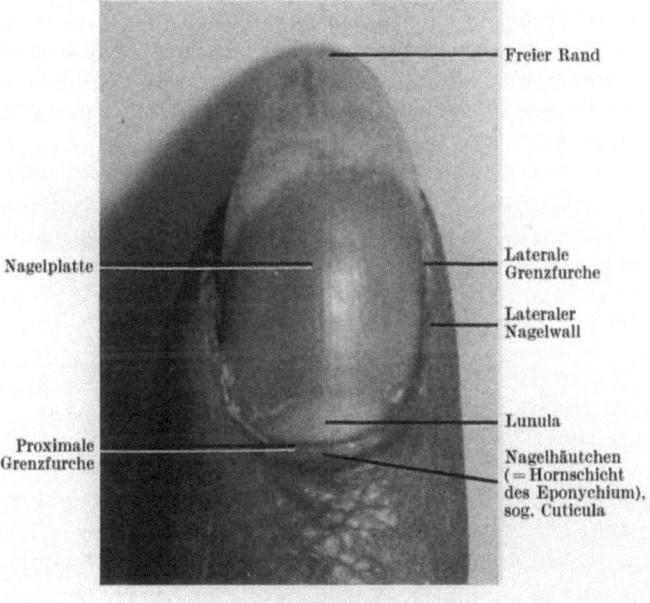

Abb. 4. Anatomie des Nagels

bei der Hand eine größere Längsachse, beim Fuß eine größere Querachse hat. Der proximale, aus der Nagelwurzel hervorgehende Teil bildet die *Lunula* des Nagels, eine weiße Zone, deren konvexes vorderes Ende in den rosafarbenen Teil der Nagelplatte übergeht. Die äußere Oberfläche des Nagels ist glatt; die innere Seite dagegen weist parallele Längsleisten auf, die genau in die Vertiefungen des Nagelbettes, auf dem der Nagel ruht, hineinpassen. Wird ein Nagel ausgerissen, dann kann man diese Striae auf seiner Innenseite sehen, so wie auf Abb. 3 beim Querschnitt durch die Fingerextremität.

2. Nagelplatte

Die Nagelplatte schiebt sich während ihres Wachstums auf das *Nagelbett* (Hyponychium, Abb. 3). Dieses wird aus der dorsalen Haut der Fingerspitze gebildet, verhornt, verstärkt dadurch die Dicke des Nagels, und hängt mit ihm eng zusammen.

3. Periunguiale Gewebe

Von dem *periunguialen Gewebe* (Abb. 3) unterscheidet man, abgegrenzt durch die Nagelfurchen, beim proximalen Teil das Eponychium und beim distalen Teil das Hyponychium (Sohlenhorn oder Terminalzone), das sich in die Fingerbeere fortsetzt.

a) Die Nagelfurchen

Die *Nagelfurchen* begrenzen den Nagel. Man unterscheidet proximale, distale und laterale Nagelfurchen. Nach Extraktion des Nagels wird auch die Nageltasche (Sinus unguis) sichtbar. Die distale Nagelfurche auf der Höhe des Sohlenhorns wird durch die Nagelplatte verdeckt. Dagegen sind die proximalen und lateralen Furchen durch die Epidermis der proximalen und lateralen Region deutlich markiert. Sie überragen den Nagel und bilden den Nagelwall. Der Nagel fügt sich in diese Taschen in ähnlicher Weise ein wie ein Uhrglas in seine Fassung (Pardo-Castello, 1960).

b) Das Eponychium

Das *Eponychium* wird durch die dorsale Oberhaut im Gebiet der proximalen Furche gebildet. Seine verhornte Schicht setzt sich auf dem proximalen Teil der Nagelplatte fort und bildet das *Nagelhäutchen*, das die Nagelplatte ein kurzes Stück weit zudeckt.

c) Das Hyponychium

Das *Hyponychium* (Sohlenhorn) liegt zwischen dem distalen Ende des Nagelbettes und der distalen Furche am Fingerende. Diese distale Furche läuft quer über das Fingerende und grenzt Nagelbett und Fingerkuppe voneinander ab (Abb. 3).

d) Die Fingerkuppe

Die *Fingerkuppe* entspricht dem konvexen Ende des Fingers. Sie ist der vordere Teil der Fingerbeere.

II. Der Altersnagel

Der Nagel verändert sich mit dem Alter (Lewis und Montgomery, 1955). Der Altersnagel hat seinen Glanz verloren, er ist matt und weniger durchsichtig, seine Längsstreifen werden immer deutlicher und zahlreicher. Er ist dünner oder dicker als der normale Nagel, und die Lunula wird vom Eponychium überdeckt. Die laterale Konvexität wird stärker, diejenige in der Längsrichtung nimmt ab. Sprünge in den Nagelrändern treten auf, das Nagelwachstum verlangsamt sich.

B. Embryologie

Mit der Untersuchung der Entwicklung des Fingerendes haben sich schon Zander (1866) und Kölliker (1888) befaßt. In jüngster Zeit haben Pinkus (1910, 1927), Lewis (1954), Achten (1959/63) und Zaias (1963) diese Forschungen im einzelnen sowohl makroskopisch wie mikroskopisch weiterverfolgt.

I. Makroskopische Untersuchung

Makroskopisch können an den Händen die ersten digitalen Anlagen beim 6wöchigen, an den Füßen beim 7—8 Wochen alten Embryo beobachtet werden. Die erste Nagelstruktur ist nach 10 Wochen an der Endphalanx des Fingers festzustellen. Eine quadratische glatte Fläche, welche durch eine kontinuierliche

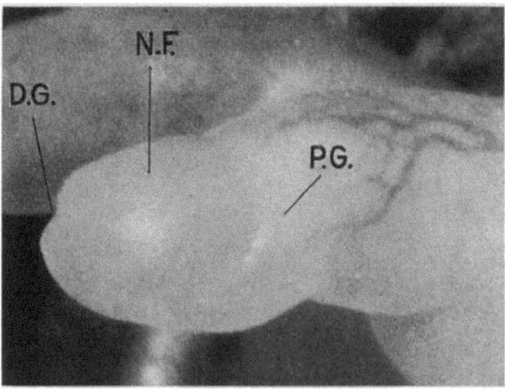

Abb. 5. Fingerende eines $2^{1}/_{2}$ Monate alten Embryos. *D.G.* Distale Grenzfurche. *N.F.* Nagelfeld. *P.G.* Proximale Grenzfurche. (Aus ZAÏAS, 1963)

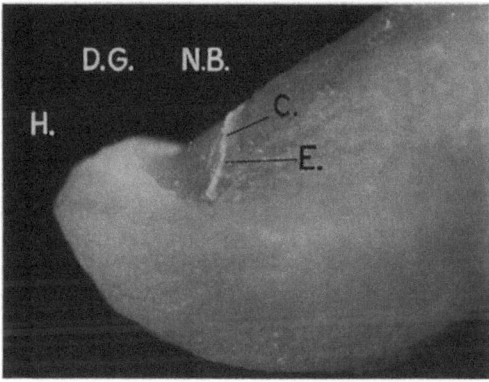

Abb. 6. Fingerende eines $3^{1}/_{2}$ Monate alten Embryos. *H* Hyponychium (Sohlenhorn). *D.G.* Distale Grenzfurche. *N.B.* Nagelbett. *C.* Cuticula (Nagelhäutchen). *E* Eponychium. (Aus ZAÏAS, 1963)

Furche an der Oberfläche abgegrenzt ist, bildet das *Nagelfeld* oder die *primäre Basis* des Nagels (Abb. 5). Nach 11 Wochen sind die proximalen sowie die lateralen Furchen deutlich entwickelt. Die distale Furche ist stärker abgegrenzt und infolge der Entwicklung der Fingerbeere besser sichtbar.

Während der Finger sich streckt und das Ende sich zuspitzt, läßt sich die Nagelplatte an ihrer glatten Oberfläche nach 14 Wochen erkennen. Sie erscheint unter der proximalen Nagelfurche (Abb. 6). Nach 16 Wochen bedeckt diese noch dünne Nagelplatte die Hälfte des Nagelbettes. Der proximale Nagelwulst, das Nagelhäutchen und die distale Nagelfurche sind gut sichtbar. Je mehr der Nagel wächst, um so flacher wird die distale Furche.

Von diesem Augenblick an bis zur Geburt sind die Veränderungen allein durch das Wachstum bedingt. Das Gebiet der Nagelwurzel und der Nagel wird breiter.

Die Nagelplatte erreicht im Bereich der 20. Woche allmählich die distale Leiste. In der 24. Woche überragt die Nagelplatte diese distale Leiste, die sich abflacht und das Hyponychium (Sohlenhorn oder Terminalzone) bildet.

Der Nagel des geburtsreifen Kindes läßt sich mit demjenigen des Erwachsenen vergleichen, nur ist er dünner und weicher. Er reicht bis zum Ende der Fingerbeere, über das er gebogen ist. Bei manchen Fingern ist die Lunula bereits vorhanden.

II. Mikroskopische Untersuchung

Dieser makroskopischen Entwicklung entsprechen histologische Veränderungen (PINKUS, 1910—1927; LEWIS, 1954; ACHTEN, 1959/63; ZAIAS, 1963).

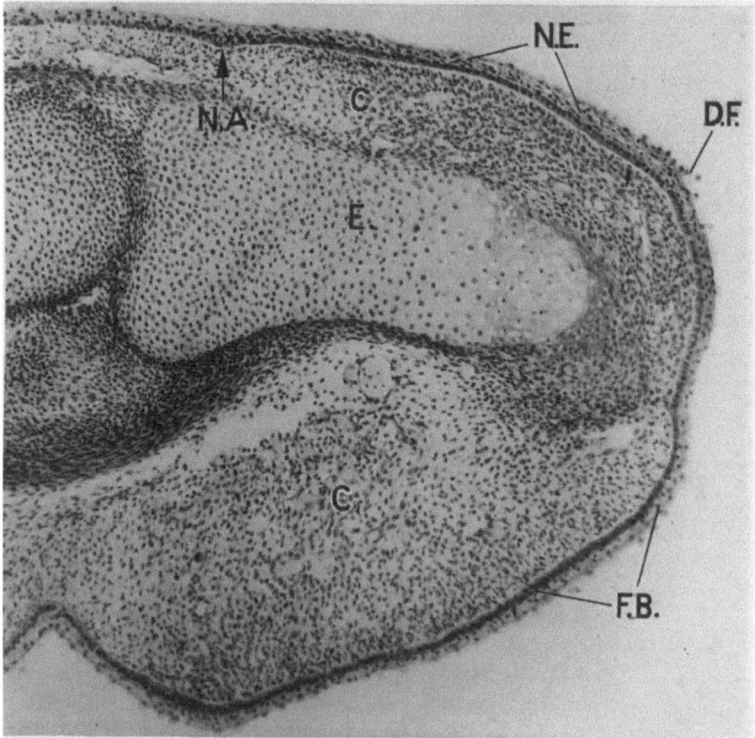

Abb. 7. Längsschnitt durch das Fingerende eines Embryos von 2¹/₂ Monaten. Nichtdifferenzierte Periode. *N.A.* Nagelanlage. *N.F.* Nagelfeld. *D.F.* Dorsale Feder (Epidermiswucherung). *F.B.* Fingerbeere. *E.* Endphalanx. *C.* Corium (nicht differenziertes)

Die Entwicklung des Fingerendes während ihrer ersten Stadien kann mit derjenigen der gesamten Haut verglichen werden. Die Epidermis besteht zuerst aus einer und dann aus zwei Zellschichten (Basalschicht und Periderm); die Lederhaut ihrerseits wird aus nichtdifferenzierten Mesenchymzellen gebildet. Diese Periode erstreckt sich über die ersten beiden Entwicklungsmonate und entspricht der nichtdifferenzierten oder afibrillären Entwicklungsperiode (Abb. 7). In der Tat sind während dieses Stadiums weder Keratin-, Retikulin-, Kollagen- noch Elastinfasern zu finden.

Erst in der 9. Woche läßt sich auf cellulärer Ebene eine Differenzierung feststellen (ZAIAS, 1963). Die Basalzellen sind mehr aneinandergehäuft und entsprechen der zukünftigen Nagelanlage. Sie bereitet die zweite Periode vor, die man als differenzierte oder fibrilläre bezeichnet und in der die verschiedenen Anhangselemente sowie die Fasern der Epidermis und der Lederhaut in Erscheinung treten (ACHTEN, 1959).

Die mikroskopische Untersuchung dieser zweiten Entwicklungsperiode ermöglicht es, die Herkunft der verschiedenen Bestandteile des Nagels und der ihn umgebenden Gewebe genau festzustellen.

1. Der Nagel und seine Matrix

Im Verlauf des 3. Schwangerschaftsmonats bildet eine Einstülpung der dorsalen Epidermis des Fingerendes die erste Andeutung des Nagels (Abb. 7). Man

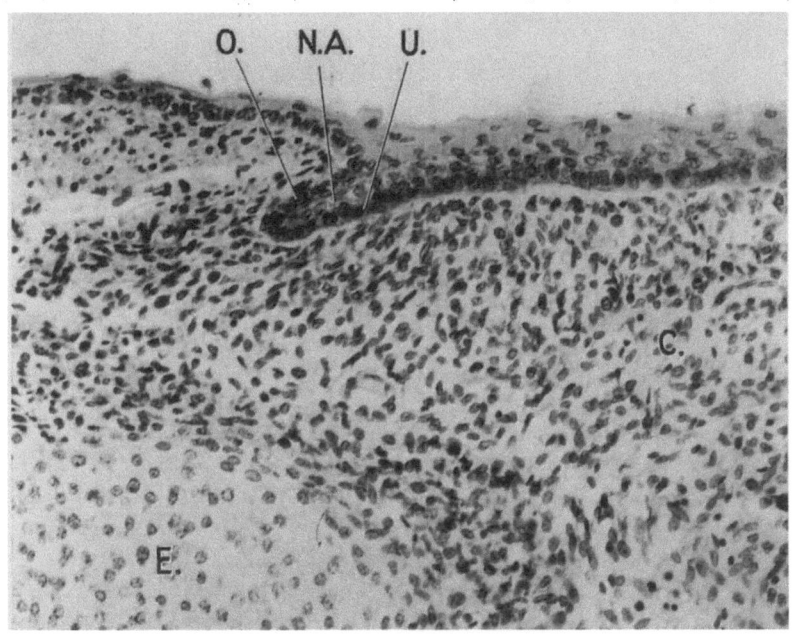

Abb. 8. Längsschnitt durch das Fingerendglied eines Embryos von 3¹/₂ Monaten mit der Anlage der Nagelmatrix (Wurzelblatt). *N.A.* Nagelanlage (Matrix). *O.* Oberlippe. *U.* Unterlippe. *C.* Corium. *E.* Endphalanx

nennt diesen Sporn aus Epidermis Wurzelblatt (nach KÖLLIKER) oder Nagelknospe (bourgeon unguéal); er besteht an der Peripherie aus stark basophilen Basalzellen und im Zentrum aus Stachelzellen.

Die Nagelknospe setzt sich aus zwei Lippen zusammen: einer oberen Lippe und einer unteren Lippe (Abb. 8). Aus der unteren Lippe und dem proximalen Teil der oberen Lippe wird die Nagelmatrix gebildet, aus der sich der eigentliche Nagel oder die Nagelplatte entwickelt. Mit dem Erscheinen des Nagels wird das Wurzelblatt zur Nageltasche (Nagelfalz, Sinus unguis). Die Nagelplatte wächst von hinten nach vorne und ruht auf dem Ende des dorsalen Teils des Fingers, den man als Nagelbett (Hyponychium) bezeichnet.

Querschnitte durch das Endglied zeigen, daß das proximale Ende der Nageltasche sich als eine horizontale Zone aus Epidermiszellen präsentiert, die in einem nach oben konvexen Bogen angeordnet sind. Dieser Bogen überspannt ein an horizontal verlaufenden Capillaren reiches Bindegewebe. Darunter befinden sich eine fibröse Verdichtung und weite, lacunäre Gefäße (LEWIS, 1954).

2. Das Nagelbett (Hyponychium)

Die Entwicklung des Nagelbettes ist mit derjenigen der Oberflächenhaut vergleichbar.

Während der ersten Entwicklungsstadien setzt sich diese Epidermis zuerst aus einer, dann aus zwei cellulären Schichten (Basalschicht und Periderm) zusammen. Während der Entwicklung der Nagelknospe treten Zwischenschichten auf, aus denen das Stratum spinosum hervorgeht.

Im Verlauf der ersten Entwicklungsstadien kann man eine Schicht von Keratohyalinkörnern beobachten. Später, gegen den 6. Monat zu, verschwindet diese Granulaschicht wieder. Die Keratinisierung erfolgt direkt, ohne Übergang; manche Zellen sind parakeratotisch, während andere ihren Kern verlieren.

Die so gebildete Schicht haftet an der Unterseite des Nagels fest, dessen Dicke sie damit leicht verstärkt (LEWIS, 1954; ZIEGLER, 1954; ACHTEN, 1959).

Am distalen Ende des Nagelbettes bildet eine Erhebung während ihres Wachsens die sog. ,,Dorsalfeder" (LEWIS, 1954), das spätere Terminalhorn — die zweite Komponente des Sohlenhorns (Abb. 7). Diese Epidermiswucherung besteht aus einer Schicht von mehreren verhornten Zellagen. Eine dichte Schicht von Keratohyalinkörnern liegt unter dieser keratinisierten Zone von kugelförmigen, nicht aneinanderklebenden Zellen, die der Desquamation anheimfallen.

Gegen den 6. Schwangerschaftsmonat erreicht die Nagelplatte diese Region der Dorsalfeder, welche abblättert und zunächst eine der distalen Nagelfurche entsprechende Vertiefung hinterläßt. Diese wird beim weiteren Wachstum des Nagels wieder flacher und bildet schließlich das Hyponychium (Terminalhorn).

3. Das periunguiale Gewebe
(Abb. 9)
a) Das Eponychium

Das *Eponychium* entspricht der Einstülpungsstelle der dorsalen Epidermis und der Oberlippe der hinteren Nagelfurche und wächst parallel zur Oberhaut und mit

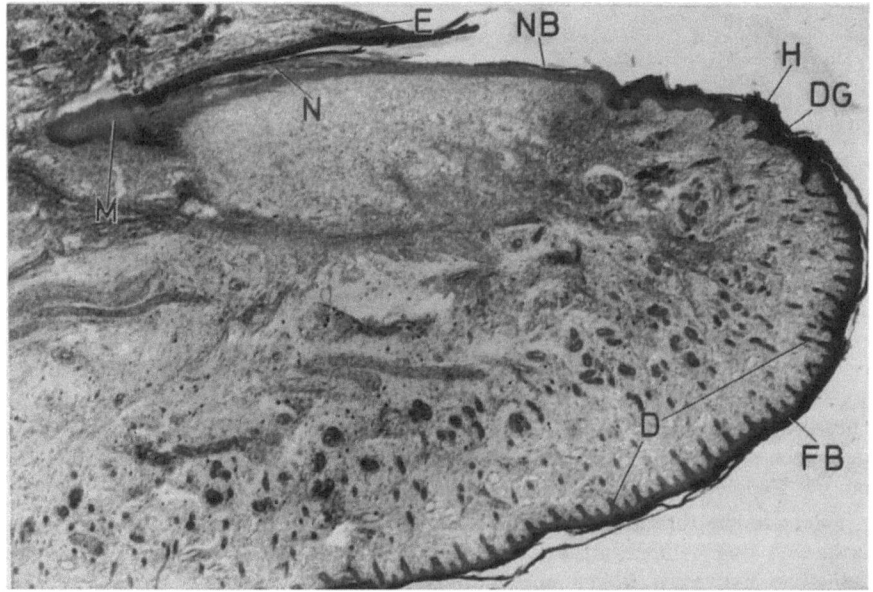

Abb. 9. Fingerende eines Embryos von 5½ Monaten. Längsschnitt. Der Bau ist derselbe wie beim Erwachsenen. *M* Matrix. *E.* Eponychium. *N* Nagel. *N.B.* Nagelbett (Hyponychium). *D.G.* Distale Grenzfurche. *H* Hyponychium (Sohlenhorn oder terminale Zone). *D* Drusenleisten. *F.B.* Fingerbeere

deren Entwicklung gleichlaufend heran. Die Anlage dazu wird im 5. Schwangerschaftsmonat gelegt. Das Eponychium verdickt sich progressiv, bedeckt zunächst die ersten Nagellamellen, dann den ganzen Nagel und bildet schließlich das Nagelhäutchen (Abb. 9).

b) Das Hyponychium

Das *Hyponychium* (Sohlenhorn oder Terminalzone) bietet während den ersten Entwicklungsstadien den Aspekt der Dorsalfeder (LEWIS, 1954). Diese Dorsalfeder aus mehreren Lagen keratinisierter Kugelzellen wird von der Nagelplatte während ihres Wachstums dissoziiert, und es entsteht die distale Nagelfurche. Gegen den 6. Entwicklungsmonat füllt sich die Furche mit Keratin des distalen Teils des Nagelbettes und bildet so das Hyponychium (Sohlenhorn) (Abb. 9).

c) Die Fingerbeere

Die *Fingerbeere* (Torus tactilis terminalis) entwickelt sich gleichzeitig mit dem Handteller. Genau wie die Epidermis des ganzen Tegumentes wird ihr Epithel aus einer, später aus zwei Zellschichten gebildet. Die Basalschicht besteht aus

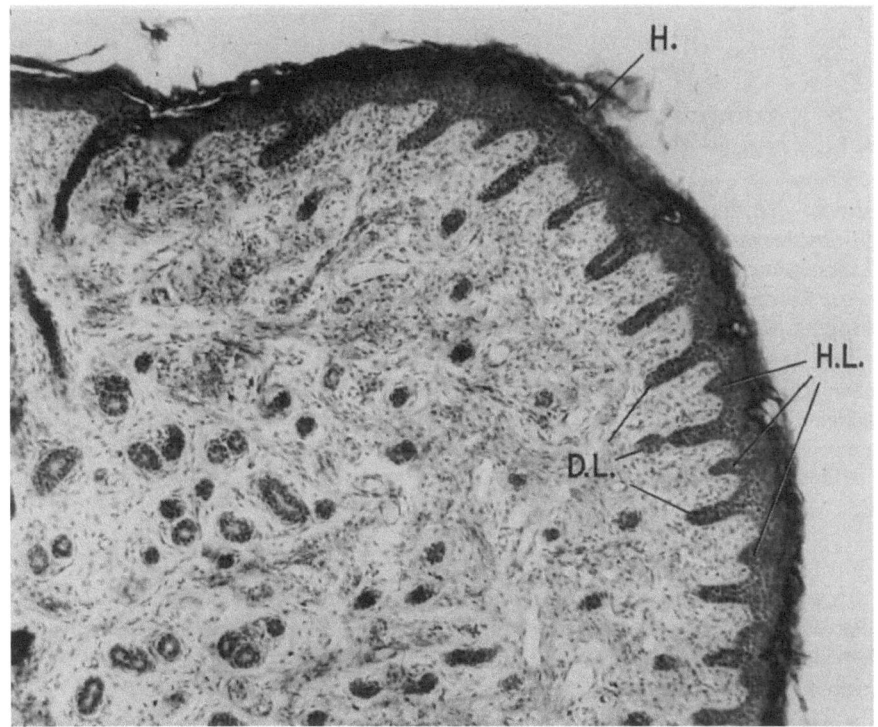

Abb. 10. Haftleisten (*H.L.*) und Drüsenleisten (*D.L.*). *H.* Hyponychium (Sohlenhorn)

kubischen Zellen und erscheint deutlicher individualisiert. Das Stratum spinosum entwickelt sich progressiv. Gegen den 5. Schwangerschaftsmonat erscheint die Granulaschicht. Ihre Dicke sowie die Zahl der Granulationen nehmen bis zum 10. Schwangerschaftsmonat zu.

Fingerbeere und Zehenballen sowie die Hand- und Fußfläche sind besonders interessante Gebiete, um die Embryologie der Schweißdrüsen und Schweiß-kanälchen zu untersuchen (Abb. 9 und 10). Diese Gebilde sind hier reichlich vorhanden, und kein anderer Epidermisanhang stört ihre Entwicklung. Die erste Anlage der Schweißdrüsen tritt zu Beginn des 4. Monats auf in Form regelmäßiger Leisten der Basalschicht. Man beobachtet darin Zellanhäufungen, welche die Anlagen für die Schweißdrüsen darstellen. Diese breiten sich aus und dringen immer tiefer in die Lederhaut ein. An ihrem Ende sind sie leicht verdickt. Der glanduläre Teil differenziert sich mit 5 Monaten: er setzt sich aus Anhäufungen von Kugelzellen zusammen, die tief im Corium liegen. Diese Gebilde zeigen erst nach $5^{1}/_{2}$ Monaten ein Lumen. Zur gleichen Zeit lassen sich Kanalzone und Drüsenzone histologisch unterscheiden.

Im 7. Monat sind Drüse und Kanal vollständig ausgebildet. Der glanduläre Teil erreicht die oberste Schicht des Unterhautfettgewebes, das sich ebenfalls im 7. Monat zu differenzieren beginnt.

Die aus den Epidermisleisten gebildeten Haftkämme, die mit den Einmündungen der Schweißdrüsen alternieren, beginnen sich zu Anfang des 6. Monats zu formen. Sie entwickeln sich zunehmend und sind im 7. oder 8. Monat vollständig ausgebildet. In der Oberhaut kommen sie in Form der Papillar- oder Tastleisten zum Ausdruck, deren Anordnung sich in den Fingerabdrücken widerspiegelt.

d) Lederhaut und Subcutis

Die Entwicklung der Lederhaut (Corium) geht in jeder Hinsicht genau gleich wie beim übrigen Tegument vor sich.

Ebenso wie bei der Epidermis unterscheidet man eine erste Periode (Abb. 7), während der die Zellen noch nicht differenziert sind (undifferenzierte Periode), von einer sowohl cellulär wie fibrillär differenzierten Periode. Vom 3. Schwangerschaftsmonat an entstehen neben den sternförmigen Mesenchymzellen Histiocyten, Fibrocyten und Lymphocyten. Zur gleichen Zeit künden sich Endothelbildungen an, die ausgedehnte Capillarschlingen hervorbringen.

Die Retikulin-, Kollagen- und Elastinfasern bilden sich während der zweiten Entwicklungsperiode. Die Subcutis taucht im 6. Monat auf, und die Fettschicht erscheint im 8. Monat deutlich differenziert. Die der Endphalanx entsprechende knorpelige Differenzierung hat bereits in der zweiten Hälfte des 3. Monats stattgefunden (ZAIAS, 1963).

4. Die drei Nagelschichten

LEWIS (1954) hat die Silberfärbung für modifizierte Proteine nach BODIAN und MOSKOWICKI angewendet und gezeigt, daß der Nagel aus drei Schichten besteht. Diese drei Lagen (Abb. 11), die auch bei anderen Färbungen beobachtet werden konnten (ACHTEN, 1959/63), umfassen:

eine Dorsalschicht, welche dem proximalen Teil der Oberlippe der Nagelanlage entspricht;

eine Intermediärschicht (oder Zwischenschicht), die der unteren Lippe der Nagelanlage entspricht;

eine ventrale Schicht, die dem Keratin des Nagelbettes entspricht und daher keinen der Nagelwurzel entstammenden Bestandteil darstellt.

Der dorsale und der ventrale Nagel haben in bezug zum Intermediärnagel ungefähr die gleiche Dicke wie die Epidermis, wenn man sie mit der Lederhaut vergleicht.

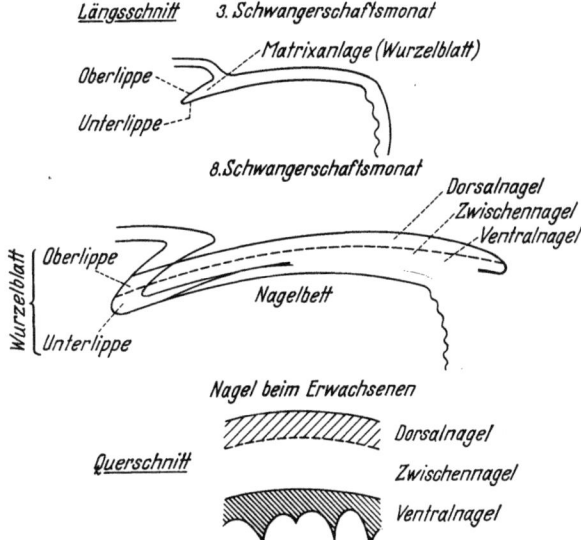

Abb. 11. Die drei Schichten des Nagels. Auftreten der Nagelanlage im 3. Schwangerschaftsmonat mit einer oberen und einer unteren Lippe. Mit dem 8. Schwangerschaftsmonat hat der Nagel seine definitive Struktur, wie man sie beim Erwachsenen beobachten kann. Der dorsale Nagel entspricht dem proximalen Teil der Oberlippe der Nagelwurzel. Der Zwischennagel entspricht der Unterlippe der Nagelwurzel. Der ventrale Nagel entspricht dem Keratin des Nagelbettes. Diese drei Schichten werden im Querschnitt durch den Nagel sichtbar

C. Histologie
I. Der Nagel und seine Matrix

Die Nagelmatrix, welche embryologisch aus der Basalschicht der Epidermis hervorgeht (Wurzelblatt), hat dieselbe Struktur wie das Oberflächenepithel allgemein. Sie enthält eine Basalschicht von nebeneinander angeordneten kubischen Zellen, die sich in der Nagelwurzelgegend nicht von den Basalzellen der Oberhaut des Fingerrückens oder denjenigen des Nagelbettes unterscheiden. Die Basalschicht ist von polyedrischen Zellen überlagert, die das Stratum spinosum (die Malpighische Schicht) bilden. Diese Zellen werden distal zunehmend länger und keratinisieren. LEWIS (1954) hat die besonderen Vorgänge bei der Bildung der Nagelzellen beschrieben. Die dorsale Nagelschicht entsteht im proximalen Teil der Oberlippe der Nagelmatrix durch einen Inflations-Deflationsprozeß: Anschwellen der Zelle (Makrocytose), Verschwinden des Kerns (Karyolyse), zuletzt Abflachung (Kollaps). Die so gebildete Zelle findet ihren Platz in der Nagelmasse. Der Zwischennagel entsteht in der Unterlippe der Nagelmatrix in einem Prozeß, welchen LEWIS als „Gradient der Parakeratose" bezeichnet hat. Während dieses Vorgangs zeigen die Epidermiszellen zuerst eine zunehmende Verbreiterung und Abflachung unter länger dauernder Erhaltung des Kerns. Man findet bei dieser Umwandlung der Basalzelle zur Ungualzelle keine Keratohyalinkörnchen (LEWIS, 1954; ACHTEN, 1959).

Die weiße Farbe der Nagellunula wurde der Tatsache zugeschrieben, daß die noch nicht ganz verhornten Zellen ihre Keratohyalinkörnchen zurückhalten. Jedoch findet BURROWS (1919) keine besondere histologische Struktur in dieser Nagelzone. Diesem Autor zufolge stammt die weiße Farbe dieser Zone von der Lichtreflexion an der Nageloberfläche, da das der Lunula entsprechende Nagelgebiet nicht mit der darunterliegenden Dermis zusammenhängt, im Gegensatz zur eng mit dem Nagelbett und der darunterliegenden Lederhaut verwachsenen rosafarbigen Zone des Nagels.

Die Wachstumsrichtung des Nagels wird durch den Blindsack bestimmt, in welchem er gebildet wird (KLIGMAN, 1961). Dieser Blindsack (Sinus unguis = Nagelfalz) (Abb. 12) gestattet das Nagelwachstum nur in einer Richtung und bewirkt damit ein Gleiten der Hornzellen gegen das distale Gebiet. Während die Hornzellen der Oberhaut über dem Teil der Basalschicht liegen, aus dem sie entstanden sind, entfernen sie sich im Bereich des Nagels in distaler Richtung von den entsprechenden Basalzellen. Wird die Wurzelregion in den Unterarm transplantiert und damit der proximale Blindsack ausgeschaltet, dann bildet sich das Nagel-

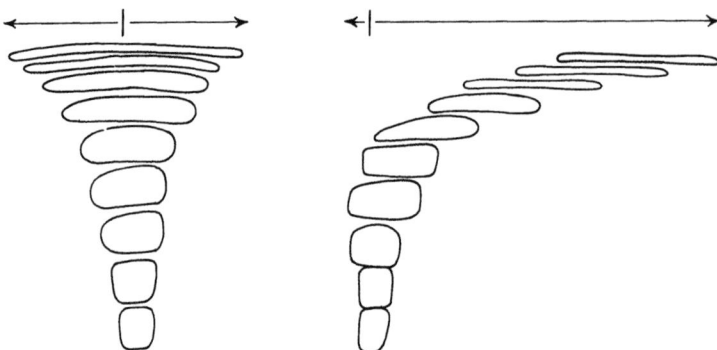

Abb. 12. Entwicklung der Hornzellen der Oberflächenhaut und der Nagelzellen, die infolge des Vorhandenseins der Nageltasche (Sinus unguis) nach distal gleiten. (Aus: KLIGMAN, 1961)

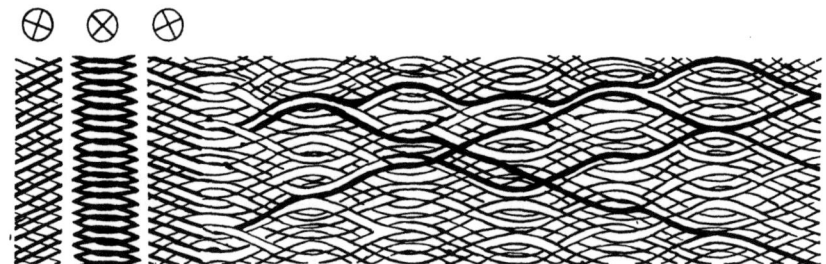

Abb. 13. Schematische Darstellung der Wellung und Verflechtung der Tonofibrillenbündel in der Nagelsubstanz am Querschnitt. Links zeigen die dicken Linien die maximal aufleuchtenden Fibrillenstrecken bei der darüber angegebenen Polarisator-Analysatorstellung. Rechts ist in dünnen Linien der bogige Verlauf der Wellen und Gegenwellen dargestellt. Die dickeren Linien kennzeichnen beobachtete stärkere durchlaufende Züge. An ihnen soll hier die Möglichkeit der Verflechtung von Fibrillenbündeln gezeigt werden. Jeder Strich ist als ein Bündel von Tonofibrillen anzusehen. (Aus: HORSTMANN, 1957)

keratin vertikal in gleicher Weise wie die Hornschicht der umgebenden Epidermis. Die quere Verteilung der Nagelmatrix-Zellen soll ebenfalls in der Orientierung des Nagelwachstums eine Rolle spielen.

Mitosen kann man im Bereich der Basalschicht und den tieferen Lagen des Stratum spinosum beobachten.

Die Tonofibrillen der Nagelsubstanz sind doppeltbrechend. Mit dem Polarisationsmikroskop haben PORT (1933) und besonders HORSTMANN (1955) ihre Anordnung untersucht. PORT zeigte, daß die Fasern des dorsalen und ventralen Nagels in Längsrichtung verlaufen, während die Fasern des Zwischennagels quergerichtet sind. HORSTMANN (1955) hat aufgrund einer genaueren Analyse festgestellt, daß die Struktur komplexer ist (Abb. 13). Die Faserbündel sind in der Tat ineinander verflochten und in Bogen oder Wellen angeordnet. Im Bereich der Nagelwurzel wird im polarisierten Licht eine feine Streifung erkennbar.

Der normale Nagel ist nicht pigmentiert, außer beim Neger (MONASH, 1932). Bei diesem erscheint die Pigmentierung in Form von Streifen; seltener ist sie diffus. Die dem Melanin zugeschriebene Pigmentierung ist besonders in den tieferen Nagelschichten verteilt. Bei der Geburt ist sie noch nicht vorhanden und nimmt mit dem Alter zu. Sie ist um so stärker, je dunkler die Hautfarbe ist.

II. Das Nagelbett (Hyponychium)

Das Nagelbett (Hyponychium), die Unterlage der Nagelplatte (früher auch „steriler Teil des Nagelbettes" genannt), weist eine Basalschicht von kubischen Zellen auf, die proximal an die Nagelmatrix und distal an die Fingerkuppe anschließen.

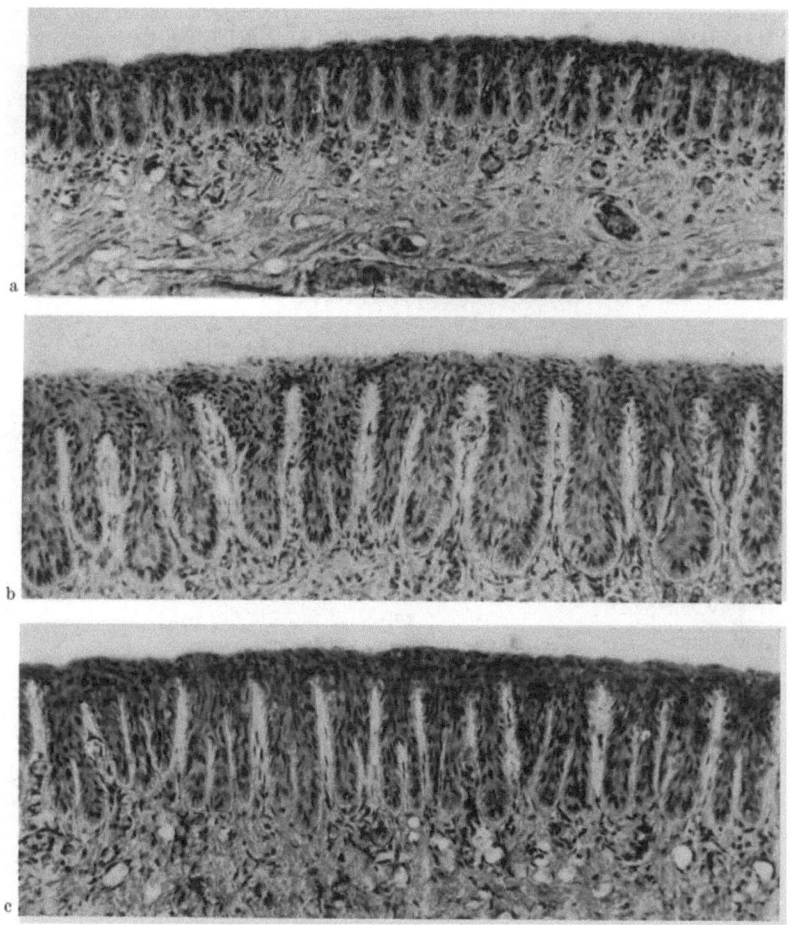

Abb. 14a—c. Querschnitte durch das Nagelbett (Hyponychium) desselben Nagels. a Unmittelbar distal der Lunula. b Mitte des Nagelbettes (Hyponychium). c Etwa 1 mm proximal vom freien Nagelrand. (Aus: MORIKE, 1954)

Diese Schicht ist von einer aus sechs bis zehn Lagen polygonaler Zellen bestehenden Stachelzellschicht überlagert. Diese Zellen werden um so flacher, je mehr sie sich der Nagelplatte nähern. Sie verlieren ihren Kern und enthalten keine Keratohyalinkörnchen. Ihr Cytoplasma wird weniger eosinophil, und die Zellmembran nimmt an Dicke ab (sog. „leere" Zelle nach LEWIS). Die Keratinisierung beruht auf einem Inflations-Deflationsvorgang und ist mit demjenigen der dorsalen Nagelschicht zu vergleichen (LEWIS, 1954).

Das so gebildete Keratin hängt eng mit der unteren Seite der Nagelplatte zusammen und begleitet den Nagel bei seinem Wachstum. Man kann dies an der Progression eines subungualen Hämatoms oder an der Markierung sehen, die eine Nagelextraktion auf dem Nagelbett hinterläßt (KRANTZ, 1939), ebenso durch subunguale Injektion von Tusche (MORIKE, 1954).

An der Unterseite des Nagelbettes (Hyponychiums) sind Längsleisten der Epidermis sichtbar, die in entsprechende Furchen der Lederhaut passen und bei einem Querschnitt durch den Finger beobachtet werden können. Die Epidermisleisten der proximalen Region (Abb. 14) sind kleiner, mehr unterteilt und daher zahlreicher als diejenigen des distalen Teils (HORSTMANN, 1957).

Dieser Autor stellt keine ausgesprochene Grenze zwischen der ventralen Lippe der Nagelmatrix und dem Epithel des Nagelbettes (Hyponychiums) fest. Hingegen haben MARTIN und PLATTS (1959) eine deutliche Demarkation beobachtet. In der Tat zeigt nur das Epithel der Matrixregion zwei verschiedene Zellzonen. Die tiefe Zone besteht aus polygonalen Zellen mit schwach eosinophilem Cytoplasma und einem rundlichen Kern, die oberflächliche Zone hingegen aus abgeflachten Zellen mit stark eosinophilem Cytoplasma und einem geschrumpften, unregelmäßigen, pyknotischen Kern. Die im Bereich dieser Zellen vorhandenen Tonofibrillen geben ihnen ein faseriges Aussehen. Die Intercellularbrücken sind hier schwerer festzustellen als beim Keimepithel des Nagelbettes. Diese beiden Zonen des Nagelwurzelgebiets haben die gleiche Dicke und werden gewöhnlich beim Schneiden getrennt.

III. Das periunguiale Gewebe
1. Eponychium

Das *Eponychium* (Abb. 15) wird von Zellen gebildet, die in einem ähnlichen Prozeß keratinisieren wie die Oberhaut. Das Eponychium ist eine Hornlamelle,

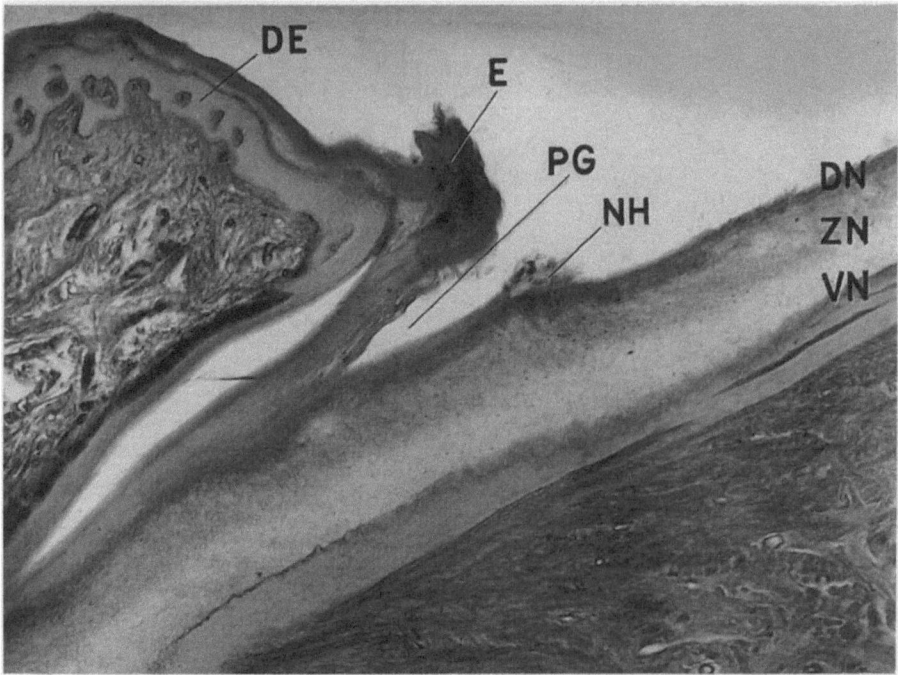

Abb. 15. Eponychium und Nagelhäutchen. *D.E.* Dorsale Epidermis. *E.* Eponychium. *P.G.* Proximale Grenzfurche. *N.H.* Nagelhäutchen (Cuticula). *D.N.* Dorsalnagel. *Z.N.* Zwischennagel. *V.N.* Ventralnagel. (PAS-Färbung)

welche die Nagelplatte auf einer kurzen Strecke bedeckt. Die verhornte Lamelle, deren Zellen ähnlich wie Dachziegel übereinander liegen, wird zunehmend dünner, denn der Nagel wächst wahrscheinlich rascher als die germinative Schicht des Eponychiums. Das ursprünglich vielschichtige Eponychium verliert Schicht um Schicht in dem Maße, wie der Nagel wächst. In der proximalen Region geht das Eponychium in die Haut des Fingerrückens über.

2. Hyponychium

Das *Hyponychium* (Sohlenhorn oder terminale Zone) (Abb. 16), der Treffpunkt des Nagelbetts und der Fingerkuppe, besteht aus einer Epidermis (Terminalmatrix), die derjenigen des Nagelbetts, mit allerdings dickerer Hornschicht, vergleichbar ist.

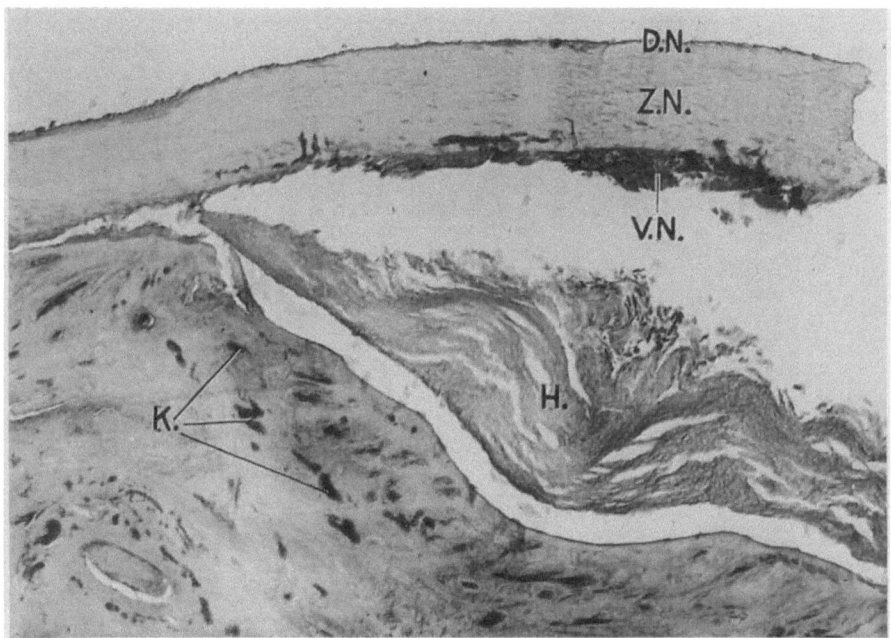

Abb. 16. Hyponychium (Sohlenhorn oder terminale Zone). *D.N.* Dorsalnagel. *Z.N.* Zwischennagel. *V.N.* Ventralnagel. *H.* Hyponychium. *K.* Capillaren

3. Fingerbeere

Die *Fingerbeere* ist durch Schweißdrüsen charakterisiert, die bis an die Terminalzone reichen. Auf der Epithelunterseite wechseln Schweißdrüsenkämme (die Einmündungszonen der exkretorischen Kanäle) mit Leisten ab, welche die „epidermocutane" Verbindung sichern; sie werden als „Haftleisten" bezeichnet. Ihnen gegenüber laufen auf der Epidermisoberseite die Papillarfurchen, die für das Muster der Fingerabdrücke verantwortlich sind.

Die Epidermis ist mit einer verhornten Schicht bedeckt, deren Keratinisierung nach Typus A von ZANDER vor sich geht. Eine Keratinisierung dieses Typs findet sich an der Hand- und der Fußfläche. Die Hornzellen bleiben bis zu einer Höhe von sieben bis zehn Zellschichten über der Granulaschicht miteinander verbunden. Die Keratinisierung dieses Typs ist dem Typus B nach ZANDER entgegengesetzt, bei welchem sich die verhornten Zellen direkt über der Granulaschicht lösen.

4. Lederhaut

Einige besondere Punkte unterscheiden die periunguiale Cutis vom übrigen Tegument. Die Kollagenfaserbündel im Bereich des Nagelbetts sind in einem Netzwerk kreuzweise angeordnet. Unter diese Bündel sind einige wenige elastische Fasern gemischt. Fibröse Bindegewebsfasern in schiefer und vertikaler Richtung verbinden das Nagelbett mit dem Periost der darunterliegenden Endphalanx (MORIKE, 1954). Die Nagelwurzelregion ist insbesondere von einer dichten Scheide aus Bindegewebe umgeben, deren Bündel mit dem Periost der lateralen Ränder der Endphalanx verwachsen sind. Im ganzen Nagelbett fehlen Schweißdrüsen.

5. Gefäßversorgung

Die Blutversorgung des Nagels geschieht durch zwei arterielle Bogen, die durch Anastomosen zwischen den beiden lateralen Arterien der Finger gebildet werden. Diese Bogen liegen in der Tiefe und haben Kontakt mit dem Periost: der eine verläuft parallel zur Lunula, der andere folgt dem freien Rand des Nagels.

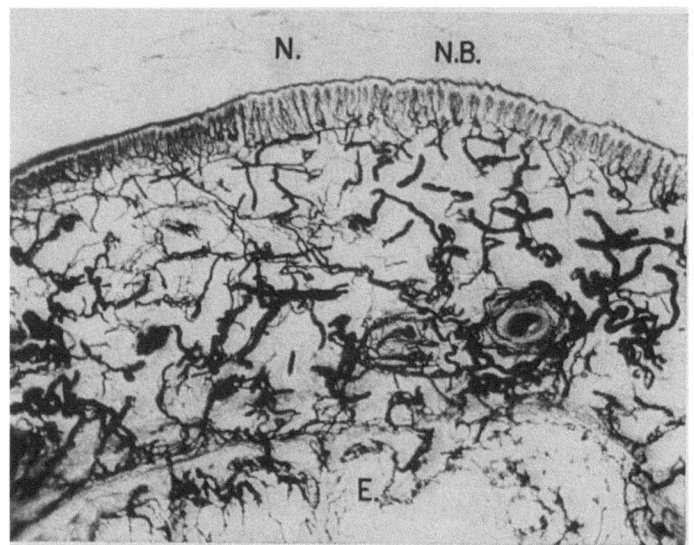

Abb. 17. Querschnitt einer Zehe mit Nagel (*N.*), Nagelbett (*N.B.*) Hyponychium) und Endphalanx (*E.*) mit Blutversorgung. Regelmäßige Anordnung des Capillarsystems in der papillären Schicht des Nagelbettes. (Aus: WINKELMANN, SCHEEN, PYKA und COVENTRY, 1961)

Von diesen beiden Bogen gehen kleine vertikale Äste nach oben und verteilen sich in ein zur Nageloberfläche paralleles Capillarnetz. In den Fingerspitzen ergänzen sich der Kreislauf der Phalanx, der Sehnen und der Cutis gegenseitig (Abb. 17).

Die Zirkulation im Fingerendglied wurde von TRUFFI (1934), FLEISCHHAUER und HORSTMANN (1955), HORSTMANN (1957), MARTIN und PLATTS (1959), ELLIS (1961) sowie von WINKELMANN u. Mitarb. (1961) untersucht. Die Gefäße wurden teils durch Tuschinjektion dargestellt, teils durch Reaktionen der alkalischen Phosphatase, welche die Wände der Capillaren und Arteriolen umgibt.

Diese Autoren zeigen, daß das Gefäßnetz bis ins subpapilläre Gebiet hinein keinen regelmäßigen Verlauf erkennen läßt. Hingegen verleihen die Epidermispapillen dem Capillarsystem eine regelmäßige Anordnung (Abb. 17), die sich je nach der untersuchten Region unterscheidet.

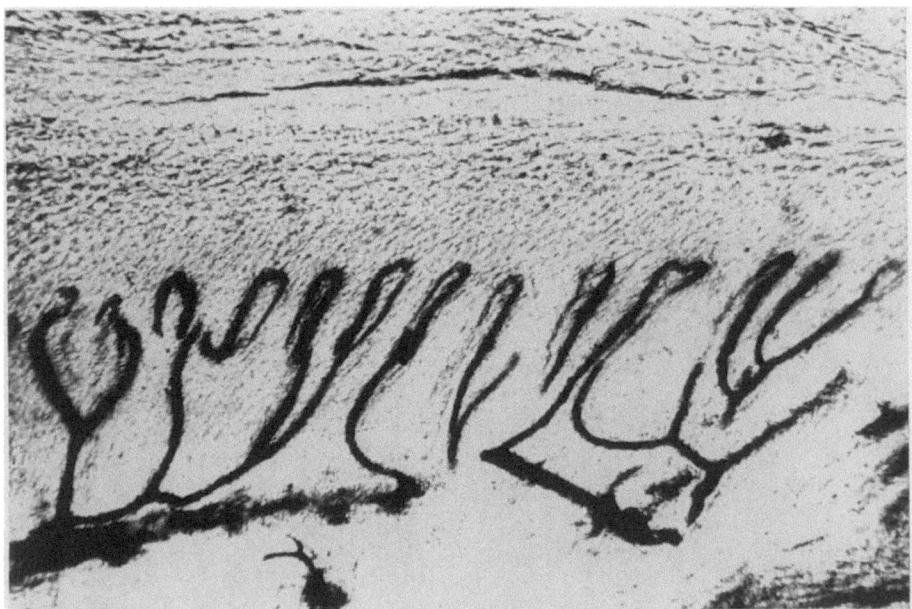

Abb. 18. Verschmälerte Capillarschlingen versehen das mittlere Feld des vasculären Nagelbettes. Dieser Aspekt ist dem Bild der Capillaroskopie identisch. (Aus: ELLIS, 1961)

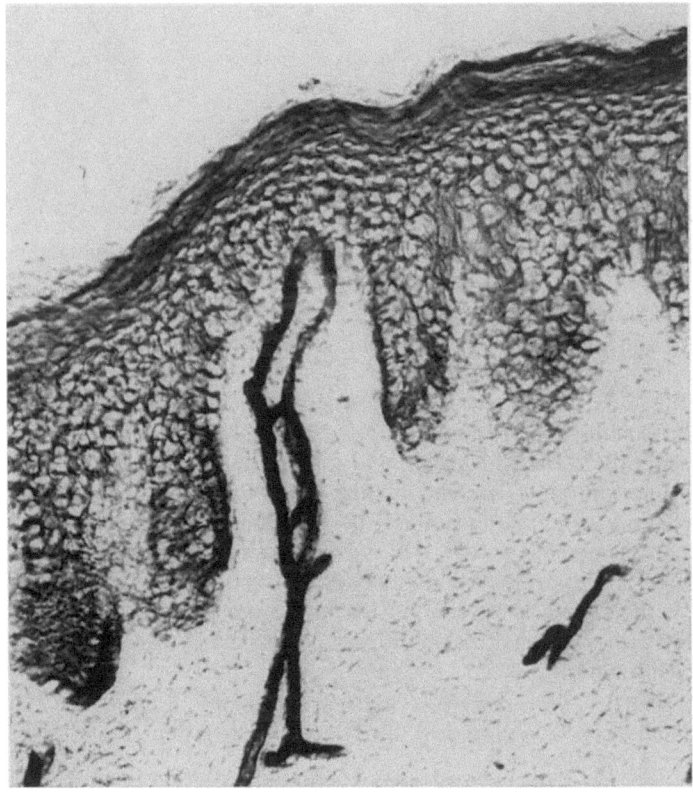

Abb. 19. Shunts zwischen den Schenkeln der Capillarschlingen. (Aus: ELLIS, 1961)

Die Capillaren im *Nagelwall* verlaufen parallel zur Oberfläche. Sie sind ungefähr 0,30 mm lang. Der arterielle Teil ist ca. 0,010—0,013 mm breit, der venöse 0,013 mm. Pro Quadratmillimeter findet man ungefähr 20 Capillaren, während man in Hand- und Fußrücken 60—70 zählt; außerdem sind sie enger als im Nagelwall (DAVIS und LAWLER, 1961). Die geringe Zahl der breiteren Capillaren ist für das Studium der makroskopischen Capillaroskopie besonders günstig (Abb. 18).

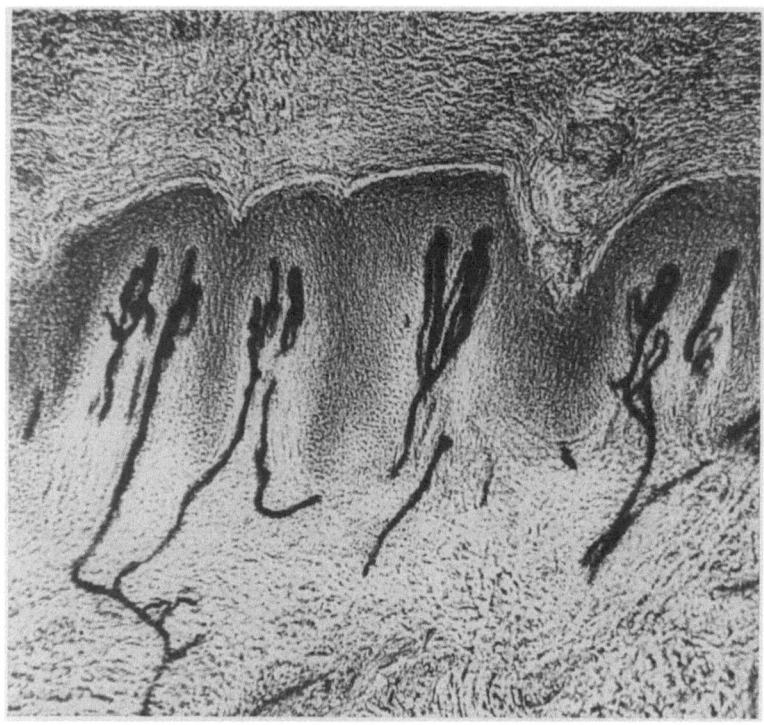

Abb. 20. Multiple Capillarschlingen dringen tief in die Hautpapillen der Fingerbeere. (Aus: ELLIS, 1961)

Im Bereich des *Nagelbetts* hält eine Gruppe von Capillarschlingen jede Papille besetzt. An einigen Stellen sind die Schlingenschenkel undeutlich und mit Shunts verbunden (Abb. 19).

Im unmittelbar unter dem *Hyponychium* (terminale Zone) befindlichen Gebiet findet man Gefäße einer besonderen Art, wie sie HORSTMANN (1957) beschrieben hat. Dort sind die Hautpapillen breit und enthalten dünnwandige Capillaren von großem Kaliber. Sie sind lang und spiralig aufgewickelt. Von diesen Capillaren aus entstehen die sog. „Splitterblutungen" bei bestimmten inneren Krankheiten. Diese Gefäßformationen sollen an der Wärmeregulierung der Fingerendglieder beteiligt sein, wobei der Blutstrom von den arteriovenösen Anastomosen des Nagelbetts gesteuert wird. Dieser besonderen Anordnung der Capillaren ist die rosa Linie zuzuschreiben, die man makroskopisch am Nagelrand ca. 4 mm hinter dem Fingerende beobachten kann.

Im Bereich der *Fingerbeere* wie an den Hand- und Fußflächen (ELLIS, 1961) sind die Capillarbogen lang und in der Haut zwischen den Epidermispapillen eingeschlossen (Abb. 20).

Die *Glomusorgane*, die von MASSON (1935) beschriebenen arteriovenösen Anastomosen, sind im Fingerendglied besonders zahlreich vorhanden (Abb. 21).

Bei diesen Gebilden ist der arterielle Ast aufgerollt und von konzentrischen Bindegewebsschichten umgeben, während die glatten Muskelzellen der Wand sich runden und dann epitheloid aussehen. Im histologischen Schnitt erscheint sein Lumen praktisch verschlossen. Man findet Glomera nicht nur in der Handfläche und im Fingerendglied, sondern auch in der Umgebung des Nagelbetts bis unterhalb der ventralen Lippe der Nagelmatrix. Sie fehlen hingegen im proximalen Nagelwall. Ihre Kontraktionsfähigkeit macht sie zu wichtigen Organen bei der Regulierung der Blutzufuhr in die Extremitäten.

Die *Venen* der Fingergegend besitzen keine besonderen Eigenschaften. Immerhin ist die Wand der Nagelvenen auffallend dünn.

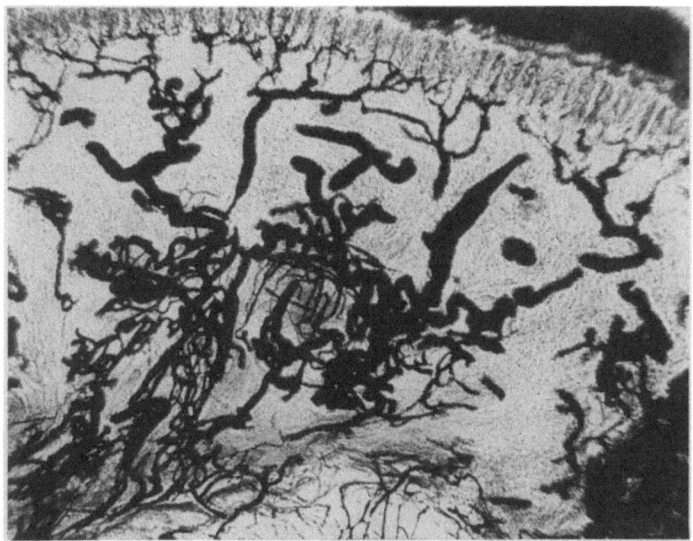

Abb. 21. Glomus in der Zehenhaut. Das Arterienlumen ist durch eine feine Linie dargestellt. Sammelvenen bilden die Hauptmasse. (Aus: WINKELMANN u. Mitarb., 1961)

Die *Lymphgefäße* der Ungualregion weisen eine eigenartige Struktur auf (TRUFFI, 1934). Das Netz ist hochentwickelt; Anastomosen finden sich nicht nur zwischen den angrenzenden Formationen der Oberfläche, sondern auch zwischen weiter entfernten, verschiedenartigen Netzen. Außerdem bestehen Verbindungen zwischen dem Oberflächensystem und den Lymphgefäßen im Periost des Fingerendglieds.

Die Anordnung des Ungualnetzes richtet sich nach dem Bau der verschiedenen Regionen der Fingerextremität. In der Matrixregion sind die terminalen Äste vertikal gestellt; im Bereich des Nagelbetts, wo Hautpapillen fehlen, hat das Netz eine horizontale Lage. Im Terminalgebiet folgen die Lymphgefäße den Papillen und sind, wie die Blutgefäße, horizontal angeordnet.

6. Innervation

Die Nervenendigungen der Haut im allgemeinen und des Fingerendglieds im besonderen wurden von folgenden Autoren untersucht: MARTINEZ PEREZ (1931), HORSTMANN (1952), CAUNA (1954), DASTUR (1955), WEDDEL (1955), RICHTER (1955), WINKELMANN (1960), MILLER u. Mitarb. (1960), DUPONT und BOURLOND (1962), LELOUP und BOURLOND (1961), BOURLOND (1962/63).

Es lassen sich in der Haut Endigungen des cerebrospinalen Nervensystems von solchen des vegetativen Nervensystems unterscheiden. Die ersteren enthalten sensible afferente Fasern, deren Endigungen nicht mehr myalinhaltig sind. Sie enden entweder frei, einzeln oder indem sie sich verästeln; ferner können sie eingekapselt sein in Form von hochdifferenzierten Strukturen.

In der Umgebung der Epidermis der Fingerbeere bilden sie zahlreiche Verzweigungen, die sich in alle Richtungen schlängeln, sich überkreuzen und so einen Plexus unter der Haut bilden, dessen Dichte und Komplexität nur in Flachschnitten gut gezeigt werden kann (BOURLOND, 1963) (Abb. 22).

Die freien Nervenfasern werden im Corium im Bereich der Hautpapille und innerhalb der Epidermis gefunden (Abb. 23). Freie Endigungen sind in der Hand zahlreicher als im Fuß und dringen tiefer in die Epidermis ein. Das Vorhandensein

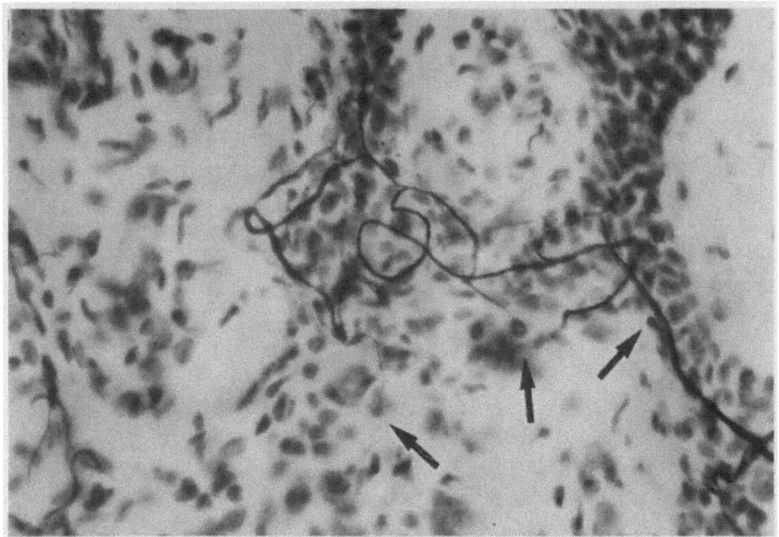

Abb. 22. Subepidermaler Plexus, feine Verzweigungen mit anulärer Endigung. Horizontalschnitt. Färbung nach BIELCHOWSKY. (Aus: DUPONT und BOURLOND, 1962/63)

dieser intraepithelialen Nervenfasern, die zwischen den Basalzellen und den Schichten der Stachel- und Granulazellen verlaufen, wird von namhaften Autoren bestritten.

Andere Fasern (MILLER u. Mitarb., 1960) enden in Form kleiner Näpfchen auf den Epithelzellen und bilden die Merkelschen Tastscheiben. Diese Tastscheiben stehen mit den Zellen der Basalschicht der Drüsenleisten und ihrer Anhänge in Beziehung; die Haftleisten sind in der Palmar-Haut praktisch ohne sensiblen Apparat im Gegensatz zu dem, was man in der Plantar-Haut beobachtet.

Die Coriumpapillen enthalten Meissnersche Körperchen. Bei jungen Menschen findet man in jeder Papille ein Körperchen. Nach dem 30. Lebensjahr nimmt ihre Zahl ab (MILLER).

Die Cutis der Hand enthält Krausesche und Ruffinische Körperchen. In der Plantar-Haut hat man sie nicht beobachtet.

Hand- und Fußrücken enthalten freie Nervenfasern, welche im Corium, vielleicht in den tiefen Zellen der Epidermis und im Bereich der Haarfollikel enden. Hier findet man auch Merkelsche Tastscheiben (MILLER).

Die von diesen Endigungen ausgehenden sensiblen Fasern werden myelinhaltig und sammeln sich zu Nervenstämmen.

Die *vegetativen* Fasern erscheinen nach Silberimprägnation als ein syncytiales Netzwerk, was man besonders bei dicken Schnitten beobachten kann (BOURLOND,

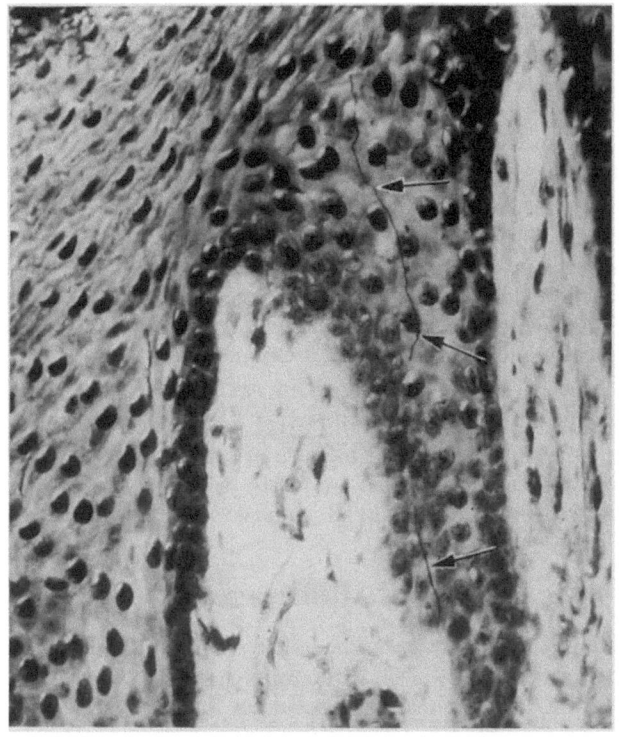

Abb. 23. Freie Endigungen in der Epidermis. Färbung nach VAN CAMPENHOUT.
(Aus: DUPONT und BOURLOND, 1962/63)

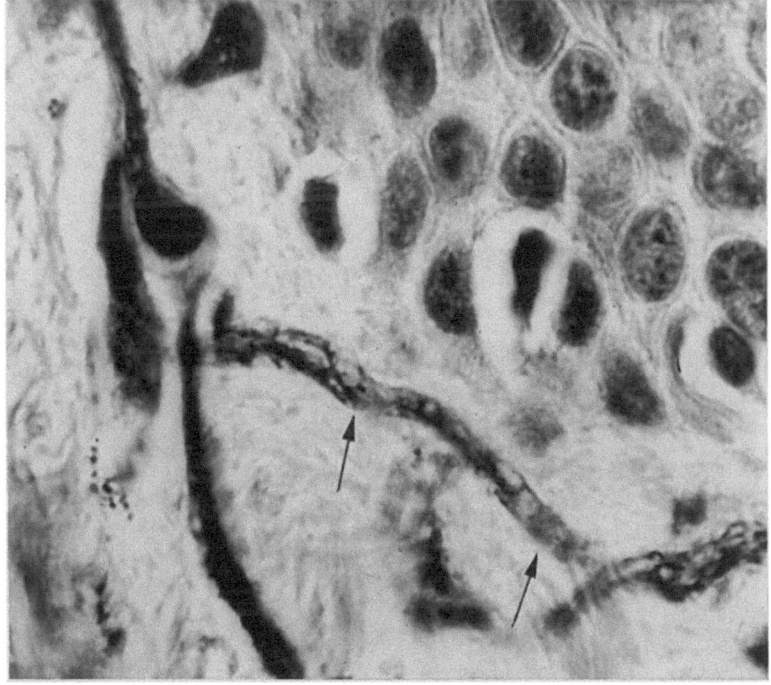

Abb. 24. Subepidermales vegetatives Netzwerk. Querschnitt. Färbung nach VAN CAMPENHOUT.
(Aus: DUPONT und BOURLOND, 1962/63)

1963). Diese Fasern enthalten Neuriten, die sich — in den verschiedensten Richtungen — untereinander mischen. Nach Durchlaufen der dicken Nervenstränge und der kleinen gemischten Nerven durch tiefe und mittlere Lederhaut senden die Endäste der sympathischen Fasern zahlreiche und immer dünner werdende Verzweigungen aus. Sie sind von einer Lemmoblastenhülle umgeben, die eine dicke Manschette aus Cytoplasma um die feinen vegetativen Neuriten bildet (Abb. 24).

In der Umgebung der Erfolgsgewebe (Gefäße, Drüsen, Epithel, glatte Muskulatur) wird das Netz besonders dicht und umgibt diese Organe mit einer Art kontinuierlichem Schleier, ohne irgendeine besondere Endigung zu zeigen. BOURLOND hat nie beobachtet, daß das Netz in die aktiven Zellen eingedrungen ist. Die Weiterleitung der Nervenreize soll durch das Freiwerden von aktivierenden Substanzen zustande kommen, die bis zu diesen Organen gelangen.

Die vegetative Fasern sollen stehen in Kontakt mit den ,,hellen'' Zellen oder sind sogar mit ihnen kontinuierlich verbunden.

An der Fingerbeere sind die myelinfreien Fasern sehr zahlreich und sehr dünn. Vermischt mit vegetativen Elementen umfassen sie als Netz die epitheloiden Zellen des Sucquet-Hoyerschen Kanals (BOURLOND, 1963).

IV. Der Altersnagel

Die Struktur der Nagelplatte verändert sich mit dem Alter (HELLER, 1927; LEWIS und MONTGOMERY, 1955). Der Altersnagel weist längsgerichtete Furchen auf (Abb. 25a), während seine Dicke im einen oder anderen Sinne variiert.

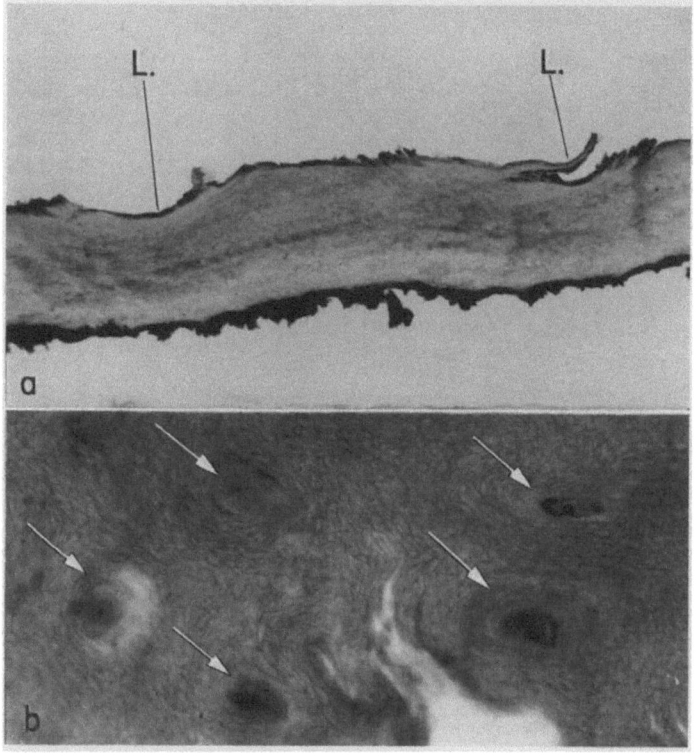

Abb. 25a u. b. Der Altersnagel (PAS-Färbung). a *L* Längsfurchen. b ↘ ,,Säulenförmige Stränge'' (organes pectinés)

Es können die sog. „säulenförmigen Stränge" KÖLLIKERS („Organes pectinés" französischer Autoren) vorkommen (Abb. 25b) in der Form cellulärer Inseln innerhalb der Nagelplatte, die im Gegensatz zu den benachbarten Zellen wirbelförmig angeordnet sind. Sie bestehen aus Zellen mit geschrumpftem Kern und sind von eosinophilem oder vacuolisiertem Material umgeben. Beide Arten können vorkommen.

Beobachtet man derartige Stränge im normalen Nagel, so weist eine Zunahme ihrer Zahl auf einen Altersnagel hin. Diesen Gebilden entsprechen Wülste in der Nagelmatrix. Sie sind besonders im Dorsalnagel zu finden und geben sich makroskopisch als Längsstreifen zu erkennen.

D. Histochemie

Über die Histochemie der Haut und des Haares sind zahlreiche Arbeiten publiziert worden. Für das digitale Endglied trifft dies jedoch nicht zu. Technische Schwierigkeiten scheinen für diese Tatsache verantwortlich zu sein. Die in der vorliegenden Arbeit beschriebenen Untersuchungen sind daher zum größten Teil an den Fingerenden menschlicher Embryonen durchgeführt worden, weil die Herstellung von Präparaten einfacher war. Es hat sich jedoch herausgestellt, daß die gegen Ende der Entwicklung gemachten Beobachtungen (7.—10. Schwangerschaftsmonat) mit den Verhältnissen am Fingerendglied des Erwachsenen vergleichbar sind.

Im Verlauf dieser histochemischen Analyse werden wir zwei Kapitel unterscheiden. Der erste Abschnitt ist der Nagelmatrix, dem Nagelbett (Hyponychium) und den periungualen Geweben gewidmet. Wir werden uns mit den Untersuchungen des Glykogens, der Mucopolysaccharide, der Ribonucleinsäure und den Enzymen befassen. Das zweite Kapitel behandelt den eigentlichen Nagel mit seinen drei hauptsächlich aus Keratin gebildeten Zonen.

Aus jedem dieser Kapitel werden wir die Schlußfolgerungen ziehen. Bei einer sich noch in voller Entwicklung befindenden Disziplin wie der Histochemie kann es sich nur um eine Zusammenfassung des aktuellen Standes der Dinge handeln, und es ist sehr wohl möglich, daß diese Ansichten teilweise schon in naher Zukunft einer Revision unterzogen werden müssen.

I. Nagelmatrix, Nagelbett (Hyponychium) und periunguiale Gewebe

1. Das Glykogen

Die Rolle des Glykogens bei der Mitose und beim Keratinisierungsprozeß der Haut wird an anderer Stelle behandelt. Die Lokalisierung dieses Kohlenhydrats in den verschiedenen Epidermisbestandteilen des Nagels, des Nagelbettes und des Periungualgewebes erlaubt die gleichen Feststellungen.

Die Basalschichten der Nagelmatrix, der Epidermis des hyponychialen Nagelbettes und der verschiedenen Epidermisbestandteile der periungualen Gewebe enthalten kein Glykogen (Abb. 26).

Im Stratum spinosum dieser Regionen und insbesondere in denjenigen des Nagelbetts (Hyponychiums) befindet sich nur wenig Glykogen, und im Gebiet der Nagelmatrix ist im allgemeinen fast keines vorhanden. Die verhornten Schichten enthalten nie Glykogen.

Das Vorkommen dieses Metaboliten während der Bildung des Fingerendgliedes wurde von ACHTEN (1959), ANDERSEN (1961) sowie SERRI, MONTAGNA und MESCON (1962) untersucht. Es zeigte sich, daß die Epidermis der verschiedenen Nagelregionen in jeder Hinsicht mit derjenigen der Deckhaut verglichen werden kann. In der Tat kann man während den frühen Entwicklungsstadien das Fehlen von Glykogen in der Basalschicht der verschiedenen Hautkomponenten und sein Vorhandensein in den Malpighischen Zellen beobachten. In dem Maß, in welchem der Keratinisierungsprozeß fortschreitet, nimmt das Glykogen in den Keratinocyten ab und verschwindet manchmal ganz. Die Hornschicht enthält nie Glykogen.

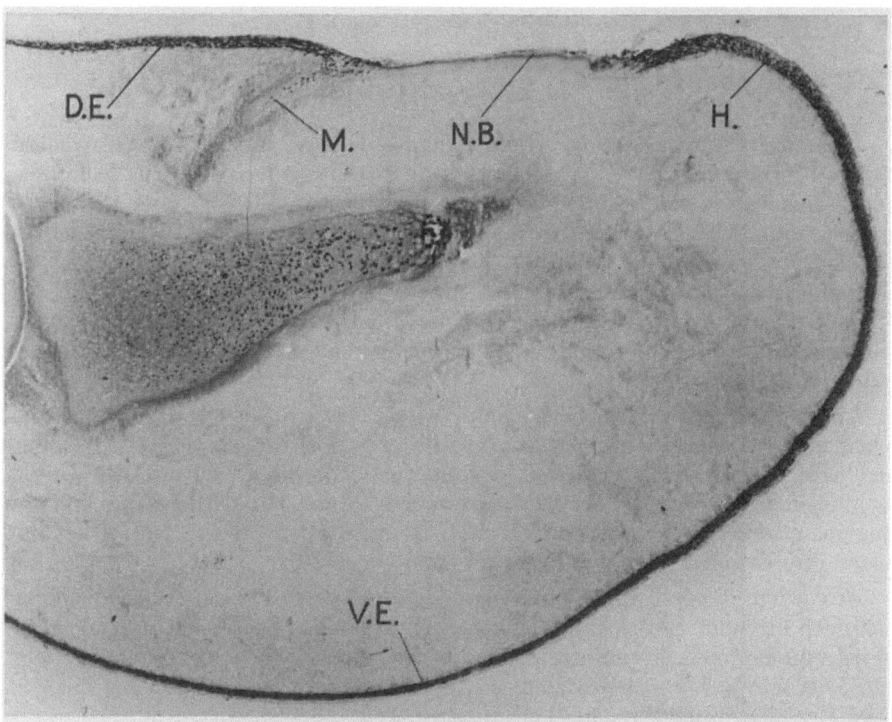

Abb. 26. Embryo von 4 Monaten. Vorkommen von Glykogen in den Zellen des Strat. spinosum der dorsalen (*D.E.*) und ventralen (*V.E.*) Epidermis und in dem Hyponychium (*H*) (Sohlenhorn) Fehlen von Glykogen in den Basalschichten, in der Matrix (*M*) und in dem Nagelbett (*N.B.*) (Hyponychium)

Diese Befunde machen die Bedeutung des Glykogens für den Zellteilungsprozess und seine Rolle bei der Bildung des Keratins offensichtlich. Zweifellos ist, wie SERRI, MONTAGNA und MESCON (1962) betonen, die stark wechselnde Menge an nachweisbarem Hautglykogen ein Beweis für die Labilität dieses Metaboliten, der sehr rasch auf- und abgebaut wird. Dies unterstreicht seine Bedeutung im Zellstoffwechsel. Das cutane Glykogen wird ständig von den Hautzellen synthetisiert und verbraucht und stellt eine Energiequelle dar, wahrscheinlich sogar eine Substanz, die als Zwischenprodukt bei der Synthese anderer Substanzen benützt werden kann. SERRI, MONTAGNA und MESCON stellen die Hypothese auf, daß das Hautglykogen bei der Synthese des Materials der Grundsubstanz beteiligt ist.

2. Mucopolysaccharide

Wir betrachten nacheinander die Basalmembran, das Corium sowie die Intercellularräume der Epidermis.

a) Basalmembran und Corium

Die Mucopolysaccharide der Basalmembran unterscheiden sich in keiner Weise von denjenigen der übrigen Haut. Es soll darum hier nicht näher darauf eingegangen werden.

ANDERSON (1961) hat saure Mucopolysaccharide in der Lederhaut von Nagelwurzel und Nagelbett festgestellt. Diese Mucopolysaccharide vom Typ der Chondroitinschwefelsäure spielen anscheinend bei der Histogenese des Nagels dieselbe Rolle wie bei der Histogenese des Haares (MONTAGNA, CHASE und HAMILTON, 1951).

b) Intercellularräume der Epidermis

Die Intercellularräume sind in der Färbung nach MACMANUS und mit Alcianblau gut erkennbar. In der Basalschicht sind sie verschwommen, werden aber bis zur Granulaschicht, wo sie stets vorhanden sind, immer deutlicher.

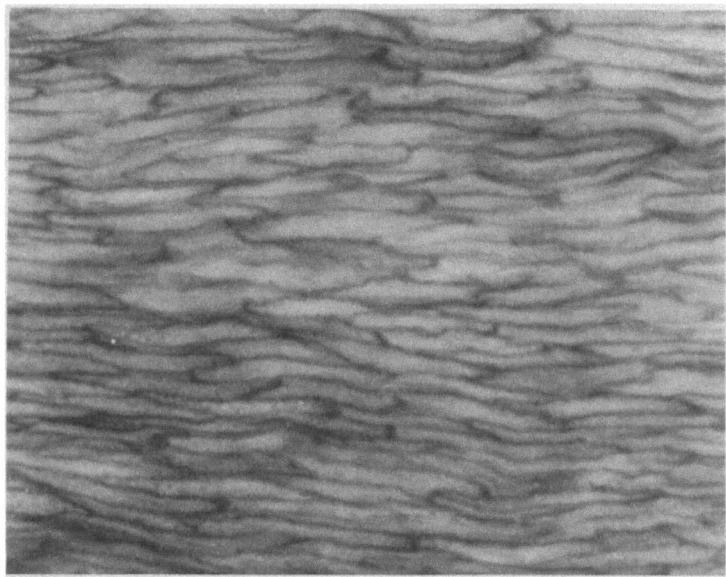

Abb. 27. Querschnitt durch den Nagel. Intercellulargebiet der Nagelzellen PAS-positiv

Bei der weichen Keratinisierung vom Typus B (Haut des Fingerrückens, Eponychium) zeigt die Hornschicht, die aus in die Länge gezogenen Zellen besteht, keine Intercellularräume mehr.

Beim weichen Keratin vom Typus A (kohärente Hornzellen: Fingerbeere, Nagelbett und Hyponychium) weisen die verhornten Zellen eine kontinuierliche PAS-positive Umrandung auf. Diese aneinandergefügten Rahmen verleihen der ganzen Hornschicht ein gitterartiges Aussehen. An der äußersten Oberfläche dieser Schicht verschwinden die Rahmen, und man spricht von „stratum disjunctum".

Bei der harten Keratinisierung des eigentlichen Nagels zeigen die Zellen des Nagelrandes an ihrer Peripherie bis an den freien Rand hin solche PAS-positiven Rahmen (Abb. 27).

Beim Embryo unterscheidet man von der 14. Woche der intrauterinen Entwicklung an in der Epidermis der Fingerbeere sehr deutlich die mit PAS und Alcianblau gefärbten Brückenknötchen der Stachelzellen. In dem Maße, in welchem der Embryo wächst, werden sie immer deutlicher und können zu Ende des 8. Schwangerschaftsmonats im Stratum spinosum und Stratum granulosum sowie in den ersten Lagen der Hornschicht beobachtet werden. Der ganze Intercellularraum färbt sich, und die Hornzelle ist von einem kontinuierlichen PAS-Rahmen umgeben. Die gleichen Knötchen finden sich später auch auf dem Fingerrücken, wo man sie aber erst etwa in der 18. Woche unterscheiden kann. Bei der Nagelanlage sind diese Bizzozeroschen Knötchen nicht sichtbar. Mit der fortschreitenden Differenzierung in Oberlippe und Unterlippe zeigen die Stachelzellen PAS-positive Knötchen. Diese verschwinden beim Beginn der Verhornung, und die Zellen lösen sich voneinander. Vom 7. Monat an persistieren die Knötchen sowohl in der von der Matrix gebildeten Hornsubstanz als auch in der keratinisierten Zone.

Man weiß, daß unter dem Elektronenmikroskop das Bizzozerosche Knötchen als eine lokalisierte Verdickung der Zellwand erscheint, wo die intracellulären Fibrillen bündelweise endigen (PORTER, 1954; WEISS und FERRIS, 1954; SELBY, 1955/56; HORSTMANN und KNOOP, 1958; ODLAND, 1958/60; HIBBS und CLARK, 1959). Es sind intercelluläre Kontaktstellen, die sich in den oberflächlichen Hautschichten so dicht nebeneinanderlegen, daß um die Epidermiszellen ein PAS-positiver Rahmen entsteht. Diese Formationen sind für die Kohäsion der Epidermiszellen in der Stachelschicht und der Hornschicht sowohl bei der Verhornung nach Typus A von ZANDER als auch beim harten Verhornungstypus der Nagelzellen verantwortlich. Im weichen Keratin verschwinden sie gleichzeitig mit dem Lockerwerden der Hornzellen.

BRAUN-FALCO (1958), STEIGLEDER und WEAKLEY (1961) sind der Ansicht, daß ihr Kittvermögen, wie es von DUPRÉ (1952) beschrieben wurde, nicht ihre einzige Funktion ist. Sie könnten auch bei der Erhaltung des Enzymmusters in der Hornschicht eine Rolle spielen. Wieweit die sauren Mucopolysaccharide der Zwischenzellbrücken als Filter für große Moleküle oder als Inhibitoren oder Aktivatoren von Enzymen wirken, ist nicht sicher bekannt.

Aufgrund aller dieser Untersuchungen lassen sich zwei Untergruppen unterscheiden:

α) Stützmucopolysaccharide, die der Gruppe der neutralen Mucopolysaccharide angehören (Basalmembran, Kittsubstanz der Lederhaut, Intercellularraum der Epidermis);

β) Mucopolysaccharide, die in den Zellstoffwechsel eingreifen, sei es in die Induktionsprozesse, sei es in den Enzymstoffwechsel. Diese Gruppe entspricht den sauren Mucopolysacchariden (Intercellularbrücken der Epidermis, Cutis der Haarpapille und der Nagelmatrix).

3. Ribonucleinsäure

Die Basalzellen der Nagelknospe sind reich an Ribonucleinsäure (RNS), ebenso die Malpighischen Zellen (ACHTEN, 1959; ANDERSEN, 1961). Die Zellen des eigentlichen Nagels enthalten keine RNS.

Die Zellen der Basalschicht und des Schleimhautanteils des Nagelbettes werden mit Pyronin gefärbt. Diese Färbung ist der Ribonuclease gegenüber resistent. Die Hornschicht färbt sich nicht.

Der RNS-Gehalt der basalen und acanthinen Schichten der periungualen Regionen ist demjenigen der übrigen Haut vergleichbar.

Beim Embryo kann man feststellen, daß die Nagelknospe im Augenblick ihrer Bildung reich an RNS ist. Mit fortschreitender Entwicklung nimmt der RNS-Gehalt der Stachelzellen zu; die keratinisierten Zellen enthalten nie RNS.

Die Rolle der RNS bei der Proteinsynthese ist seit den Arbeiten von BRACHET (1947, 1952, 1957) und CASPERSSON (1947, 1950) wohlbekannt. Diese Wechsel-beziehung zwischen RNS und Proteinsynthese kann man auch an den Hautformationen beobachten (KONING und HAMILTON, 1954, 1955, 1957; FIRKET, 1951; R. SCOTHORNE und A. SCOTHORNE, 1953). In den tieferen Zonen der Haut (Basalschicht und untere Stachelzellschicht) und ihrer Adnexe (Haarfollikel- und Nagelknospe) spielt die RNS anscheinend eine Doppelrolle: Proteinsynthese der neuen Zellen und Mitwirkung am Keratinisierungsprozeß. In den oberen Schichten der Malpighischen Zone, wo keine Zellvermehrung mehr stattfindet, beeinflußt die RNS möglicherweise die Keratinsynthese (ACHTEN, 1959).

4. Die Enzyme

Die Untersuchungen der Enzyme wurden an Fingerendgliedern von menschlichen Embryonen und Ratten durchgeführt (BECKETT, BOURNE und MONTAGNA, 1956; HURLEY und MESCOW, 1956; ACHTEN, 1959; CAUNA, 1960; ORMEA, 1961; SERRI, HUBER und MESCON, 1962; SERRI, MONTAGNA und MESCON, 1962, 1963; SERRI, 1963). Sie beschränken sich auf die Erforschung der sauren und alkalischen Phosphatasen, der Cholinesterase und der Amylo-Phosphorylase.

a) Saure Phosphatasen

Die sauren Phosphatasen (Abb. 28) sind in allen Epidermiszellen mit Ausnahme der Hornzellen vorhanden (ACHTEN, 1959; SERRI, HUBER und MESCON, 1962). Die

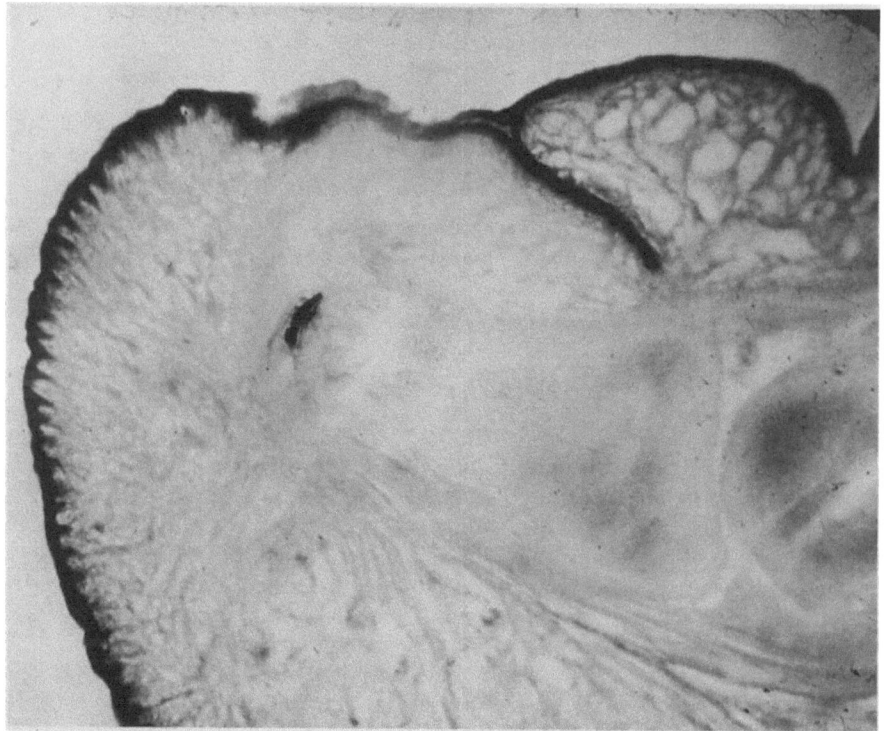

Abb. 28. Saure Phosphatasen in allen Epidermiszellen mit Ausnahme der Hornzellen. Keine Phosphatasen in der Lederhaut (Embryo 4 Monate). (Aus: SERRI, HUBER und MESCON, 1962)

Zellen des Nagelbetts enthalten deutlich weniger davon (SERRI). Keinerlei Aktivität wird in cutanen Bindegewebszellen, an Capillaren, Glomusorganen oder Nerven gefunden.

Die saure Phosphatase greift wahrscheinlich in den Allgemeinstoffwechsel der Epidermiszelle und in den Prozeß der Keratogenese ein (MORETTI und MESCON, 1956; ACHTEN, 1959; SERRI, HUBER und MESCON, 1962).

b) Alkalische Phosphatase

Die alkalische Phosphatase fehlt in den Epidermiszellen der Nagelwurzel, des Nagelbetts und der periunguialen Gewebe. Hingegen sind die Mesenchymzellen der Lederhaut dieser Region stark positiv. Zwischen dem 4. und 5. Entwicklungsmonat ist der Gehalt derart hoch, daß die umgebenden Strukturen infolge

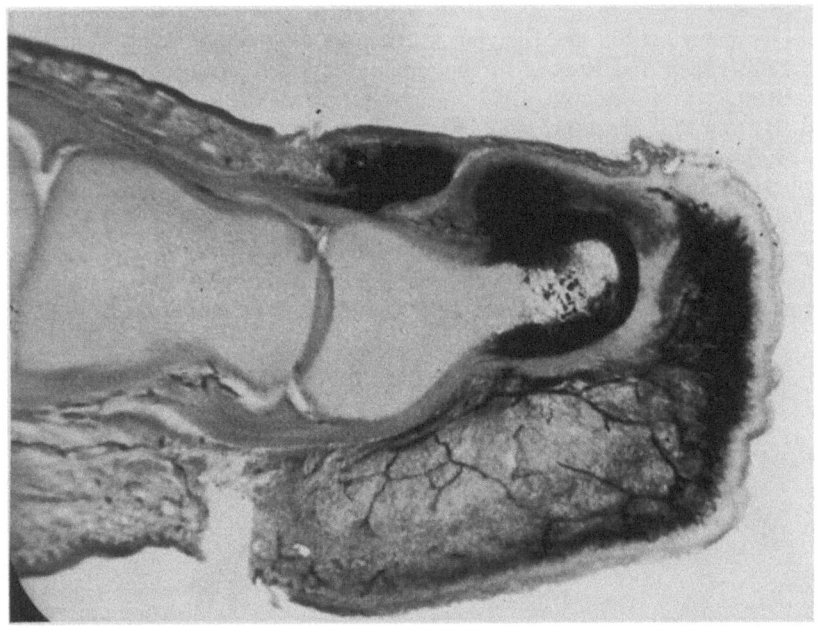

Abb. 29. Alkalische Phosphatasen (Embryo 3 Monate). Besonders intensive Reaktion der Mesenchymzellen, die das Nagelgebiet umgeben. (Aus: SERRI, MONTAGNA und HUBER, 1963)

Diffusion verwischt werden (Abb. 29). Die Intensität der Reaktion nimmt nach dem 5. Monat ab. Von diesem Zeitpunkt an kann man die alkalische Phosphatase in der Umgebung der Leder- und Unterhautcapillaren darstellen. Die Capillaren des arteriellen Kanals der Glomera sind vom 4. Monat an positiv.

Die Rolle der alkalischen Phosphatase scheint eine zweifache zu sein (ACHTEN, 1959; MONTAGNA, 1962; SERRI, MONTAGNA und HUBER, 1963). Während der frühen Entwicklungsstadien greift die alkalische Phosphatase vermutlich in die Induktions- und Differenzierungsprozesse der Hautadnexe ein (sie ist in den Mesenchymzellen in der Umgebung der Haarknospen, besonders reichlich im Bindegewebe, das Nagelwurzel und Nagelbett umgibt, vorhanden).

In den Endothelzellen könnte die alkalische Phosphatase eine Rolle beim Stoffaustausch spielen. Vom Augenblick an, in dem sich die Schichten der Gefäßwand entwickeln, sistiert die Phosphataseaktivität in den Endothelzellen und ist nur noch in den Capillarformationen vorhanden.

c) Die Cholinesterasen

Die histochemische Methode nach GOMORI hat sich für die Darstellung des Nervennetzes in den Fingerenden des Fetus als außerordentlich nützlich erwiesen

(BECKETT, BOURNE und MONTAGNA, 1956; HURLEY und MESCON, 1956; WINKELMANN, 1960; CAUNA, 1960). Sämtliche Nervenstrukturen des Fetus enthalten zugleich spezifische Cholinesterase und nichtspezifische Pseudocholinesterase.

Bei Anwendung dieser Technik erkennt man die außerordentlich reiche Versorgung der Nagelfurche mit dicken Nervensträngen, die sich bis unter die Epidermis verzweigen, sowie mit zahlreichen Nervenformationen im Fingerende und im Nagelbett (Abb. 30).

Zwischen dem Verhalten der Haut des Erwachsenen und derjenigen des Fetus besteht in bezug auf die Aktivität der Cholinesterase und der Pseudocholinesterase

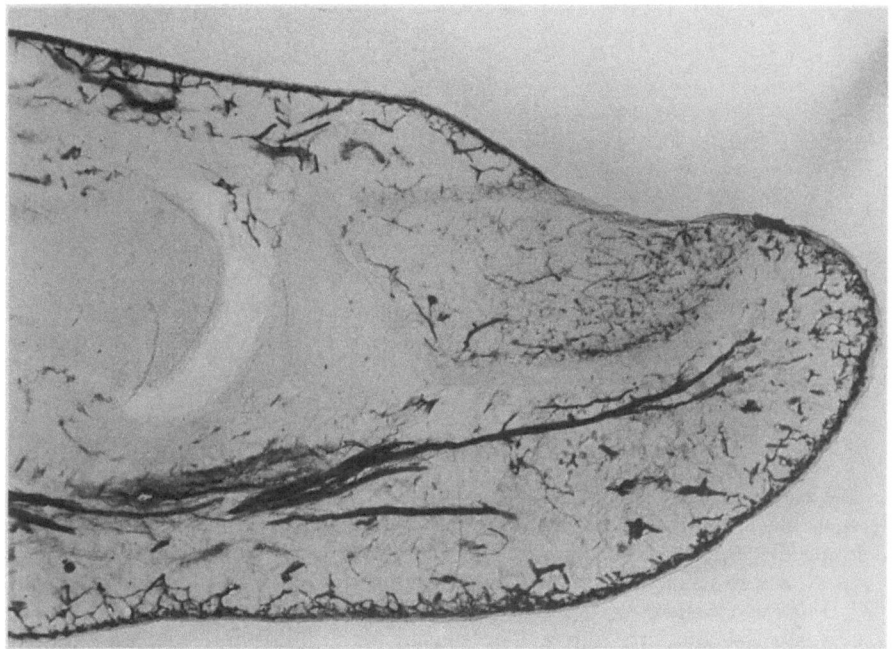

Abb. 30. Nachweis der Acetyl-Cholinesterase. Ein dicker Nervenstrang läuft durch das ganze Präparat; massenhaft Nervenfasern am Fingerende und im Gebiet des Nagelbettes. Embryo 4 Monate. (Aus: SERRI, MONTAGNA und MESCON, 1963)

ein Unterschied. Beim Erwachsenen findet man — welche Rolle man der spezifischen Cholinesterase auch zuschreiben mag — Hautnerven, in denen sie vorhanden ist, und andere, in denen sie fehlt. Im Gegensatz dazu zeigen beim Fetus alle Nervenendigungen eine Cholinesterase- und Pseudocholinesterase-Aktivität.

Trotz der jüngsten Untersuchungen über die Rolle dieser Enzyme in der Physiologie der Nerven (HURLEY und KOELLE, 1958) ist eine genaue Interpretation dieser Unterschiede zur Zeit noch nicht möglich.

d) Die Amylo-Phosphorylase

Die Phosphorylase-Aktivität wird überall dort gefunden, wo die Zellen histochemisch darstellbares Glykogen enthalten. Jedoch kann man das Enzym auch in gewissen Zellen feststellen, in denen kein Glykogen vorhanden ist, so z.B. bei den Zellen der Nagelwurzel und des Nagelbettes (SERRI, MONTAGNA und MESCON, 1962). In den Nagelzellen selbst fehlt die Phosphorylase (Abb. 31).

Die Amylo-Phosphorylase ist am Glykogenabbau beteiligt.

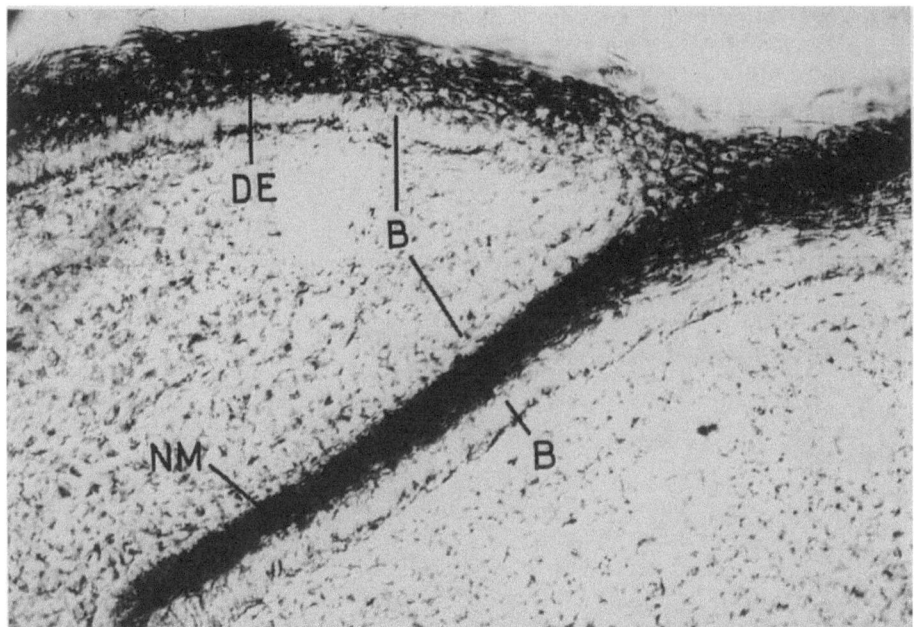

Abb. 31. Embryo von 3 Monaten. Amylophosphorylase im Stratum spinosum der dorsalen Epidermis (*D.E.*) und in den Zellen der Nagelmatrix (*N.M.*). In den Basalzellen (*B.*) ist sie nicht zu finden. (Aus: SERRI, MONTAGNA und MESCON, 1962)

Schlußfolgerungen

Die verschiedenen Beobachtungen am Nagel und an der Haut gestatten den Versuch einer Synthese der histochemischen Resultate in bezug auf die Entwicklung des Fingerendgliedes und des Prozesses der Nagelbildung.

Im 3. Schwangerschaftsmonat differenzieren sich die ersten Nagelstrukturen. Die *alkalische Phosphatase* der Dermis, welche die Nagelknospe und das Gebiet des Nagelbettes umgibt, dürfte hier sowohl als Induktions- wie als Differenzierungsfaktor dieser Nagelanlage fungieren. Die alkalische Phosphatase trägt anscheinend in den Capillaren zur Zufuhr der für das Wachstum notwendigen Materialien sowie zur Differenzierung und Bildung des Keratins bei. Dabei dürfte das *Hautglykogen* unter anderem die zur Herstellung der Grundsubstanz notwendige Energie liefern.

In den Epidermisschichten selbst liefert das Glykogen die zur Mitose erforderliche Energie. Dieses Kohlenhydrat ist auch an der Lieferung der Energie für das Leben der Zelle und für die Herstellung des Keratins beteiligt. Seine Synthese und seine Verwendung variieren von einem Augenblick zum andern und von einer Zelle zur andern. Man kann daher nie genau voraussagen, wo man es beobachten kann. Dennoch fehlt es meistens bei den aktivsten Zellen des Fingerendgliedes, nämlich denjenigen der Nagelwurzel und des Nagelbettes. Die beim Abbau der Kohlenhydrate aktiven Enzyme sind in den Epidermiszellen des Fingerendes vorhanden. Alle Enzyme des Krebs-Cyclus wurden in der menschlichen Haut gefunden.

Ohne daß man ihre Rolle genau präzisieren kann, ist die *saure Phosphatase* in allen Epidermiszellen vorhanden; wahrscheinlich greift sie in den allgemeinen Stoffwechsel der Zelle und speziell in den Keratinisierungsprozeß ein.

Die *RNS* soll bei der Synthese des Nagelkeratins eine ebenfalls wichtige Rolle spielen.

Sowohl bei der Lederhaut wie bei der Oberhaut muß man die *neutralen* Stütz-*mucopolysaccharide* von den metabolisch aktiven *sauren Mucopolysacchariden* unterscheiden. Die sauren Mucopolysaccharide scheinen bei der Differenzierung der Zellen und dem Stoffwechsel der Enzyme von Bedeutung zu sein.

In der Lederhaut zeigt die *Cholinesterase* die Entwicklung von Nervengewebe an.

Infolge der wenigen am Fingerende durchgeführten Untersuchungen ist unsere Synthese unvermeidlich skizzenhaft. Sie wird vervollständigt und wahrscheinlich in Zukunft modifiziert werden, doch gestattet sie, die histochemischen Befunde am Nagel und seinen Entwicklungsstadien übersichtlich zusammenzustellen.

II. Der eigentliche Nagel

Die histochemischen Befunde an der Hornschicht der Epidermis und des Haares wurde anderweitig behandelt. Wir befassen uns hier nur mit den besonderen Eigenschaften des Nagelkeratins.

1. PAS-positive Substanzen

Im Augenblick ihres Auftretens beim Embryo wird die Hornschicht des Nagels durch PAS rosa gefärbt. Die Färbung wird mit der fortschreitenden Entwicklung immer intensiver; man kann sie auch beim Erwachsenen beobachten.

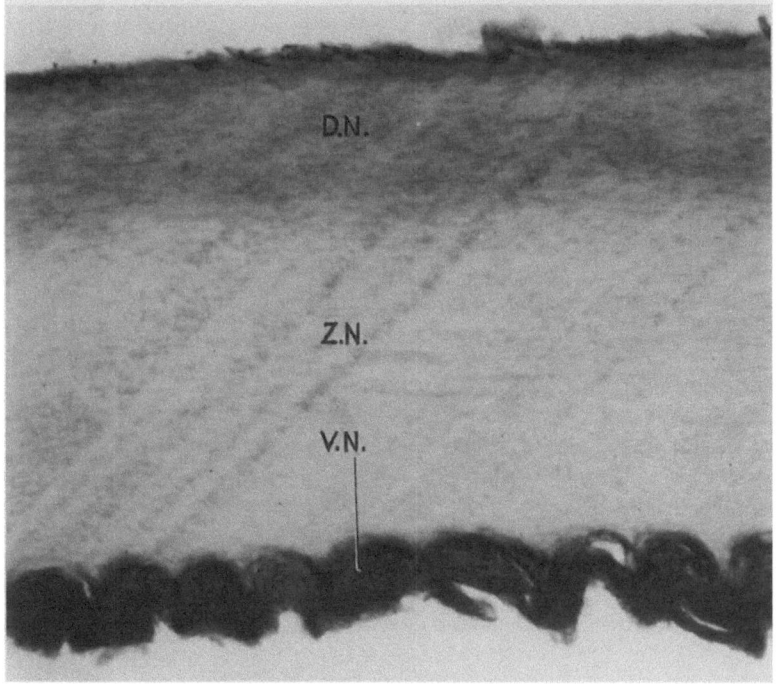

Abb. 32. Die drei Nagelschichten. *D.N.* Dorsalnagel PAS-positiv. *Z.N.* Zwischennagel negativ. *V.N.* Ventralnagel stark positiv

Die drei Nagelschichten — ihre Embryologie wurde bereits behandelt — werden durch PAS verschiedenartig gefärbt. Im Querschnitt erscheint der Dorsalnagel leicht gefärbt, der Zwischennagel ungefärbt und der Ventralnagel stark gefärbt (Abb. 32).

Im Längsschnitt erscheint der proximale Teil des Nagels zur Gänze PAS-positiv. Sobald man sich vom proximalen Teil entfernt, beobachtet man das Auftreten der leicht gefärbten Dorsalschicht und der Zwischenzone, die ihre Affinität zum PAS zunehmend verliert. Der Übergang zwischen der gefärbten und der nichtgefärbten Zone entspricht der Lunula des Nagels.

Etwa auf halber Nagellänge erscheint das Keratin des Nagelbetts (Hyponychium), welches der Unterseite des Zwischennagels anhaftet und durch PAS stark gefärbt wird.

Auch die Reaktion nach MACMANUS gestattet eine Unterscheidung der drei Nagelschichten.

Die gleichen färberischen Unterschiede, wie sie von LEWIS (1954) beobachtet wurden, ergeben sich auch mit basophilen Farbstoffen sowie mit Reagentien, welche Proteine mit Sulfhydrylgruppen sichtbar machen.

2. Basophilie

Die Färbung mit Toluidinblau in einer Lösung mit einem von 2,2—8 variierenden pH (Technik von MONTAGNA, CHASE und MELARAGNO, 1951) gestattet, drei Nagelzonen zu unterscheiden.

Bei einem pH von 5 an färbt sich der Dorsalnagel zunächst leicht, mit höherem pH immer intensiver.

Der Zwischennagel färbt sich nicht mit Toluidinblau, ganz gleich, wie hoch die pH-Werte sind.

Der Ventralnagel wird mit der gleichen Technik von pH 5 an stark gefärbt.

Im Längsschnitt erlaubt die Basophilie ebenso wie die Färbung nach MACMANUS, den proximalen vom distalen Nagel zu unterscheiden.

Auf der Höhe der Lunula wird die ganze Nagelsubstanz gefärbt, während gegen den distalen Teil die drei Schichten sichtbar werden, die man beim Querschnitt durch den Nagel beobachten kann. Die Unguialzellen des Embryo und Neugeborenen sind von pH 5 an alle basophil.

Beim Kind lassen sich nach und nach die drei Schichten wie beim Erwachsenen unterscheiden.

Der Nagel wird durch Alcianblau nicht gefärbt. Nach Oxydation mit Permanganat besteht eine Affinität zu diesem Farbstoff von pH 0,2 bis pH 8. Nach Oxydation ist auch eine Färbung mit Fuchsinaldehyd möglich. Die Zunahme der Basophilie wird Sulfongruppen ($R-SO_3H$) zugeschrieben, die aus schwefelhaltigen Gruppen entstehen.

Verschiedene histochemische Untersuchungen wurden am weichen Keratin und am Keratin des Haares durchgeführt. Man kann diese Versuche an der Nagelsubstanz reproduzieren (ACHTEN, 1959). Auf diese Befunde werden wir hier nicht weiter eingehen; es ist gewiß zweckmäßiger, wenn wir sämtliche Beobachtungen bei der Behandlung der Histochemie des Keratins zusammenfassen.

3. Proteine mit Sulfhydrylgruppen

Die Ergebnisse bei der Darstellung von Sulfhydrylgruppen (Technik von CHÈVREMONT und FRÉDÉRIC, 1943, und von BARNETT und SELIGMAN, 1952/54), sind denen mit PAS und Toluidinblau vergleichbar.

Der Dorsalnagel wird nur schwach gefärbt, der Zwischennagel gar nicht und der Ventralnagel stark. Schon beim Aufzeigen der Proteine hatte LEWIS (1954) die verschiedenartige Affinität der drei Nagelzonen beobachtet.

Schlußfolgerungen

Keratin wie auch Kollagen und Elastin sind Skleroproteine (Abb. 33), d.h. Proteine, die im kalten Wasser selbst bei Vorhandensein von Salzen oder verdünnten Basen bzw. Säuren nicht löslich sind. Diese in Fasern angeordneten Proteine sind aus Aminosäuren in regelmäßig wiederholter Anordnung gebildet, die durch peptidische Bindungen zusammenhängen (RCO-NHR') (GIROUD und CHAMPETIER, 1936; DERKSEN, HERINGA und WEIDINGER, 1937; ASTBURY, 1933/40; BEAR und RUGO, 1951; RUDALL, 1952; ROE, 1956; FLESCH, 1958; MERCER, 1961; MONTAGNA, 1962). Auf diese Weise gebildete Hauptketten sind unter sich durch Querketten verbunden.

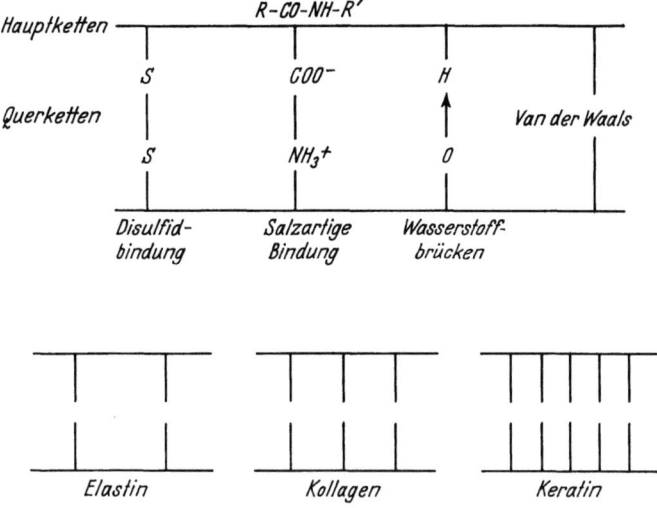

Abb. 33. Schema der Skleroproteine

Bei diesen Querketten (Abb. 33) handelt es sich im einzelnen um:

a) Disulfidbrücken, die zwischen den Sulfhydrylgruppen der Aminosäuren entstehen; solche Kovalenzbindungen sind besonders stabil.

b) Wasserstoffbrücken, die sich aus der gemeinsamen Bindung zweier elektronegativer Atome an ein Wasserstoffatom ergeben.

c) Salzartige elektrovalente Bindungen zwischen zwei ionisierten Gruppen, die Träger entgegengesetzter Ladungen sind (Untersuchung der Basophilie nach der Technik von MONTAGNA, CHASE und MELARAGNO, 1951).

d) Die van der Waalsschen Kräfte, gebildet durch residuelle Anziehungskräfte, die an die Polarisation sehr nahe beieinanderliegender Atome gebunden sind.

Die Gesamtheit dieser Querketten bildet ein mehr oder weniger dichtes Gitterwerk.

Auf diese Weise unterscheiden sich Elastin, Kollagen und Keratin in ihrer Zusammensetzung sowohl durch die Aminosäuren, welche die Hauptketten bilden, wie durch die Anzahl ihrer Querverbindungen (LLOYD, 1948; LLOYD und GARROD, 1946/48; GROSS, 1950). Querverbindungen sind im elastischen Gewebe nicht sehr zahlreich, im Kollagen sind sie häufiger, am häufigsten im Keratin (Abb. 33).

Das Keratin selbst ist keine physikalisch und chemisch einheitliche Substanz. Es gibt in der Tat nicht nur eines, sondern mehrere Keratine, welche sich voneinander durch ihre Zusammensetzung aus Aminosäuren und die Anzahl der Querketten unterscheiden. Die beiden Extreme dieser Zusammensetzung sind im weichen Keratin und im harten Keratin verwirklicht. Das weiche Keratin enthält weniger Querketten als das harte Keratin. Aus diesem Grunde läßt sich das weiche Keratin mit seinen SH-, sauren und alkalischen Gruppen nach den Methoden von CHÈVREMONT und FRÉDÉRIC, BARNETT und SELIGMAN sowie von MONTAGNA, CHASE und MELARAGNO färben.

Im Gegensatz dazu kann man das harte Keratin, das keine oder nur wenig SH-Gruppen und freie Säure-Base-Verbindungen enthält, mit diesen Methoden nicht färben.

Der Grund für die Färbung der Hornzellen durch PAS könnte eine amorphe Substanz, die Keratinfasern umgebend, sein. Diese Substanz würde im weichen

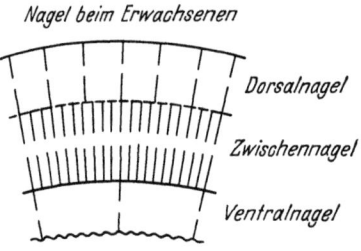

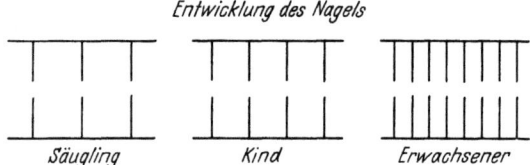

Abb. 34. Nagel des Erwachsenen und Entwicklung des Nagels

Keratin freie Hydroxylgruppen besitzen, welche eine PAS-positive Reaktion hervorrufen. Dieselben werden nicht im harten Keratin frei, welches sich deshalb durch PAS nicht färben läßt.

Diese verschiedenen Arten Keratin finden sich nun auch in den drei Schichten des Nagels (Abb. 34). Schematisch kann man unterscheiden:

1. Der Dorsalnagel zeigt eine mittlere Anzahl freier Lateralgruppen; die Seitenketten sind in mäßiger Anzahl vorhanden.

2. Der Zwischennagel hat keine oder nur wenige freie Lateralgruppen; die Querketten sind zahlreich.

3. Der Ventralnagel hat zahlreiche freie Lateralgruppen. Man kann ihn mit dem weichen Keratin der Deckhaut vergleichen. Die Querketten sind hier am wenigsten zahlreich.

Die drei verschiedenen Keratine im Nagel sind also die Ursache für den verschiedenen Färbeeffekt von Toluidinblau, der Färbung der Sulfhydrylgruppen und der Färbung nach MACMANUS.

Man beobachtet auch eine Veränderung der Färbung des Nagels mit dem Alter (Abb. 34). Tatsächlich werden die Nägel des Embryos und des Neugeborenen mit MacManus sowie Toluidinblau mit pH 4 gefärbt und enthalten Sulfhydrylgruppen. Diese Affinitäten werden während des Kindesalters kleiner und zeigen progressiv die gleichen Eigenschaften wie beim Erwachsenen.

Man kann diese Entwicklung in eine Parallele zur Zunahme der Querketten setzen. Der kindliche Nagel besteht aus weicherem Keratin als derjenige des Erwachsenen.

Aus diesen embryologischen, histochemischen und physikalisch-chemischen Daten kann man folgern, daß die Nägel des Embryos und des Kindes aus weicherem Keratin bestehen als diejenigen des Erwachsenen. Der Erwachsenennagel ist aus drei sich scharf voneinander unterscheidenden Schichten gebildet: eine Zwischenzone aus hartem Keratin, die von zwei Schichten (dorsal und ventral) aus weichem Keratin eingerahmt ist, wobei die ventrale Schicht noch weniger Querketten hat als die dorsale.

Es ist möglich, daß diese verschiedenen Affinitäten der dorsalen Wölbung des Nagels entsprechen. Bei der Kräuselung der Schafwolle z.B. besteht eine Folge von Ondulationen. Jede dieser Wellen hat eine äußere konvexe und eine innere konkave Seite. In der Konkavität zeigt das Keratin — im Gegensatz zur konvexen Seite — keine Affinität zu den basischen Farbstoffen, und die S-S-Gruppen sind zahlreicher (HORIO und KONDO, 1953; MERCER, 1953; FRASER und ROGERS, 1953/54; FRASER, LINDLEY und ROGERS, 1954).

Die Längsschnitte durch das Fingerendglied gestatten, die Färbemodifikation und demgemäß die vom Keratin durchgemachten physikalisch-chemischen Veränderungen im Verlauf des Nagelwachstums festzustellen.

In der proximalen Region wird der Nagel mit PAS, Toluidinblau sowie mit jenen Techniken gefärbt, die das Vorhandensein der SH-Gruppen aufzeigen. Je mehr man sich von der Nagelwurzel entfernt, um so stärker erscheint die Differenzierung des Dorsalnagels und des Zwischennagels: der Dorsalnagel behält seine Farbaffinitäten, während der Zwischennagel sie nach und nach einbüßt. Der Übergang vom gefärbten zum nichtgefärbten Keratin entspricht der Grenze der Lunula.

Das Keratin der Nagelwurzel hat eine Struktur, die der des weichen Keratins entspricht. Während des Nagelwachstums verändert sich diese Struktur: Die Querketten werden immer zahlreicher, insbesondere im Zwischennagel, wo das Keratin zur Gruppe des harten Keratins gehört.

Das vom Nagelbett gebildete und dem unteren Teil des Zwischennagels anhaftende Keratin unterscheidet sich in keiner Weise vom Keratin der übrigen Haut.

Die Lunula und der unsichtbare Teil der Nagelwurzel entsprechen der Zone des weichen Keratins; dieser proximale Teil ist der darunterliegenden Haut im Gegensatz zum rosa Teil des Nagels nicht adhärent.

4. Elektronen-Mikroskopie

HASHIMOTO, GROSS, NELSON und LEVER (1966) haben die Entwicklung des Nagels mit dem Elektronen-Mikroskop studiert. Sie bestätigen die mit dem Licht-Mikroskop durchgeführten Beobachtungen, hinsichtlich der Entwicklung des Nagels vom oberen und unteren Teil der Matrix und hinsichtlich der Rolle des Nagelbettes in der Konstitution des ventralen Nagels.

Der untere Teil der Matrix gibt mehr Hornzellen ab als der obere Teil. Das Keratin bildet sich nicht, bevor die Zellen ein Viertel der Distanz zwischen Apex und Matrix erreicht haben, wo sich eine Färbung der Sulfhydrylgruppen beobachten läßt. Die letzteren zeichnen ein Band, welches sich parallel zur Nagelplatte gegen die distale Seite hin verdickt. Diese Keratinschicht scheint nicht von derjenigen der oberflächlichen Epidermis different zu sein.

Die Basalzellen der Nagelmatrix enthalten dichte Lipidkörperchen. Das endoplasmatische Reticulum ist hier spärlich vorhanden, wobei gleichzeitig die RNS-Partikel sehr zahlreich sind.

Im Stratum spinosum und im Stratum granulosum, weiter gelegen als der Anfang der Keratinisationszone, beobachtet man runde Körnchen von verschiedener Dichte. Diese Formationen, „membrane coating granules" (MATOLTSY und PARAKKAL, 1965) genannt, scheinen durch den Golgi-Apparat hergestellt zu sein. Dieselben sind oft an der Plasmamembran fixiert und geben ihren Inhalt in die intercellulären Räume ab. Die Färbeaffinität von diesen Körnchen zeigt, daß sie wahrscheinlich für die amyloresistente PAS-Färbung verantwortlich sind, welche in der Nähe der Nagelplatte beobachtet wird.

Die Hornzellen bestehen aus Filamenten und aus einer amorphen Substanz, welche die Räume zwischen den Filamenten ausfüllt.

Das Ergebnis dieser histologischen und histochemischen Analyse des Nagels erlaubt somit, das Bestehen einer *Nageleinheit* zu bestätigen, die sich aus dem Nagel und seiner Wurzel, seinem Bett und dem periungualen Gewebe zusammensetzt.

Diese unitarische Konzeption, die man mit derjenigen der follikulären Einheit vergleichen kann, vermag schließlich den Zugang zu dem oft komplexen Gebiet der Pathologie des Nagels zu erleichtern.

Für die freundliche Erlaubnis, verschiedene Dokumente zu reproduzieren, danke ich den Autoren und Verlagen herzlich. Den Herren DUPONT und BOURLOND, ELLIS, HORSTMANN, KLIGMAN, MORIKE, SERRI u. Mitarb., WINKELMANN u. Mitarb., ZAIAS sowie dem Verlag Pergamon Press, spreche ich meine Dankbarkeit aus.

Literatur

ACHTEN, G.: Recherches sur la kératinisation de la cellule épidermique chez l'homme et le rat. Arch. Biol. (Liège) **70**, 1—119 (1959). — L'ongle normal et pathologique. Dermatologica (Basel) **126**, 229—245 (1963). — ANDERSEN, H.: Histochemical studies on the histogenesis of the nails. Acta morph. neerl.-scand. **3**, 322—330 (1961). — ASTBURY, W.: The X-ray interpretation of fibre structure. Science **28**, 210—288 (1933). — The hydrogen bond in protein structure. Trans. Faraday Soc. **36**, 871—880 (1940). — BARNETT, R., and A. SELIGMAN: Histochemical demonstration of protein-bound sulfhydryl group. Science **116**, 323—327 (1952). — Histochemical demonstration of sulfhydryl and disulfide group of protein. J. nat. Cancer Inst. **14**, 769—803 (1954). — BEAR, R., and H. RUGO: The results of X-ray diffraction studies on keratin fibers. Ann. N.Y. Acad. Sci. **53**, 627—648 (1951). — BECKETT, E., G. BOURNE, and W. MONTAGNA: Histology and cytochemistry of human skin. The distribution of cholinesterase in the finger of the embryo and the adult. J. Physiol. **134**, 202—206 (1956). — BOAS, J.: Ein Beitrag zur Morphologie der Nägel, Krallen, Hufe und Klauen der Säugethiere. Morph. Jb. **9**, 389—400 (1884). — BOURLOND, A.: Étude par l'impregnation argentique de l'innervation du derme superficiel et de la jonction dermo-épidermique. Bull. Soc. franç. Derm. Syph. **69**, 246—249 (1962). — Structures nerveuses du derme superficiel et de l'épiderme. Arch. belges Derm. **19**, 297—309 (1963). — BRACHET, J.: Embryologie chimique. Paris: Masson & Cie. 1947. — Le rôle des acides nucléiques dans la vie de la cellule et de l'embryon. Actual. Biochim. **16**, 1—122 (1952). — Biochem. Cytology. New York: Academic Press 1957. — BRAUN-FALCO, O.: The histochemistry of psoriasis. Ann. N.Y. Acad. Sci. **73**, 936—976 (1958). — BRUHAS, F.: Der Nagel der Halbaffen und Affen. Morph. Jb. **40**, 501—609 (1910). — BURROWS, M.: The significance of the lunula of the nail. Johns Hopk. Hosp. Rep. **18**, 357—361 (1919). — CASPERSSON, T.: Relation between nucleic acid and protein synthesis. Symp. Soc. exp. Biol. **1**, 127—151 (1947). — Cell growth and cell function. New York: Norton 1950. — CAUNA, N.: Nature and function of the papillary ridges of the digital skin. Anat. Rec. **119**, 449—468 (1954). — The distribution of cholinesterase in the cutaneous receptor organs especially tanch corpuscules of the human finger. J. Histochem. Cytochem. **8**, 367—375 (1960). — CHEVREMONT, M., et J. FREDERIC: Une nouvelle méthode histochimique de mise en évidence des substances à fonction sulfhydryle. Application à l'épiderme, au poil et à la levure. Arch. Biol. (Liège) **54**, 589—605 (1943).

Dastur, D.: Cutaneous nerves in leprosy. The relationship between histopathology and cutaneous sensibility. Brain 78, 615—633 (1955). — Davis, M., and J. Lawler: Capillary microscopy in normal and diseased human skin. Advanc. Biol. Skin. 2, 79—97 (1961). — Derksen, J., G. Heringa, and A. Weidinger: On keratin and cornification. Acta neerl. Morph. 1, 31—37 (1937). — Dupont, A., et A. Bourlond: Innervation de la jonction dermoépidermique. Arch. belges Derm. 18, 249—257 (1962). — Recherches sur les structures nerveuses de la peau humaine. Trab. Inst. Cajal Invest. biol. 54, 177—186 (1962). — Dupre, A.: Étude histochimique des glucides de la peau humaine. Toulouse: Du Viguier 1952.

Ellis, R.: Vascular patterns of the skin. Advanc. Biol. Skin. 2, 20—37 (1961).

Firket, A.: Recherches sur la régénération de la peau de mammifère. Arch. Biol. (Liège) 62, 309—351 (1951). — Fleischhauer, K., u. E. Horstmann: Der Papillarkörper und die Kapillaren des Perionychiums. Z. Zellforsch. 42, 213—228 (1955). — Flesch, P.: Chemical data on human epidermal keratinization and differenciation. J. invest. Derm. 31, 63—73 (1958). — Fraser, R., H. Lindley, and G. Rogers: Chemical heterogeneity and cortical segmentation in wool. Biochim. biophys. Acta (Amst.) 13, 295—297 (1954). — Fraser, R., and G. Rogers: Microscopic observations of the alkaline-thioglycolate extraction of wool. Biochim. biophys. Acta (Amst.) 12, 484—485 (1953). — The origin of segmentation in wool cortex. Biochim. biophys. Acta (Amst.) 13, 297—298 (1954).

Giroud, A., et G. Champetier: Recherches sur les roentgenogrammes de la kératine. Bull. Soc. chim. Biol. 18, 656—664 (1936). — Gross, J.: Connective tissue fine structure and some methods for its analysis. J. Geront. 5, 343—360 (1950).

Hashimoto, K., B. Gross, R. Nelson, and W. Lever: The ultrastructure of the nail in 16—18 weeks old embryos. J. invest. Derm. 47, 205—217 (1966). — Heller, J.: Die Krankheiten der Nägel. In: Jadassohns Handbuch der Haut- und Geschlechtskrankheiten, Bd. 13/3. Berlin-Göttingen-Heidelberg: Springer 1957. — Hibbs, R., and W. Clark: Electron microscope studies of the human epidermis. The cell boundaries and topography of the stratum Malpighi. J. biophys. biochem. Cytol. 6, 71—76 (1959). — Horio, M., and T. Kondo: Theory and morphology of crimped rayon staples. Textile Res. J. 23, 373—386 (1953). — Horstmann, E.: Über den Papillarkörper der menschlichen Haut und seine regionalen Unterschiede. Acta anat. (Basel) 14, 23—42 (1952). — Bau und Struktur des menschlichen Nagels. Z. Zellforsch. 41, 532—555 (1955). — Der Nagel. In: v. Möllendorffs Handbuch der mikroskopischen Anatomie des Menschen, Bd. III/3. Berlin-Göttingen-Heidelberg: Springer 1957. — Horstmann, E., u. A. Knoop: Elektronenmikroskopische Studien der Epidermis. I. Rattenpfote. Z. Zellforsch. 47, 348—362 (1958). — Hurley, H., and G. Koelle: The effect of inhibition of non-specific cholinesterase on perception of tactile sensation in human volar skin. J. invest. Derm. 31, 243—245 (1958). — Hurley, H., and H. Mescon: Cholinergic innervation of the digital arteriovenous anastomoses of human skin. A histochemical localization of cholinesterase. J. appl. Physiol. 9, 82—84 (1956).

Kligman, A.: Why do nails grow out instead of up? Arch. Derm. 84, 181—183 (1961). — Kolliker, A.: Die Entwicklung des menschlichen Nagels. Z. wiss. Zool. 47, 129—154 (1888). — Koning, A.: Histochemical localization of certain constituents of the developing juvenile wing feather. Amer. J. Anat. 100, 17—49 (1957). — Koning, A., and H. Hamilton: Localization of enzyme systems nucleid acids and polysaccharides during morphogenesis in the down feather of the chick. Amer. J. Anat. 95, 75—108 (1954). — Changes in the localization of alcaline, ribonucleic acid and polysaccharides during the transition from down to juvenile stage of the feather. Anat. Rec. 122, 422—423 (1955). — Krantz, W.: Beitrag zur Anatomie des Nagels. Derm. Z. 64, 239—242 (1939).

Leloup, R., et A. Bourlond: Quelques images du réseau sympathique cutané. Arch. belges Derm. 17, 223—229 (1961). — Lewis, B.: Microscopic studies of fetal and mature nail and surrounding soft tissue. Arch. Derm. Syph. 70, 732—747 (1954). — Lewis, B., and H. Montgomery: The senile nail. J. invest. Derm. 24, 11—18 (1955). — Lloyd, D.: Progress in leather science. Brit. Leather Man. Res. Ass. London 3, 1920—1945 (1948). — Lloyd, D., and M. Garrod: The rubberlike condition of the fibers of animal skin. Symp. on fibrous proteins. Soc. of Dyers and Colourists. London: Chorley & Pickersgell 1946. — A contribution to the theory of the structure of protein fibers with special reference to the socalled thermal skrinkage of collagen. Trans. Faraday Soc. 44, 441—451 (1948).

Martin, B., and M. Platts: A histological study of the nail region in normal human subjects and in those showing splinter haemorrhages of the nail. J. Anat. 93, 323—330 (1959). — Martinez Perez, R.: Contribution à l'étude des terminaisons nerveuses de la peau de la main. Trav. Lab. Rech. biol. Univ. Madrid 27, 187—226 (1931). — Masson, P.: Le glomus cutané de l'homme. Bull. Soc. franç. Derm. Syph. 42, 1174—1245 (1935). — Matoltsy, A. G., and P. F. Parakkal: Membrane-coating granules of keratinizing epithelia. J. Cell Biol. 24, 297 (1965). — Mercer, E.: The heterogeneity of the keratin. Textile Res. J. 23, 388—397 (1953). — Keratin and keratinisation. An essay in molecular biology. New York: Pergamon Press 1961. — Miller, M., H. Ralston, and M. Kasahara: The pattern of cutaneous innervation of the human hand, foot and breast. Advanc. Biol. Skin. **1**, 1—47 (1960). — MONASH, S.: Normal pigmentation in the nails of the negro. Arch. Derm. Syph. **25**, 876—881 (1932). — MONTAGNA, W.: The structure and function of the skin. New York: Academic Press 1962. — MONTAGNA, W., H. CHASE, and J. HAMILTON: The distribution of glycogen and lipids in human skin. J. invest. Derm. **17**, 147—157 (1951). — MONTAGNA, W., H. CHASE, and H. MELARAGNO: Histology and cytochemistry of human skin. Metachromasia in the mons pubis. J. nat. Cancer Inst. **12**, 591—597 (1951). — MORETTI, G., and H. MESCON: Chemical-histochemical evaluation of acid phosphatase activity in human skin. J. Histochem. **4**, 247—253 (1956); — Histochemical distribution of acid phosphatases in normal human skin. J. invest. Derm. **26**, 347—360 (1956). — MORIKE, K.: Das Verhalten des Hyponychiums beim normalen Nagelwachstum. Verh. anat. Ges. (Jena) **101**, 289—293 (1955).

ODLAND, G.: The fine structure of the interrelationship of cells in the human epidermis. J. biophys. biochem. Cytol. **4**, 529—538 (1958). — A submicroscopic granular component in human epidermis. J. invest. Derm. **34**, 11—15 (1960). — ORMEA, F.: La cute organo di senso. Minerva med. (1961).

PARDO-CASTELLO, V., and O. A. PARDO: Diseases of the nails. Springfield (Ill.): Ch. C. Thomas 1960. — PINKUS, F.: The development of the tegument. Manual of human embryology. Philadelphia: J. B. Lippincott Co. 1910. — Die normale Anatomie der Haut. In: JADASSOHNS Handbuch der Haut- und Geschlechtskrankheiten, Bd. I/1, S. 1—378. Berlin: Springer 1927. — PORT, E.: Das Auftreten von drei Schichten in der Hornsubstanz des Nagels bei der Betrachtung im polarisierten Lichte und ihre Beziehung zur Nagelmatrix. Z. Zellforsch. **19**, 110—118 (1933). — PORTER, K.: Observation on the fine structure of animal epidermis. Proc. Ed. Int. Conf. Electron. Microsc. London, p. 539 (1954).

RICHTER, R.: Über die Brauchbarkeit der Einschlußfärbung nativer Gefrierschnitte in Ehrlich's saurem Hämatoxylin nach Feyrter zur Darstellung der Nervenelemente der Haut. Z. Haut- u. Geschl.-Kr. **18**, 33—39 (1955). — ROE, D.: a) A fibrous keratin precursor from the human epidermis. J. invest. Derm. **27**, 1—8 (1956). — b) Further studies of a fibrous keratin precursor from the human epidermis. J. invest. Derm. **27**, 319—324 (1956). — RUDALL, K.: The proteins of the mammalian epidermis. Advanc. Protein Chem. **7**, 253—259 (1952).

SCOTHORNE, R., and A. SCOTHORNE: Histochemical studies on human skin autografts. J. Anat. **87**, 22—29 (1953). — SELBY, C.: An electron microscope study of the epidermis of mammalian skin in thin sections. I. Dermo-epidermal junction and basal cell layer. J. biophys. biochem. Cytol. **1**, 429—444 (1955). — Fine structure of human epidermis. J. Soc. cosmet. Chem. **7**, 584—599 (1956). — SERRI, F.: Les Cholinestérases dans le développement de la peau foetale. Arch. belges Derm. **19**, 351—352 (1963). — SERRI, F., W. HUBER e H. MESCON: Studi sulla cute del feto e del bambino. III. Attivata della fosfatasi acida nella cute del feto. Boll. Soc. ital. Biol. sper. **38**, 1169—1172 (1962). — SERRI, F., W. MONTAGNA, and H. MESCON: Studies of the skin of the fetus and the child. Glycogen and amylophosphorylase in the skin of the fetus. J. invest. Derm. **39**, 199—217 (1962). — Osservazioni sull'innervazione della cute fetale con particulare riguardo delle dita. Acta neuroveg. (Wien) **24**, 166—174 (1963). — SERRI, F., W. MONTAGNA, and W. HUBER: Studies of skin of fetus and the child. The distribution of alkaline phosphatase in the skin of the fetus. Arch. Derm. **87**, 234—245 (1963). — STEIGLEDER, G., and D. WEAKLEY: Mucopolysaccharides in human epidermis. Brit. J. Derm. **73**, 171—179 (1961).

TRUFFI, G.: Sulla vascolarizzazione degli annessi cutanei. Arch. ital. Derm. **10**, 681—728 (1934).

WEDDEL, G., E. PALMER, and W. PALLIE: Nerve endings in mammalian skin. Biol. Rev. **30**, 159—195 (1955). — WEISS, P., and W. FERRIS: Electron microscopic study of the texture of the basement membrane of larval amphibian skin. Proc. nat. Acad. Sci. (Wash.) **6**, 528—540 (1954). — WINKELMANN, R.: Nerve endings in normal and pathologic skin. Springfield (Ill.): Ch. C. Thomas 1960. — WINKELMANN, R., S. SCHEEN jr., R. PYKA, and M. COVENTRY: Cutaneous vascular patterns in studies with injection preparation and alkaline phosphatase reaction. Advanc. Biol. Skin. **2**, 1—19 (1961).

ZAIAS, N.: Embryology of the human nail. Arch. Derm. **87**, 37—53 (1963). — ZANDER, R.: Die Histogenese des Nagels beim menschlichen Foetus. Arch. Anat. Entwickl.-Gesch. 273—305 (1886). — ZIEGLER, H.: Die Bildung des menschlichen Nagels und des Pferdehufs. Z. mikr.-anat. Forsch. **60**, 556—572 (1954).

Zur Innervation der Haut

Von

E. Hagen, Bonn

Mit 47 Abbildungen

Einleitung

Die morphologischen Studien von v. Frey (1895) waren mehr als 50 Jahre grundlegend für eine Sinnesphysiologie, die bestimmten nervösen Strukturen der Haut spezifische Funktionen zuordnete.

Stöhr hatte 1928 bereits davor gewarnt, den mit den Autorennamen bezeichneten, sensiblen Endkörperchen eine unterschiedliche physiologische Deutung zu geben. Er gab zu bedenken, ,,daß das, was wir unter Krause-, Meissner-, Pacini-, Ruffini-Körperchen usw. verstehen, rein willkürlich aus einer unendlichen Formenreihe herausgegriffene Typen sind, die man aber niemals als feste, nebeneinander bestehende, unveränderliche Formengebilde ansehen darf, sondern die durch eine riesige Menge von Modifikationen alle ineinander gleichsam fließend übergehen''.

Vor etwa 15 Jahren konnten Weddell und seine Mitarbeiter (1953—1964) die alte v. Freysche Lehre durch sehr einfache Beobachtungen ins Wanken bringen. Bisher hatte man der Wahrnehmung von Berührung, Druck, Schmerz, Wärme und Kälte jeweils eine spezifisch gebaute Endigung (Grandry, Golgi-Mazzoni, Krause, Meissner, Merkel, Vater-Pacini, Ruffini usw.) zudiktiert. Hagen, Knoche, Sinclair und Weddell (1953) stellten nun fest, daß in der normalen behaarten Haut der Körperoberfläche nervöse Endkörperchen der eben genannten Typen fast gänzlich fehlen, obwohl auch behaarte Körperstellen eine ausgeprägte Empfindungsfähigkeit für Temperatur, Berührung, Schmerz usw. besitzen.

Diese histologische Beobachtung gab den Anstoß zu erneuter neurophysiologischer Überprüfung der Haut und rückte die reiche Innervation der Wurzelscheide und des Haarbalgs ins Licht. In den korbartig um das Haar gebauten Nervengittern (Manschetten), die sich nur morphologisch, nicht funktionell, von den in der unbehaarten Haut vorkommenden nervösen Endapparaten unterscheiden, liegen demnach Empfänger für alle die behaarte Haut treffenden Reize.

Auf die Problematik eines gesetzmäßigen Zusammenhangs von Struktur und Sinnesqualität im Sinne von v. Frey weisen auch Untersuchungen von Cauna (1965) und Sinclair (1967) hin. Er beobachtete, daß die überwiegende Mehrzahl in der unbehaarten Haut gelegener, spezifisch gebauter receptorischer Nervenorgane im Laufe des Lebens einem Wechsel in Form und Zahl unterworfen ist.

Morphologische und experimentell-physiologische Methoden führten bis heute nur zu einer Teillösung in der Zuordnung der Gestalt und Funktion nervöser Strukturen. Viel bleibt noch zu tun, die obige Frage zu erhellen.

Methoden

Cerebrospinale und vegetative Nerven beteiligen sich an der Versorgung der menschlichen Haut. Ihr außerordentlicher Reichtum an markhaltigen und marklosen Nervenfasern wurde schon lichtmikroskopisch durch zahlreiche Färbeverfahren gezeigt. Während die üblichen histologischen Methoden nur gröbere Nervenstrukturen zur Darstellung bringen, vermögen supravitale Methylenblau- und Rongalit-Weiß-Färbung (TAMPONI, 1938; KAMIDE, 1955; MALCOLM und MILLER, 1960) sowie Silberimprägnationen in geübter Hand Vorzügliches zu leisten. Mit Hilfe der Bielschowsky-Gros-Methode vermag man sowohl das sensible cerebrospinale Nervensystem als auch das in der Haut oft aufs engste mit ihm verquickte vegetative Nervensystem zu erfassen. Die von JABONERO, BENGOECHEA und PEREZ-CASA (1962) angegebene Silbercarbonatmethode, die Protargol-Technik (FITZGERALD, 1962) und die Osmium-Zink-Jodid-Färbung (MAILLET, 1959 und 1963) erzielen lohnende Resultate über die Nervenversorgung der Haut. Letztere Methode bringt in der Cutis gelegene Dendritenzellen besonders deutlich zum Vorschein (NIEBAUER, 1967).

Um die Endausbreitung vegetativer Nerven zu studieren, empfiehlt sich die Versilberung der Organschnitte nach RICHARDSON (1960) in der Modifikation nach NEWTON (1964). In der Haut gelingt es auf diese Weise, — vollkommener als mit allen übrigen Färbeverfahren — Gefäßnervenbündel bis in ihre Endaufzweigungen im Verlauf der Capillaren aufzufinden. Schweißdrüsen und bindegewebiger Haarbalg zeigen die Fülle sie umspinnender markloser Nervenelemente. Selbst die mit anderen Methoden kaum zu erfassenden Nervenfasern an den Talgdrüsen werden sichtbar.

Die lichtmikroskopischen Ergebnisse über die Nervenversorgung der Haut stellen die notwendige Voraussetzung zum Verständnis des ultramikroskopischen Bildes dieser Nerven dar. Wenn auch das Elektronenmikroskop die Feinstruktur der Gewebe bis in den Mikrobereich zu durchdringen vermag, so erschweren die in Ångström gemessenen Schnitte außerordentlich eine räumliche Vorstellung vor allem bei geweblichen Strukturen, die sich durch Verästelungen und Knäuelbildungen auszeichnen. So läßt sich das elektronenmikroskopische Bild eines Endkörperchens der Haut nur an Hand des lichtmikroskopischen, in Mikron gemessenen Parallelschnittes deuten und ergänzen. Daher wurde besonderer Wert darauf gelegt, die für die Elektronenmikroskopie verwendeten Abschnitte der Haut mit Hilfe des Phasenkontrastmikroskops einer exakten lichtmikroskopischen Kontrolle zu unterziehen, und ein weiteres Teilstück vergleichend mit Silbermethoden zu behandeln.

Das elektronenoptische Material wurde teils in eisgekühlter, gepufferter 1%iger Osmiumsäure mit 4,5% Saccharose-Zusatz, teils in 6,25% Glutaraldehyd und nachfolgender OsO_4-Lösung fixiert. Dehydrierung in aufsteigender Acetonreihe und Einbettung in Vestopal W. Kontrastierung durch 1% Phosphorwolframsäure und 0,5% Uranylacetatlösung nach WOHLFARTH-BOTTERMANN. Ultradünnschnitte am „Ultrotome LKB". Mikroskop: Zeiss EM 9''.

Frau PAULA SCHOLZ und Fräulein CHRISTA FRANKEN danke ich für sorgfältige Handhabung der licht- und elektronenmikroskopischen Methodik sowie für die Herstellung der Mikrophotogramme.

1. Epidermale Nerven

Seit nahezu 100 Jahren widersprechen sich die Beobachtungen über Vorkommen und Nichtvorkommen intraepidermaler Nervenfasern (BONNET, 1878; KÖLLIKER, 1889; DOGIEL, 1903; BOTEZAT, 1908; KADANOFF, 1928; LEVI, 1933; SZYMONOWICZ, 1933; WADA, 1949 und BOURLOND, 1962; DUPONT und BOURLOND, 1962 und PAWLOWSKI, 1963; KADANOFF, 1966).

Trotz ihres bisher lückenhaften morphologischen Nachweises spricht die Physiologie bereits intraepitheliale Nerven als schmerzleitende Nerven an (WEDDELL, 1957). Durch die Einwirkung chemischer Stoffe, die etwa von mechanisch oder thermisch geschädigten Epithelzellen abgegeben werden, sollen ihre Endigungen in Erregung geraten (BARGMANN, 1967).

Sucht man im Epithel behaarter oder unbehaarter menschlicher Hautstücke lichtmikroskopisch nach Nerven, so ist das ein zumeist aussichtsloses Unternehmen. Auch geeignete Färbemethoden wie Silberimprägnation oder intravitale Methylenblaufärbung lassen Zweifel aufkommen, ob nicht tangential geführte Schnittrichtungen oder optische Unzulänglichkeiten eine intercelluläre oder gar intracelluläre Lagerung der Nervenfasern im Epithel vortäuschen. Nur vereinzelt sieht man durch die Keimschicht des Epithels marklose Nervenfasern ziehen. Diese als freie, intraepithelial endigende Nervenelemente anzusprechen, schien bisher nicht gesichert, da das vermeintliche Nervenende auch der Schnittpunkt der hier umbiegenden Fasern sein könnte.

Flachschnitte durch die Schichten einer epithelialen Oberfläche zeigen senkrecht aus den Bindegewebspapillen in die Epidermis vordringende Nervenfasern meist nur im Querschnitt. Ihre Achsencylinder können lichtmikroskopisch bestenfalls als dickere Punkte erkannt werden.

Letztlich erbrachten elektronenoptische Ergebnisse den Beweis für das Vorkommen von Nerven im Epithel der menschlichen Haut (HAGEN und WERNER, 1966/67).

In ihrem Endausbreitungsgebiet innerhalb der Cutis scheinen die markhaltigen, cerebrospinalen Nervenfasern der Haut, lichtoptisch gesehen, ihre Markscheiden zu verlieren und sind dadurch von den sog. marklosen vegetativen Nerven auch elektronenmikroskopisch noch nicht eindeutig zu unterscheiden. Trotzdem erscheint eine nähere Begriffsklärung der Feinstruktur sog. ,,markhaltiger" und ,,markloser" Nervenelemente (Axone) in diesem Zusammenhang notwendig.

Elektronenoptisch bestehen die Markscheiden der klassischen Histologie aus einer mehr oder weniger großen Zahl spiralig um das Axon gewickelter Lamellen (ENGSTRÖM und WERSÄLL, 1958), die aus dem Plasmalemm (Cytomembran) der Schwannschen Zellen bestehen. Je nach Zahl der Lamellen spricht man besser von markarmen oder markreichen Nervenfasern.

Auch die aus der Lichtmikroskopie als marklos bekannten Nervenelemente zeigen elektronenoptisch eine einfache Hülle aus Plasmalemm der Schwannschen Zellen (periphere Glia oder Lemnocyten), dazu als Zeichen ihrer Einstülpung in die Schwannsche Zelle ein Mesaxon (Duplikatur des Plasmalemm). Unvollständige Umfassungen durch das Plasmalemm der Schwannschen Zelle geben das Axolemm des Axons frei, das nunmehr mit seiner Nachbarschaft in unmittelbaren Kontakt zu treten vermag. Die freigegebenen Axonabschnitte werden deswegen als ,,Neuroeffector-Gebiete" (VAN DER ZYPEN, 1967 und HAGEN und WERNER, 1966/67) gedeutet, da sie als einzige periphere Nervenstrecke wirklich einer Umhüllung des Schwannschen Plasmalemm entbehren und dadurch am ehesten die Voraussetzung zu synapsenähnlicher Wirksamkeit besitzen.

Eigene elektronenmikroskopische Beobachtungen zeigen, daß die lichtmikroskopisch gerade noch sichtbaren, subepithelial gelegenen, feineren Nervenfasern im elektronenoptischen Bild (Abb. 1) in deutlichem Zusammenhang mit Epithelzellen stehen, denen sie sich, von gemeinsamer Basalmembran umschlossen, anfügen. Die strukturarmen Axone liegen mit einem mehr oder weniger langen Mesaxon versehen im Schwannschen Cytoplasma. Die Nervenäste entstammen dem in unmittelbarer Nähe zu beobachtenden subepidermalen Plexus (Abb. 1).

Nach unseren Beobachtungen vermögen Ausläufer der Schwannschen Zellen die Oberflächenmembran basaler Epithelzellen weit in das Innere hineinzustülpen (Abb. 2), so daß nur noch ein Doppelkontur die Invaginationsstelle der Epithelzelle

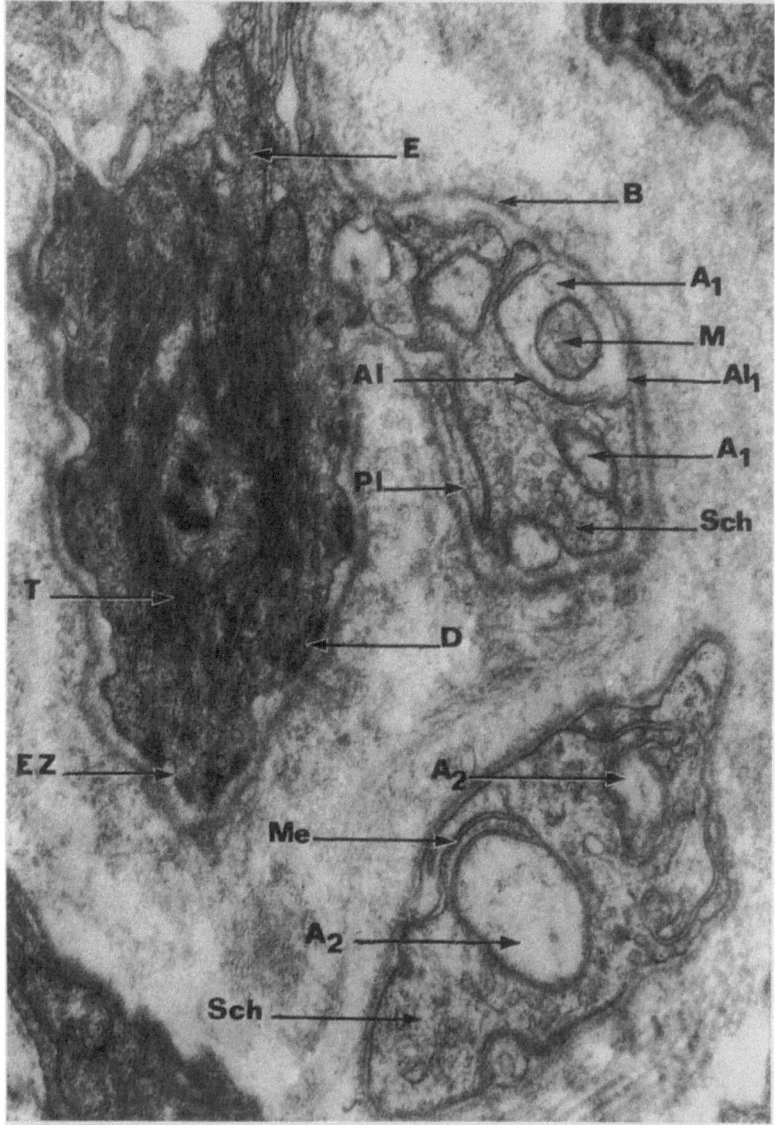

Abb. 1. Epidermale Axone (A_1) mit Schwannschem Cytoplasma (*Sch*). Behaarte Haut Mensch. *B* Gemeinsame Basalmembran umschließt Epithelzelle (*E*) und epidermale Axone (A_1), subepidermale Axone (A_2) mit Schwannschem Cytoplasma (*Sch*); *Me* Mesaxon, *EZ* Cytomembran der Epithelzelle, *D* Desmosomen, *T* Tonofibrillen, *Al* von Schwannschem Plasmalemm umhüllter Axonabschnitt, Al_1 freies Axolemm, *Pl* Plasmalemm (Cytomembran der Schwannschen Zelle), *M* Mitrochondrien im Axon. Neg. Vergr. 12 000 ×

anzeigt. Der Schwannsche Cytoplasmaausläufer umschließt quer getroffene Axone (Abb. 2). Diese sind allseitig von der Schwannschen Oberflächenmembran umhüllt.

Auch die intercellulär gelagerten Nerven des Epithels entspringen den Aufteilungen des subepidermalen Geflechtes, mit dessen Ultrastruktur sie übereinstimmen. Um eine Reizübertragung der dem subepidermalen Geflecht entstammenden, markarmen Nervenfasern auf die Epithelzellen zu ermöglichen, müssen die Schwannschen Zellen die Axone ganz (Abb. 3) oder teilweise (Abb. 4) aus ihrer membranösen Hülle freigeben. Dabei umfaßt die angrenzende Cytomembran der basalen Epithelzelle das nunmehr nackte Axon (Abb. 3), das mehr

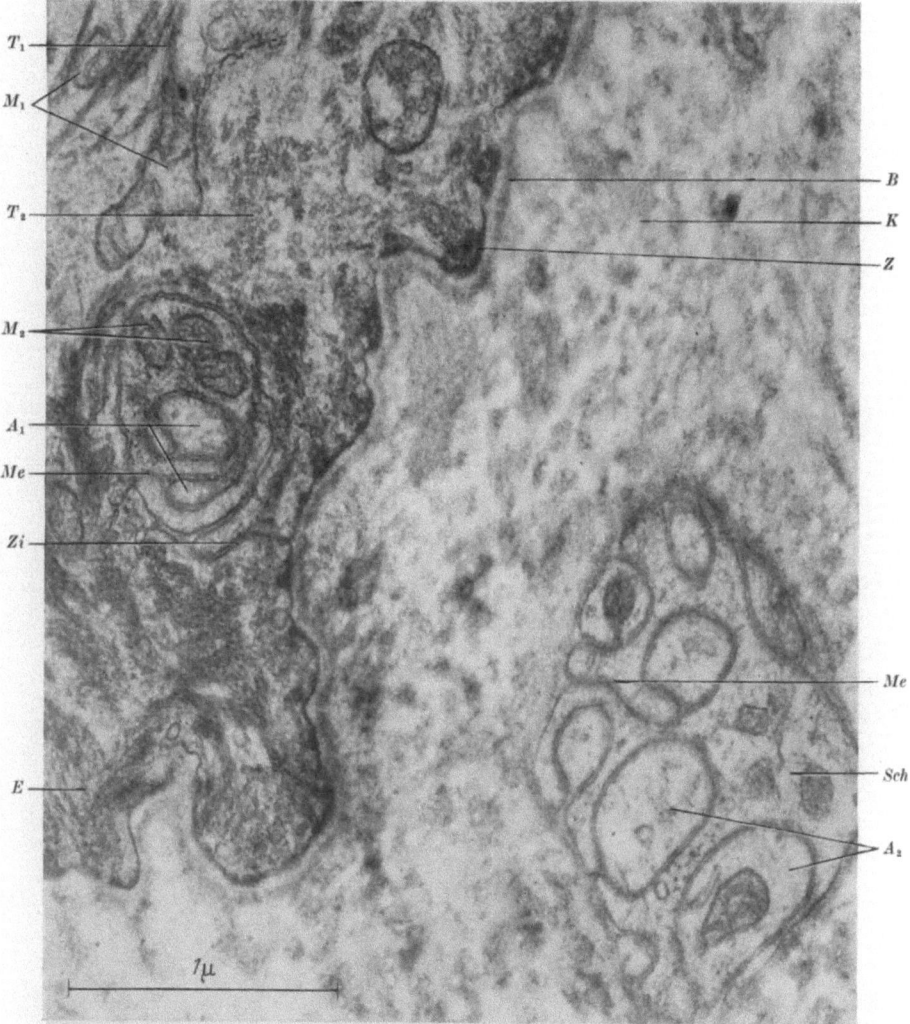

Abb. 2. Intraepitheliale Lage der in Schwannschen Zisternen gelegenen Axone (A_1). Normale Unterlippe, Affe. Cytoplasma der Epithelzelle (E) im Stratum basale; M_1 Mitochondrien der Epithelzelle, T_1 Tonofibrillen der Epithelzelle längs, T_2 Tonofibrillen der Epithelzelle quer, M_2 Mitochondrien der Schwannschen Zelle, Me Mesaxone, Z Zellmembran und Desmosomen der Epithelzelle, Zi von Schwannscher Zelle eingestülpte Oberflächenmembran der Epithelzelle, B Basalmembran, K kollagenes Bindegewebe, Sch Schwannsches Cytoplasma, A_2 subepidermale Axone. Neg. Vergr. 12200 × (HAGEN und WERNER, 1966)

oder weniger tief in den Zelleib eingelagert ist, während die Basalmembran den Rand der Epithelzellen zum Corium hin nahtlos säumt.

Wenn die Axone nur teilweise von der Schwannschen Cytomembran freigegeben werden (Abb. 4), geht die Basalmembran der basalen Epithelzellen in die Basalmembran der Schwannschen Zellen über. Wahrscheinlich durch den engen Kontakt zwischen Nervenfasern und Epithelzelle bedingt, — der Abstand zwischen den beiden Elementen mißt nur ca. 200 Ångström — treten im Axon nur selten einzelne synaptische Bläschen oder Elementargranula in Erscheinung im Gegensatz zu den synaptischen Verbindungen von Nerven in anderen Organen (PALAY und PALADE, 1955; DE ROBERTIS und BENETT, 1955; ROBERTSON, 1956; ALLEN und NICHOLS, 1961; RUSKA und RUSKA, 1961 und VAN DER ZYPEN, 1965).

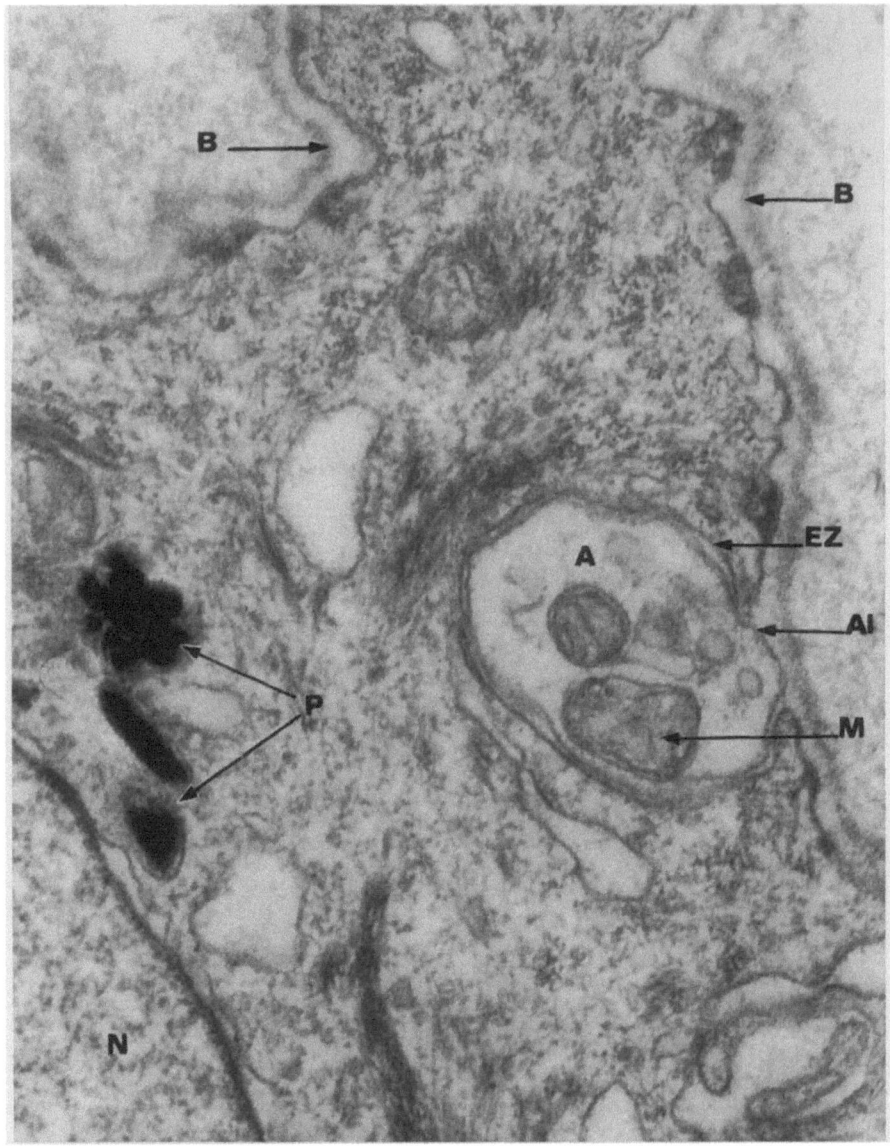

Abb. 3. In die basale Epithelzelle der Epidermis eingestülptes Axon (*A*), das von Schwannschem Cytoplasma freigegeben ist; dabei direkte Parallellagerung von Axolemm (*Al*) und epithelialer Cytomembran (*EZ*). Behaarte Haut, Mensch. *B* Basalmembran, *N* Nucleus der Epithelzelle, *P* Pigment, *M* Mitochondrien. Neg. Vergr. 15700 ×

Dieser durch keine Schwannsche Zellmembran gehinderte Kontakt zwischen Nervenfaser und Epithelzelle muß ein Gebiet effektorischer oder receptorischer Funktion mit einem synapsenähnlichen Übertragungsmodus darstellen, da nirgendwo im epidermalen oder subepidermalen Bereich eindeutig synaptische Formationen anzutreffen sind, die den sonst bekannten entsprächen.

Die ersten Axone findet ORFANOS (1965) unter der Basalmembran der menschlichen Epidermis. Er erörtert die Möglichkeit einer neuroepidermalen Verbindung im Basalmembranbereich, wo die Nervenfasern endigen sollen.

Bisher sind intracellulär gelagerte Nervenfasern des Epithels im Elektronenmikroskop nur von MUNGER (1965) in der Schnauze des Opossums gesehen worden.

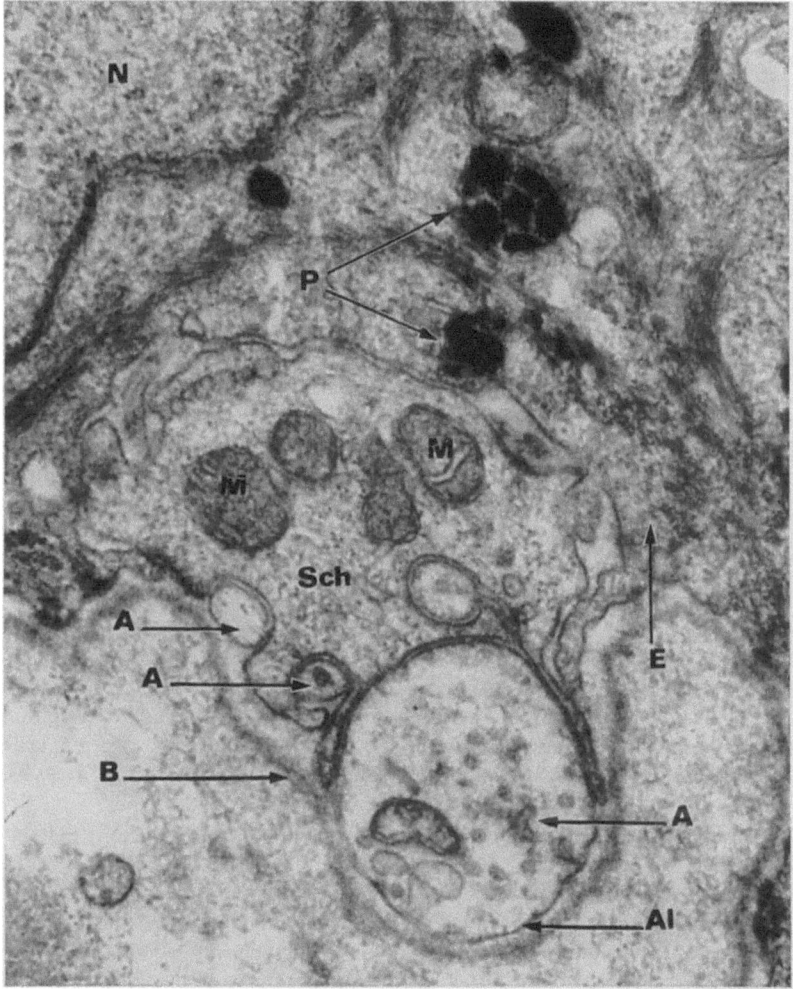

Abb. 4. Verschiedenkalibrige Axone (*A*) mit Schwannschem Cytoplasma (*Sch*) in Basalzelle der Epidermis eingelagert. Behaarte Haut, Mensch. *B* gemeinsame Basalmembran für Epithelzelle *E*, Schwannsches Cytoplasma (*Sch*) und durch die Schwannsche Zelle freigegebenes Axolemm (*Al*). *M* Mitochondrien der Schwannschen Zelle, *N* Nucleus der Epithelzelle, *P* Pigment. Neg. Vergr. 12 200 ×

Nach seinen Beobachtungen dringen zahlreiche, breite Nervenfasern unter Verlust ihrer Myelinscheide aus dem Corium in die Epidermis ein. Innerhalb des Epithels suchen die Axone den Anschluß an Zellen, die Sekretgranula enthalten. Der Autor interpretiert sie als Neuriten, die gemeinsam mit angelagerten Epithelzellen Receptororgane bilden.

Im Epithel des Lippen-Nasenbereichs verschiedener Tiere fand ONO (1956) und WALTER (1960/61) mit Silberimprägnationen freie Nervenendigungen. KADANOFF (1924) gelang eine sehr gute Darstellung intraepithelialer Nerven in der Rinderschnauze, und BOEKE (1925) bestätigte einen ungeheuren Nervenreichtum im „Eimerschen Organ" der Maulwurfschnauze.

Von intraepithelialen Nervenfasern im Vestibulum nasi der Kleinfledermäuse, dargestellt mit der Osmium-Zink-Jodidmethode, berichtet GOTHE (1965). An der Hornhaut des Auges wurden von COHNHEIM (1866), HOYER (1866), REISER (1935), PAU u. CONRADS (1957) sowie LELE u. WEDDELL (1959) Nervenfasern im Epithel beobachtet.

Nach der Entfernung der Keratinschicht von menschlicher Haut beobachteten ALLENBY, PALMER und WEDDELL (1966) die Proliferation markloser Nervenelemente und ihr Einwachsen in die untersten Epidermisschichten. Gleichzeitig kam es zur mitotischen Vermehrung der Epithelzellen. ARTHUR und SHELLEY (1959) sahen nach Abschaben der Epidermis eine Regeneration freier Nervenenden mit Knotenbildungen und borstenähnlichen Anordnungen. Ein regionales, hyperplastisches Wachstum von Nervenfasern in die Epidermis hinein ruft auch die Bepinselung der Mäusehaut mit Methylcholanthren hervor.

Zu den Nervenfasern, die eine lichtmikroskopisch sichtbare, fibrilläre Endaufsplitterung an Epithelzellen hervorbringen, gehören die in der Literatur der Haut bekannten „Merkelschen Tastscheiben". Dickere sensible Nervenfasern unter den basalen Zellschichten der Epidermis geraten nach den Beobachtungen von MARTINEZ-PEREZ (1931) in Kontakt mit den Merkelschen Tastscheiben und werden von ihm als „Plexus sousbasaux" bezeichnet. Ihnen wird allein aufgrund ihrer Struktur und Lage eine Tast- wie Schmerzempfindung zugeschrieben. Den physiologischen Beweis für die Sinnesleistung einer einzelnen Zelle anzutreten, bleibt problematisch.

An den untersten Zellschichten der Epidermis von Meerschweinchen enden kräftige Nervenfasern, die einzelne Epithelzellen korbartig umfassen (Abb. 7). Sie gleichen den von PINKUS (1903) und KAWAMURA (1954) an den „Haarscheiben" von Mensch und Tier beschriebenen intraepithelialen Endigungen von Nervenfasern, die den nach MERKEL (1880) benannten Tastzellen ähnlich sehen.

Die Mehrzahl aller intraepithelial gelagerten Nerven zeigt wenig elektronendichte Binnenstruktur. Einzelne, kleinere Mitochondrien, wenige Neurofilamente und Neurotubuli lassen das angeschnittene Axon inmitten der Epithelzellen hell erscheinen (Abb. 3).

Selten treten großkalibrige, an Mitochondrien reiche Axone unmittelbar an das Epithel heran (Abb. 5). Sie sind der Cytomembran der Epithelzellen ohne Zwischenlagerung einer Basalmembran, die unterbrochen scheint, unmittelbar angelagert und besitzen keine Markscheiden, sondern nur eine lückenhafte Umfassung durch Schwannsches Cytoplasma. Die Schwannsche Zelle zeichnet sich an diesen Nerven durch lamellär ineinandergreifende Fortsätze aus, die reichlich mit Pinocytose-Bläschen durchsetzt sind. Über lamelläre Formen und vacuolisierte Schwannsche Zellen an den Hautnerven der Menschen berichten EVANS, FINEAN und WOOLF (1965).

Der ununterbrochene Verlauf der Basalmembran parallel zur Unterfläche der Basalzellen der menschlichen Epidermis wird von STOIAN (1965) betont. Die Unterbrechung ihrer Kontinuität im Bereich der großen mitochondrienreichen Axone (sensible cerebrospinale Faser?) ist zweifellos bemerkenswert. Schließen sich kleinere, an Zellorganellen arme Axone dem Epithel an, dann geht die Basalmembran ihrer Schwannschen Zellen in die Basalmembran des Epithels über. Ob dieses Verhalten der Basalmembran einer besonderen funktionellen Bedeutung entspricht, läßt sich morphologisch nicht klären, jedoch ist der Kontakt bestimmter heller Epithelzellen des Stratum germinativum (Abb. 6) mit mitochondrienreichen Axonen auffällig. Die Cytomembran des Axons liegt nur wenige Ångström von der Cytomembran der Epithelzelle getrennt. Zwischen beiden fehlt die sonst übliche Basalmembran des Epithels. Durch helles Cytoplasma und spezifische Granula — die an Katecholamingranula erinnern — unterscheidet sich die abgebildete Zelle (Abb. 6) im Bau von anderen Epidermiszellen.

Ähnliche elektronenmikroskopische Beobachtungen machten PATRIZI und MUNGER (1966). Die Autoren beschreiben bei Ratten in den „Merkelzellen" der äußeren Wurzelscheide der Sinushaare Sekretgranula, die PAS-positiv und Diastase-resistent sind. Sie beobachten die Granula im Bereich der Kontaktstelle mit der mitochondrienreichen Nervenfaser, die sie als Mechanoreceptor deuten.

Vielleicht stellen diese unter Aufhebung der Basalmembran mit der Nervenfaser enger verknüpften Epithelzellen spezifische Tastzellen dar, wie sie für die Wurzelscheide des Sinushaares typisch sind.

Unter Berücksichtigung der lichtmikroskopischen Studien an Vater-Pacinischen und Meissnerschen Körperchen konnte die Entstehung mitochondrienreicher

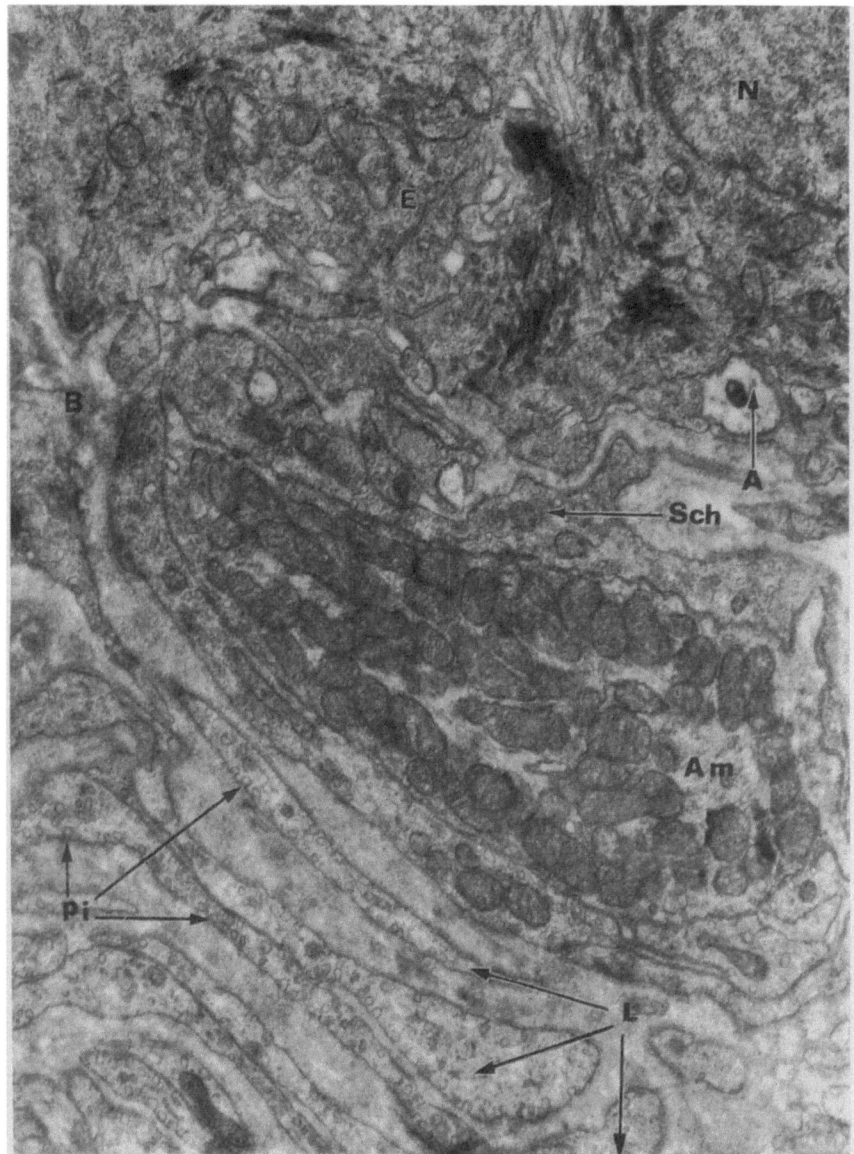

Abb. 5. Mitochondrienreiche Nervenfasern (*Am*) an Epithelzelle (*E*) in Schwannsches Cytoplasma eingelagert. Lippe, Affe. *L* lamelläre Fortsätze der Schwannschen Zelle mit Pinocytoseerscheinungen (*Pi*), *A* epidermales Axon, *N* Nucleus der Epithelzelle, *B* Basalmembran. Neg. Vergr. 7000 ×

Nervenfasern aus markhaltigen, sensiblen Nervenfasern nachgewiesen werden. Die Axone, welche die Endorgane entwickeln, zeichnen sich innerhalb der Körperchen elektronenoptisch durch einen großen Reichtum an Mitochondrien aus und haben keine Markscheiden mehr. Es liegt die Vermutung nahe, die mitochondrienreichen

25 Handb. d. Haut- u. Geschlechtskrankheiten, Erg.-Werk I/1

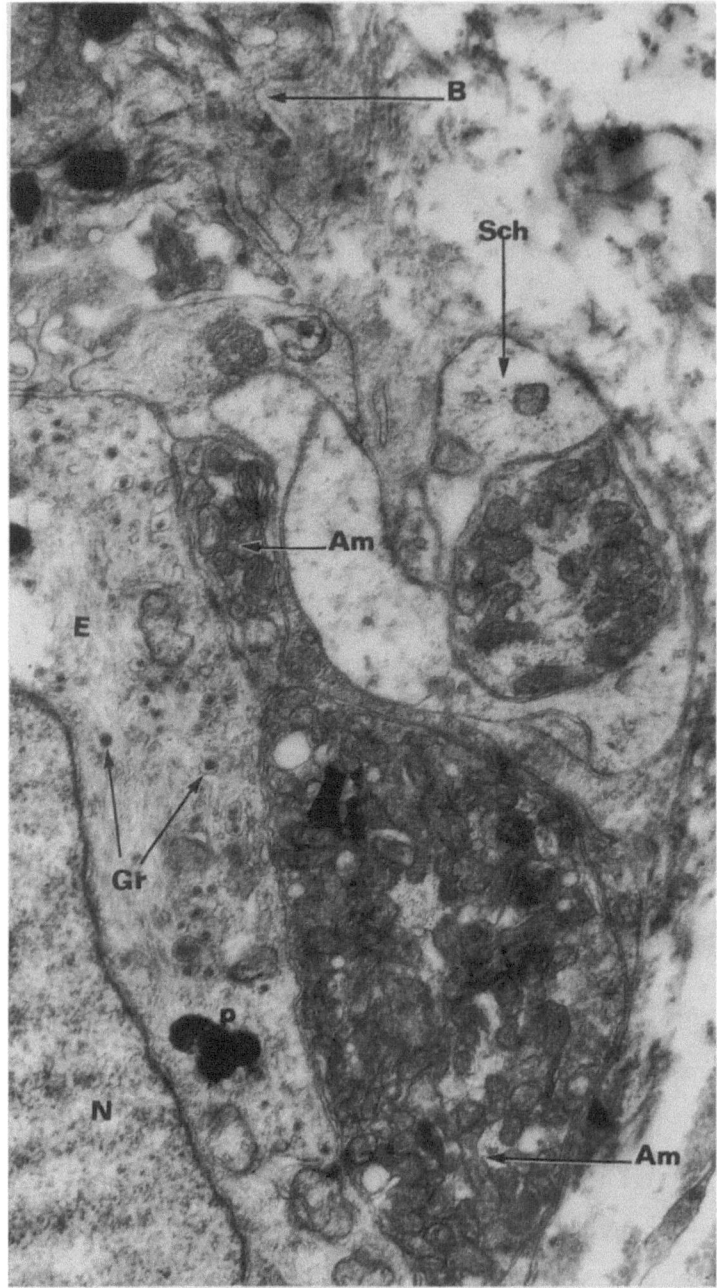

Abb. 6. Zwei mitochondrienreiche Axone (*Am*) in direktem Membrankontakt zu heller Epithelzelle (*E*) mit spezifischen Grana (*Gr*) und Pigment (*P*). Großzehenballen Affe. *Sch* Schwannsches Cytoplasma, *B* Basalmembran, *N* Nucleus der hellen Epithelzelle. Neg. Vergr. 7000 ×

Nerven, wie sie in großer Zahl an der äußeren Wurzelscheide des Haares (Abb. 35) zu finden sind, als sensible cerebrospinale Nerven zu deuten. Das Fehlen der Markscheide allein ermöglicht keine Unterscheidung gegenüber vegetativen Nervenfasern der Haut.

DUPONT und BOURLOND (1962) und FITZGERALD (1965) fanden keine intraepithelialen Nerven in der menschlichen Haut, jedoch stellten sie mit der Methode nach MAILLET (1959) ein Netz von Dentritenzellen in der Epidermis dar, das eine enge Beziehung zum subepidermalen vegetativen Nervengeflecht besitzt. AMERETTI (1965) hält den epidermalen Melanocyten für ein Neuron der „Berührungsempfindung" und konstruiert aus seinen Beobachtungen ein eigenes Funktionssystem dieser Zellen.

NIEBAUER (1967) berichtet ausführlich über die Dendritenzellen der Epidermis und stellt ihren Zusammenhang mit peripheren Nerven fest. Er hält ihre Herkunft aus der Neuralleiste für nachgewiesen. Die ersten Untersuchungen hierüber stammen von BORCEA (1909) und WEIDENREICH (1912). Eindeutige experimentelle Befunde über Dendritenzellen bei Säugetier und Mensch wurden von RAWLES (1947), ZIMMERMANN und CORNBLEET (1948), BECKER und ZIMMERMANN (1955)

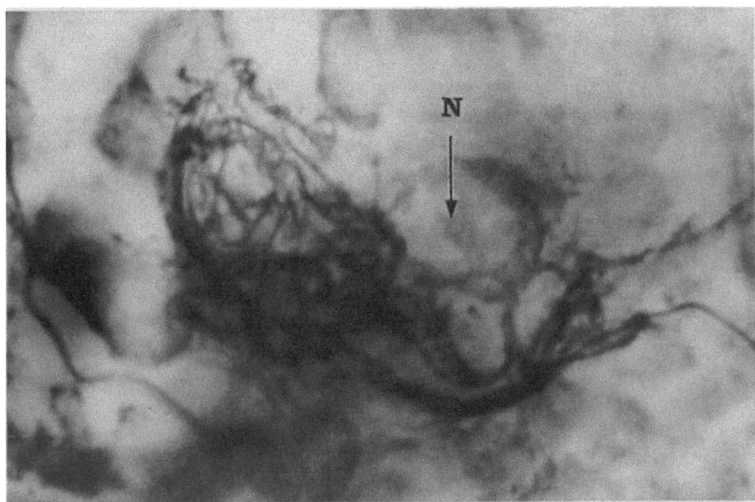

Abb. 7. Epithelzelle mit Neurofibrillenkorb. Behaarte Haut, Meerschweinchen. N Nucleus der Epithelzelle. Richardson-Newton-Methode. Präp.: W. Wittkowski. Neg. Vergr.: 640 ×

und ZIMMERMANN und BECKER (1955, 1959) erhoben. Auch im späteren Leben zeigen diese Zellen eine enge morphologische Beziehung zu den peripheren Hautnerven. Das Verhalten manifestiert sich lichtoptisch durch Kontakte zwischen den Dendriten der Melanocyten und den Nervenfasern der Haut. Auch MASSON (1926), TAMPONI (1938), FALCHI (1951), WIEDMANN (1952), NISHIHARA (1953), NIEBAUER (1956), MATSUMOTO (1961), SEKIDO (1963) und YANAZAKI (1964) haben auf die enge morphologische Beziehung hingewiesen.

Die von NIEBAUER (1952 und 1963), NIEBAUER und SEKIDO (1965) lichtmikroskopisch beobachteten Kontakte von Dendritenzellen der Epidermis mit vegetativen Nerven regten zu eigenen elektronenoptischen Untersuchungen an, die vor allem das Verhalten der Basalmembran erhellen sollten.

In der pigmentreichen Affenhaut begegnet man nicht selten Pigmentzellen in unmittelbarer Nähe des subepidermalen Plexus, der wiederum Axone in die unterste Epithelzellschicht abgibt (Abb. 8).

Langgestreckte Fortsätze der Dendritenzellen (Melanocyten) aus der Epidermis schmiegen sich oftmals dem Schwannschen Cytoplasma mit seinen eingebetteten Axonen an (Abb. 9). Dieselbe Basalmembran umschließt hierbei den Melanocytenfortsatz und die Schwannsche Zelle. Dies spricht für die oben erwähnte Hypothese einer gemeinsamen Genese. Stellenweise liegt das Axolemm frei unter der Basalmembran. In Parallelität zu den Beobachtungen über die neuroepidermalen Verknüpfungen könnte hier ein Neuroeffectorgebiet vorliegen.

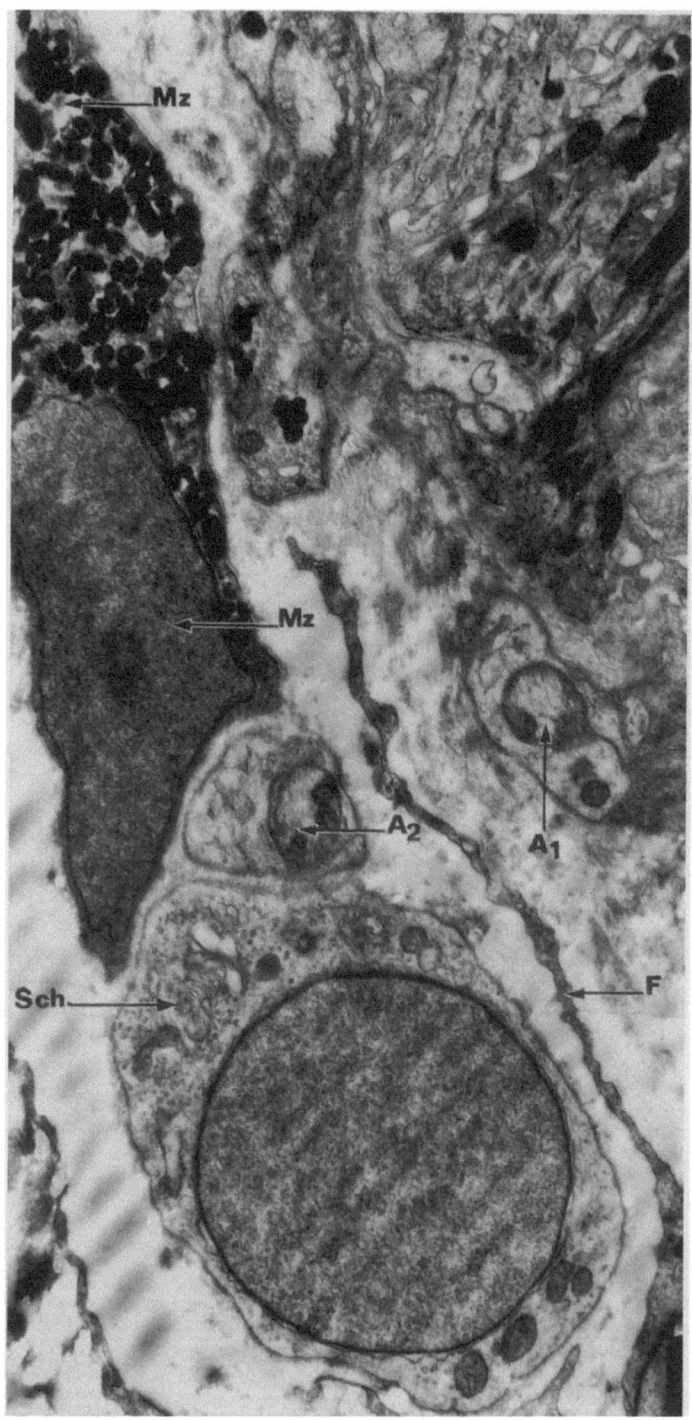

Abb. 8. Epidermales Axon (A_1), subepidermaler Melanocyt (Mz) mit anliegendem subepidermalen Axon (A_2) und benachbarter Schwannscher Zelle? (Sch). F Fibrocytenfortsatz. Großzehenballen, Affe.
Neg. Vergr. 7000 ×

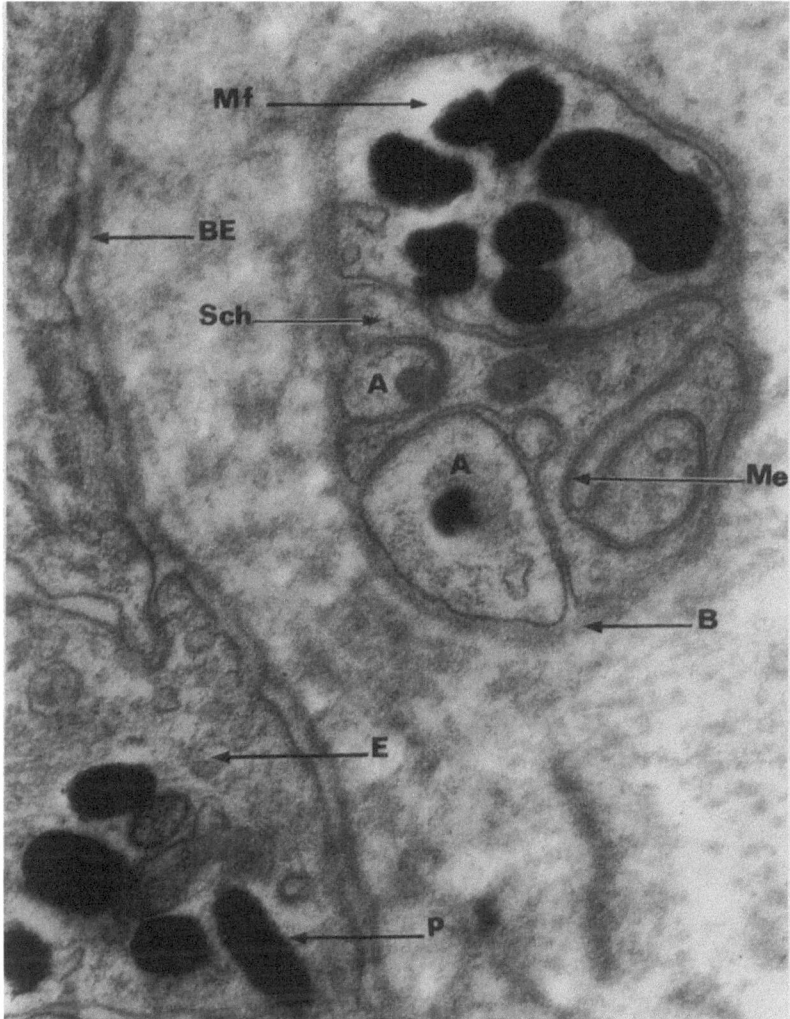

Abb. 9. Melanocytenfortsatz (*Mf*) und Schwannsches Cytoplasma (*Sch*) mit Axonen (*A*) von gemeinsamer Basalmembran (*B*) umschlossen. Normale Affenlippe. *Me* Mesaxon, *E* Epithelzelle, *BE* Basalmembran der Epithelzelle, *P* Pigment. Neg. Vergr. 12 200 ×

2. Das subepidermale Nervengeflecht

Aus der Lichtmikroskopie ist bekannt (STÖHR, 1957 und HAGEN, 1964), daß subepidermal ein besonders dichter Nervenplexus ausgebildet wird, der an der unbehaarten Haut eine flächenhafte, parallel zur Epitheloberfläche gerichtete Ausdehnung besitzt (Abb. 10). Der Plexus setzt sich bei der behaarten Haut meist aus lichtmikroskopisch marklosen Nervenelementen zusammen, die zum Teil aus markhaltigen Fasern hervorgehen.

Bei der Mehrzahl der Fasern handelt es sich jedoch um ursprünglich marklose vegetative Nerven, die mit den Blutgefäßen und den cerebrospinalen Nerven das Corium erreicht haben (LELOUP und BOURLOND, 1962/63; HAGEN, 1966). Unter fortwährender Aufteilung und Verkleinerung der Nervenbündel kommt es zu einer Durchmischung und Verflechtung sämtlicher nervöser Elemente. Elektrophysiologische Messungen von HENSEL (1964) ergaben deutliche Unterschiede in der Leitungsgeschwindigkeit der erwähnten Faserarten.

390   E. Hagen: Zur Innervation der Haut

Subepitheliale Nervengeflechte stellen sich mit der Richardson-Methode in einer Reichhaltigkeit und Vollendung dar wie kaum zuvor beobachtet, falls man der flächenhaften Ausbreitung des Geflechtes, das zumeist tangential zur Epithel-

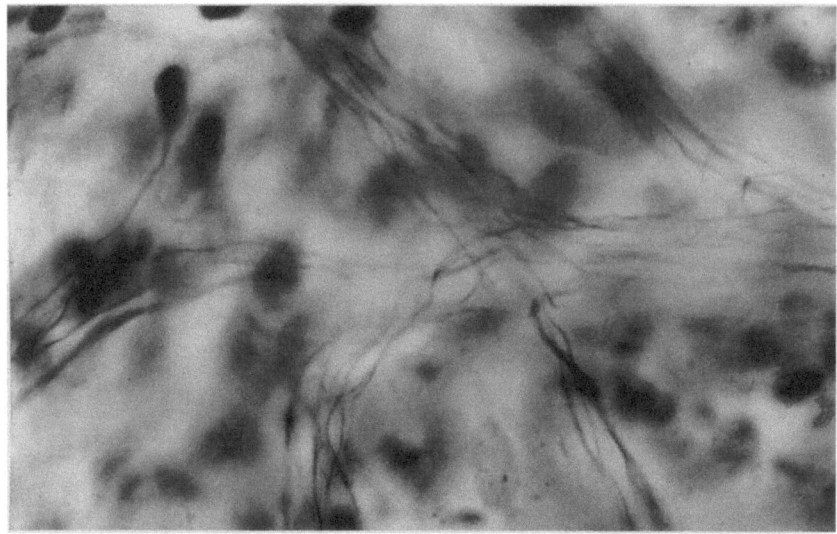

Abb. 10. Subepithelialer Nervenplexus, Mensch. Richardson-Newton-Methode. Neg. Vergr. 14 000 ×

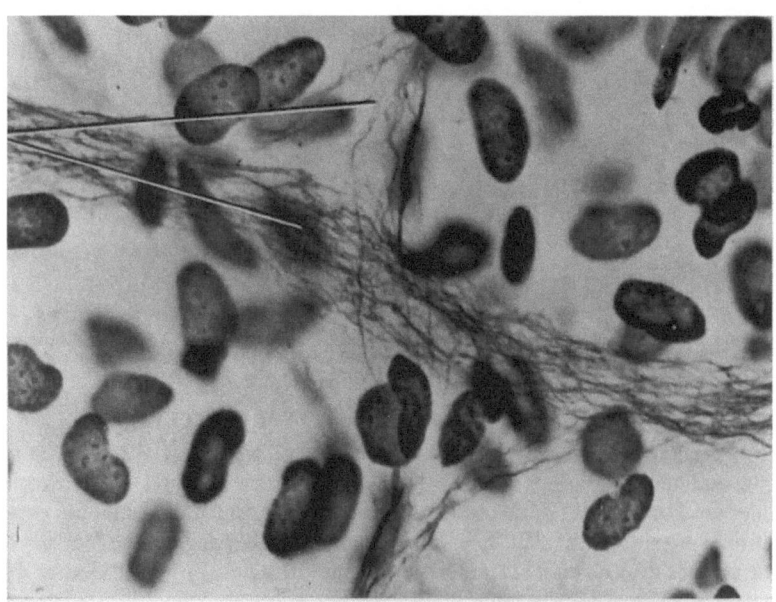

Abb. 11. Subepitheliales Nervengeflecht (*nf*) in der embryonalen Haut, Mensch. Richardson-Methode. Präp.: Dr. G. Garweg. Neg. Vergr. 1000 ×. (Hagen, 1966)

oberfläche ausgerichtet ist, durch entsprechende Schnittweise Rechnung getragen hat. Schon im 3. Embryonalmonat des Menschen fällt ein dichter, faserreicher Nervenplexus unter dem Epithel der Haut auf, bevor es zur Ausbildung spezieller, sensibler Endapparate des cerebrospinalen Nervensystems gekommen ist (Abb. 11).

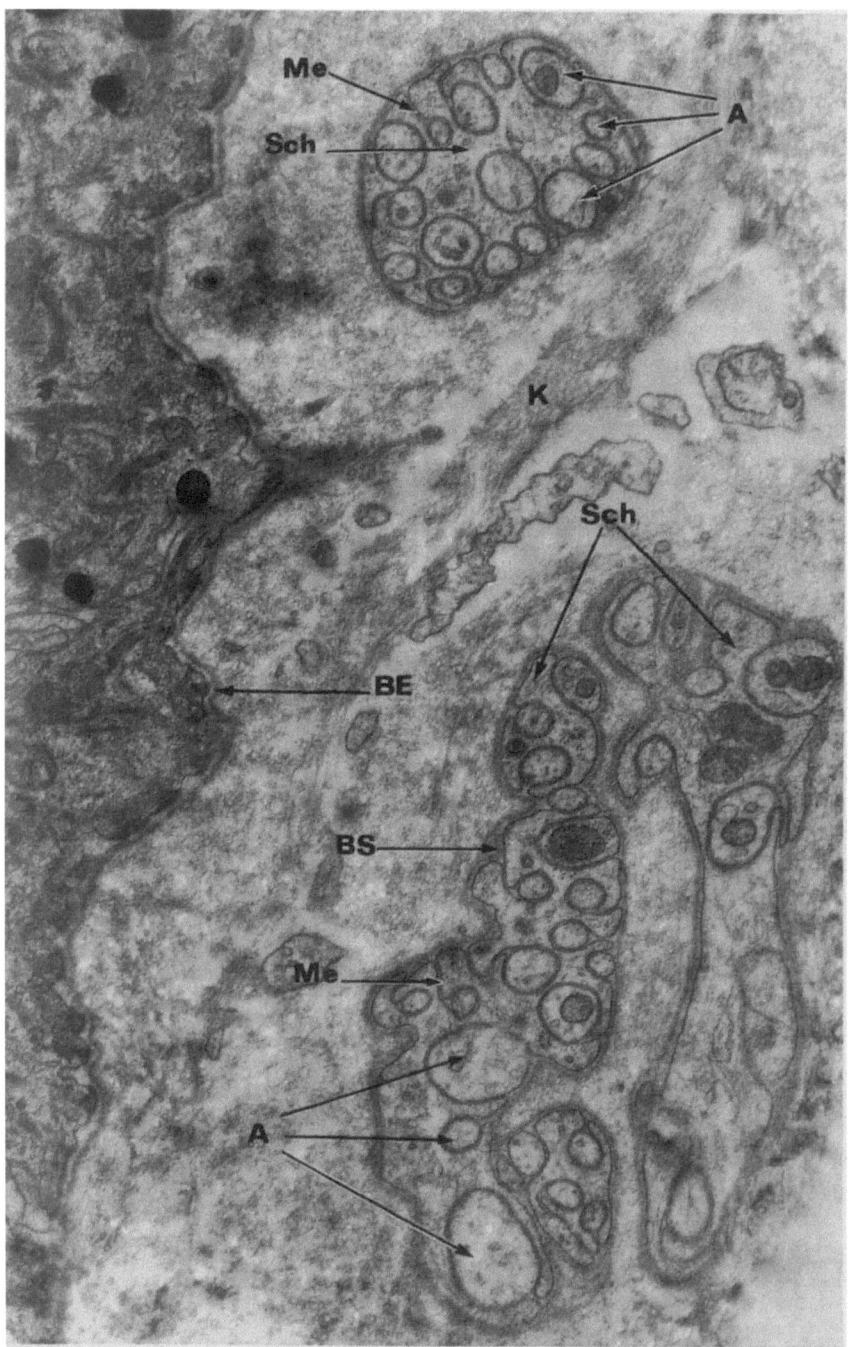

Abb. 12. Subepidermaler Nervenplexus. Lippe, Affe. Verschiedenkalibrige Axone (*A*) in Schwannsche Zellen (*Sch*) invaginiert. *Me* Mesaxone, *BS* Basalmembran der Schwannschen Zelle, *BE* Basalmembran der Epithelzelle, *K* kollagenes Bindegewebe. Neg. Vergr. 7000 ×

Der Reichtum an nervösen Elementen im subepidermalen Bindegewebe erfährt durch die elektronenmikroskopischen Untersuchungen eine Bestätigung (Abb. 12). Die Fülle der markarmen Nervenfasern mit ihren sie einhüllenden Schwannschen

Zellen formiert ein lichtmikroskopisch marklos erscheinendes, zusammenhängendes Geflecht, das sowohl mit der Epidermis — wie beschrieben — als auch mit der Subcutis nervöse Verbindungen herstellt.

Normalerweise besitzen die Schwannschen Zellen des subepidermalen Plexus (Abb. 13) einen runden bis längsovalen Kern. Das Cytoplasma wird von einer

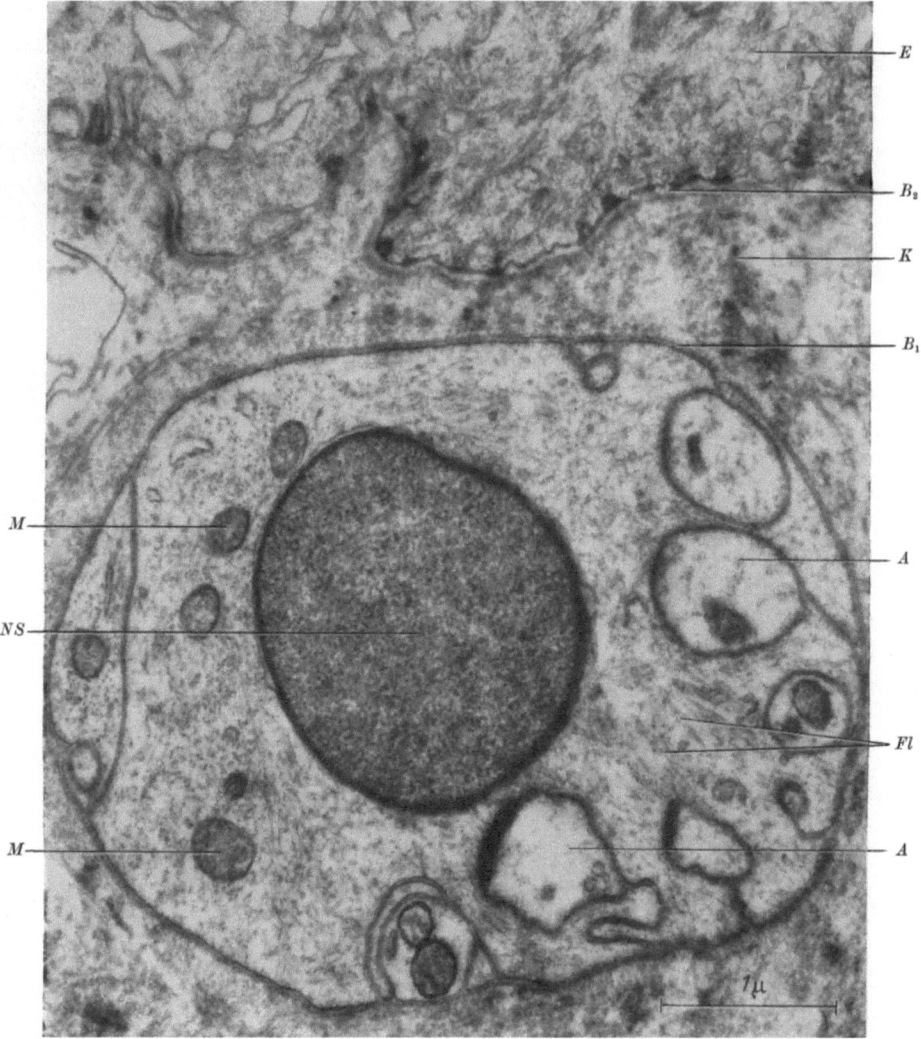

Abb. 13. Schwannsche Zelle aus dem subepidermalen Nervengeflecht. Areola mammae, Affe. NS Kern der Schwannschen Zelle, M Mitochondrien der Schwannschen Zelle, Fl Filamente der Schwannschen Zelle, A Axon mit Mesaxon, B_1 Basalmembran der Schwannschen Zelle, B_2 Basalmembran der Epithelzelle, K kollagenes Bindegewebe, E Epithelzellen. Neg. Vergr. 7000 × (HAGEN und WERNER, 1966)

mäßigen Anzahl feiner, netzförmig angeordneter Filamente durchsetzt. Die quergetroffenen Axone liegen in einer Zisterne der Schwannschen Oberflächenmembran und sind durch einen konstanten Abstand von dieser getrennt. Das mehr oder weniger gewundene Mesaxon zeigt die Invaginationsstelle der Schwannschen Oberflächenmembran an. Die Axone enthalten quergetroffene, zu kleinen Feldern gruppierte Neurotubuli und Filamente, wenige Mitochondrien und geringe

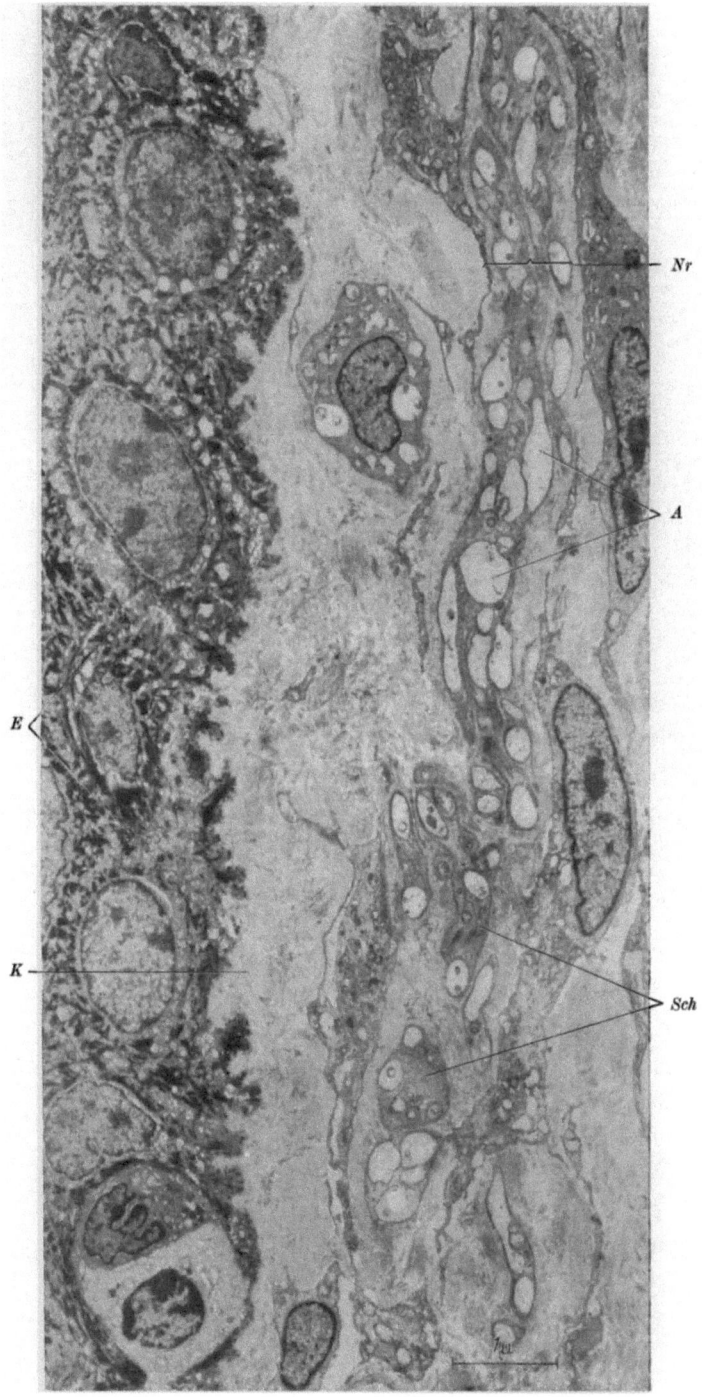

Abb. 14. Verändertes subepidermales Nervengeflecht (*Nr*). Behaarte Haut, Affe. Fraktionierte Röntgenbestrahlung. 10 Sitzungen à 200 R/O. Excision 3 Monate nach der ersten Bestrahlung. *E* pathologisch veränderte, basale Epithelzellenschicht, *K* kollagenes Bindegewebe, *A* geschwollene Axone, *Sch* Schwannsches Cytoplasma. Neg. Vergr. 1700 × (HAGEN und WERNER, 1966)

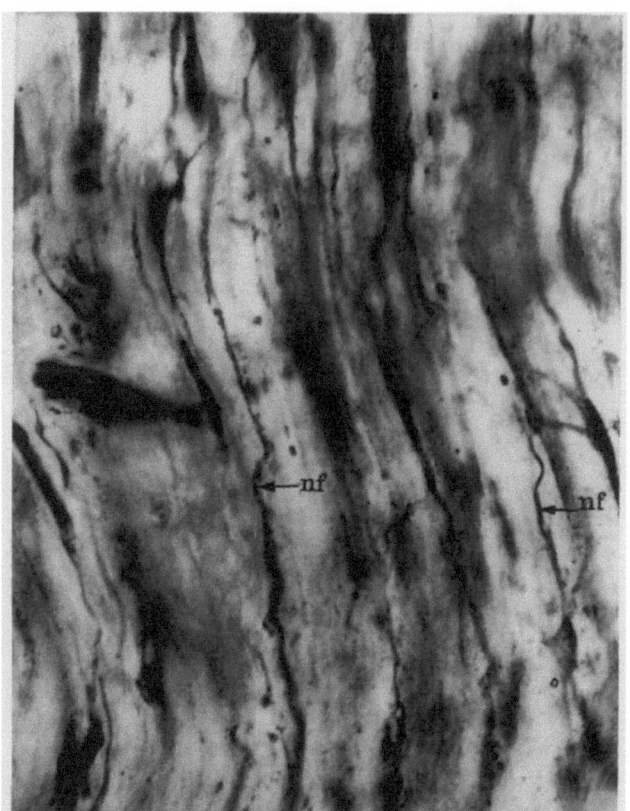

Abb. 15

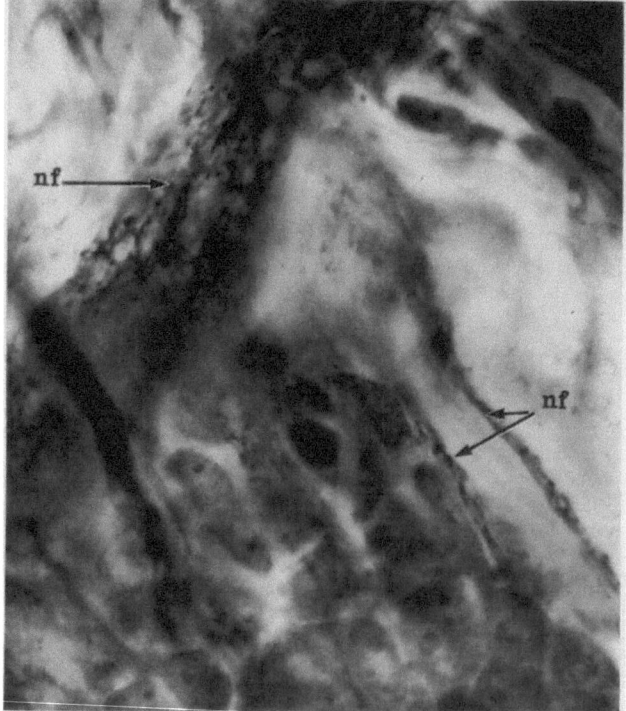

Abb. 16

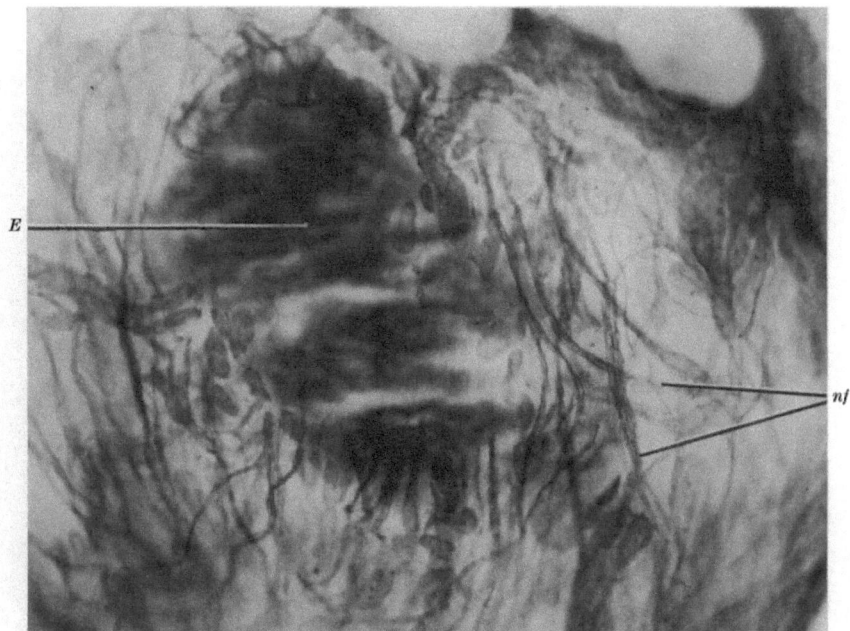

Abb. 17. Vegetatives Nervengeflecht (*nf*) an einer Schweißdrüse, Mensch. Richardson-Methode. *E* Epithel. Präp.: Dr. G. Garweg. Neg. Vergr. 350 × (Hagen, 1966)

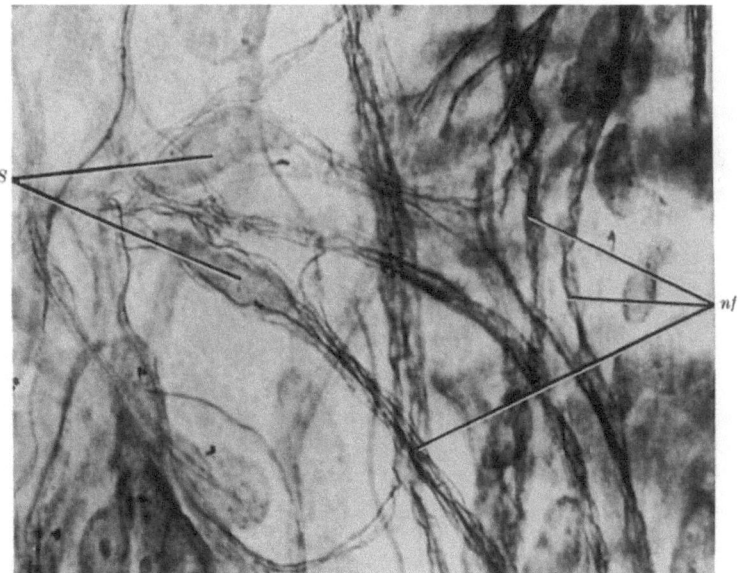

Abb. 18. Vegetatives Nervengeflecht (*nf*) an einer Schweißdrüse, Mensch. Richardson-Methode. *S* Schwannsche Zellen. Präp.: Dr. G. Garweg. Neg. Vergr. 1000 × (HAGEN, 1966)

Abb. 15. Vegetative Nervenfasern (*nf*) am M. arrector pili. Behaarte Haut, Mensch. Bielschowsky-Gros-Methode. Neg. Vergr. 160 ×

Abb. 16. Vegetative Nervenstränge (*nf*) an einer Talgdrüse. Augenlid, Mensch. Richardson-Newton-Methode. Präp.: Dr. G. Garweg. Neg. Vergr. 1100 ×

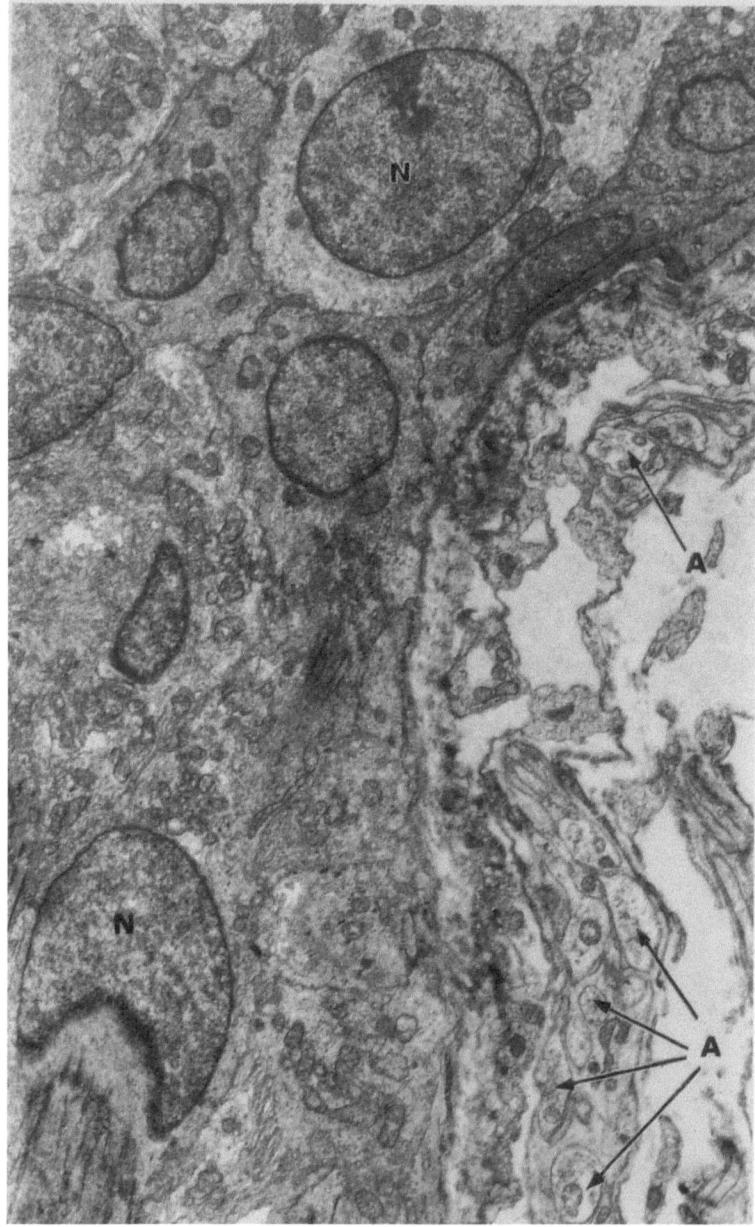

Abb. 19. Nervenplexus unter der Basalmembran einer Schweißdrüse, Mensch. *N* Nucleus von Schweißdrüsenzellen, *A* Axone. Neg. Vergr. 1700 ×

Anteile des endoplasmatischen Reticulum. Die Armut an elektronendichter Struktur ist auffällig.

Selten gelangen markreiche Nervenfasern im subepidermalen Plexus zu Gesicht, während sie in größerer Zahl in der Subcutis vertreten sind.

Die Axone des subepidermalen Plexus treten an der röntgenbestrahlten Haut besonders deutlich im Schwannschen Cytoplasma hervor. Durch die Bestrahlung erfahren die Nervenfasern eine Schwellung, verlieren ihre Neurotubuli und

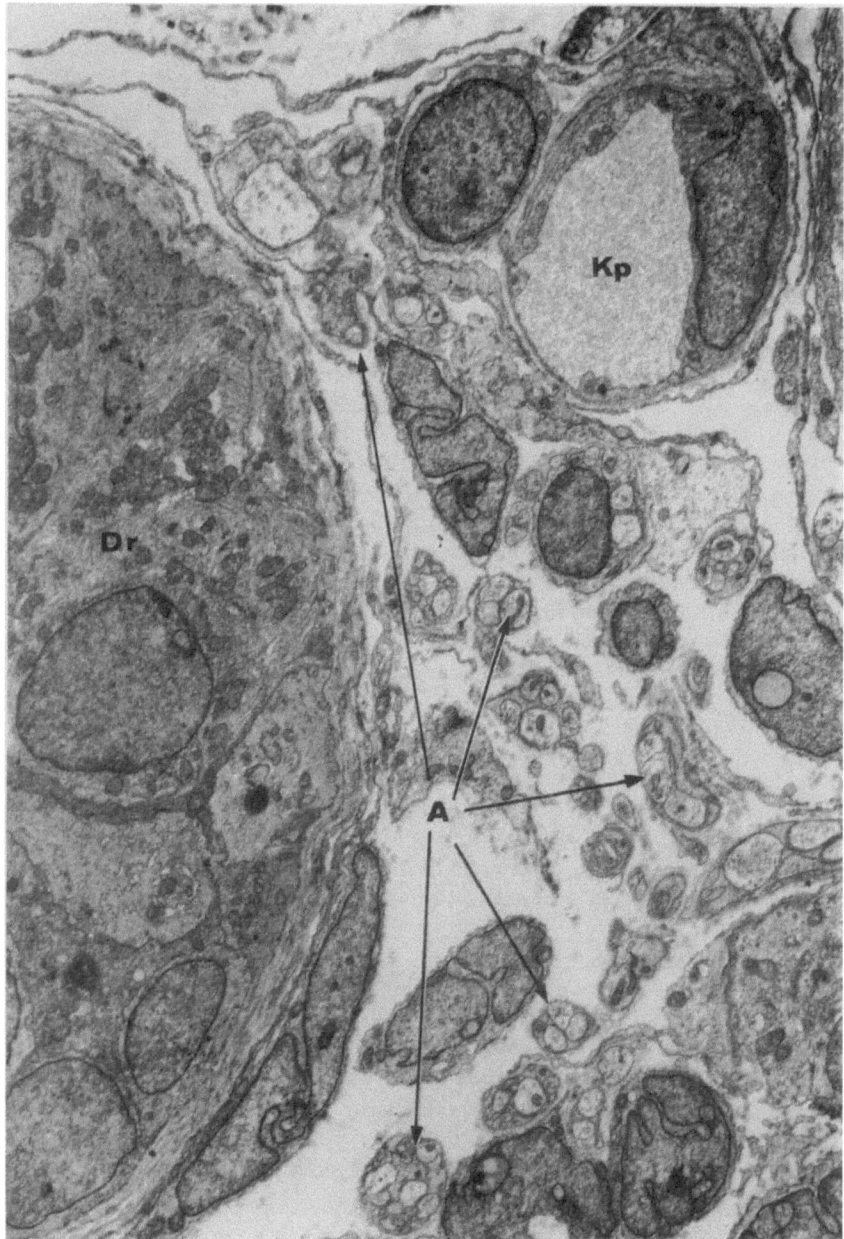

Abb. 20. Feiner Nervenplexus (*A*) an Schweißdrüse (*Dr*) und Capillare (*Kp*). Behaarte Haut, Mensch. Neg. Vergr. 1700 ×

treten durch Größe und Aufhellung deutlich in Erscheinung. Die feinen ribosomenartigen Granula im Cytoplasma der Schwannschen Zellen verdichten sich. Der subepidermale Plexus wirkt wie eine zusammenhängende nervöse Gewebsplatte, die die Epidermis unterlagert (Abb. 14).

Der Musculus arrector pili sowie Talg- und Schweißdrüsen zeigen lichtmikroskopisch Verbindungen zum vegetativen Nervengeflecht der Haut (JOHN, 1940,

1941, 1942; JABONERO, 1962; HAGEN, 1964). Die glatten Muskelzellen des Arrector pili sind von marklosen Nervenelementen begleitet (Abb. 15). Die Darstellung von Nerven an den Talgdrüsen ist färbetechnisch schwierig. Nur selten gelingt es, die strangförmigen Nervenzüge auf den Drüsenzellen zu imprägnieren. Die Nervenelemente haben meistens ihren scharf gezeichneten, welligen Kontur verloren und erscheinen granulär verändert, mit vielen Varicositäten versehen (Abb. 16).

Von einem besonders dichten, vegetativ-nervösen Flechtwerk sind die Schweißdrüsen eingeschlossen (Abb. 17). Das Geflecht enthält zahlreiche, scheinbar ungeordnet verlaufende Nervenbündel (Abb. 18). Die morphologische Anordnung der Nerven an der Schweißdrüse ermöglicht in funktioneller Hinsicht ein breites Feld sympathischer Erregungsausbreitung (ZENIN, 1962). Jedoch sind elektronenoptisch trotz der Vielzahl der die Drüse umgebenden Axone (Abb. 19) niemals echte Synapsenbildungen zu finden gewesen, eine Beobachtung, die für das gesamte Ausbreitungsgebiet der Hautnerven zutrifft. Untrennbar sind lichtmikroskopisch Gefäßnerven und Nerven an Schweißdrüsen miteinander verbunden. Auch in ihrer Ultrastruktur unterscheiden sie sich nicht (Abb. 20). Entgegen den Beobachtungen von BOEKE (1934) sahen JOHN (1940), STÖHR (1957) und VAN DER ZYPEN (1960) u.a. niemals ein Eindringen von Nervenfasern in das Protoplasma der Schweißdrüsenzellen. Diese lichtoptischen Befunde erfuhren durch die elektronenmikroskopischen Untersuchungen von YAMADA und MIYAKE (1960) sowie GANSLER (1961) eine Bestätigung. Die Autoren vermochten nicht einmal eine Unterbrechung der dem Schweißdrüsenepithel anliegenden Basalmembran zu beobachten.

3. Gefäßnerven

Die Darstellung der Gefäßnerven war von jeher für den Histologen ein besonders schwieriges Kapitel. Hier ist man heute durch die Verwendung der Richardson-Technik erfolgreicher. So sind in Abb. 21 gröbere Gefäßnervenbündel wiedergegeben, wie sie im Corium und in der Subcutis vorkommen. Sie zweigen sich in immer feiner werdende Bündel auf, um nur noch mit wenigen Nervenelementen die Capillaren zu begleiten.

Hirn- und Spinalnerven bringen wohl in der Hauptsache sympathische Nervenfasern an die Gefäßwand der Haut heran. Wenn dem segmentalen Innervationsmodus bei der Gefäßversorgung eine Hauptrolle zugesprochen wird, so besteht außerdem eine zusammenhängende Gefäßnervenbahn, die, von der Aorta ausgehend, die Gesamtheit aller Gefäße bis herunter zu den Capillaren umfaßt.

Besser als mit den bisherigen Methoden kann mit der Richardson-Methode ein plexusartig mit dem Gefäß verlaufendes Nervengeflecht der Adventitia und Periadventitia (Abb. 22) von einem Muskelgeflecht unterschieden werden.

Der flächenhaft in der Adventitia ausgebreitete Nervenplexus besitzt Faserverbindungen zum darunter liegenden Muskelgeflecht.

Der Basalmembran der Capillaren mit ihrem Porenendothel liegen feinste Axone unmittelbar auf (Abb. 20 und 23), deren Vorkommen immer wieder in Zweifel gezogen wurde. Oftmals sind Capillarendothel und Axone von lamellären Fibrocytenfortsätzen gemeinsam umschlossen (Abb. 23). Auch die pericapillären Lymphräume zeigen ihrer Wand anliegende Axone (Abb. 23), die bemerkenswerterweise keine synaptischen Strukturen entwickeln.

In der Haut der Labia maiora besitzen die arteriovenösen Anastomosen, abweichend vom übrigen Gefäßsystem der Haut, einen besonders gebauten Nervenapparat. Die Gefäße sind mit marklosen Nervenelementen dicht umwickelt und

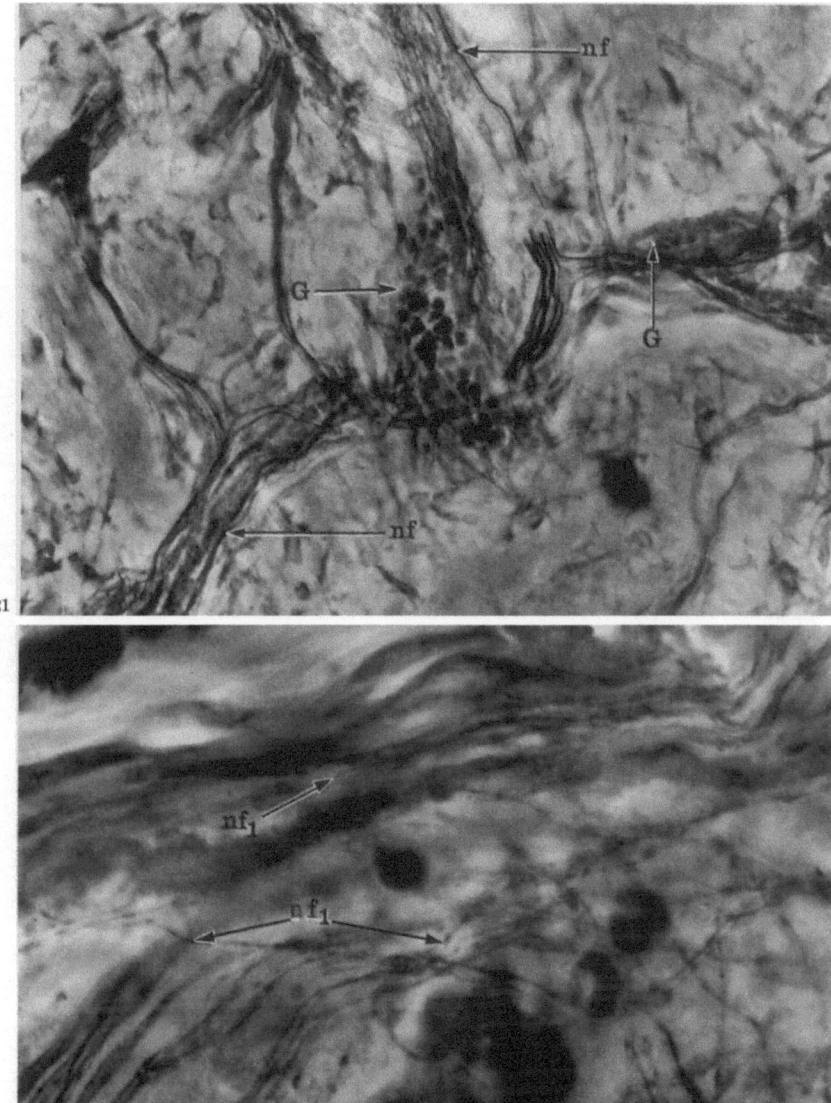

Abb. 21. Gefäßnervenbündel im Corium. Augenlid, Mensch. *nf* Nervenbündel, *G* Blutgefäße. Richardson-Newton-Methode. Präp.: Dr. G. Garweg. Neg. Vergr. 350 ×

Abb. 22. Nerven in einer Arterienwand des Corium. Augenlid, Mensch. nf_1 Nerven der Adventitia, nf_2 Nerven auf der Muscularis. Richardson-Newton-Methode. Präp.: Dr. G. Garweg. Neg. Vergr. 1100 ×

gleichen Kokons von Seidenraupen (Abb. 24). Während auf den benachbarten Gefäßen der normale Gefäßnervenplexus erhalten bleibt, scheren Nervenbündel aus (Abb. 25), um in dichten Zirkulärtouren die Gefäßanastomosen und ihre Aufgabelungen zu umwinden.

In der Adventitia arteriovenöser Anastomosen in der Fingerbeere des Menschen schildert HETT (1943) ein besonders enges Netz von Neurofibrillen; im Nagelbett von Neugeborenen sah KNOCHE (1958) sensible Formationen aus markhaltigen Fasern entstehen, die in der Adventitia arteriovenöser Anastomosen liegen. Bei gestörter Vascularisierung an den Vater-Pacinischen Körperchen und arteriovenösen Anastomosen bildet nach Beobachtungen von CAUNA und MANNAN (1959) das gleiche Axon einen neuen Receptor.

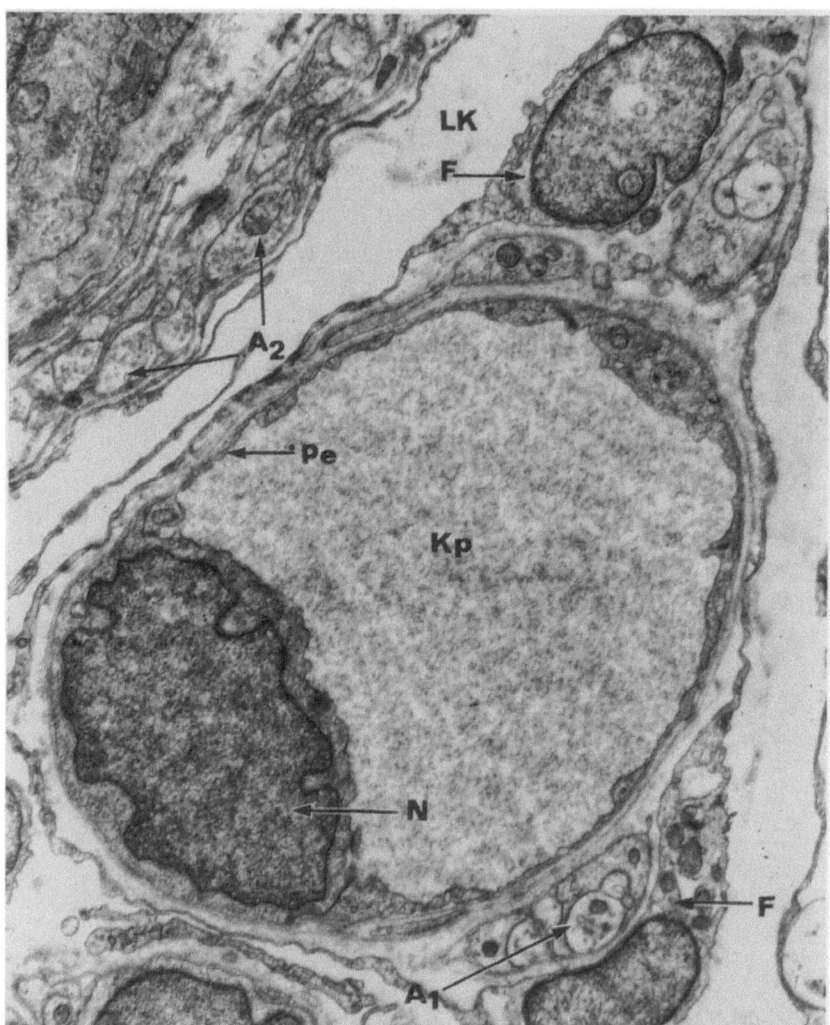

Abb. 23. Axone (A_1) an einer Capillare (Kp); Axone (A_2) am pericapillären Lymphraum (LK). Haut, Mensch. N Kern einer Endothelzelle, Pe Porenendothel, F Fibrocyten. Neg. Vergr. 5200 ×

4. Spezifisch gebaute, sensible Nervenformationen

a) Der Nervenapparat des Haares

Die größte Fläche der menschlichen Haut ist behaart. Unbehaarte Körperoberflächen finden sich an Handteller, Fußteller, Lippenrot und Brustwarze. Die viel kleineren unbehaarten Regionen zeichnen sich durch ihren Reichtum an vielgestaltigen, sensiblen Nervenbildungen im Corium und in der Subcutis aus.

Die spezifischen Nervenformationen der behaarten Haut beschränken sich auf die Hüllen des Haares. Dort fügt sich lichtmikroskopisch untrennbar die End-

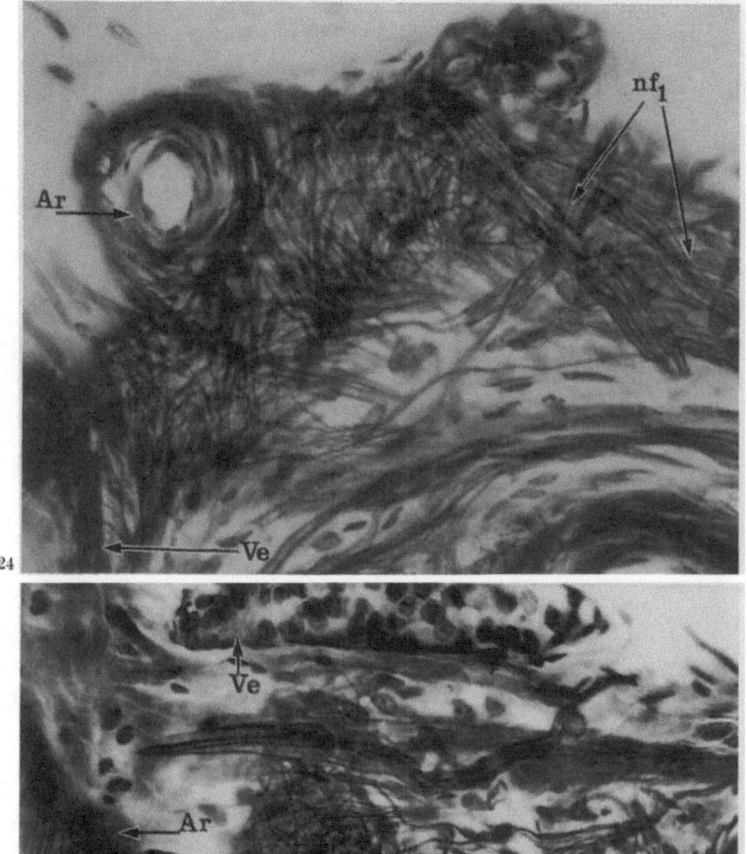

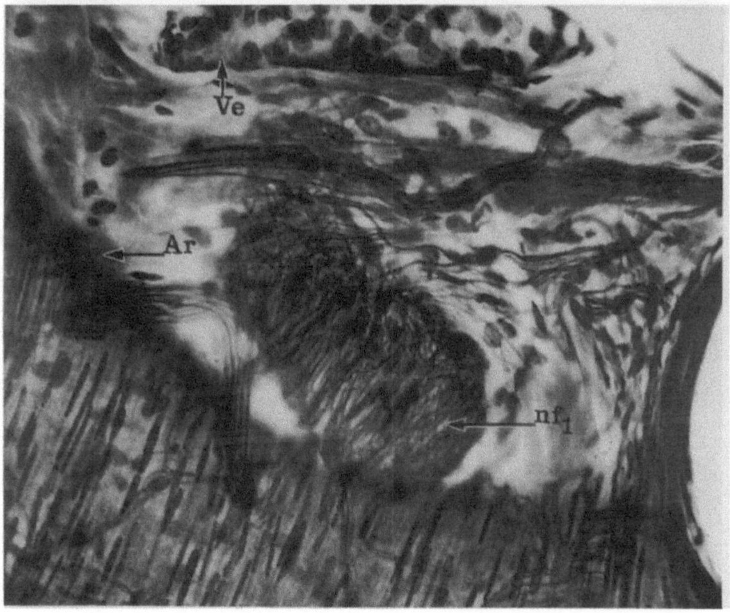

Abb. 24. Innervation (nf_1) arteriovenöser Anastomosen. Labia maiora, Hund. *Ar* Arterie, *Ve* Vene. Richardson-Newton-Methode. Präp.: Dr. G. Trossmann. Neg. Vergr. 100 ×

Abb. 25. Von Nerven (nf_1) kokonartig umsponnene, arteriovenöse Anastomose. Labia maiora, Hund. *Ar* Arterie, *Ve* Vene. Präp.: Dr. G. Trossmann. Neg. Vergr. 64 ×

ausbreitung cerebrospinaler und vegetativer Nerven in einem sensiblen Empfangsorgan zusammen (Abb. 26).

Unmittelbar um die epidermale Wurzelscheide, die das Haar mit verhornten, geschichteten Epithelzellen umgibt, formiert sich hülsen- oder manschettenartig ein nervöses Gitterwerk (Abb. 27), wie es am eindrucksvollsten an den Haaren der Labia maiora zu studieren ist. Schon 1878 wurden „gerade Terminalfasern" und „circuläre Terminalfasern" unterschieden (BONNET, 1878; LEONTOWITSCH,

1891; SZYMONOWICZ, 1909; KADANOFF, 1927/28). Das Nervengitter liegt gewöhnlich unterhalb der Einmündung der zum Haar gehörigen Talgdrüse und erreicht seine untere Grenze an der bindegewebigen Haarpapille (Abb. 28). Oftmals sind die zuführenden, das Gitter bildenden markhaltigen Nervenfasern deutlich sichtbar (Abb. 28).

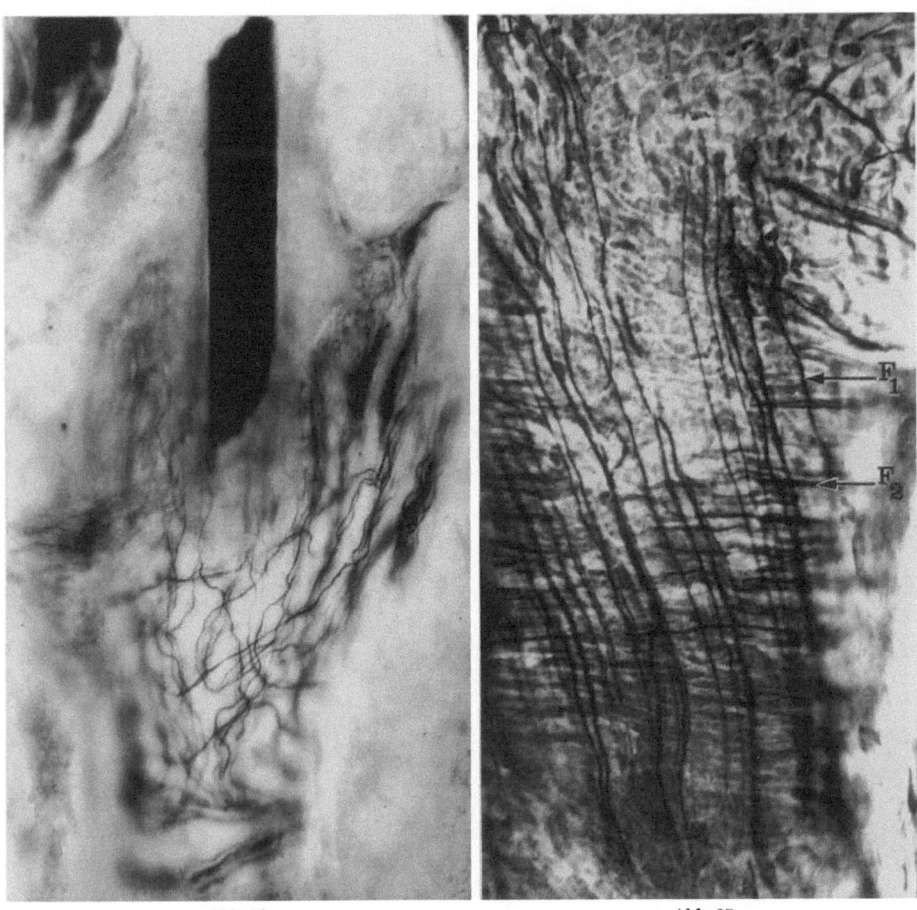

Abb. 26   Abb. 27

Abb. 26. Nervenringgeflecht und Palisaden. Lippe, Mensch. Präp.: Prof. Kadanoff. Neg. Vergr. 240 × (NIEBAUER, 1966)

Abb. 27. Nervengitterbildung an der Haarwurzelscheide, Hund. F_1 Palisadenfasern, F_2 Ringfasern. Richardson-Newton-Methode. Präp.: Dr. G. Trossmann. Neg. Vergr. 64 ×

Die epitheliale Wurzelscheide umfaßt mit einer zwiebelartigen Anschwellung die bindegewebige Haarpapille, in der Blutgefäße und Nerven zur Haarwurzel ziehen. Breite markhaltige Nervenfasern splittern sich gabelartig in dickere (Abb. 29) und feinere Äste (Abb. 30) auf und begleiten die Wurzelscheide in Richtung des Haares (Abb. 31). Ringförmig verlaufende Nervenfasern (Abb. 32) ergänzen die geraden Terminalfasern zur beschriebenen Gitterstruktur und ver-

Abb. 28. Nervengitterbildung (Manschette) an der Haarwurzelscheide mit zuführender markhaltiger Nervenfaser (F). Hp Haarpapille. Behaarte Haut, Mensch. Bielschowsky-Gros-Methode. Neg. Vergr. 325 ×

Abb. 29. Aufteilung einer Nervenringfaser (F_2) an der äußeren Haarwurzelscheide. Hund. F_1 palisadenförmig angeordnete Nervenfasern. Richardson-Newton-Methode. Präp.: Dr. G. Trossmann. Neg. Vergr. 160 ×

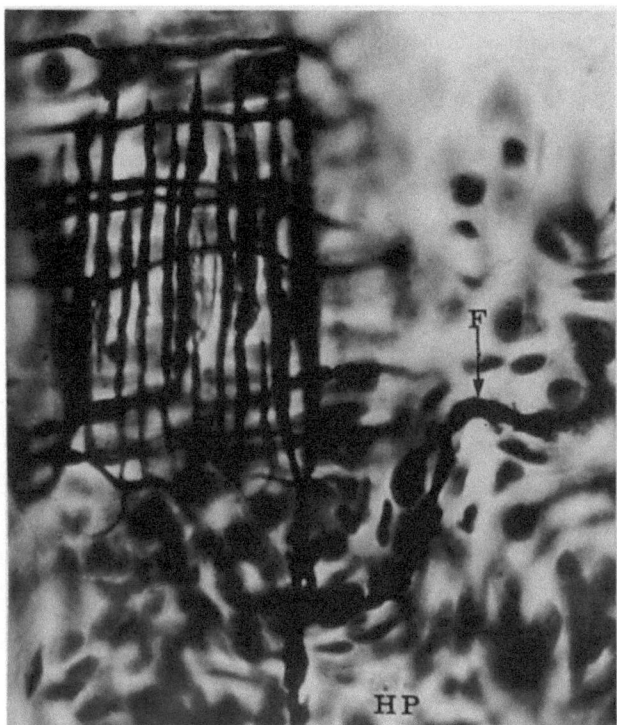

Abb. 28

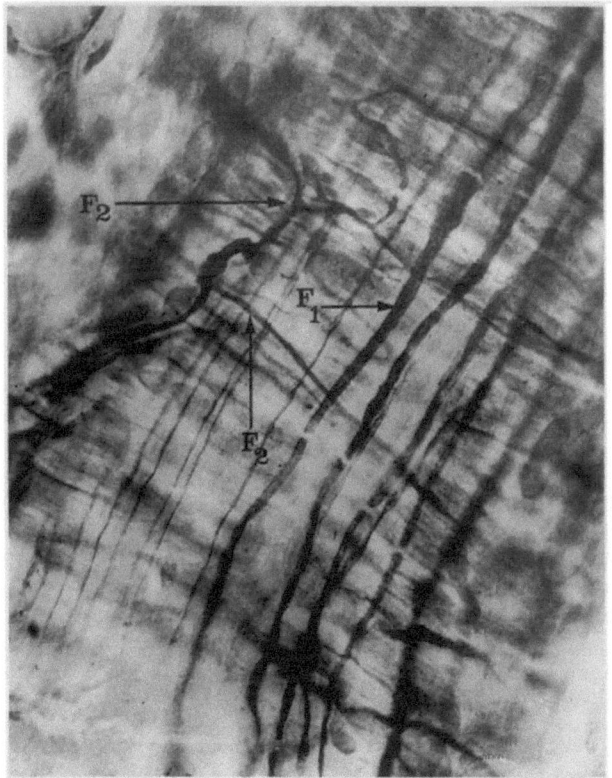

Abb. 29

vollständigen die Nervenhülse zu einem spezifischen Nervenendapparat um die Wurzelscheide des Haares. In Ermangelung andersartiger, sensibler Endformationen muß das erwähnte Organ als Receptor der die behaarte Haut treffenden Reize dienen.

Ausgezeichnete Präparate zum Studium der Haarinnervation gelangen KADANOFF (1927 und 1958). SETO (1963) schildert in der Haarwurzelscheide der

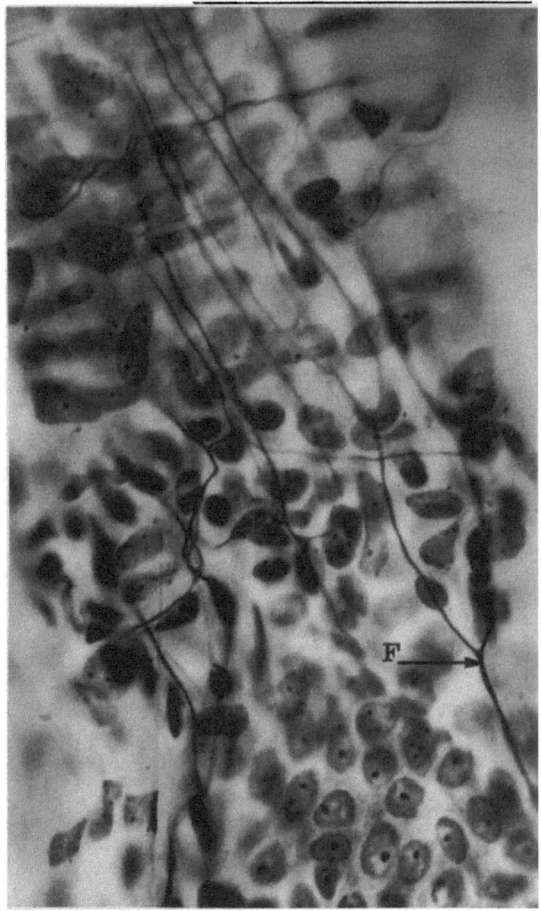

Abb. 30. Aufsplitterung feiner Nervenelemente (*F*). Haarwurzelscheide, Hund. Richardson-Newton-Methode. Präp.: Dr. G. Trossmann. Neg. Vergr. 250 ×

Kopfhaut vier Typen von sensiblen Nervenendigungen und findet hier weniger kompliziert gebaute, nervöse Formationen als z. B. an den Haaren des Lides oder des Bartes. An den Haaren des Augenlides von Kaninchen gelang JABONERO, BENGOECHEA und PEREZ-CASAS (1962) mit der Osmium-Zink-Jodid-Methode die Darstellung von Palisaden- und Ringgeflechten. Ob Lanugo- oder Terminalhaar einem unterschiedlichen Innervationsmuster unterliegen, ist ungeklärt.

Eine besonders reiche Nervenversorgung bieten die sog. Sinushaare einiger Tiere (Affe. Hund, Katze, Kaninchen u.a.). Es handelt sich um einzelne, kräftige Haare, die in der Haupt-

Abb. 31. Feine, parallel zum Haarschaft angeordnete Nervenfasern (F_1) und markhaltige Faser (mF) im bindegewebigen Haarbalg. Hund. Richardson-Newton-Methode. Präp.: Dr. G. Trossmann. Neg. Vergr. 250 ×

Abb. 32. Das cerebrospinale Ringgeflecht im Bereich des Haarwurzelhalses. Kopfhaut. Mensch. Silberimprägnation. Neg. Vergr. 400 × (NIEBAUER, 1966)

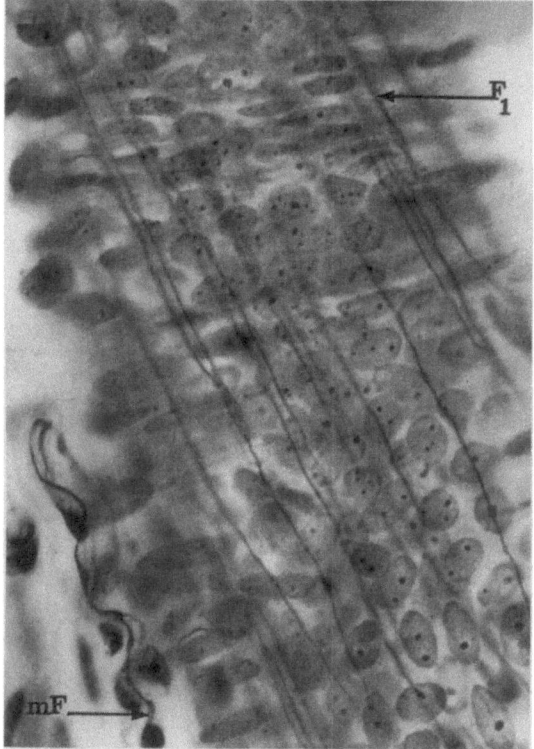

Abb. 31

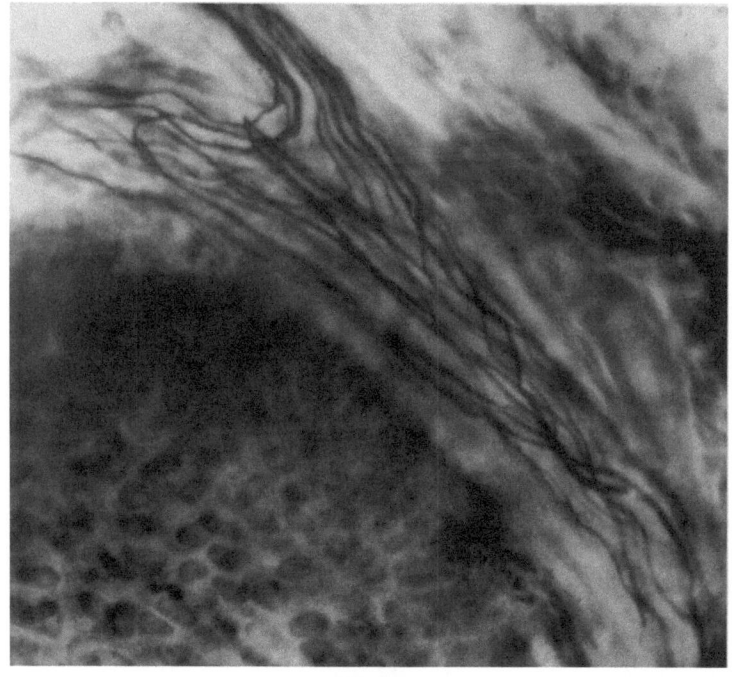

Abb. 32

sache um die Mundöffnung liegen und von weiten Venenpolstern umschlossen sind. Wegen ihres ungeheuren Nervenreichtums stellen sie ein leicht zu färbendes Studienobjekt dar (JALOWY, 1934, 1937; STEFANELLI, 1936 und SZYMONOWICZ, 1936, 1937; WALTER, 1960/61 u. a.).

Die Ultrastruktur der Nerven am Rattensinushaar untersuchte ANDRES (1966). Das Ausbreitungsgebiet der Merkelschen Tastzellen beschränkt sich nach seinen

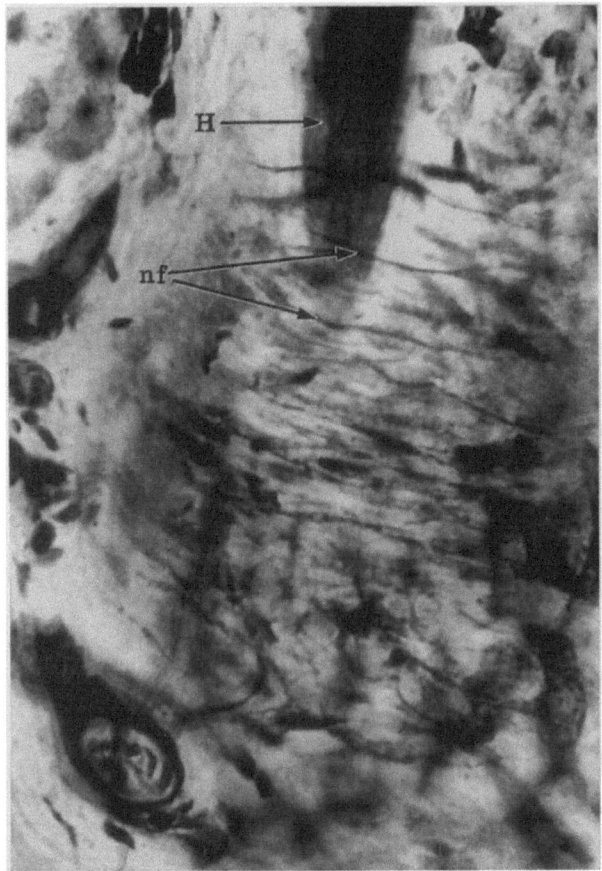

Abb. 33. Bindegewebiger Haarbalg mit Spiraltouren vegetativer Nervenfasern. Behaarte Haut, Mensch. *nf* vegetative Nervenfasern, *H* Haarschaft. Bielschowsky-Gros-Methode. Neg. Vergr. 160 ×

Ergebnissen auf den mittleren und äußeren Abschnitt der oberen Anschwellung der Wurzelscheide.

An Längs- und Tangentialschnitten der Wurzelscheide vom menschlichen Haar ist das Eindringen von marklosen Nerven in die äußere Wurzelscheide, die dem „Stratum germinativum" der Epidermis entspricht, zu beobachten. Dort scheinen sich die Nervenelemente zu verzweigen oder bilden kolbenartige Verdickungen und retikuläre Verbreiterungen ohne ein sicheres, lichtmikroskopisch nachweisbares Ende. Ring- und Längsfasern der Nervenhülse sollen in die untersten Epithelzellschichten der Haarwurzelscheide vorstoßen (AKKERINGA, 1930; BOEKE, 1934). Elektronenoptisch konnte bisher kein Beweis dafür geliefert werden.

Die Haarpapille und ihre kontinuierlich bindegewebige Fortsetzung, der Haarbalg beherbergen eine Fülle feinster, vegetativer Nervenelemente. Sie sind stellenweise eng mit den cerebrospinalen Nerven verknüpft und bilden im Haarbalg eine zweite, nur aus feinen Spiraltouren bestehende Nervenhülle (Abb. 33). Geradlinig verlaufende, feine Endaufsplitterungen cerebrospinaler Nervenfasern unterscheiden sich deutlich von den vielfach anastomosierenden Strängen vegetativer Nervenelemente (Abb. 34).

Die Hauptmenge vegetativer Nervenelemente liegt dem sensiblen Gitterwerk im Bereich des bindegewebigen Haarbalgs auf. Bezüglich der Quantität dieser

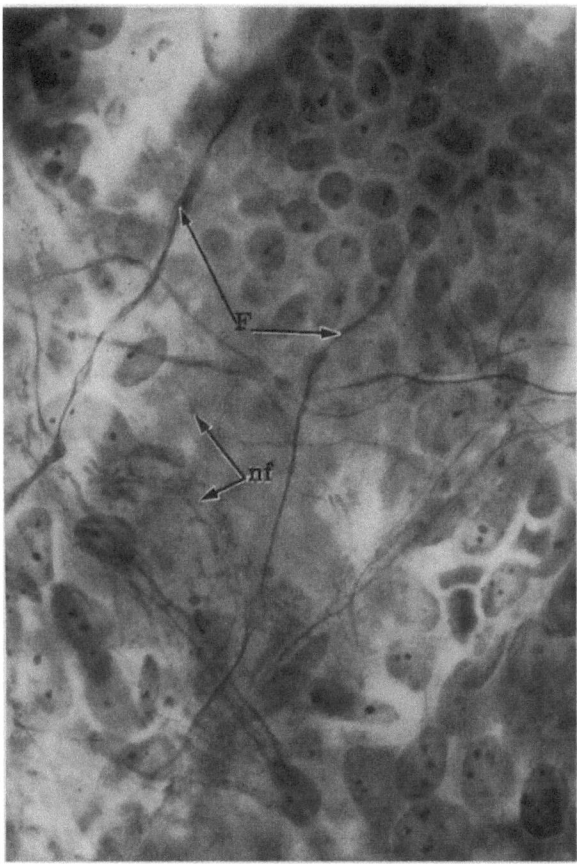

Abb. 34. Morphologisch verschiedene Nervenfaserqualitäten am bindegewebigen Haarbalg, Mensch. *F* grobkalibrige Nervenfasern (Aufsplitterungen cerebrospinaler Nervenfasern?), *nf* vegetative Nervenelemente. Richardson-Newton-Methode. Neg. Vergr. 240 ×

Nervenfasern liegen unterschiedliche Angaben vor (DROZ, 1954 und NIEBAUER, 1966).

Im Rahmen des Haarcyclus machen nach NIEBAUER (1966) die sensiblen Nerven keine gestaltlichen Veränderungen durch, während die vegetativen Fasern an den Blutgefäßen der Nachbarschaft morphologisch faßbare Veränderungen zeigen. Jedoch sind weitere Untersuchungen über die Innervationsverhältnisse beim Haarwechsel notwendig.

Ebenso bedürfen die von PINKUS (1903) beschriebenen „Haarscheiben" des Menschen, die er mit Hilfe der Methylenblau-Methode durch einen großen Nervengehalt ausgezeichnet fand, noch der elektronoptischen Untersuchung. In der Bauchhaut des Menschen werden Haarscheiben, wie KAWAMURA (1954) berichtet, von dicken „Tastfasern" versorgt, die zur Gruppe der Nerven aus dem sensiblen

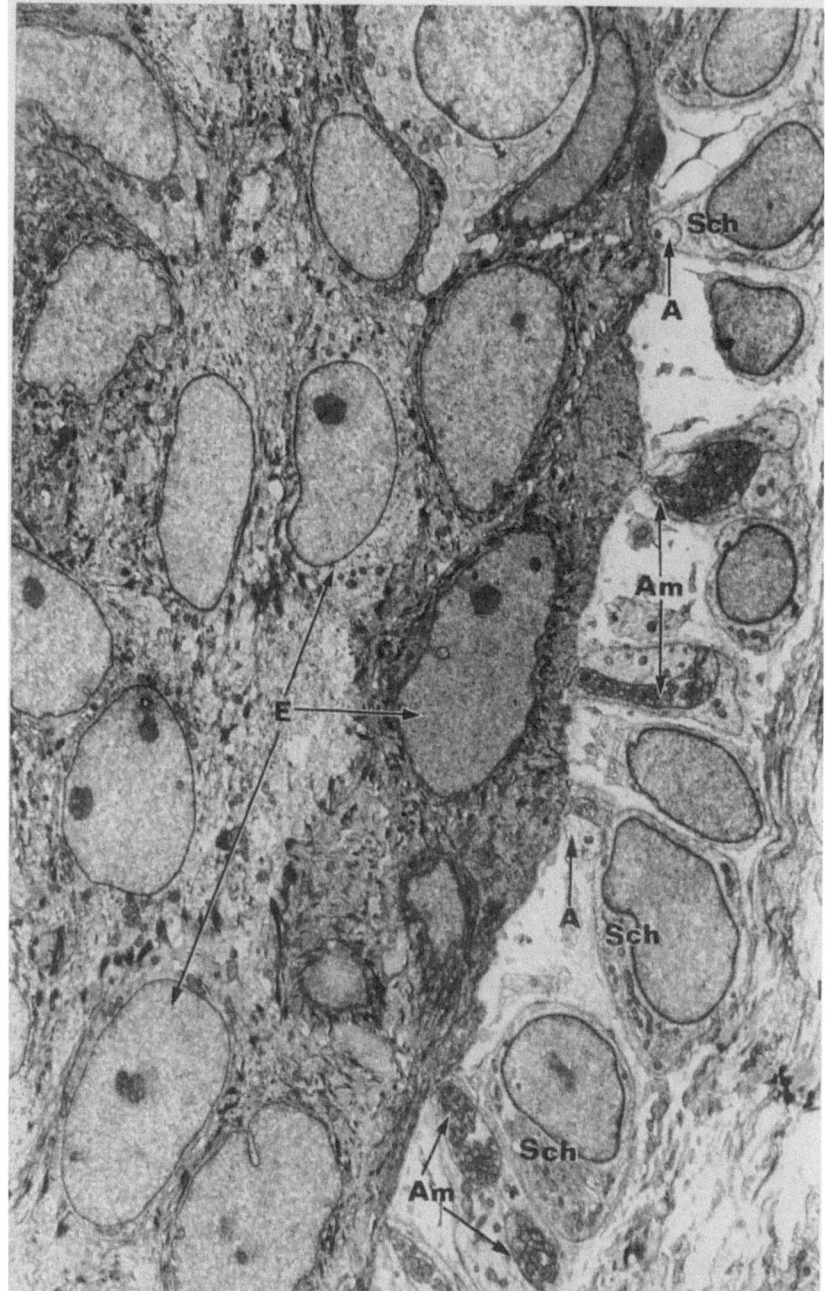

Abb. 35. Mitochondrienreiche große Axone (*Am*) und strukturarme kleinere Axone (*A*) an der äußeren Wurzelscheide des Haares. Mensch. *Sch* Schwannsche Zellen, *E* Epithelzellen der äußeren Wurzelscheide. Neg. Vergr. 1700 ×

Endapparat des Haarfollikels gehören. Es wird eine unterschiedliche Leitungsgeschwindigkeit verschiedener Faserdicken festgestellt, die besondere Arten der Tastempfindungen auslösen soll.

Das Haar ist nach lichtmikroskopischen Ergebnissen mit vegetativen und cerebrospinalen Nerven versorgt. Durch die vegetative Innervation ist das Haar, wie die Talg- und Schweißdrüsen als Anhangsgebilde der Haut, den Musculus arrector pili eingeschlossen, in den nervösen Plexus der Cutis einbezogen. Diese Beobachtungen finden Bestätigung durch Untersuchungen der behaarten Tierhaut von Kaninchen und Katze (JABONERO, BENGOECHEA und PEREZ CASAS, 1962).

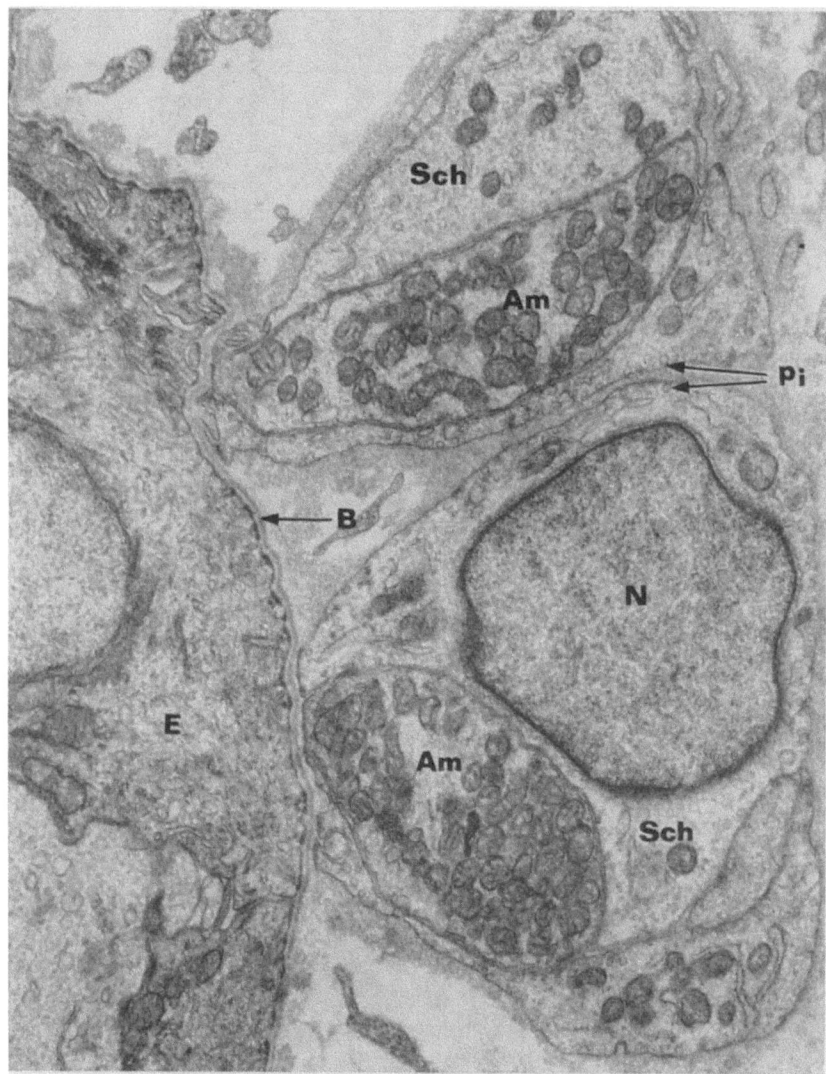

Abb. 36. Große mitochondrienreiche Nervenfasern (*Am*) (cerebrospinale Nerven?) mit Schwannscher Zelle. Haarwurzelscheide, Mensch. *N* Nucleus der Schwannschen Zelle, *Sch* Cytoplasma der Schwannschen Zelle, *Pi* Pinocytosebläschen, *B* Basalmembran der Epithelzelle (*E*) der äußeren Wurzelscheide. Neg. Vergr. 7000 ×

Elektronenmikroskopisch lassen sich an der äußeren Wurzelscheide des menschlichen Haares nicht nur sehr zahlreiche Nervenfasern, sondern darunter zwei morphologisch trennbare Typen von Nervenfasern auffinden. Eine Anzahl der Axone ist durch einen auffälligen Reichtum an Mitochondrien charakterisiert, während kleinere Axone wenig Binnenstruktur zeigen und als vegetative Fasern zu deuten sind (Abb. 35). Das beträchtliche Kaliber der mitochondrienreichen Axone spricht für ihre cerebrospinale Abkunft (HAGEN und WERNER, 1967). Die

Schwannsche Zelle vermag nur wenige dieser mächtigen Axone zu umschließen und bildet dementsprechend auch nur kurze Mesaxone aus. Stellenweise gibt die Cytomembran der Schwannschen Zelle die Axone frei; dort berührt das Axon unmittelbar die Basalmembran der Epithelzellen der äußeren Wurzelscheide

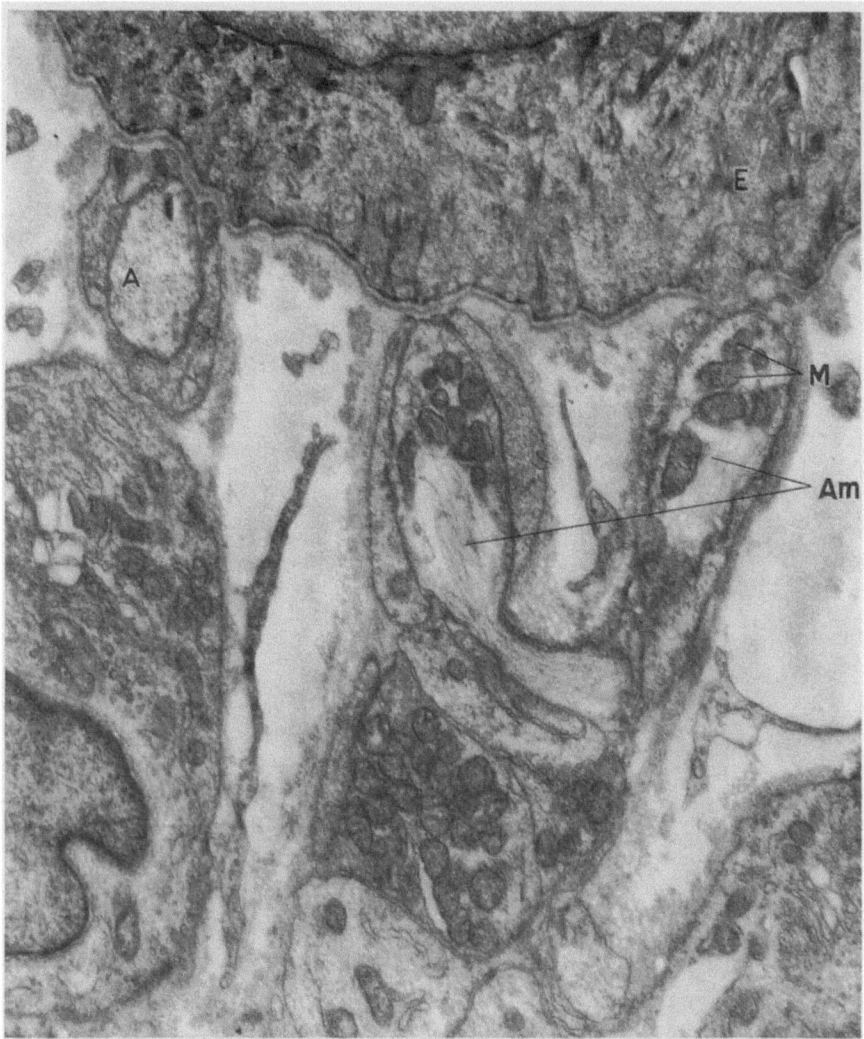

Abb. 37. Nervenfasern an der äußeren Wurzelscheide des menschlichen Haares. *M* Mitochondrien, *Am* Axone cerebrospinaler Nervenfasern(?), *E* Epithelzelle, *A* vegetatives Axon(?). Neg. Vergr. 7000 ×
(HAGEN und WERNER, 1967)

(Abb. 36). In Längsschnitten von mitochondrienreichen Nervenfasern finden sich streckenweise filamentäre Strukturen (Abb. 37). In den Axonen des aus vegetativen Nervenfasern gebildeten, subepidermalen Plexus waren Zellorganellen in dieser Fülle niemals zu beobachten.

Als „neuroepitheliale" Verbindungen bezeichnet ORFANOS (1967) mitochondrienreiche Nervenaufzweigungen an Follikelepithelzellen des menschlichen Haares. Er vermißt synaptischen Vesikel in diesen Axonen und hält sie für Mechanoreceptoren oder Startorgane der Membrandepolarisation afferenter, peritrichaler Nerven.

b) Sensible Endkörperchen

Die sensible Versorgung der Haut mit cerebrospinalen, markhaltigen Nervenfasern zeigt nur in der unbehaarten Haut eine formenreiche Endigungsweise in Gestalt von Körperchen, während, wie oben erwähnt, die receptorischen Nervenformationen der behaarten Haut im Nervengeflecht um das Haar zu suchen sind (WEDDEL, PALLIE und PALMER, 1955; WINKELMANN, 1959; KADANOFF, 1958).

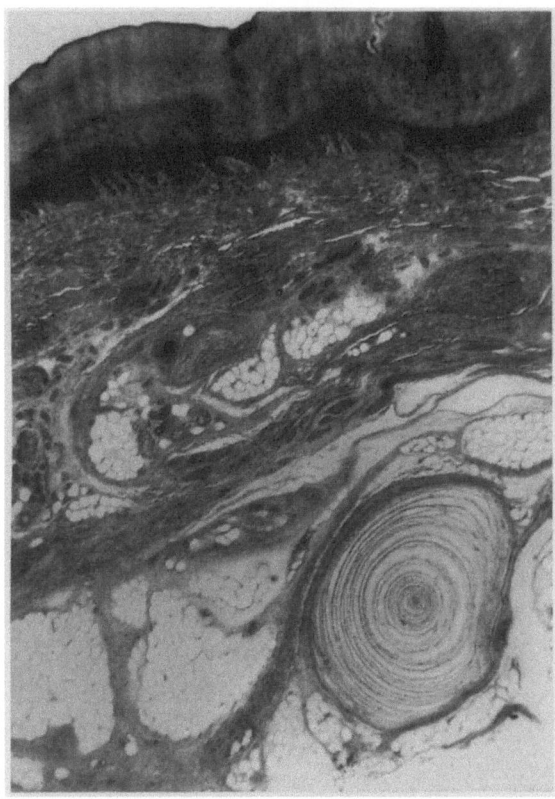

Abb. 38. Lamellenkörperchen in der Subcutis. Unbehaarte Haut, Mensch. Hämatoxylin-Eosin-Methode. Neg. Vergr. 250 ×

Subcutis und Corium der unbehaarten Haut beherbergen, zu einem Geflecht verwoben, cerebrospinale Nerven, aus denen sich eine Fülle vielgestaltiger Endstrukturen zu entwickeln vermag. Die spezifische Besonderheit der einzelnen Receptoren ist sicherlich nicht in ihrer Morphologie zu suchen, sondern in der Art und Weise der Reizaufnahme und Reizleitung (HOEPKE, 1958; BOMAN, 1960; STEIGLEDER (1958); KANTNER, 1961).

In der Subcutis des Handtellers und der Fußsohle findet man bei schwacher Vergrößerung mit den gebräuchlichen färbetechnischen Verfahren große, rundliche bis ovale Gebilde, die Lamellenkörperchen (Abb. 38).

Zwiebelschalenartig aufeinander gelagerte Bindegewebslamellen — bis zu 60 an der Zahl — umfassen die eintretende, marklos werdende Nervenfaser, der die begleitenden Schwannschen Zellen fehlen. Die Achsenfaser ist in eine plasmatische Substanz eingebettet, die als Innenkolben bezeichnet wird. Durch enge, nachbarliche Beziehung zu Blutgefäßen sowie ihre beachtliche Größe treten diese als Vater-Pacinische Körperchen benannten Bildungen aus der übrigen Schar der nervösen Endorgane hervor. Elektrophysiologische Untersuchungen (ADRIAN und UMRATH, 1929/30) deuten auf ihre Tätigkeit als Receptoren-Kontroll-Organ im Spannungs- und Druckgefälle hin.

Nach der Entstehung des vegetativen Nervensystems in der Haut des Embryo im 3. Monat bilden sich die Lamellenkörperchen als sensible Endorgane erst im 4. Monat aus und erreichen ihre endgültige Form gegen Ende der Schwangerschaft (PILATE, 1925 und CAUNA und MANNAN, 1959). Die afferenten Nervenfasern

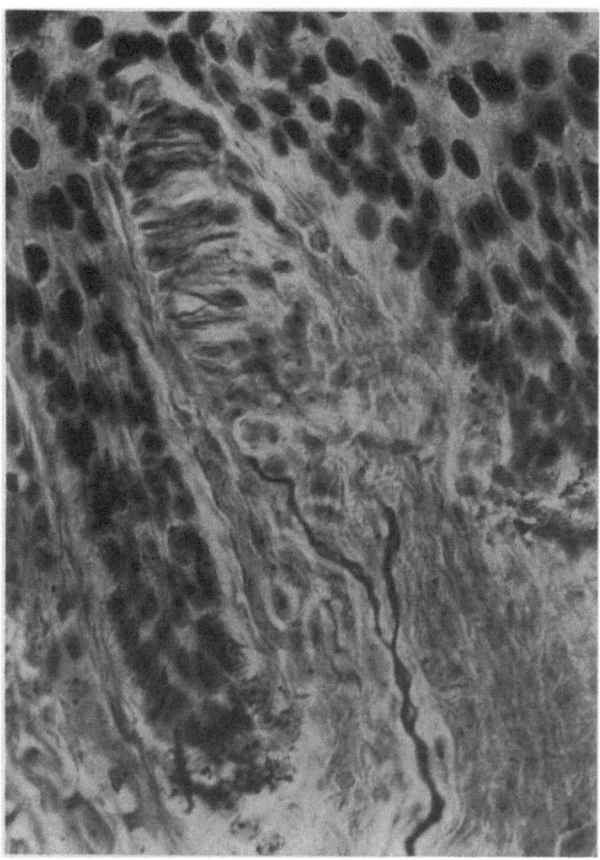

Abb. 39. Meissnersches Tastkörperchen (Schlingenkörperchen) in einer Bindegewebspapille unter dem Epithel. Unbehaarte Haut, Mensch. Präp.: Dr. G. Garweg. Bielschowsky-Gros-Methode. Neg. Vergr. 400 ×

für die Endkörperchen sollen erst später ihre selektive Empfindlichkeit erwerben, wenn sie mit spezialisierten Zellen der untersten Epidermisreihe in Zusammenhang treten. Ihr Vorkommen ist nicht nur auf die unbehaarte Haut beschränkt, sondern auch an behaarten Körperstellen, wie Kopfhaut, lassen sie sich, wenn auch selten, beobachten (IGGO, 1960/63).

KELLNER (1966) beschreibt verschiedene Typen von sensiblen Endkörperchen an Akupuncturstellen behaarter, menschlicher Haut und in Gelenknähe. Diese für die behaarte Haut außergewöhnliche Beobachtung mag vielleicht mit mechanischer Beanspruchung der Hautregion um die Gelenke in Beziehung zu bringen sein (STILWELL, 1957). SERGEEV (1963) unterstreicht im physiologischen Selbstversuch die Polyvalenz und Spezifität von Hautreceptoren. Im Bindegewebe der Bauchspeicheldrüse, dem Bauchfell (Mesenterium) und der Beinhaut (Periost) des Knochens sowie im Urogenitalbereich und an den Gefäßen treten den Lamellenkörperchen der Haut verwandte nervöse Endorgane in Erscheinung (RAUBER-KOPSCH, 1953).

Von allen übrigen Endorganen cerebrospinaler Nerven in der unbehaarten Haut tritt eine weitere Gruppe hervor: sie zeichnet sich nicht nur durch einen gewissen gleichmäßigen Bauplan aus, sondern wird auch ohne Anwendung spe-

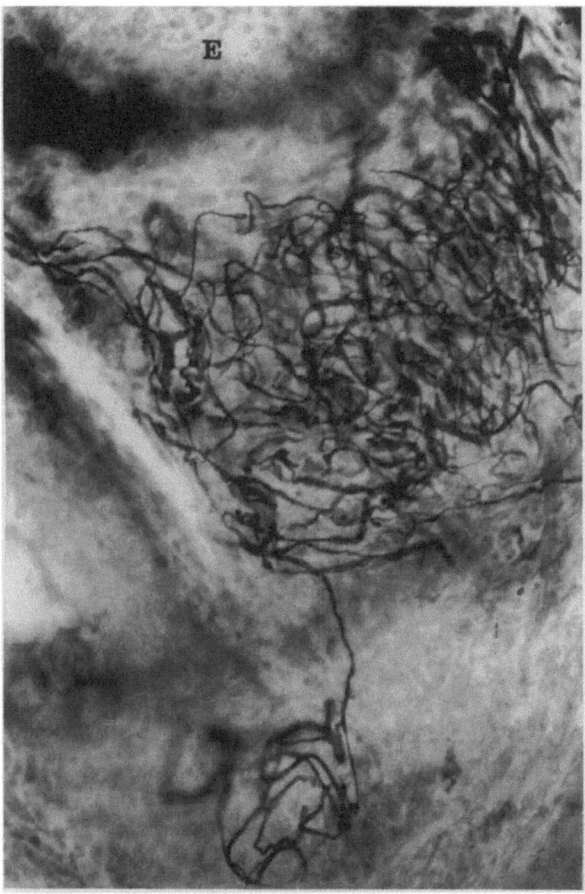

Abb. 40. Zwei zusammenhängende sensible Nervenkörperchen. Augenlid, Mensch. *E* Epithel. Richardson-Newton-Methode. Präp.: Dr. G. Garweg. Neg. Vergr. 475 ×

zieller Nervendarstellungsmethoden im histologischen Präparat sichtbar. Als kolbenförmige Bildungen liegen nervöse Endkörper in den bindegewebigen Papillen unter der Epidermis, von einer Kapsel als Fortsetzung des Perineurium umgeben. Eine spezifische Technik bringt das Vorhandensein von serpentinenartig gewundenen, marklos werdenden Nervenfasern (Abb. 39) hervor, denen besondere Zellelemente (Tastzellen) anliegen.

Trotz vieler, variierender Formen der ,,Schlingenkörperchen" unterliegen sie dem Sammelbegriff ,,Meissnersche Tastkörperchen" und werden als Druck- und Berührungsempfänger angesehen (MEISSNER, 1855; VAN DER VELDE, 1909; HERINGA, 1917; BOEKE, 1925; AIBA, 1956; WINKELMANN und OSMENT, 1956; STEIGLEDER und SCHULTIS, 1958). Sie wachsen erst nach der Geburt, und ihre Zahl nimmt im Alter, z.B. in den Papillen des Handtellers, beträchtlich ab (MILLER,

RALSTON und KASAHARA, 1958/60). CAUNA (1956) nahm mit Hilfe der Bielschowsky-Gros-Methode an der Fingerhaut von Neugeborenen bis zu Menschen im Alter von 93 Jahren eine genaue lichtmikroskopische Untersuchung Meissnerscher Körperchen vor. Meissnersche und Vater-Pacinische Körperchen entstammen nach seinen Beobachtungen verschiedenen cerebrospinalen Nervenbündeln.

Die Wandelbarkeit in der Gestalt aller übrigen im Corium der unbehaarten Haut beobachteten Nervenformationen erhellt die Abb. 40. In breiten Schleifen

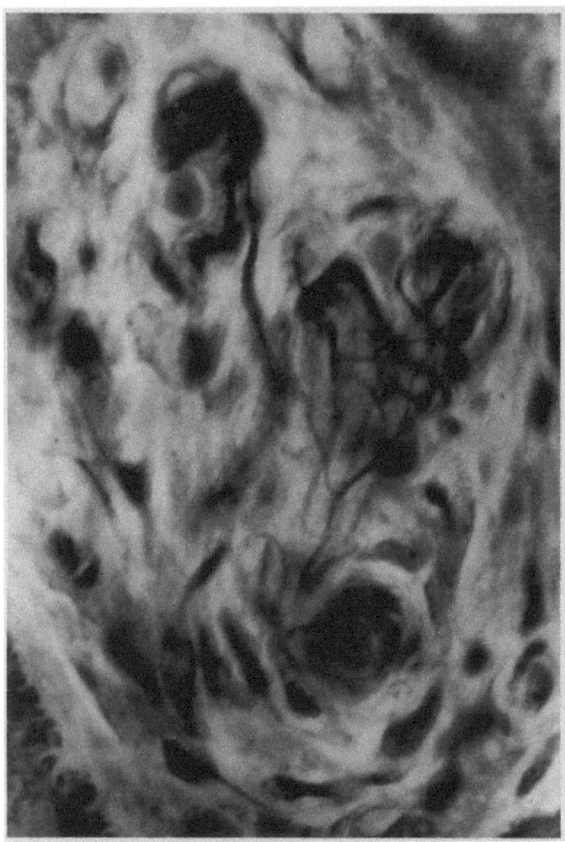

Abb. 41. Endigungen cerebrospinaler Nervenfasern. Unbehaarte Haut, Mensch. Bielschowsky-Gros-Methode. Neg. Vergr. 400 ×

einherziehende Nervenfasern formieren imponierende Endapparate auf der haarfreien Lidhaut. Zu Knäueln gewickelte Nerven, die lichtmikroskopisch keine Markscheide mehr erkennen lassen, ballen sich in Gruppen im Corium zusammen (Abb. 41). Eine einzelne Nervenfaser vermag große und kleine Knäuelbildungen nebeneinander zu entwickeln. Zum Teil sind sie ohne besondere bindegewebige Hülle im Corium zu finden. Auch ihre Verteilung unterliegt keinem gesetzmäßigen Muster (Abb. 41, 42). Die Knäuelbildungen erscheinen an allen unbehaarten Körperstellen und nur wenige überschreiten die Grenze zur behaarten Haut hin. YAMAMOTO, ITO, OHNO et al. (1958) untersuchten die Übergangsstelle von der behaarten zur unbehaarten Haut an der Affenlippe. MALINOVSKY (1966) glaubt an eine Abhängigkeit des Formenreichtums eingekapselter Endorgane von der Art der Reize, die die Körperoberfläche treffen. Er unternahm vergleichende Untersuchungen an Katzenlippe, -zunge und -fußballen. Danach hält er die meisten Nervenbildungen an diesen Stellen für Mechanoreceptoren.

In der Haut der äußeren Geschlechtsteile vermag eine einzige sensible Faser ebenfalls mehrere Endgebilde zu liefern (SETO, 1963). Trotz der großen Formenverwandtschaft mit allen übrigen Endkörperchen faßt SETO (1963) die sensiblen Endigungen von Penis, Clitoris, Scrotum und den kleinen Schamlippen als besondere Gruppe genitaler „Corpusceln" zusammen. Über ihre elektronenoptische

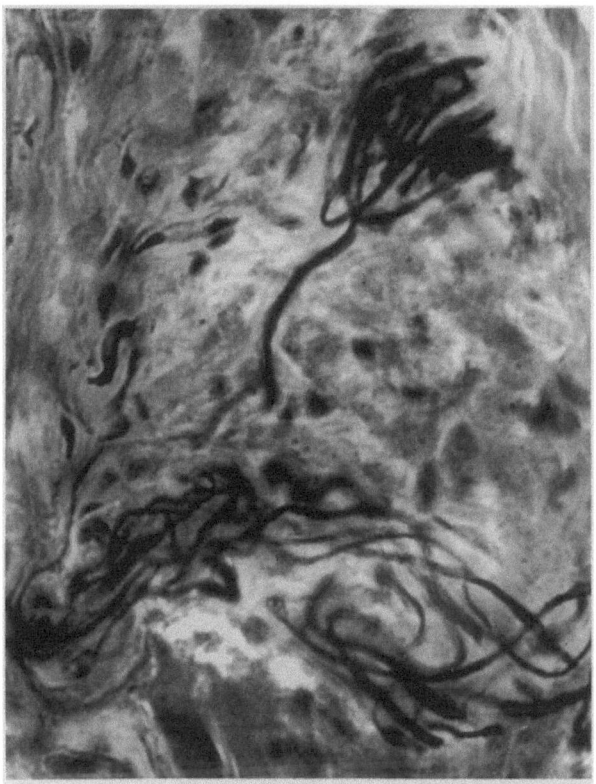

Abb. 42. Endigungsweise cerebrospinaler Nervenfasern. Unbehaarte Haut. Mensch. Bielschowsky-Gros-Methode. Neg. Vergr. 400 ×

Feinstruktur am Praeputium des Neugeborenen berichten BOURLOND und WINKELMANN (1965) sowie LAMBERTINI (1965). STÖHR (1957) und andere Autoren heben hervor, daß der Ausdruck „Endigung" im eigentlichen Sinne für das nervöse Körperchen unzutreffend sei, da es sich meist um Nervenfasern handele, die ihr starkes Längenwachstum und die damit verbundene Oberflächenvergrößerung in einer Knäuelbildung untergebracht haben, bei der ein sicheres Nervenende nicht auszumachen ist. Auf engstem Raum findet eine Vergrößerung des nervösen Apparates statt.

Unter der Vielzahl der sensiblen Endkörperchen der Haut wurde dem Vater-Pacinischen Lamellenkörperchen (Abb. 43) und dem Meissnerschen Tastkörperchen (Abb. 44) in der Elektronenmikroskopie zuerst Beachtung geschenkt, da sie wegen ihrer Größe und typischen Struktur leicht erkennbar sind.

Nach PEASE und PALLIE (1959) besitzen diese sensiblen Körperchen eine Kapsel, die sich aus einer unterschiedlichen Anzahl von Lamellen zusammensetzt.

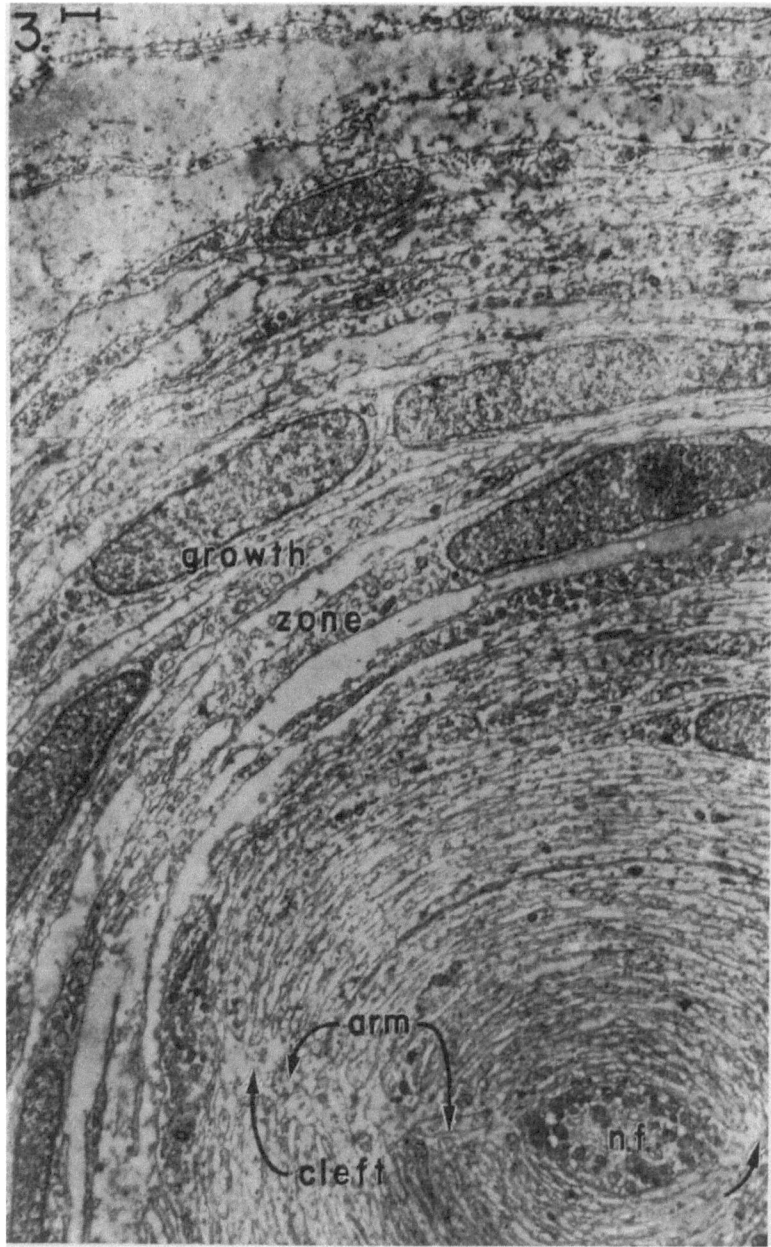

Abb. 43. The central region of a Pacinian corpuscle of a kitten at relatively low magnification. In the lower right hand corner may be seen the nerve fiber (*nf*) with its contained mitochondria. To the left is the connective tissue cleft with sectioned profiles of cytoplasmic arms (*arm*). A small portion of cleft also shows in the right corner indicated by an arrow. Note that no perikarya are to be seen deep in the core region. Nuclei are present in somes numbers, however, in the growth zone. The outer cells of the growth zone are forming definitive circumferential laminae, and there is a complete spectrum of transition from relatively unspecialized cells of the growth zone to elevated circumferential lamellae. × 5700 (PEASE and QUILLIAM, 1957)

Zentralgebiet eines Pacinischen Körperchens von einem Kätzchen bei verhältnismäßig schwacher Vergrößerung. Unten rechts ist die Nervenfaser (*nf*) mit eingeschlossenen Mitochondrien zu sehen. Links im Querschnitt zeigt sich die bindegewebige Spalte mit Profilen von cytoplasmatischen Ausläufern (*arm*). Ein kleiner Teil der Spalte ist auch rechts unten zu sehen (Pfeil). Es ist zu beachten, daß keine Perikaryen tief im Zentralbereich liegen. Mehrere Nuclei zeigen sich im Wachstumsbereich. Die äußeren Zellen dieses Wachstumsgebietes bilden definitive periphere Lamellen; sämtliche Übergangsstadien von verhältnismäßig unspezialisierten Zellen der Wachstumszone bis zu ausgebildeten peripheren Lamellen sind dargestellt. 5700 × (PEASE und QUILLIAM, 1957)

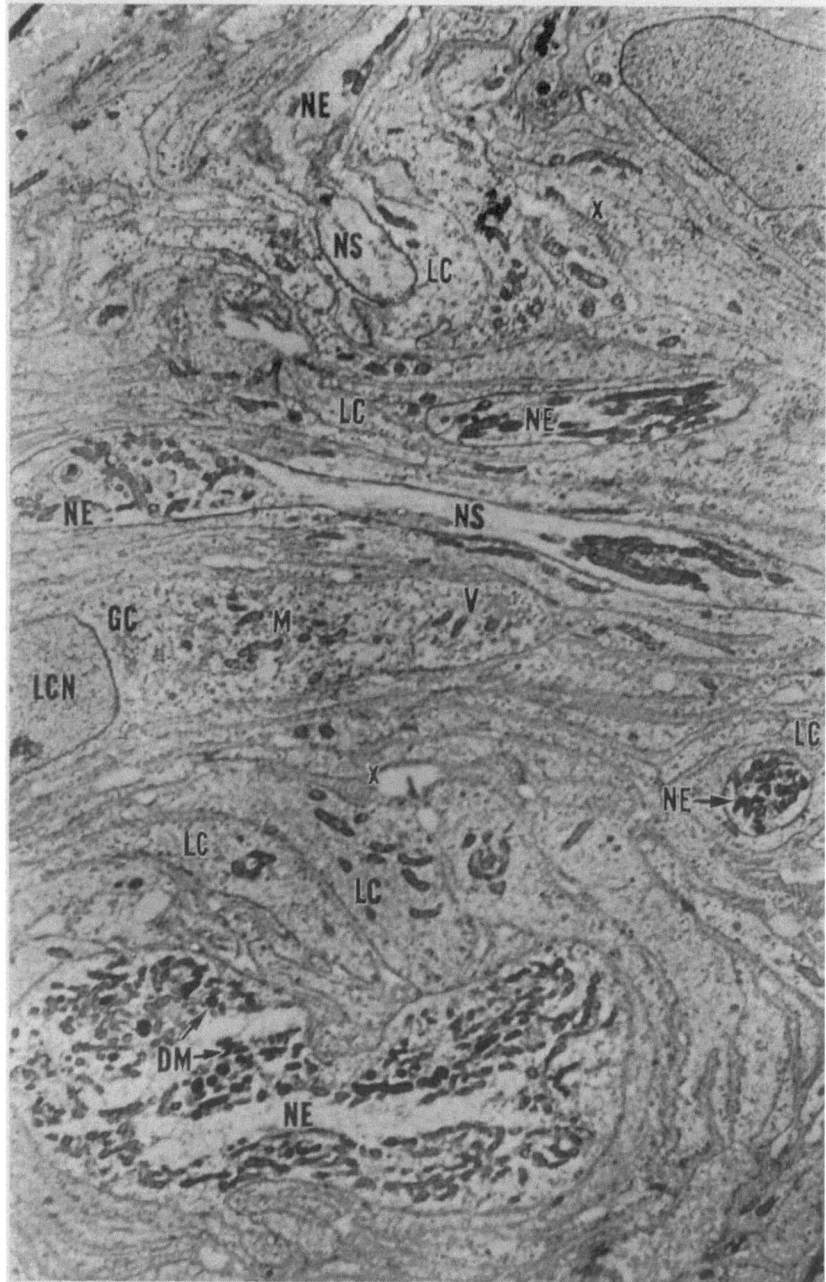

Abb. 44. A field from a transverse section of MEISSNER'S corpuscle showing the complex relationship between the laminar cells (*LC*) and nerve enlargements (*NE*). Nerve enlargements and narrow segments (*NS*) differ in structure (see text). A laminar cell with its nucleus (*LCN*) is shown in the center of the field. Its cytoplasm contains a Golgi complex (*GC*), many small vesicles (*V*), and small mitochondria (*M*). Note the dense mitochondria (*DM*) in the nerve endings. At *x* the intercellular substance is cut in such a plane that the periodic banding is shown. Female, 21 years. × 8800 (CAUNA and ROSS, 1960)

Ausschnitt eines horizontalen Querschnittes von einem Meissnerschen Körperchens, mit Laminarzellen (*LC*) und Nervenauftreibungen (*NE*). Nervenauftreibungen und schmale Abschnitte (*NS*) zeigen verschiedenartige Strukturen (s. Text). Eine Laminarzelle mit Nucleus (*LCN*) ist in der Mitte zu sehen. Ihr Cytoplasma enthält einen Golgiapparat (*GC*), mehrere kleine Vesikel (*V*) und kleine Mitochondrien (*M*). Dicht gelagerte Mitochondrien (*DM*) sind in den Nervenendigungen zu bemerken. Bei *x* läßt die Schnittführung die periodischen Bänder der Intercellularsubstanz erkennen. Frau, 21 Jahre. 8800 × (CAUNA und ROSS, 1960)

Die Kapsel und ihre Ausläufer können die Körperchen in mehr oder weniger getrennte Felder aufgliedern. Innerhalb der Felder befinden sich markhaltige und marklose Nervenfasern. Der Aufbau der sensiblen, eingekapselten Körperchen der Haut läßt sich mit dem Bau peripherer Nervenbündel vergleichen. Das Perineurium der Nervenbündel zeigt, ähnlich wie die eben beschriebene Kapsel der sensiblen Körperchen, eine lamelläre Konstruktion. Die Lamellen sind in beiden Fällen durch eine augenfällige Basalmembran charakterisiert, was sie von Fibroblasten unterscheidet.

Nach PEASE und PALLIE (1959) leiten sich die Kapselzellen bzw. die Perineuralzellen von Schwannschen Zellen her, die eine ähnliche Basalmembran besitzen. Diese Annahme gewinnt an Wahrscheinlichkeit durch die Beobachtungen von CAUNA und ROSS (1960), nach denen im Meissnerschen Tastkörperchen die Schwannschen Zellen durch lamelläre Zellen ersetzt werden. CAUNA (1956) hat einen Aufbau der Kapsel sensibler Körperchen aus elastischen Fasern angenommen und eine mechanische Funktion der Tastkörperchen postuliert. Elektronenoptisch haben sich jedoch keine elastischen Elemente nachweisen lassen (PEASE und PALLIE, 1959).

Im Cytoplasma dünner, markloser Axone der Endkörperchen finden sich elektronenoptisch kleine Bläschen, die von PALADE (1954) und PALAY (1954), PALAY und PALADE (1955), DE ROBERTIS und BENNET (1955) als „synaptic vesicles" bezeichnet werden. Nach der Vorstellung der genannten Autoren enthalten die synaptischen Bläschen Acetylcholin oder andere neurohumorale Übermittlersubstanzen. PEASE und PALLIE (1959) schreiben den Bläschen keine spezifische Bedeutung zu, da nach ihrer Auffassung das Vorkommen dieser Vacuolen nicht an einen Ort „synaptischer Natur" gebunden ist.

PEASE und QUILLIAM (1957), die diese Bläschen in Nervenfasern des Vater-Pacinischen Lamellenkörperchens beobachteten, halten sie eher für Golgi-Vacuolen und bezweifeln ihre Bedeutung für eine synaptische Übertragung. PALAY (1958) und DE ROBERTIS (1958) fanden eine zahlenmäßige Zunahme der synaptischen Bläschen bei Reizung der zugehörigen Nerven, während sich bei Denervierung die Anzahl der Vesikel in den Axonen verringern soll.

Elektronenmikroskopische Untersuchungen von PEASE und QUILLIAM (1957) haben gezeigt, daß sich am Vater-Pacinischen Lamellenkörperchen drei Zonen unterscheiden lassen. Die äußere Zone besteht aus konzentrisch angeordneten lamellären Zellen. Der Kern dieser Zellen liegt im Gegensatz zu dem der lamellären Zellen der inneren Zone in der Mitte der Zelle. Die Lamellen überlagern sich an ihren Enden häufig. Zellorganellen liegen perinucleär. Der Abstand der Lamellen nimmt nach der Peripherie hin zu. Meist zeigen die Nervenfasern in den Vater-Pacinischen Körperchen keine Aufzweigungen. Auf die äußere lamelläre Zone folgt nach innen die Wachstumszone, charakterisiert durch zahlreiche Kerne und Mitosen. Die zentrale Zone besteht wieder aus lamellären Zellen. Die konzentrischen Lamellen umfassen einen längsgerichteten Zentralkanal, in dem sich die Nervenfaser befindet. Die Anzahl der Lamellen übersteigt bei weitem die Anzahl der Zellkerne. PEASE und QUILLIAM (1957) nehmen an, daß die Zellkörper der zentralen Lamellen in dem kernreichen Verbindungsstück zwischen Wachstumszone und Zentralzone liegen. Nach Eintritt der markhaltigen Nervenfasern (QUILLIAM und SATO, 1955) in die Zentralregion des Lamellenkörperchens verliert die Faser zunächst die Markscheide, wenig später auch die letzte Umhüllung Schwannschen Cytoplasmas. Zwischen Schwannscher Scheide und proximaler „Herzlamelle" besteht ein durch undifferenzierte Zellen ausgefüllter Spaltraum. Nach Verlust der Schwannschen Scheide tritt die Nervenfaser in engen protoplasmatischen Kontakt zur innersten Zentrallamelle. Ähnlich wie beim Meissnerschen

Körperchen wird nach Eintritt der Nervenfaser in das Lamellenkörperchen im Axon ein großer Reichtum an Mitochondrien bemerkt, wie er nach den Beobachtungen von HAGEN und WERNER (1966) scheinbar den cerebrospinalen Nervenendaufzweigungen eigen ist.

An den Mitochondrien der Nervenfasern innerhalb des Meissnerschen Tastkörperchens haben CAUNA und ROSS (1960) bemerkenswerte Veränderungen beobachtet, die als degenerierende Prozesse gedeutet werden. Als beginnende Involution bezeichnen die Autoren Mitochondrien, bei denen es zur Ausbildung mehrerer konzentrisch angeordneter Lamellen kommt. Der Prozeß soll über Vacuolenbildung und Granulierung zum völligen Untergang der Mitochondrien führen. CAUNA und ROSS (1960) vermissen eine Ursache für den Zerfall der Mitochondrien im Meissnerschen Tastkörperchen. Die Autoren denken an die Möglichkeit einer extrem hohen Anforderung an den Stoffwechsel, dem die Mitochondrien erliegen. Alter und funktionelle Inanspruchnahme der Meissnerschen Körper sollen elektronenoptisch nachweisbar deren Feinbau verändern (CAUNA, 1959).

Auffallend bleibt bei allen umfangreichen sensiblen Körperchen der Haut das Fehlen der Blutgefäße innerhalb ihrer Kapsel. KELLNER (1966) fand Gefäße in einem Endkörperchen, das er dem Typ Krause zuordnet.

Die nervösen Endkörperchen, die lichtmikroskopisch zu vielgestaltig sind, um eine ihren Formen entsprechende Einteilung zu erfahren (Meissnersche und Vater-Pacinische Körperchen ausgenommen), sind nach den Untersuchungen von HAGEN und WERNER (1966) elektronenmikroskopisch nach drei Typen zu ordnen: 1. Marklose Nervenkörperchen ohne Kapsel (Abb. 45); 2. eingekapselte marklose Nervenkörperchen (Abb. 46); 3. eingekapselte, marklose und markhaltige, gemischte Nervenkörperchen (Abb. 47). Es erscheint besonders bemerkenswert, daß die unter 1. genannten marklosen Nervenkörperchen mit ihrer Beziehung zu den Schwannschen Zellen und ihrer sensiblen Funktion sich elektronenoptisch offensichtlich nicht im geringsten von vegetativen Axonen, etwa denjenigen des subepidermalen Geflechts, unterscheiden. Nur vergleichende lichtmikroskopische Untersuchungen vermögen hier klärend zu wirken und erlauben, die in Abb. 45 dargestellte Anhäufung von Axonen im Schwannschen Cytoplasma als sensibles Endkörperchen zu diagnostizieren.

Wenn die Ultrastruktur eines nervösen Gebildes eine direkte Zuordnung der Nervenelemente zum vegetativen oder cerebrospinalen Nervensystem nicht zuläßt, da den feinen Endaufsplitterungen der sensiblen Nerven der Reichtum an Mitochondrien nicht immer eigen ist, so kann man doch aus vergleichend geführten lichtmikroskopischen Serienschnitten die Zusammensetzung der Nervenkörperchen erschließen.

Nervösen Formationen im Stratum papillare der unbehaarten Haut aus ihrem ultrastrukturellen Bild heraus Receptoreigenschaften zuzuweisen, gelingt wesentlich leichter, wenn die ins Schwannsche Cytoplasma invaginierten Axone von einer besonderen Kapsel umhüllt sind (Abb. 46). Diese Kapsel setzt sich aus einer oder mehreren Lamellen zusammen. Die in ihrer Dicke stark wechselnden Lamellen stellen Fortsätze spezifischer Schwannscher Zellen dar, die keine Axone einschließen, jedoch im Gegensatz zu Fibrocyten eine Basalmembran besitzen.

In Abb. 46 wird das den lamellenförmigen Ausläufern zugehörige Perikaryon deutlich sichtbar. Genese und cytologischer Aufbau scheinen auch hier für Schwannsche Zellen der lamellären Form zu sprechen, die eigenartigerweise keine Axone invaginieren, jedoch außen von einer Basalmembran umschlossen bleiben und hierdurch ihre Sonderstellung gegenüber den Fibrocyten kundtun. Die Cytomembran der Lamellen zeigt nach innen und außen zahlreiche Vesiculationserscheinungen. Wahrscheinlich können in Form der Cytopempsis Stoffe durch die

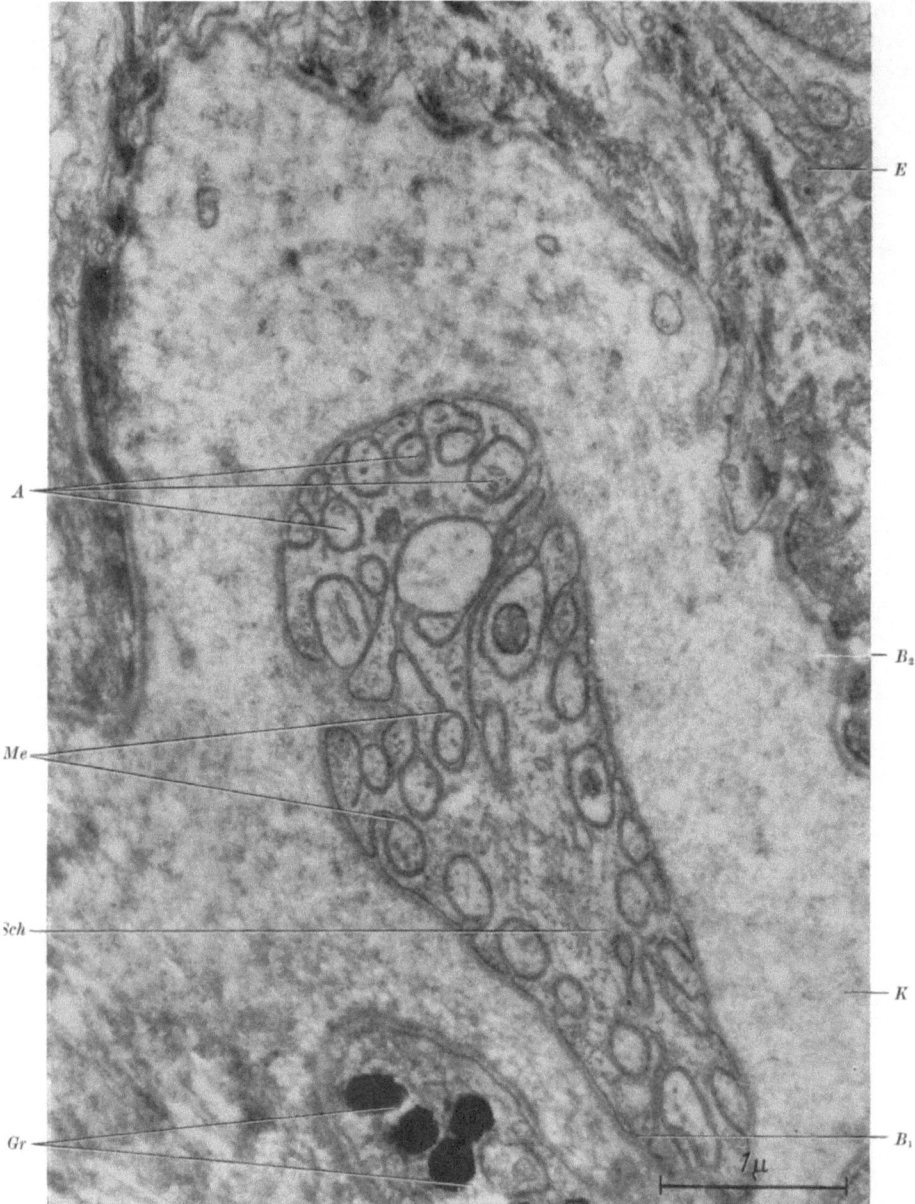

Abb. 45. Sensibles Körperchen(?) aus zahlreichen, marklosen Axonen (*A*) bestehend. Stratum papillare. Lippe, Affe. *Sch* Schwannsches Cytoplasma, *Me* Mesaxone, B_1 Basalmembran der Schwannschen Zelle, *K* kollagenes Bindegewebe, B_2 Basalmembran der Epithelzelle, *E* Epithelzelle, *Gr* Granula. Neg. Vergr. 7000 × (HAGEN und WERNER, 1966)

Lamelle in den inneren Kapselraum geschleust werden. Im Kapselraum selbst liegen, eingebettet in locker angeordnete Bindegewebsfibrillen, axonhaltige Schwannsche Zellen und lamelläre Zellen, ihrerseits wieder von einer Basalmembran umgeben. Die Axone unterscheiden sich in ihrer Beziehung zu den Schwannschen Zellen morphologisch nicht von den bereits besprochenen, nervösen Strukturen.

Die dritte Gruppe der Endkörperchen (Abb. 47) zeichnet sich von den eben geschilderten Formen durch das Auftreten markreicher Nervenfasern innerhalb

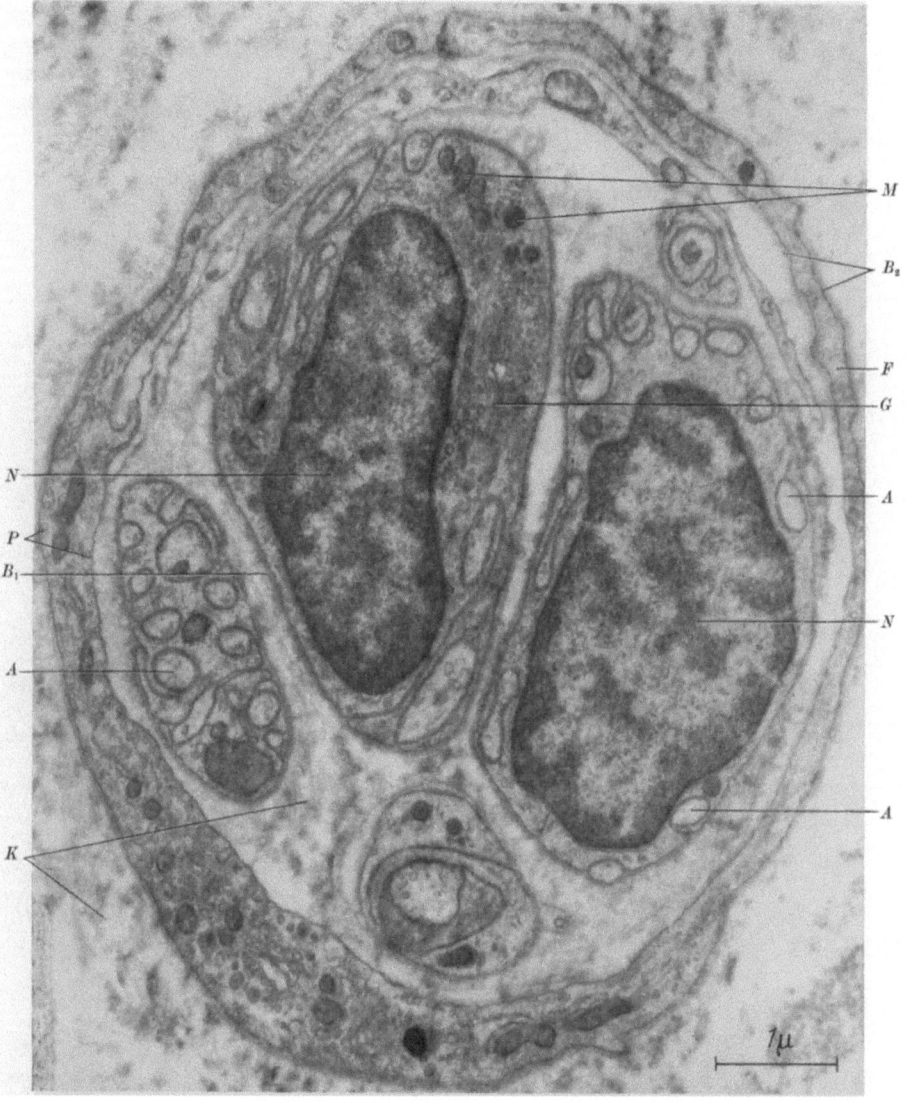

Abb. 46. Eingekapseltes (*F*) sensibles Körperchen im Stratum papillare .Unterlippe, Affe. *N* Kerne von Schwannschen Zellen, *G* Golgiapparat der Schwannschen Zelle, *A* Axone und Mesaxone, *M* Mitochondrien der Schwannschen Zelle, B_1 Basalmembran der Schwannschen Zelle, B_2 Basalmembran der Lemnocytenlamellen, *K* kollagenes Bindegewebe, *P* Pinocytose. Neg. Vergr. 7000 × (HAGEN und WERNER, 1966)

der Kapsel aus. Auch hier besteht die Kapsel der nervösen Körperchen aus einer wechselnden Zahl von Lamellen mit zwischengelagerten, bindegewebigen Spalträumen. Gelegentlich sind die beschriebenen Kapselräume mehrkammerig, wobei eine markreiche Nervenfaser und mehrere markarme Axone von der übrigen Masse markarmer Nervenformationen durch eine gesonderte Kapsel getrennt sind (Abb. 47).

Der in die Haut eingebaute Nervenapparat läßt sich folgendermaßen beurteilen: Cerebrospinale und vegetative Nerven treten nebeneinander auf. Das gilt für die vielgestaltigen Endkörperchen der unbehaarten Haut, für den Nervenapparat des Haares wie für die gesamte, im bindegewebigen Stratum subcutaneum entwickelten Nervengeflechte (STÖHR, 1957; PEREZ, 1964; HAGEN, 1966).

Somit weist die untrennbare Zusammengehörigkeit sensibler Receptoren mit den vegetativen Nerven auf die Möglichkeit einer gegenseitigen Beeinflussung des cerebrospinalen und vegetativen Nervensystems in der Körperperipherie hin. Unter solchem Befund ist eine kausale Analyse der Sinnesempfindungen der Haut, der Drüsensekretion und Blutbewegung im Gefäßgebiet zu durchdenken.

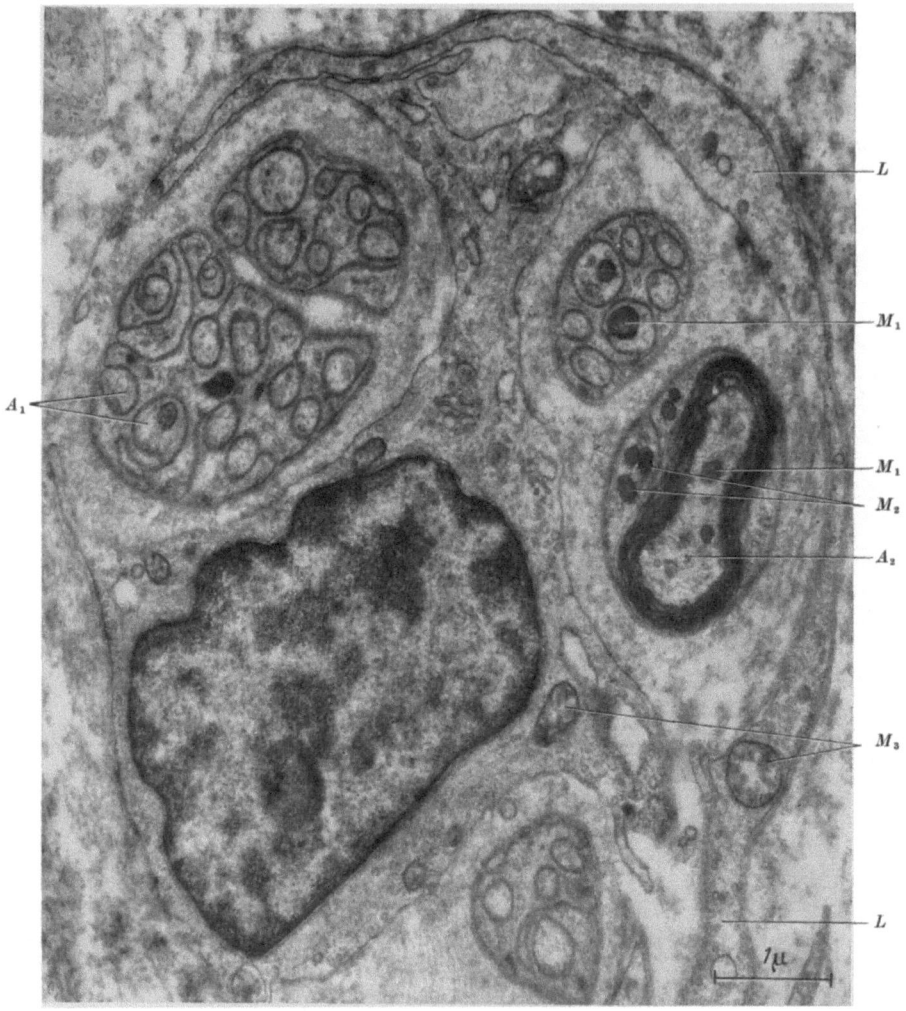

Abb. 47. Aus marklosen (A_1) und markhaltigen (A_2) Nervenfasern bestehendes sensibles, eingekapseltes Körperchen. Stratum papillare. Unterlippe, Affe. M_1 Mitochondrien der Axone, M_2 Mitochondrien der Schwannschen Zelle, M_3 Mitochondrien der Lemnocyten, L Lamellen. Neg. Vergr. 7000 × (HAGEN und WERNER, 1966)

Psychische Einflüsse, die zum Schweißausbruch, zum Erröten und Erblassen der Haut und zum Sträuben der Haare führen können, bedürfen offenbar des in der Haut verankerten, sensiblen Überwachungssystems nicht in besonderem Grade, wenn sich auch eine isolierte Funktion des cerebrospinalen und vegetativen Nervensystems in der Peripherie des Körpers nur schwer vorstellen läßt.

Demgemäß kann man bei der Klassifikation unserer Sinnesempfindungen in der Haut kaum bei den vier Qualitäten Druck, Berührung, Temperatur, Schmerz beharren. Schwer definierbare Sensationen, wie Jucken, Kitzeln, Kribbeln usw.

zeigen die Schwierigkeit einer klaren Unterscheidung zwischen cerebrospinaler und vegetativer Wirkungsweise.

So gilt für den Nervenapparat der Haut die gleiche Feststellung wie für das Zentralnervensystem: Jede gedachte Verbindung zwischen Form und Funktion ist fragwürdig und bedarf sorgfältiger Überprüfung.

Literatur

ADRIAN, E. D., and K. UMRATH: The impulse discharge from the Pacinian corpuscle. J. Physiol. (Lond.) **68**, 139—154 (1929/30). — AIBA, K.: On the sensory innervation of the foot-sole in human adults. Arch. histol. jap. **10**, 329—350 (1956). — AKKERINGA, L. I.: Die Lage der Neurofibrillen am peripheren Ende der Nervenbahn. Z. mikr.-anat. Forsch. **19**, 183—270 (1930). — ALLEN, N., and J. G. NICHOLS: Presynaptic failure of neuromuscular propagation after x-radiation. Effect of ionizing radiation on the nervous system. Proc. Symp. Vienna Atomic Agency vol. 51 (1962). — ALLENBY, C. F., E. PALMER, and G. WEDDELL: Changes in the dermis of human hairy skin resulting from stripping the keratinized layer of the epidermis. Z. Zellforsch. **69**, 566—572 (1966). — AMARETTI, A. R.: El melanocito epidermico, neurona del tacto. Hipotesis. Dermatologia (Mex.) **9**, 197—209 (1965). — ANDRES, K. H.: Über die Feinstruktur der Rezeptoren an Sinushaaren. Z. Zellforsch. **75**, 339—365 (1966). — Die Feinstruktur der sensiblen Endapparate gerader, zirkulärer und verzweigter Terminalfasern am Sinushaar. Naturwissenschaften 8, 204 (1966a). — Zur Feinstruktur des Merkelschen Tastrezeptors am Sinushaar. Naturwissenschaften (im Druck) (1966b). — ARTHUR, R. P., and W. B. SHELLEY: The innervation of human epidermis. J. invest. Derm. **32**, 397—411 (1959).

BARGMANN, W.: Histologie und mikroskopische Anatomie des Menschen. Stuttgart: Georg Thieme 1967. — BECKER jr., S. W., and A. A. ZIMMERMANN: Further studies on melanocytes and melanogenesis in the human fetus and new born. J. invest. Derm. **25**, 103—112 (1955). — BOEKE, J.: Die intrazelluläre Lage der Nervenendigungen im Epithelgewebe und ihre Beziehung zum Zellkern. Z. mikr.-anat. Forsch. **2**, 391—428 (1925). — Die Beziehung der Nervenfasern zu den Bindegewebselementen und Tastzellen. Z. mikr.-anat. Forsch. **4**, 448—509 (1925). — Innervationsstudien. 6. Der sympathische Grundplexus in seinen Beziehungen zu den Drüsen. Z. mikr.-anat. Forsch. **35**, 551—601 (1934). — BOMAN, K.: Über die Spezifität der Hautnerven. Ann. Acad. Sci. fenn A5 **73**, (1960). — BONNET, R.: Studien über die Innervation der Haarbälge der Haustiere. Gegenbauers morph. Jb. **4**, 329—398 (1878). — BORCEA, M. E.: Sur l'origine du coeleur des cellules masculins et des cellules pigmentaires chez le téléosteus. C. R. Acad. Sci. (Paris) **149**, 688—693 (1909). — BOTEZAT, E.: Über die epidermoidalen Tastapparate in der Schnauze des Maulwurfs und anderer Säugetiere mit besonderer Berücksichtigung derselben für die Physiologie der Haare. Arch. mikr. Anat. **61**, 730—764 (1903). — Die fibrilläre Struktur von Nervenendapparaten in Hautgebilden. Anat. Anz. **30**, 321—344 (1907). — Die Nerven in der Epidermis. Anat. Anz. **33**, 45—75 (1908). — Die Apparate des Gefühlsinnes der nackten und behaarten Säugetierhaut, mit Berücksichtigung des Menschen. Anat. Anz. **42**, 193—250 (1912). — BOURLOND, A.: Étude par l'imprégnation argentique de l'innervation du derme superficiel et de la jonction dermo-epidermique. Bull. Soc. franç. Derm. Syph. **69**, 246—249 (1962). — BOURLOND, A., et R. K. WINKELMANN: L'innervation du prépuce chez le nouveau-né. Arch. belges Derm. **21**, 139—153 (1965). — Study of cutaneous innervation in congenital anesthesia. Arch. Neurol. Chicago **14**, 223—227 (1966).

CAPANNA, E., and M. V. CIVITELLI: Le espansioni nervose sensitive in rapporto alle penne nel pollo. Rend. ist. Sci. Univ. Camerino **4**, 18—32 (1963). — CAUNA, N.: Nerve supply and nerve endings in Meissner's corpuscles. Amer. J. Anat. **99**, 315—336 (1956). — Structure and origin of the capsule of Meissner's corpuscle. Anat. Rec. **124**, 77—94 (1956). — The mode of termination of the sensory nerves and its significance. J. comp. Neurol. **113**, 169—199 (1959).— Functional significance of the submicroscopical, histochemical and microscopical organization of the cutaneous receptor organs. Verh. Anat. Ges. Anat. Anz. **111**, 181—198 (1962). — The effects of aging on the receptor organ of the human dermis. Advances in biology of skin, vol. 6. Aging Symp. held 1964. At the University of Oregon Medical School 1965. — CAUNA, N., and G. MANNAN: The structure of human digital Pacinian corpuscles and its functional significance. J. Anat. (Lond.) **92**, 1—14 (1958). — CAUNA, N., and G. MANNAN: Development and postnatal changes of digital Pacinian corpuscles (corpuscula lamellosa) in the human hand. J. Anat. (Lond.) **93**, 271—286 (1959). — CAUNA, N., and L. L. ROSS: The fine structure of Meissner's touch corpuscles of human fingers. J. biophys. biochem. Cytol. **8**, 467—482 (1960). — CHARLES, A.: Myelin figures occurring in the peripheral nerve bundle

of human skin. Exp. Cell Res. **14**, 440—442 (1959). — COHNHEIM, J.: Über die Endigungen der sensiblen Nerven in der Hornhaut der Säugetiere. Zbl. med. Wiss. (1866).
DANIEL, C., PH. D. PEASE, and T. ANDREWS: Electron microscopy of the pacinian corpuscle. J. biophys. biochem. Cytol. **3**, 331—342 (1957). — DARIAN-SMITH, I., P. MUTTON, and R. PROCTOR: Functional organization of tactile cutaneous afferents within the semilunar ganglion and trigeminal spinal tract of the cat. J. Neurophysiol. **28**, 682—694 (1965). — DE ROBERTIS, E.: Ultrastructure and function in some neurosecretory systems. In Proc. 3rd Int. Symp. on Neurosecretion, Bristol 1961. Mem. Soc. Endocrinol. **12**, 3—20 (1962). — DE ROBERTIS, E., and H. S. BENETT: Some features of the submicroscopic morphology of synapses in frog and earthworm. J. biophys. biochem. Cytol. **1**, 47—58 (1955). — DIXON, A. D.: The innervation of hair follicles in the mammalian lip. Anat. Rec. **140**, 147—159 (1961). — DOGIEL, A. S.: Die Nervenendigungen in Tastkörperchen. Arch. Anat. Physiol., Anat. Abt. **182**, (1891). — DROZ, B.: Recherches sur le système nerveux végétatif de la peau: innervation sympathique des poils. Arch. Anat. micr. Morph. exp. **43**, 299—309 (1954). — Recherches sur le système nerveux végétatif de la peau. II. Innervation sympathique du derme. Arch. Anat. micr. Morph. exp. **44**, 70—88 (1955). — DUPONT, A., et A. BOURLAND: Recherches sur les structures nerveuses de la peau humaine. Trab. Inst. Cajal Invest. biol. **54**, 177—186 (1962). — Innervation des dermoepidermalen Bindegewebes. Arch. belges Derm. **18**, 249—257 (1962).
EKHOLM, J.: Some properties of cutaneous sense organs during postnatal development. Acta Soc. Med. upalien. **70**, 255—258 (1965). — ENGSTRÖM, H., and J. WERSALL: Myelin sheath structure in nerve fibre demyelinization and branching regions. Exp. Cell Res. **14**, 414—425 (1958). — EVANS, M. J., J. B. FINEAN, and D. L. WOOLF: Ultrastructural studies of human cutaneous nerves with special reference to lamellated cell inclusions of Schwann cells and vacuole-containing cells. J. clin. Path. **18**, 188—192 (1965).
FALCHI, G.: Stato attuale delle nostre conoscence sola genese del pigmento melanico. Minerva derm. **26**, 14—28 (1951). — FERREIRA-MARQUES, J.: Systema sensitivum intraepidermicum. Arch. Derm. Syph. (Berl.) **193**, 191—250 (1951). — Systema intra-epidermicum. Die Langerhans'schen Zellen als Doloriceptores. Acta neuroveg. (Wien) **3**, 346—353 (1952). — FITZGERALD, M. J. T.: A protargol technique for the impregnation of cutaneous nerves. Irish J. med. Sci. **438**, 287—291 (1962). — The postnatal growth of the nerves of vibrissae. J. Anat. (Lond.) **96**, 521—525 (1962). — On the structure and life history of bulbous corpuscles (corpuscula nervorum terminalia bulboidea). J. Anat. (Lond.) **96**, 189—208 (1962). — Transmedian cutaneous innervation. J. Anat. (Lond.) **97**, 313—322 (1963). — Epidermal innervation in methylcholanthrene-painted mouse skin. Nature (Lond.) **206**, 107—108 (1965). — Perinatal changes in epidermal innervation in rat and mouse. J. comp. Neurol. **126**, 37—42 (1966). — FITZGERALD, M. J. T., and S. M. LAVELLE: Response of murine cutaneous nerves to skin painting with methylcholanthrene. Anat. Rec. **154**, 617—633 (1966). — FREY, M. v.: Beiträge zur Sinnesphysiologie der Haut. 3. Ber. Sächs. Ges. Wiss. math. phys. Kl. Leipzig Bd. 47. S. 166—184. 1895. — FUSARI, R.: Alcune osservationi di fina anatomica nel campo del sistema nervoso peripherico. 2. Su alcune apparenze di cellule nervose che si possono esservare col mezzo della reazione nera nella papille della lingua e della cute dei mammiferi. Sulla terminazion della fibre nervose nelle ghlandole sebacee dei mammiferi. G. Accad. Med. Torino **65**, 426—428 (1902).
GAMBLE, H. J.: Further electron microscope studies of human fetal peripheral nerves. J. Anat. (Lond.) **103**, 487—502 (1966). — GAMBLE, H. J., and R. A. EAMES: An electron microscope study of the connective tissues of human peripheral nerve. J. Anat. (Lond.) **98**, 655—663 (1964). — GANSLER, H.: Phasenkontrast und elektronenmikroskopische Untersuchungen zur Innervation der glatten Muskulatur. Acta neuroveg. (Wien) **22**, 192—211 (1961). — GOTHE, J.: Die intraepithelialen Nervenfasern im Vestibulum nasi der Kleinfledermäuse, dargestellt an Hand der Osmium-Zinkjodid-Methode nach Maillet. Z. mikr.-anat. Forsch. **72**, 383—402 (1965). — GOTO, M.: Innervation of pars cutanea of vestibulum nasi and nasus externus in latter half of human embryonic life. Tohoku. J. exp. Med. **61**, 77—81 (1954).
HAGEN, E.: Über die Nervenversorgung der Haut. Stud. gen. (Berl.) **17**, 513—526 (1964). — Anatomie des vegetativen Nervensystems. Akt. Fragen Psychiat. Neurol. **3**, 1—73 (1966). — HAGEN, E., u. S. WERNER: Beobachtungen an der Ultrastruktur epidermaler und subepidermaler Nerven vor und nach Röntgenbestrahlung. I. Mitt. Arch. klin. exp. Derm. **225**, 306—327 (1966). — Beobachtungen an der Ultrastruktur epidermaler und subepidermaler Nerven vor und nach Röntgenbestrahlung. II. Mitt. Arch. klin. exp. Derm. **225**, 328—334 (1966). — Zur Ultrastruktur des Nervensystems in der Haut. Verhandlungen der Anatomischen Gesellschaft. Anat. Anz. Erg.-H. **120**, 277—288 (1967). — HENSEL, H.: Spezifische und unspezifische Receptorfunktion peripherer Nervenendigungen. Pflügers Arch. ges. Physiol. **273**, 543—561 (1961). — Die Spezifität der Hautsinne. Stud. gen. (Berl.) **8**, 471—495 (1964). — HENSEL, H., A. IGGO, and I. WITT: A quantitative study of sensitive cutaneous thermo-

receptors with C afferent fibres. J. Physiol. (Lond.) 153, 113—126 (1960). — HERINGA, G. C.: Le développement des corpuscules de Grandry et de Herbst. Arch. néerl. Physiol. 3, 74—83 (1917). — HETT, J.: Zur feineren Innervation der arterio-venösen Anastomosen in der Fingerbeere des Menschen. Z. Zellforsch. 33, 151—156 (1943). — HOEPKE, H.: Neue Befunde über die sensible Innervation der Haut. Acta neuroveg. (Wien) 18, 49—59 (1958). — HORSTMANN, E.: Sinnesorgane und Innervation. In: Handbuch der mikroskopischen Anatomie des Menschen, Bd. III/3, S. 208—213. Haut und Sinnesorgane 1957. — HOYER, H.: Über den Austritt der Nervenfasern in das Epithel der Hornhaut. Arch. Anat. Physiol. 180, 165—172 (1866). — HUNT, C. C., and A. K. McINTYRE: Properties of cutaneous touch receptors. J. Physiol. (Lond.) 153, 88—98 (1960). — An analysis of fibre diameter and receptor characteristics of myelinated cutaneous afferent fibres in the cat. J. Physiol. (Lond.) 153, 99—112 (1960).

IGGO, A.: Cutaneous mechanoreceptors with afferent fibres. J. Physiol. (Lond.) 152, 337—353 (1960). — New specific sensory structures in hairy skin. Acta neuroveg. (Wien) 24, 175—180 (1963). — An electrophysiological analysis of afferent fibres in primate skin. Acta neuroveg. (Wien) 24, 225—240 (1963). — The significance of the terminal structure of efferent nerve fibres Proc. of the first intern. Symp. on Olfaction and Taste, vol. 149. Oxford-London-New York-Paris: Pergamon Press 1963.

JABONERO, V.: Mikroskopische Studien über die Morphologie und die Morphopathologie der vegetativen Innervation der menschlichen Haut. I. u. II. Acta neuroveg. (Wien) 18, 67—154 (1958). — Über die Osmium-Zinkjodid-affinen Elemente der Haut. Acta neuroveg. (Wien) 24, 154—155 (1963). — Morphologie normale et pathologique du système nerveux cutane. Arch. belges Derm. 19, 237—249 (1963). — Über die Brauchbarkeit der Osmiumtetroxyd-Zinkjodid-Methode zur Analyse der vegetativen Peripherie. Acta neuroveg. (Wien) 26, 184—210 (1964). — JABONERO, V., M. E. BENGOECHEA u. A. PEREZ-CASAS: Über die feinere Innervation der Haut. II. Die Innervation der Hautanhangsorgane. Acta neuroveg. (Wien) 23, 305—328 (1962). — JABONERO, V., u. A. PEREZ-CASAS: Über die feinere Innervation der Haut. I. Die Innervation der Epidermis, der Cutis und der Hautblutgefäße. Acta neuroveg. (Wien) 22, 360—384 (1961). — JALOWY, B.: Über die Regeneration der Nervenendigungen in den Tasthaaren des Meerschweinchens. Z. Zellforsch. 21, 149—168 (1934). — Über die Regeneration der Nervenendigungen in den Sinushaaren nach mehrfacher Durchschneidung des Nervus infraorbitalis. Z. Zellforsch. 26, 715—727 (1937). — JOHN, F.: Zur mikroskopischen Anatomie der Gefäß- und Schweißdrüsennerven in der menschlichen Haut. Z. Zellforsch. 30, 298—320 (1940). — Zur vegetativen Innervation der Talgdrüsen. Arch. Derm. Syph. (Berl.) 182, 402—411 (1941). — Zur vegetativen Nervenversorgung der menschlichen Haare und Haarmuskeln. Arch. Derm. Syph. (Berl.) 183, 1—14 (1942). — Zur vegetativen Nervenversorgung der menschlichen Epidermis. Arch. Derm. Syph. (Berl.) 185, 341—350 (1944). — Netz und Geflecht im vegetativen Nervensystem der Haut. Acta neuroveg. (Wien) 18, 41—48 (1958).

KADANOFF, D.: Beiträge zur Kenntnis der Nervenendigungen im Epithel der Säugetiere. I. und II. Z. ges. Anat. I. Abt., Z. Anat. Entwickl.-Gesch. 73, 431—452 (1924). — Über die Nerven in der äußeren Wurzelscheide der Haare des Menschen. Z. Zellforsch. 6, 631—636 (1927/28). — Über die Regeneration der hypolemmalen Nervenendigungen der Sinushaare nach Nervendurchschneidung. Ergebn. Anat. Entwickl.-Gesch. 66, 259—263 (1928). — Über die intraepithelialen Nerven und ihre Endigungen beim Menschen und bei den Säugetieren. Z. Zellforsch. 1, 553—576 (1928). — KADANOFF, D.: Die Innervation der Haare des Menschen. Acta neuroveg. (Wien) 18, 159—168 (1958). — KADANOFF, D., W. WASSILEV, and I. MATEV: Über die regenerierten Nervenfasern und Nervenendigungen in Hautnarben und Hauttransplantaten bei Menschen. Anat. Anz. 118, 503—515 (1966). — KAMIDE, J.: On the findings of skin nerves supravitally stained with methylene blue, especially in the Haarscheibe of the human skin. Jap. J. Derm. 65, 339—355 (1955). — KANTNER, M.: Neue morphologische Ergebnisse über die peripherische Nervenausbreitung und ihre Deutung. Acta anat. (Basel) 31, 397—425 (1957). — Das Nervensystem der Haut. In: Dermatologie und Venerologie, von H. A. GOTTRON u. W. SCHOENFELD, Bd. I/1, S. 104—128. Stuttgart: Georg Thieme 1961. — La morphologie des recepteurs dans la peau. Acta anat. (Basel) 60, 463—478 (1965). — Zur Morphologie der Hautrezeptoren. Zbl. Vet.-Med., Reihe A, 12, 493—500 (1965). — KAWAMURA, T.: Über die menschliche Haarscheibe unter besonderer Berücksichtigung ihrer Innervation und subepidermalen perineuralen Pigmenthülle. Hautarzt 5, 106—109 (1954). — KELLNER, G.: Über ein vaskularisiertes Nervenendkörperchen vom Typ der Krauseschen Endorgane. Z. mikr.-anat. Forsch. 75, 130—144 (1966). — KISS, F.: Innervation der Haut (Symp.). Acta neuroveg. (Wien) 18, 32—40 (1958). — KITTEL, F.: Vorkommen eines Schweißdrüsenausführungsganges innerhalb eines Nerven. Anat. Anz. 118, 140—142 (1966). — KNOCHE, H.: Untersuchungen über die feinere Innervation arteriovenöser Anastomosen. Z. Anat. Entwickl.-Gesch. 120, 379—391 (1958). — KOECKE, H. U.: Die Haut der Wirbeltiere, ihr Bau und ihre Funktionen. Stud. gen., Berlin 17, 288—322 (1964). — KÖLLIKER, A. V.: Handbuch der Gewebelehre des Menschen, Bd. 1. Leipzig: Wilhelm Engelmann 1889.

Lambertini, G.: Considerations sur les corpuscles de Pacini et l'étude morphologique des ces récepteurs dans le prépuce de l'homme. Bull. Ass. Anat. (Nancy) 126, 914—940 (1965). — Lehmann, H. J.: The epineurium as a diffusion barrier. Nature (Lond.) 172, 1045—1046 (1953). — Über Struktur und Funktion der perineuralen Diffusionsbarriere. Z. Zellforsch. 46, 232—241 (1957). — Lele, P. P., and G. Weddell: Sensory nerves of the cornea and cutaneous sensibility. Exp. Neurol. 1, 334—360 (1959). — Leloup, R., et A. Bourland: Quelques images du réseau sympathique cutané. Arch. belges Derm. 17, 223—229 (1961). — Leontowitsch, A.: Die Innervation der menschlichen Haut. Int. Mschr. Anat. Physiol. 12, 278—283 (1891). — Levi, S.: Osservazioni sullo sviluppo delle terminazioni nervose intraepiteliali, corpuscoli del Meissner e corpuscoli del Pacini. Arch. ital. Anat. Embriol. 32, 149—170 (1933). — Lindblom, U.: Excitability and functional organization within the peripheral tactile unit. Acta physiol. scand. 44, Suppl. 153, 1—84 (1958). — Phasic and static excitability of touch receptors in toad skin. Acta physiol. scand. 59, 410—423 (1963). — Properties of touch receptors in distal glabrous skin of the monkey. J. Neurophysiol. 28, 966—985 (1965). — List, C. F., and M. M. Peet: Sweat secretion in man. II. Anatomic distribution of disturbances in sweating associated with lesions of the sympathetic nervous system. Arch. Neurol. Psychiat. (Chic.) 40, 37 (1938).

Maillet, M.: Modifications de la technique de Champy au tétraoxyde d'osmiumiodure de potassium. Resultats de son application à l'étude des fibres nerveuses. C. R. Soc. biol. (Paris) 153, 939—940 (1959). — Le réactif aus tétraoxyde d'osmiumiodure du zinc. Rev. Med. Tours. 4, 247—267 (1963). Z. mikr.-anat. Forsch. 70, 397—425 (1963). — Malcolm, R., H. J. R. Miller III, and M. Kasahara: The patterns of cutaneous innervation of the human hand. Amer. J. Anat. 12, 183—192 (1958). — Malinovský, L.: The variability of encapsulated corpuscles in the upper lip and tongue of the domestic cat (Felis ocreata L., f. domestica). Folia morph. (Warszawa) 14, 175—191 (1966). — Variability of sensory nerve endings in foot pads of a domestic cat. Acta anat. (Basel) 64, 82—106 (1966). — Martinez-Perez, R.: Contribution à l'étude des terminaisons nerveuses dans la peau de la main. Trav. Lab. Rech. biol., Univ. Madrid 27, 187—226 (1931). — Maruhashi, J., K. Mizuguchi, and I. Tasaki: Action currents in single afferent nerve fibers elicited by stimulus of the skin of the toad and the cat. J. Physiol. (Lond). 117, 129—151 (1952). — Masson, P.: Innervation des glomus cutanés de l'homme. Tans. roy. Soc. Can., Sect. V. 30, 31—38 (1936). — Matsumoto, R.: Studies on skin pigment, particularly on vitiligo. Jap. J. Derm. 71, 57—63 (1961). — Meissner, G.: Bemerkungen, die Tastkörperchen betreffend. Z. wiss. Zool. 6, 296—297 (1855). — Merkel, F.: Über die Endigung der sensiblen Nerven in der Haut der Wirbeltiere. Rostock: Schmidt 1880. — Miller, M. R., H. J. Ralston III, and M. Kasahara: The pattern of cutaneous innervation of the human hand. Amer. J. Anat. 102, 183 (1958). — The pattern of cutaneous innervation of the human hand, foot and breast. Cutaneous innervation, vol. 1: Advances in biology of skin, p. 1—47. Montagna, W. (Ed.). Oxford: Pergamon Press 1960. — Miller, S., and G. Weddell: Mechanoreceptors in rabbit ear skin innervated by myelinated nerve fibres. J. Physiol. (Lond.) 187, 291—307 (1966). — Montagna, W.: Histology and cytochemistry of human skin. J. Invest. Dermat. 42, 119—129 (1964). — Montagna, W., and R. A. Ellis: Histology and cytochemistry of human skin. XII. Cholinesterases in the hair follicles of the scalp. J. invest. Derm. 29, 151—157 (1957). — Montagna, W., and S. S. Yum: The skin of primates. Amer. J. physic. Anthrop. 21, 371—381 (1963). — Munger, B. L.: The intraepidermal innervation of the snout skin of the opossum. A light and electron microscope study, with observations on the nature of Merkel's Tastzellen. J. Cell Biol. 26, 79—97 (1965).

Newton, D.: Über die Leistung der Silberimprägnationsmethode nach Richardson zur Darstellung des vegetativen Nervensystems an der Haut, am Darm und an der Gallenblase. Acta anat. (Basel) 58, 201—216 (1964). — Niebauer, G.: Der Aufbau des peripheren neurovegetativen Systems im Epidermal-Dermalbereich. Acta neuroveg. (Wien) 15, 109—123 (1956). — Neurohistologie des Haares. Arch. klin. exp. Derm. 227, 409—419 (1966). — Dendritic cells of human skin. In: Experimental biology and medicine. Basel and New York: S. Karger 1968. — Niebauer, G., u. N. Sekido: Über die Dendritenzellen der Epidermis. Arch. klin. exp. Derm. 222, 23—42 (1965). — Niebauer, G., and A. Wiedmann: Zur Histochemie des neurovegetativen Systems der Haut. Acta neuroveg. (Wien) 18, 280—296 (1958). — Niggli-Stokar, U.: Faseranalyse der Euternerven und die Nervenendformation in der Zitzenhaut des Rindes. Acta anat. (Basel) 46, 104—126 (1961). — Niizuma, S.: Histological study on the innervation of rectum and anus of bat. Arch. histol. jap. 9, 283—298 (1955). — Niizuma, S., K. Nozaki, M. Komatsu, and T. Numata: On sensory innervation of zona cutanea ani in bat. Arch. histol. jap. 9, 343—348 (1955). — Nishihara, K.: Studies on the nature of Langerhans cells and findings of the Langerhans staining method on the naevus pigmentosus and others. Jap. J. Derm. 63, 284—304 (1953).

Ono, S.: Histological study on the innervation of the snout and the nasal cavity with their surroundings in cat. Arch. histol. jap. 10, 37—52 (1956). — Orfanos, C.: Elektronenmikroskopische Befunde an epidermisnahen Nervenanteilen. Arch. klin. exp. Derm. 222,

603—612 (1965). — Der Aufbau peripherer Nervenfasern der menschlichen Haut. Eine EM-Studie. Arch. Klin. exp. Derm. **223**, 457—477 (1965). — Elektronenmikroskopischer Nachweis epithelio-neuraler Verbindungen (Mechano-Receptoren) am Haarfollikelepithel des Menschen. Arch. klin. exp. Derm. **228**, 421—429 (1967). — ORMEA, F.: Betrachtungen zur nervösen Innervation der Haut. Hautarzt **1**, 226—230 (1950). — On the problem of the relations between the innervation of the sweat-glands and of other organs of the human skin. Dermatologica (Basel) **101**, 157—166 (1950).

PALADE, G. E.: Electron microscope observations of intraneural and neuromuscular synapses. Anat. Rec. **118**, 335—336 (1954). — PALAY, S. L.: Electronmicroscope study of the cytoplasm of neurons. Anat. Rec. **118**, 366ff. (1954). — PALAY, S. L., and G. E. PALADE: The fine structure of neurons. J. biophys. biochem. Cytol. **1**, 69—88 (1955). — PATRIZZI, G., and B. L. MUNGER: The ultrastructure and innervation of rat vibrissae. J. comp. Neurol. **126**, 423—436 (1966). — PAU, H., u. H. CONRADS: Zur Morphologie der feinen Hornhautnerven. Z. Zellforsch. **46**, 96—99 (1957). — PAWLOWSKI, A.: Frei und geformte Nervenendigungen in Epidermis und oberen Hautschichten bei Mensch und Tier. Przegl. derm. **50**, 31—43 (1963). — PAWLOWSKI, A., and G. WEDDELL: The lability of cutaneous neural elements. Brit. J. Derm. **79**, 14—20 (1967). — PEASE, D. C., and W. PALLIE: Electron microscopy of digital tactile corpuscles and small cutaneous nerves. J. Ultrastruct. Res. **2**, 352—365 (1959). — PEASE, D. C., and T. A. QUILLIAM: Electron microscopy of the Pacinian corpuscle. J. biophys. biochem. Cytol. **3**, 331—342 (1957). — PILATE, M.: Contribution à l'étude de la structure et du développement des corpuscles de Vater-Pacini. Arch. Russ. Anat. histol. embryol. **3**, 225—278 (1925). — PINKUS, F.: Über Hautsinnesorgane neben dem menschlichen Haar (Haarscheiben) und ihre vergleichend anatomische Bedeutung. Arch. mikr. Anat. **65**, 121—179 (1905). — Die normale Anatomie der Haut. In: JADASSOHN Handbuch der Haut- und Geschlechtskrankheiten, Bd. 1. Berlin: Springer 1927. — PINKUS, H.: Anatomy of the skin, 1957. Dermatologica (Basel) **118**, 44—64 (1959). — POLLEY, E. H.: The innervation of blood vessels in striated muscle and skin. J. comp. Neurol. **103**, 255—267 (1955). — PRIETO, R. L., and V. JABONERO: Innervation des glandes sudoripares. Acta neuroveg. (Wien) **8**, 1—26 (1954).

QUILLIAM, Z. A., and M. SATO: The distribution of myelin on nerve fibres from Pacinian corpuscles. J. Physiol. (Lond.) **129**, 167—176 (1955).

RAUBER-KOPSCH: Lehrbuch und Atlas der Anatomie des Menschen, Bd. III. Leipzig: Georg Thieme 1953. — RAWLES, M.: Origin of pigment cells from the neural crest in mouse embryo. Physiol. Zool. **20**, 248—266 (1947). — REISER, K. A.: Über die Innervation der Hornhaut des Auges. Arch. Augenheilk. **109**, 251—280 (1935). — REITER, W.: Über das Raumsystem des endoplasmatischen Retikulums von Hautnervenfasern. Untersuchungen an Serienschnitten. Z. Zellforsch. **72**, 446—461 (1966). — RICHARDSON, K. C.: Studies on the structure of autonomic nerves in the small intestine, correlating the silver-impregnated image in light microscopy with the permanganate-fixed ultrastructure in electronmicroscopy. J. Anat. (Lond.) **94**, 457—472 (1960). — RICHTER, R.: Die Innervation der Epidermis und Cutis. Acta neuroveg. (Wien) **18**, 1—31 (1958). — RICHTER, W. H.: Über nervöse Strukturelemente der Haut. Materia Med. Nordmark **22**, 170—185 (1956). — RODRIGUEZ-PEREZ, A. P.: On the existence of accessory unmyelinated fibres in the Meissner corpuscles of the pulp of the human toe. Dermatologica (Basel) **129**, 468—474 (1964). — Ross, L. L.: Electron microscope observation of carotid body of the cat. J. biophys. biochem. Cytol. **6**, 253—262 (1959). — RUSKA, H., u. C. RUSKA: Licht- und Elektronenmikroskopie des peripheren vegetativen Systems im Hinblick auf die Funktion. Dtsch. med. Wschr. **86**, 1697—1701 (1961).

SEKIDO, N.: Epidermal melanocytes of guinea-pigs and their behaviour in experimental contact dermatitis. Jap. J. Derm., Ser. B **73**, 18—31 (1963). — SERGEEV, K. K.: Morphophysiology and physiology of the skin receptors. Vestn. Derm. Vener. **27**, Nr 3, 205—222 (1963). — SETO, H.: Studies on the sensory innervation (human sensibility), 2nd. ed. Osaka and Tokyo: Igaku Shoin 1963. — SHANTHARCERAPPA, T. R., and G. H. BOURNE: New observations on the structure of the Pacinian corpuscle and its relation to the perineural epithelium of peripheral nerves. Amer. J. Anat. **112**, 97—109 (1963). — STEFANELLI, A.: Indagini comparative sulla natura (somatica et autonoma) delle fibre nervose e dei loro apparati espansionali nella cute, cavitá orale et muscoli striati voluntari. Riv. Biol. **21**, 3—30 (1936). — Indagini comparative sulla natura (somatica e autonomia) della fibre nervose e dei loro volontasi. Riv. Biol. **21**, 48—75 (1936). — STEIGLEDER, G. K., u. K. SCHULTIS: Zur Histochemie der Meissnerschen Tastkörperchen. Acta neuroveg. **18**, 335—344 (1958). — STILWELL, D. L.: The innervation of deep structures of the foot. Amer. J. Anat. **101**, 59—73 (1957b). — The innervation of deep structures of the hand. Amer. J. Anat. **101**, 75—99 (1957c). — STOCKINGER, L.: Nervenabschnitte ohne Perineurium. Acta anat. (Basel) **60**, 244—252 (1965). — STÖHR jr., PH.: Mikroskopische Anatomie des vegetativen Nervensystems. Berlin: Springer 1928. — Handbuch mikroskopischer Anatomie, Bd. IV/5. Mikroskopische Anatomie des vegetativen Nervensystems. Berlin-Göttingen-Heidelberg: Springer 1957. — STOIAN, M.: Ultrastruktur der normalen menschlichen Haut. I. Kutis-Epidermis-Verknüpfung. Derm.-

Vener. (Buc.) **10**, 39—48 (1965). — SZYMONOWICZ, L.: Über die Nervenendigungen in den Haaren des Menschen. Arch. mikr. Anat. **74**, 622—634 (1909). — SZYMONOWICZ, M.: Vergleichende Untersuchungen über die Innervation der Sinushaare bei den Säugern. I. I. Z. Anat. Entwickl.-Gesch. **105**, 459—490 (1936). — Vergleichende Untersuchungen über die Innervation der Sinushaare bei den Säugern. II. I. Z. Anat. Entwickl.-Gesch. **106**, 85—97 (1937). — SZYMONOWICZ, W.: Beiträge zur Kenntnis der Nervenendigungen in Hautgebilden. Arch. mikr. Anat. **45**, 624—654 (1895). — Über die Entwicklung der Nervenendigungen in der Haut des Menschen. Z. Zellforsch. **19**, 356—382 (1933).

TAKINO, M.: Die Innervation der menschlichen Haut, besonders über die musculi arrectores pilorum, der Talgdrüsen, der Schweißdrüsen und der kleinen Haare. Acta Sch. med. Univ. Kioto **12**, 281—294 (1929). — Strutture nervose della cute umana. Monographia. Bologna: L. Capelli 1940. — TAMPONI, M.: Ricerche di colorazione sopravitale della cute. Arch. ital. Derm. **14**, 499—536 (1938). — TAPPER, D. N.: Input-output relationships of a skin tactile sensory unit of the cat. Trans. N.Y. Acad. Sci. **26**, 697—701 (1964). — TETZLAFF, M. J., R. A. PETERSON, and R. K. RINGER: Cutaneous and subcutaneous blood and nerve supply to the feather follicle (Aves). In: 53rd Annual Meeting of the Poultry Science Assoc. Poultry Sci. **43** (5), 1369—1370 (1964) (Abstract). — THIES, W.: Über die Morphologie des vegetativen Nervensystems in der menschlichen Haut nebst Untersuchungen über die neuropathologischen Veränderungen bei verschiedenen Hautkrankheiten. I. II. Verhalten der neurovegetativen Formationen in den oberen Schichten des Coriums und an der Epidermis-Cutis-Grenze. Z. Haut- u. Geschl.-Kr. **27**, 287—300 (1959); **28**, 37—59 (1960). — Über die Morphologie des vegetativen Nervensystems in der menschlichen Haut nebst Untersuchungen über neuropathologischen Veränderungen bei verschiedenen Hautkrankheiten. Z. Haut- u. Geschl.-Kr. **27**, 330—343 (1959). — Über die Morphologie des vegetativen Nervensystems in der menschlichen Haut nebst Untersuchungen über neuropathologische Veränderungen bei verschiedenen Hautkrankheiten. Z. Haut- u. Geschl.-Kr. **28**, 101—112 (1960). — Über die Morphologie des vegetativen Nervensystems in der menschlichen Haut nebst Untersuchungen über neuropathologische Veränderungen bei verschiedenen Hautkrankheiten. Z. Haut- u. Geschl.-Kr. **28**, 185—196 (1960).

VELDE, VAN DER: Die fibrilläre Struktur der Nervenendorgane. Mschr. Anat. Physiol. **26**, 225 (1909).

WALTER, P.: Zur Innervation der Pferdelippe. Z. Zellforsch. **43**, 459—477 (1955/56). — Die sensible Innervation des Lippen- und Nasenbereiches von Rind, Schaf, Ziege, Schwein, Hund und Katze. Z. Zellforsch. **53**, 394—410 (1960/61). — WEDDELL, G.: Axonal regeneration in cutaneous nerve plexuses. J. Anat. (Lond.) **77**, 49 (1942). — Referred pain in relation to the mechanism of common sensibility. Proc. roy. Soc. Med. **50**, 581—586 (1957). — Studies related to the mechanisms of common sensibility. Advanc. Biol. Skin **1**, 112—160 (1960). — WEDDELL, G., and S. MILLER: Cutaneous sensibility. Ann. Rev. Physiol. **24**, 199—222 (1962). — WEDDELL, G., W. PALLIE, and E. PALMER: The morphology of peripheral nerve terminations in the skin. Quart. J. micr. Sci. **95**, 483—501 (1954). — Studies on the innervation of skin. I. The origin, course and number of sensory nerves supplying the rabbit ear. J. Anat. (Lond.) **89**, 162—174 (1955). — WEDDELL, G., and E. PALMER: Die Nervenfasern und ihre Endigungen im menschlichen Integument. Acta neuroveg. (Wien) **24**, H. 1—4 (1963). — WEIDENREICH, F.: Die Lokalisation des Pigments und ihre Bedeutung in Ontogenie und Phylogenie der Wirbeltiere. Z. Morph. Anthrop., Sonderh. **2**, 59—140 (1912). — WIEDMANN, A.: Studien über das neurohormonale System der menschlichen Haut. Acta neuroveg. (Wien) **3**, 354—372 (1951). — Zur Frage der sogenannten Langerhanszellen der Haut. Hautarzt **3**, 249—252 (1952). — Neuere Untersuchungen über das neurovegetative System der Haut. Hautarzt **4**, 125—129 (1953). — Über das neurohormonale System der Haut. Hautarzt **14**, 60—64 (1963). — Structure du système nerveux vegetatif. Arch. belges Derm. **19**, 75—78 (1963). — Über die Struktur des neurovegetativen Systems. Hautarzt **15**, 13—16 (1964). — Über die nervöse Versorgung der Haut, unter besonderer Berücksichtigung der Merkelschen Scheiben. Hippokrates (Stuttg.) IV, H. 12 (1964). — WINKELMANN, R. H., and L. S. OSMENT: The Vater-Pacinian corpuscle in the skin of the human finger tip. Arch. Derm. **73**, 116—122 (1956). — WINKELMANN, R. K.: The mucocutaneous endorgan. The primary organized sensory ending in human skin. Arch. Derm. **76**, 225—235 (1957). — The sensory endings in the skin of the cat. J. comp. Neurol. **109**, 221—232 (1958). — The innervation of a hair follicle. Ann. N.Y. Acad. Sci. **83**, 400—407 (1959/60). — Similarities in cutaneous nerve end-organs. Cutaneous innervation, vol. 1: Advances in biology of skin, p. 48—62. Oxford: Pergamon Press 1960. — The end-organ of feline skin. Amer. J. Anat. **107**, 281—290 (1960a). — Nerve endings in normal and pathologic skin. Springfield (Ill.): Ch. C. Thomas 1960. — Nerve endings in the skin of the gorilla. J. comp. Neurol. **116**, 145—156 (1961). — The mammalian end-organ in oral tissue of the cat. J. dent. Res. **41**, 207—212 (1962a). — Cutaneous sensory end-organs of some anthropoid apes. Science **136**, 384—386 (1962b). — Innervation of the skin: Notes on a comparison of primate and marsupial nerve ending. In: Biology of the skin and hair growth, p. 171—182. Canberra, Australia, August 1964. New York: Elsevier Pub. Co. Inc. 1965. — YAMADA, H., and S. MIYAKE: Elektronenmikroskopische Untersuchungen an Nervenfasern in menschlichen Schweißdrüsen. Z. Zellforsch. **52**, 129—139 (1960). — YAMAMOTO, T., J. ITO, T. OHNO, T. OHYAMA, H. OMOTO, and S. SEINO: Histology and sensory innervation of transitional and mucosae parts of the lip of monkey. Arch. histol. jap. **14**, 611—624 (1958). — YAMAZAKI, K.: Cholinesterase in the skin. I. Cholinesterase in normal human skin. Fukushima J. med. Sci. **11**, 85—96 (1964). II. Cholinesterase in pigmented nevi. Fukushima J. med. Sci. **11**, 97—108 (1964). — YAMOMOTO, T.: On the sensory innervation of the hair follicle in mice, vol. 2, p. 515. 6th Int. Congr. Electronmicroscopy Kyoto, Japan (ed. R. UYEDA). Tokyo: Maruzen Co. Ltd. 1966.

ZENIN, B. A.: Innervation of sweat glands. Vestn. Derm. Vener. **36**, 10—14 (1962). — ZIMMERMAN, A. A., and S. W. BECKER jr.: Melanoblasts and melanocytes in fetal negro skin. In: Illinois monographs in medical science, vol. VI. Urbana: University of Illinois Press 1959. — ZIMMERMAN, A. A., and T. CORNBEET: The development of epidermal pigmentation in the Negro fetus. J. invest. Derm. **11**, 383—395 (1948). — ZOLLMANN, P. E., and R. K. WINKELMANN: The sensory innervation of the common North American Raccoon (Procyon lotor). J. comp. Neurol. **119**, 149—157 (1962). — ZYPEN, E. VAN DER: Über das Verhalten des Nervensystems im Narbengewebe der behaarten Haut. Acta neuroveg. (Wien) **21**, 41—78 (1960). — Vergleichende licht- und elektronenmikroskopische Betrachtungen über die Endausbreitung des peripheren vegetativen Nervensystems im normalen und pathologisch veränderten menschlichen Colon. Acta neuroveg. (Wien) **30**, 445—463 (1967).

Die normale Histologie von Corium und Subcutis

Von

Walter Schmidt, München

Mit 22 Abbildungen

An die Epidermis schließen sich als bindegewebige Schichten Corium und Subcutis an. Die Basalmembran bildet als spezialisierte Formation des Corium-Bindegewebes die verbindende Grenze. In den folgenden Ausführungen werden zuerst die einzelnen Bauelemente (Abschnitt A), dann ihr Zusammenschluß zu Geweben (Abschnitt B) und anschließend die speziellen Konstruktionsprinzipien und Texturen des cutanen und subcutanen Bindegewebes besprochen (Abschnitt C). Hierbei soll vor allem einer funktionell-morphologischen Betrachtungsweise Raum gegeben werden, soweit dies die Ergebnisse der morphologischen Forschung erlauben. Sind doch alle unsere licht- und elektronenmikroskopischen Bilder nur Momentaufnahmen aus einem biologischen Vorgang, die oft nur mit Hilfe von Vitaluntersuchungen, biochemisch-analytischen Methoden oder autoradiographischen und experimentell-cytologischen Untersuchungen ergänzend gedeutet werden können.

A. Die Bauelemente des Bindegewebes von Corium und Subcutis

Die Bauelemente von Corium und Subcutis sind, gleich den übrigen Bindegewebsformationen des Organismus, Zellen, Fasern und Grundsubstanz. Unterschiedlich sind nur die mengenmäßige Verteilung der einzelnen Elemente, die besonderen Texturen der Fasern im Gewebe und ihre mechanischen Faktoren folgende Anordnung innerhalb der verschiedenen Schichten.

I. Die zelligen Bestandteile des Bindegewebes

Man unterscheidet allgemein folgende Typen von Bindegewebszellen: Fibrocyten bzw. Fibroblasten, Histiocyten, Gewebsmastzellen, Plasmazellen, Reticulumzellen, Fettzellen, undifferenzierte Mesenchymzellen, Lymphocyten, Granulocyten und Pigmentzellen. Über die Pigmentzellen gibt der einschlägige Abschnitt von STARCK, Band I/2 dieses Handbuches Auskunft. Eine eingehende Darstellung der eosinophilen Granulocyten und Lymphocyten ist im Abschnitt „Das entzündliche Haut-Infiltrat" von MACHER, Band I/2, zu finden. Die übrigen Zelltypen werden im Folgenden in einer kurzen zusammenfassenden Übersicht abgehandelt. Genauere Auskunft ist der einschlägigen Literatur (v. MÖLLENDORFF, 1928—1932; MAXIMOW, 1929; GUSEK, 1962; MONTAGNA, 1962) zu entnehmen. Vgl. außerdem den Beitrag von MACHER, Bd. I/2.

1. Fibrocyten und Fibroblasten

Die Bezeichnungen „Fibrocyt" und „Fibroblast" sind nicht scharf voneinander abzugrenzen. Da Fasern und Grundsubstanz des Bindegewebes ständig erneuert und damit stets neugebildet werden, verdiente der Terminus „Fibroblast" den Vorzug. Dennoch wird hier, dem allgemeinen Sprachgebrauch folgend, die eine Zustandsform der Zelle, in der keine deutlichen Anzeichen einer Faserbildung zu beobachten sind, als Fibrocyt und die andere mit deutlichen Anzeichen einer produktiven Leistung als Fibroblast bezeichnet. Fibroblasten finden sich sehr zahlreich im embryonalen und fetalen Gewebe und während der Wundheilung, Fibrocyten im normalen Bindegewebe.

Lichtmikroskopisch sind die *Fibrocyten* mit ihren Ausläufern nur an Häutchenpräparaten (JASSWOIN, 1932) vollständig zu übersehen. Auf den üblichen Schnittpräparaten erhält man meist Schräg- oder Längsschnitte und damit das Bild einer langgestreckten, scheinbar spindeligen Zelle mit spindeligem Zellkern. In Wirklichkeit ist der Zelleib an seinen Enden oft lang ausgezogen oder verzweigt, an anderen Stellen membranartig ausgebreitet, und deshalb schwer färbbar. Er läßt sich infolgedessen von der Intercellularsubstanz nicht immer sicher abgrenzen. Im Cytoplasma findet man nach Spezialfärbungen oder im Phasenkontrast langgestreckte, fadenförmige Mitochondrien, verschieden große Vacuolen, in unmittelbarer Nähe des Zellkernes ein kleines Golgi-Feld und in dessen Mitte das Centriol. Fetttröpfchen und „paraplasmatische" Granula sind entsprechend nicht näher bekannten Funktionszuständen (LINDNER, 1962) entweder diffus „monoplasmatisch" über den Zelleib verteilt oder in Nähe des Zellkernes „diplasmatisch" unter dem Bild eines Ekto- und Endoplasmas konzentriert. Es ist aus Zeitrafferaufnahmen an Gewebekulturen bekannt, daß die Mitochondrien einem ständigen Ortswechsel unterliegen, dem auch die „paraplasmatischen Einlagerungen" folgen. Diese nehmen unter der Zelltätigkeit an Größe zu und ab, konfluieren und verschwinden wieder, während neue gebildet werden. Gleiches dürfte auch für die Zelle in situ gelten. Der Zellkern der Fibrocyten ist in der Aufsicht elliptisch, abgeplattet, relativ chromatinarm und enthält 1—4 Nucleolen.

Mit histochemischen Methoden wurden in den Fibrocyten bzw. Fibroblasten der Haut Cytochromoxydase, Succinodehydrogenase, Esterasen, β-Glucuronidase und Monoaminooxydase nachgewiesen (MONTAGNA, 1962). Das Reaktionsergebnis ist in den Fibrocyten des Papillarkörpers meist stärker als im Stratum reticulare. Dieses Verhalten ist besonders auffällig beim Nachweis auf Aminopeptidase. Die Fibrocyten des Stratum papillare geben allein einen positiven Ausfall; im Stratum reticulare ist er negativ (ADACHI u. MONTAGNA, 1961). Im Bereich von Wundrändern wird in den Fibroblasten auch eine positive Reaktion auf alkalische Phosphatase verzeichnet.

Das elektronenmikroskopische Bild zeigt im Cytoplasma der Fibrocyten zahlreiche Mitochondrien, ein mäßig entwickeltes englumiges endoplasmatisches Reticulum mit Ribosomenbesätzen und verschieden großen Vacuolen. Außerdem werden granuläre oder lamelläre osmiophile Einschlüsse, die von einer einschichtigen Membran umgeben sind, beobachtet. Ich möchte in Übereinstimmung mit GUSEK (1962) nach Untersuchungen an anderen Zelltypen (SCHMIDT, 1962) den Inhalt als phagocytiertes Material betrachten und mit den „paraplasmatischen" Granula identifizieren. Sie wären demnach als „Phagosomen" zu bezeichnen (vgl. „Phagocytosetätigkeit" der Histiocyten, S. 435). Die Plasmalemmoberfläche der Fibrocyten zeigt an verschiedenen Stellen pinocytotische Einsenkungen, woraus geschlossen werden muß, daß die Zelle makromolekulare Stoffe aufzunehmen vermag und außerdem ein Großteil der intracytoplasmatischen Vacuolen durch Plasmalemmvesikulation entstand. Von KARRER u. COX (1960) wurden an der Plasmalemmoberfläche Öffnungen des endoplasmatischen Reticulums beschrieben, durch die, vielleicht nur temporär, das Lumen des Reticulums mit dem extra-

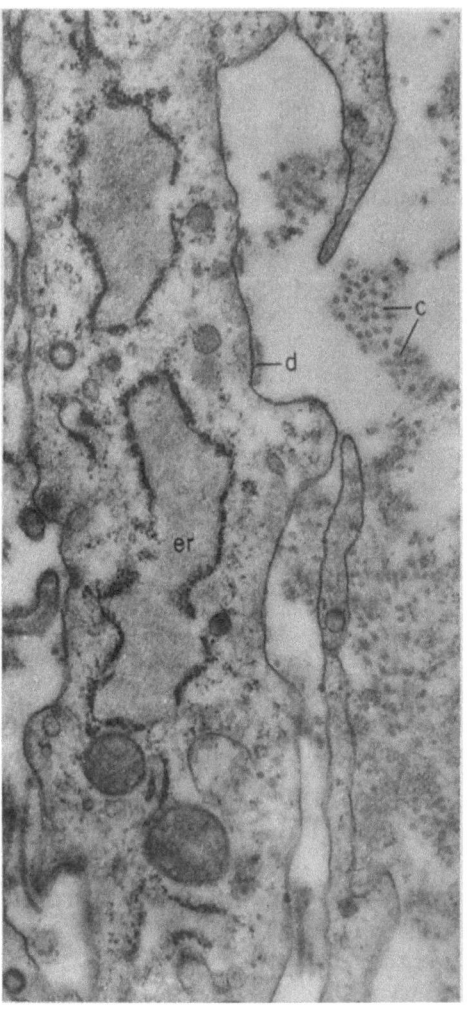

Abb. 1. Querschnitt durch einen Fibroblasten im Zustand der Kollagensynthese (Wundheilung). Das endoplasmatische Reticulum ist zisternal erweitert und enthält ein elektronendichtes, fast homogenes Material (er). An der Oberfläche der Zelle wird, dicht dem Plasmalemm angelagert, die erste extracelluläre Kondensation von kollagenen Fibrillen sichtbar (d). Weiter entfernt liegen im extracellulären Raum bereits zu Bündeln aggregierte kollagene Fibrillen (c), die quer geschnitten wurden. Sie sind in eine dichtere Matrix (Mucopolysaccharide) eingelagert. Vergr. ungef. 20000fach. (Ross u. BENDITT, 1964)

cellulären Raum in Verbindung steht. Wie anscheinend in jeder Zelle, bestehen auch Kommunikationen mit der perinucleären Zisterne (Spaltraum zwischen äußerer und innerer Kernmembran). Die Elektronenmikroskopie konnte außerdem nachweisen, daß kein syncytialer Zusammenhang innerhalb der Fibrocytennetze besteht, wie nach lichtmikroskopischen Beobachtungen verschiedentlich angenommen wurde; stets ist an den Kontaktstellen das Plasmalemm vorhanden, durch das ein jedes Zellindividuum in sich abgeschlossen ist.

Der funktionell aktive Zustand des Fibrocyten, der *Fibroblast*, ist durch die Bildung von Fasern und Grundsubstanz ausgezeichnet. Alle morphologischen Kriterien einer proteinbildenden Zelle werden jetzt sichtbar: Ein ausgeprägtes und verzweigtes endoplasmatisches Reticulum (Ergastoplasma) (MERKER, 1961; GUSEK, 1962; GOLDBERG u. GREEN, 1964) mit stellenweise außerordentlich weiten zisternalen Auftreibungen (Abb. 1) und einem dichten Ribosomenbesatz sowie eine auffällige Vergrößerung der Nucleolen. Im Lumen des endoplasmatischen Reticulums ist ein elektronendichter Inhalt nachweisbar (MERKER, KARRER, GOLDBERG u. GREEN), der jedoch keine Fibrillen erkennen läßt. Der Vermehrung des Ergastoplasmas entspricht im lichtmikroskopischen Präparat eine Zunahme der Basophilie. Biochemische Untersuchungen haben gesichert — und dies trifft auch für den Fibroblasten zu —, daß die Proteinsynthese nur mit Hilfe der RNS-

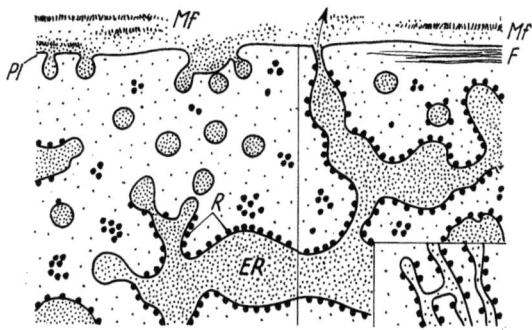

Abb. 2. Vorgang der Stoffabgabe aus einer sezernierenden Zelle, hier als Beispiel für die beiden Möglichkeiten der Kollagensekretion. Im stark erweiterten endoplasmatischen Reticulum (*ER*) werden die Bausteine für die Kollagenfibrillen (Tropokollagen und Mucopolysaccharide) bereitgestellt. An der Bildung des Tropokollagens sind die RNS-haltigen Ribosomen (*R*) beteiligt. In der linken Bildhälfte schnüren sich an der Oberfläche des endoplasmatischen Reticulums Vacuolen samt Inhalt ab und transportieren diesen an die Zelloberfläche, wo sie ihn in den extracellulären Raum entlassen. Die andere Möglichkeit der Abgabe durch Poren des endoplasmatischen Reticulums ist auf der rechten Bildhälfte dargestellt (Pfeil). Außerhalb der Zelle, im Kontakt mit dem Plasmalemm (*Pl*) beginnt die Bildung der Mikrofibrillen (*Mf*). Im Grundplasma liegen stellenweise Filamente unbekannter Bedeutung (*F*). Rechts unten vergleichsweise das endoplasmatische Reticulum eines inaktiven Fibrocyten

haltigen Ribosomen (Durchmesser 150 Å) (Abb. 2) erfolgen kann. Das Produkt wird in das Lumen des endoplasmatischen Reticulums abgegeben. Die im Stadium der aktivierten Zelleistung anfallenden großen Stoffmengen haben die zisternale Erweiterung des Schlauchsystems zur Folge (Abb. 1, 2). Der Inhalt besteht aus Tropokollagen und Mucopolysacchariden, wie der intensive Ausfall der PJS-Reaktion (KNESE u. KNOOP, 1961) und die Ergebnisse autoradiographischer Untersuchungen an Gewebekultur- und Gewebsfibroblasten nach Verabreichung von S^{35} (MANCINI et al., 1961) erkennen ließen. Für eine getrennte Produktion beider Stoffe in verschiedenen Zellen oder in verschiedenen Systemen der Fibroblasten ergaben sich bisher keine Anhaltspunkte. Mit der Stofferzeugung steht die merkliche Zunahme der Succinodehydrogenase-, β-Glucuronidase- und Aminopeptidase-Reaktion (MANCINI) in Zusammenhang. Auf welche Weise die beiden für die Kollagenfaserbildung notwendigen Bausteine aus der Zelle entlassen werden, ist eine noch offene Frage. Es liegt der Verdacht nahe, die Entleerung erfolge durch die Öffnungen des endoplasmatischen Reticulums an der Zelloberfläche. Vergleiche mit der sekretorischen Tätigkeit anderer Zellen lassen aber eher daran denken (KAJIKAWA, 1961; GOLDBERG u. GREEN, 1964), daß sich aus dem endoplasmatischen Reticulum Vacuolen samt Inhalt abschnüren, an das Plasmalemm der Zelloberfläche Anschluß bekommen, sich hier öffnen und ihren Inhalt in den extracellulären Raum abgeben (Abb. 2).

Im Grundplasma von Fibrocyten oder Fibroblasten gelegene Fibrillen stehen nach den bisherigen Beobachtungen nicht mit der Faserbildung in Zusammenhang (GOLDBERG). Eher gleichen sie Tonofibrillen oder contractilen Elementen (SCHWARZ et al., 1962).

Unter bestimmten Bedingungen besitzen auch Fibrocyten die Fähigkeit zur Speicherung (M. v. MÖLLENDORFF, 1932). Die Aufnahme der kolloidalen Modellsubstanzen Trypanblau oder Tusche erfolgt, wie man annehmen muß (SCHMIDT, 1962), durch Pinocytose. Die Farbstoffe werden dann in Vacuolen gespeichert, die durch mehrfachen Konflux zahlreicher kleiner Pinocytosebläschen zu lichtmikroskopischer Größe heranwachsen.

Durch Umwandlung können aus Fibrocyten Histiocyten (Makrophagen) entstehen, wie die Untersuchungen M. v. MÖLLENDORFFs (1932) und MAXIMOWs (1929) glaubhaft gemacht haben. Auch scheinen die Pericyten der Capillaroberfläche fibrocytärer Herkunft zu sein. Eine ausführliche monographische Zusammenfassung der Funktion der Fibroblasten findet sich bei BRANWOOD (1963).

Fibrocyten und Fibroblasten sind relativ ortsständige Zellen. Ihnen gegenübergestellt werden die mobilen Bindegewebszellen wie Histiocyten, Granulocyten, Plasmazellen, Lymphocyten und Mastzellen.

2. Histiocyten

Die Histiocyten (Makrophagen, nicht sehr glücklich „ruhende Wanderzellen", MAXIMOW, 1929) sind Zellen des Bindegewebes, die sich vor allem durch die Fähigkeit zur Lokomotion, zur Phagocytose und Speicherung auszeichnen. Im Lichtmikroskop ist die Zelle entsprechend ihrem unter der Fixation erstarrten Funktionszustand polymorph: Meist ist der Zelleib langgestreckt und endet in einigen wenigen pseudopodienartigen Fortsätzen, die im Gegensatz zum Fibrocyten gut abgrenzbar sind. Andere Zellen haben sich abgekugelt und ihre Fortsätze eingezogen, wieder andere strecken zahlreiche dünne Pseudopodien mit oft kolbigen Verdickungen aus. Ganz allgemein färbt sich das Cytoplasma der Histiocyten intensiver als das der Fibrocyten. Es enthält in sehr unterschiedlicher Menge Granula, Fetttröpfchen und Vacuolen. Bisweilen erscheint der Zelleib schaumig durch Einlagerung von massenhaft großen Vacuolen. Der Zellkern ist ovoid, manchmal auch polymorph und relativ stark färbbar. Im Innern liegen 1—3 kleine Nucleolen.

Elektronenmikroskopisch wurden im Cytoplasma der Histiocyten reichlich runde bis ovale Mitochondrien, ein spärlich entwickeltes endoplasmatisches Reticulum mit Ribosomenbesätzen und Vacuolen unterschiedlicher Größe und Menge nachgewiesen (GUSEK, 1962). Ein kleiner Golgi-Apparat findet sich in Nähe des Zellkernes. Als Oberflächendifferenzierung sind einzelne Mikrovilli, Anschnitte dünnster membranöser Cytoplasmafortsätze (ondulierende Membranen, FRÉDÉRIC u. CHÈVREMONT, 1953) neben zahlreichen pinocytotischen Einsenkungen des Plasmalemms sichtbar. Die Oberfläche des Zellkernes ist an mehreren Stellen tief eingebuchtet, wie es häufig bei stoffwechselaktiven Zellen beobachtet wird.

Die Tätigkeit der Histiocyten wurde bereits oben umrissen. Die Stoffaufnahme sowie die Speicherungs- und Abbauvorgänge können licht- bzw. elektronenmikroskopisch durch die Applikation von Fluorochromen, Trypanblau, Silicium, Tusche, Eisenverbindungen oder Hühnereiweiß (GUSEK) sichtbar gemacht werden. Niedermolekulare, lipoidlösliche Stoffe gelangen in die Zelle durch Plasmalemmpermeation. Kolloid- oder grobdisperse Stoffe werden dagegen durch Phagocytose bzw. Pinocytose vereinnahmt. Anscheinend können sich auch die ondulierenden Membranen an der Stoffaufnahme beteiligen (SCHMIDT, 1962). Bei der Pinocytose

(Abb. 3) bildet sich an der Zelloberfläche, die mit Mucopolysaccharidauflagerungen versehen ist, zuerst eine seichte Mulde, dann ein mehr und mehr sich in die Tiefe des Cytoplasmas einsenkendes Grübchen oder Bläschen. Durch Abschnürung (Plasmalemmvesikulation) wird jetzt das Bläschen abgelöst (HOLTER, 1959; STAUBESAND, 1965) und gelangt schließlich unter mehrfachem Konflux mit anderen Pinocytosebläschen und Einengung seines Inhaltes immer weiter in die Tiefe des Zelleibes, oft bis in den Bereich des Zellkernes, wo es unter dem Bild der Speicherung verharrt. Derartige Einschlüsse werden als „*Pinosomen*" oder „*Phagosomen*" bezeichnet. Im Lichtmikroskop erscheinen sie unter dem Bild der „paraplasmatischen Granula". Wie man heute aus zahlreichen histochemischen und biochemischen Untersuchungen weiß (DE DUVE, 1959; ESSNER, 1961; ESSNER u. NOVIKOFF, 1961, 1962; DANNENBERG et al., 1963; STRAUS, 1964), versucht unterdessen die Zelle, den aufgenommenen Inhalt abzubauen, indem hydrolysierende Fermente in das Pinosom abgegeben werden. Diese Fermente (saure und alkalische Phosphatase, Aminopeptidase, α-Glucosidase, β-Glucuronidase, DN-ase, RN-ase, unspezifische Esterasen, Glucose-6-Phosphatdehydrogenase) werden durch Vesikel, auch *Lysosomen* genannt (DE DUVE, 1959), an die Phagosomen herangebracht (STRAUS, 1964), verschmelzen mit diesen oder gelangen in deren Inneres und geben ihren Inhalt ab. Dieser entfaltet innerhalb des „Phago-Lysosoms" seine Tätigkeit. Erst nach der Spaltung können die resorbierbaren Stoffe, die sich ja innerhalb einer aus dem Plasmalemm entstandenen Vacuole befinden, permeieren (SCHMIDT, 1962, 1965) und in das Grundplasma übertreten. Nicht verdaubare Stoffe (z. B. Metallsole) werden wieder ausgestoßen. Die Frage, woher die Lysosomen stammen, als deren Hauptmerkmal die positive Phosphatasereaktion gilt (NOVIKOFF), ist noch nicht vollständig geklärt. Ein Teil der Bläschen hat sich offensichtlich an der Oberfläche des Golgi-Apparates abgeschnürt (Abb. 3) (ESSNER u. NOVIKOFF, 1962). Nicht alle der hier geschilderten Schritte, wohl aber das Vorkommen der genannten Fermente (MONTAGNA, 1955, 1957; BEJDL, 1954; VITRY u. PRIVAT, 1961; STEIGLEDER et al., 1962; RUDOLPH u. KLEIN, 1964) sind an den Histiocyten der Haut überprüft, jedoch darf man aus den bekannten Bildern von vergleichbaren Zelltypen auf homologe Vorgänge schließen. Mit histochemischen Methoden sind in den Phagosomen und Phago-Lysosomen auch Mucopolysaccharide und Peroxydase nachweisbar. Außerdem wurde in Histiocyten auch Adenosin-Triphosphatase festgestellt (NAKAMURA, 1960). Ein-

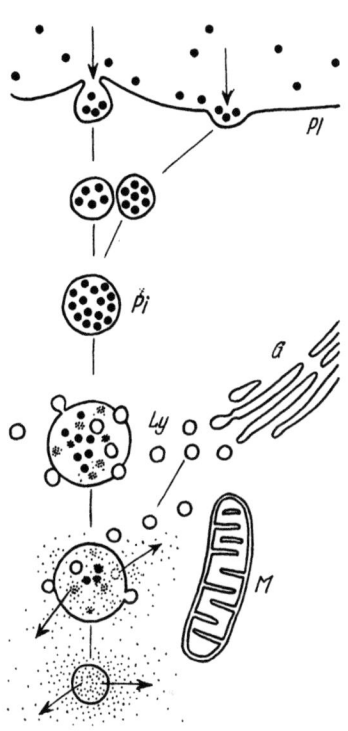

Abb. 3. Schematische Darstellung der Stoffaufnahme durch Pinocytose und der intracellulären Stoffverarbeitung. Plasmalemm (*Pl*), Pinosom (= Phagosom) (*Pi*), das aus mehreren durch Plasmalemmvesikulation abgeschnürten Pinocytosebläschen durch Konflux entstand. Lysosomen (*Ly*), die sich aus dem Golgi-Apparat (*G*) abschnürten und ihren Fermentführenden Inhalt in das Pinosom entleeren. Dieses Gebilde wird als Pino-Lysosom bezeichnet. Mitochondrium (*M*), das die Energie für diese Vorgänge liefert. Die aufgenommenen makromolekularen Stoffe sind durch große Punkte markiert, die zu niedermolekularen abgebauten, durch kleine Punkte. Sie permeieren in Pfeilrichtung durch die Membran des Pino-Lysosoms in das Grundplasma

gehender unterrichten die Arbeiten von NOVIKOFF (1961), GOLDFISCHER et al. (1964) und GORDON et al. (1965) über histochemische Befunde an den fermentführenden Lysosomen.

Die Herkunft der Histiocyten scheint nicht einheitlich zu sein. Übergangsformen zwischen Histiocyten und Fibrocyten lassen diese als wichtigste Quelle erscheinen. Offensichtlich stellt sich im cutanen Bindegewebe ein bestimmtes Fibrocyten-Histiocyten-Gleichgewicht ein, das sich erst bei Bedarf verschiebt. Beim Rind beträgt das Verhältnis 56% Fibrocyten zu 27% Histiocyten bezogen auf sämtliche Formen der Bindegewebszellen (LINDNER, 1962).

An dieser Stelle muß über einige Zelltypen berichtet werden, die nach ihrer Gestalt den Histiocyten nahestehen:

DAF-Zellen (dermal autofluorescent cells). ADAMS-RAY, BLOOM und RITZÉN (1960) fanden im Bindegewebe der Haut des Menschen (Stamm, Extremitäten, Genitalregion) Zellen mit langen Fortsätzen und granulären Einschlüssen im Cytoplasma, die sich durch eine gelbe Autofluorescenz auszeichneten. Im normalen durchfallenden Licht sind die Granula von gelbbrauner Eigenfarbe. Sie geben eine positive PJS-Reaktion und färben sich mit Sudan-Schwarz an. Aus diesem Verhalten wird von den Untersuchern auf ein Lipopigment, das dem Lipofuscin nahestehe, geschlossen. Herkunft und Bedeutung dieser Zellen sind unbekannt. Es scheint aber auch nicht ausgeschlossen, daß die Granula aus phagocytiertem Material bestehen, zumal die Zellen im Bereich von Hauttätowierungen den Farbstoff granulär gespeichert haben.

Zellen mit chromaffinen Granula (ADAMS-RAY u. NORDENSTAM, 1956; RHODIN, ADAMS-RAY u. NORDENSTAM, 1959). Diese Zellen sind beim Menschen unregelmäßig über das Corium verstreut. Gehäuft finden sie sich in der Umgebung von Gefäßen, Nervenfasern, Talg- und Schweißdrüsen und an der Oberfläche von Haarfollikeln. Der Zelleib ist langgestreckt und hat vereinzelt kleine pseudopodienartige Fortsätze. Das Cytoplasma enthält 0,2—0,3 μ große chromaffine Granula (NORDENSTAM u. ADAMS-RAY, 1957). Diese sind, wie elektronenmikroskopische Aufnahmen gezeigt haben, strukturlos und werden von einer einschichtigen Membran umgeben. Vermutlich enthalten die Granula Adrenalin und Noradrenalin und könnten damit zum enterochromaffinen System gerechnet werden.

Die von NIEBAUER u. Mitarb. (1957—1961) als „*interstitielle Zellen*" oder „neurovegetative Zellen" beschriebenen Gebilde sind vermutlich mit den DAF-Zellen identisch und ständen damit nicht, wie von ihm angenommen, mit dem peripheren vegetativen Nervensystem in Zusammenhang.

Die „*neurohormonalen Zellen*" (WIEDMANN, 1952—1963) zeigen große Ähnlichkeit mit den chromaffinen Zellen, die Noradrenalin enthalten. Der Beweis ihrer Identität steht jedoch noch aus. Von MERCANTINI (1960) wird die Existenz eines chromaffinen Zellsystems in der Haut in Abrede gestellt. Es ist aber auch nicht ausgeschlossen, daß die chromaffinen Zellen mit Mastzellen identisch sind.

Auch die *Monocyten* (Histiomonocyten) sind durch Lokomotion, Phagocytose- und Speichertätigkeit ausgezeichnet. Die 12—20 μ großen Zellen unterscheiden sich von den Histiocyten lichtmikroskopisch durch die stärkere Basophilie ihres Cytoplasmas. In Nähe des nierenförmigen oder gelappten Zellkernes liegen im Bereich des Golgi-Apparates mit Neutralrot supravital färbbare Granula. An sie ist anscheinend auch die positive Oxydase- und Peroxydase-Reaktion gebunden. Im Elektronenmikroskop stößt das Auffinden der Monocyten auf Schwierigkeiten. GUSEK (1962) beschreibt „monocytoide Histiocyten", die jedoch nach seinen Größenangaben (7 μ im Durchmesser) nicht mit den typischen Histiomonocyten wesensgleich sein können. Während entzündlicher Vorgänge wandern Monocyten aus den Capillaren in das Gewebe ein und unterstützen die Abwehrfunktion der Histiocyten (vgl. Abschnitt MACHER, S. 485).

3. Gewebsmastzellen

Gewebsmastzellen (Ehrlichsche Mastzellen, Labrocyten) finden sich in der Haut verstreut oder in kleinen Gruppen im lockeren Bindegewebe, besonders gehäuft im Bereich kleiner Gefäße. Bei den üblichen Präparationsmethoden werden die charakteristischen Granula zerstört, weshalb die Zellen dann nicht mehr in

Erscheinung treten. Der plumpe Zelleib bildet meist nur einige pseudopodienartige Fortsätze. Das Cytoplasma erscheint mit massenhaft 0,5 µ großen basophilen Granula angefüllt; nur der relativ kleine, oft exzentrisch liegende Zellkern bleibt ausgespart.

Zur histologischen und histochemischen Untersuchung werden die Granula am besten mit Bleiacetat fixiert. Sie lassen sich dann mit der PJS-Reaktion mit unterschiedlichem Ergebnis oder elektiv mit Astrablau (BLOOM u. KELLY, 1960) darstellen. Dieses Verhalten spricht dafür, daß die Granula vor allem aus sauren Mucopolysacchariden bestehen. Nach Färbung mit Toluidinblau erfolgt ein typischer metachromatischer Farbumschlag nach rot-violett (WISLOCKI, BUNTING u. DEMPSEY, 1947). Durch den negativen Ausfall der Peroxydasereaktion unterscheiden sie sich von den Granula der Granulocyten. [Nach WACHSTEIN u. MEISEL (1964) ist der Ausfall positiv beim Menschen.] Bereits JORPES, HOLMGREN und WILANDER (1937) nahmen an, die Granula enthielten Heparin. Zahlreiche neuere Untersuchungen (Lit. bei SMITH, 1963), unter anderem nach Markierung mit C^{14} und S^{35}, konnten mit hinreichender Sicherheit beweisen, daß in den Mastzellen *Heparin* gebildet und in granulärer Form gespeichert wird. Nach der z.Z. wieder verlassenen Ansicht von SYLVÉN (1951) läge es intergranulär an eine mikrosomale Fraktion des Cytoplasmas gebunden und würde erst durch die histologische Technik an der Oberfläche der eigentlich orthochromatischen Granula niedergeschlagen. Neben Heparin konnten in den Mastzellen auch beträchtliche Mengen an *Histamin* nachgewiesen werden (RILEY u. WEST, 1953). Mit einer histochemischen Fällungs- und Nachweismethode gelang SCHAUER u. WERLE (1959) mit hoher Wahrscheinlichkeit, seine Lokalisation in den Granula in Form einer Heparin-Histaminbindung zu sichern. Offensichtlich sind die Mastzellen selbst zur Bildung des Histamins befähigt. Außerdem konnte bei Maus und Ratte, jedoch nicht beim Menschen, *Serotonin* in den Mastzellen aufgefunden werden (BENDITT et al., 1955). Mit histochemischen Methoden wurden neuerdings in den Granula eine größere Anzahl von Fermenten nachgewiesen: Leucylaminopeptidase (BRAUN-FALCO u. SALFELD, 1959), saure Phosphatase (MONTAGNA, 1962) — nicht signifikant in den reifen Mastzellgranula des Menschen (SCHAUER, 1964) —, ATP-ase (SCHAUER), β-Glucuronidase (MONTAGNA, 1957; NAKAMURA, 1960), unspezifische Esterasen (SCHAUER), ein Trypsin-ähnliches Ferment (GLENNER u. COHEN, 1960) sowie Lactat- und Maltatdehydrogenase. Im Grundplasma fand sich Histidindecarboxylase (SCHAUER). Auffallend sind Unterschiede in der Stärke der Reaktionen und im Vorkommen bei den verschiedenen Tierspecies und beim Menschen. Die Histidindecarboxylase und die Aminopeptidase sind an der Bildung des Histamins aus Histidin in der Mastzelle beteiligt. Über die mögliche Bedeutung der anderen Fermente vgl. Monographie von SMITH (1963) und SCHAUER (1964).

Im elektronenmikroskopischen Bild wurden in den Mastzellen folgende Einzelheiten gefunden (STOECKENIUS, 1956; ROGERS, 1956; SMITH u. LEWIS, 1957; GUSEK, 1962): Der Zellkern ist längsoval. Der Cytoplasmaleib trägt auf der Zelloberfläche relativ lange Mikrovilli (GUSEK). Zahlreiche Vesikel in Plasmalemmnähe lassen auf pinocytotische Vorgänge schließen. Der Durchmesser der Mastzellgranula beträgt 0,5—0,7 µ. Sie bestehen aus einem feinfädigen (ROGERS, 1956) oder lamellär geschichteten Material, eingebettet in eine homogene Matrix, die von einer einschichtigen Membran umschlossen wird. Im Grundplasma liegen zahlreiche kleine Vesikel, Anschnitte eines typischen endoplasmatischen Reticulums, vereinzelt Mitochondrien und in der Nähe des Zellkernes ein kleiner Golgi-Apparat. Zwischen den charakteristischen Mastzellgranula werden auch Cytosomen-ähnliche Gebilde beobachtet, die vermutlich (GUSEK, 1962) pinocytotisch aufgenommenes Material enthalten.

Die Entstehung der Mastzellgranula ist noch unklar. ZOLLINGER (1950) und GUSEK vermuten, sie würden aus transformierten Mitochondrien hervorgehen. Vieles spricht jedoch für einen Segregationsvorgang in Vacuolen, die nach der wohl begründeten Ansicht von SCHAUER zum Golgi-Apparat gehören könnten.

Die Aufgabe der Mastzellen erscheint außerordentlich vielfältig. Sie liegt in der Produktion und Speicherung von Heparin und Histamin (evtl. Serotonin). Anscheinend sind die Mastzellen das Hauptdepot für Gewebshistamin (SCHAUER, 1964). Außerdem wird die Metachromasie des Bindegewebes auf Hyaluronsäurehaltige *saure Mucopolysaccharide* bezogen (ASBOE-HANSEN, 1950), die allem Anschein nach gleichfalls aus den Mastzellen (SYLVÉN, 1941, 1951), speziell aus den Granula, stammen. Über den Einfluß von Thyroxin, Adrenalin, Oestrogenen, Entzündungen und Hibernisation auf die Mastzellen muß wieder auf die Monographie von SMITH (1963) und SCHAUER (1964) verwiesen werden.

Die Anzahl der Mastzellen in der Haut ist unverhältnismäßig höher, als man nach Schnittpräparaten annehmen möchte. HELLSTRÖM u. HOLMGREN (1950) zählten in oberflächlichen Schichten des Coriums pro Kubikmillimeter 7000 Zellen; im Alter von 70—80 Jahren war die Zahl auf 1000 abgesunken. Zu einem übereinstimmenden Ergebnis gelangten OKONKWO et al. (1955), die im Papillarkörper ungefähr die gleiche Menge, in der Umgebung von Drüsen 10000 und im übrigen Bindegewebe nur 2400 ermittelten. Somit ist eine merkliche Häufung der Zellen im Bereich der Drüsen und der Epidermis, also im Grenzgebiet zum stoffwechselaktiveren Gewebe, zu verzeichnen.

Über die Herkunft der Gewebsmastzellen ist man heute noch nicht ausreichend orientiert. GUSEK (1962) vertritt die Ansicht, sie würden sich aus Fibroblasten, Capillarwandzellen oder den undifferenzierten Mesenchymzellen entwickeln. SCHAUER (1964) macht allein die Capillarwandzellen (Capillarmesenchymzellen) hierfür verantwortlich. Über einzelne Stadien der Entwicklung unterrichtet die Arbeit von COMBS et al. (1965).

4. Plasmazellen

Die Plasmazellen (Plasmocyt) findet man in kleineren und größeren Gruppen im lockeren Bindegewebe, meist in Nähe von Gefäßen. Der Zelleib ist kugelig bis ovoid, manchmal auch polyedrisch. Das Cytoplasma verhält sich stark basophil und läßt sehr oft einen perinucleären helleren Hof frei. Der runde Zellkern liegt meist exzentrisch. Die Chromatinschollen zeigen bevorzugt eine randständige Lage und gaben damit Veranlassung zur Bezeichnung „Radspeichenstruktur".

Elektronenmikroskopisch sind die Plasmazellen durch ein außerordentlich stark entwickeltes, fast den ganzen Zelleib einnehmendes Ergastoplasma gekennzeichnet. Seine teils zisternal erweiterten Lumina enthalten einen dichten Inhalt. Der Membranoberfläche sind massenhaft Ribosomen (sog. rauhe Form des endoplasmatischen Reticulums) aufgelagert. Daneben finden sich im Grundplasma auch freie Ribosomen. Neben dem Zellkern, der im elektronenmikroskopischen Bild massive Chromatinanhäufungen unter der Kernmembran erkennen läßt, liegt das ausgedehnte Golgi-Feld mit größeren Membranpaketen und zugehörigen Vesikeln. Hier finden sich auch zahlreiche Mitochondrien. Im Lichtmikroskop erscheint dieses Gebiet als der helle perinucleäre Hof.

Der mit histochemischen Methoden nachweisbare hohe Gehalt an RNS entspricht dem ausgedehnten Ergastoplasma mit Ribosomen. Experimentelle elektronenmikroskopische Untersuchungen mit Ferritin-Markierung (DE PETRIS et al., 1963) haben fluorescenzmikroskopisch erhobene Befunde (RIFKIND et al., 1962) bestätigt, nach denen die Plasmazellen als die Bildungsstätte von Antikörpern identifiziert werden konnte. Die γ-Globuline werden in den zisternalen Erweiterungen des Ergastoplasmas gebildet und entsprechen dem elektronendichten Inhalt (DE PETRIS). Über die Herkunft der Plasmazellen aus Hämocytoblasten, Lymphoblasten und Fibroblasten s. JORDAN (1954).

5. Die Reticulumzelle und Fettzelle

Die Reticulumzelle ist die Zelle des retikulären Bindegewebes, das sich maßgeblich am Aufbau lymphatischer Organe beteiligt. Im normalen Bindegewebe der Haut des Erwachsenen kommt der Reticulumzelle keine nachweisbare Funktion zu; anders beim Embryo und Fetus: Hier entsteht aus arealförmigen, in unmittelbarer Nähe von Capillaren gelegenen Ansammlungen von Reticulumzellen das Fettgewebe (s. dort). Die *Fettzellen* des subcutanen Bindegewebes, auch des Erwachsenen, sind also umgewandelte Reticulumzellen im Zustand extremer Speicherung (vgl. S. 455ff.).

Das lichtmikroskopische Bild der Reticulumzelle sei hier kurz umrissen: Die Zellen stehen mit Fortsätzen untereinander in Verbindung und bilden ein Raumnetz. Das Cytoplasma enthält einen ovalen, relativ großen, chromatinarmen Zellkern mit 1—2 Nucleolen auf dem Schnitt. Die Intercellularräume sind weit und mit einer dünnflüssigen Intercellularsubstanz angefüllt. Ein typisches Kennzeichen des retikulären Bindegewebes sind die Retikulinfasern, die über eine größere Strecke der Zelloberfläche folgen. Auf elektronenmikroskopischen Bildern wird deutlich, daß die Fasern oft in den Zelleib hineinverlagert sind, stets aber durch das Plasmalemm vom Grundplasma abgegrenzt werden und damit extracellulär liegen. Die argyrophilen Retikulinfasern (s. S. 443) bilden gleichfalls ein dreidimensionales Netzwerk. Die Reticulumzellen können sich aus dem Zellverband lösen und als Makrophagen oder Monocyten in das lockere Bindegewebe übertreten. Dort entfalten sie ihre Speichertätigkeit als Angehörige des RES: Sie phagocytieren, speichern und bauen die vereinnahmten Stoffe ab.

Ein mit morphologischen Methoden nur schwer definierbarer Zelltyp ist die *ruhende Mesenchymzelle* (undifferenzierte Mesenchymzelle nach MARCHAND und HERZOG). Lichtmikroskopisch ist diese Zelle keinesfalls eindeutig charakterisiert. Eigentlich kann sie nur per exclusionem von den anderen Zelltypen abgegrenzt werden. Die Basophilie ihres Cytoplasmas wird als Kennzeichen angeführt. Elektronenmikroskopisch (GUSEK, 1962) sind ein wenig differenziertes Cytoplasma, vereinzelte runde Mitochondrien und ein unterschiedlich entwickeltes Ergastoplasma sichtbar. Übergänge zu Plasmazellen und Histiocyten wurden von GUSEK (1962) und STOECKENIUS (1957) beobachtet.

II. Die Fasern des Bindegewebes

Die klassische Einteilung der Bindegewebsfasern in argyrophile, kollagene und elastische ist auch heute noch üblich und wird deshalb in den folgenden Ausführungen beibehalten, obwohl in letzter Zeit sich mehr und mehr die Ansicht bestätigt, daß zwischen kollagenen und argyrophilen Fasern kein grundsätzlicher Unterschied bestehe (BAIRATI et al., 1964). Die Bauelemente beider Fasern sind nach elektronenmikroskopischen Untersuchungen kollagene Mikrofibrillen.

Im Rahmen dieses Beitrages scheint es ratsam, zuerst einen Überblick über die derzeitigen Vorstellungen von der Entstehung des Kollagens zu geben. Gerade in diesem Punkt der Bindegewebsforschung war die Zusammenarbeit von Chemie, Biochemie und elektronenmikroskopischer Mikromorphologie besonders fruchtbar. Jedoch dürfen trotz zahlreicher Arbeiten die Ergebnisse noch nicht als abgeschlossen betrachtet werden.

Entstehung des Kollagens und Bildung der kollagenen Fibrille

Mit chemisch-analytischen Untersuchungsmethoden ließen sich aus dem Skleroprotein Kollagen folgende Aminosäuren isolieren: Glykokoll (ungefähr $1/3$), Prolin, Hydroxyprolin, Alanin, Glutaminsäure, in geringen Mengen Valin, Leucin, Hydroxylysin, Arginin und Spuren anderer Aminosäuren (FLASCHENTRÄGER u. LEHNARTZ, 1951; ENGSTRÖM u. FINEAN, 1958). Hinzu kommen noch Zucker als Bausteine für die Mucopolysaccharide, die sich auf ungefähr 0,6% belaufen (GRASSMANN, 1960). Wasser ist als Quellungswasser eingebaut.

Aus den Aminosäuren, aus den Bausteinen für die Mucopolysaccharide und Quellungswasser wird das lichtmikroskopisch scheinbar so einfache Gebilde der kollagenen Faser aufgebaut. Über den submikroskopischen Feinbau wurden zahlreiche Theorien aufgestellt. Sichere Ergebnisse brachten zuerst physikalische Untersuchungsmethoden. Sie zeigten übereinstimmend, daß die Faser aus fibrillären Bauelementen absteigender Größenordnung zusammengesetzt sein muß, die einem bestimmten Ordnungssystem folgen. Wie man aus Röntgendiffraktionsdiagrammen (BEAR, 1944, 1952) schloß, besteht die Faser aus sehr langen Fadenmolekülen, den Polypeptidketten, die innerhalb des kristallinen Raumgitters bevorzugt parallel zur Fibrillenachse, jedoch in einer spiraligen Anordnung orientiert sein müssen und die untereinander durch Seitenketten über Wasserstoffbrücken verbunden sind. Der Abstand der einzelnen Polypeptidketten beträgt je nach Quellungsgrad ~ 2 Å. Mit diesen Vorstellungen von der Anordnung der Moleküle stimmen auch die Ergebnisse der Polarisationsmikroskopie überein (W. J. SCHMIDT, 1924); denn die positive einachsige Anisotropie (Eigendoppelbrechung) der kollagenen Faser konnte gleichfalls nur als Ausdruck einer bis in den micellaren Bereich reichenden Längsorientierung der Bauteile gedeutet werden. Schließlich brachte die Elektronenmikroskopie (WOLPERS, 1943; F. O. SCHMITT u. Mitarb., 1942—1960; GROSS, 1948—1956) eine Bestätigung im morphologisch sichtbaren Bereich.

Die aufgeführten Befunde sagen jedoch nichts über den Bildungsort und über den Bildungsmechanismus der kollagenen Fibrille aus. In diesem Punkt standen sich vor allem 3 Theorien gegenüber: 1. Die klassische Theorie der *intracellulären Fibrillogenese* wurde auch noch in neuerer Zeit von WASSERMANN (1954) und GIESEKING (1959) vertreten. Die von beiden Untersuchern im elektronenmikroskopischen Bild intracytoplasmatisch beobachteten Mikro- oder Elementarfibrillen (WASSERMANN) waren jedoch vermutlich Täuschungen, die auf die seinerzeit noch unzulängliche Präparationstechnik zurückzuführen sind. Auch ist es nicht ausgeschlossen, daß sie mit den in jüngster Zeit (GOLDBERG und GREEN, 1964) im Cytoplasma nachgewiesenen Fibrillen identisch sind, denen jedoch das charakteristische Kennzeichen der kollagenen Fibrille, das Querstreifungsphänomen, fehlt.

Die 2. Theorie, nach der die Fibrillen und Fasern an der Oberfläche der Fibroblasten durch Umwandlung des Cytoplasmas — *Exoplasmatheorie* STUDNICKAs — entstehen würden, scheint heute endgültig widerlegt zu sein.

3. Argumente für eine *extracelluläre Genese* der Faser wurden bereits früher angeführt. Sehr einleuchtend war die Beobachtung, daß sich die Fibrillen in Gewebekulturen auch in größerer Entfernung von den Fibroblasten bilden können, ja daß sogar in Abwesenheit von Zellen aus einer Essigsäurelösung von Kollagen einzelne Fibrillen auszusalzen waren (NAGEOTTE, 1927; HUZELLA, 1932), die sich nicht von den ursprünglichen genuinen Kollagenfibrillen unterscheiden. Dieses Phänomen wurde neuerdings durch elektronenmikroskopische Kontrollen (BAHR, 1950; KEECH, 1961) bestätigt. Für die extracelluläre Genese sprechen auch auto-

radiographische Untersuchungen (HARKNESS et al., 1954; JACKSON u. BENTLEY, 1960), bei denen C^{14}-markiertes Glykokoll intraperitoneal appliziert wurde und sich bereits nach 8 Std im extrahierbaren, dann im citratlöslichen und schließlich im reifen Kollagen der Haut wiederfand. Für die Entstehung der kollagenen Fibrille und Faser scheint demnach die Zelle nicht notwendig zu sein.

Die Elektronenmikroskopie führte nun zu einem Kompromiß zwischen den Theorien: Sie konnte nämlich zeigen, daß der erste Schritt, die Verarbeitung der Bausteine bis zu einer Vorstufe, dem Tropokollagen, intracellulär abläuft, die Bildung der Fibrillen und Fasern dagegen extracellulär. Im einzelnen stellt man sich den ersten Schritt dieses Vorganges wie folgt vor: Im stark vermehrten, dicht mit Ribosomen besetzten endoplasmatischen Reticulum (GIESEKING, 1959; PORTER u. PAPPAS, 1959; SCHWARZ et al., 1962) der Fibroblasten findet unter Mitwirkung der für die Proteinsynthese wichtigen Ribosomen die Synthese der Aminosäuren in einer typischen Sequenz zu Polypeptidketten statt und aus diesen die Zusammenlagerung zu den Tropokollagen-Fadenmolekülen (GROSS et al., 1953, 1954; F. O. SCHMITT et al., 1953). Das Tropokollagen wird in den zisternal erweiterten Lumina des endoplasmatischen Reticulums angereichert (Abb. 2) (SCHWARZ, 1960; MERKER, 1961). Die wasserlöslichen Tropokollagenmoleküle, die noch kein Querstreifungsphänomen zeigen, haben eine Länge von 2800 Å und einen Durchmesser von 14 Å. Ein solches Molekül ist aus drei Polypeptidketten in einer α-Helix aufgebaut (RICH u. CRICK, 1955). Wegen des geringen Durchmessers wurde es in dem elektronendichten homogen-granulären Inhalt des endoplasmatischen Reticulums der Fibroblasten bisher noch nicht sicher nachgewiesen. Über den Abgabemechanismus in den extracellulären Raum besteht noch keine volle Übereinstimmung. Eine direkte Abgabe durch das Plasmalemm stellt KAJIKAWA (1961) zur Diskussion. Das Fadenmolekül könne durch Plasmalemmporen (die noch niemals nachgewiesen wurden) ungehindert ausgeschleust werden. SCHWARZ (1960), KARRER u. COX (1960) u.a. halten die Abgabe des Tropokollagens durch Öffnungen des endoplasmatischen Reticulums an der Zelloberfläche für wahrscheinlicher (Abb. 2). GOLDBERG u. GREEN (1964) sind der Ansicht, daß sich aus dem endoplasmatischen Reticulum mit dem tropokollagenhaltigen Inhalt Vacuolen abschnüren. Sie würden dann, wie es allgemein in sezernierenden Zellen beobachtet wurde, an die Zelloberfläche wandern, dort mit dem Plasmalemm verschmelzen, sich nach außen öffnen und ihren Inhalt in den extracellulären Raum entlassen (Abb. 2). Die Bezeichnung Kollagen-Sekretion (GOLDBERG) wäre für diesen Vorgang gerechtfertigt. Ob und in welcher Weise der Golgi-Apparat an der Kollagenbildung beteiligt ist (SHELDON u. KIMBALL, 1962), bleibt noch offen. Als Bildungsstätte der für die Fibrillen- und Faserbildung notwendigen Mucopolysaccharide werden allgemein die Fibroblasten (GERSH et al., 1949; SCHWARZ, 1960) und als Bildungsort gleichfalls die Erweiterungen des endoplasmatischen Reticulums oder Vacuolen unbekannter Herkunft verantwortlich gemacht (KNESE u. KNOOP, 1961; MERKER, 1961). Für die Polymerisation, Ausrichtung und „Verkittung" (JACKSON, 1953, 1960; KEECH, 1961) der Fibrillen haben die Mucopolysaccharide eine im einzelnen noch nicht völlig übersehbare Bedeutung.

Sind die Tropokollagenmoleküle und die Mucopolysaccharide in den extracellulären Raum abgegeben, beginnt der 2. Schritt der Faserbildung, der über die Polymerisation der Tropokollagenmoleküle zu den an Umfang zunehmenden Mikrofibrillen bis zur reifen Kollagenfibrille führt. Sie werden schließlich zu kollagenen bzw. argyrophilen Fasern aggregiert. Die Aufklärung dieser Vorgänge ist vor allem das Verdienst von F. O. SCHMITT, GROSS, HODGE und GRASSMANN. Sie haben in außerordentlich einfallsreichen, logisch aufgebauten Experimenten Struktur und Entstehung des Kollagens weitgehend geklärt. Über die inzwischen immens angewachsene Literatur kann an dieser Stelle nur eine knappe Übersicht gegeben werden. Zusammenfassende Arbeiten (GROSS, 1956; F. O. SCHMITT u. HODGE, 1960; GRASSMANN, 1960; KÜHN et al., 1960; GIESEKING, 1962; KÜHN, 1962; RAMACHANDRAN, 1963; OLSEN, 1963/64) müssen im Originaltext nachgelesen werden.

Der Aufbau der kollagenen Fibrille erfolgt also außerhalb der Zelle, jedoch meist in engstem Kontakt mit der Oberfläche der Fibroblasten (PORTER u. PAPPAS, 1959). Die Orientierung der Zellen ist für die Richtung der zu bildenden Fibrille bestimmend. So verlaufen die ersten elektronenmikroskopisch sichtbaren, bereits

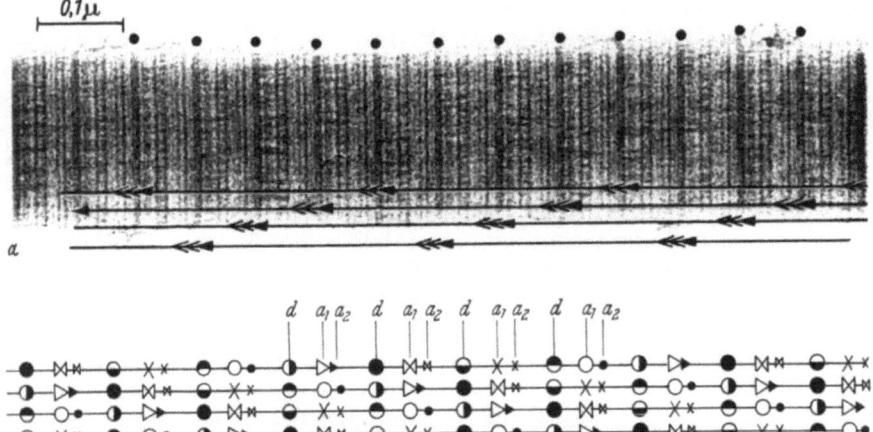

Abb. 4. a Kollagene Mikrofibrille nach Kontrastierung mit Phosphorwolframsäure. Durch die oberhalb der Fibrille stehenden Punkte sind die großen Perioden (640 Å) gekennzeichnet. Im unteren Bereich ist die Aggregation der Tropokollagenmoleküle durch Pfeilsymbole eingetragen. Hiermit soll die Seit-zu-Seit-Polymerisation mit einer Verschiebung um je ¹/₄ der Länge des Moleküls gezeigt werden. Von den Unterperioden sind auf der Reproduktion 10 zu erkennen, die längsverlaufenden Tropokollagenmoleküle nur zu ahnen. (Aus HODGE, 1960). b Schematische Darstellung des Zustandekommens der Periodizität der kollagenen Mikrofibrille. Auch hier sind die Tropokollagenmoleküle durch Pfeile symbolisiert, jedoch ist die Pfeilspitze nach rechts gerichtet. Die verschiedenen Zeichen markieren die Stellen einiger Phosphorwolframsäure-bindender Seitenkettengruppen, die bei der Verschiebung um ein Viertel der Länge und der Seit-zu-Seit-Polymerisation das Bild der Unterperioden erzeugen. Die Buchstaben d, a_1 und a_2 sind zur Kennzeichnung eines bestimmten Bandes allgemein gebräuchlich.
(Aus F. O. SCHMITT u. HODGE, 1960)

periodisch strukturierten Fibrillen parallel zu den Fibroblasten. Die Fibrillen sind in eine homogene Matrix eingelagert, die aus Mucopolysacchariden besteht (Abb. 1). Nach Ansicht von GRASSMANN (1960) sind neben Neutralzucker vor allem glucosaminhaltige saure Mucopolysaccharide in die Fibrillen als integrierenden Bestandteil eingebaut, und zwar können anscheinend ihre kettenförmigen Moleküle für die Ausrichtung des Tropokollagens eine Bedeutung haben und ein zu schnelles, ungeordnetes Polymerisieren verhindern.

Der Vorgang der Kollagenfibrillenbildung kann auf folgende vereinfachte Form gebracht werden: Das wasserlösliche *Tropokollagenmolekül* besitzt, wie man experimentell geschlossen hat, in einer bestimmten Folge Häufungen polarer basischer und saurer Seitenketten, von denen die basischen Phosphorwolframsäure, die sauren Chrom adsorbieren und sich damit distinkt markieren lassen. Das 2800 Å lange Molekül ist strukturell polarisiert, d.h. die Enden sind physikalisch-chemisch nicht gleichwertig (am Pfeilsymbol in Abb. 4a als Pfeilspitze bzw. Fiederung), was für die lineare Polymerisation und für die Ausrichtung der einzelnen Moleküle von Bedeutung ist. Während der Polymerisation entsteht nun durch End-zu-End- und Seit-zu-Seit-Anlagerung die *Mikrofibrille* (Protofibrille, Elementarfibrille, unit fibril), die, elektronenmikroskopisch bereits sichtbar, durch eine typische Periodizität charakterisiert ist. Dieses Merkmal kommt dadurch zustande, daß bei der Polymerisation die einzelnen Tropokollagenmoleküle um ein Viertel ihrer Länge verschoben werden (Abb. 4a, b), wodurch die grobe Periode von 640 Å (bis 700 Å) (Abb. 5) und die 10—14 Unterperioden entstehen. Die Unterperioden sind also das Produkt der in ganz bestimmten Abständen liegenden, mit Phosphorwolframsäure gefärbten Seitenketten der Tropokollagenmoleküle, die durch ihre gestaffelte Anordnung dunklere Querbänder bilden. Der Abstand der einzelnen Tropokollagenmoleküle innerhalb einer Mikrofibrille wurde auf 15—18 Å berechnet; der Durchmesser beträgt, wenn der stationäre Zustand (Reifezustand) der Mikrofibrille erreicht ist, durchschnittlich 600—*700*—1000 Å. Es wurden aber auch schon 2000 Å (0,2 μ) im Sehnengewebe (GIESEKING, 1962) ermittelt. Im Bindegewebe der menschlichen Haut beträgt er bis 1000 Å (GROSS u. SCHMITT, 1948). Der Durchmesser der *lichtmikroskopisch definierten kollagenen Fibrille* beträgt 0,2 μ und weniger (PETERSEN, 1935), liegt also unter dem Auflösungsvermögen des Mikroskops. Anscheinend sind Mikrofibrille und die lichtmikroskopisch beobachtete Kollagenfibrille bereits identisch oder es wurden im Lichtmikroskop mehrere nebeneinander liegende Fibrillen nicht aufgelöst und als eine gedeutet. Die Aggregation und parallele Bündelung zahlreicher kollagener Fibrillen mit ihrer Kittsubstanz wird als *kollagene Faser* bezeichnet. Ihr Durchmesser beträgt 1—12 μ.

Der Durchmesser der kollagenen Mikrofibrille bleibt keinesfalls zeitlebens konstant. Beim Feten und Neugeborenen sind die Fibrillen dünn, nehmen dann beim Jugendlichen an Dicke zu und im hohen Alter wieder ab (LINKE, 1955). Gleichfalls führt eine ständige Zugbeanspruchung zu einer Verdickung (INGELMARK, 1948; WOLPERS, 1950). Sie erfolgt jedoch nicht durch Zusammenlagerung mehrerer dünner Fibrillen (MERKER, 1961), sondern durch Anlagerung weiterer monomerer Tropokollagenmoleküle (HODGE u. SCHMITT, 1960; GROSS et al., 1955).

1. Die argyrophile Faser

Die lichtmikroskopisch nachweisbare argyrophile Faser (Gitterfaser, präkollagene Faser, Retikulinfaser) hat einen Durchmesser von ungefähr 0,2—1 μ. Sie ist durch Imprägnierbarkeit mit Silbersalzen (nach BIELSCHOWSKY und Modifikationen) und durch die Bildung von Netzen (Gittern) unter Verzweigung der einzelnen Faser gekennzeichnet. Mit den üblichen Färbungsmethoden und im polarisierten Licht ist die argyrophile Faser nicht von der kollagenen zu unterscheiden. Der kontinuierliche Übergang beider Faserarten in Versilberungspräparaten (Abb. 11) ist mehrfach beobachtet worden (PLENK, 1927; HERINGA, 1931; ENGHUSEN, 1957). Die Bezeichnung präkollagene Faser besagt, daß sie auch als eine Vorstufe der kollagenen aufgefaßt wird (MAXIMOW, 1929; PLENK, 1927). Dies trifft für die Faserentwicklung beim Embryo und Fetus zu. Hier sind zunächst ausschließlich argyrophile Fasern (schon im 2. Monat, MERKER, 1961) nachweisbar und in der weiteren Entwicklung (ab 33 cm Gesamtlänge, LINKE, 1955) treten kollagene Fasern auf. Im fertigen Organismus erfolgt die Kollagenfaserbildung — ausgenommen die Vorgänge bei der Wundheilung — nicht über ein argyrophiles Zwischenstadium. Für die Bildung der argyrophilen Faser werden außer Fibroblasten auch Pericyten, Endothelzellen, Reticulumzellen und ihre spezialisierte Sonderform, die Fettzellen, verantwortlich gemacht (PLENK, 1927).

Über die mechanischen Eigenschaften der argyrophilen Faser und über ihre beträchtliche Beständigkeit gegenüber chemischen Reagenzien und Fermenten unterrichtet die einschlägige Literatur, vor allem das Übersichtsreferat von PLENK (1927) und ENGHUSEN (1957). Auch heute haften noch der färberischen Abgrenzung von argyrophilen und elastischen Fasern Unsicherheitsfaktoren an. Unter nicht näher bekannten Bedingungen färben sich argyrophile Fasern mit Orcein (PLENK, 1927; JALOWY, 1927; FULLMER u. LILLIE, 1957). Neuerdings konnten auch PUCHTLER und SWEAT (1964) zeigen, daß es möglich ist, argyrophile Fasern mit Resorcin-Fuchsin anzufärben.

Elektronenmikroskopisch besteht die argyrophile Faser aus Bündeln der gleichen periodisch strukturierten Mikrofibrillen wie die kollagene (GROSS, 1950; PORTER, 1952; v. HERRATH u. DETTMER, 1951; DETTMER, NECKEL u. RUSKA, 1951; BAIRATI et al., 1964). Echte Verzweigungen der Fibrillen konnten auch hier nicht beobachtet werden (BAIRATI et al., 1964). Die Fibrillendicke wird mit 400 bis 650 Å angegeben (DETTMER, 1951; GROSS u. SCHMITT, 1948) und liegt damit unterhalb der Dicke der Fibrillen der kollagenen Faser. Entsprechend dem unterschiedlichen Verhalten bei der Versilberung im lichtmikroskopischen Bereich wurde elektronenmikroskopisch nach einer besonderen Perjodsäure-Silbersalz-Methode der Silberniederschlag bei der argyrophilen Faser in grober Verteilung *auf* der Fibrillenoberfläche, bei der kollagenen Fibrille in feiner Verteilung *im Innern* der Fibrille festgestellt (DETTMER u. SCHWARZ, 1953). Dieses Verhalten kann den unterschiedlichen Imprägnationseffekt — braun für kollagene, schwarz für argyrophile Fasern — ausreichend erklären, bedarf aber noch weiterer Bestätigung. Da alle Übergänge der einen Art in die andere elektronenmikroskopisch gefunden wurden, schloß DETTMER auf einen geringeren „Reifungsgrad" der Retikulinfaser. Hiermit würde übereinstimmen, daß kollagene Fasern aus argyrophilen hervorgehen können (LINKE, 1955). Außerdem geht nach anderen Beobachtungen (s. oben) die Umwandlung der „unreifen" präkollagenen in die „reife" kollagene mit einer merklichen Zunahme des Fibrillendurchmessers einher. Der unterschiedliche Ausfall der Versilberung nach DETTMER u. SCHWARZ kann auch mit den lichtmikroskopisch-histochemischen Untersuchungsergebnissen in Einklang gebracht werden. Man kennt schon seit den Untersuchungen von LILLIE (1947), CLARA (1952), GERSH u. CATCHPOLE (1949) die stark positive PJS-Reaktion der argyrophilen Faser. Sie beruht, wie GRAUMANN (1954) nachweisen konnte, auf einem relativ hohen Gehalt an Mucopolysacchariden (ungefähr 4,5%). Er vertritt die Ansicht, bei der argyrophilen Faser lägen die PJS-positiven Mucopolysaccharide als „Kittsubstanz" zwischen, und nach der Isolierung *auf* den Fibrillen. Dies würde mit den elektronenmikroskopisch erhobenen Befunden von DETTMER u. SCHWARZ (1953) und SCHWARZ u. MERKER (1959) über die Verteilung der Silberniederschläge übereinstimmen. Das zu einem Proteinkomplex verbundene Mucopolysaccharid könnte nach diesen Feststellungen mit dem von PLENK (1927) aufgefundenem Retikulin identisch sein. Nach diesen Befunden und Überlegungen läge der Unterschied zwischen den beiden Faserarten nicht in den mikrofibrillären Bausteinen, die in der argyrophilen Faser zwar etwas dünner sind, sondern in der Verteilung und in der Menge der Kittsubstanz (GRAUMANN, 1964) sowie in der Anzahl der zu einer Faser verbundenen Fibrillen. Ganz allgemein nimmt die Kittsubstanz bei einer Zunahme der Faserdicke ab (LINKE, 1955). Jedoch lassen sich durch die Verschiebung der Faser-Kittsubstanz-Relation nicht alle Unterschiede der beiden Faserarten erklären, wie verschiedene Quellbarkeit, Löslichkeit oder fermentative Andaubarkeit.

Zu einem anderen Ergebnis über die Natur der argyrophilen Faser gelangten HERINGA (1931) und JALOWY (1927), dieser nach Untersuchungen an pathologisch veränderter Haut, und neuerdings auch ENGHUSEN (1950—1959) an Gewebe, das in vitro gezüchtet wurde. HERINGA und JALOWY machten aufgrund ihrer Beobachtungen eine Veränderung der Stoffwechsellage des Gewebes für die Argyrophilie verantwortlich. Sie sahen nämlich im Bereich entzündlicher Exsudate und in der Nähe von Ansammlungen von Eiterzellen die Umwandlung typischer kollagener Fasern in argyrophile. Diese Veränderung erwies sich nach Abklingen des Prozesses als reversibel. JALOWY stellte fest, daß sogar elastische Fasern hierbei vorübergehend Tendenz zur Argyrophilie angenommen hatten. Hieraus schlossen sie, die Argyrophilie würde durch die Stoffwechselprodukte der Eiterzellen oder durch Stauung des Lymphabflusses hervorgerufen. Zu einem ähnlichen Ergebnis gelangte ENGHUSEN nach Untersuchungen an Gewebekulturen. Er stellte fest, daß bei einer Veränderung der Stoffwechsellage (z.B. innerhalb eines veränderten Gewebeabschnittes) eine Verschiebung des pH in Richtung einer sauren Reaktion resultiere. Hierdurch würde aus der Grundsubstanz ein Stoff ausgefällt, das Retikulin, das sich als Silber reduzierender Belag auf der Oberfläche von benachbarten kollagenen Fasern niederschlage. Eine innere Veränderung der Faser erfolge dabei nicht. Allein dieser Überzug sei für den Versilberungseffekt und auch für die hohe Resistenz gegenüber tryptischer Verdauung verantwortlich zu machen. Es gelang ENGHUSEN (1957) schließlich auch, aus dem Gewebe bei pH 7 einen Stoff zu fällen und zu isolieren, den er als Retikulin bezeichnet. Dieser stellt nach seiner Ansicht das native Produkt des von PLENK (1927) und FOOT (1928) nach tryptischer Verdauung erhaltenen Retikulins dar. Als Bildungsort dieser Substanz werden in den Fibroblasten besondere Vacuolen vermutet (ENGHUSEN, 1959). Von seiner chemischen Zusammensetzung weiß man nur so viel, daß in hoher Konzentration Galaktose, Glucose und Mannose (GLEGG et al., 1953) enthalten sind.

Das Für und Wider beider Theorien abzuwägen, ist zur Zeit noch schwierig. Die Enghusenschen Untersuchungen wurden an Gewebekulturen vorgenommen. Die Beobachtungen von HERINGA und JALOWY erfolgten an Geweben, die pathologisch verändert waren. Beide Befunde sind also nicht unbedingt miteinander vergleichbar, ebensowenig wie ein Vergleich mit dem Verhalten von argyrophilen Fasernetzen in der Basalmembran oder im retikulären Bindegewebe des normalen, gesunden Organismus ohne Einschränkung zulässig ist.

2. Die kollagene Faser

Von den Eigenschaften der kollagenen Faser soll hier nur ihre große Zugfestigkeit hervorgehoben werden, die 5—10 kg/mm^2 beträgt. Bei Einwirkung von Zug wird zunächst die charakteristische Wellung der Faser ausgeglichen (2,5—3% Verlängerung). Sie trägt auch zu einer gewissen Elastizität der kollagenen Faser bei. Die Dehnbarkeit der gespannten Faser wird mit 5% (WÖHLISCH et al., 1927; BARGMANN, 1964; 10% nach ROLLHÄUSER) angegeben; dann beginnt die Faser unter dem Phänomen des „Fließens" zu zerreißen. Über die Beständigkeit der Faser gegenüber Temperatur, Säuren, Laugen oder Fermenten gibt der Handbuchartikel von PINKUS (1927) sowie die einschlägige neuere Literatur Auskunft (BARGMANN, 1964; BUCHER, 1965).

Im lichtmikroskopischen unfixierten Präparat erscheint die Faser opak-farblos, schwach lichtbrechend und gewellt. Über die grundsätzlichen Unterschiede im Verhalten gegenüber Farbstoffen und Versilberungsmethoden von kollagenen und argyrophilen Fasern wurde bereits im vorangehenden Abschnitt berichtet. Mit Silbersalzen imprägniert sich die kollagene Faser braun bis gelb. Vom Feinbau der Faser sind im Lichtmikroskop die Fibrillen mit einem Durchmesser von 0,2 µ eben noch erkennbar. Sie sind unverzweigt und laufen in der Faser annähernd parallel. Die Zahl der Fibrillen, die zu einer Faser gebündelt sind, bestimmt die Dicke der Faser. Sie schwankt zwischen 2—15 µ. Auf dem Querschnitt erscheint die Faser meist oval. Verzweigungen entstehen dadurch, daß zwei oder mehrere Fibrillenbündel ausscheren und sich benachbarten Fasern wieder zugesellen (Abb. 8a). Die Fibrillen selbst bleiben aber stets unverzweigt.

Im Polarisationsmikroskop verhält sich die Faser einachsig doppelbrechend. Mit histochemischen Methoden lassen sich z.T. die am Aufbau des Kollagens beteiligten Aminosäuren nachweisen (GÖSSNER, 1961). Wie der mäßige Ausfall der PJS-Reaktion schließen läßt, ist der Anteil der Mucopolysaccharide mit 1% (GRASSMANN, 1960) geringer als bei der argyrophilen Faser.

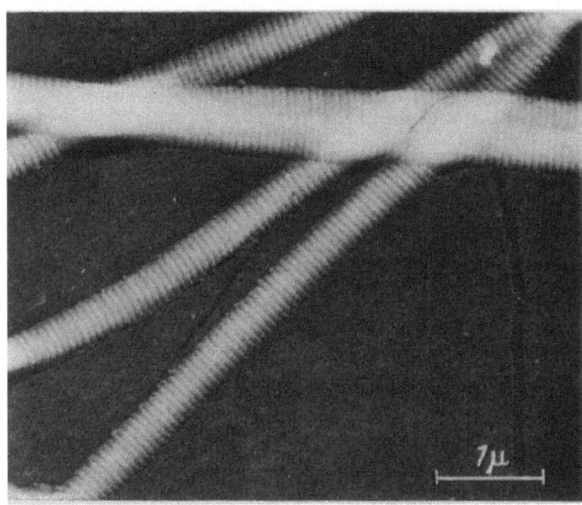

Abb. 5. Fünf schrägbedampfte kollagene Mikrofibrillen, die das typische Bild der Periodizität erkennen lassen. Die Isolation der Fibrillen aus der Faser erfolgte durch Ultraschall

Im elektronenmikroskopischen Bereich sind die kollagenen Mikrofibrillen an ihrer typischen Periodizität erkennbar (S. 442 und Abb. 5). Von der Kittsubstanz ist allerdings bei der normalen elektronenmikroskopischen Technik nur wenig zu sehen. Wie DETTMER u. SCHWARZ (1953) und PAHLKE (1954) mit Hilfe einer besonderen Versilberungsreaktion zeigen konnten, die als histochemische Reaktion auf die Glykolgruppen ausgerichtet ist und damit die Mucopolysaccharide erfaßt, liegen diese bevorzugt innerhalb der kollagenen Fibrille. BLINZINGER u. MATUSSEK (1966) glauben, mit einer speziellen Bariumchloridfärbung elektronenmikroskopisch auch saure Mucopolysaccharide im Innern der Fibrillen nachgewiesen zu haben.

Man ist allgemein geneigt, die Fasern zu statisch zu betrachten. Sie sind aber, wie alle lebendigen Substanzen, einem ständigen Auf- und Abbau und einem Austausch ihrer molekularen Bausteine unter Beibehaltung ihrer Gestalt unterworfen, wie Markierungsversuche mit C^{14} (SLACK, 1953) bewiesen haben. Hiermit hängt auch die Beobachtung zusammen, daß bei Inaktivität die kollagene Faser schrumpft und durch Aktivität erst wieder die notwendige Länge hergestellt wird. Auch sind Fasern in mechanisch auf Zug beanspruchten Geweben dicker als in weniger beanspruchten (INGELMARK, 1948). Eine Schrumpfung der kollagenen Faser tritt bei Einwirkung sehr hoher Temperatur ein. Bei 80°C ist im elektronenmikroskopischen Bild eine deutliche Verkürzung des Bänderabstandes um $^1/_3$ zu verzeichnen. Bei 170—200°C erfolgt eine irreversible Degeneration (ISHIMOTO, 1955).

Altersunterschiede manifestieren sich gleichfalls in der Dicke der Fibrillen. Sie sind beim Jugendlichen auffallend dünner als beim Erwachsenen. Hiermit läßt sich gut in Einklang bringen die zunehmende Zugfestigkeit kollagenen Materials mit fortschreitendem Alter. ROLLHÄUSER (1950a) stellte bei Messungen an Sehnen fest, daß sie sich im Laufe des Lebens auf das Dreifache erhöht. Ähnliche Beobachtungen liegen auch an der Haut vor (ROLLHÄUSER, 1950b). Eine Altersdegeneration der kollagenen Faser wird von TELLER et al. (1957) nach elektronenmikroskopischen und histochemischen Untersuchungen beschrieben. Eine konstitutionelle Minderwertigkeit des kollagenen Bindegewebes ist nicht nur klinisch, sondern auch experimentell gesichert (ROLLHÄUSER, 1950b). Jedoch liegen m.W. keine Untersuchungen darüber vor, wo diese „Schwäche" zu suchen ist. Hinsichtlich Altersveränderungen und degenerativen Veränderungen des Kollagens muß auf den Handbuchbeitrag von BRAUN-FALCO, Bd. I/2, verwiesen werden.

3. Die elastische Faser

Wie überall im Körper, so sind auch in der Haut elastische Fasern nicht selbständig, sondern Anteile eines dreidimensionalen Netzwerkes. Hinsichtlich ihres Verhaltens gegenüber Chemikalien und Fermenten muß auf die einschlägigen Lehr- und Handbücher (PINKUS, 1927; BARGMANN, 1964; BUCHER, 1965; DEMPSEY u. LANSING, 1954) verwiesen werden. Die Dicke der im Gewebsverband gestreckt verlaufenden Faser schwankt zwischen 0,5 und 3 μ. Wird das Gewebe zur Untersuchung aus dem Zusammenhang ohne vorherige geeignete Fixation herausgeschnitten, dann ziehen sich die stets unter Spannung stehenden Fasern infolge ihrer Elastizität zusammen und verlaufen unterschiedlich stark gewellt. Ihre reversible Dehnbarkeit wird allgemein mit 100—150% angegeben (WÖHLISCH et al., 1927; BARGMANN, 1964). In elastischen Sehnen fand PETRY (1951a) sogar eine wesentlich höhere Elastizität (bis 250%).

Über die Entstehung der elastischen Faser sind wir heute nur mangelhaft unterrichtet, obwohl es nicht an Untersuchungen fehlte. Bestimmte Zellen, die für die Bildung allein verantwortlich gemacht werden könnten, sog. „Elastoblasten" (KROMPECHER, 1928), oder ein mit der Kollagenfaserbildung vergleichbarer Mechanismus wurden nicht gefunden. Sicher ist, daß die ersten elastischen Elemente in unmittelbarer Nähe von Fibroblasten (KARRER u. COX, 1960), oft zwischen Kollagenfaserbündeln, in Erscheinung treten. KEECH et al. (1956, 1957) vermuten sogar Zwischenstufen zwischen Kollagen und Elastin, ja sie fanden bei Versuchen in vitro, daß sich Kollagen in Elastin umwandeln könne. Auch wurde bereits die Meinung vertreten (HALL et al., 1952), Elastin könne aus Zwischenprodukten im Aufbau des Kollagens entstanden sein. Eine enge Beziehung in der Kollagen- und Elastin-Bildung ist unbestritten. SCHWARZ (1964) konnte die Elastinbildung in Gewebekulturfibroblasten sicher nachweisen. Die ersten mit Orcein färbbaren elastischen Fasern sind bei menschlichen Keimlingen vom 5. Fetalmonat an, also in einem späteren Entwicklungsstadium als Kollagen, beobachtet worden (LYNCH, 1934). Allerdings finden sich auch schon in frühen Entwicklungsstadien Fasernetze, die durch ihre hohe Lichtbrechung elastischen Elementen gleichen (DEMPSEY u. LANSING, 1954). SCHWARZ (1964) fand die ersten elastischen Elemente an der Oberfläche von Fibroblasten in Form von Perlen oder Tropfen von 100 bis 500 mμ Durchmesser und 200—1000 mμ Länge, die dann zu Bändern konfluieren.

Mit chemisch-analytischen Untersuchungsmethoden wurde aus dem elastischen Gewebe vor allem Glykokoll und Prolin (FLASCHENTRÄGER-LEHNARTZ, 1951), aber auch Valin und Leucin (DEMPSEY u. LANSING, 1954; ENGSTRÖM u. FINEAN, 1958) isoliert, jedoch kein Histidin und Tryptophan. Die unterschiedlichen Prozentangaben lassen vermuten, daß die Zusammensetzung nicht generell gleichartig ist oder daß z.T. verunreinigte Lösungen als Ausgangsmaterial vorlagen. Außerdem fanden sich noch die Bausteine der sauren Mucopolysaccharide (ROBB-SMITH, 1952; MOORE u. SCHOENBERG, 1959).

Die Aminosäuren sind zu langen Polypeptidketten verbunden, die, wie Röntgendiffraktionsbilder (BEAR, 1944; ASTBURY, 1950) erkennen ließen, innerhalb der Protofibrille ziemlich ungeordnet liegen müssen. Werden die Fasern und damit auch die Protofibrillenbündel gedehnt, dann erfolgt eine zunehmende Längsorientierung der Polypeptidketten (vgl. FLASCHENTRÄGER-LEHNARTZ, Abb. 16).

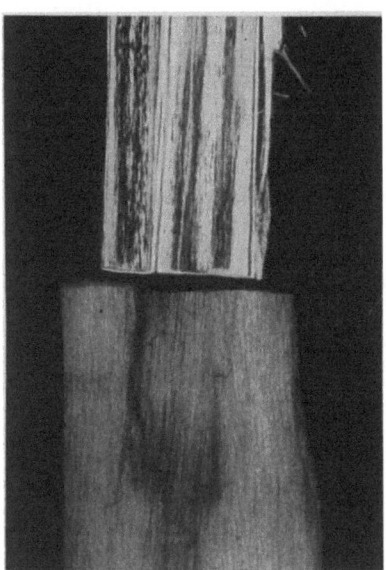

Abb. 6. Elastisches Band vom Rind im gedehnten Zustand (oben) und im ungedehnten (unten). Bei der Untersuchung im polarisierten Licht wird die Zunahme des Doppelbrechungsphänomens während der Dehnung deutlich. (Nach W. J. SCHMIDT, 1939; aus BARGMANN, 1964)

Mit diesen Modellvorstellungen lassen sich auch die polarisationsmikroskopischen Beobachtungen in Einklang bringen, wie auch die von BAHR (1951) vertretene Ansicht, die Molekülketten des Elastins verfügten nur über eine geringe Anzahl von Seitenketten. Aufgrund dieses strukturchemischen inneren Baues würden sie nach Aufhören des Zuges wieder in ihre Ausgangslage zurückkehren. Im Polarisationsmikroskop gibt die Faser im ungedehnten Zustand (Abb. 6) ein relativ schwaches Doppelbrechungsphänomen, das sich mit zunehmender Dehnung verstärkt. Aus diesem Verhalten schloß bereits W. J. SCHMIDT (1939), daß während der Dehnung eine zunehmende Ausrichtung der submikroskopischen Bauelemente erfolgen müsse.

Für die lichtmikroskopische Untersuchung sind die Fasern nach den klassischen Färbungsmethoden mit Orcein oder Resorcin-Fuchsin, aber auch mit Aldehyd-Fuchsin elektiv erfaßbar. Das geeignetste Fixationsmittel ist nach PETRY (1951b, 1952) 1%ige Phosphormolybdänsäure. Sie führt zu einer vollständigen Blockierung der Elastizität, also zu einer echten Fixation. Anschließend läßt sich die Faser sogar mit Hämatoxylin anfärben. In den üblichen Fixationsgemischen verliert dagegen die Faser ihre Elastizität nicht. Sie wird auch nicht durch einen vorübergehenden Trocknungsprozeß verändert; nach Übertragen in Wasser quillt die Faser und die Elastizität stellt sich unvermindert wieder ein (PETRY, 1951b). Im frischen Zupfpräparat fallen die elastischen Fasern durch ihr hohes Lichtbrechungsvermögen auf. Sie erscheinen bei allen lichtmikroskopischen Untersuchungen homogen und nicht, wie die kollagene Faser, aus einzelnen Fibrillen aufgebaut. Bei Veränderungen der Stoffwechsellage, z.B. im Bereich entzündlicher Exsudate, kann sich auch eine reversible Argyrophilie einstellen (ENGHUSEN, 1957). Hierfür wird von ENGHUSEN die Auflagerung einer Silber reduzierenden Substanz (s. S. 445), die sich im Gewebe infolge einer pH-Verschiebung bildet, verantwortlich gemacht. Unter bestimmten Bedingungen, z.B. durch Blockierung polarer Gruppen, lassen sich auch kollagene Fasern mit Elasticafarbstoffen darstellen (BRAUN-FALCO, 1956; FULLMER u. LILLIE, 1957) und sind damit histologisch nicht von elastischen sicher abzugrenzen.

Histochemisch verhalten sich die elastischen Fasern verschiedener Tierspecies aber auch aus den verschiedenen Organen recht unterschiedlich (GRAUMANN, 1964). Mit der PJS-Reaktion wird ein noch nicht genauer analysiertes, dem Chondroitin-Sulfat nahestehendes Glykoproteid erfaßt, das vermutlich als Grund- oder „Kittsubstanz" die submikroskopischen Proteinfilamente verbindet und maskiert (KARRER, 1961; HALL et al., 1952). Außerdem zeigt das elastische Gewebe eine merkliche Sudanophilie (DEMPSEY u. LANSING, 1954; BRAUN-FALCO, 1957; WOLMAN, 1964), die vermutlich auf einer Lipoprotein-Verbindung beruht.

Im elektronenmikroskopischen Bild (WOLPERS, 1944; GROSS, 1949; BAHR, 1950; LANSING et al., 1952) besteht die elastische Faser aus Protofibrillen ohne Querstreifung, die als kleinstes bisher sichtbares Bauelement eine Länge von

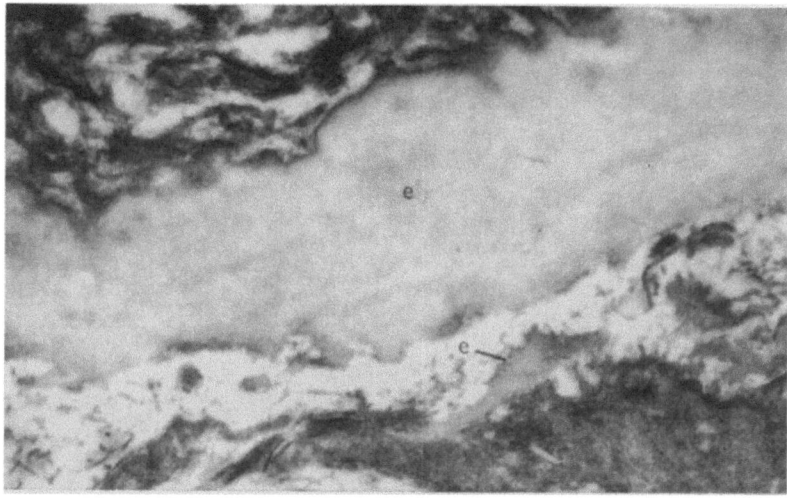

Abb. 7. Elektronenmikroskopische Aufnahme des elastischen Gewebes (*e*) zwischen Quer- und Schrägschnitten kollagener Fasern. Die elastische Faser ist weniger kontrastreich und unregelmäßig begrenzt. Die Protofibrillen sind nicht erkennbar. Vergr. ungefähr 15000fach. (Nach KARRER, 1961)

ungefähr 1 μ und einen Durchmesser von 70—80 Å aufweisen. 10—15 solcher Fibrillen sind zur Elastinfibrille (BAHR, dessen Nomenklatur ich weiterhin folge) mit einer Dicke von 350 Å vereinigt. Verzweigungen dieser Fibrillen wurden von WOLPERS (1944) beschrieben. Mehrere Elastinfibrillen sind zu elastischen Strängen von 800—1200 Å Durchmesser vereinigt (BAHR). Innerhalb der Stränge sind die Elastinfibrillen anscheinend verflochten und in eine unterschiedliche Menge einer amorphen Grundsubstanz eingelagert. Sie dürfte für den positiven Ausfall der PJS-Reaktion und für die Färbbarkeit mit Elasticafarbstoffen verantwortlich sein. Die „Verzwirnung" zweier oder mehrerer Protofibrillen (GROSS, LANSING et al.) hält BAHR für ein Artefakt. Jedoch lassen die von LANSING vorgelegten Bilder schwerlich auf eine artifizielle Entstehung schließen. Die Angaben einer periodischen Strukturierung der Fibrillen (TURNBRIDGE et al., 1952; SCHWARZ u. DETTMER, 1953) fanden keine weitere überzeugende Bestätigung. Im elektronenmikroskopischen Schnittpräparat (KEECH, 1960a; KARRER, 1961; SEIFERT, 1962) erscheint die elastische Faser kontrastarm (Abb. 7), nach Färbungen mit Phosphor-Molybdänsäure kontrastreich, homogen und nur von vereinzelten, oft schwer erkennbaren Fibrillen längs durchzogen. Durch Andauung mit Elastase (KEECH, 1960b) werden die Fibrillen deutlicher. Ihr Durchmesser soll 160—190 Å betragen. SCHWARZ (1964) ermittelte in neugebildeten elastischen Elementen eine Fibrillendicke von 80—100 Å. Die relativ hohe Widerstandsfähigkeit der elastischen

Faser gegen Säure- und Fermenteinwirkung ist seit langem bekannt. Von BALÓ und BANGA (1950) wurde aus dem Pankreastrypsin ein elastolytisches Ferment Elastase abgetrennt, das anscheinend spezifisch auf das Elastin wirkt (BANGA, 1952; LANSING et al., 1952).

III. Die Grundsubstanz

Zellen und Fasern sind in eine amorphe, wäßrig-viscöse Grundsubstanz (MAXIMOW, 1929; DORFMAN, 1955) eingelagert. Aus ihr konnten mit chemisch-analytischen Methoden reines lösliches Kollagen (BENSLEY, 1934; ROBB-SMITH, 1952, 1953), Plasmaproteine sowie neutrale und saure Mucopolysaccharide isoliert werden, bzw. als Bausteine der sauren Mucopolysaccharide Hyaluronsäure und Chondroitin-Sulfat A, B und C (MEYER u. RAPPORT, 1951; LOEWI u. MEYER, 1958; STROUGHTON u. WELLS, 1950; DORFMAN, 1963). Beim erwachsenen Tier überwiegen die neutralen Mucopolysaccharide, die sauren treten quantitativ zurück (LOEWI u. MEYER, 1958). Vermutlich liegen im Gewebe die Mucopolysaccharide als kettenförmige Proteinkomplexe (MEYER, 1954) unterschiedlichen Polymerisationsgrades vor. Von diesem ist der Grad der Viscosität abhängig. Außerdem enthält die Grundsubstanz in nicht bestimmbaren Mengen Hyaluronidase, Kollagenase und Elastase, also Fermente, die mit dem physiologischen Auf- und Abbau der Intercellularsubstanzen in Zusammenhang stehen. Die Konzentration von Mineralsalzen und Glucose wurde in der Grundsubstanz sogar höher als im Blutplasma gefunden (COWDRY, 1939).

Bei den üblichen lichtmikroskopischen Untersuchungen ist von der Grundsubstanz nicht viel zu sehen, denn ein Großteil ihrer Bestandteile wird schon durch ungeeignete Fixation herausgelöst (BENSLEY, 1934), der Rest anscheinend bei der Entwässerung unter dem Einbettungsvorgang auf der Oberfläche der Fasern niedergeschlagen und schließlich sind die Mucopolysaccharide nur mit besonderen histochemischen Methoden elektiv zu erfassen. Entsprechend der unterschiedlichen Dichte der Fasertextur ist die mengenmäßige Verteilung der Grundsubstanz in den verschiedenen Schichten der Haut nicht gleich.

Für histochemische Untersuchungen ist das Fixationsgemisch nach HELLY oder Bleiacetat besonders geeignet. Sehr gute Ergebnisse liefern Kryostatschnitte (NIEBAUER u. RAAB, 1961) und die Gefriertrocknung. Danach erscheint die Grundsubstanz homogen, oft etwas wolkig. Sie verhält sich bei der PJS-Reaktion schwach positiv. Dieser Ausfall beruht auf dem Nachweis von 1,2-Glykolgruppen in neutralen wie sauren Mucopolysacchariden. Die sauren Mucopolysaccharide sind außerdem durch einen metachromatischen Effekt und durch die Färbbarkeit mit Astra- oder Alcianblau gekennzeichnet (Fermentteste s. S. 453). Eine merkliche Metachromasie läßt sich im Bereich des Mammabindegewebes (GRAUMANN, 1953), des Papillarkörpers (WISLOCKI et al., 1947; VITRY u. PRIVAT, 1961; MANCINI et al., 1961; NIEBAUER u. RAAB, 1961), des perivasculären und periglandulären Bindegewebes (GRAUMANN, 1953) feststellen. Im übrigen lockeren Bindegewebe ist der Ausfall negativ oder äußerst schwach. Nachfixieren der Kryostatschnitte mit Alkohol verstärkt die Reaktion (STEIGLEDER, 1959). Es tauchten Bedenken auf (MEYER, 1954), ob die Reaktion allein durch Hyaluronsäure bedingt sein könne. Von GRAUMANN werden auch Sulfomucopolysaccharide hierfür verantwortlich gemacht, da die ohnedies nur in geringen Mengen in der Grundsubstanz vorhandenen Hyaluronsäuren nicht als freie, reaktive Gruppen vorliegen, sondern an Proteine gebunden sind (latente Metachromasie). Hierfür spricht, daß nach Einwirkung von proteolytischen Fermenten der metachromatische Effekt sofort zutage tritt (FOLLIS, 1951).

Mit dem Elektronenmikroskop ist in der lichtmikroskopisch amorphen Grundsubstanz ein Netzwerk kollagener Mikrofibrillen nachweisbar (DETTMER, 1951; WASSERMANN, 1956). Da diese zweifellos zu den geformten Bestandteilen des Gewebes gehören, dürfte nur die zwischen den Mikrofibrillen gelegene „Flüssigkeit" als Grundsubstanz bezeichnet werden. Sie enthält aber die heute elektronenmikroskopisch noch nicht quantitativ erfaßbaren Mucopolysaccharidmoleküle und die wegen ihrer geringen Größe nicht auflösbaren Tropokollagenmoleküle. Doch auch diese sind zweifellos typisch strukturierte Gebilde. Sollte man also nur noch die Flüssigkeit und die Mucopolysaccharide als Grundsubstanz bezeichnen? Ja gibt es überhaupt „freies Wasser" in der Grundsubstanz, oder ist es vollständig als Quellungswasser gebunden? An diesem Beispiel wird deutlich, in welch hohem Grad die Terminologie und die Grenzziehung zwischen Begriffen vom momentanen Stand der Technik bestimmt wird, und wie sich heute mehr und mehr die Grenzen verschieben. Vor kurzem gelang durch eine Blei-Färbung der histochemische Nachweis der PJS-positiven Substanzen (DAEMS u. PERSIJN, 1962) im elektronenmikroskopischen Bereich. Von dieser Methode sind noch weitere Aufschlüsse zu erwarten, ebenso von der Mitteilung (BLINZINGER u. MATUSSEK, 1966) über den elektronenmikroskopischen Nachweis von sauren Mucopolysacchariden.

Die Frage nach der Herkunft der Grundsubstanz ist zwar noch Gegenstand wissenschaftlicher Diskussionen, doch darf man aus dem bisher Bekannten folgern: Kollagen und neutrale Mucopolysaccharide werden von Fibroblasten erzeugt (GERSH u. CATCHPOLE, 1949; MANCINI et al., 1961). Von den Mastzellen werden die granulär gespeicherten metachromatischen Stoffe in die Grundsubstanz abgegeben (SYLVÉN, 1941; ASBOE-HANSEN, 1950; SCHAUER, 1964). So ist es naheliegend, den Gehalt an sauren Mucopolysacchariden auf die Tätigkeit der Mastzellen zurückzuführen (BENSLEY, 1950; ASBOE-HANSEN, 1950, 1954; NIEBAUER u. RAAB, 1961), zumal ihre Zahl in der Haut wesentlich höher ist, als man nach der Durchsicht von Schnittpräparaten vermuten möchte. Wurden doch bis zu 7000 Zellen pro mm^3 Gewebe gezählt (HELLSTRÖM u. HOLMGREN, 1950). Auch enthalten Gewebsregionen mit einem hohen Gehalt an metachromatischen sauren Mucopolysacchariden auffallend viele Mastzellen. Andererseits ist nicht auszuschließen, daß auch aus dem Blut metachromatische Substanzen übertreten (KLEMPERER, 1953). Dies trifft sicherlich zu für die wäßrige Flüssigkeit mit den gelösten Mineralsalzen, Aminosäuren, Plasmaproteinen und Glucose, die nicht nur für den Betriebsstoffwechsel der Bindegewebszellen, sondern auch als Bausteine für die Bildung von Fasern und Grundsubstanz an die Zellen herangebracht werden und hierzu die Grundsubstanz passieren müssen; sie bilden damit keinen integrierenden Bestandteil wie die Mucopolysaccharide.

Damit ist bereits auch die Frage nach der funktionellen Bedeutung der Grundsubstanz angeschnitten. Sie stellt das flüssigkeitsreiche Verkehrsfeld dar, durch das der Elektrolyt-Stoff- und Gasaustausch vom Gefäßsystem zum Epithel und zu den Bindegewebszellen und der Abtransport von Stoffwechselschlacken stattfindet. An der Grenze von Epithel und Gefäßen ist die Grundsubstanz zur Basalmembran verdichtet (GERSH u. CATCHPOLE, 1949). In dieses Verkehrsfeld des Stoffwechsels werden aber auch die Tropokollagenmoleküle abgegeben, aus denen sich Fibrillen und Fasern formieren. In der „Gewebsflüssigkeit" etwas Stagnierendes zu sehen, wäre unbiologisch gedacht. Sie unterliegt vielmehr, wie die praktische Erfahrung von der Applikation intracutan applizierter Stoffe lehrt, einem ständigen Austausch. Die Drainage erfolgt über das Lymphgefäßsystem oder über die Blutcapillaren. Auf welche Weise die Auswahl getroffen wird, ist unbekannt. Aber auch die Mucopolysaccharide unterliegen, wie autoradiographische Untersuchungen zeigten (SCHILLER et al., 1955), einem ständigen Umbau. In nicht ganz 2 Tagen sind die Moleküle der Hyaluronsäure zur Hälfte ausgetauscht. Allerdings ist von den Austausch- und Transportvorgängen in der Grundsubstanz mit rein morphologischen Methoden nicht viel zu erfassen. Die Stoffe sind bis zu einer Molekülgröße abgebaut (vgl. Fettspeicherung, S. 460), die unter dem Auflösungsvermögen des Elektronenmikroskopes liegt oder sie werden, weil wasser- bzw. lipoidlöslich, bei der Präparation herausgelöst. Eine wichtige, in den letzten Jahren mehr und mehr an wissenschaftlichem Interesse gewinnende Funktion erfüllen die Mucopolysaccharide (vgl. GRAUMANN, 1964). Durch den Gehalt an Hyaluronsäuren vermögen sie Wasser zu binden (MEYER u. RAPPORT, 1951; MEYER, 1954) und bilden damit einen bestimmenden Faktor für die Aufrechterhaltung des Hautturgors. Dieser sinkt bekanntlich proportional mit ihrer physiologischen Abnahme im Alter ab. Entsprechend dem ubiquitären Vorkommen von neutralen Mucopolysacchariden an resorbierenden Zelloberflächen (z.B. Bürstensäume, Fettzellen, Protozoen) müssen diese mit den Vorgängen bei der Stoffaufnahme in Zusammenhang stehen. Sie wurden deshalb auch als „Resorptionsvermittler" (SCHMIDT, 1962) oder „Überträgergewebe" (GRAUMANN, 1953) bezeichnet. Andererseits wirkt die Grundsubstanz als Ganzes auch als Barriere oder „kontrollierende Schranke" vor allem gegen eingedrungene kolloidale Partikelchen oder Bakterien. Dies wird aus den folgenden Ausführungen verständlich: Die Fermente Hyaluronidase, Kollagenase (ROBB-SMITH, 1953) und Elastase sind an den ständig ablaufenden Umbauvorgängen von Fasern und Grundsubstanz beteiligt. Die depolymerisierende Wirkung der Hyaluronidase (spreading factor) macht man sich zunutze bei der Injektion von Stoffen in die Haut, die in der depolymerisierten und damit weniger viscösen Grundsubstanz schneller und besser verteilt werden (DURAN-REYNALS, 1942, 1949). Infolgedessen können sich auch Bakterien, die selbst Hyaluronidase bereiten, in der Grundsubstanz schneller ausbreiten. Die reversible Polymerisation und Depolymerisation der Mucopolysaccharide (GERSH u. CATCHPOLE, 1949) wird von GRAUMANN (1953) auch mit dem physiologischen Stofftransport in Zusammenhang gebracht. Gleichfalls scheint sie in Beziehung zu stehen zur Regulation und Konstanterhaltung des osmotischen Druckes. Schließlich bildet die flüssigkeitsreiche Grundsubstanz ein plastisches Druckpolster, und das Verschieben der Fasern bei Zugwirkung wird erst in einem Gleitmedium wie dem Mucopolysaccharidsol ohne wesentliche Reibung möglich.

Auffällig sind auch die vom Lebensalter abhängigen unterschiedlichen Mengen von Mucopolysacchariden in der Grundsubstanz und die Veränderungen ihrer Zusammensetzung während des Lebens. Beim Embryo ist der Gehalt an Mucopolysacchariden außerordentlich hoch. Er nimmt bis zur Geburt und dann im postfetalen Leben mehr und mehr ab (BENSLEY, 1934; MANCINI et al., 1961), während die Menge der Fasern zunimmt. Durch die Verringerung der Mucopolysaccharide wird die wasserbindende, den Turgor der Haut bestimmende Komponente des Bindegewebes der Haut herabgesetzt (KIERLAND u. O'LEARY, 1953). Während der Fetalentwicklung und im Laufe des Lebens verschiebt sich außerdem das relative Verhältnis von sauren zu neutralen Mucopolysacchariden (bestimmt in der Haut embryonaler, fetaler und erwachsener Schweine; LOEWI u. MEYER, 1958). Beim Embryo wurden 25—37% saure Mucopolysaccharide ermittelt, beim erwachsenen Tier nur noch 0,11%. In der embryonalen Haut bestehen die Mucopolysaccharide zu 80% aus Hyaluronsäure, zu 5—12% aus Chondroitin-Sulfat B und zu 20% vermutlich aus Chondroitin-Sulfat C. Beim erwachsenen Tier überwiegt dagegen Chondroitin-Sulfat B mit 64% gegenüber 30% Hyaluronsäure und 0,1% Chondroitin-Sulfat C. Über die Bedeutung dieser Verschiebung lassen sich, solange man über die Funktion dieser Stoffe noch keine fundierten Kenntnisse besitzt, nur Spekulationen anstellen. Sollten sie die Ursache dafür sein, daß der stoffwechselaktive Zustand das Bindegewebe beim Feten und Kind mit zunehmendem Alter in einen „bradytrophen" Zustand übergeht? Der Rückgang der als Produzenten in Frage kommenden Mastzellen würde hierfür sprechen, ebenso wie die erneute lokale Zunahme während der Wundheilung. Die Lokalisation der sauren Mucopolysaccharide im Grenzgebiet von Epidermis, epidermalen Anhangsgebilden und Gefäßen läßt daran denken, daß sie maßgeblich an Stoffwechselvorgängen teilnehmen. Außerdem ist ihre Beteiligung am Aufbau der kollagenen Faser weitgehend gesichert, sowohl im embryonalen Gewebe wie auch während der Wundheilung (SYLVÉN, 1941). Über Einflüsse von Vitaminen, Hormonen und Strahlwirkungen auf die Grundsubstanz unterrichten die Handbuchbeiträge von ASBOE-HANSEN (1963), GRAUMANN (1964) und der Beitrag von BRAUN-FALCO in diesem Handbuch (Bd. II/2).

Die verschiedenen bekannten *Hyaluronidasen* verhalten sich nicht gleichartig. Bakterienhyaluronidase greift nur Hyaluronsäure an, während aus Testes gewonnene Hyaluronidase auch noch Chondroitinsulfat A und C depolymerisiert, Chondroitinsulfat B und Heparin jedoch unbeeinflußt läßt. Hierdurch ist es möglich, die verschiedenen Mucopolysaccharide auch histochemisch zu unterscheiden (BENSLEY, 1950; MEYER u. RAPPORT, 1951).

B. Aggregationsweise der Bauteile und Gewebebildung

Die Art und Weise, wie die einzelnen Bauteile, Zellen und Fasern, in den verschiedenen Schichten der Haut in die Grundsubstanz eingelagert sind, wird in den einschlägigen Abschnitten abgehandelt. Ganz allgemein kann man feststellen, daß die zugfesten kollagenen Fasern überwiegen. Im Gewebe durchflechten sie sich mattenartig (Abb. 8a), jedoch nicht wie bei einem der bekannten Stoffgewebe in einer, sondern in zwei Ebenen: sie bilden eine dreidimensionale Textur. Innerhalb dieser überschneiden sich die Fasern im spitzen Winkel, wodurch ein rautenförmiges Muster entsteht. Bei Einwirkung von Zug ändert sich dieser Winkel (Abb. 8b) und die Fasern gleiten etwas aneinander vorbei, jedoch nur wenig, denn sie sind durch abzweigende Faserzüge untereinander verbunden. Die flüssige Grundsubstanz, die das ganze Gewebe durchtränkt, spielt nicht nur für den Quellungszustand der Faser, sondern auch für diese Verschiebungen eine bedeutsame Rolle (ROLLHÄUSER, 1951). Da bei Einsetzen einer Zugwirkung die Wellung der kollagenen Fasern erst ausgeglichen werden muß, ist ein „elastischeres" Anziehen möglich. In die Kollagenfasertextur sind die elastischen Netze eingebaut, und zwar so, daß sie nach Aufhören des Zuges die Kollagenfasern wieder in die Ausgangslage zurückführen helfen, wozu auch der Quellungszustand der Faser beitragen mag. Ein Teil der elastischen Fasern verläuft infolgedessen schräg zur bevorzugten Verlaufsrichtung der kollagenen Fasern (Abb. 8a, rechte Bildhälfte). Die Fibroblasten liegen der Oberfläche der Fasern dicht an und sind vorwiegend parallel zur Faserrichtung orientiert. Dieses Grundkonzept der Textur wird in den verschiedenen Hautregionen und -schichten entsprechend den funktionellen Anforderungen modifiziert.

Der Frage, wie die Ausrichtung der Fibrillen und Fasern entsprechend den mechanischen Anforderungen erfolgt, waren die grundlegenden experimentellen Untersuchungen von WEISS (1929) und HERINGA (1931) gewidmet. Den beiden gelang es, im Zuchtmedium der Gewebekultur definierte Spannungsverhältnisse zu erzeugen. Sie bewirken, wie man schließen muß, eine Ausrichtung von „Ultramikronen", Fibrinmicellen oder anderen fadenförmigen Makromolekülen (JARRETT, 1958), vielleicht auch von sauren Mucopolysacchariden. Parallel zu diesen submikroskopischen Leitstrukturen ordnen sich die Fibroblasten an und bilden dann entsprechend orientierte Fibrillen und Fasern. Flüssigkeitsverschiebungen, die notwendigerweise im Zuchtmedium auftreten, werden gleichfalls für die Aus-

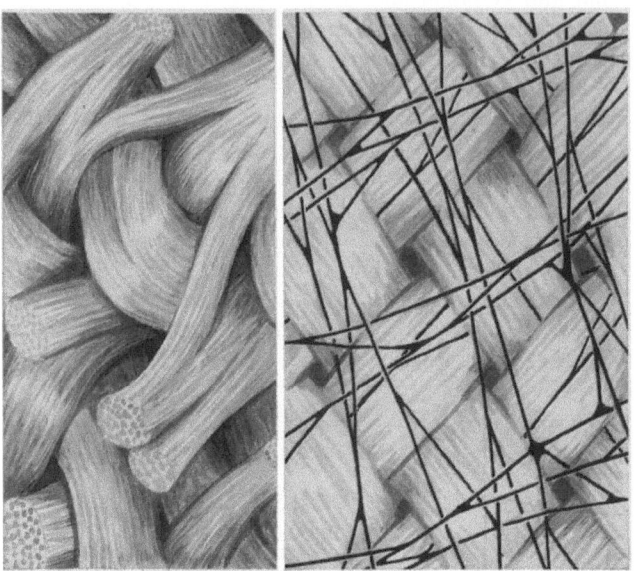

Abb. 8a. Halbschematische Darstellung der Textur kollagener und elastischer Fasern (rechte Bildhälfte) in der Haut. Das dreidimensionale elastische Netz und das kollagene Fasergeflecht sind in der rechten Bildhälfte nur in einer Ebene gezeichnet

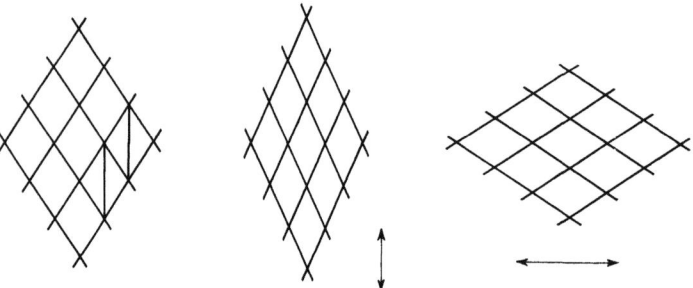

Abb. 8b. Schematische Darstellung der Veränderungen der Textur unter verschiedenen Zugrichtungen (Pfeile). In der ersten Zeichnung ist durch die beiden senkrechten Striche die Richtung der Spaltlinien eingetragen

richtung verantwortlich gemacht. Zu vergleichbaren Ergebnissen gelangte BENNINGHOFF (1931). Er untersuchte Veränderung und Anpassung der Bindegewebstextur nach Narbenbildung an der Rückenhaut der Maus. Auffallend war eine tiefgreifende Umordnung der Faseranordnung im Bereich der gesamten Rückenhaut, die sich in einer entsprechenden Veränderung des Spaltlinienverlaufes äußerte. In Übereinstimmung mit den Beobachtungen von WEISS machte auch BENNINGHOFF die Ausbildung primärer Leitstrukturen im regenerierenden Narbengewebe für die Orientierung der Fibroblasten und damit auch der Fasern verantwortlich. Als solche dienen z.B. Fibrinfäden, die sich entsprechend den gegebenen Zugspannungen des noch intakten Hautüberzuges oder, was wahrscheinlicher ist, entsprechend der Resultate dieser Spannungen ausrichten.

Die charakteristische Textur der kollagenen Fasern im Corium ist beim geburtsreifen Kind noch nicht ausgebildet (ROLLHÄUSER, 1951). Die Faserbündel verlaufen noch vorzugsweise parallel und durchflechten sich wenig. Die Festigkeit des Gewebes ist dementsprechend gering. Beim Kleinkind tritt allmählich eine stärkere Bündelung und Durchflechtung ein und mit zunehmendem Alter werden die Bündel dicker, die Texturen typischer.

Fettgewebe und Fettorgane

Das Fettgewebe, das in der Haut so gut wie ausschließlich als subcutanes Fettgewebe in Erscheinung tritt, muß als eine spezialisierte und organisierte Sonderform des retikulären Bindegewebes aufgefaßt werden (WASSERMANN, 1926). Nach Füllung der Zellen mit Fett tritt der zellige Charakter in den Vordergrund, während der Intercellularraum zumindest lichtmikroskopisch weitgehend schwindet. Im Gebiet der Haut sollen nirgendwo einzelne Fettzellen vorkommen, sondern nur Zellaggregate in Gestalt unterschiedlich großer Läppchen, den „*Fettorganen*" WASSERMANNs.

Über die Entstehung des Fettgewebes sind wir durch zahlreiche Untersuchungen (WASSERMANN, 1926; BECKER, 1930; HAUSBERGER, 1934; HOFFMANN, 1951; DABELOW, 1958, u.a.) gut unterrichtet. Die einzelnen Läppchen bilden sich beim Menschen vom 4. Fetalmonat an (Keime von 11—12 cm Scheitel-Steißlänge, HOFFMANN) aus umschriebenen Anhängen des Gefäßbindegewebsapparates, den Primitivorganen.

1. Die Primitivorgane (WASSERMANN)

Sie bestehen aus lokalen Verdichtungen retikulären Bindegewebes an der Oberfläche von Capillaren und sind zunächst an der Bildung von Blutzellen beteiligt. Funktionell und morphologisch zeigen sie Ähnlichkeit mit den „Milchflecken" des Omentums. Durch progressive intracytoplasmatische Ablagerung zunächst kleinster Fetttröpfchen, die an Zahl und Größe zunehmen und allmählich konfluieren, entwickeln sich aus den Reticulumzellen, die unterdessen auch ihre Fortsätze eingezogen haben, plurivacuoläre Fettzellen. Sie kugeln sich schließlich ab und wandeln sich in die univacuoläre Form um. Hiermit schwindet auch die Fähigkeit der Fettorgane, Blutzellen zu bilden. Fettzelle liegt jetzt neben Fettzelle; der Intercellularraum ist nur noch als feiner zwickelförmiger Spalt zu erkennen. Das für das retikuläre Bindegewebe charakteristische Netzwerk argyrophiler Fasern (Retikulinfasern) umschließt, wesentlich dichter geworden, ballonnetzartig die prall gefüllten, nur noch aus einer dünnen Cytoplasmahaut bestehenden Fettzellen. Neben der univacuolären Form bleibt zeitlebens in bestimmten Regionen auch die plurivacuoläre bestehen.

2. Das Gewebe univacuolärer Fettzellen

In dem schmalen Cytoplasmasaum der einzelnen Fettzelle finden sich im elektronenmikroskopischen Bild kleine Vesikel und besonders im Bereich des Zellkernes in großer Menge Mitochondrien. Die Zelloberfläche ist annähernd glatt konturiert, abgegrenzt von einem typischen Plasmalemm. Verstreut werden auch Anschnitte des endoplasmatischen Reticulums (rauhe Form) und ein kleiner, nur aus wenigen langgestreckten Bläschen bestehender Golgi-Apparat gefunden (NAPOLITANO, 1963). Der zentral gelegene große Fetttropfen muß als Paraplasma aufgefaßt werden. Allerdings unterscheidet er sich von den übrigen paraplasmatischen Einlagerungen durch das Fehlen einer membranösen Abgrenzung vom Grundplasma (WASSERMANN u. McDONALD, 1960; NAPOLITANO, 1963). Der stark abgeplattete Zellkern ist mit dem Cytoplasma an die Zelloberfläche verlagert. Jede Fettzelle wird von einer elektronenmikroskopisch und histochemisch nachweisbaren Basalmembran (CHASE, 1959) umhüllt. Im Gewebsverband sind die 40—120 µ großen Zellen meist gegeneinander etwas abgeplattet. Entgegen früheren Ansichten (WASSERMANN, 1926) bilden sie keinen syncytialen Verband. Die sich netzförmig verzweigenden argyrophilen Faserhüllen (PLENK, 1927) liegen, wie die Elektronenmikroskopie bestätigte, extracellulär, außerhalb der Basalmembran. Ihr Feinbau unterscheidet sich nicht von anderen argyrophilen Fasern. An dicken Gewebsschnitten ist in lichtmikroskopischen Versilberungspräparaten zu beobachten, daß die argyrophilen Fasern ein das ganze Fettläppchen durchziehendes zusammenhängendes Raumnetz bilden (LAUBINGER, 1938), das an der Läppchengrenze in deren Scheidewände (S. 474) einstrahlt, indem die Silberfasern kontinuierlich in die Kollagenfasern übergehen. Damit sind die Fettzellen untereinander durch die Kontinuität der Faserkörbe und -netze verbunden. In das argyrophile Netzwerk sind auch die Grundhäutchen der Capillaren eingewebt. Innerhalb eines jeden Läppchens breitet sich ein Geflecht vegetativer Nervenfasern aus (HAUSBERGER, 1934).

3. Das Gewebe plurivacuolärer Fettzellen

Beim Erwachsenen kommt im Bereich der Rückenhaut, der Achselhöhle und der Halsregion zeitlebens plurivacuoläres Fettgewebe vor, das wegen seiner Eigenfarbe auch als braunes Fett bezeichnet wird. Das Cytoplasma der einzelnen Fettzelle ist lichtmikroskopisch stark granuliert und enthält in unterschiedlicher Menge sudanophile Tröpfchen, oft in rosettenförmiger Anordnung. Elektronenmikroskopisch wurden massenhaft Mitochondrien, kleine Vacuolen, freie Ribosomen und in unterschiedlicher Menge und Häufung Glykogengranula gefunden. Ergastoplasmatische Strukturen sind äußerst spärlich oder fehlen vollständig (LEVER, 1957; NAPOLITANO und FAWCETT, 1958). Die von einer einschichtigen Membran umgebenen kleinen Fetttröpfchen (LEVER, 1957; NAPOLITANO und FAWCETT, 1958) liegen meist in unmittelbarer Nähe von Mitochondrien. Der zentral gelegene Zellkern enthält mehrere Nucleolen. Im Gewebsverband grenzen die einzelnen Zellen unter Facettierung ihrer Oberfläche so dicht aneinander, daß nur ein schmaler Intercellularraum frei bleibt. Er wird von einem amorphen Material ausgefüllt, das der Basalmembran der univacuolären Zelle völlig gleicht. In diese Substanz sind die lichtmikroskopisch nachweisbaren Gitterfasern und Blutcapillaren eingelagert. Braunes Fett ist außerordentlich reich capillarisiert (HOFFMANN, 1951).

4. Cyto- und histochemische Unterschiede von weißem und braunem Fett

Das *Cytoplasma* der Fettzellen enthält je nach Funktionszustand Esterasen, Succinodehydrogenase, alkalische Phosphatase, β-Glucuronidase (MONTAGNA, 1957). Die Esterasen (Lipasen) stehen zweifellos mit den ana- und katabolen Vorgängen während der Fettspeicherung und Entspeicherung in Zusammenhang. Die Phosphatasen greifen vermutlich in den Glucose-Stoffwechsel ein. Glykogen wurde licht- und elektronenmikroskopisch (HAUSBERGER, 1934; NAPOLITANO, 1963, u.a.) in sehr verschiedenen Mengen nachgewiesen.

Das in den *univacuolären Zellen* enthaltene *weiße Fett* besteht vor allem aus Triglyceriden, nämlich Glycerinestern der Palmitin-, Stearin-, Olein- und Linolsäure.

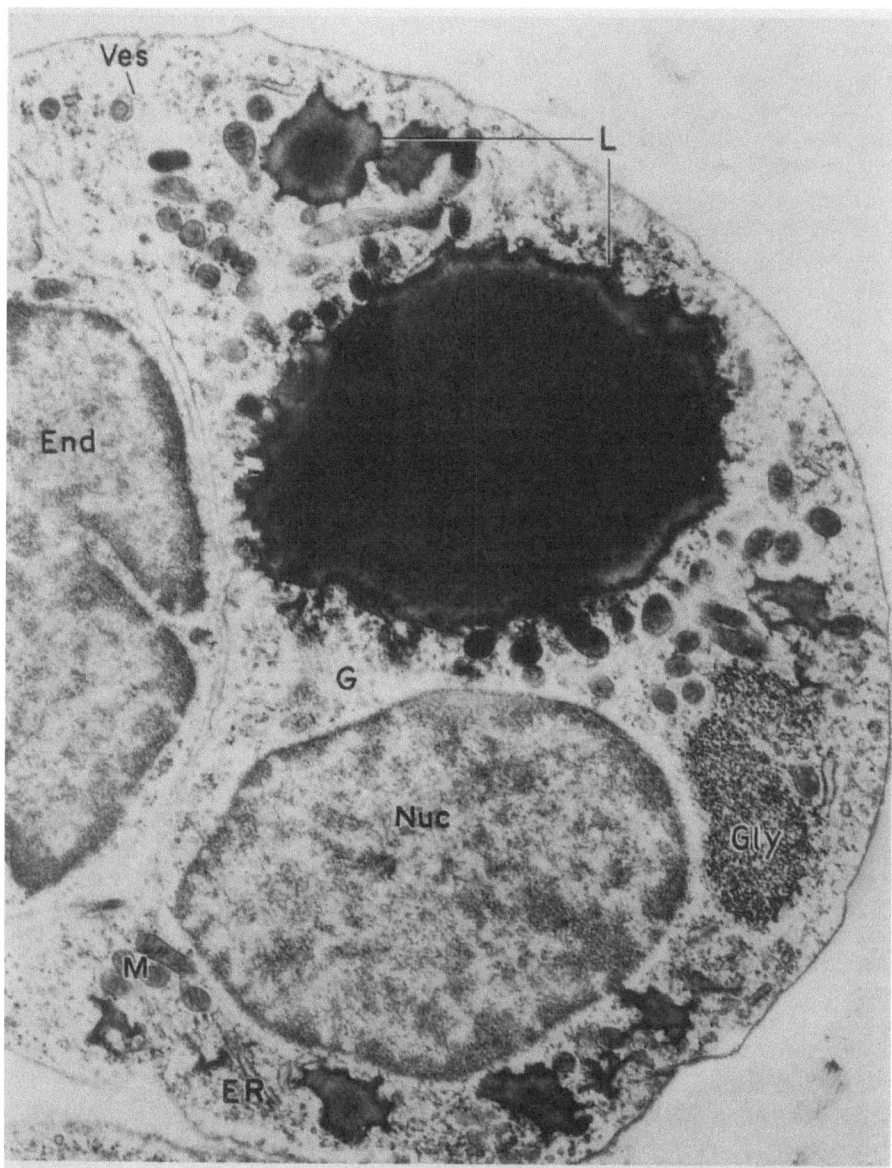

Abb. 9. Fettzelle während der Speicherung (weißes Fett). An der Oberfläche des großen Tropfens liegen zahlreiche kleine, die inkorporiert werden. Kern einer Endothelzelle (*End*), Ergastoplasma (*ER*), Glykogen (*Gly*). Golgi-Apparat (*G*), Lipidtröpfchen (*L*), Mitochondrien (*M*), Kern der Fettzelle (*Nuc*), kleine Vacuolen (*Ves*). Vergr. ungefähr 15000fach. (Nach NAPOLITANO, 1963)

Die Zusammensetzung ist in den verschiedenen Fettlagern des gleichen Organismus, gemessen an der Jodzahl, unterschiedlich (Untersuchungen am Schwein s. FLASCHENTRÄGER u. LEHNARTZ, 1951). Das Hautfett hat einen niedrigeren Schmelzpunkt als z. B. das Nierenfett und befindet sich im Leben im flüssigen Zustand. Die Eigenfarbe beruht auf Beimischungen von Lipochromen (vgl. WOLMAN, 1964).

Vom weißen Fett unterscheidet sich das in den *plurivacuolären Zellen* enthaltene *braune Fett* durch einen höheren Gehalt an Phospholipiden und Plasmalogen (FAWCETT, 1947), Mucoproteinen, Cholesterin (MENSCHIK, 1953) und Lipochromen. Auch im Verlauf der Bildung univacuolärer Zellen enthalten die an der Oberfläche der großen Neutralfettvacuolen liegenden kleinen Vacuolen (Abb. 9) reichlich Phospholipide (LEVER, 1957; FAWCETT, 1952). In der Fetalentwicklung des Menschen soll gleichfalls das zuerst gebildete Fett besonders reich an Lipoiden sein; erst später treten Neutralfette auf. Beim Säugling sollen noch Fettsäuren mit höherem Schmelzpunkt als beim Erwachsenen überwiegen (BECKER, 1930).

Die Bedeutung des braunen Fettes beim Menschen und die Frage, in welchem Umfang plurivacuoläres in univacuoläres Fettgewebe übergehen kann, ist zwar für Tiere (HAUSBERGER, 1934, 1937), jedoch noch nicht für den Menschen befriedigend geklärt. Außerdem ist nicht ausgeschlossen, daß das plurivacuoläre braune Fett der Nagetiere und das des Menschen verschieden sind. Es wurden jedoch die meisten bisherigen Untersuchungen an den aus plurivacuolärem Fettgewebe bestehenden „Interscapularkörpern" von Versuchstieren ausgeführt. Für diese Gebilde liegen Beobachtungen vor, die einen Zusammenhang mit dem Winterschlaf (Winterschlafdrüse, RASMUSSEN, 1924) wahrscheinlich machen. Weitere Untersuchungen müssen klären, inwieweit das beim Menschen zeitlebens bestehende braune Fett mit dem gleichnamigen der Nagetiere Verwandtschaft zeigt. Ohne Zweifel wird in der Entwicklung des Menschen die plurivacuoläre Form durchlaufen. Es scheint mir aber nicht entschieden, ob das plurivacuoläre Fettgewebe des Erwachsenen nur ein stehengebliebenes Entwicklungsstadium oder eine besonders stoffwechselaktive Form (HOFFMANN, 1951) darstellt, die nur unter besonderen Bedingungen in die univacuoläre Form übergehen kann. Auffällig ist die enge Lagebeziehung von Lymphknoten und braunem Fettgewebe (WASSERMANN, HOFFMANN).

5. Fettgewebe oder Fettorgane?

Diese Frage ist keinesfalls eindeutig zu entscheiden. Im subcutanen Bindegewebe ist das Fettgewebe zu einzelnen Läppchen zusammengefaßt, die von WASSERMANN (1926 ff.) ganz allgemein und nicht nur in der Subcutis als „Fettorgane" bezeichnet werden. Er geht von der Ansicht aus, jedes Läppchen sei eine in sich geschlossene entwicklungsgeschichtliche, funktionelle und morphologische Einheit, die von einer kapselähnlichen Umhüllung von ihrer Umgebung abgegrenzt würde. Diese ist auch auf den Abbildungen des von WASSERMANN (1926) bearbeiteten Materials vom Kind sichtbar. Beim Erwachsenen konnte ich jedoch in Übereinstimmung mit HOFFMANN (1951) und LAUBINGER (1938) diese Abgrenzung nicht feststellen, sondern es zeigte sich vielmehr, daß die dem Fettgewebe angehörenden argyrophilen Fasern kontinuierlich in das Bindegewebe der Scheidewände übergehen. In jedes Läppchen treten an mehreren Stellen, und nicht etwa an einem Hilus, Blutgefäße ein, verzweigen sich und tangieren anscheinend eine jede Fettzelle. Außerdem durchzieht das Läppchen ein Netz vegetativer Nervenfasern. Trotz dieser inneren Organisation möchte ich mich nicht ohne Einschränkung der von WASSERMANN vorgeschlagenen Bezeichnung „Fettorgan" anschließen, sondern eher der von DABELOW (1958) benutzten „organähnliche Komplexe". Zweifellos stellt das Fettläppchen eine ganz besonders organisierte Form des Bindegewebes dar (s. auch Bd. I/2, S. 724).

6. Die funktionelle Bedeutung des subcutanen Fettgewebes

Die Bedeutung des subcutanen Fettgewebes kann schematisch auf folgende Punkte bezogen werden: Es wirkt 1. als mechanisches Druckpolster (Baufett), 2. als Energiedepot (Depotfett), 3. als Wasserspeicher, 4. als Wärmeschutz, 5. ist die Bedeutung des „braunen Fettes" noch als unklar zu bezeichnen.

Über die *mechanische Bedeutung* des Fettgewebes als elastisches Druckpolster durch die Kombination wasserkissenartig wirkender Fettzellen, argyrophiler Faserkörbe und -netze und dem Läppchenbau innerhalb eines nachgiebigen, gekammerten Systems wird auf S. 475 am Beispiel des Fersenpolsters berichtet. Von dieser Art Baufett, das auch in Hungerzuständen nicht oder nur unwesentlich angegriffen wird, unterscheidet sich nur funktionell (nicht histologisch) das *Depotfett*. Dieses bildet die Masse des Panniculus adiposus. Dies soll jedoch nicht besagen, daß er nicht auch eine mechanisch-polsternde Funktion zu erfüllen hätte. Für den Grad der Fettspeicherung im Panniculus adiposus sind nicht allein, wie die tägliche Erfahrung lehrt, die Menge der zugeführten Nahrung verantwortlich, sondern auch Rassen-Konstitutions- und Geschlechtsunterschiede sowie die hormonelle Steuerung. Nicht unbedeutend sind auch topographische Unterschiede: Ein aus der Bauchdecke auf den Handrücken transplantiertes Hautstück bleibt, was die Ausbildung seines subcutanen Fettpolsters betrifft, Bauchhaut. Bei einer allgemeinen Vermehrung der Fettdepots entwickelt sich auf dem Handrücken ein „Bäuchlein" (HOFF, 1953). *Rassenunterschiede* in der Ausbildung des subcutanen Fettpolsters sind gleichfalls gut bekannt. Es braucht nur an die Steatopygie der Hottentottinnen (auch Bantu, Somali) erinnert zu werden, die, entsprechend anderen Landessitten, als Schönheitsmerkmal gewertet wird. *Konstitutionsbedingte Unterschiede* manifestieren sich augenfällig beim Pykniker und Leptosomen (GÜNTHER, 1955). Beispiele, wie *hormonelle Umstellungen* sich auf den Fettansatz auswirken können, kennt man schon lange, wie den zum Fettansatz neigenden Kapaun oder im Klimakterium die überschießende Polsterung, die der Volksmund als „Matronenspeck" bezeichnet. Die physiologisch stärkere Fettpolsterung des weiblichen Organismus wird als sekundäres Geschlechtsmerkmal (SALLER, 1954) gewertet, das zweifellos in Abhängigkeit zur hormonellen Steuerung steht. Zufuhr vermehrter Insulinmengen bedingen einen gesteigerten Speichereffekt (Insulinmast), der sich auch in vitro elektronenmikroskopisch verifizieren ließ (BARRNETT u. BALL, 1960). Hypophysektomie und Adrenalektomie führen dagegen eine Entspeicherung herbei (WERTHEIMER u. SHAPIRO, 1948). Einen im einzelnen noch nicht genauer bekannten regulierenden Einfluß übt das vegetative Nervensystem aus (HAUSBERGER, 1934, 1937). Nicht zur Zufriedenheit geklärt scheint mir die Frage, wo im Fettgewebe *Wasser retiniert* werden kann. Nach Überlegungen, die sich aufgrund histologischer Beobachtungen anstellen lassen, kommt hierfür der Intercellularraum in Betracht, der wasserbindende Mucopolysaccharide enthält. BECKER (1930) fand bei Kleinkindern, die in einem hydropischen Zustand verstorben waren, die Intercellularräume auffallend erweitert. Nach anderer Ansicht tritt das Wasser in das Cytoplasma der Fettzellen ein und wird dort retiniert (BARGMANN, 1964). Der *Wärmeschutz* durch Fettgewebe ist so bekannt, daß sich eine weitere Besprechung erübrigt. Wenn oben hinsichtlich der *Funktion des braunen Fettes* festgestellt wurde, hierüber hätte man nur völlig unzureichende Vorstellungen, so trifft dies ganz besonders für den Menschen zu. In Tierexperimenten (Nagetiere) konnte gezeigt werden (SMITH, 1961; CAMERON u. SMITH, 1964), daß in Abhängigkeit von Kälteeinwirkung eine vermehrte Fetteinlagerung in den interscapulären Fettorganen erfolgt. Auf Zusammenhänge mit dem Winterschlaf wurde von RASMUSSEN (1924) hingewiesen.

7. Vorgänge bei der Speicherung und Entspeicherung

Die Vorgänge während der Speicherung und Entspeicherung des Fettgewebes sollen aus didaktischen Gründen nach folgenden Gesichtspunkten abgehandelt werden, die im Leben freilich kontinuierlich ineinander übergehen: 1. Fettspeicherung in der Reticulumzelle und Bildung der plurivacuolären Fettzelle, 2. Umwandlung der plurivacuolären in die univacuoläre Fettzelle, 3. Fettstoffwechsel der univacuolären Fettzelle, 4. Entspeicherung der univacuolären Fettzelle. Grundsätzlich kann die Zelle aus Kohlenhydraten Fett synthetisieren oder sie nimmt es bereits als Fett bzw. dessen Spaltprodukte mittels eines heute noch nicht restlos geklärten Mechanismus in das Cytoplasma auf. Beide Vorgänge sind mit morphologischen Methoden nicht sichtbar zu machen.

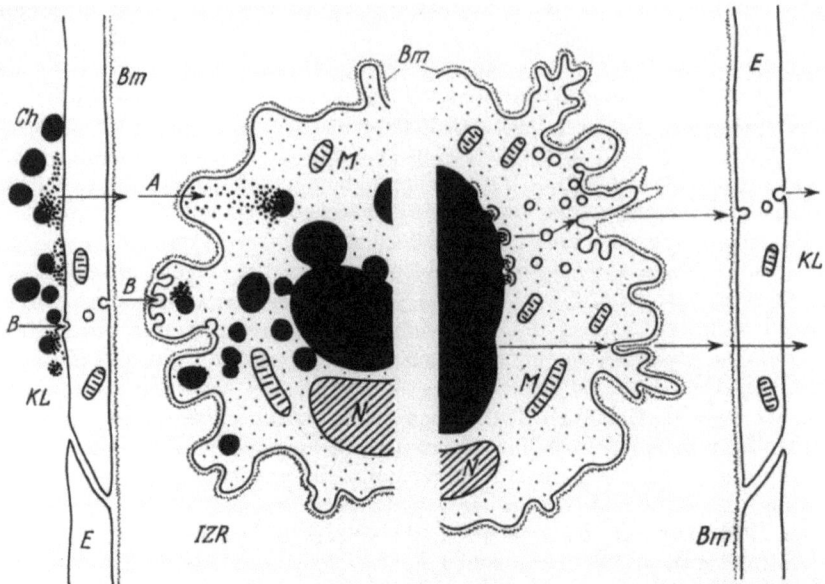

Abb. 10. Vorgänge bei der Fettspeicherung (li) und Entspeicherung (re). Auf der Zeichnung sind 2 nur scheinbar verschiedene Aufnahmemechanismen dargestellt, nämlich durch direkte Plasmalemmpermeation (A) und durch Pinocytose (B). Beide Vorgänge schließen sich nicht aus. Basalmembran (Bm), Chylomikronen (Ch), Endothel (E), Intercellularraum = Interstitium (IZR), Capillarlumen (KL), Mitochondrien (M), Lipide schwarz, Zellkern (N). Die Richtung der Aufnahme und Abgabe durch Pfeile markiert. Unter Benutzung der Abbildungen von WASSERMANN u. McDONALD (1963) und WILLIAMSON (1964)

1. Bei der Entstehung des Fettgewebes treten im Cytoplasma der mesenchymalen *Reticulumzelle* vereinzelt unregelmäßig begrenzte osmiophile Einlagerungen auf. NAPOLITANO (1963) fand, daß sich diese Stammzellen des Fettgewebes elektronenmikroskopisch nicht von Fibroblasten unterscheiden. Nach den Untersuchungen von HAUSBERGER (1938) sind sie jedoch als Lipoblasten bereits determiniert. Während der Fetteinlagerung bildet sich an der Zelloberfläche eine Basalmembran aus. Das endoplasmatische Reticulum ist anscheinend nicht an der Fettsynthese beteiligt; es bildet sich zurück. Vielleicht wird das erste Fett durch Ab- und Umbau von Glykogen gebildet (HAUSBERGER, 1934). Die enge Nachbarschaft von Fetttröpfchen und Mitochondrien läßt vermuten, daß diese mit der Bereitstellung von Energie und Fermenten in den Prozeß direkt eingreifen. Das neugebildete Fett wird in das Grundplasma eingelagert, nicht in eine membranös abgegrenzte Vacuole (NAPOLITANO u. a.). Währenddessen laufen an der Zelloberfläche pinocytotische Vorgänge ab, die vermutlich mit der weiteren Stoffaufnahme in Zusammenhang stehen, bis schließlich eine *plurivacuoläre Fettzelle* entstanden ist (Abb. 10).

2. Durch progressive Fettspeicherung wandelt sich die plurivacuoläre Zelle in die *univacuoläre Fettzelle* um. Über diesen Mechanismus liegen mehrere, im einzelnen nicht völlig übereinstimmende Beobachtungen vor.

a) Das Fett kann gleichfalls wieder aus abgebautem Glykogen synthetisiert worden sein (FAWCETT, 1947; WERTHEIMER u. SHAPIRO, 1948), das auch elektronenmikroskopisch im Grundplasma reichlich gefunden wird (Abb. 9) (NAPOLITANO, 1963). Der Nachschub von Glucose erfolgt aus dem Blut durch den extracellulären Raum. Bei einer experimentell durch Insulin in vitro erhöhten Speicherbereitschaft beobachteten BARRNETT u. BALL (1960) an der Zelloberfläche eine auffällige Ausbildung von Cytoplasmafortsätzen mit Pinocytosetätigkeit. Offensichtlich steht diese erhöhte Zellaktivität mit der Aufnahme von Glucose in Zusammenhang. Unter physiologischen Bedingungen dürften die Vorgänge weniger ausgeprägt sein, aber grundsätzlich gleichartig ablaufen. Bei der Bildung und Segregation des Neutralfettes spielen Phospholipide eine im einzelnen noch nicht näher bekannte Rolle. So geben auch die kleinen, dicht an der Oberfläche großer Neutralfetteinschlüsse gelegenen Tröpfchen (Abb. 9) eine positive Phospholipid-Reaktion (Bakerscher Hämateintest) (LEVER, 1957; FAWCETT, 1952). Die Vermutung, sie würden durch Transformation aus Mitochondrien hervorgehen, hat sich nicht bestätigt.

b) Über den Mechanismus der Speicherung von experimentell über den Verdauungsapparat angebotenen Neutralfetten in Depot-Fettzellen sind wir durch die Untersuchungen von WASSERMANN u. McDONALD (1963) und WILLIAMSON (1964) gut orientiert. Die nach enteraler Resorption im Blut suspendierten Fett-Chylomikronen (0,5—1,5 µ Durchmesser; Bestandteile: 80% Triglyceride + Phospholipide, Cholesterin und Proteine) werden anscheinend nach fermentativer Spaltung an der Endotheloberfläche (oder allerfeinster Verteilung?) in elektronmikroskopisch unsichtbarer Form durch die Capillarwand durchgeschleust und in das Interstitium abgegeben (Abb. 10, A). WILLIAMSON möchte Pinocytosevorgänge (eigentlich Cytopempsis) für diese transcelluläre Passage nicht ausschließen. Auch im Interstitium ist noch kein Fett nachweisbar. Es tritt erst wieder im Cytoplasma der Fettzellen in Erscheinung, und zwar in Gestalt massenhaft kleinster Tröpfchen (50—300 Å Durchmesser) (WASSERMANN). Man muß also annehmen, daß erst nach Aufnahme der Spaltprodukte in die Fettzelle die Resynthese stattfand. Für den Aufnahmemechanismus halten WASSERMANN und McDONALD Pinocytosevorgänge nicht für notwendig, während WILLIAMSON an der Zelloberfläche Protuberanzen und zahlreiche Pinocytosebläschen nachweisen konnte. Beide Untersucher sind sich darüber einig, daß die im Cytoplasma erscheinenden osmiophilen Tröpfchen nicht von Membranen umgeben sind (wie dies nach einer pinocytotischen Aufnahme der Fall sein müßte!). Unter ständigem Konflux vergrößern sich die Tröpfchen und werden schließlich in die großen Tropfen inkorporiert (Abb. 9, 10). Inwieweit auch bei diesem Mechanismus Phospholipide eine Rolle spielen, muß weiteren Untersuchungen vorbehalten bleiben.

Experimentell läßt sich eine Umwandlung plurivacuolärer Fettzellen in die univacuoläre Form nach Durchschneidung der versorgenden vegetativen Nervenfasern erreichen (HAUSBERGER, 1934). Die vermehrte Fetteinlagerung äußert sich in einer Gewichtszunahme der Fettläppchen. Stellt sich die Innervation wieder ein, dann erfolgt eine Entspeicherung unter Rückbildung zu plurivacuolären Zellen (HAUSBERGER, 1937).

3. Man muß annehmen, daß die gespeicherten Fette nur beschränkte Zeit in der Fettzelle deponiert bleiben und ständig ausgetauscht werden. Allerdings blieb der Nachweis dieses Stoffwechsels Markierungsversuchen mit Isotopen vorbehalten. SCHOENHEIMER u. RITTENBERGER (1935) gelang es damit nachzuweisen, daß markiertes Öl nach der Verfütterung zuerst umgebaut und in den Depots abgelagert wird, bevor es im Organismus der weiteren Verarbeitung zugeführt wird.

4. Die Entspeicherung der Fettzelle erscheint elektronenmikroskopisch wie die Umkehrung des Speicherungsvorganges (Abb. 10), nur sind die in das Capillarlumen abgegebenen mobilisierten Fette bzw. ihre Spaltprodukte nicht darzustellen (WASSERMANN u. McDONALD, 1963). WILLIAMSON (1964) stellte an der Oberfläche des abzubauenden Fettropfens eine rege Bläschenbildung fest (Abb. 10), die als Transportvacuolen an der Oberfläche der Zelle ihren Inhalt (freie Fettsäuren?) in den extracellulären Raum entlassen. In schweren Hungerzuständen werden die Fettdepots fast vollständig abgebaut. Bei der Säuglingsatrophie entwickelt sich das plurivacuoläre Fettgewebe so weit zurück, daß nur noch Reticulumzellen in Gestalt der Primitivorgane zurückbleiben (WASSERMANN, 1926). Eine solch vollständige Rückbildung wird indessen von HOFFMANN (1951) bestritten. Sie findet mehr einen epithelialen Charakter des Zellverbandes. Beim Erwachsenen ist die Differenzierung der Zelle offensichtlich schon so weit fortgeschritten (HOFFMANN), daß der ursprüngliche Zustand retikulären Bindegewebes nicht mehr angenommen werden kann. Es entsteht die „seröse Fettzelle", eine Zelle, in der anstelle des Fettes eine seröse Flüssigkeit trat. Einzelne univacuoläre, noch mit Fett gefüllte Zellen bleiben eingestreut liegen. Von diesen Abbauvorgängen wird bekanntlich bevorzugt das Depot-Fett betroffen. Weshalb gerade dieses und nicht das Baufett, wissen wir nicht, ebensowenig wie der hierzu notwendige Steuerungsmechanismus funktioniert. Die Entspeicherung des braunen Fettes führt zu kompakten, epithelartigen Zellkomplexen (HOFFMANN).

C. Mikroskopische und submikroskopische Anatomie von Corium und Subcutis
I. Die Basalmembran

An der Grenze zwischen Epidermis und Corium bildet sich, wie überall dort, wo epitheliale und mesenchymale Elemente verbunden sind, eine Basalmembran aus, deren Zugehörigkeit zum Bindegewebe als weitgehend gesichert gelten darf.

Eine entsprechende Membran umhüllt auch Fettzellen, Nerven und Blutgefäße. Sie grenzt damit das Interstitium, durch dessen Grundsubstanz der Stoffaustausch stattfindet, von den angrenzenden und eingelagerten Geweben ab. Ganz allgemein kann die Basalmembran als eine Verdichtung der Grundsubstanz mit einem eingelagerten argyrophilen Faserfilz betrachtet werden. Ohne Basalmembran sind alle integrierenden Bestandteile des Interstitiums, wie Zellen und Fasern.

Die Bezeichnung „Basalmembran" wird heute in der Histologie nicht einheitlich verwendet. Die Lichtmikroskopie versteht darunter eine 0,5 μ dicke Schicht, die aus den oben genannten Bestandteilen, argyrophilen Fasern und homogener Grundsubstanz, besteht, während in der Nomenklatur der Elektronenmikroskopie unter „Basalmembran" eine 200—350 Å (VOGEL, 1958; SELBY, 1955) dicke, unter der Epithelzellbasis gelegene homogene Lamelle verstanden wird, für die verschiedentlich auch Bezeichnungen wie „Dermalmembran" oder „lamina densa" eingeführt wurden. Die faserigen Elemente rechnet die Elektronenmikroskopie nicht zur Basalmembran, wie sie auch die argyrophile Faser nicht als besonderen Fasertyp anerkennt (vgl. S. 444 und Abb. 12).

Da die Basalmembran den Verzahnungen von Epidermis und Papillarkörper folgt, ist ihre Gestalt von Region zu Region entsprechend unterschiedlich kompliziert. Sie erscheint im lichtmikroskopischen Bereich bei Rutinefärbungen annähernd homogen. Die Azanfärbung bringt jedoch ein Geflecht von Fasern zur Darstellung, das nach Versilberung noch deutlicher hervortritt. Es imponiert in der Flächenansicht als Netzwerk (Abb. 11c), in dessen Maschen die Basalfüßchen der Epidermiszellen eingelassen sind. Auf Querschnitten erscheinen diese Anteile des Netzes als Leisten (PLENK, 1927) oder keulenförmige Fortsätze (HOMMA, 1922). Es handelt sich aber, wie ODLAND (1950) klären konnte, um bügelförmig verlaufende argyrophile Fasern, die sich zwischen die Basalfüßchen einschieben und wieder in das basale Grundnetz zurückkehren (Abb. 12). Durch die Verprojizierung erscheinen die Bügel als Zapfen oder keulenförmige Endauftreibungen. Im Bereich der seitlichen Abhänge der Bindegewebspapillen tritt anstelle der netzartigen eine bevorzugt parallele Anordnung der Fasern. Hieraus kann geschlossen werden, daß die basalen Zelldifferenzierungen leistenförmig gestaltet sind. Am Boden der Täler zwischen den Papillen oder im Bereich der Haarbälge fehlen solche basalen Zelldifferenzierungen anscheinend weitgehend. An den Versilberungspräparaten wird außerdem deutlich, daß die argyrophilen Fasern der Basalmembran kontinuierlich in die kollagenen Fasern des Papillarkörpers übergehen (Abb. 11a), oder anders formuliert, die Fasern der Basalmembran sind die durch eine argyrophile Substanz besonders imprägnierbaren, in sich vernetzten, Endaufzweigungen der Kollagenfasern des Coriums. Im Bereich der Basalmembran endet außerdem das feine Netzwerk der elastischen Fasern des Coriumbindegewebes. Weder an gefärbten Präparaten noch im polarisierten Licht ist mit Sicherheit zu entscheiden, ob das terminale elastische Netz bis an das argyrophile Fasernetz reicht und sich mit diesem durchflicht oder unterhalb von diesem endet. Nach den Untersuchungen von DICK (1947) und BRAUN-FALCO (1954, 1955) sind elastische Elemente nicht am Aufbau der Basalmembran beteiligt, während COOPER (1956) dies bejaht. Da durch die Versilberung unter besonderen Umständen (S. 445) auch elastische Fasern erfaßt werden, dürfte die Entscheidung hierüber elektronenmikroskopischen Untersuchungen vorbehalten bleiben. Nirgendwo ließen sich die elastischen Fasern bis in die Räume zwischen den Basalfüßchen verfolgen.

Histochemische Untersuchungen im lichtmikroskopischen Bereich (vgl. BRAUN-FALCO, Bd. I/2; GRAUMANN, 1964) haben im gesamten Bereich der Basalmembran einen unterschiedlich starken Ausfall der PJS-Reaktion (Abb. 11b) zu verzeichnen (MCMANUS, 1946; GERSH u. CATCHPOLE, 1949, speziell Haut), der auf einen hohen Gehalt an neutralen Mucopolysacchariden (BRAUN-FALCO, 1955) zu beziehen ist. Sie durchtränken und umschließen das argyrophile Fasernetz (MCMANUS, 1954). Saure Mucopolysaccharide oder Glykogen, Lipide und Proteine wurden in der Basalmembran nicht gefunden (STROUGHTON u. WELLS, 1950; BRAUN-FALCO, 1955, 1957). Auffallend ist ihre hohe Beständigkeit gegen Fermente. Nach der Einwirkung von Testis- oder Streptokokkenhyaluronidase, Diastase, proteolytischen Fermenten wird keine Veränderung beobachtet. Nur Pektinase

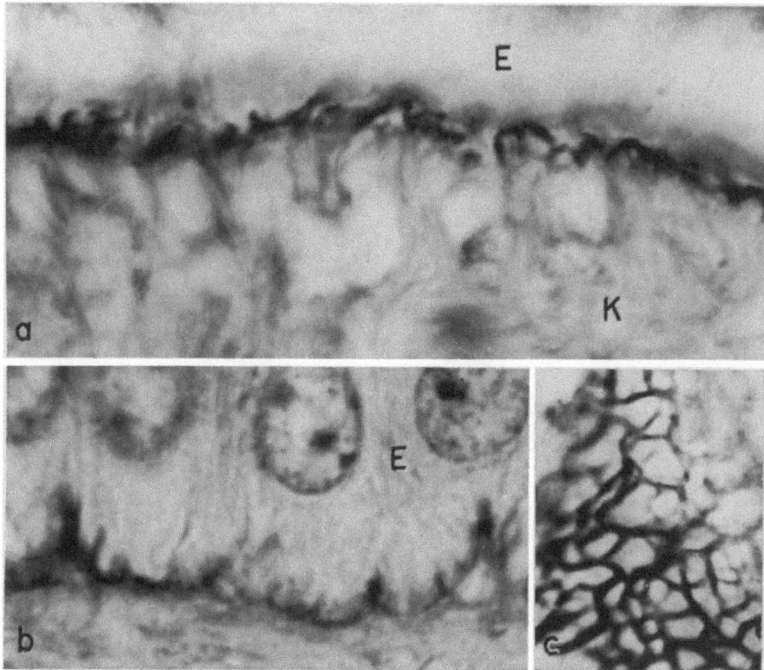

Abb. 11a—c. a Argyrophile Fasern der Basalmembran. Der arkadenförmige Verlauf ist stellenweise sichtbar. Epidermis (*E*), Kollagene Fasern (*K*), die in die argyrophilen der Basalmembran (schwarz) übergehen. Versilberung nach BIELSCHOWSKY-GÖMÖRI. Vergr. 2000fach. b Basalmembran nach der PJS-Reaktion und Gegenfärbung mit Hämatoxylin. Vergr. 2000fach. c Flachschnitt durch das Netzwerk der argyrophilen Fasern. (Gleiches Präparat wie a)

und eine Kollagenase (aus Clostridium welchii) sind in der Lage, die Mucopolysaccharide der Basalmembran zu lösen (BRAUN-FALCO, 1955; nach GERSH u. CATCHPOLE, 1949, vermag dies auch Trypsin und Pepsin).

Für die Bildung der Mucopolysaccharide der Basalmembran dürften Fibroblasten verantwortlich gemacht werden (S. 433). Jedoch scheint es nicht ausgeschlossen, daß die Lamina densa von den basalen Epidermiszellen erzeugt wird, wie BRAUN-FALCO (1955) und PIERCE et al. (1963) vermuten. Diese dünne Schicht, die im elektronenmikroskopischen Bild allein sichtbar ist, kann mit dem Lichtmikroskop nicht aufgelöst werden. Sie hat eine Dicke von ungefähr 350 Å (SELBY, 1955) und folgt in einem Abstand von 300—400 Å allen Einbuchtungen und füßchenförmigen Ausläufern der basalen Epidermiszellen. Elektronenmikroskopisch erscheint sie amorph, manchmal, vielleicht in Abhängigkeit vom Funktionszustand oder der Art der Fixation, feingranulär oder filamentös.

Von der lichtmikroskopisch definierten Basalmembran ist im Elektronenmikroskop nur wenig auszumachen. Die Stränge des Fasernetzes sind wegen der außerordentlich geringen Schnittdicke nur vereinzelt getroffen. Die Mikrofibrillen, aus denen die Fasern aufgebaut sind, unterscheiden sich außer ihres etwas geringeren Durchmessers (SELBY, 1955) nicht von den übrigen kollagenen Fasern (vgl. Abschnitt A, II). Von der PJS-positiven Grundsubstanz können, ausgenommen die Lamina densa, nur spärliche Reste nachgewiesen werden. Entweder wurden die Mucopolysaccharide zum Großteil herausgelöst oder sie geben bei der üblichen Präparationsmethode keinen ausreichenden Kontrast. Entscheidend konnte die Elektronenmikroskopie in die Streitfrage eingreifen, ob die Bindegewebsfasern des Stratum papillare kontinuierlich in die fibrillären Elemente der Epidermis-

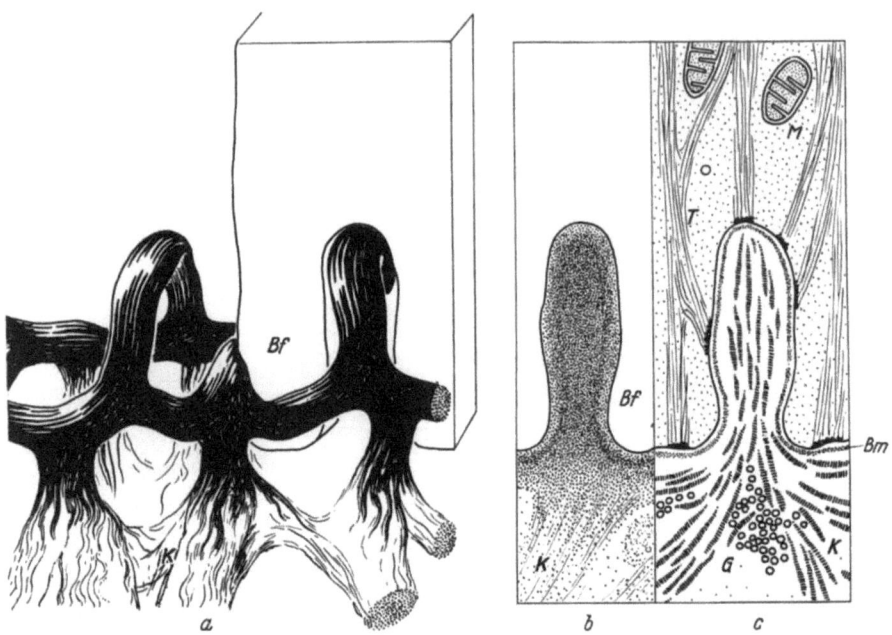

Abb. 12a—c. Schema zum Begriff „Basalmembran" in der Anwendung der klassischen Lichtmikroskopie a, in der Histochemie b und in der Elektronenmikroskopie c, erläutert an einem Epidermisabschnitt mit zahlreichen Basalfüßchen (Bf). b und c sind im Schnitt gezeichnet. Elektronenmikroskopisch sichtbare Basalmembran (Bm), Grundsubstanz (G), Kollagenfibrillenbündel (K), Mitochondrien (M), Tonofilamente mit Befestigungen am Plasmalemm (T). In a argyrophile Fasern massiv schwarz, in b Darstellung der Mucopolysaccharide durch PJS-Reaktion

zellen übergehen. Nirgendwo wurde eine Kontinuität beobachtet; stets war die Basalmembran zwischengeschaltet (PEASE, 1951; SELBY, 1955).

Experimentell erarbeitete Argumente für die funktionelle Bedeutung der Basalmembran im Bereich der Haut stehen noch aus. Wir sind also in diesem Punkt auf Überlegungen, Folgerungen und Analogien angewiesen. Zweifellos dient das aus argyrophilen Fasern aufgebaute Netz der Befestigung der Epidermis, deren basale Zellen mit ihren Basalfüßchen in den Netzmaschen stecken. Auch ist die klassische Auffassung von der „Kittmasse", also einem mechanisch wirksamen Faktor der Mucopolysaccharide bei der Befestigung der Zellen, nicht grundsätzlich abzulehnen. Nicht minder wichtig ist jedoch ihre Bedeutung für den Stoffwechsel. Alle Stoffe, Baustoffe und Schlacken, O_2 und CO_2 müssen auf ihrem Weg zwischen Epithel und Gefäßsystem diese Basalmembran passieren. Im Modellbeispiel der Darmschleimhaut, wo resorbierte Stoffe in solchen Mengen anfallen, daß sie ohne Schwierigkeit elektronenmikroskopisch nachgewiesen werden können, drängen sie das elektronendichte Material der Basalmembran auseinander, das sich sofort hinter den Resorbaten wieder schließt. Silbernitrat wird jedoch z. T. zurückgehalten und in relativ hoher Konzentration in der Basalmembran angereichert (eigene Untersuchungen). Diese letzte Beobachtung darf nicht dazu verleiten, die Basalmembran nur als eine semipermeable, statische Membran, etwa als eine Dialysiermembran aufzufassen. Sie ist vielmehr eine biologisch aktive Mucopolysaccharidschicht, in der bisher niemals präformierte Poren nachgewiesen wurden, die dem Stoffdurchtritt dienen könnten. Über die Bedeutung der neutralen Mucopolysaccharide können wir heute nicht viel mehr als Spekulationen anstellen. Da man sie an Bürstensäumen resorbierender Zellen, im Bereich pinocytotischer Einsenkungen oder an der Oberfläche von Protozoen sehr reichlich findet, stehen sie vermutlich mit den Vorgängen der Stoffaufnahme in Beziehung. Welche Funktion sie hierbei zu erfüllen haben, ist unsicher.

Regionale Unterschiede im Bau der Basalmembran, die vor allem die Dicke der argyrophilen Fasern betreffen, wurden von DICK (1947) beobachtet. Im Bereich des mechanisch weniger beanspruchten Handrückens fand er die Fasern dünner als im Bereich des Handtellers. Auch der Grad der Befestigung der basalen Epidermisschicht ist nicht überall gleich. An Hand- und Fußsohle findet man langgestreckte Basalfüßchen und entsprechend lange „Basalmembranzapfen" bzw. hohe argyrophile Faserschlingen, im Bereich von Hand- und Fußrücken ist diese Verbindung wesentlich schwächer ausgebildet (DICK, 1947, und eigene Beobachtungen).

II. Das Corium

1. Das Stratum papillare

Die Unterlage der Epidermis bildet das Stratum papillare bzw. der Papillarkörper, wie man auch die Gesamtheit der Papillen zu bezeichnen pflegt. Die Grenzfläche ist zur Basalmembran differenziert. Die zwischen Papillarkörper und Stratum reticulare liegende Schicht trägt auch die Bezeichnung Stratum subpapillare. Sie ist hinsichtlich ihrer Struktur nicht vom Papillarkörper abgesetzt, sondern bildet eigentlich den basalen Anteil des Stratum papillare.

Die Strukturanalyse dieser Schichten stößt lichtmikroskopisch wegen des sehr komplizierten Oberflächenreliefs und wegen der verwickelten Textur ihrer faserigen Bauelemente auf beträchtliche Schwierigkeit. Das normale histologische Schnittpräparat ist zur Klärung der Verhältnisse völlig unzureichend. Sie gelang an Totalpräparaten, bei denen die Epidermis durch Maceration entfernt war. Eine weitere Schwierigkeit kann nur dadurch umgangen werden, daß die Haut noch an der Leiche fixiert wird. Im unfixierten Zustand herausgeschnittene Hautstückchen erfahren besonders durch den Einbau elastischer Elemente unkontrollierbare Veränderungen ihrer Textur.

Die Gestalt des Papillarkörpers wurde von BLASCHKO (1887), GREB (1940), HORSTMANN u. Mitarb. (1950—1957) und FLEISCHHAUER (1951—1955) an Totalpräparaten genauer untersucht. GREB macerierte das Epithel und stellte isoliert die Bindegewebspapillen dar, während HORSTMANN und FLEISCHHAUER den Papillarkörper entfernten und die Unterseite der Epidermis, also das Negativbild des Papillarkörpers, nach Trocknung (nach SEMPER) studierten. Alle Untersucher konnten auffällige Gestaltunterschiede des Papillarkörpers in Abhängigkeit von mechanischer Beanspruchung einer Hautregion und vom Lebensalter feststellen. In den ersten Lebensjahren bildet sich der Papillarkörper erst vollständig aus (FLEISCHHAUER). Bei einem 6jährigen Kind fand GREB (1940) Hautzonen, die noch nicht dem Bild des Erwachsenen entsprachen. Im jugendlichen und mittleren Lebensalter sind folgende Formen und Aggregationstypen der Papillen zu beobachten (Abb. 13): 1. Im Bereich der Kopfhaut, des Nasenrückens, der Schläfe, der Stirn, der Rhaphe perinei und der Scrotalhaut sind sehr spärlich niedrige, in kleinen Gruppen stehende Papillen zu finden. Größere Flächen sind frei von Papillen. 2. Schlanke, niedrige, fingerförmige Papillen finden sich in der Haut der Extremitäten. 3. Plattenförmige, oft breitbasige Papillen, deren Oberfläche bisweilen kammförmig gezackt ist, bilden die subepidermale Lage im Bereich des

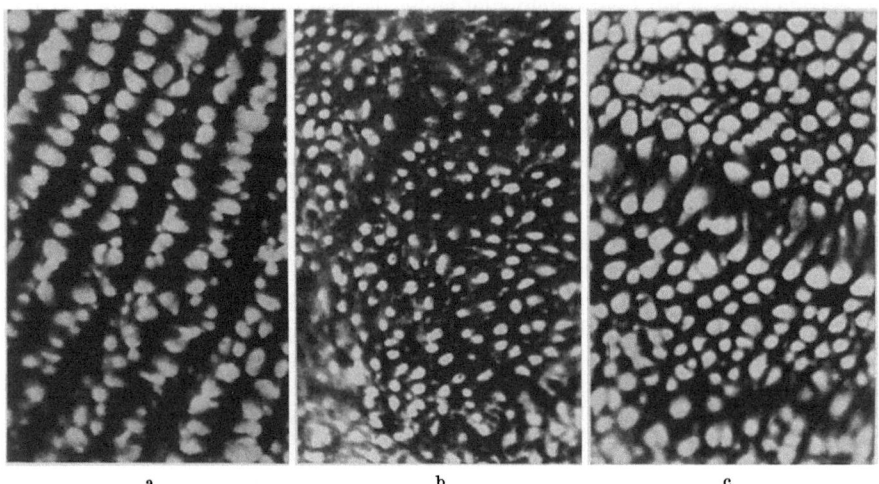

Abb. 13 a—c. Papillarkörper der Haut nach Entfernung der Epidermis in der Ansicht von oben. a Leistenhaut der Vola manus, b Streckseite des Unterarmes eines 59jährigen Mannes, c aus dem Gebiet über der Patella des gleichen Mannes. Vergr. ungefähr 25fach. (Nach GREB, 1940; Abb. a nach BRAUS, 1960)

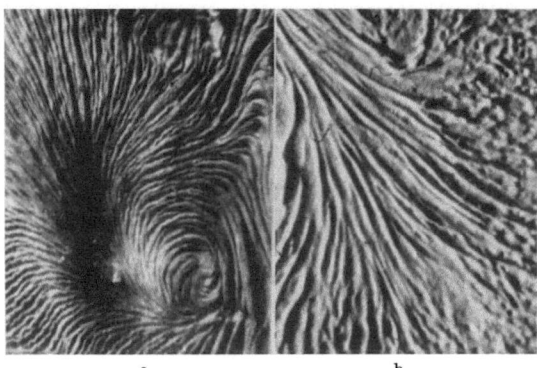

Abb. 14a u. b. Unterfläche der abgelösten Epidermis mit Negativbild der Papillarleisten (Sempersches Trockenpräparat). a Aus dem Gehörgang eines 7 Monate alten Feten (Vergr. 40fach). b Von der Glans penis eines 28jährigen (Vergr. 30fach). (Aus HORSTMANN, 1957)

Rumpfes. 4. Hohe, dicke, oft keulen- und pilzförmige Papillen in dichtgedrängter Anordnung sind typisch für mechanisch besonders stark beanspruchte Hautregionen wie Olecranon und Patella. 5. Meist in Doppelreihen stehende, große und massive Papillen, mit Papillenbüschel an der Oberfläche, findet man in der Leistenhaut der Hohlhand und Fußsohle. Die Höhe der Papillen beträgt hier 0,2 cm. 6. Reine Papillarleisten beobachteten HORSTMANN (1952) und BUTTGE (1959) im Bereich der Glans penis, der Labia minora (Abb. 14), des Gehörganges, des Anus und, wie bereits bekannt, im Hyponychium. Im Bereich der Felderhaut fehlen unter den die Felder begrenzenden Furchen die Papillen oder sie sind gespalten (Abb. 13c) oder sehr niedrig. Um das 60. Lebensjahr beginnt allmählich die Rückbildung des Papillarkörpers. GREB fand bei einem 80jährigen die Haut der medialen Seite des Oberarmes frei von Papillen und glattkonturiert. HORSTMANN (1952) stellte eine besondere und im Prinzip immer wiederkehrende Zuordnung der Papillen zu Haarbälgen und Schweißdrüsenausführungsgängen fest, die er als „Motivbildung" bezeichnet. Er unterscheidet eine rosetten- und eine kokardenförmige Anordnung (Abb. 15). Abweichungen von diesem Muster finden sich vor allem in der Genital- und Analregion (BUTTGE, 1959). Die Rosetten und Kokarden kommen dadurch zustande, daß sich um die epidermalen Anhangsgebilde konzentrisch besonders starke oder plattenförmige Papillen gruppieren und an der Epidermisunterseite ein korrespondierendes Negativbild hinterlassen. Um ein Haar oder eine Haargruppe ordnen sich kreisförmig die Schweißdrüsenausführungsgänge, die dann als „zifferblattförmige" Ausprägung (HORSTMANN) imponieren (Abb. 15c). Die „Motivbildung" fehlt in Hautregionen, wo keine Anhangsgebilde vorhanden sind. EICHNER (1954) stellte fest, daß die Motive in

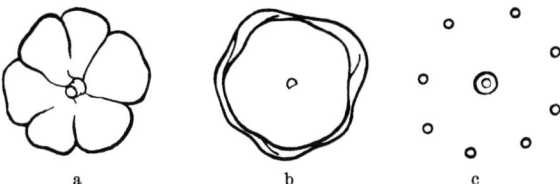

Abb. 15a—c. Schematische Zeichnung der „Motivbildung" nach HORSTMANN. a Rosettenförmig um ein Haar oder Schweißdrüsenausführungsgang angeordneter Epithelwall mit radiär stehenden Furchen. b Kokardenförmig angeordnete Epithelleisten. c Zifferblattförmige Anordnung der Schweißdrüsenausführungsgänge um ein Haar. (Aus HORSTMANN, 1957)

den tieferen Schichten der Cutis nicht streng beibehalten werden, indem Schweißdrüsenausführungsgänge ihren Motivbezirk verlassen und sich anderen Bezirken anschließen.

Die Entwicklung des Papillarkörpers und seine Beziehungen zur Entstehung des Haarstriches (vgl. PINKUS, Bd. II/1) wurde von FLEISCHHAUER (1953) untersucht. Er konnte einen direkten Zusammenhang zwischen der Ausbildung der Papillen und der Anordnung der Haare bestätigen (LUDWIG, 1921). Das bestimmende Element ist auch hier die Epidermis, in der in einer typischen Anordnung bestimmte Zellgruppen als Haar- und Papillenanlagen vorgegeben sind.

Der Papillarkörper stellt eine nicht unbedeutende Oberflächenvergrößerung dar, die von KATZBERG (1957, 1958) an der Bauchhaut in verschiedenen Lebensaltern genauer bestimmt wurde. Es ergaben sich, bezogen auf 1 mm² äußere Hautoberfläche, folgende Mittelwerte: bis 20. Lebensjahr 2,75 mm², vom 20.—40. Lebensjahr 2,67 mm², vom 40.—60. Lebensjahr 2,15 mm², vom 60.—80. Lebensjahr 1,9 mm², über 80. Lebensjahr 1,16 mm². Die Untersuchungen ergaben außerdem, wie auch die von GREB und HORSTMANN über die Gestalt des Papillarkörpers, keinen Anhalt für Geschlechtsunterschiede.

Im lichtmikroskopischen Bild besteht das Stratum papillare aus einem sehr locker gefügten Gewebe relativ dünner kollagener Fasern, elastischer Netze und aus argyrophilen Fasergeflechten, die an der Epidermisgrenze, an der Oberfläche von Capillaren und Nervenfasern, Drüsenausführungsgängen und Haarbälgen die Basalmembranen bzw. das Capillargrundhäutchen bilden. Grundsubstanz ist entsprechend der lockeren Textur reichlich vorhanden. An Zellen sind außer Fibroblasten, besonders im Bereich von Capillaren, Mastzellen und Histiocyten zu beobachten, außerdem vereinzelt eingestreute Pigmentzellen.

Über die Textur der Fasern in den Papillen liegen bisher keine erschöpfenden Untersuchungen vor. Wie Übersichtsaufnahmen im polarisierten Licht (Abb. 16) zeigen, besteht hier eine unterschiedlich starke Durchflechtung der kollagenen

Fasern, die vorzugsweise senkrecht zur Epidermisunterseite orientiert sind (Untersuchung an Achselhaut und Fußsohle). Im Stratum subpapillare sind die Fasern gröber und durchflechten sich, wie Flachschnitte erkennen ließen, unter fast rechtwinkliger Überkreuzung (PETERSEN, 1935; SCHREIBER, 1942). Auf Querschnitten durch die Haut wird deutlich (Abb. 16), daß die Fasern zum Großteil schräg zur Oberfläche verlaufen (PETERSEN). Der Steigungswinkel ist im Bereich der Stirnhaut ganz besonders flach. An Stellen, wo der Papillarkörper fehlt, ziehen die Fasern sogar fast parallel zur Epidermisoberfläche. Der Anteil der elastischen Elemente und die Dicke der einzelnen Faser sind regional außerordentlich verschieden (DICK, 1951). Im allgemeinen haben breite Papillen stärkere Fasern als schlanke (SCHALLWEGG, 1942). Die bevorzugte Verlaufsrichtung fällt nur ungefähr mit der der kollagenen Fasern zusammen. So steigen im Bereich der Fingerbeere auch die elastischen Fasern fast senkrecht zur Epidermis auf, verzweigen sich und bilden im Bereich der Basalmembran ein aus dünnsten elastischen Fasern bestehendes flächenhaftes Netzwerk (vgl. Handbuchbeitrag PINKUS, 1927, Abb. 68). An der Oberfläche von Capillaren und Ausführungsgängen der Schweißdrüsen vernetzen sich gleichfalls die Fasern, wodurch diese Gebilde im Gewebe elastisch verspannt sind. Fettgewebe fehlt in allen Schichten des Coriums völlig.

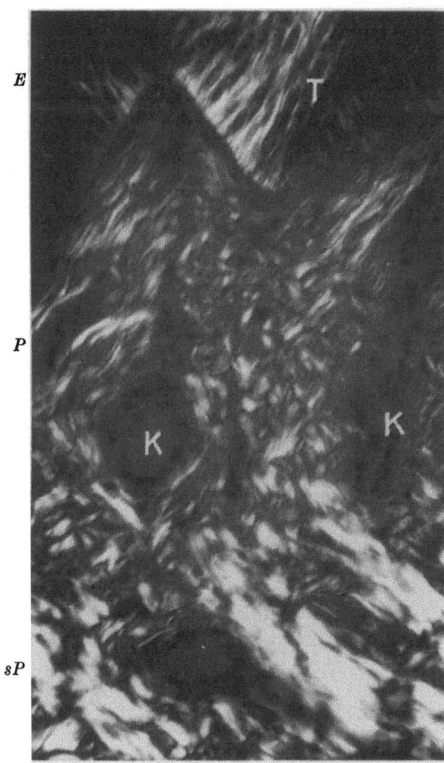

Abb. 16. Querschnitt durch Epidermis (E), Stratum papillare (P) und subpapillare (sP) im polarisierten Licht zur Darstellung des Faserverlaufes (Achselhaut). Im Stratum papillare ist die geflechtartige Textur deutlich sichtbar. Im Stratum subpapillare verlaufen die wesentlich dickeren Faserzüge schräg zur Epidermisoberseite. In der Epidermis Tonofibrillen (T), deren Verlaufsrichtung sich in die der kollagenen Fasern des Coriums fortsetzt. Capillaren (K). Vergr. 600fach

Wenn man auch für die feine Felderung der Haut das morphologische Substrat in der besonderen Gestaltung des Papillarkörpers, im Fehlen von Papillen, gespaltenen oder besonders niedrigen Papillen gefunden hat (PÄTZOLD, 1932; GREB, 1940) (Abb. 13b, c), so stehen entsprechende Beobachtungen für die groben Faltenbildungen noch aus (BETTMANN, 1928).

Die Ausbildung des Papillarkörpers wird meist funktionell als eine „Verzahnung" und Befestigung der Epidermis auf ihrer Unterlage gedeutet. Von ELZE (1960) wird diese Interpretation z. T. in Frage gestellt mit dem Hinweis, daß in der Greisenhaut der Papillarkörper so gut wie völlig fehle, die Haftfestigkeit jedoch nicht merklich geringer sei. Allerdings liegen meines Wissens keine vergleichenden Untersuchungen über die Abscherfestigkeit von Hautgebieten mit hohem, niedrigem oder fehlendem Papillarkörper vor. Hier könnte man einwenden, daß in Gebieten, die einer besonderen mechanischen Beanspruchung ausgesetzt sind, wie Ellenbogen- oder Knievorderseite, besonders hohe Papillen gefunden werden (GREB, 1940). Sie haben aber offensichtlich eine andere Bedeutung (s. unten). Die mechanische Beanspruchung des Papillarkörpers bei Verschiebung der Haut steht ungeachtet dessen außer Frage. Die Fortsetzung des Tonofibrillenverlaufes in der Epidermis in die Verlaufsrichtung der kollagenen Fasern des Stratum papillare (Abb. 16) beweist, daß der bei Verschiebung der Epidermis entstehende Zug auf das Bindegewebe der Papillen übertragen und von hier aus über die schräg verlaufenden Fasern des Stratum subpapillare auf das Stratum reticulare fortgeleitet wird. Ohne Zweifel stellt der innige verzahnende Kontakt von Basalmembran und Epidermisbasis den mechanisch wichtigsten Faktor für die Verbindung beider Schichten dar (Abb. 12a).

Sieht man von der mechanischen Bedeutung des Papillarkörpers ab, so erfüllt er durch die beträchtliche Vergrößerung der Austauschoberfläche zwischen Bindegewebe und Epidermis eine oft nicht genügend beachtete trophische Funktion. Nimmt im Alter die Höhe der Papillen ab, so verringert sich im gleichen Maße auch die Dicke der Epidermis (KATZBERG, 1958). Die Korrelation zwischen den beiden Komponenten, Austauschoberfläche und Epidermisdicke, zu bestimmen, erscheint wünschenswert, ebenso die Beziehung zur Zahl der Mitosen und zur Mitoserate. Bei solchen funktionellen Betrachtungen ist zu bedenken, daß mit der Verringerung der Papillarhöhe die capillare Endstrecke und damit auch die Austauschoberfläche kleiner wird. Für die hohe Stoffwechselaktivität des Stratum papillare sprechen die histochemischen Befunde an den Bindegewebszellen, die hier eine stärkere Fermentaktivität entwickeln (s. S. 431) als im Stratum reticulare, die große Zahl von Mastzellen, wie auch die relativ höhere Konzentration von sauren Mucopolysacchariden (Hyaluronsäure und Chondroitinsulfat) in der Grundsubstanz (SYLVÉN, 1941; BUNTING, 1950; KAWASE u. SUNAHARA, 1952; NIEBAUER u. RAAB, 1961), die nach der geltenden Ansicht als „Überträgerstoffe" fungieren. Sie machen in der menschlichen Haut ungefähr 25 mg-% aus (PEARCE u. WATSON, 1949). Vermehrt findet man sie in den als mechanisch besonders beansprucht bezeichneten Hautgebieten, also an Stellen, an denen ein großer Zellabrieb erfolgt und damit ein größerer Nachschub mit vermehrtem Stofftransport notwendig wird (SYLVÉN, 1941; ELZE, 1960). An einer ausgedehnten basalen Oberfläche können eben mehr Mitosen ablaufen als an einer kleinen. Hierin dürfte also die Bedeutung des Papillarkörpers zu suchen sein und nicht in einer mechanischen Bedürfnissen entsprechenden „Verzahnung".

Auf die mögliche Bedeutung einer für die Tastempfindung wichtigen Wechselwirkung zwischen den relativ festen basalen Epidermiskämmen an der Fingerbeere und den leicht verformbaren, flüssigkeitsreichen Bindegewebspapillen, in denen die nervösen Endapparate liegen, wird von CAUNA (1954) hingewiesen. Bei Druck auf die Epidermisoberfläche würde das im Bereich der Leisten liegende nachgiebigere Stratum corneum verformt, der darunterliegende epitheliale Mittelkamm nach einer Seite ausweichen und eine Erregung des ihn umspinnenden Nervenplexus auslösen, außerdem auch auf die benachbarten Meissnerschen Tastkörperchen einwirken.

Altersveränderungen, die sich am Papillarkörper sichtbar äußern, wurden bereits oben ausführlich behandelt, so daß hier eine Zusammenfassung ausreichend erscheint. Die Veränderungen betreffen eine zunehmende Atrophie der Papillen, eine kompensatorische Verbreiterung der Epithelkämme verbunden mit einer progressiven Atrophie der Epidermis, eine Verdichtung und Zunahme des Polymerisationsgrades der Mucopolysaccharide, aber auch eine mengenmäßige Abnahme der sauren Mucopolysaccharide und damit eine Herabsetzung des Turgors, Verdichtung und schließlich Degeneration der kollagenen Fasern und eine scheinbare Zunahme elastischer Elemente mit teilweise schlolligem Zerfall (GREB, 1940; MONTGOMERY, 1940; SCHALLWEGG, 1942; KIERLAND u. O'LEARY, 1953; KATZBERG, 1958; LINKE, 1955).

2. Das Stratum reticulare

Das Stratum subpapillare geht ohne Grenze in das Stratum reticulare (Stratum compactum) über. Dieses besteht vorwiegend aus kollagenen und elastischen Fasern, die in wenig Grundsubstanz eingelagert sind. Zellen treten an Zahl zurück.

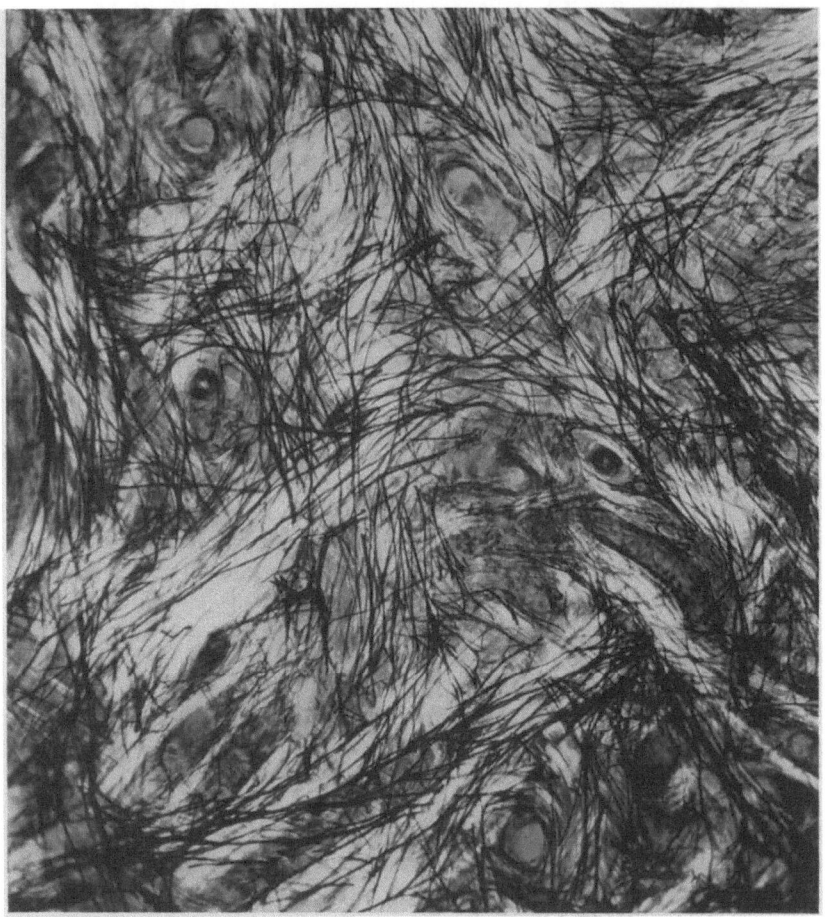

Abb. 17. Flachschnitt durch das Stratum reticulare des Fingerrückens nach Färbung der elastischen Fasern mit Orcein (schwarz) und Darstellung der kollagenen Fasern durch polarisiertes Licht (vgl. hierzu das Konstruktionsschema Abb. 8a). Die runden Gebilde in den Maschenräumen zwischen den Fasern sind Querschnitte durch Blutgefäße oder Ausführungsgänge von Schweißdrüsen (schwarz mit kleinem helleren Lumen). (Nach PETERSEN, 1935; aus BRAUS, 1960)

Es finden sich hier vorwiegend Fibroblasten. Die kollagenen Fasern bilden je nach Körperregion eine unterschiedlich dicke Matte sich überkreuzender und in drei Dimensionen durchflechtender Faserzüge (vgl. Abschnitt B, S. 453). Die Verlaufsrichtung der Fasern steht schräg aufeinander. Dadurch entsteht ein rhombisches Texturmuster (Abb. 8, 17). Die Fasern sind so dicht aneinandergefügt, daß im lichtmikroskopischen Präparat keine Maschenräume sichtbar sind, es sei denn, artifiziell durch Wasserentzug. Lediglich im Bereich der Durchtrittsstellen von Blutgefäßen, Schweißdrüsen und Haarbälgen bleibt eine Lücke, die durch konzentrische Faserzüge abgerundet wird. Die Faserbündel der tiefen Schichten sind wesentlich dicker als die der oberflächlichen (ELZE, 1960). Die Länge der einzelnen Faser beträgt in den tiefen Schichten schätzungsweise einen bis mehrere

Zentimeter (ELZE, 1960). Die Mikropräparation stößt auf beträchtliche Schwierigkeit, da die Textur dreidimensional angelegt ist und sich größere Faserbündel abspalten, um in andere wieder einzustrahlen. Infolgedessen lassen sich einzelne Fasern kaum herauspräparieren. Die elastischen Fasern sind zu Netzen verbunden und stehen an Masse wesentlich hinter dem Geflecht der kollagenen zurück. Innerhalb der Fasermatte bilden sie ein zweites, zwischen den kollagenen Fasern eingeflochtenes, dreidimensionales Netzwerk. Auf Flachschnitten ist zu beobachten (Abb. 17), daß die Verlaufsrichtung beider Faserarten nicht immer kongruent ist (ELZE, 1960), sondern die Hauptzugrichtungen sich oft in einem spitzen Winkel überschneiden, einige elastische Fasern sogar quer zur allgemeinen Verlaufsrichtung der kollagenen Fasern ziehen. Auf die Bedeutung dieses Konstruktionsprinzips wurde bereits auf S. 453 hingewiesen. Es wird in so gut wie allen Hautregionen grundsätzlich beibehalten mit Ausnahme des Nagelbettes. Große individuelle und topographische Unterschiede zeigt das elastische Material, nicht nur hinsichtlich seiner Menge, sondern auch der Verschiedenheit der Dicke der einzelnen Fasern. Unterschiede bei den beiden Geschlechtern, wie sie von LINDHOLM (1931) erhoben wurden, konnte DICK (1947) nicht bestätigen.

3. Das Corium als Ganzes

Stratum papillare und Stratum reticulare gehen kontinuierlich ineinander über und bilden eine mechanische Einheit, in der das Stratum reticulare an Masse überwiegt. Die oben geschilderte Gefügeordnung ist keinesfalls zeitlebens festgelegt und statisch. Narbenbildungen führen zu einer tiefgreifenden Umordnung der Textur in beiden Schichten (BENNINGHOFF, 1931; KÖNIG, 1942; HORSTMANN, 1957), je nach Grad des Defektes. Die Textur reagiert also recht empfindlich auf veränderte mechanische Bedingungen. Auch ist sie beim Neugeborenen noch nicht endgültig ausgebildet, sie entwickelt sich vielmehr erst im Laufe der Kindheit.

Die geflechtartige Textur der Fasern im Stratum subpapillare und reticulare wird schon seit geraumer Zeit mit dem Auftreten des Phänomens der *Spaltlinien* (vgl. auch PINKUS, Bd. II/2, Abb. 26) in Zusammenhang gebracht. Diese verlaufen bekanntlich in Richtung der geringsten Dehnbarkeit der Haut (VOSS, 1937) bzw. senkrecht zu den Linien größter Dehnbarkeit (Abb. 18). Eine restlos einleuchtende Erklärung für das Zustandekommen der Spaltlinien steht jedoch heute noch aus. Man vermutet, daß sie den Resultanten des Rautengitters (Abb. 8b) entsprechen und damit mit den Hauptspannungslinien der Haut zusammenfallen. Anscheinend verlaufen parallel mit ihnen auch die langgezogenen Scheidewände der subcutanen Druckpolster (VOSS, 1937). Mit den Spaltlinien stimmt weitgehend, jedoch nicht überall am Körper, die Ausrichtung der feinen rhombischen Hautfelder überein (PINKUS, 1927). Einen vom Erwachsenen abweichenden Spaltlinienverlauf beschreiben HUTCHINSON u. KOOP (1956) und ELZE (1960) beim Neugeborenen. Hier sind sie an Rumpf und Extremitäten zirkulär angeordnet (vgl. PINKUS, Bd. II/2, Abb. 27).

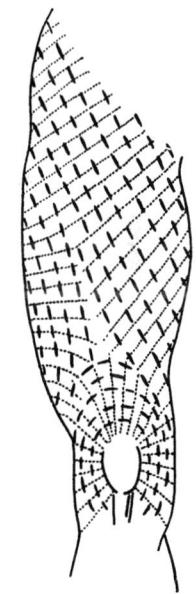

Abb. 18. Spaltlinien (gestrichelt) und Linien größter Dehnbarkeit (punktiert) am Beispiel der Haut des Oberschenkels. Kombination zweier Abbildungen aus VOSS (1937)

Durch die Art der Textur und die Verwendung zugfesten und elastischen Materials findet die *reversible Dehnbarkeit und Verschieblichkeit* der Cutis, speziell des Stratum reticulare, eine einleuchtende Erklärung: Sie beruht auf einer Verstellung der Rautengitter, wobei der spitze Winkel der sich kreuzenden Fasern entweder größer oder bei entgegengesetztem Zug kleiner wird (Abb. 8b). Die größte Dehnbarkeit ist, wie die Untersuchung der Spaltlinien bereits vermuten ließ, senkrecht zur Längsachse der „Raute" gegeben. Bei diesen Vorgängen erfolgt in geringem Grad auch eine Verschiebung der Fasern in der flüssigen Grundsubstanz gegeneinander. Bei Zugwirkung werden außerdem die Wellen der Kollagenfasern zunehmend ausgeglichen und die elastischen Fasern gespannt. Nach Aufhören der Krafteinwirkung kehrt das Gewebe wieder in seine Ausgangslage zurück. Die kollagenen Fasern haben die Tendenz, ihre im Molekülbau begründete Wellung wieder anzunehmen und die elastischen Fasern ziehen sich zusammen. Die rückläufige Stellungsänderung des Rautengitters wird, durch die Dichte des Gewebes an sich (wie bei der Elastizität eines dicht geschlagenen Textilgewebes) und durch die quer oder schräg zur Rautenlängsachse verlaufenden elastischen Fasern (Abb. 8a) herbeigeführt. Sicherlich spielen bei dem komplizierten dreidimensionalen Netz der elastischen Fasern auch wieder die Resultanten der durch den Faserverlauf gegebenen Zugrichtungen eine wesentliche Rolle. Schließlich hängt die Dehnbarkeit vom Durchmesser und vom Zustand der elastischen Fasern ab (DICK, 1951). Dicke, lange Fasern setzen dem Zug schon sehr schnell einen merklichen bremsenden Widerstand entgegen. Altersveränderungen der Fasern vermindern die Elastizität. Hinzu kommt die unterschiedliche regionale Verteilung. So fand SCHALLWEGG (1942) an der Vorderseite der Extremität mehr elastische Elemente als an der Rückseite. Schließlich sprechen seine Untersuchungen auch dafür, daß bei den verschiedenen Konstitutionstypen eine unterschiedliche Ausbildung der elastischen Elemente erfolgt.

Wird die äußerste Grenze der Dehnbarkeit überschritten, zerreißt die Haut. Die *Zug- und Reißfestigkeit* ist vor allem eine Funktion der kollagenen Fasern des Coriums, ihrer Textur, Menge und Festigkeit. Die mechanische Belastbarkeit wurde von ROLLHÄUSER (1950b) am Beispiel der Bauchhaut (Corium-Epidermis-Streifen) für verschiedene Lebensalter überprüft. Hierbei kann die Festigkeit der Epidermis vernachlässigt werden. Er gelangte zu folgenden Ergebnissen:

Altersklasse	Gruppe I Mens 7—3 Jahre	Gruppe II		Gruppe III 50—80 Jahre
		15—30	30—50 Jahre	
Zugfestigkeit kg/mm^2	$0{,}75 \pm 0{,}16$	$1{,}61 \pm 0{,}08$		$2{,}05 \pm 0{,}11$
Verlängerung in %	47	34,3		30,5
Elastizitätsmodul	$2{,}9 \pm 0{,}45$	$6{,}7 \pm 0{,}29$	$8{,}1 \pm 0{,}34$	$11{,}0 \pm 0{,}47$

Mit zunehmendem Lebensalter steigt also der Dehnungswiderstand der Haut an, d.h. die Dehnbarkeit wird geringer. Die Ursachen hierfür sind verschieden. Einmal wird das Gewebe mit zunehmenden Lebensjahren ärmer an Flüssigkeit infolge der Abnahme der Mucopolysaccharide; folglich rücken die Fasern näher zusammen, es kommen auf den Querschnitt mehr zugfeste Fasern (ROLLHÄUSER). Bekanntlich nimmt aber auch mit zunehmendem Alter die Dicke der einzelnen kollagenen Fibrillen und Fasern zu und damit ihre Zugfestigkeit. Bei abnorm geringer Festigkeit liegt, wie auch andere Symptome erkennen ließen, eine konstitutionelle Minderwertigkeit der Kollagenfasern vor (ROLLHÄUSER, 1950b), für die jedoch noch keine befriedigende kausale Erklärung gegeben wird. Signifikante

Unterschiede zwischen weiblichem und männlichem Geschlecht konnten von ROLL-HÄUSER bei der mechanischen Prüfung im Gegensatz zu den Befunden von WENZEL (1950) nicht erhoben werden. Dies überrascht um so mehr, als das Corium bzw. die Haut im histologischen Schnittpräparat beim Mann dicker als bei der Frau gefunden wird (SCHALLWEGG, 1942; LEE, 1957). Regionale Unterschiede lassen sich aus den Befunden von SCHALLWEGG ableiten. Er beobachtete an der Dorsalseite der Extremitäten zahlreichere und dickere Kollagenfaserbündel als an der Ventralseite, wo hingegen die elastischen Elemente stärker vertreten sind. Auffällige regionale Unterschiede in Abhängigkeit vom Lebensalter fand auch LEE (1957). Er registrierte an der Haut des Vorderarmes (Chinese) bis zum 30. Lebensjahr einen merklichen Anstieg der Zugfestigkeit, dann einen allmählichen Rückgang, verbunden mit einer entsprechenden Zu- bzw. Abnahme der Dicke der Haut. Hiervon völlig abweichend verhielt sich die Stirnhaut. Sie zeigte, wie die Bauchhaut bei den Untersuchungen ROLLHÄUSERs, nach der Geburt einen stetigen Rückgang ihrer Dehnbarkeit. Auch WENZEL (1950) fand die Zugfestigkeit der Bauchhaut größer als der Haut im Bereich der Extremitäten. Zusammenfassend muß festgestellt werden, daß die bisherigen Untersuchungen noch kein vollständiges Bild von den Zusammenhängen von mechanischen Eigenschaften und anatomischem Substrat ergeben. Erschwerend für die Deutung sind auch noch die von der Konstitution abhängigen Unterschiede im Bau des Coriums, die von SCHALLWEGG (1942) an einem großen Material aufgedeckt wurden. Demnach besitzt der Papillarkörper des Asthenikers in der Jugend zahlreiche Papillen. Sie atrophieren mit zunehmendem Lebensalter schneller als beim Pykniker, so daß dessen Papillarkörper in einem vergleichbaren höheren Lebensalter papillenreicher erscheint. Auch bleiben beim Pykniker die mechanisch wirksamen elastischen Elemente länger erhalten. Der Astheniker verfügt zwar in jungen Jahren über ein ausgedehntes elastisches Fasersystem. Allein es fällt nach dem 40. Lebensjahr schneller der Degeneration anheim als beim Pykniker.

Für den *Stoffwechsel der Cutis* ist das Stratum papillare der wichtigste Anteil. Hier finden Stoffaustausch und Stofftransport statt, während dem Stratum reticulare vorwiegend mechanische Aufgaben zufallen. Morphologisches Kennzeichen hierfür ist auch die Gefäßverteilung. Das Stratum reticulare durchziehen größere Arterien- und Venenstämme, von denen sich nur hie und da Capillaren abzweigen. Ganz anders das Bild im Stratum papillare! Hier setzt sich der subpapilläre Plexus in die Capillaren der zahlreichen Papillen fort, die je nach Höhe der Papillen eine unterschiedlich lange Austauschoberfläche bieten (vgl. Gefäßsystem der Haut, S. 491 ff.). Auch die große Zahl aktiver Bindegewebszellen wie Histiocyten, Plasmazellen oder Gewebsmastzellen sind morphologische Kennzeichen dieser am Stoffwechselgeschehen aktiv beteiligten Bindegewebsschicht. Der Stofftransport geht von den Blutcapillaren durch die Grundsubstanz zur Epidermis mit ihren Anhangsgebilden und zu den Zellen, die Grundsubstanz und Fasern bilden; Stoffwechselendprodukte laufen größtenteils wieder zurück zu den Blut- und Lymphcapillaren, um über diese abtransportiert zu werden. Über das Stoffwechselfeld der Grundsubstanz wurde bereits eingehend in dem Abschnitt A, III, S. 451, berichtet. Wie ich dort ausgeführt habe, ist mit normalen licht- und elektronenmikroskopischen Methoden von den Stoffen nicht viel auszumachen. Einen Fortschritt bedeutete die Applikation radioaktiv markierter Stoffe, mit deren Hilfe über die Entstehung der kollagenen Fasern und der Grundsubstanz bereits einige Erkenntnisse gewonnen wurden. Hinsichtlich der integrierenden Bestandteile wie Skleroproteine und Mucopolysaccharide muß hier auf das einschlägige Kapitel verwiesen werden. Dort wurde auch dargelegt, daß die Stoffe wie Kohlenhydrate, Lipide und Proteine die Grundsubstanz offensichtlich in niedermolekularer Form passieren als Monosaccharid, Aminosäuren, Fettsäuren und Glycerin. Hierfür sprechen auch die Befunde von BRAUN-FALCO (1956), der speziell für Polysaccharide mit hinreichender Sicherheit nachweisen konnte, daß die für die Glykogensynthese notwendige Phosphorylase im Epithel selbst (Epidermis, Schweißdrüsen, Haarbalg) lokalisiert ist, so daß dort erst aus dem Monomer das polymere Polysaccharid aufgebaut wird. Es ist wahrscheinlich, daß Gleiches auch für die Synthese der anderen Stoffe gilt. Was brachten sonst histochemische und fermentchemische Untersuchungen im Bereich des Coriums? Die Ausbeute war ausgesprochen mager. Die höchste Fermentaktivität stellten sämtliche Untersucher übereinstimmend in den epithelial-epidermalen Gebilden fest, eine merklich geringere Aktivität in den Bindegewebszellen (vgl. S. 431 und S. 437). Im Bereich des bindegewebigen Haarbalges wurden unspezifische Esterasen (MONTAGNA, 1955), β-Glucuronidase (MONTAGNA, 1957), Aminopeptidase (STEIGLEDER et al., 1962), Phosphorylasen (BRAUN-FALCO, 1956), auch alkalische Phosphatase nachgewiesen. Aminopeptidase findet sich gleichfalls in der Bindegewebshülle der Schweißdrüsen. So gut wie frei von Fermenten sind die Grundsubstanz und die Fasern, bzw. die Fermente liegen in so niedriger Konzentration vor (Kollagenase, Hyaluronidase, Elastase), daß sie mit histochemischen Methoden nicht zu erfassen sind. Auch quantitative Fermentuntersuchungen nach Gefriertrocknung (HERSHEY et al., 1960) bestätigen die minimalen Enzymaktivitäten im Corium. Dabei wurde im Papillarkörper eine doppelt so hohe Aktivität ermittelt wie im Stratum reticulare. Es bleibt bei diesen Untersuchungen offen, ob die nachgewiesenen Fermente (Aldolase, saure Phosphatase, Glucose-6-Phosphatase) an Zellen gebunden waren oder in der Grundsubstanz lagen. Ein weiteres Argument für die besonders hohe Stoffwechselleistung des Papillarkörpers ist der von RILEY u. WEST (1956) nachgewiesene hohe Gehalt an Gewebshistamin, der sich in der Haut fast proportional zu der Zahl der Mastzellen verhält.

III. Die Subcutis

An das Corium schließt sich in der Schichtenfolge die Subcutis (Tela subcutanea) an. Sie bildet die wichtige druckelastische Verschiebe- und Verbindungsschicht zwischen der Unterlage (Periost oder Muskelfascie) und der Cutis. Über ihre Gefügeordnung gibt das übliche histologische Schnittpräparat nur unzureichend Auskunft. Es zeigt unregelmäßige Areale von Fettgewebe, die von den Retinacula cutis begrenzt werden (TIETZE, 1921). Diese gehen kontinuierlich in das Stratum reticulare des Coriums über. Erst die plastische Rekonstruktion (BLECHSCHMIDT, 1931, 1934; BOCHUD, 1954) konnte die räumliche Anordnung der einzelnen Bauelemente aufklären. Sie zeigte, daß die Retinacula Querschnitte durch die Wände teils vollständig, teils unvollständig unterteilter Kammern darstellen (Abb. 19), die mit Fettgewebe ausgefüllt sind. Die Anordnung der Kammern, die Dicke und die Stellung der Kammerscheidewände sind entsprechend den mechanischen Bedingungen in den verschiedenen Regionen der Haut sehr unterschiedlich (Abb. 20). Für die Ausbildung dieses Systems ist nicht allein die mechanische Beanspruchung beim Erwachsenen verantwortlich zu machen, sondern die Kammerung wird, wenn auch wesentlich weniger kompliziert, bereits beim Fetus im 6. Monat (BLECHSCHMIDT, 1934) entsprechend den späteren mechanischen Erfordernissen angelegt.

Die Scheidewände der Kammern bestehen aus mattenartigen Geflechten kollagener und elastischer Fasern nach den bekannten Konstruktionsprinzipien (vgl. S. 453). Größere Bindegewebssepten dienen den Gefäßen und Nerven als Verkehrsräume. Im Corium-nahen Abschnitt sind die Knäueldrüsen eingelagert. Die

Kammern werden von Fettläppchen, den Fettorganen WASSERMANNS (1926), vollständig ausgefüllt. Nach den Untersuchungen LAUBINGERs (1938) und nach eigenen Beobachtungen gehen die argyrophilen Fasernetze des Fettgewebes kontinuierlich in das Geflecht der kollagenen Fasern der Scheidewände über, sind also mit diesen verbunden (vgl. S. 456). Abweichend von diesem Konstruktionsprinzip durchziehen im distalen Ende der Großzehe (untersucht beim Neugeborenen, BOCHUD, 1954) nur einzelne Bindegewebsstränge das subcutane Fettgewebe und befestigen sich an der Tuberositas unguicularis. Weiter proximal wurde das typische Druckkammersystem nachgewiesen.

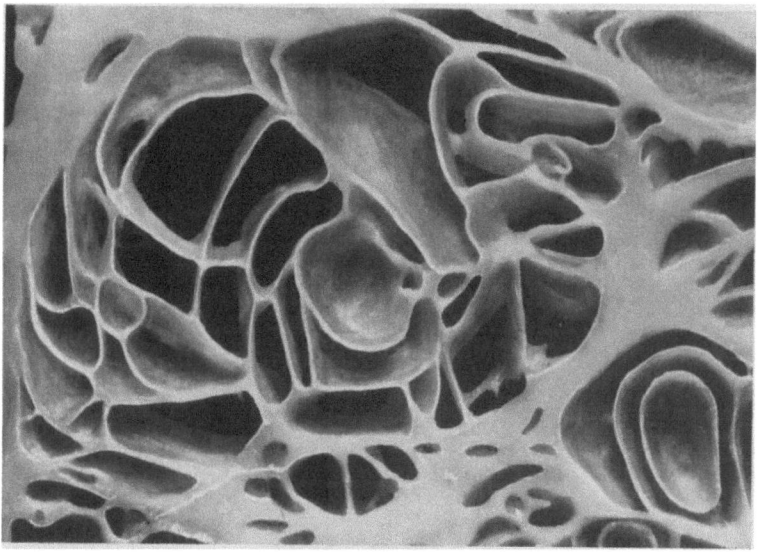

Abb. 19. Rekonstruktion der Druckkammern in der Tiefe des Fersenpolsters des Menschen. Fettgewebe herauspräpariert gedacht. Auffällig ist hier die konzentrische, spiralige Anordnung der Kammerscheidewände.
(Nach BLECHSCHMIDT, 1934; aus HORSTMANN, 1957)

Die Konstruktion der Subcutis muß in erster Linie von mechanischen Gesichtspunkten aus betrachtet werden (TIETZE, BLECHSCHMIDT, BOCHUD). Sie stellt ein enkaptisches System von Druckpolstern dar, deren kleinstes Element der inkompressible, plastisch verformbare Fetttropfen ist. Das Cytoplasma der Fettzelle wird außen von einem Gespinst argyrophiler Fasern umgeben. Diese sind zu einem zusammenhängenden, das gesamte Läppchen durchziehenden Netzwerk und über dieses mit der Kammerscheidewand verbunden. Bei Druckeinwirkung verformen sich die Zellen und verschieben sich geringfügig innerhalb des Läppchens, wobei die Gitterfasern einer senkrecht zur Druckeinwirkung verlaufenden Zugwirkung ausgesetzt werden. Nach Aufhören des Druckes nehmen die Zellen durch die hohe Oberflächenspannung des Fetttropfens und der Elastizität der Gitterfaserhülle ihre ursprüngliche Form wieder an und kehren durch die Zugwirkung der gedehnten argyrophilen Fasern in ihre Ausgangslage zurück. Für die Verlagerung spielen sicherlich die mit einer solartigen Flüssigkeit gefüllten Intercellularräume eine wesentliche Rolle. Durch die dichte Packung der Fettzellen wird die Druckwirkung, gleichzeitig aber auch die regional auftretende Zugspannung, über die im Läppchen verlaufenden Fasern auf die Kammerscheidewände übertragen und von deren Fasermatten aufgefangen, bzw. über ein größeres Gebiet des in sich zusammenhängenden Systems weitergeleitet. Die Bremsung der Zugwirkung erfolgt durch die elastischen Fasern und durch die zunehmende

Entwellung der kollagenen Fasern. Eine wesentliche Bedeutung des Fettpolsters besteht demnach, wie auch BOCHUD (1954) feststellt, in der Umwandlung von Druckspannungen z.T. in Zugspannungen. Hierbei spielt sicherlich die Mehrschichtigkeit der Polster eine mechanisch nicht genauer analysierbare Rolle. In gleicher Weise werden auch Scherwirkungen, die auf die Haut einwirken, gebremst.

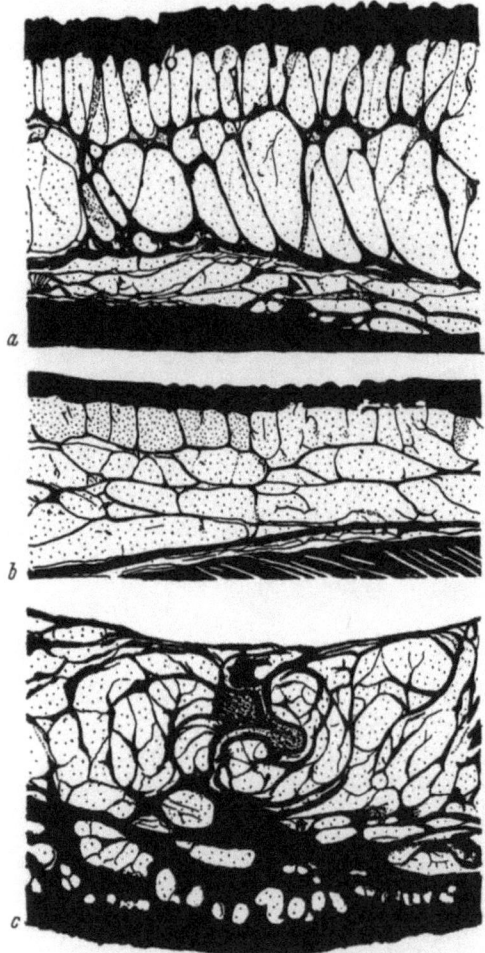

Abb. 20a—c. Schnittbilder des gekammerten Fett-Bindegewebes der Subcutis. a Gesäßregion (Neugeborenes), b seitliche Rumpfwand (Erwachsener), c Fersenpolster (Erwachsener). Umzeichnungen nach BLECHSCHMIDT, (1931, 1934)

Auffallend ist, daß in Hautzonen, die bevorzugt Druckeinwirkungen ausgesetzt sind, die Kammerwände annähernd senkrecht zur Oberfläche orientiert sind, während in Zonen, auf die bevorzugt Scherkräfte einwirken, die Wände der mittleren Kammern horizontal verlaufen (Abb. 20b). Stets sind die oberflächlich liegenden Kammern kleiner als die tiefer gelegenen. Im Bereich des Fersenpolsters fand BLECHSCHMIDT (1934) eine spiralige Anordnung (Abb. 19, 20c) der am Periost befestigten Septen. Beim Aufsetzen der Ferse werden, wie sich aus Röntgenaufnahmen entnehmen ließ, die Kammerwände nicht gestaucht, sondern in der im Ruhezustand angedeuteten Schräglage weiter umgelegt. Hieraus leitet BLECHSCHMIDT ab, die Scheidewände würden beim Aufsetzen des Fußes auf Verwindung beansprucht. Über die Verformung der Kammern im Bereich des Gesäßes während der Streckung und Beugung im Hüftgelenk stellte NOETZEL (1936) Untersuchungen an, die jedoch nur bedingten Aussagewert haben, da sie an der Leiche ausgeführt wurden. Im Bereich des Fingers bestehen auffallende Unterschiede im Bau der Subcutis. Sie wird auf der Dorsalseite von einem Gleitgewebe gebildet, auf der Volarseite von einem typischen Druckkammersystem (SCHREIBER, 1942). Die Ausbreitung unter Druck injizierter Flüssigkeit erfolgt in den Septen, woraus SCHREIBER auf eine gleichartige Ausbreitung entzündlicher Prozesse schließt. Die Kammerwände der Volarseite sind mit den osteofibrösen Kanälen der Sehnenscheiden verbunden (GRAYSON, 1940).

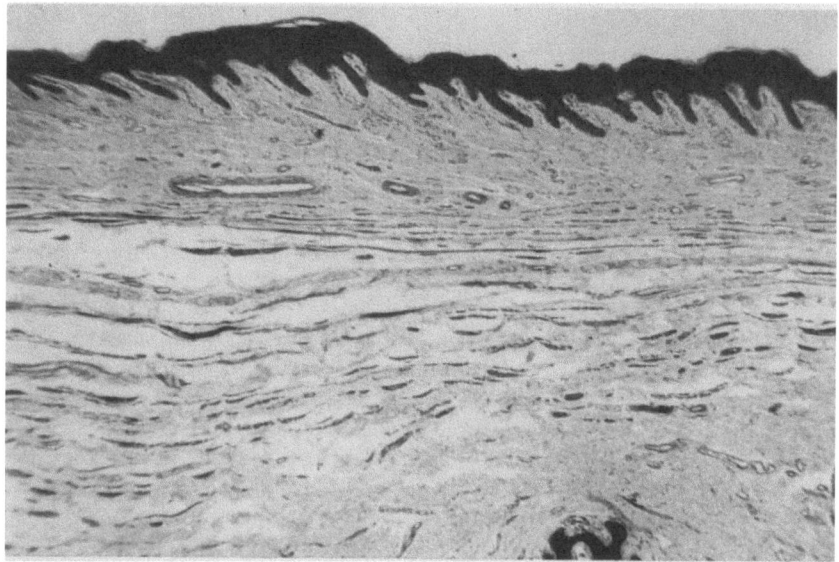

Abb. 21. Längsschnitt durch das Praeputium penis. Unter dem kompakten Stratum reticulare liegt eine lamellär gebaute, lockere Verschiebeschicht. Die langgestreckten mehr oder weniger spindeligen Einlagerungen (dunkel) sind Längsschnitte durch glatte Muskelzellen der Tunica dartos. Färbung H.-E., Grünfilter, Vergr. 75fach

Nicht überall im Körper ist der Druckkammertyp der Subcutis vorhanden. Im Bereich der Streckseite der Finger und Zehen, am Penisschaft liegt ein *lamellärer Bautyp* vor, der durch mehrere übereinander liegende und gegeneinander verschiebliche Schichten faserigen Bindegewebes (Abb. 21) gekennzeichnet ist (NAGEL, 1939; SCHREIBER, 1942).

Eine typische Subcutis mit Fettgewebe oder lamellärer Schichtung fehlt im Bereich des Scrotums, der Ohrmuschel, des Gehörganges und über dem Augenlid. Dennoch ist die Cutis über dem Lid außerordentlich gut verschieblich. Dies beruht auf dem sehr lockeren Bau des Coriums, das überaus reich an Flüssigkeit gefunden wird, und auf der leichten Verschieblichkeit der einzelnen Fasern des Musculus orbicularis oculi.

Eine besondere Verschiebeeinrichtung sind die *Bursae synoviales subcutaneae*. Die bekannteste Bursa dieser Kategorie ist die Bursa synovialis praepatellaris subcutanea. Entsprechende Bursae können aber unter besonderer Beanspruchung an den verschiedensten Stellen entstehen (ELZE, mündliche Mitteilung; BAMMER, 1947). Histologisch findet sich im subcutanen Bindegewebe ein Spaltraum, der von einem flachen einschichtigen Epithel ausgekleidet ist. Das Epithel unterscheidet sich nicht von der synovialen Auskleidung der Gelenkinnenräume und vermag wie diese eine mucinartige Flüssigkeit, die Synovia, zu bilden. Sie besteht vorwiegend aus Wasser mit 1—2% an Hyaluronsäure reichen Mucopolysacchariden (MEYER, 1950; GRAUMANN, 1964) und Proteinen.

Die Verschieblichkeit der Cutis auf ihrer Unterlage wird also von folgenden Faktoren bestimmt: 1. gute Verschieblichkeit: typisches subcutanes Bindegewebe, lamelläres Verschiebegewebe, sehr lockerer Bau des Coriums, Schleimbeutel. 2. geringe Verschieblichkeit: starke Retinacula cutis mit bevorzugt senkrechtem Verlauf, Fehlen einer Subcutis. Neben der mechanischen Bedeutung der Subcutis kann hier nur auf die sonstigen Funktionen des Fettgewebes hingewiesen werden, über die bereits an anderer Stelle berichtet wurde (S. 459). Außer dem Fersenpolster und dem Fettgewebe des Handtellers dient der Panniculus adiposus ganz besonderls der Fettspeicherung (Depotfett). Erfolgt ein zu schneller Abbau der Depots, dann wird die Cutis zu weit. Auch im hohen Alter nimmt die Masse des Fettgewebes ab. Dieser Schwund gemeinsam mit der Muskelatrophie und den oben genannten Veränderungen (S. 469) führt zu der schlaffen, faltigen Haut des Greises (BRAUS u. ELZE, 1960).

Der Einbau der Gefäße in Subcutis und Corium

Die in Subcutis und Corium verlaufenden Gefäße lassen entsprechend der Textur der jeweiligen Schicht besondere Prinzipien des Einbaues erkennen. In der *Subcutis* steigen größere Arterien zur Oberfläche auf und Venen verlassen diese. In Hautgebieten, die wenig verschieblich sind, wie z.B. Fußsohle oder Fingerbeere, benutzen diese Gefäße die bindegewebigen Scheidewände der Druckkammern, wodurch sie offensichtlich bei Belastung vor Verlagerung geschützt werden. Einzelne Äste zweigen zu den Fettläppchen und Schweißdrüsen ab. An Schnittpräparaten zeigt sich im polarisierten Licht, daß die kollagenen Fasern der Kammerscheidewände in die Fasern der Adventitia übergehen, ja es fällt schwer, die Adventitia überhaupt abzugrenzen. Dies gelingt erst nach einer Elasticafärbung, bei der zumindest an den von mir untersuchten Objekten (Hand, Fuß) eine besondere Verdichtung der elastischen Netze in der Adventitia zu beobachten war. Wie der eigentliche Einbau erfolgt, kann aus Schnittpräparaten nicht erschlossen werden. In diesem Punkt genauer bekannt ist der Einbau subcutaner Venen (V. saphena magna, parva) durch mikropräparatorische Untersuchungen v. LANZs (1936). Er fand ein rautengitterförmiges Verspannungssystem von Fasern, die aus der oberflächlichsten Schicht der Fascia cruris und von den Fettläppchen aus der Vene zustreben, dann in die Richtung der Gefäßachse einbiegen und schließlich in die Adventitia einstrahlen. Ein anderes Prinzip des Einbaues stellte FREERKSEN (1938) für die Venen des Handrückens fest. Hier liegen die Gefäße innerhalb der Fettläppchen und werden durch zarte Bänder gehalten, die in die Bindegewebsumhüllung des Fettläppchens übergehen. Die darunterliegenden Läppchen wirken wie Polster und gestatten die außerordentlich große Verschieblichkeit der Venen des Handrückens. Eine ähnliche Auffassung wird von BOCHUD (1954) für den Gefäßeinbau in der großen Zehe vertreten. Im Bereich des *Stratum reticulare* treten die Gefäße senkrecht oder schräg durch die Lücke zwischen „Kette und Schuß" (Abb. 17). Der Spalt wird durch konzentrisch um die Oberfläche des Gefäßes verlaufende kollagene Fasern abgerundet, die in die Adventitia einstrahlen und gemeinsam mit dünnen elastischen Fasern das Gefäß verschieblich befestigen. Im Bereich des *Stratum subpapillare* breitet sich oberflächenparallel der subpapilläre Gefäßplexus aus. Er läßt einen ähnlichen Einbau erkennen. Die Capillaren des *Papillarkörpers* sind durch die argyrophilen Fasern des Grundhäutchens (eigentlich Basalmembran) mit den kollagenen Fasern der Umgebung kontinuierlich verbunden und dort verankert. Um die Capillaren bildet sich außerdem eine sehr weitmaschige elastische Netzhülle, die gleichfalls mit dem grobfaserigen Netz der Umgebung im Zusammenhang steht, wodurch die kleinen Gefäße elastisch im Gewebe verspannt werden. Eine besondere Bedeutung scheint auch den elastischen Sehnen zuzukommen. NAGEL (1939) beobachtete, wie Gefäße von elastischen Sehnen überbrückt werden, so daß sie nicht ins Spannungsfeld der Muskulatur (z. B. Tunica dartos) geraten. Nicht ohne Bedeutung für den Einbau der Gefäße ist die flüssigkeitsreiche, viscöse Grundsubstanz, deren Turgor zu einer plastischen Fixierung beiträgt.

IV. Die Muskulatur der Haut

In der Konstruktion der Haut mit ihren Anhangsgebilden finden drei Arten von Muskulatur Verwendung: glatte Muskulatur, quergestreifte oder Skeletmuskulatur und Epithelmuskelzellen.

1. Glatte Muskulatur

Glatte Muskulatur findet sich stets im Bereich der Mamille, der Genital- und Analregion und, im Zusammenhang mit Haarbälgen, als Musculi arrectores pilorum. Das contractile Bauelement ist die glatte Muskelzelle mit einem zentral gelegenen, länglichen Zellkern und den polarisations- sowie elektronenoptisch sichtbaren Myofibrillen. Innerhalb des Gewebes sind die Muskelzellen durch Gitterfasern verbunden, die sich an der Oberfläche einer jeden Zelle zu einem Netz verflechten (PLENK, 1927). Die Zellen sind entweder zu kleinen Muskeln gebündelt (z. B. Mm. arrectores) oder zu Strängen vereinigt, die untereinander ein Netzwerk bilden (z. B. Mamille). Die Kontraktion wird über elastische Sehnen auf das umliegende Gewebe übertragen (NAGEL, 1939, 1942; HÄGGQVIST, 1931, 1956; PETRY, 1942, 1951a). Diese Sehnen lassen sich mit „Elastica-Farbstoffen" unter bestimmten Bedingungen (NAGEL, 1939) elektiv darstellen. Ob sie wie die elastischen Fasern aufgebaut sind, kann an den üblichen Färbungspräparaten nicht entschieden werden. Elektronenmikroskopische Untersuchungen liegen noch nicht vor. Anscheinend gehen die Sehnen aus dem argyrophilen Faserstrumpf hervor, der eine jede Zelle umhüllt. Das Ende der Sehne strahlt in die Bindegewebsfaserhülle des Haarbalges oder des Coriums ein. Auch scheinen hier erst wieder kollagene bzw. argyrophile Fasern zwischengeschaltet zu sein. BENNINGHOFF (1929) faßte elastische Sehnen und Muskulatur als eine funktionelle und morphologische Einheit auf und bezeichnete sie als „elastisch-muskulöses System". Freilich bedarf heute sein Konzept einer gewissen Einschränkung: das Elektronenmikroskop hat den „einheitlichen syncytialen" Verband der glatten Muskulatur widerlegt.

Für die Erigierbarkeit der *Mamille* ist, wie man schon seit geraumer Zeit weiß, ein Geflecht glatter Muskulatur verantwortlich. Wie NAGEL (1942) zeigen konnte, besteht der mechanisch wirksame Apparat aus einem spiralig-netzförmigen System elastisch-muskulöser Elemente in kegelförmiger Anordnung (Abb. 22). Bei der Kontraktion übertragen die elastischen Sehnen (in der Zeichnung dunkel) den Muskelzug auf die Fasergeflechte des Coriums. Außerdem wird der Durchmesser des Muskelkegels verringert und dadurch die Mamille erigiert. Die Hauptmasse des Muskelnetzes breitet sich in der Subcutis und in den tiefen Schichten der Cutis aus. Von NAGEL wird das elastisch-muskulöse System auch für den Entleerungsmechanismus beim Lactieren verantwortlich gemacht, indem durch den Zug an der Mamille während des Saugens die in das Verspannungssystem eingebauten Milchgänge entgegen dem entstehenden Unterdruck offengehalten werden. Gleichzeitig werden auch die in das System eingebauten Venen erweitert. Damit findet die Ansicht, die Venenfüllung sei für den Erektionsmechanismus der Mamille mitverantwortlich, eine weitere Stütze. In der Brust-

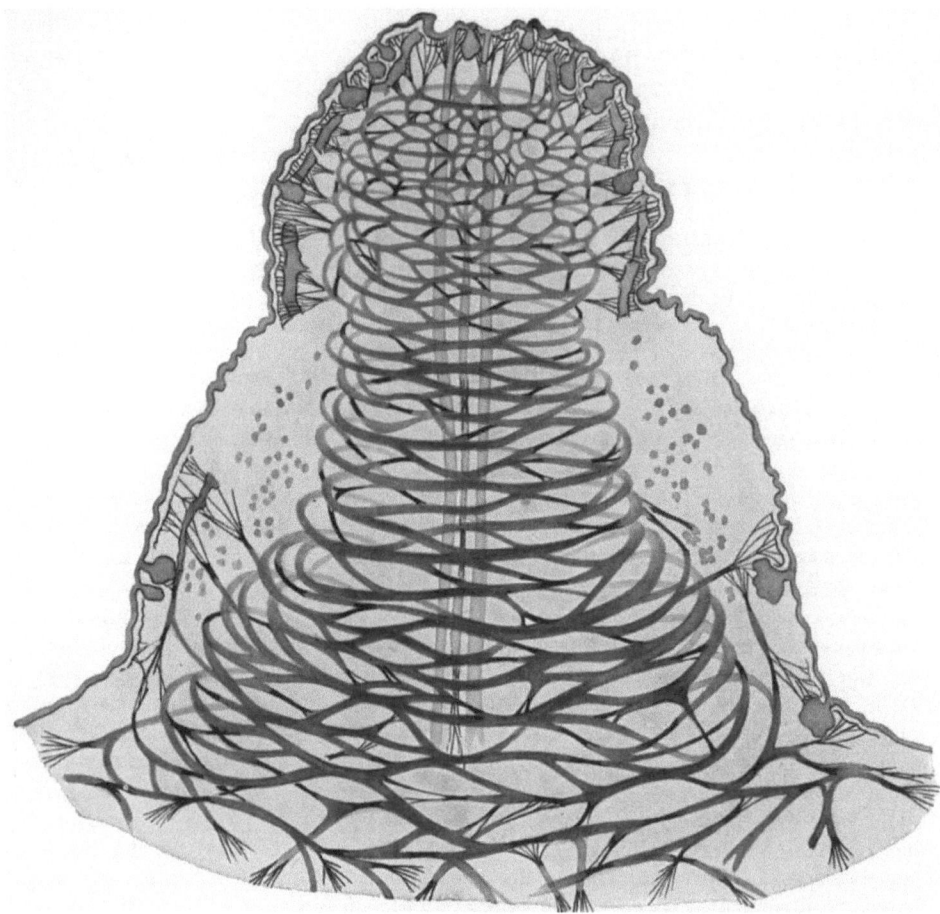

Abb. 22. Schema des elastisch-muskulösen Systems der Mamille im Zustand der Erektion. Elastische Zwischensehnen und Sehnenpinsel schwarz, Muskulatur grau. Im Innern des Muskeltrichters 2 Milchgänge. Beachte den schraubigen Verlauf der glatten Muskelbündel, deren Endsehnen z.T. an der Haut ansetzen. (Nach NAGEL, 1942; aus BARGMANN, 1964)

warze des Mannes fand sich ebenfalls ein „elastisch-muskulöses" System, wenn auch von sehr viel einfacherer Bauweise (QUAST, 1922).

Unter der Bezeichnung *Musculus sexualis* (SCHIEFFERDECKER, 1917) wird die Gesamtheit der glatten Muskulatur zusammengefaßt, die in der Haut der Genital- und Analregion zu finden ist. Sie geht entwicklungsgeschichtlich aus dem Blastem der Geschlechtsfalten und des Genitalhöckers hervor. Hierzu gehört vor allem die *Tunica dartos* (Muskelhaut). Diese Bezeichnung findet auf beide Geschlechter Anwendung, wird jedoch meist für die in das Stratum reticulare und in die Subcutis des Scrotums eingelagerte Muskulatur benutzt. Sie setzt sich kontinuierlich bis in den Penisschaft und in das Praeputium fort (NAGEL, 1939; QUAST, 1922) und breitet sich in der Perineal- und Analregion aus. Die Tunica dartos ist ein in sich geschlossenes Muskelnetz, das im Bereich des Scrotums eine deutliche Schichtung erkennen läßt (NAGEL, 1939). Im Penisschaft ist das Netzwerk lockerer und die Schichtung oft nicht so deutlich (Abb. 21). Freie Muskelbündelchen wurden von NAGEL nirgendwo gefunden. Der Muskelansatz ist die Cutis. Die Schichtung wird von NAGEL als ein Gleitgewebe gedeutet (vgl. auch Abschnitt Subcutis), in dem die für die Erektion notwendige Hautreserve verschoben wird. Die elastischen Sehnen sollen nach der Ansicht NAGELs außerdem verhindern, daß bei der mit der Erektion verbundenen Gewebsverschiebung Gefäße abgeknickt oder zu sehr verlagert werden (vgl. Einbau der Gefäße, S. 478). Auf die allgemein bekannte wärmeregulatorische Funktion der Tunica dartos braucht hier nur hingewiesen zu werden.

Als *Tunica dartos labialis* wird bei der Frau ein wesentlich schwächer entwickeltes Netzwerk glatter Muskelzellen dicht unter dem Stratum reticulare im Bereich der großen Labien bezeichnet, das auch auf das Perineum und auf den Mons pubis übergreift (MORITA, 1953). Eine genaue Untersuchung der Anordnung seiner Muskelbündel steht noch aus.

Nur durch eine andere regionale Verteilung unterscheiden sich die *Musculi cutis diagonales* von der Tunica dartos. Es sind gleichfalls dickere oder dünnere Muskelzüge, die sich in den drei Richtungen des Raumes im Corium oder der Subcutis (SCHIEFFERDECKER, 1917) netzartig verbinden. Auch sie haben keinen Kontakt zu den Haarbälgen, wodurch sie von den Musculi arrectores pilorum abgegrenzt werden können. Offensichtlich bestehen große individuelle Verschiedenheiten hinsichtlich Lage, Verteilung und Menge der contractilen Elemente. QUAST (1922) findet ein ausgedehntes flächenhaftes Muskelnetz, das nach den oben genannten Kriterien als Musculus cutis diagonalis bezeichnet werden muß, im Stratum reticulare der Wangenhaut, der Achselhaut, im Bereich der Stirnhaut und auf der Streckseite der Extremität. Von anderer Seite wurden diese Befunde noch nicht bestätigt.

Von den bisher genannten glatten Muskelelementen der Haut unterscheiden sich die *Musculi arrectores pilorum* durch ihre funktionelle Beziehung zum Haarbalg (Haarbalgmuskeln) und zu den Talgdrüsen (expressor sebi). Ging das Haar zugrunde, bleiben die Muskeln dennoch erhalten. Sie fehlen im Bereich des Knies, des Handtellers und der Fußsohle, der Lippe, der Stirn, der Augenlider, des Nasenrückens, an den Vibrissae und an den Augenwimpern (BRAUS u. ELZE, 1960; BUCHER, 1965). Unregelmäßig sollen sie an den Barthaaren, Achselhaaren und an den Haaren der Augenbraue vorkommen. Sie entspringen mit elastischen Sehnen im Stratum subpapillare und reticulare (HÄGGQVIST, 1931) und setzen über elastische Sehnen (KANAIZUKA, 1926) am bindegewebigen Haarbalg an. Die Gestalt der einzelnen Muskelchen ist außerordentlich variabel. Wachsplattenrekonstruktionen (KANAIZUKA, 1926) gestatteten, in die Vielfalt Einblick zu gewinnen. So zweigt sich der Muskel bisweilen vor dem Ansatz am Haarbalg in 2—5 kleine Muskelbäuche auf oder es bilden sich Anastomosen zu benachbarten Muskeln, oder es finden sich abnorme Ansätze an Schweißdrüsen und Talgdrüsen. Augenfällig ist die charakteristische Zuordnung zu Haargruppen. Eine Gruppe von 5—6 Haaren mit den zugehörigen Haarbälgen besitzt zumindest zwei Muskeln. OKAJIMA et al. (1933a, b) bestimmten den Haar-Arrectorwinkel β, durch den auch die Stellung des Haares definiert ist. Beziehungen zwischen Haarstrich und Stellung der Haarbalgmuskeln sind m.W. bisher noch nicht untersucht.

Mit histochemischen Methoden wurde in den Musculi arrectores alkalische Phosphatase und β-Glucuronidase (BRAUN-FALCO, 1956; MONTAGNA, 1957), Succinodehydrogenase (MONTAGNA u. FORMISANO, 1955) sowie eine positive Plasmalreaktion (BANDMANN u. SPIER, 1957) nachgewiesen. Bei der PJS-Reaktion verhalten sie sich stark positiv (BRAUN-FALCO u. RATHJENS, 1954).

2. Skeletmuskulatur

Von der *Skeletmuskulatur*, die allein der Haut angehört, findet man beim Menschen nur noch im Kopf-Halsbereich Reste, nämlich die mimische Muskulatur und das Platysma. Sie sind stammesgeschichtlich nahe verwandt und gehen aus den beiden Schichten des Sphincter colli hervor. Auf ihn folgt caudalwärts der Panniculus carnosus, der noch bei vielen rezenten Säugetieren (Erdferkel, Maulwurf, Pferd) den gesamten Rumpf überzieht. Beim Embryo entwickelt sich die Muskelmasse aus einem gemeinsamen Blastem im Bereich des Hyoidbogens und wird dementsprechend vom 2. Kiemenbogennerv, dem Nervus facialis, innerviert.

Die unterschiedlich dicken Bündel der mimischen Muskulatur entspringen von Fascien (z.B. Fascia parotideomasseterica), vom Periost (z.B. die tiefe Schicht der mimischen Muskulatur) oder sie bilden in sich geschlossene Ringlagen (z.B. Musculus sphincter oris). Die Muskelbündelchen, die über keine Fascie verfügen, verlaufen durch das subcutane Bindegewebe und strahlen unter pinselförmiger Aufspaltung der Endsehnen in das Stratum reticulare des Coriums ein. Die Befestigung an dem mattenartigen Geflecht des Coriums führt dazu, daß der Muskelzug auf eine größere Hautfläche wirksam wird, während sonst an der Stelle der Insertion eine grübchenförmige Einsenkung entstehen würde.

3. Die myoepithelialen Zellen

Die *myoepithelialen Zellen* (Korbzellen, Epithelmuskelzellen) werden nur der Vollständigkeit halber hier aufgeführt. Sie stammen aus dem Ektoderm und gehören damit nicht dem Bindegewebskörper der Haut an. Entsprechend ihrer Herkunft liegen sie zwischen Basalmembran und Basis der Drüsenzellen, in die sie sich in entsprechende Kannelierungen einfügen. Man findet sie regelmäßig an der Oberfläche von Duftdrüsen, Endstücken der Schweißdrüsen, Glandulae ceruminales und Endstücken der Brustdrüse. Sie setzen sich nicht auf den Ausführungsgang der Drüse fort.

Die Gestalt der einzelnen Zelle ist spindelförmig langgestreckt (Duft- und Schweißdrüsen). Die myoepithelialen Zellen der Mamma und Speicheldrüsen sind dagegen oft verzweigt und umgeben körbchenförmig das Endstück (DABELOW, 1957). Der längsovale Zellkern liegt meist etwas exzentrisch in einer Cytoplasmaverdichtung. Der Zelleib enthält längsorientierte, relativ dicke Myofibrillen, die im polarisierten Licht und mit Eisenhämatoxylin nachweisbar sind. Das Cytoplasma gibt einen positiven Ausfall bei der Reaktion auf alkalische Phosphatase (BUNTING et al., 1948; LEESON, 1960), auf β-Glucuronidase (MONTAGNA, 1957) und Monoaminooxydase (YASUDA u. MONTAGNA, 1960). Die Verbindung der einzelnen Zellen untereinander und mit dem Drüsenendstück erfolgt, wie lichtmikroskopische Beobachtungen erkennen lassen, über argyrophile Fasern, die anscheinend mit den Faserkörpern der Basalmembran in Zusammenhang stehen. Infolge ihrer Kontraktilität vermögen die myoepithelialen Zellen das Drüsenendstück zu komprimieren (LEESON, 1960) und damit bei der Entleerung der Sekrete mitzuwirken. Vitalmikroskopische Untersuchungen konnten diesen Vorgang verifizieren (HURLEY u. SHELLEY, 1954). Darüber hinaus obliegt ihnen anscheinend im Stofftransport für die Drüsenzellen (LEESON) eine noch nicht genauer bekannte Bedeutung, mit dem die bisher nachgewiesenen Fermente in Zusammenhang gebracht werden. Über ihre Innervation durch das vegetative Nervensystem liegen Untersuchungen von JOHN (1940) vor.

Literatur*

ADACHI, K., and W. MONTAGNA: Histology and cytochemistry of human skin. XXII. Sites of leucine aminopeptidase (LAP). J. invest. Derm. **37**, 145—147 (1961). — ADAMS-RAY, J., G. BLOOM, and M. RITZÉN: Cells with autofluorescent granules in dermis of human skin and their correlation to degree of pigmentation. Acta morph. neerl.-scand. **3**, 131 (1960). — ADAMS-RAY, J., et H. NORDENSTAM: Un système de cellules chromaffines dans la peau humaine. Lyon chir. **52**, 125 (1956). — ASBOE-HANSEN, G.: A survey of the normal and pathological occurence of mucinous substances and mast cells in the dermal connective tissue in man. Acta derm.-venerol. (Stockh.) **30**, 338 (1950). — Connective tissue in health and disease. Kopenhagen: Munksgaard 1954. — The hormonal control of connective tissue. In: Int. Rev. connect.

---

* Abgeschlossen im September 1966.

tiss. Res., vol. 1. New York and London: Academic Press 1963. — ASTBURY, W. T.: The molecular structure of skin, hair, and related tissue. Brit. J. Derm. **62**, 1 (1950).

BAHR, F. G.: The reconstitution of collagen fibrils as revealed by electronmicroscopy. Exp. Cell Res. **1**, 603 (1950). — Über die Feinstruktur elastischer Fasern. Z. Anat. Entwickl.-Gesch. **116**, 134 (1951). — BAIRATI, A., L. AMANTE, ST. DE PETRIS, and B. PERNIS: Studies on the ultrastructure of the lymph nodes I. The reticular network. Z. Zellforsch. **63**, 644 (1964). — BALÓ, J., and J. BANGA: The elastolytic activity of pancreatic extracts. Biochem. J. **46**, 384 (1950). — BAMMER, H. G.: Untersuchung über die Bursa suprapatellaris und die angrenzenden Nebenschleimbeutel des Kniegelenks. Inaug.-Diss. Joh. Wolfg. Goethe-Universität Frankfurt 1947. — BANDMANN, H. J., u. H. W. SPIER: Histochemische Darstellung der Plasmalreaktion an gesunder und krankter Haut. Dermatologica (Basel) **115**, 444 (1957). — BANGA, J.: Isolation and crystallization of elastase from cattle pancreas. Acta physiol. Acad. Sci. hung. **3**, 317 (1952). — BARGMANN, W.: Histologie und mikroskopische Anatomie des Menschen, 6. Aufl. Stuttgart: Georg Thieme 1967. — BARRNETT, R. J., and E. G. BALL: Metabolic and ultrastructural changes induced in adipose tissue by insulin. J. biophys. biochem. Cytol. **8**, 83 (1960). — BEAR, R. S.: X-ray diffraction studies on collagen fibres. I. The large fibre axis period of collagen. J. Amer. chem. Soc. **66**, 1297 (1944). — The structure of collagen fibrils. Advanc. Protein Chem. **7**, 69 (1952). — BECKER, J.: Über Eigentümlichkeiten des Fettgewebes in der frühen Kindheit. Z. Anat. Entwickl.-Gesch. **92**, 814 (1930). — BEJDL, W.: Die saure Phosphatase in Haut und Vagina des Menschen und ihre Bedeutung für die Verhornung. Z. Zellforsch. **40**, 389 (1954). — BENDITT, E. P., R. L. WONG, M. ARASE, and E. ROEPER: 5-Hydroxytryptamine in mastcells. Proc. Soc. exp. Biol. (N.Y.) **90**, 303 (1955). — BENNINGHOFF, A.: Über die Beziehungen zwischen elastischem Gerüst und glatter Muskulatur in der Arterienwand und ihre funktionelle Bedeutung. Z. Zellforsch. **6**, 348 (1929). — Funktionelle Anpassung im Bereich des Bindegewebes. Verh. Anat. Ges. 1931. Anat. Anz., Erg.-H. **72**, 95 (1931). — BENSLEY, S. H.: On the presence, properties and distribution of the intercellular ground substance of loos connective tissue. Anat. Rec. **60**, 93 (1934). — Histological studies of the reaction of cells an intercellular substance of loos connective tissue to the spreading factor of testicular extracts. Ann. N.Y. Acad. Sci. **52**, 983 (1950). — BETTMANN, S.: Felderungszeichnung der Bauchhaut und Schwangerschaftsstreifen. Z. Anat. Entwickl-Gesch. **85**, 658 (1928). — BLASCHKO, A.: Beiträge zur Anatomie der Oberhaut. Arch. mikr. Anat. **30**, 495 (1887). — BLECHSCHMIDT, E.: Zur Anatomie des Subcutangewebes. Z. Zellforsch. **12**, 284 (1931). — Die Architektur des Fersenpolsters. Morph. Jb. **73**, 20 (1934). — BLINZINGER, K., u. N. MATUSSEK: Die Dünnschichtkontrastierung mittels Bariumchlorid: Eine Methode für den topochemischen Nachweis von Stoffen mit unvollständig veresterten Schwefelsäuregruppen im submikroskopischen Bereich. Histochemie **6**, 173 (1966). — BLOOM, G., and J. W. KELLY: The copper phtalocyanin dye „Astrablau" and its staining proprieties especially the staining of mast cells. Histochemie **2**, 48 (1960). — BLOOM, G., and E. M. RITZÉN: Autofluorescent granules in cells of human dermis. II. Histochemical observations. Z. Zellforsch. **61**, 841 (1964). — BOCHUD, J. M.: Contribution à l'étude de la fonction mécanique du tissu conjectif dans la planque distale du gros orteil chez le nouveau né. Acta anat. (Basel) **22**, 345 (1954). — BRANWOOD, A. W.: The fibroblast. In: Intern. Rev. of Conn. tiss. Res., vol. 1. New York and London: Academic Press 1963. — BRAUN-FALCO, O.: Histochemische und morphologische Studien an normaler und pathologisch veränderter Haut. Arch. Derm. Syph. (Berl.) **198**, 111 (1954). — Weitere histochemische Untersuchungen am homogenen Anteil des subepidermalen Grenzstreifens normaler menschlicher Haut. Arch. klin. exp. Derm. **201**, 521 (1955). — Zur Histotopographie der β-Glucuronidase in normaler menschlicher Haut. Arch. klin. exp. Derm. **203**, 61 (1956). — Zur Frage des Mechanismus der Resorcin-Fuchsin- und Aldehyd-Fuchsin-Färbung elastischer Fasern. Arch. klin. exp. Derm. **203**, 256 (1956b). — Über die Fähigkeit der menschlichen Haut zur Polysaccharidsynthese, ein Beitrag zur Histochemie der Phosphorylase. Arch. klin. exp. Derm. **202**, 163 (1956c). — Histochemie des Bindegewebes. Arch. klin. exp. Derm. **206**, 319 (1957). — BRAUN-FALCO, O., u. R. RATHJENS: Beitrag zum Studium histochemischer Reaktionen an Keratin und anderen cutanen Gewebsanteilen. Acta histochem. (Jena) **1**, 82 (1954). — BRAUN-FALCO, O., and K. SALFELD: Leucine aminopeptidase activity in mast cells. Nature (Lond.) **183**, 51 (1959). — BRAUS: Anatomie des Menschen, fortgef. von C. ELZE, 2. Aufl., Bd. 3. Berlin-Göttingen-Heidelberg: Springer 1960. — BUCHER, O.: Histologie und mikroskopische Anatomie des Menschen, 4. Aufl. Bern u. Stuttgart: Hans Huber 1965. — BUNTING, H.: The distribution of acid mucopolysaccharides in mammalian tissues as revealed by histochemical methods. Ann. N.Y. Acad. Sci. **52**, 977 (1950). — BUNTING, H., G. B. WISLOCKI, and E. W. DEMPSEY: The chemical histology of human eccrine and apocrine sweat glands. Anat. Rec. **100**, 61 (1948). — BURCH, G. E., and J. H. PHILLIPS: Chromaffin reacting cells in human digital skin. Circulat. Res. **6**, 416 (1958). — BUTTGE, U.: Morphologie der Grenzfläche zwischen Epithel und Bindegewebe der weiblichen Genital- und Analregion sowie der Vagina. Z. Zellforsch. **50**, 598 (1959).

Cameron, I. L., and R. E. Smith: Cytological responses of brown fat tissue in cold-exposed rats. J. Cell Biol. 23, 89 (1964). — Cauna, N.: Nature and functions of the papillary ridges of the digital skin. Anat. Rec. 119, 449 (1954). — Chase, W. H.: Fine structure of rat adipose tissue. J. Ultrastruct. Res. 2, 283 (1959). — Clara, M.: Beiträge zur Kenntnis der Gitterfasern. Z. Zellforsch. 37, 389 (1952). — Combs, J. W., D. Lagunoff, and E. P. Benditt: Differentiation and proliferation of embryonic mast cells of the rat. J. Cell Biol. 25, 577 (1965). — Cooper, J. H.: The basement membrane-elastica system of the dermo-epidermal junction. Nature (Lond.) 178, 643 (1956). — Cowdry, E. v.: Principles of ageing. London: H. Kempton 1939.

Dabelow, A.: Die Milchdrüse. In: v. Möllendorffs Handbuch der mikroskopischen Anatomie des Menschen. Ergänzung zu Bd. III/1. Berlin-Göttingen-Heidelberg: Springer 1957. — Die Entwicklung der Fettorgane (Wassermann) im subcutanen Gewebe menschlicher Feten (nach Untersuchungen an dicken Schnitten mit Gefäßinjektion). Anat. Anz. Erg.-H. 104, 83 (1958). — Daems, W. Th., and J. P. Persijn: Demonstration of PAS-positive material in electron microscopy with lead-staining. Histochemie 3, 79 (1962). — Dannenberg, A. M., M. S. Burstone, D. D. S. Paul, C. Walter, and J. W. Kinsley: A histochemical study of phagocytic and encymatic functions of rabbit mononuclear and polymorphonuclear exsudate cells and alveolar macrophages. J. Cell Biol. 17, 465 (1963). — Dempsey, E. W., and A. J. Lansing: Elastic tissue. Int. Rev. Cytol. 3, 437 (1954). — Dettmer, N., J. Neckel u. H. Ruska: Elektronenmikroskopische Befunde an versilberten kollagenen Fibrillen. Z. wiss. Mikr. 60, 290 (1951). — Dettmer, N., u. W. Schwarz: Die qualitative elektronenmikroskopische Darstellung von Stoffen mit der Gruppe CHOH—CHOH. Ein Beitrag zur Elektronenfärbung. Z. wiss. Mikr. 61, 423 (1953). — Dick, J. C.: Observations on the elastic tissue of the skin with an note on the reticular layer at the junction of the dermis and epidermis. J. Anat. (Lond.) 81, 201 (1947). — The tension and resistance to stretching of human skin and other membranes, with results from a series of normal and oedemtous cases. J. Physiol. (Lond.) 112, 102 (1951). — Dorfman, A.: Metabolism of the mucopolysaccharides of connective tissue. Pharmacol. Rev. 7, 1 (1955). — Polysaccharides of connective tissue. J. Histochem. Cytochem. 11, 2 (1963). — Duran-Reynals, F.: Tissue permeability and the spreading factors in infection. Bact. Rev. 6, 197 (1942). — Ground substance of the mesenchyme and hyaluronidase. Science 110, 74 (1949). — Duve, C. de: Lysosomes, a new group of cytoplasmic particles. In: Subcellular particles (ed. Thayashi). New York: Ronald Press 1959. — Funktionelle und morphologische Organisation der Zelle. Berlin-Göttingen-Heidelberg: Springer 1963.

Eichner, F.: Zur Frage der Motivbildung in der menschlichen Haut. Anat. Anz. 100, 303 (1954). — Elze, C.: Die Haut, Integumentum commune. In: H. Braus, Anatomie des Menschen, fortgef. von C. Elze, 2. Aufl., Bd. 3. Berlin-Göttingen-Heidelberg: 736—800 1960. — Enghusen, E.: Über die Bildung der argyrophilen Fibrillen. Acta anat. (Basel) 11, 664 (1950/51). — Über die Bildung der kollagenen Fibrillen in vitro. Acta anat. (Basel) 20, 94 (1954). — Über Reticulin, Kollagen und die Interzellularsubstanz des Bindegewebes. Acta anat. (Basel) 31, 46 (1957). — Über die Entwicklung der Reticulins in vitro. Acta anat. (Basel) 36, 264 (1959). — Engström, A., and J. B. Finean: Biological ultrastructure. New York: Academic Press 1958. — Essner, E., and A. B. Novikoff: Localization of acid phosphatase activity in hepatic lysosomes by means of electron microscopy. J. Cell Biol. 9, 773 (1961). — Essner, E., and A. B. Novikoff: Cytological studies on two functional hepatomas. Interrelation of endoplasmic reticulum, golgi apparatus, and lysosomes. J. Cell Biol. 15, 289 (1962).

Fawcett, D. W.: Differences in physiological activity in brown and with fat as revealed by histochemical reactions. Science 105, 123 (1947). — A comparison of the histological organisation and cytochemical reactions of brown and white adipose tissue. J. Morph. 90, 363 (1952). — Flaschenträger, B., u. E. Lehnartz: Physiologische Chemie. Berlin-Göttingen-Heidelberg: Springer 1951. — Fleischhauer, K.: Über die Morphogenese des Haarstrichs und der Papillarleisten. Z. Zellforsch. 38, 50 (1953). — Fleischhauer, K., u. E. Horstmann: Untersuchungen über die Entwicklung des Papillarkörpers der menschlichen Palma und Planta. Z. Zellforsch. 36, 298 (1951). — Der Papillarkörper und die Kapillaren des Perionychium. Z. Zellforsch. 42, 213 (1955). — Follis, R. H.: Effect of proteolytic encymes and fixation on metachromasia of skin collagen. Proc. Soc. exp. Biol. (N.Y.) 76, 272 (1951). — Foot, N. C.: Chemical contrasts between collagenous and reticular connective tissue. Amer. J. Path. 4, 525 (1928). — Frédéric, J., et M. Chèvremont: Recherches sur les chondriosomes des cellules vivantes par la microscopie et la microcinématographie. Arch. Biol. (Liège) 63, 109 (1953). — Freerksen, E.: Die Venen des menschlichen Handrückens. Z. Anat. Entwickl.-Gesch. 108, 82 (1938). — Fullmer, H. M., and R. D. Lillie: The staining of collagen with elastic tissue stains. J. Histochem. Cytochem. 5, 11 (1957).

Gerald, G. B., L. R. Miller, and K. G. Bensch: Studies on the intracellular digestive process in mammalian tissue culture cells. J. Cell Biol. 25, 41 (1965). — Gersh, J., and H. R. Catchpole: The organization of ground substance and basement membrane and its significance in tissue injury, disease and growth. Amer. J. Anat. 85, 457 (1949). — GIESEKING, R.: Über die faserige Differenzierung des Mesenchyms in frühen Stadien der Entwicklung. Verh. dtsch. Ges. Path. 43, 56 (1959). — Elektronenmikroskopische Beobachtungen zur Anordnung der kollagenen Elementarfibrillen in der Sehnenfaser. Z. Zellforsch. 58, 160 (1962). — GLEGG, R. E., E. EIDINGER, and C. P. LEBLOND: Some carbohydrate components of reticular fibers. Science 118, 614 (1953). — GLENNER, G., and L. A. COHEN: Histochemical demonstration of a species specific trypsin-like enzyme in mast cells. Nature (Lond.) 185, 846 (1960). — GÖSSNER, W.: Vergleichende histochemische Untersuchungen über die Proteinkomponente von Amyloid, Hyalin und Kollagen. Histochemie 2, 199 (1961). — GOLDBERG, B., and H. GREEN: An analysis of collagen sekretion by established mouse fibroblast lines. J. Cell Biol. 22, 227 (1964). — GOLDFISCHER, S., E. ESSNER, and A. B. NOVIKOFF: The localization of phosphatase activities at the level of ultrastructure. J. Histochem. Cytochem. 12, 72 (1964). — GORDON, G. B., L. R. MILLER, and K. G. BENSCH: Studies on the intracellular digestive process in mammalian tissue culture cells. J. Cell Biol. 25, 41 (1965). — GRASSMANN, W.: Unsere heutige Kenntnis des Kollagens. Leder 6, 241 (1955). — Kollagen und Bindegewebe. Svensk lem. T. 72, 275 (1960). — GRAUMANN, W.: Mikroskopische Anatomie der männlichen Brustdrüse. Z. mikr.-anat. Forsch. 59, 523 (1953). — Die histochemische Perjodatreaktion der Reticulin- und Kollagenfasern. Acta histochem. (Jena) 1, 116 (1954). — Polysaccharide, II. Teil. In: Handbuch der Histochemie. Stuttgart: Gustav Fischer 1964. — GRAYSON, J.: The cutaneous ligaments of the digits. J. Anat. (Lond.) 75, 164 (1940/41). — GREB, W.: Untersuchungen über die Gestalt des Papillarkörpers der menschlichen Haut. Z. Anat. Entwickl.-Gesch. 110, 247 (1940). — GROSS, J.: The structure of elastic tissue as studied with the electron microscope. J. exp. Med. 89, 699 (1949). — A study of certain connective tissue constituents with the electron microscope. Ann. N.Y. Acad. Sci. 52, 964 (1950). — The behavior of collagen units as model in morphogenesis. J. biophys. biochem. Cytol. 2, Suppl., 261 (1956). — GROSS, J., J. H. HIGHBERGER, and F. O. SCHMITT: Extraction of collagen from connective tissue by neutral salt solutions. Proc. nat. Acad. Sci. (Wash.) 41, 1 (1955). — GROSS, J., and F. O. SCHMITT: The structure of human skin collagen as studied with the electron microscope. J. exp. Med. 88, 555 (1948). — GÜNTHER, H.: Das subcutane Fettpolster als konstitutionelles Merkmal und seine endokrinen und neurovegetativen Regulationen. Endokrinologie 33, 9 (1955). — GUSEK, W.: Submikroskopische Untersuchungen zur Feinstruktur aktiver Bindegewebszellen. Veröffentlichung aus der Morphologischen Pathologie. Stuttgart: Gustav Fischer 1962.

HÄGGQVIST, G.: Gewebe und Systeme der Muskulatur. In: Handbuch der mikroskopischen Anatomie des Menschen. Berlin: Springer 1931. — Gewebe und Systeme der Muskulatur. Handbuch der mikroskopischen Anatomie des Menschen, Bd. 2, 4. Teil. Berlin-Göttingen-Heidelberg: Springer 1956. — HALL, D. A., R. REED, and R. E. TURNBRIDGE: Structure of elastic tissue. Nature (Lond.) 170, 264 (1952). — HARKNESS, R. D., A. M. MARKO, H. M. MUIR, and A. NEUBERGER: Metabolism of collagen and other proteins of skin of rabbits. Biochem. J. 56, 558 (1954). — HAUSBERGER, F. X.: Über die Innervation der Fettorgane. Z. mikr.-anat. Forsch. 36, 231 (1934). — Über die Wachstums- und Entwicklungsfähigkeit transplantierter Fettgewebskeimlager von Ratten. Virchows Arch. path. Anat. 302, 640 (1938). — HAUSBERGER, F. X., u. O. GUJOT: Über die Veränderungen des Gehaltes an Fett-, Wasser-Glykogen und Trockensubstanz im wachsenden Fettgewebe junger Ratten. Naunyn-Schmiedebergs Arch. exp. Path. Pharmak. 187, 647 (1937). — HELLSTRÖM, B., and H. J. HOLMGREN: Numerical distribution of mast cells in the human skin and heart. Acta anat. (Basel) 10, 81 (1950). — HERINGA, G. C.: Funktionelle Anpassung im Bereich des Bindegewebes. Verh. anat. Ges. 40, Vers., Erg.-H. Anat. Anz. 72, 123 (1931). — HERRATH, E. v., u. N. DETTMER: Elektronenmikroskopische Untersuchungen an Gitterfasern. Z. wiss. Mikr. 60, 282 (1951). — HERSHEY, F. B., CH. LEWIS, J. MURPHY, and TH. SCHIFF: Quantitative histochemistry of human skin. J. Histochem. Cytochem. 8, 41 (1960). — HILL, W. R., and H. MONTGOMERY: Regional changes and changes caused by age in the normal skin. J. invest. Derm. 3, 231 (1940). — HODGE, A. J.: Principles of ordering in fibrous systems. 4. Int. Kongr. Elektronenmikroskopie, Berlin, S. 119. Berlin-Göttingen-Heidelberg: Springer 1960. — HODGE, A. J., and F. O. SCHMITT: End chain and side chain interactions in the ordered aggregation of modified collagen macromolecules. In: 4. Int. Kongr. Elektronenmikroskopie, Berlin, S. 343. Berlin-Göttingen-Heidelberg: Springer 1960. — HOFF, F.: Beobachtungen an Hauttransplantaten. Klin. Wschr. 31, 56 (1953). — HOFFMANN, A.: Die Entwicklung des Fettgewebes beim Menschen. Z. mikr.-anat. Forsch. 56, 415 (1951). — HOLTER, H.: Pinocytosis. Int. Rev. Cytol. 8, 480 (1959). — HOMMA, H.: Über Gitterfasern in normaler menschlicher Haut. Wien. klin. Wschr. 35, 149 (1922). — HORSTMANN, E.: Über den Papillarkörper der menschlichen Haut und seine regionalen Unterschiede. Acta anat. (Basel) 14, 23 (1952). — Morphologie und Morphogenese des Papillarkörpers der Schleimhäute in der Mundhöhle des Menschen. Z. Zellforsch. 39, 479 (1954). — Die Haut. In: Haut und Sinnesorgane, Handbuch der mikroskopischen Anatomie des Menschen, Erg.-Bd. zu Bd. III/1. Berlin-Göttingen-Heidelberg: Springer 1957. — HURLEY,

W. J., and W. S. Shelley: The rôle of the myoepithelium of the human apocrine sweat gland. J. invest. Derm. 22, 143 (1954). — Hutchinson, C., and C. E. Koop: Lines of cleavage in the skin of the newborn infant. Anat. Rec. 126, 299 (1956). — Huzella, T.: Formation des constructions fibrillaires de la trame conjonctive par les forces de la cristallisation. C.R. Soc. Biol. (Paris) 109, 415 (1932).

Ingelmark, B. E.: The structures of tendons at various ages and under different functional conditions. Acta anat. (Basel) 6, 193 (1948). — Ishimoto, Y.: Studies on the collagen fibre of the skin. Report 2: Study on the effect of heat on the collagen fiber by means of electron microscopy. Jap. J. Derm. 65, 521 (1955).

Jackson, D. S.: Chondroitin sulfuric acid as a factor in the stability of tendon. Biochem. J. 54, 638 (1953). — Jackson, D. S., and J. P. Bentley: On the significance of the extractable collagen. J. biophys. biochem. Cytol. 7, 37 (1960). — Jalowy, B.: Kollagen, Elastin und Retikulin der Haut. (Ein Beitrag zur Erklärung des Wesens der Fasernargyrophilie.) Z. Zellforsch. 27, 667 (1927). — Jarrett, A.: The structures of collagen and elastic tissues in unprocessed skin. Brit. J. Derm. 70, 343 (1958). — Jasswoin, G. W.: Beiträge zur vergleichenden Histologie des Blutes und des Bindegewebes. Z. mikr.-anat. Forsch. 19, 513 (1930). — Eine zuverlässige Herstellungs- und Färbungsmethode der Häutchen des lockeren Bindegewebes. Z. wiss. Mikr. 49, 191 (1932). — John, F.: Zur mikroskopischen Anatomie der Gefäß- und Schweißdrüsennerven in der menschlichen Haut. Z. Zellforsch. 30, 297 (1940). — Jordan, H. E.: The origin and fate of plasmacytes. Anat. Rec. 119, 325 (1954). — Jorpes, E., H. Holmgren u. O. Wilander: Über das Vorkommen von Heparin in den Gefäßwänden und in den Augen. Z. mikr.-anat. Forsch. 42, 279 (1937).

Kajikawa, K.: The fine structure of fibroblasts of mouse embryo skin. J. Electronmicr. 10, 131 (1961). — Kanaizuka, Z.: Beiträge zur Morphologie des Musculus arrector pili. Folia anat. jap. 4, 141 (1926). — Karrer, H. E.: An electron microscope study of the aorta in young and aging mice. J. ultrastruct. Res. 5, 1 (1961). — Karrer, H. E., and J. Cox: Electron microscope study of developing chick embryo aorta. J. Ultrastruct. Res. 4, 420 (1960). — Katzberg, A. A.: The surface area of the dermal-epidermal junction as a factor in the renewal of the epidermis. Anat. Rec. 127, 471 (1957). — The area of the dermo-epithelial junction in human skin. Anat. Rec. 131, 717 (1958). — Kawase, O., and K. Sunahara: On the membran-like architectures in dermal connective tissue: a histochemical study on hyaluronic acid, a substrate of the spreading factor. Acta Sch. med. Univ. Kioto 29, 192 (1952). — Keech, M. K.: Electron microscope study of the normal rat aorta. J. biophys. biochem. Cytol. 7, 533 (1960a). — Electron microscope study of elastase-digested rat aorta. Gerontologia (Basel) 4, 1 (1960b). — The formation of fibrils from collagen solutions. J. biophys. biochem. Cytol. 9, 193 (1961). — Keech, M. K., and R. Reed: Enzymatic elucidation of the relationship between collagen and elastin. Amer. rheumat. Dis. 16, 35 (1957). — Keech, M. K., R. Reed, and W. J. Wood: Further observations on the transformation of collagen fibrils into „elastin". J. Path. Bact. 71, 477 (1956). — Kierland, R. R., and P. A. O'Leary: The ageing skin. J. Amer. Geriat. Soc. 1, 676 (1953). — Klemperer, P.: The significance of the intermediate substances of the connective tissue in human disease. Harvey Lect. 49, 100 (1953). — Knese, K. H., u. A. Knoop: Über den Ort der Bildung des Mukopolysaccharid-Proteinkomplexes im Knorpelgewebe. Z. Zellforsch. 53, 201 (1961). — König, J.: Über die Wirkung von Hautnarben, Amputationen und Gelenkversteifungen auf das Gefüge der umgebenden Lederhaut. Morph. Jb. 88, 81 (1942). — Krompecher, St.: Die Entwicklung der elastischen Elemente der Arterienwand. Z. Anat. Entwickl.-Gesch. 85, 704 (1928). — Kühn, K.: Die Struktur des Kollagens. Leder 13, 73 (1962). — Kühn, K., W. Grassmann u. U. Hofmann: Über den Aufbau der Kollagenfibrille aus Tropokollagenmolekeln. Naturwissenschaften 47, 258 (1960).

Lansing, A. I., T. B. Rosenthal, M. Alex, and E. W. Dempsey: The structure and chemical charakterization of elastic fibers as revealed by elastase and by electron microscopy. Anat. Rec. 114, 555 (1952). — Lanz, T. v.: Über den funktionellen Einbau peripherer Venen. Anat. Anz. 83, 51 (1936/37). — Laubinger, W.: Über den systemartigen Zusammenhang der Gitterfasern in den Fettorganen und seine funktionelle Bedeutung. Morph. Jb. 81, 230 (1938). — Lee, M. M.: Physical and structural age changes in human skin. Anat. Rec. 129, 473 (1957). — Leeson, R.: The histochemical identification of myoepithelium, with particular reference to the Harderian and exorbital lacrimal glands. Acta anat. (Basel) 40, 87 (1960). — Lever, I. D.: The fine structure of brown adipose tissues in the rat with observations on the cytological changes fallowing starvation and adrenal ectomy. Anat. Rec. 128, 361 (1957). — Lillie, R. D.: Reticulum staining with Schiff reagent after oxidation by acidified sodium periodate. J. Lab. clin. Med. 32, 76 (1947). — Lindholm, E.: Über die Schwankungen in der Verteilung der elastischen Fasern in der menschlichen Haut als Beitrag zur Konstitutionspathologie. Frankfurt. Z. Path. 42, 394 (1931). — Lindner, D.: Zur vergleichenden Zellmorphologie des lockeren Bindegewebes I. Das Zellbild der Subcutis des Rindes. Z. mikr.-anat. Forsch. 69, 153 (1962). — Linke, K. W.: Elektronenmikroskopische Untersuchung über die Differenzierung der Interzellularsubstanz der menschlichen Lederhaut. Z. Zellforsch. 42,

331 (1955). — LOEWI, G., and K. MEYER: The acid mucopolysaccharides of embryonic skin. Biochim. biophys. Acta (Amst.) 27, 453 (1958). — LUDWIG, E.: Morphologie und Morphogenese des Haarstrichs. Z. Anat. Entwickl.-Gesch. 62, 59 (1921). — LYNCH, F. W.: Elastic tissue in fetal skin. Arch. Derm. 29, 57 (1934).

MANCINI, R. E., O. VILAR, E. STEIN, and H. FIORNI: A histochemical and autoradiographic study of the participation of fibroblasts in the production of mucopolysaccharides in connective tissue. J. Histochem. Cytochem. 9, 278 (1961). — MAXIMOW, A.: Bindegewebe und blutbildende Organe. In: v. MÖLLENDORFs Handbuch der mikroskopischen Anatomie, Bd. II/1, S. 232. Berlin: Springer 1929. — MCMANUS, J. F.: Histological demonstration of mucin after perjiodic acid. Nature (Lond.) 158, 202 (1946). — Histochemistry of connective tissue. In: ASBOE-HANSEN, Connective tissue in health and disease. Kopenhagen: Munksgaard 1954. — MENSCHIK, Z.: Histochemical comparison of brown and white adipose tissue in guinea pigs. Anat. Rec. 116, 439 (1953). — MERCANTINI, E. S.: Failure to show the presence of a chromaffin system of cells in the human skin. J. invest. Derm. 34, 317 (1960). — MERKER, H. J.: Elektronenmikroskopische Untersuchungen über die Fibrillogenese in der Haut menschlicher Embryonen. Z. Zellforsch. 53, 411 (1961). — MEYER, K.: Chemistry of connective tissue; polysaccharides. Trans. Conf. Connect. Tiss. (Jos. Macy Found.,ed. RAGAN) 1, 88 (1950). — The chemistry of the ground substance of connective tissue. In: ASBOE-HANSEN, Connective tissue in health and disease. Kopenhagen: Munksgaard 1954. — Struktur und Biologie der Polysaccharidsulfate im Bindegewebe. In: Struktur und Stoffwechsel des Bindegewebes (Hrsg. W. H. HAUSS u. H. LOSSE). Stuttgart: Georg Thieme 1960. — MEYER, K., and M. M. RAPPORT: The mucopolysaccharides of the ground substance of connective tissue. Science 113, 596 (1951). — MÖLLENDORFF, M. v.: Bindegewebsstudien VI. Die Wirkung der künstlichen Höhensonnenbestrahlung auf das subcutane Bindegewebe der weißen Maus. Z. Zellforsch. 6, 151 (1928). — Phagocytoseversuche mit Fibrocyten. Z. Zellforsch. 15, 160 (1932). — MÖLLENDORFF, W. v.: Bindegewebsstudien V. Die Ableitung der entzündlichen Gewebsbilder aus einer den Bindegeweben gemeinsamen Zellbildungsfolge. Z. Zellforsch. 6, 61 (1928). — Das Mutterstück von Bindegewebskulturen. Ein Beitrag zur Frage, wie konstruktive Fasersysteme und Hartsubstanzen entstehen. Z. Zellforsch. 15, 131 (1932). — MONTAGNA, W.: Histology and cytochemistry of human skin. IX. The distribution of non-specific esterases. J. biophys. biochem. Cytol. 1, 13 (1955). — XI. The distribution of β-glucuronidase. J. biophys. biochem. Cytol. 3, 343 (1957). — The structure and function of skin, sec. ed. New York: Academic Press 1962. — MONTAGNA, A., and V. FORMISANO: Histology and cytochemistry of human skin. VII. The distribution of succinic dehydrogenase activity. Anat. Rec. 122, 65 (1955). — MOORE, R. D., and M. D. SCHOENBERG: The relation of mucopolysaccharides of vessel walls to elastic fibres and endothelial cells. J. Path. Bact. 77, 163 (1959). — MORITA, S.: Morphologische Untersuchungen der glatten Muskulatur in der Unterbauchhaut bei den japanischen Frauen. Folia anat. jap. 25, 95 (1953).

NAGEL, A.: Das elastisch-muskulöse System der Tunica dartos und seine Beziehungen zum Blutgefäßnetz. Morph. Jb. 83, 201 (1939). — Das elastisch-muskulöse System der Brustwarze und seine funktionelle Bedeutung. Gegenbaurs morph. Jb. 87, 216 (1942). — NAGEOTTE, J.: Action des sels neutres sur la formation du caillot artificiel de collagène. C. R. Soc. Biol. (Paris) 96, 828 (1927). — NAKAMURA, S. H. K.: A new method for histochemical observation of the subcutaneous connective tissue. J. Histochem. Cytochem. 8, 72 (1960). — NAPOLITANO, L.: The differentiation of white adipose cells. J. Cell Biol. 18, 663 (1963). — NAPOLITANO, L., and D. FAWCETT: The fine structure of brown adipose tissue in the newborn mouse and rat. J. biophys. biochem. Cytol. 4, 685 (1958). — NIEBAUER, G.: Der Aufbau des peripheren neurovegetativen Systems im Epidermal-Dermalbereich. Acta neuroveg. (Wien) 15, 109 (1957). — Über Zellen mit eigenfluoreszierenden Granula in der Haut des Menschen. Derm. Wschr. 144, 773 (1961). — NIEBAUER, G., u. W. RAAB: Histochemische Untersuchungen des Hautbindegewebes nativer Gefrierschnitte (Kryostatschnitte). I. Der Einfluß der Vorbehandlung. Acta histochem. (Jena) 12, 26 (1961). — NIEBAUER, G., u. A. WIEDMANN: Zur Histochemie des neurovegetativen Systems der Haut. Acta neuroveg. (Wien) 18, 280 (1958). — NOETZEL, H.: Die Architektur des subcutanen Bindegewebes in der Gefäßgegend. Morph. Jb. 78, 523 (1936). — NORDENSTAM, H., and ADAMS-RAY: Chromaffin granules and their cellular location in human skin. Z. Zellforsch. 45, 435 (1957). — NOVIKOFF, A. B.: Lysosomes and related particles. In: The cell (ed. J. BRACHET and A. E. MIRSKY), vol. 2. New York: Academic Press 1961.

ODLAND, G. F.: The morphology of the attachment between the dermis and the epidermis. Anat. Rec. 108, 399 (1950). — OKAJIMA, K., u. K. YAMADA: Über die Haar-Arrektor-Winkel beim japanischen Erwachsenen. Folia anat. jap. 11, 83 (1933). — Über die Haar-Arrektor-Winkel beim Deutschen. Folia anat. jap. 11, 95 (1933). — OKONKWO, B., S. RUST u. G. K. STEIGLEDER: Die Verteilung der Mastzellen in der gesunden menschlichen Haut. Arch. klin. exp. Derm. 223, 99 (1955). — OLSEN, B. R.: Electron microscope studies on collagen. I. Native collagen fibrils. Z. Zellforsch. 59, 184 (1963). — II. Mechanism of linear polymerization of tropokollagen Molecules. Z. Zellforsch. **59**, 199 (1963). — III. Tryptic digestion of tropocollagen macromolecules. Z. Zellforsch. **61**, 913 (1964).

PÄTZOLD, A.: Die Hautfelderung des Menschen und ihre Beziehung zum Corium. Z. Anat. Entwickl-Gesch. **97**, 794 (1932). — PAHLKE, G.: Elektronenmikroskopische Untersuchungen an der Interzellularsubstanz des menschlichen Sehnengewebes. Z. Zellforsch. **39**, 421 (1954). — PEARCE, R. H., and E. M. WATSON: The mucopolysaccharides of human skin. Canad. J. Res. **27**, 43 (1949). — PEASE, D. C.: Electron microscopy of human skin. Amer. J. Anat. **89**, 469 (1951). — The electron microscopy of human skin. Anat. Rec. **112**, 373 (1952). — PETERSEN, H.: Histologie und mikroskopische Anatomie. München: J. F. Bergmann 1935. — PETRIS, S. DE, G. KARLSBAD, and B. PERNIS: Localization of antibodies in plasma cells by electron microscopy. J. exp. Med. **117**, 849 (1963). — PETRY, G.: Das elastisch-muköse System der Plica lata uteri. Morph. Jb. **87**, 85 (1942). — Beitrag zur Kenntnis der elastischen Fasern und Sehnen. Anat. Anz. **98**, Erg.-H. 183 (1951a). — Die Dehnbarkeit der unfixierten und „fixierten" elastischen Faser. Z. Zellforsch. **36**, 333 (1951b). — Über die Färbung elastischer Fasern mit Haematoxylin. Z. wiss. Mikr. **61**, 66 (1952a). — Zur Fixation elastischer Fasern. Z. wiss. Mikr. **61**, 121 (1952b). — PIERCE, G. B., A. R. MIDGLEY, and J. SRI RAM: The histogenesis of basement membranes. J. exp. Med. **117**, 339 (1963). — PINKUS, F.: Die normale Anatomie der Haut. In: JADASSOHN, Handbuch der Haut- und Geschlechtskrankheiten, Bd. I/1. Berlin: Bergmann 1927. — PLENK, H.: Über argyrophile Fasern (Gitterfasern) und ihre Bildungszellen. Ergebn. Anat. Entwickl.-Gesch. **27**, 302 (1927). — PORTER, K. R.: Repair processes in connective tissues. 2. Conf. on Connect. Tiss., p. 126 (Jos. Macy jr. Foundation). New York 1952. — PORTER, K., and G. D. PAPPAS: Collagen formation by fibroblasts of the chick embryo dermis. J. biophys. biochem. Cytol. **5**, 153 (1959). — PUCHTLER, H., and F. SWEAT: Histochemical specifity of staining methods for connective tissue fibres: Resorcin-fuchsin and van Gieson's picro-fuchsin. Histochemie **4**, 24 (1964).

QUAST, P.: Über das Vorkommen, Verhalten und die Verbreitung von glatter Muskulatur in der Haut des Menschen. Z. Anat. Entwickl.-Gesch. **66**, 385 (1922).

RAMACHANDRAN, G. N.: Molecular structure of collagen. In: Int. Rev. Connect. tiss., vol. 1. New York and London: Academic Press 1963. — RASMUSSEN, A. T.: The so-called hibernating gland. J. Morph. **38**, 147 (1924). — RHODIN, J., J. ADAMS-RAY, and H. NORDENSTAM: Electron microscopy of human skin cells containing chromaffin granules. Z. Zellforsch. **49**, 275 (1958/59). — RICH, A., and F. H. CRICK: The structure of collagen. Nature (Lond.) **176**, 915 (1955). — RIFFKIND, R. A., E. F. OSSERMAN, K. C. HSU, and C. MORGAN: The intracellular distribution of gamma globulin in a mouse plasma cell tumor (X 5563) as revealed by fluorescence and electron microscopy. J. exp. Med. **116**, 423 (1962). — RILEY, J. F., and G. B. WEST: The presence of histamin in tissue mast cells. J. Physiol. (Lond.) **120**, 528 (1953). — Skin histamine. Its location in the tissue mast cells. Arch. Derm. **74**, 471 (1956). — ROBB-SMITH, A. H. T.: The nature of reticulin. In: Connective tissue Transact. of 3nd Conf. (ed. RAGAN). New York: Jos. Macy Found. 1952. — Significance of collagenase. In: Nature and structure of collagen (ed. I. F. RANDALL). London: Butterworth & Co. 1953. — ROGERS, G. E.: Electron microscopy of mast cells in the skin of young mice. Exp. Cell Res. **11**, 393 (1956). — ROLLHÄUSER, H.: Konstitutions- und Altersunterschiede in der Festigkeit kollagener Fibrillen. Morph. Jb. **90**, 157 (1950/51a). — Die Zugfestigkeit der menschlichen Haut. Morph. Jb. **90**, 249 (1950/51b). — ROSS, R., and E. P. BENDITT: Wound healing and collagen formation. IV. Distortion of ribosomal patterns of fibroblasts in scurvy. J. Cell Biol. **22**, 365 (1964). — RUDOLPH, G., u. H. J. KLEIN: Histochemische Darstellung und Verteilung der Glukose-6-phosphat-Dehydrogenase in normalen Rattenorganen. Histochemie **4**, 238 (1964).

SALLER, K.: Zur Anatomie der Geschlechter beim Menschen. Acta anat. (Basel) **20**, 62 (1954). — SAMS, W. M., J. G. SMITH, and E. A. DAVIDSON: The connective tissue histochemistry of normal and some pathological skin. J. Histochem. Cytochem. **10**, 710 (1962). — SCHALLWEGG, O.: Die menschliche Haut in ihrer Beziehung zu Alter, Geschlecht und Konstitution (eine morphologische Studie). Z. Konstit.-Lehre **25**, 206 (1942). — SCHAUER, A.: Die Mastzelle. In: Veröffentlichungen aus der morphologischen Pathologie. Stuttgart: Gustav Fischer 1964. — SCHAUER, A., u. E. WERLE: Zur histochemischen Darstellung des Histamins der Mastzellen. Z. ges. exp. Med. **131**, 100 (1959). — SCHIEFFERDECKER, P.: Die Hautdrüsen des Menschen und der Säugetiere, ihre biologische und rassenanatomische Bedeutung, sowie die Muscularis sexualis. Biol. Zbl. **37**, 534 (1917). — SCHILLER, S., M. B. MATHEWS, L. GOLDFABER, J. LUDOWIEG, and A. DORFMAN: The metabolism of mucopolysaccharides in animal. J. biol. Chem. **212**, 531 (1955). — SCHMIDT, W.: Licht- und elektronenmikroskopische Untersuchungen über die intrazelluläre Verarbeitung von Vitalfarbstoffen. Z. Zellforsch. **58**, 573 (1962). — Morphologische Aspekte der Stoffaufnahme und intrazellulären Stoffverarbeitung. In: Sekretion und Exkretion. Berlin-Heidelberg-New York: Springer 1965. — SCHMIDT, W. J.: Die Bausteine des Tierkörpers in polarisiertem Lichte. Bonn: F. Cohen 1924. — Einige Unterrichtsversuche zur Doppelbrechung der Elastinfaser. Kolloid-Z. **89**, 333 (1939). — SCHMITT, F. O., J. GROSS, and J. H. HIGHBERGER: A new particle type in certain connective tissue extracts. Proc. nat. Acad. Sci. (Wash.) **39**, 459 (1953). — SCHMITT, F. O., E. HALL, and M. A. JAKUS: Electron microscope investigations of the structure of collagen. J. cell. comp. Physiol. **20**, 11 (1942). — SCHMITT, F. O., and A. J. HODGE: Das Tropokollagen-Molekül und die Eigenschaften seiner geordneten Aggregationsform. Leder **11**, 74—91 (1960). — SCHOENHEIMER, R., and D. RITTENBERG: Deuterium as an indicator in the study of intermediary metabolism. III. The rôle of the fat tissues. J. biol. Chem. **111**, 175 (1935). — SCHREIBER, H.: Das Gefüge des cutanen und subcutanen Bindegewebes der Finger in seiner Bedeutung für die Ausbreitung entzündlicher Prozesse. Langenbecks Arch. klin. Chir. **203**, 496 (1942). — SCHWARZ, W.: Electron microscopical studies in the fibrillogenesis in the human cornea. VII. Int. Cong. of Anatom. New York. Anat. Rec. **136**, 275 (1960). — Elektronenmikroskopische Untersuchungen über die Bildung elastischer Fasern in der Gewebekultur. Z. Zellforsch. **63**, 636 (1964). — SCHWARZ, W., u. N. DETTMER: Elektronenmikroskopische Untersuchung des elastischen Gewebes in der Media der menschlichen Aorta. Virchows Arch. path. Anat. **323**, 243 (1953). — SCHWARZ, W., H. J. MERKER u. A. KUTSCHE: Elektronenmikroskopische Untersuchungen über die Fibrillogenese in Fibroblastenkulturen. Z. Zellforsch. **56**, 107 (1962).— SCHWARZ, W., u. H. J. MERKER: Elektronenmikroskopische Untersuchungen über die Innenversilberung der Sehnenfibrillen. Histochemie **1**, 225 (1959). — SEIFERT, K.: Elektronenmikroskopische Untersuchungen der Aorta des Hausschweines. Z. Zellforsch. **58**, 331 (1962). — SELBY, C. C.: An electron microscope study of the epidermis of mammalian skin in thin sections. I. Dermo-epidermal junction and basal cell layer. J. biophys. biochem. Cytol. **1**, 429 (1955). — SHELDON, H., and F. B. KIMBALL: Studies on cartilage. III. The occurence of collagen within vacuoles of the golgi apparatus. J. biophys. biochem. Cytol. **12**, 599 (1962). — SLACK, H. G. B.: Metabolism of collagen in the rat. In: Nature and structure of collagen (ed. RANDALL). London: Butterworth & Co. 1953. — SMITH, D. E.: The tissue mast cell. In: Int. Rev. Cytol. **14**, 327—386 (1963). — SMITH, D. E., and Y. S. LEWIS: Electron microscopy of the tissue mast cell. J. biophys. biochem. Cytol. **3**, 9 (1957). — SMITH, R. E.: Thermogenetic activity of the hibernating gland in the cold-acclimatized rat. Physiologist. **4**, 113 (1961). — STAUBESAND, J.: Cytopempsis. In: Sekretion und Exkretion. Berlin-Heidelberg-New York: Springer 1965. — STEIGLEDER, G. K.: Zum Verhalten der Grundsubstanz, der Basalmembran und der Schweißdrüsen in der menschlichen Haut, zugleich eine Bemerkung zum Phänomen der Glykogenflucht. Klin. Wschr. **36**, 389 (1958). — Neue Befunde zur Phanerose der Grundsubstanz in der Cutis. Dermatologica (Basel) **118**, 154 (1959). — STEIGLEDER, G. K., R. KUDICKE u. Y. KAMEI: Die Lokalisation der Aminopeptidasenaktivität in normaler Haut. Arch. klin. exp. Derm. **215**, 307 (1962). — STOECKENIUS, W.: Zur Feinstruktur der Granula menschlicher Gewebsmastzellen. Exp. Cell Res. **11**, 656 (1956). — Weitere Untersuchungen am lymphatischen Gewebe. Verh. dtsch. path. Ges. **41**, 304 (1957). — STOUGHTON, R., and G. WELLS: A histochemical study on polysaccharid in normal and diseased skin. J. invest. Derm. **14**, 37 (1950). — STRAUS, W.: Cytochemical observations on the relationship between lysosomes and phagosomes in kidney and liver by combined staining for acid phosphatase and intravenously injected horseradish peroxidase. J. Cell Biol. **20**, 497 (1964a). — Occurence of phagosomes and phagolysosomes in different segments of the nephron in ration to the reabsorption, transport, digestion, and extrusion of intravenously injected horseradish peroxidase. J. Cell Biol. **21**, 295 (1964b). — SYLVÉN, B.: Über das Vorkommen von hochmolekularen Esterschwefelsäuren im Granulationsgewebe und bei der Epithelregeneration. Acta chir. scand. **86**, Suppl. 5, 5—151 (1941). — On the cytoplasmic constituents of normal tissue mast cells. Exp. Cell Res. **2**, 252 (1951).

TELLER, H., G. VESTER u. L. POHL: Elektronenmikroskopische Untersuchungsergebnisse an der Interzellularsubstanz des Coriums bei Altersatrophie. Z. Haut- u. Geschl.-Kr. **22**, 67 (1957). — TIETZE, A.: Über den architektonischen Aufbau des Bindegewebes in der menschlichen Fußsohle. Bruns' Beitr. klin. Chir. **123**, 493 (1921). — TURNBRIDGE, R. E., R. N. TATTERSALL, D. A. HALL, W. T. ASTBURY, and R. REED: The fibrous structure of normal and abnormal human skin. Clin. Sci. **11**, 315 (1952).

VITRY, G., et Y. PRIVAT: Phosphatases et métachromasie dans la peau humaine. C. R. Soc. Biol. (Paris) **154**, 2358 (1961). — VOGEL, A.: Zelloberfläche und Zellverbindung im elektronenmikroskopischen Bild. Verh. dtsch. Ges. Path. 41. Tgg., 284—298 (1958). — Voss, M.: Die Struktur von Haut und Fascie des Oberschenkels in ihrer Beziehung zu den Bewegungen des Beins. Morph. Jb. **79**, 209 (1937).

WACHSTEIN, M., and E. MEISEL: Demonstration of peroxidase activity in tissue sections. J. Histochem. Cytochem. **12**, 538 (1964). — WASSERMANN, F.: Die Fettorgane des Menschen. Entwicklung, Bau und systematische Stellung des sogenannten Fettgewebes. Z. Zellforsch. **3**, 235 (1926). — Über die derzeitige Kenntnis vom Feinbau und der Bildung der intrazellulären Strukturen des Bindegewebes. Verh. anat. Ges. (Jena) **101**, 97 (1954). — The intercellular components of connective tissue: Origin, structure and interrelationship of fibers and ground substance. Ergebn. Anat. Entwickl.-Gesch. **35**, 240 (1956). — WASSERMANN, F., and T. F. MCDONALD: Electron microscopic investigation of the surface membrane structures of the fat-cell and their changes during depletion of the cell. Z. Zellforsch. **52**, 778 (1960). — Electron microscopic study of adipose tissue (fat organs) with special reference to the transport of lipids between blood and fat cells. Z. Zellforsch. **59**, 326 (1963). — WEISS, P.: Erzwingung elementarer Strukturverschiedenheiten am in vitro wachsenden Gewebe. Arch. Entwickl.-Mech. Org. **116**, 438 (1929). — WENZEL, H. G.: Untersuchungen einiger mechanischer Eigenschaften der Haut, insbesondere der Striae cutis distensae. Virchows Arch. path. Anat. **317**, 654 (1950). WERTHEIMER, E., and B. SHAPIRO: The physiology of adipose tissue. Physiol. Rev. **28**, 451 (1948). — WIEDMANN, A.: Studien über das neurohormonale System der menschlichen Haut. Acta neuroveg. (Wien) **3**, 354 (1952). — Über das neurohormonale System der Haut. Hautarzt **14**, 60 (1963). — WILLIAMSON, J.: Adipose tissue. Morphological changes associed with lipid mobilization. J. Cell Biol. **20**, 57 (1964). — WISLOCKI, G. B., H. BUNTING, and E. W. DEMPSEY: Metachromasia in mammalian tissues and its relationship to mucopolysaccharides. Amer. J. Anat. **81**, 1 (1947). — WÖHLISCH, E., R. DU MESNIL DE ROCHEMONT u. H. GERSCHLER: Untersuchungen über die elastischen Eigenschaften tierischer Gewebe. Z. Biol. **85**, 379 (1927). — WOLMAN, M.: Lipides. Histochemistry of lipids. In: Handbuch der Histochemie, Bd. V/1. Stuttgart: Gustav Fischer 1964. — WOLPERS, C.: Kollagenquerstreifung und Grundsubstanz. Klin. Wschr. **22**, 624 (1943). — Zur elektronenmikroskopischen Darstellung elastischer Gewebselemente. Klin. Wschr. **23**, 196 (1944). — Elektronenmikroskopische Kollagenbefunde. Leder **1**, 3 (1950).

YASUDA, K., and W. MONTAGNA: Histology and cytochemistry of human skin. XX. The distribution of monoamine oxidase. J. Histochem. Cytochem. **8**, 356 (1960).

ZOLLINGER, H. U.: Gewebsmastzellen und Heparin. Experientia (Basel) **6**, 384 (1950).

The Blood Vessels of the Skin

By

Giuseppe Moretti M. D., Genova/Italy

With 165 Figures, of which are 10 in Colour

A. Introduction

I. General Considerations

The epidermis has an avascular circulation[1], probably similar to that of the cornea and cartilage (COMEL, 1961); the other layers are traversed by hematic (arteries, capillaries, veins) and lymphatic vessels.

We know little about the latter. It now appears almost certain that the arteriocapillary-venous system is composed of an unbroken network of blood vessels of different calibre anastomosed into meshes of varying width and more closely knit at particularly important cutaneous levels more or less parallel to the superficial epidermis or situated around the appendages.

Superficially, the distribution of all these blood vessels does not seem to differ noticeably from that of other organs having parenchyma and stroma (BIANCHI, 1961). In these, from a capsule or fascia of dense lamellar connective tissue originate small septa which subdivide the organ into units and advance by means of reticular fibers until the parenchyma is reached. The larger blood vessels penetrate from the hilus and the periphery, branching out along the septa and into the loose connective structure that surrounds the capillaries almost to the point of contact with the parenchyma.

Similarly, in the skin, the subcutaneous tissue and the deepest dermis, roughly corresponding to the loose pericapsular connective tissue as well as to the capsule, and the connective periappendageal bands, apparently corresponding to the septa, are perforated by fairly large blood vessels that subdivide progressively and create a terminal capillary network immediately below the epidermal parenchyma.

In this network especially, the cutaneous vessel circuit in bodily circulation is characterized by unmistakable quantitative and qualitative features.

On the quantitative level, the skin is thinly supplied with capillaries in contrast to the muscles, intestine, kidneys, and other organs. Even allowing for variations, the supporting muscle structure to the skin, according to KROGH (1929), has about 2,000 capillaries per square mm, a figure at least 6 times greater than the 150 per square mm we counted on the cutaneous surface of the face, one of the most richly supplied areas[2] (MORETTI et al., 1959).

---

[1] Some authors, however, do not agree (FERREIRA-MARQUES et al., 1965).

[2] Since the subpapillary venous network plays an important role in the normal functioning of the capillaries (WETZEL and ZOTTERMANN, 1926), it is probable that the vascularization of the skin is greater than is indicated by the number of capillaries. Furthermore it should be kept in mind that only 75%, perhaps less, of the capillary loops are open and therefore visible (LEWIS, 1927; KROGH, 1929; DAVIS and LAWLER, 1961).

According to other calculations, the vascular volume in the muscle is 7:1 in relation to that in the skin (SCHROEDER, 1959). Besides, on the functional level, the amount of blood in the muscles of a man of 60 kg represents 13.2% of the total, whereas that of the skin comes to only 4.5%[3] (GROSSE-BROCKHOFF and SCHOEDEL, 1957).

On the static-morphological qualitative level, the typical cytology of the cutaneous vessels is obvious. One immediately thinks of the exceptional height of the endothelial capillary in the dermis (HIBBS, 1958; MAJNO, 1965), of its peculiar histochemical behaviour, and of its relative poverty in cytoplasmic vesicles in comparison with the endothelium in the muscle and lung (ODLAND, 1961; MAJNO, 1965).

On the dynamic-morphological qualitative level, the skin capillary system is characterized by periodic phases of growth and involution of the hairs and sebaceous glands, which imply the necessity for many vessels, particularly the capillaries, to reach and supply tissue zones apparently abandoned at other times.

This means the organization and possible degeneration of sometimes highly specialized vasal networks (ELLIS and MORETTI, 1959) and in some circumstances, the increased development of the vessels in one appendage to the detriment of those in another (ELLIS, 1958). In fact, very often the vessel architecture in the skin is indicative only of a particular biological moment.

The characteristics not only of the capillaries but of the whole hematic network are determined by several factors. Among these are the intrinsic structural qualities of the skin and its broad local differentiation.

The varying contours of the dermal-epidermal line, the different consistency of the tissue levels, the presence or absence of appendages, have, for example, elaborated local capillary design to such an extent that each papilla has its own type of capillary.

Contemporaneously, the greater or lesser mobility of the tegument over the underlying tissues, the presence of a more or less consistent and flat deep tissue on which to rest have so modified some vasal architectures, as to enable them to roll up or unroll when stretched out; and other vessels to be flattened almost parallel to the dermoepidermal line in the lower dermis of cutaneous areas overlying osseous levels.

The blood vessels in the human skin then, in their inner structure and organization, possess as many elements clearly referable to the general vascular pattern of body tissues as characteristics which reflect the physiological and anatomic condition of the organ in which they live and function. This could not be otherwise.

So, for the skin too the old distinction between "public vessel" and "private vessel" is still valid: the former has prevailingly thermo-regulatory and pressure value; the latter, merely local functions of nutrition and differentiation (HAVLICEK, 1929).

According to most authors, the duplicate function of the cutaneous vessels does not however mean teleological parity; the primary task of cutaneous circulation is not the maintenance of the metabolic requirements of the parenchymal structures (private vessel) (WINKELMANN, 1961) but rather the thermic and pressor regulation of the blood (public vessel) (BURTON, 1959).

---

[3] The real state of cutaneous blood supply must, therefore, be assessed only in those areas which have no underlying muscular structure (behind the knee in dogs, the forehead and the region above the femoral condyles in man). On the other hand, it must be remembered that in man the minimum blood supply necessary to satisfy the O_2 needs of the skin is 0.8 ml/min per 100 gr of cutaneous tissue (BURTON, 1961).

The disproportion between the development of the adult vascular network and its utility for the nourishment of the skin is therefore scarcely apparent (MONTAGNA, 1962), and it becomes less so when we consider the possible dangers (traumatic, thermic, radiant, etc.) to which the vessels of the skin are exposed.

II. Historical Considerations

This introductory phase, besides being informative, should provide a brief historical survey as a tribute to the men who have contributed most to the study of the vessels of the skin.

Examination of the vessels of the skin began in the 17th century when, in 1663, with the aid of a microscope, J. C. KOLHAUS noticed the presence of very small vessels in the nail fold. Other findings were made in 1665 by PIETRO BORELLO, physician to Louis XIV, soon after the discovery of the circulation of the blood (HARVEY, 1628) and of the capillaries (MALPIGHI, 1661).

Only towards the end of the 17th century, however, were injection techniques used to give the first visual idea of cutaneous circulation (SWAMMERDAMM, 1666; MONRO, 1741; RUYSCH, 1695—1713; LIEBERKUEHN, 1748; CASSEBOHM, 1740; cit. by HYRTL, 1886).

"The special blood supply to the skin", shown in the figures in the Opera Postuma (1821) by PAOLO MASCAGNI (1752—1815), was described as a dense network of minute venous vessels mingled with some fine "arteries" in a more or less extensive mesh work. The close network in contact with the hair follicles was also identified.

In the same century, LEALE LEALI (1707) identified an arterio-venous anastomosis for the first time, while COWPER (1704) devoted his attention to the problem of whether the vessels of the skin are able to contract.

In the first half of the 19th century, research became more detailed until in the second half it was following comparatively specific lines.

HENLE (1841) described the smooth musculature of the vessels and the general appearance of some skin capillaries. TODD and BOWMAN (1845) studied the vascularization of the eccrine sweat glands and even distinguished between the blood supply to the glomerulus and the excretory duct. KOELLIKER (1856) gave surprisingly exact illustrations of the papillary capillaries and the vessels which surround the adipose lobules. SUCQUET (1862) examined the vascularization of some appendages (according to him, supplied with a venous network originating from the superficial capillary network) and gave the first proof of arteriovenous anastomosis in the skin. HOYER (1865) recognized the endothelial nature of the capillaries; HYRTL (1862—1864), ARNOLD (1867), and HOYER (1872—1877) studied arteriovenous anastomoses.

In 1873 TOMSA published the first really important work on the subject, which is still substantially valid. He gave such an accurate description of the vascular network on the levels of the dermis and around the appendages that the continuity of the vascular circuit and its wide morphological differentiation around nourished structures became evident. In 1879 HUETER referred to the capillaries of the lips in a work considered by some to be the first real treatise on capillaroscopy (GILJE et al., 1953).

In 1888 KÜLCZYCKI ascertained in the dog the symmetrical distribution of the cutaneous arteries. In 1889 MANCHOT identified the deep origins of cutaneous arteries and suggested that a pseudo-metameric distribution of arteries may exist in man.

Spalteholz (1888—1893) and Renaut (1897) climaxed the work of the 19th century. Spalteholz, after having clearly classified cutaneous arteries into "direct" and "mixed" arteries, was the first to synthesize earlier opinions and the results of wide personal research into the scheme of horizontal and overlapping vascular levels. Furthermore, he gave the first description of the regional appearances of deep vessels in great detail. Renaut's greatest contribution was the isolation of cone-like areas in the skin ("vascular cones") with rich blood supply alternating with intermediate areas of lesser hematic flow.

The beginning of the 20th century was characterized by the re-elaboration of the data previously collected, by outstanding advances in the study of capillaries and arteriovenous anastomoses, and, above all, by the extensive application of capillaroscopy.

Darier (1900), and Koelliker (1902) reviewed and then modified previous research. The blood supply to the hair and the sweat glands was attributed to the deep venous system by Darier, but to the superficial by Koelliker; Darier ascribed that of the sebaceous glands and the arrectores pilorum to the superficial network.

Grosser (1901—1902) and Vastarini-Cresi (1902—1903) continued the structural analysis of arteriovenous anastomoses begun by Hoyer and accurately described the anastomoses in the wings of bats as well as in many other regions of various animals.

Dieulafé and Durand (1906) for the first time examined the vascularization of the nails and isolated particular territories which are directly nourished by an artery coming from the subcutaneous tissue.

Unna jun. (1908) noted the rhombic appearance of the perifollicular network and attributed the difference between fetal and adult vascularization to the appendages.

Also in 1907, Schumacher isolated typical muscular cells with epithelioid differentiation in arteriovenous anastomosis.

In 1912 Lombard (90 years after Purkinje, 1823) again took up direct examination of ungual capillaries and was soon followed by the school of Mueller (1921—1939) which in the course of long clinical research made capillaroscopic studies of the vessels in the ungual folds and other places.

The next 20 years, 1920 to 1940, were characterized by a large number of findings, often capillaroscopic but prevailingly histologic, which mainly concerned pathology as well as the analysis of the capillary structure and of arteriovenous anastomosis and also the regional appearances of the network. Discussion among these authors was, however, always within the limits of the scheme set down by Spalteholz.

Versari (1923) gave a clear picture of the differentiated vascularization around the various parts of a follicle; Bellocq (1925) using a combined injective-radiological method (much criticized by Spalteholz in the 1927 Handbuch) differentiated, on a circulatory basis, between those regions of the skin which divide into isolated areas without dermal and hypodermal anastomoses and those which are provided with only dermal or dermal and hypodermal anastomoses.

Monacelli (1924) and Chiale (1927) investigated the modifications that occur in cutaneous vessels with the aging process. In Freiburg, the School of O. Müller and his pupils — Weiss (1916—1921), Nickau (1920—1925), Parrisius (1921—1923) — meanwhile pursued systematic regional analysis of capillary morphology. Nesterow (1925), Wetzell and Zotterman (1926), Bettmann (1929—1930), Scolari (1933), and Bordley (1938) did likewise, but their work, because of the insuperable limitations of capillaroscopy, did not lead to any important findings.

Meanwhile, studies on arteriovenous anastomoses continued. CLARA (1927) verified the existence of epithelioid modifications to muscular cells and the complete lack of an internal elastic lamina in the arteriovenous anastomoses of different birds and mammals. GRANT and BLAND (1929—1931) calculated the population; MASSON (1935, 1936a, b, 1937) described the nerve fibers; POPOFF (1935) definitively linked the concept of arteriovenous anastomoses with that of thermoregulation.

After World War II and as a result of CHAMBERS and ZWEIFACH's new outlook on the capillary network in 1944, research on the vascularization of the skin was vigorously renewed.

Further interesting work on capillaroscopy was carried on by GOLDMAN and KOUNKER (1947), GILJE et al. (1954), and especially by DAVIS and LORINCZ (1957), who introduced useful technical modifications. BUCCIANTE's analysis (1948—1950) of arterial blocking mechanisms was generally confined to the appendages and the dynamic aspects of the vessel network.

RYDER (1953—1955a, b), DURWARD and RUDALL (1949—1958), and others, after careful examination of perifollicular networks in various animals, came to a fundamental conclusion about the mutability of these networks which, in accordance with the development stages of the follicle, exhibit definite periods of expansion or degeneration.

MONTAGNA et al. (1957—1958) applied an alkaline phosphatase technique to a thorough revision of the periappendageal vessels in man; their work culminated in that of ELLIS and MORETTI (1959) on the behavior of the perifollicular network in catagen and telogen and of MORETTI et al. (1959) on the "vascular units" situated around the upper part of the follicle.

Other noteworthy research was carried out by KLINGMUELLER (1959), CORMIA (1961), and RAMPINI and MORETTI (1963) who used the same method.

The most significant results in the 60's seem to be dependent upon the use of new methods. DE SAUNDERS (1957—1961), through contact microradiography and intravasal injection of radiopaque substances in vivo advanced a new hypothesis on circulation. ODLAND (1961), HIBBS (1958), MACHER and VOGELL (1962), ELLIS (1965), and ZELIKSON (1966), by means of electron microscopes, defined the structural characteristics of cutaneous capillaries.

ILLIG condensed into a remarkable book (1961) the facts he himself had acquired, as well as those in the literature on the anatomic-functional qualities of the arterioles, capillaries, and venules.

CLARA did the same thing with arteriovenous anastomoses and also summed up current knowledge in a monumental monograph (1956). This was further expanded in 1956 by MESCON et al., who gave the first histochemical description of anastomoses and observations on the surrounding colinergic nerve fibers. Valuable results were also obtained by WINKELMANN (1961) and ORMEA (1961) on nerve fibers.

III. Technical Considerations

Both the advances and the limitations in cutaneous angiology have been due to the kind and quality of the techniques used. Some are old, some of recent or very recent date, often cleverly combined with old methods. They can be classified as follows:

1. Capillaroscopic methods. These almost correspond to true biopsies, revealing in vivo the flow of red cells, i.e., the material "injected" naturally into the capillaries (ILLIG, 1961). Applied particularly to the skin in some regions (ungual folds, lips, ears), they may follow the classic technique (MÜLLER, 1939) or variations of it which improve visibility.

2. Injection methods. These show clearly arteries, arterioles and capillaries, venules and veins. They require various substances of differing colors and densities to be expertly introduced into the vascular network.

3. Histologic methods. These are the most suitable for illustrating the inner morphology of the vessels by well-known techniques which indicate the presence of endothelium, muscle, collagen, elastic fibers, etc.

4. Histochemical methods. These trace the course of arterioles, capillaries, and venules by reacting specifically upon their walls or upon the blood content. At the same time, they give important information on the biochemical structures of the vessels.

5. Physical methods. These supplement the information gained by methods 3. and 4. taking advantage of modern research methods which supply information on the submicroscopic cellular structure, including chemico-physical properties (mass density, for instance).

6. Combined methods. These consist of a more or less successful combination of some of the techniques listed above.

Let us now examine in greater detail these methods:

1. Capillaroscopic Methods

This technique applies to the skin illuminated by the incidental light of the objective lens of a microscope which shows some of the underlying capillaries through an immersion fluid.

The capillary loops of the ungual folds or the pretibial regions are usually chosen for study. Being parallel or oblique to the surface of the epidermis, they exhibit their arterial and venous parts on the same level. Oral mucous from the genital and other regions has also been used with success (BETTMANN, 1930; SCHÖNFELD, 1939).

Even under ideal conditions, only a minute part of the cutaneous network is visible; beyond the capillary loops, only small collector venules interposed between capillaries, the subpapillary layer and veins of the first subpapillary network, plus some of the more superficial arterioles (the latter on the bulbar conjunctiva) may be revealed. All this depends on the state of the underlying vessel network and against a yellowish-white or reddish-yellow background.

Capillaroscopic methods need considerable technological knowledge and present disadvantages. It is enough to say about the former, that in spite of the numerous variations of the original apparatus (ILLIG, 1961; RAPP, 1963) above all of photomicrography (electronic flash as source of light, stereoscopic capillary microscopy with photographs, etc.) a fixed apparatus is preferred, with the optical part suspended above the skin as steadily as possible (ILLIG, 1961).

Concerning the technical disadvantages, let us bear in mind the diffused reflection of light on the skin, which prevents deep observation, and the varying thickness of the cornified layer, which very much affects the visibility of capillary loops (usually perpendicular to the cutaneous surface and, therefore, not very large entities in themselves).

Because of these inconveniences, attempts have been made to remove the epidermis first by means of cantharide plaster (LEWIS, 1928; cf. ILLIG, 1961; WETZEL and ZOTTERMANN, 1926); burn blisters (LEWIS, 1928); the application of strips of scotch tape (DAVIS and LORINCZ, 1957) which, when peeled off one after the other for 30 or 40 applications, take away enough layers of the skin to create a window through which the capillaries can be directly observed.

Other disadvantages in capillaroscopy come 1. from the practical impossibility of finding ungual folds and, therefore, capillaries in perfectly normal condition on account of traumatic, cosmetic, and household reasons (YAMINE, 1931); 2. from the existence of histomechanical factors like pressure or traction (BETTMAN, 1931) which influence the capillaroscopic picture; 3. from its enormous variations in the skin of one particular individual (WALLS and BUCHANAN, 1956) and that of other individuals of different constitution (ILLIG, 1961; WERTHEIMER and WERTHEIMER, 1955) as well as with the region, age, and other factors (BETTMANN, 1931; WERTHEIMER and WERTHEIMER, 1955; ALLEN, BARKER and HYNES, 1955).

Despite this, the capillaroscopic picture of one finger would be constant and characteristic of the individual, like finger prints (BRAASCH and NICKSON, 1948) for quite long periods, even up to one year (WALLS and BUCHANAN, 1956).

2. Injection Methods

They have been used for several centuries (see HYRTL, 1886) and make use of the introduction into the vessel circuit of substances able to delineate it with the same color or other colors in the arterial or venous portions. Results are often notable because of the precision and wealth of detail achieved.

Injections are performed into the vascular system of the live animal (by intracardiac injection) or into corpses of mammals, including man, with previous total washing-out of the vasal circuit with hypertonic salt or other solution until the liquid introduced comes out clear (MESCON et al., 1956).

Afterwards, substances, different in composition and color but resistant to common solvents, are introduced into the vascular system with or without cannulation of large arteries or veins, in order to trace the outline of the vasal network on a three dimensional level. The usual histological techniques follow this process.

The injection compound used varies: TOMSA (1873) used soluble berlin blue, for example ferrous hydroxide, and copper ferrocyanide with glue; KÜLCZYKY (1889) a mixture of barium carbonate and minium (cf. BELLOCQ, 1925); SPALTEHOLZ (1893) glue and gelatin mixed with various mineral substances according to the type of vessel; RENAUT (1897; cf. BELLOCQ, 1925) prussian blue and gelatin; DIEULAFÉ and DURAND (1906; cf. BELLOCQ, 1925) minium with turpentine essence, etc. China ink, pure or mixed with gelatin, has been used with success as was recently proved by DURWARD and RUDALL (1958), GOODALL and YANG (1954), MESCON et al. (1956), WINKELMANN (1961), and finally the use of a special silicone rubber to the skin has been proved effective (SOBIN, FRASHER and TREMER, 1962; DEMIS and BRIM, 1965).

Injection methods are useful also when combined with other techniques. BELLOCQ (1925), as had DIEULAFÉ and DURAND (1906), benefited from the radiopacity of a mixture of minium and turpentine essence for simple radiographic and stereoscopic studies of the injected vessels. For X-ray microscopy DE SAUNDERS first made intravasal injection of a radiopaque mass, which easily combined with the blood and was composed of such small particles ($0.5\,\gamma$) (Micropaque: DE SAUNDERS, 1957—1961) that it passed through the capillaries. Others like RYDER (1954) added some substances reactive with hemoglobin, like Cyanol, to the effects made by china ink and thus prevented any vessel from escaping notice.

Another promising technique, which seems to combine histochemical reactions with injection method characteristics, was perfected in our laboratory by CROVATO and RAMPINI (1965) and consists mainly in injecting into a rat's arterial system the usual substrate for alkaline phosphatase histochemistry (GOMORI, 1952).

3. Histological Methods

They are undoubtedly most used in routine work and are relatively classic. Apart from hematoxylin and eosin, van Gieson and Mallory-Azans' techniques are used frequently, since they are particularly suitable for revealing the connective and muscular tissue; Masson's trichrome stain demonstrates collagen and muscular fibers; the techniques of UNNA-TANZER-LIVINI, WEIGERT and VERHOEFF reveal the elastic fibers, and silver methods show the reticular fibers.

4. Histochemical Methods

These consist of numerous techniques of fairly recent date and of varying efficiency in revealing the anatomical and functional state of the vasal structure. As we have already mentioned, some show up the walls or the blood content of the vessels.

Of all the methods for making the walls visible, Gomori's alkaline phosphatase is undoubtedly the most important and most widely used (1952). In frozen sections, this technique provides a sufficiently complete and reasonably exact image of the capillary-arterial network by taking advantage of the high enzyme concentration within the endothelium of the arterioles and capillaries of many mammals. According to some investigators (CORMIA and ERNYEY 1961), this method should be completed by further treatment of the section with toluidine blue, which would trace the entire vasal course by making the larger arterioles visible too.

Since we shall refer later to the other histochemical techniques, particularly to the enzymatic ones which are able to demonstrate the cutaneous capillaries and sometimes the arterioles, here let us just mention the TPN reductase, succinic-dehydrogenase, and aminopeptidase (STEIGLEDER, 1962; BRAUN-FALCO and PETZOLDT, 1964; MORETTI and CROVATO, 1965), all sufficiently suitable techniques for revealing the capillary network.

On the other hand, widely used and currently better fitted for the purpose are the methods based on the chemical reaction of hemoglobin with benzidine or with substances, like Cyanol, which stain hemoglobin by forming a precipitate (RYDER, 1953). Techniques of this kind, especially PICKWORTH's (RIGGIO, 1952) are relatively easy and give worthwhile results.

5. Physical Methods

These are basically contact microradiography, X-ray microscopy, and electron microscopy.

Contact microradiography was widely used by TOSTI (1964) and is based on exposure to X-rays of thin sections of injected skin stretched over a very fine grain photographic film; the resulting picture is then analyzed under a microscope. With this method, resolution of the smaller cutaneous vessels is limited, mostly because of the dimensions of the source of the X-rays and, therefore, of the probably indistinct picture which is the result and partly because of the size of the recording grain itself; furthermore this resolution cannot exceed that of the optic system used to enlarge the X-ray negative.

X-ray microscopy (DE SAUNDERS and MONTAGNA, 1964) is based on the principle that the smaller the source of radiation, the sharper will be the edges of the shadow projected by an illuminated object. In practice, electronic lenses are used to reduce the size of a minute beam of electrons which, on hitting a metallic target, effect a very small point source of X-rays; as a result, a body situated between the target and a screen will give a larger shadow the nearer it is to the X-ray source and a resolution which is approximately equal to its diameter.

In X-ray microscopy the magnification obtained is, therefore, calculated from the ratio between two elements which are both inconstant: the distance of the body from the target and the distance of the target from the screen. Further enlargements of the first picture are obtained photographically. Especially in the hands of DE SAUNDERS (1961) this technique has produced noteworthy results.

The electron microscopy methods used are, although varied, the well-known ones. The skin samples are fixed in buffered osmium tetroxide, then dehydrated, and after being put through propylene oxide, infiltrated with epoxy resins (which are more satisfactory than metacrylate), then embedded and polymerized. Finally from the hardened tissue block thin sections are cut and stained with a solution of 3% uranyl acetate (WATSON, 1958; ODLAND, 1961), or uranyl acetate followed by lead citrate.

With this technique, knowledge of vessel morphology has drawn appreciably nearer to its biochemical-physiological basis.

B. Notes on Comparative Anatomy, Embryology, and Prenatal and Postnatal Development of Cutaneous Blood Vessels [4]

I. General Observations

Even a brief phylogenetic and ontogenetic analysis of the cutaneous blood vessel network will throw light on its many aspects in adult man. This is because comparative anatomy and embryology of mammals clearly display definite characteristics of their own which at the same time suggest certain capabilities of this network. For example, the constant and necessary presence of more or less numerous well-supplied networks at various depths in the skin (Fig. 1) which are in contrast to the inconstant and relatively precarious networks which nourish the appendages and which probably developed later and in a less complicated way. This is in spite of the apparently increasing tendency in some groups (primates) towards ever more specialized and elaborate perifollicular vascularization networks and especially of the strict and obvious interdependence between the complexity of vessel organization and the morphology of the ectodermic-mesodermic structure of the skin in which it lies.

---

[4] The differentiation of the endothelium from mesodermal cells, which are usually called "angioblasts" or "vasoformative" cells (see HIS, 1900; MAXIMOW, 1909; RUECKERT and MOLLIER, 1906; cf. BENNINGHOFF, 1930; see also, HERTIG, 1935; WILLIER, WEISS and HAMBURGER, 1955), the subsequent formation of "blood islands" (BENNINGHOFF, 1930) and of "angioblastic" plexuses (FINLEY, 1922), the organization and canalization of primitive endothelial tubules, the starting point for the future capillaries, as of the more specialized arterial and venous structures (WILLIER, WEISS and HAMBURGER, 1955) and the events connected with the construction of a hematic network in mammals in general — man included — are well known occurrences for which one should refer to more appropriate texts (CHIARUGI, 1929; BENNINGHOFF, 1930; AREY, 1963).

The morphogenesis of these characteristics in vessel architecture is completely unknown to us. A partial explanation, however, may perhaps lie in the influence upon the neoformation of vessels by the growth and metabolic rate of the tissues which contain them.

In the embryo, the construction of new vasal germs, in fact, besides genetic, chemical and mechanical factors (THOMA, 1893; cf. AREY, 1963; WILLIER, WEISS and HAMBURGER, 1955) will be influenced (CLARK, 1918; cf. WILLIER, WEISS and HAMBURGER, 1955) by the existence of the biochemical changes occurring through the vessel walls, in the blood and surrounding tissue.

The predominant development of the cutaneous vessel network at particular points rather than at others may, therefore, coincide with the site of the skin's greatest metabolic activities. Hypothetically, a typical manifestation of this would be the constant large quantity of vessels in the papillary dermis (Fig. 1), wherever it is well developed. Another example would be the marked vascular development in the boundary zone (Fig. 1) wich is rich in glands between two very different tissues, dermis and hypodermis.

II. Indications from Comparative Embryology and Comparative Anatomy in Mammals (Excluding Man)

Comparatively little complete information exists on this subject, apart from that on primates and the usual run of laboratory animals. The knowledge we have of the *comparative embryology* of the blood network in mammalian skin is fragmentary (HARDY, 1951; GOODALL and YANG, 1954; RYDER, 1955a, b; DURWARD and RUDALL, 1958) and appears to suggest an elaboration of the perifollicular vessel network which may be slower than that of the networks in the tissue layers which lie parallel to the epidermis.

When, for example, in a sheep fetus, a "subepidermal", a "dermal", a "cutaneous", and various deeper networks (Fig. 1) are already present (RYDER, 1955; DURWARD and RUDALL, 1958), the follicles do not yet have their own vasal network (RYDER, 1955a, b) (even in each group of 3 hairs a single vessel, coming from the dermal network, has been observed to be replaced afterwards by the individual blood supply to the follicles).

We know much more about *comparative anatomy*. In outline, the skin of adult mammals is traversed by a continuous vessel reticulum primarily made up of *permanent horizontal hematic networks* (the classical "plexuses[5]" [SPALTEHOLZ, 1893]) situated at different depths (RYDER, 1955a, b; DURWARD and RUDALL, 1958; etc.) and in overlapping layers roughly parallel to the surface of the skin (Fig.1).

These networks have meshes of varying breadth, which besides being connected by vessels of different direction are crossed by *longitudinal networks, partly permanent and partly transient*, specialized to supply blood to the hair follicles[6] (Fig. 2 and 3) or by vessels directed to the other appendages (Figs. 4—7). *Several arteriovenous anastomoses* complete the vascular apparatus in the skin.

---

[5] The continuity of the skin's vessel organization inevitably implies a relatively lesser preeminence of the "plexuses". The latter, without altering their embryological significance (GRAY and LEWIS, 1936) lose the greater part of the supremacy hitherto enjoyed, because they are rich in anastomoses (SCHAEFER, 1912). The word "plexus" therefore becomes a synonym for a particularly rich "network" (AREY et al., 1957) and we have always used it in this sense.

[6] There does not exist any direct relationship between the distribution of the horizontal network and the growth of hair; it is, however, well to remember that when hairs grow, in animals the dermis vessels seem to increase in diameter (DURWARD and RUDALL, 1958).

The authors (SPALTEHOLZ, 1893; RYDER, 1955; DURWARD and RUDALL, 1958; etc.) have never made it clear how far their terminology for horizontal vascular layers coincides[7]; nevertheless, it is probable they may be defined in this way (Fig. 1): from a "deep" arteriovenous network (f)[8], situated in the connective tissue, interposed between the striated muscles in the skin (panniculus carnosus) and the body wall, the blood goes to the arterial and venous vessels of one or two networks of the fascia, i.e., above or below the panniculus carnosus (e, d) (when present).

PERMANENT BLOOD NETWORKS OF MAMMALS

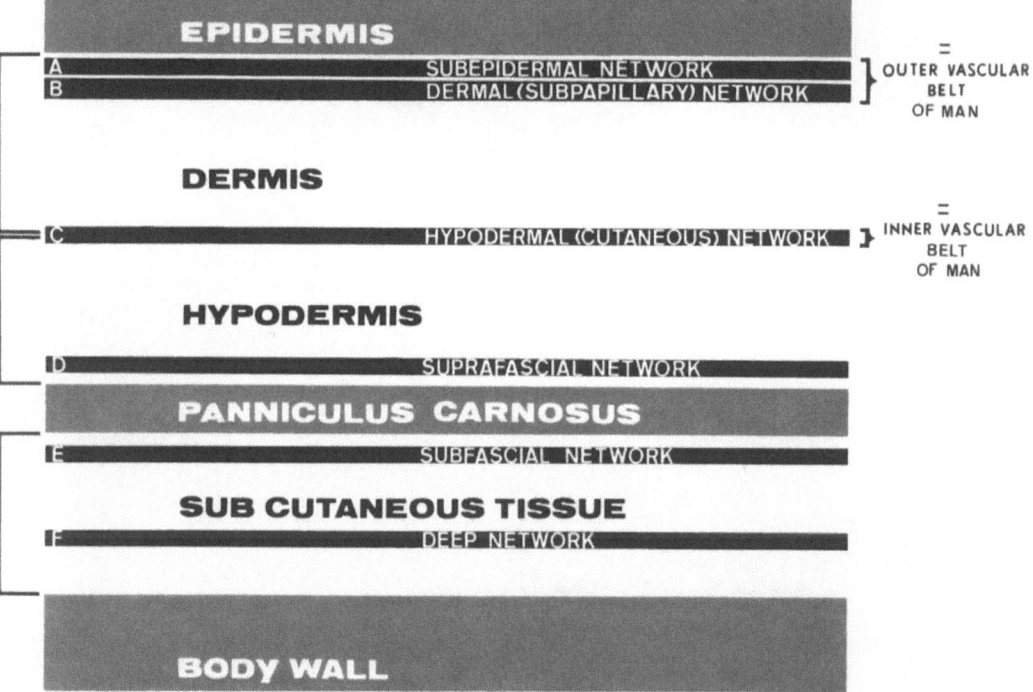

Fig. 1. A scheme of the permanent horizontal hematic networks in the skin of mammals (see text and compare with Figs. 160, 161, 164)

From this network different branches reach the boundary zone between dermis and hypodermis and form a "cutaneous" network (c) containing the principal arterial and venous vessels of the corium and acting as a connecting level between the different vascular areas of the skin (RYDER, 1955a, b).

From the "cutaneous" network some vertical vessels ascend and at the same time diminish in diameter and in muscle-coat thickness, possibly passing through the vascular level of the middle dermis (RYDER, 1955a, b), to the "dermal" network

---

[7] In this connection, there is an interesting list of synonyms used by German, French, and Anglo-Saxon authors, in the works of SPALTEHOLZ (1927) and DURWARD and RUDALL (1958).

[8] This seems to us to be the most practical term for indicating a network, which, since it is immediately above the bodily, muscular, bony and cartilagineous layers is the deepest (DURWARD and RUDALL, 1958).

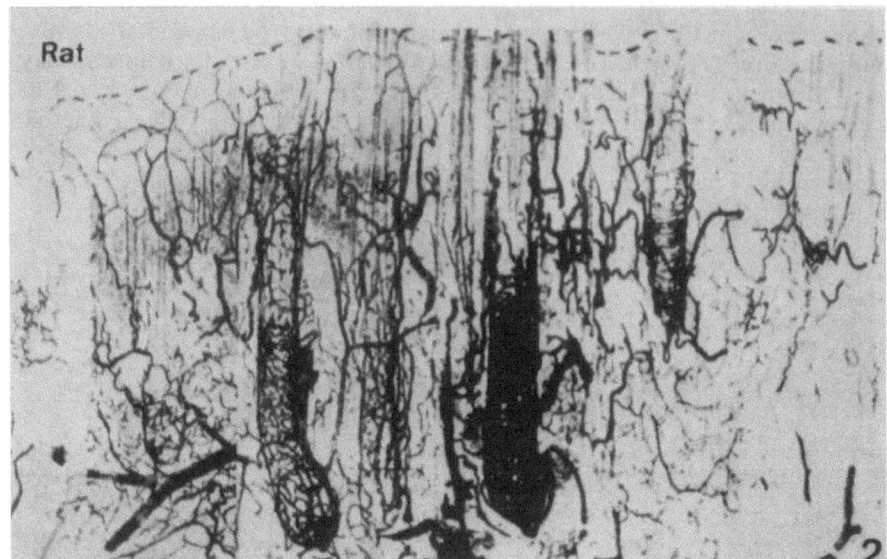

Fig. 2. Skin of rat

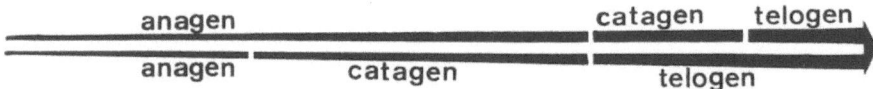

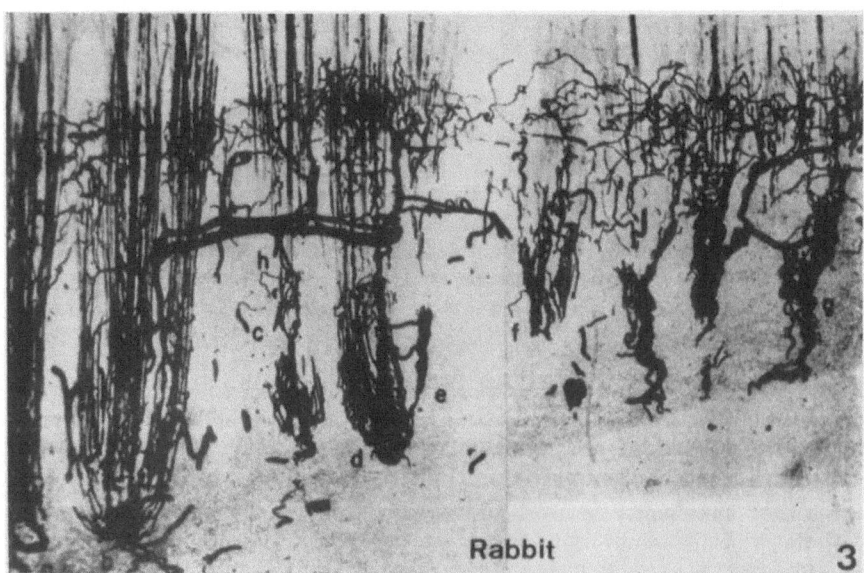

Fig. 3. Skin of rabbit

Figs. 2 and 3. Expansion and contraction of the longitudinal perifollicular vascular networks during the various phases of hair cycle. The transition from dilation and lengthening (Anagen) to dwindling calibre, degeneration, and finally permanent reduction of the vessel bed (catagen, telogen) is evident. (DURWARD, A., and K. M. RUDALL, courtesy of the Academic Press in: W. MONTAGNA, The structure and function of the skin, 1st ed., p. 201. 1956)

(b) which lies in the external half of the corium (SPALTEHOLZ, 1893; DURWARD and RUDALL, 1958) and is composed of rather wide venous meshes and arteries. From this level the vessels reach the papillary zone and there, together with the corresponding venules, form a fine and intricate "subepidermal network" (a) rich in terminal capillary loops (RYDER, 1955a, b; DURWARD and RUDALL, 1958).

The arterial perifollicular networks are longitudinal, more or less oblique in relation to the surface of the skin, and of different types (three, according to RYDER, 1958).

Above these the upper or "permanent" portion of the follicles, as well as the adjacent sebaceous glands, are nourished by the vessels (Figs. 2 and 3) from the subepidermal (a) or dermal (d) networks (RYDER, 1955a, b)[9], while the lower "transient" portion of the follicle is supplied by the dermal (b) and cutaneous (c) networks connected by vessels which are parallel to the length of the hair (DURWARD and RUDALL, 1958).

In relation to its size, the papilla is occupied by a single loop or by a true vessel coil (Figs. 147—150), which usually originates in the perifollicular but sometimes in the dermal network (b) (RYDER, 1955a, b).

In the same animal, on the other hand (DURWARD and RUDALL, 1958), extension and elaboration of the perifollicular networks, which greatly vary in development with the type of hair, affect the size of the hair (RYDER, 1955a, b); the follicles with larger hairs exhibit a dense vessel mesh, while those with smaller hairs have only a few vessels.

As for veins, the perifollicular networks drain into the veins of the upper and lower dermis (a, b, c) through vessels structurally very like the arterial ones [save that in the papilla, afferent and efferent vessels are indistinguishable because of their shape (RYDER, 1955a, b)].

During the hair cycle, all the vessels of the perifollicular networks periodically undergo more or less extensive expansion and contraction, involving dilation and lengthening first and then dwindling calibre and degeneration of the vessel bed, which is particularly clear around the lower part of the follicle [transient network (Figs. 2 and 3) (DURWARD and RUDALL, 1958)].

The sweat glands, which are generally apocrine, are surrounded by not very elaborate vessel designs (RYDER, 1955a, b; MORETTI and FARRIS, 1963), coming from the perifollicular, subpapillary (b), and perhaps cutaneous (c) networks (Figs. 4—7) (MORETTI and FARRIS, 1963).

Arteriovenous anastomoses, "blocking arteries", and "blocking veins" (see Part III of this Chapter) are more or less numerous and vary structurally. In the ungulates, they are situated in regions of particular functional importance (the distal regions of the limbs, breasts, etc.) where they represent a constant vascular element (GROSSER, 1902).

Since we have no data concerning cutaneous vascularization in the animals belonging to the orders of Insectivora, Dermoptera, Edentata, Pholidota, Tubulidentata, Proboscidea, Sirenia, and Hyracoidea (MONTAGNA, 1959), let us examine here the few species of placental mammals that are considered in the literature.

1. The Order Chiroptera

In these animals venous drainage of the wing skin seems to be facilitated by a characteristic pulsation, as yet unexplained (SCHUMACHER, 1931).

---

[9] Given the absence of a true papillary dermis in many species of mammals, it seems more suitable to us to talk of a "dermal" network (RYDER, 1955a, b; DURWARD and RUDALL, 1958) rather than of a "subpapillary" one.

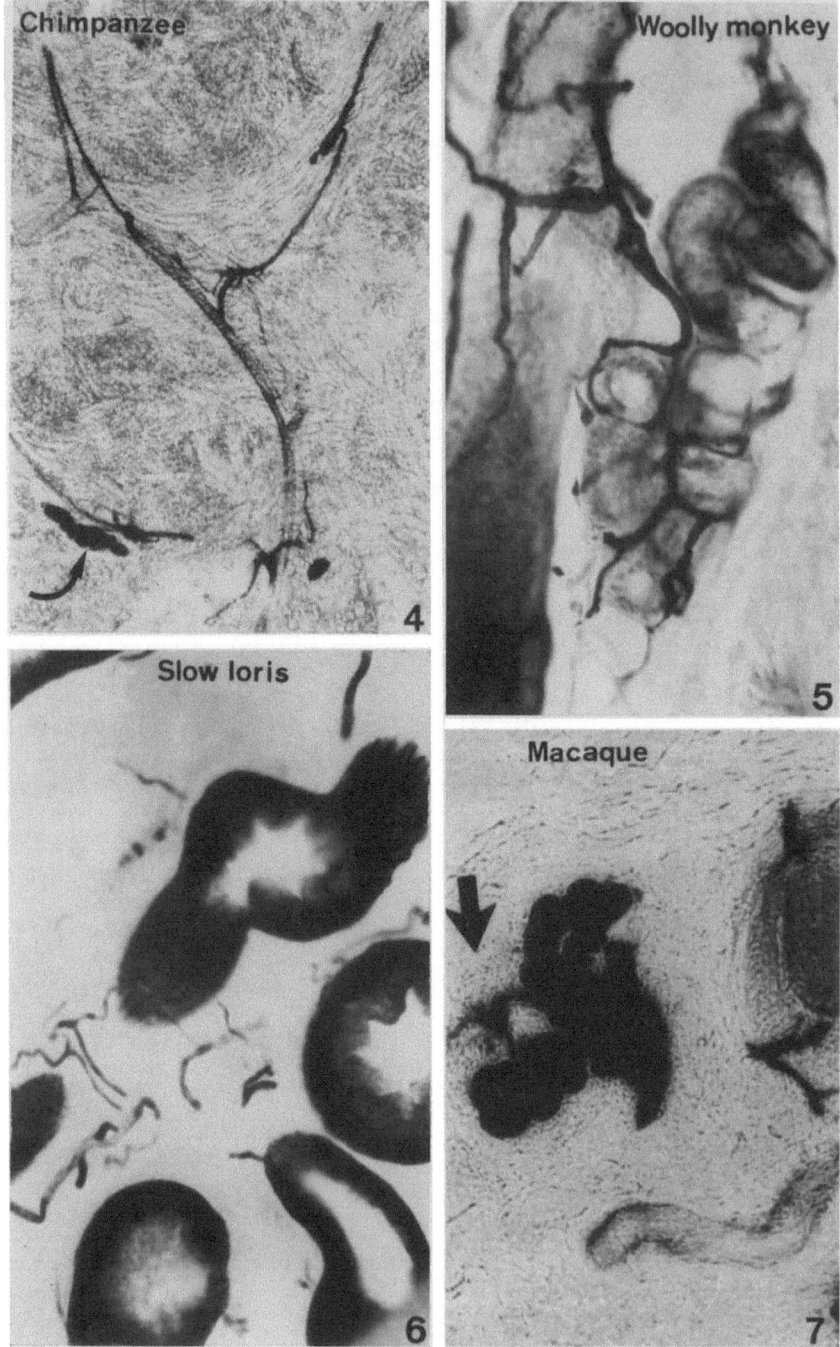

Figs. 4—7. Some aspects of the periglandular networks

Fig. 4. A thick artery from the deep networks of a chimpanzee (Pansatyrus) before subdividing releases branches supplying the eccrine sweat glands (arrow). [MORETTI and FARRIS, courtesy of the Z. Haut- u. Geschl.-Kr., Die alkalischen Phosphatasen in den Blutgefäßen der Haut bei einigen Primaten **34**, 165 (1963)]

Fig. 5. Active hair follicle and adjacent apocrine sweat gland from the eyebrow of a woolly monkey (*Lagotrix lagotricha*). Both structures are scantily vascularized, in contrast to those found in human skin. (Courtesy of W. MONTAGNA)

Fig. 6. Poor vascularization of the glands in the brachial organ of the slow loris (*Nycticebus coucang*). (Courtesy of W. MONTAGNA)

Fig. 7. A group of eccrine sweat glands (arrow) of the macaque (*Macaca fuscata*) with some of their vessels. [MORETTI and FARRIS, courtesy of the Z. Haut- u. Geschl.-Kr., Die alkalischen Phosphatasen in den Blutgefäßen der Haut bei einigen Primaten **34**, 165 (1963)]

2. The Order Primates

The information collected by different authors is largely based on the alkaline phosphatase method and may be criticized because of the well-known species variability of this reaction. In the animals studied, furthermore, the complexity

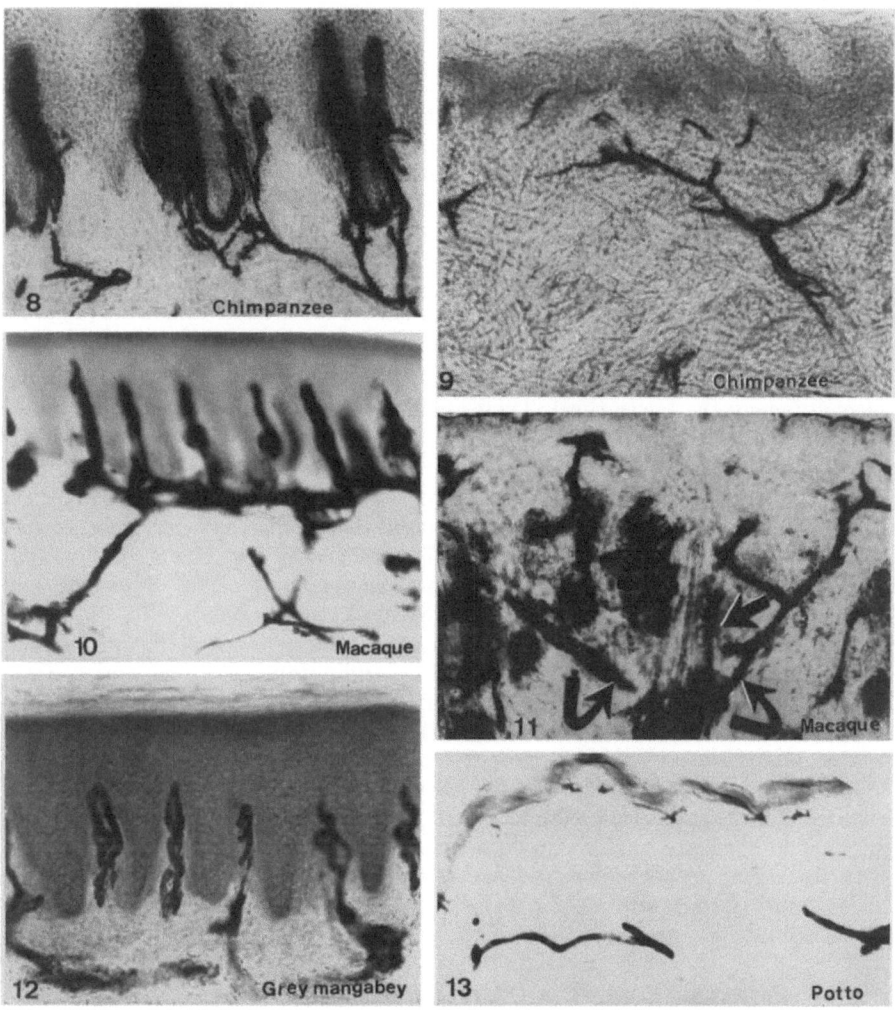

Figs. 8—13. Development of the papillary dermis and state of the vessel network in primates

Fig. 8. Plantar skin of a chimpanzee (Pan-Satyrus) revealing narrow capillary bifurcations from which straight vessels ascend to well-pronounced papillae. [MORETTI and FARRIS, courtesy of the Z. Haut- u. Geschl.-Kr., Die alkalischen Phosphatasen in den Blutgefäßen der Haut bei einigen Primaten 34, 166 (1963)]

Fig. 9. Sacral skin of a chimpanzee (Pan-satyrus) showing the wide bifurcations of vessels supplying the rather flat papillae of the upper dermis. [MORETTI and FARRIS, courtesy of the Z. Haut- u. Geschl.-Kr., Die alkalischen Phosphatasen in den Blutgefäßen der Haut bei einigen Primaten 34, 166 (1963)]

Fig. 10. Intense development of blood vessels within the thin and high papillae of ischial callosities of the rhesus monkey (Macaca mulatta). (Courtesy of W. MONTAGNA)

Fig. 11. Widely diverging deep branches (arrow) and practically no superficial vessels lie under the scarcely developed papillaris dermis of the upper lip of a macaque (Macaca fuscata). [MORETTI and FARRIS, courtesy of the Z. Haut- u. Geschl.-Kr., Die alkalischen Phosphatasen in den Blutgefäßen der Haut bei einigen Primaten 34, 167 (1963)]

Fig. 12. Twisted loops in the "terminal" papillae between the epithelial ridges of ischial callosities of a grey mangabey (Cercocebus fuliginosus). These vessels are similar to those found in other friction surfaces. (Courtesy of W. MONTAGNA)

Fig. 13. Poor development of papillae and paucity of arterial branches in the skin on the back of a Potto (Perodicticus Potto). (Courtesy of W. MONTAGNA)

of the vessel organization changes considerably, possibly for evolutionary reasons; for example, a chimpanzee has a network which is richer in fine vessels, branching out into thinner capillaries (MORETTI and FARRIS, 1963) than the somewhat coarse ones of the macaque.

In any case, development of the papillary dermis is important for the state of the vessel network (Figs. 8—13); where the papillae are pronounced (Figs. 8, 10 and 12), at least one subepidermal and dermal (a, b) network is always seen (MONTAGNA and YUN, 1963; MORETTI and FARRIS, 1963); when there are few or no papillae (MONTAGNA and YUN, 1962a, b), as for instance, in Lorisiformes (Fig. 11) (MONTAGNA and ELLIS, 1959—1960); analogous networks do not appear to exist. In an animal which is sparsely provided with papillary dermis, on the other hand, the regions which have well-developed papillae and epidermal ridges exhibit a more or less elaborate vascular design; gibbons and other primates have numerous capillaries which are often sinous and react well to alkaline phosphatase (PARAKKAL et al., 1962; MACHIDA et al., 1965) only in the soles, palms, lips, and the friction areas (Figs. 8—13).

The hair follicles in the anthropoid Hominoidea (SIMPSON, 1945) usually have, in addition, a well-developed vascular network along their whole length and especially along the lower third. Their glands also have a reasonably good blood supply (Fig. 4) (ELLIS and MONTAGNA, 1962; MONTAGNA and YUN, 1963; MORETTI and FARRIS, 1963). On the contrary, in the greater part of the Old World anthropoid apes, as in some New World monkeys and Prosimii (SIMPSON, 1945) there are fewer arterioles and capillaries visible round the follicles, and the blood supply to the glands is distinctly poor (Figs. 5—7) (MONTAGNA and ELLIS, 1959—1960; MONTAGNA and YUN, 1962a, b, 1963; MONTAGNA et al., 1962; MORETTI and FARRIS, 1963; IM and MONTAGNA, 1965; MACHIDA et al., 1965).

The macaque has, nevertheless, a rich perifollicular network made up of vessels coming from two rather rich subepidermal (a) and cutaneous (c) networks. From the latter, the arteries allocated to the papilla of the hair, the arrectores pilorum, the sebaceous glands, and the sweat glands arise as well (Fig. 7) (MORETTI and FARRIS, 1963)[10].

Finally, one must keep in mind the characteristic changes in the "sex skin" of primates (PARVIS and UGO, 1960a, b). In the subpapillary dermis of the Hamadryad, when not in heat, are numerous spiral-shaped or coiled vessels which are temporarily thickened deeper down and are characterized by unusually wide lumen. During heat these features of the hematic network disappear because of an increase of mucopolysaccharides and the rectilinear stretching of the vessels.

3. The Order Lagomorpha

A rabbit's skin has a subepidermal network (a) and a predominant dermal network (b).

Between the dermis and the hypodermis there is a scarcely developed cutaneous network (c), which is composed of thick branches anastomosed into a wide mesh. The majority of these vessels originate in an arteriovenous network overlying the panniculus carnosus (d). Finally, another network lies under this muscle (e) (DURWARD and RUDALL, 1958).

In the rabbit each group of hairs is supplied with blood by a vasal system which is distinct from, even if connected with, other groups. With the hair cycle

---

[10] In the stumptailed macaque vascularization of the scalp and face dermis is very rich in both arterioles and venules, which are alkaline phosphatase positive, and under the epidermis forms sponge-like cavernous systems by means of large branching sinusoidal venous arcades (MONTAGNA et al., 1966).

this undergoes profound changes; while with the growth process, anagen, it is rather thick, perhaps because of the stretching of the perifollicular vascular meshes as well as of vessels previously contorted; or because of the appearance of numerous stout vessels running along the follicles. Throughout the phases of transition and rest, catagen and telogen, this system becomes extremely impoverished and in the end shrinks to a tuft of capillaries hanging from the lower third of the hair follicle (DURWARD and RUDALL, 1958) (Fig. 3).

In the ungual bed (CLARA, 1959) and in the skin of the cephalic extremity (HOYER, 1877), some arteriovenous anastomoses may exist. In the ear various types have been described ranging from the contractile arterial anastomotic bridge to numerous anastomoses of epithelioid type, with some smooth muscle cells, and rhythmic contraction besides (STAUBESAND and GENSCHOW, 1952).

4. The Order Rodentia

In the mouse and the rat a subepidermal network (a) is visible and well developed, but a true dermal network (b) does not seem to exist (Fig. 2).

The most important vasal element in the rat, however, is a network situated just above the panniculus carnosus (d). This is characterized by the presence, on the same layer, of both afferent vessels and the anastomotic branches originating therefrom. Below the panniculus carnosus one finds another thick network (e) of somewhat serpiginous vessels, under which there is probably a deeper network (DURWARD and RUDALL, 1958).

In the rat (DURWARD and RUDALL, 1958), as in the mouse, each follicle in anagen is surrounded by a dense capillary network (which, however, in the rat does not encroach upon the dermal papillae (HARDY, 1952) bound to degenerate during each successive phase of catagen and telogen (Fig. 2).

The hamster exhibits some alkaline phosphatase positive vessels in the external part of the dermis and especially in the subepidermal region and others on the level of the panniculus carnosus [pertaining to networks a, b, e, d? (MORETTI and RAMPINI, 1965)].

The guinea pig has a subepidermal (a), a dermal (b), and a cutaneous (c) network, the latter composed of quite large vessels from which smaller vessels join to form a rather dense mesh and two deep networks, one above (d) and the other below (e) the panniculus carnosus (DURWARD and RUDALL, 1958).

5. The Order Carnivora

The most detailed observations are still those made on the dog (SPALTEHOLZ, 1893). This animal possesses a dermal network (b) at half the height of the corium and a deeper cutaneous network (c). The last is composed of extraordinarily long branches, analogous to those overlying the panniculus carnosus in the rat, through which the greater part of the blood flow reaches the skin. In the house cat, the lion, the tiger, and other felines, the presence of a subepidermal capillary network has been ascertained, although the vessels are not reactive to alkaline phosphatase (WINKELMANN, 1961).

A dog's pad has no arteriovenous anastomoses (GROSSER, 1902); but arteriovenous anastomoses are present in the Zibet or Civet-cat's extremities (HYRTL, 1864; cf. CLARA, 1959).

The seal, whose dermis is perforated by a complex of sinusoid vasal cavities, has a subepidermal (a) and dermal (b) network and possibly other deeper ones.

Besides the capillaries, numerous venules appear (Fig. 14) which have thin walls and are so dilated as to be separated from the base of the epidermal cells by only a very small amount of connective tissue.

The perifollicular network is highly developed and has long vessels parallel to the course of the follicles as well as numerous capillaries reaching as far as the center of the dermal papillae (MONTAGNA and HARRISON, 1957).

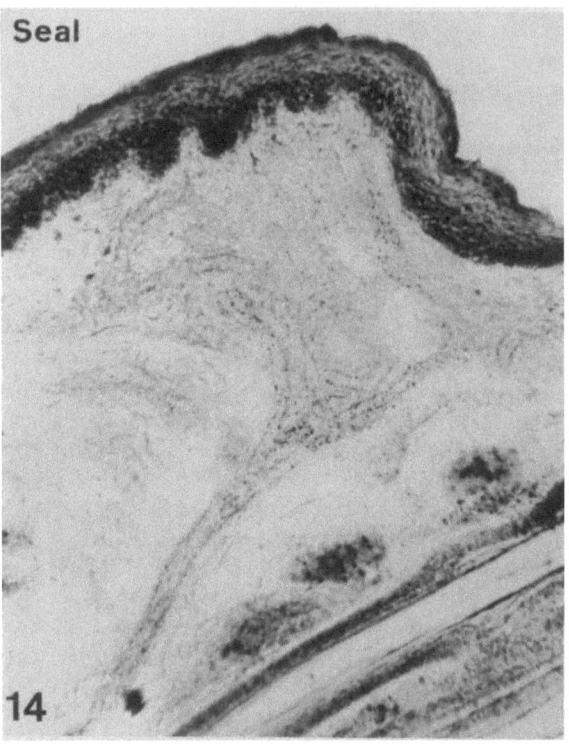

Fig. 14. Capillaries and venules in the dermis of the seal (*Phoca vitulin*) reveal a strong succinic-dehydrogenase activity. [MONTAGNA, W., and R. J. HARRISON, courtesy of the Amer. J. Anat., Specialization in the skin of the seal (*phoca vitulina*) **81**, 100 (1957)]

6. The Order Cetacea

In whales, as in other animals, the extensive development of the papillary body is accompanied by the presence of enormous capillary coils [subepidermal network (a) (SCHUMACHER, 1931)].

As regards papillary vessels, the dolphin resembles the whale. In fact, in a cephalic region characterized by long narrow papillae we observed a subepidermal (a) and a dermal network (b) which was reactive for alkaline phosphatase (MORETTI and RAMPINI, 1964) (Figs. 15 and 16).

7. The Order Perissodactyla

In the cervical region of the horse, we noticed alkaline phosphatase positive vessels in the papillary and middle dermis (network b ?) as well as in the perifollicular zone (MORETTI and RAMPINI, 1965).

In the hoof, besides a dense fine meshed capillary network which is just subepidermal (a), the papillary arteries push forward up to the tips of the papillae and continue in the corresponding veins.

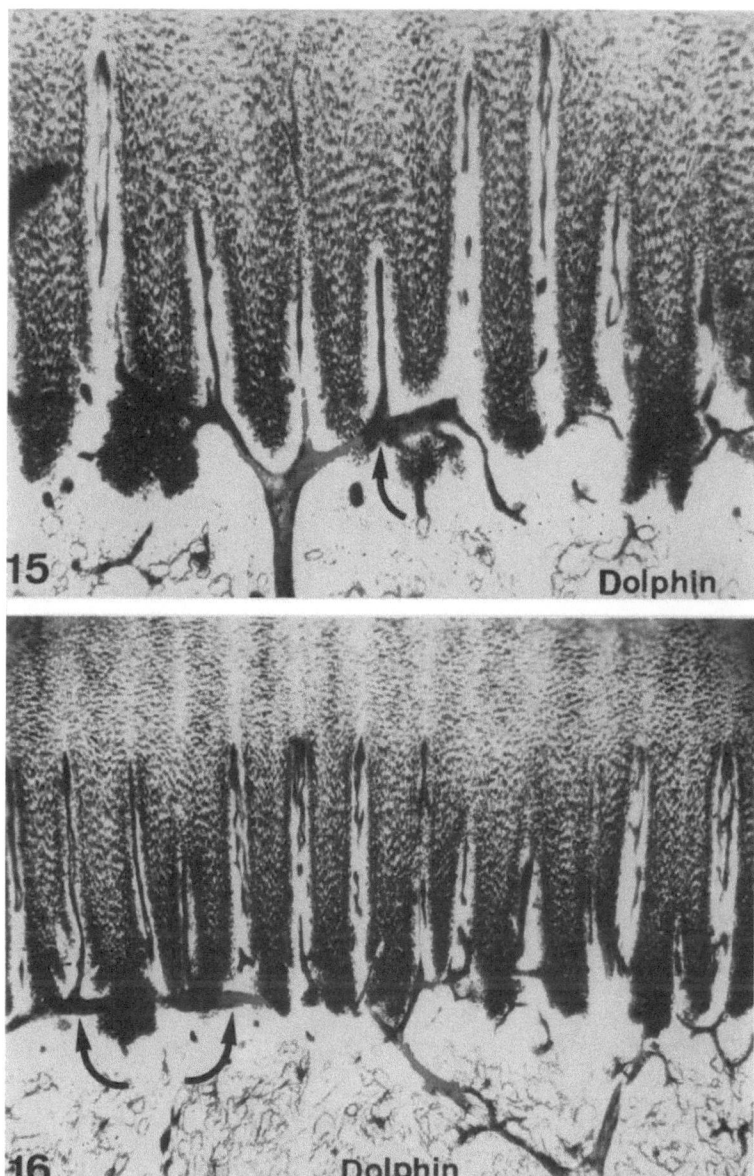

Figs. 15 and 16. Long capillaries rise from the robust "dermal" network (arrow) and perforate the tall, narrow papillae of the dolphin (*Delphinus delphis*)

These vessels, therefore, function as arteriovenous anastomoses and save the blood from having to pass through a capillary network (SCHUMMER, 1951). Other anastomoses with a more or less convoluted course and coated with epithelioid cells are found in the dermis of the zone underlying the hoof matrix, in the papillary body of the bladed dermis, and in the sole cushion (CASTIGLI and MORICONI, 1949).

In the horse, furthermore, the arteriovenous anastomosis is associated with the sweat glands (ROSATI, 1955) in the breast, perineum, inguinal, and tail skin.

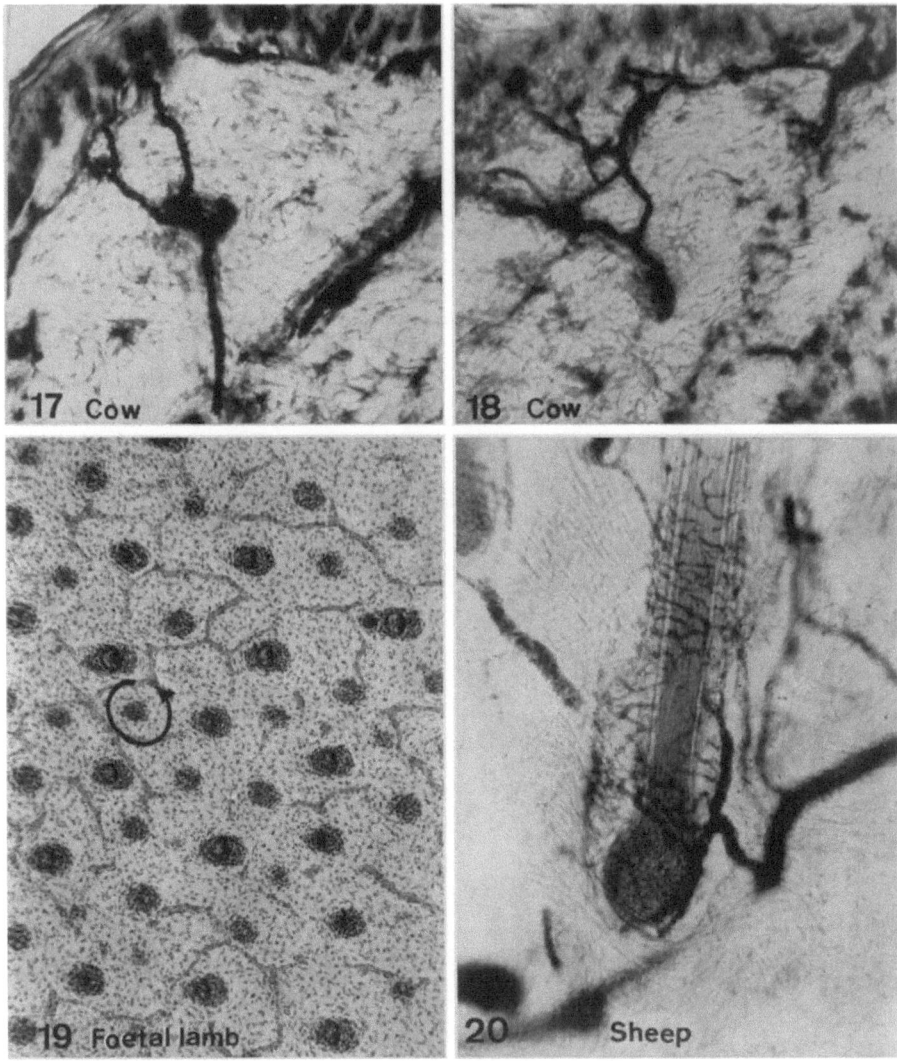

Figs. 17 and 18. Alkaline phosphatases-positive capillaries belong to the "subepidermal" and "dermal" networks of the cow

Fig. 19. "Vascular-unit" like horizontal spreading of the meshes (arrow) in the "subepidermal" network of a 75-day old foetal lamb. (RYDER, M. L., courtesy of the Comm. Scient. and Industr. Res. Organiz. Australia. In: Proceedings of the Int. Wool Textile Research Conference, Australia 1955, vol. F, p. 5)

Fig. 20. Vascular connections between two follicles and drainage into a vein of the "dermal" network of Border Leicester foetal sheep. (RYDER, M. L., courtesy of the Comm. Scient. and Industr. Res. Organiz. Australia. In: Proceedings of the Int. Wool Textile Research Conference, Australia 1955, vol. F, p. 2)

8. The Order Artiodactyla

In the pig, within the deep papillary body and enclosed by strong epidermal ridges, the superficial capillaries and the true vascular coils which they form make up a sort of plexus corresponding to the subepidermal network (a).

Compared with man's, the rest of the dermis is thinly vascularized. The same can be said of the glands of the hair and of the dermal papillae (despite a few capillaries visible around the follicles in anagen) (MONTAGNA and YUN, 1964).

In the pig the subpapillary connective tissue contains some arteriovenous anastomoses (HOYER, 1877; cf. CLARA, 1959).

The hippopotamus has many capillary coils in its tall papillae which are very much like those in the pig (SCHUMACHER, 1931). Interposed between the valves of the thin-walled veins in the dermis of its ears are coarse thicknesses of annular musculature presumably designed to prevent stasis in the venous network (SCHUMACHER, 1931).

The skin of the ox has apparently at least three of the vascular layers described as subepidermal, dermal (Figs. 17 and 18), and cutaneous (a, b and c).

In the hoof, the epidermal ridge level is distinguished by a considerable meshwork of vertical and horizontal capillaries (network a), which react to alkaline phosphatase (WINKELMANN, 1961). In the ungual dermis there also exist blocking arteries from 70 to 200 micron in diameter (CASTIGLI and MORICONI, 1949). Thick-walled arteriovenous anastomoses without internal elastic lamina are also found, 10—20 cm^2 of skin, in the ears of "Ayrshire bull calves" (GOODALL, 1955).

Although a sheep's skin has almost all the known vascular layers (a—d), it is nourished mostly by blood from a fascial network (e) below the panniculus carnosus (f) (RYDER, 1955a, b).

The perifollicular networks in this animal are also very extensive and significant because of their "vascular unit" like (see afterwards) horizontal spreading (Figs. 19 and 20). There are at least 3 types of design while the papilla is almost always richly vascularized (RYDER, 1955b). On the contrary, the apocrine sweat glands (WILDMAN, 1932) have few vessels. Besides the arteries and block veins, numerous typical arteriovenous anastomoses are present in the long mammae of the sheep (as in the cow, goat, and other ungulates (CLARA, 1959).

III. Embryology, Prenatal, and Postnatal Development of the Vessel Network in Man

The embryology, as also the comparative anatomy, and the pre and postnatal development of the hematic network in the human skin are known only relatively (SPALTEHOLZ, 1893—1927; PINKUS, 1910—1927; FINLEY, 1922; LYNCH, 1934; HORSTMANN, 1957).

By supplementing previous data, however, recent researchers have reconstructed the greater part of embryogenesis (SERRI, 1963—1965).

In subepidermal regions particularly, the accumulation of mesenchymal vasoformative cells reacts vigorously to alkaline phosphatase; this activity, however, is common (SERRI, 1965) to all the undifferentiated cells in the embryonic dermis and hypodermis (Figs. 21 and 22).

The development of true vessels is rather precocious and is probably linked with topographical, structural, genetic (AREY, 1963) mechanical, and chemical factors (LOEB, 1893; EVANS, 1912; cf. AREY, 1963), among which are circulation, tension exercised on the walls by surrounding tissues, and blood pressure (THOMA, 1893; CLARK and CLARK, 1940; cf. AREY, 1963).

In the finger dermis of a 9-week embryo, a wide-meshed arteriovenous reticulum is seen, with vessels rich in vascular sprouts. In the finger skin at the 11th week of life, there is an outline of vascular tubules, which are, however, missing in the face and chest (SERRI, 1965).

In any case, at the 3rd fetal month, deep vessels of a certain caliber exist in the skin of the hands, feet, and fingers, while a vascular dermal network is not yet clearly delineated (SERRI, 1965) (Fig. 23).

This begins to show in the dermis and around the appendages between the 3rd and 4th month (Figs. 25 and 26). Some of the future perifollicular meshes (Fig. 32) develop from small branches of a network situated in the upper dermis (like some of the capillaries, which surround and perforate the sebaceous glands); they become larger and begin to function just at this period (SERRI, 1963a, 1965) (Figs. 24 and 26). Under the dermis, at the same time, the incomplete outline of the incipient arterial and venous network on the cutaneous level becomes visible (Lo CASCIO, 1913).

After the 4th month several important developments can be seen (SERRI, 1963a, 1965): 1. a network of wide polygonal mesh becomes evident (Lo CASCIO, 1913); 2. around the lumen of the more important vessels in the dermis and hypodermis, rather similar in structure to those in the adult (Lo CASCIO, 1913), the connective and muscular tunics differentiate; 3. the endothelium loses most of its ability to react to alkaline phosphatase, which, as it disappears from the arteries and arterioles of larger calibre, can be seen in ever-increasing degree in the arterioles and the capillaries (Figs. 27 and 28); 4. in the dermal areas of intense phosphatase activity underlying the cellular columns which will form hairs and papillae, the perifollicular vessels[11] connected with the vessels of the more superficial dermis or with the deeper ones (Lo CASCIO, 1913) of the glomerular region of the future eccrine sweat glands (SERRI, 1965) become continually more visible (Figs. 29—31). The differentiation of the dermal papillae and penetration of the vessels into them has also begun (Lo CASCIO, 1913) (Fig. 32).

The veins, which up till now were less developed and distinct, have become fairly obvious (Lo CASCIO, 1913).

After the 5th month in the dermis and hypodermis in the ungual region, the intense diffuse phosphatase reactivity present before diminishes to give way to numerous small reactive vessels (SERRI, 1963a) (Fig. 33).

Some derangements in the differentiation of the vessel network persist into the second half of fetal life, however complete the network may be. Perhaps local factors are partly responsible for this despite the high degree of organization and even the presence of future candelabra-shaped arterioles (Figs. 34 and 36) in some regions at about the 5th—6th month; in other zones (thighs and chest) (SERRI, 1965) the vasal network is still scarcely discernible.

Halfway through the 5th month, beneath the basement membrane of the epidermis a finely-meshed reticular layer is noticeable. At the end of the same month, the cutaneous network is almost fully formed, the arteries insinuate into the dermis, bend and ramify, and thus form the dermal vessels' plot. They continue to develop and differentiate most of the networks which circle the follicles (Fig. 35), the sebaceous glands, the eccrine sweat glands, and the adipose lobules (Lo CASCIO, 1913).

Perhaps there are other important factors in this period of intrauterine life. The capillary loops have a tendency to become taller and wider, like the papillae that they perforate (SERRI, 1965) (the height and calibre of a loop, always more easily recognizable in the ascending part, is not, however, always strictly comparable with the size of the relative papillae). Vascularization of the plantar and palmar regions is always greater where the outlines of the future secretory and excretory parts of the sweat glands are present. These outlines unlike those of the hairs, are without alkaline phosphatase and nourished by thin straight branches coming from the deep dermis (SERRI, 1963a, 1965).

---

[11] Some authors have recently stated that the vessel-supply to the fetal lanugo-hairs comes only from the "cutaneous" network (JOSTOCK and KLINGMUELLER, 1966).

The formation of the vasal network is doubtless more rapid in the regions rich in hair follicles and sebaceous glands, even if an authentic periappendageal network is not recognizable before the 6th month[12].

In the 6th month, on the other hand, one can recognize from the surface to the depth of the dermis several horizontal vascular levels and particularly a series of meshes, which surround the whole hair follicle, the peribulbar area, the sebaceous, and the rather pronounced sweat gland networks with vessels of different origin (Lo Cascio, 1913).

Other parts of the original perifollicular network are completed (Serri, 1965) with vessels both from the dermal papilla and from other bifurcations of the arterioles going to the epidermis.

At the 7th month (Fig. 37), the principal ramifications of the dermal arteries form large arcades in the deep half of the tissue, whose convexity faces towards the skin surface. Afterwards these arcades anastomose forming, in their turn, a wide-meshed network whose rami create a second closer meshed network (Lo Cascio, 1913).

After the 7th month, the so-called "Vascular Unit" may be seen (Serri, 1965).

In conclusion, the fetal skin in man is well vascularized, even though characterized by a vessel design which is generally more simple than that of the adult because of the scarcity of tortuous vessels and above all of anastomoses (Serri, 1965).

As for Sucquet-Hoyer's arterial tracts of arteriovenous anastomoses of glomic type, they appear in the fingers and in the nail bed between the 4th and the 5th month (Rotter and Wagner, 1952; Beckett, et al., 1956; Serri et al., 1963b) (Fig. 38); at this period they already have a thick wall lined with epithelioid cells (Masson, 1937).

According to some authors, arteriovenous anastomoses, however well developed at the 5th month of fetal life, do not achieve the "topographical and numerical distribution" characteristic of the adult before the 4th year of life (Gasparini and Bucciante, 1950); other authors state that they appear only after birth (Vastarini-Cresi, 1903; Popoff, 1935).

The hypothesis advanced by Vastarini-Cresi in 1903 about the histogenesis of arteriovenous anastomoses with epithelioid walls seems to be confirmed, since it is now certain that arteriovenous anastomosis comes from periendothelial apposition of elements to the capillaries that are mesenchymal in nature (Schumacher, 1907—1915; Clara, 1959); myocytes and epithelioid elements, therefore, would have the same cellular origins (Clara, 1959).

The appearance of an arteriovenous anastomosis would be heralded by the crowding together of a considerable number of nuclei outside the basement membrane; these produce a considerable thickening of the vessel by forming a syncytial mass of homogenous cytoplasm.

The succeeding formation in the syncytium of perinuclear vacuoles thus brings about the isolation of a single cell, even if the existence of an epithelioid cell does not appear certain until the 24th week of fetal life.

To begin with, the arteriovenous anastomoses sink into a mucous-like material. After birth they acquire a true capsula, which is in part supplied with nerves (Rotter and Wagner, 1950; cf. Clara, 1959).

---

[12] The dermal network of the forehead is further proof of the organizing influence of the hairs; at the 8th month this is still scarcely delineated and extended, perhaps because of the tendency of the terminal follicles in these areas to regress in the early months into lanugo follicles soon after birth (Moretti, 1965; Serri, 1965).

11th →14th WK about

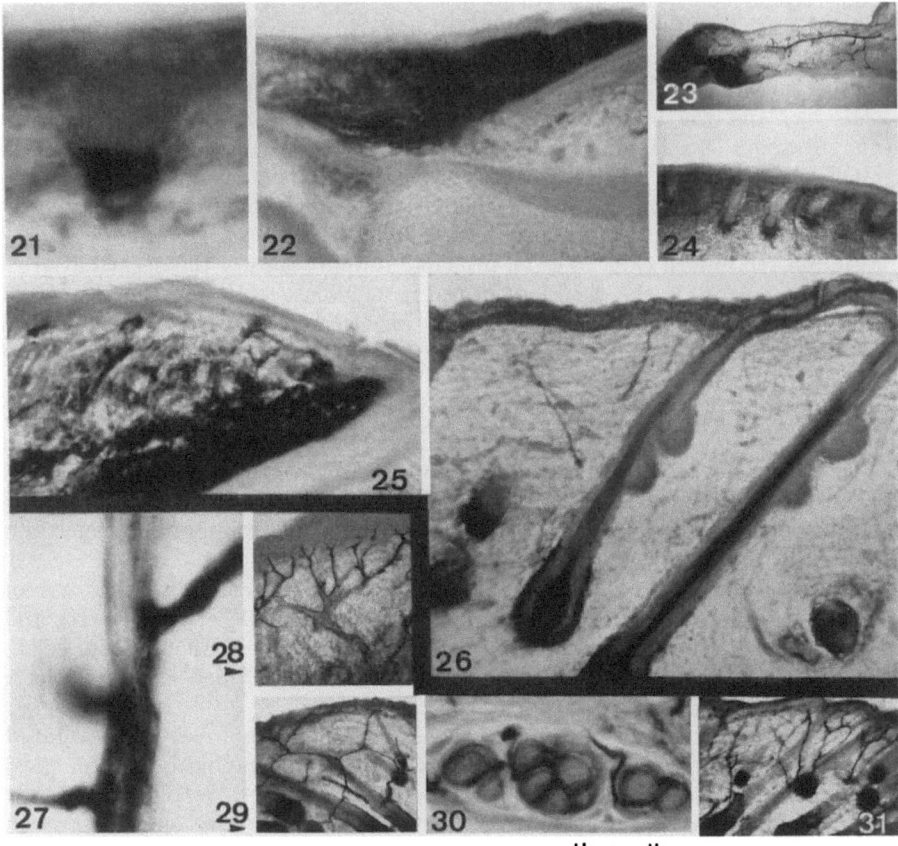

15th →20th WK about

Figs. 21—37. Embryology and prenatal development of the vessel network in man. (The thick black stripes separating. Figs. 21—26 from Figs. 27—32 and Figs. 27—32 from Figs. 33—37 aim to stress the existence of three basically different phases of prenatal development of vessels.) (Figs. 21—37 and Figs. 22, 33: [SERRI, F., W. MONTAGNA, and W. M. HUBER, courtesy of the Arch. Derm., Studies of skin of fetus and the child **87**, 234 (1963) and of the Minerva derm., Lo sviluppo e l'organizzazione vascolare nella cute del feto umano **40**, 180, 181, 182, 184, 185 (1965)

Figs. 21 and 22. In "dermal" regions underlying the germs of hair and nails, the accumulations of mesenchymal vasoformative cells react vigorously to alkaline phosphatases (11—14 wks.-old fetus)

Fig. 23. Deep vessels of a certain caliber already exist in the skin of the fingers while a "dermal" network is not yet clearly delineated (11 wks.-old fetus)

Fig. 24. Thin vessels begin to surround the developing hairs between the 3rd and 4th month (12 wks.-old fetus)

Fig. 25. A vascular "dermal" network appears at the same time in the ungual area (12 wks.-old fetus)

Fig. 26. Parts of the future perifollicular meshes develop from small branches situated in the upper dermis (13 wks.-old fetus)

Fig. 27. The endothelium of arterioles loses most of its reactivity to alkaline phosphatases, that of the capillaries does not (15 wks.-old fetus)

Fig. 28. A weakly alkaline-phosphatases positive arteriole releases progressively thinner rami which react to alkaline phosphatases in everincreasing degree (17 wks.-old fetus)

Fig. 29. The perifollicular vessels finally link up with the vessels of the more superficial dermis (17 wks.-old fetus)

Fig. 30. The deeper vessels of the glomerular region of the future eccrine sweat glands become constantly more visible (17 wks.-old fetus)

Fig. 31. Capillaries extend from the papillary dermis downwards to the region of the hair bulbs (17 wks.-old fetus)

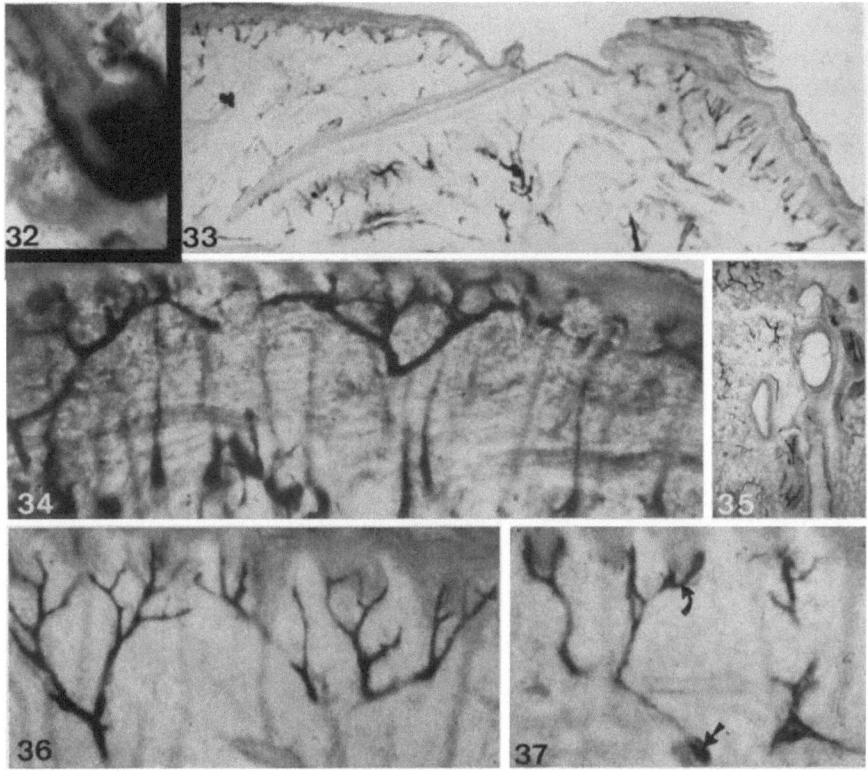

20th→30th WK about

Fig. 32. The differentiation of the "dermal" papillae and penetration of the vessels into them has begun (12 wks.-old fetus)

Fig. 33. In the ungual region the previously intense enzymatic reactivity has given way to numerous small reactive vessels (25 wks.-old fetus)

Fig. 34. Some of the future "candelabra"-shaped arterioles appear in the palms (20 wks.-old fetus)

Fig. 35. The endothelial lining of the larger vessels reveal a mild alkaline phosphatases-activity while the smaller vessels react intensely (23 wks.-old fetus)

Fig. 36. An alkaline phosphatases positive "candelabrum" shaped arteriole and its capillaries (25 wks.-old fetus)

Fig. 37. Some vessels circle the eccrine sweat glands' glomeruli straight (arrow) as well as the epidermal ridges curved (arrow) from which the sweat-ducts leave (25 wks.-old fetus)

The data and conclusions of those studying the postnatal development of the blood cutaneous network differ.

Some authors (BELLOCQ, 1925) held that the skin of the newborn child is characterized by reduced vascularization of the type maintained by "independent areas"; that is, by arteries that nourish isolated territories, and before the age of 5 diffusion of this type temporarily increases in certain regions of the body.

Changes in the postnatal vessel network still must be ascertained, since the authors examined the capillaroscopic behavior of capillary loops instead of the whole network (HOLLAND and MEYER, 1919; JAENSCH, 1929; STEFKO, 1931; GRIGOROVA, 1933; etc.).

In this connection, let us remember that JAENSCH et al. (1929) observed that in some capillaries in the primitive subpapillary network interesting changes (e.g., archicapillaries, intermediate forms, neocapillaries) occurred in an infant's life between the 2nd and 5th week and sometimes continued to the 6th month.

Vessels which were initially "horizontal" and of uniform calibre, i.e., more or less parallel to the surface of the epidermis, were gradually transformed into capillary loops, continually growing longer and in a vertical direction and easily identifiable by their arterial and venous parts. In this regard dermatologists should note that the progressive advance of the capillary towards the surface is accompanied by an increasing undulation of the corresponding dermal-epidermal border, which was initially flat.

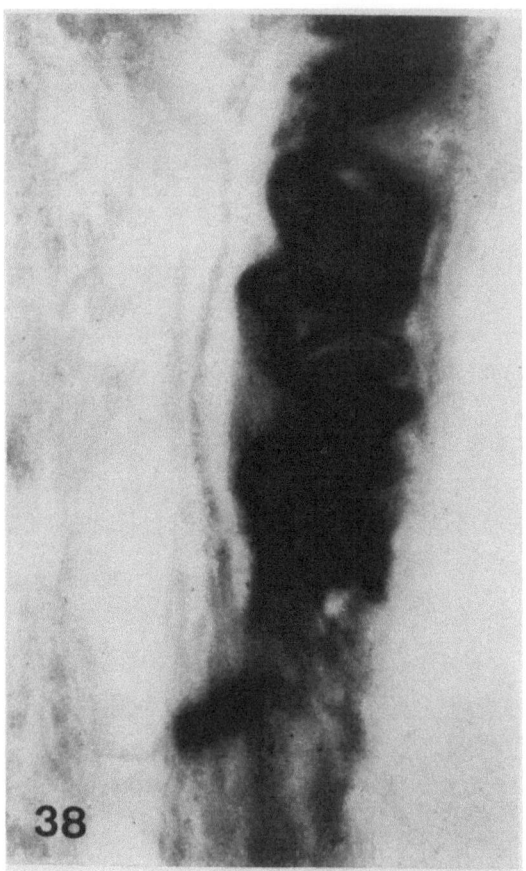

Fig. 38. A glomus body reacts intensely to alkaline phosphatases in the skin of the finger (16 wks.-old fetus) [SERRI, F. courtesy of the Minerva derm., Lo sviluppo e l'organizzazione vascolare nella cute del feto umano 40, 182 (1965)]

On the contrary, many other authors (LO CASCIO, 1913; SPALTEHOLZ, 1927; SALMON, 1936; MENEGHINI, 1942) think that really important morphological differences between the newborn child's and the adult's vessel layout do not exist.

For them the variations in the course, number, and richness of anastomoses of the newborn child's vessels do not exceed those in the adult (including regional ones (SPALTEHOLZ, 1927)), nor do the vessel walls differ in structure in any way (CHIALE, 1927).

At this juncture it should be remembered that in postnatal development the surface of the tegument at the cephalic extremity increases three times but that it enlarges about ten times on the rest of the body (BOYD, 1935); furthermore, it thickens considerably.

Although SPALTEHOLZ (1927) held that everything, including the possible intervention of external factors, only emphasizes the hereditary differences in construction in the dermal network, which are less apparent in a baby, nevertheless it does not seem possible to us that at least some changes do not occur in postnatal life. According to some authors, for example, the sweat glands of the scalp are at first supplied by the cutaneous network; with the development of the dermis, the glomeruli end up enclosed in the middle dermis, henceforth nourished by vessels which link the dermal and cutaneous network (ELLIS and MONTAGNA, 1958). In the first year of life (MORETTI, 1965), the majority of "primary" fetal hairs are changed into secondary "lanugo" hairs; this must have some effect upon the perifollicular networks; the same may be said at puberty of the later transformation of the glandular apparatus in particular areas (pubis, armpits, etc.).

C. Building Stones for the Cutaneous Blood Vessel Network

I. Introductory Observations

In the preceding pages we have outlined the development and the principal locations of the cutaneous vascular networks in various kinds of mammals and, in greater detail, their morphogenesis in the human fetus.

Let us now examine the fundamental cytological features and the relative spatial positions of all the elements which compose the cutaneous networks in the adult, keeping some dominant characteristics in mind:

1. The extraordinary adaptability of the skin for particular exigencies. Because of the skin's mobility over the underlying layers and malleability into folds, its arteries have a winding course and can be considerably distended without affecting blood supply (COMEL, 1933);

2. The obvious plastic dependence of vasal morphology upon the structures which they nourish and in which they are contained;

3. A marked biological capacity of self-modification that permits extensive temporary or definitive phenomena (cycles of pilosebaceous unit, aging, grafts, etc.), of degeneration or disappearance, regeneration and reconstruction in many parts of the network.

II. Arteries and Arterioles

1. Artery Types

The building stones that we wish to discuss are often spread around in the vast quantity of literature without being clearly defined or named (ILLIG, 1961). This obviously renders identification more complicated (see, for example, ILLIG's interesting pages (1961) on the confused nomenclature of small cutaneous vessels).

There is no doubt that numerous arteries, the number and calibre of which display considerable regional changes, come from many directions to reach the vast surface of the skin.

Only in the thigh, for instance, would there be many voluminous arteries; numerous and of medium calibre in the finger and plantar region; of medium calibre and fairly frequent on the outer surface of the leg, and small and rather rare on the inner side (DIEULAFÉ and DURAND, 1906).

The cutaneous arteries are of two types: a) "pure" cutaneous arteries (Fig. 39), and b) the so-called "mixed" cutaneous arteries (Fig. 40).

The "pure" cutaneous arteries are direct branches from the large arterial trunks (the superficial epigastric artery, for example (Fig. 41)) that come directly to the skin and divide and subdivide themselves, completely or almost completely, in the skin and its appendages.

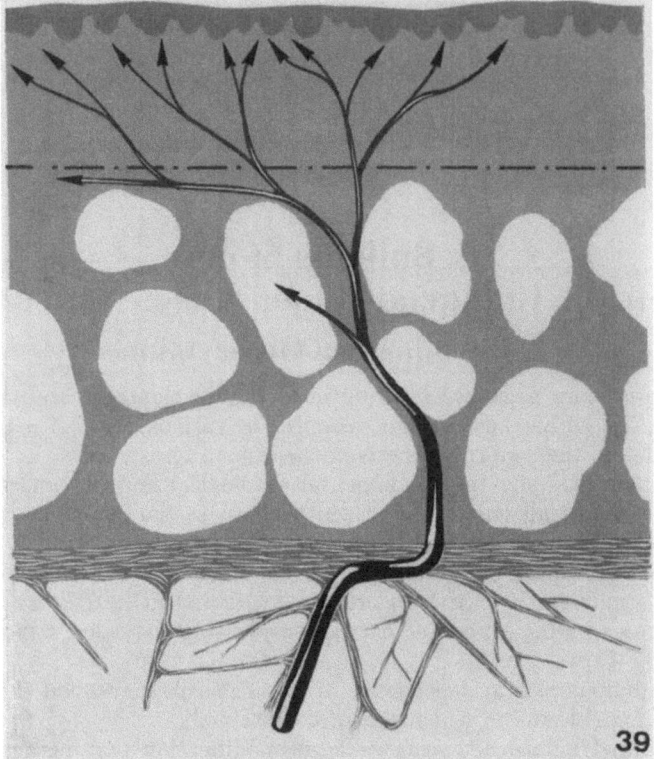

Fig. 39. Schematic drawing of the path followed from a "pure" cutaneous artery to reach the skin

These vessels usually come from the connective intermuscular spaces and move into the subcutaneous tissues which they traverse in a direction oblique or parallel to the surface (SPALTEHOLZ, 1927) (Fig. 39).

The "mixed" cutaneous arteries, before reaching the skin, provide larger or smaller branches for other organs and especially for the muscles (musculo-cutaneous artery); a very large part of the skin's vascular organization, therefore, is indirectly tied to that of the underlying muscles.

"Mixed" arteries are commonly associated with the larger muscles which they often perforate in a transverse or oblique direction to the muscular fibrils. They come out from the fibrils in a direction perpendicular to their surface, then cross, with a slight loop, the muscular fascia, and thereafter enter directly into the skin (SPALTEHOLZ, 1927) (Fig. 40).

Independent of type, the distribution of arteries over the trunk is so segmentary as to suggest metameric distribution (MANCHOT, 1889; GROSSER, 1905; cf. SPALTEHOLZ, 1927) (Figs. 41 and 42).

Because of the almost consistent number and arrangement of the vessels, moreover, the vascular pattern often seems extraordinarily similar on the two halves of the body (SPALTEHOLZ, 1927).

On the other hand, once they have penetrated the subcutaneous tissue, the arteries and the vessels which originate from them turn toward the epidermis, which they reach after having released branches going to the periappendageous networks, at various levels, which are anastomosed with those nearby into a

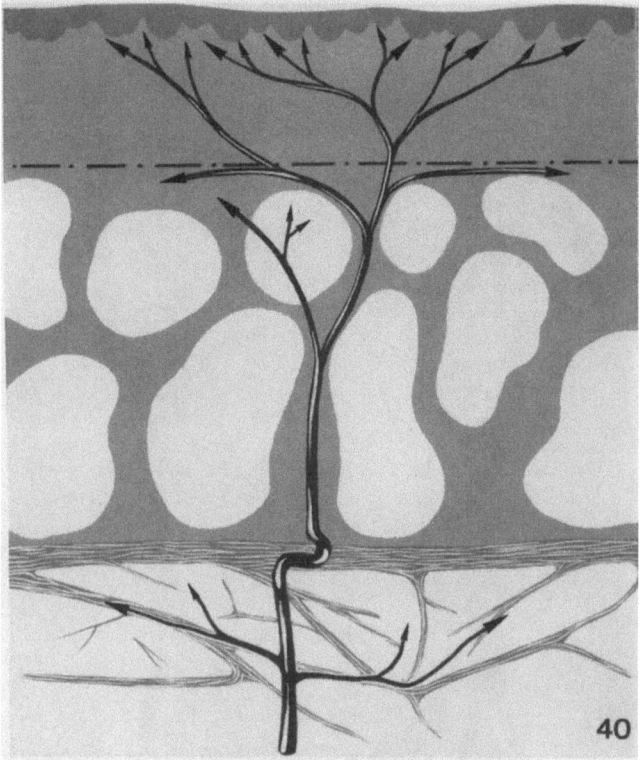

Fig. 40. Schematic drawing of the path followed from a "mixed" cutaneous artery to reach the skin

"fascial," a "cutaneous," a "subpapillary[13]," a "dermal," and a "subepidermal" network, about which we shall speak more fully later on.

Now it is enough to point out that the most characteristic examples of the first three networks are to be seen in the trunk, neck, and limbs (SPALTEHOLZ, 1927).

2. Arterioles: Types and Distributive Characteristics

From the arteries numerous arterioles gradually originate which occupy a large part of the dermis with their branches, until they reach the immediately subpapillary region, if the so-called capillary arteries are included therein (SPALTEHOLZ, 1927).

In crossing the corium, the arterioles move in the most varying directions, depending on their task; there are some with a more or less parallel orientation (horizontals) (Figs. 43—46) and some oblique (Fig. 44) or even perpendicular to

---

[13] In man it seems to us more appropriate to talk of the "subpapillary" rather than the "dermal" network, either because of the wide-spread use of the term or because of greater adherence to anatomic reality.

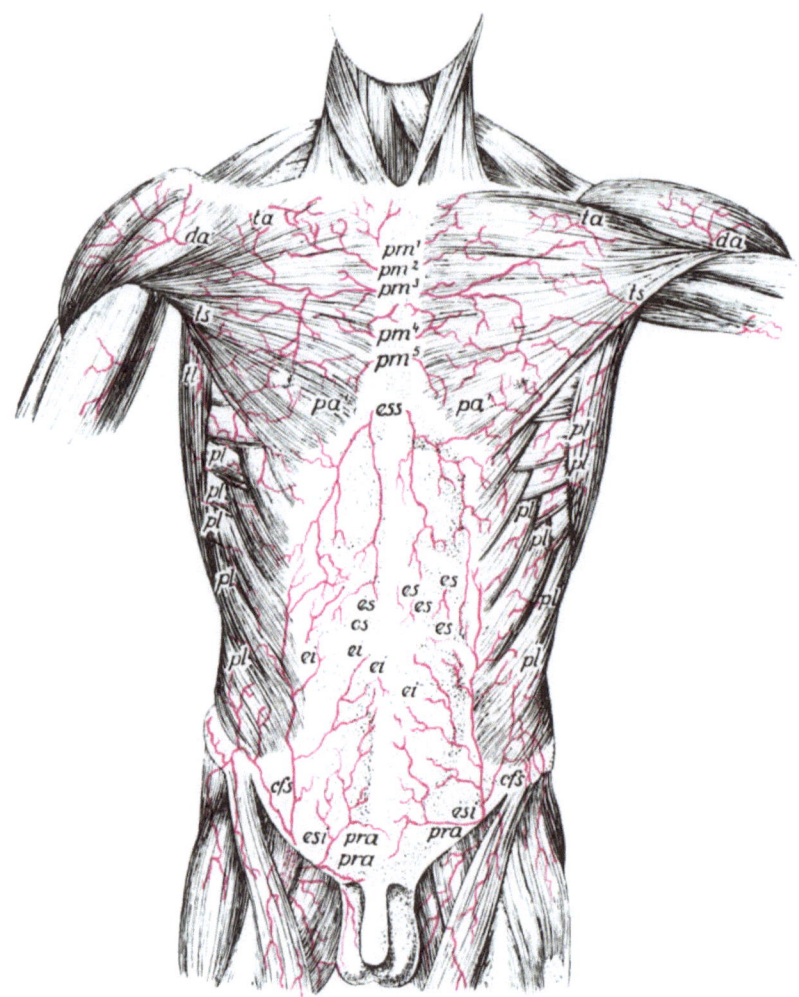

Fig. 41. Cutaneous arteries of the anterior surface of the trunk (from MANCHOT as reproduced from SPALTEHOLZ, 1927). Explanation of drawing: *cfs.* A. circumflexa ilium superficialis; *da* A. subcutanea deltoidea anterior; *ei* Rr. cutanei der A. epigastrica inferior; *es* Rr. cutanei der A. epigastrica superior; *esi* A. epigastrica superficialis inferior; *ess* A. epigastrica superficialis superior; *pa'* Rr. perforantes der Aa. intercostales anteriores; *pl* Rr. perforantes laterales der Aa. intercostales et lumbales; *pm* Rr. perforantes der A. mammaria interna; pm^1, pm^2 doppelter R. perforans secundus (1. Intercostalraum); pm^3 R. perforans tertius (2. Intercostalraum); *pra* R. abdominalis der A. pudenda externa superior; *ta* R. thoracicus der A. thoracoacromialis; *tl* A. thoracalis longa; *ts* A. thoracalis superficialis. (Reproduced from W. SPALTEHOLZ and the 1st issue of this Handbuch 1927)

the surface of the epidermis. There are others which form true vascular arcades (Figs. 43—46), still others (recurrent ones) which go downwards (Fig. 45), e.g., from the meshwork of the cutaneous network or from branches arching from it in the direction of the adipose lobules or the sweat gland glomeruli (HORSTMANN, 1957; MORETTI and MONTAGNA, 1959; RAMPINI and MORETTI, 1963).

Because of their plasticity in relation to the anatomy of the surrounding tissue, those arterioles are particularly worthy of note which, in man and in some primates (WINKELMANN, 1961; MORETTI and FARRIS, 1963), lie either horizontally over deep layers or above important muscular, fascial, or osseous tissues.

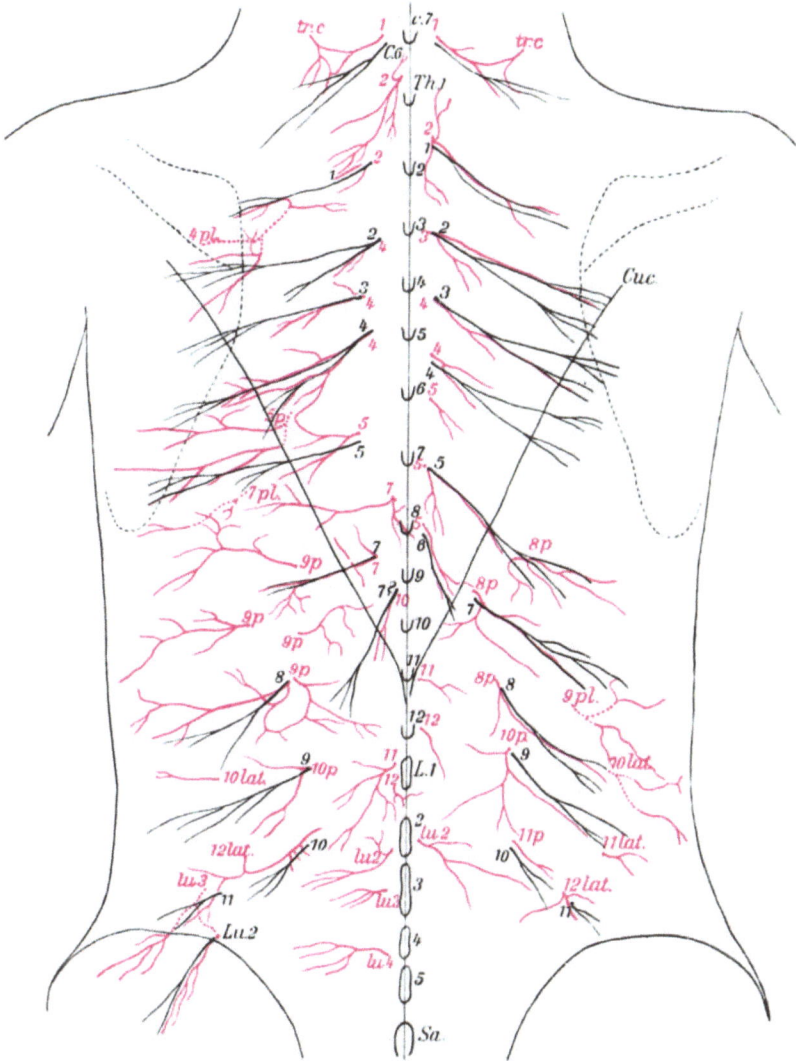

Fig. 42. Cutaneous arteries of the posterior surface of the trunk (from GROSSER as reproduced from SPALTEHOLZ, 1927). Explanation of drawing: The black numbers beside the black-drawing of nerves indicate a segmentary distribution. The vessels are distingued otherwise and precisely: thus the "Rami posteriores mediales" of the intercostal arteries with the number of the artery from which they originate; the "Rami perforantes posteriores mediales" with an annexed "*p*"; the "Rami perforantes posteriores laterales" with the letters "*ph*"; the "lumbar arteries" with the letters "*lu*". Finally tr. c. corresponds to the "A. transversa colli. Cuc. Rand. to the "musc. cucullaris". (Reproduced from W. SPALTEHOLZ and the 1st issue of this Handbuch 1927)

Some robust arterioles, originating in the cutaneous network, have outstanding characteristics. They cross the dermis, anastomizing among themselves by means of arcades in the compact part of this tissue; and, despite numerous successive ramifications with their principal trunk, they penetrate below the papillae, which they supply with various smaller terminal rami.

These arterioles are called "candelabra arteries" because of the appearance of their method of distribution (PETERSEN, 1935; HORSTMANN, 1957) (Fig. 47).

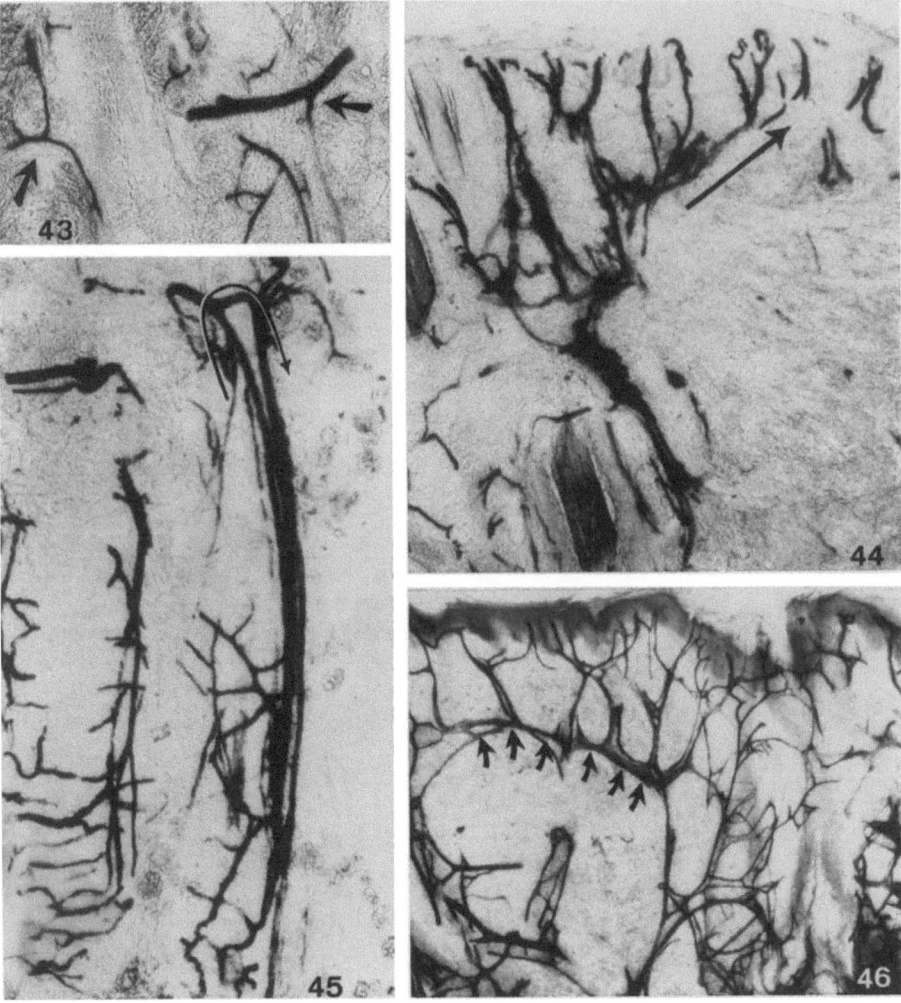

Figs. 43—46. Arteriole types and distributive characteristics

Fig. 43. Branches of the arterial arcades (arrow) divide into perifollicular vessels, both ascending and descending along the follicle. [RAMPINI, MORETTI and REBORA, courtesy of the Minerva derm., Arteriole e capillari della cute ed alopecia areata. Atti SIDES **38**, 301 (1963)]

Fig. 44. Some vessels oblique to the surface of the epidermis (arrow) link up arterioles from the lower dermis with capillaries of the upper dermis. [RAMPINI, MORETTI and REBORA, courtesy of the Minerva derm., Arteriole e capillari della cute ed alopecia areata. Atti SIDES **38**, 301 (1963)]

Fig. 45. Recurrent vessels belonging to the "transient perifollicular network" descend from some arcades lying on the "dermal-hypodermal junction". [RAMPINI, MORETTI and REBORA, courtesy of the Minerva derm., Arteriole e capillari della cute ed alopecia areata. Atti SIDES **38**, 301 (1963)]

Fig. 46. Some vascular arcades (arrows) are clearly visible in the dermis. [CORMIA, F., and A. ERNYEY, courtesy of the Arch. Derm., Vasculature of the normal scalp **88**, 699 (1963)]

Inside the dermis there is very wide distribution of arterioles; according to some observations, their terminal branches reach a height no less than 214 micron from the dermal-epidermal line (MIKHAIL, 1965; see SPALTEHOLZ, 1927, also).

A vast part of the stromal blood supply and, particularly, that of the perifollicular and periglandular networks and an integral part of dermal vascularization is, consequently, made up of the arterioles.

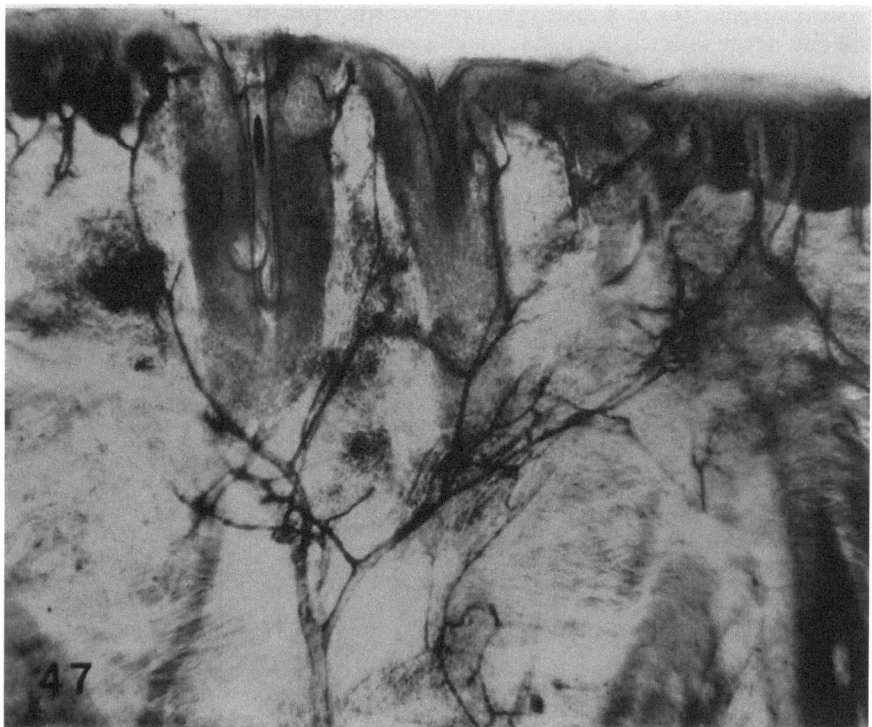

Fig. 47. A robust "candelabrum" arteriole crosses the dermis releasing numerous successive ramifications and various smaller terminal rami. [CORMIA, F., and A. ERNYEY, courtesy of the Arch. Derm., Vasculature of the normal scalp 88, 699 (1963)]

3. The Structure of the Arteries and Arterioles

The histology of the small (or very small) arteries, that go to the skin is well known (BENNINGHOFF, 1930).

Under the endothelium (Figs. 48—50) the intima reveals an internal elastic lamina which is largely composed of longitudinal, sometimes spiral-shaped, elastic fibers; the divisions are not absolutely clear between these and the endothelium and the muscular cells; on the transverse level it may even be that they form a spiral, which, after leaving the intima, penetrates into the media (BENNINGHOFF, 1930).

The muscular cells in this tunic are arranged circularly and are still adjacent to each other with no spaces between (Figs. 48—50).

Generally they are short fibers with oval nuclei and intracytoplasmic fibrils, the delicate edges of which seem to indicate the existence of a meshwork of interstitial fibrils. Suitable stains disclose a fine structure of elastic and reticular fibers around the smooth muscular fibers ("Gitterfasern," BENNINGHOFF, 1930).

The adventitia, which is made up of sporadic collagen fibers, having little connection with the media, has some elastic fibers also (BENNINGHOFF, 1930).

The arteries described gradually become terminal arterioles, between 40 and 15 micron in diameter (ILLIG, 1961; MIKHAIL, et al., 1965), which, in their turn, are destined to continue as the capillaries.

The intima of the arterioles (Figs. 52 and 53) has an endothelium similar to that in the capillaries. It is, however, devoid of an internal elastic lamina which is replaced by a delicate "gitterfasern" membrane (BENNINGHOFF, 1930).

In the media, the muscular cells are somewhat primitive; their nuclei are still oval and not necessarily perpendicular to the tube axis.

At the arteriole branching points some of these particularly strong elements constitute "closure" muscles, which are rather important in vessel dynamics (BENNINGHOFF, 1930).

In the orientation to the lumen, the muscle fibers (Figs. 52 and 53) of the arterioles may be circular, slightly oblique, or spiral, and joined together in a continuous layer or in groups separated by spaces of varying width or entirely isolated (SPALTEHOLZ, 1927; BENNINGHOFF, 1930).

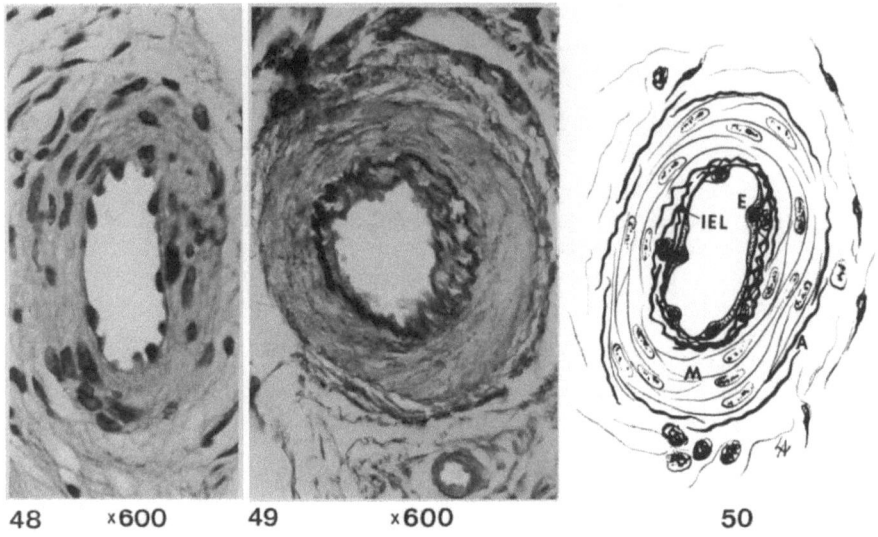

Figs. 48—50. The structure of arterioles

Fig. 48. An arteriole reveals prominent endothelial nuclei and a consistent media with oval nuclei (Hematoxylin-eosin stain)

Fig. 49. The same arteriole still possesses a fairly developed internal elastic lamina (Weigert-stain)

Fig. 50. A schematic drawing of the anatomy of the same arteriole. *E* endothelium; *IEL* internal elastic lamina; *M* media; *A* adventitia

4. The Transition of the Arteries into Arterioles and of These into Capillaries

Progressive diminution of the thick muscular tunic of the arterial vessels finally reduces them, at the height of half the corium, to a single stratum of muscular cells (Fig. 51) (SPALTEHOLZ, 1927); from this point it loses its continuity and is gradually replaced as far as the subpapillary network by evermore separated groups of cells (Fig. 51).

From the level where the muscular cells are discontinued, it then passes to another higher level (100—400 micron from the dermal-epidermal line) (WIMTRUP, 1923, cf. SPALTEHOLZ, 1927), in which there are isolated muscular elements, more or less oblique or circular, that are destined to disappear in the capillaries[14].

Consequently, it seems logical to consider as arterioles (ILLIG, 1961) all the transition vessels included among the arteries, which are vessels with continuous muscular walls, and capillaries, which are without muscular elements.

---

[14] According to SPALTEHOLZ (1927), circular or oblique fibers joined in groups are present almost up to the beginning of the papillary capillary and then vanish suddenly.

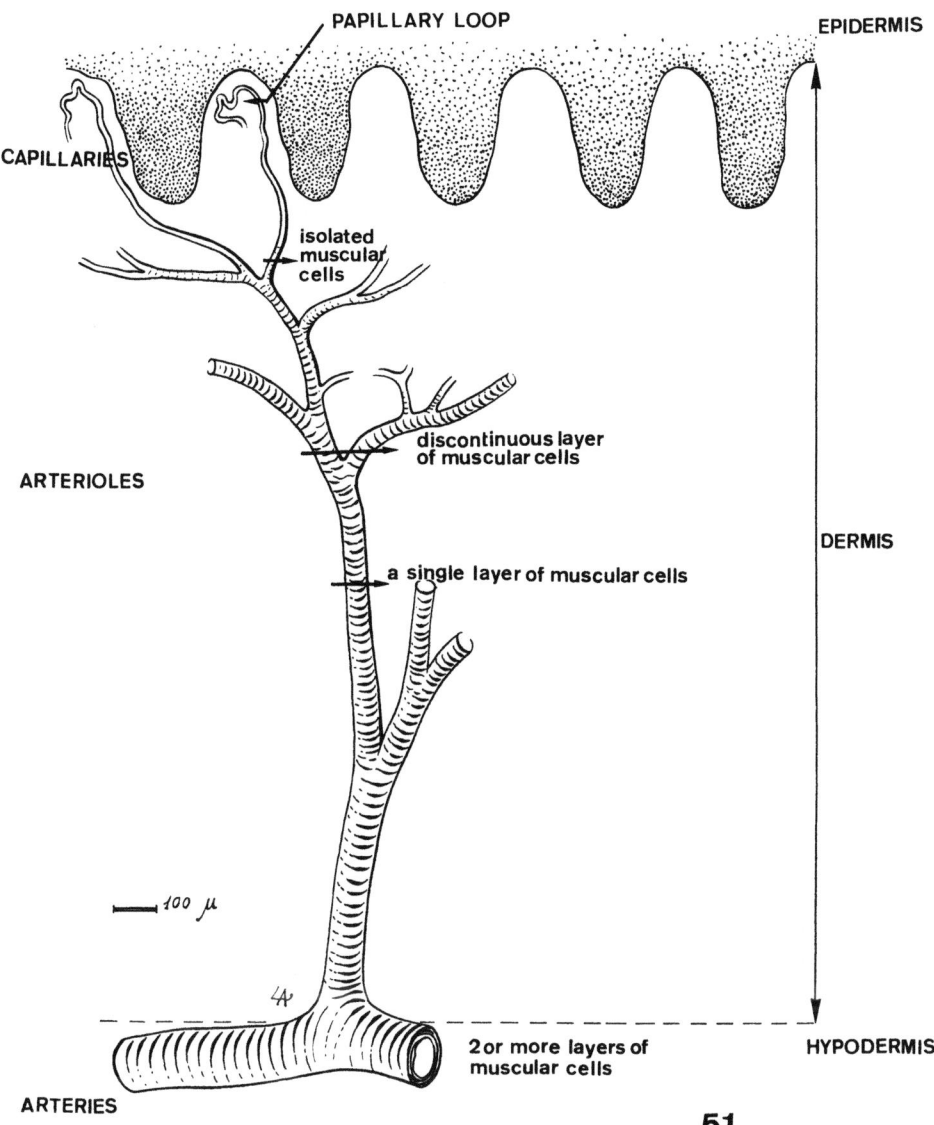

Fig. 51. The transition of the arteries into arterioles and of these into capillaries

5. The Histochemistry and Electron Microscopy of the Arterioles

There is not much information on either of these subjects as far as the skin is concerned; we shall, therefore, treat it rather sketchily (Table 2).

The presence of carbohydrates of the glycogen type in the endothelial cells of the arteriolar walls seems to be revealed by means of the periodic acid Schiff reaction not resistant to amylase (MORETTI and CROVATO, 1965). Glucose may be visible with MÜLLER's method (SACCHI, 1957).

The existence of both neutral and acid mucopolysaccharides in the wall of arterioles, is generally shown by means of metachromasia; PAS and Alcian blue methods, after papain and hyaluronidase; and the colloidal iron reaction (ZUGIBE, 1962).

Nucleoproteins (DNA) were found with the Feulgen technique in the smooth muscle nuclei as well as in other nuclei (MESCON et al., 1956); protein-bound sulfhydryl groups revealed with BARNETT and SELIGMAN's technique (MESCON et al., 1956) were however absent in the media[15]. Histamine has been detected (JUHLIN and SHELLEY, 1966) in the muscle cells of cutaneous arterioles[16].

Neither Sudan IV nor Sudan Black B reveals the slightest presence of fatty acids or esters of fatty acids or phospholipids in the same media (MESCON et al., 1956).

On the subject of enzymes there is little data. Of oxidative enzymes it would seem almost certain that the arterioles undoubtedly contain in the endothelium

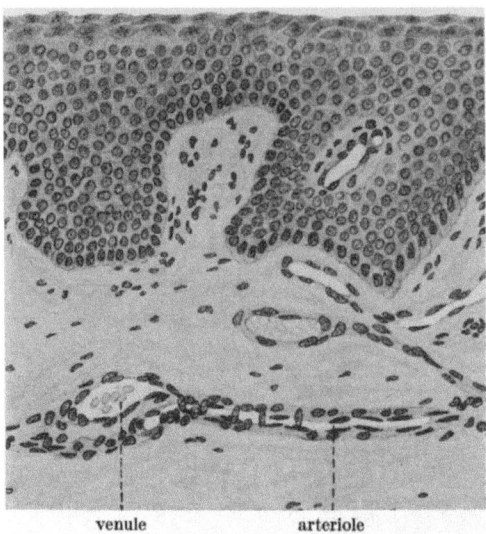

Fig. 52. Arterioles and venules in the skin of the finger-tips. (Reproduced from W. SPALTEHOLZ and the 1st issue of this Handbuch 1927)

a clearly reactive succinodehydrogenase[17] (BRAUN-FALCO and RATHJENS, 1955; MONTAGNA and FORMISANO, 1955) a weakly positive or an indefinite cytochrome oxidase activity (BRAUN-FALCO, 1961; MONTAGNA and YUN, 1961) and NAD and NADP reductase which are also rather reactive in the muscle structures of the media (BRAUN-FALCO and PETZOLDT, 1964). A reactive dehydrolipoic dehydrogenase is present in the smooth muscle cells (BALOGH, 1964).

Hydrolases, and particularly the group of the nonspecific esterases in the endothelium of arterioles, react weakly to both α-naphthyl and indoxyl esterase (MONTAGNA, 1955; STEIGLEDER and LOEFFLER, 1956; BRAUN-FALCO, 1956d).

In the group of phosphatases, the absence of acid phosphatase in the tunica media of the arterioles seems certain, while the progressively decreasing reactivity of alkaline phosphatase in the endothelium with the increase in diameter of the vessels is well known.

---

[15] The extracellular metachromatic staining with Toluidin blue of loose connective tissue immediately around the blood vessels of the dermis suggests on the other hand the presence of acid mucopolysaccharides around the adventitia (WISLOCKI et al., 1947).

[16] A specific fluorescence characteristic of a primary catecholamine was shown in varicose nerve fibres around blood vessels (arteries? veins?) in the deeper parts of animal corium (FALCK and RORSMAN, 1963 cit. MOELLER, 1964).

[17] The endothelium and the smooth muscle cells in the wall of cutaneous arterioles of the Rhesus monkey show moderate activity in dehydrogenases (IM, 1966).

On this subject, the important fact to be stressed is that the reactivity of the arteriole endothelium is particularly intense at the vessels' point of bifurcation, so that the branches usually show stronger reactivity at the beginning.

This particular site of maximum activity might, according to some, indicate an active function of transport of metabolites from the blood through the endothelium "as a system for sampling continuously the chemical content of the blood for the purpose of regulation of the lumen of the artery" (ROMANUL and BANNISTER, 1962).

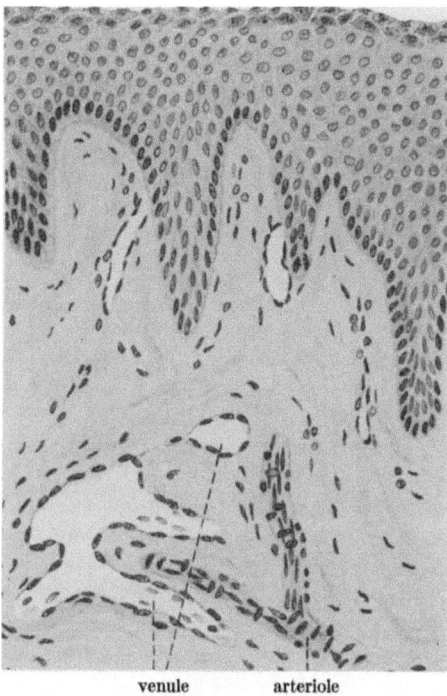

Fig. 53. Arterioles and venules in the skin of the finger-tips. (Reproduced from W. SPALTEHOLZ and the 1st issue of this Handbuch 1927)

This does not at all disagree with the usual observation that enzyme activity in the endothelial cell is very great, chiefly in the terminal arterioles and the arteriolar part of the capillary loop, two essential zones for the transfer of chemicals from the blood to the tissues (ELLIS, 1959).

Other important phosphatases, particularly reactive in the arterioles, are 5-nucleotidase (BRADSHAW, 1963), adenosinetriphosphatase and adenosinemonophosphatase, both present in lesser quantity in the endothelium and in greater amount in the tunica media (especially the AMP); the reaction to β-glycerophosphatase is, however, absolutely negative (BRADSHAW, 1963; WOLFF, 1963).

With β-glucuronidase, both the endothelial cells and the smooth muscle fibers of arterioles are moderately reactive (MONTAGNA, 1957).

Also studied, but not found in the arterioles, are aminopeptidases (STEIGLEDER et al., 1962), nonspecific, and specific cholinesterases (MESCON et al., 1956) (Table 2).

On the subject of electron microscopy of the arterioles (Figs. 54 and 55), we know that these vessels in the finger tips, like the capillaries, can be divided into two types (HIBBS et al., 1958). The first type visible in the deep subcutaneous tissue is practically indistinguishable from most arterioles in the other organs. The intima apparently possesses endothelial cells flattened when the vessels are dilated; wrinkled and deeply folded when the vessels are contracted, so that the cytoplasm protrudes in the lumen together with the nucleus (HIBBS et al., 1958).

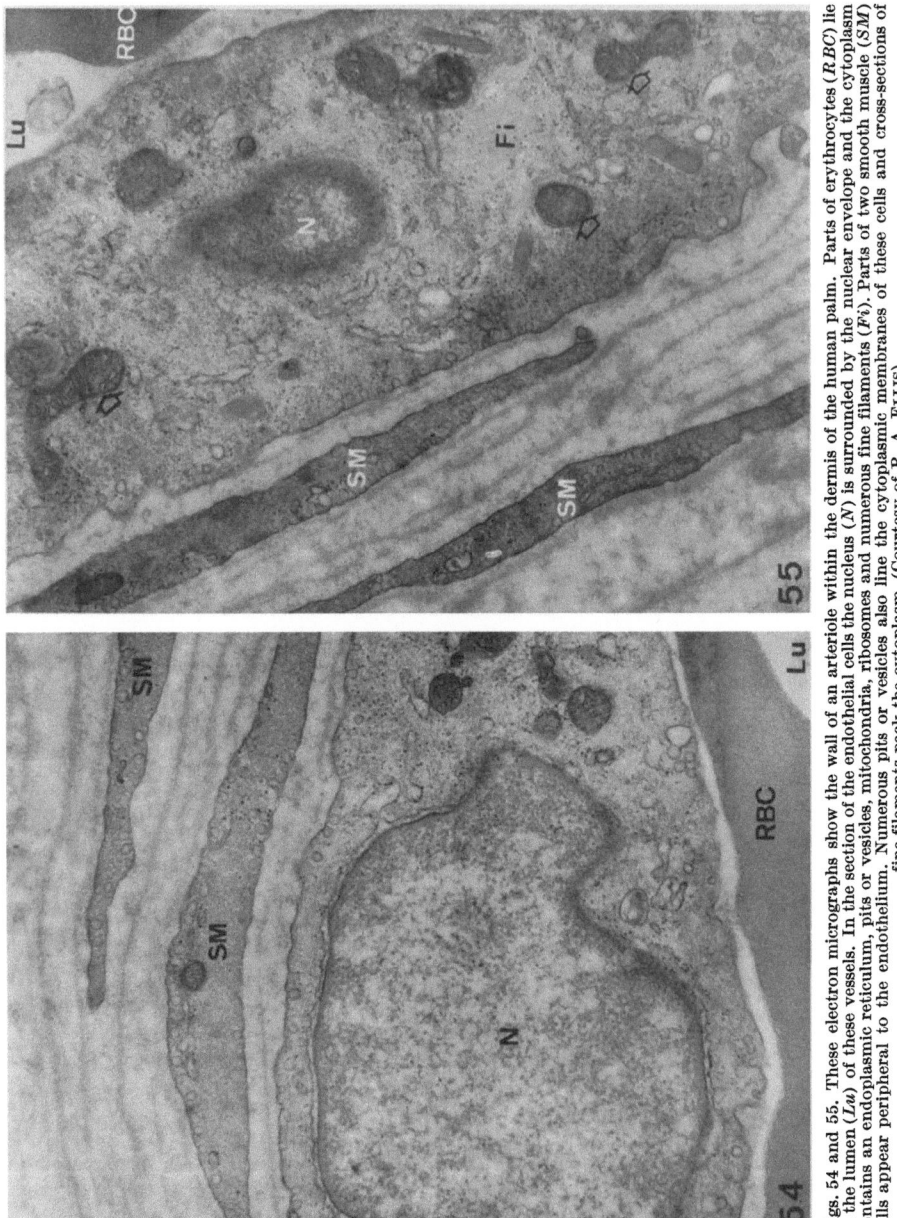

Figs. 54 and 55. These electron micrographs show the wall of an arteriole within the dermis of the human palm. Parts of erythrocytes (*RBC*) lie in the lumen (*Lu*) of these vessels. In the section of the endothelial cells the nucleus (*N*) is surrounded by the nuclear envelope and the cytoplasm contains an endoplasmic reticulum, pits or vesicles, mitochondria, ribosomes and numerous fine filaments (*Fi*). Parts of two smooth muscle (*SM*) cells appear peripheral to the endothelium. Numerous pits or vesicles also line the cytoplasmic membranes of these cells and cross-sections of fine filaments pack the cytoplasm. (Courtesy of R. A. ELLIS)

In addition, these cells possess a cytoplasm with numerous "pinocytotic" vesicles similar to those of the first type of capillaries (see afterwards). Between the endothelium and the muscles of the tunica media a thick elastic membrane of 0.1 and 0.3 micron is found, while the media is composed of one or more layers of smooth muscle cells (Figs. 54 and 55) with the innermost ones lying in close contact with the lamina. The arterioles of the second type are generally more superficial than those just described and are found in the dermis and in the subcutaneous stratum. The endothelial cells lining their intima closely resemble the thick ones of the second type of capillary (see afterwards) and also contain filaments. In any case, when they are observed in a cross section, the large number of nuclei of the endothelium seems to be characteristic of these vessels; on the other hand, if the arterioles are contracted, these endothelial cells become pyramidal or columnar even while retaining the smooth contours of their free edges (HIBBS et al., 1958)[18].

In the cytoplasm these cells contain (Figs. 54 and 55) the same kind of filaments, rod-shaped granules, and vascular bodies, though less than in the capillary endothelium. Arterioles of this type are without elastic lamina and their muscle cells are separated from the endothelium and from one another by rather thick layers of connective tissue (HIBBS et al., 1958).

III. The Capillaries

1. Definition and General Characteristics

The capillaries are extremely narrow vessels with a diameter similar to that of the red globules, or possibly even smaller[19], which put a minimum blood content into maximum contact with the walls.

It is easily understandable, therefore, why the circulatory system culminates, both anatomically and conceptually (MAJNO, 1965), at the level of the capillary wall; the whole vascular system is, in fact, dependent on this tenuous barrier (histangic zone)[20] (COMEL, 1955) which, while presiding over the exchanges between the blood, tissues, and interstitial fluids (MAJNO, 1965), is characterized by conspicuous physico-chemical differences in species and organ.

Having developed in fixed relationship and in close contact with the parenchyma (KROGH, 1924), the capillary system begins where the smooth muscular elements cease to surround the endothelial cell, i.e., at the site where the vessel is reduced to a simple endothelial tube. The morphofunctional characteristics of the capillaries are sufficiently clear for precise classification (BENNET, LUFT and HAMPTON, 1959).

The development of this system in the skin (in some regions from 100 to 150 capillaries per square mm) (MORETTI et al., 1959; BACCAREDDA-BOY et al., 1961) is certainly not, as we have said before, comparable with the enormous one

---

[18] Other important electron microscopy details have been supplied by STAUBESAND (1959). In the walls of arterioles in general, some prolongations of the endothelial cells penetrate through openings in the elastic lamina (see also FAWCETT, 1956) as far as the body of the smooth muscle fibers; as is suggested by vesicles in the protrusion and in the cytoplasm of the muscle cells, this might indicate the probability of an ultramicroscopic transfer of metabolites from the blood, through the endothelium, and as far as the muscle of the vessel.

[19] Here we are referring, of course, to the vessels of the capillary loops only, even if in the text we apply the term "capillaries" more loosely to vessels of larger diameter, provided that they have walls of "capillary thickness" (MAJNO, 1965). Therefore, we do not follow those authors (LEVI, 1927) who hold that the capillary diameter varies between 6.7 to 11 micron in the tegument and the mucosae.

[20] Here and elsewhere we have used this word [derived from the Greek "histos" (tissue) and "angeion" (vessel)], because we consider it the most suitable to indicate the anatomical-functional unity formed by the territory enclosed between the wall of the very last vascular structures and the immediately surrounding tissue (see also COMEL and MIAN, 1961).

already observed in other organs. In the cardiac ventricle, for example, it is 5.550 per square mm (WEARN, 1928; KROGH, 1929) and in the muscle, 2,000 mm² (KROGH, 1929). The entity of the capillary network in the skin is, moreover, evident in some data; one capillary loop supplies between 0.04 and 0.27 square mm of surface (SPALTEHOLZ, 1927); the average distance between one papillary loop and another is 50—100 micron (CARRIER, cf. COMEL, 1933); their vascular surface is 1—2 square cm per square cm of cutaneous surface (KROGH, 1929).

In the rest of the skin, the concentration of capillary population, although not so vast as at the subepidermal level, is nevertheless sizable and varies according to the area around and across the papillae, the appendages and all the tissue layers, so as to permeate every part of the dermis and its structures.

The capillaries also vary considerably in shape:

a) With the state of vessel distension; in some cases, for example, the mere passing of a red cell is enough to deform the surface (KROGH, 1929).

b) With the morphofunctional location of the tissue units supplied with blood and, therefore, with the mechanical quality of its structure, its anatomical and biochemical consistency, and the metabolic state of the tegument. Particularly important from this point of view are the papillae (HORSTMANN, 1962), the appendages, and the tissue levels. For example, in the extremely mobile skin on the back of the hand, the feet, and the prepuce the papillary capillaries may be twisted into knots, an arrangement which gives elastic movement to the skin and protects the vessels at the same time (WINKELMANN, 1961 b); in the high narrow papillae, the capillary bifurcations appear to be numerous and usually at acute angles; in the papillae which are short and wide there are few and usually at wide angles to each other (BACCAREDDA-BOY et al., 1960; HORSTMANN, 1962); beneath an almost flat dermal-epidermal line, the capillaries practically disappear (ELLIS, 1961); in the areas characterized by many sweat ducts and hairs, these appendages are surrounded by true capillary rings; on the forehead, the capillaries separate the numerous appendages (in a septum-like way) (ILLIG, 1964).

c) With the location of the vessel; even in the fingers of the same person there are intercurrent differences in the shape of the capillaries. Later on we shall speak of the considerable differences in number.

d) With the exposure of the cutaneous area; the covered regions of the trunk generally exhibit more constant types of capillaries than those observed in the fingers of the hand for example (WEISS and NICKAU, 1921; cf. MUELLER, 1921).

e) With the constitution (WERTHEIMER and WERTHEIMER, 1955); a marked similarity exists in the capillaroscopic picture of parents and their children (KUKLOVA-STUROVA, 1941): whatever the deviation in the capillary development of the former, it will be inevitably reflected in the capillary picture of the latter. In the region above the sternum in the newly born child, different types of capillaries are visible which are probably hereditary (SCHWALM, 1934; SCHNITZER, 1937). In monochorial twins, the capillaroscopic picture is identical in corresponding cutaneous areas (MAYER-LIST and HÜBENER, 1925). In a large group of normal adults, more than 90% exhibit a capillaroscopic picture (Fig. 56) belonging to one of 4 kinds of open or closed nail loop. There is no doubt that the capillaries in neurasthenic subjects have a typical appearance (GRIFFITH, 1932; LOVETT-DOUST, 1955). This is a question of a peculiar tortuosity of the loops, which is sometimes found in the nail folds of normal people (LANDIS, 1938).

f) With age; in the lips and the nail wall, young peoples' capillary loops are shorter than those of the old (BETTMAN, 1930); in old peoples' walls, the loops are more tortuous (WRIGHT and DURJEE, 1933). Between the 3rd and the 6th decades of life, the diameter of the arterial part of the capillary loop diminishes considerably (ALLEN, BARKER and HYNES, 1955)[21].

g) With the season of the year and with diet (PISCHZEK and SCHMIDT, 1926). On quantitative capillary distribution, possibly correlated to the size of single vessels in the various parts of the skin (DAVIS and LAWLER, 1961), considerable divergence of opinion exists, whether because of the techniques used [cantharide

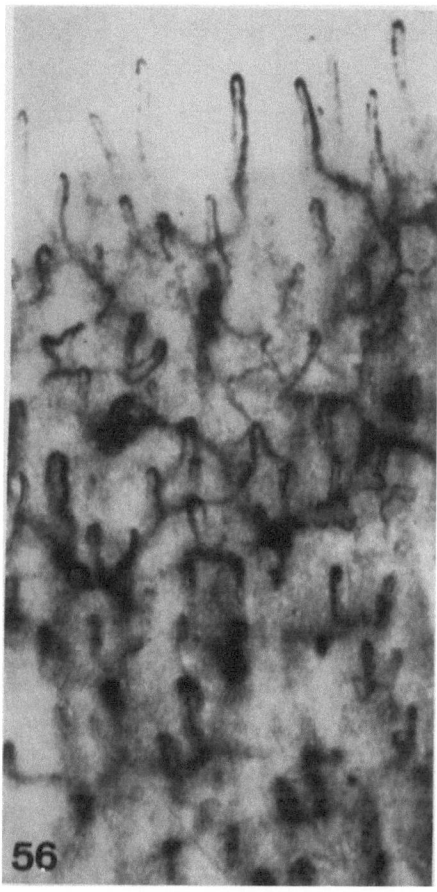

Fig. 56. Capillarascopic view of nail-fold terminal capillaries with marked blood sludging of the normally smooth axial stream. (DAVIES, M. J., and J. C. LAWLER, courtesy of the Pergamon Press. In: Advances in biology of skin, vol. 2, p. 81. 1961)

blister (WETZEL and ZOTTERMANN, 1926); capillaroscopy after application of Scotch Tape (DAVIS and LAWLER, 1961); serial or nonserial sections (BACCAREDDA-BOY et al., 1961; etc.)] in studying diverse cutaneous areas, or because the number of capillaries which are open [22] and therefore visible depends upon the functional state of the organ and may vary from one moment to the next (BORDLEY, et al. 1938).

From this originate the appreciable differences in the "range" of the values collected (Table 1 and Figs. 57—59 and 60a, b).

---

[21] Other authors, however, deny that age (and sex) can influence loop morphology (WETZELL and ZOTTERMANN, 1926; WEISS and FRAZIER, 1930; ZIMMER and DEMIS, 1962).

[22] Only 15—70% of cutaneous capillaries will be open at the same time, with wide individual differences (LEWIS, 1927; KROGH, 1929; LANDIS, 1938; ROBERTS and GRIFFITH, 1937; cf. ILLIG, 1961).

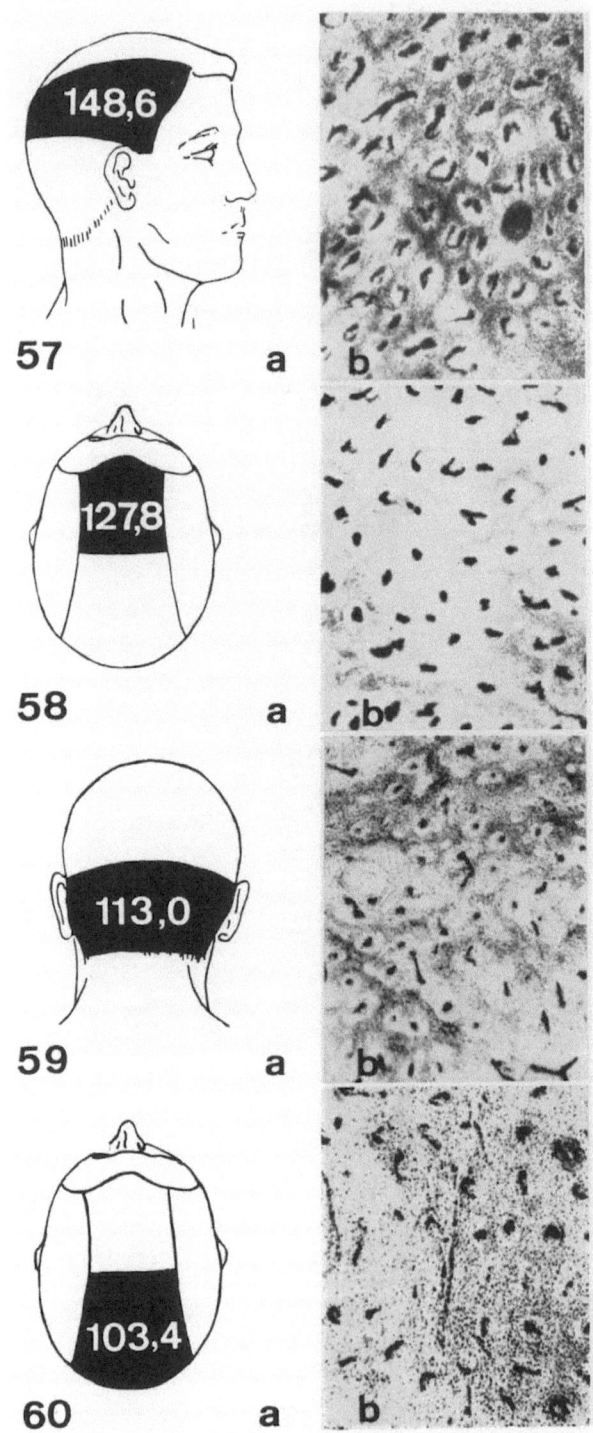

Figs. 57—60a and b. The capillary-papillary concentration of various areas of the scalp and a horizontal view of the corresponding capillary loops at the level of the "subepidermal" network

Table 1. *The regional frequency of papillary capillary distribution*

Region[b]	Mean Value[a]	Region	Mean Value[a]	Region	Mean Value[a]
Nape	113 (B)	Eyelids	127 (M)	Mandibular	149 (M)
Posterior vertex	94 (B)	Ear lobe	38 (W)	Chin	158 (M)
Anterior vertex	117 (B)	Ear pavillion	120 (M)	Hand, foot (dorsum)	65 (W); 15—40 (BG); 60—70 (D); 40 (C)
Frontal	128 (B)	Nose[c]	100 (M); 16 (W)	Ungual fold	20 (D)
Temporal	149 (B)	Philtrum	141 (M)	Knuckles	20—70 (D); 58 (W); 41 (BS); 30 (BR)
Frontal (glabr.)	157 (M)	Cheek	131 (M)	Forearm	35 (WF); 47 (W); 42 (Z); 51 (L)
Temporal (glabr.)	145 (M)	Perioral	130 (M); 20 (W)	Other areas	intermediate values (D)
Orbital, infra-orbital	126 (M)	Lips	88 (M)		

Legenda. B: Baccaredda, Moretti, Rebora (1961); BG: Brown, Giffin (1922, 1926); BR: Brown, Roth (1927); BS: Brown, Sheard (1926); C: Carrier (quoted by Comel, 1933); D: Davis, Lawler (1958); L: Lawler, Lumpkin (1961); M: Moretti, Mescon, Montagna (1959); W: Wetzel, Zottermann (1926); WF: Weiss, Frazier (1930); Z: Zimmer, Demis (1962).

[a] per mm^2 of skin surface.

[b] In the scalp (region not specified) of adult individuals (20—90 Y.O) Giacometti (1964) found 102—130 capillaries/mm^2.

[c] on blister floor: 58 (W).

2. Papillary Loops

The loops of the papillae represent the culmination of the capillary system in the skin.

One capillary loop usually goes to each papilla, even if more loops may originate at an angle of 90° from the same branch of the subpapillary network (Davis and Lawler, 1961).

Usually perpendicular to the cutaneous surface and parallel in the ungual folds and sometimes pretibial regions, the loops exhibit an arterial afferent tract, an intercalary tract or crest (Gilje et al., 1953), and an efferent or venous one. The last two have the same diameter[23].

The ascending or afferent tract has fewer endothelial cells than the descending or efferent one which, however, is slightly wider and has a denser pericyte network (Macher and Vogell, 1962).

Furthermore the structure of the afferent part is analogous to the efferent part which, being without muscular cells as well as adventitia (principal characteristics of the veins), is composed of the same elements that constitute the arterial fraction (endothelium, basement membrane and pericytes) and is, therefore, to be considered venous only on a hemodynamic basis (Macher and Vogell, 1962).

The length of one entire loop oscillates between 0.2 and 0.4 mm according to the region (Krogh, 1929; Deutsch, 1941); on the nail folds, for example, it is

---

[23] The shape of the intercalary tract varies considerably and sometimes is very characteristic: corkscrew, onion, spiral, curl, coil, spindle and spirochete like forms, etc. (Gilje et al., 1953).

0.30 mm long (DAVIS and LAWLER, 1961). The other dimensions also vary with the area[24]; the arterial fraction of the nail loop has a diameter of 0.010—0.013 mm, the venous one, 0.013—0.020 mm; on the back of the hands the diameter is 0.010 micron for the arterial part, and 0.015 micron for the venous one (DAVIS and LAWLER, 1961). The ratio existing between the two fractions is 1:1.5 (DAVIS and LAWLER, 1958a).

The surface occupied by the capillaries (cm^2 of skin surface) also changes with the region. On the cheeks and knuckles of the finger it is maximal; on the ear lobe and back of the hands it is 50% less than on the former and on the forearm and back of the finger it is the least among those areas studied or about a sixth of that on the cheeks. As a whole, the entire capillary population covers from 9 to 22% of the total vascular surface (WETZEL and ZOTTERMANN, 1926).

Finally, it should be kept in mind that quite independently of the walls, the blood contained in the loop frequently changes in color, in circulatory speed, and in the type of blood column formed.

The only visible flow in man is axial (DAVIS and LANDAU, 1960). In the arterial-capillary tract one can see, for example, agglutination phenomena of erythrocytes in varying granular accumulations, up to the point of forming the so-called "blood sludge," which may even block the flow for 30 seconds (DAVIS and LANDAU, 1960). This blood column sometimes appears separated from the wall by a clear plasmatic zone and interrupted by conglomerations of leukocytes (GILJE et al., 1953).

3. Structure of the Capillaries

In spite of the marked differences between one organ and another, the inmost structure of the capillaries of the skin, like all others, consists of the following elements:

a) the endothelial cells which form the true and proper luminal walls;

b) the pericyte cells which are freely anastomosed by themselves and are afterwards present at the bifurcations;

c) the basement membrane (Figs. 61, 62 and 63).

The endothelial cell of the dermal capillary is rather "high" (2—4 microns) (MAJNO, 1965) in comparison with the majority of other organs (0.2 micron in the adipose tissue, in the central nervous system (MAJNO, 1965), in the striated musculature, in the smooth musculature of the digestive and reproductive systems (PALADE, 1961; cf. MAJNO, 1965)). In the capillaries in the deep subcutaneous tissue, nevertheless, the endothelium goes back to the "short" type (about 0.2 micron) that is common to the rest of the body (HIBBS, 1958).

Under the optical microscope, the endothelial cell appears to be thin and flat and has a tendency to adopt a polygonal shape (LEVI, 1927; BARGMANN, 1956; MAJNO, 1965).

This cell has a nucleus, which is usually so large and prominent as sometimes to occlude the vessel lumen (Figs. 61—63). Its appearance varies with the degree of flattening of the capillaries; more or less stretched out in the cell's lengthwise direction and often round along the vessel axis (BENNINGHOFF, 1930) whenever it lies close to the venules.

Structurally, the nuclei of the endothelium are similar to those of fibrocytes except for denser chromatin zones and smaller nucleoli (BENNINGHOFF, 1930).

---

[24] For the same type of loop, interesting indications on the variability of reports are given by ILLIG (1961): total length, 0.42 mm (BROWN, 1925); 0.20—0.40 (DEUTSCH, 1941); arterial fraction diameter, 0.007 mm (BROWN, 1925); 0.009—0.012 (DEUTSCH, 1941; WALLS and BUCHANAN, 1956); venous fraction diameter, 0.009 mm (BROWN, 1925); 0.02 (DEUTSCH. 1941); 0.009—0.02 (WALLS and BUCHANAN, 1956).

The cytoplasm is of varying density. It looks thicker around the nucleus, where it has a granular thickening with minute striae (BENNINGHOFF, 1930), and thinner on the cell's periphery[25]. In the contact region with the other endothelial cells, the cytoplasm possesses a zone of greater specialization, of which we shall speak later.

Here let us just recall that endothelial cells, if treated with $AgNO^3$, have dark peripheral or wavy or zigzag edges up to now considered (MAJNO, 1965) indicative of the cementing substances or basal membrane which surrounds them.

The endothelial cells altogether are arranged parallel to the longitudinal axes of the vessel (Figs. 61—63) and with the lengthening of the capillary, tend to

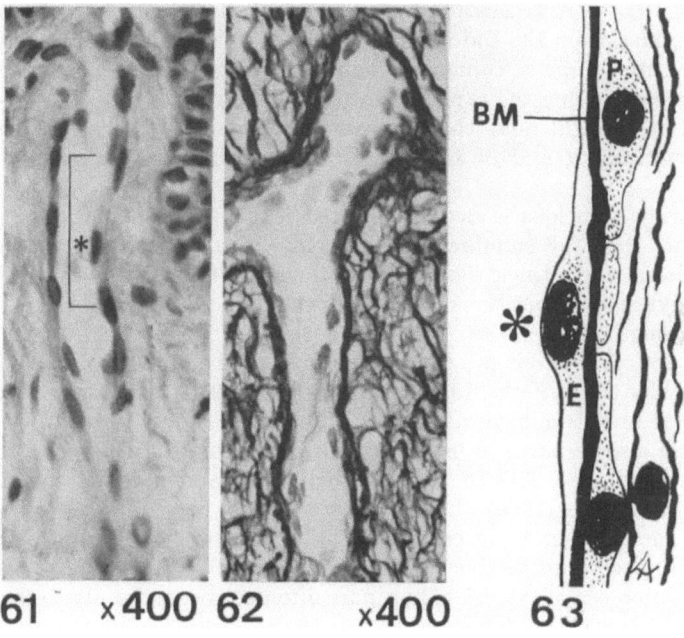

Figs. 61—63. The structure of capillaries

Fig. 61. A capillary reveals the large and prominent nuclei of endothelial cells, and the pericytes arranged lengthwise along the vessels (Hematoxylin-eosin stain)

Fig. 62. Another aspect of the capillary (Gomori's silver stain)

Fig. 63. Schematic drawing of the anatomy of a capillary: E the endothelial cells; P the pericytes; BM the basement membrane

become more oblique if not to arrange themselves in a spiral around the vasal tubule (MACHER and VOGELL, 1962).

The lumen of this tubule is, as a rule, reinforced by two cells. It is not, however, unusual to find capillaries composed of 4—6 cells (HIBBS, 1958), while the existence of capillaries with unicellular walls is not confirmed in the rat (HIBBS et al., 1958). The vasal tube thus constructed appears to be continuous and resting on an apparently amorphous membrane, the basal membrane, which is interposed between the endothelial cells and the pericytes and fills up all the intervening spaces and surrounds the latter (Figs. 62 and 63).

According to histology, it is essentially an elastic-connective membrane even though it contains extremely fine argyrophil fibrils (Gitterfasern) that are usually

---

[25] In a state of apparent contraction, the endothelial cell and its nucleus change morphologically (LEVI, 1927); the nucleus becomes spindle-shaped, the cellular body shorter and thinner, and the outline saw-edged.

circular (BARGMANN, 1956) and sometimes spiral (BENNINGHOFF, 1930) with a layer of more delicate amorphous ground substance between them (BARGMANN, 1956).

The pericytes (Figs. 61—63), or ROUGET's cells, or ZIMMERMANN's pericytes form a true "adventitia capillaris" (AUERBACH, 1865; EBERTH, 1871; cf. BENNINGHOFF, 1930). Differing, in the transition zone, from the arteriole to the capillary and from the capillary to the venule (MAJNO, 1965) and subject to great differences in organs and species (ZIMMERMANN, 1923) from time to time, the pericytes have been considered: 1) cells endowed with contractile activity (WIMTRUP, 1922—1923; ZIMMERMANN, 1923); 2) noncontractile adventitial elements stemming from the endothelial cell (MARCHAND, 1923); 3) an integral part of an adventitial tunic of connective lamellar reticular tissue (VOLTERRA, 1925); and 4) fibrocytes along the capillary surface (BENNINGHOFF, 1930).

Now it is thought that they possess the structural characteristics both of smooth musculature and of the endothelium with probably some phagocytic qualities.

The pericyte nucleus is ovoid, arranged lengthwise along the vessel and in close contact with the endothelial tube from which it separates with difficulty. The cytoplasm is less thick than the endothelial cell and has considerable protoplasmic argyrophile projections with which the pericyte contacts the endothelium while enclosing it.

Under optical microscope, the cytoplasm has the ability to hold vital colors like trypan blue (BARGMANN, 1956; BENNINGHOFF, 1930) while it lacks myofibrils. Sometimes it reveals mitoses (ZELIKSON, 1966).

It should also be borne in mind, in this connection, that the pericyte tends to elongate when it lies close to the endothelial cell and becomes round when at a distance (ZELIKSON, 1966).

Furthermore, around the endothelial cells the pericytes form an incomplete tunic which, according to the position of the capillary, may be as long as the whole circumference of the vessel but more often corresponds only to the diameter (MACHER and VOGELL, 1962).

4. Histochemistry of the Capillaries

Adequate treatment of the subject, besides being complicated in itself, is rendered difficult by the absence of any work exclusively dedicated to the histochemistry of cutaneous capillaries.

Hence, what we shall here set down is the result mainly of personal observations which complement those of other authors. It should be borne in mind, however, that these refer primarily to the capillaries of the papillary and immediately subpapillary regions of the skin (Table 2).

On the subject of carbohydrates, the presence of glycogen in the endothelial cells may be proved by their positive reaction to the PAS method and non resistance to amylase (Figs. 64—65) (MORETTI and CROVATO, 1965).

Glucose was be demonstrated with MUELLER's method (SACCHI, 1957) and neutral and acid mucopolysaccharides have also been shown with various techniques (HOLLANDER et al., 1954; MORETTI and CROVATO, 1965) (Figs. 64—65).

Concerning proteins, we know practically nothing except that the nuclei of these cells contain nucleoproteins.

The endothelial cells have sulfhydryl-containing aminoacids demonstrable both by the nitro-prusside and by BARNETT and SELIGMAN's method (SANNICANDRO, 1932; HOLLANDER et al., 1954). Tryptophane is shown by the dimethylamino-

Table 2. *A comparison between the histochemical properties of arterioles, capillaries and venules* [a]

Studied substances		Reactivity		
		Arterioles	Capillaries	Venules
Carbohydrates	Glycogen	Doubtful	Doubtful	Doubtful
	Glucose	Doubtful	Doubtful	Doubtful
	MPS, AMPS	Present	Present	Present
Proteins	DNA	Present	Present	Present
and Amines	-SS; -SH groups	Present	Present	—[b]
	Tryptophan	—	Present	—
	Histamine	Present	Present	—
Lipids	Fatty acids and esters	Absent	Doubtful	—
	Phospholipids	Absent	Present	—
	Acetalphosphatides	—	Present	Doubtful
	Enzymes			
Reductases	SDH	Present	Present	Present
	Dehydrolipoic-DH	Present	—	—
	Cytochrome oxidases	Present	Present	—
	MAO	—	Doubtful	—
	Ubiquinone	—	—	Doubtful
Esterases	α-naphthyl esterases	Present	Present	Doubtful
	Indoxyl esterases	Present	Present	Doubtful
	AS esterases	—	Present	Doubtful
	Tween esterases	—	Absent	Doubtful
	Cholinesterases	Absent	—	—
β-glucuronidases		Present	Present	—
Aminopeptidases		Absent	Present	—
	AMP, ADP, ATPases	Present	Present	Present
	Acid phosphatases	Absent	Doubtful	—
	Alkaline phosphatases	Present	Present	Present
Phosphatases	NAD, NADPases	Present	Present	Present
	5-nucleotidases	Present	—	—
	β-glycerophosphatases	Absent	—	Absent
Phosphorylases		—	Doubtful	—

[a] For Authors, see text.
[b] Unknown.

benzoaldehyde method (BACCAREDDA-BOY et al., 1958). Histamine is present (JUHLIN and SHELLEY, 1966).

As regards fats, we have not found glycerol, cholesterol esters, or fatty acids either with Nile blue sulphate or with oil red O (MORETTI and CROVATO, 1965). Instead, stainable granules of lipid were seen inside the endothelial cells with Sudan III, Nile blue sulphate, and other methods (SANNICANDRO, 1934). In the endothelial cells the plasmal technique also reveals strong quantities of acetalphosphatides (BRAUN-FALCO, 1961; MORETTI and CROVATO, 1965) (Fig. 66) but no esterphosphatides (CRAMER, 1964). Much more is known about oxidative enzymes; succinic dehydrogenase activity is clearly recognizable in the endothelium of the capillaries of man and of animals (Fig. 67). In some species the reaction follows the outline of the vessels (MONTAGNA and FORMISANO, 1955); also, there is considerable reactivity of the capillaries in general, and particularly in the endothelium of arterial and venous tracts, to NAD and NADP reductase (BRAUN-FALCO and PETZOLDT, 1964) (Fig. 68). Reactivity to cytochromeoxidase appears on the contrary to be rather weak in the whole capillary loop (MONTAGNA and YUN, 1961) while monoamino oxidase seems to be present (MORETTI and CROVATO, 1965).

Concerning hydrolases, a vast group of nonspecific esterases, according to some authors, are almost all present (SERRI, 1959). Other authors besides ourselves have noticed an excellent reactivity of the capillaries both to α-naphthyl and to AS-esterase (Fig. 69), a weak response to the 5-indoxylesterase and no reaction to Tween-esterase (MORETTI and CROVATO, 1965; MONTAGNA, 1955; STEIGLEDER and LOEFFLER, 1956; BRAUN-FALCO, 1956a).

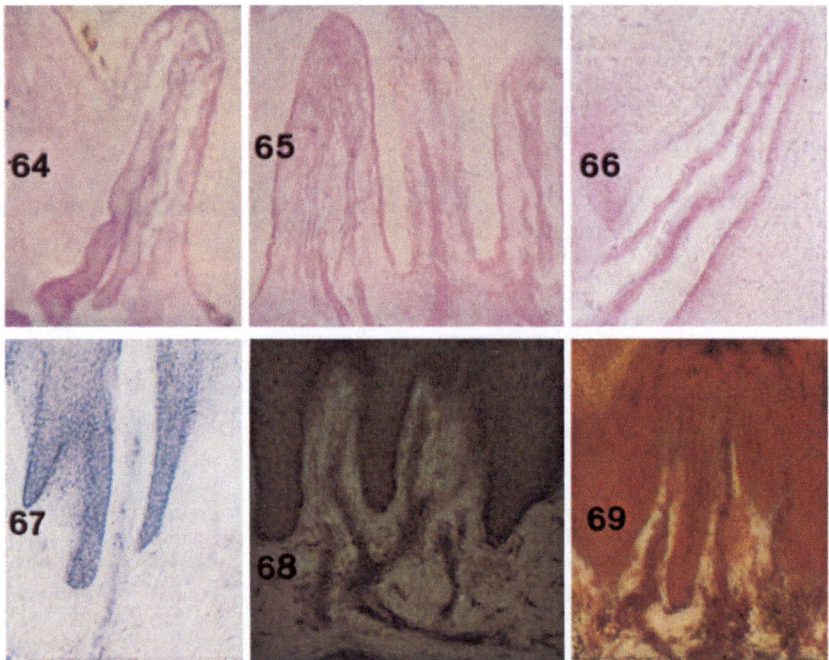

Figs. 64—69. Some histochemical properties of capillaries

Figs. 64 and 65. Positive reaction to the PAS method and sensitivity to amylase of capillaries immediately below the epidermis

Fig. 66. Strong reactivity of the endothelial cells with the plasmal technique

Fig. 67. A succinic-dehydrogenase activity is clearly recognizable

Fig. 68. There is considerable reactivity of papillary capillaries to NAD reductase

Fig. 69. The reactivity of capillaries to AS-esterase is excellent

Over phosphatases, while it is doubtful that the dermal blood vessels and capillaries, in particular, are positive to the acid phosphatase method (SERRI, 1959), there is no need to dwell further upon the intense reactivity of the endothelium to the alkaline phosphatase technique (see Part 1 of this Chapter). Let us remember that it is notable in the whole capillary environment and more intense in the arterial and intercalary tract of the terminal loops and localized at the inside of the endothelial cells, while the pericytes remain negative (CORMIA and ERNYEY, 1961).

A rather good technique for tracing the course of the capillaries, of which we have already spoken, is another phosphatase method, the adenosinetriphosphatase and adenosinemonophosphatase reaction (see afterwards Figs. 98—104), developed by several authors (BRADSHAW, et al., 1963; WOLFF, 1963b) and used successfully by us (MORETTI and CROVATO, 1965). Over glucosidases, the β-glucuronidase technique is positive in the arterial part of the capillary loops and probably in the pericytes (MONTAGNA, 1957; MORETTI and CROVATO, 1965).

As regards proteases, several authors observed rather intense leucil-aminopeptidase activity in the capillary endothelial cells and especially in the arterial tract of the loops (STEIGLEDER et al., 1962; ISHIKAWA and KLINGMUELLER, 1963; WOLFF, 1963a). As for transferases, the presence of phosphorylase in the capillaries seems to us rather doubtful, notwithstanding some data in the literature (SERRI, 1959).

In spite of numerous studies (GERSH and CATCHPOLE, 1949; NIESSING and ROLLHAUSER, 1954; RINEHART and FARQUHAR, 1955; LEBLOND, et al., 1957; PEASE, 1958; PUCHTLER and LEBLOND, 1958), the histochemistry of the basement membrane too is incompletely known. Nevertheless, its generally evident stainability with the PAS and PAS-amylase methods suggests the presence of a proteincarbohydrate complex (LEBLOND et al., 1957; PUCHTLER and LEBLOND, 1958; GARRACHON et al., 1964).

Inside the protein skeleton there are isolated lamellar accumulations of lipoids (NIESSING and ROLLHAUSER, 1954; BARGMANN, 1956) and, according to some authors, the protein precursors of elastin, embedded in a mucopolysaccharide matrix (PEASE and MOLINARI, 1960; PEASE and PAULE, 1960).

Definitive conclusions about the histochemistry of the papillary and subpapillary capillaries seem premature at this time (Table 2). In the vessels studied, however, the wall has probably reached a high degree of organization in carbohydrate metabolism. This involves the capillaries' capacity for the rapid liberation of energy, used in the metabolization of a variety of organic substances. The presence in the endothelial cells of a great deal of hydrolases may be rather significant in this connection.

5. Electron Microscopy of the Capillaries

Much of the information collected up to now on their histology and histochemistry has been partially completed, if not elucidated entirely, by electron microscopy.

Recent classification of the capillaries (BENNETT, LUFT and HAMPTON, 1959)[26] based on the variability of the basal membrane of the endothelium and the pericytes has, in fact, enabled classification of the capillaries of the skin as Type A 1 α vessels (MACHER and VOGELL, 1962).

This means that they are capillaries with a completely continuous basal membrane, with an endothelium lacking intracellular fenestrations, intercellular spaces, and a partially surrounding pericyte barrier.

Electron microscopy has also ascertained the existence of two models of the cutaneous endothelial cell (HIBBS et al., 1958): the first composed of an extremely flat smooth cell, except for the protruding nucleus, even when the vessel is dilated; the second, of a cell with high cytoplasm which is voluminous, gnarled, and more or less pyramid-shaped in a closed vessel.

---

[26] According to these authors, the capillaries can be catalogued thus: a) Type A: if they have a complete continuous basal membrane; Type B: if they are without this; b) Type 1: when the endothelial wall is continuous and without "holes" and "spaces" Type 2: when they have "windows" or intercellular "holes" Type 3: when "windows" and "intercellular holes" are present; c) Type α: without a complete pericyte barrier interposed between capillaries and parenchyma: Type β: whenever a barrier of this kind exists (MAJNO, 1965).

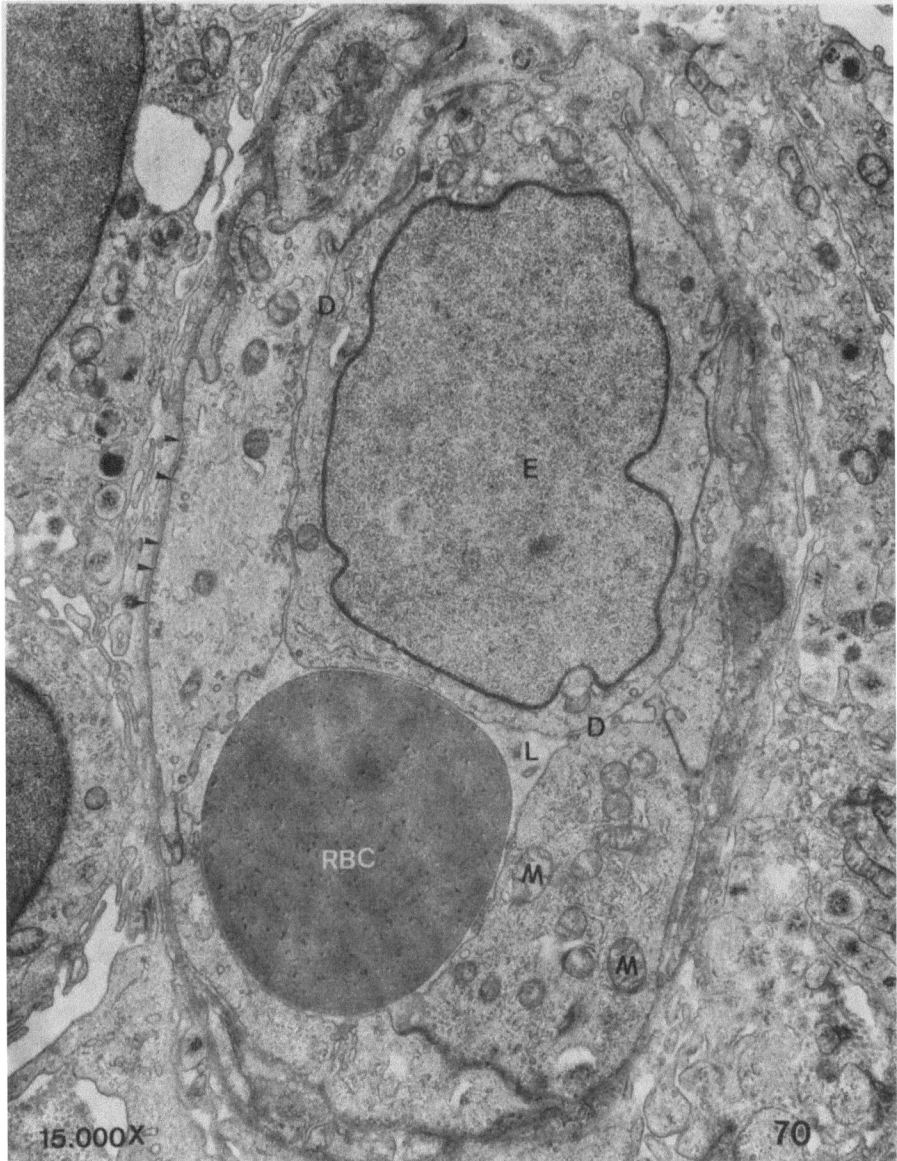

Figs. 70—77. Electron microscopy of the capillaries

Fig. 70. Electron microscopy of a capillary of the superficial dermis. Note within lumen (L) an erythrocyte (RBC) in the endothelial cells, nucleus (E), desmosomes (D), some cytoplasmic vesicles (arrow) and mitochondria (M) with their "cristae". (Courtesy of G. F. ODLAND)

The first model, as already mentioned (0.2 micron in height), predominates in the superficial and in the deep subcutaneous tissue; the second (2—4 micron high) in the dermis (MAJNO, 1965).

The nucleus of each of these cells contains inside its envelope, nuclear pores excluded (ODLAND, 1961), a uniform material about 300 Å thick, studded with particles of 150—200 Å in diameter (Figs. 70, 71 and 72).

There are numerous elements in the cytoplasm. Among these are a thick interlacing of filaments of 75—100 Å in diameter each prevalently concentrated in the perinuclear zone and lacking on the internal surface of the desmosomes (ODLAND, 1961); an endoplasmic reticulum with both rough and smooth surfaces (ZELICKSON, 1966); vesiculae of the Golgi complex; centrioles; numerous round and spheroid mitochondria, some up to a micron in length and variously distributed; in certain cases, some round structures of dimensions similar to the mitochondria and characterized by a double wall and by a dense matrix bursting with granules of unknown function (HIBBS, 1958; ODLAND, 1961) (Figs. 70, 71 and 72). Finally, in the endothelium are the so-called "vesiculae" described for the first time by PALADE (1953).

These vesicles (Figs. 70, 71, 74 and 75) are present along the whole length of the endothelial cell and joined together in groups which are more or less numerous in the cytoplasm, especially that which faces the lumen or that facing towards the basement membrane; each group of these vesicles is surrounded by a membrane, without openings, and has a total diameter of 200—500 Å (HIBBS, 1958; ODLAND, 1961; MACHER and VOGELL, 1962).

A good deal of argument exists on their functional significance; according to some (BENNETT, 1956; MOORE and RUSKA, 1957), they should have a transport function controlling metabolic material passing through the capillary walls.

The plasma membrane of the endothelium, although provided with a variable number of pseudopodic projections and microvilli (Figs. 72 74 and 75), has never revealed continuous solutions, openings, fissures, or cuts (ODLAND, 1961; MAJNO, 1965).

The plasma membrane is more or less equivalent to the desmosomes (Figs. 71 and 72) or intercellular bridges in the prickle cell layer (ODLAND, 1961) and is a truly specialized structure which serves as a barrier between the capillary lumen and the pericapillary space and at the same time binds the endothelial cells to the adjacent cells.

In joining these (Figs. 71, 72 and 77), it becomes more dense (though never absolutely tight[27]; there is a distance of 150—200 Å between the plasma membrane of two neighboring endothelial cells (ODLAND, 1961)) while the contact surface behaves in different ways; sometimes it engages another cell, sometimes overlaps it[28], and at other times merely approaches it (MACHER and VOGELL, 1962).

Along the intercellular contact line besides, lengthwise thickenings are enclosed on both sides somewhat recalling the structure of the plasmadesmosomes, without however achieving their level of organization (MACHER and VOGELL, 1962).

The intralumenal protein coat adhering to the endothelium as described by CHAMBERS and ZWEIFACH (1947) has not been observed with an electron microscope (MACHER and VOGELL, 1962), but it may exist nevertheless (MAJNO, 1965).

As a fundamental characteristic, the basement membrane interposed between endothelial cells and pericytes runs over the endothelial surface without any interruption (Figs. 72, 73, 74 and 75) (ODLAND, 1961; MAJNO, 1965).

According to electron microscopy, its organization is simple; often only 100 Å at the thinnest points adjacent to the endothelium and 300 Å at the furthest

---

[27] It is well to state two facts on this subject: 1. the term "desmosome", although in current use (ODLAND, 1961), should be reserved more correctly to the border structures which are buttonshaped (MAJNO, 1965); 2. the intercellular space is completely occluded on the side of the lumen by the partial fusion of the two adjacent plasma membranes ("tight junction") (MAJNO, 1965). Exact details of this "zonula occludens" are obtainable only under favorable technical conditions (MAJNO, 1965).

[28] A dark reduced silver line probably becomes visible in this case with $AgNO^3$ (FLOREY, POOLE and MECK, 1959). This does not, however, explain the presence of an analogous line between nonoverlapping cells, which are close or engaged in contact.

(ODLAND, 1961; MACHER and VOGELL, 1962), it fills and surrounds all the cavities between the various types of cells (Figs. 72, 73, 74 and 75) and the periphery of the pericytes with a double or even multiple layer of intercellular material (MACHER and VOGELL, 1962).

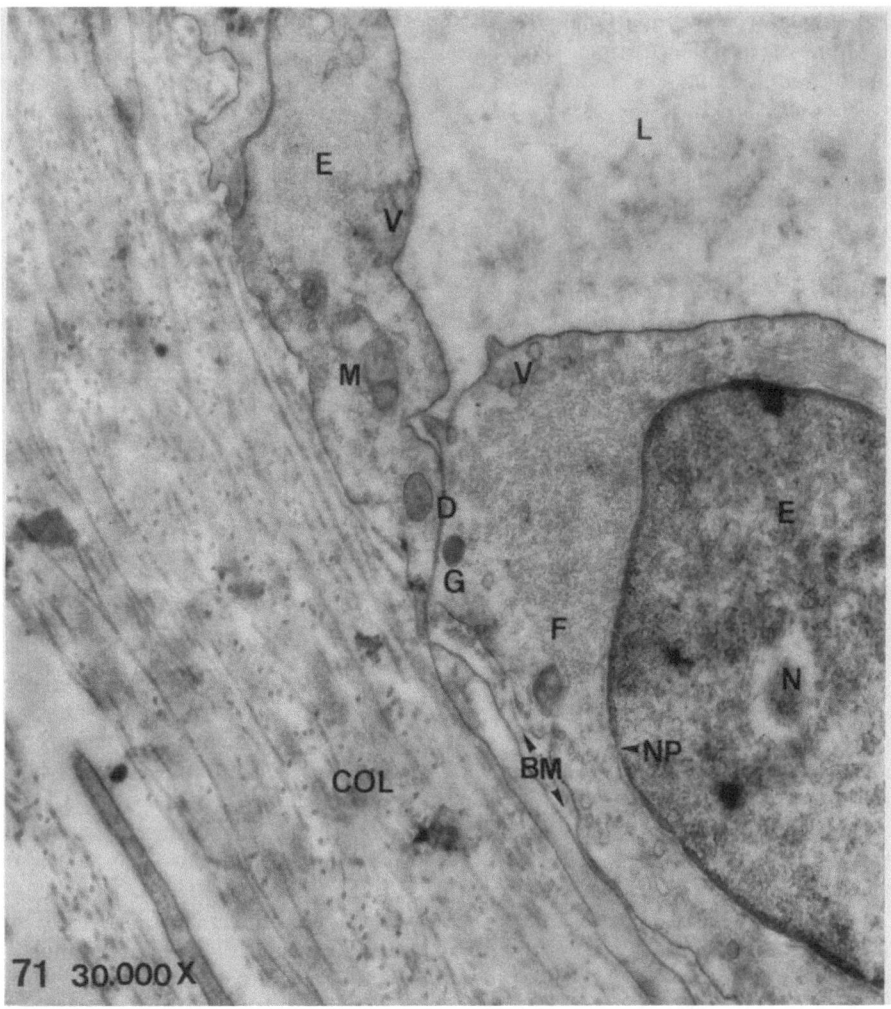

Fig. 71. Other important details of electron-microscopy of the "dermal" capillary. Within two endothelial cells (*E*) surrounding the lumen (*L*) of the vessel are clearly visible a nucleus (*N*), a nuclear pore (*NP*), intracytoplasmic filaments (*F*), mitochondria (*M*), vesicles (*V*), unidentified granules (*G*) and desmosomes (*D*); outside the cells the lamellar appearance of collagen fibres (*Col*) cut into two directions, and part of basement membrane (*BM*) are to be seen. (ODLAND, G. F., courtesy of the Pergamon Press. In: Advances in biology of skin, vol. II, p. 62. 1961)

Sometimes, however, it reveals alternate thick or thin layers or fibrillar filaments in 3 layers with two large interposing strips rich in sponge-like cavities (MACHER and VOGELL, 1962).

As for the pericytes (Figs. 72, 73, 74, 75, and 76) adhering to the surface of the vessel, they are more or less thick and quite like the endothelial cell especially in the region of the nucleus (ODLAND, 1961).

Its most apparent cytological characteristics are: less cytoplasm than the endothelial cell[29], but not so dense as that of the smooth muscle cell (ODLAND, 1961; MACHER and VOGELL, 1962); the presence of vesicles (Figs. 74 and 75) on the

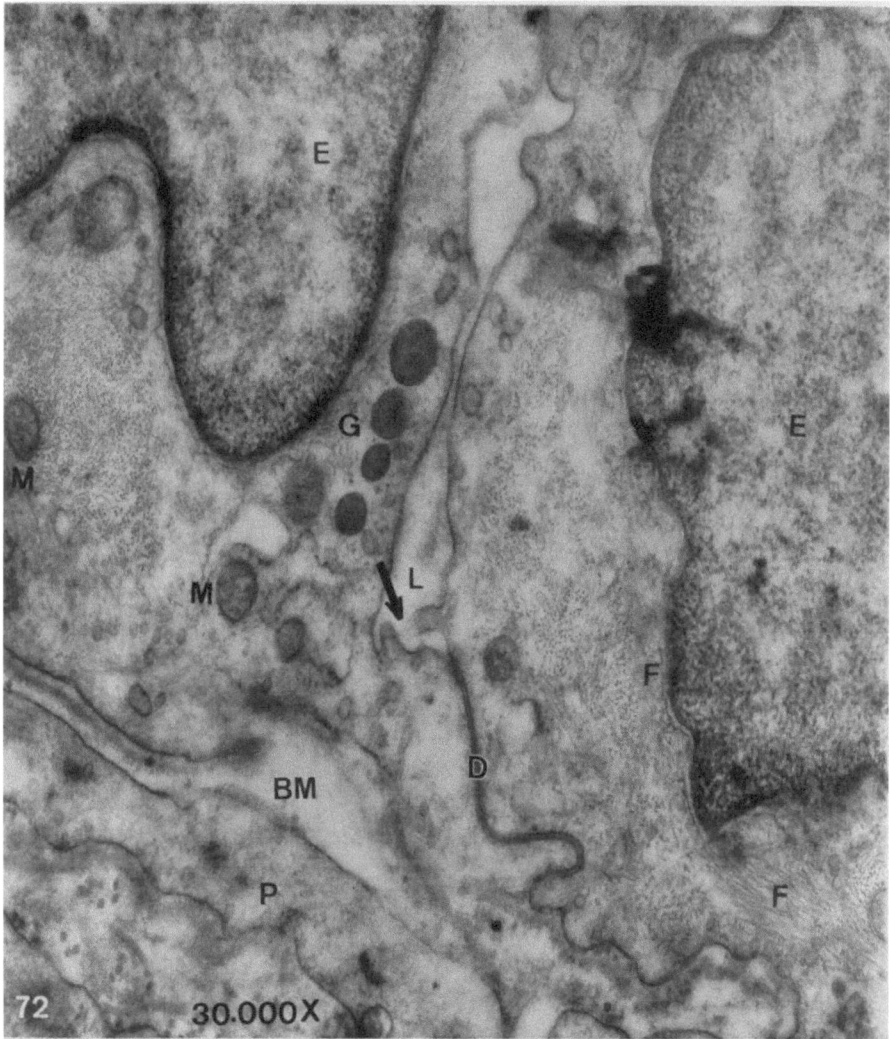

Fig. 72. Another illustration of the electron microscopy of the "dermal" capillary. About two adjacent endothelial cells (E) note dense granules (G) of a size similar to mitochondria (M), filaments (F), desmosomes (D) microvilli projecting into lumen near desmosomes (arrow). The lumen of vessel (L) is largely collapsed. The basement membrane (BM) and a pericyte (P) are also visible. (ODLAND, G. F., courtesy of the Pergamon Press. In: Advances in biology of skin, vol. II, p. 63. 1961)

cell membrane, which are more numerous than on the endothelial cell; the presence of rod-shaped tubular formations isolated in the cytoplasm and similar to those of the endothelium (ZELICKSON, 1966) and the absence of a conspicuous tangle of filaments (ODLAND, 1961).

---

[29] Because of the presence of fibrils and other characteristics (MISSOTTEN, 1962), these cells would have a smooth muscle fine structure that is incompletely developed (MAYNARD, et al., 1957).

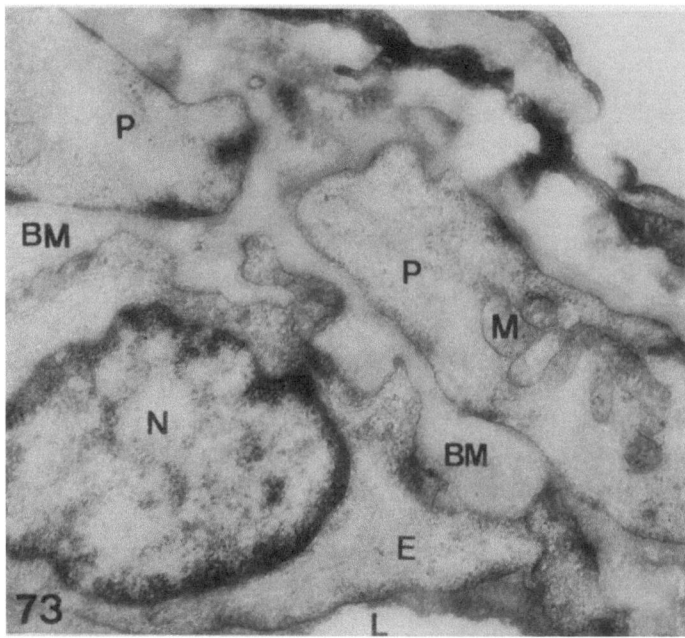

Figs. 73—75. Other views of the electron microscopy of capillaries

Fig. 73. In this figure observe lumen of vessel (*L*), endothelial cell (*E*) with its nucleus (*N*), pericytes with its mitochondria (*M*) and chiefly basement membrane (*BM*) filling and surrounding all cavities between the various types of cells. [MACHER, E., and W. VOGELL, courtesy of the Dermatologica (Basel), Elektronenmikroskopische Untersuchungen an Hautkapillaren. **124**, 119 (1962)]

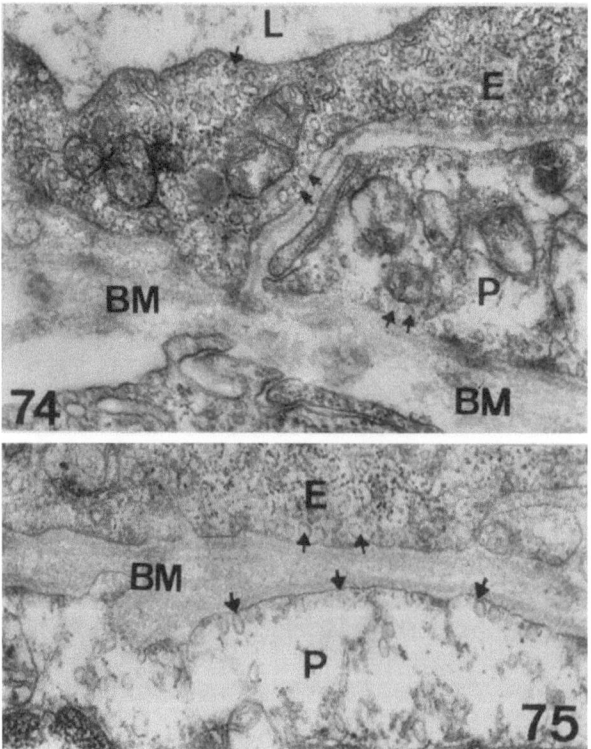

Figs. 74 and 75. These figures illustrate the lumen (*L*) of a capillary; the intracytoplasmic vesicles and invaginations (arrows) of the cytoplasmic membranes of endothelial cells (*E*); the pericytes (*P*); the basement membranes (*BM*) interposed between the cells. [MACHER, E., and W. VOGELL, courtesy of the Dermatologica (Basel), Elektronenmikroskopische Untersuchungen an Hautkapillaren. **124**, 117 (1962)]

The pericytes, although usually embracing (Fig. 76) a region corresponding to the vessel diameter, surround no less than 90° of the periphery of the ascending capillaries and about 180° of the larger descending portion and the whole circumference of the deeper vessels in the subpapillary network (MACHER and VOGELL, 1962).

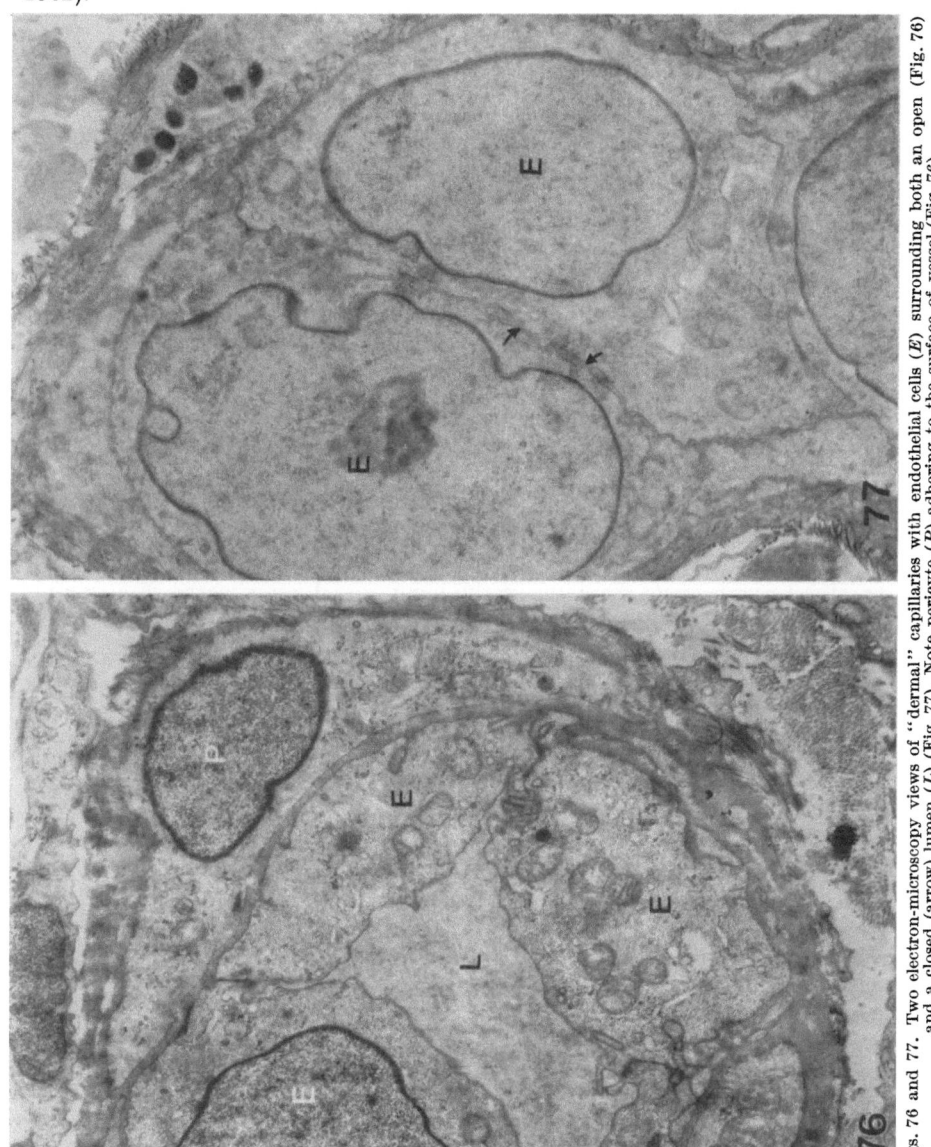

Figs. 76 and 77. Two electron-microscopy views of "dermal" capillaries with endothelial cells (*E*) surrounding both an open (Fig. 76) and a closed (arrow) lumen (*L*) (Fig. 77). Note pericyte (*P*) adhering to the surface of vessel (Fig. 76)

In this case, too the pericyte layer is incomplete and reveals the existence of large spaces of 0.5—1 micron between its cells that are filled by the basement membrane (MACHER and VOGELL, 1962).

Besides being surrounded by the basement membrane, the pericyte may be in contact with the collagen fibers that thread their way between pericytes and endothelial cells (ODLAND, 1961).

This cell and pericyte are, on the other hand, surrounded by a special connective sheath, 0.3—1 microns in thickness, which separates them from the remaining collagen (ODLAND, 1961). The collagen fibrils which compose it are quite distinct from one another and arranged in layers, alternately oriented either in the direction of the circumference or longitudinal to the vessel axis and enclosed in a matrix analogous to the basement membrane (Fig. 71) (ODLAND, 1961).

To sum up, electron microscopy has produced notable results. Above all, it has defined many of the characteristics of the endothelial cell. Other observations e.g. the abundance of basement membrane which is roughly equivalent to a real "micro-skeleton" (PEASE, 1958) as well as the solidity of the collagen sheath (ODLAND, 1961) have warranted some interesting hypotheses of a morpho-functional kind on skin capillaries. These hypotheses are that the vessel is so solidly anchored to the surrounding dermal tissue as to face the various sharing forces to which the skin is exposed; the capillaries probably have an "intrinsic capacity to close at critical times" probably linked to thermoregulatory phenomena (ODLAND, 1961); but through its wall metabolic exchange may be small. We realize, of course, that this last assumption is partly in contrast with the histochemical data which we have just put forward.

IV. The Venules and Veins of the Skin

1. Types of Venules and Veins

The total number and diameter of the venules and veins in the skin are undoubtedly much greater than those of the arteries (SPALTEHOLZ, 1927).

The venous system which they form begins, in theory, at the efferent loop of the papillary capillary. This, as we have seen, is indistinguishable from the other parts of the loop (MACHER and VOGELL, 1962); some of the venules of the upper dermis can be recognized as such only when they are open (ODLAND, 1961).

True venules, in any case, cross the corium in various ways; they are completely isolated; or they are fine vessels accompanying the bigger veins; or in their descent from the superficial levels to the deeper ones they flank the arteries (SPALTEHOLZ, 1927).

In the various layers of the skin the direction in which they move varies. Some venules and veins have a course more or less parallel or oblique to the surface epidermis; others form arcades (DE SAUNDERS, 1961); others subdivide into vast arborizations coming from the subpapillary venous network and from other dermal levels. These are called "candelabra venules" on account of their similarity to arterial ones (Fig. 78). Finally, some venules developed in spirals or even arranged in a circle are frequently visible around the sweat gland glomeruli and ducts.

The diameter of the venules and veins increases progressively from 40—60 micron in the dermis to 100—400 micron in the subcutaneous (MIANI and RUBERTI, 1958a, b).

After having formed, at various levels, a whole series of periappendageal and horizontal overlying networks (Fig. 79) more or less similar to the arterials, these vessels empty themselves into progressively more substantial deep veins some of which are considered "terminal" veins, i.e., capable of draining a whole area of subcutaneous tissue without anastomizing themselves with other veins (DODD and COCKETT, 1956).

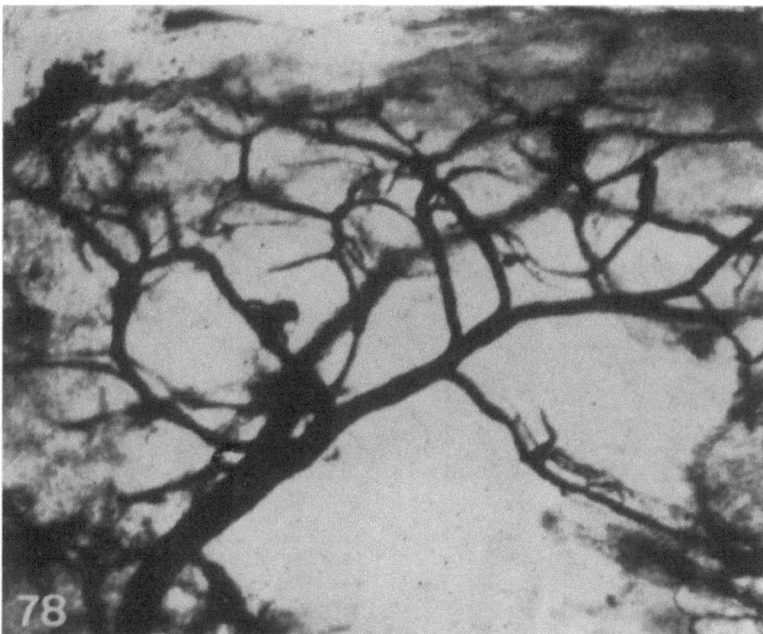

Fig. 78. "Candelabra" venules in an oblique section of the dorsum of the toe. (Courtesy of R. K. WINKELMANN and of the Pergamon Press. In: Advances in biology of skin, vol. II, p. 6. 1961)

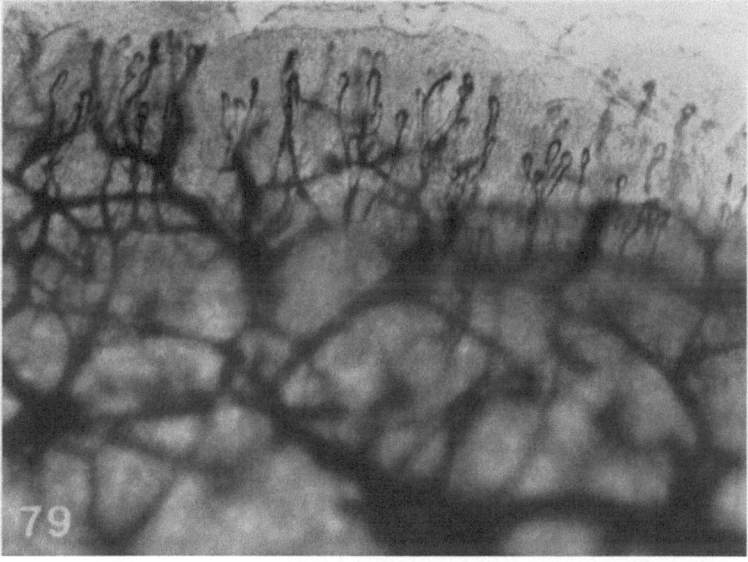

Fig. 79. An oblique view of a subpapillary venous "plexus" and of some of its tributary capillaries in the dorsum of the toe. (Courtesy of R. K. WINKELMANN and of the Pergamon Press)

2. The Structure of the Venules and Veins

A vein wall is usually thinner than that of an artery and less clearly divided especially in the smaller vessels (BARGMANN, 1956) into its three classic layers

The postcapillary venules are formed of endothelial cells, which are somewhat more rhombic than those of the capillaries, generally with an oval, or sometimes circular, nucleus, a basement membrane and pericytes, which vary slightly in shape because of irregular transverse expansion, being either star-shaped or zigzag (BENNINGHOFF, 1930).

Venules of this type, therefore, on account of their large size and absence of muscle, are not very different from the capillaries and, in fact, SPALTEHOLZ (1893) considered the subpapillary venules as no more than gigantic capillaries. Still, at a certain point, some muscular fibers appear around the vessel[30]. Short initially, with long or round nuclei placed transversally to the axis of the vessels and separated by vast intercellular spaces (Figs. 52, 53, 80 and 82), these cells become

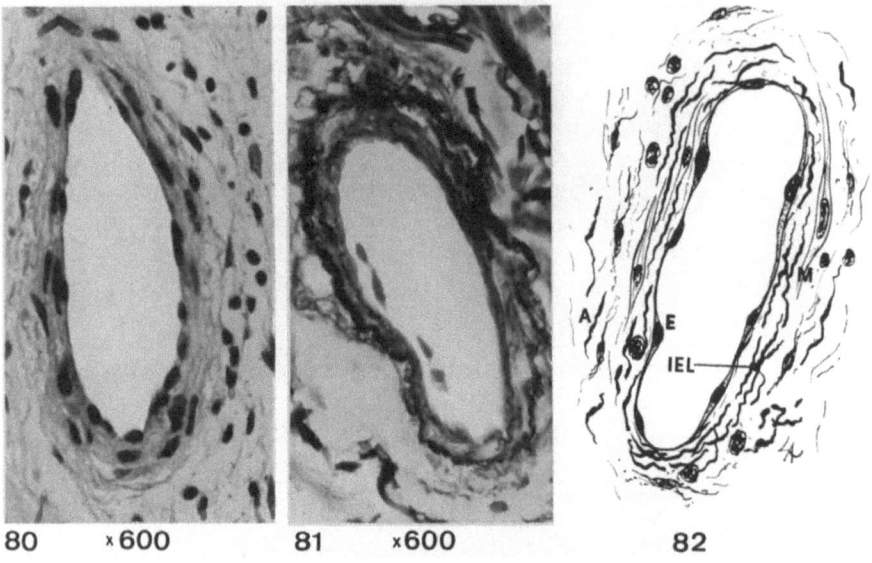

Figs. 80—82. The structure of venules

Fig. 80. The oval nuclei of the endothelial cells and the thin wall of a venule may be easily observed (Hematoxylin-eosin stain)

Fig. 81. The same venule reveals the presence in its wall of fairly abundant elastic fibers (Weigert-stain)

Fig. 82. A schematic drawing of the anatomy of the already-mentioned venule. *E* endothelium; *IEL* internal elastic lamina; *M* media; *A* adventitia

continually more frequent and longer until they form a continuous muscle layer around the endothelium. Longitudinal muscular elements gradually appear beside the circular ones (BENNINGHOFF, 1930).

The increase in vessel calibre is accompanied by an increase of the muscle fibers. The internal circular and external longitudinal fibers together manage to organize a kind of loose network over a vast area; at the same time the elastic fibers come into close contact with them, but without creating an authentic internal elastic membrane (BENNINGHOFF, 1930).

With successive development of the muscle layers, the elastic network, on the other hand, expands from the external surface of the muscle layer to the whole width of the wall; medium-sized veins thus end by having an internal elastic lamina underlying the endothelium (Figs. 80, 81 and 82) (BENNINGHOFF, 1930; BARGMANN, 1956).

---

[30] For SPALTEHOLZ, venous vessels with muscular fibers of this type are observed as far as the depths of the venous cutaneous network ("capillary veins" (SPALTEHOLZ, 1927); for FREERKSEN (1938), BRAUS and ELZE (1940), on the contrary, these vessels in this network are without muscle elements.

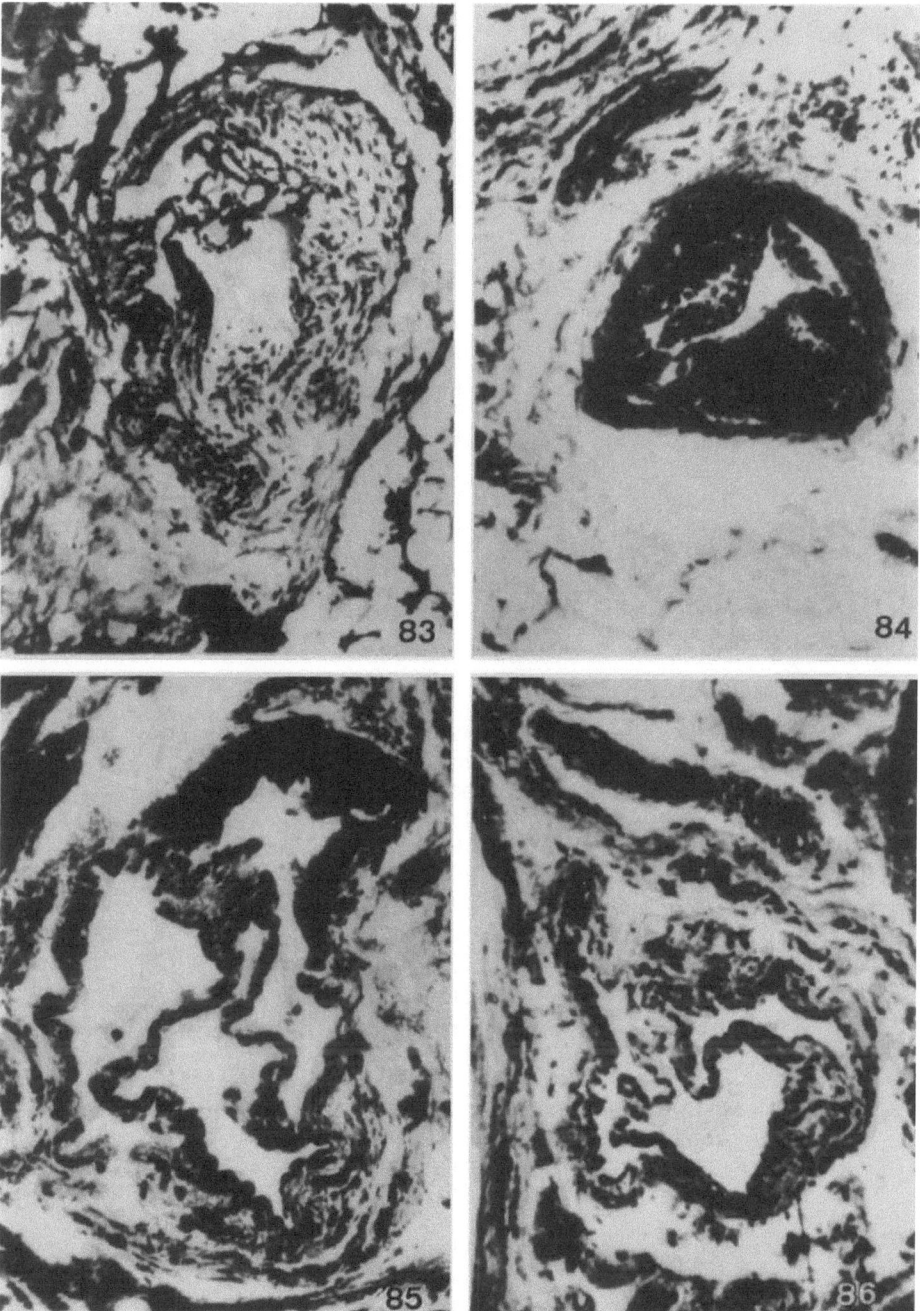

Figs. 83—86. Some valvulae in the venules provided with muscle fibers of the skin on the foot

Fig. 83. The number of muscle fibers in this type of valvula is modest. [MIANI, A., and U. RUBERTI, courtesy of the Minerva cardioangiol., Sulla morfologia degli apparati valvolari delle venule effluenti delle AVA della pianta del piede **6**, 542 (1958)]

Fig. 84. Another example of valvula. [MIANI, A., and U. RUBERTI, courtesy of the Minerva cardioangiol., Sulla morfologia degli apparati valvolari delle venule effluenti delle AVA della pianta del piede **6**, 542 (1958)]

Fig. 85. The amount of muscle fibers in this type of valvula is rather large. [MIANI, A., and U. RUBERTI, courtesy of the Minerva cardioangiol., Sulla morfologia degli apparati valvolari delle venule effluenti delle AVA della pianta del piede **6**, 542 (1958)]

Fig. 86. Both the walls of the venule and the insertion muscles may be weak. [MIANI, A., and U. RUBERTI, courtesy of the Minerva cardioangiol., Sulla morfologia degli apparati valvolari delle venule effluenti delle AVA della pianta del piede **6**, 542 (1958)]

The veins of the skin never go beyond the level of the subcutaneous layer and vary somewhat in structure (FREERKSEN, 1938). Without substantial variations in the endothelial type, they have: 1) a media containing chiefly circular muscle fibers, but occasional longitudinal fibers especially in medium sized vessels; 2) a considerable adventitia (BENNINGHOFF, 1930) composed of abundant muscle fibers that give the vessels of the cutaneous network the typical "arterial" appearance first described by DARIER et al. (1936), plus elastic and connective tissue (LEVI, 1927; BENNINGHOFF, 1930; BARGMANN, 1956).

As regards the valves, another important element in venous histology, while some authors (SPALTEHOLZ, 1927; HORSTMANN, 1957) state that only the veins in the cutaneous network possess isolated valves, other research workers affirm their existence in the subcutaneous and reticular dermis in the plantar region (MIANI and RUBERTI, 1958a, b) and even in post-capillary vessels of 20 microns in diameter (DZIALLAS, 1949, cit. BARGMANN, 1956).

Generally more frequent in the efferent venules in all kinds of arteriovenous anastomoses, these valvulae (Figs. 83, 84, 85 and 86) are both "birds' nest" type with 2—3 edges and divisible into two types according to the number of muscle fibers present; when these are numerous, the venular walls and the insertion muscle display great strength (MIANI and RUBERTI, 1958a, b).

3. Histochemistry and Electron Microscopy of Venules

Unfortunately the data on the histochemistry of the venules and veins in the skin are still less than those on the arterioles and capillaries (Table 2).

Apart from the presence of endothelial glucose (SACCHI, 1957), mucopolysaccharides (MORETTI and CROVATO, 1965) and nucleoproteins, the only fairly reliable data seem to be the reactivity of the tunica intima with succinic-dehydrogenase (MONTAGNA and FORMISANO, 1955); the marked reaction of the venules' smooth muscles to NAD and NADP reductase (BRAUN-FALCO and PETZOLDT, 1964); possibly that of the same wall with ubiquinone (BRAUN-FALCO, 1965), nonspecific esterases and tween-esterase (STEIGLEDER and LOEFFLER, 1956); the moderate alkaline-phosphatase staining of the beginning of the post-capillary venule (CORMIA and ERNYEY, 1961); and the positive reaction with adenosine-triphosphatase (less in the endothelium than in the tunica media) opposed to the doubtful response to adenosine-monophosphatase and the negative response to betaglycero-phosphatase (Table 2) (WOLFF, 1963b).

The data are equally scarce on the electron microscopy of the venules (Fig. 87). These vessels are generally lined by the same type of cell, an endothelial one containing the filaments already described in arterioles and capillaries (HIBBS et al., 1958).

This usually means pyramidal cells with the apex towards the lumen. They contain large bundles of filaments, several of which have rod-shaped granules and vesicular bodies like those of the capillaries.

Just beyond the basement membrane, furthermore, a lamella of collagen fibers pressed against one another and occasional fragments of smooth muscle cells can be seen (HIBBS et al., 1958).

On the other hand, the venule lumen is somewhat larger than that of the capillaries and is made up of several endothelial cells (Fig. 87). Electron microscopy facilitates the distinction between venules and capillaries, but only when they are open. When they are closed, it is quite difficult to distinguish one from the other, since the intimal structure of the endothelial cell and of the perivascular collagen sheath seem identical (ODLAND, 1961).

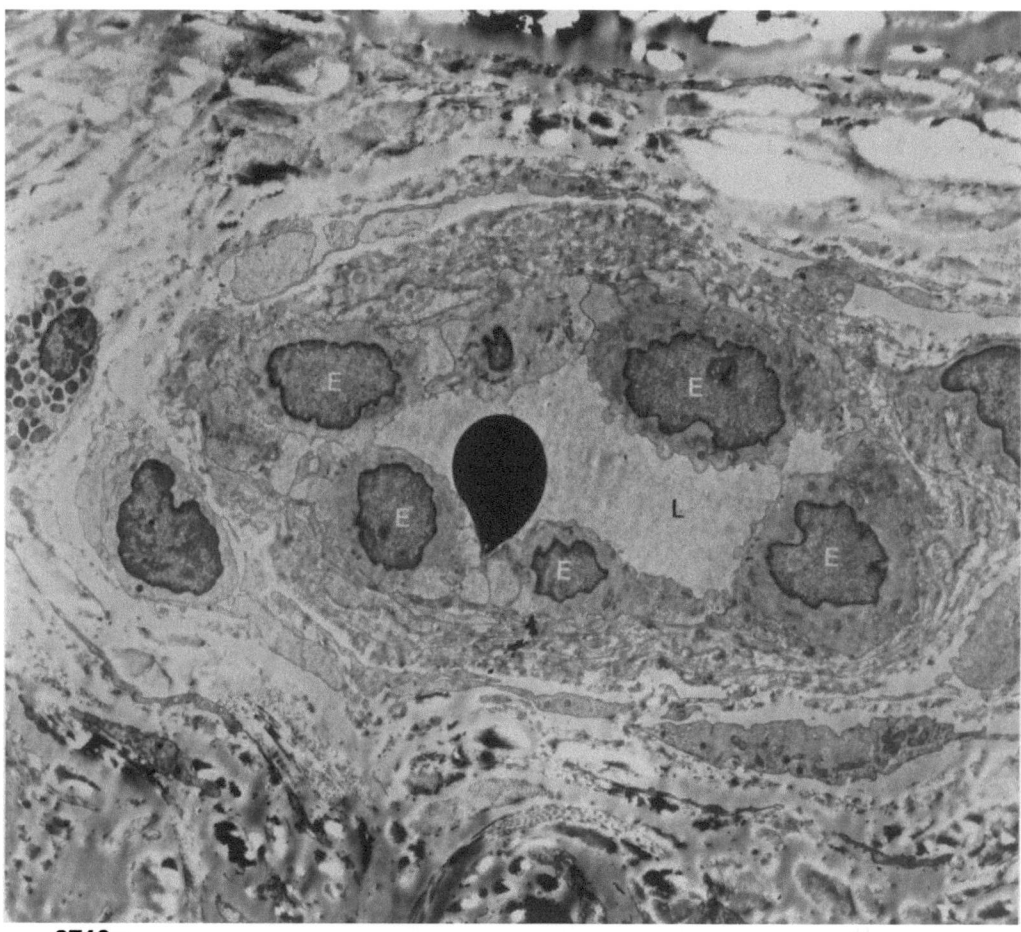

3760 x

Fig. 87. The electron microscopy of venules reveals a lumen (L) larger than that of the capillaries and made up of several endothelial cells (E). (Courtesy of G. F. ODLAND)

V. Arteriovenous Anastomosis (AVA)

1. Types of Anastomoses[31]

In the skin, as in the rest of the organism, various devices can greatly simplify normal hematic flow. Among these are the "blocking arteries" and "blocking veins," which, combined with the AVA, are present in the arteries and probably in the veins of the armpit, the finger tips, etc. (GROSSER, 1902; VASTARINI-CRESI, 1903; WATZKA, 1936; BARGMANN, 1956; CLARA, 1959). In the arteries, for example, the block device, situated below the intima and within the internal lamina, is composed, in addition to circular elastic fibers, of more layers of smooth longitudinal muscle cells capable of protruding into the lumen to the point of occlusion. There are different kinds of such arteries: sphincters, a variably organized musculature belonging to the intima, and polypoid cushions (BUCCIANTE, 1950;

---

[31] For the classification of arteriovenous anastomosis into two types i.e. with or without intercalary tracts and for an explanation of the existence of the two aspects of this, rectilinear or glomerular and of their distribution in the tissues, one should refer to the authors who studied the matter thoroughly (CLARK and CLARK, 1934; BUCCIANTE, 1945).

ORMEA et al., 1959). There are still others: vessels of doubtful histological demonstration interpreted by ZWEIFACH (1949) as arteriovenous anastomoses of the cutaneous capillary system (CLARA, 1959); those problematical ones described by SPALTEHOLZ (cit. CLARA, 1959) as superficial arteriovenous anastomoses of certain terminal arteries, which release very fine capillary loops; contractile and superficial ones, which according to HEIMBERGER (1930), link up arterioles and venules.

The most important, however, are undoubtedly the arteriovenous anastomoses (AVA), which, usually in the middle and deep dermis, join up directly by means of variations in their caliber, high pressure arterial system and low pressure venous system, which promotes the insertion or disconnection of the capillary bed from the two systems (CLARA, 1959).

2. Number and Size of Anastomoses

Because of their thermoregulatory qualities, the AVA are concentrated in particular regions of the skin. In the finger tips, they are found (HOYER, 1877; CLARA, 1959) in the surface zones of the reticular dermis above the level of the sweat glands, sometimes in the deeper regions, sometimes even above and within

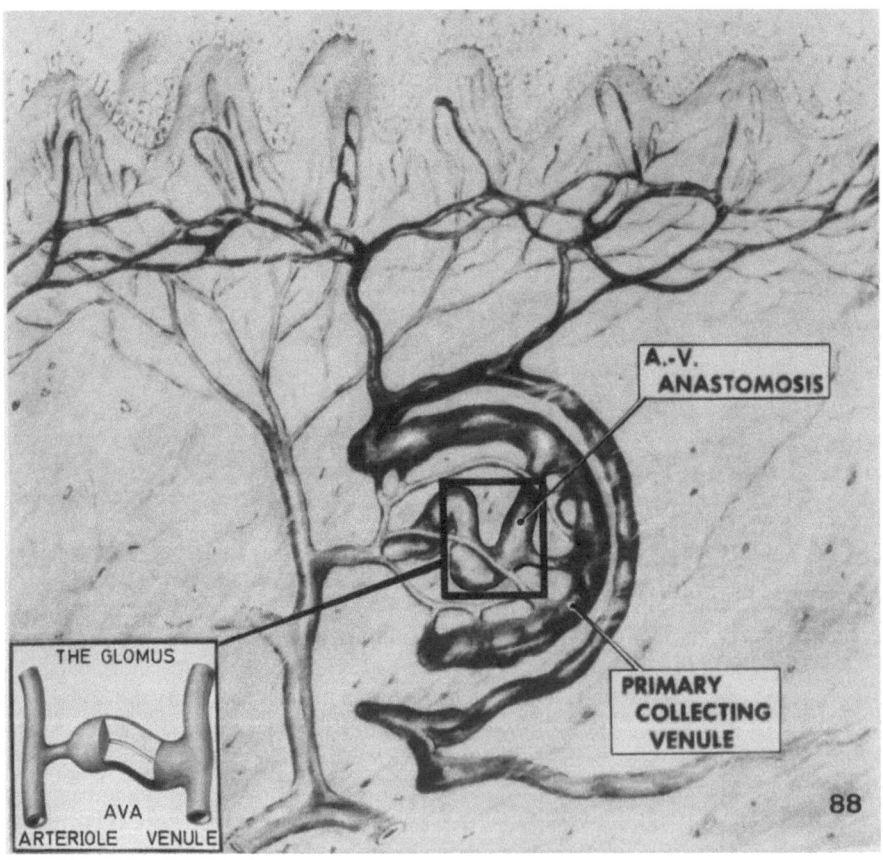

Fig. 88. Schematic drawing of main vessels in a digital glomus. Thick walls and narrow lumen of the intercalary tract, are represented within squares. [MESCON, HURLEY, MORETTI (modified and reprinted by permission of J. invest. Derm.), The anatomy and histochemistry of the arteriovenous anastomosis in human digital skin 27, 136 (1956)]

the periost (CLARA, 1959). Other AVA have been described in the nail bed, in the tenar and hypotenar eminence (SUCQUET, 1862; VASTARINI-CRESI, 1903; GRANT and BLAND, 1931; etc.) in the ears, on the tip of the nose (SUCQUET, 1862) on the cubital prominence (SUCQUET, 1862; VASTARINI-CRESI, 1903), in the armpits (CAVAZZANA, 1945—46), and in the gluteal region (CLARA, 1959).

The considerable disagreement about the population of the AVA is due mostly to the technique used in observing them. According to MESCON and others (1956), there are between 20 and 25/cm² in the finger tip[32]; POPOFF (1935) counted 18 AVA in the center surface of the same region, 10 in the lateral surface besides 24 AVA (per cm²) in the nail bed and 12 in the nail matrix.

These findings, which more or less agree, contrast strongly with others. GRANT and BLAND (1931) counted a good 236 AVA in the finger tip even finding 593 in the nail bed, whereas MASSON (1937) counted only 3—4 cm² (1—2/cm² on the cutaneous surface of the other phalanges). Finally, BIANCHI (1961) found not more than 19 in 25 cm² of skin.

The external diameter of the AVA in the fingers of the hand goes as high as 150 micron (GROSSER, cit. CLARA, 1959); it is 120—220 micron in the toes and between 60 and 150 micron in the anastomoses of the finger nail bed (POPOFF, 1935, cit. CLARA, 1959).

On the other hand, the thickness of the walls in the fingers is 20—60 micron (MESCON et al., 1956; GROSSER, cit. CLARA, 1959) and the diameter of the lumen between 10 and 30 micron (HOYER, GROSSER, cit. CLARA, 1959); in the ears, however, it is normally no more than 10 micron (PRITCHARD and DANIEL, 1956).

3. Structure of the Arteriovenous Anastomoses (AVA)

The most complete arteriovenous anastomoses can usually be seen in the finger tips and the nail bed, as a continuation of arterial branches of 50 to 150 micron in diameter (CLARA, 1959).

These arterial branches have varied courses: rather serpentine in a baby (HOYER, 1877), they are almost glomerular in an adult, sometimes with italic "S" loops in the anastomotic segment tract (SCHORN, 1955). Again, they are rectilinear (VASTARINI-CRESI, 1903; CLARA, 1959) or even undulating with sporadic hook-shaped vessels (CLARA, 1959).

The AVA found in the finger tips (Figs. 88 and 91) (organs of Hoyer-Grosser) and the nail bed in their classic form are composed of an ascending arteriole[33] which sends out the afferent arteriole of the anastomoses laterally; after 30—40 micron it sprouts several arterioles, which will nourish the glomus, it then continues[34] with 1—4 tortuous vessels as the "intercalary tracts" or as "true anastomoses." They empty into a primary collecting venule which first functions as a reservoir, then arches over, circles around, and drains into a subpapillary vein (Figs. 88 and 91) (MESCON et al., 1956).

---

[32] According to GROSSER (GROSSER, 1902 cit. by CLARA, 1959) in this region the glomic AVA would not be more than 1—2 mm one from another and would dwindle progressively from the center towards the periphery (MASSON, 1937; CLARA, 1959).

[33] The "vasa-vasorum" (capillaries) in the AVA originate (POPOFF, 1935) from small branches from the afferent artery itself, at the point of departure of the intercalary and anastomotic tract.

[34] This arteriole rises perpendicularly at the level of the anastomosis from vessels starting deeper down (cutaneous network, SPALTEHOLZ, 1927) and parallel to the surface of the epidermis.

According to Hoyer (1877) and Clara (1959), the efferent venous system in the ungual bed, like that in the finger tips, is represented, instead, by a dense network of channels, which are more or less wide and tortuous with simple walls, which form a vascular angle round the individual anastomotic segments.

In the fingers and toes, afferent arterial branches, anastomotic segments, and efferent venous vessels, whether plexiform or not, are in any case enclosed in a connective capsule of concentric lamellar layers which because of its "organoid" appearance conferred the name of "Hoyer and Grosser's organs", or "cutaneous glomi "or" digital glomi" [by analogy with the "coccygeous glomus" (Clara, 1959)].

The anastomoses of the nail bed are by contrast without capsula (Schorn, 1955). Even more simple would be the anastomosis of the ears, composed of more or less tortuous vessels connecting arteries and veins.

On the histological level, the anastomotic segments of the finger and of the nail bed are generally similar, even if not so neatly separated into layers as in other animals.

In the anastomotic segment, the endothelium has 2 or 3 layers of cells instead of the sole stratum present in the afferent arterioles and the efferent venules (Fig. 90). The considerable protrusion of the endothelium makes the lumen of the AVA rather narrow and scarcely visible (Mescon et al., 1956; Clara, 1959) (Figs. 94, 95 and 97). Under the endothelium is a fine reticulum of argentophile fibrils, which are also stainable with elastic fiber methods (Mescon et al., 1956; Clara, 1959).

The middle tunic of the afferent arterial branches has an internal elastic membrane which in the myoepitheliod intercalary segment progressively dwindles in thickness until it reaches the immediate vicinity of the venous outlet (Clara, 1959). At the same time the elastic fibers also change their position. They are thicker near the lumen and distributed over the whole wall of the zone near the intercalary tract; in the more distal zone of the latter, they are mainly concentrated in the outer layers of the wall (Schorn, 1955). According to some authors (Mescon et al., 1956), the intercalary tract is entirely devoid of elastic membrane. This membrane is also absent in arteriovenous anastomosis of the ear (Pritchard and Daniel, 1956).

The muscular tunic in the afferent arterial branches is robust and composed of a circular external layer of smooth muscle cells and an internal layer of longitudinal ones.

In the anastomotic segment, these layers remain, though they often forego their normal arrangement and, according to some authors (Grosser cit. Clara, 1959), are often separated in the initial tract of the anastomosis by a parvicellular layer of smooth muscle cells that are thinner and shorter than typical ones and densely packed with intensely stainable nuclei.

The fundamental cytological characteristic of the anastomotic segment is, however, the gradual and almost total substitution just before the outlet into the efferent vein of all the smooth muscle elements with the myoepitheloid cells (Figs. 89, 90, 93, 95 and 97) described by Schumacher (1907; Clara, 1959).

In transverse section these large cells exhibit a polyhedric shape, their cytoplasm which is voluminous and clear, an ovoid nucleus which is barely stainable (Benninghoff, 1930) and some myofibrils (Masson, 1937; Mescon et al., 1956); between the subendothelial reticulum the external loose connective tissue contains up to 6 layers of nuclei with no obvious cellular demarcations (Mescon et al., 1956).

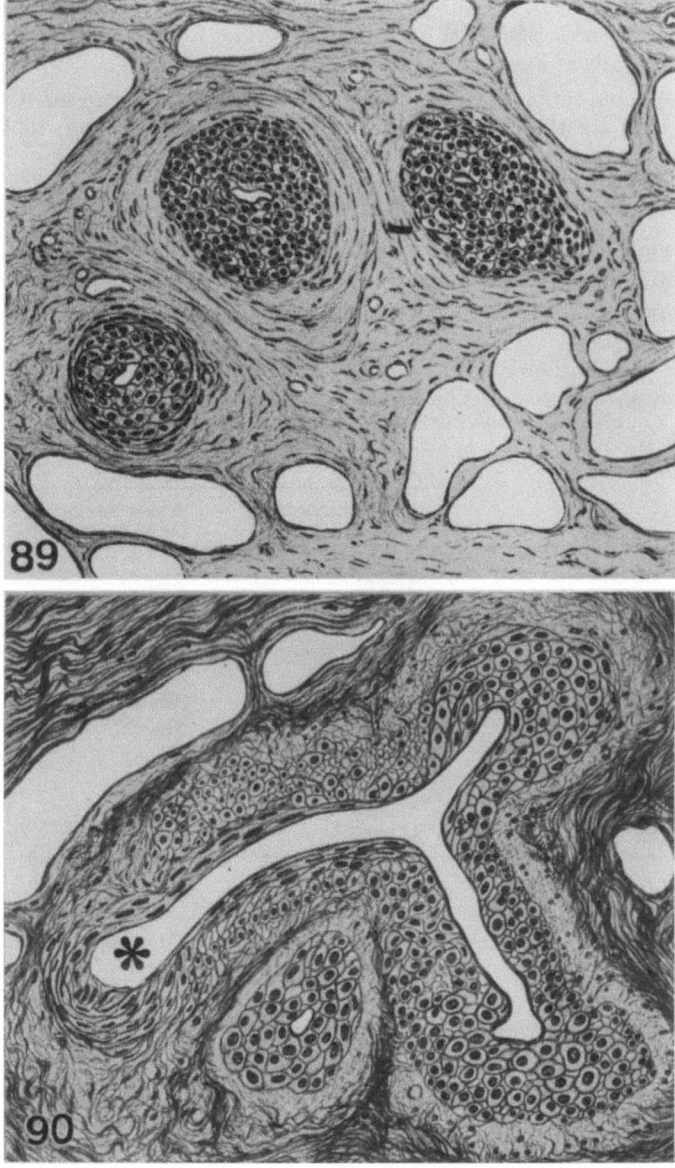

Fig. 89. The wall of the anastomotic segments is thick, made only of myoepithelioid cells and devoid of elastic membrane. The lumen of the thin surrounding veins is wide (Hoyer and Grosser's organ of the finger). (CLARA, M., courtesy of the Vallardi Ed. in: Le anastomosi arteriovenose, p. 29. 1956)

Fig. 90. The anastomotic segment originated from an artery (*) initially shows longitudinal smooth muscular cells later substituted by myoepithelioid cells. The whole structure is surrounded by a loose connective tissue sheath (Hoyer and Grosser's organ of the finger). (CLARA, M., courtesy of the Vallardi Ed. in: Le anastomosi arteriovenose, p. 26. 1956)

The anastomotic tract with epithelioid walls, instead of being enclosed by a sort of adventitia, is surrounded by concentric layers of a loose connective sheath, reacting differently from the surrounding connective tissue either with ordinary stain or with particular techniques, and containing a rather well-developed network of fine nerve fibers (Fig. 96), numerous mast-cells, and capillaries (MESCON et al., 1956; CLARA, 1959).

Furthermore, according to some authors (MESCON et al., 1956), this region is particularly important both as an expansion zone for dilating AVA and for the metabolic changes of anastomosis (SCHORN, 1955).

In the venous section of the AVA, the vessels with epithelioid mantle transform into veins with a rather large lumen and very thin walls (CLARA, 1959).

4. Histochemistry of the Arteriovenous Anastomoses (AVA)

Some important data on the functioning and biochemistry of the AVA have been gathered from histochemical research.

In a series of observations, in fact, the data shown in table 3 (MESCON et al., 1956) were collected.

Table 3. *A comparison between some of the histochemical properties of the AVA and corresponding properties of other cutaneous structures* (MESCON et al., 1956)

Studied substances	Reactivity		
	Smooth muscle in the AVA	Smooth muscle in the arterioles	Epidermis and eccrine ducts
Glycogen	Absent	Absent	Present
Lipid	Absent	Absent	Absent
Metachromasia	Present	Absent	Absent
Nucleic acids	Present	Present	Present
Protein-bound sulfhydryl groups	Minimal to absent	Absent	Present
Alkaline phosphatases	Minimal to absent	Absent	Absent
Acid phosphatases	Absent	Absent	Present
Cholinesterases			
Specific	Absent	Absent	Absent
Non-specific	Absent	Absent	Absent

The subendothelial connective tissue of the AVA and the arterioles exhibit PAS-positive material, which is resistant to diastasis (Fig. 94); hence we are not dealing with glycogen but with mucopolysaccharides.

This reactivity, less diffuse and less intensive in the arterioles, shows itself with pink staining which under higher magnification reveals red fiber-like concentrations.

With toluidine blue (Fig. 93) the AVA media takes on a diffuse pink staining (probably from the acid mucopolysaccharides) and sometimes reddish pink strand-like concentrations appear between the nuclei in the media (MESCON et al., 1956).

The media of the AVA with stains for the sulfhydryl groups is barely positive (BARNETT and SELIGMANN, 1952). Nucleoproteins and nucleic acids are present in the smooth muscular cells of the arterioles as in the AVA.

The AVA does not seem to be reactive to acid phosphatase (Fig. 92) (GOMORI, 1941; BURTON, 1954), or, if they are (RUTENBURG and SELIGMANN, 1955), the reaction is very slight.

On the contrary, the endothelial cells of the AVA exhibit an intense black reaction for alkaline phosphatase (GOMORI, 1941) but the media does not.

Specific and nonspecific cholinesterases are missing from the AVA wall. Nerve fibers, which are intensely positive to acetylcholinesterases (KOELLE, 1951) and negative to butyryl-cholinesterases (Fig. 96), are to be seen instead all around the AVA (Table 3) (MESCON et al., 1956).

As for electron microscopy, unfortunately we have no information about arteriovenous anastomosis.

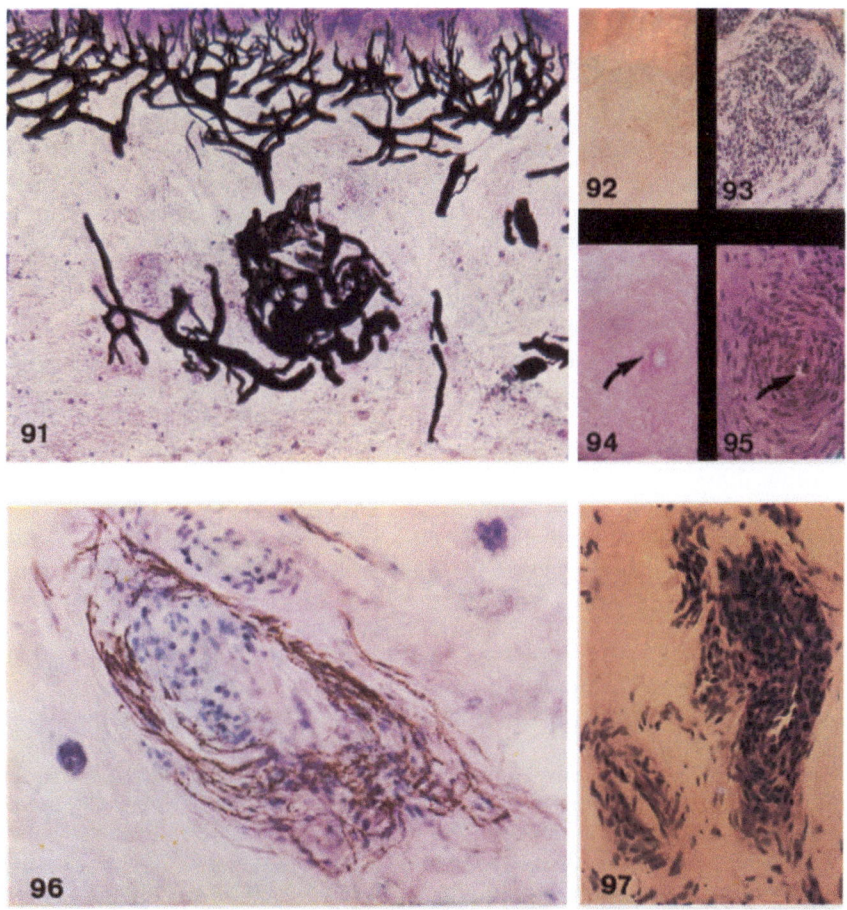

Figs. 91—97. Histology and histochemistry of the AVA

Fig. 91. Capillary loops of papillae and subpapillary plexus, above; ball-shaped configuration of glomal vessels below. (Injected dermal vessels, counterstaining with hematoxylin-eosin.) [MESCON, HURLEY and MORETTI, courtesy of the J. invest. Derm., The anatomy and histochemistry of the arteriovenous anastomosis in human digital skin 27, 136 (1956)]

Fig. 92. No acid phosphatases-staining in AVA; heavy staining in eccrine sweat duct. [MESCON, HURLEY and MORETTI, courtesy of the J. invest. Derm., The anatomy and histochemistry of the arteriovenous anastomosis in human digital skin 27, 141 (1956)]

Fig. 93. Intensely stained nuclei of myoepithelioid cells of the AVA (toluidine-blue). [From MESCON, HURLEY and MORETTI 1956 (Reprinted by permission of J. invest. Derm.)]

Fig. 94. Diastase-resistant positive reaction to periodic acid-Schiff stain in subendothelium (arrow) but not in media. [MESCON, HURLEY and MORETTI, courtesy of the J. invest. Derm., The anatomy and histochemistry of the arteriovenous anastomosis in human digital skin 27, 139 (1956)]

Fig. 95. Narrow lumen, endothelium with two nuclei, media densely packed with nuclei and surrounding loose, collagenous reticulum (hematoxylin-eosin). [MESCON, HURLEY and MORETTI, courtesy of the J. invest. Derm., The anatomy and histochemistry of the arteriovenous anastomosis in human digital skin 27, 138 (1956)]

Fig. 96. The AVA is surrounded by dark strands of copper sulfide precipitated by the cholinesterase in nerve fibers. [MESCON, HURLEY and MORETTI, courtesy of the J. invest. Derm., The anatomy and histochemistry of the arteriovenous anastomosis in human digital skin 27, 142 (1956)]

Fig. 97. Another view of the intercalary tract shows oblong nuclei of the media, narrow lumen and perianastomotic collagen of AVA. [From MESCON, HURLEY and MORETTI 1956 (Reprinted by permission of J. invest. Derm.)]

VI. Notes on the Biological Modifications of the Blood Vessels in the Skin

1. Indications on the Periodic or Permanent Regeneration of Cutaneous Vessels

The vasal structures described above are capable, if necessary, of more or less complete regenerative or degenerative phenomena, either temporary or permanent. The literature on the subject is rather vast; here, however, we shall touch upon only the facts of major biological interest.

Our knowledge of the neoformative qualities of the vessels and of the capillaries in particular comes from observation with the so-called transparent chamber technique of their development in vivo in the rabbit's ear (SANDISON, 1928) or in other similar preparations (ALGIRE, 1943; FULTON, JACKSON, and LUTZ, 1946); from electron microscopy (SCHOEFL, 1962, 1963); and from analysis, especially in animals, of the healing of wounds, the taking of grafts, etc.

This research showed the endothelial cells to be capable not only of ameboid motions (MAJNO, 1965) which explain their migratory speed of 0.10—0.15 mm/24 h, higher than that for the fibroblasts (MACKENZIE and LOEWENTHAL, 1960) but also of spreading into the surrounding tissues when there is no basement membrane (MAXIMOW, 1902; LEWIS, 1931).

On the other hand, vessel neoformation and differentiation follow the same steps as embryogenesis. From a preexistent network endothelial germs originate and are transformed into syncytia of endothelial cords; after acquiring a lumen (SCHOEFL and MAJNO, 1964), they reveal cells of varying thicknesses and a very thin, or almost entirely absent, basement membrane.

Afterwards these cords, on meeting and amalgamating or simply lengthening the preexistent vessels, form a constantly changing network from which some channels regress. Others form the capillaries while still others differentiate into arteries or veins perhaps on account of apposition to the endothelium of pluripotential fibrocytes, individual or organized into syncytium that are able later on to transform themselves into pericytes, adventitial cells or, in the case of an artery, into smooth muscle cells (BENNINGHOFF, 1926). In the view of some authors (MAXIMOV, 1902; ALLGOWER, 1956), the vascular tissue included in the healing process of a wound does not come from the injured tissue but from monocytic blood elements (CONVERSE and BALLANTYNE, 1962).

The neoformed capillaries, however, have unmistakable characteristics. In the rabbit, for example, the walls are generally dilated, sometimes even aneurysmatic (COGAN, 1949), extremely fragile, and characterized by increased permeability (COGAN, 1949; MAJNO, 1965).

We shall only mention now the capacity for self-reconstruction of entire sections of the cutaneous network such as that periodically and temporarily established by the hair cycle, since we shall have occasion to reconsider it. In man and many other mammals, with every new anagen inside the connective sheath and the dermal papilla of the newly-formed follicle, a thick network of perpendicular and horizontal vessels reappears and stays until the beginning of the next catagen (ELLIS and MORETTI, 1959).

The changes induced in the skin by various trauma, such as wound-healing, experimental or otherwise, are, on the contrary, more complex and lasting. In these cases we frequently see an unexpected neogenesis of the vasal structures; this happens, for example, in the skin of the rat after prolonged hyperemia

(HORSTMANN, 1957) and after ultraviolet radiation (RAIGROTZKI, 1938), similarly, perhaps, to what has been already observed in man (MUELLER, 1937).

The course of the wound repairing network also[35] never quite follows that of the initial one (HOPPE-SEYLER, 1941; TIEDEMANN, 1949) since the vessels try to reach the center of the damaged zone by the shortest route. In linear scars the neoformed capillaries, arterioles, and venules turn towards the center of the scar tissue in a direction which is roughly perpendicular to the larger axis of the scar (HORSTMANN, 1957).

Finally, in grafts the dynamics of restoration in a normal blood network are not at all clear. According to some authors, the host vasal network and the graft network (CONWAY et al., 1952; CONWAY et al., 1957; cit. WOLFF, 1965) anastomize ("inosculation"); according to others, either the graft is invaded by vessels coming from the host (BELLMANN and VERLANDER, 1957; CONVERSE and BALLANTYNE, 1962) or both mechanisms occur (CONVERSE and RAPAPORT, 1956; BALLANTYNE and CONVERSE, 1958). CLEMMESEN (1962) believes that some anastomosis occurs between new vessels which have penetrated from the host and some of the older vessels of the graft.

The literature[36] describes several examples of the reconstructive capabilities of the blood circuit: the hamster's cheek pouch if grafted keeps most of its original blood network (HALLER and BILLINGHAM, 1964); in an autograft, the vessels are initially collapsed and empty and remain so for 6—12 or even 24 hours postoperatively although hyperemia and dilation follow; only the formation of new vessels reestablishes normal circulation (HYNES, 1954). In man in both homografts and autografts, the anatomic picture of deep and superficial vessels generally conforms to that seen in the surrounding skin (except for the papillary capillaries); while the junction region between the two tissues is crossed by rather large vessels (MACGREGOR, 1955). In the rat, this area is penetrated by a series of more numerous branched and distended perpendicular vessels than is normal (CONVERSE and BALLANTYNE, 1962).

2. Notes on the Histochemistry and Electron Microscopy of Neoformed Vessels

Although there is not much information on the subject (RAEKALLIO, 1960, 1961; RAEKALLIO and LEVONEN, 1963) histochemical techniques and electron microscopy have revealed the existence of particular characteristics in neoformed capillaries.

In the guinea pig, after an experimental wound, the granulation tissue, enclosed between capillaries and fibroblasts, histochemically revealed a small amount of acid mucopolysaccharides (RAEKALLIO, 1961). In the rat, 7 days after an experimental wound, the newly-formed dermal vessels showed obvious alkaline phosphatase activity (CARRANZA-CABRINI, 1963) and slight beta glucuronidase activity. In the same animal, the capillaries of the autograft rapidly lost their NAD

---

[35] There is a correlation between the consistency of the injury and the type of neoformed vessel; usually after a mild stimulus there follows eventual formation of loops through the gradual lengthening of the preexistent network, or of new sprouts with more serious stimulus (SCHOEFL, 1962—1963). In a rabbit's ear, furthermore, after resection the arteriovenous anastomoses would reform, starting from preexistent arteriovenous-capillary connections (ROSSATI, 1956).

[36] In man the time of reappearance of the vascular network is uncertain; even if two or three days are enough for the beginning of its reconstruction, after only 9—12 days the graft should be well nourished (CLEMMESEN, 1962).

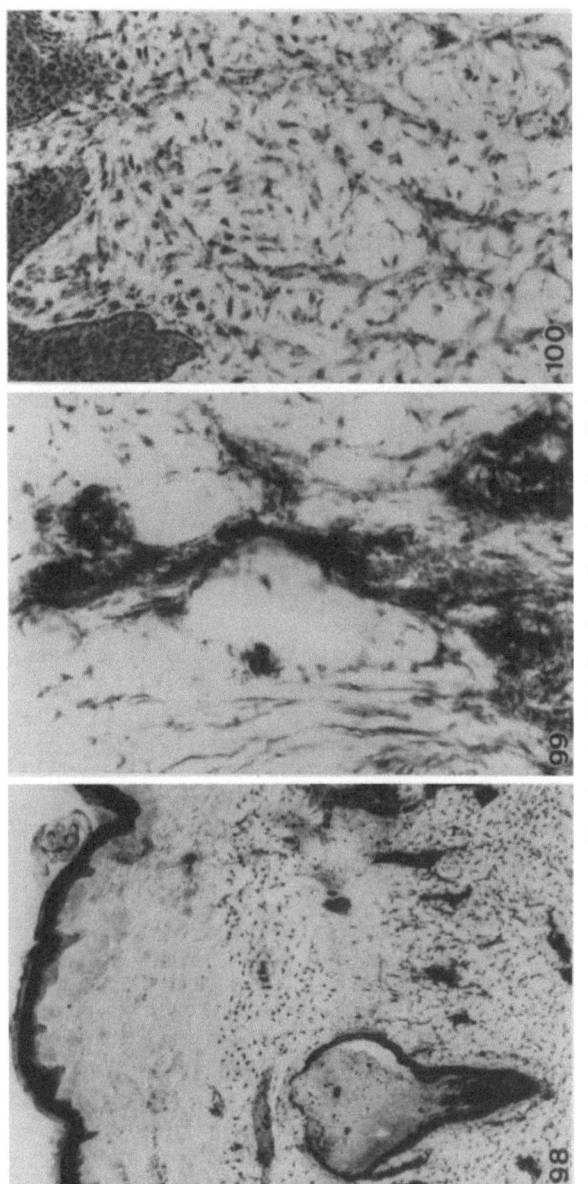

Figs. 98—104. Histochemistry of neoformed capillaries

Fig. 98. NAD-reductase, autograft; 2nd p.o. day (phase of regression). The vessels of the graft have lost most of their activity while those of the recipient tissue exhibit strong enzymatic reactions. [WOLFF, K., and F. G. SCHELLANDER, courtesy of the J. invest. Derm., Enzyme-histochemical studies on the healing process of split skin grafts **45**, 40 (1965)]

Fig. 99. NAD-reductase, autograft; 12th p.o. day (phase of recovery). A vessel with strong enzymatic reactivity invades the graft. [WOLFF, K., and F. G. SCHELLANDER, courtesy of the J. invest. Derm., Enzyme-histochemical studies on the healing process of split skin grafts **45**, 42 (1965)]

Fig. 100. NAD-reductase, autograft; 8th p.o. day (phase of recovery). Enzymatic activity in fibroblasts and ingrowing capillaries. (K. WOLFF and F. G. SCHELLANDER, courtesy of the J. invest. Derm.)

reductase activity but regained it later when the new vessels penetrated from the surrounding tissue (CONVERSE and BALLANTYNE, 1962).

In particular breeds of pigs, the granulation tissue between autograft and host, after an initial diminution ("regression" phase) of NAD reductase (Fig. 98), amino peptidase and succinic-dehydrogenase activity revealed capillaries with intense enzymatic reaction which penetrated and invaded the graft ("recovery" phase) (Figs. 99 and 100) (WOLF and SCHELLANDER, 1965). In the same animal, the behavior of other enzymes of the vascular network is also interesting. With adenosine-triphosphatase the graft vessels revealed variable activity in the "regression" phase (Fig. 101). In the "recovery" phase (Figs. 102—104), on the

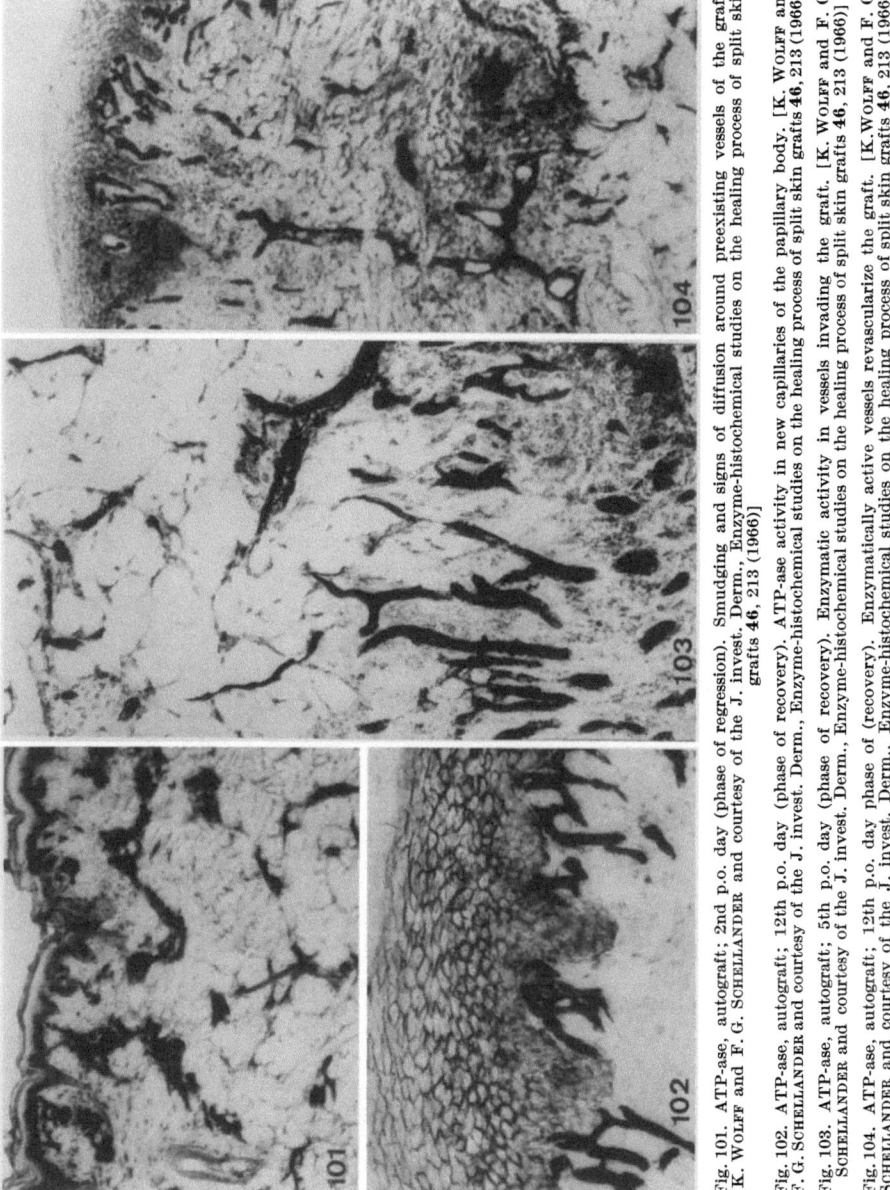

Fig. 101. ATP-ase, autograft; 2nd p.o. day (phase of regression). Smudging and signs of diffusion around preexisting vessels of the graft. [K. WOLFF and F. G. SCHELLANDER and courtesy of the J. invest. Derm., Enzyme-histochemical studies on the healing process of split skin grafts **46**, 213 (1966)]

Fig. 102. ATP-ase, autograft; 12th p.o. day (phase of recovery). ATP-ase activity in new capillaries of the papillary body. [K. WOLFF and F. G. SCHELLANDER and courtesy of the J. invest. Derm., Enzyme-histochemical studies on the healing process of split skin grafts **46**, 213 (1966)]

Fig. 103. ATP-ase, autograft; 5th p.o. day (phase of recovery). Enzymatic activity in vessels invading the graft. [K. WOLFF and F. G. SCHELLANDER and courtesy of the J. invest. Derm., Enzyme-histochemical studies on the healing process of split skin grafts **46**, 213 (1966)]

Fig. 104. ATP-ase, autograft; 12th p.o. day phase of (recovery). Enzymatically active vessels revascularize the graft. [K.WOLFF and F. G. SCHELLANDER and courtesy of the J. invest. Derm., Enzyme-histochemical studies on the healing process of split skin grafts **46**, 213 (1966)]

other hand, the histochemical technique for this enzyme makes it possible to follow the course of the vessel perfectly. Since they penetrate the graft from the host, these vessels confirm their true origin. In the endothelium of newly-formed vessels, there is no-5 nucleotidase; alkaline phosphatase, contrary to the norm, is found to some extent in the newly-formed vessels. In a homograft, after the "regression" and "recovery" phases, which are similar to those in an "autograft", one may observe in addition a "rejection" phase characterized by the sudden disappearance of most of the enzymatic activities mentioned above, particularly in succinic dehydrogenase and diphosphopyridine nucleotide diaphorase. The vascular structures thus seem to be injured earlier than the other cutaneous structures by the factors causing the "rejection" (CONVERSE and BALLANTYNE, 1962; WOLF and SCHELLANDER, 1966).

Recent electron microscopy studies (Figs. 105—108) on the regenerating capillaries in the cornea (SCHOEFL and MAJNO, 1965) revealed pseudopodial cytoplasmic processes and a variable and rather loose contact (MAJNO, 1965)

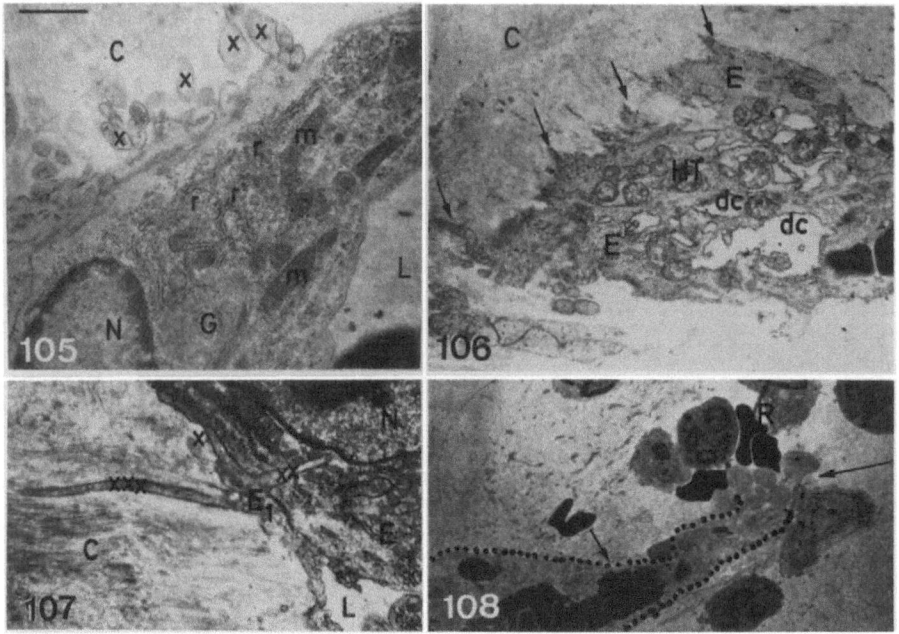

Figs. 105—108. Electron microscopy of neoformed capillaries

Fig. 105. The regenerating capillaries of the cornea reveal pseudopodial cytoplasmic processes (×) and a cytoplasm rich in mitochondria, ribosomes, a prominent Golgi apparatus (G). The basement membrane is not visible (N nucleus; L lumen; C collagen). (SCHOEFL, G. I., and MAJNO, G. courtesy of the Pergamon Press. In: Advances in biology of skin, vol. 5, p. 180. 1964)

Fig. 107. A vascular sprout whose lumen is visible at lower right (L) reveals various pseudopodial cytoplasmic processes (×—×× —×××) projecting into surrounding structures, the loosened collagen fibrils (C) included (N nucleus). (SCHOEFL, G. I., and MAJNO, G. courtesy of the Pergamon Press. In: Advances in biology of skin, vol. 5, p. 185. 1964)

Figs. 106 and 108. An open ended-sprout of the cornea shows a cytoplasm containing dilated cisternae (dc) and rounded mitochondria while red blood cells (R) are pouring into the corneal stroma (arrow) [Dotted line = contour of endothelial cells (E); C collagen]. (SCHOEFL, G. I., and G. MAJNO, courtesy of the Pergamon Press. In: Advances in biology of skin, vol. 5, p. 187. 1964)

between the growing endothelial cells. In addition, the cytoplasm was rich in mitochondria and cisterns, and free ribosomes were evident in the endoplasmic reticulum; but vesicles were scant or absent (SCHOEFL and MAJNO, 1965).

The endothelium of the growing vessels, therefore, seems to be characterized both by high metabolic activity (abundance of endoplasmic reticulum and mitochondria) and by slight differentiation [many free ribosomes and few vesicles (SCHOEFL and MAJNO, 1964)].

Around the apices of the more recently formed vessels, the basement membrane was fragmentary or missing, but it thickened progressively with the age of the vessel (SCHOEFL and MAJNO, 1965); these data agree with those of GERSH and CATCHPOLE (1949).

3. Indications of Degenerative Phenomena in the Cutaneous Blood Network

As we have already said, these degenerative phenomena may be temporary or permanent. The disappearance during catagen (ELLIS and MORETTI, 1959) of the greater part of the perifollicular and papillary network is temporary. However, changes due to age are permanent. DIEULAFÉ and DURAND (1906) were the first to notice the apparent diminution in the number of anastomoses between vessels and progressive appearance of vascular territories, apparently independent of each other, caused by aging.

BELLOCQ (1925) and SPALTEHOLZ (1927), while they seem to agree that cutaneous circulation decreases in these circumstances disagree about the interpretation of the phenomenon. For BELLOCQ, aging alone causes the disappearance of some vasal sectors (networks of "independent area" type) in regions like the scalp; but SPALTEHOLZ attributes, probably correctly, the greater part of BELLOCQ's data either to technical effects or to arteriosclerotic changes (BELLOCQ, 1925; SPALTEHOLZ, 1927).

Other authors (LO CASCIO, 1913—1914; CHIALE, 1927; SALMON, 1936; MENEGHINI, 1942) appear convinced of the substantial inaccuracy in DIEULAFÉ's, DURAND's, and BELLOCQ's hypotheses.

CHIALE (1927) for example, noticed in subjects over 30 years of age progressive sclerotic alterations in the arterial intima, particularly in the subcutaneous vessels. MENEGHINI (1942) using a radiographic technique, found fewer anastomoses in addition to tortuous or sclerotic arteries in the skin of the aged, perhaps because of secondary mechanical phenomena in the senile cutis. PIETRZYKOWSKA observed senile widening of the lumen and stiffness of the arterioles (PIETRZYKOWSKA, 1966). The veins, although less affected (PANEBIANCO, 1942), also became flexuous, angular, and varicose (MENEGHINI, 1942).

The degenerative changes in the blood network of an old person, on the other hand, cannot be explained simply by arteriosclerotic phenomena, because of the impossibility of separating the anatomic alterations of the vascular apparatus from that of the ground substance (MANGANOTTI, 1965) and of the confusion caused by contradictory reports.

According to MONACELLI (1924) only the vessels in the hypodermal network are affected by arteriosclerosis. CHIALE (1927) and MUSUMECI (1961), on the contrary, hold that the latter are involved in the degenerative processes caused by arteriosclerosis even if these phenomena were topographically limited and not absolutely identifiable with that disease [both calcification and intimal lipids would be lacking (REITANO, 1959 cit. MUSUMECI, 1961)].

Here the importance of the wall structure must be kept in mind. In the precapillary arterioles of the subpapillary network, which are seldom affected (WATANABE, 1921) and are radically diminished after 40 (BERRES, 1957), hyaline degeneration is prevalent. In the small arteries provided with elastic structures of the middle and deep dermis, granulosis (BERRES, 1957) and hyperplasia of the internal elastic lamina (WIEDMANN, 1936) prevail.

Finally, a curious and apparently paradoxical phenomenon should be remembered. In the senile scalp, despite the relative rarity of a blood network (as in baldness), the capillary networks surrounding the sebaceous and eccrine glands remain intact and may even become richer in vessels (ELLIS, 1958; MONTAGNA, 1962).

VII. The Nerves of the Cutaneous Blood Vessels

1. General Principles

While the satellite arteries to the nerves (SALMON'S "relay" arteries) are so numerous that one might almost describe a neurocutaneous network next to an independent arterial network, opinions on the nerves of vessels are contradictory and certainly not definitive, probably also because of the organ specificity of vessel nerve supply (ILLIG, 1961).

Generally the number of the axons accompanying the vessels change per surface unit with the cutaneous region, and the number of vessel nerves are more or less proportional to that of the vessels, capillaries excepted (in the palmar region, for example) (WEDDELL, 1961).

In man and in some other mammals (felines, rodents, and lagomorphs), usually small bundles of nerve fibers come from the cutaneous network; approach the arteries, veins, arterioles (Figs. 109 and 110), and venules (WEDDELL, 1961); and then disappear. With proper techniques, however, some nerve fibers may be observed even in the neighborhood of the capillaries (Fig. 111) (JABONERO, 1958; ORMEA, 1961).

The nerve fibers advancing towards the various sections of the blood network, on the other hand, are not completely independent; in fact, the nerve elements of the different vasal parts sometimes end up by being rather close. On the premise that the nerves running along a vessel are not necessarily responsible for its innervation, let us bear in mind that a fine small trunk with typical reticular arrangement of the neurofibrillar elements spreading first over the capillary walls can pass under the arteriole which it contacts so as to reach the vein in the end (ORMEA, 1961).

Despite this knowledge, we have not solved the fundamental problem of the sensory or vegetative nature of the perivasal nerves. Most authors maintain that the majority are composed of amyelinic vegetative fibers flanked by some sensory fibers (DOGIEL, 1898; BOEKE, 1949; STÖHR, 1957; JABONERO, 1958; MILLER et al., 1960; WINKELMANN, 1960; HERXHEIMER, 1960; WEDDELL et al., 1961)[37]. The somatic fibers sometimes seem to follow, beside arteries and arterioles, veins and venules, rather close to the capillary walls (WEDDELL, 1961). The greater part of the sympathetic vegetative fibers supply arterioles and venules (KUNTZ and HAMILTON, 1938); some may even enwrap the capillaries (BOEKE, 1949; STÖHR, 1957; JABONERO, 1958).

The manner in which these fibers terminate in the vessels is also debatable. According to most (BOEKE, 1949; STOEHR, 1957; JABONERO, 1958; ORMEA, 1961; WEDDELL, 1961; etc.) this occurs by means of a so-called "terminal reticulum", or "pre-terminal network" or "vegetative end formation" stretched to surround arteries, arterioles, veins, venules, and probably capillaries. The nature of this reticulum, however, remains somewhat obscure (ORMEA, 1961; WEDDELL, 1961). Some authors maintain that it is a syncytial lemmoblastic meshwork in simple relation to the vessel (BOEKE, 1949; WEDDELL, 1961); others refute its syncytial tendency, describing it as a plexus in which the fine vegetative nerve filaments are totally independent (BAIRATI, 1961). Some axons beside the adventitia layer would reach the muscle layer of some vessels directly (JABONERO, 1958; ORMEA, 1961).

The cytoneural junction is achieved by submicroscopic buttons, which establish contact between the axonal membrane and sarcolemma of the smooth muscle cells.

---

[37] It is certainly not easy, in any case, with certain techniques at least, to distinguish the S.N.C. fibers from the S.N.V. ones (MONTAGNA, 1960; WINKELMANN, 1960).

Except for the capillaries, the action of the sympathetic and parasympathetic vegetative fibers finally act as vasoconstrictors and as vasodilators over all the vessels, in a vasoconstricting as well as dilating direction (ILLIG, 1961).

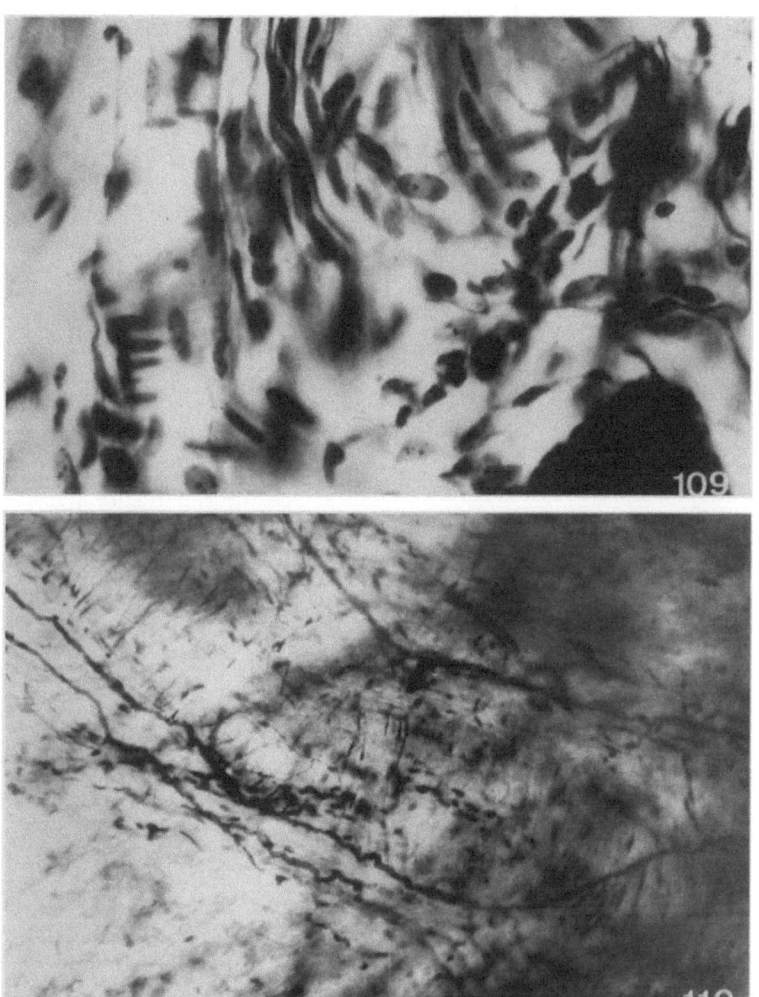

Figs. 109—111. Some aspects of the nerves of the cutaneous blood vessels

Fig. 109. Innervation of an arteriole (Rabbit skin; Silver stain). (Courtesy of G. WEDDELL)

Fig. 110. Branches from trunks supplying an artery. (Rabbit skin; methylene-blue vital staining). (Courtesy of G. WEDDELL)

2. The Nerves of the Arteries and Arterioles, Veins and Venules and Arteriovenous Anastomoses (AVA)

The existence of somatic fibers in the walls of arterioles and arteries is mainly indicated by experimental data (POLLEY, 1955; WEDDELL, 1961); however, different authors have observed plexuses of fibers coming from the posterior roots in the adventitia of these vessels (WEDDELL and PALLIE, 1954).

Unmyelinated fibers coming from the cutaneous plexus accompany the arteries and arterioles for long tracts (Figs. 110 and 119), later forming continuous networks between the adventitia and the tunica media (KUNTZ and HAMILTON, 1948; JOHN, 1940; RICHTER, 1955; POLLEY, 1955; ORMEA, 1961; WEDDELL, 1961).

From a pharmaco-dynamic point of view, the fibers of the posterior spinal root are the basis for the axon reflex (ROTHMANN, 1954); the vegetative, on the other hand, are essentially adrenergic and therefore vasoconstricting (HERXHEIMER, 1960) even though colinergic fibers have been clearly seen in the media of some vessels (MONTAGNA and ELLIS, 1957).

Since veins and venules are accompanied by some sensory fibers and reached by sympathetic fibers, they normally have an innervation that is practically analogous to that of the corresponding arterial vessels (STÖHR, 1938; JOHN, 1940; WEDDELL, 1961; ORMEA, 1961).

A terminal vegetative meshwork is, in effect, visible in veins with and without muscles, the nerve plexus when present penetrating from the adventitia region into that of the media (ORMEA, 1961).

The innervation of the AVA, besides that of the other surrounding vessels (CAUNA, 1956) is different from one tract to another in the same anastomosis.

The arterial tract, in fact, is richly innervated, while the venous tract has few nerves (JABONERO cit. ORMEA, 1961); in addition, the former possesses nerves of the cerebro-spinal and of the neurovegetative systems (JABONERO cit. ORMEA, 1961).

We have already mentioned the colinergic fibers which surround the AVA (MESCON et al., 1956); on the other hand, fibers, unmyelinated and anastomotic or perivasal, about one micron in diameter have been observed from the intercalary segment to the start of the vein (MASSON, 1953). Since the cutaneous AVA receive fibers which are probably adrenergic, from adjacent arterioles and venules (MESCON et al., 1956), their double vegetative innervation does not seem impossible.

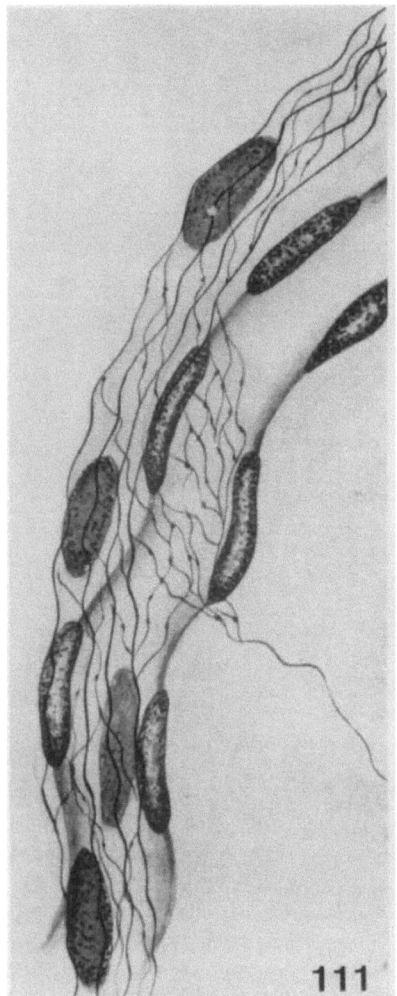

Fig. 111. The vegetative nerve network skirts past the vessel without actually touching it (human skin). (ORMEA, F., courtesy of the Minerva Medica Ed. In: La cute organo di senso, p. 256. 1961)

3. The Problem of Capillary Innervation

The general ambiguity and uncertainty on capillary innervation is especially evident in the literature. Apart from the question, still moot, whether they possess vegetative or somatic innervation (WEDDELL, 1961), the existence of vegetative fibers around the papillary or subpapillary vessels is doubted by some authors (POLLEY, 1955). However, the presence of pericapillary vegetative fibers seems to be generally accepted (RUFFINI, 1905; WOOLLARD, 1926; STOEHR, 1932; REISER,

1933; JOHN, 1940; WEDDELL and PALLIE, 1954, ORMEA, 1961) although the manner of this innervation remains uncertain.

According to SUNDER-PLASMANN, STÖHR, REISER, and others (cit. ORMEA, 1961), the capillary wall is reached by a terminal vegetative meshwork[38]. ORMEA (1961), although he had occasionally observed actual contact between capillary and nerve, sometimes had the impression that the nerve network skirts (Fig. 111) past the vessel without actually touching it[39].

D. The Architecture of the Cutaneous Blood Network
I. General Observations

The elements just described constitute the complex architecture of the arterial capillary-venous reticulum in the human skin which, as in other mammals, is developed through the dermis and hypodermis into a single vessel circuit within which each vessel district, while maintaining its morphological unity, is closely connected with the others: the vascular system which supplies the follicles is linked to that which nourishes both the sebaceous and apocrine glands; vessels directed towards the epidermis will provide for the hair follicles, together with the eccrine sweat gland ducts and so on.

II. The Distribution of the Arterial Vessels in the Subcutaneous and in the Dermis (apart from the Appendages)

1. Networks Formed in the Subcutaneous

As we have already pointed out, the arteries coming from the deep layers form in the fascia (Fig. 112), or immediately above it, a "fascial" network mostly of wide mesh (SPALTEHOLZ, 1927). In the subcutaneous layer the anastomoses between big branches (chiefly in the plantar region) and smaller ones are frequent (DIEULAFÉ and DURAND, 1906). The vast majority of vessels, however, rise to the border between the subcutaneous adipose tissue and the corium and there form a "cutaneous network" (Figs. 113, 161 and 164) of wide regular mesh, generally parallel to the epidermal surface but located at varying depths (SPALTEHOLZ, 1927; HORSTMANN, 1957).

The fatty tissue (Fig. 155) lying between these two networks, is, therefore, divided into two different, somewhat indistinct arterial territories: the upper is nourished by the "cutaneous network" and the lower by the "fascial" one. If the adipose panniculum is not fully developed, blood reaches it only in the recurrent arterioles from the overlying "cutaneous" network; when developed, from the underlying "fascial" network also (SPALTEHOLZ, 1927).

In the coarse connective trabeculae, which separate the adipose lobules, the vessels divide repeatedly and branch out into arterioles of different shapes and caliber; the smaller lobules, if not each adipose cell (SPALTEHOLZ, 1927), thus

---

[38] KROGH had already suggested the existence of nerve control of pericytes (KROGH, 1929).

[39] In the pericapillary space, ODLAND (1961) occasionally observed nerves structurally equivalent to the unmyelinated fibers of light microscopy, which he did not however consider associated with vascular function.

become perforated or surrounded by an extremely fine capillary network. The ascending arterioles originating from the cutaneous network supply the true dermis with blood.

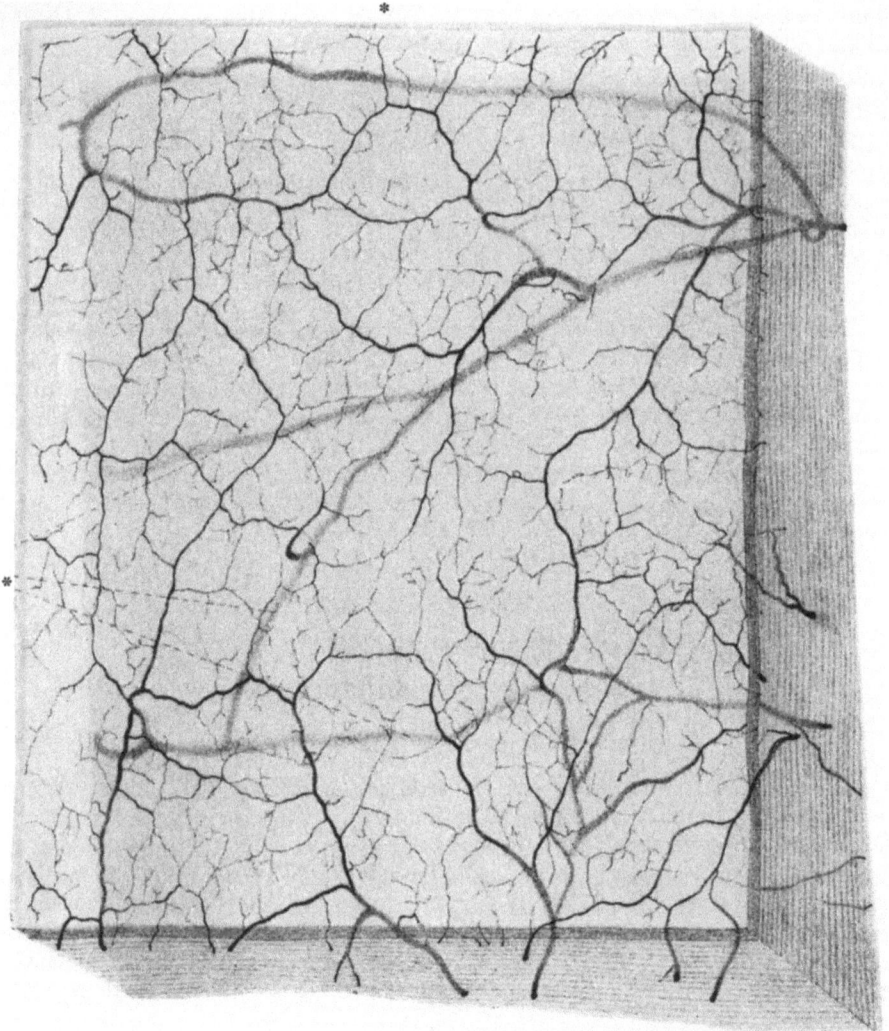

Fig. 112. An horizontal over-all view of the arterial vascularization of the skin of the thigh reveals the presence of anastomoses (*) in the fascia. (Reproduced from W. SPALTEHOLZ and the Arch. Anat. Physiol. 1893)

2. Regional Aspects of the "Cutaneous" and "Fascial" Network

The "fascial" and "cutaneous" networks above described are usually found in the skin of the trunk, neck, and limbs, with variations caused by mobility in the structure and thickness of the tegument.

The regional differences between these networks can be reduced to two (SPALTEHOLZ, 1927). In the first (glutei, plantar regions, etc.), many musculocutaneous arteries of similar diameter perforate the muscular layer perpendicularly; having formed with finer branches, an extensive "fascial" network, they penetrate the fatty layer. Here the vessels divide into branches which are somewhat twisted and almost equally thick. Later on these divide and form convex arcades at the lower edges of the dermis. At this level, by a series of numerous coarse anastomoses (anastomosis of the "first order"), thinner vessels originate which, together with other divisions and anastomoses (anastomosis of the "second order"), compose a "cutaneous" network with meshes that are generally uniform in size (SPALTEHOLZ, 1927).

In the second case, especially apparent on the chest and abdomen and more frequent than the first, a lesser number of vessels penetrate the subcutaneous layer leaving rather thin branches there which by anastomizing with the surrounding ones build up a well-developed "fascial" network.

Some small branches, after having travelled along tracts of varying length in the subcutaneous layer release many smaller vessels which, by subdivision and anastomosis, form at the dividing line between the subcutaneous layer and the dermis the rather coarse reticulum of a "cutaneous" network that is later fragmented into meshes by fine connective vasal elements (SPALTEHOLZ, 1927).

On the premise that the rich arterial supply in the cutaneous regions matches that in the nerve fibers (SALMON, 1936), some of the regional[40] characteristics of the two arterial networks described should now be considered (BELLOCQ, 1925[41]; SPALTEHOLZ, 1927; SALMON, 1936; etc.).

In the head, the cutaneous blood supply is more abundant than in most of the other body areas. It is, however, somewhat different in various parts of the head because of the presence or absence of terminal hairs (BELLOCQ, 1925; SPALTEHOLZ, 1927; TRUFFI, 1934; SALMON, 1936) and because of the number of vessels and their method of branching.

The hairy epicranial regions are nourished by four thick "mixed" arteries-frontal, temporal, auricular, and occipital all moving like meridians towards the region of the vertex (BELLOCQ, 1925).

After penetrating the "galea capitis" or frontal or occipital muscle with their branches, these vessels create a "fascial" network of fine branches. It is wide and entirely isolated in the galea. The muscles appear to be enclosed between two networks, anastomized between them and with other lesser vessels, one lying on the lower surface and the other on the upper surfaces of the muscle (SPALTEHOLZ, 1927).

Having passed the muscles and the galea, the principal vessels, which in the temporal region are already tortuous in youth, penetrate the subcutaneous layer and converge in the region of the vertex, and to a lesser degree, in the temporal regions, in a rather wide "subcutaneous" network, typical of the skull (SPALTEHOLZ, 1927). From this network numerous straight or oblique vessels rise to the surface where they branch and form a "cutaneous network" together with arched rami. This is less dense on the galea, and in the temporal region[42] it has a close meshwork and vessels of equal thickness in the frontal region and finer in the nuchal region (SPALTEHOLZ, 1927).

The face is also well supplied. Arteries which are partly "cutaneous" and partly "mixed" reach it from the superficial temporal, ophthalmic, and internal maxillary arteries. After penetrating to the deep layers of the skin, they leave

---

[40] With the cutaneous territory the average ratio between wall and lumen of the arterioles would also vary in the skin of the arm, leg and lumbar region; it would be 1:2.13; 1:2.10; 1:2.66 respectively (FARBER et al., 1947).

[41] Since BELLOCQ's three known types, more or less correspond to the so-called "scarce", "rich", and "very rich" vascularization of SALMON (1936), we shall use the latter's simpler terminology when the regional evaluation of the authors is not in question.

[42] The works of OTTAVIANI (1941) and MENEGHINI (1942) should be consulted on this and are especially important on the subject of the large vessels.

numerous branches similar in caliber to those of the principal trunk, either through dichotomy or monopodic division perpendicular to it (BELLOCQ, 1925).

In specific facial areas, greater detail is noted. In the region of the parotid gland and the masseter, a "fascial" and a "cutaneous" network are seen, the latter of coarse meshwork subdivided into close regular meshes (SPALTEHOLZ, 1927). In the eyebrows, there is a strong "fascial" network above which lies a narrow meshwork of thick subcutaneous vessels; thinner vessels arise from this and divide to form an even closer "cutaneous" network with their anastomosis (SPALTEHOLZ, 1927). Vessels also arise from the palpebral and neighboring arteries (SPALTEHOLZ, 1927). In the region of the M. quadratus labii superioris, the vessels, after forming a strong supraperiosteal "fascial" network, cross the muscle anastomizing with other vessels in the subcutaneous layer. Here they form a close "subcutaneous" network of thick vessels and higher up a "cutaneous" network of very close mesh with vessels of almost equal diameter (SPALTEHOLZ, 1927). On the nose, the "fascial" network is barely noticeable, while on the nostrils rather strong "cutaneous" and "subcutaneous" networks of close mesh are plainly visible (SPALTEHOLZ, 1927). On the lips, more twisted arterioles emerging from the deep layers and generally perpendicular to the free edge of the lip anastomize to form a sort of "subcutaneous" network with the vessel arcades constructed by the upper and lower labial arteries. From this, some arterioles move towards the lower edge of the dermis, where they anastomose with the surrounding ones and form a fine "cutaneous network" (SPALTEHOLZ, 1927).

In the area of the M. triangularis and the chin, the vessels are generally twisted and the "cutaneous" network is close meshed (SPALTEHOLZ, 1927). There are numerous arterioles on the outer ear muscle; and on the lobule there is a "subcutaneous" network of serpiginous branches, among which one that is parallel to the lobule edge joins branches from different directions. From all these vessels the finer vessels of the "cutaneous" network originate (SPALTEHOLZ, 1927). In the cartilage, the vessels extend over both surfaces, particularly the convex one, forming networks corresponding to the "cutaneous" plexus (SPALTEHOLZ, 1927).

In the skin of the neck, the arteries terminate at certain specific sites (WALSH, 1963). They are partly "direct" and the "cutaneous" network is well developed; in the upper part, the latter has rather close meshes and the vessels are often spiral.

On the dorsal side of the trunk, the arteries are essentially "muscular-cutaneous", the "fascial" network has vessels of varying diameter and wide meshwork, and the "cutaneous" network is similar to that in some parts of the abdominal walls. On the ventral side, vascularization is considerable in some regions (mammary regions, for example) and somewhat reduced elsewhere (BELLOCQ, 1925).

The upper part of the back is well vascularized (SALMON, 1936) by arteries which, without achieving a true metameric arrangement, nevertheless have a rather regular and symmetrical disposition.

The vascularization of the upper limbs is generally considerable (BELLOCQ, 1925; SALMON, 1936) although there are perceptible differences in the extensor and flexor surfaces (BELLOCQ, 1925; SALMON, 1936). The former is apparently supplied with a greater number of hypodermal anastomoses (BELLOCQ, 1925).

The deltoid area is well vascularized (BELLOCQ, 1925) and the manner in which the vessels branch out and the frequency and strength of the anastomoses resemble those of the abdominal skin.

The arteries of the arm are also almost all "cutaneous" with rather long vessels in the longitudinal direction, and short ones generally in the transverse direction.

The vascularization of the forearm is considerable and is characterized by the same differences between flexor and extensor surfaces that characterize the arm (BELLOCQ, 1925; SALMON, 1936). In the dorsal area of the wrist, the branches of a rather rich "fascial" network with varying diameter but essentially parallel to the longitudinal axis of the limb originate from short vessels. Hence branches reach the subcutaneous layer that are transverse or serpiginous, and which, together with others, form (sometimes at right angles) a rich "cutaneous" network of vessels of varying diameter and meshes of irregular width (SPALTEHOLZ, 1927).

In some parts of the forearm like that overlying the olecranon process (SPALTEHOLZ, 1927) and on the back of the hand, vascularization is reduced (BELLOCQ, 1925; SALMON, 1936). Furthermore, the vasal picture is characterized by extreme tortuosity, by the spiral movement of the smaller vessels, and by the close proximity of the two deep networks caused by the moderate thickness of the fatty tissue.

The palmar region, unlike the dorsal region, is generally rich in vessels (BELLOCQ, 1925; SALMON, 1936). In the dorsal region, the vascularization of the finger surface presents a wide-meshed "subcutaneous" network from which, in addition to the thin vessels that form the "cutaneous" network in the dermis, three arcades spring. The proximal one goes a few millimeters under the free edge of the nail wall, while the other two remain under the posterior and anterior part of the ungual bed. Fine vessels rise from the proximal arcade and radiate (SPALTEHOLZ, 1927) to the free edge of the nail wall whence the pre-capillary vessels later originate (SPALTEHOLZ, 1927). The nail bed and matrix are nourished by the two sublaminar vascular arcades that arise from the digital arteries (SAMMAN, 1965). Each of these arcades provides robust vessels, generally parallel to the finger axis, which when meeting branches from the plantar region form the "cutaneous" network from which smaller vessels go to the longitudinal ridges of the nail bed (Fig. 127) (SPALTEHOLZ, 1927).

In the region of the matrix, these minor vessels often run perpendicularly to the finger axis whereas in the bed they are tortuous (SPALTEHOLZ, 1927).

In the lower limbs, the skin is well vascularized (BELLOCQ, 1925) with substantial differences between the anterior and posterior surfaces and the inside and the outside of the thighs and legs (BELLOCQ, 1925; SALMON, 1936) and perhaps with some hypovascularized zones — the dorsal face of the foot, tibial crest, etc. In the lower limbs, however, regional variations in the blood network are less obvious than in the upper limbs, and in regions with little adipose tissue the vessel design seems rather like that of the forearm (SPALTEHOLZ, 1927). From this point of view, the upper and lower thighs are similar to the forearm; their blood supply is entrusted to rather long thick branches, prevalently belonging to "cutaneous", sometimes to "mixed" arteries (SPALTEHOLZ, 1927).

The "fascial" network of the lower limb is better developed than in any other part of the tegument. It is composed of a close meshwork of thin or thick branches, usually running parallel to the length of the limb, but sometimes perpendicular (SPALTEHOLZ, 1927).

Another important characteristic of this zone is that the frequently tortuous vessels that leave the fascia and traverse the subcutaneous layer for long tracts form therein a "subcutaneous" network by anastomizing. From this network some terminal branches move in a perpendicular direction to the lower edge of the corium. There they form with their arched divergent branches a "cutaneous" network further subdivided into very fine branches (SPALTEHOLZ, 1927). This network seems to have the same characteristics everywhere, even in the knee region (BELLOCQ, 1925; SPALTEHOLZ, 1927).

In the thigh the "primary order" anastomoses at the base of the "cutaneous" network are thicker and closer than in the leg. The anastomoses of the "subcutaneous" and "cutaneous" networks, on the other hand, are robust in the anterior part of the knee (Fig. 113) (SPALTEHOLZ, 1927). On the foot, the vascularization of the front part may be said to be relatively light (BELLOCQ, 1925; SALMON, 1936). That in the plantar region is rather rich in the heel and the anterior third, while it is less so in the middle third (BELLOCQ, 1925; SALMON, 1936).

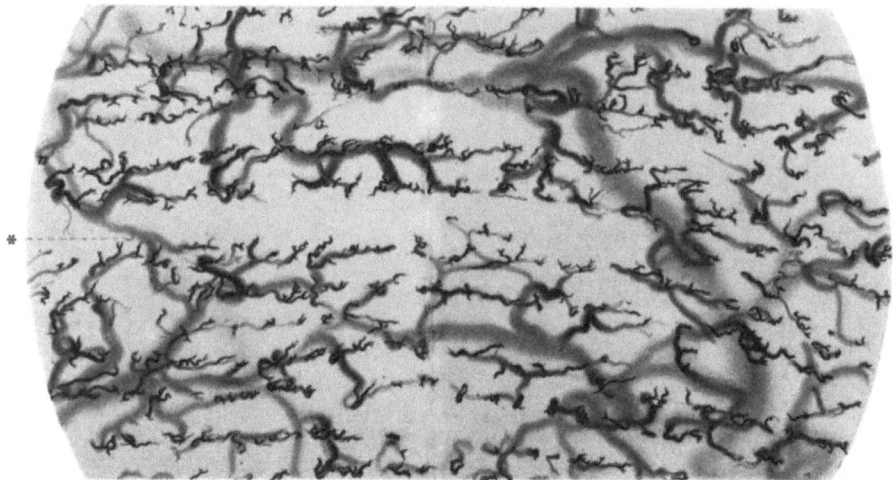

Fig. 113. An horizontal but partial view of the arteries belonging to the "cutaneous" "network" (background) indicates the presence of some anastomatic (*) vessels reaching the level of the "subpapillary" network (Foreground). Skin of the big toe. (Reproduced from W. SPALTEHOLZ and the Arch. Anat. Physiol. 1893)

3. Networks Formed in the Dermis

From the "cutaneous" network[43] (Fig. 113) originate both thin branches, moving mainly parallel to the epidermis, and thick vessels perpendicular to the epidermis (HORSTMANN, 1957). The former link again with the "cutaneous" network (Figs. 161 and 164) according to some (HORSTMANN, 1957), after a rather lengthy course during which they send arterioles to the adipose lobules and to the sweat glomerules (Fig. 114). The thick vessels rise in the dermis in a characteristic manner, dividing at various heights into the "candelabra" (Fig. 47) (PETERSEN, 1935; HORSTMANN, 1957) already described and then reaching the papillae. Here their terminal branches enclose a certain number of papillae into vascular districts which are probably intercommunicating (PETERSEN, 1935; HORSTMANN, 1957). Moreover, branches of "candelabra" vessels anastomize among themselves, creating vascular arcades on other levels that are convex in relation to the epidermis, and each is on the same level as the adjacent one (Fig. 114) (SPALTEHOLZ, 1927; MORETTI and MONTAGNA, 1959; MORETTI, et al. 1959). There exists in the face, for example, a primary order stretching between the maximum and minimum depths of 1.6 and 1.3 mm, a second of 1.3 and 1 mm in depth (Fig. 114) (MORETTI et al., 1959), and still others which appear to be located between the upper and middle third of the dermis. The deeper arcades are often less frequent than the more superficial ones (SPALTEHOLZ, 1927; HORSTMANN, 1957).

---

[43] The vast number of structures nourished by branches from the same vessel is characteristic of this network (CORMIA and ERNYEY, 1961; CORMIA, 1963).

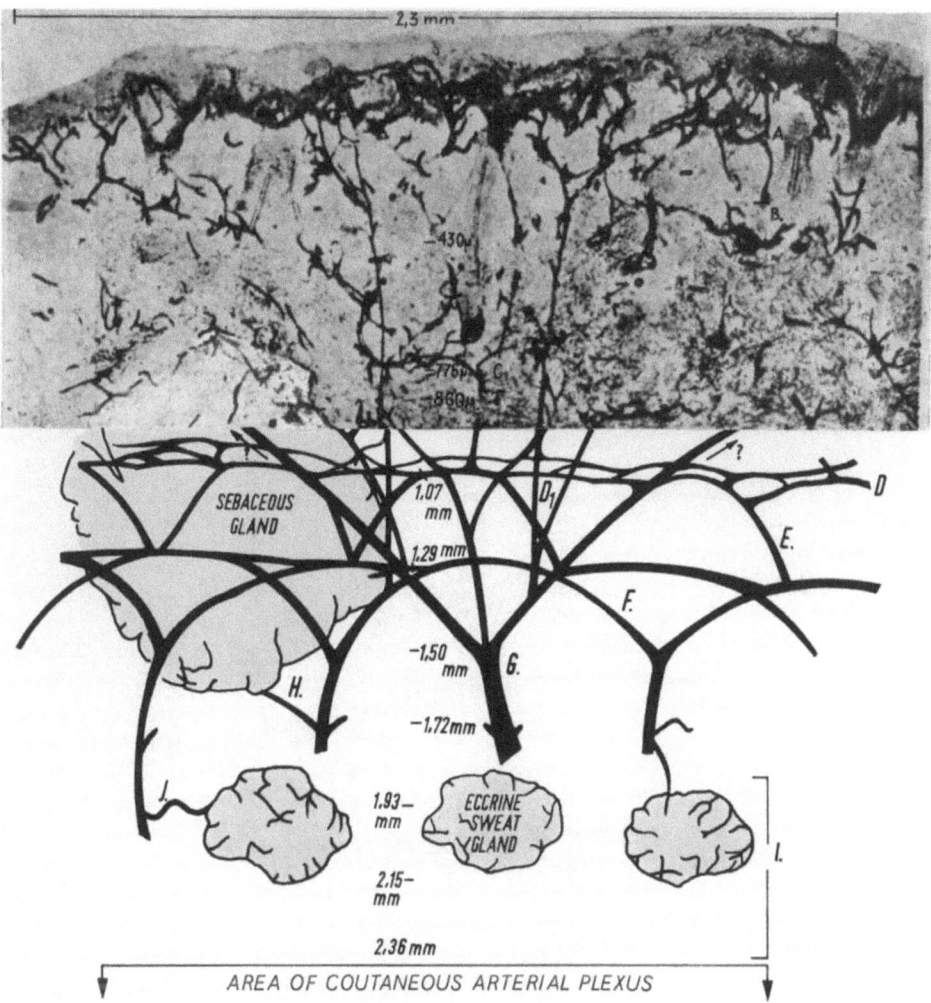

Fig. 114. A partly micro-photographic (superimposed film), partly graphic reconstruction (from serial sections) of the main blood networks in the skin of the parotideo-masseteric region. [MORETTI and MONTAGNA, courtesy of the G. ital. Derm., Le unità vascolari **3**, 247 (1959).] *A* The "subpapillary" or "dermal" network, about 235 μ deep. *B* The level of the vascular arcades linking the "vascular units" (This is also the approximate level of the section shown in Figure 151). *C* The apex of the "vascular units" is 775 μ deep. *D* The so-called "arterial plexus of the middle dermis". D_1 A "candelabrum" arteriole crossing the upper half of the dermis. *E* A primary order of vascular arcades. *F* A second order of vascular arcades. *G* A fairly thick arteriole bifurcates to enclose 2 or 3(?) "vascular units". *H* An arteriole supplying the sebaceous gland. *I* The vascular level of the eccrine sweat glands. *J* An arteriole supplying eccrine sweat glands

From the higher anastomotic arcades therefore the "dermal" (RYDER, 1955; DURWARD and RUDALL, 1958) or "subpapillary" network (Figs. 115, 116, 161 and 164)[44] is born (SPALTEHOLZ, 1927). This is present everywhere and is constructed of a more or less close mesh (always closer than the underlying networks (HORSTMANN, 1962) according to the body region. In plantary skin (Figs. 115, 116, 161 and 164) the meshworks seem to be rather regular and stretched in the direction of the cutaneous furrows, each being as wide as the distance between 1—2 of the furrows with an average surface of 0.31 mm² (SPALTEHOLZ, 1927). In the leg,

---

[44] "Dermal" and "cutaneous" plexuses are also linked by the capillaries which enwrap the eccrine sweat glands' duct (EICHNER, 1954).

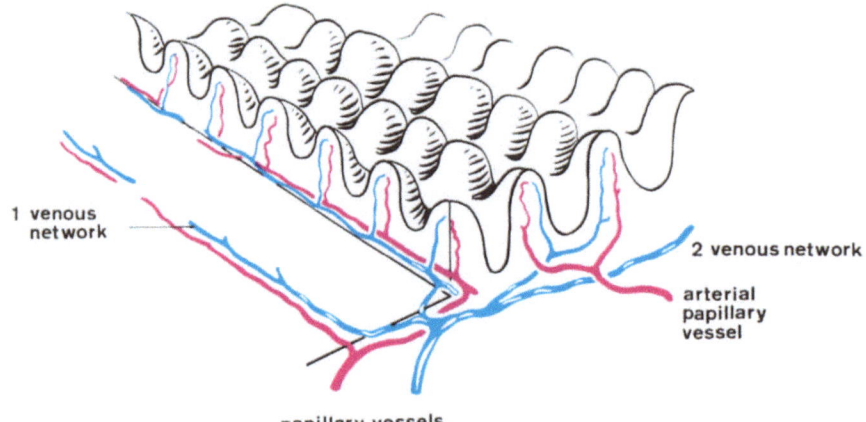

Fig. 115. Distribution of the terminal arterial branches going to the papillary body and venous vessels' drainage in the plantar region. (Modified from W. SPALTEHOLZ and the 1st issue of this Handbuch 1927)

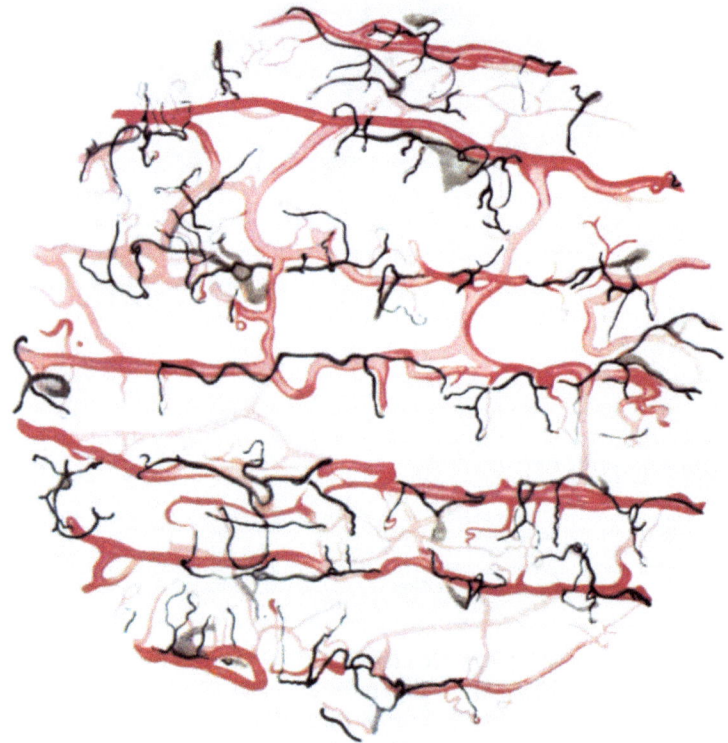

Fig. 116. An horizontal view of the arterial (black) and venous (red) networks immediately under the papillary body of the skin on the heel. (Reproduced from W. SPALTEHOLZ and the Arch. Anat. Physiol. 1893)

the meshes are transversely irregular, often quadrangular, without clear orientation and with an average surface of 0.91 mm². In the gluteal region, their surface is 1,53 mm² (SPALTEHOLZ, 1927).

From the subpapillary "dermal" network, terminal branches of varying diameter and length go to the papillary body (Figs. 115, 116, 161 and 164), below which they divide in various ways until they supply two to four or even more papillae. According to some authors, they may supply as many as eighteen papillae which flank one cutaneous furrow (SPALTEHOLZ, 1927). In any event, it is clear that from this point the papillary body is penetrated by a compact group, which sometimes almost reaches the dermoepidermal line (MORETTI et al., 1959), of capillaries directed upwards and of various shapes and diameters (see part III of this chapter).

The papillary body, which constitutes a considerable part of the total volume of the dermis, thus harbors a vasal mass (Figs. 57—60a and b) which not only is very thick and undoubtedly greater in surface area than the overlying epidermis but also provided with anastomosis (CORMIA and ERNYEY, 1961; CORMIA, 1963). Because of these characteristics and the existence (DURWARD and RUDALL, 1958) of other mammals with true networks in the same place, a "subepidermal" network (CORMIA and ERNYEY, 1961) seems plausible.

4. Regional Aspects of the Dermal Networks

This section will detail the predominant characteristics of dermal vessels and will consider the general appearance of arterial-capillary design in the various regions insofar as this is feasible without serial sections (MORETTI et al., 1959, 1960; BACCAREDDA-BOY et al., 1960a, b; 1961). In addition, the type of branching prevalent at papillary and subpapillary levels and the number and depth of the horizontal vascular elements that are roughly parallel to the dermoepidermal line will be discussed[45].

On the skull, the predominant impression is the thickness of the arteriole capillary network which is greater in the dermis of the temporal and frontal regions than in the occipital region and the vertex (BELLOCQ, 1925; MORETTI et al., 1960). This impression is confirmed by the calculation of the capillary-papillary concentration (BACCAREDDA-BOY et al., 1961; see also Part 3 of this chapter).

In the temporal and frontal (Fig. 121) regions arterioles and capillaries are seen (by means of alkaline phophatase preparations), which react rather well and which are often thick, frequently bifurcating at acute angles and sometimes almost straight or candelabra in type (MORETTI et al., 1960).

On the contrary, in the occipital and vertex regions, the arterioles are usually less reactive, sparse and thinner and bifurcating into multiple arborizations that end with more variously twisted capillaries (MORETTI et al., 1960).

Dermal vascularization is notable upon the face (BELLOCQ, 1925; MENEGHINI, 1942), and there are numerous, rather large arterioles (MORETTI et al., 1959) or capillaries which are reactive for alkaline phosphatase.

There is also considerable variety in the shape of the capillaries which adapt themselves to the varying architecture of different parts. In the nasolabial furrow (Fig. 117) and the upper labial (Fig. 122) and frontal regions, many straight capillaries send out bilateral frond-like branches with rather sharp angles or ascend close to the surface epidermis. In the buccal, oral (Fig. 118), mental (Fig. 119) and parotideo-masseteric (Fig. 120) regions, lesser branches separate from the capillaries almost at right angles; in the orbital and infraorbital regions, there are various ramifications of the two patterns just described (MORETTI et al., 1959).

---

[45] The capillary-papillary concentration and the development of the "subpapillary" and "cutaneous" networks lying below are directly correlated: see f.i. the skin of the eyelids, ear-lobules and back of hands (HORSTMANN, 1962).

Other differences are noticeable in the subepidermal tissue that are sometimes supplied with anastomized loops or with papillae each of which is supplied by a true tuft of independent capillaries, as in the parotid and masseteric regions (Fig. 120) (MORETTI et al., 1959).

In addition to the fundamental networks with classic nomenclature, vessels parallel to the epidermal surface are to be found at practically all depths.

On the face, an unbroken vascular ribbon of capillaries penetrates into the papillae. They are joined together at about 45 microns from the epidermal surface. At 270, 360, and 470 microns in depth, other rather thick vessels cross the hair follicles or the excretory sweat ducts. At 775 and 560 micron, horizontal branches link the oblique vessels of some large bifurcations, of which we shall speak later.

Finally at about 1.07 mm, a series of meshes and thick ramifications form halfway below the vertex of the vascular unit (see afterwards) and roughly between the surface of the epidermal papillae and the hypodermis forming a true arterial network of the middle dermis (MORETTI et al., 1959; MORETTI and MONTAGNA, 1959).

The apparent density of the dermal network in the trunk region is less than on the cephalic extremity and greater than that of the limbs, except for the plantar region (Figs. 123—126) (BELLOCQ, 1925; BACCAREDDA-BOY et al., 1960a); on the other hand, its development is greater in the upper limbs than in the lower (BACCAREDDA-BOY et al., 1960a).

On the trunk, the mammary regions (both at the second intercostal level and the periareolar zone) (Fig. 124) are better vascularized than the scapular (Fig. 123) and interscapular regions (BACCAREDDA-BOY et al., 1960a); the latter possesses the greater number of reactive vessels (BACCAREDDA-BOY et al., 1960b).

The anterior regions of the trunk and the interscapular region also have vessels that are reactive for alkaline phosphatase at almost all depths of the dermis, but in the scapular region only the superficial dermis seems well provided with arterioles and reactive capillaries (BACCAREDDA-BOY et al., 1960b).

In the periumbilical region a considerable number of capillaries rise to the papillae surrounding the sweat gland ducts (BACCAREDDA-BOY et al., 1960a).

As for the papillae, the types of vessel encountered on the trunk may be of two different patterns, with some variations. In the first, which is particularly apparent in the olecranon region, the same terminal arteriole divides at an acute angle into thin branches, so that the capillaries are indented in tufts one beside the other. In the second, the vessel divides at a wide and almost ovoid angle; the width of the branches springing from this arteriole is considerable and the different groups of the capillaries are widely separated. This pattern is seen in the mammary regions (Fig. 124) including the periareolar zone, the axillary region, and the extremities (BACCAREDDA-BOY et al., 1960a, b). The vessels are "grosso modo" parallel to the dermal-epidermal line in the mammary regions; and especially in the periareolar skin, at 154, 286, 658 and 798 microns, some horizontal vessels can be seen (BACCAREDDA-BOY et al., 1960a).

In the periumbilical, scapular, and interscapular regions, vessels roughly parallel to the epidermis, were observed at depths of 154, 220 and 275 microns but seldom farther down.

In the pubic regions, reactive vasal structures are not seen below 220 micron deep; the sacral region is similar (BACCAREDDA-BOY et al., 1960a). In the upper limbs and particularly in the regions of the olecranon and antecubital fossa, the dermis is well supplied with reactive capillaries and arterioles (BACCAREDDA, BOY et al., 1960a).

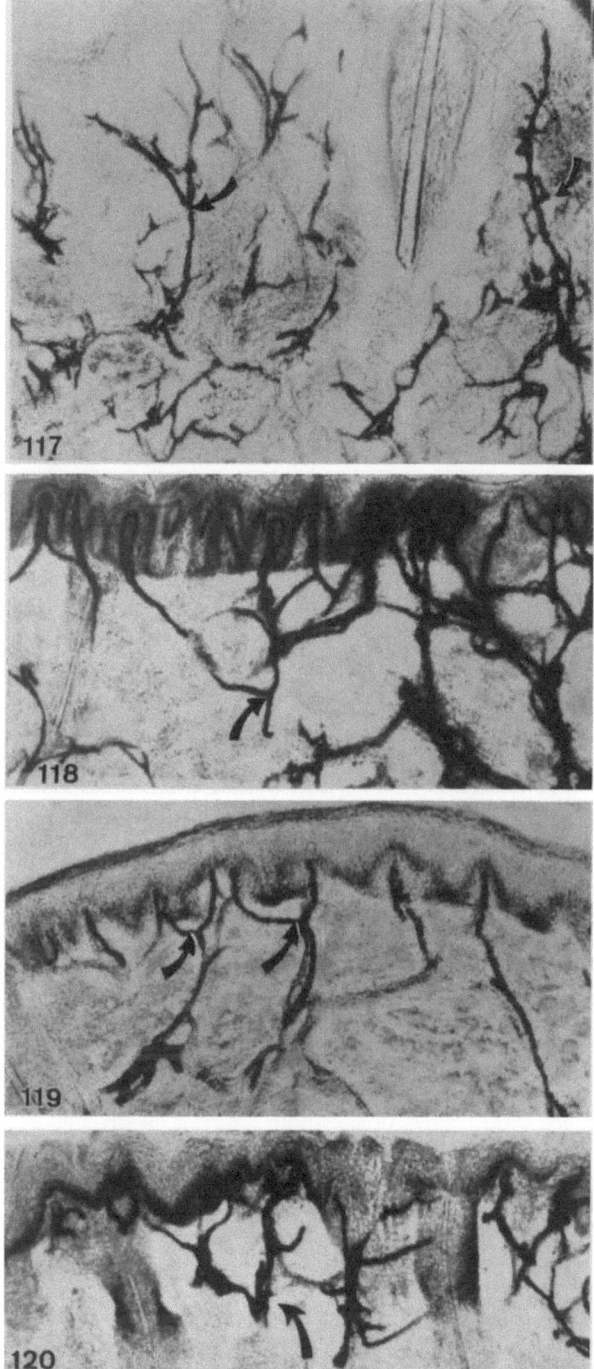

Figs. 117—120. The considerable variety in the shape of the papillary capillaries

Fig. 117. Straight capillaries (arrow) send out bilateral frond-like branches (nasolabial furrow)

Fig. 118. Lesser branches separate from the main capillaries almost at right angles (arrow) (oral region). [MORETTI and MONTAGNA, courtesy of the G. ital. Derm., Le unità vascolari **3**, 245 (1959)]

Fig. 119. Rounded capillary bifurcations (arrows) embrace the epidermal ridges (mental region). [MORETTI and MONTAGNA, courtesy of the G. ital. Derm., Le unità vascolari **3**, 245 (1959)]

Fig. 120. Each papilla is supplied by a true tuft (arrow) of independent capillaries (parotideo-masseteric region). [MORETTI and MONTAGNA, courtesy of the G. ital. Derm., Le unità vascolari **3**, 245 (1959)]

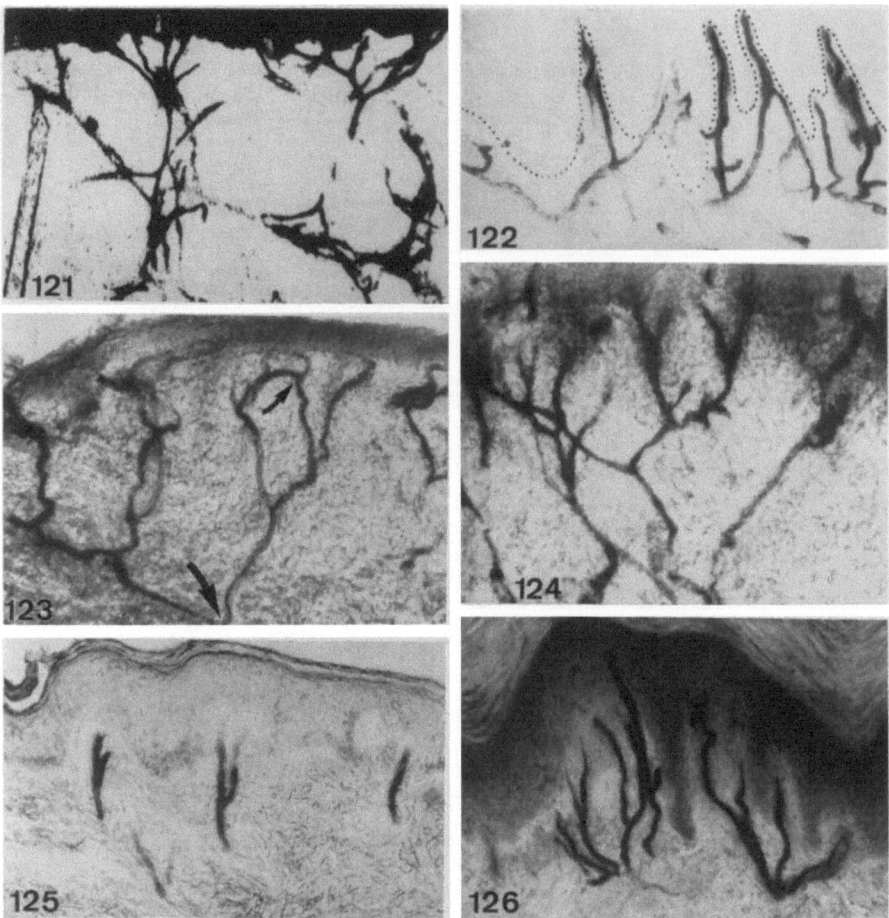

Figs. 121—126. Some regional aspects of the dermal networks

Fig. 121. Thick arterioles and capillaries frequently bifurcate at acute angles (frontal region). [MORETTI, ELLIS and MESCON, courtesy of the J. invest. Derm., Vascular patterns in the skin of the face **33**, 107 (1959)]

Fig. 122. Long straight capillaries ascend close to the surface epidermis (upper labial region). [MORETTI, ELLIS and MESCON, courtesy of the J. invest. Derm., Vascular patterns in the skin of the face **33**, 109 (1959)]

Fig. 123. Slightly tortuous capillaries (thin arrow) ascend from a deep wide bifurcation (thick arrow) (scapular region)

Fig. 124. A vessel divides at a wide and almost ovoid angle (arrow). The different groups of springing capillaries are widely separated (periareolar zone)

Fig. 125. The blood supply may be extremely poor (dorsum of the foot)

Fig. 126. The papillary capillary supply numerous branches perpendicular to the apex, dividing at a rather narrow angle into smaller branches which sometimes almost enclose the interposed epidermal ridges (palmar and plantar regions). [BACCAREDDA-BOY, MORTETI and FARRIS, courtesy of the Ann. ital. Derm. Sif., Varietà topografiche della reazione per la fosfatasi alcalina nel circolo superficiale cutaneo **1—2**, 189 (1960)]

The subpapillary network is usually the vascular layer most reactive in these cutaneous segments. With alkaline phosphatase, other reactive layers have, however, been discerned farther down, but only on the medial face of the arm and in the elbow.

In the upper limbs, the vessels usually found in the papillae seem to correspond to those previously described in the trunk.

On the lower limbs, the thighs, and legs, the number of vessels is rather small, being restricted to the subpapillary dermis. The pre-tibial area also has an extre-

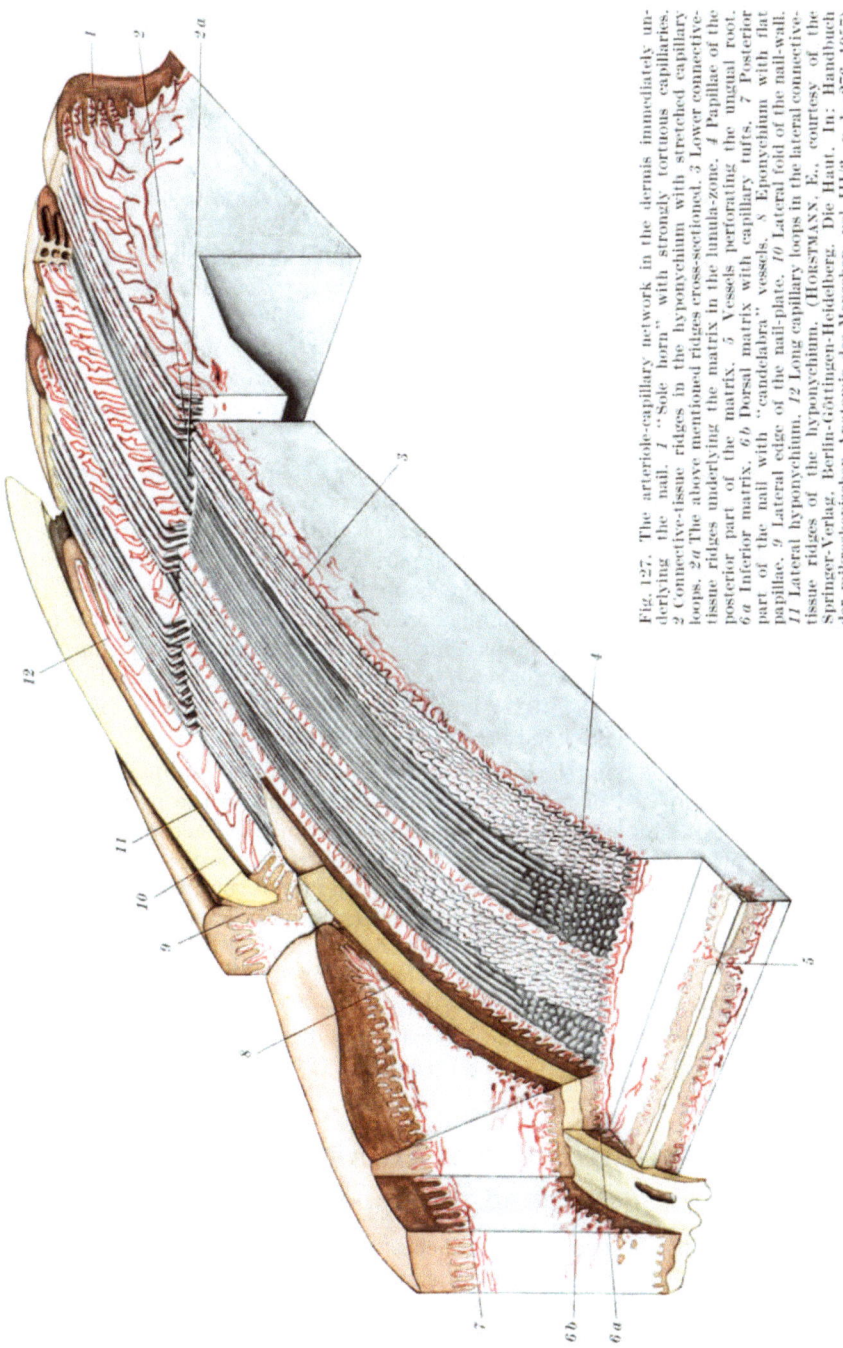

Fig. 127. The arteriole-capillary network in the dermis immediately underlying the nail. *1* "Sole horn" with strongly tortuous capillaries. *2* Connective-tissue ridges in the hyponychium with stretched capillary loops. *2a* The above mentioned ridges cross-sectioned. *3* Lower connective-tissue ridges underlying the matrix in the lunula-zone. *4* Papillae of the posterior part of the matrix. *5* Vessels perforating the ungual root. *6a* Inferior matrix. *6b* Dorsal matrix with capillary tufts. *7* Posterior part of the nail with "candelabra" vessels. *8* Eponychium with flat papillae. *9* Lateral edge of the nail-plate. *10* Lateral fold of the nail-wall. *11* Lateral hyponychium. *12* Long capillary loops in the lateral connective-tissue ridges of the hyponychium. (HORSTMANN, E., courtesy of the Springer-Verlag, Berlin-Göttingen-Heidelberg. Die Haut. In: Handbuch der mikroskopischen Anatomie des Menschen. vol. III/3, p. 1—276. 1957)

mely poor blood supply (BACCAREDDA-BOY et al., 1960a) and actually seems to constitute a "hypovascularized" zone [like the flexor surface of the wrist, dorsum of the foot (Fig. 125) and other surfaces (SALMON, 1936)]. For the lower limbs too the types of vessels in the papillae seem to vary between the two models observed in the trunk; we have no precise information about their possible levels parallel to the dermo-epidermal line (BACCAREDDA-BOY et al., 1960a).

The dermis of the palmar and plantar regions however exhibits such peculiar vasal qualities as to merit separate description. In these vascular districts, the arterio-capillary network is very rich (BELLOCQ, 1925; BACCAREDDA-BOY et al., 1960a), especially on the papillary level and around the sweat glands (BACCAREDDA-BOY et al., 1960a) even though a hypovascularized zone may be present in the median part of the palm, for example (SALMON, 1936).

In these areas the papillae capillaries supply numerous branches (Fig. 126) perpendicular to the apex, dividing at a rather narrow angle into more small branches which sometimes almost enclose the interposed epidermal ridges (BACCAREDDA-BOY et al., 1960a).

The arteriole-capillary network in the dermis immediately underlying the nail (Fig. 127) is another subject which deserves attention and has been well described by HORSTMANN (1957). To recapitulate, the capillary loops go from bottom to top when there are papillae, parallel to the epidermis in the region of the ridges, and from bottom to top again in the more distal zone of the bed (Fig. 127) (TRUFFI, 1934). It should be borne in mind furthermore that the posterior ungual wall is nourished by loops which, by rising in a candelabrum from the "dermal" network ("subpapillary"), continually lengthen out (up to 1—2 mm; DIETER and SUNG-SHENG, 1922) in the direction of the lamina (Fig. 127) (an orientation which is made good use of by capillaroscopy).

In the rest of the nail, the vessels originating from the "subpapillary dermal" network are composed of tufts of short capillary loops in the matrix and in the hyponychium of simple loops which, in the posterior part, accompany the ridges proximally while in the anterior part they cross them in a distal direction, up to some millimeters in distance from the horny plantar layer (Fig. 127). In a single ridge, especially in those on the nail edge, more layers of loops can be found, each one being up to 1.5 mm in length including its arterial fraction. The venous segment is often 15—35 microns thick (HORSTMANN, 1957).

In the region characterized by the large digitiform papillae of the plantar horny layer, the long hyponychial loops are substituted by strongly tortuous capillaries taking sometimes up to 8 turns (Fig. 127) (HORSTMANN, 1957).

III. The Distribution of Arterioles and Capillaries around the Appendages

Instead of distributing their branches inside one of the more or less rich vascular levels or plexuses just described and finally anastomizing and forming a meshwork there, many arterioles and capillaries move at different depths and in different directions to the cutaneous appendages which they supply with special, more or less complex, networks.

These networks have some characteristics in common: above all they have a capacity to receive arterioles and capillaries at the same time from several horizontal underlying and overlying vascular levels. The individual branches are extremely adaptable to even the most sinuous shape of each appendage, the

1. Periglandular Networks

The architecture of the arteriole-capillary network which enwraps the sebaceous glands (Figs. 128—130 and 164) is an integral part of the hair follicle and often, therefore, reflects its changeable nature. The origins of the arterial vascularization of the sebaceous glands, in any case, seem to be multiple. It must be made clear that this vascularization is not necessarily secondary and dependent upon the follicular network (Figs. 128—130) (TRUFFI, 1934) originating from several points in the vessel circuit, from dermal collateral vessels of the candelabra arterioles (HORSTMANN, 1957) or from branches coming from anastomotic branches and directed to the glands (TRUFFI, 1934), or opened up into bifurcations which at the same time send out vessels to the follicles and to the glands (TRUFFI, 1934). In children, they may originate from a small capillary network usually coming from vessels connected with the perifollicular network and finally, from my observations, branches reach at least to the sebaceous glands of the face both from the second vessel arcade system and the first deeper system (Figs. 114 and 138) (MORETTI and MONTAGNA, 1959).

The result is that each glandular acinus finds itself wrapped in a particularly thick vessel mesh (Figs. 128—130). This is exceptionally tight and composed of thicker capillaries than the surrounding ones [no more than 10—12 μ thick (BIMTS, 1960)] around the bigger sebaceous glands (SPALTEHOLZ, 1927). These vessels follow the glandular perimeter and the excretory duct penetrating the connective septa between lobes and lobules, or even into the sebaceous acini (ELLIS, 1961).

The eccrine sweat glands are also enwrapped by a characteristic vasal network (Figs. 132 and 164) which, by following the contours, models its shape. According to the type of gland and the degree to which it is enclosed, its elaboration is different: when the glandular tubules are slightly contorted as in the skull, armpit, and arm, for example (MONTAGNA, 1962), the meshes are dense and rolled up. The blood flow to the eccrine sweat glands varies then with the dimensions and with the part of the gland nourished.

The small glands have, around the secretory portion and the tortuous part of their duct, capillaries which frequently originate from the same vessel (ELLIS et al., 1958; BIMTS, 1960) [perhaps a medium calibre artery coming from the deep fatty tissue (CORMIA and ERNYEY, 1961; CORMIA, 1963)]. On the contrary, the large glands possess a pluriarteriolar network (ELLIS et al., 1958) with capillaries coming from anastomotic arcades situated at 1.9—2.3 mm deep in the dermis (Fig. 114) (MORETTI and MONTAGNA, 1959).

In these glands both the secretory portion and tortuous part are nourished as much by the so-called vascular level of the gland (HORSTMANN, 1957), that is, by the "cutaneous" network (HEYNOLD, 1874; SPALTEHOLZ, 1927), as by the "candelabra" arterioles (HORSTMANN, 1957) or vasal arcades which spring out from it (MORETTI et al., 1959). The upper part of the duct (Fig. 131) is supplied by the subepidermal and dermal networks (ELLIS et al., 1958) by means of vertical and possibly recurrent branches (SPALTEHOLZ, 1927) contained in the vascular unit (MORETTI and MONTAGNA, 1959; BERTAMINO and RAMPINI, 1963) and also from transverse branches which enwrap the straight and terminal part of the tubule in a sort of mesh (Fig. 131) (ELLIS et al., 1958; ELLIS, 1961). At the base of the papillary body, on the other hand, the vessels at the side of the duct bifurcate,

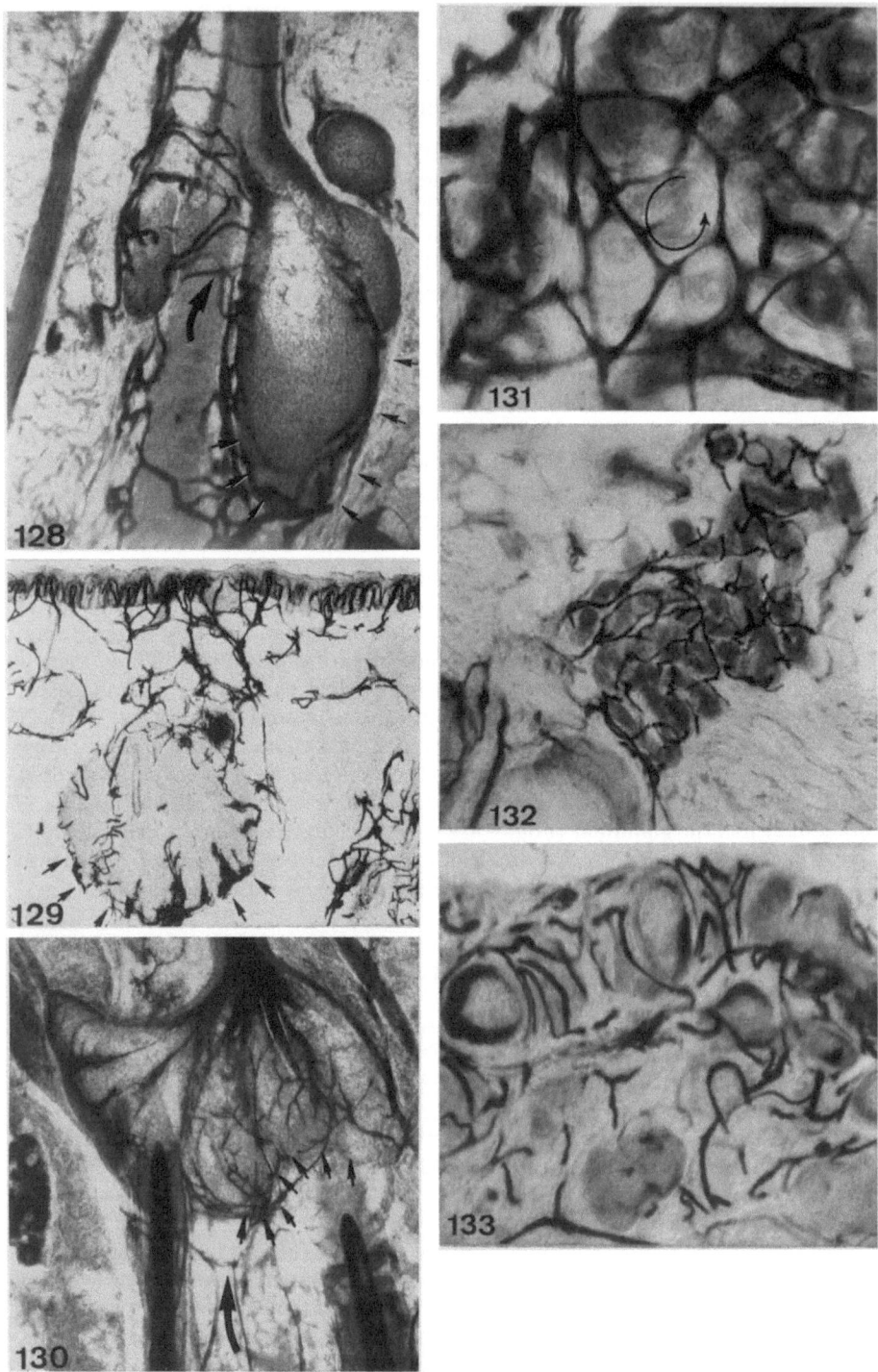

Figs. 128—133. For Legends see p. 583

sending out capillary loops which are arranged in a sort of cone below the parenchyma which surrounds the intraepidermal tract, the epidermal sweat duct unit (LOBITZ, 1954) and in turn is enclosed in the wider system of the vascular unit (ELLIS et al., 1958; MORETTI and MONTAGNA, 1959; MORETTI et al., 1959; MONTAGNA, 1961)[46].

The capillary bed of the eccrine sweat glands like that of the sebaceous glands becomes richer with aging (ELLIS, 1958).

Concerning their secretory part, around the apocrine glands there are elaborate vasal systems without any difference between the narrow and dilated segments, with interconnecting loops and branches, bifurcations and peritubular anastomoses (ELLIS et al., 1958) (Fig. 133); the duct is accompanied only by some capillaries as far as its outlet in the hair follicle (ELLIS et al., 1958).

Like the vessels of most eccrine glands, those going to these glands originate from arterioles found at the boundary between hypodermis and dermis (ELLIS, 1961); in the armpit, however, in spite of the fact that the eccrine and apocrine glands are found together, the capillary beds of the two types of gland are completely separated (ELLIS et al., 1958).

2. Perifollicular Networks, their Static and Dynamic Aspects

Even in man (see part II of this chapter) the morphology and function of the perifollicular network depends entirely upon the type and stage of the development of the hair.

In fact, one can say in summary that while in the anagen (or growth) phase of any terminal hair, the perifollicular network has an apparently unitary structure and maximum development; in catagen and telogen phases (transition and rest phases), the progressive disappearance of the lower two-thirds of the network points to the existence, on the inside of the same perifollicular network, of the two different vessel sectors which are distinctive because of the origin of their branches and because one is preserved and the other perishes.

When a terminal hair is growing (Figs. 134, 138, 140 and 164), its upper part is supplied by "grosso modo" longitudinal vessels descending along its perimeter from the horizontal meshes at the papillary level and its lower third is surrounded around the base and hair bulb by a rich network of longitudinal parallel vessels flanking the follicle and connected by horizontal branches (Figs. 134, 138 and 164) (MONTAGNA and ELLIS, 1957; MONTAGNA and ELLIS, 1958; CORMIA and ERNYEY, 1961; CORMIA, 1963). Of these vessels, the longitudinal ones come from the "subepidermal" and the "dermal (subpapillary)" network (TOMSA, 1873; UNNA, 1908; SPALTEHOLZ, 1927; TRUFFI, 1934; CORMIA and ERNYEY, 1961; CORMIA, 1963) as well as from arterioles originating in the deep adipose tissue and going to the

---

[46] The spiral and straight part of the excretory duct is, therefore, rather better vascularized than a simple excretory task would seem to require (ELLIS, 1961).

Figs. 128—130. The arteriole-capillary network which enwraps the sebaceous glands. Note the particularly dense vessel meshes surrounding the acini of each gland (thin arrows) and the vessels (thick arrows) joining the glands' vascularization to the follicular network. [Fig. 128: courtesy of R. A. ELLIS. Fig. 130: CORMIA, F., courtesy of the Arch. Derm., Vasculature of the normal scalp 88, 697 (1963)]

Figs. 131—133. The vascularization of sweat glands

Fig. 131. The upper part of the duct (arrow) is supplied by meshes of the "subepidermal" and "dermal" networks. [CORMIA, F., courtesy of the Arch. Derm., Vasculature of the normal scalp 88, 698 (1963)]

Fig. 132. The eccrine sweat glands are enwrapped by a characteristic vasal network which, by following the contours, molds its shape. (Courtesy of R. A. ELLIS)

Fig. 133. Vascular coils surrounding an apocrine gland. (Courtesy of R. A. ELLIS)

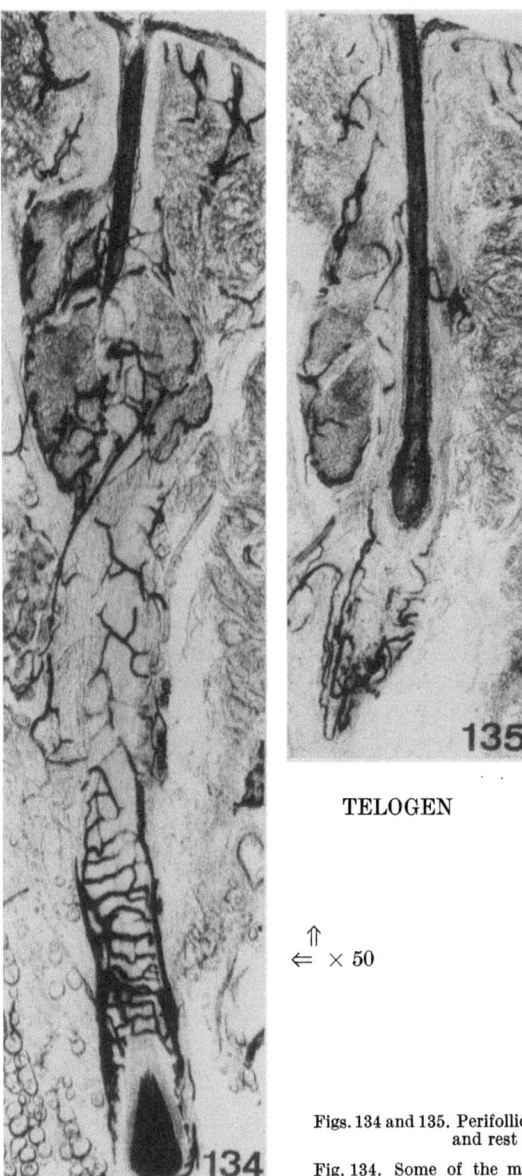

TELOGEN

⇑
⇐ × 50

Figs. 134 and 135. Perifollicular networks in growth and rest phases

Fig. 134. Some of the major vessels of the rich perifollicular network of anagen

Fig. 135. A view of the vessels surrounding the follicle in telogen

lower part of the follicle and to the papilla (TRUFFI, 1934; MONTAGNA and ELLIS, 1957; MONTAGNA and ELLIS, 1958). When they reach the junction point between the middle and the lower third of the follicle, these latter vessels bend sharply, dividing themselves into branches that go upwards and downwards (CORMIA and ERNYEY, 1961; CORMIA, 1963).

Some of the longitudinal or palisade vessels have a larger diameter than the horizontal ones and follow the connective sheath of the follicle which they nourish along its entire length; when ascending, however, they end up by vanishing at the

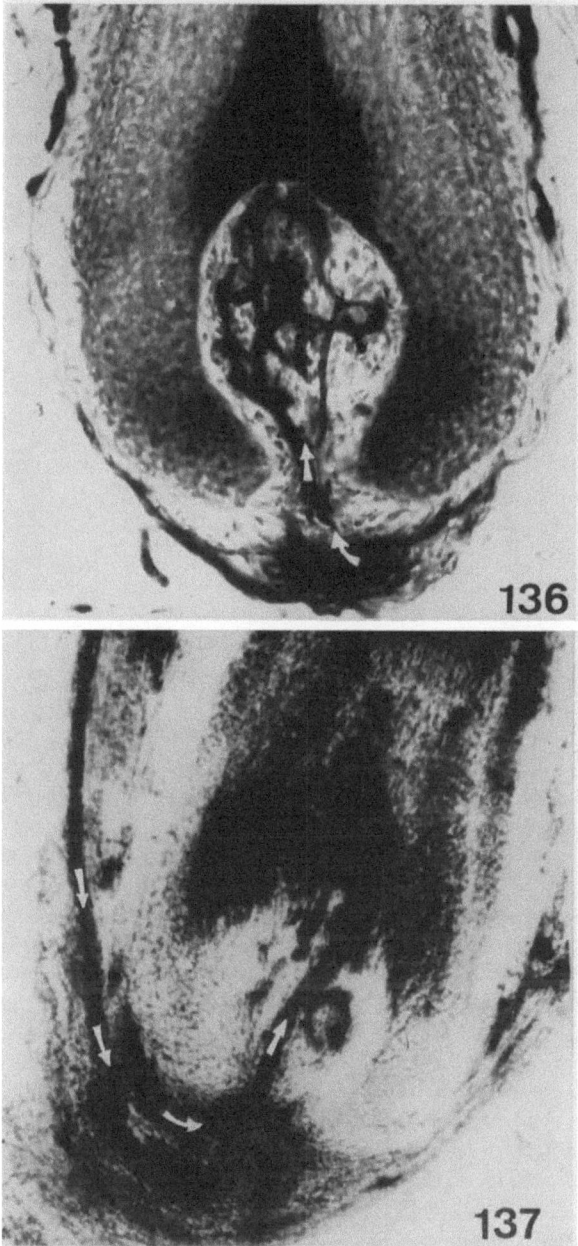

Figs. 136 and 137. Some vessels curl around the pore of the papillary cavity (arrow), penetrating the papilla itself (arrow) and reaching its apex. (Fig. 136: Courtesy of Dr. F. ALLEGRA)

height of the follicle neck in a rather large meshed network and hence in a capillary ring encircling the hair (MONTAGNA and ELLIS, 1958; ELLIS, 1961)[47].

Other longitudinal vessels descend as we have seen and curl around the pore of the papillary cavity, penetrating the papilla itself (Figs. 136, 137, 147—150

---

[47] According to some a strict relationship exists between the stage of subepidermal vascularization and development (lanugo or terminal hair) of the follicle (MONTAGNA, 1958).

and 164). Here they form a tuft of capillaries, some of which go to the apex of the papilla, while others practically touch the bulb walls (Montagna and Ellis, 1957; Montagna and Ellis, 1958; Montagna, 1962).

A further source of blood flow to this essential part of the follicle also comes (Tomsa, 1873; Spalteholz, 1927; Cormia and Ernyey, 1961; Cormia, 1963) from vessels of the cutaneous network, or from the deep fatty tissue, going exclusively to the papilla.

As for the so-called horizontal vessels that are all more or less sinuous, the greater part are concentrated around the lower third of the follicle. In this area they form around the hair a rough capillary checkwork design with the help of secondary anastomotic elements (Montagna and Ellis, 1957; Montagna, 1962).

Other "grosso modo" horizontal vessels are found at the level of the sebaceous glands, i.e. at the level of a system of vessels which at the same time embraces sebaceous glands and pilary canals (Fig. 128) (Montagna and Ellis, 1957; Montagna, 1962).

To conclude, the perifollicular network of the hair in anagen results from branches coming from various directions that are hooked into the "subepidermal" and dermal networks ("sub-papillary" and "cutaneous") above and below (Fig. 139 and 164). It supplies an adequate blood flow to the various parts of the hair at the different depths that are successively encountered by the follicle in its descent.

Hair vascularization therefore constitutes a "wide supplementary anastomotic meshwork interposed between the deep and the superficial networks of the skin" (Truffi, 1934).

On the other hand, this implies that the continuous vasal unity formed from the dermal papilla to the peri-infundibular area and including the vessels which supply the sebaceous gland (Montagna and Ellis, 1957; Montagna, 1962) is more apparent than real.

On the inside of the perifollicular network of the terminal hair two fractions (Fig. 139) potentially exist: a "permanent" one, that is composed of vessels arranged around the upper third of the hair; and another one that shows up in the following phases of transition (catagen) and rest (telogen) and is "transient" and made up of branches which surround the underlying two-thirds of the follicle (Ellis and Moretti, 1959; Rampini et al., 1963).

In catagen (Figs. 141—144), however, even after the characteristic phenomena of corrugation of the external sheath and the thickening of the glassy and connective membrane (Montagna, 1962), the vessels of the perifollicular network and of the papilla are apparently intact, well reactive to alkaline phosphatase and open until the contraction of the connective sheath and the partial disintegration of the outer epithelial sheath overlying the bulb and the bulb itself (Fig. 141) (Ellis and Moretti, 1959).

Only with the progress of the alterations in the connective sheath and the almost total destruction of the peribulbar epithelial sheath do the reactive papillary capillaries begin to lose their crisp outlines and tend to disappear from the dermal papilla, which is still rich in phosphatase. The longitudinal perifollicular vessels, nevertheless, remain intact (Fig. 142) (Ellis and Moretti, 1959); and the vasal network of the epithelial sheath is also apparently whole despite the fact that after catagen the two lower thirds of the follicle are almost totally reabsorbed.

Thus, at this point, vasal meshes entirely devoid of parenchymal content are rendered visible (Ellis and Moretti, 1959) and the phosphatase activity diffuses into the surrounding tissue (Ellis and Moretti, 1959; Rampini et al., 1963).

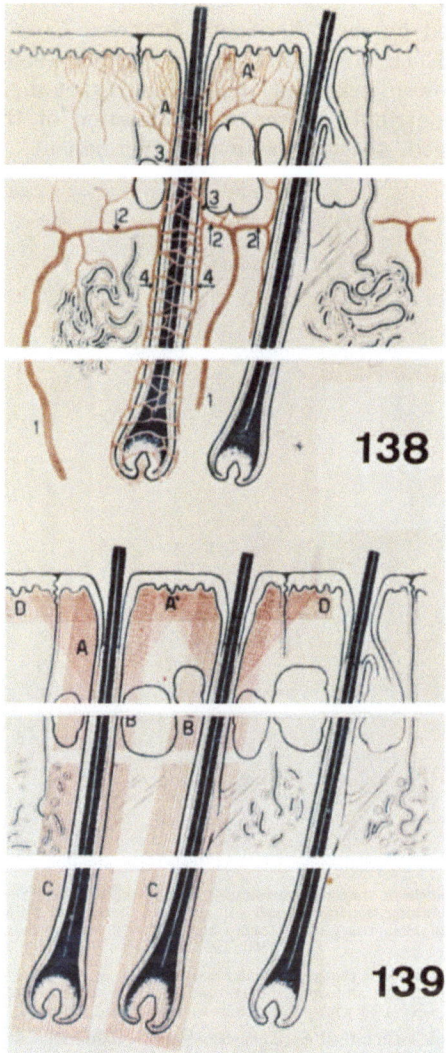

Fig. 138. Schematic drawing of a portion of the arteriole-capillary network in the scalp: *1* vessels ascending within the retinacula cutis arcades (*2*) releasing longitudinal rami flanking the follicle both ascending (*3*) or descending (*4*) and vessels supplying the sebaceous and eccrine sweat glands. [RAMPINI, MORETTI and REBORA, courtesy of the Minerva derm., Arteriole e capillari della cute ed'alopecia areata. Atti SIDES **38**, 301 (1963)]

Fig. 139. Schematic drawing of a portion of the arteriole-capillary network in the scalp: *A—A'* Territory of the "vascular unit". *B* "Permanent" perifollicular network. *C* "Transient" perifollicular network. *D* "External vascular belt". [RAMPINI, MORETTI and REBORA, courtesy of the Minerva derm., Arteriole e capillari della cute ed alopecia areata. Atti SIDES **38**, 301 (1963)]

At the end of catagen, however, the longitudinal vessels seem to collapse too (Fig. 143) and under the dermal papilla (now without vessels but rich in phosphatase activity that spreads into the surrounding tissue) a thin ribbon of reactive longitudinal vessels is left (Fig. 144) (ELLIS and MORETTI, 1959) which trails the route followed by the follicle in its ascent toward the epidermis (MONTAGNA, 1962).

In telogen (Fig. 135 and 145), the dermal papilla, faintly reactive and entirely free from the mass of epithelial tissue, shows underneath a characteristic bundle of capillaries connected by short horizontal branches hanging down for a long way (MONTAGNA and ELLIS, 1957; ELLIS and MORETTI, 1959; MONTAGNA, 1962). The remnants of the lower "transient" tract (RAMPINI et al., 1963) of the perifollicular network may contribute to the vascularization of the sebaceous gland, probably left unchanged, together with the "permanent" tract of the upper

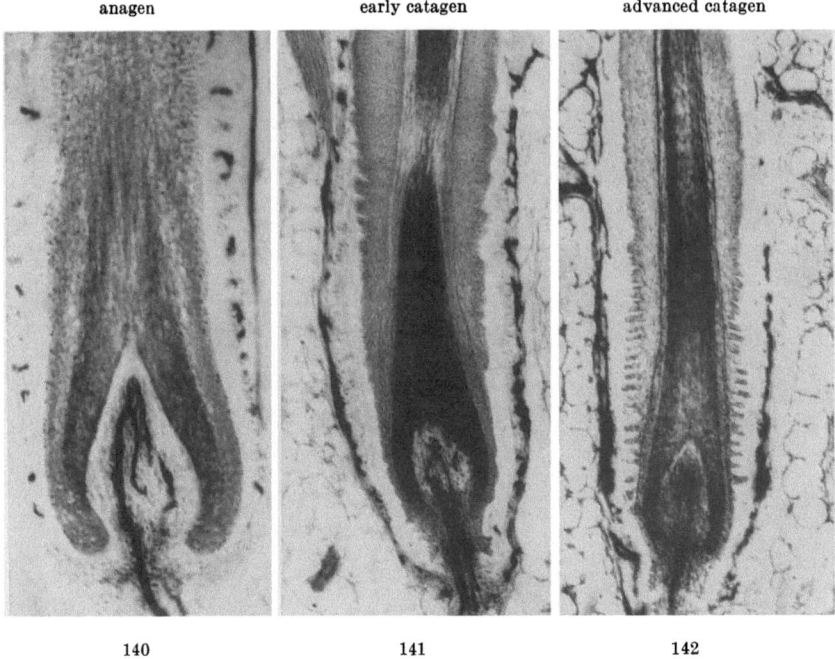

anagen   early catagen   advanced catagen

140   141   142

Figs. 140—145. Perifollicular networks, their static and dynamic aspects

Fig. 140. The lower third of follicle in anagen is surrounded around the base and hair bulb by a rich network of longitudinal parallel vessels flanking the follicle and connected by horizontal branches. [ELLIS and MORETTI, courtesy of the Ann. N.Y. Acad. Sci., Vascular patterns associated with catagen hair follicles in the human scalp **83**, 450 (1959)]

Fig. 141. In early catagen the vessels of the perifollicular network and of the papilla are still apparently intact, well reactive to alkaline phosphatases, and open. [ELLIS and MORETTI, courtesy of the Ann. N.Y. Acad. Sci., Vascular patterns associated with catagen hair follicles in the human scalp **83**, 450 (1959)]

Fig. 142. Later in catagen the longitudinal perifollicular vessels remain intact while capillaries are no longer discernible in the "dermal" papilla. [ELLIS and MORETTI, courtesy of the Ann. N.Y. Acad. Sci., Vascular patterns associated with catagen hair follicles in the human scalp **83**, 451 (1959)]

third of the follicle (RAMPINI et al., 1963). The epithelial sack, which enwraps the keratinic club, is surrounded by a rather scanty bundle of collapsed vessels at its base (MONTAGNA and ELLIS, 1957; MONTAGNA, 1962).

On the reestablishment of the growth phase, the new bulb develops inside the bundles of subpapillary vessels already described (MONTAGNA, 1962).

Up to now we have considered the arteriole-capillary organization of the most complex terminal follicle; the smaller the follicle, on the other hand, the simpler is its vascularization (MONTAGNA, 1962).

Through many transition grades one thus passes from the type of network just described to the vasculature of the lanugo follicle (Fig. 146), that consists only of some capillaries coming from the dermal network (CORMIA and ERNYEY, 1961; CORMIA, 1963) that surrounds the lower part of a follicle (MONTAGNA et al., 1962), whose dermal papilla is very reactive to alkaline phosphatase.

Sometimes the supply to a terminal hair and a lanugo hair is linked; a vessel of moderate caliber going to the terminal follicle and a very small one to the lanugo can, in fact, leave from the same arteriole (CORMIA and ERNYEY, 1961).

Although we have already spoken of the perifollicular networks in other mammals, it now seems opportune to refer again to some observations of com-

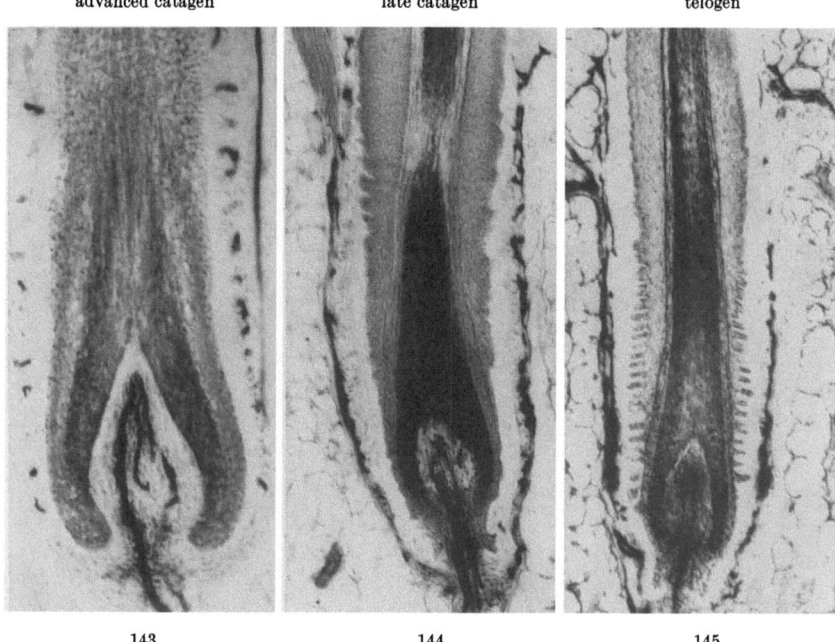

Fig. 143. In advanced catagen the longitudinal vessels seem to collapse too but the lower plexus is intact. [ELLIS and MORETTI, courtesy of the Ann. N.Y. Acad. Sci., Vascular patterns associated with catagen hair follicles in the human scalp **83**, 453 (1959)]

Fig. 144. In late catagen under the "dermal" papilla, now without vessel a thin ribbon of reactive longitudinal vessels is left. [ELLIS and MORETTI, courtesy of the Ann. N.Y. Acad. Sci., Vascular patterns associated with catagen hair follicles in the human scalp **83**, 455 (1959)]

Fig. 145. In telogen the "dermal" papilla shows underneath a characteristic bundle of capillaries hanging down for a long way

parative anatomy, because they may also have an important relationship to the pilary system in man.

First of all, in many animals a definite relationship exists between the size of the dermal papilla and the quantity of vessels contained therein[48] (Figs. 147—150) (RYDER, 1955). The shape, size and even duration of the growth period of the hair produced depend upon the degree of richness and on the type of perifollicular and papillary vascularization (RYDER, 1955; DURWARD and RUDALL, 1958). Some of these characteristics in certain rodents, bovines, and ovines suggest that the peribulbar vasal plot may have a compensatory function for papillary vascularization and the task of maintaining the outer epithelial sheath may be delegated to the vessels overlying the external sheath (DURWARD and RUDALL, 1958).

A further aspect of the appendageal supply concerns the probability that in some animals the regions showing simultaneous growth of the follicles may have a single vessel network quite different from the individually growing hairs having

---

[48] To this can be opposed the negative relationship between the phosphatase activity of the papilla and its wealth of capillaries (MONTAGNA and Ellis, 1958).

separate perifollicular networks (DURWARD and RUDALL, 1958). Although small in diameter, these vessels continue to communicate among various groups of hairs even during the resting phase (DURWARD and RUDALL, 1958).

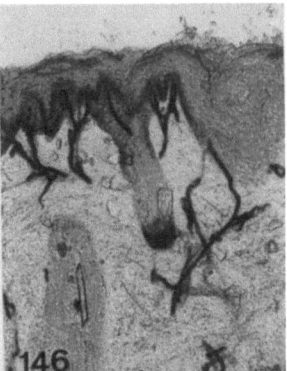

Fig. 146. The vasculature of the "lanugo" follicle consists only of some capillaries from the "dermal" network that surrounds the lower part of a follicle whose "dermal" papilla is highly reactive to alkaline phosphatase

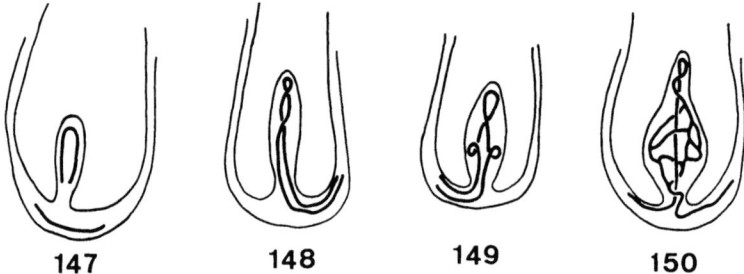

Figs. 147—150. Four drawings which indicate that a definite relationship exists between the size of the "dermal" papilla and the quantity of vessels contained therein i.e. the broader the papilla, the more vessels it contains. (RYDER, M. L., courtesy of the Comm. Scient. and Industr. Res. Organiz. Australia. In: Proceedings of the Int. Wool Textile Research Conference, Australia 1955, vol. F, 77)

3. The Vascular Unit

Some special structures, termed "vascular units" by us (MORETTI et al., 1959), complete the picture of vessel architecture just set down. Interposed (Fig. 164) between the horizontal vessel levels of the subepidermal and papillary regions and the higher ones of the perifollicular networks which they link up; the "vascular units" (Figs. 151—154a, b) probably correspond (MORETTI et al., 1959), at least in part, to the "vascular area" (BELLOCQ, 1925) and to the subpapillary vessel "cones" (SPALTEHOLZ, 1927) already described in the literature.

On vertical sections of facial skin treated with the alkaline phosphatase technique (MORETTI and MONTAGNA, 1959), the presence of two vascular bifurcations can be seen, which are open towards the epidermis and join with their

Fig. 151. An horizontal view of some adjoining "vascular units". Note ellipses containing some peripilary vascular ring (hair follicle: curved arrows), slight overlapping of the ellipses at the apices, narrow intermediate areas apparently supplied with fewer vessels (straight arrows). [MORETTI and MONTAGNA, courtesy of the G. ital. Derm., Le unità vascolari **3**, 249 (1959)]

Figs. 152—154a and b. Three photomicrographs of "vascular units" and their graphic reconstruction from serial sections. The inverted coneshaped structure, equal depth of lower apices and different "subepidermal" diameter are evident (Fig. 152a and b: skin of the nasolabial furrow. Fig. 153a and b: skin of the oral region. Figs. 154a and b: skin of the parotideo-masseteric region). [MORETTI and MONTAGNA, courtesy of the G. ital. Derm., Le unità vascolari **3**, 248 (1959)]

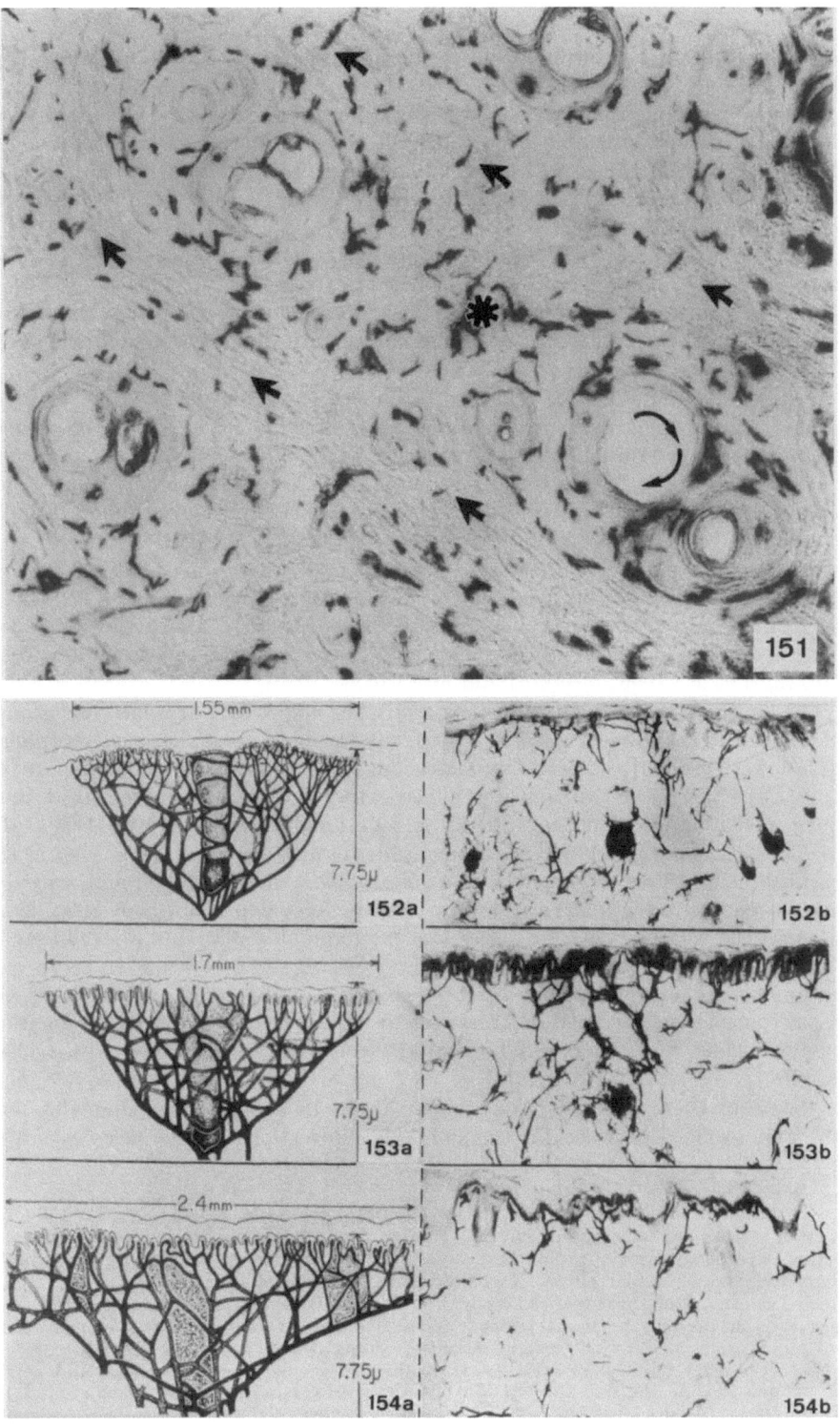

Figs. 151—154a and b. The "vascular unit". (For Legends see p. 590)

apices on the axis of terminal follicles or just under the papilla of lanugo type hairs (Figs. 152—154a, b).

When detaching themselves bilaterally from forks of this kind, some principal branches ascend to the epidermis and form in vertical sections two more or less triangular dermal areas with bases and upper subepidermal vertices almost touching; the lower vertex is 560 or 775 micron from the surface of the tegument (Figs. 152—154a, b).

At the two sides of the central axis formed by the hair follicle (either alone or accompanied by lateral hairs), two concentric triangles can thus be observed. From the principal branches 5 or 7 symmetrical branches arise from the double fork and go to the epidermis; each of these in turn divides and subdivides into various tertiary branches.

Altogether these oblique branches (primary, secondary and tertiary) with the arterioles and capillaries which cross them in a direction either parallel or perpendicular to the epidermis end up by forming above the 775 micron level a complicated vascular meshwork, that is roughly cone-shaped. This "vascular unit" surrounds one or more hair follicles, each of which is nourished by its own minor vascular circles (MORETTI et al., 1959; MORETTI and MONTAGNA, 1959).

On sections parallel to the cutaneous surface, at a depth of about 400 micron, especially in the chin, the "vascular units" appear as vascular elipses of varying lengths containing some peripilary vessel rings (Fig. 151). Depending upon the zone of the face, their widest diameter may range from one to two millimeters[49] (MORETTI et al., 1959; MORETTI and MONTAGNA, 1959).

Still on sections parallel to the epidermis, the ellipses are arranged like groups of hairs in alternate lines, with the narrow intermediate areas apparently supplied with fewer vessels. Inside the lines, adjoining ellipses that slightly overlap at the apices, the vessels of two touching ellipses cross and become entangled at their point of contact (MORETTI et al., 1959; MORETTI and MONTAGNA, 1959) (Fig. 151).

The "vascular units," on the other hand, are intercommunicating even in the vertical plane, either by means of horizontal vessels or perhaps through vascular arcades coming directly from the deep dermis. At a depth of about 800 micron beneath the surface epidermis, they lose their complex plan and are reduced to single rings around the hairs[50].

In this region around the excretory channels of the sweat glands, there are dense conical capillary networks arranged at regular intervals and joined together on the surface by branches of horizontal vessels and, deeper down, by arched vessels.

Some of these vascular areas, about 1 mm in subepidermal diameter, are probably grouped between the arms of wide bifurcations, visible below one mm in depth (BACCAREDDA-BOY et al., 1960a).

---

[49] The more medial regions of the face (frontal, oral, nasal, labial (Figs. 152, 153a, b), mental, orbital and infraorbital) having vascular units of lesser diameter seem to possess better superficial vascularization than that of the more lateral regions, (Figs. 153a, b) characterized by vascular elipses of greater width (MORETTI et al., 1959).

[50] The conic structures described by SPALTEHOLZ (1927) have a round or oval subepidermal base, with the apex on the dermal network and an average surface of about 0.16 mm². As they are ramifications of terminal arterioles, these, at first sight, would not seem to coincide with the vascular units, in relation to which they are smaller, more superficial, and above all not referable to the hair follicles. SPALTEHOLZ's data, however, do not really seem to be contradictory to ours since the skin he used was most likely glabrous skin from the plantar regions (SPALTEHOLZ, 1927). The smaller diameter may be due to the fact that his observations are always on a more superficial level. On the same plantar region, furthermore, our studies would seem to complement those of SPALTEHOLZ (1927).

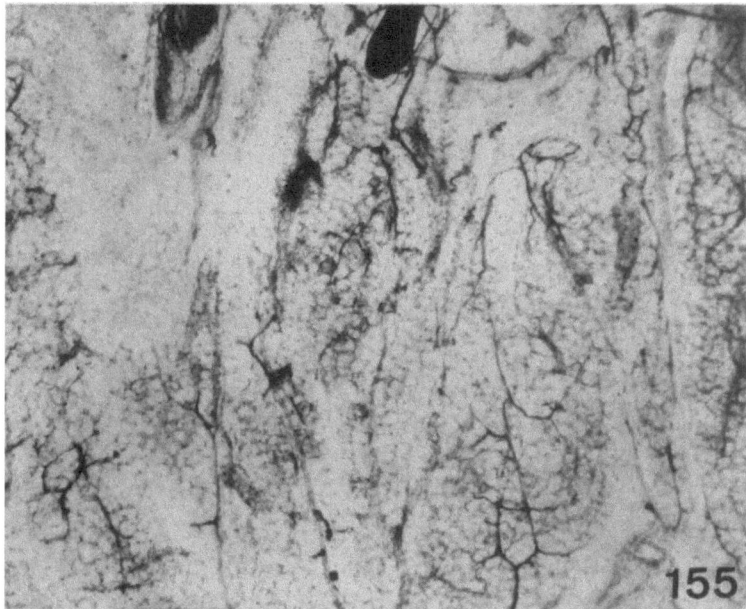

Fig. 155. Vessels in the "subcutaneous-fat". [CORMIA, F., courtesy of the Arch. Derm., Vasculature of the normal scalp **98**, 699 (1963)]

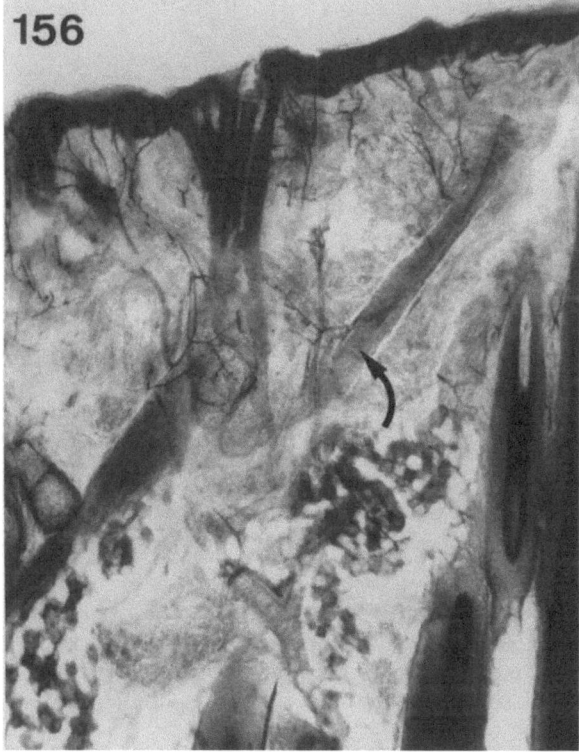

Fig. 156. The "arrectores pilorum" (curved arrow) are supplied by vessels insinuating themselves into the angle formed by the point of attachment of the muscle to the follicle. [CORMIA, F., courtesy of the Arch. Derm., Vasculature of the normal scalp **98**, 699 (1963)]

4. Smooth Muscles

The "arrectores pilorum" are supplied by capillary networks dependent on papillary vascularization or directly by hypodermal vessels (Fig. 155) (CORMIA and ERNYEY, 1961; CORMIA, 1963). According to TRUFFI (1934) in common with the hair follicle and the sebaceous gland, a small trunk insinuates itself into the angle formed by the point of attachment of the muscle to the bulbar portion of the follicle (Fig. 156). The "dartos tunic" depends instead upon capillaries originating from special branches of the cutaneous arteries (TOMSA, 1873; SPALTEHOLZ, 1927).

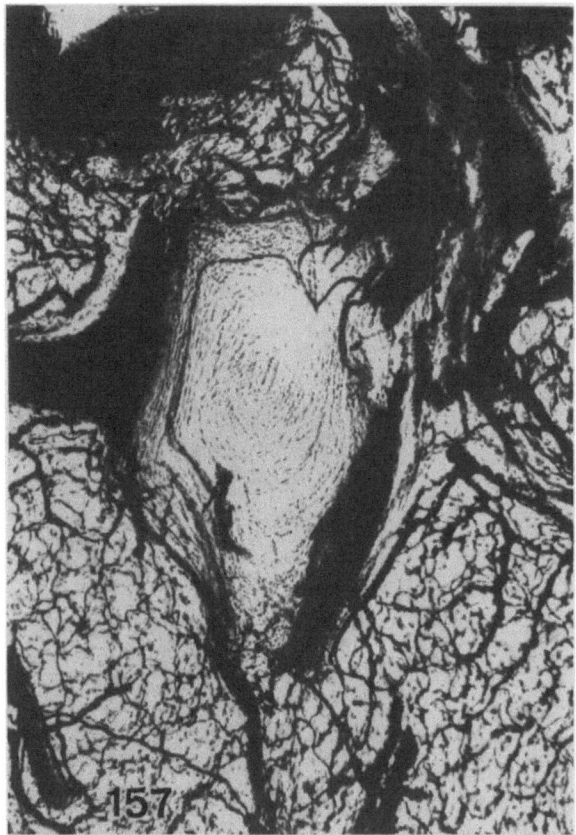

Fig. 157. The Vater-Pacini complex is provided with capillaries which supply the periphery of the outer capsula and chiefly one side of the inner layers. (WINKELMANN, R. K., courtesy of the Pergamon Press. In: Advances in biology of skin, vol. 2, p. 10. 1961)

5. Nerve Structures

The sensory nerve fibres are nourished, as far as the terminal corpuscles, by a capillary network (coming from vessels of the cutaneous network) with a mesh more or less closely adherent to the fibre, depending on its thickness (SPALTEHOLZ, 1927).

We have more detailed information on the vascularization of the Vater-Pacini complex. This is provided with capillaries which supply the various parts of the capsula and chiefly one side of the inner layers (Fig. 157) (WINKELMANN, 1961).

IV. The Distribution of the Venous Vessels in the Dermis and Subcutaneous (Appendages Included)

1. Networks Formed in the Dermis and Subcutaneous Tissue

In the descending tract of the papillary capillary loop, the blood is conveyed to the venous system. This is composed, like the arterial one, of more overlying horizontal networks anastomized in all directions as well as by periappendageal networks.

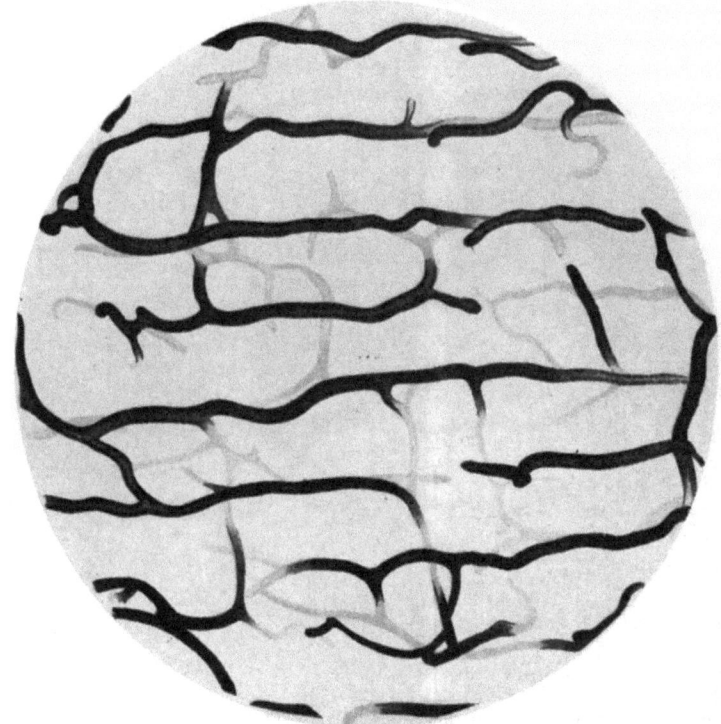

Fig. 158. An horizontal view of the "first venous or subpapillary dermal" network in the plantar region. [See also Figs. 116, 159. Reproduced from SPALTEHOLZ, W., courtesy of the Arch. Anat. Physiol., Die Verteilung der Blutgefäße in der Haut (1893)]

In the plantar region (Fig. 115), for example, the venous tract of the capillary drains, at the level of the bases of the cutaneous ridges, into a superficial venous network composed of vessels of wide diameter arranged parallel to the longitudinal axis of the cutaneous furrows and interconnected by oblique or transverse vessels. Each of these veins runs below a line of papillae and at the same time interweaves in the same direction with the downward arterial branches (SPALTEHOLZ, 1927).

The network thus created has extremely fine venules (a few hundredths of a millimeter in diameter) which offer a vast surface for the exchange of water and solutes between the tissue and the blood circulation: this is the "first venous or subpapillary dermal" network (Figs. 158, 161 and 164) (WETZEL and ZOTTERMANN, 1926).

From this first network a series of vessels sinking obliquely (Fig. 79) lead to a second venous dermal network of wide and regular polygonal meshwork (WINKELMANN, 1961) usually resting on the anastomotic arches of the underlying subpapillary arterial network (Figs. 159, 161 and 164) (SPALTEHOLZ, 1927).

Since it is close to the upper one, this network is, on the horizontal level, barely distinguishable from the first venous network, and many authors (DE SAUNDERS, 1961; DAVIS and LAWLER, 1961) talk of a single "subpapillary venous plexus" or "principal network" composed of wide or narrow venules connected by a network of venous arcades. The study of vertical sections, however, clearly indicates that one is dealing with two different overlying networks (SPALTEHOLZ, 1927).

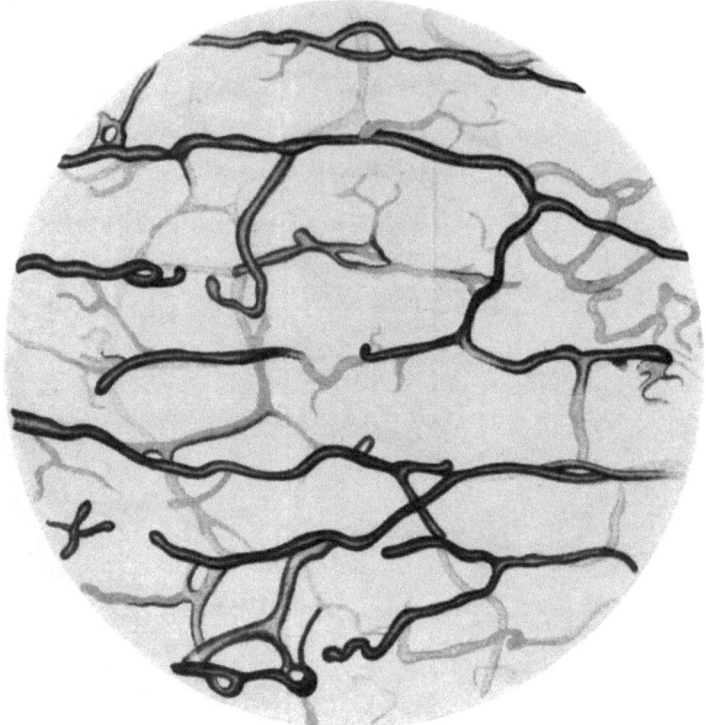

Fig. 159. A horizontal view of the "second venous dermal" network in the plantar region [see also Figs. 116, 158. SPALTEHOLZ, W., courtesy of the Arch. Anat. Physiol., Die Verteilung der Blutgefäße in der Haut (1893)]

Below the imposing venous development in the superficial dermis [because of the greater thickness of the vessels in comparison with the arterial network (DAVIS and LAWLER, 1961)] other venous networks follow in the deeper layers that are connected with the upper ones by candelabra venules (Fig. 78) (WINKELMANN, 1961) even though they are rather far apart. These networks possess venules and veins strongly anastomized and of progressively increasing diameter.

A third venous network is present between them in the middle dermis of the plantar region (SPALTEHOLZ, 1927). This is placed between the arterial "dermal (subpapillary)" and "cutaneous" networks and is composed of veins which, having left the vessel levels of the upper half of the dermis behind, often anastomize themselves forming a practically flat network of branches with no particular direction and meshes of varying dimensions that are sometimes more extensive than those of the subpapillary arterial network (SPALTEHOLZ, 1927).

It is characteristic of this meshwork that a large number of its vessels are made up of fine veins "which accompany the veins coming down from the upper layers" (SPALTEHOLZ, 1927). These accompanying vessels anastomize themselves, on the inside of the network, with similar or thicker branches. Sometimes they flank a vessel in pairs or run down separately; at other times they rest on other vessels or even open into them. These small accompanying veins, in their descent from the papillary layer to the deeper levels, often lean on arteries from which, on the contrary, the large veins separate (SPALTEHOLZ, 1927). In the corium, on the other hand, there are many more veins than arteries. Many veins, therefore, certainly do not accompany the arteries (SPALTEHOLZ, 1927). In the meantime, as we have said, the diameter of the venules increases steadily.

On the lower edges of the dermis, at about the height of the gland layer, the largest network is finally found, the fourth venous network, or so-called "venous cutaneous network" (Figs. 161 and 164), into which all the branches draining the fatty tissue, the hairs and the sweat glands (HORSTMANN, 1957) empty simultaneously. Of closer mesh than the corresponding arterial network, it is composed both of fine vessels lying almost on the same level as the arteries and above the glandular apparatus and of thick branches underlying the appendages (vascular level of the glands).

On the inside of the cutaneous network, the veins run separately from the arteries and are almost regularly surrounded by an elongated meshwork of thin vessels, which are likewise predominantly venous (SPALTEHOLZ, 1927)[51].

From the cutaneous network the veins flow down, sinking into a "subcutaneous" network. According to some (DODD and COCKETT, 1956) each subcutaneous tissue area thus discharges its venous blood into a nonanastomized "terminal" vein unconnected with the surrounding ones.

We have already spoken about the presence and debated location of valvules in the venous networks in the skin.

2. The Veins and Venules of the Appendages

For obvious drainage reasons, there is greater development of the veins in hairy than in glabrous skin, especially in the middle and lower levels of the dermis and the upper part of the hypodermis where the majority of the appendages are. From an architectural point of view, the interweaving of veins coming from the appendages usually corresponds to the arterial ones, even though they are external and provided with larger vessels (Fig. 164) (TRUFFI, 1934; BIMTS, 1960). As a result, around the follicle the veins form periappendageal networks which discharge into branches destined for the superficial venous plexus or to the deeper venous one (BIMTS, 1960). Furthermore, in catagen before the venous branches disappear around the lower two-thirds of the arterial peri-follicular net they take part of the catabolites, originating from the destruction of the hair, to the deep veins. The venous network supplying the upper third of the follicle remains intact and is directed surfacewards.

As for the papilla, the venous out-flow of the numerous capillary loops which penetrate the pore of the dermal papilla are collected by a very small afferent vein of the venous follicular system (SPALTEHOLZ, 1927; TOMSA, 1873).

The sebaceous gland is enveloped in a venous network which presumably empties at the venous subpapillary level.

The sweat glands have a periductal capillary network which conveys the blood to elongated veins that are slightly serpentine and not infrequently looped and go to the superficial venous networks and veins entrusted with the drainage of the glomerular region (WINKELMANN, 1961) which then connect with the cutaneous network (SPALTEHOLZ, 1927).

---

[51] The latter are probably the same "vasa vasorum" recently observed (WINKELMANN, 1961) around the deep collector veins.

In the nail, the venous tract of the capillary loops in the hyponychium is dilated and serpiginous (RENAUT, 1897 cit. HORSTMANN, 1957).

3. Regional Aspects and Factors which May Influence the Appearance of the Veins and Cutaneous Venules

We know almost nothing about the regional appearances of the venous system. According to WETZEL and ZOTTERMANN (1926), the average diameter of the subpapillary venules varies with the region; 63 microns on the cheek, 37 microns on the ears, 17 microns on the forearm, 32 microns on the finger knuckles. Another regional aspect was described by SPALTEHOLZ (1927) who remarked the frequent accompaniment of many large and small subcutaneous veins with numerous thin or thick anastomatic chains of the "fascial" arterial network, in the upper and lower limbs.

Further information has been obtained with a microangiographic method: in the eyelids venous vessels reach the commissure perpendicularly and form long arches; in the scalp their network has wide meshes; in the ear it follows a shrublike pattern; on the dorsum of the nose their configuration recalls that of birds' nests (DE SOUSA and RODRIGUES, 1962).

The condition of the adipose tissue, on the other hand, also influences the venous system. As long as, for any reason, there is little subcutaneous fat, the venous blood that flows from it pours into the "cutaneous" network (SPALTEHOLZ, 1927). When, on the contrary, the fatty tissue increases (as, for example, in embryonic life), the venous blood is emptied into the veins of the "fascial" network. The adipose tissue, from a venous as well as from an arterial point of view is, therefore, divided into two layers, the lower belonging to the deeper vascular districts, the upper to the ones nearer the surface (SPALTEHOLZ, 1927).

Depending on the volume of the adipose lobule, the distribution scheme of the vein which accompanies the arteries perforating the "retinaculum" also varies. In the small lobules, the arteries enter from one side and the veins go out at the other; in the larger lobules the arteries perforate the axis of the lobule from which the veins come out, in pairs and from several points (SPALTEHOLZ, 1927).

4. Smooth Muscles

The venous blood coming from the "arrectores pilorum" like that of the "dartos tunic" pours into the papillary venous system (TOMSA, 1873; SPALTEHOLZ, 1927).

5. Nerve Structures

According to the site of the nerve, its venous blood goes to the fatty tissue, the glandular papillary, or the "cutaneous" network (RUFFINI, 1900 cit. SPALTEHOLZ, 1927).

V. Arteriovenous Anastomosis of the Dermis

We have already mentioned the characteristic construction of the cutaneous arteriovenous anastomoses. Let us recall that in the tips of the toes and in the finger tips of the upper and lower limbs typical glomic structures are usually integrated into the vasal architecture at depths averaging between 1 and 1.5 mm from the surface. Consequently they are at about the height of the second order of arterial arcades and a little above the cutaneous venous network (MESCON et al., 1956).

The existence of anastomotic channels between arterial and venous circulation at the level of the subpapillary network seems a moot point (DAVIS and LAWLER, 1961).

E. An Outline of the Blood Cutaneous Network Design
I. Preliminary Remarks

Elsewhere in these pages we have outlined a history of the people concerned in these studies and the progress of their research, which demonstrates how in science an advance may be followed by a reversal and how ideas are rediscovered sooner or later. These inevitable shifts can probably be imputed to the prevailing scientific thought of the time, to the techniques available, and sometimes even to illustrations which concentrate attention for decades on hypotheses which are not entirely valid.

From this review it would nevertheless appear that since the known facts outnumber the unknown (above all as regards functional significance) a scheme of the blood network in the skin which conforms to reality can now be traced.

Leaving aside events of slight current interest, we shall endeavor to isolate the fundamental results, in the history of our subject, which have enabled us to reach the present day functional anatomical concept of the vascular cutaneous network.

II. How the Blood Vessel Cutaneous Network was Envisaged before Spalteholz

Between the end of the 18th and 19th centuries, those interested in cutaneous vascularization did not distinguish between the vessels which nourish the surface of the epidermis and the vessels of the appendages.

Before plexuses were detected, the authors applied themselves to the glands' blood supply and to that of the follicles, the adipose lobules, the arteriovenous anastomoses (TODD and BOWMAN, 1845; KOELLIKER, 1856; SUCQUET, 1862; etc.) or to the type of vessels which reach the skin (MANCHOT, 1889) as unconnected facts without coordinating them into one complete anatomic framework.

In spite of this, the work of TOMSA (1873), the most noteworthy of his time, made it possible for the dynamic aspects and extraordinarily modern morphofunctional observations to emerge. The circulation of the pilosebaceous unit is seen as a continuation of that of the papillary body. Some of his figures illustrating the peripilary capillary network and the vessels which sometimes (in catagen) surround the swollen and wrinkled glassy membrane are the first indirect recognition of the network's capacity for cyclical mutation. An articulated blood supply for some glands is recognized and the vessels from different parts are seen to supply different parts of the sweat glands. The existence of a direct relationship between metabolic requirement and blood nutrition of tissue is also suggested by both the strict correlation between the development of the overlying epidermis and the amount of blood flow to the papillary region and the fact that, in the latter, the total capillary diameter is in inverse proportion to the surface supplied by a single vessel.

The same author, on the other hand, while completing his work with some tables (Fig. 160) which suggest the plexuses and describe some of them does not greatly concern himself with, nor considers absolutely essential, the presence of plexuses or networks in which the blood is collected before being sent to or after returning from the epidermis or the appendages.

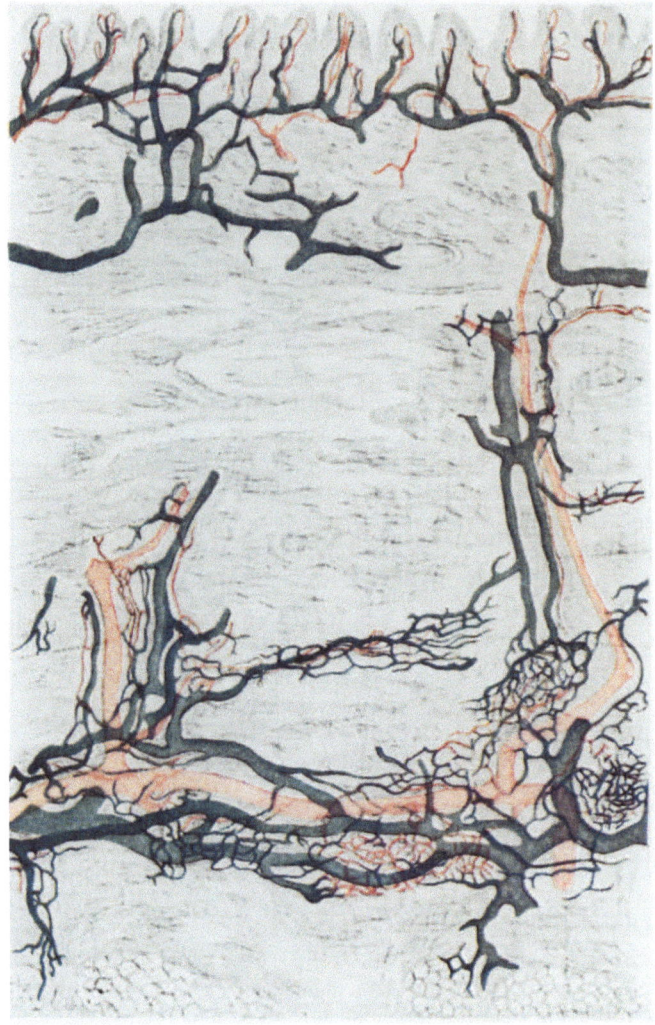

Fig. 160. Tomsa's extraordinarily modern observations. The vessels of "subepidermal", "dermal", "cutaneous" plexues and the elaborate systems surrounding the eccrine glands' duct and secretory portion are clearly evident (reproduction of a table published by the author in 1873). [TOMSA, W., courtesy of the Arch. Derm. Syph. (Berl.), Beiträge zur Anatomie und Physiologie der menschlichen Haut 1, 5 (1873)]

III. Spalteholz's View of the Blood Network

In contrast with his predecessors, SPALTEHOLZ gave a really systematic and detailed, even though static, picture.

The whole course of the blood network is crystallized by the author into different specified vessel levels, as the points of arrival and departure, of a progressively increasing or decreasing series of arterial or venous vessels. Furthermore he describes more or less strong meshworks and networks, which are of varying amplitude, but at the same time pays little attention to elements which are characteristic from a descriptive point of view, such as arcades. Other features that are even more pretentious like, "candelabra" venules and arterioles, entirely

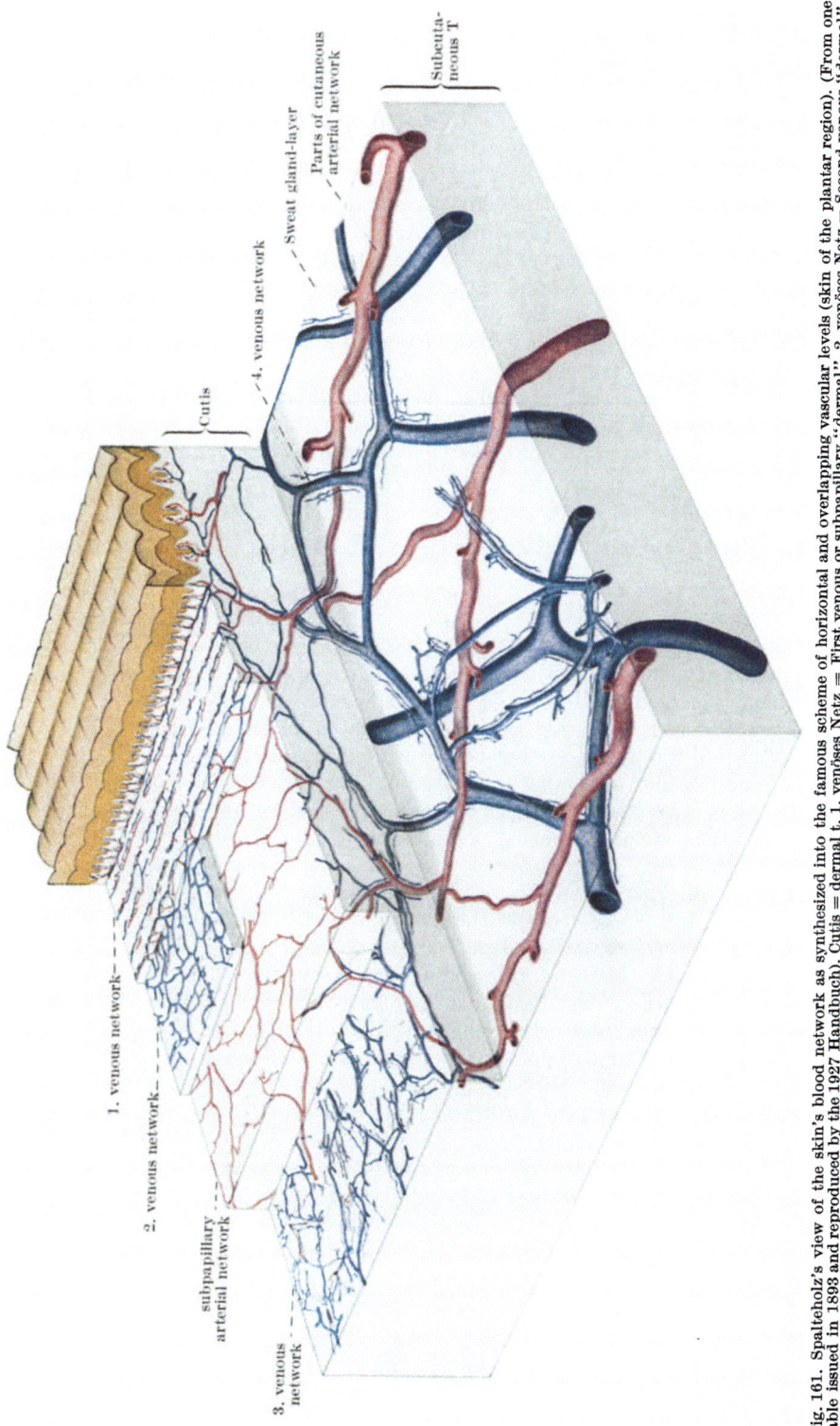

Fig. 161. Spalteholz's view of the skin's blood network as synthesized into the famous scheme of horizontal and overlapping vascular levels (skin of the plantar region). (From one table issued in 1893 and reproduced by the 1927 Handbuch). Cutis = dermal t. 1. venöses Netz = First venous or subpapillary "dermal". 2. venöses Netz = Second venous "dermal". Subpapillares arterielles Netz = Subpapillary or "dermal" arterial network. 3. venöses Netz = Third venous "dermal" network. 4. venöses Netz = "Cutaneous" venous network. Schweißdrüsenschicht = Sweat glands' vascular level. Teile des cutanen arteriellen Netzes = "Cutaneous" arterial network (part of). Subcutis = Subcutaneous t. [SPALTEHOLZ, W., courtesy of the Arch. Anat. Physiol., Die Verteilung der Blutgefäße in der Haut (1893)]

escape him. This is all well shown in his illustrations, especially in one table (Fig. 16, 1893; Fig. 8, 1927) issued for the first time in 1893 and reproduced in the 1927 Handbuch which in its numerous later editions probably influenced authors of several generations, since it represented the most valid graphic synthesis of our knowledge and theories on the subject of that time (Fig. 161).

His viewpoint seems to exclude the necessity for "ad hoc" networks for the nourishment of the appendages. It is, therefore, almost surprising that SPALTEHOLZ was interested in the periappendageal networks even though he dedicated only 2 of the 55 pages in the Handbuch[52] to them and completely ignored the fact that the perifollicular network, by no means an unimportant part of vascular architecture, is subject to profound cyclic modifications.

Although almost a century old, SPALTEHOLZ's work is still the accepted basis for current knowledge of cutaneous vascularization and for the attention brought to bear upon its regional aspects.

One need only recall that any consideration of thermoregulation among the other tasks of cutaneous circulation would be unacceptable without his preliminary description of the site and the progressive approach of the plexuses to the epidermis.

IV. The Modern Conception of the Cutaneous Blood Network

SPALTEHOLZ's work and that of his predecessors made available a vast series of data for research workers, which was later synthesized into a solid background.

The majority of authors today seem basically to agree, both on the continuity of the arterial capillary venous network and on the static and dynamic organization scheme repeatedly described in previous pages.

Certain aspects of these two points still have to be examined and clarified chiefly because of the prospects that they open for future research.

Concerning the first, it should be pointed out that the traditional view of the constantly branching vessel tree is now supplanted by new hypotheses, each one giving recognition to the increasing complexity of the arterial capillary-venous circuit[53].

CHAMBERS and ZWEIFACH, for example, considered the possibility that in animals at least, the blood bypasses the normal arterial-capillary-venous circuit, by flowing into "preferential central" or peripheral "axial" channels which shorten the distance between artery and vein. Granting that, these central channels are contractile "vascular bridges" from which capillaries provided with muscle sphincters branch out (pre-capillary sphincters). The blood supply to the true capillaries thus depends upon the functional state of these vascular bridges (CHAMBERS and ZWEIFACH, 1949).

More recently, DE SAUNDERS (DE SAUNDERS et al., 1957; DE SAUNDERS, 1961) by means of X-ray microradiography, singled out another type of capillary network in man, more or less between those described in the post-malpighian period and after CHAMBERS and ZWEIFACH. In addition to the "central" or "axial" channels which directly connect the arteries with the veins, the arteriolar and venular meshes are linked either by a capillary reticulum or by small arteriovenous

---

[52] A possible reason for this may be found in the method used: SPALTEHOLZ usually worked on injected glabrous skins, stretched on boards, and so cut into parallel sections (SPALTEHOLZ, 1893).

[53] This seems to rule out most of the hypothesis stated by BELLOCQ (1925), SALMON (1936) and others; even if, as we shall see, the existence of "vascular units" seems to suggest the presence of vessel districts, in that some areas at least are connected to the surrounding ones in a particular way.

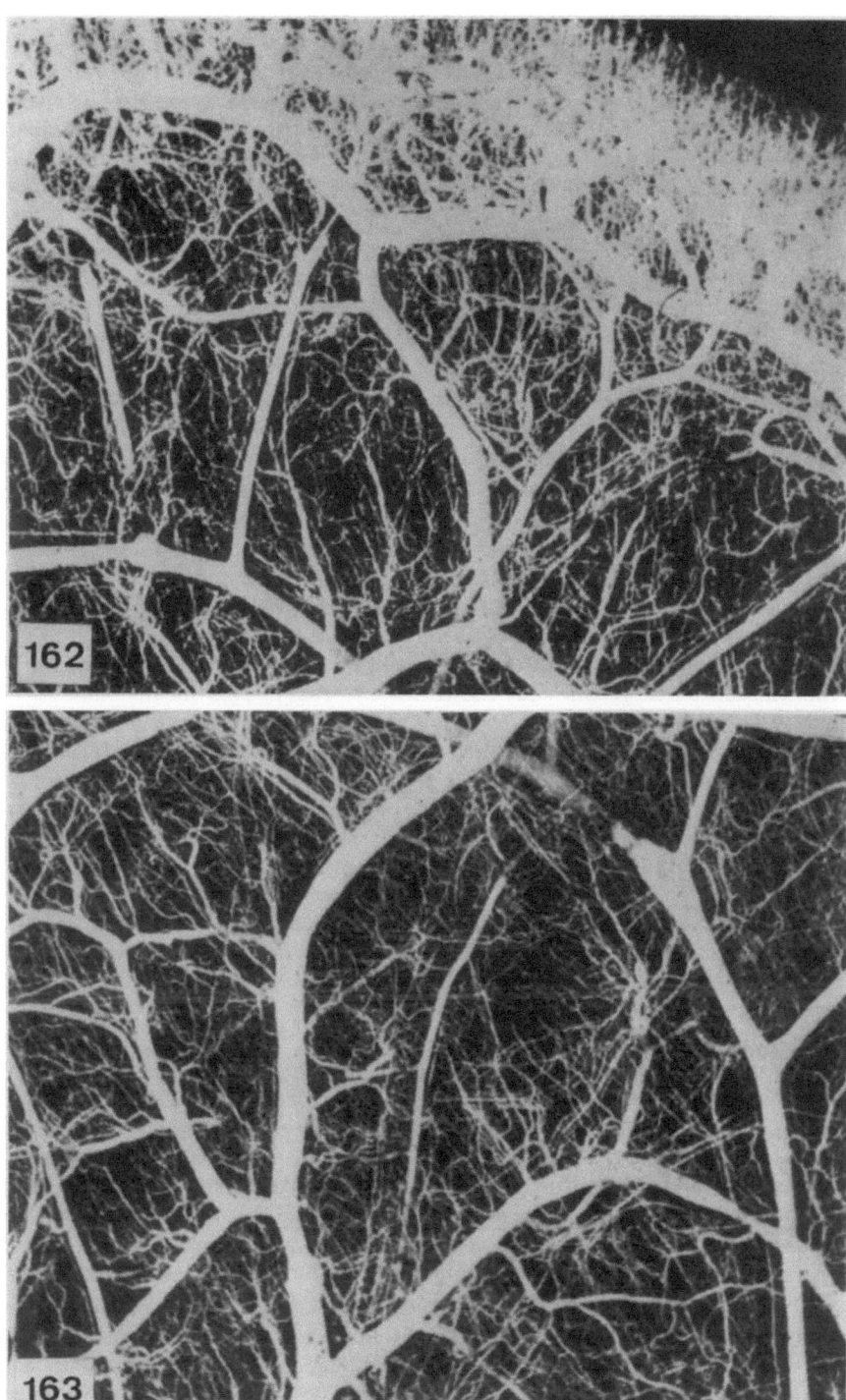

Figs. 162 and 163. In the rabbit's ear two micro-angiograms show an extremely developed continuous vascular network with either fine or coarse meshes (macromeshes and micromeshes), robust arcades and details of the capillary bed. (DE SAUNDERS, R. L. courtesy of the Pergamon Press. In: Advances in biology of skin, vol. 2, p. 51. 1961)

anastomoses. This model is also true of other animals. In the rabbit's ear (Figs. 162 and 163), for example, a rather wide continuous network of varying-sized vessels provided with either fine or coarse meshes, has small arteries connected by a series of arcades that form first a coarse meshwork (macromesh) containing in its turn a second finer meshwork (micromesh) of arterioles, capillaries, and venules. There are also frequent arteriovenous anastomoses directly linking the small arterioles to the larger veins (DE SAUNDERS, 1961).

These two types of meshwork, the small as well as the large, function as a reservoir and a distributor as well as a pressure equalizator for the blood. They can provoke at the same time both "high level" anastomotic circulation and "low level" nutritive circulation for the enclosed tissue islands (DE SAUNDERS, 1961).

Concerning the development scheme, I wish to emphasize that as far as the dermis is concerned, because of the already stated reasons of comparative and normal anatomy (see part IV of this chapter) there should be definitively introduced into the nomenclature, in addition to the series of "fascial," "cutaneous" [middle dermis in some regions (MORETTI et al., 1959)], and "dermal or subpapillary" plexuses, the "subepidermal or papillary" plexus as well.

Some important distinctions between the networks should then be traced. While it is the "fascial" network that chiefly supplies the well developed subcutaneous fat (SPALTEHOLZ, 1927), it is the wide meshworks, as well as the strong muscular vessels of the "cutaneous," arterial, and venous networks, which in man [and in animals (RYDER, 1955)] have the task of distributing the blood suitably to the various parts of the skin (SPALTEHOLZ, 1927). This means that at the boundary between dermis and hypodermis an "internal vascular belt" (Figs. 1 and 164) exists as a junction between extracutaneous and cutaneous circulation and, at the same time, as a control over the latter. On the upper layer of the dermis, the arterial "dermal" or "subpapillary" network, with its close meshes and delicate vessels, the subepidermal capillaries which depend on it for numerous rami and the two interposed venous networks all together nourish the epidermal structures. The extreme closeness of each of these networks to one another is, however, conspicuously opposed to the distance which separates them from other networks the "cutaneous," the "fascial," and the "deep one." In the skin "in toto" therefore the vascular development of the last hundreds of microns of the subepidermal structures is quantitatively more vast and more elaborate than that lying millimeters deeper down.

The vessel region contained in the space between the dermo-epidermal line and the lower limits of the papillary layer is distinguished, therefore, very neatly from the underlying dermis. Thus, immediately under the ectodermal cover, the tegument in mammals possesses a true "external vascular belt" which contains in its venous section 70% of the blood vital for thermoregulation (PETERSEN, 1935) and to which we owe, to a great extent, the color of the skin (WETZEL and ZOTTERMAN, 1926; WINKELMANN et al., 1961) and in which can be noticed characteristic cutaneous vessel phenomena of defense and adaptation (ROTHMAN, 1954).

The existence of such an "external vascular belt," on the other hand, throws a ray of light on some aspects of the perifollicular and perisebaceous networks hitherto obscure. The division of the former into two fractions, "permanent" and "transient" (see part IV of this chapter), results from the vascular organization of the permanent part and of the external vascular belt being practically identical; the former appears to be the natural continuation of the latter just as the connective papillary tissue continues into the connective tissue which surrounds the upper third of the pilosebaceous follicle.

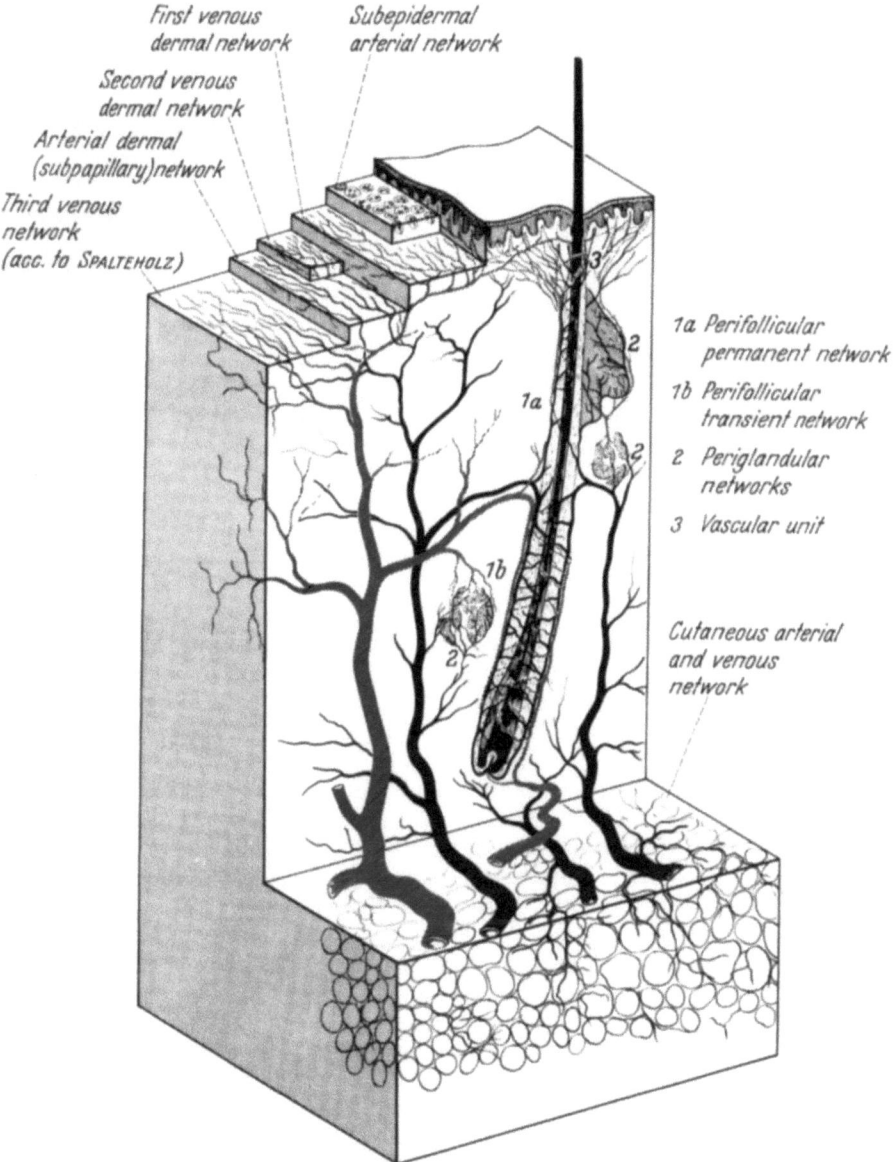

Fig. 164. Our conception of the cutaneous blood network. (Compare with Figs. 1, 160, 161 and 164)

From this point of view, the upper part of the longitudinal perifollicular vessels would have a value substantially equivalent to that of the subpapillary vascular levels, while those anastomotic horizontals and the other branches that depend on them would correspond to the vessels of the subepidermal network. The same concept holds good for the hyponychial loops of the nails which lie in the ridges parallel to the lamina and correspond to the subpapillary network (HORSTMANN, 1957).

This interpretation of a part of the perifollicular network renders the organization scheme of cutaneous vessel tissue clearer, and simplifies the explanation of other phenomena: 1) that in aging (ELLIS, 1958) in alopecia areata (GANS and STEIGLEDER, 1955; KLINGMULLER, 1955) and in seborrheic hairfall according to some, the sebaceous glands of the scalp are enlarged, suggesting that the vascularization of the sebaceous gland may be independent of that of the hair follicles (TRUFFI, 1934) and after the involution of the hair and its vascular network, the gland may draw more heavily than before upon the increased reserves of the external vascular belt; 2) that in catagen (ELLIS and MORETTI, 1959) the horizontal and longitudinal anastomotic vessels surrounding the follicle remain intact for a long time, even when the peribulbar vessel mesh and the capillaries of the dermal papilla are already degenerating or have disappeared, may mean that their temporary maintenance is from blood coming in some way from the external vascular belt (through the sebaceous circuit, for example) while the papilla essentially supplied by deep vessels (CORMIA and ERNYEY, 1961) would suffer greatly (from unknown antivessel factors?) during the transition phase; 3) finally, it is very likely that the regression observed in all subepidermal vessels, when for some reason the terminal follicles transform themselves into lanugo ones (MONTAGNA, 1958), may be due to a large reduction in the functional load of the external vascular belt normally used for the bigger follicles.

Regarding the vasal organization scheme, "the vascular unit" (Fig. 164) still remains to be exactly defined.

Without repeating ourselves (see part IV of this chapter), here let us recall that the "units" observed in some regions of the tegument and especially those related to the hairs are not at all new. The literature shows, in fact, that the recognition of well- and poorlysupplied vascular territories occurred long ago. According to UNNA, the more superficial skin regions are occupied by "vessel cones" the size of a lentil, connected by collateral capillaries (UNNA, 1894). RENAUT maintained that the skin was divided into numerous areas or "vascular units" supplied by a deep artery (RENAUT, 1897, cit. SPALTEHOLZ, 1927). The cutaneous surface is divided into territories with rounded or oval bases, each one composed of a superficial vascularization cone connected to the adjacent ones by arteriovenous anastomoses through which the blood does not pass easily. Round or elliptical "fields of complete blood supply" united by arteriovenous anastomosis, however, alternate with "fields of anastomotic supply." SPALTEHOLZ criticized UNNA's and RENAUT's hypotheses: the former did not notice the existence of anastomosis between the cutaneous arteries, and the latter did not consider that the apex of the vessel cone being below the dermis necessarily ended by being connected with the surrounding cones not from one but from two levels of anastomosis. At least two anastomotic networks exist one above the other in the dermis, of which the "cutaneous" network is provided with far from narrow anastomotic channels.

If, instead, the vessel cone began above the cutaneous network, the anastomosis in question could only be that of the "dermal" network even though these are rather narrow in relation to the other vessels of the network [54].

However incomplete anatomists' information may be, the hypothesis that the organization of the more superficial layers of the vessel network include vasal

---

[54] IRAGUE (cit. LO CASCIO, 1913) encountered areas of full circulation in the face, palmar and plantar regions — those, that is, supplied with structures of the vascular unit type (SPALTEHOLZ, 1927; MORETTI et al., 1959) which are connected by means of intradermal ramifications only. Furthermore, still according to IRAGUE, areas of full circulation formed by apparently independent vascular territories are found in the dorsal regions of the hand and foot. In fact, I saw a subject burned on the back of the hand who presented hyperpigmented circular spots some millimeters in diameter and separated by thin depigmented tracts.

architecture of the "unit" type seems to be supported by wide clinical and experimental data. The injection of colored substances into a cadaver immediately produces minute round or oval patches (the bases of vessel cones and, therefore, areas of maximum circulation?) initially separated by tracts of normal skin color (area of reduced circulation comparable to the areas between the various ellipses?) (UNNA, 1894; RENAUT, 1897[55]).

With injections of trypan blue one can obtain spots and rings, depending on the skin area, caused by infiltrate reactive at the center of the injected zone. If the ring were caused by the mass of the infiltrate which mechanically pushes the coloring back to the periphery, then the central vessels from which the infiltrate repels the colorant must have a circular arrangement (PERRUCCIO, 1935). In the early stage of scarlet fever and in septic infections, characteristic patches appear with dimensions corresponding to the capillary territories supplied by terminal branches (SPALTEHOLZ, 1927). Petecchiae have an average diameter of between one to five millimeters (PILLSBURY et al., 1956). The smallest of the vascular units described by us therefore expands as much as the smallest purpuric lesion. The anemic nevus is circular in shape (SUTTON, 1956). In MAJOCCHI's purpura, a purpuric ring is formed (RADAELLI, 1911; LEVER, 1949). The papular telangiectases (REDISCH and PELZER, 1949) are round, etc.

Finally, the existence of structures of the "vascular unit" type seem largely justified in theory since in establishing the simplest connection between the "external vascular belt" and the individual perifollicular networks (Fig. 164) they guarantee the best possible supply to the infundibular region while enclasping at the same time more pilary appendages, even of various types, in the same vascular system.

F. Conclusions

Notwithstanding the obvious task of nourishing an organ constituting 10% of body weight and an area, in the adult, of approximately 1.8 square meters, the venous arterial capillary network in the skin, as in other organs, is certainly not absolutely indispensable. This is indicated directly or indirectly by 1. the formations of subepidermal and periappendageal networks when a moderate degree of development already exists in the structures supplied (see part II of this chapter); 2. the avascular development and differentiation in tissue culture of the hair follicles (HARDY, 1951); 3. the apparent degeneration of the latter structures in catagen whenever the perifollicular network is still mostly intact (ELLIS and MORETTI, 1959); 4. the appearance in healing alopecia areas, still without vessels, of absolutely normal follicles (Fig. 165) (RAMPINI et al., 1963); 5. the appearance of a subpapillary blood supply in the dermal papilla in the eyelash only after the formation of the entire structure (ENGEL, 1907; cit. LO CASCIO, 1913).

The hair follicle that we see developed in vitro, on the other hand, produces keratin in a much smaller quantity than the follicle in vivo, while the hairs regrowing in alopecia patches initially present a thin and scarcely pigmented hair.

---

[55] On the substances capable of coloring first some and then other parts of a cadaver's skin, SPALTEHOLZ (1927) contends that these deductions are not valid for living subjects. Even admitting that his objections have weight, the fact remains that by using a histochemical technique which was entirely different we too have reached conclusions more or less similar to those of UNNA.

If, then, survival of the skin and its appendages and vascularization are not proportional phenomena, to a certain extent the functional capability of the cutaneous structure and the development of the vascular network may be proportional.

On closer observation, the way in which the capillaries introduce and divide in the dermal papilla in man and other mammals is, in fact, similar to if not exactly the same as, that of a narrow superficial papilla (RYDER, 1955; BACCA-REDDA-BOY et al., 1960a; MORETTI and FARRIS, 1963).

On a purely morphological level, furthermore, it is well substantiated that for all the sites of intense keratogenesis a particular type of vascularization of the papilla exists in mammals. In man a marked development of superficial

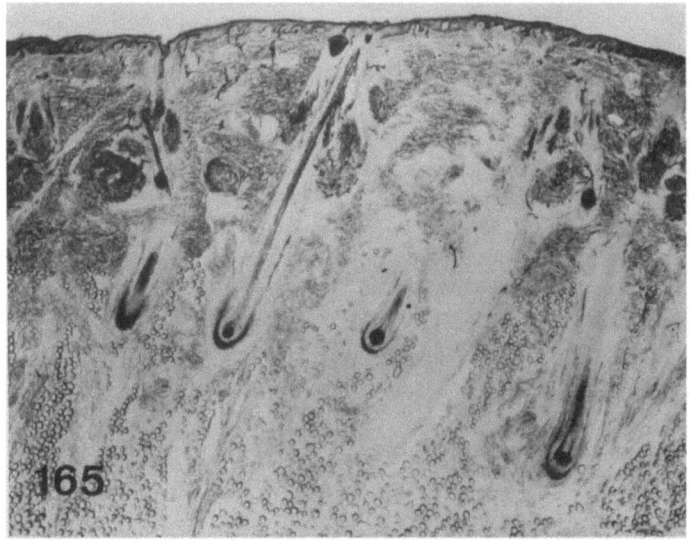

Fig. 165. Healing alopecia areata patches: absolutely normal follicles are still without vessels. [RAMPINI, MORETT and REBORA, courtesy of the Minerva derm., Arteriole e capillari della cute ed alopecia areata. Atti SIDES **38** 303 (1963)]

and dermal papilla corresponds to the high keratogenesis of the epidermis or hair as well as an abundant capillary network; similarly in the hippopotamus, the pig, the dolphin, the whale, and many other animals with a very strong keratinic mantle, the abundant mesoderm enclosed by the ectodermal structures is penetrated by a very thick meshwork and sometimes by a true capillary coil (see part II of this chapter). Further confirmation of these hypotheses lies in the existence of a close relationship between the development of the papilla and of the capillary network on the one hand and the diameter of the hair produced on the other (RYDER, 1955).

At this point, at any rate, the limits of these phenomena go far beyond the vessel, since in any hystangic zone (see note, page 24) both the metabolic and respiratory processes are true processes of correlation between vessels and tissues (COMEL and MIAN, 1961).

Information on the intimate structure and biochemical organization of the capillary (of which, as we have said, each organ possesses one type) takes on consequent importance in understanding the functional anatomy of the organ which contains it. In zones of mesodermal-ectodermal interaction like the papillae for instance, the capillary indirectly supplies information on the tegument also [56].

The strict capillary-tissue correlation, furthermore, in the skin takes on particular values for thermoregulatory purposes. A good example of this are the nails (Fig. 127): at no other point in the skin do the morpho-functional capacities of the cutaneous vessel network betray their predominant significance so clearly.

In the region of the matrix, the papillae having disappeared, the low mounds visible are supplied only by capillary tufts; lengthened masses follow, in the long connective ridges of the hyponychium, arranged in parallel and sometimes overlying tubes. These are gradually supplanted by the pronounced spirals of capillaries which literally throng the robust papillae of the plantar region whenever the dermal epidermal line again becomes undulating (Fig. 127).

This variety of vessel structures emphasizes, according to HORSTMANN (1957), their predominant thermoregulatory task; in the ridges of the anterior part of the hyponychium, a site covered by an abundant keratinic mantle, the shape and site of the capillary roughly corresponds to those of a cooling apparatus, the function of which they perform; in the acral region at the beginning of the plantar horny layer, the capillary serpentines instead perform the task of true heating spirals (HORSTMANN, 1957).

Before closing this chapter, it may be profitable to repeat that, besides keeping alive the covering of the human body, the primary task of the vascularization of the skin is probably thermoregulatory. Within its structure the skin, in fact, includes a truly poikilothermic structure, the epidermis, which forms part of an otherwise homeothermic system. The underlying layers must, therefore, interpose a sort of vascular protective zone between the epidermis and the deeper tissues and keep the body temperature constant. For this purpose, there is a preponderant richness of vessels in the layers immediately under the epidermis, the distribution of the network into overlying plexuses which separate tissue levels of different insulating materials (epidermis, subcutaneous adipose tissue, and muscle layer), the probably secondary importance of the periappendageal vessel apparatus and other facts, among which are included the regional differences of the varying blood supplies from the very abundant one on the face to the relatively poor one in areas like the knee and the tibia (HERTZMANN, 1938).

More extensive and deeper knowledge on the percentage of blood used for thermoregulation, which adapts, on the one hand, to the external world, and on the other, to the internal environment, will come only from functional studies and dynamic biochemistry. This belongs to the future, whose shadowy outlines these pages may in some measure help to define.

The author wishes to aknowledge the precious collaboration of Mrs. MARY COTTON for translation the work and of Mr. ARNALDO LEPRINI for the drawings.

References [57]

A. Introduction

ALLEN, E. V., N. W. BARKER, and E. A. HYNES: Peripheral vascular diseases, p. 871. London: W. B. Saunders Co. 1955. — ARNOLD, J.: Über die Glomeruli caudales der Säugetiere. Virchows Arch. path. Anat. **36**, 497 (1867).

BELLOCQ, P.: Étude anatomique des artères de la peau chez l'homme. Paris: Masson & Cie. 1925. — BETTMANN, S.: Steuerungsbefunde im Gefäßenabschnitt der Haut. Arch. Derm.

---

[56] In the skin the correlation between metabolic activity of the endothelium and surrounding tissue is stressed by the fact that the number of vessels contained in one papilla is as small as the phosphatase capacity of the endothelium is great (MONTAGNA and ELLIS, 1957; MONTAGNA, 1962; RYDER, 1955). We can deduce that the metabolic power of one unit of endothelium surface (admitting that the phosphatase reactivity has this meaning) is as great as the whole endothelial surface of which an enzyme may dispose is small.

[57] References are given up to the end of 1966.

Syph. (Berl.) **157**, 105 (1929). — Capillarmikroskopische Untersuchungen an der Lippenschleimhaut. Arch. Derm. Syph. (Berl.) **162**, 480 (1930). — BIANCHI, L.: Connettivo e vasi in ambito cutaneo. Minerva derm. **36**, 309 (1961). — BORDLEY, J., M. H. GROW, and W. B. SHERMAN: Intermittent blood flow in the capillaries of human skin. Bull. Johns Hopk. Hosp. **62**, 1 (1938). — BORELLO, P.: Quoted from Microfotografie in vivo, vol. 2 (L. ILLIG and H. CONRATHS, eds.). Ingelheim a. Rh.: Boehringer 1960. — BRAASCH, N. K., and M. J. NICKSON: A study of the hands of radiologists. Radiology **51**, 719 (1948). — BRAUN-FALCO, O., u. D. PETZOLDT: Über die Histotopie von NADH- und NADPH-Tetrazoliumreduktase in menschlicher Haut. Arch. klin. exp. Derm. **220**, 455 (1964). — BUCCIANTE, L.: Referto bioptico nell'uomo di arteriole provviste di cuscinetti peduncolati. Monit. zool. ital. **56** (Suppl.), 208 (1948). — Anastomosi arterio-venose e dispositivi regolatori del flusso sanguigno. Monit. zool. ital. **57** (Suppl.), 3 (1949). — La morfologia dei vasi sanguiferi sulla base di moderne acquisizioni. Atti III Giorn. Ital. Med. Triest 1950. — BURTON, A. C.: Physiology of cutaneous circulation, thermo-regulatory functions. In: The human integument normal and abnormal (S. ROTHMAN, ed.). Amer. Ass. Adv. Sci., Washington D. C. 1959. — Special features of the circulation of the skin. In: Advances in biology of skin, vol. II. Blood vessels and circulation, p. 117 (W. MONTAGNA and R. A. ELLIS, eds.). New York: Pergamon Press 1961.

CASSEBOHM, J. F.: Quoted by J. HYRTL. In: Manuale di dissezione pratica. Bologna 1886. — CHAMBERS, R., and B. W. ZWEIFACH: Topography and function of the mesenterie capillary circulation. Amer. J. Anat. **75**, 173 (1944). — CHIALE, C.: Delle modificazioni dei vasi cutanei inerenti all'età. G. ital. Derm. Sif. **682**, 163 (1927). — CLARA, M.: Die arteriovenösen Anastomosen der Vögel und Säugetiere. Ergebn. Anat. **27**, 246 (1927). — Die arteriovenösen Anastomosen. Wien: Springer 1956. — COMEL, M.: Phlêbologie et histangéiologie, dans le cadre de l'angéiologie generale. Folia angiol. (Pisa) **8**, 4, 363 (1961). — CORMIA, F. E., and A. ERNYEY: Circulatory changes in alopecia. Arch. Derm. **84**, 772 (1961). — COWPER, W.: An account of diverse schemes of arteries and veins dissected from adult human bodies, etc. Phil. Trans. **23**, 1177 (1704). — CROVATO, F., and E. RAMPINI: Una nuova tecnica di visualizzazione della rete ematica cutanea con la reazione per le fosfatasi alcaline. Riv. Istochim. norm. pat. **11**, 4, 523 (1965).

DARIER, J.: Anatomie de la peau. In: Pratique dermatologique. Paris: Masson & Co. 1900. — DAVIS, M. J., and F. C. LAWLER: Capillary microscopy in normal and diseased human skin. In: Advances in biology of skin, vol. VI. Blood vessels and circulation, p. 79 (W. MONTAGNA and R. A. ELLIS, eds.). New York: Pergamon Press 1961. — DAVIS, M. J., and A. L. LORINCZ: An improved technic for capillary microscopy of the skin. J. invest. Derm. **28**, 283 (1957). — DEMIS, D. J., and J. BRIM: A method of preparing three-dimensional casts of the microcirculation of the skin. J. invest. Derm. **45**, 324 (1965). — DIEULAFÉ et DURAND: Sur les vaisseaux de la peau. C. R. Ass. Anat. Bordeaux 1906. — DURWARD, A., and K. M. RUDALL: Studies on hair growth in the rat. J. Anat. (Lond.) **83**, 325 (1949). — The vascularity and patterns of growth of hair follicles. In: The biology of hair growth, p. 189 (W. MONTAGNA and R. A. ELLIS, eds.). New York: Academic Press 1958.

ELLIS, R. A.: Ageing of the human male scalp. In: The biology of hair growth, p. 469 (W. MONTAGNA and R. A. ELLIS, eds.). New York: Academic Press 1958. — Personal communication 1965. — ELLIS, R. A., and G. MORETTI: Vascular patterns associated with catagen hair follicles in the human scalp. Ann. N.Y. Acad. Sci. **83**, 448 (1959).

FERREIRA-MARQUES, J., E. O. BITTAR u. J. F. LEONFORTE: Zum Studium der Blutzirkulation im allgemeinen in der Brustwarze des Menschen und in der verschiedener Tiere, insbesondere über die Beziehungen zwischen der Epidermis, ihren Anhangsorganen und Blutcapillaren. Arch. klin. exp. Derm. **223**, 568 (1965).

GILJE, O., R. KIERLAND, and E. J. BALDES: Capillary microscopy in the diagnosis of dermatologic diseases. J. invest. Derm. **23**, 199 (1954). — GILJE, O., P. A. O'LEARY, and F. J. BALDES: Capillary microscopic examination in skin diseases. Arch. Derm. Syph. (Chic.) **68**, 136 (1953). — GOLDMANN, L., and W. KOUNKER: Studies in microscopy of the surface of the skin: preliminary report of technic. J. invest. Derm. **9**, 11 (1947). — GOMORI, M. D.: Microscopic histochemistry principles and practice, p. 37. Chicago: Chicago University Press 1952. — GOODALL, A.M., and S. H. YANG: The vascular supply of the skin of the Ayrshire calves and embryos. J. Agricult. Sci. **44**, 1 (1954). — GRANT, R. T., and E. F. BLAND: Observations on the arterio-venous anastomoses in human skin and the bird's foot with special reference to reaction to cold. Heart **15**, 385 (1929—1931). — GROSSER, O.: Zur Anatomie und Entwicklungsgeschichte des Gefäßsystems der Chiropteren. Anat. H. **17**, 203 (1901). — Über arterio-venöse Anastomosen in den Extremitätenenden beim Menschen und den krallentragenden Säugetieren. Arch. mikr. Anat. **60**, 191 (1902). — GROSSER-BROCKHOFF, F., u. W. SCHOEDEL: Physiologie und Pathologie des Kreislaufes. In: Handbuch der Thoraxchirurgie. Berlin 1957.

HARVEY, H.: Exercitatio anatomica de motu cordis et sanguinis in animalibus. Frankfurt 1628. — HAVLICEK, H.: Vasa privata und vasa publica neue Kreislaufprobleme. Hippokrates

(Stuttg.) **2**, 105 (1929). — HENLE, F.: Allgemeine Anatomie, Lehre von den Mischungs- und Formbestandsteilen des menschlichen Körpers. Leipzig: Voss 1841. — HIBBS, R. G., G. E. BURCH, and G. H. PHILLIPE: The fine structure of the small blood vessels of the normal human dermis and subcutis. Amer. Heart. J. **56**, 662 (1958). — HOYER, H.: Ein Beitrag zur Histologie bindegewebiger Gebilde. Arch. Anat. Physiol. **9**, 445 (1865). — Über die unmittelbare Verbindung zwischen Arterien und Venen. Tageblatt der Naturforscher 149. Versammlung zu Leipzig 1872. — Über unmittelbare Einmündung kleinster Arterien in Gefäßäste venösen Charakters. Arch. mikr. Anat. **13**, 603 (1877). — HUETER, C.: Die Cheiloangioskopie, eine neue Untersuchungsmethode zu physiologischen und pathologischen Zwecken. Zbl. med. Wiss. **17**, 225 (1879). — HYRTL, J.: Manuale di dissezione pratica. Bologna 1886. — Quoted from M. CLARA. In: Le anastomosi arteriovenose, p. 6. Milano: Vallardi 1959.

ILLIG, L.: Die terminale Strombahn. Berlin-Göttingen-Heidelberg: Springer 1961

JAMINE, F.: Nagelfalzkapillaren und konstitutionelle Eigenart. Z. ges. Neurol. Psychiat. **131**, 114 (1931).

KLINGMÜLLER, G.: Über alkalische Phosphatase und ihre histochemische Darstellung in Kapillaren. Habil.-Schr. Bonn 1959. — KOELLIKER, A.: Elements d'histologie humaine. Paris: Masson & Cie. 1856. — KOLHAUS, J. C.: Quoted from Microfotografie in vivo, 2 (L. ILLIG and H. CONRATHS, eds.). Ingelheim a. Rh.: Boehringer 1930. — KROGH, A.: Anatomie und Physiologie des Capillaren. Berlin: Springer 1929. — KÜLCZYCKI, W.: Die Hautarterien des Hundes. Anat. Anz. **4**, 276 (1889).

LEALE-LEALI: De partibus semen confic. Leyden 1707. Quoted from M. CLARA. In: Le anastomosi arteriovenose, p. 1. Milano: Vallardi 1959. — LEWIS, T.: The blood vessels of the human skin and their responses. London: Shaw 1927. — Die Blutgefäße der menschlichen Haut und ihr Verhalten gegen Reize. Berlin: S. Karger 1928. — LIBERKÜHN, J. N.: Quoted from J. HYRTL. In: Manuale di dissezione pratica. Bologna 1886. — LOMBARD, W. P.: The blood pressure in the arterioles, capillaries and small veins of the human skin. Amer. J. Physiol. **29**, 335 (1912).

MACHER, E., u. W. VOGEL: Elektronenmikroskopische Untersuchungen an Hautkapillaren. Dermatologica (Basel) **124**, 110 (1962). — MAJNO, G.: Ultrastructure of the vascular membrane. In: Handbook of physiology, Sect. 2, Circulation, III. Amer. Physiol. Soc., ed. 1965. — MALPIGHI, M.: De pulmonibus. Epistola II ad Borellium. Bologna 1661. In: Opera Omnia, p. 140. London: Scott & Wells 1686. Quoted from Microfotografie in vivo, 2 (L. ILLIG and H. CONRATHS, eds.). Ingelheim a. Rh.: Boehringer 1960. — MANCHOT, C.: Die Hautarterien des menschlichen Körpers. Leipzig 1889. — MASCAGNI, P.: Prodromo della grande anatomia. "Opera Postum" II. Milano 1821. — MASSON, P.: Les glomus cutanés de l'homme. Bull. Soc. Franç. Derm. Syph. **42**, 1174 (1935). — Innervation des glomus cutanés de l'homme. Trans. Roy. Soc. Can., Sect. V **3**, 37 (1936a). — L'appareil nerveux des glomus cutanés. Bull. Histol. appl. **13**, 209 (1936b). — Les glomus neuro-vasculaires. Paris: Hermann & Cie. 1937. — MAXIMOW, A.: Untersuchungen über Blut und Bindegewebe. I. Die frühesten Entwicklungsstadien der Blut- und Bindegewebezellen beim Säugetierembryo bis zum Anfang der Blutbildung in der Leber. Arch. mikr. Anat. **73**, 444 (1909). — MESCON, H., J. HURLEY, and G. MORETTI: The anatomy and histochemistry of the arteriovenous anastomosis in human digital skin. J. invest. Derm. **27**, 133 (1956). — MONACELLI, M.: Contributo allo studio dell'arteriosclerosi cutanea. G. ital. Derm. Sif. **65**, 1793 (1924). — MONROE, A.: Quoted from J. HYRTL. In: Manuale di dissezione pratica. Bologna 1886. — MONTAGNA, W.: Summary. In: The biology of hair growth, p. 487 (W. MONTAGNA and R. A. ELLIS, eds.). New York: Academic Press 1958. — The structure and function of skin. New York: Academic Press 1962. — MONTAGNA, W., and R. A. ELLIS: Histology and cytochemistry of human skin. XIII. The blood supply of the hair follicle. J. nat. Cancer Inst. **19**, 451 (1957). — MORETTI, G., and F. CROVATO: Unpublished data 1965. — MORETTI, G., R. A. ELLIS, and H. MESCON: Vascular patterns in the skin of the face. J. invest. Derm. **33**, 103 (1959). — MÜLLER, O.: Mein Kapillarmikroskop. Med. Klin. **17**, 1148 (1921). — Die feinsten Blutgefäße des Menschen in gesunden und kranken Tagen. Stuttgart: Ferdinand Enke 1939.

NESTEROW, A. J.: Über Kontraktilität der Blutcapillaren beim Menschen. Pflügers Arch. ges. Physiol. **209**, 465 (1925). — NICKAU, B.: Anatomische und klinische Beobachtungen mit dem Hautkapillarmikroskop (ausführliche Darstellung der anatomischen Voraussetzungen). Dtsch. Arch. klin. Med. **131**, 301 (1920). — Kinematographische Beobachtung der Kapillarbeweglichkeit am Menschen. Klin. Wschr. **4**, 620 (1925).

ODLAND, G. F.: The fine structure of cutaneous capillary. In: Advances in biology of skin, II. Blood vessels and circulation, p. 57 (W. MONTAGNA and R. A. ELLIS, eds.). New York: Pergamon Press 1961. — ORMEA, F.: La cute organo di senso. Torino: Minerva Medica 1961.

PARRISIUS, W.: Zur Frage der Kontraktilität der menschlichen Hautkapillaren. Pflügers Arch. ges. Physiol. **191**, 217 (1921). — PARRISIUS, W., u. WITTERLIN: Der Blutstrom in den Hautkapillaren in verschiedenen Körperregionen bei Wechseln der Konjelage. Dtsch. Arch. klin. Med. 141, 243 (1923). Quoted from Microfotografie in vivo, 2 (L. ILLIG and H. CONRATHS, eds.). Ingelheim a. Rh.: Boehringer 1960. — POPOFF, N. W.: Recherches sur l'histologie des anastomoses arterioveineuses des extrémités et sur leur rôle en pathologie vasculaire. Bull. Histol. appl. **12**, 156 (1935). — PURKINJE, J. E., Ritter v.: Commentatio de examine physiologico organi visus et systematis cutanei. Breslau 1823.

RAMPINI, E., G. MORETTI e A. REBORA: Arteriole e capillari della cute ed alopecia areata. Atti S.I.D.E.S. 46. Congr. Naz. Derm., Genova 1963. — RAPP, Y., F. S. GLICKMAN, and L. FRANK: Capillary microscopy in induced skin inflammation. Arch. Derm. **88**, 257 (1963). — RENAUT, J.: Traité d'histologie pratique, 2, 1. Paris 1897. — RIGGIO, T.: Saggio del metodo istochimico di Pickworth nello studio della vascolarizzazione della pelle normale e patologica. G. ital. Derm. Sif. **4**, 291 (1952). — RUYSCH, F.: Quoted from J. HYRTL. In: Manuale di dissezione pratica. Bologna 1886. — RYDER, M. L.: Use of cyanol in the study of blood vessels in sheep skin. Nature (Lond.) **172**, 125 (1953). — Med. Sci. Thesis University of Leeds 1954. — Studies of nutrition of wool follicles in sheep: the anatomy of the general blood supply to the skin. J. Agricult. Sci. **45**, 311 (1955a). — The blood supply to the wool follicle. Proceedings of the Int. Wool Textile Research Conf., vol. F. Australia 1955b.

SAUNDERS, C. H. DE: X-ray microscopy of human dental pulp vessels. Nature (Lond.) **180**, 1353 (1957). — X-ray projection microscopy of the skin. In: Advances in biology of skin, II. Blood vessels and circulation, p. 38 (W. MONTAGNA and R. A. ELLIS, eds.). New York: Pergamon Press 1961. — SAUNDERS, C. H. DE, and W. MONTAGNA: X-ray microscopy and microangiography. Arch. Derm. **89**, 451 (1964). — SCHÖNFELD, W.: Capillarmikroskopie und Capillarphotogramme der äußeren männlichen Geschlechtsteile. Arch. Derm. Syph. (Berl.) **178**, 276 (1939). — SCHROEDER, W.: Eine einfache Methode zur festlaufenden Registrierung von Änderungen der Haut, bzw. des Muskeldurchbluten des Menschen und des wachen Hundes (Capillardruckmessung). Z. ges. exp. Med. **130**, 513 (1959). — SCHUMACHER, S.: Über das Glomus coccygicum des Menschen und die Glomeruli caudales der Säugetiere. Arch. mikr. Anat. **71**, 58 (1907). — SCOLARI, E.: Gli aspetti della irrorazione sanguifera cutanea alla luce della capillaroscopia a forte ingrandimento. Ricerche ed osservazioni. G. ital. Derm. Sif. **74**, 1117 (1933). — SOBIN, S. S., W. G. FRASHER, and H. M. TREMER: Vasa vasorum of the pulmonary artery of the rabbit. Circulat. Res. **9**, 257 (1962). — SPALTEHOLZ, W.: Die Verteilung der Blutgefäße im Muskel. Abh. sächs. Ges. Wiss., math.-phys. Kl. **14**, 509 (1888). — Die Verteilung der Blutgefäße in der Haut. Arch. Anat. u. Physiol. Anat. Abt. 1893. — Blutgefäße der Haut. In: Handbuch der Haut- und Geschlechtskrankheiten, vol. I/1, p. 379. Berlin: Springer 1927. — STEIGLEDER, G. K., R. KUDICKE u. Y. KAMEI: Die Lokalisation der Aminopeptidasenaktivität in normaler Haut. Arch. klin. exp. Derm. **215**, 307 (1962). — SUCQUET, J. P.: Anatomie et physiologie. Circulation du sang. D'une circulation derivative dans les membres et dans la tête chez l'homme. Paris: A. Delahaye 1862. — SWAMMERDAM, J.: Quoted from J. HYRTL. In: Manuale di dissezione pratica. Bologna 1886.

TOMSA, W.: Beiträge zur Anatomie und Physiologie der menschlichen Haut. Arch. Derm. Syph. (Berl.) **5** (1873). — TODD and BOWMANN: Quoted from G. TRUFFI, Sulla vascolarizzazione degli annessi cutanei. Arch. ital. Derm. **10**, 681 (1934). — TOSTI, A.: Microradiografia da contatto della cute umana. Ann. Ital. Derm. Clin. Sperim., Palermo 1964.

UNNA jr., P.: Untersuchungen über die Lymph- und Blutgefäße der äußeren Haut mit besonderer Berücksichtigung der Haarfollikel. Arch. J. mikr. Anat. u. Entwickl.-Gesch. **72** (1908).

VASTARINI-CRESI, G.: Comunicazioni dirette tra le arterie e le vene (anastomosi arterovenose). Nota preliminare. Monit. zool. ital. **13**, 136 (1902). — Le anastomosi artero-venose nell'uomo e nei mammiferi. Studio Anatomo-Istologico, Napoli 1903. — VERSARI, A.: Contributo alla conoscenza della fine circolazione sanguigna del cuoio capelluto. Ric. morf. **3**, 1 (1923).

WALLS, E. W., and T. J. BUCHANAN: Observations on the capillary blood vessels of the human skin. J. Anat. (Lond.) **90**, 529 (1956). — WATSON, M. L.: Staining of tissue sections for electron microscopy with heavy metals. J. biophys. biochem. Cytol. **4**, 475 (1958). — WEISS, E.: Das Verhalten der Hautkapillaren bei akuter Nephritis. Münch. med. Wschr. **63**, 925 (1916). — WEISS, E., u. M. HOHANEL: Zur Morphologie und Topographie der Hautkapillaren. Z. exp. Path. **22**, 108 (1921). — WERTHEIMER, N., and M. WERTHEIMER: Capillary structure: its relation to psychiatric diagnosis and morphology. J. nerv. ment. Dis. **122**, 14 (1955). — WETZEL, N. C., and Y. ZOTTERMANN: On differences in the vascular coloration of various regions of the normal human skin. Heart **13**, 358 (1926). — WINKELMANN, R. K.: Nerve endings in the skin of gorilla. J. comp. Neurol. **116**, 145 (1961).

ZELIKSON, A. S.: A tubular structure in the endothelial cells and pericytes of human capillaries. J. invest. Derm. **46**, 167 (1966).

B. Notes on Comperative Anatomy, Embryology and Prenatal and Postnatal Development of Cutaneous Blood Vessels

AREY, L. B.: The development of peripheral blood vessels. In: The peripheral blood vessels (J. LOWELL ORBISON and D. E. SMITH, eds.). Baltimore: Williams & Wilkins Co. 1963. — AREY, L. B., W. BURROWS, J. P. GREENHILL, and R. M. HEWITT: Dorland's illustrated medical dictionary. Philadelphia: W. B. Saunders Co. 1957.

BECKETT, E. B., G. H. BOURNE, and W. MONTAGNA: The distribution of cholinesterase in the finger of the embryo and the adult. J. Physiol. (Lond.) 134, 202 (1956). — BELLOCQ, PH.: Étude anatomique des artères de la peau chez l'homme. Paris: Masson & Cie. 1925. — BENNINGHOFF, A.: Blutgefäße und Herz. In: Handbuch der mikroskopischen Anatomie der Menschen (A. BENNINGHOFF, A. HARTMANN u. T. HELLMAN, eds.). Berlin: Springer 1930. — BOYD, E.: The growth of the surface area of the human body, p. 145. Minneapolis: University Minnesota Press 1935.

CASTIGLI, C., e A. MORICONI: Dispositivi di blocco in arterie del piede di bue. Atti Soc. ital. Sci. vet. 3, 1, 411 (1949). — CHIALE, C.: Delle modificazioni dei vasi cutanei inerenti all'età. G. ital. Derm. Sif. Vener. 682, 163 (1927). — CHIARUGI, G.: Trattato di Embriologia. Milano: Società Editrice Libraria 1929. — CLARA, M.: Le anastomosi arteriovenose. Milano: Vallardi 1959. — CLARK, E. R.: Studies on the growth of blood vessels in the tail of the gray larva by observation and experiment on the living animal. Amer. J. Anat. 23, 37 (1918). — CLARK, E. R., and E. L. CLARK: Microscopic observations on the extra-endothelial cells of living mammalian blood vessels. Amer. J. Anat. 66, 1 (1940).

DURWARD, A., and K. M. RUDALL: The vascularity and patterns of growth of hair follicles. In: The biology of hair growth, p. 189 (W. MONTAGNA and R. A. ELLIS, eds.). New York: Academic Press 1958.

ELLIS, R. A., and W. MONTAGNA: Sites of phosphorylase and amylo-1-6-glucosidase activity. J. Histochem. Cytochem. 6, 201 (1958). — The skin of the gorilla (Gorilla gorilla). Amer. J. phys. Anthrop. 20, 70 (1962). — EVANS, A. M.: The development of the vascular system. In: Manual of human embryology II, p. 570 (F. KEIBEL and F. P. MALL, eds.). Philadelphia: J. B. Lippincott Co. 1912.

FINLEY, E.: The development of the subcutaneous vascular plexus in the head of the human embryo. Contr. Embryol. 14, 71, 155 (1922).

GASPARINI, F., e G. BUCCIANTE: Sulla morfogenesi delle anastomosi arterio-venose delle dita dell'uomo. Atti Soc. med.-chir. Padova 28, 198 (1950). — GOODALL, A. M., and S. H. YANG: The vascular supply of the skin of Ayrshire calves and embryos. J. Agricult. Sci. 44, 1 (1954). — GOODALL, H. M.: Arterio-venous anastomoses in the skin of the head and ears of the calf. J. Anat. (Lond.) 89, 100 (1955). — GRAY, H., and W. H. LEWIS: Grays anatomy, p. 494. Philadelphia: Lea & Febiger 1936. — GRIGOROVA, O. P.: Zur Frage der Genese der Capillaren. Z. menschl. Vererb.- u. Konstit. Lehre 17, 428 (1933). — GROSSER, O.: Über arterio-venöse Anastomosen in den Extremitätenenden beim Menschen und den krallentragenden Säugetieren. Arch. mikr. Anat. 60, 191 (1902).

HARDY, M. H.: The histochemistry of hair follicles in the mouse. Amer. J. Anat. 90, 285 (1952). — HERTIG, A. T.: Angiogenesis in the early human chorion and in the primary placenta of the macaque monkey. Contr. Embryol. Carneg. Instn 25, 37 (1935). — HIS, W.: Lecithoblast und Angioblast der Wirbeltiere. Abh. math.-nat. Wiss. Klin., Kgl. sächs. Ges. 26 (1900). — HOLLAND, M., u. L. MEYER: Beobachtungen an den Hautcapillaren bei Kindern mit exsudativer Diathese. Münch. med. Wschr. 1919. — HORSTMANN, E.: Die Haut. In: Handbuch der mikroskopischen Anatomie der Menschen, vol. III/3, p. 198 (W. v. MÖLLENDORFF u. W. BARGMANN, eds.) Berlin-Göttingen-Heidelberg: Springer 1957. — HOYER, H.: Über unmittelbare Einmündung kleinster Arterien in Gefäßaste venösen Charakters. Arch. mikr. Anat. 13, 603 (1877). — HYRTL, J.: Neue Wundernetze und Geflechte bei Vögeln und Säugetieren. Denkschr. Kais. Akad. Wiss., Wien, math. nat. Kl. 22, 113 (1864).

IM, M. J. C., and W. MONTAGNA: The skin of primates. XXVI. Specific and nonspecific phosphatases in the skin of the rhesus monkey. Amer. J. phys. Anthrop. 23, 131 (1965).

JAENSCH, W.: Die Hautkapillaren. In: ABDERHALDENs Handbuch der biologischen Arbeitsmethoden, vol. IX, p. 3. Berlin: Urban & Schwarzenberg 1930. — JAENSCH, W., W. WITTNEBEN, TH. HOEPFNER, G. LEUPOLD u. O. GUNDERMANN: Die Hautkapillarmikroskopie. Halle: Carl Marhold 1929. — JOSTOCK, P. J., u. G. KLINGMÜLLER: Histochemische Untersuchungen zur Morphogenese des menschlichen Haares. Arch. klin. exp. Derm. 224, 285 (1966).

LO CASCIO, G.: La morfogenesi dei vasi sanguiferi nella cute dell'uomo: Ricerche fatte nel Laboratorio di Anatomia Normale della R. Università di Roma ed altri Laboratori Biologici, pubblicate dal Prof. F. TODARO, XVII, Roma 1913/14. — LOEB, J.: Über die Entwicklung von Fischembryonen ohne Kreislauf. Pflügers Arch. ges. Physiol. 54, 525 (1893). — LYNCH, F. W.: Elastic tissue in fetal skin. Arch. Derm. Syph. (Chic.) 29, 57 (1934).

MACHIDA, H., E. PERKINS, W. MONTAGNA, and L. GIACOMETTI: The skin of the white-crowned mangabey (Cercocebus otys). Amer. J. Physiol. Anthrop. **23**, 1 (1965). — MASSON, P.: Les glomus neuro-vasculaires. Paris: Hermann & Cie. 1937. — MAXIMOW, A.: Untersuchungen über Blut und Bindegewebe. I. Die frühesten Entwicklungsstadien der Blut- und Bindegewebszellen beim Säugetierembryo bis zum Anfang der Blutbildung in der Leber. Arch. mikr. Anat. **73**, 444 (1909). — MENEGHINI, N.: Osservazioni anatomoradiografiche sulle reti arteriose e venose della faccia dell'uomo nelle varie epoche della vita. Arch. ital. Derm. **18**, 62 (1942). — MONTAGNA, W.: Comparative anatomy. New York: John Wiley & Sons 1959. — MONTAGNA, W., and R. A. ELLIS: The skin of the potto (periodicticus potto). Amer. J. phys. Anthrop. **17**, 137 (1959). — The skin of the sleuder loris (Loris tardigraders). Amer. J. phys. Anthrop. **18**, 19 (1960). — MONTAGNA, W., and R. J. HARRISON: Specialization in the skin of the seal (phoca vitulina). Amer. J. Anat. **100**, 81 (1957). — MONTAGNA, W., H. MACHIDA, and E. PERKINS: The stump-tail macaque (macaca speciosa). Amer. J. phys. Anthrop. **24**, 71 (1966). — MONTAGNA, W., and J. S. YUN: The skin of the anubis baboon (papio doguera). Amer. J. phys. Anthrop. **20**, 131 (1962a). — The skin of primates. VII. The skin of the great bush-baby (Galaga crassicaudatus). Amer. J. phys. Anthrop. **20**, 149 (1962b). — The skin of the chimpanzee (pan satyrus). Amer. J. phys. Anthrop. **21**, 189 (1963). — The skin of the domestic pig. J. invest. Derm. **43**, 11 (1964). — MORETTI, G.: Das Haar. In: Die normale und pathologische Physiologie der Haut, p. 506 (G. STÜTTGEN, ed.). Stuttgart: Gustav Fischer 1965. — MORETTI, G., u. G. FARRIS: Die alkalischen Phosphatasen in den Blutgefäßen der Haut einiger Primaten. Z. Haut- u. Geschl.-Kr. **34**, 6 (1963). — MORETTI, G., and E. RAMPINI: Unpublished data 1964. — Unpublished data 1965.

PARAKKAL, P., W. MONTAGNA, and R. A. ELLIS: The skin of the white browed gibbon (hylobates hoolock). Anat. Rec. **143**, 169 (1962). — PARVIS-PRETO, V., e A. UGO: Studio morfologico ed istochimico della cute sessuale della scimmia. G. ital. Derm. **4**, 290 (1960a). — La cute sessuale della scimmia. Contributo allo studio delle correlazioni endocrine-cutanee. Boll. Soc. med.-chir. Varese **15**, 1 (1960b). — PINKUS, F.: The development of the integument. In: Manual of human embryology, vol. 1, p. 243 (F. KEIBEL and F. P. MALL, eds.). Philadelphia: J. B. Lippincott Co. 1910. — Die normale Anatomie der Haut. In: Handbuch der Haut- und Geschlechtskrankheiten, vol. 1/1. Berlin: Springer 1927. — POPOFF, N. W.: Recherches sur l'histologie des anastomoses arterio-veineuses des extrémités et sur leur rôle en pathologie vasculaire. Bull. Histol. appl. **12**, 156 (1935).

ROSATI, P.: Su alcune particolarità morfologiche e strutturali dei vasi cutanei e del loro probabile significato funzionale. Boll. Soc. ital. Biol. sper. **31**, 1, 70 (1955). — ROTTER, W., u. L. WAGNER: Über die Entwicklung der subungualen Glomera (sog. arteriovenöse Anastomosen) der Zehen. Arch. Kreisl.- Forsch. **18**, 68 (1952). — RUCKERT, J., u. S. MOLLIER: Die erste Entstehung der Gefäße und des Blutes bei Wirbeltieren. In: Handbuch der vergleichenden und experimentellen Entwicklungslehre der Wirbeltiere. Jena: von Hertwig 1906. — RYDER, M. L.: Studies of nutrition of wool follicles in sheep: the anatomy of the general blood supply to the skin. J. Agricult. Sci. **45**, 311 (1955a). — The blood supply to the wool follicle. Proc. Intern. Wool Text. Res. Conf. p. 63, Australia 1955b, vol. F. — Nutritional factors influencing hair and wool growth. In: The biology of hair growth, p. 305 (W. MONTAGNA and R. A. ELLIS, eds.). New York: Academic Press 1958.

SALMON: Artères de la peau. Étude anatomique et chirurgicale. Paris: Masson & Cie. 1936. — SCHAEFER, E. A.: Textbook of microscopic anatomy. New York: Longmans, Green & Co. 1912. — SCHUMACHER, S.: Über das Glomus coccygicum des Menschen und die Glomeruli caudales der Säugetiere. Arch. mikr. Anat. **71**, 58 (1907). — Arteriovenöse Anastomosen in den Zehen der Vögel. Arch. mikr. Anat. **87**, 309 (1915). — Integument der Mammalier. In: Handbuch der vergleichenden Anatomie der Wirbeltiere, vol. 1/3, p. 449. Berlin: Urban & Schwarzenberg 1931. — SCHUMMER, A.: Blutgefäße und Zirkulationsverhältnisse im Zehenendorgan der Pferdes. Morph. Jb. **91**, 568 (1951). — SERRI, F.: Lo sviluppo e l'organizzazione vascolare nella cute del feto umano. Minerva med. **40**, 179 (1965). — SERRI, F., W. MONTAGNA, and W. M. HUBER: Studies of skin of fetus and the child. The distribution of alkaline phosphatase in the skin of the fetus. Arch. Derm. **87**, 234 (1963). — SERRI, F., W. MONTAGNA, and H. MESCON: Osservazioni sull'innervazione della cute fetale con particolare riguardo alle dita. Acta neuroveg. (Wien) **24**, 163 (1963). — SIMPSON, G. G.: The principles of classification and classification of mammals. Bull. Amer. Museum Nat. Hist. **85** (1945). — SPALTEHOLZ, W.: Die Verteilung der Blutgefäße in der Haut. Arch. Anat. u. Physiol. Anat. Abt. **1**, 54 (1893). — Blutgefäße der Haut. In: Handbuch der Haut und Geschlechtskrankheiten, vol. 1/1, p. 379. Berlin: Springer 1927. — STAUBESAND, J., u. G. GENSCHOW: Die arterio-venösen Anastomosen in Löffel des Kaninchens nach graphischen Rekonstruktionen. Z. Anat. Entwickl.-Gesch. **116**, 446 (1952). — STEFKO, W.: Die Entwicklung der Hautcapillaren im Kindesalter (0—16 Lebensjahr). Ein Altersschema für die Kinderärzte. Kinderärztl. Prax. **2**, 468 (1931).

Thoma, R.: Untersuchungen über die Histogenese und Histomechanik des Gefäßsystems, 91. Stuttgart: Ferdinand Enke 1893.
Vastarini-Cresi: Le anastomosi artero-venose nell'uomo e nei mammiferi. Studio Anatomo-istologico Napoli 1903.
Wildman, A. B.: Coat and fibre development in some british sheep. Proc. zool. Soc. (Lond.) **2**, 257 (1932). — Willier, B., P. Weiss, and V. Hamburger: Analysis of development. Philadelphia: W. B. Saunders Co. 1955. — Winkelmann, R. K.: Nerve endings in the skin of gorilla. J. comp. Neurol. **116**, 145 (1961).

C. Building Stones for the Cutaneous Blood Vessel Network

Algire, G. H.: An adaptation of the transparent-chamber techniques to the mouse. J. nat. Cancer Inst. **4**, 1 (1943). — Allen, E. V., N. W. Barker, and E. A. Hynes: Peripheral vascular disease, p. 871. London: W. B. Saunders Co. 1955. — Allgower, M.: The cellular basis of wound repair, vol. III. Springfield (Ill.): Ch. C. Thomas 1956. — Auerbach: Über die feinere Struktur der Saugadern und der Blutcapillaren. Breslau Ztg 1865. Quoted from A. Benninghoff, A. Hartmann u. T. Hellman in: Blutgefäße- und Lymphgefäßapparat-Atmungsapparat und innersekretorische Drüsen. Berlin: Springer 1930.
Baccaredda-Boy, A., e G. Moretti: Fattori patogenetici cooperanti coll'insufficienza venosa alla sindrome da stasi degli arti inferiori. Folia angiol. **5**, 1 (1958). — Baccaredda-Boy, A., G. Moretti e G. Farris: Varietà topografiche della reazione per la fosfatasi alcalina nel circolo superficiale cutaneo. Atti del II. Simposium di Derm. Sperim. Ann. ital. Derm. Sif. **15**, 186 (1960). — Baccaredda-Boy, A., G. Moretti e B. Filippi: Il circolo superficiale in rapporto alle zone elettive di trapianto cutaneo. Minerva derm. **35**, 9, 345 (1960). — Baccaredda-Boy, A., G. Moretti e A. Rebora: Densità capillare e istamina nel cuoio capelluto. Minerva derm. **36**, 337 (1961). — Baccaredda-Boy, A., G. Moretti, S. Zocchi e F. Crovato: Sul contenuto in triptofano in diverse regioni cutanee. Ann. ital. Derm. Sif. **13**, 95 (1958). — Bairati, A.: Quoted from F. Ormea. In: La cute organo di senso. Torino: Minerva Medica Ed., 1961. — Ballantyne jr., D. L., and J. M. Converse: Vascularization of composite auricular grafts transplanted to the chorio-allantois of the chickembryo. Transplant. Bull. **6**, 373 (1958). — Balogh, K.: Dihydrolipoic dehydrogenase activity: a step in formation of acyl-coenzyme A, demonstrated histochemically. J. Histochem. Cytochem. **12**, 404 (1964). — Bargmann, W.: Histologie und mikroskopische Anatomie des Menschen. Stuttgart: Georg Thieme 1956. — Barnett, R. J., and A. M. Seligman: Histochemical demonstration of proteinbound sulphydryl groups. Science **116**, 323 (1952). — Bellmann, S. B., and E. Vercander: Trans. Int. Soc. Plast. Surg. Finst. Congr. p. 493. Baltimore: Williams & Wilkins Co. 1957. — Bellocq, Ph.: Étude anatomique des artères de la peau chez l'homme. Paris: Masson & Cie. 1925. — Bennett, H. S.: The concepts of membrane flow and membrane vesiculation as mechanism for active transport and ions pumping. J. biophys. biochem. Cytol. **2**, Suppl., 99 (1956). — Bennett, H. S., J. H. Luft, and J. C. Hampton: Morphological classification of vertebrate blood capillaries. Amer. J. Physiol. **196**, 381 (1959). — Benninghoff, A.: Über die Formenreihe der glatten Muskulatur und die Bedeutung der Rougetschen Zellen in den Capillaren. Z. wiss. Biol., Abt. B. Z. Zellforsch. u. mikr. Anat. **4**, 41, 125 (1926). — Blutgefäße und Herz. In: Blutgefäß- und Lymphgefäßapparat — Atmungsapparat und innersekretorische Drüsen (A. Benninghoff, A. Hertmann u. T. Hellman, (eds.). Berlin: Springer 1930. — Berres, H. H.: Die Histologie der Altersveränderungen der menschlichen Haut. Arch. klin. exp. Derm. **206**, 751 (1957). — Bettmann, S.: Capillarmikroskopische Untersuchungen an der Lippenschleimhaut. Arch. Derm. Syph. (Berl.) **162**, 480 (1930). — Bianchi, L.: Connettivo e vasi in ambito cutaneo. Minerva derm. **36**, 309 (1961). — Boeke, J.: The sympathetic end formation its synaptology, the interstitial cell, ect. Acta anat. (Basel) **8**, 18 (1949). — Bordley, J., M. H. Grow, and W. B. Sherman: Intermittent blood flow in the capillaries of human skin. Bull. Johns Hopk. Hosp. **62**, 1 (1938). — Bradshaw, H., M. Wachsteim, J. Spence, and S. M. Elias: Adenosine-triphosphatase activity in melanocytes and epidermal cells of human skin. J. Histochem. Cytochem. **11**, 465 (1963). — Braun-Falco, O.: Über die Fähigkeit der menschlichen Haut zur Polysaccharidsynthese, ein Beitrag zur Histotopochemie der Phosphorylase. Arch. klin. exp. Derm. **202**, 163 (1956a). — Zur histochemischen Darstellung von Glukose-6-Phosphatase in normaler Haut. Derm. Wschr. **1956b**, 134. — Zur Histotopographie der β-Glucuronidase in normaler menschlichen Haut. Arch. klin. exp. Derm. **203**, 61 (1956c). — Beitrag zum histochemischen Nachweis von Esterasen in normaler und psoriatischer Haut. Arch. klin. exp. Derm. **202**, 153 (1956d). — Die Histochemie der Haut. In: Dermatologie und Venerologie (H. A. v. Gottron u. W. Schönfeld, eds.). Stuttgart: Georg Thieme 1961. — Personal communication 1965. — Braun-Falco, O., u. D. Petzoldt: Über die Histotopie von NADH- und NADPH-Tetrazoliumreduktase in menschlicher Haut. Arch. klin. exp. Derm. **220**, 455 (1964). — Braun-Falco, O., u. B. Rathjens: Über die histochemische Darstellung der Kohlensäureanhydratase in normaler Haut. Arch. klin. exp. Derm. **201**, 73 (1955). — Braus, H., u. C. Elze: Anatomie des

Menschen, IV. Berlin: Springer 1940. — Brown, G. E.: The skin capillaries in Raynaud's disease. Arch. intern. Med. **35**, 56 (1925). — Brown, G. E., and H. Z. Giffin: Studies of the vascular changes in polycythemia vera. Amer. J. med. Sci. **171**, 157 (1926). — Brown, G. E., and G. M. Roth: Biomicroscopy of the surface capillaries in normal and pathologic subjects. Med. J. Aust. **1**, 496 (1927). — Brown, G. E., and C. Sheard: Measurements on the skin capillaries in cases of polycythemia vera and the role of these capillaries in the production of erythrosis. J. clin. Invest. **2**, 423 (1926). — Bucciante, L.: Sulla struttura dei vasi prostatici dell'uomo. Atti Soc. med.-chir. Padova **23**, 5 (1945). — La morfologia dei vasi sanguigni sulla base di moderne acquisizioni. Atti III Giorn. Ital. Med. Triestina, Sept. 1950. — Burton, J. F.: Histochemical demonstration of acid phosphatase by an improved azodye method. J. Histochem. Cytochem. **2**, 88 (1954).
Carranza, F. A., and R. L. Cabrini: Histoenzymic behavior of healing wounds. J. invest. Derm. **40**, 27 (1963). — Carrier, E. B.: Studies on the physiology of capillaries. The reaction of human skin capillaries to drugs and other stimuli. Amer. J. Physiol. **61**, 528 (1922). Quoted by M. Comel 1933. — Cauna, N.: Structure and origin of the capsule of Meissner's corpuscle. Anat. Rec. **124**, 77 (1956). — Cavazzana, P.: Dispositivi di blocco e cellule epitelioidi nei vasi della cute ascellare e perianale dell'uomo. Atti Soc. med.-chir. Padova **23**, 3 (1945). — Dispositivi di chiusura, anastomosi artero-venose e cellule muscolo-epitelioidei nei vasi cutanei. Ric. Morf. **22**, 1 (1946). — Chambers, R., and B. W. Zweifach: Intercellular cement and capillary permeability. Physiol. Rev. **27**, 431 (1947). — Chiale, C.: Delle modificazioni dei vasi cutanei inerenti all'età. G. ital. Derm. Sif. **682**, 163 (1927). — Clara, M.: Le anastomosi arteriovenose. Milano: Vallardi 1959. — Clark, E. R., and E. L. Clark: Observation on living arterio-venous anastomoses as seen in transparent chambers introduced into the rabbit's ear. Amer. J. Anat. **54**, 229 (1934). — Clemmesen, T.: The early circulation in split grafts. Acta chir. scand. **124**, 11 (1962). — Cogan, D. G.: Vascularization of the cornea, its experimental induction by small lesions and a new theory of its pathogenesis. Arch. Ophthal. **41**, 406 (1949). — Comel, M.: Fisiologia normale e patologica della cute umana, 1, p. 650. Milano: Treves Ed. 1933. — L'architettura strutturale e la prassi funzionale nel circolo dei piccoli vasi. Folia angiol. **2**, 3, 181 (1955). — Comel, M., et E. Mian: Corrélations histangiques et métabolisme de la paroi vasculaire. Folia angiol. **8**, 4, 371 (1961). — Converse, J. M., and D. L. Ballantyne: Distribution of diphosphopyridine nucleotide diaphorase in rat skin autografts and homografts. Plast. reconst. Surg. **30**, 415 (1962). — Converse, J. M., and F. T. Rapaport: The vascularization of skin autografts and homografts. Ann. Surg. **143**, 3, 306 (1956). — Conway, H.: Reexamination of the transparent chambre technique as applied to the study of circulation in autografts and homografts of the skin. J. Plast. reconstr. Surg. **20**, 103 (1957). — Conway, H., D. Joslin, T. D. Rees, and R. B. Stark: Observations on the development of circulation in skin grafts. III Morphologic changes observed in homologous skin grafts. J. Plast. reconstr. Surg. **9**, 557 (1952). — Cormia, F. E., and A. Ernyey: Circulatory changes in alopecia. Arch. Derm. **84**, 772 (1961). — Cramer, H. J.: Histochemische Untersuchungen mit dem sauren Hämateintest nach Baker an normaler und pathologisch veränderter Haut. I. Normale Haut. Arch. klin. exp. Derm. **218**, 191 (1964).
Darier, J., A. Civatte, C. Flandin et A. Tranck: Anatomie de la peau. In: Nouvelle pratique dermatologique, p. 31 (J. Darier et al., eds.). Paris: Masson & Cie. 1936. — Davis, E., and J. Landau: The small blood vessels of the conjuntiva and nailbed in arteriosclerosis. Angiology **11**, 173 (1960). — Davis, M. J., and J. C. Lawler: The capillary circulation of the skin. Arch. Derm. **77**, 690 (1958a). — Capillary alterations in pigmented purpuric disease of the skin. Arch. Derm. **78**, 723 (1958b). — Capillary circulation of skin: some normal and pathological findings. Arch. Derm. **77**, 690 (1958c). — Capillary microscopy in normal and diseased human skin. In: Advances in biology of skin II. Blood vessels and circulation, p. 79 (W. Montagna and R. A. Ellis, eds.). New York: Pergamon Press 1961. — Deutsch, F.: Capillary studies in Raynaud's disease. J. Lab. clin. Med. **26**, 1729 (1941). — Dieulafé et Durand: Sur les vaisseaux de la peau. C.R. Ass. Anat. Bordeaux 1906. — Dodd, H., and F. B. Cockett: The pathology and surgery of the veins of the lower limb. Edinburgh: Livingston 1956. — Dogiel, A. S.: Die sensiblen Nervendigungen im Herzen und in den Blutgefäßen der Säugetiere. Arch. mikr. Anat. **52**, 44 (1898). — Dziallas, P.: Über das Vorkommen von Klappen in kleinsten Venen beim Menschen. Z. Anat.-Entwickl.-Gesch. **114**, 309 (1949).
Eberth, C. J.: Von den Blutgefäßen. In: Strickers Handbuch der Lehre von den Geweben, S. 191. Leipzig 1871. — Ellis, R. A.: Ageing of the human male scalp. In: The biology of hair growth, p. 469 (W. Montagna and R. A. Ellis, eds.). New York: Academic Press 1958. — Circulatory patterns in the papillae of the mammalian tongue. Anat. Rec. **133**, 579 (1959). — Vascular patterns of the skin. In: Advances in biology of skin II. Blood vessels and circulation, p. 20 (W. Montagna and R. A. Ellis, eds.). New York: Pergamon Press 1961. — Ellis, R. A., and G. Moretti: Vascular patterns associated with catagen hair follicles in the human scalp. Ann. N.Y. Acad. Sci. **83**, 448 (1959).

FALCK, B., and H. RORSMAN: Experientia (Basel) **19**, 205 (1963). Quoted from H. MÖLLER in: The catecolamines of the skin. Acta derm.-venereol. (Stockh.) **42**, 386 (1962). — FAWCETT, D. W.: Observations on the submicroscopic structure of small arteries, arterioles and capillaries. Amer. Ass. Anat. 1956, p. 69. Abstract. in Anat. Rec. **124**, 401 (1956). — Comparative observations on the fine structure of blood capillaries, p. 17. In: The peripheral blood vessels (J. L. ORBISON and D. SMITH, eds.). Baltimore: Williams & Wilkins Co. 1963. — FLOREY, H. W., J. C. F. POOLE, and G. A. MEEK: Endothelial cells and "cement" lines. J. Path. Bact. **77**, 625 (1959). — FREERKSEN, E.: Die Venen des menschlichen Handrückens. Z. Anat. **108**, 82 (1938). — FULTON, G. P., R. G. JACKSON, and B. R. LUTZ: The use of the cheek pouch of the hamster, cricetus auratus, for the cinephotomicroscopy of small blood vessels. Anat. Rec. **96**, 554 (1946).

GARRACHON, J., J. MUNOZ y M. ORTEGA: Estudio mediante biopsia de los capillares dermicos del diabético. Rev. Clin. esp. **94**, 268 (1964). — GERSH, I., and H. R. CATCHPOLE: The organization of ground substance and basement membrane and its significance in tissue injury, disease and growth. Amer. J. Anat. **85**, 457 (1949). — GIACOMETTI, L.: The anatomy of the human scalp. In: Advances in biology of skin VI. Ageing, p. 97 (W. MONTAGNA, ed.). New York: Pergamon Press 1964. — GILJE, O.: Capillary microscopy in the differential diagnosis of skin diseases. Acta derm.-venereol. (Stockh.) **33**, 304 (1953). — GILJE, O., P. A. O'LEARY, and E. J. BALDES: Capillary microscopic examination in skin diseases. Arch. Derm. Syph. (Chic.) **68**, 136 (1953). — GOMORI, G.: Distribution of phosphatase in normal organs and tissues. J. cell. comp. Physiol. **17**, 71 (1941). — GRANT, R. T., and E. F. BLAND: Observations on the arterio-venous anastomoses in human skin and in the bird's foot with special reference to the reaction to cold. Heart **15**, 385 (1931). — GRIFFITH jr., J. O.: The frequent occurrence of abnormal cutaneous capillaries in constitutional neurasthenic states. Amer. J. med. Sci. **183**, 180 (1932). — GROSSER, O.: Über arterio-venose Anastomosen an den Extremitätenenden bei den Menschen und den krallentragenden Säugetieren. Arch. mikr. Anat. **60**, 191 (1902). — Zur Frage der segmentalen Gefäßversorgung der Haut beim Menschen. Gegenbaurs morph. Jb. **33** (1905). — Quoted from "Le anastomosi arteriovenose" p. 25 (M. CLARA). Milano: Vallardi 1959.

HALLER jr., A. J., and R. E. BILLINGHAM: Preliminary studies on the origin of the vasculature in free skin grafts. In: Advances in biology of skin III. Wound healing, p. 165 (W. MONTAGNA and R. E. BILLINGHAM, eds.). New York: Pergamon Press 1964. — HEIMBERGER, H.: Mikrokapillarpuls und arterio-venöse Verbindungen. Z. Kreisl.-Forsch. **22**, 313 (1930). — HERXHEIMER, A.: The autonomic innervation of the skin. In: Advances in biology of skin I. Cutaneous innervation, p. 63 (W. MONTAGNA, ed.). New York: Pergamon Press 1960. — HIBBS, R. G., G. E. BURCH, and W. P. PHILLIPE: The fine structure of the small blood vessels of the normal human dermis and subcutis. Amer. Heart J. **56**, 662 (1958). — HOLLANDER, A., S. C. SOMMERS, and A. E. GRIMWADE: Histochemical and ultraviolet microscopic studies of chronic dermatoses and the corium membrane. J. invest. Derm. **22**, 335 (1954). — HOPPE-SEYLER, H.: Das Verhalten der Gefäße bei Hautwunden und Narben in der Rückenhaut der weißen Maus. Morph. Jb. **86**, 123 (1941). — HORSTMANN, E.: Die Haut. In: Handbuch der mikroskopischen Anatomie der Menschen, vol. III/3, p. 198 (W. v. MÖLLENDORFF u. W. BARGMANN, eds.). Berlin-Göttingen-Heidelberg: Springer 1957. — Das Muster der Blutgefäße. Sonderdruck aus Bad Oeynhausener Gespräche VI, October 1962. — HOYER, H.: Über unmittelbare Einmündung kleinster Arterien in Gefäßäste venösen Charakters. Arch. mikr. Anat. **13**, 603 (1877). — HURLEY jr., H. J., and H. MESCON: Cholinergic innervation of the digital arteriovenous anastomoses of human skin. A histochemical localization of cholinesterase. J. appl. Physiol. **9**, 82 (1956). — HYNES, W.: The early circulation of skin grafts. Brit. J. plast. Surg. **6**, 257 (1954).

ILLIG, L.: Die terminale Strombahn, p. 458. Berlin-Göttingen-Heidelberg: Springer 1961. — Die Topographie der peripheren Zirkulation der Haut. Arch. klin. exp. Derm. **219**, 101 (1964). — ISHIKAWA, H., u. G. KLINGMÜLLER: Capillardarstellung im Papillarkörper insbesondere bei Psoriasis vulgaris durch die Leucin-aminopeptidase-Reaktion. Arch klin. exp. Derm. **217**, 340 (1963).

JABONERO, V.: Mikroskopische Studies über die Morphologie und die Morphopathologie der vegetativen Innervation der menschlichen Haut. Acta neuroveg. (Wien) **18**, 69 (1958). — Quoted from F. ORMEA in: La cute organo di senso. Torino: Minerva Medica ed. 1961. — JOHN, F.: Zur mikroskopischen Anatomie der Gefäß- und Schweißdrüsennerven in der menschlichen Haut. Allg. Zellforsch. **30**, 297 (1940). — JUHLIN, L., and W. B. SHELLEY: Detection of histamine by a new fluorescent o-Phthaldehyde stain. J. Histochem. Cytochem. **14**, 525 (1966).

KOELLE, G. B.: The elimination of enzymatic diffusion artifacts in the histochemical demonstration of cholinesterases and survey of their cellular distribution. J. Pharmacol. exp. Ther. **103**, 153 (1951). — KROGH, A.: Anatomie und Physiologie der Capillaren. Berlin: Springer 1929. — KUKLOVA-STUROVA: Beziehungen zwischen den Capillaren der

Eltern und der Kinder. Čas. Lék. čes. **1941**, 585, [Tschechisch]. Quoted from Zbl. Haut- u. Geschl.-Kr. **68**, 619 (1942). — KUNTZ, A., and J. W. HAMILTON: Afferent innervation of the skin. Anat. Rec. **71**, 387 (1938).
LANDIS, E. M.: The capillaries of the skin. J. invest. Derm. **1**, 295 (1938). — LAWLER, J. C., and L. R. LUMPKIN: Cutaneous capillary changes in lupus erythematosus. Arch. Derm. **83**, 636 (1961). — LEBLOND, C. P., R. E. GLEGG, and D. EIDINGER: Presence of carbohydrates with free 1,2-glycol groups in sites stained by the periodic acid-Schiff technique. J. Histochem. Cytochem. **5**, 445 (1957). — LEVI, G.: Trattato di istologia. Torino: Unione Tipografica Editrice Torinese 1927. — LEWIS, T.: The blood vessels of the human skin and their responses. London: Shaw & Sons 1927. — LEWIS, W. H.: The vascular pattern of tumors. Bull. Johns Hopk. Hosp. **41**, 156 (1927). — The outgrowth of endothelium and capillaries in tissue culture. Bull. Johns Hopk. Hosp. **48**, 242 (1931). — Lo CASCIO, G.: La morfogenesi dei vasi sanguiferi nella cute dell'uomo. Ricerche fatte nel Laboratorio di Anatomia Normale della R. Università di Roma ed altri Laboratori biologici, pubblicate dal Prof. F. TODARO, XVII, Roma 1913/14. — LOVETT-DOUST, J. W.: The capillary system in patients with psychiatric disorder. J. nerv. ment. Dis. **121**, 516 (1955).
MACGREGOR, I. A.: The vascularization of homografts of human skin. Brit. J. plast. Surg. **7**, 331 (1955). — MACHER, E. V., u. W. VOGEL: Elektronenmikroskopische Untersuchungen an Hautkapillaren. Dermatologica (Basel) **124**, 110 (1962). — MACKENZIE, D. G., and J. LOWENTHAL: Endothelial growth in nylon vascular grafts. Brit. J. Surg. **48**, 212 (1960). — MAJNO, G.: Ultrastructure of the vascular membrane. In: Handbuch of Physiology. Section 2, Circulation, III, Am. Physiol. Soc. Ed. 1965. — MANCHOT, C.: Die Hautarterien des menschlichen Körpers. Leipzig 1889. — MANGANOTTI, G.: Contributo allo studio dei fenomeni di senescenza della cute umana. V. Congr. Soc. Ital. Geront. Ger., Mattioli, Fidenza 1955. — MARCHAND, F.: Über die Contractilität der Capillaren und die Adventitiazellen. Münch. med. Wschr. **70**, 385 (1923). — MASSON, P.: Les glomus cutanés de l'homme. Bull. Soc. franç. Derm. Syph. **42**, 1174 (1935). — Les glomus neuro-vasculaires. Paris: Hermann & Cie. 1937. — MAYER-LIST, R., u. G. HÜBENER: Die Kapillarmikroskopie und ihre Bedeutung zur Zwillingsforschung. Münch. med. Wschr. **72**, 2185 (1925). — MAYNARD, E. A., R. L. SCHULTZ, and D. C. PEASE: Electron microscopy of the vascular bed of rat cerebral cortex. Amer. J. Anat. **100**, 409 (1957). — MAXIMOW, A.: Experimentelle Untersuchungen über die entzündliche Neubildung von Bindegewebe. Jena: Gustav Fischer 1902. — MENEGHINI, N.: Osservazioni anatomoradiografiche sulle reti arteriose e venose della faccia dell'uomo, nelle varie epoche della vita. Arch. ital. Derm. **18**, 62 (1942). — MESCON, H., J. HURLEY, and G. MORETTI: The anatomy and histochemistry of the arteriovenous anastomosis in human digital skin. J. invest. Derm. **27**, 133 (1956). — MIANI, A., e U. RUBERTI: Sulla morfologia degli apparati valvolari delle venule affluenti dalle anastomosi artero-venose della pianta del piede. Minerva cardioangiol. **41**, 541 (1958a). — La morfologia normale delle anastomosi artero-venose e dei dispositivi di blocco. Rass. ital. Chir. Med. **7**, 2 (1958b). — MIKHAIL, G. R., M. S. W. FARRIS, and N. S. GIMBEL: The pattern of superficial blood vessels in healing skin donor sites. J. invest. Derm. **44**, 75 (1965). — MILLER, M. R., H. J. RALSTON, and M. KASAHARA: The pattern of cutaneous innervation of the human hand, foot and breast. In: Advances in biology of skin I. Cutaneous innervation, p. 1 (W. MONTAGNA, ed.). New York: Pergamon Press 1960. — MISSOTTEN, L.: Étude des capillaries de la rétine et de la choriocapillarie au microscope electronique. Ophthalmologica (Basel) **144**, 1 (1962). — MONACELLI, M.: Contributo allo studio della arteriosclerosi cutanea. G. ital. Derm. Sif. **65**, 1793 (1924). — MONTAGNA, W.: The distribution of nonspecific esterases. J. biophys. biochem. Cytol. **1**, 13 (1955). — The distribution of β-glucoronidase. J. biophys. biochem. Cytol. **3**, 343 (1957). — Cholinesterases in the cutaneous nerves of man. In: Advances in biology of skin I. Cutaneous innervation, p. 74 (W. MONTAGNA, ed.). New York: Pergamon Press 1960. — The structure and function of skin. New York: Academic Press 1962. — MONTAGNA, W., and R. A. ELLIS: The blood supply of the hair follicle. J. Cancer Inst. **19**, 451 (1957). — MONTAGNA, W., and V. R. FORMISANO: The distribution of succinic dehydrogenase activity. Anat. Rec. **122**, 65 (1955). — MONTAGNA, W., and J. S. YUN: The distribution of cytochrome oxydase. J. Histochem. Cytochem. **9**, 694 (1961). — MOORE, D. M., and H. RUSKA: Fine structure of capillaries and small arteries. J. biophys. biochem. Cytol. **3**, 457 (1957). — MORETTI, G., and F. CROVATO: Unpublished data 1965. — MORETTI, G., R. A. ELLIS, and H. MESCON: Vascular patterns in the skin of the face. J. invest. Derm. **33**, 103 (1959). — MORETTI, G., u. G. FARRIS: Die alkalischen Phosphatasen in den Blutgefäßen der Haut einiger Primaten. Z. Haut- u. Geschl.-Kr. **34**, 6 (1963). — MORETTI, G., e W. MONTAGNA: Le unità vascolari. G. ital. Derm. Sif. **100**, 243 (1959). — MÜLLER, O.: Die feinsten Blutgefäße des Menschen in gesunden und kranken Tagen. Stuttgart: Ferdinand Enke 1937. — MUSUMECI, V.: Aspetti della rete vasale nella cute senile. Minerva derm. **36**, 209 (1961).
NIESSING, K., u. H. ROLLHAUSER: Über den submikroskopischen Bau des Grundhäutchens der Hirnkapillaren. Z. Zellforsch. **39**, 431 (1954).

ODLAND, G. F.: The fine structure of cutaneous capillaries. In: Advances in biology of skin II. Blood vessels and circulation, p. 577 (MONTAGNA, W. and R. A. ELLIS, eds.). New York: Pergamon Press 1961. — ORMEA, F.: La cute organo di senso. Torino: Minerva Medica 1961. — ORMEA, F., M. VISETTI e F. ALBERTAZZI: Sui dispositivi di blocco delle arterie cutanee. Atti S.I.D.E.S. Minerva derm. 34, 559 (1959).

PALADE, G. E.: Fine structure of blood capillaries. J. appl. Phys. 24, 1424 (1953). — Blood capillaries of the heart and other organs. Circulation 24, 368 (1961). — PANEBIANCO, G.: Studio sistematico sulla arteriosclerosi dei distretti cutanei e musculari. Pathologica 34, 109 (1942). — PEASE, D. C.: The basement membrane: substratum of histological order and complexity. Proc. IV. Int. Conf. Electron Microscopy 2, 139, Berlin 1958. — PEASE, D. C., and S. MOLINARI: Electron microscopy of muscular arteries; pial vessels of the cat and monkey. J. Ultrastruct. Res. 3, 447 (1960). — PEASE, D. C., and W. J. PAULE: Electron microscopy of elastic arteries; the thoracic aorta of the rat. J. Ultrastruct. Res. 3, 469 (1960). — PETERSEN, H.: Histologie und mikroskopische Anatomie (W. BARGMANN, ed.). München 1935. — PIETRZYKOWSKA, A.: Some function tests in senile skin. Przegl. derm. 52, 6, 581 (1965). — PISCHZEK, F., u. P. SCHMIDT: Über Capillarbeobachtungen an Schwangeren. Zbl. Gynäk. 50, 578 (1926). — POLLEY, E. H.: The innervation of blood vessels in striated muscle and skin. J. comp. Neurol. 103, 253 (1955). — POPOFF, N. W.: The digital vascular system. Arch. Path. 18, 295 (1934). — Recherches sur l'histologie des anastomoses arterio-veneuses des extrémités et sur leur rôle en pathologie vasculaire. Bull. Histol. appl. 12, 156 (1935). — PRITCHARD, M., and P. DANIEL: Arteriovenous anastomoses in the human external ear. J. Anat. (Lond.) 90, 309 (1956). — PUCHTLER, H., and C. P. LEBLOND: Histochemical analysis of cell membranes and associated structures as seen in the intestinal epithelium. Amer. J. Anat. 102, 1 (1958).

RAEKALLIO, J.: Enzymes histochemically demonstrable in the earliest phase of wound healing. Nature (Lond.) 188, 234 (1960). — Histochemical studies on vital and post-mortem skin wounds. Ann. Med. exp. Fenn. 39, Suppl. 6 (1961). — RAEKALLIO, J., and E. LEVONEN: Histochemical demonstration of transglycosylases and glycogen in the "lag phase" of wound healing. Exp. molec. Path. 2, 69 (1963). — RAIGROTZKI, J.: Über den Einfluß von Hyperämiemitteln auf das Gefäßsystem der weißen Maus. Morph. Jb. 81, 213 (1938). — RAMPINI, E., G. MORETTI e A. REBORA: Arteriole e capillari della cute e alopecia areata. Atti S.I.D.E.S. 46. Congr. Naz. Derm., Genova 1963. — REISER, K. A.: Über die Endausbreitung des vegetativen Nervensystems. Z. Zellforsch. 17, 610 (1933). — REITANO, R.: Sul problema dell'arteriosclerosi. In: Scritti in onore di Franco Flarer. Torino: Minerva Medica 1959. — RICHTER, R.: Über die Brauchbarkeit der Einschlußfärbung nativer Gefrierschnitte in Ehrlich's saurem Hämatoxylin nach Feyrter zur Darstellung der Nervenelemente der Haut. Z. Haut- u. Geschl.-Kr. 18, 33 (1955). — RINEHART, J. F., and M. G. FARQUHAR: The fine vascular organization of the anterior pituitary gland. An electron microscopic study with histochemical correlations. Anat. Rec. 121, 207 (1955). — ROBERTS, E., and J. A. GRIFFITH: A quantitative study of cutaneous capillaries in hyperthyroidism. Amer. Heart J. 14, 598 (1937). — ROMANUL, F. C. A., and R. G. BANNISTER: Localized areas of high alkaline phosphatase activity in endotheliums of arteries. Nature (Lond.) 195, 611 (1962). — ROSSATTI, B.: Rabbit's ear and new formation of arteriovenous anastomoses. J. Anat. (Lond.) 90, 318 (1956). — ROTHMANN, S.: Non-nervous vascular reactions. In: Physiology and biochemistry of the skin IV, p. 79. Chicago: Chicago University Press 1954. — RUFFINI, A.: Les dispositifes anatomiques de la sensibilité cutanée: sur les expansions nerveuses de la peau. Lyon: A. Storck 1905. — RUTENBURG, A. M., and A. M. SELIGMAN: The histochemical demonstration of acid phosphatase by a post incubation coupling technique. J. Histochem. Cytochem. 3, 455 (1955).

SACCHI, S.: Contributo alla conoscenza istotopochimica del glucosio e dei suoi rapporti col glicogeno nella cute umana normale e patologica. Riv. Istochim. norm. Pat. 3, 179 (1957). — SALMON: Artéres de la peau. Étude anatomique et chirurgicale Paris: Masson & Cie. 1936. — SANDISON, J. C.: Observations on the growth of blood vessels as seen in the transparent chamber introduced in the rabbit's ear. Amer. J. Anat. 41, 475 (1928). — SANNICANDRO, G.: La reazione nitroprussica nello studio della cheratinizzazione epidermica. Arch. ital. Derm. 8, 647 (1932). — I lipidi della cute. G. ital. Derm. 75, 495 (1934). — SAUNDERS, C. H. DE: X-ray projection microscopy of the skin. In: Advances in biology of skin II. Blood vessels and circulation, p. 38 (W. MONTAGNA and R. A. ELLIS, eds.). New York: Pergamon Press 1961. — SCHNITZER, K. L.: Ist das Hautcapillarbild beim Neugeborenen als Reifezeichen verwertbar. Mschr. Geburtsh. Gynäk. 107, 19 (1937). — SCHOEFL, G. I.: Growing capillaries. Their fine structure and permeability (Doctoral Thesis). Radcliffe College, Cambridge (Mass.) 1962. — Studies on inflammation. III. Growing capillaries: their structure and permeability. Arch. Path. Anat. Physiol. 337, 97 (1963). — SCHOEFL, G. I., and G. MAJNO: Regeneration of blood vessels. In: Advances in biology of skin III. Wound healing, p. 173 (W. MONTAGNA and R. E. BILLINGHAM, eds.). London: Pergamon Press 1964. — SCHORN, J.:

Zur normalen und pathologischen Anatomie der Hoyer-Grosserschen Organe, der sogenannten "Arterio-venösen Anastomosen" in den Endgliedern der Finger und Zehen des Menschen. Habil.-Schr. Gießen 1955. — SCHUMACHER, S. V.: Über das Glomus coccygium des Menschen und die Glomeruli caudales der Säugetiere. Arch. mikr. Anat. 71, 58 (1907). — SCHWALM, H.: Die Hautcapillaren bei Neugeborenen. Arch. Kinderheilk. 103, 129 (1934). — SERRI, F.: Apporto dell'istotopochimica alla conoscenza delle attività enzimatiche cutanee. Atti S.I.D.E.S., Minerva derm. 465 (1959). — SPALTEHOLZ, W.: Die Verteilung der Blutgefäße in der Haut. Arch. Anat. u. Physiol. Anat. Abt. (1893). — Blutgefäße der Haut. In: Handbuch der Haut- und Geschlechtskrankheiten, vol. I/1, p. 379. Berlin: Springer 1927. — STAUBESAND, J.: Über die Versorgung der Arterienwand. Anat. Anz. 107, 332 (1959). — STEIGLEDER, G. K., R. KUDICKE u. Y. KAMEI: Die Lokalisation der Aminopeptisenaktivität in normaler Haut. Arch. klin. exp. Derm. 215, 307 (1962). — STEIGLEDER, G. K., u. H. LÖFFLER: Zum histochemischen Nachweis unspezifischer Esterasen und Lipasen. Arch. klin. exp. Derm. 203, 41 (1956). — STÖHR jr., P.: Mikroskopische Anatomie des vegetativen Nerven-Systems. In: Handbuch der mikroskopischen Anatomie des Menschen, vol. IV/5, p. 516 (1957). — STÖHR jr., P.: Nerves of the blood vessels, heart, etc. Quoted from R. K. WINKELMANN in: Nerve endings in normal and pathologic skin, p. 114. Springfield (Ill.): Ch. C. Thomas 1960. — Quoted from F. ORMEA in: La cute organo di senso. Torino: Minerva Medica 1961. — SUCQUET, J. P.: Anatomie et physiologie, circulation du sang. D'une circulation derivative dans les membres et dans la tête chez l'homme. Paris: A. Delahaye 1862. — SUNDER-PLASMANN, P.: Quoted from F. ORMEA in: La cute organo di senso. Torino: Minerva Medica 1961.

TIEDEMANN, A.: Über Gefäßversorgung von Haut- und Lebertransplantaten. Virchows Arch. path. Anat. 317, 461 (1949).

VASTARINI-CRESI, G.: Le anastomosi artero-venose nell'uomo e nei mammiferi. Napoli: Studio Anatomo-istologico 1903. — VOLTERRA, M.: Einige neue Befunde über die Struktur der Capillaren und ihre Beziehungen zur "sogenannten" Contractilität derselben. Zbl. inn. Med. 46, 876 (1925).

WALLS, E. W., and T. J. BUCHANAN: Observations on the capillary blood vessels of the human blood. J. Anat. (Lond.) 90, 329 (1956). — WATANABE, S.: Über die Arteriosklerose der Hautgefäße. Schweiz med. Wschr. 51, 34, 780 (1921). — WATZKA, M.: Über Gefäßsperren und arterio-venöse Anastomosen. Z. mikr. anat. Forsch. 39, 521 (1936). — WEARN, J. T.: The extent of the capillary bed of the heart. J. exp. Med. 47, 273 (1928). — WEDDELL, G.: The innervation of cutaneous blood vessels. In: Advances in biology of skin II. Blood vessels and circulation, p. 71 (W. MONTAGNA and R. A. ELLIS, eds.). New York: Pergamon Press 1961. — WEDDELL, G., and W. PALLIE: Observations on the neurohistology of cutaneous blood vessels. In: Peripheral circulation in man. Ciba Foundation Symposium (G. E. W. WOLSTENHOLME, ed.). London: Churchill 1954. — WEISS, S., and W. R. FRAZIER: The density of the surface capillary bed of the forearm in health, in arterial hypertension and in arteriosclerosis. Amer. Heart J. 5, 511 (1930). — WEISS, S., and B. NICKAU: Quoted from O. MÜLLER in Verh. dtsch. Kongr. inn. Med. 211 (1921). — WERTHEIMER, N., and M. WERTHEIMER: Capillary structure: its relation to psychiatric diagnosis and morphology. J. nerv. ment. Dis. 122, 1 (1955). — WERTHEMANN, A.: Über den Aufbau der Blutgefäßwand in entzündlichen Neubildungen, insbesondere in Pleuraschwarten (Histologische Studie zur Frage mesenchymaler Differenzierungen). Habil.-Schr. Virchows Arch. path. Anat. 270 (1928). — WETZEL, N. C., and Y. ZOTTERMANN: Differences in the vascular coloration of venous regions of the normal human skin. Heart 13, 357 (1926). — WIEDMANN, A.: Beiträge zur Pathologie der Gefäßerkrankungen der Haut. Derm. Z. 73, 241 (1936). — WINKELMANN, R. K.: Nerve endings in normal and pathologic skin. Springfield (Ill.): Ch. C. Thomas 1960. — Cutaneous vascular patterns in studies with injection preparation and alkaline phosphatase reaction. In: Advances in biology of skin II. Blood vessels and circulation, p. 1 (W. MONTAGNA and R. A. ELLIS, eds.). New York: Pergamon Press 1961. — WIMTRUP, B.: Beiträge zur Anatomie der Capillaren. Z. Anat. 68, 469 (1923). Quoted by W. SPALTEHOLZ 1927. — WISLOCKI, G. B., H. BUNTING, and E. W. DEMPSEY: Metachromasia in mammalian tissues and its relationship to mucopolysaccharides. Amer. J. Anat. 81, 1 (1947). — WOLFF, K.: Zur Orthotopie der histochemisch erfaßbaren Aminopeptidasenaktivität der menschlichen Haut. Arch. klin. exp. Derm. 217, 534 (1963a). — Histologische Beobachtungen an der normalen menschlichen Haut bei der Durchführung ferment-histochemischer Untersuchungen mit Adenosintriphosphat als Substrat. Arch. klin. exp. Derm. 216, 1 (1963b). — WOLFF, K., and F. G. SCHELLANDER: Enzyme-histochemical studies on the healing-process of split skin grafts. I. Aminopeptidase, diphosphopyridine-nucleotide-diaphorase and succinic-dehydrogenase in autografts. J. invest. Derm. 45, 38 (1965). — Enzyme-histochemical studies on the healing process of split skin grafts. III. Oxidative and hydrolytic enzymes in homografts. J. invest. Derm. 46, 213 (1966). — WOOLLARD, H. H.: Innervation of blood vessels. Heart 13, 319 (1926). — WRIGHT, I. S., and A. W. DURJEE: Human capillaries in health and disease. Arch intern. Med. 52, 545 (1933).

ZELICKSON, A. S.: A tubular structure in the endothelial cells and pericytes of human capillaries. J. invest. Derm. **46**, 67 (1966). — ZIMMER, J. G., and D. J. DEMIS: Studies on the microcirculation of the skin in disease. J. invest. Derm. **39**, 501 (1962). — ZIMMERMAN, K. W.: Der feinere Bau der Blutkapillaren. Z. Anat. Entwickl.-Gesch. **68**, 29 (1923). — ZUGIBE, F. T.: Mucopolysaccharides of the arterial wall. J. Histochem. Cytochem. **2**, 35 (1963). — ZWEIFACH, B. W.: Basic mechanisms in peripheral vascular homeastasis. Tr. 3rd conf. on factors regulating blood pressure. New York: Macy J. Jr. Foundation, 1949.

D. The architecture of the Cutaneous Blood Network

BACCAREDDA-BOY, A., G. MORETTI e G. FARRIS: Varietà topografiche della reazione per la fosfatasi alcalina nel circolo superficiale cutaneo. Ann. ital. Derm. Sif. **15**, 186 (1960a). — BACCAREDDA-BOY, A., G. MORETTI e B. FILIPPI: Il circolo superficiale in rapporto alle zone elettive di trapianto cutaneo. Minerva derm. **35**, 345 (1960b). — BACCAREDDA-BOY, A., G. MORETTI e A. REBORA: Densità capillare e istamina nel cuoio capelluto. Minerva derm. **36**, 337 (1961). — BELLOCQ, PH.: Étude anatomique des artères de la peau chez l'homme. Paris: Masson & Cie 1925. — BERTAMINO, R., E. RAMPINI e C. RUFFINI: Osservazioni sulla capacità funzionale delle ghiandole sudoripare eccrine nell'alopecia areata. Atti XLVI Congr. Naz. S.I.D.E.S. 1963, p. 342. — BIMTS, K. N.: Veins of human cutaneous appendages. Vestn. Derm. Vener. **34**, 24 (1960).

CORMIA, F. E.: Vasculature of the normal scalp. Arch. Derm. **88**, 692 (1963). — CORMIA, F. E., and A. ERNYEY: Circulatory changes in alopecia. Arch. Derm. **84**, 772 (1961).

DAVIS, M. J., and J. C. LAWLER: Capillary microscopy in normal and diseased human skin. In: Advances in biology of skin II. Blood vessels and circulation, p. 79 (W. MONTAGNA and R. A. ELLIS, eds.). New York: Pergamon Press 1961. — DE SOUSA, A., and S. RODRIGUES: Angioarchitecture of the skin. Microangiographie studies. Amer. J. Röntgenol. **88**, 1, 112 (1962). — DIETER, W., u. C. SUNG SHENG: Zur Physiologie und Morphologie der Capillaren am Nagelwall bei gesunden Personen. Z. ges. exp. Med. **28**, 234 (1922). — DIEULAFÉ et DURAND: Sur les vaisseaux de la peau. C. R. Ass. Anat. Bordeaux 1906. — DODD, H., and F. B. COCKETT: The pathology and surgery of the veins of the lower limb. Edinburgh: Livingstone 1956. — DURWARD, A., and K. M. RUDALL: The vascularity and patterns of growth of hair follicles. In: The biology of hair growth, p. 189 (W. MONTAGNA and R. A. ELLIS, eds.). New York: Academic Press 1958.

EICHNER, F.: Zur Frage der Motivbildung in der menschlichen Haut. Anat. Anz. **100**, 303 (1954). — ELLIS, R. A.: Vascular pattern of the skin. In: Advances in biology of skin II, p. 20 (W. MONTAGNA and R. A. ELLIS, eds.). London: Pergamon Press 1961. — ELLIS, R. A., W. MONTAGNA, and H. FANGER: The blood supply of the cutaneous glands. J. invest. Derm. **30**, 137 (1958). — ELLIS, R. A., and G. MORETTI: Vascular pattern associated with catagen hair follicles in the human scalp. Ann. N.Y. Acad. Sci. **83**, 448 (1959).

FARBER, E. M., E. A. HINES jr., H. MONTGOMERY, and K. McCRAIG: The arterioles of the skin in assential hypertension. J. invest. Derm. **9**, 285 (1947).

HARDY, M.: The development of pelage hairs and vibrissae from the skin in tissue culture. Ann. N.Y. Acad. Sci. **53**, 546 (1951). — HEYNOLD, H.: Über die Knäueldrüsen der Menschen. Virchows Arch. path. Anat. **61** (1874). — HORSTMANN, E.: Die Haut. In: Handbuch der mikroskopischen Anatomie der Menschen, vol. III/3, p. 198 (W. v. MÖLLENDORFF u. W. BARGMANN, eds.). Berlin-Göttingen-Heidelberg: Springer 1957.

LOBITZ, W. C., J. B. HOLYOKE jr., and W. MONTAGNA: The epidermal eccrine sweat duct unit. A morphologic and biologic entity. J. invest. Derm. **22**, 157 (1954).

MENEGHINI, N.: Osservazioni anatomo-radiografiche sulle reti arteriose e venose della faccia dell'uomo, nelle varie epoche della vita. Arch. ital. Derm. **18**, 62 (1942). — MESCON, H., J. HURLEY, and G. MORETTI: The anatomy and histochemistry of the arteriovenous anastomosis in human digital skin. J. invest. Derm. **27**, 133 (1956). — MONTAGNA, W.: Summary. In: The biology of hair growth, p. 487 (W. MONTAGNA and R. A. ELLIS, eds.). New York: Academic Press 1958. — The structure and function of skin. New York: Academic Press 1962. — MONTAGNA, W., and R. A. ELLIS: The blood supply of the hair follicle. J. nat. Cancer Inst. **19**, 451 (1957). — MONTAGNA, W., and J. S. YUN: The skin of the great bush-baby (galago crassicaudatus). Amer. J. phys. Anthrop. **20**, 149 (1962a). — The skin of the anubis baboon (papio doguera). Amer. J. phys. Anthrop. **20**, 131 (1962b). — MORETTI, G., R. A. ELLIS, and H. MESCON: Vascular patterns in the skin of the face. J. invest. Derm. **33**, 103 (1959). — MORETTI, G., e W. MONTAGNA: Le unità vascolari. G. ital. Derm. Sif. **100**, 243 (1959). — MORETTI, G., A. REBORA, C. GIACOMETTI e F. CROVATO: Arteriole e capillari nel cuoio capelluto. Minerva derm. **35**, 43 (1960).

OTTAVIANI, G.: Annotazioni anatomoradiografiche della vascolarizzazione arteriosa e venosa della faccia dell'uomo. Morph. Jb. **85** (1941).

PETERSEN, H.: Histologie und mikroskopische Anatomie. München: J. F. Bergmann 1935.

Rampini, E., G. Moretti e A. Rebora: Arteriole e capillari della cute ed alopecia areata. Atti S.I.D.E.S. 46. Congr. Naz. Derm., Genova 1963. — Renaut, J.: Traite d'histologie pratique, 2, 1. Paris 1897. — Ruffini, A.: Contributo allo studio della vascolarizzazione della cute umana con proposta di una classificazione più razionale dei suoi diversi strati. Monit. zool. ital. 11 (1900). — Ryder, M. L.: The blood supply to the wool follicle. Proc. Int. Wool. Text. Res. Conf., vol. F, p. 63. Australia 1955.
Salmon: Artères de la peau. Étude anatomique et chirurgicale. Paris: Masson & Cie. 1936. — Samman, P. D.: The nails in disease. London: Heinemann W. Medical Books Ltd. 1965. — Saunders, C. H. de: Microradiographic studies of the vascular patterns in muscle and skin. In: X-ray microscopy and microradiography (V. E. Cosslett, A. Engstrom, and H. H. Patteeya). New York: Academic Press 1957. — X-ray projection microscopy of the skin. In: Advances in biology of skin II. Blood vessels and circulation, p. 38 (W. Montagna and R. A. Ellis, eds.). New York: Pergamon Press 1961. — Spalteholz, W.: Blutgefäße der Haut. In: Handbuch der Haut- und Geschlechtskrankheiten, Bd. I/I, S. 379. Berlin: Springer 1927.
Tomsa, W.: Beiträge zur Anatomie und Physiologie der menschlichen Haut. Arch. Derm. Syph. (Berl.) **5** (1873). — Todd and Bowmann (1845): Quoted from G. Truffi in: Sulla vascolarizzazione degli annessi cutanei. Arch. ital. Derm. **10**, 681 (1934). — Truffi, G.: Sulla vascolarizzazione degli annessi cutanei. Arch. ital. Derm. **10**, 681 (1934).
Unna jr., P.: Untersuchungen über die Lymph- und Blutgefäße der äußeren Haut mit besonderer Berücksichtigung der Haarfollikel. Arch. mikr. Anat. Entwicklungsgesch. **72** (1908).
Walsh jr., T. S.: The dermal arteries of the neck and shoulder. Quoted from Excerpta med. (Amst.), Sect. XIII **18**, 493 (1964). — Wetzel, N. C., and Y. Zottermann: On differences in the vascular coloration of venous regions of the normal human skin. Heart **13**, 358 (1926). — Winkelmann, R. K.: Cutaneous vascular patterns. In: Advances in biology of skin II. Blood vessels and circulation, p. 1 (W. Montagna and R. A. Ellis, eds.). New York: Pergamon Press 1961.
Zika, K., and E. Kominkora: The blood supply of Vater-Pacini corpuscles. Folia morph. (Warszawa) **13**, 394 (1965).

E. An Outline of the Blood Cutaneous Network Design

Bellocq, Ph.: Étude anatomique des artères de la peau chez l'homme. Paris: Masson & Cie. 1925.
Chambers, R., and B. W. Zweifach: Intercellular cement and capillary permeability. Physiol. Rev. **27**, 431 (1947). — Cormia, F. E., and A. Ernyey: Circulatory changes in alopecia. Arch. Derm. **84**, 772 (1961).
Ellis, R. A.: Ageing of the human male scalp. In: The biology of hair growth, p. 469 (W. Montagna and R. A. Ellis, eds.). New York: Academic Press 1958. — Ellis, R. A., and G. Moretti: Vascular patterns associated with catagen hair follicles in the human scalp. Ann. N.Y. Acad. Sci. **83**, 448 (1959).
Gans, O., u. G. K. Steigleder: Histologie der Hautkrankheiten, vol. I, p. 48. Berlin-Göttingen-Heidelberg: Springer 1955.
Horstmann, E.: Die Haut. In: Handbuch der mikroskopischen Anatomie der Menschen, vol. III/3, p. 198 (W. v. Möllendorf u. W. Bergmann, eds.). Berlin-Göttingen-Heidelberg: Springer 1957.
Irague: Disposition generale des artères de la peau. Quoted from G. Lo Cascio, La morfogenesi dei vasi sanguiferi nella cute dell'uomo. Ricerche fatte nel Laboratorio di Anatomia Umana Normale della R. Università di Roma ed in altri Laboratori biologici, pubblicate dal Prof. F. Todaro, XVII, 1 (1913/14).
Klingmüller, G.: Neue Beobachtungen zur Ätiologie der Alopecie. Arch. Derm. Syph. (Berl.) **200**, 448 (1955). — Koelliker, R. A.: Elements d'histologie humaine. Paris: Masson & Cie. 1856.
Lever, W.: Histopathology of the skin, p. 243. Philadelphia: J. B. Lippincott Co. 1949.
Manchot, C.: Die Hautarterien des menschlichen Körpers. Leipzig 1889. — Montagna, W.: Summary. In: The biology of hair growth, p. 487 (W. Montagna and R. A. Ellis, eds.). New York: Academic Press 1958. — Moretti, G., R. A. Ellis, and H. Mescon: Vascular patterns in the skin of the face. J. invest. Derm. **39**, 103 (1959). — Moretti, G., e W. Montagna: Le unità vascolari. G. ital. Derm. Sif. **100**, 243 (1959).
Perruccio, L.: Sul comportamento del trypan-blau iniettato intradermicamente nelle varie regioni del corpo. G. ital. Derm. Sif. **76**, 171 (1935). — Petersen, H.: Histologie und mikroskopische Anatomie. München: J. F. Bergmann 1935. — Pillsbury, D. M., W. B. Shelley, and A. M. Kligmann: Dermatology, p. 755. Philadelphia: W. B. Saunders Co. 1956.
Radaelli, F.: Sopra un caso di "Purpura annularis teleangiectodes". G. ital. Derm. **52**, 381 (1911). — Redisch, W., and R. H. Pelzer: Localized vascular dilatations of the human

skin. Capillary microscopy and related studies. Amer. Heart J. **37**, 106 (1949). — RENAUT, J.: Traité d'histologie pratique, 2, 1. Paris 1897. — ROTHMAN, S.: Physiology and biochemistry of the skin. Chicago: Chicago University Press 1954. — RYDER, M. L.: The blood supply to the wool follicle. In: Proc. Int. Wool Text. Res. Conf. F, 63, Australia 1955.
SALMON: Artères de la peau. Étude anatomique et chirurgicale. Paris: Masson & Cie. 1936. — SAUNDERS, C. H. DE: X-ray microscopy of dental pulp vessels. Nature (Lond.) **180**, 1353 (1957). — X-ray projection microscopy of the skin. In: Advances in biology of skin II. Blood vessels and circulation (W. MONTAGNA and R. A. ELLIS, eds.). New York: Pergamon Press 1961. — SPALTEHOLZ, W.: Die Verteilung der Blutgefäße in der Haut. Arch. Anat. u. Physiol. Anat. Abt. (1893). — Blutgefäße der Haut. In: Handbuch der Haut- und Geschlechtskrankheiten, vol. 1/1, p. 379. Berlin: Springer 1927. — SUCQUET, J. P.: Anatomie et physiologie. Circulation du sang. D'une circulation derivative dans les membres et dans la tête chez l'homme. Paris: Delahaye 1862. — SUTTON, R. L.: Diseases of the skin, p. 735. St. Louis: C. V. Mosby Co. 1956.
TOMSA, W.: Beiträge zur Anatomie und Physiologie der menschlichen Haut. Arch. Derm. Syph. (Berl.) **5** (1873). — TODD and BOWMANN: Quoted from G. TRUFFI, Sulla vascolarizzazione degli annessi cutanei. Arch. ital. Derm. **10**, 681 (1934). — TRUFFI, G.: Sulla vascolarizzazione degli annessi cutanei. Arch. ital. Derm. **10**, 681 (1934).
UNNA, P.: Quoted from J. ORTH, Lehrbuch der speziellen pathologischen Anatomie, Erg.-Bd. 2, Die Histopathologie der Hautkrankheiten. Berlin 1894.
WETZEL, N. C., and Y. ZOTTERMANN: On differences in the vascular colouration of venous regions of the normal human skin. Heart **13**, 358 (1926). — WINKELMANN, R. K., S. R. SCHEEN, R. A. PYKA, and M. B. COVENTRY: Cutaneous vascular patterns in studies with injection preparation and alkaline phosphatase reaction. In: Advances in biology of skin II, p. 1 (W. MONTAGNA and R. A. ELLIS, eds.). Oxford: Pergamon Press 1961.

F. Conclusions

BACCAREDDA-BOY, A., G. MORETTI e G. FARRIS: Varietà topografiche della reazione per la fosfatasi alcalina nel circolo superficiale cutaneo. Ann. ital. Derm. Sif. **15**, 3 (1960).
COMEL, M., et E. MIAN: Correlation histangiques et métabolisme de la paroi vasculaire. Folia angiol. **8**, 4, 371 (1961).
ELLIS, R. A., and G. MORETTI: Vascular patterns associated with catagen hair follicles in the human scalp. Ann. N.Y. Acad. Sci. **83**, 448 (1959). — ENGEL: Lo sviluppo dei vasi sanguiferi nelle palpebre dell'uomo. Quoted from G. LO CASCIO, La morfogenesi dei vasi sanguiferi nella cute dell'uomo. Ricerche fatte nel Laboratorio di Anatomia Umana Normale della R. Università di Roma ed in altri Laboratori biologici, publicate dal Prof. F. TODARO, XVII, 1 (1913/14).
HARDY, M. H.: The development of pelage hairs and vibrissae from the skin in tissue culture. Ann. N.Y. Acad. Sci. **53**, 546 (1951). — HERTZMANN, A. B.: Blood supply of various skin areas as estimated by the photoelectric plethysmograph. Amer. J. Physiol. **124**, 328 (1938). — HORSTMANN, E.: Die Haut. In: Handbuch der mikroskopischen Anatomie des Menschen, vol. III/3, p. 198 (W. v. MÖLLENDORF u. W. BARGMANN). Berlin-Göttingen-Heidelberg: Springer 1957.
KUWABARA, T., and D. G. COGAN: Mural cells of the retinal capillaries. Arch. Ophthal. **69**, 492 (1963).
LANDERS, J. W., J. L. CHASON, J. E. GONZALES, and W. PALUTKE: Morphology and enzymatic activity of rat cerebral capillaries. Lab. invest. **11**, 1253 (1962).
MONTAGNA, W.: The structure and function of skin. New York: Academic Press 1962. — MONTAGNA, W., and R. A. ELLIS: The blood supply of the hair follicles. J. nat. Cancer Inst. **19**, 451 (1957). — MORETTI, G., and F. CROVATO: Unpublished data 1965. — MORETTI, G., and G. FARRIS: Die alkalischen Phosphatasen in den Blutgefäßen der Haut einigen Primaten. Z. Haut- u. Geschl.-Kr. **34**, 161 (1963).
RAMPINI, E., G. MORETTI e A. REBORA: Arteriole e capillari della cute e alopecia areata. Atti S.I.D.E.S. 46. Congr. Naz. Derm., Genova 1963. — RYDER, M. L.: The blood supply to the wool follicle. In: Proc. Int. Wool Text. Res. Conf., vol. F. p. 63. Australia 1955.

Die Embryologie der Haut

Von

H. Pinkus und A. Tanay, Detroit

Mit 37 Abbildungen

Einleitung

Die Entwicklung der menschlichen Haut wurde zum erstenmal ausführlich im Keibel-Mallschen Lehrbuch von F. Pinkus (1910) behandelt. Derselbe Autor brachte embryologische Daten in seiner Anatomie der Haut (1927) im Jadassohnschen Handbuch. Etwa gleichzeitig gaben Pernkopf und Patzelt eine kurze, klare Darstellung im Arzt-Zielerschen Werk. Schließlich stellte Horstmann neue und ältere Befunde in seinem Beitrag zum Möllendorff-Bargmannschen Handbuch (1957) zusammen und gab auch eine kurze Übersicht im Gottron-Schönfeldschen Werk (1961).

Unsere Darstellung, die ja den Beitrag von F. Pinkus ergänzen soll, wird versuchen, Ergebnisse der letzten 40 Jahre aufgrund der Weltliteratur und eigener Untersuchungen so zusammenzufassen, daß sich ein übersichtliches, modernes Bild ergibt.

Für die Grundlagen verweisen wir auf F. Pinkus und Horstmann. Untersuchungen an tierischer Haut werden nur ausnahmsweise berücksichtigt werden.

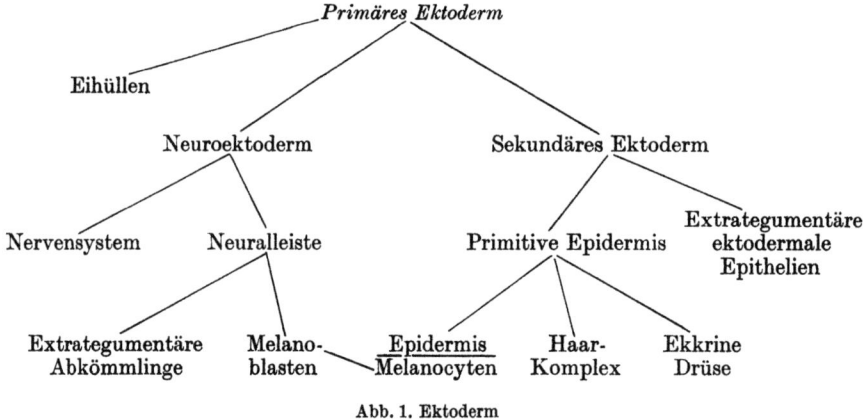

Abb. 1. Ektoderm

An der Entwicklung der Haut beteiligen sich Ektoderm und Mesoderm. Die Epidermis und der epitheliale Teil der Anhangsgebilde entstehen aus dem nach Absonderung der Medullarplatte und der Neuralleiste übrigbleibenden Ektoderm (sekundäres Ektoderm, s. Abb. 1). Tatsächlich geht fast das ganze sekundäre Ektoderm in der Haut auf, mit Ausnahme der verhältnismäßig kleinen Teile, die das Ohrbläschen bilden, die Mundrachenhöhle, die Nase und den Conjunctivalsack auskleiden, die Cornea und Linse des Auges liefern und sich an den Übergangszonen des Urogenital- und Analgebietes beteiligen. Der äußere Gehörgang und das Trommelfell gehören im eigentlichen Sinne zur Haut.

Die Lederhaut (Corium, Cutis, Dermis) entwickelt sich teils aus ungegliedertem Mesenchym, teils aus den Urwirbeln, und zwar aus der lateralen oder Cutislamelle (Abb. 2). Die dadurch verursachte Metamerie geht aber schnell verloren und ist später nicht mehr im Bau des Bindegewebes, sondern nur noch in der Verteilung von Nerven und Gefäßen nachzuweisen.

Zwei wichtige Bestandteile der Haut wandern nachträglich vom Neuroektoderm her ein. Die eine dieser Komponenten ist das System der sensorischen und

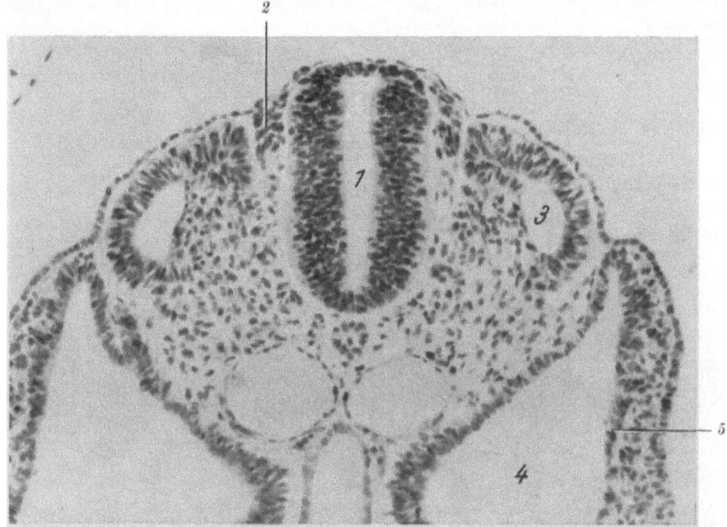

Abb. 2. Querschnitt durch einen menschlichen Embryo von 2,5 mm. *1* Neuralrohr, unter dem ventralen Pol die Chorda dorsalis; *2* Neuralleiste in Auswanderung begriffen; *3* Ursegmente; Sklerotom in Auflösung, Dermatom unterlagert als solide Lamelle die Epidermis; *4* Cölom; *5* Somatopleura. (Aus TÖNDURY, 1964)

autonomen Nerven, die andere ist das Pigmentsystem der Haut, das Melanocyten der Epidermis, der Haare und des Coriums und Langerhanssche Zellen einschließt.

Im folgenden wird die morphologisch faßbare Entwicklung der Epidermis und des Coriums zuerst gesondert besprochen werden. Dann werden wir versuchen, das Zusammenwirken dieser innig aufeinander eingestellten Teile zu skizzieren. Das wird die darauffolgende Schilderung der Hautanhangsgebilde erleichtern. Schließlich werden neuroektodermale Abkömmlinge kurz besprochen werden. Von diesen ist die Entstehung der Pigmentzellen schon von STARCK in Band I/2 behandelt worden, und es werden hier nur einige ganz neue Arbeiten berücksichtigt werden.

A. Entwicklung der Epidermis

1. Allgemeines

Eine ausführliche Beschreibung der Frühentwicklung der Epidermis wurde von STERNBERG (1927) aufgrund der Untersuchung eines menschlichen Embryos mit vier Ursegmenten gegeben. Bei diesem war der ektodermale Anteil der Embryonalanlage in zwei Abschnitte gegliedert: das Epithel der späteren Körperoberfläche und das Epithel der Medullaranlage. Am erstgenannten waren schon verschieden gebaute Partien zu erkennen. Im Bereiche der Perikardialplatte stimmte sein Bau mit dem Epithel des Amnion überein. Die Zellen waren flach und einschichtig angeordnet. Zellgrenzen waren in den mit Hämatoxylin-Eosin gefärbten Schnitten nicht zu erkennen. An einigen Stellen waren aus mehreren Zellen bestehende Nester eingelagert, welche keilförmig gegen die darunter gelegene Wand der Perikardialhöhle vorsprangen und gelegentlich Mitosen enthielten. An der Unterseite des abgehobenen Kopfteils war das Epithel prismatisch, 26—28 μ hoch, mit zweireihig angeordneten, länglichen Kernen. Zahlreiche Zell-

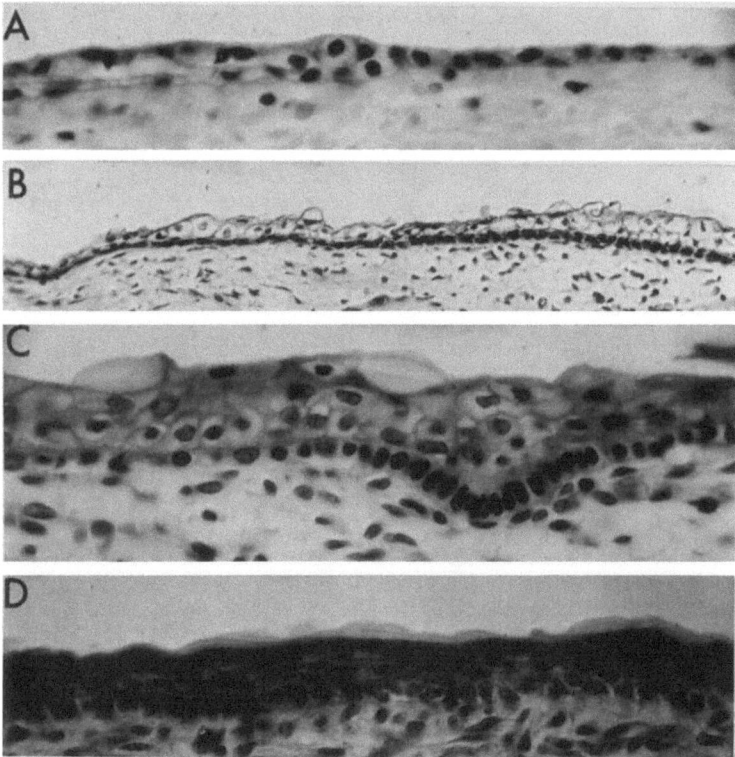

Abb. 3. Phasen der Entwicklung der Epidermis. *A* Übergang von einschichtigem zu zweischichtigem Epithel an der lateralen Rumpfwand eines jungen Embryos. *B* Ausbildung der Basalschicht und des Periderms und einiger Zellen des Stratum intermedium. *C* Mehrschichtige Epidermis, noch ohne Verhornung. Rechts ein frontal geschnittener Haarkeim mit typischen pyknotischen Zellkernen im Zentrum (s. S. 647). *D* Beginn der Verhornung. Oberste Zellschicht kernfrei

teilungsfiguren lagen durchweg in der oberen Zellreihe. Dieses hohe Epithel setzte sich auf die seitliche Kopfwand fort und war scharf von der Bekleidung des Embryonalschildes abgesetzt, das aus einem nur 8—10 μ hohen einschichtigen Epithel bestand. Caudalwärts wurde der Streifen zweireihigen Epithels allmählich schmaler und flacher und verschwand im Bereich des Rückenmarks ganz. Hier grenzte einschichtiges flaches Epithel direkt an die Medullarplatte. Noch weiter hinten nahm das Ektoderm an der Bildung des Primitivknotens teil.

Die Epidermis weist also schon sehr frühzeitig regionäre Unterschiede auf, die teils mit späterer Spezialentwicklung verknüpft sind, teils auf phylogenetischer Grundlage erklärt wurden, während für noch andere entwicklungsmechanistische Deutungen gegeben worden sind. Darauf werden wir unter A. 4 und C zurückkommen. Als Schema der Allgemeinentwicklung (Abb. 3) kann gelten, daß das einschichtige Ektoderm, das flach, kubisch oder prismatisch sein kann, nach einiger Zeit zweischichtig und später mehrschichtig wird. Dies geschieht offenbar durch stärkere mitotische Aktivität, die mehr Zellen liefert als nötig sind, um mit dem Körperwachstum Schritt zu halten. Mehrschichtigkeit ist eine grundlegende Eigenschaft des Ektoderms, die sich nicht nur im Bau der Epidermis und dem mindestens zweischichtigen Epithel ektodermaler Drüsen ausdrückt, sondern sich auch in der Gewebekultur offenbart (PINKUS, 1932).

Traditionell wird beim Embryo die mesoderm-nahe Schicht als Basalschicht, die äußere als Periderm bezeichnet. Wenn weitere Zellagen dazukommen, werden diese Stratum intermedium genannt. Mitosen kommen anfangs in allen Lagen vor

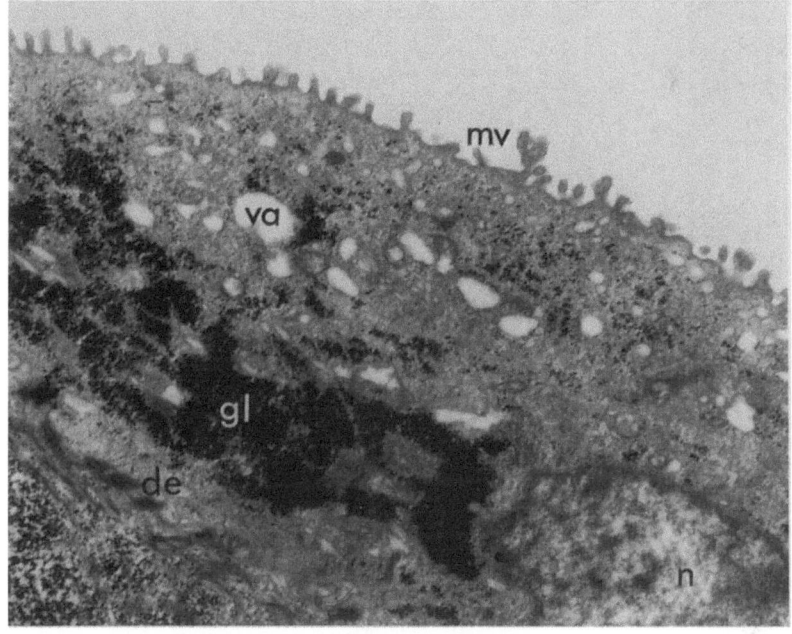

Abb. 4. Peridermzelle eines 12 Wochen alten Fetus mit Mikrovilli und Glykogen. Elektronenoptische Aufnahme, 16400mal, fixiert mit Osmium, gefärbt mit Bleihydroxyd. *de* Desmosomen, die die Zelle mit der darunterliegenden Zelle des Stratum intermedium verbinden; *gl* Glykogen; *mv* Mikrovilli; *n* Nucleus; *va* cytoplasmatische Vacuolen.
(Aus BREATHNACH, 1965)

(HÄGGQVIST, 1921; EICHENLAUB und OSBOURN, 1951), aber Versuche, sie als selbständig organisierte Einheiten aufzufassen, sind überholt (PINKUS, 1954; KOHAN, 1965).

Die Basalschicht wird zum Stratum germinativum, von dem die äußeren Lagen gebildet und ersetzt werden, wenn sie an der Körperoberfläche verlorengehen. Vom 5. Monat an (OLIN, 1942; ACHTEN, 1957) wird das Periderm an der allgemeinen Körperoberfläche von Keratohyalin und Hornschicht abgelöst. Handflächen und Fußsohlen eilen 1—2 Monate voraus.

Daß das Periderm eine funktionelle Anpassung der fetalen Haut an das Leben im Fruchtwasser darstellt, wurde schon durch CHLOPINs (1933) Gewebekulturen embryonaler Menschenhaut wahrscheinlich gemacht (PINKUS, 1932), die zu vorzeitiger Hornschichtbildung führten. Ganz ähnlich berichten PULLAR und LIADSKY (1965), daß die Epidermis menschlicher Feten sich in der Gewebekultur innerhalb von 4 Tagen vom Peridermstadium auf Verhornung umstellt, mit entsprechenden Änderungen im Enzymgehalt. Weitere Hinweise auf spezifische Austauschfunktionen der Peridermzellen finden sich in ZASTAVAs (1951) schönen

Oberflächenbildern mit der Bildung von Bläschen. Am überzeugendsten sind die elektronenoptischen Befunde (BREATHNACH, 1965; BONNEVILLE, 1965; RIEGEL, 1965; HASHIMOTO et al., 1966), die die Anwesenheit von Mikrovilli auf der freien Oberfläche des Periderms nachwiesen (Abb. 4).

2. Ultrastruktur

Untersuchungen mit dem Elektronenmikroskop haben überhaupt manche alten Fragen über die Organisation der embryonalen Epidermis geklärt und ganz

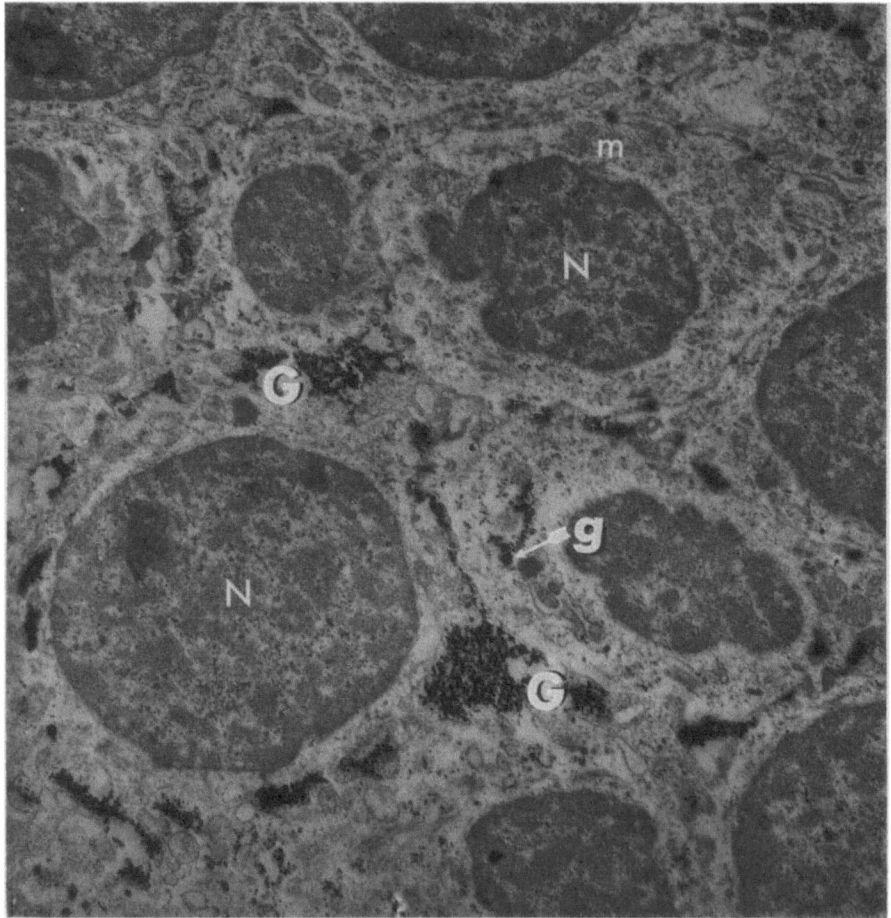

Abb. 5. Zellen der Basalschicht und des Stratum intermedium der Sohlenepidermis eines Fetus von 70 mm Scheitel-Steißlänge in der Gegend einer Schweißdrüsenanlage. Osmium, Bleihydroxyd, 5750mal. Das Corium ist links unten gerade außerhalb des Bildes. G Glykogen in den Zwischenzellenräumen; g intracelluläres Glykogen; m Mitochondrien; N Kern. (Aus HASHIMOTO et al., 1965)

neue Erkenntnisse vermittelt. Während sich KRAUCHER (1931) und SAJNER (1933) noch mit klassischen Methoden bemühten, Zellgrenzen nachzuweisen und FRIEBOES' Ansichten (1920) über Plasmodien und Epithelfasermutterzellen zu widerlegen, herrscht jetzt kein Zweifel mehr über das Vorhandensein von Zellgrenzen, Desmosomen und Tonofilamenten (SELBY, 1955; HASHIMOTO et al., 1965, 1966), wenn auch Brücken und Tonofibrillen nicht immer lichtmikroskopisch nachweisbar sind.

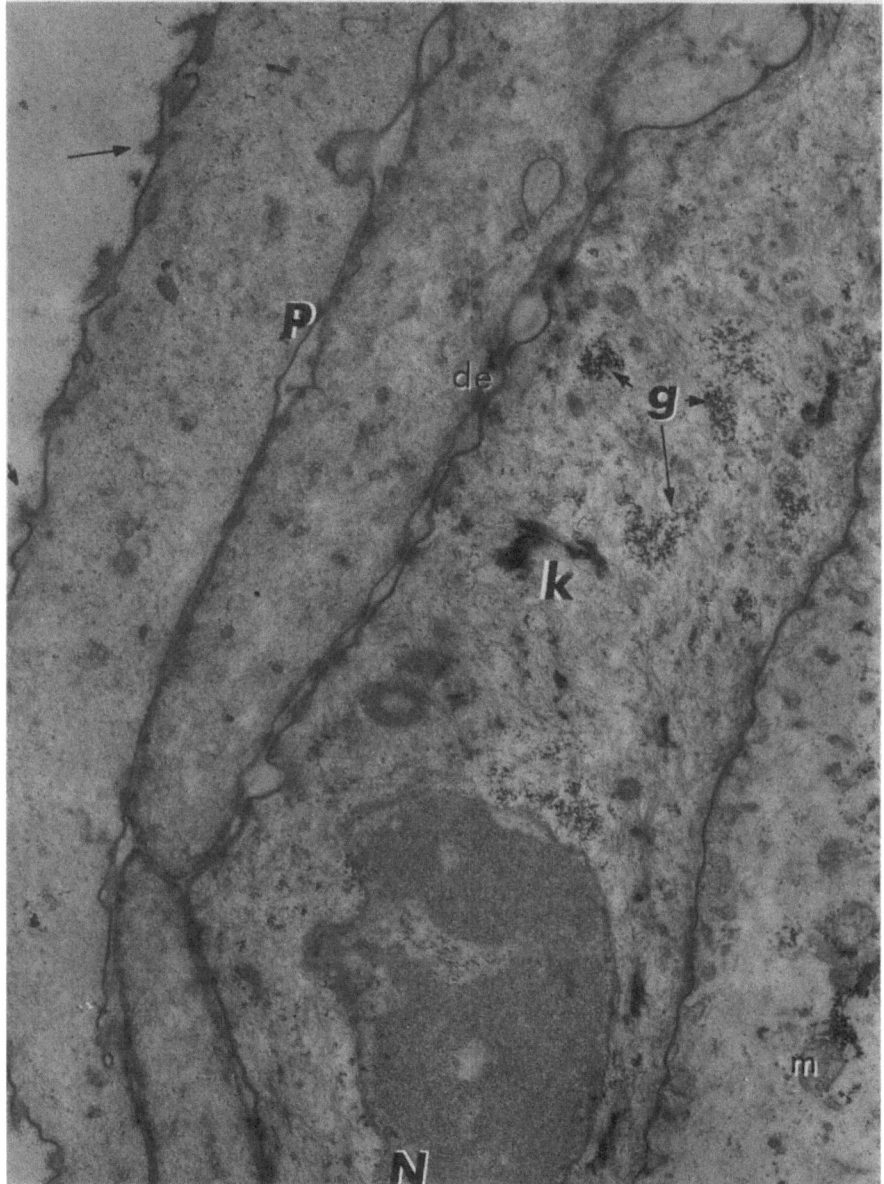

Abb. 6. Äußere Zellschichten der Kopfepidermis eines Fetus von 100 mm Scheitel-Steißlänge, 14500mal. Die Mikrovilli (Pfeile) der Peridermzellen (P) sind in Zahl und Ausbildung gegenüber jüngeren Stadien reduziert und von einer feinkörnigen Substanz bedeckt. Die Peridermzellen enthalten kein Keratohyalin und kaum Glykogen. Der ganze Zelleib ist von feinsten Fäserchen erfüllt. Sie sind durch Desmosomen (de) mit darunterliegenden Zellen verbunden, die sowohl Glykogen (g) wie Keratohyalin (k) und auch ein Geflecht von feinen Tonofilamenten enthalten. N Kern einer Keratohyalinzelle; m Mitochondrien. Freundlichst von Dr. KEN HASHIMOTO zur Verfügung gestellt

Die erste gründliche elektronenoptische Arbeit wurde von BRODY und LARSSON (1965) an Mäuseembryonen durchgeführt. Sie fanden, daß zwischen dem 15. und 17. Tag die Peridermzellen unter Entwicklung von Keratohyalin sich direkt in Hornzellen umwandeln. Mikrovilli wurden nur während eines kurzen Übergangsstadiums an der freien Oberfläche der Peridermzellen beobachtet.

Menschliches Material wurde von RIEGEL (1965) und von HASHIMOTO et al. (1966) in zwei Veröffentlichungen verwendet, die sich insofern recht gut ergänzen, als RIEGEL Embryonen von 25—60 mm SSL untersuchte, während HASHIMOTO Früchte von 60—180 mm benutzte[1]. Nach RIEGEL zeigen die einzelnen Zellen der Ulnargegend des Handtellers bei 25—30 mm großen Embryonen eine basale und antibasale Verschiedenheit. Der Kern befindet sich im oberen Teil der Zelle, von

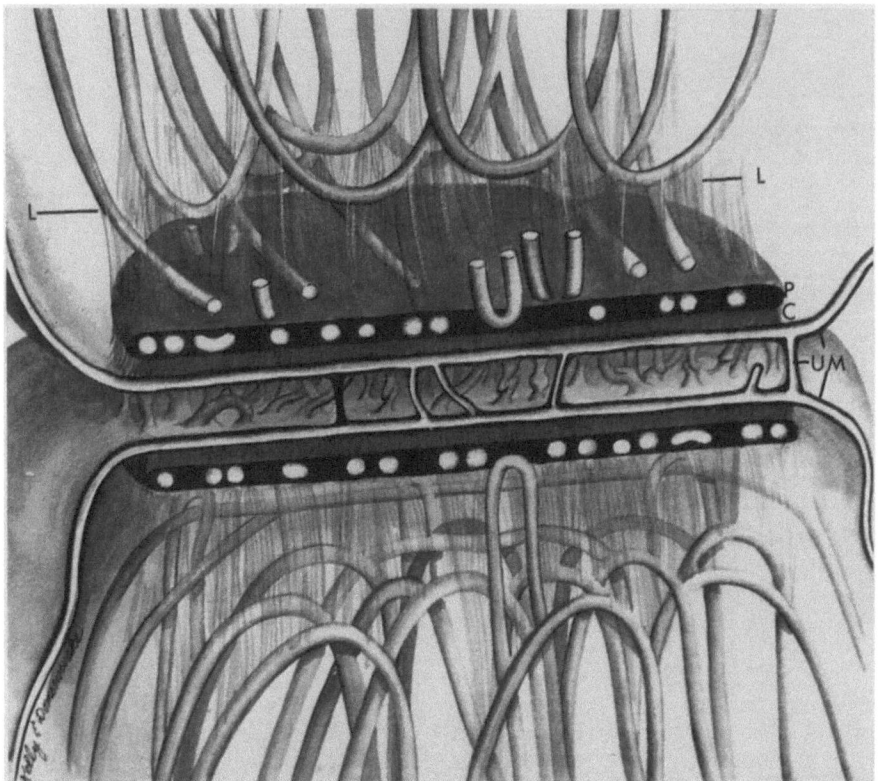

Abb. 7. Zeichnerische Interpretation des Desmosom-Tonofilament-Komplexes in der Epidermis von Urodelenlarven. Durchschnitt durch das Desmosom mit je einer dichten Platte (P) hinter der Zellmembran (unit membrane = UM) der aneinandergrenzenden Zellen. Die Platten sind mit dem Innenblatt der Zellmembran durch eine Zementsubstanz (C) verbunden. Der Intercellularraum ist überbrückt von Material, das entweder eine direkte Fortsetzung des äußeren Blattes der Zellmembran ist oder auf ihm deponiert ist. Verschiedene mögliche Konfigurationen dieses Materials sind illustriert, und der Autor nimmt an, daß Unterschiede in der Dichtigkeit des Intercellularraums, die so häufig in Elektronenmikrogrammen gesehen werden, sich durch Kreuzung, Aufeinanderprojektion, Vereinigung oder Faltung dieser Bänder erklären lassen. Die meisten Tonofilamente biegen in einiger Entfernung vom Desmosom um in einer durch L—L bezeichneten Ebene. Andere biegen erst in der Platte (P) oder zwischen diesen beiden Ebenen um. Wahrscheinlich existiert eine elektronendichtere Substanz zwischen den Platten und den in der Ebene L—L sich befindenden Schleifen. Diese ist in der Zeichnung eingetragen, aber kann z.Z. noch nicht näher charakterisiert werden. (Aus KELLY, 1966)

der Basalmembran durch reichliches Cytoplasma getrennt, das Mitochondrien, osmiophile Körnchen und zusammenhängende glykogenreiche Felder aufweist. Später wird auch über dem Kern Cytoplasma angereichert, und der Kern rückt mehr nach unten, während der Glykogengehalt abnimmt. Die Basalschicht enthält beim 60 mm-Embryo vermehrt endoplasmatisches Reticulum, das dicht von Ribosomen besetzt ist. Die Peridermzellen zeigen in allen Stadien, aber mit dem Alter zunehmend, ins Fruchtwasser vorspringende Mikrovilli.

---

[1] Wo immer möglich, wird in diesem Abschnitt die von den Autoren angegebene Scheitel-Steißlänge (SSL) benutzt, da die Altersberechnungen nicht immer übereinstimmen. Für Formeln zur Alters- und Längenberechnung menschlicher Früchte s. AREY (1925).

HASHIMOTO et al. (1966) untersuchten neben der Palmarhaut auch Fußsohle, Augenbrauenregion und behaarten Kopf. Sie beschreiben die Epidermis 60 mm langer Embryonen als aus Basalschicht, 1—3 Lagen von Stratum intermedium und einer Lage von Peridermzellen bestehend. Die letzteren haben eine bis zu 160 A dicke äußere Membran und tragen reichlich Mikrovilli, die von einem feinfaserigem Filz überzogen erscheinen. Glykogen ist in der Basalschicht mehr in weiten Zwischenzellräumen als in den Zellen selbst vorhanden (Abb. 5) und verschwindet bis zum 120 mm-Stadium ganz. Alle Zellen enthalten Tonofilamente, aber die Basalzellen relativ weniger als die oberen Schichten. Das Stratum intermedium besteht aus erheblich größeren Zellen als die Basalschicht. Sie enthalten Glykogen und lose gebündelte Tonofilamente, die mit Desmosomen in Verbindung stehen. Peridermzellen zeigen in ihrem Innern einen Filz von feinen Fasern nahe der Oberfläche, ähnlich dem der postnatalen Mundschleimhaut, aber sie enthalten kein Keratohyalin und behalten im allgemeinen ihren Kern. Die Fasern sind bei 120 mm-Feten dicker, steifer und kürzer und füllen den ganzen Zelleib der abgeflachten Peridermzellen. Die Autoren nehmen an, daß diese noch Mikrovilli tragenden Zellen schließlich abgestoßen und durch mit Keratohyalin verhornende Zellen unterer Lagen ersetzt werden (Abb. 6). Dieser Vorgang ist mit 130 mm SSL abgeschlossen und von da an ähnelt die fetale Epidermis der des Erwachsenen.

An den viel größeren Zellen der Epidermis von Urodelenlarven hat KELLY Einzelheiten der Desmosomenstruktur aufgezeigt, die in Abb. 7 erläutert sind.

3. Histochemie

Von histochemischen Erkenntnissen sind hauptsächlich die Verteilung von Glykogen und Enzymen zu erwähnen. Als Leitmotiv dieser Befunde sei an STREETERs (1951) Betrachtungen erinnert, daß Embryonen sich nicht nur entwickeln, sondern auch leben müssen. Um sich auf seinem jeweiligen biologischen Niveau erhalten zu können, muß die Struktur eines Embryos in jeder Entwicklungsperiode so geplant sein, daß sie eine genügende physiologische Leistung gewährleistet. Es ist gut, diesen Gedanken auch für viele der im folgenden zu besprechenden Morphen im Gedächtnis zu behalten.

Schon CLAUDE BERNARD (1859) und LIVINI (1927) wiesen auf den hohen Glykogengehalt der fetalen Epidermis hin, der hauptsächlich für das „helle", „plasmaarme" Aussehen der Zellen in gewöhnlichen Präparaten verantwortlich ist. In frühen Stadien enthalten sowohl Basalzellen wie obere Schichten (McKAY et al., 1955; PINKUS, 1958; PRIDVIZHKIN und BERLIN, 1964; BERLIN und PRIDVIZHKIN, 1965; SERRI et al., 1962; RIEGEL, 1965) viel Glykogen, so daß in PAS gefärbten Schnitten oft weder Kerne noch andere Einzelheiten zu erkennen sind (Abb. 17). Der erste Ort, der glykogenfrei wird, ist der Haarkeim (Abb. 16) (PINKUS, 1958). Mit etwa 16 Wochen verliert die Basalschicht in charakteristischer Weise ihr Glykogen (Abb. 18, 26) und bleibt so durch das ganze Leben, mit Ausnahme einiger ungewöhnlicher Situationen. LOBITZ und seine Mitarbeiter (PASS et al., 1965) wiesen nach, daß leichtes Trauma, wie Entfernung der Hornschicht, Ultraviolettbestrahlung oder Einspritzung von Kininen, zum temporären Auftreten von Glykogen in den Basalzellen führt. Wenn die Basalzellen ihr Glykogen verlieren, nimmt ihr Gehalt an RNS und damit ihre Basophilie zu (PRIDVIZHKIN u. BERLIN, 1964). Daß sie orthochromatisch sind, spricht für geringen Gehalt an Mucopolysacchariden (ALLEGRA, 1961).

Die oberen Schichten, Stratum intermedium und Periderm, enthalten Glykogen noch für längere Zeit (SERRI et al., 1962a), wenn es auch in manchen Periderm-

Tabelle 1. *Glykogen und Phosphorylase in embryonaler menschlicher Haut, modifiziert nach* SERRI *et al.*

Gewebsbestandteil[a]	Glykogen (Monat)			Phosphorylase (Monat)		
	1—3	3—6	6—9	1—3	3—6	6—9
Epidermis						
Periderm-Hornschicht	+++	++bis+	0[b]	++	++bis+	0
Körnerzellen	—[b]	+bis0	0	—	++	+bis0
Stachelzellen	+++	++	++bis0	++	++	++bis+
Basalzellen	++bis+	+bis0	+bis0	+bis0	+bis0	+bis0
Corium, Subcutis						
Mesenchym, Fibroblasten	0bis++	0bis+	+bis0	++bis+	++bis0	+bis0
Histiocyten	—	0bis++	0	—	0bis+	0
Mastzellen	—	0bis++	0	—	+	0
Grundsubstanz	++	++	+bis0	0	0	0
Fettzellen	—	++	+	—	+	+
Haarzapfen						
Basale Cylinderzellen	0bis++	0bis++	0bis++	++	++	++
Zentrale Zellen	++	++	++	+++	+++	+++
Wulst	+++	+++	+++	++	++	++
Aktiver Haarfollikel						
Äußere Wurzelscheide	—	++bis+++	++bis+++	—	++bis+++	++bis+++
Musculus arrector pili	—	++	+	—	++	++
Talgdrüse						
Anlage	+	+++	+++	+	++	++
Spätere Basalzellen	+	++	++	+	++	++
Ausführungsgang	—	+bis0	+bis0	—	++bis0	++bis0
Apokrine Drüse						
Ausführungsgang	—	+	++bis0	—	+bis0	+bis0
Ekkrine Drüse						
Anlagen, Hand und Fuß	Spur	Spur	Spur	++	++	++
Sekretorisches Epithel	—	+bis0	+	—	++	++
Intradermaler Gang	—	+bis0	+bis++	—	++bis+++	++
Nagel						
Hintere Nagelfalte	++	++	+	++	++	++
Eponychium	+	++	+	+	++	++
Nagelwall	+	++	+	+	++	+
Matrix, proximal	+bis0	+	+bis0	+bis0	++	+
Matrix, distal	+++	+++	++bis0	++	++	+
Distale Grenzfurche	+	+++	+bis0	+	++	+

[a] Folgende Strukturen waren immer fast oder ganz negativ für beide Reaktionen: Basalmembran, Reticulum-, Kollagen- und elastische Fasern, Blutgefäße, Nerven, Haarkeim, Haarbulbus und Haarpapille, keratogene Zone des Haares, innere Wurzelscheide, Anlage und sekretorisches Epithel der apokrinen Drüse, reife Talgdrüsenzellen, ekkrines Acrosyringium, Nagelbett und Nagelplatte.

[b] 0 bedeutet negative Reaktion, — bedeutet, daß der Gewebsbestandteil zu dieser Zeit noch nicht ausgebildet ist.

zellen ausgelaugt erscheint. Erst wenn die Epidermis schon der postnatalen ähnelt, verlieren auch die Stachelzellen ihr Glykogen. Die Körner- und Hornschichten enthalten gewöhnlich kein Glykogen (ACHTEN, 1957).

Die Verteilung verschiedener Enzyme in der Haut des menschlichen Fetus vom 4. bis zum 10. Monat wurde von MACHIDA in einer breit angelegten Studie 1964 untersucht. Wir folgen seiner Darstellung unter Erwähnung der Resultate anderer Autoren.

Vorher jedoch müssen MORIs Befunde (1959) über alkalische Phosphatase bei ganz jungen Embryonen berücksichtigt werden. Dieser Autor untersuchte 3 Embryonen im 5,8- und 14-Somitenstadium. Im jüngsten Stadium (gerade etwas älter als das von STERNBERG [1927] untersuchte) wiesen Neurektoderm und somatisches Ektoderm starke Phosphataseaktivität auf und setzten sich scharf von dem schwach reagierenden Amnionepithel ab. Die beiden älteren Embryonen zeigten ähnliche Verhältnisse, und es wird besonders betont, daß die auswandernden Zellen der Neuralleiste sich scharf von den schwach gefärbten Mesodermzellen absetzten. Am Ende der 4. Woche fanden MCKAY et al. (1955) Enzymaktivität nur noch im Periderm, abgesehen von Gliedmaßenanlagen und Pharyngealgegend, wo alle Epithelzellen positiv reagierten. Diese Befunde sind interessant, weil übereinstimmend von MACHIDA (1964) und SERRI et al. (1963) berichtet wird, daß von der 4. Woche bis zum Ende der Schwangerschaft die Epidermis nie alkalische Phosphataseaktivität aufweist, während Mesenchymzellen mäßig positiv sind. Dagegen ist eine starke saure Phosphataseaktivität in der Epidermis besonders in den höheren Lagen nachzuweisen (SERRI et al., 1962b; MACHIDA, 1964).

MACHIDA fand Bernsteinsäuredehydrogenase, Cytochromoxydase und Monoaminooxydase ziemlich schwach im 4. Monat. Mit dem Alter stieg die Aktivität an, wobei Handflächen- und Fußsohlenepidermis der übrigen Haut außer im 5. Monat vorauseilte. Interessant ist es, daß PULLAR und LIADSKY (1965) in ihren Gewebekulturen von 11—15 Wochen alter Haut fanden, daß alle Dehydrogenasen im Anfang fehlten, aber innerhalb von 4 Tagen, in denen das Epithel zu verhornen begann, mehr oder weniger stark aktiv wurden.

Es scheint, daß der Enzymstoffwechsel im Embryo regulativ auf einer unreifen Stufe gehalten wird, während die Zellen, sich selbst überlassen, dem erwachsenen Typ zueilen.

MACHIDA fand Phosphorylaseaktivität sehr stark im 5. und 6. Monat, dann allmählich abnehmend. Nach dem 7. Monat ist dies Enzym nur noch in der Axilla und im Rand der Augenlider nachweisbar. Es verschwindet vor der Geburt ganz. Die Befunde von SERRI et al. (1962a), die ihre Untersuchungen schon im 1. Monat begannen und Glykogen und Amylophosphorylase verglichen, sind in Tabelle 1 wiedergegeben.

Esterasen verhalten sich wie folgt: Die Naphthol-AS-esterase-Methode gibt kräftige Resultate unabhängig vom Alter, die α-Naphthol-esterasen-Aktivität nimmt allmählich zu. Cholinesterasen sind nur in intraepidermalen Nervenendigungen nachzuweisen.

4. Topographische Unterschiede

Unterschiede in der Morphologie des Epithels verschiedener Hautregionen bei jungen menschlichen Früchten wurden eingehend von STEINER (1929, 1930) untersucht, der die von HÄGGQVIST (1921) bei Fledermäusen erhobenen Befunde weitgehend bestätigen konnte, aber die Verhältnisse in anderer Weise erklärte. Embryonen mit 4—27 Urwirbelpaaren aus der 3. und 4. Schwangerschaftswoche besitzen 3 Formen ektodermalen Epithels. Typ I ist ein prismatisch mehrreihiges Epithel an der Unter- und Vorderseite des Kopfes, Typ II ein flaches einschichtiges Epithel über der Herz- und Zentralnervensystemanlage, und Typ III ein einschichtiges kubisches Epithel am übrigen Embryonalkörper. Typ III wird als der ursprüngliche aufgefaßt, während Typ I hauptsächlich in den Gegenden sich findet, die später Entwicklungen verbunden mit starker Zellvermehrung durchmachen. Das sind die Gesichts- und Kiemenbogengegend, die Gliedmaßenanlagen und die Urogenital- und Aftergegend. Ohne auf entwicklungsmechanische Fragen einzugehen (s. unter C) seien hier die Veränderungen, die sich im Gebiet des Typs I abspielen, kurz geschildert.

Der schon auf S. 626 beschriebene Streifen hohen Epithels zwischen der flachzelligen Membrana reuniens anterior und ähnlichen Membrana reuniens posterior wird allmählich in mehrere Inseln zerlegt, und das Gebiet des Typ I bleibt relativ im Flächenwachstum zurück. Dagegen steigert sich das Dicken-

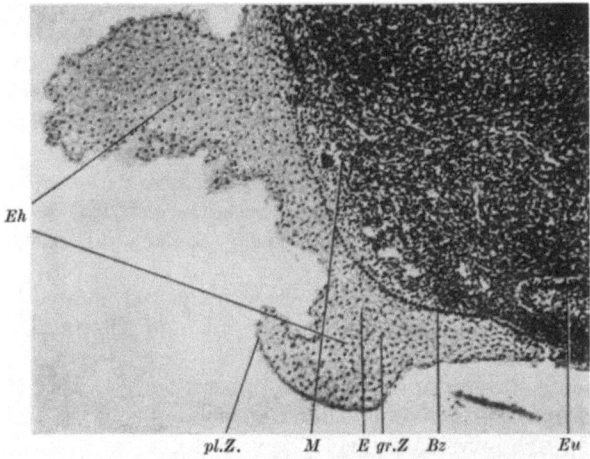

Abb. 8. Längsschnitt durch das Epithelhörnchen der Eichel eines menschlichen Embryos von 105 mm Scheitel-Fersenlänge. *Bz* Basalzellen; *gr.Z.* große, plasmaarme, blasige Zellen der Intermediärschicht; *pl.Z.* platte Peridermzellen; *Eh* Epithelhörnchen; *E* Epithel; *M* Mesoderm; *EU* Epithel der Urethra; Vergrößerung 80mal. (Aus STEINER, 1932)

wachstum, und es entstehen epitheliale Hörnchen, Pfröpfe, Platten, Nähte und Wülste. Hierher gehören die Epithelhörnchen der embryonalen Eichel (Abb. 8), die Epithelpfröpfe der Nase und Gehörgänge, die Gehörgangs- und Präputialplatte und die Nähte an Lidern, Wangen, Penis, Scrotum und Damm. Auch die Lidfalten, Ohrhöckerchen, Genito-Analhöcker und Geschlechtswülste entstehen nach STEINER (1950) im Gebiet des Hauttyp I. In seiner späteren Ausbildung ist das Epithel hier charakterisiert durch eine Lage kubischer oder zylindrischer Basalzellen und viele Schichten unregelmäßig angeordneter blasiger Zellen, die von wenigen Lagen platter Zellen bedeckt werden.

STEINERs Befunde wurden von späteren Untersuchern (KATZBERG, 1953; GRENBERG, 1957, 1958; PRIDVIZHKIN und BERLIN, 1964) bestätigt und erweitert.

Es gibt aber noch andere Besonderheiten während des Embryonallebens der Epidermis. So beschrieb INGALLS (1929) symmetrische Verdickungen des Ektoderms über den Spinalganglien bei zehn 4—12,5 mm langen Embryonen, die er weder früher noch später finden konnte. Ursache und Zweck sind unbekannt. Von großer Bedeutung sind dagegen die als Milchstreifen und Milchleiste bekannten Bildungen, die von DABELOW (1957) sehr ausführlich aufgrund der Literatur und eigener Untersuchungen behandelt wurden. In ihrem Gebiet entstehen die Brustdrüse und überzählige Mamillen; ob sich aber ihre Bedeutung in dieser phylogenetisch-ontogenetischen Aufgabe erschöpft, ist nicht sicher. So weist GRAU-

MANN (1950) darauf hin, daß ein ringförmiger Streifen von hohen Epithelzellen sich auch bei Nicht-Säugern zwischen Gesicht und Urogenitalsinus ausbildet. Nach GRAUMANN absorbieren diese hohen Zellen Flüssigkeit aus einer darunterliegenden Saftspalte und geben sie ans Fruchtwasser ab. Dadurch werde die Bildung der Körperwand beeinflußt. Wir werden auf die Anschauungen der Blechschmidtschen Schule noch später zurückkommen.

Auf jeden Fall ist dieser seit langem bekannte Milchstreifen nicht identisch mit der sich später in seinem Gebiet entwickelnden Milchleiste. Nach der Darstellung DABELOWS (1957), auf die für Einzelheiten hingewiesen wird, tritt der Milchstreifen bei menschlichen Feten von 6—8 mm SSL auf und läuft seitlich am Rumpf im Bereich der dorsoventralen Grenzfurche zwischen vorderer und hinterer Extremitätenanlage entlang. Er besteht aus einer unscharf begrenzten Epithelverdickung, die sich aus zuerst einschichtigen, später bis vierschichtigen kubischen Zellen zusammensetzt (THÖLEN, 1949). Cranial und caudal setzt er sich in das Epithel des Sinus praecervicalis, des Geschlechtshöckers und der Extremitäten fort. Er scheint demnach zum Teil mit der Verteilung von STEINERs Hauttyp I übereinzustimmen. Der Milchstreifen verschwindet langsam durch allmähliche Abflachung bei gleichzeitiger Verbreiterung, aber in einigen seiner Abschnitte wird das Epithel mehrschichtig und wird zur Milchleiste, aus der sich je nach der Tierart eine oder viele Milchdrüsen entwickeln.

Nachdem GRÜNEBERG (1952) eine ektodermale Leiste an der Ventralseite der Schwanzanlage von Mäuseembryonen in Fehlbildungen der Uro-ano-caudalregion impliziert hatte, fand LANDOLT (1959) eine ähnliche Schwanzleiste bei menschlichen Embryonen von 3,5—7 mm SSL, die sich dann wieder zurückbildet. Untersuchungen über ihre funktionelle Bedeutung fehlen noch, doch mögen hier einige Daten über die Entwicklung des Anus angeschlossen werden, eines Gebietes, das doch von beträchtlichem Interesse für den Dermatologen ist.

Wenn sich das Schwanzende des Embryos vom Embryonalschild abhebt, bleiben in einer begrenzten Region Entoderm des Enddarms und Ektoderm in Berührung, ohne daß sich Mesoderm dazwischenschiebt (STERNBERG, 1927; TENCH, 1936; STARCK, 1965). Diese Stelle wird zur Kloakenmembran. Wenn sie bei 14 mm langen Embryonen beginnt sich zu verdünnen und einzureißen, bleibt das Rectum noch bis etwa 22 mm Länge verschlossen (TENCH) und öffnet sich dann nicht direkt nach außen, sondern in die Kloake, die erst durch das Herunterwachsen des Urogenitalseptums in eine vordere und hintere Partie getrennt wird. Auf diese Weise wird ektodermales Material in den Analkanal einbezogen. Ob die Grenze zwischen Ektoderm und Entoderm der späteren Grenze zwischen geschichtetem Epithel und Cylinderepithel entspricht, ist nicht sicher. Diese Verhältnisse sind für die Pathogenese des extramammären Paget von Wichtigkeit. Auch schon im Embryonalleben wachsen von den Analkrypten Gänge aus, die, meist in der hinteren Hälfte des Rectums gelegen (KRATZER u. DOCKERTY, 1947), oft durch den Sphincter hindurchwachsen und später für Entzündungen und Fisteln von Bedeutung sind.

Die Vereinigung und Wiedertrennung von geschichtetem Epithel an verschiedenen Körperöffnungen ist wohlbekannt. Die Trennung dieser epithelialen Verwachsungen kommt durch Verhornung der mittleren Partien zustande, ohne daß Näheres über die Ursache bekannt ist. BURROWS (1945) führt aus, daß bei mehreren Tierarten, insbesondere Katzen und Nagern, die Trennung zwischen Vorhaut und Eichel normalerweise erst bei Geschlechtsreife zustande kommt und durch Kastration verhindert wird. Zuführung von Androgen verursacht Verhornung und Lösung der Verwachsung. Der Effekt ist auf dieses eine Epithel beschränkt. Die angrenzende Urethra z.B. wird nicht zur Verhornung angeregt. Es ist dies ein ausgezeichnetes Beispiel epithelialer Spezifität, auf die wir auf S. 642 zurückkommen werden.

Andere topographische Unterschiede in der Entwicklung der Epidermis, z.B. zwischen Volarhaut und behaartem Kopf (ACHTEN, 1956), sind zu wohlbekannt, um hier Besprechung zu erfordern, besonders da sie schon von F. PINKUS (1927) dargestellt wurden. Daten über die Entwicklung der Hand- und Fußleisten und der Papillarmuster finden sich im makroskopischen Teil (Band I/2). Hier mag nur der ganz neue Befund erwähnt werden (ACHS et al., 1966), daß Kinder, die in utero mit Rubellavirus infiziert wurden, Affenfurchen, distal verlagerte Palmartriradii und Radialschleifen an den Fingern mit erhöhter Häufigkeit aufweisen. Diese zuerst als ererbte Stigmata bei Mongoloiden beschriebenen Entwicklungsabweichungen brauchen also nicht genetisch bedingt zu sein. Andere topographische Unterschiede werden später bei der Entwicklung der Hautanhangsgebilde und Nerven erwähnt.

5. Epidermis des Neugeborenen

Die Epidermis ist bei der Geburt von der Vernix caseosa bedeckt, die ein Gemisch von Talg, Hornfett und den Leibern der abgeschilferten Hornzellen ist (REISS, 1932). In allen wesentlichen Eigenschaften gleicht die neugeborene Epidermis der im späteren Alter, nur die Mitosenrate wird gewöhnlich höher angegeben. So fand COOPER (1939) 14—68 Mitosen pro 10000 Zellen in der Vorhaut 6—10 Tage alter Knaben. THURINGER und KATZBERG (1959) berichten allerdings den niedrigen Wert von 16 Mitosen unter 100000 Zellen der Bauchhaut eines 2 Tage alten Kindes. EMERY und McMILLAN (1954) fanden das Geschlechtschromatin in der Epidermis von Frühgeburten im allgemeinen gut erkennbar. CERESA (1936) und ZELEZNIKOW (1957) gaben die in Tabelle 2 zusammengestellten Werte für Epidermisdicke bei Feten und Neugeborenen.

Tabelle 2. *Epidermisdicke in μ beim Neugeborenen* (ZELEZNIKOW) *und bei Feten* (CERESA)

Körpergegend	Minimum	Maximum	Körpergegend	Minimum	Maximum
Scheitel	37,9	100,4	Hüfte, flex.	54,1	119,4
Stirn	52,7	105,4	Hüfte, ext.	56,6	130,6
Nase	58,2	106,5	Fußrücken	70,5	162,2
Oberlippe	48,0	107,9	Fußsohle	113,0	242,9
Brust	48,8	120,8	Gesäß	58,9	114,8
Bauch	42,8	117,3	Pubis	44,1	102,9
Rücken	52,6	117,1	Analregion	42,6	141,4
Oberarm, flex.	43,9	102,7	Labium majus	58,2	108,2
Oberarm, ext.	46,6	107,7	Penis	40,9	104,7
Handrücken	59,7	113,1	Scrotum	37,4	82,8
Handfläche	105,1	225,5	Axilla	40,9	109,5
	5 Monate		6 Monate	8 Monate	Neugeboren
Genitalgegend	15		17	20	27

B. Entwicklung des Coriums und des Fettgewebes

1. Allgemeines

STERNBERG (1926) gab eine ausführliche Beschreibung des Mesoderms bei einem menschlichen Embryo mit 4 Ursegmenten. Neben diesen findet sich das unsegmentierte embryonale Bindegewebe des Embryonalschildes und die schon aus dem Mesoderm entstandenen Differenzierungen, die Perikardialhöhle und das Gefäßsystem. Das Ektoderm ist überall von Mesoderm unterlagert, aber die Menge wechselt von einzelnen Zellen zwischen Perikard und zukünftiger Epidermis bis zu dicht gefügten Zellplatten in der Region zwischen vorderer Darmpforte und dem Vorderrand des ersten Urwirbels, der sich von dem unsegmentierten Teil mehr oder weniger deutlich absetzt. Ventral vom Kiemendarm ist das Mesoderm lockerer gefügt. Caudal von den Urwirbeln finden sich auch dicht gefügte mesodermale Platten, in denen sich das nächste Ursegment durch örtlich vermehrte Mitosen anzeigt. Das embryonale Bindegewebe, wo es lockerer angeordnet ist, besteht aus sternförmigen Zellen mit unregelmäßigen Fortsätzen, die mit den Fortsätzen der Nachbarzellen in Verbindung stehen. Dazwischen findet sich stellenweise eine mit Hämatoxylin bläulich gefärbte Zwischensubstanz von wabigem Aussehen. Karyokinesen sind in wechselnder Zahl vorhanden, und gleichzeitig finden sich auch im Untergang begriffene Zellen, deren Kerne pyknotisch oder fragmentiert sind. Nach SERRI et al. (1962) enthalten die mesenchymalen Zellen stets Glykogen.

Eine übersichtliche Darstellung der Frühentwicklung des mesodermalen Hautanteils wurde 1964 von TÖNDURY gegeben. Corium und Subcutis der Rückenregion entstehen aus den Ursegmenten, das Corium der lateralen und ventralen Rumpfwand stammt aus Zellen der nie segmentalen Somatopleura, die das Cölom umgibt. Auch das Blastem der Extremitätenknospen stammt aus der Somatopleura, während Kopf- und Gesichtshaut aus dem ebenfalls ungegliederten Kopfmesoderm sich entwickeln. Wenn man die Verhältnisse bei Amphibien auf den Menschen übertragen kann (s. STARCK, Bd. I/2, S. 146), sollte in dieser Gegend auch Material des Mesektoderms aus der Kopfganglienleiste dazukommen. Die zunächst epitheliale Cutisplatte (das Dermatom) der Urwirbel löst sich durch Wanderung ihrer Zellen auf, und die segmentale Ordnung wird rasch verwischt. Sie bleibt nur in den Arteriae intersegmentales erhalten, die aus den primitiven Aorten entspringen und ursprünglich zwischen den Urwirbeln verlaufen.

Die zunächst morphologisch undifferenzierbaren Zellen des so gebildeten Hautmesenchyms liegen in einer dünnen Matrix, die neben Wasser und löslichen Substanzen wohl hauptsächlich Mucopolysaccharide (HOLMGREN, 1939, 1940; MANCINI und BACARINI, 1951) und Glykogen (SERRI et al., 1962) enthält. GRENBERG (1958) fand schon mit 3 Wochen argyrophile Fasern. Erst im 2. Monat treten Kollagenfasern in nennenswertem Maße auf, elastische Fasern viel später. Die Intersegmentalarterien bilden bald ein Capillarnetz in der dorsalen Rumpfhaut, während in anderen Körperteilen nach TÖNDURY (1964) das Gefäßsystem in Form geflechtartiger Capillaren entsteht, aus welchen sich erst sekundär Arterien und Venen herausbilden. Wie wir später sehen werden, bilden sich aus dem primitiven cutanen Mesenchym auch die mesodermalen Anteile der Hautadnexe, insbesondere die Haarmuskeln und auch die übrige glatte Muskulatur der Haut. Weiterhin ist zu bemerken, daß das Corium zu bestimmten Zeiten des intra-uterinen Lebens ein hämatopoetisches Organ ist (POPOFF u. POPOFF, 1958) und zeitlebens aktives Reticuloendothel enthält.

Die Ausdifferenzierung und Reifung des Mesoderms geht in verschiedenem Tempo und zu verschiedenen Zeiten vor sich. Man denke nur daran, daß die Extremitäten sich erst entwickeln, wenn die Rumpf- und Kopfhaut schon wichtige Schutzfunktionen für die darunterliegenden Organe erfüllt. Nach STEINER (1929) und HOLMGREN und JOHANSON (1933) ist das über dem Herzwulst gelegene Gewebe früher fibrillär und relativ zellarm als z.B. das des Gesichtes, wo sich noch weitgehende Formwandlungen vollziehen. Außerdem ist, wie beim Epithel, ein cranio-caudales Gefälle vorhanden.

2. Fasern und Zellen

Die ersten Fasern der Dermis sind argyrophil (ORLOVSKAJA, 1949; LINKE, 1955; GRENBERG, 1958; BERLIN u. PRIDVIZHKIN, 1965). Im Elektronenmikroskop zeigen Kollagenfibrillen des 4. Monats eine Periodizität von 310—450 A (ISHIMOTO, 1955), die sich allmählich bis zum 8. Monat auf Zahlen des reifen Gewebes umstellt (560—800 A). Zu dieser Zeit erreicht auch die Verteilung von Silberpartikeln auf der Faser das reife Muster. Länge und Breite der Fibrillen nehmen allmählich zu (BANFIELD, 1955), der Durchmesser von einem Durchschnitt von 10—20 mµ bis zu 50 mµ (LINKE, 1955). Das Verhältnis von Fasern zu Grundsubstanz verschiebt sich zugunsten der Fasern, was sich auch im Anstieg des Hydroxyprolins und in der Abnahme des Hexosamins nachweisen läßt (SERRI et al., 1963). Eine interessante Beobachtung ist die von LEITAN (1961), daß in 5—13 Wochen alten Früchten, die von thyreotoxischen Müttern stammten, das mit PAS, Hale und Toluidinblau färbbare Material entschieden gegenüber Kontrollfeten vermindert war.

Die Fasern des Coriums reiften auch in embryonaler Haut aus, die in die Backentaschen von Hamstern homotransplantiert war (HAMBRICK u. BLOOMBERG, 1959). Weiterhin wies ZELICKSON (1963) elektronenoptisch nach, daß embryonale menschliche Fibroblasten in der Gewebekultur kollagene Fasern bilden können. 80 A dicke Fäserchen entstehen in der Zelle, werden ausgeschleust und legen sich außerhalb zu 200 A dicken Fibrillen zusammen, die dann die typische Periodizität erkennen lassen.

Elastische Fasern treten anscheinend in verschiedenen Körperteilen zu sehr verschiedenen Zeiten auf. ORLOVSKAJA (1949) fand sie im Gesicht eines 3monatigen Fetus, SAMEJIMA (1956) sah sie an Knie und Ellenbogen in der zweiten Hälfte des 3. Monats, in der Planta im 4. Monat, in der Handfläche im 5. Monat. Ähnlich beschreibt sie GEIGER (1926) in der Planta mit $4^1/_2$ Monaten, mit $5^1/_2$ Monaten überall. LYNCH (1934) fand elastische Fasern früher in den Blutgefäßen der Haut als im Corium selbst. Der Gehalt an elastischen Fasern nimmt auch sicher noch nach der Geburt zu. Nach den elektronenoptischen Untersuchungen von SCHWARZ (1964) an Fibroblastenkulturen von Hühnerembryonen werden elastische Fasern von Zellen gebildet, die sich nicht von anderen Fibroblasten unterscheiden. Die Vorstufen entstehen nach ihm in der Zelle, aber die eigentliche Faser außerhalb.

Es scheint, daß alles Bindegewebe der Haut während des intra-uterinen Lebens Umformungen durchmacht, die sich z.B. im Wechsel der Spaltlinienrichtungen ausdrücken. Das wurde schon von F. PINKUS (1927) ausführlich aufgrund älterer Untersuchungen besprochen. Histologisch wiesen GARDNER und RAYBURN (1954) nach, daß kollagene und elastische Fasern auch beim menschlichen Embryo parallel zu den Spaltlinien laufen. Deren Änderung während des Fetallebens bedeutet also Umordnung der Fasern und wahrscheinlich Wechsel der Wachstumsrichtungen der Haut.

Mastzellen treten in der Haut bei 19 cm langen Feten auf, früher als in manchen anderen Organen (HOLMGREN, 1946). Dies geht einem ansteigenden Histamingehalt (ZACHARIAE, 1964) und Histaminstoffwechsel (LINDBERG et al., 1963) der Haut parallel. Beim Neugeborenen fanden HELLSTRÖM und HOLMGREN (1950) 7000 Mastzellen im Kubikmillimeter, das Mehrfache von Zahlen im höheren Alter.

In einer Studie an 86 Embryonen verfolgten POPOFF und POPOFF (1958) Hämatopoiese in der embryonalen Haut. Vom Ende des 2. Monats an (8 cm Gesamtlänge) fanden sie erythroblastische Herde, andere Formen der Blutbildung erst im 5. Monat. Rote Blutzellenbildung verschwand in den 2 letzten Fetal-monaten. Die blutbildenden Zellen entstehen lokal durch Umwandlung von Mesenchymzellen.

Zahlen betreffend die Dicke des Coriums beim Fetus und Neugeborenen sind in Tabelle 3 nach ZELEZNIKOW (1957) und CERESA (1936) zusammengestellt.

Tabelle 3. *Dicke des Coriums in μ beim Neugeborenen (ZELEZNIKOW) und bei Feten (CERESA)*

Körpergegend	Minimum	Maximum	Körpergegend	Minimum	Maximum
Scheitel	608	845	Hüfte, flex.	855	1008
Stirn	570	845	Hüfte, ext.	906	1026
Nase	855	1102	Fußrücken	513	798
Oberlippe	1083	1387	Fußsohle	418	789
Brust	598	950	Gesäß	674	988
Bauch	693	1130	Pubis	503	1045
Rücken	735	1320	Analregion	627	1178
Oberarm, flex.	693	992	Labium majus	1045	1520
Oberarm, ext.	760	1007	Penis	589	667
Handrücken	418	807	Scrotum	325	410
Handfläche	342	731	Axilla	427	616
	5 Monate		6 Monate	8 Monate	Neugeboren
Sternalgegend	580		640	660	680
Fußsohle	230		220	450	570
Genitalgegend	520		600	850	660

3. Die Basalmembran

Obwohl durch moderne histochemische und elektronenoptische Befunde viele der älteren Fragestellungen auf diesem Gebiet überholt sind, waren die Ansichten von STEINER (1928) und LAPIÈRE (1939) nicht so weit vom Ziel, die die Basalmembran aus einem verdichteten Exoplasma (Zellmembran) und feinen mesodermalen Fasern hervorgehen sahen. Neuere Arbeiten (GRENBERG, 1959; PRIDVIZHKIN und BERLIN, 1964) beschrieben schon bei 3 Wochen alten Embryonen eine deutliche Basalmembran, der sich bald argyrophile Fibrillen zugesellen. Nach eigenen Beobachtungen (1958) findet sich eine PAS-positive Membran zuerst um die frühesten Haarkeime, erst etwas später an der Epidermis selbst. BECKER und ZIMMERMANN (1957) nehmen eine Ausreifung der Basalmembran erst im 6. Monat an und folgern dies daraus, daß erst dann eine enzymatische Trennung von Epidermis und Corium gelingt.

Nach MCLOUGHLIN (1963) besteht die Basalmembran aus drei Komponenten: der nur elektronenmikroskopisch nachweisbaren ad-epidermalen Membran, einem tiefer gelegenen Filz von kollagenen Fibrillen und neutralen Mucopolysacchariden, die beide Teile durchtränken. Alle diese Befunde, die für einen rein dermalen Ursprung der in der Basalzone vereinigten Elemente sprechen, werden aber wieder in Frage gestellt durch ganz neue Berichte, daß eine immunochemisch spezifische Substanz von normalen und neoplastischen Epithelzellen gebildet wird, die sich in allen Basalmembranen nachweisen läßt (HAY, 1965; PIERCE, 1965).

4. Blut- und Lymphgefäße

Die embryonale Entwicklung von Blutgefäßen ist teils mit Injektionsmethoden (TRUFFI, 1934; SAUNDERS u. MONTAGNA, 1964), teils färberisch verfolgt worden. Besonders eignet sich nach SERRI (1965) die auch beim Erwachsenen so erfolgreich angewendete Methode, Capillarendothelien durch die alkalische Phosphatase-reaktion sichtbar zu machen. Entsprechend den Angaben TÖNDURYs (1964, s. S. 637) konnte SERRI zeigen, daß im jungen Mesenchym sich lokal Capillaren ausbilden. Junge Bindegewebszellen sind immer reich an Phosphatase. Sie legen sich zusammen und die so entstandenen Capillaren gewinnen allmählich Anschluß an die von tieferen Geweben auswachsenden Gefäße. Wenn die Gefäße eine Media erwerben, geht der Enzymgehalt der Endothelien zurück. Capillarentwicklung dieser Art ist in den Fingern von der 12. Woche an nachzuweisen, an anderen Körperteilen etwas später.

Die Entwicklung arterio-venöser Anastomosen, über die einige Angaben schon von MASSON (1937) und CLARA (1939) vorliegen, wurde eingehend von ROTTER und WAGNER (1952) an den subungualen Glomera der Zehen untersucht. Sie beschreiben deren Entwicklung als ganz allmählich bei Feten von etwa 16 cm Länge einsetzend. Zunächst vermehren sich die dem Grundhäutchen der Capillarwand aufsitzenden Zellkerne und lassen eine relativ dicke Gefäßwand entstehen. Die Kerne liegen zuerst dichtgepackt in einem homogenen Symplasma, das allmählich vacuolisiert wird. Die Kerne scheinen dann in hellen Blasen zu schwimmen, zwischen denen ein zartes, scharf konturiertes lineares Gitterwerk Zellgrenzen vortäuscht. Die epitheloidzellige Modifikation der Gefäßwand beginnt bei Feten von 27—30 cm Länge. Während der frühen Entwicklungsphasen sind die anastomotischen Gefäßstrecken von einem schleimigen Bindegewebe umgeben. Eine eigentliche, zum Teil nervale Kapsel bildet sich erst nach der Geburt.

Mit Ausnahme von TRUFFI (1934), der die Lymphbahnen eines 7monatigen Fetus injizierte, scheinen sich nur OTTAVIANI und LUPIDI (1941) mit der Entwicklung der Lymphgefäße in der menschlichen Haut befaßt zu haben. Sie untersuchten 25 Embryonen von 28—380 mm Länge, die sie mit gefärbter Masse injizierten. Nach diesen Autoren entwickelt sich schon zwischen 28 und 35 mm Länge ein primäres Netz durch Zusammenfließen von Lacunen, und zwar zuerst in den Jugular-Axillar- und Inguinalgegenden. Diese Netze breiten sich auch durch Knospung aus und werden schließlich zur Bildung von Sammelgefäßen in und unter der Haut benutzt. Schon bei 47 mm langen Feten finden sich Klappen in den Lymphbahnen. Später bildet sich ein zweites Netz, und schließlich, bei 380 mm langen Feten, findet sich ein reiches Lymphcapillarnetz in den Papillen der Haut.

5. Subcutanes Fettgewebe

In makroskopischen Mengen entwickelt sich das subcutane Fettgewebe erst recht spät (s. Band I/2, S. 7). Es ist ja bekannt, daß Frühgeborene sehr wenig Unterhautfett besitzen. Die mikroskopische Entwicklung der Fettorgane wurde schon von F. PINKUS (1927) aufgrund der Befunde von WASSERMANN (1926) ausführlich dargestellt, und es ist nichts Neues hinzuzufügen (vgl. Abb. 15).

Eine Studie des braunen Fettes bei Frühgeburten und Neugeborenen unternahmen LERNE und HULL (1964) aufgrund der Beobachtung, daß menschliche ebenso wie tierische Neugeborene bei Abkühlung Hitze produzieren können, ohne fröstelnd zu zittern. Aufgrund von Röntgenaufnahmen dreier Kinderleichen stellten sie fest, daß Venen aus dem interscapulären braunen Fettpolster zusammen mit Venen aus Muskeln und Rückenhaut einen Plexus vertebralis posterior externus bilden, der zur Vena jugularis oder Vena azygos abfließt. Auf diese Weise mag Abkühlung des Rückens direkt die Temperatur des Rückenmarks beeinflussen. Histologische Untersuchung des braunen Fetts von 187 Kleinkindern ergab, daß der Fettgehalt in den ersten 4 Tagen abnimmt. Drei Kinder, die in Hypothermie gestorben waren, zeigten starke Fettverarmung der Zellen.

6. Histochemie

Es wurde schon erwähnt, daß embryonale Bindegewebszellen und die Grundsubstanz zwischen ihnen ziemlich viel Glykogen enthalten (SERRI et al., 1962). MANCINI und BACARINI (1951) fanden auch Mucoproteine in fetalen Fibroblasten. MACHIDA (1964) gab einen Überblick über verschiedene Enzymreaktionen.

Die Endothelien der fetalen Blutgefäße, das unreife Fettgewebe und die Hautmuskulatur haben positive Reaktionen für Bernsteinsäuredehydrogenase, Cytochromoxydase und Monoaminoxydase. Während die letzteren ziemlich konstant sind, nimmt die erstere im Muskel vom 4.—10. Monat zu. Phosphorylase ist stark positiv in der Media von Blutgefäßen und anderen Muskeln. Dieses Enzym nimmt im Fettgewebe allmählich ab, und die Reaktivität wird im 10. Monat Null. Cholinesteraseaktivität ist auf Nerven beschränkt, während andere Esterasen nahe dem Lumen der Blutgefäße vorhanden sind. Das Fettgewebe reagiert schwach oder gar nicht, von Muskeln reagiert nur der Sphincter ani. MACHIDA bestätigt die allgemeinen Befunde, daß das Capillarendothel eine starke alkalische Phosphatase-Aktivität hat, während größere Gefäße negativ reagieren. Fettgewebe und Muskeln sind negativ. SERRI et al. (1963) bemerken, daß auch junge Mesenchymzellen und Fibroblasten regelmäßig positiv reagieren, daß aber in älteren Feten die Reaktion schwächer und unregelmäßig wird. Saure Phosphatase konnte MACHIDA nirgends nachweisen. Schließlich fand er Leucinaminopeptidase in den lumennahen Teilen der Blutgefäße und ein wenig in Muskeln, aber nicht im Fettgewebe.

C. Entwicklungsmechanik der menschlichen Haut

Entwicklungsmechanische Erkenntnisse im Gebiet der menschlichen Haut sind stark behindert durch die Unmöglichkeit, Hypothesen experimentell nachzuprüfen. Mit wenigen Ausnahmen gilt das für alle Säuger. Die Häute der Vögel und Amphibien, die eher experimentell angegangen werden können, sind doch so verschieden vom menschlichen Integument, daß Rückschlüsse nur mit großer Vorsicht erlaubt sind. Am humanen Material kann selbst die sorgfältigste Untersuchung und Beschreibung immer nur das „post hoc" ermitteln, das „propter hoc" bleibt hypothetisch. Diese Unsicherheit und die Subjektivität aller entwicklungsmechanischen Schlüsse muß stets im Auge behalten werden.

Wohl der erste, der mechanistische Betrachtungen in die Embryologie der Säugerhaut einführte, war HÄGGQVIST (1921), der bei Fledermausembryonen die lang bestehende Einschichtigkeit platten Epithels über Herz, Leber und Nervensystem auf den Druck dieser schnell wachsenden Organe zurückführte, mit dem die mitotische Vermehrung des Ektoderms nur gerade Schritt halten könne. STEINER (1929) bestritt diese Erklärung, da das Epithel dieser Regionen schon flach sei, bevor die darunterliegenden Organe stark wachsen. Er zog es vor, die spezifische Ausbildung des Ektoderms verschiedener Regionen auf unbekannte innere Ursachen (Selbststeuerung) zurückzuführen und betrachtete weiterhin das platte Epithel als das mehr ausgereifte, weil es regelmäßig mit mehr ausgereiftem, fibrillenreichen Bindegewebe assoziiert ist. Dem wurde von HOLMGREN und JOHANNSSON (1933) entgegengehalten, daß das platte Epithel sich später in ein zweischichtiges, kubisches verwandelt, sobald eine stärkere Ausbildung des darunterliegenden Coriums es vom Innendruck der großen Organe schützt. Wie gesagt, müssen alle diese Schlüsse spekulativ bleiben, solange keine experimentellen Nachprüfungen vorliegen.

Auf jeden Fall muß aber der Begriff der embryologischen Differenzierung im Sinne von Determinierung und Potenzbeschränkung streng von rein morphologischer „Differenzierung" im Sinne der Ausreifung der Zellen und Gewebe getrennt werden. Die Gleichstellung und Verwechslung dieser zwei völlig verschiedenen Begriffe, die auch in STEINERS Schriften angedeutet ist, hat zu mehr unklarem Denken und Mißverständnissen der im Schrifttum niedergelegten Befunde geführt, als vielleicht irgendein anderer Faktor. Das gilt nicht nur im Gebiet der Anatomie, sondern noch viel mehr im Gebiet der Onkologie, wie an anderer Stelle ausgeführt wurde (PINKUS, 1966).

Die embryologische Differenzierung (Determinierung) der Epidermis ist im großen ganzen mit der Abtrennung des Neuroektoderms und der Absonderung der ektodermalen Schleimhäute beendet. Später werden weitere Unterteilungen eintreten, wenn Haare, Drüsen und Nägel sich entwickeln. Es ist jedoch nicht richtig, diese Ereignisse als vollwertige Determinierungen anzusehen, da unter besonderen physiologischen Bedingungen, besonders bei der Wundheilung, die scheinbar differenten Epithelien sich als pluripotent und modulationsfähig (WEISS, 1939) erweisen, und die teilungsfähigen Zellen der verschiedenen Adnexe wieder Epidermis bilden können (PINKUS, 1953; MONTAGNA, 1956). Ob die verschiedenen Regionen der Haut spezifische Epidermis haben, ist bisher unbewiesen, da Verpflanzung reiner Epidermis ohne Mesoderm äußerst schwierig ist. Nur für definitiv von der Haut abgesonderte Teile des Ektoderms, wie Zunge und Cornea (BILLINGHAM und MEDAWAR, 1950), scheint die Fixation ihrer spezifischen Eigenschaften bewiesen (s. BILLINGHAM und SILVERS, 1963). Es sei hier auch noch einmal auf BURROWS' (1945) Erfahrungen mit der hormongesteuerten Trennung des Nagerpraeputiums hingewiesen (s. S. 636).

Topographische Differenzierung des Bindegewebes ist bei Hauttransplantaten oft beobachtet worden. So behält auf die Hand transplantierte Bauchhaut ihre herkunftsgemäßen Eigenschaften bei und mag später im Leben z.B. stark Fett ansetzen (s. PINKUS, Band I/2, S. 9). Doch wird natürlich in solchen Fällen immer auch Epidermis mitverpflanzt, und wir müssen erst die Frage beantworten, wieweit die beiden Gewebe einander beeinflussen und welches der leitende Teil ist.

In dieser Hinsicht haben Experimente der letzten Jahre einige klare Antworten gebracht, wenn auch mehr für die Adnexe als für die Epidermis selbst. Auch müssen wir uns dabei auf Tierversuche verlassen. Fast die einzige Arbeit, die wenigstens einen Weg weist, solche Untersuchungen auf menschliche Haut auszudehnen, ist die von HAMBRICK und BLOOMBERG (1959), die fetale Menschenhaut in die Backentaschen von Hamstern verpflanzten und regelrechte Differenzierung von Epidermis, Drüsen und Bindegewebe nachwiesen.

Ohne auf Einzelheiten einzugehen, kann gesagt werden, daß bei der Haar- und Federentwicklung Ektoderm und Mesoderm zusammenarbeiten; werden sie in frühen Stadien getrennt, so ereignet sich nichts. Für neue Übersichten und Literaturangaben s. MCLOUGHLIN (1963), BILLINGHAM und SILVERS (1963), SENGEL (1964), RAWLES (1965). Es scheint, daß zuerst das Mesoderm die induzierende Führerrolle spielt und z.B. beim Huhn Ektoderm zur Bildung entweder von Federn oder Schuppen anregen kann. Später ist die Epidermis determiniert und kann sogar sekundär die Entwicklung des Mesoderms beeinflussen. Man kann hoffen, daß die nächsten Jahre weitere Klärung bringen werden.

Seit einer Reihe von Jahren haben BLECHSCHMIDT und seine Schüler neuartige Gedankengänge in die beschreibende Embryologie auf Grund entwicklungsmechanistischer Deutungen eingeführt. BLECHSCHMIDT schenkte den „Entwicklungsbewegungen" des ganzen Körpers und seiner Organe besondere Aufmerksamkeit und unterschied Lageentwicklung, Formentwicklung und Strukturentwicklung. Hier können wir nur einige der mit der Haut sich befassenden Arbeiten kurz skizzieren und wollen dabei noch einmal auf den prinzipiell unbeweisbaren Charakter aller an menschlichem Material gezogenen Schlüsse hinweisen (s. S. 641).

Folgend auf eine strukturelle Analyse der Septen und Maschen des subcutanen Fettgewebes beim Neugeborenen (BLECHSCHMIDT, 1930) ergab eine Untersuchung von GASTGEBER (1936) eine architektonische Beziehung zwischen Haarkleid und Subcutis. Bei Feten und Neugeborenen ließ sich nachweisen, daß die Haut durch

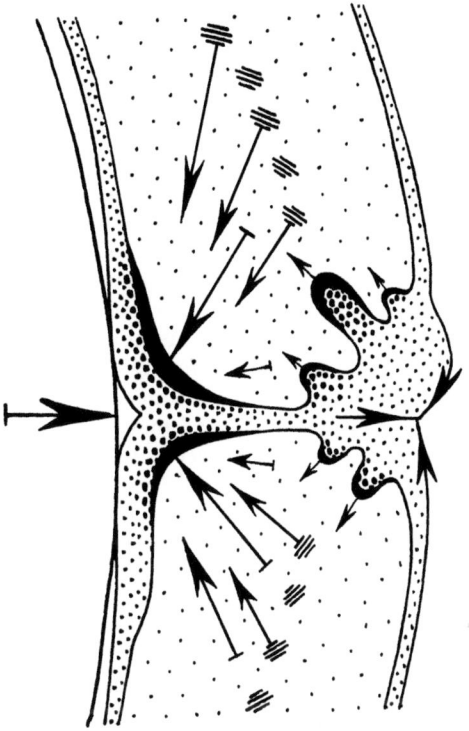

Abb. 9. Schematische Darstellung der bei der Entwicklung von Wimpern und Drüsen am Lidrand wirkenden Kräfte. Die schraffierten Felder in der Substanz der Lider bedeuten Querschnitte der Bündel des M. orbicularis oculi. (Aus BLECHSCHMIDT, 1950)

das Septensystem schräg an die oberflächliche Fascie angeheftet ist, und daß diese Schrägstellung durch die Stellung der Haare äußerlich angezeigt wird. Daraus wurde auf einen konstruktiven Zusammenhang geschlossen. In weiterer Analyse schloß FÜHRERS (1940), daß der Haarstrich dadurch zustande kommt, daß die Haut schräg in Beziehung zu ihrer Unterlage wächst, und daß dies darauf beruht, daß der ganze Organismus vom Primitivknoten aus exzentrisch in cranialer Richtung wächst. 1950 analysierte dann BLECHSCHMIDT selbst die Wachstumsbewegungen der Hautorgane bei menschlichen Embryonen und unterstellte auch stoffwechselmechanische Leistungen des Fetus als wichtigen Faktor in Entwicklung und Differenzierung. Die an Einzelheiten und entwicklungsmechanischen Deutungen der histologischen Befunde überreiche Arbeit läßt sich kaum referieren. Als Beispiel sei BLECHSCHMIDTs Analyse der unterschiedlichen Entwicklung von Wimperhaaren am äußeren und Meibomschen Drüsen am inneren Lidrand angeführt (Abb. 9). Der Tonus der Fasern des sich entwickelnden M. orbicularis oculi wirkt als Kompresse der hinteren Lidkante. Dort werden die Epithelzellen vor der prallgespannten Bulbuswand zusammengepreßt. Die unter Druck heranwachsenden jungen Zellen werden hier, wo ihre Vermehrung besonders behindert wird, nach BLECHSCHMIDTs Meinung zu besonderer Differenzierung veranlaßt, die das Aussprossen von Haarkeimen verhindert. Es finden sich hier frühzeitig relativ degenerative Prozesse, die Epithelzellen verfetten und werden zu sog. Talgzellen An der vorderen Lidkante werden die kräftiger heranwachsenden Zellen des Stratum germinativum während der Flächenspannung des mager gebliebenen, plattgespannten Periderms nur daran gehindert, nach außen vorzudringen, behalten dagegen den Weg nach innen in Richtung auf das lockere Bindegewebe offen. Wir finden Haarkeime an der Innenseite der vorderen Lidkante etwa in Richtung der Winkelhalbierenden nach innen vorwachsen. BLECHSCHMIDT schließt, daß die Entwicklungsprodukte ihren konstruktiven Einbau in das Körperganze direkt der Wachstumsmechanik verdanken.

GRAUMANNs (1950) Deutung der Milchstreifen als eines wichtigen Faktors in der Stoffwechselmechanik der sich entwickelnden Körperwand wurde schon auf S. 635 erwähnt. BLECHSCHMIDT analysierte später in ähnlicher Weise die Entwicklung der Gliedmaßen (1951a, b, c), der Zahnleiste (1955) und der Ohrmuschel (1955).

Weitere Arbeiten behandelten die Schichtenbildung des Integuments (1963a), die Entstehung des Papillarkörpers der Fingerbeere (1963b) und die der Tastballen (SCHMIDT, 1964). BLECHSCHMIDTs Auffassungen wurden schließlich in zwei kürzlich erschienenen Artikeln dahin zusammengefaßt, daß die Organe, die alle aus derselben Eizelle stammen, lokale Wachstumsmodifikationen des Zellgewebes des einheitlichen Organismus sind (1964), daß man ein Organ des Menschen nicht phylogenetisch mit dem einer anderen Species vergleichen kann, und daß HAECKELs biogenetisches Grundgesetz durch ein auf die Erkenntnisse der kinetischen Anatomie begründetes genetisches Grundgesetz (1965) ersetzt werden muß.

D. Der Haarkomplex

Der menschliche Haarkomplex setzt sich aus dem Haarfollikel selbst, der Talgdrüse, der apokrinen Drüse und dem M. arrector pili zusammen. In seiner Anlage und Entwicklung spielen Ektoderm und Mesoderm in vorbildlicher Weise zusammen, um ein kompliziertes kleines Organ zu bilden, das seinen eigenen, noch recht undurchsichtigen Gesetzen folgt. Die von MARKS (1895) eingeführte Bezeichnung „primärer Epithelkeim" für die erste Anlage dieses fibro-epithelialen Organs war daher ein Rückschritt gegen die ältere Benennung „Haarkeim". Die Entwicklung des menschlichen Haarkomplexes wurde 1958 von PINKUS nach modernen Gesichtspunkten nachuntersucht, und die folgende Schilderung hält sich meist an diese Arbeit.

Da die von STÖHR (1904) veröffentlichten Zeichnungen zur Entwicklung des Haares in ihrer Klarheit auch heute noch unübertroffen sind, werden sie hier als Abb. 12, 15 und 18 wiedergegeben.

I. Morphologische Entwicklung des Haarkomplexes

1. Frühe Stadien

Das erste Zeichen der Haaranlage ist ein näheres Zusammentreten hoher Cylinderzellen in der Basalschicht, der von F. PINKUS (1910) sogenannte Haarvorkeim. Der Vorgang ist derselbe, ob die Epidermis zweischichtig oder mehrschichtig, mit Periderm bedeckt oder verhornt ist, und er wiederholt sich ebenso in der schon viel reiferen Haut, wenn neben den Primärfollikeln Seitenhaare

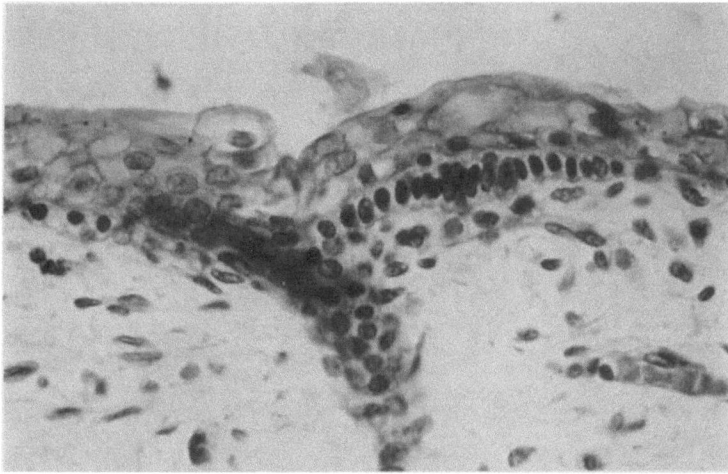

Abb. 10. Vorkeimstadium eines Sekundärhaares rechts von einem schräg angeschnittenen Primärfollikel, von dem ein Teil der Haarkanalanlage in der Epidermis und das tangential getroffene Infundibulum im Corium sichtbar sind. Der Haarvorkeim besteht aus hohen, dicht gedrängten Basalzellen, unter denen sich große Fibroblasten sammeln. Die oberen Lagen der Epidermis erscheinen ungestört. Rückenhaut eines Fetus von 150 mm Scheitel-Steißlänge. Hämatoxylin-Eosin, 465mal. (Aus PINKUS, 1958)

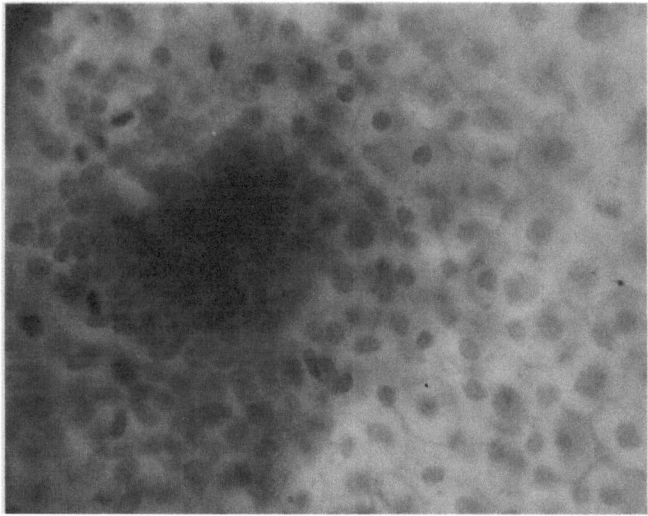

Abb. 11. Früher Haarkeim im Flächenpräparat. Drei Mitosen am linken und oberen Rand sichtbar, andere in der dichten Zellansammlung des Zentrums nicht erkennbar. Infolge einer leichten Wölbung des Präparats sind in der rechten Seite des Bildfeldes Peridermzellen scharf eingestellt. Hämatoxylin, 600mal

entstehen (Abb. 10). Wie FLEISCHHAUER (1953) zeigte, ist dieses Stadium besser in Flachpräparaten als in Schnitten zu sehen. Die Kerne des Stratum germinativum und in geringerem Grade die des Stratum intermedium stehen enger zusammen, haben kleineren Querschnitt und färben sich dunkler in einer runden Zone, die etwa 8—12 Zellen breit ist. Oft kann man um den Haarvorkeim eine zuerst dichtere, dann lichtere Corona erkennen, die FLEISCHHAUER so deutete, daß Zellen in den Haarkeim hineingezogen werden. Es ist richtig, daß nicht nur im Keim selbst, sondern auch in seiner Umgebung Mitosen gehäuft auftreten (Abb. 11), aber von einer wirklichen Invagination ist nichts zu sehen. Der Haar-

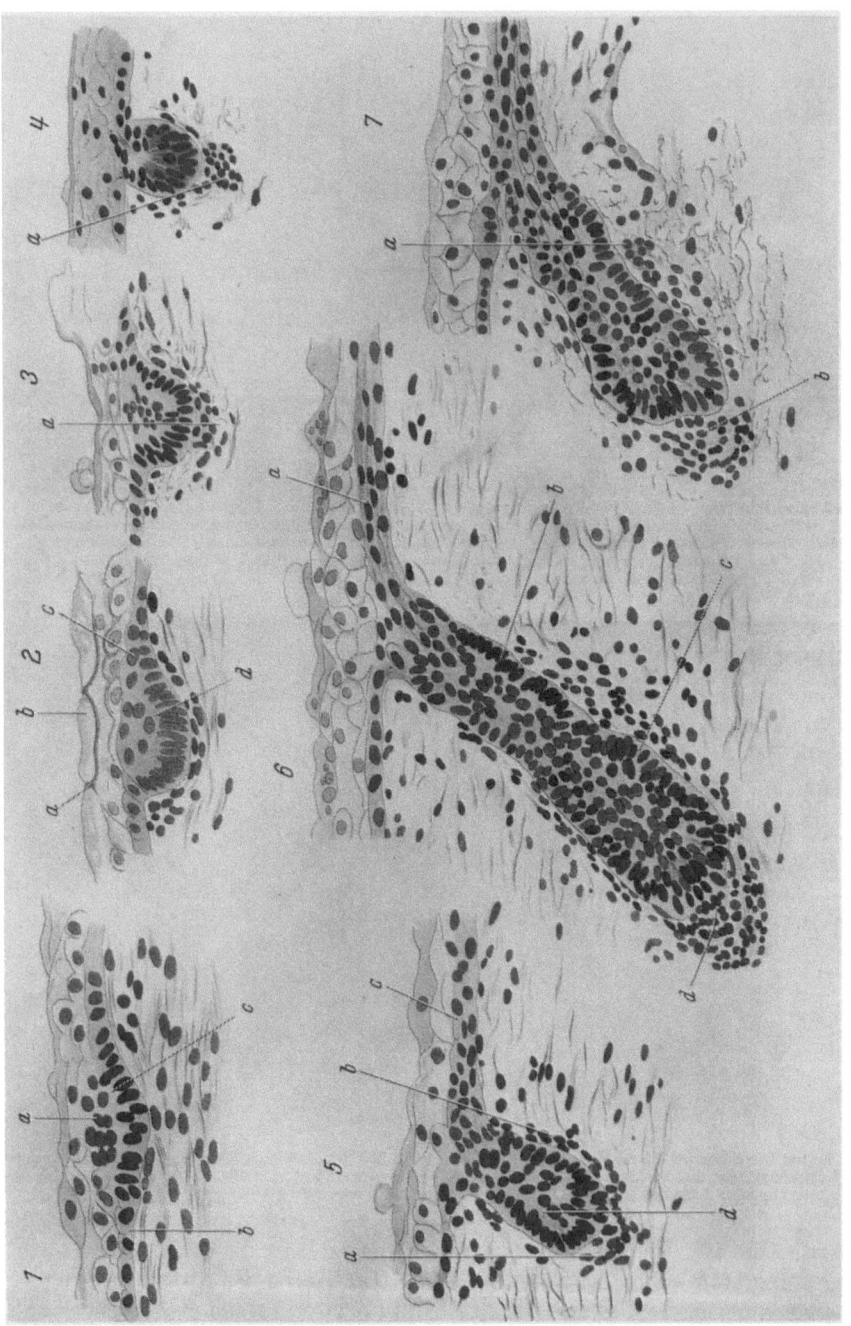

Abb. 12. Frühe Stadien der Haarentwicklung nach STÖHR. Schwarz-weiß-Reproduktion der Buntlithographien, Tafeln III und IV aus STÖHR, 1904. Teilbild 1. *a* Vermehrte Zellen des stratum intermedium, *b* Haarkeim. Teilbild 2. *a* Schlußleisten, *b* Periderm, *c* Haarkanalzellen, *d* Haarkeim. Teilbilder 3—5. *a* Papillenanlage, *b* bindegewebige Balganlage, *c* Haarkanalzellen, *d* Haarzapfen. Teilbild 6. *a* Haarkanalzellen, *b* Talgdrüsenanlage, *c* Wulstanlage, *d* Papillenanlage. Teilbild 7. *a* Arrectoranlage, *b* Papillenanlage

keim ist eine neue Bildung in der Basalschicht, und wenn er sich nach unten vorzuwölben beginnt, geschieht das, weil seine eigenen Zellen sich mitotisch vermehren, während die oberen Schichten der Epidermis ungestört bleiben. Schon unter dem noch schildförmigen Epithelkeim sammeln sich mesodermale Zellen, und von da an ist die Haaranlage ein fibro-epitheliales Gebilde (PINKUS, 1959).

Wie schon auf S. 642 ausgeführt, sprechen Tierversuche dafür, daß das Ektoderm unter der Induktionswirkung des Mesoderms Haare bildet, wenn auch die primäre Veränderung des Coriums morphologisch nur bei den Sinushaaren der Tiere faßbar ist (DAVIDSON und HARDY, 1952). Es ist hier nicht der Platz, auf diese entwicklungsmechanischen Fragen näher einzugehen, aber es ist gut, sich daran zu erinnern, daß die dermale Haarpapille während des ganzen Lebens die

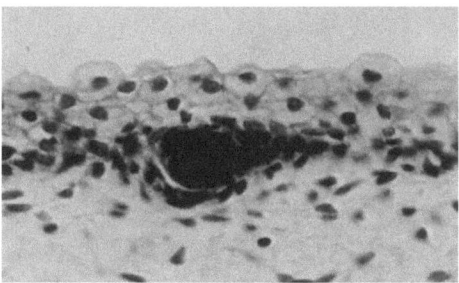

Abb. 13. Haarkeim im Sagittalschnitt. Steile Vorderkante links. Gut ausgebildete mesodermale Kappe. Keine Invagination der Epidermis. Kopfhaut eines Fetus von 110 mm Scheitel-Steißlänge. Hämatoxylin-Eosin, 370mal. (Aus PINKUS, 1958)

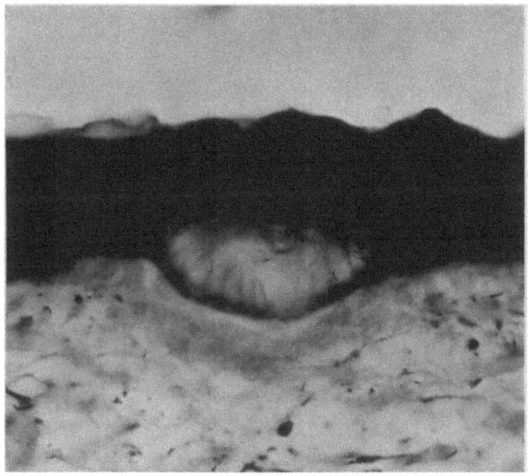

Abb. 14. Haarkeim in mit PAS-Lichtgrün gefärbtem Schnitt der Rückenhaut eines Fetus von 110 mm Scheitel-Steißlänge. Alle Lagen der Epidermis so voll Glykogen, daß sie im Druck schwarz erscheinen. Epithelzellen des Haarkeims haben fast alles Glykogen verloren. Sie sind von der mesodermalen Kopfkappe durch eine PAS-positive Linie, die Basalmembran, getrennt. 600mal

leitende Rolle beim Haarcyclus zu führen scheint, und daß ihre Zerstörung mit der elektrolytischen Nadel dauernde Verödung des Haarfollikels zur Folge hat, während das Ausreißen eines lebenden Haares, das oft alles Epithel einschließlich der Matrix und Wurzelscheiden entfernt, prompt vom Wiederwachsen des Haares gefolgt ist.

Sowie der Stöhrsche Haarkeim (Abb. 12) sich genügend ins Bindegewebe vorwölbt, ist er bilateral symmetrisch (Abb. 13). Er hat im Sagittalschnitt eine steile Vorderkante und eine schräge Hinterwand, und er wächst, dieser Neigung folgend, schräg nach unten vorwärts. Diese Benennung von ,,vorne" und ,,hinten" bedeutet, daß später das Haar sich nach ,,hinten" neigt und daß der Teil der Haut, der vom Haar beschattet wird, hinter ihm liegt (s. Bd. I/2, S. 77). Die Zellen der Hinterseite des Haarkeims bilden bald eine sich verlängernde Kolonne, die in die Epidermis schräg hineinwächst und das Primordium des Haarkanals ist.

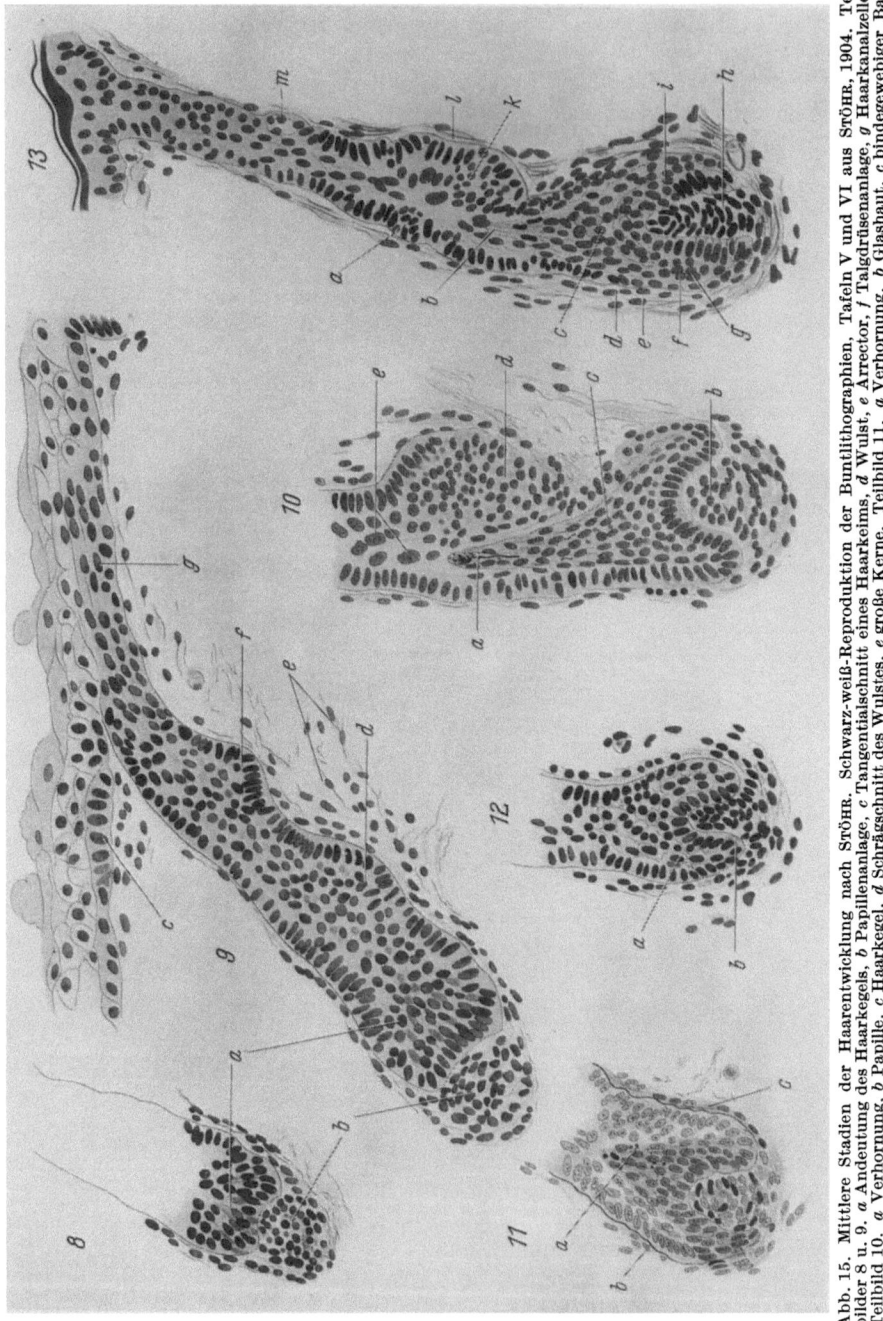

Abb. 15. Mittlere Stadien der Haarentwicklung nach STÖHR. Schwarz-weiß-Reproduktion der Buntlithographien, Tafeln V und VI aus STÖHR, 1904. Teilbilder 8 u. 9. *a* Andeutung des Haarkegels, *b* Papillenanlage, *c* Tangentialschnitt eines Haarkeims, *d* Wulst, *e* Arrector, *f* Talgdrüsenanlage, *g* Haarkanalzellen. Teilbild 10. *a* Verhornung, *b* Papille, *c* Haarkegel, *d* Schrägschnitt des Wulstes, *e* große Kerne. Teilbild 11. *a* Verhornung, *b* Glashaut, *c* bindegewebiger Balg. Teilbild 12. *a* Henle's Schicht, *b* Umschlag. Teilbild 13. *a* Äußere Wurzelscheide, *b* Haarkegelspitze, *c* Anlage der Haarrinde, *d* und *e* innere und äußere Lage des bindegewebigen Balges, *f* Henle's Schicht, *g* Huxley's Schicht, *h* Papille, *i* Bulbus

In Frontalschnitten erscheint der Haarkeim selbstverständlich symmetrisch. In seinem Zentrum sind oft ein paar pyknotische Zellkerne zu finden (Abb. 3C), die im Kalliusschen Sinne andeuten, daß Zelltod ebenso wie Zellvermehrung im Entwicklungsgeschehen eine Rolle spielt. Färbt man die Haut, die gerade die ersten Haarkeime hat, auf Glykogen (PAS), so erscheint die ganze Epidermis einschließlich der Basalzellen leuchtend rot. Nur die Zellen des Haarkeims verlieren ihr Glykogen (Abb. 14) und die distalsten Zellen, die Vorläufer der späteren Matrix, werden nie wieder Glykogen enthalten. Gleichzeitig zeigt sich zwischen dem epithelialen Keim und seiner mesodermalen Kopfkappe eine dünne rote Linie, die erste Anlage der PAS-positiven Basalmembran.

Der nach unten wachsende Epithelzapfen mit seiner Hülle von jungen Bindegewebszellen heißt nun der Haarzapfen und ein wenig später der Bulbuszapfen (Abb. 15). Die äußerste Zellage ist zylindrisch und radiär zur langen Achse angeordnet. Die inneren Zellen richten sich bald parallel zur Längsachse aus. Sie enthalten früh wieder Glykogen, und etwas später taucht dies auch wieder in den Basalzellen hinter dem kolbenförmigen Vorderende auf (Abb. 16). Dies Vorderende wird breiter, bekommt erst eine flache Endplatte und wird dann von dem Ball der prospektiven Papillenzellen eingedellt oder, wohl richtiger, es wächst glockenförmig um sie herum. Der Ball wird dadurch in die im Bulbuszapfen gelegene eiförmige Papille und das mit ihr durch einen dünner werdenden Hals verbundene Papillenpolster zerlegt. Dies wiederum geht kontinuierlich in die sich differenzierende mesodermale Wurzelscheide über. Früh sind auch schon Melanoblasten auf der Außenseite des Haarzapfens vorhanden (ZIMMERMANN, 1954), die dann zwischen Papille und Matrix zu liegen kommen.

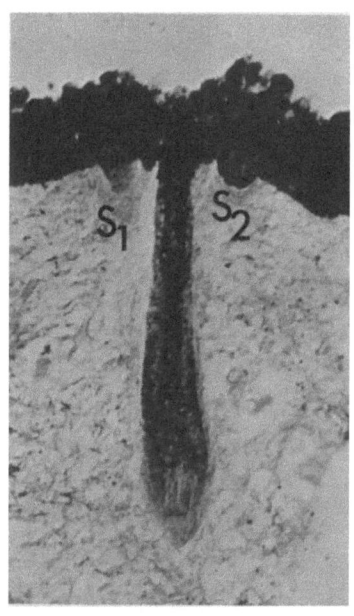

Abb. 16. Übergang vom Haarzapfen zum Bulbuszapfen in der Kopfhaut eines Fetus von 110 mm Scheitel-Steißlänge. Frontalschnitt eines Primärfollikels mit symmetrischen Anlagen von zwei Sekundärfollikeln (S_1 und S_2). Die zukünftige Haarmatrix ist hell, weil sie kein Glykogen enthält. Die radial eingestellten peripheren Zellen des Follikels enthalten weniger Glykogen als die längsgerichteten inneren. Zu beachten sind die mesodermalen Kopfkappen aller drei Follikel und die mesodermale Hülle des Primärfollikels. Alle Lagen der Epidermis voll von Glykogen. PAS-Lichtgrün, 225mal

Im Stadium des Bulbuszapfens treten weitere Differenzierungen auf (Abb. 17). An der Hinterwand des Follikels, also der Seite, die mit der Epidermis einen stumpfen Winkel bildet, entwickeln sich ziemlich gleichzeitig zwei epitheliale Knospen. Die untere, die stets solide und glykogenreich bleibt, wird der Wulst. Er zeigt später die untere Grenze des permanenten Follikels an, das „Haarbeet", bis zu dem das Telogenhaar aufsteigt. Er ist auch die Stelle, wo gewöhnlich der Haarmuskel mit einer elastischen Sehne ansetzt. Die obere Knospe wird zur Talgdrüse, verliert bald ihr Glykogen und entwickelt reife Talgzellen in ihrem Innern. Ferner wächst das obere Ende des Follikels, das jetzt glykogenfrei wird, als eine solide Zellsäule in schräger Richtung durch die Epidermis, um später den Haarkanal zu bilden. In einem etwas späteren Stadium bildet der untere glykogenreiche Teil des Follikels einen merkwürdigen Kontrast zu dem glykogenfreien oberen. Die Resultate histochemischer Enzymreaktionen werden später zusammengefaßt werden.

Ein weiterer wesentlicher Teil des Follikelkomplexes legt sich um diese Zeit an. Seitlich und in einiger Entfernung von der Talgdrüse erscheint eine mit basischen Farben metachromatische Stelle im Corium, und in ihr legen sich junge Mesenchymzellen parallel zueinander, wachsen in die Länge und werden zum M. arrector pili.

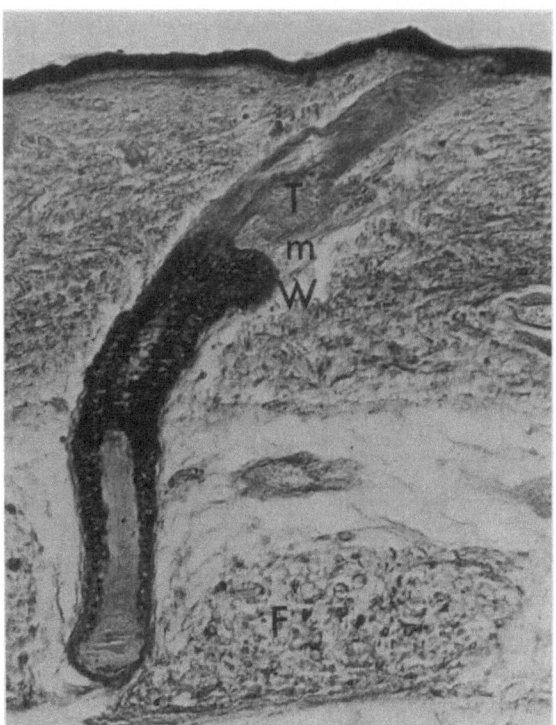

Abb. 17. Leicht gekrümmter Haarfollikel in der Rückenhaut eines Negerfetus von 180 mm Scheitel-Steißlänge. Der Bulbus ist bis ins subcutane Fettgewebe vorgewachsen. Der obere glykogenfreie Abschnitt einschließlich der Talgdrüse (*T*) kontrastiert mit dem den Wulst (*W*) einschließenden unteren Abschnitt. Haarmatrix und ihre Abkömmlinge sind ebenfalls frei von Glykogen. *m* Fasern des M. arrector. *F* Primitives Fettläppchen mit reicher Blutversorgung. Die Basalschicht der Epidermis ist frei von Glykogen im Gegensatz zu den oberen Lagen. PAS-Lichtgrün, 135mal. (Aus Pinkus, 1958)

2. Entwicklung der verschiedenen Teile

In der Weiterentwicklung des Haarkomplexes (Abb. 18) scheinen alle Teile in organischer Weise aufeinander abgestellt zu sein. Doch müssen wir die einzelnen Teile getrennt besprechen. Es sind deren zehn.

a) Der Bulbus mit der Matrix und der Papille.
b) Der untere Follikelabschnitt oberhalb des Bulbus bis zum Wulst.
c) Der Wulst.
d) Der Isthmus.
e) Die Talgdrüse.
f) Das Infundibulum.
g) Der Haarkanal.
h) Das Haar mit den inneren Wurzelscheiden.
i) Der Arrector-Muskel.
k) Die inkonstante apokrine Drüse.

a) Der Bulbus

Die das Zentrum des Bulbus einnehmende fetale Papille besteht aus dicht gepackten Bindegewebszellen, die gewöhnlich etwas Glykogen enthalten. Sie unterscheidet sich in zwei Dingen scharf von der des Erwachsenen. Während Blut-

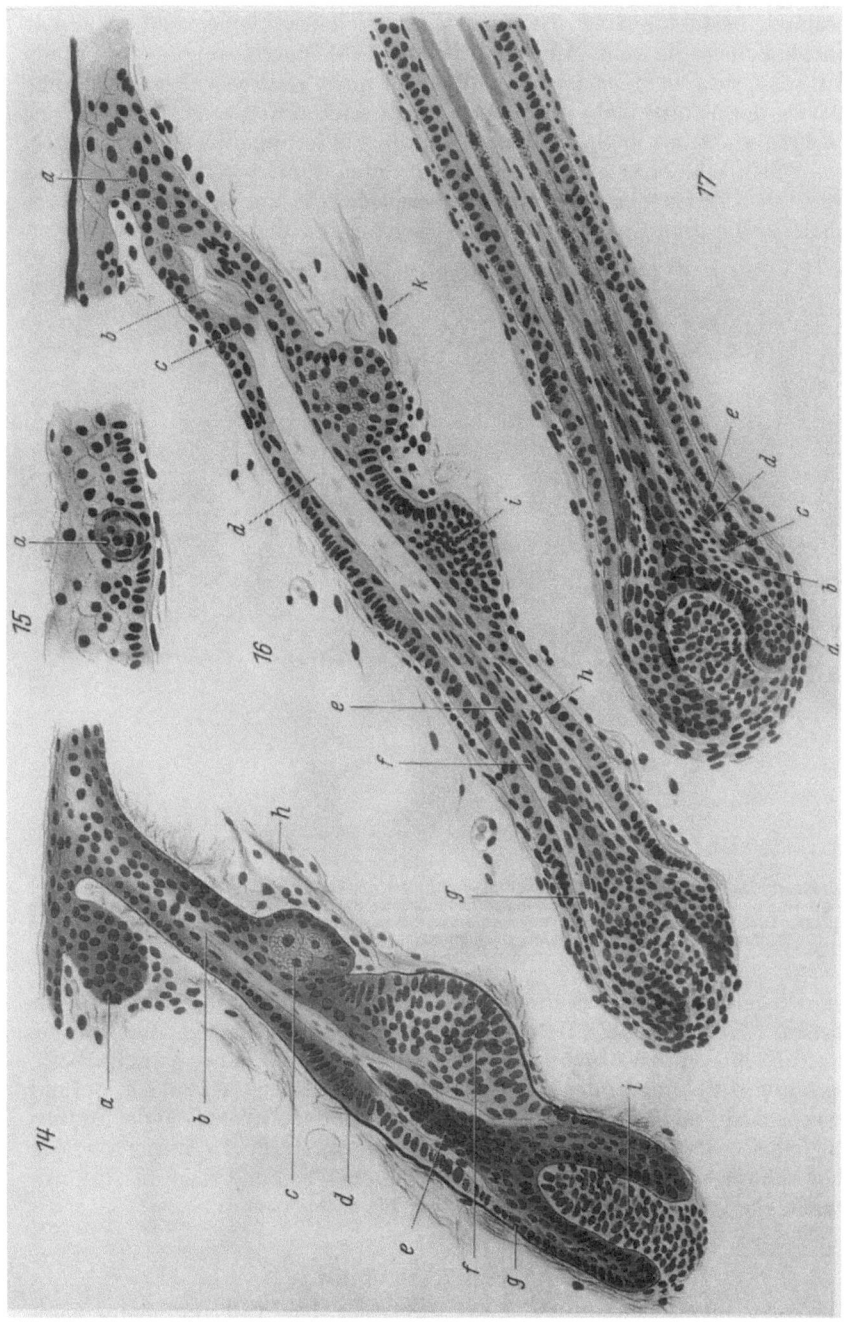

Abb. 18. Spätere Stadien der Haarentwicklung nach STÖHR. Schwarz-weiß-Reproduktion der Buntlithographien, Tafeln VII und VIII aus STÖHR, 1904. Teilbild 14. *a* Tangentialschnitt eines Haarzapfens, *b* Spitze der inneren Wurzelscheide, *c* Talgdrüse, *d* Glashaut, *e* indifferente Zellen des Haarkegels, *f* Wulst, *g* äußere Wurzelscheide, *h* Arrector, *i* Papille. Teilbild 15. *a* Haarkanalstrang. Teilbild 16. *a* Verhornende Zellen des Haarkanals, *b* zerfallende innere Wurzelscheide, *c* Tangentialschnitt der äußeren Wurzelscheide, *d* innere Wurzelscheide (verhornt), *e* Scheidencuticula, *f* Huxley's Schicht, *g* Henle's Schicht, *h* Haar, *i* Wulst, *k* Arrector. Teilbild 17. *a* Haar, *b* Haarcuticula, *c* Scheidencuticula, *d* Huxley's Schicht, *e* Henle's Schicht

capillaren im Papillenpolster vorhanden sind, treten keine durch den Papillenhals. Ferner fehlt die beim Erwachsenen so sehr charakteristische Metachromasie. Erst in den ältesten Stadien der eigenen Serie (150 mm SSL) war sie angedeutet. Dagegen ist stets eine PAS-positive Basalmembran als dünne scharfe Linie zwischen Papille und Matrix zu sehen.

Die epitheliale Matrix, die in jüngeren Stadien aus einer Lage hoher Cylinderzellen bestand, besteht später aus einer Masse ziemlich kleiner und scheinbar ungeordneter Zellen, die viele Mitosen aufweisen. Die Matrix umgibt die Papille wie eine Haube, sie gleicht im Längsschnitt einer nicht ganz geschlossenen Zange (Abb. 19). Da der Papillenhals gewöhnlich direkt nach unten zeigt, während der Follikel schräg steht, ist in Sagittalschnitten die Vorderlippe der Matrix länger. Auf ihrer Außenfläche erstreckt sich eine nach unten dünner werdende Lage von glykogenhaltigen Zellen der äußeren Wurzelscheide, die am tiefsten Punkt am Papillenhals in die glykogenfreie Matrix umschlägt. In den früh pigmentierten

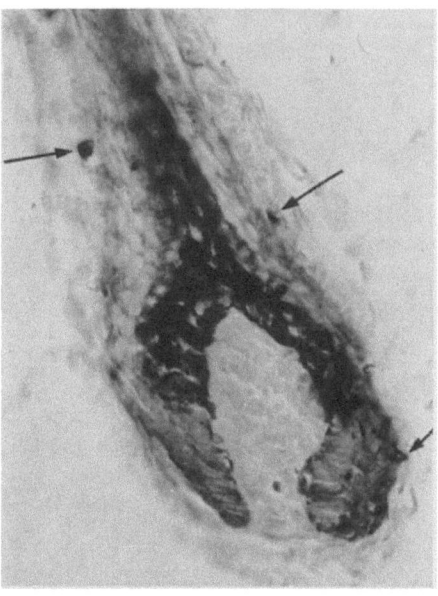

Abb. 19. Kopfhaarfollikel eines Negerfetus im Sagittalschnitt. Der epitheliale Bulbus erscheint als Zange mit stärkerer Vorderlippe. Melanocyten und beginnende Pigmentierung der Haarrinde oberhalb der Auberschen kritischen Ebene. Drei Melanocyten (Pfeile) zwischen äußerer Wurzelscheide und bindegewebigem Haarbalg. Zellreiche Papille ohne Blutgefäße. Toluidinblau, 370mal. (Aus PINKUS, 1958)

Haaren der Neger (für neueste Befunde bei Japanern s. unter G. 3.) sieht man mit gewöhnlichen Färbemethoden Melanocyten sich zwischen Matrix und Papille sammeln (Abb. 19), und zwar meist oberhalb der kritischen Ebene (AUBER, 1952), die dem größten Durchmesser der Papille entspricht. Im Gegensatz zu dem Befund beim Erwachsenen sind einzelne Melanocyten auch auf der Außenwand des Bulbus und etwas höher entlang der äußeren Wurzelscheide verstreut. Im übrigen ist der Bulbus von zahlreichen jungen Bindegewebszellen umgeben und zeigt die Anfänge der Glashaut, die im nächsten Abschnitt näher besprochen wird.

b) Unterer Follikelabschnitt

Der untere Follikelabschnitt des Fetus entspricht dem Teil, der später beim Haarwechsel wieder aufgelöst und neu gebildet wird. Dieser Teil des Follikels verlängert sich stark, während die Matrix schon anfängt, die innere Wurzelscheide zu bilden, wie später (S. 655) besprochen wird. Man kann sagen, daß die sich hier entwickelnde äußere Wurzelscheide von Anfang an einen Hohlzylinder um die Haaranlage bildet. Das Epithel wird bald mehrschichtig und besteht aus einer Lage radiär angeordneter hoher Basalzellen und mehreren Lagen von polyedrischen Zellen, die später zu Stachelzellen werden, aber nie Anzeichen der Verhornung aufweisen. Alle diese Zellen sammeln so viel Glykogen an, daß sie mit gewöhnlichen Färbungen hell und plasmaarm erscheinen.

Die Bindegewebszellen beginnen sich in Ring- und Längsschichten zu ordnen und bilden die fibröse Wurzelscheide. Zwischen ihr und dem Epithel erscheint bald eine bis zu 2—3 μ dicke hyaline Schicht, die Glashaut. Sie ist nicht wie beim Erwachsenen metachromatisch und färbt sich nicht klar mit PAS, sondern nimmt in den mit Lichtgrün gegengefärbten Schnitten eine grünblaue bis violette Tönung an. VAN GIESONS Färbung zeigt Züge feiner roter Fibrillen in ihr. Meine Präparate erlaubten es nicht, die Art ihrer Bildung zu entscheiden.

c) Wulst

Am oberen Ende des zylindrischen unteren Follikelabschnittes wird die bilaterale Symmetrie wieder deutlich. Der Wulst steht als eine oft halbkugelige Masse auf der Hinterseite heraus. Er ist an vielen Follikeln das hervorstechendste Gebilde, oft ebenso groß wie der Bulbus und größer als die Talgdrüsen (Abb. 17, 18). Manchmal reicht er um den Follikel herum und verursacht eine Verdickung auch der Vorderwand. Gelegentlich hat er eine schräge Unterseite und eine flache Oberseite. Obwohl seine Zellen fast ebensoviel Glykogen zu enthalten scheinen wie die Zellen der äußeren Wurzelscheide, sehen sie in gewöhnlichen Färbungen immer solide, niemals hell aus. Die Glashaut reicht um den Wulst herum (Abb. 18) und endet abrupt an seiner oberen Kante. Später entwickeln sich hier dichte Bindegewebszüge und elastische Fasern in Zusammenhang mit dem Haarmuskel. Bei älteren Feten wird der Wulst relativ kleiner und fällt am erwachsenen Follikel oft wenig auf.

d) Isthmus

Zwischen dem Wulst und der Einmündung der Talgdrüse liegt der Isthmus, der beim Fetus wenige spezifische Eigenschaften aufweist. Die Glashaut ist hier nicht vorhanden. Die innersten Zellen werden pyknotisch, bevor die Haarspitze sich durchbohrt, aber sie verhornen nicht. Die Außenwand, die aus 2—3 Reihen ziemlich flacher Zellen besteht, zeigt einen merkwürdigen Wechsel der Richtung der Kernachsen an der Hinterseite. Die Kerne des unteren Teiles zeigen schräg aufwärts und nach außen, die des obersten Teiles schräg abwärts (Abb. 23). Dazwischen sind Kerne quer zur Achse des Follikels angeordnet. Die Zellen des Isthmus enthalten wenig Glykogen und kontrastieren scharf mit denen der unteren Abschnitte. Später im Leben ist der Isthmus von einer charakteristischen elastischen Hülle umgeben und um seinen obersten Teil, im Winkel zwischen Follikelwand und Talgdrüse, findet sich konstant ein Ring von sauren Mucopolysacchariden.

e) Talgdrüse

Wenn die Talgdrüsenzellen anfangen auszureifen, verliert die Drüse temporär ihr Glykogen. Später taucht es in den Basalzellen wieder auf. Anfangs bilden talghaltige Zellen einen Teil der Follikelwand und grenzen direkt an das Follikellumen. Ein aus verhornendem Plattenepithel bestehender Gang formt sich erst später. Die Vorderwand des Follikels gegenüber der zunächst auf die Hinterwand beschränkten Drüse ähnelt der des gleich zu besprechenden Infundibulums und verhornt frühzeitig.

f) Infundibulum und g) Haarkanal

Oberhalb der Talgdrüsenmündung ändert sich das Follikelepithel drastisch. Es wird jetzt ein geschichtetes Plattenepithel, das gewöhnlich früher als die

Epidermis mit Keratohyalinbildung verhornt. Dieses Epithel erstreckt sich als ein zunächst solider Strang in die Epidermis hinein (Abb. 20) und schräg durch sie hindurch bis zur Oberfläche. Wenn die zentralen Zellen verhornen, entsteht der Haarkanal (Abb. 21), der gewöhnlich nur ein potentielles Lumen hat, da er mit verhornten Zellen gefüllt ist. Der Kanal mag kurz sein, aber oft ist er sehr lang und verläuft beinahe waagerecht in der Epidermis. Er öffnet sich schließlich durch völlige Verhornung seiner Oberfläche und setzt so die Haarspitze, die in ihn ein-

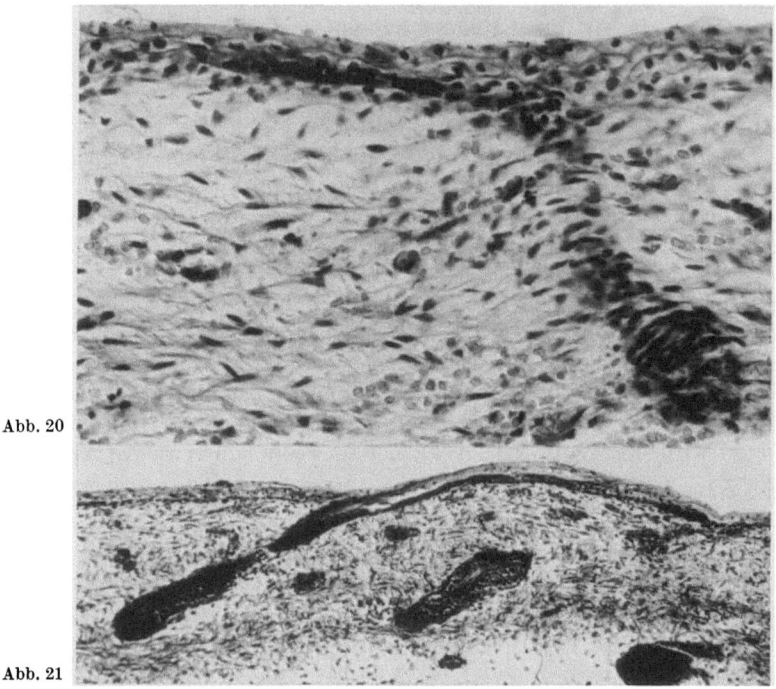

Abb. 20. Anlage des Haarkanals bei einem Fetus von 115 mm Scheitel-Steißlänge. Ein solider Epithelstrang erstreckt sich vom Haarfollikel schräg nach hinten in die Epidermis hinein. Hämatoxylin-Eosin, 280mal. (Aus PINKUS, 1958)

Abb. 21. Sehr langer Haarkanal mit verhorntem Zentrum in einer Epidermis, die noch im Peridermstadium ist. Brusthaut eines Fetus von 180 mm Scheitel-Steißlänge. Hämatoxylin-Eosin, 90mal. (Aus PINKUS, 1958)

gedrungen ist, frei. Auf diese Weise geht der größte Teil des Kanals noch im fetalen Leben verloren. Der kürzere untere Teil, zusammen mit dem intradermalen Abschnitt, bildet dann das endgültige Infundibulum, das die Epidermis beinahe senkrecht durchsetzt (Acrotrichium, DUPERRAT u. MASCARO, 1963). Seine Zellen sind dem geschichteten Plattenepithel der Epidermis so ähnlich und sind so eng mit ihm verbunden, daß die noch in vielen Lehrbüchern vertretene Ansicht entstand, die Epidermis stülpe sich hier ein (ACHTEN, 1957). Näheres über die biologische und pathologische Bedeutung der hier vertretenen Auffassung findet sich bei PINKUS (1959). Übrigens kam DANNEEL (1931) bei der Ratte auch zu dem Schluß, daß der Haarkanal follikulären Ursprungs ist.

Die Einheitlichkeit der subepidermalen und intraepidermalen Teile des Infundibulums ist in fetaler Haut besonders augenfällig in PAS-gefärbten Schnitten. Die Zellen des Infundibulums und Haarkanals enthalten zunächst viel weniger Glykogen (Abb. 17) als die Epidermis, und man kann ihren Pfad durch die Epidermis hindurch verfolgen. Später, wenn die Basalzellen der Epidermis glykogenfrei werden, sammeln die Zellen des Follikels wieder Glykogen an, und zwar in allen Lagen, von der äußersten zur innersten. Dadurch entsteht zwischen Epidermis und Follikelepithel eine zellscharfe Grenze, an der sich glykogenfreie epidermale Basalzellen um den Follikel anordnen und ihn wie einen Kragen umgeben (Abb. 22).

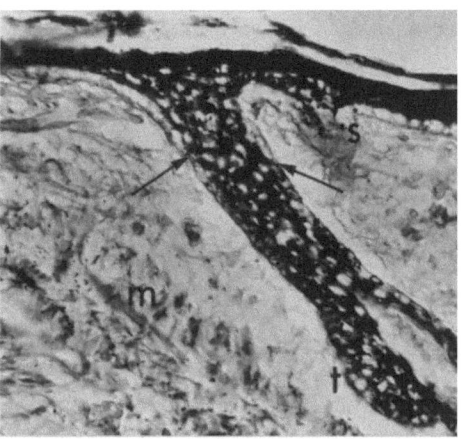

Abb. 22. Kontrast zwischen Basalschicht der Epidermis und Infundibulum. Die glykogenfreien Basalzellen umgeben den Follikel wie ein Kragen, dessen untere Grenze durch Pfeile angegeben ist. Rechts vom Follikel ist ein Nebenhaar angeschnitten (s). t Talgdrüse, deren Basalzellen jetzt Glykogen enthalten; m M. arrector. PAS-Lichtgrün, 280mal. (Aus PINKUS, 1959)

h) Haar und innere Wurzelscheide

Wir kommen nun zu dem Inhalt und wichtigsten Teil des Follikels, dem Haar und seiner inneren Wurzelscheide. Diese entstehen aus dem unreifen und mitosereichen Epithel der Matrix, das sich nach unerschütterlichen Regeln in fünf ganz verschiedene Endprodukte verwandelt. Die Matrixzellen nächst der äußeren Wurzelscheide beginnen zuerst Trichohyalin zu formen, verhornen schon im Gebiet des Bulbus und bilden die gefensterte Membran der Henleschen Schicht, die wie ein starres röhrenförmiges Netz die weicheren Innenteile umgibt. Mehrere konzentrische Ringe von Matrixzellen beginnen auf einer etwas höheren Ebene unter Trichohyalinbildung zu verhornen. Dies ist die Huxleysche Schicht, die sich zusammen mit der Henleschen in Giemsa-Präparaten ganz spezifisch dunkelblau färbt. An der Innenseite dieser dickeren Röhre entwickelt sich die dritte Schicht der inneren Wurzelscheide, die Cuticula, deren Schuppen mit den freien Rändern der Cuticula des Haares verhakt sind. Die innerste solide Säule ist dann die Haarrinde, da fetale Lanugo kein Mark besitzt. Tatsächlich ist der Durchschnitt des Haares im Verhältnis zur inneren Wurzelscheide klein, oft nicht mehr als ein Drittel des ganzen Inhalts der Follikelröhre. Der Haarschaft mag schon bei der ersten Anlage regelmäßige Reihen von Melaninkörnchen enthalten, die von den Melanocyten der Matrix gebildet werden. Im Gegensatz zum Haar des Erwachsenen enthält bei Negern auch die Huxleysche Schicht oft Pigmentklumpen und manchmal Klumpen von PAS-positivem Material.

Dadurch, daß die Matrix die innere Wurzelscheide vor dem eigentlichen Haar bildet, ist dessen feine Spitze von einer konischen Hülle von Wurzelscheidenmaterial geschützt, ähnlich dem jungen Schoß einer Tulpenzwiebel. Jedoch ist das Bild des die Erde durchbohrenden Pflanzenschosses falsch. Zur Zeit der ersten Anlage liegt der Haarscheidenkegel dicht am Niveau des Wulstes. Tatsächlich wächst die Matrix von ihm weg nach unten. Erst wenn der untere Follikelabschnitt seine völlige Länge erreicht hat und der Bulbus im Unterhautfettgewebe liegt, beginnt ein wirkliches Nach-oben-Wachsen der Haarspitze, und jetzt ist ihr im Isthmus, Infundibulum und Haarkanal ein Weg vorgezeichnet dadurch, daß die innersten Zellen dieser Teile entweder degenerieren, vertalgen oder verhornen.

In seinem ersten Trieb zur Oberfläche ist, wie gesagt, die fadenförmige Haarspitze von der Wurzelscheide geschützt, die oft auch im Haarkanal erscheint. Manchmal jedoch, wie auch beim Erwachsenen, ist das Haar oberhalb der Talgdrüsenöffnung frei. MONTAGNAs Hypothese (1956, S. 190), daß die Wurzelscheide enzymatisch verdaut wird, wird durch Befunde an Negerfeten gestützt. Man kann

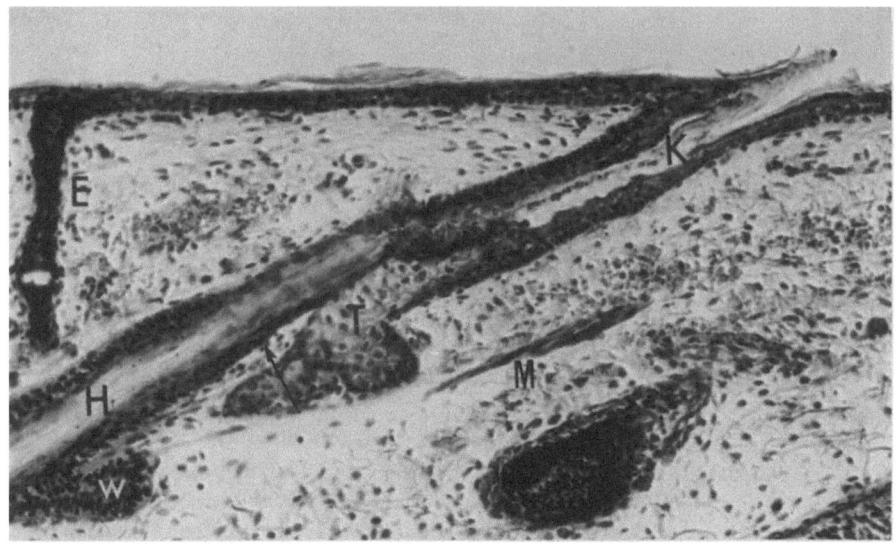

Abb. 23. Schräg gestellter Kopfhaarfollikel und senkrecht absteigende ekkrine Drüse (*E*) bei einem Fetus von 150 mm Scheitel-Steißlänge. Das Haar (*H*) ist fast bis zur Talgdrüsenmündung vorgedrungen. Gerade oberhalb ist das Follikellumen nicht im Schnitt getroffen, aber erscheint wieder im Infundibulum und dem durch Verlust seines Daches ganz kurz gewordenen Haarkanal. Im Infundibulum sind körnige Reste der inneren Wurzelscheide und Melaninkörnchen (*K*) sichtbar. Wechsel der Achsenrichtung der peripheren Kerne im Isthmus ist durch einen Pfeil bezeichnet. *T* Talgdrüse; *W* Wulst; *M* M. arrector. Hämatoxylin und Eosin, 180mal. (Aus PINKUS, 1958)

hier sehen, daß die noch solide Wurzelscheide gerade unterhalb der Talgdrüse ihre Färbbarkeit mit Giemsa einbüßt. Oberhalb des Drüseneingangs verschwinden geformte Zellen, und man sieht eine Mischung von Melaninkörnchen und PAS-positivem Material, als ob diese Bestandteile nach Auflösung der Hornzellen zurückgeblieben wären (Abb. 23).

i) Arrector-Muskel

Der M. arrector pili entsteht, wie schon erwähnt, in einer metachromatischen Zone des embryonalen Bindegewebes ungefähr auf dem Niveau der Talgdrüse hinter dem Haarfollikel. Dort legen sich Zellen parallel zueinander, wachsen in die Länge, nehmen an Zahl zu und erstrecken sich schräg aufwärts nach der Epidermis hin und schräg abwärts beinahe parallel zum Follikel (Abb. 23), bis sie die Spitze des Wulstes erreichen. Manchmal ziehen sie aber auch an ihm vorbei zum unteren Follikelabschnitt. Der Muskel tritt in Verbindung mit der bindegewebigen Wurzelscheide. Elastische Fasern treten erst später auf, wenn sie sich auch sonst in der Haut entwickeln. Die glatten Muskelfasern des Arrector erwerben Glykogen sehr viel später als die quergestreifte Muskulatur.

Daß Haarbalgmuskeln bei manchen spezialisierten Haaren nicht ausgebildet werden, wurde schon von F. PINKUS (1927, S. 256) erwähnt. Ihr Fehlen an den Wimpern und den kleinen Haaren der Lider wurde von IKADA (1953) bei japanischen Feten bestätigt. TAKEDA (1952) vermißte sie auch am Nasenflügel und der Nasenspitze.

k) Apokrine Drüse

Die Embryonalentwicklung der apokrinen Drüsen ist natürlich hauptsächlich in der Axilla untersucht worden (STEINER, 1926; BORSETTO, 1951; MONTAGNA, 1959). Obwohl, wie in Bd. I/2 ausgeführt, erheblich größere Körperregionen regelmäßig oder potentiell apokrine Drüsen besitzen, ist es nach eigenen Untersuchungen zweifelhaft, ob die Majorität der Haarfollikel je morphologisch faßbare

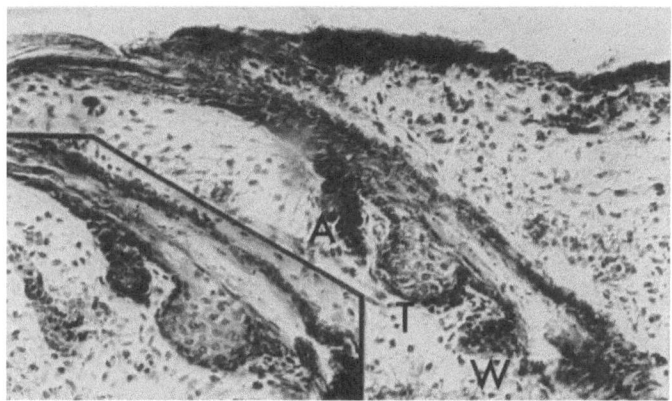

Abb. 24. Apokrine Drüsenanlagen an 2 Kopfhaarfollikeln eines Fetus von 190 mm Scheitel-Steißlänge. Typische Anordnung von apokriner Drüse (*A*), Talgdrüse (*T*) und Wulst (*W*)

Drüsenanlagen entwickelt. Doch hat SERRI (1962) Anlagen apokriner Drüsen an Kopf, Gesicht, Hals, Thorax, Rücken und Oberschenkel gefunden.

Die apokrine Drüse entsteht immer oberhalb der Talgdrüse und ebenfalls an der Hinterwand des Follikels (Abb. 24). Ihr erster Anfang ist ein solider Knopf, der sich in einen keulenförmig oder spitz zulaufenden Epithelstrang verlängert. Nach MONTAGNA (1959) legt sie sich in der Axilla im 5. Monat an, aber nicht in allen Follikeln gleichzeitig, so daß man nebeneinander kleine Knospen, Stränge mit keulenförmigem Ende und schon aufgeknäuelte Drüsen finden kann. Im 6. Monat sind alle Drüsen an der Basis aufgerollt, einige beginnen ein Lumen zu zeigen. Sie liegen in derselben Tiefe wie die lange vor ihnen entwickelten ekkrinen Drüsen, und einige zeigen einen größeren Durchmesser des Drüsenschlauchs als diese. Im 9. Monat sind die apokrinen Achseldrüsen voll entwickelt und zeigen ein weiteres Drüsenlumen als die ekkrinen, obwohl sie im ganzen kleiner sind.

Nach ENDO (1939) beträgt das Durchschnittsvolumen individueller a-Drüsen in der Axilla des Neugeborenen 0,0024 mm^3, das der e-Drüsen 0,0020. Pro Quadratzentimeter Hautoberfläche sind 0,89 mm^3 a-Drüsen und 2,62 mm^3 e-Drüsen vorhanden.

Das Lumen enthält oft Glykogen und diastaseresistentes Material, das auf PAS reagiert. Andererseits fand KARRENBERG (1929) bei Neugeborenen nur solide Zellkomplexe und selbst bei einjährigen Kindern noch keine Sekretion. MONTAGNA stimmt nicht mit BORSETTO (1951) überein, daß sich um diese Zeit die Ausführungsgänge der apokrinen Drüsen auf die Hautoberfläche verlegen. Er meint, daß die sehr dünnen Ausführungsgänge der Drüsen leicht in dünnen Schnitten übersehen werden können, daß aber dicke Gefrierschnitte immer die Gangmündung in den Haarfollikeln oberhalb der Talgdrüse zeigen. Nach SERRI et al. (1962) enthalten die frühen Anlagen der apokrinen Drüsen kleine Mengen Glykogen. Dies verschwindet, wenn die Primordien länger werden, aber taucht wieder auf, sobald der sekretorische Teil sich ausbildet.

II. Topographische Entwicklung der Haare

Die Anordnung der Haare und Haargruppen in regelmäßigen Mustern ist oft betont worden. FLEISCHHAUER fand in gefärbten Macerationspräparaten (1953), daß die ersten Haarkeime zwar nicht in Reihen, aber doch in ziemlich regelmäßigen

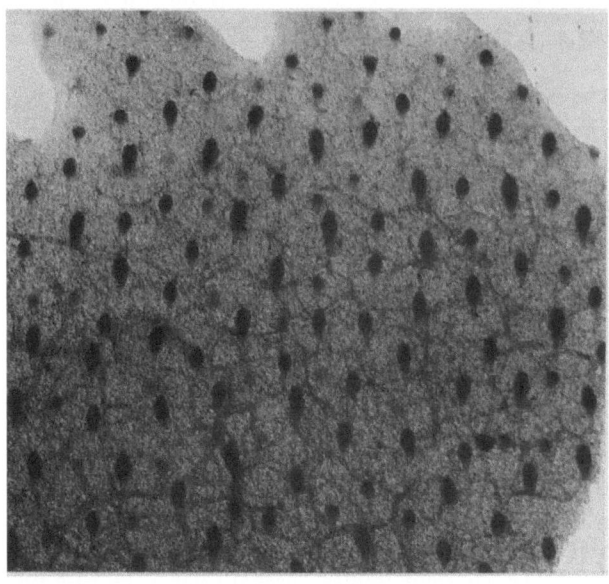

Abb. 25. Verteilung der Haaranlagen, gezeigt im Flachschnitt der Armhaut eines Fetus von 115 mm Scheitel-Steißlänge. Die älteren Follikel haben Tropfenform, das breite Ende entspricht dem Bulbus, der Schwanz der Haarkanalanlage. Die Achsen sind parallel ausgerichtet. Dazwischen jüngere runde Anlagen bis zu ganz jungen, die gerade als Zellverdichtung angedeutet sind. Blutgefäßnetz des Coriums ist sichtbar. Hämatoxylin, 28mal

Abständen angelegt werden. Verteilungskurven zeigten mittlere Werte von 274 bis 350 µ in verschiedenen Gegenden. Wenn die Anlagen beim weiteren Wachstum der Haut über einen kritischen Abstand auseinander gerückt werden, entstehen weitere primäre Haarkeime zwischen ihnen (Abb. 25). Die kritische Distanz ist kleiner in den Körperteilen, wo die ursprünglichen Keime näher beieinander standen. Von etwa 12 cm SSL an beginnen Sekundärhaare neben den Primärfollikeln aufzutreten, und die Bildung von Primärhaaren hört allmählich auf.

Der Haarstrich ist auch nach FLEISCHHAUER (1953) in der Richtung der Kerne der Epidermis vorgezeichnet, und diese deutet vielleicht im Sinne FÜHRERS' (1940) die allgemeine Richtung des Hautwachstums an. Wenn der Haarstrich plötzlich wechselt, wie es in Wirbeln und an Konvergenzlinien vorkommt, wechselt auch die Seite, an der sich Wulst und Talgdrüsen anlegen. Trotz dieser Allgemeinregeln gibt es aber Situationen, wo dem einzelnen Follikel innewohnende Tendenzen eine starke Rolle spielen. Das ist besonders wieder bei Negerhaar deutlich, wo der Follikel sich im Abwärtswachsen krümmt (Abb. 17), und der Bulbus oft wieder unter die Stelle zu liegen kommt, von wo er von der Epidermis auswuchs.

Sekundärhaare legen sich meist symmetrisch zu beiden Seiten des Primärfollikels an, gelegentlich entwickelt sich ein einzelner Follikel hinter dem ersten.

III. Histochemie

Das Verhalten des Glykogens wurde schon bei der allgemeinen Morphogenese des Haarkomplexes geschildert, weil die Fluten und Ebben dieser Substanz so ausgezeichnet in der Unterscheidung der verschiedenen Teile in ihren verschiedenen Entwicklungsstufen helfen. Weitere und allgemein ähnliche Daten werden von MONTAGNA (1959), SERRI et al. (1962) und BERLIN u. PRIDVIZHKIN (1965) beigebracht.

Betreffs der Enzyme folgen wir auch hier MACHIDA (1964). Er fand im vierten Monat schwache Reaktionen für Bernsteinsäuredehydrogenase, Cytochromoxydase und Monoaminoxydase in allen Teilen des Komplexes. Vom fünften Monat an werden die ersten beiden Enzyme im Haarfollikel, der Talgdrüse und der apokrinen Drüse fortlaufend stärker. In den Drüsen reagiert der sekretorische Teil mehr als die Gänge, und im ganzen reagiert die apokrine Drüse weniger stark als die ekkrine. Die Aktivität für Monoaminoxydase zeigt größere Schwankungen während der Entwicklungsmonate, doch steigt sie im letzten Monat an. Die Meibomschen Drüsen verhalten sich wie andere Talgdrüsen.

Nach MACHIDA ist Phosphorylase-Aktivität im Follikel stärker im fünften Monat als im vierten, und in der äußeren Wurzelscheide stärker als in der inneren. Später ist die Reaktion besonders stark im Apex des Follikels, und im zehnten Monat wird sie besonders im Mittelteil konzentriert. Während die Primordien der Talgdrüsen stark reagieren, ist Aktivität später auf die Peripherie beschränkt. Doch bestehen regionale Unterschiede. Die Talgdrüsen der Lider, Lippen und Achsel bleiben länger positiv als andere. In der Meibomschen Drüse reagiert vom fünften bis zehnten Monat nur der Ausführungsgang. Die Anlagen der apokrinen Drüsen zeigen Phosphorylase-Aktivität, später ist im allgemeinen der Gang stärker positiv als der sekretorische Teil, aber die Reaktivität im ganzen wird allmählich geringer. Mollsche Drüsen der Lider zeigen eine schwache Reaktion.

Nach SERRI et al. (1962) zeigt sich die erste Phosphorylase-Aktivität im Follikelkomplex schon früher, sobald Wulst und Talgdrüse sich abzuzeichnen beginnen, und ist stark in beiden Anlagen. Später geht die Reaktion dem Glykogengehalt der verschiedenen Teile mit einigen Ausnahmen parallel.

MACHIDA und ähnlich SERRI et al. (1963) bemerken, daß alkalische Phosphatase-Aktivität im ganzen Haarkomplex in umgekehrtem Verhältnis zum Fortschritt der Entwicklung steht. Sie ist in Talgdrüsen und Meibomschen Drüsen stets negativ. Saure Phosphatase-Aktivität, anfangs schwach, ist vom fünften bis zum zehnten Monat stark, besonders in der inneren Wurzelscheide. Talgdrüsen und Meibomsche Drüsen reagieren unregelmäßig. In apokrinen Drüsen ist die Reaktion im letzten Teil der Schwangerschaft auf den follikelnahen Teil des Ganges beschränkt.

Die Reaktionen auf unspezifische Esterasen sind verschieden, je nach der Methode, die zur Anwendung kommt. So ist die Naphthol-AS-Esterasenreaktion nach PEARSE im Haarfollikel und in der Talgdrüse während der ganzen Fetalzeit stationär. Apokrine Drüsen reagieren erst vom achten Monat an stark. Auf der anderen Seite ist GOMORIS α-Naphthol-Reaktion in Follikel und Talgdrüse und apokriner Drüse bis zum sechsten Monat schwach, um dann stark zu werden.

Leucinaminopeptidase läßt sich vom vierten bis sechsten Monat besonders im apikalen Teil des Follikels und in der inneren Wurzelscheide nachweisen. Dann wird die Reaktion schwächer und ist in der Talgdrüse stets schwach oder negativ. Im sekretorischen Teil der apokrinen Drüsen wird die Reaktion ebenso wie in den Mollschen Drüsen im achten Monat stärker.

IV. Quantitative Daten über fetale Haarkomplexe

Die Schüler OKAJIMAs haben in Japan eine Fülle von Zahlen über alle möglichen Eigenschaften der Hautanhangsgebilde zusammengetragen. Einige dieser Daten sind in Band I/2 im Abschnitt über makroskopische Anatomie tabellarisch zusammengestellt. Hier folgen einige Angaben über fetale Verhältnisse. Auch Werte aus OLINs (1942) Arbeit über die Follikelkomplexe am Tragus beim Neugeborenen sind wiedergegeben (Tabelle 4a—c).

Tabelle 4a. *Talgdrüsen*

Körpergegend	mm³ Volumen pro cm² bei einem			
	8monatigen Fetus (KOSAKA)	9monatigen Zwilling 1 (MOCHIZUKI)	9monatigen Zwilling 2 (MOCHIZUKI)	Neugeborenen (TANIGUCHI)
Kopf	1,29	2,56	4,13	2,43
Gesäß	0,24	0,14	0,20	0,74
Rücken	0,38	0,98	0,79	1,00
Brust	0,19	1,60	1,26	0,87
Bauch	0,05	0,26	0,18	0,17
Oberarm, Extensor	0,11	0,54	0,56	0,81
Oberarm, Flexor	0,14	0,50	0,64	0,47
Vorderarm, Extensor	0,26	0,45	0,52	0,48
Vorderarm, Flexor	0,05	0,15	0,06	0,27
Oberschenkel, Lat.	0,24	0,14	0,10	0,18
Oberschenkel, Med.	0,18	0,29	0,38	0,33
Unterschenkel, Ext.	0,26	0,06	0,06	0,08
Unterschenkel, Flex.	0,10	0,09	0,09	0,12
Axilla (ENDO)				4,61

	5 Monate	6 Monate	7 Monate	8 Monate	9 Monate	10 Monate
Augenbraue (BYON)	3,74	2,68	2,51	1,78	2,51	3,23

Kleinste und größte Werte der zu einer Haargruppe gehörenden Drüsen

	8 Monate	9 Monate (1)	9 Monate (2)	Neugeboren
Minimum	0,0002	0,0002	0,0003	0,0004
Maximum	0,0063	0,0138	0,0197	0,0130

Tabelle 4b. *Arrector-Muskel*

Körpergegend	Volumen in mm³ pro cm² bei einem			
	8monatigen Fetus (KOSAKA)	9monatigen Zwilling 1 (MOCHIZUKI)	9monatigen Zwilling 2 (MOCHIZUKI)	Neugeborenen (TANIGUCHI)
Kopf	1,57	1,69	1,67	2,45
Gesäß	0,34	0,16	0,18	0,97
Rücken	0,58	0,21	0,31	0,61
Brust	0,42	0,38	0,44	0,42
Bauch	0,10	0,18	0,16	0,21
Oberarm, Extensor	0,34	0,31	0,49	0,67
Oberarm, Flexor	0,26	0,10	0,18	0,35
Vorderarm, Extensor	0,42	0,74	0,49	0,94
Vorderarm, Flexor	0,26	0,09	0,02	0,42
Oberschenkel, Lat.	0,63	0,13	0,09	0,70
Oberschenkel, Med.	0,49	0,19	0,16	0,28
Unterschenkel, Ext.	0,57	0,24	0,18	0,29
Unterschenkel, Flex.	0,16	0,14	0,08	0,25

Kleinste und größte Werte der zu einer Gruppe gehörenden Haarbalgmuskeln

Minimum	0,0004	0,00012	0,00006	0,0008
Maximum	0,0089	0,0117	0,0808	0,013

Tabelle 4c. *Meßwerte in μ der Haarkomplexe am Tragus Neugeborener* (OLIN)

Kind No.	Haarfollikel				Haar		Talgdrüse	
	Länge		Breite		Dicke		Größte Durchmesser	
	Min.	Max.	Min.	Max.	Min.	Max.	Min.	Max.
1	340	820	40	60	8	15	22×33	150×190
2	370	540	42	75	9	12	22×22	150×190
3	370	490	42	77	8	20	33×35	190×290
4	460	720	44	66	7	21	22×51	200×270
5	410	680	44	68	9	13	11×33	77×150
6	270	610	31	77	9	20	18×44	200×270
7	340	570	35	50	7	13	45×90	88×170
8	420	820	35	81	6	13	26×42	120×180
9	350	580	37	44	11	11	13×33	40×100
10	420	820	33	150	9	22	20×70	140×260
11	340	840	55	88	9	15	26×44	130×350
12	340	640	44	62	11	17	18×33	160×340
13	420	710	44	66	11	15	22×33	120×190
14	410	990	44	68	11	15	22×55	110×160
15	460	700	53	92	11	16	15×20	150×170
16	570	950	40	84	7	15	33×66	340×470
17	420	630	44	81	11	13	33×97	90×200
18	600	1010	44	70	9	18	24×110	230×420
19	460	910	40	92	11	19	29×35	170×340
20	480	820	37	40	11	13	35×110	140×350

V. Spezialisierte Drüsen

Es gibt einige Körperstellen, an denen sich Talgdrüsen und apokrine Drüsen ohne Zusammenhang mit Haaren entwickeln. Andere Stellen haben spezialisierte Drüsen.

1. Freie und spezialisierte Talgdrüsen

Die am höchsten entwickelte Form freier Talgdrüsen sind die hochspezialisierten Meibomschen Drüsen der Augenlieder. Es scheinen keine besonderen Untersuchungen über ihre Embryonalentwicklung vorzuliegen, doch ist es wohl nicht angängig, die Entwicklung eines so komplizierten Mikro-Organs, das in die Tarsi beider Lider hineinwächst, einfach auf Raumbeengung zurückzuführen (BLECH-SCHMIDT, 1950), besonders da Talgbildung ja eine biochemische Spezialfunktion darstellt, die nichts mit degenerativer Verfettung zu tun hat. Im übrigen sind die Orte mit freien Talgdrüsen im makroskopischen Abschnitt (Bd. I/2) besprochen und brauchen hier nicht behandelt zu werden, da die Drüsen sowieso meist erst nach der Geburt auftreten.

2. Mammaregion

Die primitivsten Milchdrüsen, die Mammardrüsen der Echidna, stehen in engem räumlichen und wohl auch genetischem Zusammenhang mit einem Haarfollikel. Die menschliche Brustdrüse dagegen (DABELOW, 1957) entwickelt sich als erst linsenförmiges, dann kugelig eingesenktes Gebilde aus Teilen der Milchleiste und hat wenig Ähnlichkeit mit dem sich entwickelnden Haarkomplex. Wenn aber die Primäranlage Sprossen treibt, bilden sich manche derselben nicht zu Milchgängen, sondern zu Haaranlagen, Talgdrüsen oder Schweißdrüsen aus (Abb. 26). Haar- und Schweißdrüsenanlagen bilden sich meist bald wieder zurück, aber freie Talgdrüsen sind recht häufig in der Mamille zu finden.

Die Drüsen der Areola, gewöhnlich Montgomerysche Drüsen genannt, wurden hauptsächlich von v. EGGELING (1904) untersucht und von F. PINKUS (1927) mit

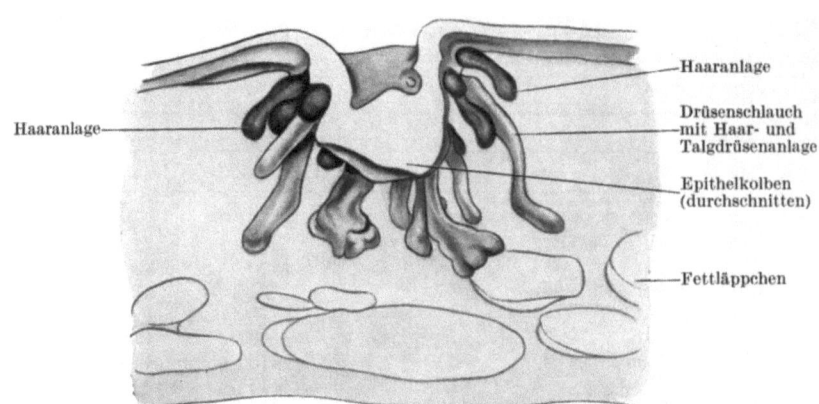

Abb. 26. Rekonstruktion der Milchdrüsenanlage eines weiblichen Fetus von 135 mm Länge nach SPULER (1930). Das Modell ist durchgeschnitten und man sieht den massiven zentralen Epithelkolben, von dem eine ganze Reihe Sprossen ausgehen. Diese sind teils Drüsenschläuche (hell), teils Haar- und Talgdrüsenanlagen (dunkel). (Aus DABELOW, 1957)

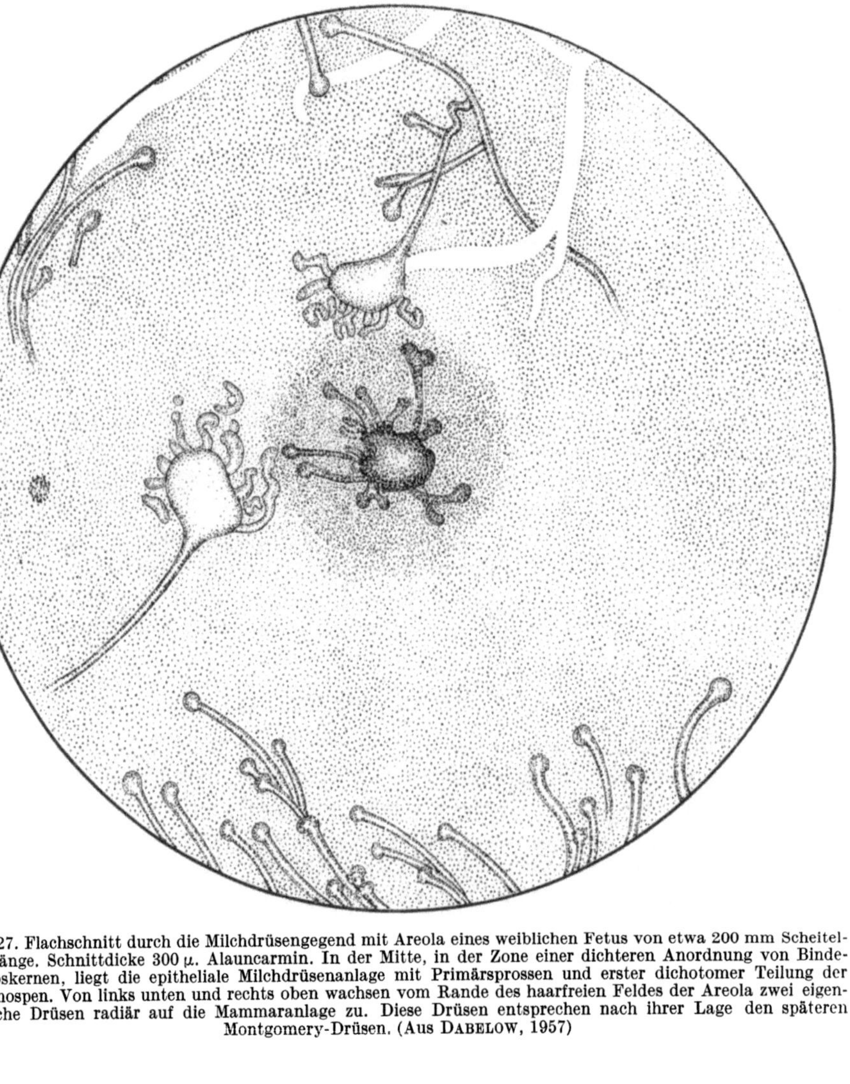

Abb. 27. Flachschnitt durch die Milchdrüsengegend mit Areola eines weiblichen Fetus von etwa 200 mm Scheitel-Steißlänge. Schnittdicke 300 μ. Alauncarmin. In der Mitte, in der Zone einer dichteren Anordnung von Bindegewebskernen, liegt die epitheliale Milchdrüsenanlage mit Primärsprossen und erster dichotomer Teilung der Endknospen. Von links unten und rechts oben wachsen vom Rande des haarfreien Feldes der Areola zwei eigentümliche Drüsen radiär auf die Mammaranlage zu. Diese Drüsen entsprechen nach ihrer Lage den späteren Montgomery-Drüsen. (Aus DABELOW, 1957)

einem eigenen Plattenmodell abgebildet. DABELOW beschreibt ihre Fetalentwicklung ausführlich nach eigenen Präparaten. Bei Embryonen von 180—200 mm SSL entwickeln sie sich am Rande des haarfreien Feldes, das die Milchdrüsenanlage umgibt (die spätere Areola). Die Mammaranlage zeigt um diese Zeit beginnende dichotome Teilung ihrer Primärsprossen. Die Montgomeryschen Drüsen wachsen radiär von der Peripherie auf die Mammaranlage zu. DABELOW vermutet, daß es sich dabei eher um chemotrope Reaktion als um eine morphologisch faßbare Führung handelt. Die Drüsen dieses Stadiums stellen meist einfache Schläuche dar, an deren blindem Ende eine Erweiterung sitzt, die offenbar durch Flüssigkeit gebläht ist. Aus einer Enderweiterung wachsen bis zu 10 sekundäre zylindrische Knospen aus, die sich gelegentlich noch einmal verzweigen. Die Drüsen sind tatsächlich länger und in ihrem Endkomplex größer als die Sprosse der Mamma selbst. Beim Neugeborenen (Abb. 27) liegen die Drüsen wie ein Kranz um das Bündel der Milchgänge in der Warzenzone herum. Auch dann sind sie noch im Verhältnis zu den Einzeldrüsen der Mamma recht groß.

Nach dieser Schilderung unterscheiden sich also die Montgomeryschen Drüsen erheblich von Beginn an, sowohl von der Milchdrüse wie von apokrinen oder ekkrinen Schweißdrüsen. Sie sind und bleiben auch später etwas Besonderes, scheinen jedoch, mindestens beim Neugeborenen, dem hormonalen Sekretionsimpuls zu folgen. Es ist auch Milchzucker in ihrem Sekret nachgewiesen worden (NAESLUND, 1957).

3. Gehörgang und Nasenvorhof

Die Haut des äußeren Gehörgangs enthält spezialisierte apokrine Drüsen, die Ceruminal- oder Ohrschmalzdrüsen. ZORZOLI (1948) erwähnt, daß sie beim Neugeborenen schon sezernieren. TAKEDA (1951), fußend auf der bekannten Differenz zwischen dem krümeligen hellen Cerumen der Orientalen und dem weichen bräunlichen Produkt der Europäer und Neger (s. Bd. I/2), untersuchte eingehend die Entwicklung der Drüsen bei Mischlingsfeten im Vergleich mit rein japanischen Früchten. Er fand keine sicheren Unterschiede in ihrer Verteilung und Form. Doch entwickelten sich die Kanäle bei Europäer-Japaner-Feten schon früher, im 6. Monat. Die Zahl der Drüsen war am größten bei Neger-Japaner-Mischlingen, am kleinsten bei reinen Japanern.

Mehr den gewöhnlichen apokrinen Drüsen ähnelnde Formen entwickeln sich nach ALVERDEZ (1934), MOGI (1938) und YANAGISAWA (1957) im 5. Monat im Vestibulum Nasi. ALVERDEZ zählte etwa 35 in jeder Seite und beschrieb helle und dunkle Zellen im sekretorischen Abschnitt.

E. Ekkrine Drüsen

1. Allgemeines

Die ekkrinen Drüsen entwickeln sich im Gegensatz zu den apokrinen direkt aus der Epidermis. An der behaarten Haut (Abb. 23) entstehen sie im 5.—7. Monat, erheblich später als die Haarfollikel. Obwohl sie in keinem direkten Zusammenhang mit diesen stehen, erwähnte schon F. PINKUS (1927), daß sie gewisse räumliche Beziehungen zu den Haaren haben, eine Anordnung, die von FLEISCHHAUER (1953) und HORSTMANN (1957) besonders betont wurde (Zifferblattmotiv).

An der haarlosen Haut der Hände und Füße sprossen ekkrine Drüsen schon im 4. Monat, nach FLEISCHHAUER und HORSTMANN (1951) von 13,5 cm Länge an, von den vorher angelegten epidermalen Drüsenleisten (cristae intermediae) aus, und die letztgenannten laufen vielfach in Verlängerung des Haarstrichs. Seit 1927 sind mehrere Untersuchungen mit den klassischen Methoden gemacht worden

(HORN, 1935; AURELL, 1938; UEDA, 1939; BORSETTO, 1951; TSUCHIYA, 1954), und manches Neue ist mit histochemischen und elektronenmikroskopischen Untersuchungen beigesteuert worden. Die meisten Autoren fanden sich in recht guter Übereinstimmung und eigene, nicht veröffentlichte Erfahrungen zeigten keine Abweichungen (Abb. 28). Nur BORSETTO meint, daß ekkrine und apokrine Drüsen näher verwandt sind und nimmt sogar an, daß sie sich ineinander verwandeln können. Die allerjüngste Anlage einer ekkrinen Drüse sieht dem Haarvorkeim zum Verwechseln ähnlich und besteht wie dieser aus einer dichten Sammlung von Basalzellen. Doch bilden sich schnell Unterschiede aus. Der Drüsenkeim ist auf einen kleinen Raum beschränkt, er wächst meist ziemlich senkrecht nach unten (Abb. 23) und läßt keine zweiseitige Symmetrie erkennen. Seine Form ist mehr

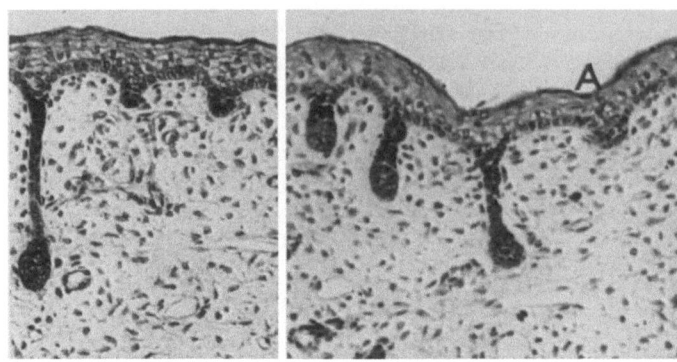

Abb. 28. Ekkrine Drüsen der Fußsohle in verschiedenen Entwicklungsstadien. *A* Anlage des Acrosyringiums. Hämatoxylin-Eosin, 180mal

flaschen- als kolbenförmig, mit einem sich stetig verlängernden dünnen Hals, dem Gang, an dem nur am Ende eine rundliche Auftreibung sitzt. Die mesodermale Kopfkappe des Haarfollikels, aus der sich später die Papille bildet, fehlt, und nur bei genauerer Untersuchung sieht man, daß auch die Drüsenanlage von einer dünnen mesodermalen Hülle umgeben ist. Die Anlagen verlängern sich durch mitotische Teilung ihrer Zellen schnell und dringen durch das nun meist schon recht gut entwickelte Corium bis ins subcutane Fettpolster vor, wo sie sich aufzurollen beginnen.

Gleichzeitig wächst der Gang auch nach außen durch die Epidermis hindurch und bildet, analog dem Haarkanal, das Acrosyringium (PINKUS et al., 1956), dessen Bau beim Erwachsenen 1939 von PINKUS beschrieben wurde, und das von LOBITZ et al. (1955) als selbständige biologische Einheit (epidermal eccrine sweat duct unit) bestätigt wurde.

Im Corium besteht der Gang von vornherein aus einer zweischichtigen Zellsäule, in der sich gegen Ende des 7. Monats ein Lumen entwickelt (Näheres unter Ultrastruktur, S. 665). Außen ist der Gang von einer PAS positiven Basalmembran und einer Hülle von feinen argyrophilen und kollagenen Fasern begleitet, die wohl von parallel angeordneten Bindegewebszellen stammen. Nach TSUCHIYA (1954) können die prospektiven Drüsenzellen schon im Stadium der linsenförmigen Anlage von den prospektiven Gangzellen unterschieden werden. Die ersteren bilden eine Kappe von größeren helleren Zellen. Im 7. Monat sind die später als „helle" und „dunkle" sekretorische Zellen benannten Elemente unterscheidbar, und die Myoepithelzellen zeigen Fibrillen. Sekretkörnchen treten in den Zellen im 6. bis 7. Monat auf und intercelluläre Saftkanälchen im 8. Monat. Nach BECKET et al. (1956) und MACHIDA (1964) ist das prospektive sekretorische Epithel des ekkrinen Knäuels von Anfang an von cholinesterasepositiven Nervenfasern eingehüllt.

2. Ultrastruktur

Elektronenoptisch konnten HASHIMOTO et al. (1965, 1966b) den ekkrinen Vorkeim schon bei 6—7 cm SSL Embryonen an der Fußsohle erkennen. Er bestand aus einer Anzahl dicht zusammenstehender hoher Basalzellen, die eine leichte Welle im Kontur der Drüsenleiste hervorriefen. Im Gehalt an Mitochondrien, Tonofilamenten und endoplasmatischem Reticulum glichen sie ganz den übrigen Zellen des Stratum germinativum. Glykogen war hauptsächlich in den intercellulären Spalten vorhanden (Abb. 5). Bei 8—10 cm langen Früchten waren die Drüsen schon tief in das Corium ausgewachsen, und die Anlage des intraepidermalen Gangteils war als eine Säule eigentümlicher Zellen zu erkennen. Jedes Acrosyringium bestand aus zwei konzentrischen Zellagen, von denen die innere ein Lumen dadurch entstehen ließ, daß sich intracelluläre Vacuolen bildeten (Abb. 29), die zusammenflossen und durch Ruptur der Zellmembranen extracellulär zu liegen kamen. Selbst in der Höhe des Stratum granulosum, wo auch die inneren Zellen der Ganganlage Keratohyalinkörner enthielten, kam die Lichtung auf dieselbe Weise zustande, d.h. durch Zusammenfließen mehrerer intracellulärer Vacuolen, die dann die Zellmembranen durchbrachen. Vergleiche ELLIS' Artikel in diesem Bande.

Im Gegensatz hierzu entstand die Lichtung des intradermalen Gangteils (Abb. 30) durch Auseinanderweichen der Zellen der inneren Lage, deren Desmosomen verschwanden. Ein besonders merkwürdiger Befund war das gelegentliche Auftreten von Cilien, einzeln oder in Paaren. Sie bestanden in typischer Weise aus einem Basalkörper, von dem 7—9 periphere Fibrillen ausgingen. Die Wimpern ragten ins Lumen vor. So merkwürdig dieser Befund ist, steht er nicht vereinzelt da. Es sind Cilien in verschiedenen, gewöhnlich nicht Wimpern tragenden tierischen Epithelien gesehen worden, und beim Menschen in normalen Basalzellen der Epidermis und im Basalzellenepitheliom (WILSON u. MCWHORTER, 1963).

Die lumenbegrenzenden Zellen enthielten auch reichlich Tonofilamente und besaßen Mikrovilli an der freien Oberfläche. Von 16 cm SSL an begann die Ausbildung von sekretorischen Zellen, und von 18 cm an waren myoepitheliale Zellen zu erkennen.

3. Histochemie

Der für ekkrine Drüsen beim Erwachsenen so charakteristische Gehalt an Glykogen ist nicht von Anfang an vorhanden. Sowohl nach eigenen Beobachtungen wie nach denen von GOTO et al. (1961) und SERRI et al. (1962) sind die ekkrinen Anlagen gewöhnlich frei von Glykogen, obwohl die zentralen Zellen kleine Mengen enthalten können. Nur MONTAGNA (1959) sagt, daß in der Axilla sowohl apokrine wie ekkrine fetale Drüsen stets Glykogen enthalten. Das enge Lumen der reiferen Drüsen enthält manchmal diastaseunverdauliches Polysaccharid, und zu dieser Zeit beginnen Knäuel und Gang auch mehr Glykogen aufzuweisen. Der intraepidermale Teil bleibt aber stets frei. YASUI u. KAGEMOTO (1961) und GOTO et al. (1961) berichten über granuläres diastaseresistentes Material in fetalen Drüsen der Axilla und der Volarhaut.

Nach SERRI et al. (1962) enthalten die ekkrinen Drüsen während ihrer ganzen Entwicklung reichlich Amylophosphorylase, mehr im Knäuel als im Gang. MACHIDA (1964) berichtet etwas größere Variabilität der Phosphorylasereaktion. Er betont, daß die myoepithelialen Zellen immer negativ sind, und findet meist stärkere Aktivität im Gangepithel als im Drüsenepithel.

SERRI et al. (1963) fanden die allerersten Primordia der ekkrinen Drüsen frei von alkalischer Phosphatase entsprechend der Basalschicht, in der sie sich entwickeln. Später enthält der zentrale Teil der ausgewachsenen Anlage Aktivität,

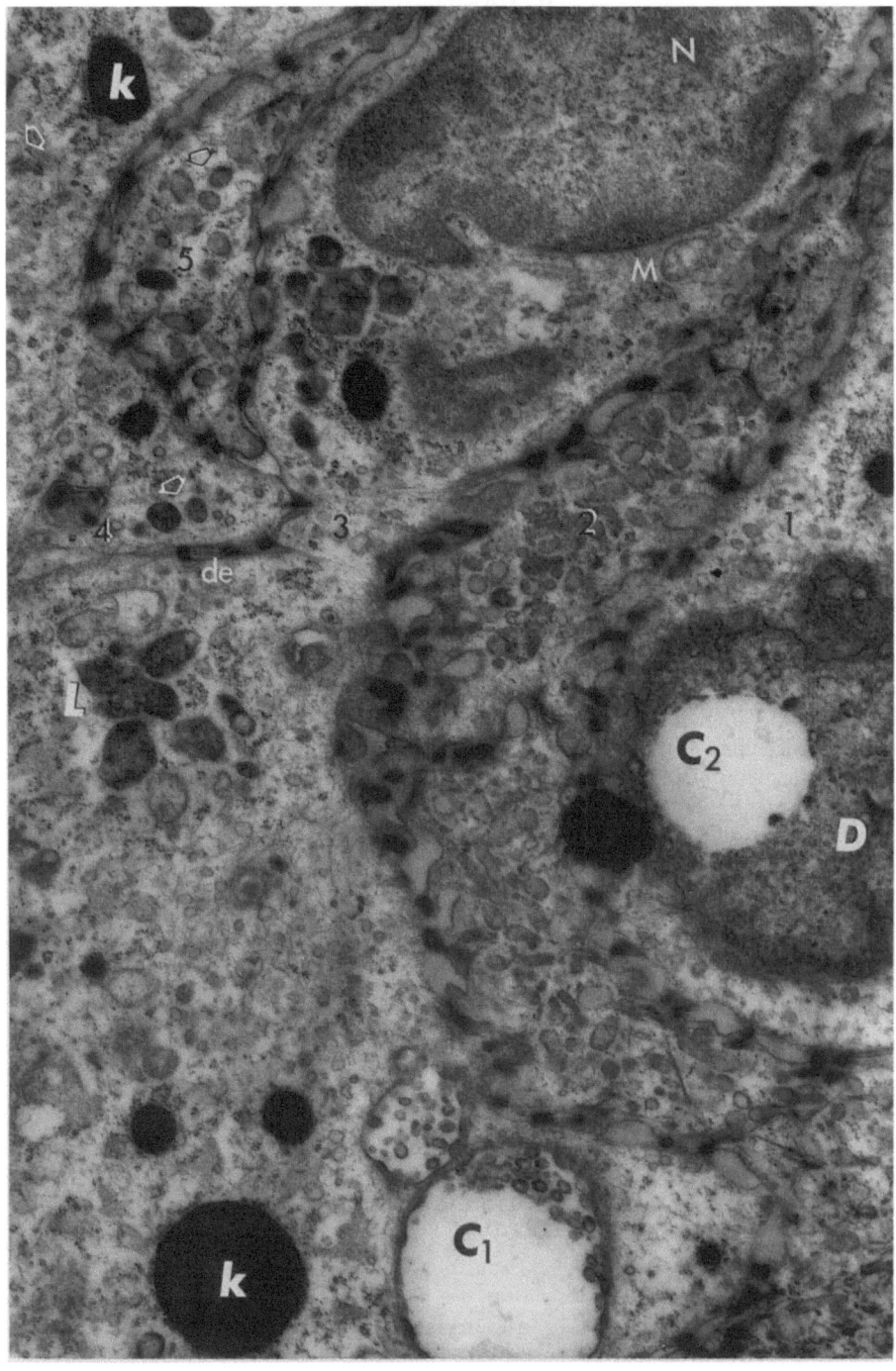

Abb. 29. Elektronenoptischer Flachschnitt durch mehrere Innenzellen (1—5) des Acrosyringiums von der Fußsohle eines Fetus von 115 mm Scheitel-Steißlänge in der Höhe der Keratohyalinschicht. Lumenbildung deutet sich in zwei intracellulären Höhlungen (C_1 und C_2) an, von denen C_1 ein ganz frühes Stadium darstellt und nur abgeschnürte Teilchen des Cytoplasmas enthält. C_2 enthält Zelltrümmer (D) und die Wand der Höhlung besitzt Mikrovilli. Die Zellen sind miteinander durch Desmosomen (de) verbunden und enthalten Mitochondrien (M), Lysosomen (L) und Keratohyalinkörnchen (K). N Kern der Zelle 3. Pfeile zeigen auf ganz junge Lysosomen.
Aufnahme freundlichst von Dr. KEN HASHIMOTO zur Verfügung gestellt. 20000mal

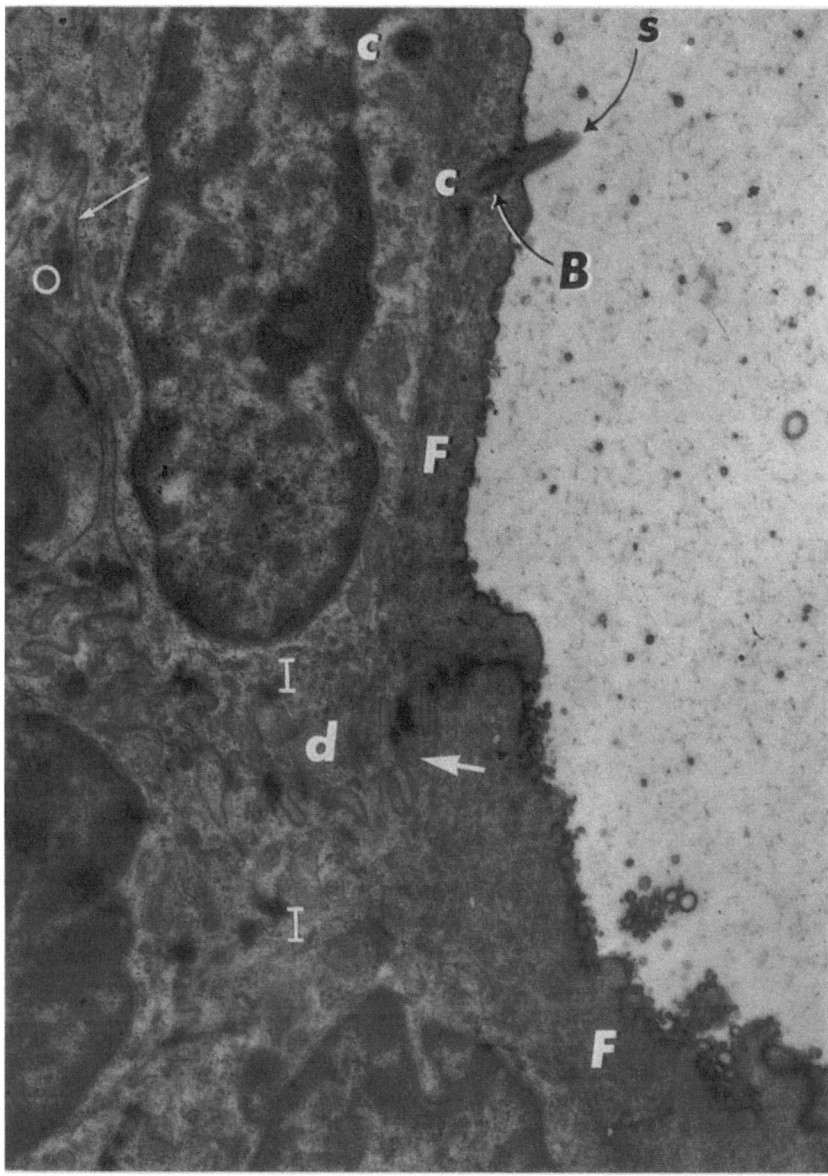

Abb. 30. Embryonaler ekkriner Gang im Corium. Innere Zellen (*I*) sind eng miteinander verhakt (dicker Pfeil) und durch gelegentliche Desmosomen (*d*) verbunden. Sie zeigen Mikrovilli und eine dichte filamentöse Zone (*F*) unter der Oberfläche. In der oberen Zelle sind 2 Cilien (*c*) zu sehen, die eine im Querschnitt, die andere im Längsschnitt. Die letztere zeigt einen dem Centriol entsprechenden Basalkörper (*B*), ihr Schaft (*S*) ragt ins Lumen vor. Die Grenze zwischen inneren und äußeren (*O*) Gangzellen ist verhältnismäßig glatt (dünner Pfeil). Aufnahme freundlichst von Dr. KEN HASHIMOTO zur Verfügung gestellt. 14 500mal

was auch MACHIDAs Befunden entspricht. Noch später verschwindet das Enzym außer im sekretorischen Epithel einiger Körperteile, von denen MACHIDA die Perianalregion, SERRI et al. die Volarhaut erwähnen. Dagegen berichten GOTO et al. (1961) von Beginn an über viel stärkere Reaktionen in den Drüsen der Volarhaut. Nach MACHIDA findet sich wenig oder gar keine saure Phosphatase, nur etwas mehr im Gang gerade unter der Epidermis. Dagegen berichten SERRI et al. (1962) über mäßig starke Reaktivität in allen Teilen der Drüse.

MONTAGNA (1959) erwähnt schwache Esterasenaktivität in den ekkrinen Drüsen der Axilla. MACHIDA (1964) fand ein wechselndes Bild, je nachdem ob GOMORIs Technik für α-Naphthol-Esterase oder PEARSEs Methode für Naphthol-AS-Esterase benutzt wurde. Die letztere war schwach positiv im 4. Monat und wurde stärker in den Drüsenepithelien der Volarhaut, aber nicht an anderen Körperstellen. α-Naphthol-Esterase wurde erst im 6. Monat stärker positiv, und zwar nach dem 7. Monat am ganzen Körper, obwohl die Drüsen der Volarhaut immer am meisten reagierten. Die Myoepithelien waren negativ.

MACHIDAs Untersuchungen über Bernsteinsäure-dehydrogenase, Cytochromoxydase und Monoaminoxydase zeigten diese schwach positiv in den frühen Anlagen. Die Aktivität stieg allmählich an, besonders in den apikalen Teilen der Primordia, nur die Monoaminoxydase zeigte eine temporäre Schwächung im 6. und 7. Monat. Alle drei Enzyme reagierten sehr kräftig in den sezernierenden Teilen der reiferen Drüsen, besonders denen der Volarhaut. Nach demselben Autor ist die Reaktion auf Leucinaminopeptidase kräftig im Apex der volaren Schweißdrüsenprimordien des 4. Monats. Später bleibt die Aktivität auf den Drüsenteil beschränkt während der Gang schwach reagiert. Die sekretorischen Teile der übrigen Körperhaut werden erst nach dem 7. Monat stärker reaktiv.

KAGA et al. (1961) benutzten Bromphenolblau zur Darstellung von Protein und mehrere Methoden zur unterschiedlichen Färbung von DNS und RNS. Alle Reaktionen erwiesen sich als stark positiv, wie zu erwarten war.

4. Quantitative Daten und Drüsen des Neugeborenen

OKAJIMAs Schüler haben auch über die Schweißdrüsenentwicklung viele sorgfältige Untersuchungen gemacht und sie zahlenmäßig belegt. Einige dieser Daten sind in Tabelle 5a und b zusammengestellt.

Tabelle 5a. *Ekkrine Drüsen*

Körpergegend	Volumen in mm³ pro cm² bei einem			
	8monatigen Fetus (KOSAKA)	9monatigen Zwilling 1 (MOCHIZUKI)	9monatigen Zwilling 2 (MOCHIZUKI)	Neugeborenen (TANIGUCHI)
Kopf	1,7	1,9	2,4	3,7
Gesäß	1,5	2,5	2,9	5,2
Rücken	1,5	2,6	3,1	4,9
Brust	1,2	3,3	3,4	3,5
Bauch	0,7	2,1	2,4	2,7
Oberarm, Extensor	1,3	4,4	3,6	7,6
Oberarm, Flexor	1,0	4,5	3,8	6,2
Vorderarm, Extensor	1,1	4,4	4,6	7,1
Vorderarm, Flexor	1,3	3,5	2,4	8,0
Oberschenkel, Lat.	1,3	3,8	3,7	8,6
Oberschenkel, Med.	1,3	4,0	4,8	5,0
Unterschenkel, Ext.	1,4	5,2	4,2	5,9
Unterschenkel, Flex.	1,8	4,2	3,9	8,9
Einzeldrüse, Min.	0,0004	0,0012	0,0015	0,0026
Einzeldrüse, Max.	0,0015	0,0032	0,0034	0,0046

Augenbraue nach BYON	5 Monate	6 Monate	7 Monate	8 Monate	9 Monate	10 Monate
mm³ pro cm² Oberfläche	2,20	1,72	0,65	0,59	1,03	2,20
Einzeldrüse, Durchschnitt	0,0016	0,0004	0,0006	0,0006	0,0007	0,0035

Tabelle 5b. *Ekkrine Drüsen, Durchschnittswerte individueller Drüsen in mm³*

Körpergegend	7 Monate (Morita)	8 Monate (Morita)	8 Monate (Kosuka)	9 Monate (Morita)
Kopf, behaart	0,0015	0,0016	0,0012	0,0016
Stirn	0,0014	0,0015	0,0015	0,0015
Brust	0,0008	0,0008	0,0007	0,0009
Bauch	0,0007	0,0007	0,0007	0,0008
Rücken	0,0005	0,0006	0,0005	0,0007
Oberschenkel, Med.	0,0005	0,0006	0,0005	0,0006
Unterschenkel, Ext.	0,0005	0,0005	0,0005	0,0006
Oberarm, Flexor	0,0005	0,0005	0,0004	0,0006
Vorderarm, Ext.	0,0007	0,0007	0,0006	0,0007

Körpergegend	9 Monate 1 (Mochizuki)	9 Monate 2 (Mochizuki)	10 Monate (Morita)	Neugeboren (Taniguchi)
Kopf, behaart	0,0026	0,0025	0,0017	0,0034
Stirn	0,0012	0,0015	0,0017	0,0032
Brust	0,0032	0,0030	0,0010	0,0034
Bauch	0,0017	0,0028	0,0009	0,0027
Rücken	0,0021	0,0024	0,0010	0,0035
Oberschenkel, Med.	0,0024	0,0025	0,0007	0,0027
Unterschenkel, Ext.	0,0026	0,0024	0,0007	0,0028
Oberarm, Flexor	0,0030	0,0023	0,0007	0,0032
Vorderarm, Ext.	0,0028	0,0024	0,0009	0,0039
Handteller (Kuriki)	bei 10 Zwillingspaaren im Alter von 5—9 Monaten (fetal) variierte das Volumen pro cm² Hautoberfläche von 3,8—7,4 mm³, das Volumen der Einzeldrüse von 0,0004—0,0019 mm³			
Fußsohle (Kuriki)	bei denselben Zwillingspaaren waren die entsprechenden Werte: 2,2—7,9 mm³ und 0,0002—0,0015 mm³			

Ellis (1958) erwähnt, daß die ekkrinen Knäuel des Kopfes beim Neugeborenen genau in der Ebene des hypodermalen Gefäßplexus liegen und ihre Capillaren von ihm beziehen. Zeleznikow (1957) konstatiert, daß der Durchmesser des Ausführungsgangs bei der Geburt 23,7—38,2 μ beträgt. Die Zellkerne messen von 5,5 × 4,5 μ bis 6,4 × 5,5 μ. Die Drüsen sind bei der Geburt voll funktionsfähig, aber ihre durchschnittliche Größe nimmt noch erheblich zu.

F. Der Nagel

1. Allgemeines

Obwohl die Entwicklung des Nagels seit über 100 Jahren wiederholt bearbeitet worden ist, hat sie auch in neuester Zeit wieder die Aufmerksamkeit mehrerer Forscher auf sich gelenkt. Wir werden uns hier auf die Arbeiten von Lewis (1954), Fleischhauer u. Horstmann (1955), Eberl-Rothe u. Langegger (1957), Achten (1963) und Zaias (1963) stützen, sowie die histochemischen Angaben von Serri et al. (1962). Alkiewicz (1951) beschrieb als allererstes Zeichen der Nagelanlage eine nur mikroskopisch sichtbare Epithelverdickung an der Grenze zwischen ventraler und dorsaler Haut der Fingerspitze bei einem 7 Wochen alten Embryo. Später liegt die Nagelanlage dorsal, und die sie distal begrenzende Furche scheidet dorsale und ventrale Teile des Fingers. Lewis beschrieb die Embryologie des Nagels sehr ausführlich, doch ist es leichter, die neueste Darstellung von ZAIAS (1963) für unsere Zwecke zu benutzen.

Bei einem 9 Wochen alten (2,75 cm SSL) Embryo war äußerlich nichts von einer Nagelanlage zu sehen. Ein Längsschnitt des Daumens zeigte gedrängtere Stellung der Basalzellen in der allgemein zweischichtigen Epidermis der Dorsalfläche nahe dem Fingerende (Abb. 31). Mit 10 Wochen (4.5 cm) sieht man schon ein glattes, glänzendes, rechteckiges Feld, das durch kontinuierliche flache Gräben

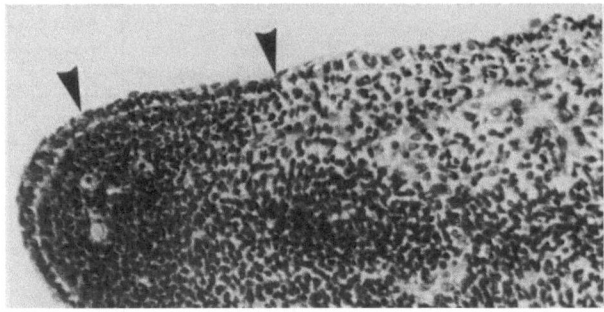

Abb. 31. Daumenende eines Embryo von 27,5 mm Scheitel-Steißlänge mit zweischichtigem Epithel. Nagelanlage (zwischen Pfeilen) an der gedrängten Stellung der Basalzellen erkennbar. Hämatoxylin und Biebrich-Scharlach, 210mal. (Aus ZAIAS, 1963)

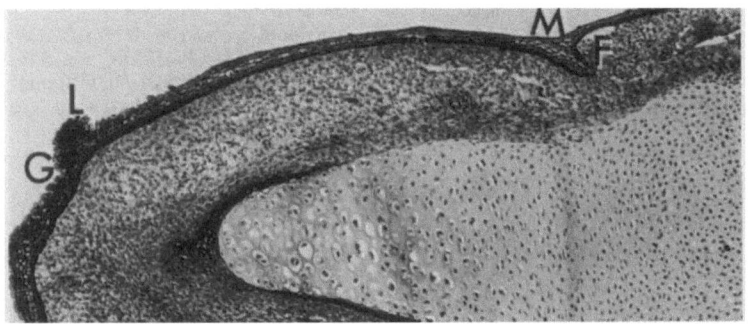

Abb. 32. Daumenende eines Fetus von 52,5 mm Scheitel-Steißlänge. Die proximale Matrix (M) beginnt schräg rückwärts ins Mesenchym einzuwachsen, wodurch die Anlage der proximalen Nagelfalte (F) geschaffen wird. Das Epithel des Nagelfeldes ist mehrschichtig und verdickt sich zur distalen Leiste (L), die von der distalen Grenzfurche (G) abgesetzt ist. Hämatoxylin und Biebrich-Scharlach, 80mal. (Aus ZAIAS, 1963)

abgegrenzt ist, das primäre Nagelfeld. Histologisch hat die Epidermis jetzt ein Stratum intermedium, und die Anlage der Nagelmatrix beginnt sich als solide Platte proximalwärts unter den dadurch entstehenden proximalen Nagelwall zu schieben. In diesem Stadium beginnt auch die knorpelige Phalanx sich abzusetzen. Mit 11 Wochen (5,25 cm) sind die Finger schon gut geformt, Phalangen und Gelenke sind erkennbar, und der Tastballen hat sich ausgebildet. Das primäre Nagelfeld mit seinen begrenzenden Furchen ist gut erkennbar. Histologisch (Abb. 32) zeigt sich eine erhebliche Verdickung des Stratum intermedium, gerade proximal zu der distalen Grenzfurche. Es besteht hier aus 6—8 Schichten. Dies ist die Anlage der distalen Leiste, die von LEWIS (1954) mit dem unglücklich gewählten Namen „dorsal plume" belegt und als pilzförmig beschrieben wurde. Pleureusen- oder schirmartig ist das Gebilde natürlich nur im histologischen Sagittalschnitt. Räumlich gesehen ist es eher einer T-Schiene vergleichbar. Ein weiteres, sehr unglückliches Mißverständnis ergibt sich daraus, daß LEWIS das Sohlenhorn, das tatsächlich später an dieser Stelle entsteht, mit „hyponychium" übersetzte, und daß diese Bezeichnung von SERRI et al. (1962) und ZAIAS (1963) angenommen wurde. In der deutschen Literatur, z.B. bei HORSTMANN (1957), bedeutet Hyponychium das Nagelbett, für das die Amerikaner „nail bed" benutzen. So erklärt sich HORSTMANNs Bemerkung, daß LEWIS der Ansicht sei, die distale Leiste entspräche dem Hyponychium und nicht dem Sohlenhorn. Es ist zu hoffen, daß diese Verwechslung wieder ausgemerzt werden kann, vielleicht dadurch, daß man dies Gebiet mit dem auch gebräuchlichen Ausdruck „terminale Matrix" bezeichnet, „Hyponychium" vergißt, und Nagelbett bzw. „nailbed" für die zwischen proximaler und terminaler Matrix liegende Epidermis benutzt.

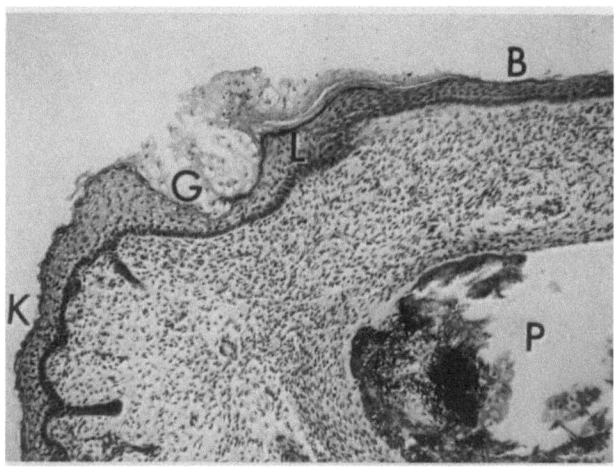

Abb. 33. Gegend der terminalen Matrix im Sagittalschnitt bei einem etwas älteren Fetus. Epithel der Fingerkuppe (K) und des Nagelbettes (B) noch von Periderm bedeckt. Die distale Leiste (L) setzt sich scharf durch ihr Stratum granulosum vom Nagelbett und der distalen Grenzfurche (G) ab. Die der distalen Leiste aufsitzenden kernhaltigen Zellen entsprechen den Resten von LEWIS' „dorsal plume". Weitere Einzelheiten im Text. P verknöchernde Phalanx. Hämatoxylin und Eosin, 280mal

Die distale Leiste, der Vorläufer der terminalen Matrix, ist jedenfalls die erste Stelle der Nagelgegend, die verhornt, und zwar unter Bildung von Keratohyalin (Abb. 33). Die Platte der proximalen Matrixanlage, bestehend aus mehreren Schichten von Stratum intermedium zwischen zwei Basallagen, schiebt sich inzwischen weiter nach hinten und erreicht schließlich beinahe das interphalangeale Gelenk, mit dem das die Platte umgebende verdickte Mesenchym und seine Blutgefäße in Verbindung treten.

Schließlich, bei Feten von 13 Wochen (8 cm SSL), wenn auch das Nagelbett schon Stratum spinosum und granulosum mit Verhornung aufweist, beginnt am distalen Ende der proximalen Matrix die erste Nagelbildung. Es bildet sich ein der Parakeratose ähnlicher Prozeß aus, bei dem die suprabasalen Zellen gebläht werden, ihre Kerne behalten und schließlich flach werden. Sie zeigen eine positive Reaktion für Sulfhydrylgruppen. Der Nagelbildungsprozeß erstreckt sich allmählich proximal in die hintere Nageltasche, das Matrixprimordium wird zur Matrix. Die hier gebildeten Nagelzellen werden aus dem Blindsack der Nageltasche einfach dadurch herausgedrängt, daß sie viel mehr Fläche einnehmen als die Basalzellen der Matrix (s. Bd I/2). Wenn die sich nach vorne schiebende Nagelplatte die distale Leiste erreicht, die inzwischen breiter und flacher geworden ist, schert sie

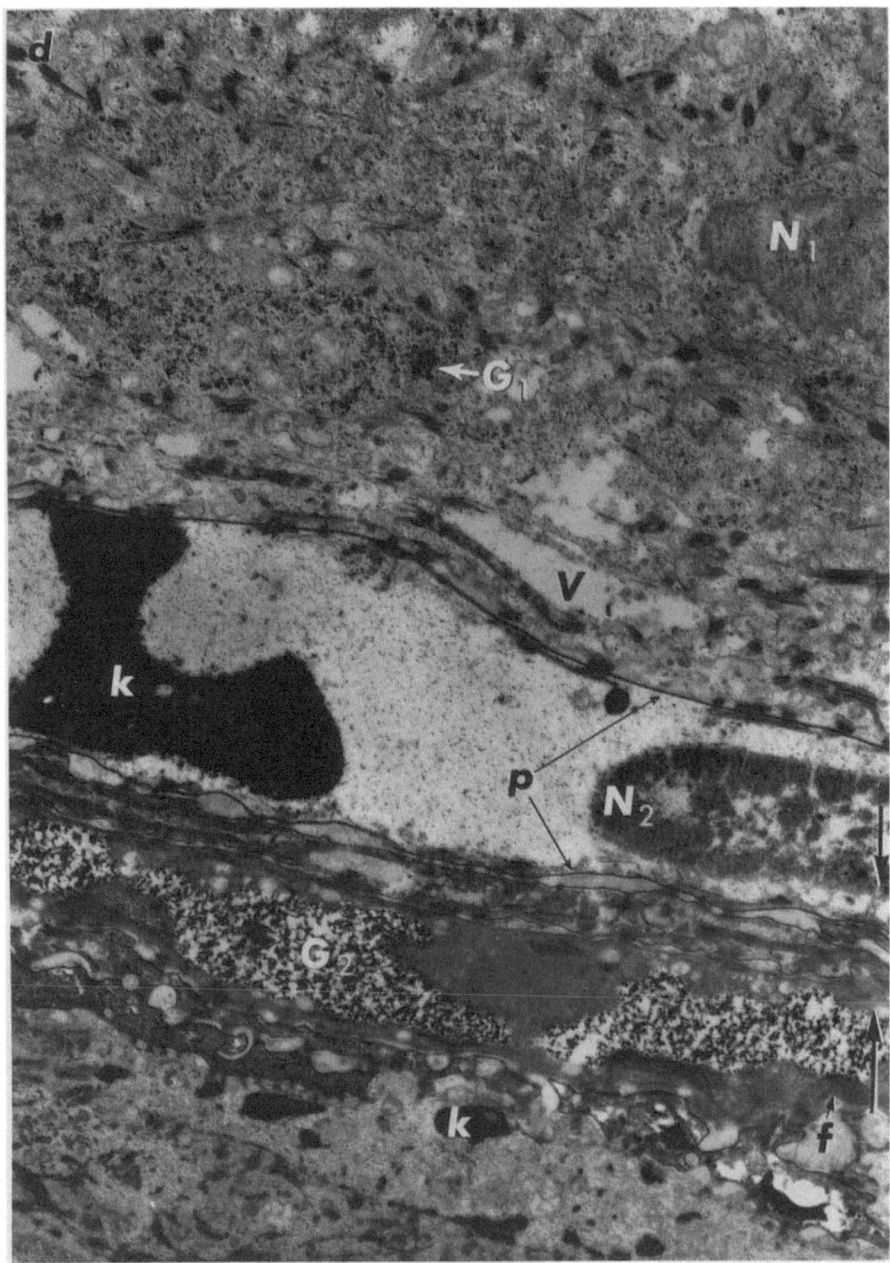

Abb. 34. Zentrum des proximalen Matrixprimordiums bei einem Fetus von 110 mm Scheitel-Steißlänge im Sagittalschnitt. N_1 und N_2 sind Kerne von Zellen des dorsalen Teils der Matrix. Zelle 1 enthält Glykogen (G_1) und Vacuolen (V). Zelle 2 enthält Keratohyalin (K) und hat eine verdickte Plasmamembran (p). Darunter liegen flache Hornzellen der Nagelplatte und am unteren Rand des Bildes Zellen des ventralen Matrixteiles, die Keratohyalin (K), Hornfilamente (f) und Glykogen (G_2) enthalten. Die Pfeile rechts unten zeigen die Richtung der Verhornung an. 8500mal. Abbildung freundlichst von Dr. KEN HASHIMOTO zur Verfügung gestellt

nach ZAIAS die hochragende Hornschicht ab und begräbt die lebende Epidermis unter sich, die nun zur terminalen Matrix wird. Damit ist die endgültige Form des Nagels beim Neugeborenen erreicht.

2. Histochemie

Die verschiedenen Teile der Nagelanlage behalten für geraume Zeit das Glykogen, das auch sonst in der fetalen Epidermis vorhanden ist. EBERL-ROTHE u. LANGEGGER (1957) machen darauf aufmerksam, daß in der terminalen Matrix sogar Zellen, die schon Keratohyalin enthalten, auch Glykogen haben, während dies im allgemeinen aus verhornenden Zellen verschwindet. Später enthält nach SERRI et al. (1962) das Epithel des Nagelbetts verhältnismäßig wenig Glykogen. Die Basalzellen sind, wie auch sonst in der Epidermis, regelmäßig frei. Phosphorylase ist von Anfang an im Matrixprimordium und den umgebenden Teilen vorhanden, und die Reaktion kann so stark werden, daß sie alle Einzelheiten verdeckt (SERRI et al., 1962). Alkalische Phosphatase erscheint nach EBERL-ROTHE und LANGEGGER (1957) für kurze Zeit während der größten Aktivität der Nagelentwicklung.

ZAIAS (1963) fand, daß sich die frühesten verhornenden Zellen der Nagelplatte von der Hornschicht der umgebenden Teile durch ihre positive Sulfhydrylreaktion unterscheiden. Die ausgebildete Platte des fetalen Nagels bleibt reich an Sulfhydrylgruppen, während die Disulfidreaktion nur mäßig positiv ist.

3. Ultrastruktur

HASHIMOTO et al. (1966a) untersuchten Fingerspitzen von drei 15 cm SSL Feten und bestätigten im allgemeinen die oben beschriebenen Befunde. Die höhere Resolution des Elektronenmikroskops zeigte aber, daß die Matrixzellen doch Keratohyalin bilden (Abb. 34). Im proximalen Teil der Matrix wird Nagelsubstanz von den dorsalen und ventralen Zellen des Primordiums geliefert. Einige Zellen degenerieren hier auch, und das sind nach HASHIMOTO u. GROSS (1964) die von ZAIAS und LEWIS beschriebenen geblähten Zellen.

G. Nerven und andere Neuralleisten-Abkömmlinge

1. Frühstadium

Eine kurze klare Übersicht der Frühentwicklung des Nervensystems in seiner Beziehung zur Haut wurde von TÖNDURY (1963) gegeben. Das Nervenrohr ist niemals segmentiert. Auch die Neuralleiste (Ganglienleiste) wird erst sekundär durch ihre Beziehungen zu den Ursegmenten in kleine Zellhaufen zerlegt, die sich zu Spinalganglien weiter entwickeln. Die Neuroblasten der Ganglien liefern den afferenten Teil des peripheren Nervensystems, indem sie zentrale Fortsätze in das Rückenmark und periphere Fortsätze in die Haut entsenden. Diese vereinigen sich mit den aus dem Rückenmark vorwachsenden motorischen Neuriten zum Spinalnerven. Der Nervus spinalis teilt sich nach kurzem Verlauf in dorsale und ventrale Äste, die das Rückengebiet bzw. die laterale und ventrale Rumpfwand versorgen. Der Innervationsbereich eines segmentalen Nerven ist daher das Kriterium der Zugehörigkeit eines Gewebsteiles zu einem bestimmten *Segment*. Das von einem Nerven versorgte Hautgebiet wird in übertragenem Sinne als *Dermatom* bezeichnet (s. Bd I/2, S. 30—31). Ein Dermatom im ursprünglichen Sinne ist die Cutislamelle eines Urwirbels (s. S. 637).

Die Kopfganglienleiste ist nie im Sinne der Rumpfleiste segmentiert, sondern wird durch das Ohrbläschen in einen cranialen und caudalen Teil zerlegt. Aus dem caudalen Teil entstehen die Ganglien der Nn. facialis, glossopharyngeus und vagus, der craniale Teil liefert Material für das Ganglion semilunare des Nervus trigeminus. Experimentelle Untersuchungen an Amphibien, Vögeln und Säugern haben gelehrt, daß die Neuralleiste noch viele andere Gewebe und Zellen liefert (HÖRSTADIUS, 1950). Von ihr stammen u. a. alle Schwann-Zellen (CAUSEY, 1960), zum Teil die Zellen des truncus sympathicus und alle Melanocyten und Langerhansschen Zellen (s. auch STARCKs Lehrbuch der Embryologie, 1965).

Da die Verteilung der Nerven in der Haut und die Struktur der Nervenendigungen an anderer Stelle dieses Bandes behandelt werden, und die Entwicklung der Pigmentzellen von STARCK in Bd I/2 vor wenigen Jahren dargestellt wurde, soll hier nur kurz auf einige Arbeiten über Entwicklung der Nerven in der Volarhaut und auf neueste Forschungen bezüglich der Melanocyten eingegangen werden. Es sei hier auch auf WINKELMANNs (1960) Monographie verwiesen, die kurze Bemerkungen über die Entwicklung der verschiedenen Nervenendigungen enthält.

2. Nerven der Finger- und Zehenbeeren

Für die Untersuchung der Nervenentwicklung in der Haut scheint die Methylenblaumethode den Silberfärbungen überlegen zu sein, weil sie einerseits Gebrauch lebensfrischen Materials gewährleistet und andererseits mit dickeren Schnitten arbeiten kann, die besser räumliche Beziehungen erkennen lassen. Der Nachteil der dünnen Schnitte bei den Silberimprägnationen ist erst von WINKELMANN (1960) teilweise überwunden worden. Ganz kürzlich haben SERRI et al. (1966) WINKELMANNs Methode mit der Cholinesterasereaktion kombiniert. Mit der Methylenblaumethode liegen zwei sich ergänzende Arbeiten von SZYMONOWICZ (1933) und JALOWY (1939) vor, aus denen wir folgendes entnehmen.

Am Ende des 3. Monats sind in den Finger- und Zehenbeeren noch keine Terminalformen darzustellen. Dünne, aus mehreren marklosen Fasern bestehende Nervenstämme beginnen sich in der Nähe der schwach ausgeprägten Epithelleisten zu verästeln. Gewöhnlich zieht ein dichotomisch sich teilender Nervenstamm zu den Bindegewebsleisten zu beiden Seiten einer Epithelleiste (Prospektive Drüsenleiste). Hier und da treten einzelne Nervenfäserchen ins Epithel über.

Gegen Ende des 4. Monats, wenn die ersten Schweißdrüsenanlagen in den Drüsenleisten sichtbar werden, und die cristae limitantes sich andeuten, ziehen reich verzweigte Nervenstämme zur Epidermis und senden Nervenfasern ins Epithel nahe dem Gipfel der bindegewebigen Leiste (Abb. 35). Diese verzweigen sich baumartig zwischen den Epithelzellen und zeigen oft rosenkranzförmige varicöse Auftreibungen und an ihren Enden kleine Verdickungen. Diese frei endigenden Fasern scheinen gleich im 4. Monat ihre höchste Ausbildung zu erfahren und halten später mit der Flächenvergrößerung der Epidermis nicht Schritt. Sowohl SZYMONOWICZ wie JALOWY geben an, daß die Zehenhaut gegenüber der Fingerhaut zeitlich im Rückstand ist.

Gleichzeitig mit der Entwicklung der freien Endigungen dringen andere Nervenfasern von vielen Seiten in die unteren Partien der Cristae intermediae ein. An diesen Stellen sind zentral zu den Basalzellen Zellen erkennbar, die größer, heller, stark lichtbrechend und kugelig sind. Dies sind die Merkelschen Tastzellen, die kleine Nester bilden und an die sich die Nervenfasern mit meniscusartigen Verbreiterungen (hederiforme Endigungen) anlegen. SZYMONOWICZ legt besonderen Wert auf die Feststellung, daß die hellen Zellen sich aus suprabasalen Epithelzellen entwickeln, und daß gewöhnlich ein Merkelsches Körperchen im tiefsten Teil der Leiste zwischen den Anlagen zweier Schweißdrüsengänge liegt. Es ist dies interessant, weil neue Befunde gezeigt haben, daß Melanocyten normalerweise vorwiegend die Cristae intermediae bevölkern (KAWAMURA et al., 1956; KITAMURA, 1963). Es taucht die Frage nach einer möglichen Beziehung zwischen diesen Abkömmlingen der Neuralleiste und den von SZYMONOWICZ beschriebenen Elementen auf. Jedoch hat HAYASHI, der 1964a eine eingehende Studie der Entwicklung der Melanocyten bei japanischen Feten nach modernen Gesichtspunkten veröffentlichte, die älteren Befunde insofern bestätigt, als er mit supravitaler Methylenblaufärbung im 7. Monat helle rund-ovale Zellen in der von SZYMONOWICZ beschriebenen Lokalisation nachweisen konnte. Einige Nervenfasern enden an diesen Zellen mit scheibenartigen Verbreiterungen, während andere höher in der Epidermis frei enden. HAYASHI (1964b) betont, daß diese Zellen nicht Melanocyten sind. Er glaubt, sie könnten Schwann-Zellen sein. Bei 9monatigen Feten sind sowohl sie wie intraepidermale Nervenfasern in der Zahl verringert.

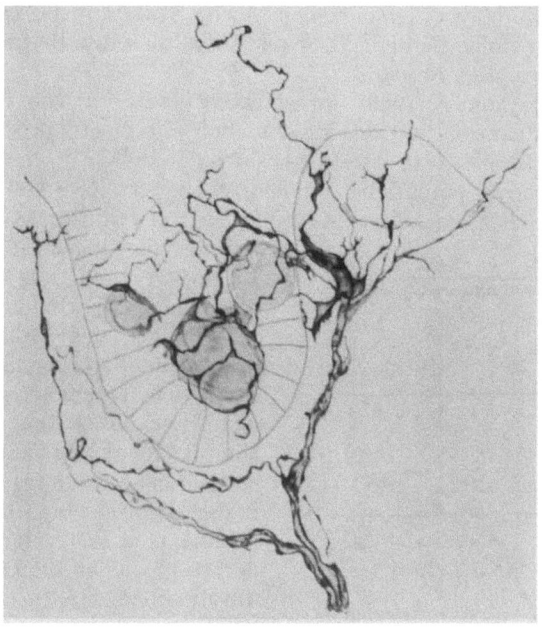

Abb. 35. Von einem senkrechten Schnitt durch die Fingerbeere eines menschlichen Fetus vom Ende des 4. Monats. Von der rechten Seite gelangt in den Unterteil der Epidermisleiste eine Nervenfaser, welche zerfällt und eine Gruppe von Zellen umflicht. Diese Zelle gibt dem Merkelschen Körperchen den Ursprung. Von außen bilden andere undifferenzierte Epithelzellen die Bedeckung. Andere Nervenfasern gehen in freie intraepitheliale Fasern über. Methylenblau, Vergrößerung etwa 1100mal. (Aus SZYMONOWICZ, 1933)

JALOWY sah schon im 4. Monat Nervenfasern in den obersten Partien mancher Bindegewebsleisten pinselartige Verzweigungen bilden, die er als die ersten Anlagen der Meissnerschen Körperchen auffaßt. Gleichzeitig entstehen nach ihm tiefer im Gewebe die ersten Anlagen der Vater-Pacinischen Körperchen. Diese Ansicht wird von TORSUEV (1940) mit Silberimprägnationen und von SERRI (1963) mit der Cholinesterasereaktion unterstützt. Nach SZYMONOWICZ dringen erst im 6. Monat, wenn die Bindegewebsleisten schon Papillen entwickeln, neue Nervenfasern in diese ein und bilden den Anfang der Meissnerschen Körperchen. Da die endgültige Ausbildung der geformten Endkörper erst in der postnatalen Periode beendet wird, werden wir sie hier nicht weiter besprechen (vgl. PÉREZ, 1931; PÉREZ u. PÉREZ, 1933; RACHMATULLIN, 1936; CAUNA, 1953; WINKELMANN, 1956; PAWLOWSKI, 1963; SERRI et al., 1966).

Nach SUGA (1951), der die Satosche Silbermethode benutzte, verbreiten sich sensorische Nerven in der behaarten Haut vom 6. Monat an hauptsächlich um die Haarzapfen, während das Stratum papillare erst im 10. Monat reichlicher versorgt erscheint. Im Lippenrot finden sich einfache und verzweigte Nervenendigungen schon im 6. Monat in den Papillen und auch im Epithel. In der letztgenannten Lage sind sie im 10. Monat fast wieder verschwunden.

Histochemisch scheint allgemeine Übereinstimmung zu herrschen, daß die Cholinesterasereaktion ein ausgezeichnetes Mittel ist, embryonale Nerven aller Arten darzustellen (BECKETT et al., 1956; SERRI, 1963; MACHIDA, 1964; SERRI et al., 1966), und daß sowohl die Acetyl- wie die Butyrylreaktion positive Ergebnisse liefert.

3. Melanocyten und Langerhanssche Zellen

Die Entwicklung der Pigmentzellen ist von STARCK in Bd I/2 dargestellt, und es sollen hier nur einige Befunde, die nach Abschluß seines Beitrages veröffentlicht wurden, berücksichtigt werden.

MISHIMA u. WIDLAN (1966) untersuchten eine Serie von japanischen Feten mit der Dopa-Reaktion und der Massonschen Silbermethode, die nach MISHIMA (1964) die strukturelle Basis des Melanosoms darstellt (,,Prämelanin'') und daher auch Dopa-negative potentielle Pigmentzellen aufzeigt (Abb. 36, 37). Sie beschreiben eine schon von ZIMMERMANN (1954) erwähnte zunächst diffuse Verteilung von jungen Melanocyten in allen Lagen der Epidermis und der sich entwickelnden Haarfollikel. Erst wenn ein Haarfollikel das Bulbuszapfenstadium durchlaufen hat, lokalisieren die Melanocyten sich in mehr typischer Weise. Auch das Alter des Fetus spielt eine Rolle. Vom 6. Monat an zeigt die Epidermis die endgültige Anordnung von Melanocyten in der Basalschicht. Im Haarfollikel sind Melanocyten wie beim Erwachsenen in der Basalschicht des Infundibulums und um die obere Hälfte der Papille herum lokalisiert. Weiterhin gibt es aber auch Melanosomen-haltige Zellen im Bulbusepithel unterhalb des kritischen Niveaus (s. auch unter D.I/2, S. 652).

HASHIMOTO et al. (1966) erwähnen in ihrer elektronenmikroskopischen Untersuchung der Epidermis, daß sie bei dem jüngsten ihrer Embryonen (120 mm SSL) Melanocyten in der Dermis entlang den

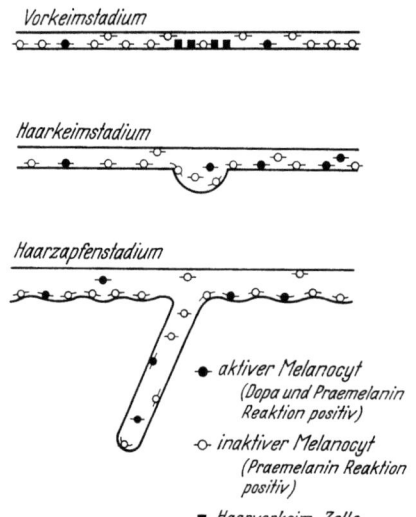

Abb. 36. Verteilung aktiver und inaktiver Melanocyten in embryonaler Epidermis und jungen Stadien des Haarfollikels. (Aus MISHIMA und WIDLAN, 1966)

Capillaren und in der Basalschicht der Epidermis fanden. Die letzteren waren dendritisch, enthielten Melanosomen in allen Stadien der Reifung, sehr hervorstechendes endoplasmatisches Reticulum mit Ribosomen, eine filamentöse Substanz und einige Mitochondrien. BREATHNACH u. WYLLIE (1965) untersuchten die Haut eines 14 Wochen alten weißen Fetus und fanden Melanocyten mit nicht melanisierten Prämelanosomen in der Basalschicht und im unteren Stratum intermedium der Epidermis. Diese Zellen waren Dopanegativ. Die beiden Autorenn sahe keine Melanocyten im Corium. Dagegen waren spärliche, aber typisch entwickelte Langerhans-Zellen mit charakteristischen scheibenförmigen Organellen in der Epidermis vorhanden, ein Befund, der stark gegen die Annahme spricht, daß Langerhans-Zellen abgenutzte alte Melanocyten sind.

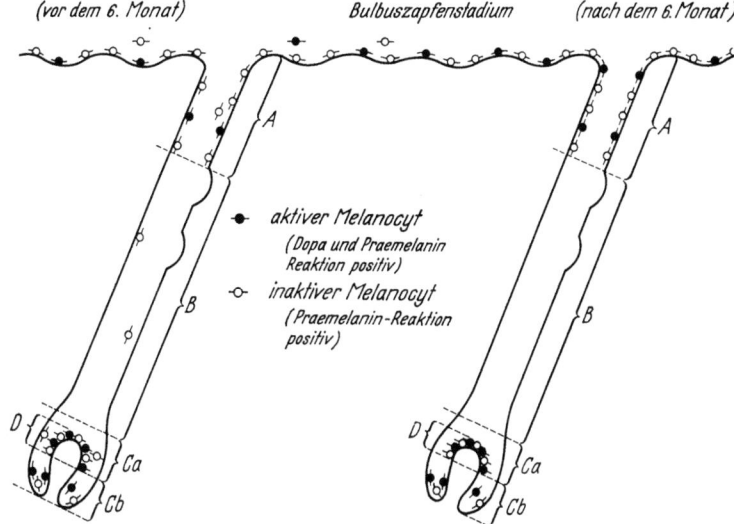

Abb. 37. Verteilung aktiver und inaktiver Melanocyten in Epidermis und Haarfollikel vor und nach dem 6. Fetalmonat. (Aus MISHIMA und WIDLAN, 1966)

H. Schlußbemerkungen

Diese Übersicht zeigt, daß Untersuchungen besonders der letzten 10 Jahre die Entwicklungsgeschichte der menschlichen Haut mit vielen neuen Erkenntnissen bereichert haben, die nicht nur um ihrer selbst willen, sondern auch zum Verständnis des erwachsenen Organs unter gesunden und pathologischen Bedingungen wichtig sind. Es kann zuversichtlich erwartet werden, daß Elektronenmikroskopie und Histochemie noch viel zu unserem Wissen beisteuern werden. Man kann auch hoffen, daß entwicklungsmechanische Experimente, trotz aller Speciesunterschiede, manche Spekulationen in sicheres Wissen verwandeln werden.

Literatur

ACHS, R., R. G. HARPER, and M. SIEGEL: Unusual dermatoglyphic findings associated with rubella embryopathy. New Engl. J. Med. 274, 148 (1966). — ACHTEN, G.: Chronologie du développement de l'épiderme de la main, du pied et du cuir chévelu chez l'homme. Arch. belges Derm. 12, 107 (1956). — Contribution à l'étude des hydrates de carbone de l'épiderme. Arch. belges Derm. 13, 456 (1957). — L'ongle normal et pathologique. Dermatologica (Basel) 126, 229 (1963). — AHERNE, W., and D. HULL: The site of heat production in the newborn infant. Proc. roy. Soc. Med. 57, 1172 (1964). — ALKIEWICZ, J.: On the original location of the germ of human nails. Bull. Soc. Amis Sci. Poznan-Ser. C 2, 56 (1951). — ALLEGRA, F.: Metacromasia dell'epidermide; ipotesi sul significato in base al comportamento dopo jaluronidasi. Arch. ital. Derm. 30, 369 (1961). — ALVERDES, K.: Die Entwicklung der Glandulae vestibulares nasi des Menschen. Z. mikr.-anat. Forsch. 35, 119 (1934). — AREY, L. B.: Simple formulae for estimating the age and size of human embryos. Anat. Rec. 30, 289 (1925). — AUBER, L.: The anatomy of follicles producing wool-fibres, with special reference to keratinization. Trans. roy. Soc. Edinb. 62, 191 (1952). — AURELL, G.: Studien über den Bau und die Entwicklung der Schweißdrüsen der menschlichen Fußsohle. Z. mikr.-anat. Forsch. 44, 56 (1938).

BANFIELD, W. S.: Width and length of collagen fibrils during the development of human skin, in granulation tissue, and in the skin of adult animals. J. Geront. 10, 13 (1955). — BECKER jr., S. W., and A. A. ZIMMERMANN: Development of the basement membrane in human skin. J. invest. Derm. 28, 195 (1957). — BECKETT, E. B., G. H. BOURNE, and W. MONTAGNA: Histology and cytochemistry of human skin; the distribution of cholinesterase in the finger of the embryo and the adult. J. Physiol. (Lond.) 134, 202 (1956). — BERLIN, L. B., u. I. G. PRIDVIZHKIN: Histochemische Untersuchung von Glykogen in der Haut des menschlichen Embryo. [Russ.]. Dokl. Akad. Nauk SSSR, Moskau 160, 213 (1965). — BILLINGHAM, R. E., and P. B. MEDAWAR: A note on the specificity of the corneal epithelium. J. Anat. (Lond.) 84, 50 (1950). — BILLINGHAM, R. E., and W. K. SILVERS: The origin and preservation of epidermal specificities. New Engl. J. Med. 268, 477, 539 (1963). — BLECHSCHMIDT, E.: Zur Anatomie des Subkutangewebes. Z. Zellforsch. 12, 284 (1930). — Über die Wachstumsbewegungen der Hautorgane bei menschlichen Embryonen. Z. Anat. Entwickl.-Gesch. 115, 224 (1950). — Die frühembryonale Lageentwicklung der Gliedmaßen (Entwicklung der Extremitäten beim Menschen, Teil I). Z. Anat. Entwickl.-Gesch. 115, 529 (1951a). — Die frühembryonale Formentwicklung der Gliedmaßen (Entwicklung der Extremitäten beim Menschen, Teil II. Z. Anat. Entwickl.-Gesch. 115, 597 (1951b). — Die frühembryonale Strukturentwicklung der Gliedmaßen (Entwicklung der Extremitäten beim Menschen, Teil III. Z. Anat. Entwickl.-Gesch. 115, 617 (1951c). — Die Entwicklungsbewegungen der Zahnleiste. Arch. Entwickl.-Mech. Org. 147, 474 (1955a). — Entwicklungsfunktionelle Untersuchungen an der menschlichen Ohrmuschel. Acta anat. (Basel) 25, 204 (1955b). — Die Gestaltungsfunktionen der menschlichen Oberhaut. I. Die Schichtenbildung des Integuments. Arch. klin. exp. Derm. 215, 567 (1963a). — Die embryonalen Gestaltungsfunktionen der menschlichen Oberhaut. II. Die Entwicklung des Papillarkörpers in den proximalen und distalen Abschnitten der Fingerbeere. Z. Morph. Anthrop. 54, 163 (1963b). — Organe als lokale Wachstumsmodifikationen des Zellgewebes. Dtsch. med. Forsch. 2, 93 (1964). — Das genetische Grundgesetz. Stimmen der Zeit Heft 1, 40 (1965). — BONNEVILLE, M. A.: The periderm of human fetal skin. Proc. 3rd Europ. Regional Confer. Electron Mic., Czechoslovak Acad. Sci. p. 565 (1964). — BORSETTO, P. L.: Osservazioni sullo sviluppo delle ghiandole sudoripare nelle diverse regioni della cute umana. Arch. ital. Anat. Embriol. 56, 322 (1951). — BREATHNACH, A. S., and L. M. WYLLIE: Electron microscopy of melanocytes and Langerhans cells in human fetal epidermis at fourteen weeks. J. invest. Derm. 44, 51 (1965a). — Fine structure of cells forming the surface layer of the epidermis in human fetuses at fourteen and twelve weeks. J. invest. Derm. 45, 179 (1965b). — BRODY, I., and K. S. LARSSON: Morphology of the mammalian skin: embryonic development of the epidermal sub-layers. In: A. G. LYNE and B. F. SHORT (eds.), Biology of the skin and hair growth. Sydney: Angus & Robertson 1965. — BURROWS, H.: The union and separation of living tissues as influenced by cellular differentiation. Yale J. Biol. Med. 17, 397 (1945). — BYON, S.: Quantitative Untersuchung der Anhangsorgane der Augenbrauenhaut bei den japanischen Feten. Okajimas Folia anat. jap. 37, 93 (1961).

CAUNA, N.: Some observations on the structure and development of Meissner's corpuscle. J. Anat. (Lond.) 87, 440 (1953). — CAUSEY, G.: The cell of Schwann. Baltimore: Williams & Wilkins Co. 1960. — CERESA, F.: Trasformazioni del tegumento dell'uomo durante la vita fetale e post-natale. Arch. ital. Anat. Embriol. 36, 101 (1936). — CHLOPIN, N. G.: Über einige Wachstums- und Differenzierungserscheinungen an der embryonalen menschlichen Epidermis im Explantat. Arch. Entwickl.-Mech. Org. 126, 69 (1932). — CLARA, M.: Die arterio-venösen Anastomosen, 2. Aufl. Wien: Springer 1956. — CLAUDE BERNARD, M.: De la matière glycogène considerée comme condition de développement de certains tissus, chez le foetus, avant l'apparition de la fonction glycogénique du foie. C. R. Acad. Sci. (Paris) 48, 673 (1859). — COOPER, Z. K.: Mitotic rhythm in human epidermis. J. invest. Derm. 2, 289 (1939).

DABELOW, A.: Die Milchdrüse. In: v. MÖLLENDORF-BARGMANN, Handbuch der mikroskopischen Anatomie des Menschen, Bd. 3, III, S. 276. Berlin-Göttingen-Heidelberg: Springer 1957. — DANNEEL, R.: Die Entwicklung der Haare bei der Ratte. Z. Morph. Ökol. Tiere 20, 733 (1931). — DAVIDSON, P., and M. H. HARDY: The development of mouse vibrissae in vivo and in vitro. J. Anat. (Lond.) 86, 342 (1952). — DUPERRAT, B., et J. M. MASCARO: Une tumeur bénigne développée aux dépens de l'acrotrichium ou partie intraépidermique du follicule pilaire: porome folliculaire (acanthome folliculaire intraépidermique; acrotrichoma). Dermatologica (Basel) 126, 291 (1963).

EBERL-ROTHE, G., u. P. A. LANGEGGER: Über Glykogen und Keratohyalin im embryonalen Nagel. Z. mikr.-anat. Forsch. 63, 212 (1957). — EGGELING, H. V.: Über die Drüsen des Warzenhofes beim Menschen. Jena. Z. Med. Naturw. 39, 423 (1904). — EICHENLAUB, F. J., and R. A. OSBOURN: Studies in the histogenesis of the epidermis. Arch. Derm. Syph. (Chicago) 64, 700 (1951). — ELLIS, R. A.: Ageing of the human male scalp. In: W. MONTAGNA and R. A. ELLIS, The biology of hair growth. New York: Academic Press 1958. — EMERY, J. L., and M. McMILLAN: Observations on the female sex chromatin in human epidermis and on the value of skin biopsy in determining sex. J. Path. Bact. 68, 17 (1954). — ENDO, M.: Über die Größe der apokrinen Schweißdrüsen an der Achselhaut bei den Japanischen Kindern. Okajimas Folia anat. jap. 17, 121 (1938). — Quantitative Untersuchung der Anhangsorgane der Achselhaut bei den japanischen Kindern. Okajimas Folia anat. jap. 17, 425 (1939a). — Beiträge zur Kenntnis der apokrinen Schweißdrüsen an der Achselhaut bei den japanischen Kindern. Okajimas Folia anat. jap. 17, 607 (1939b).

FLEISCHHAUER, K.: Über die Morphogenese des Haarstrichs und der Papillarleisten. Z. Zellforsch. 38, 50 (1953a). — Über die Entstehung der Haaranordnung und das Zustandekommen räumlicher Beziehungen zwischen Haaren und Schweißdrüsen. Z. Zellforsch. 38, 328 (1953b). — FLEISCHHAUER, K., u. E. HORSTMANN: Untersuchungen über die Entwicklung des Papillarkörpers der menschlichen Palma und Planta. Z. Zellforsch. 36, 298 (1951). — Der Papillarkörper und die Kapillaren des Perionychiums. Z. Zellforsch. 42, 213 (1955). — FRIE-

Boes, W.: Beiträge zur Anatomie und Biologie der Haut, II. u. III. Derm. Z. 31, 57, 32, 1 (1920). — Führers, M.: Über die konstruktive Entwicklung des kranio-kaudalen Haarstriches. II. Der Haarstrich beim Menschen. Z. Zellforsch. 30, 52 (1940).

Gardner, J. H., and H. F. Raybuck: Development of cleavage line patterns in the human fetus. Anat. Rec. 118, 745 (1954). — Gastgeber, W.: Über eine architektonische Beziehung zwischen Haarkleid und Subkutis. Anat. Anz. 83, 32 (1936). — Geiger, R.: Zur Frage der Entwicklung der elastischen Fasern in der Haut. Wien. med. Wschr. 76, 858 (1926). — Zur Frage der Entwicklung der elastischen Fasern in der Haut. Arch. Derm. Syph. (Berl.) 154, 108 (1928). — Goto, T., T. Kaga, and T. Oono: Cytochemical studies of alkaline phosphatase and glycogen in eccrine sweat glands in the palm and sole of the human embryo. Okajimas Folia anat. jap. 37, 246 (1961). — Graumann, W.: Entwicklung des Milchstreifens. Z. Anat. Entwickl.-Gesch. 114, 500 (1950). — Grenberg, T. F.: A comparative histological study of the development of the epidermis in vertebrates and man. Arkh. Anat. (Moskva) 34, 79 (1957) [Russ.]. — Embryohistogenesis of the epidermis in man. Tr. Leningrad. sanit. hyg. med. Inst. 42, 23 (1958) [Russ.]. — Grüneberg, H.: A ventral ectodermal ridge of the tail in mouse embryos. Nature (Lond.) 177, 787 (1952).

Häggqvist, G.: Einige Beobachtungen zur Entwicklung der Epidermis. Arch. Derm. Syph. (Berl.) 130, 231 (1921). — Hambrick jr., G. W., and R. Bloomberg: The differentiation of human fetal skin following heterotransplantation. J. invest. Derm. 33, 177 (1959). — Hashimoto, K., et G. Gross: Étude de la structure ultramicroscopique de l'ongle de l'embryon humain. Rapport preliminaire. Arch. Biochim. Cosmetol. 81, 11 (1964). — Hashimoto, K., B. Gross, R. J. Di Bella, and W. F. Lever: The ultrastructure of the skin of human embryos. IV. The epidermis. J. invest. Derm. 47, 310 (1966). — Hashimoto, K., B. G. Gross, and W. F. Lever: The ultrastructure of the skin of human embryos. I. The intraepidermal eccrine sweat duct. J. invest. Derm. 45, 139 (1965). — The ultrastructure of human embryo skin. II. The formation of the intradermal portion of the eccrine duct and of the secretory segment during the first half of embryonic life. J. invest. Derm. 46, 513 (1966). — Hashimoto, K., B. G. Gross, R. Nelson, and W. F. Lever: The ultrastructure of the skin of human embryos. III. The formation of the nail in eighteen weeks old embryos. J. invest. Derm. 47, 205 (1966). — Hay, E. D.: Secretion of a connective tissue protein by developing epidermis. In: W. Montagna and W. C. Lobitz jr.: The epidermis, p. 97. New York: Academic Press 1964. — Hayashi, T.: Studies on the development of the skin elements originating from the neural crest in the Japanese fetus. I. On melanoblasts and melanocytes. Jap. J. Derm., Ser. B 74, 298—304 (1964a). — Studies on the development of the skin elements originating from the neural crest in the Japanese fetus. II. On Merkel's tactile cells and nerve endings. Jap. J. Derm., Ser. B 74, 305—308 (1964b). — Hellström, B., and H. Holmgren: Numerical distribution of mast cells in the human skin and heart. Acta anat. (Basel) 10, 81 (1950). — Hörstadius, S.: The neural crest. New York and London: Oxford University Press 1950. — Holmgren, H.: Über das Vorkommen und die Bedeutung der chromotropen(metachromatischen) Substanz in menschlichen Feten. Anat. Anz. 88, 246 (1939). — Studien über Verbreitung und Bedeutung der chromotropen Substanz. Z. mikr.-anat. Forsch. 47, 489 (1940). — Beitrag zur Frage der Genese der Ehrlichschen Mastzellen. Acta anat. (Basel) 2, 40 (1946). — Holmgren, H., u. H. Johansson: Beitrag zur Kenntnis der Entwicklung der Epidermis. Anat. Anz. 75, 449 (1933). — Horn, G.: Formentwicklung und Gestalt der Schweißdrüsen der Fußsohle des Menschen. Z. mikr.-anat. Forsch. 38, 318 (1935). — Horstmann, E.: Die Haut. In: v. Möllendorff-Bargmann, Handbuch der mikroskopischen Anatomie des Menschen, Bd. 3, III, S. 1. Berlin-Göttingen-Heidelberg: Springer 1957. — Anatomie der Haut und ihrer Anhangsorgane. I. Entwicklung. In: H. A. Gottron u. W. Schönfeld, Dermatologie und Venerologie, I, 1, S. 42. Stuttgart: Georg Thieme 1961.

Iidaka, T.: Die Haar- und Haargruppendichtigkeit bei den Mischlingsfeten. Okajimas Folia anat. jap. 25, 263 (1954). — Ikada, M.: Das Vorkommen und die Verteilung des M. arrector pili in der Augenlidhaut bei den japanischen Feten. Okajimas Folia anat. jap. 25, 79 (1953). — Ingalls, N. W.: Symmetrical, segmental thickenings in the dorsal ectoderm of human embryos. Amer. J. Anat. 44, 455 (1929). — Ishimoto, Y.: Studies on the collagen fibre of the skin, report I. Electron microscopical observations on the collagen fibre of the skin from the healthy adults, fetus and patients with cutaneous diseases. Jap. J. Derm. Vener. 65, 237 (1955).

Jalowy, B.: Über die Entwicklung der Nervenendigungen in der Haut des Menschen. Z. Anat. Entwickl.-Gesch. 109, 344 (1939).

Kaga, T., T. Goto, and T. Ieta: A cytochemical study on protein and nucleic acids of the eccrine sweat gland in the palm and sole of human embryos. Okajimas Folia anat. jap. 37, 147 (1961). — Kan, M.: Histologische und histo-entwicklungsgeschichtliche Untersuchungen der Schweißdrüsen der Achselhaut von Japanern. Nagoya Ikakkai Z. 56, 365 (1941) [Japanisch]. — Karrenberg, C. L.: Histologische Untersuchungen von Achselhöhlenhaut bei beiden Geschlechtern und in verschiedenen Lebensaltern. Derm. Wschr. 87, 1275 (1929). — Katzberg, A. A.: Regional differences in the developing epidermis of early human embryos. Anat. Rec. 115, 397 (1953). — Kawamura, T., K. Nichihara, and H. Nakajima: On the nevoid spots of palms and soles. Jap. J. Derm. **66**, 75 (1956). — KELLY, D. E.: Fine structure of desmosomes, hemidesmosomes, and an adepidermal globular layer in developing newt epidermis. J. Cell Biol. **28**, 51 (1966). — KITAMURA, K.: Peutz-Jeghers' syndrome, incontinentia pigmenti Bloch-Sulzberger and some other pigment anomalies in Japan. Exc. Med. Internat. Congr. Ser. **55**, 137 (1963). — KOHAN, A. B.: Embryologie de la peau. Bull. Soc. franç. Derm. Syph. **72**, 390 (1965). — KOSAKA, Y.: Quantitative Untersuchung der Anhangsorgane der Haut bei einem japanischen Foetus. Folia anat. jap. **10**, 753 (1932). — KRATZER, G. L., and M. B. DOCKERTY: Histopathology of the anal ducts. Surg. Gynec. Obstet. **84**, 333 (1947). — KRAUCHER, G.: Die Histogenese der menschlichen Scrotalhaut. Z. mikr.-anat. Forsch. **26**, 281 (1931). — KURIKI, S.: Quantitative Untersuchung der Schweißdrüse der Handtellerhaut bei den Zwillingen. Okajimas Folia anat. jap. **14**, 685 (1936). — Quantitative Untersuchung der Schweißdrüse der Fußsohlenhaut bei den Zwillingen. Okajimas Folia anat. jap. **15**, 91 (1937).

LANDOLT, A. M.: Über eine ektodermale Leiste des Schwanzes menschlicher Embryonen. Z. Anat. Entwickl.-Gesch. **121**, 337 (1959). — LAPIÈRE, S.: La zone limite entre l'épiderme et le derme chez l'homme et chez l'embryon de mouton. Arch. Biol. (Paris) **50**, 343 (1939). — LEDOUX-CORBUSIER, M.: Le tissue élastique cutané. Rev. Med. Pharm. **18**, 329 (1962). — LEITAN, V. P.: Changes in embryonic cutaneous connective tissue under hyperthyreosis in pregnant women. Arkh. Anat. **40**, 24 (1961) [Russ.]. — LEWIS, B. L.: Microscopic studies of fetal and mature nail and surrounding soft tissues. Arch. Derm. Syph. (Chic.) **70**, 732 (1954). — LINDBERG, S., S. E. LINDELL, and H. WESTLING: Formation and inactivation of histamine by human foetal tissues in vitro. Acta obstet. gynec. scand. **42**, Suppl. 1, 49 (1963). — LINDE, K. W.: Elektronenmikroskopische Untersuchung über die Differenzierung der Interzellularsubstanz der menschlichen Lederhaut. Z. Zellforsch. **42**, 331 (1955). — LIVINI, F.: Riassunto di osservazioni su la presenza e la distribuzione del glicogeno, in embrioni e feti umani. Boll. Biol. Esper. **2**, 625 (1927). — LOBITZ jr., W. C., J. B. HOLYOKE, and W. MONTAGNA: The epidermal eccrine sweat duct unit, a morphologic and biologic entity. J. invest. Derm. **22**, 157 (1955). — LYNCH, F. W.: Elastic tissue in fetal skin. Arch. Derm. Syph. (Chic.) **29**, 57 (1934).

MACHIDA, H.: A histochemical study on the skin of human embryos. Okajimas Folia anat. jap. **39**, 213 (1964). — MANCINI, R. E., y E. BACARINI: Mucoproteinas del tejido conectivo adulto y embrionario. Rev. Soc. argent. Biol. **27**, 27 (1951). — MARKS, P.: Untersuchung über die Entwicklung der Haut, insbesondere der Haar- und Drüsenanlagen bei den Haussäugetieren. Inaug.-Diss. Berlin: W. Buxenstein 1895. — MASSON, P.: Les glomus neurovasculaires. Paris: Hermann & Cie. 1937. — MCKAY, D. G., E. C. ADAMS, A. T. HERTIG, and S. DANZIGER: Histochemical horizons in human embryos. Anat. Rec. **122**, 125 (1955). — MCLOUGHLIN, C. B.: Mesenchymal influences on epithelial differentiation. In: Symp. of the Soc. for Experimental Biology No 17, Cell differentiation, p. 359. New York: Academic Press 1963. — MISHIMA, Y.: Electronmicroscopic cytochemistry of melanosomes and mitochondria. J. Histochem. Cytochem. **12**, 784 (1964). — MISHIMA, Y., and S. WIDLAN: Embryonic development of melanocytes in human hair and epidermis. J. invest. Derm. **46**, 263 (1966). — MOCHIZUKI, D.: Quantitative Untersuchung der Anhangsorgane der Haut bei einpaarigen japanischen eineiigen Zwillingsfoeten. Okajimas Folia anat. jap. **15**, 59 (1937). — MOGI, E.: Beiträge zur Entwicklung der apokrinen Schweißdrüsen im Vestibulum nasi bei den japanischen Feten. Okajimas Folia anat. jap. **16**, 147 (1938). — MONTAGNA, W.: Histology and cytochemistry of human skin. XIX. The development and fate of the axillary organ. J. invest. Derm. **33**, 151 (1959). — The structure and function of skin, 2nd ed., p. 427. New York: Academic Press 1962. — MORI, T.: Histochemical studies on the distribution of alkaline phosphatase in the early human embryos: I. Observations on two embryos in early somite stage, Streeter's horizon X. Arch. histol. jap. **16**, 169 (1959a). — Histochemical studies on the distribution of alkaline phosphatase in early human embryos. II. Observations on an embryo with 13—14 somites. Arch. histol. jap. **18**, 197 (1959b). — MORITA, S.: Quantitative Untersuchung der Schweißdrüsen bei den japanischen Feten. Okajimas Folia anat. jap. **27**, 81 (1955).

NAESLUND, J.: The function of Montgomery's tubercles. Acta obstet. gynec. scand. **36**, 460 (1957).

OLIN, T. E.: Untersuchungen über die Follikelkomplexe am Tragus. Arb. Pathol. Inst. Helsingfors (Jena) **10**, 357 (1942a). — Untersuchungen über die Breite der Körnerschicht an verschiedenen Hautstellen und über ihr Verhältnis zur Breite der übrigen Epidermisschichten. Arb. Pathol. Inst. Helsingfors (Jena) **10**, 431 (1942b). — ORLOVSKAYA, G. V.: Development of, and changes with age in, the fibrous structure of the connective tissue of the skin of the face. Arch. Pat. (Moskau) **11**, 51 (1949). Zit. aus Excerpta med. (Amst.) Abt. XIII 4, 1569 (1950). — OTTAVIANI, G., e I. LUPIDI: Ricerche sullo sviluppo dei vasi linfatici cutanei dell' uomo. Arch. ital. Anat. Embriol. **45**, 123 (1941).

PASS, F., D. BROPHY, M. L. PEARSON, and W. C. LOBITZ jr.: Human epidermis and glycogen after inflammatory stimuli. J. invest. Derm. **45**, 391 (1965). — PAWLOWSKI, A.: Free and encapsulated nerve endings in epidermis and superficial layers of the skin in human and animals. II. Comparative studies of the skin innervation in animals and human foetus in embryonal development, in some skin disorders and naevi. Przegl. derm. **50**, 183 (1963). — PÉREZ, R. M.: Contribution à l'étude des terminaisons nerveuses dans la peau de la main. Trav. Lab. Rech. Biol. Madrid **27**, 187 (1931). — PÉREZ, R. M., et A. P. R. PÉREZ: L'évolution des terminaisons nerveuses de la peau humaine. Trav. Lab. Rech. Biol. Madrid **28**, 61 (1933). — PERNKOPF, E., u. V. PATZELT: Die Entwicklung der Haut und ihrer Anhangsgebilde. In: L. ARZT u. K. ZIELER, Die Haut- und Geschlechtskrankheiten, Bd. 1, S. 100. Berlin u. Wien: Urban & Schwarzenberg 1934. — PIERCE jr., G. B.: Basement membranes. VI. Synthesis by epithelial tumors of the mouse. Cancer Res. 25, 636 (1965). — PINKUS, F.: Die Entwicklungsgeschichte der Haut. In: F. KEIBEL u. F. P. MALL, Handbuch der Entwicklungsgeschichte, Bd. 1, S. 185. Leipzig: S. Hirzel 1910. — Die normale Anatomie der Haut. In: J. JADASSOHN, Handbuch der Haut- und Geschlechtskrankheiten, Bd. I, 1, S. 1. Berlin: Springer 1927. — PINKUS, H.: Über Gewebekulturen menschlicher Epidermis. Arch. Derm. Syph. (Berl.) **165**, 53 (1932). — Note son structure and biological properties of human epidermis and sweat gland cells in tissue culture and in the organism. Arch. exp. Zellforsch. **22**, 47 (1938). — The wall of the intraepidermal part of the sweat duct. J. invest. Derm. **2**, 175 (1939). — Premalignant fibroepithelial tumors of skin. Arch. Derm. Syph. (Chic.) **67**, 598 (1953). — Biology of epidermal cells. In: S. ROTHMAN, Physiology and biochemistry of the skin, p. 584. Chicago: Chicago University Press 1954. — Embryology of hair. In: W. MONTAGNA and R. A. ELLIS, The biology of hair growth, p. 1. New York: Academic Press 1958. — Zur Entwicklung des Haarfollikels beim Menschen, insbesondere des Infundibulums und des bindegewebigen Anteils. Hautarzt **10**, 146 (1959). — Adnexal tumors, benign, not-so-benign, and malignant. In: W. MONTAGNA, Advances in biology of skin. VII. Carcinogenesis, p. 255. Oxford and New York: Pergamon Press 1966. — PINKUS, H., J. R. ROGIN, and P. GOLDMAN: Eccrine poroma; tumors exhibiting features of the epidermal sweat duct unit. Arch. Derm. (Chic.) **74**, 511 (1956). — POPOFF, L., et N. POPOFF: L'hémopoïèse cutanée au cours de la vie intra-uterine. Ann. derm. syph. Paris 85, 157 (1958). — PRIDVIZHKIN, I. G., u. L. B. BERLIN: Über die embryonale Histogenese der Epidermis und ihrer Derivate. Dokl. Akad. Nauk SSSR **158**, 199 (1964) [Russ.]. — PULLAR, P., and C. LIADSKY: Dehydrogenase systems of human foetal skin. Brit. J. Derm. **77**, 314 (1965).

RACHMATULLIN, Z. C.: Die Entwicklung der Meissnerschen Körperchen in der Menschenhaut. Z. mikr.-Anat. Forsch. **40**, 445 (1936). — RAWLES, M. E.: Tissue interactions in the morphogenesis of the feather. In: A. G. LYNE and B. F. SHORT, Biology of the skin and hair growth, p. 105. Sydney: Angus & Robertson 1965. — REISS, H.: Beitrag zur Histogenese der Talgdrüsen und des Hornfettes beim menschlichen Fetus. Arch. Derm. Syph. (Berl.) **166**, 30 (1932). — RIEGEL, P.: Die Frühentwicklung der Ultrastruktur in der Epidermis menschlicher Embryonen. Z. Morph. Anthrop. **56**, 195 (1965). — ROTTER, W., u. L. WAGNER: Über die Entwicklung der subungealen Glomera (sog. arteriovenöse Anastomosen) der Zehen. Arch. Kreisl.-Forsch. 18, 68 (1952).

SAJNER, J.: Beiträge zur Histogenese der Epidermis der Vertebraten. Spiny lék. Fak. Masaryk Univ. Brno **12**, 211 (1933) [Tschech.]. — SAMEJIMA, T.: Studies on the human skin tissues. Jap. J. Derm. **66**, 192 (1965) [engl. Zusammenfass.]. — SAUNDERS, R. L. DE C. H., and W. MONTAGNA: X-ray microscopy and microangiography. Arch. Derm. **89**, 451 (1964). — SCHMIDT, S.: Die Entstehung der digitalen Tastballen. Z. Morph. Anthrop. 55, 1 (1964). — SCHWARZ, W.: Elektronenmikroskopische Untersuchungen über die Bildung elastischer Fasern in der Gewebekultur. Z. Zellforsch. **63**, 636 (1964). — SELBY, C. C.: An electron microscope study of the epidermis of mammalian skin in thin sections. I. Dermo-epidermal junction and basal cell layer. J. biophys. biochem. Cytol. 1, 429 (1955). — SENGEL, P.: The determination of the differentiation of the skin and the cutaneous appendages of the chick embryo. In: W. MONTAGNA and W. C. LOBITZ jr., The epidermis, p. 15. New York: Academic Press 1964. — SERRI, F.: Studi sulla cute del feto e del bambino. I. Peculiarità nello sviluppo e nella struttura della cute fetale. Boll. Soc. ital. Biol. sper. **38**, 1165 (1962). — Les cholinesterases dans le developpement de la peau foetale. Arch. belges Derm. **19**, 351 (1963). — Le sviluppo e l'organizzazione vascolare nella cute del feto umano. Minerva derm. **40**, 179 (1965). — SERRI, F., W. M. HUBER e H. MESCON: Studi sulla cute del feto e del bambino. III. Attività della fosfatasi acida nelle cute del feto. Boll. Soc. ital. Biol. sper. **38**, 1169 (1962). — Studi sulla cute del feto e del bambino. V. Distribuzione e significato delle colinesterasi nelle cute del feto. G. ital. Derm., Suppl. **7**, 1 (1966). — SERRI, F., W. MONTAGNA, and W. M. HUBER: Studies of skin of fetus and the child. The distribution of alkaline phosphatase in the skin of the fetus. Arch. Derm. **87**, 234 (1963). — SERRI, F., W. MONTAGNA, and H. MESCON: Studi sulla cute del feto e del bambino. II. Glycogen and amylophosphorylase in the skin of the fetus. J. invest. Derm. **39**, 199 (1962). — Osservazioni sull'innervazione della cute fetale con particolare riguardo alle dita. Acta neuroveg. (Wien) **24**, 166 (1963). — SERRI, F., M. L. SPERANZA e H. MESCON: Il rapporto mucopolisacaridi/collagene in aree ed età differenti della cute de feto umana. Boll. Soc. ital. Biol. sper. **39**, 1288 (1963). — SPULER, A.: Abriß der Entwicklungsgeschichte der Milchdrüse. In: W. STOECKEL, Handbuch der Gynäkologie, Bd. I. 1. Hälfte, 490—510, München: J. F. Bergmann 1930. — STARCK, D.: Herkunft und Entwicklung der

Pigmentzellen. In: J. JADASSOHNs Handbuch der Haut- und Geschlechtskrankheiten, Erg.-Werk Bd. I, 2, S. 139. Berlin-Göttingen-Heidelberg: Springer 1964. — Embryologie. Ein Lehrbuch auf allgemeinbiologischer Grundlage, 2. Aufl. Stuttgart: Georg Thieme 1965. — STEINER, K.: Über die Entwicklung der großen Schweißdrüsen beim Menschen. Z. Anat. Entwickl.-Gesch. 78, 83 (1926). Über die Entwicklung der Basalmembran des Hautepithels. II. Die Entwicklung der Basalmembran beim Menschen. Z. Zellforsch. 7, 577 (1928). — Über die Entwicklung und Differenzierungsweise der menschlichen Haut. I. Über die frühembryonale Entwicklung der menschlichen Haut. Z. Zellforsch. 8, 691 (1929a). — Über örtliche Verschiedenheiten des Aufbaues der Hautanlage junger menschlicher Embryonen. Arch. Derm. Syph. (Berl.) 157, 446 (1929b). — Über die Entwicklung und Differenzierungsweise der menschlichen Haut. II. Die embryonale Entwicklung der Hautgebiete mit frühzeitiger Mehrschichtigkeit des Epithels. Z. Anat. Entwickl-Gesch. 93, 750 (1930). — Über Hautbezirke mit starker Zellvermehrung bei menschlichen Embryonen. Arch. Derm. Syph. (Berl.) 162, 577 (1931). — STERNBERG, H.: Beschreibung eines menschlichen Embryos mit vier Ursegmentpaaren, nebst Bemerkungen über die Anlage und früheste Entwicklung einiger Organe beim Menschen. Z. Anat. Entwickl.-Gesch. 82, 142 (1927). — STÖHR, P.: Entwicklungsgeschichte des menschlichen Wollhaares. Anat. Hefte, Abt. 1, 23, 1 (1904). — STREETER, G. L.: Developmental horizons in human embryos. Age groups XI—XXIII. Carnegie Institution of Washington, D. C. 1951. — SUGA, Y.: Histological pictures of the lip and its innervation in the human embryo by Seto's silver impregnation. Tohoku med. J. 45, 437 (1951). — SZYMONOWICZ, W.: Über die Entwicklung der Nervenendigungen in der Haut des Menschen. Z. Zellforsch. 19, 356 (1933).

TAKEDA, S.: Über die Ohrenschmalzdrüsen bei Mischlingsfeten. Okajimas Folia anat. jap. 23, 357 (1951). — Über die Verteilung des M. arrector pili in der Haut der äußeren Nase. Okajimas Folia anat. jap. 24, 55 (1952). — TANIGUCHI, T.: Quantitative Untersuchung der Anhangsorgane der Haut bei dem japanischen Neugeborenen. Folia anat. jap. 9, 215 (1931). — TENCH, E. M.: Development of the anus in the human embryo. Amer. J. Anat. 59, 333 (1936). THÖLEN, H.: Das embryonale und postnatale Verhalten der männlichen Brustdrüse beim Menschen. I. Das Mammarorgan beim Embryo und Säugling. Acta anat. (Basel) 8, 201 (1949). — THURINGER, J. M., and A. A. KATZBERG: Effect of age on mitosis in human epidermis. J. invest. Derm. 33, 35 (1959). — TÖNDURY, G.: Embryologie und Hauttopographie. Arch. klin. exp. Derm. 219, 12 (1964). — TORSUEV, N. A.: Histologie, Embryogenese und Pathohistologie der Wagner-Meissnerschen Körperchen in der menschlichen Haut. Sborn nauk. rabot. klin.-kozh.-ven. Bolez, Krymskogo Gos. Med. Inst. No 1, 88 (1940) [Russ.]. — TRUFFI, G.: Sulla vascolarizzazione degli annessi cutanei. Arch. ital. Derm. 10, 681 (1934). — TSUCHIYA, K.: Über die ekkrine Schweißdrüse des menschlichen Embryo, mit besonderer Berücksichtigung ihrer Histo- und Cytogenese. Arch. histol. jap. 6, 403 (1954) [Jap.].

UEDA, M.: Beiträge zur Entwicklungsgeschichte der Haut und ihrer Anhangsorgane bei den Japanern. I. Über die Entwicklung und Differenzierung der Epidermis. Nagasaki Igakkai Zasshi 17, 1666 (1939a) [Jap.]. — Beiträge zur Entwicklungsgeschichte der Haut und ihrer Anhangsorgane bei den Japanern. II. Über die Entwicklung der ekkrinen Schweißdrüsen. Nagasaki Igakkai Zasshi 17, 2278 (1939b). — Beiträge zur Entwicklungsgeschichte der Haut und ihrer Anhangsorgane bei den Japanern. I. Über die Entwicklung und Differenzierung der Epidermis. Acta Med. Nagasakiensa 1, 107 (1939c) deutsche Zusammenfass.

WASSERMANN, F.: Die Fettorgane des Menschen. Z. Zellforsch. 3, 235 (1926). — WEISS, P.: Principles of development; a textbook of experimental embryology. New York: Henry Holt 1939. — WILSON, R. B., and C. A. MCWHORTER: Isolated flagella in human skin. Electron microscopic observations. Lab. Invest. 12, 242 (1963). — WINKELMANN, R. K.: The cutaneous innervation of human newborn prepuce. J. invest. Derm. 26, 53 (1956). — Nerve endings in normal and pathological skin. Springfield (Ill.): Ch. C. Thomas 1960.

YANAGISAWA, N.: Die Entwicklung der Hautanhangsorgane im Nasenvorhof und in der Außenhaut der Nase, insbesonders unter Berücksichtigung der apokrinen, ekkrinen und Talgdrüsen. Okajimas Folia anat. jap. 30, 124 (1957). — YASUI, I., and H. KAGEMOTO: Histochemical investigation on the axillary sweat glands during childhood in Japanese, especially on the PAS positive substances and iron. Okajimas Folia anat. jap. 37, 215 (1961).

ZACHARIAE, H.: Histamine and mast cells in human fetal skin. Proc. Soc. exp. Biol. (N.Y.) 117, 63 (1964). — ZAIAS, N.: Embryology of the human nail. Arch. Derm. 87, 37 (1963). — ZASTAVA, V.: Vesikulosni povrch peridermu embryonalni kůže člověka. Biol. Listy 31, Suppl. 2, 215 (1951). — ZELESNIKOW, I. G.: Histologische Struktur und topographische Besonderheiten der Haut im frühen Kindesalter. Izv. Akad. Nauk Kazah. S.S.R., Ser. Fiziol. Med. 8, 63B (1957). — ZELICKSON, A. S.: Fibroblast development and fibrogenesis; a histochemical and electron microscope study. Arch. Derm. 88, 497 (1963). — ZIMMERMANN, A. A.: Die Entwicklung der Hautfarbe beim Neger vor der Geburt. Mitt. Thurgauischen Naturforsch. Ges. Heft 37, 33 (1954). — ZIMMERMANN, A. A., and S. W. BECKER jr.: Melanoblasts and melanocytes in fetal negro skin. Illinois Monogr. Med. Sci. 6, No 3, 1 (1959). — ZORZOLI, G.: Ricerche sulla morfologia della ghiandole ceruminose dell'uomo nelle varie età. Arch. ital. Anat. Embriol. 53, 117 (1948).

Die Altersveränderungen der Haut

Von

Hans-Joachim Cramer, Erfurt

Mit 7 Abbildungen

Einleitung

Durch die erheblichen Fortschritte der Medizin in den letzten Jahrzehnten sowie durch die verbesserten Lebensbedingungen, die mit Hilfe der modernen Technik erreicht werden konnten, ist das durchschnittliche Lebensalter der Menschen in vielen Gebieten der Erde bedeutend verlängert worden. Damit treten zwangsläufig Probleme der Geriatrie immer stärker in das Aufgabengebiet der Medizin hinein. Auch die Dermatologie kann sich dieser Entwicklung nicht entziehen.

Da die Kenntnisse der normalen Anatomie von jeher eine der wesentlichen Grundlagen für die medizinische Tätigkeit und Forschung waren, erscheint es angebracht, das derzeitige Wissen über die normalen morphologischen Altersveränderungen der menschlichen Haut zusammenfassend darzustellen. Es sei dazu auch auf die Arbeiten mit gleichartiger Thematik von COOPER, SCHALLWEGG, STRÖBEL und insbesondere WAGNER verwiesen. Leider müssen wir vermerken, daß diese Kenntnisse nicht sehr umfangreich und nicht sicher begründet sind. Die Literatur zu diesem Thema ist im Vergleich zu anderen Gebieten recht spärlich. Dies ist sicher zum Teil so zu erklären, daß die wissenschaftliche Dermatologie bisher mehr ihr Augenmerk auf ausgesprochen krankhafte Veränderungen der Altershaut gerichtet hat und die Probleme der normalen Hautalterung eher den Kosmetiker und die kosmetische Industrie beschäftigt haben. Die hauptsächlichen Gründe dürften aber anderer Natur sein.

Um die Aussage machen zu können „was ist normal", benötigt man auch bei Heranziehung moderner Methoden der Statistik ein relativ großes Untersuchungsgut, um die individuelle Streubreite, die Einflüsse durch topographische Besonderheiten, Geschlecht, Rasse und Konstitution ausgleichen bzw. erfassen zu können.

Hinzu kommt noch, daß eine Haut untersucht werden muß, die Jahrzehnte zahlreichen exogenen Einflüssen unterschiedlichster Art ausgesetzt war. Es soll das Bild der „normalen Altershaut" analysiert werden. Das bedeutet, es sollen Veränderungen, die durch spezielle oder extreme Klima- und Witterungsbedingungen, durch Beruf oder persönliche Lebensbedingungen verursacht wurden, ausgeschlossen werden. Und nicht zuletzt dürfen keine Folgen einer überstandenen oder noch bestehenden Erkrankung irgendwelcher Art erfaßt werden. Ein bioptisches Untersuchungsmaterial zu erlangen, das diese Bedingungen auch nur angehend erfüllt, ist ungeheuer schwierig. Man muß sich daher bei der Wertung der hier aufgeführten Untersuchungsergebnisse und den manchmal widersprechenden Angaben immer der Zufälligkeiten bewußt sein, die sich aus dem Fehler der kleinen Zahl ergeben. So stützen sich z. B. die Aussagen von MONTES, BAKER u. CURTIS über das Verhalten der apokrinen Schweißdrüsen in der Menopause auf 2 Beobachtungen (davon einmal Zustand nach Ovariektomie). Den sehr wesentlichen Untersuchungen von TELLER, VESTER u. POHL über die submikroskopischen Befunde an Bindegewebsfasern liegen 4 Gewebsexcisionen zugrunde.

Die einschlägigen Ergebnisse, die sich auf ein größeres Zahlenmaterial stützen können (z.B. BERRES; SCHALLWEGG; STRÖBEL u.a.), sind daher verständlicherweise meist an Leichenmaterial gewonnen worden. Dieses Untersuchungsgut ist dafür mit der Fehlerquelle postmortaler Autolysevorgänge behaftet, die bei einzelnen Strukturen (z.B. apokrinen Schweißdrüsen) sehr erheblich die Beurteilung stören können.

Sieht man die recht umfangreiche Literatur über die Histochemie der normalen Haut nach Aussagen über Altersabweichungen durch, so ist das Ergebnis enttäuschend. Obwohl von den meisten Autoren angegeben wird, daß Material von verschiedenen Altersstufen untersucht wurde, fehlt fast immer eine entsprechende Auswertung der Ergebnisse. Dies dürfte überwiegend seine Ursache darin haben, daß evtl. vorhandene Abweichungen nicht grob morphologischer Natur, sondern höchstens quantitativer Art sind. Das Problem der exakten Messung von unterschiedlichen Farbintensitäten bei histochemischen Reaktionen und ihre Wertung als Ausdruck einer quantitativen Änderung des Reaktionssubstrates ist jedoch bisher noch nicht gelöst. Zahlreiche Erkenntnisse über Altersveränderungen bestimmter Gewebe erwiesen sich nach Heranziehung der Originalliteratur als nicht auf Untersuchungen an menschlicher Haut basierend und wurden daher nicht berücksichtigt, um das an sich schon sehr inhomogene Material nicht noch mehr in seiner Aussagekraft für die Dermatologie zu mindern.

1. Über Unterschiede der Altersveränderungen an bedeckter und unbedeckter Haut

Wie gezeigt wurde, gibt es viele Faktoren, die die Beurteilung eines Befundes in Hinblick darauf, ob darin eine reine Altersveränderung der Haut zu erblicken ist oder nicht, erheblich erschweren können. Besonders wichtig erscheint auch, ob das zur Untersuchung vorliegende Hautstück von einem überwiegend bedeckten Körperteil stammt oder von einer Stelle, an der die Haut über größere Zeiträume exogenen Einflüssen ungeschützt ausgesetzt war. GANS u. STEIGLEDER unterscheiden daher zwischen der einfachen Altersatrophie, die am reinsten an konstant geschützter Haut ausgebildet ist, und der degenerativen Altersatrophie, wie sie besonders im Gesicht oder im Nacken ausgeprägt ist.

Die nachfolgenden Ausführungen müßten sich in erster Linie auf Untersuchungen beziehen, die an Hautgewebe von bedeckten Körperstellen durchgeführt wurden. Es ist jedoch zu bedenken, daß es nur wenige Hautbereiche gibt, die diese Bedingung weitgehendst erfüllen und nicht andererseits durch spezielle topographische Verhältnisse (z.B. Ano-Genital-Bereich, Achselhöhlengegend) wieder andere Besonderheiten aufweisen. Viele Körperstellen dürfen nur als fakultativ bedeckte Regionen gelten und können durch Beruf oder besondere Lebensweise einer Person erheblich von der Norm abweichen. Es ist sehr schwer, derartige Umstände bei der Auswahl des Untersuchungsgutes zu erfassen und zu berücksichtigen.

Das bisher in der Literatur zum Thema „Altersveränderungen der Haut" vorliegende Material ist zu gering und inhomogen, um eine derart strenge Auswahl oder Trennung durchführen zu können. Es wurde aber versucht, durch entsprechende Hinweise diese topographischen Probleme zu berücksichtigen (s. auch Tabelle 1).

Tabelle 1. *Topographie der Untersuchungsstellen häufiger zitierter Autoren*

Autoren	Biopsiestellen
BERRES	Bauch
DICK	Fußsohle, Fußrücken, Oberschenkel, Unterschenkel, Arm
EJIRI	Kopf, Gesicht, Arm, Hand, Fuß u.a.
EVANS, COWDRY, NIELSON	Ellenbeuge
GOLDZIEHER u. Mitarb.	Oberschenkel
HILL u. MONTGOMERY	Interdigitalraum, Schamgegend, Achselhöhle, Brust, Kopf
MA u. COWDRY	Ellenbeuge
NELKE	Bauch
SCHALLWEGG	Oberarm (Beuge- und Streckseite)
SOUTHWOOD	s. Tabelle 2 und 4
STRÖBEL	Bauch, Oberschenkel, Oberarm

Ganz allgemein gesehen läßt sich sagen, daß die Unterschiede zwischen den Altersveränderungen bedeckter und unbedeckter Haut — von einigen Ausnahmen abgesehen — mehr quantitativer als grundsätzlicher morphologischer Art sind. In der Regel sind die Altersveränderungen an bedeckter Haut geringer ausgebildet. Der Alterungsprozeß bleibt hier häufig um etwa ein Jahrzehnt zurück.

Die Epidermis ist an unbedeckter Haut meist etwas breiter. Dieses Verhältnis wird auch während der Altersinvolution beibehalten. Morphologisch-celluläre Unterschiede finden sich nicht (MURTULA). Die Rückbildung der Reteleisten erfolgt an bedeckter Haut langsamer. Das Stratum corneum ist an unbedeckten Körperstellen im allgemeinen dicker, läßt aber sonst im Alterungsprozeß keine Abweichungen von anderen Regionen erkennen.

Dagegen sind die Differenzen am Bindegewebe der Haut zum Teil erheblich. Insbesondere trifft dies für die Veränderungen zu, die als „senile oder aktinische Elastose" bezeichnet werden und die an konstant bedeckten Hautstellen nicht zu finden sind. (Ausführliche Darstellung s. bei BRAUN-FALCO, Handbuch-Ergänzungswerk, Bd I/2, S. 606.) Abgesehen von diesen Erscheinungen, bei denen immer noch nicht endgültig geklärt ist, ob sie auf Veränderungen der elastischen oder kollagenen Fasern beruhen — vielleicht wird ein minderwertiges Bindegewebe produziert, was teils das Kollagen, teils die Elastica imitiert (STEIGLEDER) — weisen die kollagenen Fasern keine wesentlichen Unterschiede im Alterungsprozeß an bedeckten und unbedeckten Körperstellen auf.

Deutliche Abweichungen bestehen auch in Hinblick auf den Pigmentgehalt der Haut. Dieser läßt an den in der Regel nicht belichteten Hautstellen kaum Änderungen im Alter erkennen, während an belichteten Stellen häufig eine Pigmentvermehrung zu verzeichnen ist. Als Besonderheit dieser Alterspigmentierung ist die ungleichmäßige fleckige Verteilung des Pigmentes zu erwähnen, die auf gewisse Störungen in der Pigmentbildung schließen läßt. Die Grenzen zwischen dieser „normalen Alterspigmentierung" der belichteten Haut und der eher als pathologische Hautveränderung einzuordnenden Lentigo senilis sind fließend.

Auch an den Blutgefäßen scheinen Strukturveränderungen, die als Alterserscheinungen aufgefaßt werden können, an unbedeckten Körperstellen stärker ausgebildet zu sein. Allerdings ist zu bedenken, daß diese Regionen häufig besonderen Kreislaufbedingungen unterliegen.

Alle übrigen Strukturen der Haut lassen nach den bis jetzt vorliegenden Untersuchungen keine besonderen erwähnenswerten Differenzen des Alterungsprozesses an bedeckten und unbedeckten Körperbereichen erkennen.

2. Dicke der Haut

Eine der auffälligsten Altersveränderungen der Haut ist ohne Zweifel die Altersatrophie, also die Dickenabnahme des Hautorgans im höheren Lebensalter. Entsprechende Messungen an der Gesamthaut gehören in das Gebiet der makroskopischen Anatomie und werden daher von H. PINKUS im Bd I/2, S. 4 dieses Handbuch-Ergänzungswerkes abgehandelt. Es interessieren hier nur die mikroskopisch durchgeführten Messungen an den einzelnen Hautschichten. Es sei darauf hingewiesen, daß gerade diese Untersuchungen nicht einfach sind, da sie mit schwer zu beeinflussenden Fehlerquellen belastet sind. So kommt es bei der Verarbeitung der Präparate zu erheblichen Schrumpfungsvorgängen des Gewebes, die je nach der Methode und dem verwendeten Fixierungsmittel stark variieren können. EVANS, COWDRY u. NIELSON machen vor allem darauf aufmerksam, daß die unterschiedliche Retraktionsfähigkeit des Gewebes (besonders des Coriums) auf Grund der physikalisch-chemischen Veränderungen während des Alterungsprozesses bedeutenden Einfluß auf die Dicke einer Hautschicht im fertigen Präparat haben kann. So retrahiert sich die Haut der Ellenbeuge im Alter von 20 bis 25 Jahren nach der Excision um etwa 38—58% und zwischen 80—90 Jahren nur um 12—20%. Durch die starke Coriumschrumpfung in der jugendlichen Haut zieht sich auch die Epidermis zusammen und erscheint im gefärbten Schnitt dicker.

3. Epidermis

Es darf wohl als gesichert angesehen werden, daß mit zunehmendem Alter eine Atrophie der Epidermis stattfindet, die oft schon um das 30. Lebensjahr meßbar einsetzt (STRÖBEL). Nach EJIRI ist diese Atrophie an einzelnen Hautbezirken unterschiedlich stark, während SOUTHWOOD betont, daß diese Differenzen — abgesehen von Finger und Fußsohle — nur gering sind (Tabelle 2). Die Verschmälerung der Epidermis geht vor allem auf Kosten der Reteleisten vor sich (GOLDZIEHER, RAWLS, ROBERTS u. GOLDZIEHER; HILL u. MONTGOMERY; STRÖBEL u.a.), die im mittleren Lebensalter dünner und länger ausgezogen sind und schließlich völlig verschwinden, so daß die Epidermis-Corium-Grenze fast als gerade Linie verläuft (Abb. 1 und 2).

Eine gewisse Rückbildung zeigt jedoch auch das Stratum spinosum (EJIRI, HIMMEL, RONCHESE, SCHALLWEGG, STRÖBEL, VIGNOLI-LUTATI), das nach GOLDZIEHER, RAWLS, ROBERTS u. GOLDZIEHER von durchschnittlich 6—7 auf 3—4 Zellschichten reduziert ist. Dieser Ansicht stimmen allerdings FREEMAN, COCKERELL, ARMSTRONG u. KNOX, HILL u. MONTGOMERY sowie SOUTHWOOD nicht bei. Die Größe der Zellen nimmt ab, wobei sowohl das Cytoplasma als auch der Zellkern an Masse verlieren (Tabelle 3).

Die Zellen zeigen eine verstärkte basophile Anfärbbarkeit (SCHALLWEGG), die nach STRÖBEL teilweise durch eine engere Kernstellung bedingt ist. Ferner ist eine vermehrte Vacuolisierung festzustellen (EJIRI), eine Erscheinung, die eigenartigerweise auch bei der kindlichen und jugendlichen Haut bis etwa zum 25. Lebensjahr zu beobachten ist (HILL u. MONTGOMERY; SCHALLWEGG).

An dem Alterungsprozeß sind selbstverständlich auch die übrigen Schichten der Epidermis beteiligt. Hier sind jedoch stärker ins Auge fallende morphologische Veränderungen oft nicht vorhanden. Am wenigsten davon betroffen scheint dabei das Stratum basale zu sein, das bis ins hohe Greisenalter weitgehend unverändert bleibt. Die morphologischen Differenzierungen zwischen Basal- und Stachelzellen werden jedoch verwischt (GOLDZIEHER, RAWLS, ROBERTS u. GOLDZIEHER; STEIGLEDER u. GANS). BERRES fand im jugendlichen Alter gehäuft besondere Zellformen im Stratum basale, die er als schmal, oval, senkrecht zur Hautoberfläche stehend

Tabelle 2. *Die Dicke der Epidermis in μ nach* Southwood (1955)

Biopsiestelle	männlich/ weiblich	Alter												
		0—5	6—10	11—15	16—20	21—25	26—30	31—35	36—40	41—45	46—50	51—55	56—60	61—65	66—70
Oberschenkel, innen	M	27		84	54		71	53	62		50	51		37	39
	F	50			44		18		55		46	38	39	34	40
Oberschenkel, außen	M	27		83	59		78	60	39		70	69	51	43	37
	F	44			46		63		55		48	45		47	35
Oberschenkel, Rückseite	M	56		86	74		91	58	37		59	54	51	45	33
	F	23					35		48		58	60		53	43
Unterschenkel, innen	M	52		69	53		52	49	55	38	53	51		51	38
	F	73			53		35		113		57	48	47	48	49
Unterschenkel, außen	M	48		80	73		78	61	60	55	72	69		53	42
	F	24			52		39		40		56	51	51	53	55
Unterschenkel, Rückseite	M	43		77	70		80	63	47	57	57	58		55	37
	F						39		57		59	52	49	69	36
Fußsohle	M				864			940	1061		1170	1377	944	1282	529
	F				619				850		1094	1020		707	
Bauch	M	23		51	42		49	46	39		34	43	37	38	31
	F	41			37		34		42		46	41		47	33
Brust	M	57		55	48		62	41	58		39	40	25	33	32
	F	38			35		26		47		46	42		38	
Achsel	M	39			45			43	44		43			45	
	F	22			75						51			50	
Rücken	M	46		67	58		85	53	92		49	50	47	47	44
	F						45		61		56	49			
Schamgegend	M	37			55			48	48		42				
	F				47						43				
Oberarm, innen	M	41		59	42		45	37	52		49	51	34	38	34
	F	23			40				36		42	43		53	30
Oberarm, außen	M	44		57	59		71	46	41		48	49	47	39	35
	F				46		40		54		53	51		42	46
Unterarm, Rückseite	M	53			60			49	65		49	59	55	56	37
	F	29			50		65				53	55		50	
Unterarm, Vorderseite	M	44		79	63		39	56	34		54	57	53	62	38
	F				41				59		61	59		52	46
Finger	M	384			673		567	420	673		432	384	539	532	580
	F				395				539		413			503	
Gesicht	M								52						

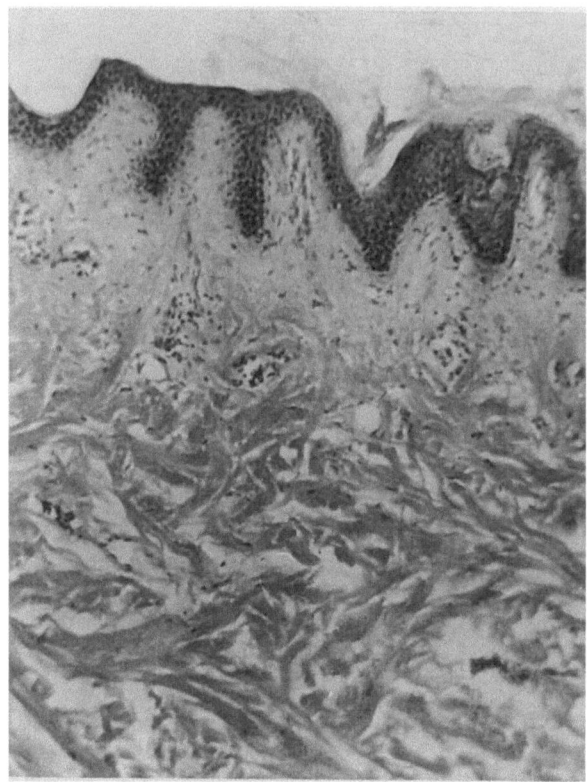

Abb. 1. Epidermis, Stratum reticulare und oberes Corium. Rückenhaut einer 28jährigen Frau. H.-E. Vergr. 150:1

und etwas stärker ins Stratum spinosum vorspringend beschreibt. Dieser Zelltyp soll mit zunehmendem Alter verschwinden.

Das Stratum granulosum wird in seinem Verhalten unterschiedlich beurteilt. Nach RONCHESE und STRÖBEL ist es oft völlig geschwunden, während EVANS, COWDRY u. NIELSON sowie SAALFELD nur eine Verschmälerung feststellten. GOLDZIEHER, RAWLS, ROBERTS u. GOLDZIEHER beobachteten eine Reduzierung der Kerato-Hyalin-Granula. Nach EJIRI ist diese Epidermisschicht meist nicht verändert, während HILL u. MONTGOMERY sogar eine gewisse Verbreiterung mit zunehmendem Alter andeuten. Diese Widersprüche finden vielleicht in den Hinweisen von SCHALLWEGG und SOUTHWOOD eine Erklärung, wobei SCHALLWEGG die Ansicht vertritt, daß im allgemeinen die Unterschiede zu gering sind, um daraus Schlüsse ziehen zu können, während SOUTHWOOD nur einen Zusammenhang mit der Stärke der Hornschicht fand.

Über Veränderungen des Stratum lucidum im Alterungsprozeß liegen noch keine verbindlichen Angaben vor, da diese Schicht an den meisten Körperstellen, die zu den hier interessierenden Untersuchungen herangezogen werden, nicht oder nur zu gering ausgebildet ist. Wahrscheinlich besteht aber nur ein Zusammenhang mit der Intensität der Hornbildung (HILL u. MONTGOMERY).

Das Stratum corneum läßt im allgemeinen eine Aufteilung in eine kompakte und in eine lockere, lamelläre Hornschicht erkennen. Die Alterungsveränderungen spielen sich im wesentlichen in einem unterschiedlichen Verhältnis dieser beiden Bereiche zueinander ab. Nach SCHALLWEGG ist im 1.—5. Lebensjahr der kompakte

Epidermis

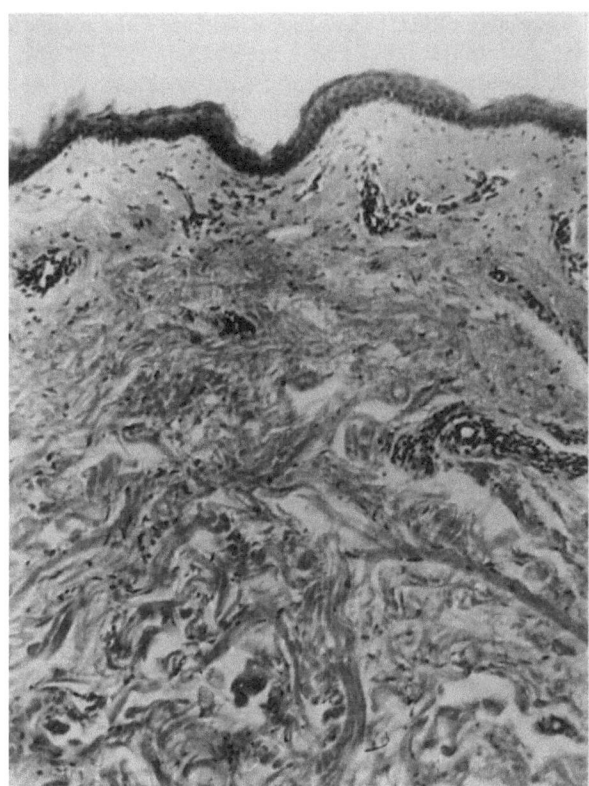

Abb. 2. Epidermis, Stratum reticulare und oberes Corium. Rückenhaut einer 83jährigen Frau. H.-E. Vergr. 150:1

Tabelle 3. *Durchmesser der Zellen im Stratum spinosum (in μ) nach* MURTULA *(1953)*

Alter	Fall-Nr.	Abdomen	Handrücken	Gesicht (Jochbein)
30—40	22	11/13 × 10/12	14/16 × 12/14	14/16 × 10/12
	23	14/16 × 11/13	14/16 × 12/14	16/18 × 15/17
40—50	8	12/14 × 10/12		
	16	10/12 × 8/10		
	20	12/14 × 9/11	18/20 × 14/10	16/18 × 10/12
	9	12/14 × 8/10		
50—60	1	11/13 × 8/10		
	6	12/14 × 10/12		
	17	10/12 × 8/10		
	11	12/14 × 10/12	10/12 × 8/10	12/14 × 10/12
	14	12/14 × 9/11	16/18 × 14/16	14/16 × 10/12
	15	12/14 × 9/11		
	19	11/13 × 8/10		
	21	11/13 × 8/10	16/18 × 12/14	16/18 × 10/12
	10	12/14 × 8/10		
60—70	2	12/14 × 8/10		
	5	14/16 × 12/14	20/22 × 16/18	14/16 × 12/14
	4	12/14 × 10/12		
	7			14/16 × 10/12
	13	10/12 × 8/10		
	12	—		
70—80	3	12/14 × 8/10		
	18	10/12 × 8/10	14/16 × 9/11	14/16 × 11/13

Teil dünn und die lamelläre Abschilferungszone breit. Mit steigendem Alter wird der kompaktere Anteil immer breiter und erreicht mit etwa 30 Jahren seine größte Dicke. Dann setzt wieder eine Rückbildung dieser Schicht ein, und die Abschilferung des Stratum corneum nimmt zu. Im ganzen gesehen ergibt sich in der Regel eine Verschmälerung der Hornschicht in höheren Lebensjahren. Diese Darstellung entspricht auch den Ansichten von EVANS, COWDRY u. NIELSON; HIMMEL; SOUTHWOOD und STRÖBEL. HILL u. MONTGOMERY konnten sich dagegen nicht von altersbedingten Veränderungen des Stratum corneum überzeugen. Histochemische Befunde, die auf einen anderen Ablauf der Verhornungsprozesse im Alter hindeuten, liegen bisher nicht vor (MANGANOTTI; SILVESTRI, 1960). Sie sind aufgrund unserer zur Zeit auf diesem Gebiet selbst bei der normalen Verhornung noch unbefriedigenden Kenntnisse auch kaum zu erwarten.

Als ein Schlüssel zur Klärung der Prozesse, die zu einer Altersatrophie des Hautoberflächenepithels führen, wurde von vielen Untersuchern die Regenerationsfähigkeit der Epidermis betrachtet. Es finden sich daher in der Literatur relativ eingehende Studien über die *Anzahl der Mitosen* in der Epidermis in den verschiedenen Lebensaltern. Es sei jedoch darauf aufmerksam gemacht, daß BERRES und NELKE die Ansicht vertreten, daß die Regeneration der Epidermis überwiegend durch eine amitotische Zellteilung erfolgt und somit die Zahl der gefundenen Mitosen nicht unbedingt ein Ausdruck der Regenerationsfähigkeit ist.

Die Untersuchungen stellten zunächst einmal klar, daß Mitosen nicht nur im Stratum basale und den untersten Lagen des Stratum spinosum vorkommen, sondern auch noch im mittleren Drittel der Stachelzellschicht zu finden sind. Die Mitosehäufigkeit ist dabei in diesen 3 Bereichen in den einzelnen Lebensaltern unterschiedlich. Die Zellteilungsaktivität des Stratum basale steigt von Geburt bis ins hohe Alter gleichmäßig an. Die Zahl der Mitosen im unteren Drittel des Stratum spinosum bleibt weitgehend konstant, während diese im mittleren Drittel auf etwa 65% abfällt (KATZBERG; THURINGER u. KATZBERG). Damit übernehmen die Zellen des Stratum basale im Alter mehr und mehr die Regeneration der Epidermis. Gleichzeitig steigt aber auch die Mitosenzahl von 1:4840 in der 1. Lebensdekade auf 1:2222 in der 8. Lebensdekade. Dies bedeutet eine Abnahme der Lebenszeit der Zellen von etwa 101 auf 46 Tage. Die Gesamtzahl der Zellen pro Flächeneinheit wird somit geringer. Insgesamt ist die Abschilferungsquote größer als die Regenerationsrate, so daß es zwangsläufig zu einer Verschmälerung der Epidermis kommen muß (KATZBERG; MANGANOTTI, 1955a). Zu ähnlichen Ergebnissen gelangten MEYER, MARWAH u. WEINMANN bei ihren Untersuchungen an der Mundschleimhaut.

Die Zahl der Epidermiszellen mit dem sog. Barrschen Geschlechtschromatin geht im Alter deutlich zurück, wobei bei Frauen eine erhebliche Streubreite der Häufigkeitszahlen auftritt (SILVESTRI, 1956c).

Mit dem Verhalten der Epidermis der Zehenzwischenräume in verschiedenen Lebensaltern beschäftigt sich OBRUČNIK. Der Alterungsprozeß läuft hier ähnlich ab, jedoch finden sich im Vergleich zu anderen Körperstellen mehr hyperkeratotisch-acanthotische Erscheinungen.

Die Veränderung der Epidermis am Penis mit seinen topographischen Besonderheiten untersuchte KANTNER. Er fand mit zunehmendem Alter einen Rückgang der Epidermisstärke an der Facies dorsalis und der Facies lateralis, während die Epidermis der Facies urethralis sich verdicken soll.

Eine auffällig, altersabhängige Erscheinung zeigt das Epithel der Mundschleimhaut. Im Säuglings- und Kindesalter finden sich hier gehäuft große blasige Zellen mit reichlich hellem Protoplasma. Diese Zellform geht mit zunehmendem Alter zurück und ist im Senium verschwunden. Eine ähnliche Entwicklung zeigt auch der Glykogengehalt der Schleimhautepithelzellen (BIZZOZERO u. DOGLIOTTI).

4. Pigmentierung

Es ist eine sehr verbreitete Ansicht, daß im Alter eine verstärkte Pigmentierung der Haut zu finden ist. Nach den bisher vorliegenden objektiveren Untersuchungen kann dies aber durchaus nicht generell behauptet werden. Diese Konzeption scheint keineswegs für die Haut an üblicherweise bedeckten Körperstellen zu gelten, an der man allein genauere Aussagen über reine Altersveränderungen der Haut machen kann; es können sonst zahlreiche Befunde mit erfaßt werden, die mehr durch exogenen Faktoren — insbesondere Witterungs- und UV-Einflüsse — bedingt sind.

Eine Veränderung der Zahl der Melanocyten scheint im Alter weder an belichteter noch an unbelichteter Haut zu erfolgen, wenn man die unterschiedliche topographische Anhäufung dieser Zellen mitberücksichtigt (STARICCO u. PINKUS). Diese Feststellung muß aber nicht unbedingt entscheidend für die Beurteilung einer evtl. verstärkten Alterspigmentierung sein, da die Hautfarbe mehr vom Pigmentgehalt als von der Zahl der Melanocyten abzuhängen scheint. Nach BECKER, FITZPATRICK u. MONTGOMERY ist z.B. die Zahl dieser Zellen in der Haut von Negern, Albinos und in Vitiligoherden etwa gleich.

SCOLARI betont daher auch eine Erhöhung der Pigmentkinese und des Pigmentstoffwechsels in der Altershaut. Dies trifft aber wohl nur für die regelmäßig belichtete Haut zu und wurde hier auch von EJIRI mikroskopisch bestätigt. Eine Pigmentzunahme an meist unbelichteter Haut (z.B. Bauchhaut) wird von HILL u. MONTGOMERY sowie STRÖBEL entschieden abgelehnt. NELKE gibt für diesen Hautbereich sogar eine Verminderung des Pigments im Alter an. An fakultativ belichteten Körperstellen (z.B. Oberarm) fand SCHALLWEGG eine mäßig verstärkte, meist nur an den Enden der Reteleisten zu beobachtende Pigmentierung.

Eine verstärkte Alterspigmentierung scheint jedoch an topographisch-anatomisch besonders gelagerten Körperstellen vorzukommen, wie einschlägigen Untersuchungen an der weiblichen Genital- und Analhaut von BUTTGE zu entnehmen ist.

5. Corium

Es wird allgemein behauptet, daß die Dicke des Coriums von der Geburt bis zum 20.—30. Lebensjahr zunimmt und dann allmählich wieder zurückgeht (SCHALLWEGG, SOUTHWOOD). Das vorliegende Zahlenmaterial ist aber noch nicht ausreichend, um exakte Angaben unter Berücksichtigung der Rasse, des Geschlechtes, der Konstitution und der Körperregion machen zu können. Auch sind gerade die Dickenmessungen der Lederhaut durch deren erhebliche Elastizität und Schrumpfungsneigung äußerst schwierig. Zur Orientierung sind die von SOUTHWOOD ermittelten Werte in Tabelle 4 angegeben.

Während HIMMEL und VOHWINCKEL den Standpunkt vertreten, daß die Altersverschmälerung des Coriums überwiegend durch die Atrophie des Kollagens bedingt sei, dürfte wohl die Annahme einer Reduzierung aller Gewebsstrukturen (EJIRI, SCHALLWEGG) eher zutreffen.

Grobstrukturell macht sich mit zunehmendem Alter ein Verwischen der Unterschiede zwischen dem feinfaserigen Stratum reticulare und dem breitfaserigen eigentlichen Corium bemerkbar (STRÖBEL). Die in das subcutane Fettgewebe einstrahlenden Bindegewebssepten werden in der Altershaut immer dünner, kürzer und spärlicher bis schließlich im hohen Senium eine fast gerade verlaufende Corium-Subcutis-Grenze ausgebildet ist. Die netzförmige Verflechtung der Bindegewebsfasern wird während des Alterungsprozesses zunehmend in eine parallele Schichtung der Fasern umgewandelt. BERRES und NELKE machen ferner darauf aufmerksam, daß die Altersveränderungen im Corium oft ausgesprochen herdförmig entwickelt sind.

Tabelle 4. *Die Dicke des Coriums in μ nach* Southwood (1955)

Biopsiestelle	männlich/weiblich	Alter 0—5	6—10	11—15	16—20	21—25	26—30	31—35	36—40	41—45	46—50	51—55	56—60	61—65	66—70
Oberschenkel, innen	M	636					1258	1312	1295		1161	1125		1037	1027
	F	510		576	1083		1071		978		941	877	833	841	796
Oberschenkel, außen	M	561		638	1226		1802	1547	1537		1161	1472		1284	1199
	F	814			996		1367		1229		1351	1314	949	913	851
Oberschenkel, Rückseite	M	863		1056	1278		1314	1168	1217		1071	1101	1153	1020	1013
	F	527					1088	1151	1017	857	1102	1071		1176	1180
Unterschenkel, innen	M	828		913	957		1634		1887		957	1122		879	1187
	F	440			578		816	1136	757	1217	706	714	694	622	505
Unterschenkel, außen	M	692		913	1375		1573		1683		923	1115		1037	1095
	F	506			802		634	1365	694	1081	741	1005	865	758	530
Unterschenkel, Rückseite	M	532		536	1404		1672		1173		1209	984		1029	901
	F						1071		847		826	833	731	865	638
Fußsohle	M	575			996				1805		1263	1593		1561	1346
	F	710			867				1535					1571	1008
Bauch	M	536		1020	1741		2015	1933	2584		1741	1862	1491	1516	1363
	F	860		655	1195		1088		1289		1174	1494		1394	
Brust	M	466			1418		1683	1960	1752		1392	1499		1027	
	F	527			1307		867		1532		1261	1224	1083		
Achsel	M	840		1102	1230			1296	1188		1076			1006	2242
	F				1292						1091			1972	
Rücken	M				2458		2159	2492	2193		2397	2300	1559	1666	
	F	932					1930	969	1535		1456	1583			
Schamgegend	M				826				1107		921				
	F				859						867				
Oberarm, innen	M	510		558	855		1275	1246	796		1173	1190	689	1103	976
	F	464			615						727	743		645	563
Oberarm, außen	M	901		806	1314		1430	1843	1941		1284	1522	672	1301	1029
	F				961		1097		1252		996	918		974	1224
Unterarm, Rückseite	M	935			1197			1234	1020		1013	1018	706	972	852
	F	561		551	1071		1107	1148	1248		827	833		681	
Unterarm, Vorderseite	M	757			1042		918		845		976	1043	668	1003	940
	F				850						812	774		689	692
Finger	M								1326		1207			1200	
	F											894			
Gesicht	M								2271						1411

Seit Einführung der PAS-Reaktion in die Dermato-Histologie liegen zahlreiche Befunde über die *Basalmembran* vor, jedoch scheinen sich bisher noch keine Untersuchungen speziell mit dem Verhalten dieses Hautanteils im Alter befaßt zu haben. Im Greisenalter dürfte aber häufiger eine Verdichtung und Verbreiterung des subepidermalen Grenzstreifens eintreten. Ferner wird durch eine Anhäufung PAS-positiver Substanzen im subepidermalen Bereich des Stratum reticulare die Abgrenzung nach dem Bindegewebe zu unschärfer (MANGANOTTI, 1955b; SOMMERS). Nach HILL u. MONTGOMERY finden sich an der Basalmembran im Senium keine Besonderheiten.

Über das Verhalten der *Bindegewebsgrundsubstanz* im Alter lassen sich noch keine sicheren Aussagen machen, da die wenigen darüber vorliegenden Angaben widersprüchlich und zum Teil auch nur sehr allgemein formuliert sind (BANFIELD; DAY; HORSTMANN; MA u. COWDRY; MANGANOTTI, 1955b; SILVESTRI u. MAURIZI).

Die *kollagenen Fasern* werden dünner, teils liegen sie gestreckter, teils aber auch wirr und ungeordneter und zeigen eine zunehmende Homogenisierung (HILL u. MONTGOMERY; STEIGLEDER; STRÖBEL u.a.) (Abb. 3 und 4).

Zu ähnlichen Ergebnissen führten auch elektronenmikroskopische Untersuchungen. So nimmt die Fibrillendicke an unbedeckter Haut im Mittelwert um 4,68 mµ ab, während an bedeckter Haut dieser Wert geringer und nicht statistisch signifikant ist (TELLER, VESTER u. POHL). Außerdem sind die Fibrillen starr, häufig frakturiert und liegen enger zusammen. Nach LINKE betragen die Fibrillenstärken im Erwachsenenalter 30—100 mµ und im Greisenalter 20—80 mµ. Die Fibrillen zeigen ferner im Senium überwiegend eine unregelmäßige Außenversilberung. Die interfibrilläre Kittsubstanz nimmt zu, maskiert die Periodizität der Fibrillen und ist oft flächenhaft sowie spinnennetzartig angeordnet (LINKE; TELLER, VESTER u. POHL).

Während TELLER, VESTER u. POHL glauben, daß diese Vermehrung der interfibrillären Kittsubstanz auch ihren Ausdruck in einer stärkeren Toluidinblau-Metachromasie findet, konnte diese LINKE nicht beobachten. Er schließt daraus auf eine andere histochemische Zusammensetzung dieser Substanz als beim Embryo, wo eine starke Metachromasie zu verzeichnen sei. Das PAS-reaktive Verhalten der kollagenen Fasern scheint sich im Alter nicht auffällig zu verändern.

Die bekannte Änderung des Elastizitätsmoduls (s. WAGNER) der Haut hat verständlicherweise den Anlaß dazu gegeben, bei mikroskopischen Untersuchungen der Altershaut ein besonderes Augenmerk auf die *elastischen Fasern* zu richten, die man in erster Linie für dieses Phänomen verantwortlich machte. Insgesamt gesehen sind aber die morphologischen Alterserscheinungen an diesen Fasern im Bereich der bedeckten Haut keineswegs so erheblich, wie man vielleicht erwarten könnte. Im Gegensatz dazu findet man in der überwiegend lichtexponierten Haut massive Erscheinungen, die als sog. senile oder actinische Elastose bekannt sind. Über die Altersveränderungen der elastischen Fasern an bedeckter und unbedeckter Haut findet sich von BRAUN-FALCO eine ausführliche Darstellung unserer derzeitigen Kenntnisse im Bd. I/2, S. 604 und 606 dieses Handbuch-Ergänzungswerkes, so daß auf diese Abschnitte verwiesen werden muß.

Die Morphologie der *argyrophilen Fasern* in der Altershaut wurde bisher wenig beachtet. Nach TELLER, VESTER u. POHL sowie STRÖBEL erscheinen sie kaum verändert. Sie liegen — wie auch die anderen Bindegewebsfasern — dichter, gestreckter und sind in der Gesamtzahl vermindert.

Die Zahl der *Fibrocyten* nimmt während des Alterungsvorganges konstant ab, so daß die senile Haut kernarm ist (BERRES; STEIGLEDER u.a.). Die auch in den Fibrocyten nachweisbaren Barrschen Chromatinkörperchen sind in ihrer Zahl

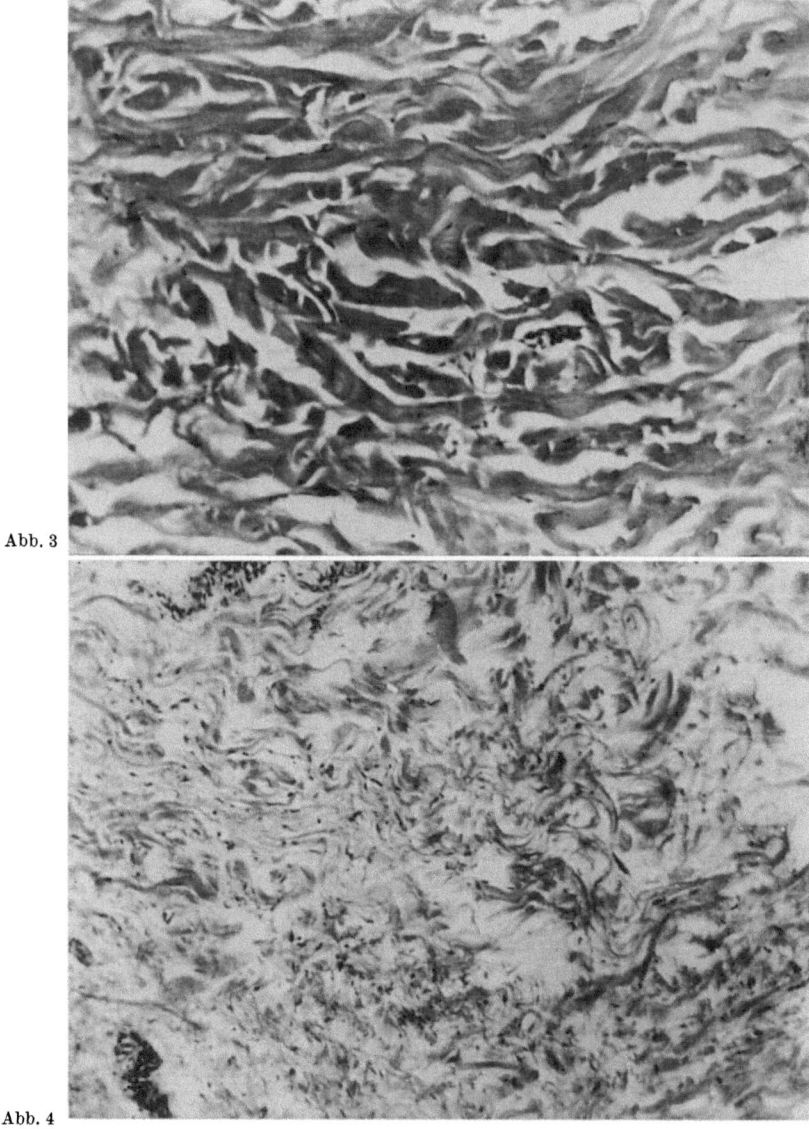

Abb. 3. Bindegewebsfasern des Corium. Rückenhaut einer 28jährigen Frau. H.-E. Vergr. 150:1
Abb. 4. Bindegewebsfasern des Corium. Rückenhaut einer 83jährigen Frau. H.-E. Vergr. 150:1

wenig altersabhängig. Erst bei Personen über 80 Jahren ist eine Verminderung nachweisbar (SILVESTRI, 1959a).

Als weitere zellige Bestandteile der normalen Haut sind die *Mastzellen* zu erwähnen. Über deren Häufigkeit in verschiedenen Altersstufen liegen genauere Zahlen vor. HELLSTRÖM u. HOLMGREN ermittelten bei 40 Personen die Anzahl der Mastzellen in der Haut (Bauch, Unterschenkel, Fußrücken) und fanden bei Neugeborenen 7000 Mastzellen pro mm^3. Bei 70—80jährigen waren nur noch 1000 Zellen pro mm^3 nachweisbar. Gleichzeitig waren häufiger Mastzellen anzutreffen, die eine sehr schwache Metachromasie der Granula zeigten. Zu einem ähnlichen Ergebnis kamen BRACK sowie MONTAGNA u. MELARAGNO. Zwischen dem 27. und 50. Lebensjahr sahen jedoch MIKHALL u. MILLER-MILINSKA in ihrem Untersuchungsmaterial keine signifikanten Änderungen der Mastzellenzahlen. Nach NELKE ist die Zahl der Mastzellen in der Haut weitgehend von dem Ausmaß der Vascularisation abhängig. Mit der Verminderung der Gefäße im Alter ist somit zwangsläufig auch eine Abnahme der Mastzellen verbunden. Außerdem werden die Zellen kleiner, sind weniger gestreckt, die Granula werden gröber und liegen gehäuft in der Zellperipherie, so daß ein perinucleärer Hof entsteht.

In der Altershaut finden sich schließlich noch häufig geringe *Rundzell-Infiltrate*, die meist in der Umgebung der Gefäße und Hautanhangsgebilde liegen. Es ist noch nicht endgültig geklärt, ob diese Zellen im Zusammenhang mit den Abbau- und Umbauvorgängen der senilen Haut stehen oder nur die Folge entzündlicher Reaktionen auf irgendwelche exogene Reize sind. Im allgemeinen wird ihnen wenig Bedeutung beigemessen, da sie auch bei jugendlichen Personen gefunden werden (EJIRI; GANS u. STEIGLEDER; HIMMEL; SCHALLWEGG).

6. Glatte Muskulatur

Ob und in welchem Umfange Altersveränderungen an der glatten Muskulatur der Haut vorkommen, ist noch recht umstritten. EJIRI sowie HILL u. MONTGOMERY sind derartige Zustände nicht aufgefallen. Nach SCHALLWEGG ist die Anzahl der Muskelbündel vom 2.—70. Lebensjahr fast konstant; erst dann ist eine deutliche Abnahme zu verzeichnen. Demgegenüber stellte HIMMEL eine Vermehrung der glatten Muskulatur fest. Jedoch kann diese Zunahme auch nur durch die Atrophie des Bindegewebes vorgetäuscht sein (VIGNOLI-LUTATI). Die Muskelbündel sind im Kindesalter relativ dünn, nehmen dann bis etwa 40 Jahre an Dicke zu und sinken schließlich wieder im Durchmesser konstant ab (HIMMEL, SCHALLWEGG).

Die Länge der Muskelfasern soll keine Veränderung dabei zeigen (SCHALLWEGG). Die von NEUMANN beobachtete Trübung des Muskelcytoplasmas im Alter konnte von HIMMEL nicht bestätigt werden. SCHALLWEGG fand nach dem 75. Lebensjahr eine Hyalinisierung der Fasern, sowie deformierte, spindelförmige Kerne mit Chromatinolyse und schlechter Anfärbung.

Weitere Ausführungen über Altersveränderungen der glatten Muskulatur der Haut s. bei ANDRADE (Handbuch-Ergänzungswerk Bd. I/2, S. 661).

7. Talgdrüsen

Die Trockenheit und Sprödigkeit der Altershaut wird häufig auf eine Atrophie der Talgdrüsen zurückgeführt. Jedoch scheinen dafür noch keine gesicherten Angaben auf Grund überzeugender Untersuchungen vorzuliegen. EJIRI sowie HILL u. MONTGOMERY konnten im Gegensatz zu SILVESTRI (1959b) keine Altersatrophie in ihrem Material beobachten. Nach BRILLANTI u. BENEFENATI, die sich jedoch nur auf Untersuchungen an 7 Personen stützen können, ist die Zahl der Talgdrüsen mit der Geburt festgelegt, so daß die Häufigkeit und Dichte der Talgdrüsen in der menschlichen Haut im wesentlichen durch das Größen- und Flächenwachstum des Körpers bestimmt wird. Aus diesem Grund sind die Talgdrüsen z. B. im 3. Lebensjahr recht gleichmäßig verteilt und liegen relativ dicht. Dann erfolgt eine Auflockerung durch das Körperwachstum und erst nach dem 60. Jahr soll eine geringe echte Atrophie vorkommen. Aufgrund klinischer Beobachtungen muß aber darauf aufmerksam gemacht werden, daß die Talgdrüsen in den einzelnen Körperregionen wahrscheinlich eine unterschiedliche Entwicklung durchmachen dürften.

Befunde über spezielle morphologische Veränderungen an den Talgdrüsen im Senium liegen bisher in der Literatur nicht vor. SILVESTRI (1959) bestimmte die Zahl der Barrschen Geschlechtschromatin-Körperchen in den Talgdrüsenzellen der Rückenhaut und beobachtete im Senium gegenüber dem mittleren Lebensalter eine Zunahme dieser Strukturen. Dies steht im Gegensatz zu den Befunden an den Epidermiszellen und den Fibrocyten und könnte mit der Funktion der Talgdrüsen in Beziehung zu bringen sein.

8. Ekkrine Schweißdrüsen

Die Zahl der ekkrinen Schweißdrüsen dürfte bei Kindern und Jugendlichen pro Flächeneinheit etwa 3—4fach höher liegen als bei Erwachsenen (PINKUS, SCHALLWEGG). Im höheren Alter ist eine weitere Rückbildung zu verzeichnen (BERRES; KALANTAEVSKAYA u. GURINA), jedoch ist unter Berücksichtigung der erheblichen topographischen Unterschiede deren Ausmaß noch nicht durch genügende Untersuchungen klar belegt. SCHALLWEGG konnte z. B. an der Bauchhaut keine eindeutige Abnahme dieser Drüsen feststellen, auch war eine Größenreduzierung nicht auffällig. Durch die Atrophie der Haut liegen die Drüsen etwas höher (HIMMEL, SCHALLWEGG).

Nach EJIRI ist im Senium eine Hornpfropfbildung in den Mündungen der Ausführungsgänge zu verzeichnen, wogegen HILL u. MONTGOMERY derartige Erscheinungen gerade bei Kindern als sehr auffällig herausstellen.

Die histomorphologischen Altersveränderungen an den Endstücken dieser Drüsen dürften im allgemeinen klarer und eindeutiger ausgebildet sein als bei den apokrinen Drüsen, wie man den weniger widersprüchlichen einschlägigen Beobachtungen entnehmen kann. Die ekkrinen Drüsenzellen vacuolisieren im Alter schneller als die apokrinen und lösen sich auch leichter aus dem Zellverband (IWASHIGE, SCHALLWEGG). Der Lipidgehalt im Cytoplasma der sezernierenden Zellen ist bei Kindern geringer als bei Erwachsenen und kann bei alten Personen sehr erheblich sein (KANO, KUSNETZ). Das in den gleichen Zellen vorkommende gelbbraune Pigment fehlt bei Kindern und ist im Alter meist reichlich eingelagert. Die PAS-positiven Zellsubstanzen scheinen dagegen nicht altersabhängig zu sein (MONTAGNA). Nach den Untersuchungen von IWASHIGE sind die in der Jugend meist fadenförmigen Mitochondrien im Alter stäbchenförmig oder körnig. Die Aktivität der Aminopeptidasen soll nach ADACHI u. MONTAGNA im Senium deutlich zurückgehen. Über ein ähnliches Verhalten anderer Enzyme liegen in der Literatur keine eindeutigen Angaben vor. Das Gefäßnetz der ekkrinen Schweißdrüsen ist bis ins hohe Alter relativ unverändert (MONTAGNA).

9. Apokrine Schweißdrüsen

Untersuchungen über Altersveränderungen der apokrinen Schweißdrüsen sind nicht einfach, da die Materialbeschaffung Schwierigkeiten bereitet und selbst auf dem Gebiet der normalen Anatomie dieser Drüsen noch erhebliche Meinungsverschiedenheiten bestehen. So wird von manchen Untersuchern das normale Vorkommen dieser Glandulae auf recht umschriebene Körperteile begrenzt, und Drüsen an anderen Stellen werden als ektopisch bezeichnet, während H. PINKUS die möglichen normalen Verteilungszonen recht weit zieht. Bei der mikroskopischen Beurteilung dieser Drüsen ist die erhebliche Formvariabilität ihrer Zellen im Rahmen der Sekretion zu beachten. Dies hat z. B. dazu geführt, daß bis heute noch keine Einigung erzielt werden konnte, welche beim Morbus Fox-Fordyce als charakteristisch beschriebenen Veränderungen an den Drüsenzellen evtl. noch als völlig normale Funktionszustände angesehen werden müssen (siehe z. B. NIKOLOWSKI u. WITTIG; HEITE u. ZAUN). Zu beachten ist auch die sehr große Anfälligkeit des sekretorischen Zellanteils für postmortale Veränderungen (MONTAGNA; CANEGHEM), die leicht zu Fehlbeurteilungen Anlaß geben können.

Die apokrinen Drüsen sind bis etwa zum 4. Lebensjahr nur sehr schwer von ekkrinen Drüsen zu unterscheiden. Um das 7.—8. Lebensjahr setzt in der Regel eine rapide Entwicklung der apokrinen Drüsen ein, so daß sie mit 10—11 Jahren meist die Strukturen normaler Erwachsenen-Drüsen erreicht haben (MONTAGNA; MONTES, BAKER u. CURTIS). Eine Rückbildung der apokrinen Drüsen im Alter wird häufig erwähnt, scheint jedoch kaum zahlenmäßig exakt belegt. Die Flächengröße des Verteilungsareals geht nach GLOOR-RUTISHAUSER im Senium nicht zurück.

Äußerst problematisch ist die Aussage über histologisch-morphologische Altersveränderungen. Als solche könnten gedeutet werden: Atrophie der Epithelzellen (ITO u. IWASHIGE), cystische Erweiterungen der Lumina, mukoide Metaplasie (WINKELMANN u. HULTIN). MONTAGNA fand derartige Erscheinungen bei Frauen schon im Alter von 20—30 Jahren. Er bestätigt auch deren Zunahme im späteren Lebensalter, wobei sie in der Menopause am häufigsten vorkommen, zweifelt aber daran, daß es sich hier um echte Altersveränderungen handelt. Es finden sich nämlich bis ins höchste Alter auch eine große Anzahl von völlig unveränderten Drüsenkörpern.

Dies soll auch für die bei älteren Personen häufiger in den Sekretzellen anzutreffenden Einlagerungen von Pigmentgranula, Lipiden, Eisen und den PAS-positiven und Diastase-resistenten Körperchen gelten. Der Glykogengehalt ist meist vermindert (ITO u. IWASHIGE). Falls man überhaupt von irgendwelchen „spezifischen" Altersveränderungen reden kann, so will MONTAGNA diese nur in der Tatsache sehen, daß auch die noch gut erhaltenen Drüsenzellen sehr leicht geschädigt werden und daher wie schlecht fixiert oder autolytisch wirken. Derartige Erscheinungen sah dieser Autor nie bei jugendlichen Personen.

Eine Erklärung für die Diskrepanz, die in diesen Befunden und ihrer Wertung liegt, deutet VAN CANEGHEM an. Er untersuchte die Strukturen „heterotoper" apokriner Drüsen (meist aus dem Gesichtsbereich) und kam in Übereinstimmung mit BRANCA und HOLMGREEN zu dem Ergebnis, daß es nicht nur typische, rein apokrine Drüsen gibt, sondern auch solche, die nach dem Ausführungsgang zu Segmente enthalten, die aus flachen, hellen, mehrschichtigen, nach dem Drüsenlumen wenig gefransten Zellen bestehen (sog. „intermediäre" Drüsen). Außerdem soll es auch reine Intermediär-Drüsen geben. Folgt man den Gedanken von CANEGHEM, so wäre es möglich, daß z. B. die von WINCKELMANN u. HULTIN beschriebene „mucoide Dysplasie" in Wirklichkeit Intermediärdrüsen-Partien darstellen, die immer vermischt mit reinen apokrinen Drüsen vorkommen. Es würde dann in diesen Strukturen kein Alterungsprozeß der Drüsen vorliegen, sondern höchstens eine Verschiebung des Verhältnisses dieser Drüsen bzw. Drüsenanteile zueinander.

Die gegebene Darstellung der Altersveränderungen der apokrinen Drüsen stützt sich auf Untersuchungen derartiger Drüsen aus der Achselhöhle oder Schamgegend. Es besteht aber bisher kein Grund zur Annahme, daß sich diese Drüsen im Bereich der Nase, des Gehörganges und der Mamille wesentlich anders verhalten.

Von den Ceruminaldrüsen ist vielleicht die Erweiterung der Drüsengänge dicht unterhalb der Epidermis erwähnenswert, die im Alter besonders auffallen soll (HORSTMANN).

10. Die Brustdrüse

Kurz umrissen seien noch die Altersveränderungen der weiblichen und männlichen Brustdrüse, die zwar auch in der Haut gelegene Drüsen darstellen, deren Erkrankungen aber den Dermatologen in der Regel wenig beschäftigen. Da sich jedoch in der letzten Zeit die Fertilitätsdiagnostik und -therapie beim Manne zu einem wichtigen Teilgebiet der Dermatologie entwickelt haben, damit zwangsläufig auch ein erhöhtes Interesse an hormonell-andrologischen Problemen verbunden ist, dürfte in der Zukunft wahrscheinlich gerade der männlichen Brustdrüse in der Dermatologie stärkere Beachtung geschenkt werden.

Mit der Altersinvolution der *weiblichen Brustdrüse* haben sich vor allem DABELOW und WALCHSHOFER beschäftigt. Nach ihren Untersuchungen setzt diese Rückbildung schon im 3. Lebensjahrzehnt ein. Sie beginnt mit der Proliferation von Fettgewebe in den peripheren Drüsenanteilen, das sich dann immer mehr nach dem Zentrum zu ausbreitet. Mit dieser Fettgewebsproliferation geht eine in der Peripherie beginnende Reduktion der Acini und Lobuli parallel. Das perilobuläre Bindegewebe verdichtet sich. Die Alveolen verlieren ihre Lumina und werden zu acinösen Drüsenbeeren. Das Bindegewebe ist von Rundzellinfiltraten einschließlich phagocytierender Wanderzellen durchsetzt. Einzelne Epithelbereiche färben sich schlecht an, sind unscharf konturiert und werden von diesen Zellinfiltraten durchdrungen. Um den Zeitpunkt der Menopause sind häufig cystische Dilationen der Drüsengänge festzustellen. Nach der Menopause geht der Abbau der epithelialen Gewebsanteile weiter, jedoch finden sich jetzt kaum noch Zellinfiltrate. Noch verbliebene Drüsenläppchen sitzen an großen Gängen der ersten Verzweigungsordnung. Das Bindegewebe zeigt Sklerosierung, Homogenisierung und manchmal herdförmige Verkalkungen. Die elastischen Fasern sind insbesondere nach dem 65. Lebensjahr zahlenmäßig vermehrt, zeigen Körnelung, Schollenbildung und Klumpung.

Unsere Kenntnisse über die Altersveränderungen der *männlichen Brustdrüse* beruhen im wesentlichen auf den Untersuchungen von GRAUMANN, GUSNAR und PFALTZ. Nach diesen Autoren verläuft die Entwicklung für beide Geschlechter bis zur Pubertät etwa gleichartig. Dann bleibt die männliche Brustdrüse jedoch weitgehend auf diesem Stadium stehen. Gewisse Proliferationsphasen sind aber beim Mann wieder im 3. und 7. Lebensjahrzehnt festzustellen. Die in der Kindheit vorwiegend gestreckt verlaufenden Milchgänge zeigen mit zunehmendem Alter eine Schlängelung. Das Kaliber der Gänge wird deutlich größer. Etwa ab dem 4. Lebensjahrzehnt treten echte Erweiterungen auf, die nach dem Senium zu an Zahl ansteigen. Neben diesen cystischen Veränderungen sind dann auch Atrophie-Erscheinungen häufiger anzutreffen. Bis ins höchste Alter hinein finden sich aber Drüsenzellen mit Anzeichen einer sekretorischen Aktivität. Vom 4. Lebensjahrzehnt an sind als besonders auffällig Zellproliferationen zu beobachten, die nach den Lumina der Milchgänge gerichtet sind. Auch nach dem 60. Lebensjahr kommt es nach GRAUMANN nicht zu einer massiven Altersatrophie der männlichen Brustdrüse. Über das Verhalten spezieller Zellformen der Brustdrüse sei auf die oben zitierten Originalarbeiten verwiesen.

11. Haar und Haarfollikel

Die Behaarung und in einem gewissen Umfang auch das Haar als solches sind im Laufe des Lebens erheblichen Wandlungen unterzogen. Die meisten bekannten Tatsachen über die Altersveränderungen an diesem Hautanhangsgebilde finden sich in dem Abschnitt „Die makroskopische Anatomie der Haut" von H. PINKUS

(Bd. I/2). Weitere Einzelheiten sind bei RICHTER (Bd. I/3) nachzulesen. Hier sei daher nur kurz auf einige Befunde eingegangen, die speziell in den Bereich der mikroskopischen Anatomie der Haut gehören.

Die Haare sind im 1. Lebensjahr am dünnsten und am ehesten als rund zu bezeichnen. Sie nehmen dann bis zum 30. Lebensjahr an Dicke und Größe zu. Später bleiben diese Werte weitgehendst konstant. Erst im Greisenalter setzt eine Stärkeabnahme ein, die mit einer leichten Abflachung verbunden ist. Dieser Ablauf geht an den einzelnen Körperstellen nicht einheitlich und im gleichen Umfang vor sich (SEIBERT u. STEGGERDA; SILVESTRI, 1956a; TROTTER; WYNKOOP).

Unser Wissen über Altersveränderungen an den Haarfollikeln ist nicht umfangreich. An Stellen normaler Körperbehaarung ist ihre Zahl bis ins 4. Lebensjahrzehnt fast konstant, dann sinkt diese jedoch ab, so daß im hohen Alter nur spärlich Haarfollikel gefunden werden (SCHALLWEGG). Während dieses Alterungsprozesses erfolgt eine geringe Verkürzung des Follikels (MARON; SCHALLWEGG). Sichtbare degenerative Veränderungen konnten von zahlreichen Untersuchern nicht festgestellt werden (HILL u. MONTGOMERY; HIMMEL; SCHALLWEGG; VIGNOLI-LUTATI).

Eine Erweiterung der Follikel und eine Hornpfropfbildung in der Mündung wird jedoch häufiger beschrieben (EJIRI, SCHALLWEGG). Als Ursache dieses Phänomens werden verschiedene Möglichkeiten diskutiert. So könnte eine Änderung in der Talgsekretion eine Retention dieses Materials im Follikel zur Folge haben, was dann zu einer Erweiterung dieses Hautanteils führt. Andererseits könnte auch die Atrophie des Bindegewebes verbunden mit einem gewissen Verlust des Hautturgors zu einer Erweiterung der Follikel führen, in denen dann Talg- und Hornsubstanzen vermehrt liegen bleiben.

12. Nägel

Die Nägel zeigen im Alter ein verlangsamtes Wachstum, jedoch scheint die Gesamthornproduktion nicht verringert zu werden, da dafür oft eine Verdickung der Nagelplatte eintritt. Sie sind häufig am freien Ende aufgesplittert und von feinen Längsstreifen durchzogen. (Einzelheiten hierzu s. bei H. PINKUS, Handbuch-Ergänzungswerk, Bd. I/2.)

Mikroskopische Untersuchungen des Nagels und vor allem des Nagelbettes im Senium liegen kaum vor. Dies ist bei der Schwierigkeit der Materialbeschaffung und der Verarbeitung nicht allzu verwunderlich. Der Nagel des Neugeborenen und des Kindes ist aus weniger dichten Maschen von Keratin-Polysaccharid-Komplexen gebildet als der des Erwachsenen (ACHTEN u. SIMONART). Nach LEWIS u. MONTGOMERY sind im Alter die Gefäße im Nagelbereich oft verändert, insbesondere zeigen diese eine Frakturierung der Elastika. Auch die elastischen Fasern des Bindegewebes weisen deutliche Abwegigkeiten in Richtung einer sog. senilen Elastose auf. Diese Veränderungen sind am stärksten unterhalb des „rosafarbigen" Nagelteiles, geringer unter der Lunula und fehlen im Gebiet des Nagelfalzes. Die epitheliale Regenerationszone des Nagels, die Matrix nach HORSTMANN, zeigt einen unregelmäßigen und gestörten Zellaufbau. Die Zellen sind oft in wirbelartigen Strukturen angeordnet. Aus diesen Bezirken heraus entwickeln sich die charakteristischen Längsrillen des senilen Nagels. Ferner finden sich vermehrte Anhäufungen von sog. „Pertinax"-Körperchen, und gelegentlich ist histochemisch Kalk in der Nagelplatte nachweisbar.

Mit der Längsstreifung des Altersnagels haben sich auch ALKIEWICZ u. GORNY eingehender beschäftigt. Nach ihren Untersuchungen sind die Vorwölbungen durch darunterliegende Gefäßveränderungen (Vermehrung, Erweiterung, perivasculäre Fibrose) bedingt. Im Gebiet der Längsrillen fanden sie konzentrische Zellanhäufungen mit teils kernhaltigen und kernlosen Zellen, die durch eine unregelmäßige Verhornung entstehen.

13. Blutgefäße

Alle Untersucher sind sich darüber einig, daß die Altersveränderungen an den Blutgefäßen der Haut im Vergleich zu solchen an den großen Gefäßen des Körpers und in manchen inneren Organen auffällig gering und unbedeutend sind. HILL u. MONTGOMERY konnten bei ihren Untersuchungen derartige Erscheinungen überhaupt nicht eindeutig beobachten.

Es steht bisher nach WAGNER noch nicht einmal genau fest, ob die individuell und regional stark schwankende Zahl der Capillaren der Haut mit höherem Alter absinkt, wie dies z. B. von GOLDZIEHER, RAWLS, ROBERTS u. GOLDZIEHER angegeben wird. CORMIA fand im Bereich der Kopfhaut einen Rückgang der Anzahl der Gefäße. Zu gleichen Ergebnissen kam POPOFF für die arterio-venösen Anastomosen in den Fingern. ELLIS, MONTAGNA u. FANGER beobachteten im Senium ein dichteres Capillarnetz im Bereich der Talgdrüsen des Kopfes mit einer vermehrten Zahl von Arteriolen. Sie hatten jedoch den Eindruck, als ob nur eine Umverteilung der Gefäße stattfindet, indem die Gefäßversorgung von den Haarfollikeln weg und nach den Talgdrüsen hin ausgerichtet wird.

Kein Zweifel dürfte daran bestehen, daß ein völliger Wandel des Verlaufs des Capillarnetzes stattfindet. Die in der Jugend lang ausgezogenen und geordnet in die Papillen ziehenden Capillarschlingen werden im Alter zunehmend kürzer, zeigen eine unregelmäßige Schlingenbildung und erscheinen erweitert. Dieser Prozeß geht weitgehend mit der Rückbildung der Reteleisten bzw. der Papillen parallel (MONTAGNA u. ELLIS; Abb. 5 und 6).

STEIGLEDER fiel an Unterschenkeln bei älteren Personen ein mehr paralleler als senkrechter Verlauf der Gefäße zur Hautoberfläche auf. Mit Hilfe röntgenologischer Methoden der Gefäßdarstellung ermittelte MENEGHINI in der Gesichtshaut eine Verminderung der Gefäßanastomosen. Auch fanden sich Gefäßveränderungen, die von ihm als Folge einer Sklerosierung gedeutet wurden. Auffällig waren ferner Gefäßektasien und glomerulusartige Bildungen. EJIRI; HIMMEL; KRZYSTALOWICZ und VIGNOLI-LUTATI fanden ab etwa dem 50. Lebensjahr eine Erweiterung der Hautgefäße, jedoch beziehen sich diese Untersuchungen teilweise auf Material von lichtexponierter Haut.

Eine Gefäßwandverdickung bemerkte SCHMIDT. Nach den Untersuchungen von FARBER, HINES, MONTGOMERY u. CRAIG verändert sich das Verhältnis Gefäßwand zu Lumen von 1:2,27 bei 10—19jährigen Personen auf 1:1,95 bei 70- bis 79jährigen (s. Tabelle 5). Auch CORMIA stellte einen Rückgang des Durchmessers der Gefäße fest. STEIGLEDER kam zu keinem eindeutigen Ergebnis, sah aber auch im Alter häufiger dickere Gefäßwandungen. Sämtliche Untersuchungen über die Gefäßwanddicke sind mit der schwierig zu beantwortenden Frage belastet, ob eine Wandverbreiterung eine echte Verdickung darstellt oder ob nur ein Kontraktionsphänomen vorliegt.

Noch spärlicher und zurückhaltender sind in der Literatur Angaben über feinere Gefäßveränderungen. So scheint es an den Hautgefäßen kaum Veränderungen im Sinne einer Arteriosklerose zu geben, wobei höchstens die Gefäße der Füße und Unterschenkel eine Ausnahme machen (FARBER, HINES, MONTGOMERY u. CRAIG; MUSUMECI; SAALFELD). Die von ORBANT angegebene hyaline Degeneration der Gefäßwände wurde von den nachfolgenden Untersuchern nicht

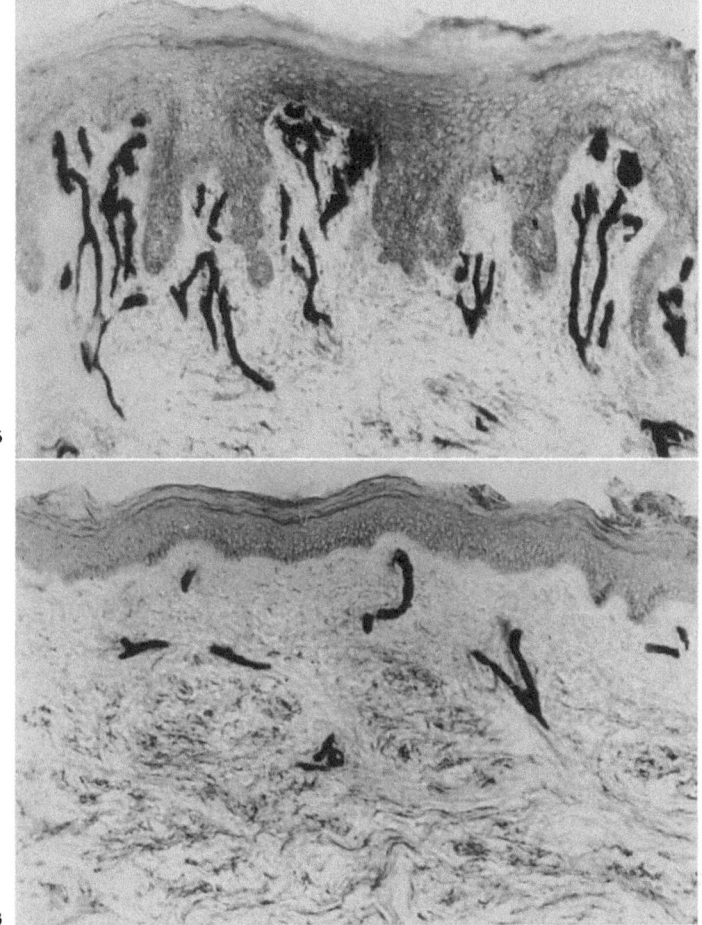

Abb. 5

Abb. 6

Abb. 5. Subepidermaler Capillarplexus. Unterschenkelhaut eines 18jährigen Mannes. Alkalische Phosphatase. Vergr. 150:1

Abb. 6. Subepidermaler Capillarplexus. Unterschenkelhaut einer 70jährigen Frau. Alkalische Phosphatase. Vergr. 150:1

Tabelle 5. *Verhältnis der Gefäßwanddicke zum Durchmesser der Arteriolen-Lichtung bei gesunden Personen und Hypertonikern unter Berücksichtigung des Lebensalters nach* FARBER, HINES, MONTGOMERY u. CRAIG *(1948)*

Alter Jahre	Normal-Personen		Hypertoniker	
	Anzahl	Verhältnis Gefäßwand/-lichtung	Anzahl	Verhältnis Gefäßwand/-lichtung
10—19	1	1:2,27	0	
20—29	7	1:2,17	3	1:2,21
30—39	9	1:2,08	17	1:1,68
40—49	15	1:2,18	32	1:1,59
50—59	14	1:2,22	11	1:1,44
60—69	3	1:1,87	5	1:1,09
70—79	2	1:1,95	1	1:1,21
80—89	1	1:2,01	1	1:1,70

bestätigt oder nicht erwähnt. ROTTER gibt eine zunehmende Sklerose der Polsterarterien der Kreislaufperipherie im höheren Alter an. Auffällige Elastica-Veränderungen sah SCHALLWEGG am Oberarm nicht, während STEIGLEDER am Unterschenkel eine Zunahme an Elastica-positivem Material feststellte.

Vom gleichen Autor wurde eine Vermehrung der Hale-positiven Schicht im Bereich der Elastica interna mit ungleichmäßiger Verteilung beobachtet. CORMIA und SILVESTRI (1956b) stellten einen Rückgang des Gehaltes an alkalischer Phosphatase in den Capillaren im höheren Alter fest.

Von zahlreichen Untersuchern wird auf die Bedeutung der Gefäßversorgung für die Altersveränderungen hingewiesen. BERRES hat dies am klarsten formuliert, indem er schreibt: „Der Altersvorgang ist ein optimales Einstellen der einzelnen Gewebselemente auf ein reduziertes Gefäßsystem", wobei man diese Reduzierung allerdings wohl auch mit auf funktionelle Leistungen beziehen muß. In diesem Zusammenhang sei darauf aufmerksam gemacht, daß die morphologisch faßbaren Altersveränderungen sehr häufig herdförmig — vermutlich in Abhängigkeit von einem Gefäßversorgungsbereich — beginnen und erst allmählich das Hautgewebe gleichmäßiger umgestalten (NELKE).

Wenn in den bisherigen Ausführungen immer nur von Gefäßen gesprochen und nicht zwischen Arterien und Venen unterschieden wurde, dann hat dies seinen Grund darin, daß auch in der Literatur fast nie eine derartige Differenzierung vorgenommen wurde bzw. kein unterschiedliches Verhalten dieser beiden Gefäßarten herausgestellt wurde. Nach STEIGLEDER verlaufen die Altersumbauvorgänge in Arterien und Venen ähnlich, wobei es jedoch dann zu Schwierigkeiten kommt, in der Altershaut Venen und Arterien zu unterscheiden.

14. Lymphgefäße

Über Altersveränderungen an den Lymphgefäßen der Haut ist bisher nichts bekannt.

15. Nerven

Untersuchungen, die eine exaktere Aussage über die Altersveränderungen an den Nerven der Haut zulassen, liegen anscheinend nicht vor.

Über gröbere nervale Strukturen finden sich einige Angaben. So sahen HERRMANN und RONGE bei Kindern eine größere Zahl von Meißnerschen Körperchen. Die Verminderung im Erwachsenenalter könnte nach HERRMANN darauf zurückzuführen sein, daß zwar ein Wachstum der Haut stattfindet, aber keine entsprechende Vermehrung der Meißnerschen Körperchen erfolgt. RONGE vermutet jedoch auch eine echte Altersinvolution und sah eine Auflösung der inneren Strukturen und einen Verlust der Nervenfasern. KANTNER beobachtete bei seinen Untersuchungen über den sensiblen Nervenapparat in der Glans penis mit zunehmendem Alter ein Tieferrücken der Nervenelemente. Die als Netz- und Schlingenkörperchen bezeichneten Strukturen weisen in der Jugend mehr langgestreckte und schlauchartige Formen auf, während im Senium kleine, runde Formen vorherrschen.

Nach WEDDELL u. PALMER sind die sog. Krauseschen Endkolben keine spezifischen Nervenendorgane, sondern „sterile" Endkolben, die immer dann entstehen, wenn eine Nervenfaser einen erfolglosen Regenerationsversuch unternommen hat. In der Altershaut finden sich nach ihren Untersuchungen zahlreiche degenerierte und regenerierende Nervenfasern sowie vermehrt solche Endkolben, die das Ergebnis gehäufter aber nicht mehr regelrecht ablaufender Regenerationsvorgänge sind.

16. Fettgewebe

Über Altersveränderungen am subcutanen Fettgewebe ist bisher wenig bekannt. Nach LAUTER u. TERHECHEBRÜGGE zeigt dieser Hautanteil im Alter in der Regel eine Zunahme, die dann im hohen Senium in eine stärkere Atrophie übergehen kann. Meist ist das Unterhautfettgewebe am Bauch bei dieser Entwicklung am stärksten beteiligt. Jedoch sind die individuellen Schwankungen so erheblich, daß man kaum allgemeingültige Aussagen machen kann.

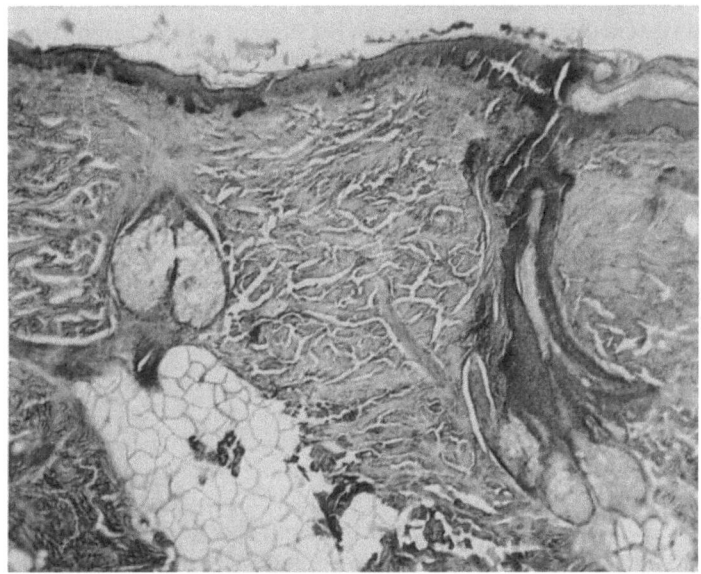

Abb. 7. Follikelatrophie mit „Vakat-Wucherung" des subcutanen Fettgewebes. Oberarmhaut eines 70jährigen Mannes. H.-E. Vergr. 45:1

HILL u. MONTGOMERY bemerkten histologisch keine Alterserscheinungen am Fettgewebe. Bei den zahlreichen anderen in diesem Kapitel zitierten Autoren finden sich keine Angaben darüber.

Die Grenze zwischen dem Corium und dem subcutanen Fettgewebe, die im jugendlichen Alter durch einstrahlende Bindegewebszüge sehr unregelmäßig verläuft, bildet mit zunehmendem Alter mehr und mehr eine gerade Linie (STEIGLEDER). Es können sich aber auch sehr hochgelegene Fettzellkomplexe finden, die vielleicht als eine Art Vakat-Wucherung gedeutet werden können, um die Atrophie der Haarfollikel und der Drüsen auszugleichen (Abb. 7).

17. Unterschiede durch Geschlecht, Konstitution und Rasse

Es besteht kein Zweifel daran, daß sich der *Unterschied der Geschlechter* auch an der Haut manifestiert, die ja im weiteren Sinne zu den sekundären Geschlechtsmerkmalen gerechnet werden kann. Dies beweisen zahlreiche einschlägige Passagen in der erotischen Literatur oder in Liebesliedern. Morphologisch ist dieser Unterschied jedoch nicht sehr eindrucksvoll faßbar. Dementsprechend sind Angaben über einen differenten Ablauf des Alterungsprozesses der Haut bei Mann und Frau nur spärlich und sehr allgemein gehalten in der Literatur zu finden.

Die Gesamthaut ist bei der Frau auf Grund eines kräftiger entwickelten Unterhautfettgewebes dicker (COMEL) und zeigt daher im ganzen eine weniger auffällige Altersatrophie. Die Epidermis bleibt dagegen beim Mann breiter (SOUTHWOOD) oder erscheint breiter, weil bei der Frau die Reteleisten sich eher zurückbilden (SCHALLWEGG). Die weibliche Hornschicht schilfert im Senium weniger schnell ab. Das Corium bleibt auch im Alter beim Manne dicker. Die Größe und Stärke der kollagenen Bindegewebsfasern läßt jedoch keine unterschiedliche Rückbildung erkennen (SCHALLWEGG). Das Verhalten der elastischen Fasern wird nicht einheitlich beurteilt. GEIGER und VOHWINKEL fanden keine Unterschiede, während EJIRI und LINDHOLM bei den Frauen mehr und besser erhaltene elastische Fasern sahen. SCHALLWEGG fiel nur ein dichteres Elasticanetz beim weiblichen Geschlecht im Stratum reticulare auf. Die glatte Muskulatur ist im Alter beim Manne meist besser erhalten. Die Haare sind beim Manne dicker und flachen während des Alterungsvorganges eher ab (SEIBERT u. STEGGERDA). Die Anzahl der Haarfollikel ist in jungen Jahren bei Frauen größer. Im Alter liegt diese Zahl jedoch bei Männern deutlich höher (SCHALLWEGG). Bei den ekkrinen Schweißdrüsen und den Talgdrüsen scheint kein Geschlechtsunterschied im Alterungsprozeß bisher festgestellt worden zu sein. Das gleiche geben GLOOR-RUTISHAUSER sowie WAY u. MEMMESHEIMER für die apokrinen Drüsen an. Nach BAKER u. CURTIS; MONTAGNA und MONTES sind gewisse Veränderungen, die evtl. als Alterungserscheinungen dieser Drüsen angesehen werden könnten (s. hierzu S. 697) beim Manne weniger stark ausgebildet.

Die Anzahl der Mastzellen scheint bei der Frau etwas schneller abzunehmen, jedoch sind diese Werte nicht signifikant (HELLSTRÖM u. HOLMGREN).

Untersuchungen über den Einfluß der *Konstitution* auf die anatomischen Altersveränderungen der Haut liegen meines Wissens nur von SCHALLWEGG vor. Danach nimmt die Hautdicke beim Astheniker schneller ab und auch die Abschilferung des Stratum corneum ist ausgeprägter. Die Haut des Asthenikers besitzt weniger elastische Fasern und glatte Muskulatur, so daß die Altersatrophie dieser Strukturen stärker hervortritt. Die Pigmentierung scheint bei diesem Körpertyp sich intensiver zu entwickeln. Der Pykniker zeigt im mittleren Alter eine stärkere Reduzierung der Körperbehaarung, die jedoch im höheren Alter durch eine stärkere Follikelatrophie beim Astheniker wieder ausgeglichen wird. An den Schweiß- und Talgdrüsen sowie in Hinblick auf die Mitosezahl sollen keine Unterschiede bestehen.

Aussagen über evtl. *rassebedingte Unterschiede* beim Alterungsprozeß der Haut können bis jetzt nicht gemacht werden, da dazu verwertbare Untersuchungen noch nicht vorliegen. Zahlreiche Faktoren erschweren derartige Forschungen. So müßte ein recht großes Untersuchungsgut zur Verfügung stehen, um die in der Einleitung zu diesen Ausführungen aufgezeigten Fehlerquellen möglichst gering zu halten. Eine gleichmäßige Verarbeitung und Beurteilung (gleiche Untersucher!) müßten gewährleistet sein, und nicht zuletzt erscheint es fast unmöglich, die Einflüsse der in manchen Ländern extremen Klima-, Ernährungs- und Lebensbedingungen auszuschalten.

Die vorstehenden Ausführungen können nicht den Anspruch auf Vollständigkeit in der Erfassung des gesamten einschlägigen Schrifttums erheben. Dies gilt insbesondere für solche Literaturstellen, die in Arbeiten völlig anderer Thematik als Teilergebnisse, Hinweise oder nebensätzliche Bemerkungen vorliegen und bibliographisch kaum zu erfassen sind. Möge aber diese Darstellung dazu anregen, die Probleme der normalen Alterung der Haut stärker als bisher in der dermatologischen Forschung zu berücksichtigen, denn "this is a fruitful field for further investigation" (COOPER).

Nachtrag

Weitere Angaben zur Morphologie der Altershaut finden sich bei MONTAGNA, W.: Advances in biology of skin. Vol. VI. Aging. Oxford-London-Edinburgh-New York-Paris-Frankfurt: Pergamon Press 1965. Da dieses Buch bei der Fertigstellung des Manuskriptes noch nicht vorlag, konnten diese Befunde nicht mehr mitberücksichtigt werden.

Literatur

ACHTEN, G., et J. M. SIMONART: L'ongel: Étude histochimique et mycologique. Ann. Derm. Syph. (Paris) **90**, 509 (1963). — ADACHI, K., and W. MONTAGNA: Histology and cytochemistry of human skin. Sites of leucine-aminopeptidase (LAP) XXII. J. invest. Derm. **37**, 145 (1961). — ALKIEWICZ, J., u. W. GORNY: Histologische Studien über die senilen Längswälle (Längsstreifen) der Nagelplatte. Arch. Derm. Syph. (Berl.) **174**, 63 (1936).

BANFIELD, W. G.: Aging of connective tissue. In ASBOE-HANSEN: Connective tissue in health and disease. Copenhagen 1954. — BECKER, S. K., T. G. FITZPATRICK, and H. MONTGOMERY: Human melanogenesis: Cytology and histology of pigment cells (melanodendrocytes). Arch. Derm. Syph. (Chic.) **65**, 511 (1952). — BERRES, H. H.: Die Histologie der Altersveränderungen der menschlichen Haut. Arch. klin. exp. Derm. **206**, 751 (1957). — BIZZOZERO, E., e M. DOGLIOTTI: Sulla senescenza della mucosa orale. Minerva derm. **30**, 277 (1955). — BRACK, E.: Über Bindegewebsmastzellen im menschlichen Organismus. Folia haemat. (Lpz.) **31**, 202 (1925). — BRANCA, A.: Sur la structura des glandes sudoripores. Ann. Derm. Syph. (Paris) **8**, 1 (1927). — BRILLANTI, F., e A. BENEFENATI: Sulla distribuzione della ghiandole sebacee nella cute del corpo umano. Boll. Soc. ital. Biol. sper. **13**, 810 (1938). — BUTTGE, U.: Die Morphologie der Grenzfläche zwischen Epithel und Bindegewebe der weiblichen Genital- und Analregionen sowie der Vagina. Z. Zellforsch. **50**, 598 (1959).

CANEGHEM, P. VAN: Über die Struktur der heterotopen apokrinen Drüsen. Hautarzt **10**, 552 (1959). — COMEL, M.: La cute nei suoi rapporti con la costituzione dell'individuo. G. ital. Derm. **71**, 2090 (1930). — COOPER, Z. K.: Ageing of the skin. In: A. I. LANSING, Cowdry's problems of ageing. Biological and medical aspects, 3. ed. Baltimore: Williams & Wilkins Co. 1952. — CORMIA, F. E.: Vasculature of the normal scalp. Arch. Derm. Syph. (Chic.) **88**, 692 (1963).

DABELOW, A.: Die Milchdrüse. In: W. v. MÖLLENDORFF u. W. BARGMANN, Handbuch der mikroskopischen Anatomie des Menschen, Bd. III, S. 3. Berlin-Göttingen-Heidelberg: Springer 1957. — DAY, F. D.: The nature and significance of cementing substance in interstitiel connective tissue. J. Path. Bact. **59**, 567 (1947).

EJIRI, J.: Studien über die Histologie der menschlichen Haut. IV. Mitt. Über das Wesen der Altersveränderungen der Haut. Jap. J. Derm. Urol. **41**, 64 (1937). — Studien über die Histologie der menschlichen Haut. V. Mitt. Über die Histologie der menschlichen Haut bei verschiedenen Hautkrankheiten, mit besonderer Berücksichtigung der Altersveränderungen der elastischen Fasern. Jap. J. Derm. Urol. **41**, 95 (1937). — ELLIS, R. A., W. MONTAGNA, and H. FANGER: Histology and cytochemistry of human skin. XIV. The blood supply of the cutaneous glands. J. invest. Derm. **30**, 137 (1958). — EVANS, R., E. V. COWDRY, and P. E. NIELSON: Ageing of human skin. I. Influence of dermal shrinkage on appearance of the epidermis in young and old fixed tissues. Anat. Rec. **86**, 545 (1943).

FARBER, E. M., E. A. HINES, H. MONTGOMERY, and W. MCCRAIG: The arterioles of the skin in essential hypertension. J. invest. Derm. **9**, 285 (1947). — FREEMAN, R. G., E. G. COCKERELL, J. ARMSTRONG, and J. M. KNOX: Sunlight as a factor influencing the thickness of epidermis. J. invest. Derm. **39**, 295 (1962).

GANS, O., u. G. K. STEIGLEDER: Histologie der Hautkrankheiten, 2. Aufl. Berlin-Göttingen-Heidelberg: Springer 1955 u. 1957. — GEIGER, W.: Diss. Erlangen 1930. Zit. SCHALLWEGG. — GLOOR-RUTISHAUSER, N.: Zur makroskopischen Anatomie der apokrinen Achseldrüsen. Acta anat. (Basel) **19**, 197 (1953). — GOLDZIEHER, J. W., W. B. RAWLS, I. S. ROBERTS, and M. A. GOLDZIEHER: Studies on aging: correlation of skin morphology with age and hormone excretion. J. Geront. **7**, 47 (1952). — GRAUMANN, W.: Beitrag zur Kenntnis der Brustdrüse alter Männer. Inaug.-Diss. Göttingen 1945. — Mikroskopische Anatomie der männlichen Brustdrüse. I. Kindheit und Pubertät. Z. mikr.-anat. Forsch. **58**, 358 (1952). — Mikroskopische Anatomie der männlichen Brustdrüse. II. Mannesalter und Senium. Z. mikr.-anat. Forsch. **59**, 523 (1953). — GUSNER, K. V.: Histologische Untersuchungen an männlichen Brustdrüsen. Langenbecks Arch. klin. Chir. **153**, 253 (1928).

HEITE, H. J., u. H. ZAUN: Zur Kenntnis der Fox-Fordyceschen Krankheit und ihrer Pathogenese. Hautarzt **12**, 307 (1961). — HELLSTRÖM, B., and H. J. HOLMGREN: Numerical distribution of mast cells in the human skin and heart. Acta anat. (Basel) **10**, 81 (1950). — HERRMANN, H.: Über die nervösen Endkörperchen in der Haut der menschlichen Hand.

Z. Haut- u. Geschl.-Kr. 14, 277 (1953). — HILL, W. R., and H. MONTGOMERY: Regional changes and changes caused by age in the normal skin. J. invest. Derm. 3, 231 (1940). — HIMMEL, J. M.: Zur Kenntnis der senilen Degeneration der Haut. Arch. Derm. Syph. (Berl.) 64, 47 (1903). — HOLMGREN, E.: Die Achsendrüsen des Menschen. Anat. Anz. 55, 553 (1922). — HORSTMANN, E.: Die Haut. In: W. v. MÖLLENDORFF u. W. BARGMANN, Handbuch der mikroskopischen Anatomie des Menschen, Bd. III/3. Berlin-Göttingen-Heidelberg: Springer 1957.
ITO, T., u. K. IWASHIGE: Zytologische und histologische Untersuchungen über die apokrinen Achselschweißdrüsen von gesunden Menschen höheren Alters. Arch. histol. jap. 5, 455 (1953). — IWASHIGE, K.: Zytologische und histologische Untersuchungen über die ekkrinen Schweißdrüsen der Achselhaut vom gesunden Menschen höheren Alters. Arch. histol. jap. 4, 75 (1952).
KALANTAEVSKAYA, K. G., and I. G. GURINS: Certain morphological and functional peculiarities of the skin in aged persons. Vestn. Derm. Vener. 35, 8 (1961). — KANO, K.: Zytologische und histologische Untersuchungen über die Schweißdrüsen im Greisenalter. Beobachtungen der ekkrinen Schweißdrüsen bei den an Krankheit verstorbenen Fällen. Arch. histol. jap. 4, 91 (1952). — KANTNER, M.: Studien über den sensiblen Apparat in der Glans penis (II). Z. mikr.-anat. Forsch. 59, 439 (1953). — KATZBERG, A. A.: The influence of age on the rate of desquamation of human epidermis. Anat. Rec. 112, 418 (1952). — KRZYSTALOWICZ, F.: Inwieweit vermögen alle bisher angegebenen Färbungen des Elastins auch Elazin zu färben. Mh. prakt. Derm. 30, 265 (1900). — KUSNETZ, M.: Über die Veränderungen der senilen Haut. Ukrain. med. Arch. 8, 1, 91 (1932). Ref. Zbl. Haut- u. Geschl.-Kr. 45, 689 (1933).
LAUTER, S., u. A. TERHECHEBRÜGGE: Über Fettansatz und Fettverteilung beim normalgewichtigen Menschen. Dtsch. Arch. klin. Med. 181, 181 (1937). — LEWIS, B. L., and H. MONTGOMERY: The senile nail. J. invest. Derm. 24, 11 (1955). — LINDHOLM, E.: Über die Schwankungen in der Verteilung der elastischen Fasern in der menschlichen Haut als Beitrag zur Konstitutionspathologie. Frankfurt. Z. Path. 42, 394 (1931). — LINKE, K. W.: Elektronenmikroskopische Untersuchungen über die Differenzierung der Intercellularsubstanz der menschlichen Lederhaut. Z. Zellforsch. 42, 331 (1955).
MA, C. K., and E. V. COWDRY: Aging of elastic tissue in human skin. J. Geront. 5, 203 (1950). — MANGANOTTI, G.: Rilievi generali e considerazioni sulla cute senile. I. Epidermide. G. Geront., Suppl. 5, 10 (1955a). — Rilievi generali a considerazioni sulla cute senile. II. Derma. G. Geront., Suppl. 5, 39 (1955b). — MARON, H.: Die Tiefe der Haarzwiebel in der menschlichen Kopfhaut. Derm. Wschr. 143, 8 (1961). — MENEGHINI, N.: Osservazioni anatomoradiografiche sulla reti arteriose e venose delle faccia dell'uomo nelle varie epoche della vita. Arch. ital. Derm. 18, 62 (1942). — MEYER, J., A. S. MARWAH, and J. P. WEINMANN: Mitotic rate of gingival epithelium in two age groups. J. invest. Derm. 27, 237 (1956). — MIKHAIL, G. R., and A. MILLER-MILINSKA: Mast cell population in human skin. J. invest. Derm. 43, 249 (1964). — MONTAGNA, W.: Histology and cytochemistry of human skin. XIX. The development and fate of the axillary organ. J. invest. Derm. 33, 151 (1959). — MONTAGNA, W., and R. A. ELLIS: Advances in biology of skin, Vol. II. Blood vessels and circulation. Oxford-London-NewYork-Paris: Pergamon Press 1961. — MONTAGNA, W., and H. P. MELARAGNO: Histology and cytochemistry of human skin. III. Polymorphism and chromotropy of mastcells. J. invest. Derm. 20, 257 (1953). — MONTES, L. F., B. L. BAKER, and A. C. CURTIS: The cytology of the large axillary sweat glands in man. J. invest. Derm. 35, 273 (1960). — MURTULA, G.: Sulle modificazioni dell'epidermide in relazione all'eta con particolare riguardo alle differenze tra cute coperta e cute scoperta. Minerva derm. 28, 231 (1953). — MUSUMECI, V.: Aspetti della rete vasale nella cute senile. Minerva derm. 36, 209 (1961).
NELKE, A.: Die Altersveränderungen der menschlichen Bauchhaut. Inaug.-Diss. Köln 1956. — NEUBER, E.: Über das Verhalten der elastischen Fasern der Haut mit spezieller Berücksichtigung des Hautkrebses. Arch. Derm. Syph. (Berl.) 94, 3 (1909). — NEUMANN, J.: Arch. Derm. Syph. (Berl.) 1 (1896), zit. nach SCHALLWEGG. — NIKOLOWSKI, W., u. R. WITTIG: Morbus Fox-Fordyce und Interrenalismus. Derm. Wschr. 151, 263 (1955).
OBRUČNIK, M.: Changes in the normal histological structure of the skin of the interdigital spaces of the foot in man and their relationship to the pathogenesis of skin disease in these regions. Čs. Derm. 28, 112 (1953). — ORBANT: Diss. Petersburg (1896). Zit. nach SCHALLWEGG.
PFALTZ, C. R.: Das embryonale und postnatale Verhalten der männlichen Brustdrüse beim Menschen. II. Das Mammaorgan im Kindes-, Jünglings-, Mannes- und Greisenalter. Acta anat. (Basel) 8, 293 (1949). — PINKUS, H.: Die makroskopische Anatomie der Haut. In: J. JADASSOHN, Handbuch der Haut- und Geschlechtskrankheiten, Erg.-Werk Bd. I/2. Berlin-Göttingen-Heidelberg-New York: Springer 1964.—POPOFF, N. W.: The digital vascular system. Arch. Path. 18, 295 (1934).
RICHTER, R.: Die Haare. In: J. JADASSOHN, Handbuch der Haut- und Geschlechtskrankheiten, Erg.-Werk Bd. I/3. Berlin-Göttingen-Heidelberg: Springer 1963. — RON-

Chese, F.: The senile and prematurely senile skin. Geriatrics **1**, 144 (1946). — Ronge, H.: Altersveränderungen der Meissnerschen Körperchen in der Fingerhaut. Z. mikr.-anat. Forsch. **54**, 167 (1947). — Rotter, W.: Altersvorgänge in der Kreislaufperipherie. Z. Alternsforsch. **9**, 372 (1955/56).
Saalfeld, E.: Zur pathologischen Anatomie der Haut im Alter mit Berücksichtigung der Arterienveränderungen. Arch. Derm. Syph. (Berl.) **132**, 1 (1921). — Schallwegg, O.: Die menschliche Haut in ihren Beziehungen zum Alter, Geschlecht und Konstitution. Z. menschl. Vererb.- u. Konstit.-Lehre **25**, 206 (1941). — Schmidt, M. B.: Über die Altersveränderungen der elastischen Fasern in der Haut. Virchows Arch. path. Anat. **125**, 239 (1891). — Scolari, E. G.: Rass. Derm. Sif. **8**, Nr 1 (1956). Zit. nach Wagner. — Seibert, H. C., and M. Steggerda: J. Hered. **35**, 345 (1944). Ref. Dermatologica (Basel) **95**, 19 (1948). — Silvestri, U.: I. Faneri nella etá senile. Studio del capello e dei peli ambosessuali. G. Geront., Suppl. **5**, 203 (1955). — Sui peli terminali del tronco nell'eta senile. I. peli del petto. Arch. ital. Derm. **28**, 141 (1956a). — Prime osservazioni sulla fosfatasi alcalina nella cute senile. Minerva derm. **12**, 646 (1956b). — Osservazioni sulle cellule a „cromatina positiva" e a „cromatina negativa" in cute umana dell'eta senile. Arch. ital. Derm. **28**, 341 (1956c). — Beobachtungen über das Chromatin von Barr in den Fibrozyten der menschlichen Haut. Minerva derm. **34**, 612 (1959a). Ref. Derm. Wschr. **143**, 589 (1961). — Osservazioni istologiche su la ghiandola sebacea del vecchio. G. Geront. **7**, 113 (1959b). — In tema di istochimica della cute senile. Ricerca dei gruppi sulfirilici legati celle proteine. Arch. ital. Derm. **30**, 307 (1960). — Silvestri, U., e M. de Maurici: Osservazioni istologiche, istochimiche ed istofisiche nella cute del capillizio e dell'ascella in gerontologia. Pathologica **48**, 1 (1956). — Sommers, G. C.: Basement membranes, ground substance and lymphytic aggregates in aging organs. J. Geront. **11**, 251 (1956). — Southwood, W. F. W.: The thickness of the skin. Plast. reconstr. Surg. **15**, 423 (1955). — Staricco, R. J., and H. Pinkus: Quantitative and qualitative dates on the pigment cells of adult human epidermis. J. invest. Derm. **28**, 33 (1957). — Steigleder, G. K.: Verhalten von Gefäßen und Bindegewebe in der Haut des menschlichen Unterschenkels in verschiedenen Altersperioden. Zbl. Phlebol. **3**, 231 (1964). — Steigleder, G. K., u. O. Gans: Pathologische Reaktionen in der Epidermis. In: J. Jadassohn, Handbuch der Haut- und Geschlechtskrankheiten, Erg.-Werk, Bd. I/2. Berlin-Göttingen-Heidelberg-New York: Springer 1964. — Ströbel, H.: Die Gewebsveränderungen der Haut im Verlauf des Lebens. Arch. Derm. Syph. (Berl.) **186**, 636 (1948).
Teller, H., G. Vester u. L. Pohl: Elektronenmikroskopische Untersuchungsergebnisse an der Interzellularsubstanz des Koriums bei Altersatrophie. Z. Haut- u. Geschl.-Kr. **22**, 67 (1957). — Thuringer, J. M., and A. A. Katzberg: The effect of age on mitosis in the human epidermis. J. invest. Derm. **33**, 35 (1959). — Trotter, M.: The life cycles of hair in selected regions of the body. Amer. J. phys. Anthrop. **7**, 427 (1924). — The form, size and color of head hair in American whites. Amer. J. physic. Anthrop. **14**, 433 (1930).
Vignolo-Lutati, C.: Die glatte Muskulatur in den senilen und praesenilen Atrophien der Haut. Arch. Derm. Syph. (Berl.) **74**, 213 (1905). — Vohwinkel, K. H.: Über die Alterserscheinungen des Hautbindegewebes und über die sogenannte „Elastica mimica" bei verschiedenen Rassen. Derm. Z. **62**, 95 (1931).
Wagner, G.: Altersveränderungen der Haut, Altersdermatose. In: H. A. Gottron u. W. Schönfeld: Dermatologie und Venerologie, Bd. IV. Stuttgart: Georg Thieme 1960. — Walchshofer, E.: Über Rückbildungsvorgänge in der alternden Mamma. Dtsch. Z. Chir. **224**, 137 (1930). — Way, St. C., and A. Memmesheimer: The sudoriporis glands. II. The apocrine glands. Arch. Derm. Syph. (Chic.) **38**, 373 (1938). — Weddell, G., u. E. Palmer: Die Nervenfasern und ihre Endigungen im menschlichen Integument. Acta neuroveg. (Wien) **24**, 139 (1962). — Winkelmann, R. K., and J. V. Hultin: Mucinous metaplasie in normal apocrine glands. Arch. Derm. Syph. (Chic.) **78**, 309 (1958). — Wynkoop, E. M.: A study of the age correlations of the cuticular scales, medullas and shaft diameters of human head heir. Amer. J. physic. Anthrop. **13**, 177 (1929).

Hautveränderungen an Leichen

Von

G. Dotzauer und L. Tamáska, Köln

Mit 22 Abbildungen (davon 5 farbig)

Einleitung und Problemstellung

Man könnte geneigt sein, das Problem der Leichenhaut lediglich anhand von makro- wie mikroskopischen Befunden aufzuzeigen, d.h., den Übergang von bio- zu nekrochemischen Vorgängen darzulegen. Eine Betrachtungsweise aufgrund morphologischer Substrate wäre unvollkommen. Die Problematik setzt erst mit folgenden Fragen ein:

Welche Befunde gestatten eine Aussage darüber, ob das Integument unmittelbar vor dem Tode, während des Sterbens, in der supravitalen Phase oder erst während der Leichenzersetzungsvorgänge einer exogenen Schädigung ausgesetzt war?

Wie steht es mit der Beweiswürdigung morphologischer Befunde?

I. Die Haut der frühen Leichenzeit

1. Algor

Körpertemperatur und damit auch die der Haut gleichen sich nach dem Tode der Umgebungstemperatur an. — Bei hoher Umgebungstemperatur und geringer Luftfeuchtigkeit sinkt jedoch die Hauttemperatur nach dem Tode *unter die der Umgebung*. — Je größer das Temperaturgefälle zwischen Hauttemperatur im Augenblick des Todes und Umgebung ist, desto augenscheinlicher wird der Temperaturverlust.

Die Haut unbekleideter Körperpartien wird betastet; man faßt auch unter die Kleidung. Das Tastgefühl ist Gradmesser des Temperaturverlustes. Warmen Händen, die einen bereits abgekühlten Körper betasten, wird das Temperaturgefälle deutlich. Betasten mit kühlen Händen vermittelt bei der gleichen Leiche u.U. einen gegensätzlichen Eindruck.

Die Abkühlung der Leichenhaut wird forensisch gelegentlich als Gradmesser für die Spanne zwischen Tod und Untersuchung gesehen. Postmortale Hauttemperaturen unterliegen aber einer Vielzahl physikalischer, d.h. exogener, wie endogener Einflüsse, die diese Methode der Todeszeitbestimmung fragwürdig machen. Nur die Temperatur im Körperkern vermittelt gewisse Anhaltspunkte.

Die Temperatur im Augenblick des Todes kann, je nach Todesursache, sehr unterschiedlich sein. Nach Gewalttaten, d.h. bei plötzlichen, aber auch natürlichen, unerwarteten Todesfällen, haben wir mit größter Wahrscheinlichkeit von normalen Meßwerten auszugehen.

Das läßt sich aber nicht ohne weiteres auf jeden forensisch wichtigen Fall übertragen.

Der Kachektische besitzt, in Relation zu seinem Körpergewicht, eine verhältnismäßig größere Körperoberfläche. Die Leichentemperatur gleicht sich hier rascher der Umgebungstemperatur an und zwar nicht nur an der Körperoberfläche, sondern auch im Körperinnern. Die Stärke des Unterhautfettgewebes spielt dabei keine wesentliche Rolle. Aus gleichen Gründen sinken die Hauttemperaturen bei Säuglingen und kleinen Kindern sehr rasch.

Die postmortale *Hyperthermie* soll bei folgenden Erkrankungen auftreten: Nach schweren Krampfzuständen, nach Vergiftungen, beim Tetanus, nach schweren Infektionskrankheiten, weiter nach Cholera. Nicht genügend geklärt sind die Fragen des Temperaturanstieges bei Erkrankungen des zentralen Nervensystems bzw. bei Verletzungen des Gehirns und des verlängerten Markes. Bei größerem Blutverlust, besonders bei verzögertem Todeseintritt, in Verbindung mit einer Unterkühlung, sprechen wir von agonalen oder postmortalen foudroyanten Hypothermien.

Ein Wort noch zum Tod im Brandherd. Ein toter Körper, der extremen Temperaturen ausgesetzt blieb, bewahrt diese sehr lange. Deshalb geht er nach Bergung aus dem Brandherd erstaunlich rasch in Fäulnis über, falls nicht die ganze Körperoberfläche verkohlt, wobei die inneren Organe gewissermaßen isoliert werden (GRÄFF).

Je größer das Gefälle zwischen Ausgangs- und Umgebungstemperatur ist, desto deutlicher stellt sich der Temperaturverlust in einer Exponentialkurve dar. Ein unmittelbar nach dem Tode winterlichen Temperaturen ausgesetzter Körper kühlt rasch ab; gleiches gilt für Tod im strömenden, kühlen Wasser oder in durchnäßter Kleidung, bei stärkerer Bewegung in kalter Luft. Wir sehen, von welchen extrem differenten Faktoren das Sinken der Hauttemperaturen abhängt. Deshalb ist es schwierig, aus dem Ergebnis einer Einzelmessung, sei es durch Handauflegung oder durch exakte Temperaturmessungen, auf die Todeszeit rückzuschließen.

Folgendes: Ein Leichenbeschauer betritt den Raum, orientiert sich an der Umgebungstemperatur und versucht, diese in Relation zur Hauttemperatur zu bringen, um in etwa die Todeszeit zu schätzen. Er setzt voraus, daß vom Augenblick des Todes an ein kühler Luftstrom durch den Raum ging. Infolge der bewegten Luft müßte der Körper rascher an Temperatur verlieren. Fenster und Türen wurden aber nach Auffinden der Leiche geöffnet, der Körper jetzt erst aufgedeckt.

Die Haut fühlt sich an unbedeckten Teilen 4—5 Std nach dem Tode deutlich abgekühlt, nach 10—12 Std p.m. kalt.

MUELLER schreibt: „3—4 Std nach dem Tode fühle sich der Körper ‚kälter' an, 10—12 Std nach dem Tode ‚kalt'. Nach 24 Std erfolgt der Ausgleich mit der Umgebung."

Ein weiteres Zitat findet sich bei PONSOLD: Hände, Füße und Gesicht sind 1—2 Std nach dem Tode abgekühlt, in den anderen unbekleideten Partien nach 4—5 Std.

SEYDELER hat anläßlich Temperaturmessungen in der Achselhöhle von gefallenen Soldaten nach der Schlacht bei Königgrätz gefunden, daß ein Ausgleich mit der Umgebungstemperatur innerhalb von 16—38 Std nach dem Tode erfolgte, im Durchschnitt nach 20 Std. Diese Differenz erklärt sich aus individueller Beschaffenheit von Leiche und Fundsituation.

Fassen wir zusammen: Nicht nur aus biochemischen bzw. nekrochemischen, sondern auch aus forensischen Gründen ist die Frage des Verhaltens der Temperaturen im Kern wie an der Oberfläche von Bedeutung.

Bei einem Dahinsiechen infolge schwerer, zugleich zehrender Erkrankung fallen die Körpertemperaturen bereits ante finem unter die Norm. Gleiches gilt für die Unterkühlung, d.h., falls ein Sterbender niedrigen Umgebungstemperaturen ausgesetzt ist. Andererseits gibt es Erkrankungen, bei denen die Temperaturen nach dem Tode noch steigen.

Der Ausgangswert einer jeden Nekrothermometrie ist also sehr unterschiedlich. In concreto wird man zunächst versuchen müssen, die vitalen Hauttemperaturen ante finem zu schätzen bzw. einen Nullwert zu bestimmen. Da nicht immer von normalen Hauttemperaturen auszugehen ist, wir aber Hyperthermien aus physikalischer oder endogener Ursache und andererseits Hypothermien aus ähnlichen Gründen kennen, ergeben sich Schwierigkeiten; handelt es sich doch bei dem zu untersuchenden Material stets um unbekannte Situationen, auf die rückzuschließen wäre; unbekannt in bezug auf den primären Zustand des Lebenden wie auch auf Ereignisse, die zum Tode führten; u.a. auch die Länge der Todeszeit und vieles andere mehr. Ein Faktor sei nur genannt: Die Verdunstung. Wir kennen den Einfluß der Verdunstung auf Hauttemperaturen. Die schweißnasse Körperhaut — sei es durch finale Hyperthermie, sei es Ausdruck eines akuten Kollapszustandes, sowohl feuchter wie kalter Schweiß, beide werden entsprechend der Ausgangssituation bereits ante finem Einfluß auf die Hauttemperatur nehmen. Hinzu treten Umweltsbedingungen: Raumtemperatur, Luftfeuchtigkeit, bewegte Luft; Kleidung, mit dem dadurch geschaffenen Privatklima, etc.

2. Palor

Da Blut nach Beendigung der Herz- und Kreislauftätigkeit — physikalischen Gesetzen folgend — in den Gefäßen sinkt, blassen Haut und sichtbare Schleimhäute in dieser Zone der *nicht abhängigen* Körperpartien ab. Die Reduzierung des Blutgehaltes der Capillaren in Haut und Unterhautfettgewebe, sowie der Pigmentgehalt der Haut und des Unterhautfettgewebes, aber auch die Stärke des Unterhautfettpolsters, tönen die Haut für unser Auge. Bei pigmentreicher Haut werden Palor — wie Livores — später auftreten bzw. sie heben sich schlechter ab. Bei stark pigmentierter Haut sind die sichtbaren Schleimhäute zu betrachten, da hier eine bessere Befunderhebung vorliegt.

Ein stärkerer Pigmentgehalt läßt übrigens ebenfalls CO-Vergiftungen oder Intoxikationen durch MetHb-bildende Gifte schwerer erkennen. Bei gleichzeitigem Ikterus z.B., wäre eine Met-Hb-Vergiftung kaum bei der Leichenschau zu diagnostizieren.

3. Livores

Totenflecke sind forensisch von großer Bedeutung (Todeszeitbestimmung, Körperlage nach dem Tode, Umlagerung, bekleidet oder unbekleidet, Todesursache).

Bei langer Agone bilden sich bereits an dem noch Lebenden intravitale „Totenflecke". Der Volksmund nennt sie „Kirchhofrosen". Bei plötzlichen Todesfällen werden die Totenflecke erst eine geraume Zeit post mortem erkennbar. Im Moment einer Leichenschau wissen wir nicht, ob es sich um einen langsamen oder perakuten Todeseintritt gehandelt hat.

Wir unterscheiden:
1. hypostatische und
2. Diffusionstotenflecke.

Nach Zusammenbruch von Herz- und Kreislauf unterliegt das Blut der Gravitation. Die Haut im Bereich der abhängigen Partien rötet sich zunächst zart; die Blutfülle nimmt mit der Zeit in den Gefäßen zu, Totenflecke breiten sich aus, werden farbintensiver.

Etwa 20—30 min nach plötzlichem Tod sind Livores zunächst im Nacken, dann aber auch an den seitlichen, rückwärtigen Brustkorbpartien zu entdecken (MERKEL).

Die Totenflecke zeichnen sich bei Rückenlage nach 15—20 min an den Brustkorbseiten und nach 20—40 min am Nacken und Hals ab. Wenn sie nach 2 Std zusammenfließen, fallen sie auf (PONSOLD).

Die Daten sind abhängig von der Menge des, flüssigen, Blutes: Je mehr Erythrocyten in die Hautcapillaren der abhängigen Körperteile sinken, desto rascher treten intensive Totenflecke auf. Die p. m. verstrichene Zeit, Menge des flüssigen Blutes sowie die Stärke der Hautpigmentierungen, wirken sich aus. — Bei gewissen Intoxikationen — z. B. Alkohol, nach schweren Infektionserkrankungen, wie Lobärpneumonie, ist das Blut in den Gefäßen jedoch geronnen; Cruor wie Speckhaut lassen die Totenflecke nicht nur spärlicher, sondern auch verzögert erscheinen. Beim fulminanten Tod mit Flüssigbleiben des Blutes (z. B. Blausäure- oder Kohlenmonoxydvergiftung) zeigen sich Totenflecke schnell und intensiv. Bei primärer oder sekundärer Anämie sind Haut wie Totenflecke blaß bzw. spärlich vorhanden (Tubarruptur, innere Verblutung nach Berstung eines Aortenaneurysmas etc.).

Ähnlich wie Körner einer Sanduhr rinnen, werden sich Totenflecke nach gewisser Zeit in einer Ebene, entsprechend der zwischen Tod und Untersuchung verstrichenen Zeit, einstellen. Das Ausmaß der Totenflecke wurde durch Messung des Spiegels bestimmt. Bei Rückenlage wurden im Bereich des Schwertfortsatzes Umfang und anteilig die Höhe der Livores gemessen.

Eine weitere Möglichkeit, die *Todeszeit* zu schätzen, besteht in ihrer Wegdrückbarkeit oder Umlagerungsfähigkeit. Bei noch flüssigem Blut werden sich die Hautgefäße auf Daumendruck, oder bei Kompression mit dem Rücken eines Messers, weitgehend von Blut leeren und dies bis zur Ausbildung von Diffusionstotenflecken. Jetzt sind die Gefäßschranken für den Blutfarbstoff zusammengebrochen, er imbibiert das umgebende Gewebe. Bis zu 10—12 Std nach dem Tode sind die Totenflecke noch fortdrückbar; soweit eine Erkrankung mit innerer vitaler Hämolyse zum Tode geführt hat, reduziert sich selbstverständlich diese Spanne erheblich; gleiches gilt für die rasch einsetzende Fäulnis.

In jüngerer Zeit hat MUELLER die Totenflecke systematisch studiert. Vergleichende Untersuchungen zwischen Wegdrückbarkeit und histologischen Befunden an den Totenflecken wurden vorgenommen.

1. 1—5 Std nach dem Tode verschwinden die Totenflecke auf Fingerdruck vollständig. Mikroskopisch finden sich hier bereits Hämoglobinwolken um die Hautgefäße.

2. 6—10 Std nach dem Tode verschwinden die Totenflecke bei Fingerdruck noch gleichfalls, doch werden mikroskopisch die Hämoglobinhöfe um die Gefäße größer.

3. 10—30 Std nach dem Tode sind die Totenflecke nicht mehr durch Druck zu beseitigen, mikroskopisch: konfluierte Hämoglobinwolken; unter dem Epithel hatte sich eine kontinuierliche Hämoglobinschicht angesammelt und das Epithel diffus imbibiert. Diffusionstotenflecke!

Bleiben wir bei dem Beispiel der Sanduhr: An den abhängigen Körperpartien bilden sich Totenflecke und dokumentieren damit die *Körperhaltung*. Ähnlich wie die Körner einer Sanduhr durch Kippen in Bewegung gesetzt werden, bilden sich — nach Änderung der primären Körperhaltung — solange das Blut flüssig bleibt und die Haut nicht durch Diffusion imbibiert wurde — sekundäre Totenflecke. Nach Umlagerung werden wir bis zur 12. Stunde nach dem Tode evtl. sekundäre zarte Totenflecke erkennen, die primären sind noch deutlich zu sehen. Wurde der Körper 6 Std nach dem Tode umgelagert, sieht man einerseits deutliche Livores in der primären Tiefstlage, andererseits solche in den jetzt abhängigen Partien. Die primären Totenflecke sollen nach HOFMANN bis zu 30 Std nach Wendung der Leiche noch gering abblassen; Erfordernis einer zweiten Leichenschau.

Tabelle 1. *Übersicht nach* BERTHOLD MUELLER *über makroskopische wie mikroskopische Befunde an Livores, geordnet nach zeitlichen Gesichtspunkten*

Zeit nach dem Tode Std	Ergebnis
1	Völlige Wegdrückbarkeit des Totenfleckes, rote Blutkörperchen gut erhalten. Hyperämie der Capillaren unter dem Epithel. Hämoglobin gelegentlich in den Gefäßwänden
4	Verschwinden auf Fingerdruck, bei Hochkanten der Leiche sofortiges Abblassen. Vereinzelt kleine Hämoglobinaustritte um die Gefäße
5	Verschwinden auf Fingerdruck. Abblassen beim Hochkanten. Hämoglobinwolken um Gefäße. Epithel noch ungefärbt
6	Verschwinden auf Fingerdruck. Abblassen bei Hochkanten erst nach einigen Minuten. Unterhautgewebe makroskopisch schwach rot gefärbt. Hyperämie der Capillaren unter dem Epithel. Hier und da beginnende Hämolyse. Hämoglobinwolken um die Gefäße. Ablagerung von nicht konfluierenden Hämoglobinwolken unter dem Epithel. Mm. arrectores pilorum um Gefäßwände mitunter braun gefärbt
8	Auf Fingerdruck kein Verschwinden der Flecke, sondern nur ein Abblassen. Bei Hochkanten der Leiche kein Abblassen mehr. Makroskopisch kleine Hautblutungen im Bereich der Hypostase, auch mikroskopisch Blutungen in der Lederhaut und im Unterhautfettgewebe sowie in den Scheiden der Talgdrüsen. Das Blut in den Gefäßen ist zum Teil hämolytisch. Große Hämoglobinwolken um die Gefäße. Muskeln und Drüsen braun gefärbt
8	Befund makroskopisch der gleiche, jedoch keine Blutungen. Auch mikroskopisch keine Blutungen. Große Hämoglobinwolken um die Gefäße
9	Nur geringes Abblassen auf Fingerdruck. Mikroskopisch sind die Capillaren unter dem Epithel strotzend mit zum Teil hämolytischem Blut gefüllt. Ziemlich ausgedehnte Hämoglobinwolken um die Gefäße und unter dem Epithel. Im Bereiche der Wolken geringe Braunfärbung des Epithels
10	Abblassen bei Fingerdruck, aber auffälligerweise auch geringes Abblassen beim Umdrehen der Leiche. Ausgedehnte Hämoglobinwolken. Epithel hier und da schwach braun. Keine Blutungen
11	Verschwinden bei Fingerdruck. Keine Blutungen. Hämoglobinwolken beginnen gerade zu konfluieren
13	Geringes Abblassen auf Fingerdruck. Kein Abblassen beim Umdrehen. Konfluierende Hämoglobinwolken. Braunfärbung des Epithels nicht sehr deutlich und schwer vom Pigment unterscheidbar
14	Abblassen auf Fingerdruck. Makroskopisch kleine Blutungen, mikroskopisch große konfluierende Hämoglobinwolken um die Gefäße. Keine Blutungen im Bereiche der Schweißdrüsen. Epithel hier und da schwach braun gefärbt, doch ist es schwierig, die Braunfärbung von dem Pigment des Epithels abzugrenzen.
14	Befund wie oben, doch keine Blutungen
15	Kein Abblassen mehr auf Fingerdruck, wohl aber auf Druck mit Pinzette. Ausgedehnte Hämolyse. Blutungen in Lederhaut und Unterhautgewebe. Hämoglobinwolkenschicht unter dem Epithel. Epithel durchgängig stellenweise braun gefärbt
17	Kein Abblassen auf Fingerdruck. Kontinuierliche Hämoglobinwolken unter dem Epithel. Drüsen und Muskeln intensiv braun gefärbt
19	Noch geringes Abblassen auf Fingerdruck, aber nicht mehr beim Umdrehen. Keine Blutungen. Mikroskopisch Blutungen unter dem Epithel und in der Tiefe. Ausgedehnte Hämoglobinwolken. Epithel hier und da braun
23	Geringes Abblassen auf Fingerdruck. Mikroskopisch Hämolyse. Ausgedehnte Hämoglobinwolken unter zum Teil braun gefärbtem Epithel. Keine Blutungen
24	Fast kein Abblassen auf Fingerdruck. Ausgedehnte Hämoglobinwolken unter braun gefärbtem Epithel
28	Angedeutetes Abblassen auf Fingerdruck. Mikroskopischer Befund wie oben
29	Geringes Abblassen auf Fingerdruck. Starke Hyperämie. Ausgedehnte Hämolyse. Kontinuierliche Hämoglobinwolken unter braun gefärbtem Epithel

Tabelle 1 (Fortsetzung)

Zeit nach dem Tode Std	Ergebnis
30	Kein Abblassen auf Fingerdruck, wohl aber auf Druck mit der Pinzette. Mikroskopisch kontinuierliche braune Epithelfärbung
32	Ganz geringes Abblassen auf Fingerdruck. Mikroskopisch kontinuierliche Wolke unter dem braun gefärbten Epithel
32	Befund wie oben. Auch Muskeln und Drüsen braun gefärbt. Ausgedehnte Hämolyse. Epithel braun gefärbt
33	Kein Abblassen auf Fingerdruck, wohl aber auf Druck mit der Pinzette. Mikroskopischer Befund wie oben
39	Makroskopischer und mikroskopischer Befund wie oben
41	Befund wie oben
46	Noch geringes Abblassen auf Fingerdruck. Sonst Befund wie oben
48	Deutliches Abblassen auf Fingerdruck (die Leiche kam sofort nach dem Tode in eine Temperatur von etwa 0°). Mikroskopisch konfluierende Wolken von Hämoglobin. Keine deutliche Braunfärbung des Epithels
48	Kein Abblassen auf Fingerdruck. Mikroskopische Befunde wie bei 32 Std
52	Befund wie oben
55	Befund wie oben. Keine Blutungen
57	Befund wie oben. Keine Blutungen
3 Tage	Kein Abblassen auf Fingerdruck, wohl aber Abblassen bei Druck mit der Pinzette. Makroskopisch keine Blutungen. Mikroskopisch Blutungen in der Lederhaut und in der Tiefe. Ausgedehnte Hämoglobinwolken. Epithel durchgängig braun
5 Tage	Befunde wie vorstehend
6 Tage	Befunde wie vorstehend. Mikroskopisch sind geborstene Capillaren sichtbar. Reichlich Blutpigment. Eisenreaktion negativ. Im Bereiche einer innerhalb des Totenfleckes liegenden Hautnarbe keine Hämoglobinwolken, auch keine Epithelfärbung
8 Tage	Kein Abblassen auf Fingerdruck, wohl aber auch jetzt noch schwaches Abblassen auf Druck mit der Pinzette. Mikroskopischer Befund wie oben. (Leiche lag in Kühlanlage)

Bei Kühllagerung (0°) waren Totenflecke sogar bis zu 48 Std post mortem auf Fingerdruck zum Abblassen zu bringen (MUELLER).

Beschränkt auf den Bereich der Totenflecke können postmortale bis erbsgroße, z.T. scharf, z.T. aber auch unscharf begrenzte p.m. Rhexisblutungen entstehen. Der Druck der auf die Hautcapillaren lastenden Blutsäule läßt die Gefäße reißen, Blut dringt ins Gewebe.

In der Hypostase sind nicht nur Haut-, sondern auch Schleimhautgefäße strotzend mit Blut gefüllt. Es kann somit auch zu Schleimhautblutungen kommen. Typisches Beispiel: Hanglage des Kopfes: Bindehäute mit flächigen Blutungen, Nasenbluten aus den Conchae. Aus diesen Blutungen sind jedoch keine Rückschlüsse auf die Todeszeit möglich.

Wird eine Leiche gefunden und zeigt sie sowohl über der Bauch- als auch über der Rückfläche Livores, wurde der Körper zu einer bestimmten Zeit nach dem Tode umgelagert! Unternahm man den Versuch einer *Beseitigung* der Leiche, den eines *Leichentransportes* ?

Die *Todesursache* läßt sich mitunter direkt oder indirekt über die Totenflecke ablesen.

Letztere sind zunächst blaß-rot, später nehmen sie intensiv die Farbe des reduzierten Hämoglobins an. Wenn jedoch Kohlenmonoxydvergiftung oder Intoxikation durch Met-Hb-bildende Gifte vorliegen, werden wir die Todesursache entsprechend deuten.

Ähnliches gilt indirekt auch für die Frage: Erhängungstod. Wir erkennen vitale Reaktionen (Stauungsblutungen in die Conjunctiven, in die Haut des Gesichtes), sehen ferner zirkulär um die unteren Extremitäten ausgebreitete, intensive Totenflecke, evtl. auch noch an Händen und Unterarmen; man wird folgern, daß einerseits die Vitalzeichen einer Stauung im Kopfbereich und andererseits die Verteilung der Totenflecke für Erhängungstod, die freie Hanglage des Körpers, sprechen. Wird die Leiche einer gesunden jungen Frau gefunden, sprechen extrem blasse Totenflecke für die Verdachtsdiagnose: Tubarruptur. Vielfältige, forensisch wichtige Aussagen gestattet die Untersuchung der Haut. Konnten sich Totenflecke wegen eng anliegender Kleidungsstücke nicht ausbilden, wird sich das Muster dieser Kleidung deutlich abzeichnen. Man erkennt ein bestimmtes Textilmuster. Ferner ist aus Lage und Verteilung der Aufliegestellen, die ja ebenfalls kein abgesunkenes Blut haben aufnehmen können, auf die Körperhaltung rückzuschließen.

a) Differentialdiagnose zwischen Cyanose und Totenflecken

Stirbt der Mensch nach oberer Einflußstauung, bei Strangulation, Drosselung oder Würgeakt mit partiellem Verschluß der arteriellen Gefäße, verfärbt sich die enorme Capillarblutfülle der Gesichtshaut intensiv bläulich. Das sich hier vital oder agonal demonstrierende, reduzierte Hämoglobin unterscheidet sich selbstverständlich in der Tönung nicht von dem der Totenflecke. Man müßte sich fragen, ob diese vital gesichert entstandene Cyanose nach dem Tode noch erhalten bleibt. Auch hier stehen viele Dinge in Abhängigkeit zueinander. Bleibt der Körper im Strang eine gewisse Zeit hängen, vergeht die Cyanose des Gesichtes nicht. Wenn die Leiche dagegen rasch aus der Schlinge befreit wird, ist es durchaus möglich, daß die vitale Cyanose postmortal abblaßt. Auf der anderen Seite wissen wir, daß häufig gerade im Gesicht jene fleckigen, zunächst rötlichen, später blau-violetten Totenflecken auftreten, selbst wenn das Gesicht sich nicht in Tieflage befindet. Sobald diese Totenflecke zusammengeflossen sind — besonders bei Hanglage des Kopfes — ist es kaum möglich, eine vitale, von der postmortalen Cyanose zu unterscheiden.

b) Postmortale Reoxydation der Livores
(Percutane Permeation von Gasen)

Die Totenflecke geben die Farbe des reduzierten Hämoglobins wieder. Wird jedoch eine Leiche — z.B. in einen kühlen Raum bei $+4°$ — gebracht, schlägt sich Feuchtigkeit auf der Körperoberfläche nieder. Wo Luft an die von Totenflecken eingenommene Haut kommt, wird Sauerstoff permiieren und das reduzierte Hämoglobin reoxydieren. Beim Wenden der Leiche sieht man dann rote Reoxydationsstreifen zumeist im Randgebiet der sonst blau-violetten Totenflecke. Man möge bei der Prüfung nicht vergessen, das Nagelbett zu betrachten, denn hier dokumentiert sich — Sauerstoff kann ja nicht hinzutreten — stets am besten die Tönung des Blutfarbstoffes.

Gehen wir einen Schritt weiter: Es ist möglich, daß andere Gase percutan permiieren; man wird aus differentialdiagnostischen Gründen Blut aus Hautcapillaren und Herzkammern asservieren und untersuchen; CO-Hb ließ sich im Hautblut feststellen, CO hat jedoch nicht in die Tiefe permiieren können! (Abb. 1).

c) Differentialdiagnose vitaler und postmortaler Blutungen

Von den postmortalen Rhexisblutungen in den Totenflecken wurde gesprochen. Sie können vereinzelt, zumeist jedoch in großer Zahl, vorkommen. Sie sind stecknadelkopfgroß, gelegentlich — besonders bei freihängenden Körpern — an den unteren Extremitäten bis zu 2-DM-Stück groß. Liegt der Mensch in Rückenlage, entstehen die Vibices in der Rückenhaut, der Rückfläche der Gliedmaßen, des Nackens; bei Bauchlage dann entsprechend über der Vorderfläche des Körpers, häufig bandförmig von den Schultern über die obere Brust gehend. Hängt z.B. der Kopf aus dem Bett, werden Rhexisblutungen auch in Gesichtshaut und

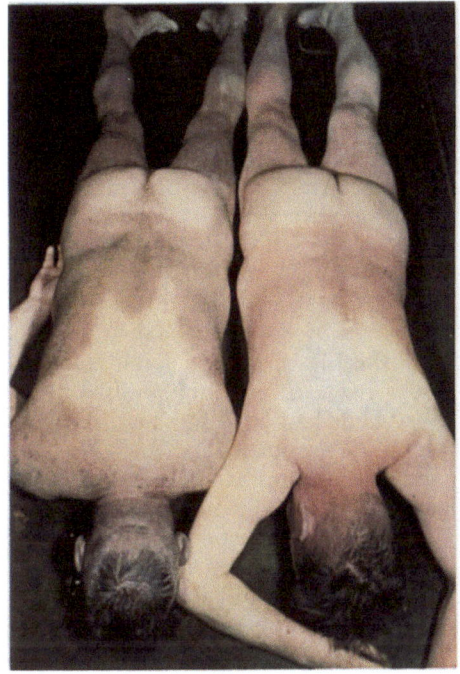 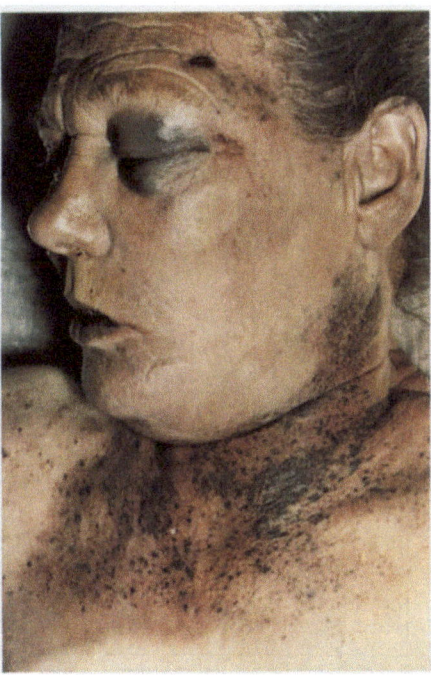

Abb. 1   Abb. 2

Abb. 1. Differente Farbtönungen der Livores. Links: reduziertes Hb. Rechts: CO-Hb

Abb. 2. Kopftieflage einer Leiche mit Rhexisblutungen nebst Blutungen in die Lider

Schleimhäuten zu sehen sein. Nasenbluten nach postmortalen Rhexisblutungen aus den Schleimhäuten der Nasenöffnungen und solche nach Rupturen der Trommelfellgefäße können nicht nur nach vitaler mechanischer Behinderung der äußeren Atmung entstehen, sondern sich auch bei Kopfhanglage an der Leiche ausbilden (PONSOLD, STICHNOTH, BSCHOR). Cave: Verwechslung mit vitalen Blutungen, mit Ekchymosen beim Erhängungstod oder nach Blutdruckkrisen etc.

Vitale neben postmortalen Blutungen haben sich evtl. ausgebildet. Ohne Obduktion ist es nicht möglich zu klären, welchen Ursprungs diese Blutungen sind. Außerhalb der Hypostase sieht man postmortale Rhexisblutungen natürlich nicht. Die Fundlage der Leiche muß bekannt sein.

Hatten sich Vibices bereits gebildet, wurde der Körper dann erst umgelagert, verblassen zwar — in Abhängigkeit von der Zeit — die Totenflecke, so bleiben jedoch postmortale Hautblutungen bestehen, heben sich noch deutlicher von der jetzt blasseren Umgebung ab. Auf der einen Körperseite finden sich Vibices, auf der Gegenseite haben sich erneut Totenflecke gezeigt. Rücken- wie Bauchfläche sind durch Livores gezeichnet.

Daß *postmortale Hautblutungen* dort fehlen, wo äußerer Druck Totenflecke nicht entstehen ließ, weist auf An- bzw. Aufliegeflächen des Körpers; ebenfalls auf Hautkompression in Körperfalten, im Bereich von Kleider- oder Schmuckaussparungen etc.!

Blutungen aus den Körperöffnungen oder in der Haut sind nicht immer vital entstanden. Zum Teil handelt es sich um agonale Sturzverletzungen. Wir denken an die ausgedehnten Schürfungen, Kopfschwarten- und Weichteilblutungen, evtl. sogar Schädelbrüche, die dann entstehen, wenn ein Mensch agonal zu Boden stürzt. Oder aber an schwerste agonale Krampfabläufe. Die krampfenden Glieder, z.B. die seitlichen Flächen der Arme, Beine und der Kopf, schlagen gegen feste Gegenstände. Auf das Verteilungsmuster dieser Blutungen und Schürfungen, wie Platzwunden, ist zu achten; Skizzen sind zu fertigen.

Aus dem Munde — später aus den Nasenöffnungen — ist ein feinstblasiges hämorrhagisches Lungenödem gequollen. Die Blasen platzen dann. Aus dem Munde scheint eine blutige Flüssigkeit ausgelaufen zu sein. Der Verdacht entsteht, es würde sich um einen Zustand nach Gewalteinwirkung handeln. Hier demonstriert sich lediglich das postmortal verflüssigte, hämorrhagische Lungenödem. Daneben kann sich ein primäres nicht hämorrhagisches Lungenödem, ein Schaumpilz vor Nasen- und Mundöffnung, sekundär verfärben. Anfangs ist der Schaumpilz des zuvor Ertrunkenen schneeweiß, dann wird der Stiel rosa, später rot, zuletzt ist der Schaum insgesamt eingefärbt und beginnt sich zu verflüssigen.

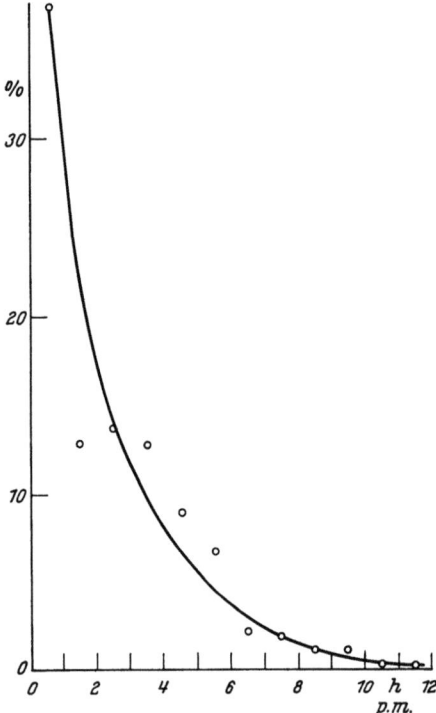

Abb. 3. Auslösung cutaner und subcutaner Blutung p.m. — 467 Ergebnisse an 176 Leichen — in Abhängigkeit von der Zeit p.m. [G. DOTZAUER, Dtsch. Z. ges. gerichtl. Med. **46**, 761—771 (1958)]

Zu leicht unterliegt man dem Fehlschluß, die vitale Entstehung von Blutungen in Haut- und Unterhautfettgewebe wäre gesichert. Im Rahmen der Auslösung des idiomuskulären Wulstes wurde festgestellt, daß sowohl in der Cutis als auch in der Subcutis nach mechanischer Irritierung Blutungen entstehen. Die Blutungsfähigkeit in das Gewebe nach p.m. Traumatisierung erlischt vor Verlust der Bildung eines idiomuskulären Wulstes (Abb. 3).

Wann blutet es postmortal in die Haut? Nach der Traumatisierung entstanden in $^2/_3$ jener Fälle mit ausgebildetem idiomuskulären Wulst postmortale Hautblutungen. — Bei welchen Leichen sind diese Blutungen sehr intensiv? Bei welchen schwach? Das *Lebensalter* scheint von Bedeutung zu sein; soweit unser relativ einheitliches Beobachtungsgut Rückschlüsse zuläßt, fehlt im höheren Alter häufig die Hautblutung nach einer Traumatisierung. Andererseits entstehen gelegentlich bei alten Menschen sehr flächenhafte Blutungen ohne Ausbildung der typischen Doppelstreifen, wenn man mit einem stabförmigen Gegenstand einen

Schlag auf die Haut über dem Bicepsmuskel führt. Ein weiteres Ergebnis zeigte sich: denn in 31% der Testungen *ohne* Hautblutungen hat es sich um *Verblutungstodesfälle* gehandelt.

Das Ausmaß der Blutung ist unterschiedlich stark. Die Rhexisblutungen sind in ihrer Ausdehnung nicht nur durch die Größe des direkt angreifenden Traumas bestimmt, sondern sie verdanken ihre Intensität z.T. sicherlich auch der supravitalen Erregbarkeit der Muskulatur. Postmortale Blutungen in das Gewebe lassen sich mit dem Messer ausstreifen.

Postmortale Rhexisblutungen in der Haut des Hodensackes sahen wir bei Erhängungstodesfällen, Hypostase wegen freier Hanglage, bei schweißmaceriertem Hodensack. Aus rupturierten Venen tritt flüssiges Blut aus, rinnt an den Beinen ab.

Vitale Blutungen werden nach Eingriffen, zum Zwecke der Wiederbelebung, vorgetäuscht. Zumeist sind zwar derartige Thorakotomiewunden sowohl schon im Unterhautfettgewebe als auch in der Haut frei von typischen Blutungen. Wenn jedoch in der ersten Zeit nach dem Tode gerade in jener interessierenden, wichtigen Periode für die Anlegung der Thorakotomie ein Operationsschnitt geführt wird, entstehen gelegentlich dünnstreifige Blutungen auch im Haut- bzw. Unterhautfettgewebsschnitt. Über die Verhältnisse im Bereich der Lungenquetschungen bzw. des Herzbeutels, des Epikards und des Myokards wurde an anderer Stelle berichtet.

Ein Mensch wird verschüttet oder unterliegt einer schweren breitflächigen, im Bereich des Oberleibes oder auch des Brustkorbes angreifenden, stumpfen Gewalt, so bilden sich die Perthesschen Blutungen in Haut, Schleimhaut, Körper- bzw. Organhöhlen außerhalb der Kompressionszone. Ist ein Leichnam in der frühen Leichenzeit einer starken breiten Kompression ausgesetzt, wird auch jetzt noch flüssiges Blut in den Hals- und Kopfbereich gepreßt, so daß sich Blutungen, ähnlich den Perthesschen Stauungsblutungen, ausbilden können.

Das Ausmaß postmortaler Blutungen ist von Todesursache und der verstrichenen Zeit nach dem Tode abhängig. Wir finden Blutungen im Bereich aller Körperteile. Sie sind nach einer gesicherten, postmortalen Einwirkung in der Zone der Totenflecke stärker als außerhalb derselben, sie bilden sich im zarten Gewebe intensiver aus, sind aber eher am Bauch als am Rücken zu sehen (RAUBER, KOPSCH, WEINIG und ZINK).

Vielleicht wäre einmal die Frage aufzuwerfen, ob Blutungen erst postmortal während der Verstümmelung eines Körpers, wie z.B. durch Verkehrsunfall, entstehen; unterstellen wir: Ein Mensch stirbt eines natürlichen Todes auf der Straße und wird sofort von einem Lkw überrollt: Schwere Traumatisierung einer Leiche.

Daß bei einem engen zeitlichen Intervall zwischen Tod und postmortaler Verletzung Haut- und Unterhautblutungen gesetzt werden, ist verständlich. Der Befund des Zustandes nach Überfahren verführt leider zu leicht zu der Folgerung, daß es sich zwangsläufig um Tod nach Verkehrsunfall handelt.

Man könnte das Problem aufzeigen, ob nicht Blutungen aus Hautwunden Auskunft darüber gäben, wann die Wunde entstanden ist. Wir stehen unter der Vorstellung, das Blut einer Leiche würde nicht mehr gerinnen. Bei 102 Leichen mit bekannter Todeszeit wurden 379 Herzpunktionen durchgeführt, es gelang bei allen plötzlichen Todesfällen flüssiges Blut zu asservieren. Das in corpore noch flüssige Blut gerann in Minutenfrist nach Einfüllen in ein Becherglas en bloque. Etwa 2 Std nach dem Tode war die spontane Gerinnung nicht mehr so augenscheinlich; wurde Blut erst mehrere Stunden post mortem entnommen, trat zwar Gerinnung ein, aber zeitlich verzögert und unvollkommen. Zwischen Todesursache und Gerinnungszustand in vitro konnte bei diesen plötzlichen Todesfällen keine Beziehung gefunden werden. Dies gilt auch für die sofort tödlichen Unfälle.

Ausnahmen bildeten einige Intoxikationen, z.B. Alkoholvergiftungen oder Thrombose wie Embolien, etc.

Blut gerinnt in vitro bis etwa zur 6. Std p.m. Dieser Befund ist von entscheidender Bedeutung. Wenn also ein Mensch in der Lache geronnenen Blutes gefunden wird, ist es durchaus möglich, daß die Verletzung, d.h. damit auch die Blutung, erst nach dem Tode entstanden ist.

4. Postmortale Gewebswasserverschiebung

Zu Lebzeiten ausgebildete Ödeme flachen gegebenenfalls nach dem Tode ab, besonders dann, wenn sie außerhalb der Zone der Hypostase gelegen haben; zumeist sind sie zu tasten.

Im Gewebe abhängiger Körperpartien, damit auch in der Haut, entstehen nicht nur Livores, sondern Haut wie Unterhautfettgewebe werden infolge Flüssigkeitswanderung aus physikalischen Gründen, ferner wegen Zusammenbruchs der Gewebsschranken, also aus nekrochemischer Verursachung, flüssigkeitsreicher.

5. pH-Wasserstoffionenkonzentration

Die H-Ionenkonzentration der Haut ist beim Lebenden von verschiedenen Faktoren abhängig:

Morphologischer Aufbau der Haut,

Funktionszustand,

Sekundäre Einflüsse wie Reinigung (Waschmittel, Kosmetika), Verschmutzungen u.a. durch Berufsarbeit.

Agonal werden sich, in Abhängigkeit von der Länge des Todeskampfes, in enger Verbindung mit den Kreislaufverhältnissen, bereits an der Körperoberfläche (Todesschweiß) Einflüsse auf die Wasserstoffionenkonzentration zeigen.

Intracutane pH-Messungen, besonders während der entscheidenden agonalen Phase, liegen unseres Wissens nicht vor.

Die Wasserstoffionenkonzentration der Leichenhaut ist in der frühen wie späten Leichenzeit von Umweltbedingungen bzw. der Art der Zersetzung des menschlichen Körpers abhängig. Da die Bakterienflora in Verbindung mit dem Ab- bzw. Umbau der Haut direkt oder indirekt über weitere Stoffwechselprodukte auf die Wasserstoffionenkonzentration Einfluß nimmt, werden wir zwangsläufig in den verschiedenen Zeiten nach dem Tode, aber auch in den einzelnen Körperregionen, sehr differente Ergebnisse zu erwarten haben.

Postmortale Verdunstung, die Austrocknung der Körperoberfläche, wirken sich aus. Feste Stoffe werden bei den auf der Körperoberfläche bestehenden Temperaturen nicht in Dampfzustand gebracht; deshalb bleiben sie zurück und ihr ionogenes Verhalten wird sich steuernd auf den pH-Wert auswirken.

Gerät die noch warme Leiche sehr rasch in eine kühle Umgebung, wird sich Feuchtigkeit auf der Körperoberfläche niederschlagen. Auch jetzt kann sich die H-Ionenkonzentration ändern.

6. Autolyse

Die Autolyse ist das Resultat komplexer, vital auslaufender, biochemischer bzw. beginnender nekrochemischer Stoffwechselprozesse. Zu differenzieren ist die Start- von der progressiven Autolyse.

Bei ersterer sind morphologische Veränderungen nicht zu erwarten, sie spielen sich im submikroskopischen Raume ab. Die Trennung gegenüber der progressiven Autolyse ist unscharf; die Stoffwechsellage, das Redoxpotential der Zelle im Augenblick des Todes sind entscheidend, damit u. a. der Glykogen- und Eiweiß- bzw. Fettgehalt der Zellen. Wegen fehlender Resynthese dirigieren katabole, in den ersten Schritten noch den zellgebundenen Sauerstoff verwertende, dann aber im wesentlichen anaerob verlaufende Prozesse die abakterielle Selbstauflösung des intra- wie extracellulären Raumes. Der Zusammenbruch der Permeabilität, der Schrankenfunktionen, läßt aus den Gefäßen nicht nur Serum, sondern auch Elektrolyte treten. Die intravasale Hämolyse, die Imbibition der Gefäßwand und des umgebenden Gewebes, leiten zur Fäulnis über.

Glykolyse, Proteolyse sowie Lipolyse durch körpereigene Enzyme bauen Gewebe ab. Da der Bakterienbefall der Körperoberfläche *vor*, aber auch *nach* dem Tode mittels bakterieller Fremdenzyme in die Zersetzung eingreift, verwischt sich die Grenze zwischen abakterieller Autolyse und bakteriellen Fäulnisvorgängen.

Wovon hängen Art wie Ausmaß kataboler Stoffwechselprozesse ab?

Nach dem Tode gleicht sich die *Temperatur* des Körpers — damit auch der Haut — der Umgebungstemperatur an. Die Autolyse ist bei Temperaturen von 37—42° am stärksten, deshalb setzt sie bei warmen Umgebungstemperaturen — Bettleiche — rascher ein als bei entblößter Haut einer im Freien, im Schnee, liegenden Leiche. Tritt der Tod unter hohem Fieber ein, befindet sich der Körper über längere Zeit in einem Autolyse-Optimum. Die Haut wird eine raschere und intensivere Autolyse zeigen. Die *Anoxybiose* wird die Autolyse in den Zellen durch gewebseigene Enzyme steuern (MÜLLER, LETTERER). Da die biochemische Ausgangslage einer jeden Zelle im Augenblick des Todes in Abhängigkeit vom Grundleiden, von der

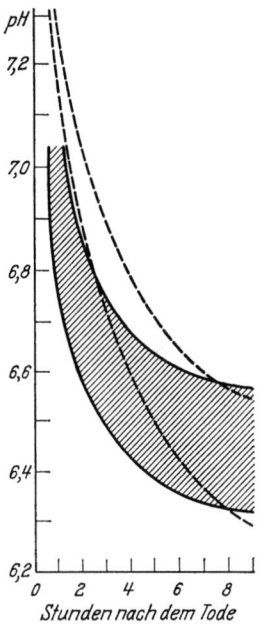

Abb. 4. pH-Messungen des Liquors (———) und des Blutes der rechten Herzkammer (------). Plötzliche Todesfälle, 140 Meßpunkte bei Zisternenpunktion, 300 Meßpunkte bei Herzpunktion. (DOTZAUER und NAEVE, 1959)

Todesursache, der Länge der Agone sehr unterschiedlich ist, sind bei Autolyse bzw. späterer Fäulnis differente Ergebnisse in einzelnen Hautbezirken zu erwarten.

Zu Beginn der 50er Jahre haben eine Reihe von Untersuchern dem Problem der postmortalen Säuerung des Gewebes ihre Aufmerksamkeit geschenkt (O. SCHMIDT u. Mitarb., SCHLEYER, SCHOURUP). An einzelnen Organen und Körperflüssigkeiten wurde in Abhängigkeit von der Glykolyse, der Milchsäureanreicherung in den Organen, eine in Relation zur Milchsäurekonzentration stehende Säuerung des Gewebes gesehen. Während der Glykolyse wird, wie wir es z. B. am Blute darstellen konnten, innerhalb von wenigen Stunden eine Säuerung bis auf pH 6 eintreten (Abb. 4).

Viele Versuche wurden unter aeroben Bedingungen durchgeführt, sie sind nicht einfach zu übertragen, denn im Gewebe interessiert die anaerobe autolytische Zellzersetzung. Die Säuerung dürfte langsamer als in vitro oder unter Sauerstoffzutritt ablaufen, gleiches gilt für die spätere — als Folge der Proteolyse sich einstellende und der Fäulnis zuzuordnende — Alkalisierung des Gewebes.

Über die Aktivierung cellulärer Enzyme mit einem Aktivitätsoptimum im Sauren liegen Untersuchungen vor. Die morphologisch faßbaren Veränderungen der Zellstruktur, des Cytoplasmas wie auch des Kernes, finden sich bei Befunden von MÖNNINGHOFF, ZOLLINGER, LETTERER, TERBRÜGGEN, SCHÜMMELFEDER, ALTMANN, MÜLLER, GREUER, CAESAR, HECHT, KORB und DAVID.

Wenige Arbeiten gibt es über die *Autolyse der Haut*. In den letzten Jahren hat sich besonders BRAUN-FALCO dieses Problems angenommen und normale menschliche Haut einer Untersuchung zugeführt: Sterile Entnahme, Unterbringung in einer feuchten Kammer bei 37°. Kontrollen bei +4° im Kühlschrank. Entnahme im Abstand von 3—48 Std und nach 3, 4 und 5 Tagen. Fixierung in neutralem Formol, Paraffineinbettungen.

a) Morphologische Befunde. Bei 37° sind am stärksten Epidermis, Haarfollikel mit Talgdrüsen betroffen, während ekkrine Schweißdrüsen und deren Ausführungsgänge gegenüber der Autolyse resistent sind. Das Bindegewebe ist nur gering, relativ spät erst, betroffen. Der Zeitpunkt erster faßbarer Veränderungen scheint in Beziehung zum Grundleiden, selbst bei „sonst normaler" Haut, zu stehen. BRAUN-FALCO und WINTER sahen initiale Befunde bei normaler Haut nach 15 Std, dagegen schon nach 3 Std in der „normalen" Haut eines wegen Endangitis obliterans amputierten Unterschenkels. In der ersten Phase wirkt die *Epidermis* stärker eosinophil. Im oberen *Stratum Malpighi* sind die Zellkerne wie kondensiert mit heller perinuclearer Zone, das *Stratum granulosum* scheint stellenweise schwächer angefärbt. Keratohyalingranula außerhalb der Zelle. Die Grenze zwischen Stratum granulosum und dem Corneum ist verwaschen.

Die zweite Phase setzt bei normaler Haut 18—25 Std, bei dem Endangitis obliterans-Fall bereits nach 6 Std ein. Zunehmende Eosinophilie des Cytoplasmas der *Epidermis*. Im *Stratum spinosum* Pyknose der Kerne mit perinucleären Vacuolen, zumindest aber Chromatin-Verklumpungen innerhalb der Kerne. Gelegentlich sind diese nur durch fädige oder unregelmäßige Chromatinverdichtungen angedeutet bzw. schwächer angefärbt. Eine Reduzierung der Basophilie wird vermerkt. Ähnliche Befunde am *Stratum granulosum*. Keine bemerkenswerten Veränderungen an den epithelialen Anhangsgebilden. Capillarendothelien o. B. Ebenfalls das Bindegewebe der Haut.

Die dritte Phase setzt nach 24—48 Std bzw. bei der Endangitis obliterans nach 9—12 Std ein. Deutlicher Verlust der Kernstruktur und der Anfärbbarkeit, bevorzugt im *Stratum spinosum und granulosum*. Auflösung der Keratohyalinkörperchen. Einzelne Zellkerne der Epidermis zeigen Pyknose bei erhaltener Anfärbbarkeit.

Im Cytoplasma des Stratum basale Vacuolen und beginnende spaltförmige Lösungen von Epidermis und Cutis.

Pyknose und Karyolyse der Zellkerne in der äußeren Wurzelscheide und der Haarmatrix — Auflösung der verfetteten Talgzellen unter Kernschwund. Die Talgdrüsen-Mutterzellen sind morphologisch resistenter. — Die Membrana propria und die Myoepithelien der ekkrinen Schweißdrüsen bleiben gut erhalten; die Schweißdrüsenendstücke zeigen eine fortschreitende Desintegration des Epithels nach Auflösung des Cytoplasmas: pyknotische Zellkerne, schlierenähnliche Cytoplasmareste. Die Ausführungsgänge und ihr intradermaler Anteil sind wenig berührt. BRAUN-FALCO unterscheidet zwei weitere Phasen:

In der vierten ist das epidermisnahe Corium bakteriendurchsetzt. Wegen der Fremdenzyme ist jetzt nicht mehr von abakterieller Autolyse, sondern von bakterieller Fäulnis zu sprechen.

b) Chemische und histochemische Befunde. Welche *chemischen* bzw. *histochemischen* Befunde in der Leichenhaut wurden bekannt? MONACELLI konstatierte einen raschen Abfall der nach HAGEDORN-JENSEN bestimmten Reduktionswerte mit einem späteren Wiederanstieg. Der Glykogengehalt war bereits nach einer

Autolyse von $1^1/_2$ Std — Haut in physiologischer Kochsalzlösung bei $+37°C$ — auf ca. 20% des Ausgangswertes gesunken, Glykogen war nach 5 Std nicht mehr darzustellen.

In den Zellen der *Endstücke* ekkriner Schweißdrüsen der *Abdominalhaut* war Glykogen 2—5 Std p.m., jedoch der *Palmar- wie Plantarhaut*, erst 14—52 Std p.m. nicht mehr nachweisbar. Aus den Zellen der *Schweißdrüsenausführungsgänge* ist Glykogen 15—30 Std p.m. verschwunden, es hält sich lange in den äußeren Wurzelscheiden der Haarfollikel (LEE).

Bei allen Testungen ist mit topischen Differenzen zu rechnen.

Was besagen die Experimente von BRAUN-FALCO und WINTER über die Histochemie der Haut während der Autolyse? In ihrer Zusammenfassung schreiben sie u.a.: Die Mitochondrien-gebundene Cytochromoxydase- und Bernsteinsäuredehydrogenase-Aktivität erlischt frühzeitig; es könnte ein Strukturabbau der Mitochondrien vorliegen.

In den Kernen erfolgt der DNS-Abbau später als der RNS, wie er sich durch den Verlust der Pyroninophilie von Nucleolen und Cytoplasma andeutet. *Verlust der Pyroninophilie ist das erste Zeichen des Zelltodes.*

Hydrolytische Enzymaktivitäten (unspezifische Esterasen, saure Phosphatasen, alkalische Phosphatasen) bleiben relativ lange erhalten. Auffällig ist eine vielleicht auf Diffusionsphänomene zu beziehende Aktivität unspezifischer Esterasen in den basalen Zellagen der Epidermis. Proteolytische Enzyme, soweit sie mit der Aminopeptidase-Reaktion faßbar sind, scheinen für die Autolyse der Haut nicht von Bedeutung zu sein.

Leider haben auch die sehr schönen histochemischen Untersuchungen von RAEKALLIO, PIOCH u.a. über diese Probleme keine Aussagen bringen können.

Ein spezieller Fall betrifft die abakterielle Maceration einer Frucht nach intrauterinem Fruchttod bei unversehrter Fruchtblase und Verbleiben im feuchten Milieu. SEITZ unterscheidet zwei Grade der Maceration:

Im ersten Grad läßt sich die Oberhaut etwa 1—3 Tage nach dem Fruchttod in Blasen lösen oder stößt sich fetzig ab.

Die Oberhaut kann noch unverfärbt sein. Ist jedoch beim Tod, besonders älterer Früchte, Meconium abgegangen, verfärben sich Oberhaut und Nabelschnur schmutzig-grünlich oder grau-grün. Nach Ausstoßung dieser Früchte vertrocknet das Corium im Bereich geplatzter Blasen, der Blasengrund verfärbt sich düster braun-rot.

Im zweiten Grad wird die Haut durch Hämolyse grau-braun bis schmutzigrot-braun. Hinzu kommt auch hier die etwaige Verfärbung durch Gallenfarbstoffe des Meconiums. Die weiß-schmierige Haut ist schlaff, die Oberhaut verschiebbar. Da durch die Hämolyse auch das Fruchtwasser rötlich oder rot-braun gefärbt wird, nimmt die Nabelschnur eine trüb-rote bis grünliche Farbe an. Die intrauterine Autolyse verläuft bei einem Fruchttod junger Schwangerschaften rascher und intensiver. Kleinere Früchte, so schreibt HABERDA, können infolge Verflüssigung der Weichteile schon in 1—2 Wochen skelettiert sein. Der Befund einer intrauterinen Mazeration läßt an natürlichen Tod denken. Liegt lediglich eine Frucht zur Untersuchung vor, sind differentialdiagnostische Überlegungen: intrauterine Maceration oder Fäulnisvorgänge nach Abtreibungshandlungen anzustellen. Ein intrauteriner Fruchttod ist ebenfalls ohne äußeren Eingriff infolge von Intoxikationen, durch Gifte, die zum Zwecke einer Fruchtabtreibung eingenommen wurden, möglich. Eine macerierte Frucht läßt nicht in jedem Fall auf einen natürlichen Vorgang schließen.

Die postmortale Autolyse fetaler menschlicher Haut untersuchte ANDERSON. Innerhalb von 6 Std trat eine Reduzierung metachromasiegebundener Substanzen oder eine Verminderung PAS-reaktiver Polysaccharide und SH-gruppenhaltiger Proteine nicht auf, gleich, ob die Haut bei +4° oder bei Zimmertemperatur gehalten wurde.

7. Rigor

Beginn wie Stärke der Totenstarre quergestreifter Muskulatur werden zur Todeszeitbestimmung eingesetzt. In der Haut wird der Rigor der Arrectores pilorum geprüft. Wir kennen die typische Gänsehautbildung beim Lebenden, wissen, daß sich ante finem häufig eine Gänsehaut ausbildet, wie wir ja auch an anderen Teilen der glatten Muskulatur Kontraktionen sehen, Kontraktionen, die

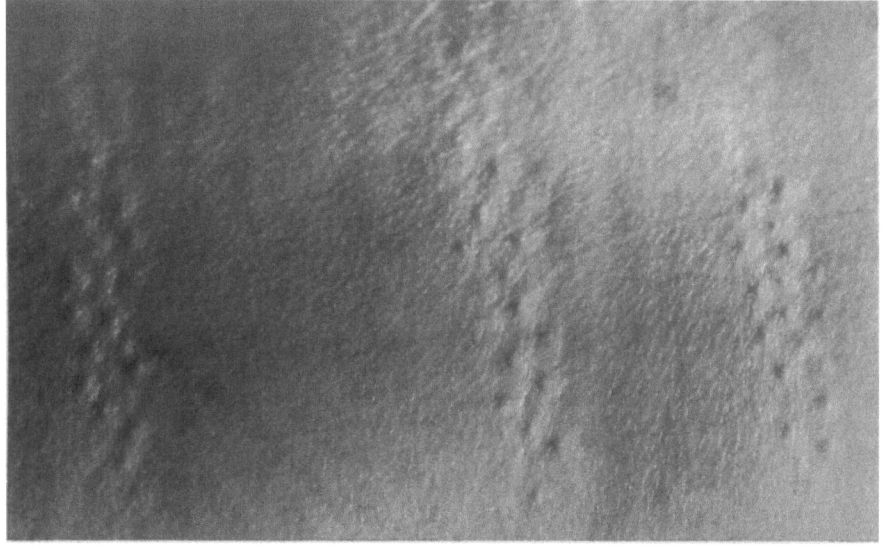

Abb. 5. Mechanische Erregbarkeit der Mm. arrectores pilorum nach drei im Abstand geführten Schlägen

zur Teilentleerung des Darmes (Kotabgang) und selbst zum Austritt des feuchten Tropfens an der Harnröhrenmündung führen. Die Totenstarre der Arrectores ist kein eigentliches Todeszeichen! Bei Prüfung des idiomuskulären Wulstes (IMW), der ja ebenfalls sowohl vital als supravital auszulösen ist, wurde nach mechanischer Irritierung ebenfalls eine „Gänsehaut" hervorgerufen. Der Kliniker Hoff faßt den vital ausgelösten IMW als Folge einer Stoffwechselstörung mit einer Glykogenverarmung und Kreatinurie auf. (Morbus Addison, Ruhr mit starker Kachexie, stark abgemagerte Fleckfieberkranke, hochgradiger Salzverlust mit Hypochlorämie, Hungerzustände, maligne Tumoren, allgemein schwere Kachexien verschiedenster Herkunft.) Ein sehr starkes subcutanes Fettpolster erschwert die Auslösbarkeit. Die Haut müßte zudem dünn und atrophisch sein, um auf mechanischen Reiz hin einen länger dauernden, idiomuskulären Wulst entstehen zu lassen. So der Kliniker. Wir können dagegen auch bei Adipösen oder bei nichtatrophischer Haut den IMW an der Leiche ausgezeichnet prüfen.

Wenn wir über die p.m. Reaktionsfähigkeit der glatten Muskulatur, speziell der Arrectores pilorum als Ausdruck der supravitalen Reaktion, etwas auszusagen versuchen, ist folgendes zu bedenken:

Der lebende Muskel läßt Kontraktionen — je nach Schwere der Stoffwechselstörung — bzw. im Sterben selbst entstehen. Art und Länge der Agone gehen als differente Ausgangspositionen in diese Testung ein. Sie sind bei den meisten gewaltsamen, d. h. akuten Todesfällen aus voller Gesundheit gegenstandslos. Im Sterben bricht der Mensch zusammen, die Muskulatur erschlafft, verformt sich, flacht ab; dieses ist besonders deutlich an den Aufliegestellen.

Zur Prüfung der p.m. Erregbarkeit wird man mit der Flachseite des Messers oder eines Lineals auf die Haut z. B. des Oberschenkels, einen kurzen Schlag ausführen. Anschließend bildet sich die „Gänsehaut" streifenförmig im Schlagbereich. Nicht nur mechanische, sondern ebenfalls faradische, chemische und thermische Reize können die Muskulatur nach dem Tode zur Kontraktion bringen.

Aus einer Serie von Untersuchungen wurden Ergebnisse von Prüfungen des IMW zusammengestellt. In der ersten Phase wird sich die „Gänsehaut" ausbilden können (Abb. 6).

Wenn wir bei Einlieferung einer Leiche eine Gänsehaut sehen, werden wir uns also nicht ohne weiteres auf vitale oder postmortale Entstehung festlegen.

Wir sprachen die Rhexisblutungen nach postmortaler Traumatisierung der Körperoberfläche an. Die Ausdehnung mag mit der supravitalen Erregbarkeit der Muskulatur in Beziehung stehen. In den ersten Stunden nach dem Tode ist nach Setzung eines mechanischen Traumas ein scharf abgegrenzter Streifen von Gänsehaut zu sehen. Dieser ist zunächst sogar wesentlich breiter als die Breite des Schlagwerkzeuges, langsam verschmälert sich der Streifen Gänsehaut bis auf die Breite des Schlaginstrumentes (DOTZAUER). Die Muskelfasern der Arrectores gehen vom Haarbalg aus,

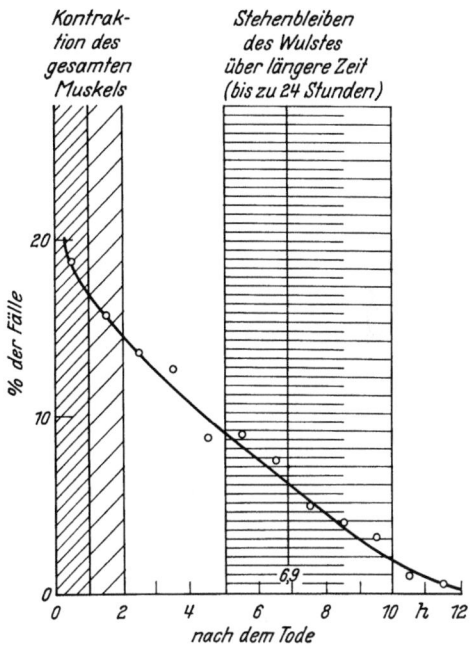

Abb. 6. Idiomuskulärer Wulst, 595 Prüfungen an 176 Leichen. [G. DOTZAUER, Dtsch. Z. ges. gerichtl. Med. **46**, 761—771 (1958)]

überbrücken den stumpfen Winkel zwischen Haar und Unterfläche der Epidermis. Im Stratum papillare endet die Muskelfaser in elastischen Fasern. Durch die Kontraktionen könnten sich die postmortalen Rhexisblutungen (Doppelstreifen z.B.), über den direkt irritierten Bezirk hinausgehend, verstärken. Die in dieser gesamten Zone liegenden Gefäße werden durch die sich kontrahierenden Arrectores pilorum komprimiert; Blut entleert sich entsprechend der Intensivierung der Rhexisblutungen. Dies trifft besonders in der ersten Zeit nach dem Tode zu.

Zwei weitere Auffälligkeiten in engem Zusammenhang mit dem Rigor: Gelegentlich fällt bei der äußeren Besichtigung einer Leiche auf, daß die Halshaut wegen der kontrahierten Muskelstränge des *Platysmas* wie in Falten gelegt erscheint. Dies wird nicht häufig registriert, d.h., trotz Einsetzens der Totenstarre in der gesamten Muskulatur braucht die Kontraktion des Platysma für das bloße Auge nicht deutlich zu werden; sicherlich sind Stärke der Muskulatur und Dicke des Unterhautfettpolsters von Bedeutung.

In den ersten Stunden nach dem Tode kontrahiert sich die *Tunica dartos*, der Hodensack hebt sich, die Haut legt sich in Falten.

8. Fettstarre

Die Konsistenz des Fettgewebes steht nach BARGMANN in Abhängigkeit von der Zusammensetzung der Fette und von der Körpertemperatur.

Das weiße Fett in den Fettzellen des menschlichen Gewebes setzt sich in erster Linie aus Neutralfetten, also Gemischen von Glycerinestern der Olein-, der Palmitin-, der Stearinsäure zusammen. Das weiße Fett enthält ferner in wechselnder Menge Lipoide, freie Fettsäuren, ihre Kalksalze und Lipochrome. Die Konsistenz der Fette wechselt je nach den Mengenverhältnissen der Ester in den verschiedenen Fettsäuren. Bei Körpertemperatur finden sich die Palmitin- und Stearinsäureester in *halbflüssigem*, die Oleinsäureester in *flüssigem* Zustande. Ein weiteres Unterscheidungsmerkmal steht in Abhängigkeit vom Alter. In den Fettzellen der Säuglinge überwiegen die festeren Fettsäuren, bei Erwachsenen die flüssigen Oleinsäuren. Nach dem Tode und damit dem Absinken der Körpertemperaturen, verändert sich auch die Konsistenz des Unterhautfettgewebes. Die Haut wird bis zum Eintritt der Fäulnis infolge der Verhärtung des Fettes etwas fester. Diese postmortale Fettstarre ist bei Neugeborenen bzw. Säuglingen wegen der relativen Vermehrung der Palmitin- und Stearinsäureester besonders ausgeprägt. Nach WALCHER kann die Fettstarre des Unterhautfettgewebes bei Kinderleichen diagnostische Schwierigkeiten bieten:

Bei entsprechender Lagerung wird die Haut bizarr in Falten gelegt, diese bleiben stehen, am Halse vermeint man, eine Pseudo-Strangfurche zu erkennen.

Weiterhin ist durch die Kälteerstarrung des Fettgewebes auch die Untersuchung des Vorhandenseins der Totenstarre erschwert. Der Rigor ist zwar schon verschwunden, man glaubt, eine totstarre Muskulatur zu tasten, dabei handelt es sich lediglich um die Fettstarre. Wir kennen ferner eine umschriebene postmortale Hautveränderung im Gefolge der Fettstarre, die sog. Acanthosis sebacea nach ORSÓS. Bei der sog. „Gänsehaut" handelt es sich nicht nur um eine Totenstarre der Arrectores, sondern sie wird nach Expression des Talgdrüseninhaltes mit anschließender Verhärtung des Talgs vorgetäuscht; eine „Gänsehaut" kann auch noch nach Lösung der Totenstarre vorgetäuscht werden, dies besonders bei Neugeborenen oder Säuglingen.

9. Vertrocknungen der Haut

a) Regulation des Wassergehaltes der intakten Haut, der sichtbaren Schleimhäute

Über den Wassergehalt der Haut und die normalen physiologischen Regulationen berichtete STÜTTGEN. Die Untersuchungen von HERRMANN über Fettfilm, den Fettmantel der Hautoberfläche, sind für unsere Betrachtungen von Wichtigkeit. Die Haut nimmt, in Abhängigkeit vom Feuchtigkeitsgehalt der atmosphärischen Luft, Wasser auf oder gibt dieses ab. Trotz erheblicher Verdunstung (Perspiration) bleibt der Wassergehalt der Haut unter physiologischen Bedingungen ziemlich konstant. Die gesunde Haut des Lebenden vertrocknet nicht.

α) Vertrocknungen der intakten Haut und der sichtbaren Schleimhäute in der Agone

Vertrocknungserscheinungen treten bereits zu Lebzeiten an der Körperoberfläche, der intakten Haut und den Schleimhäuten unter besonderen Bedingungen auf. Bei langdauernder Agonie, bei Bewußtseinsverlust usw., trocknen Lippen oder auch Teile der Schleimhaut der Mundhöhle, der Zungenspitze, aus. Es fehlen Lippenschluß und Befeuchtung durch die Zunge. — Der fehlende Lidschlag läßt die Bindehäute ebenfalls vertrocknen. Neben dem Mangel an mechanischer Befeuchtung treten bei Nachlassen der Herztätigkeit Folgen von Durchblutungsstörungen der Haut auf. Das durch Perspiration verlorengegangene Wasser wird der Haut nicht dementsprechend wieder zugeführt. Die Funktion der Schweiß- und Talgdrüsen kann ebenfalls gestört sein. — Liegt ein Mensch bewegungslos in der Agone, entstehen Druckstellen mit deutlicher Eintrocknung schneller, wenn der Körper auf einer saugfähigen Unterlage gelagert ist.

In der Agone gibt der Körper u. U. Flüssigkeiten ab, Todesschweiß bildet sich auf der Haut. Neben diesem Wasserverlust der noch lebenden Haut müssen wir jenen Wasserniederschlag auf die Haut des kürzlich Verstorbenen erwähnen: Die noch warme Körperoberfläche wird in eine kühle Umgebung (Kühlraum eines Pathologischen Institutes) verbracht. Wasser schlägt sich auf der Körperhaut nieder. Dieses Wasser wird nach Hervorziehen der Bahre aus dem Kühlraum entweder verdunsten oder aber auch percutan resorbiert.

β) Vertrocknungen der intakten Haut und der Schleimhäute post mortem

Die Haut unterliegt nach dem Tode den Gesetzen der unbelebten Welt als physikalisches Objekt. Durch Perspiration wird sehr rasch eine große Menge an Wasser abgegeben. Physiologische Regulationen ergänzen den Wasserverlust nicht mehr. Der postmortale Wasserverlust des gesamten Körpers führt unter günstigen Bedingungen letztlich zur Mumifikation (III, 4). Uns bewegen zunächst Vertrocknungserscheinungen der einzelnen Körperteile und zwar der intakten wie der vital oder postmortal versehrten Haut.

Bei der postmortalen Vertrocknung spielen anatomische und physikalische Bedingungen eine entscheidende, örtlich determinierte Rolle.

Deshalb treten postmortale Vertrocknungen an typischen Stellen auf. Für die Differentialdiagnose gegenüber vitalen Vorgängen ist dies von Bedeutung.

Die Acren — relativ große Oberfläche bei kleinem Volumen und Flüssigkeitsgehalt — werden rasch vertrocknen. Gleiches gilt für jene Teile der Körperoberfläche, wo die Epidermis sehr dünn ist.

Der Wassergehalt des Stratum corneum liegt bei 2%. Die gesamte Haut, und zwar vorwiegend das Corium, enthält demgegenüber 69—74% Wasser. Die Epidermis und besonders das Stratum corneum schützen die Haut vor Wasserverlust. Zu Lebzeiten würde der Wasserverlust ohne den Schutz der Epidermis nicht täglich 2 Liter, sondern das Zehnfache betragen. Eine dünne Epidermis mit schmalem Stratum corneum vertrocknet rascher. Dies gilt auch für Schleimhäute, sobald die mechanische Befeuchtung (Lidschlag, Zungenbefeuchtung) aussetzt bzw. physiologische Regulationsmechanismen — wie an den Conjunctiven bei offenen oder halb geschlossenen Lidern — bereits ante mortem zusammenbrechen. Dann entstehen dreieckförmige, bräunliche bis schwärzliche Streifen, die vom Rande der Cornea nach dem äußeren Augenwinkel ziehen. Diese postmortale Schleimhauteintrocknung als Zeichen des Todes wird nach einem französischen Autor (LARCHER) bezeichnet. SOMMER hatte diese Erscheinung jedoch zuerst (1833) beschrieben, worüber SIEBENHAAR in seinem Enzyklopädischen Handbuch der gerichtlichen Medizin (1840) ausführlich berichtete. Er schreibt: ,,Soweit das Auge des Gestorbenen geöffnet bleibt, wurde die der Luft ausgesetzte Stelle der Sklera, besonders nach dem äußeren Winkel zu, nach 1—3 Std gelb und nach 5—6 Std geht dieses Gelbe näher an der Hornhaut ins Bläuliche oder Schwärzliche über.''

LARCHER publizierte 1862 hierüber. Er faßte diese Vertrocknungserscheinungen seltsamerweise als Imbibition auf und bezeichnete sie als Initialerscheinung der Fäulnis. Es handelt sich aber um Vertrocknungsvorgänge. Die Sklera wird transparent, das Stratum pigmentosum der Retina schlägt durch. Es wäre also richtig, diese Flecken nicht nach LARCHER, sondern nach SOMMER zu benennen.

Die Mundlippen, besonders bei Neugeborenen und Säuglingen, verfärben sich nach dem Tode sehr rasch bräunlich, sie trocknen ein. Der Anatom LUSCHKA sowie der Gerichtsmediziner MASCHKA berichteten hierüber im Jahre 1863. Die postmortalen Hautveränderungen sollten nicht mit den Folgen der Verätzungen oder von Gewalteinwirkungen verwechselt werden. Gelegentlich findet man auch heute noch Stellungnahmen, in denen allein aufgrund der bräunlichen Eintrocknungen der Lippen ein Verschluß der Atemöffnungen eines Kindes durch Hände oder weiche Tücher, Kissen etc. unterstellt wird. LUSCHKA beschrieb, daß anschließend an der schmalen glatten Zone der Pars glabra ein breiter, weicher, mit langen Papillen versehener Saum, Pars villosa, an den Lippen der Kinder zu finden ist. Diese Pars villosa vertrocknet schon wenige Stunden nach dem Tode, sie wird dunkelbraun, schwarz und ist von lederartiger Konsistenz.

Die intakte Haut der Nasenspitze, der Nasenflügel und auch der näheren Umgebung der Nasenöffnungen wird wenige Stunden nach dem Tode bei entsprechend trockener und bewegter Luft wegen des Wasserverlustes bräunlich bis schwarz-braun austrocknen. Dies kann natürlich auch dadurch zustande kommen, daß sich evtl. eine mechanische Excoriation oberflächlichster Hautpartien während eines Geburtsaktes am Nasenrücken, bzw. der Nasenspitze, abzeichnete. Gerade diese Partien können bei Neugeborenen auch ohne äußere mechanische Gewaltanwendung rascher vertrocknen.

Aber nicht nur Lippen und Nasenspitze von Neugeborenen oder Säuglingen, sondern bei langer Agone auch die der Erwachsenen, können rasch nach dem Tode Vertrocknungserscheinungen bieten und damit Probleme aufwerfen.

Die Nabelschnur fällt zwischen dem 2. und 8. Tag nach der Geburt ab. Etwa 1—2 Std nach der Geburt bildet sich am Übergang vom Hautnabel zur Nabelschnur ein zirkulärer, rötlich-schmaler Demarkationsring. Stirbt ein Neugeborenes kurz nach oder unter der Geburt, so entsteht diese vitale Demarkationszone nicht. Es kann sich allerdings ein postmortaler Pseudodemarkationsring, zumeist nur sektoren- oder halbkreisförmig, in Abhängigkeit von der Lage der Nabelschnur zum Körper und damit in Abhängigkeit von der Möglichkeit des Luftzutritts, ausbilden. Sobald die Nabelschnur völlig von Zellstoff oder saugfähigem Material eingehüllt ist, wird die vorhandene Flüssigkeit rasch aufgesogen. Es kann sich somit postmortal ein kreisförmiger, schmaler, rötlich- bis rotbrauner Ring abzeichnen, der sich makroskopisch kaum von der vitalen Demarkation unterscheidet. Histologisch sollte der Versuch einer Differenzierung gemacht werden, s. KOCKEL, GLINSKI und HOROSZKIWICZ, FRITZ, KOPF und KOLLMANN. Wie man sieht, ist die histologische Aussagemöglichkeit sehr eingeschränkt.

Bei Kleinkindern kann man auf der Höhe der Hautfalten des Halses ebenfalls Vertrocknungsbezirke erkennen, die Ähnlichkeit mit Würge- oder Drosselspuren haben können, sie sind jedoch postmortal entstanden (E. HOFMANN).

Die Haut des Erwachsenen vertrocknet post mortem vorwiegend an jenen Stellen, bei denen eine größere Feuchtigkeitsabgabe rein physiologisch bestand und zwar dann, wenn jene Hautbezirke post mortem einem freien Luftzutritt ausgesetzt sind. Zu Lebzeiten erscheint die Haut völlig unversehrt. Urin- oder Schweißmacerationen bei Männern z.B. am Hodensack, bei Frauen an den Schamlippen oder unterhalb sehr fettreicher Brüste, lassen die Haut bereits etwa 12 Std nach dem Tode gelb-bräunlich bis schwarzbraun verfärben, sie tastet sich dann pergamentartig hart. Nach 24—48stündigem Liegen in trockener bewegter Luft kann sich die Austrocknung am Hodensack nicht nur auf die Oberhaut beschränken, sondern sogar die Tunica albuginea ergreifen. In der ersten Stunde nach dem

Tode vertrocknet der Hodensack dort, wo er nicht den Oberschenkeln anliegt, bzw. vom Membrum abgedeckt ist, auf den Höhen der Falten bräunlich. Es handelt sich hier gewissermaßen bei der Faltenbildung des Hodensackes um ein Kühlrippensystem. Die Faltung und Runzelung vergrößert die Oberfläche und erleichtert zu Lebzeiten die Verdunstung mit dem Zweck einer Abkühlung. Deshalb vertrocknet der Hodensack nach dem Tode sehr rasch. Wenn in der späten Leichenzeit die Scrotalhaut nicht nur im Bereich der Faltenhöhen rot-bräunlich verfärbt ist, wird dieser Befund als Zeichen einer Gewalteinwirkung gewertet, und zwar besonders dann, wenn z.B. eine Person im Polizeigewahrsam stirbt.

Histologisch erkennt man an der vertrockneten Scrotalhaut eine Verschmälerung mit Abflachung der Papillarleisten. Das Stratum corneum ist stellenweise zu Verlust gegangen, die Zellen des Stratum germinativum sind palisadenförmig angeordnet, z.T. oval, z.T. rundlich. In der Haut der Leistenbeuge sieht man eine Abflachung der basalen Schichten des Stratum germinativum (MUELLER). Bei Kleinkindern finden sich hier streifige Vertrocknungszonen.

Die Fingerbeeren vertrocknen regelmäßig, sie schrumpfen; die Fingernägel wirken hierdurch länger. Es kommt zu der Fehlmeinung, postmortal wären die Fingernägel gewachsen. — Die Haut des Gesichtes vertrocknet, zieht sich vom Haarschaft zurück, dadurch scheinen die Barthaare gewachsen. Bei einem Bergwerksunglück wurden Menschen nach längerer Zeit geborgen. Man glaubte, aus der Länge der Barthaare rückschließen zu können, wie lange diese Menschen nach dem Unglück noch unter Tage lebten. Hier wird man jene Phänomene mit berücksichtigen müssen.

b) Vertrocknung der versehrten Haut

α) Vertrocknung der Epidermis nach vitalen Verletzungen

Nach jeder Exkoriation, jeder Hautverletzung, wird bei entsprechender Überlebenszeit, ein histologischer Befund Auskunft über das vitale Geschehen geben können, s. hierzu RAEKALLIO, PIOCH und viele andere.

Je nach Tiefe der Hautschädigung wird sich diese wegen der nach dem Tode einsetzenden Vertrocknung gelblich, gelb-bräunlich oder bei Betroffensein der gefäßführenden Schichten, auch rötlich bis rot-bräunlich verfärben. Auch diese Vertrocknungen entstehen erst innerhalb von Stunden nach dem Tode. Man wird sie evtl. unmittelbar nach dem Ableben noch nicht sehen können.

Für das bloße Auge ist eine Differenzierung zwischen vitalen, kurzfristig überlebten Hautverletzungen und gesicherten postmortalen mechanischen Schädigungen, kaum möglich. Hier wird nur der histologische bzw. histochemische Befund weiterhelfen. Die Länge der vitalen Reaktionszeit ist ausschlaggebend. Bei den meisten Gewalteinwirkungen ist jene interessierende Spanne jedoch so kurz, daß sich vitale Reaktionen noch nicht haben ausbilden können.

Ein Beispiel: Würgemerkmale werden gesetzt, unmittelbar nach dem Würgeakt verstirbt der Mensch: Weder makroskopisch noch mikroskopisch wird man u.U. alleine aus der Befunderhebung der Hautveränderungen erklären können, ob es sich um eine vitale Verletzung mit nachfolgendem Tod oder um einen Angriff unmittelbar p.m. gehandelt hat.

β) Vertrocknungen der Haut nach agonalen Verletzungen

Die Haut wird an der Grenze zwischen Leben und Tod versehrt, z.B. bei Wiederbelebungsversuchen. Mit Händen, mit nassen Tüchern, werden die seitlichen Partien des Brustkorbes bei extrathorakaler Herzmassage traumatisiert. Die oberen Schichten der Epidermis gehen zu Verlust, die freigelegte Fläche trocknet später ein.

Bei der Mund-zu-Mund-Beatmung wird man in der Umgebung der Mund-Nasenöffnungen gleiche Hautveränderungen entstehen sehen. — Bei Wiederbelebungsversuchen mit Hausmitteln wie Essig oder Salmiakgeist tropfen diese Flüssigkeiten auf Gesicht, Hals, Brustkorb und verätzen die Haut. Anschließend werden Vertrocknungsspuren deutlich, die, für das bloße Auge, auf vitale Gewalteinwirkungen verdächtig sein können.

Ähnliches gilt für Erbrechen von Magensaft mit nachfolgenden Vertrocknungen der Mundumgebung.

γ) Vertrocknungen nach postmortalen Verletzungen

Nach dem Tode wird bei der Leichentoilette, durch Rasur, eine oberflächliche Hautschürfung gesetzt, diese trocknet rasch ein. — Beim Ankleiden, dem Transport der Leiche, werden, vorwiegend an den oberen und unteren Gliedmaßen, aber auch in Höhe der Hüfte, Hautschürfungen verursacht. Läuft die Autolyse bzw. Fäulnis bereits an, wird die Epidermis leicht abgeschoben, sogar abgelöst. Der postmortale Verlust der Epidermis führt zu einer raschen Vertrocknung einer im Fäulsniszustand versehrten Haut.

Das Corium nimmt eine citronengelbliche Farbe an. Selbstverständlich ist diese Tönung im Bereich der Hypostase schmutzig-rötlich bis braunfarben, sofern sich nicht Fäulnisblasen in der Zone der tiefsten abhängigen Körperpartien ausgebildet hatten.

Vitale Epidermisverletzungen mit Lymphaustritt bzw. Mikroblutungen durch Freilegung gefäßführender Schichten sind gegenüber Fäulnisvertrocknungen auch für das bloße Auge zu unterscheiden. In einer irrigen Beurteilung postmortaler Hautveränderungen mögen manche Fehlurteile begründet sein.

c) Vertrocknungen der Haut nach Einwirkung von Nekrophagen

Auch Leichenzehrer rufen Hautverletzungen mit nachfolgender Vertrocknung hervor. Vorwiegend handelt es sich um verschiedenste Käferarten. — Die von Mäusen, Ratten, Katzen, Hunden, Hasen, Füchsen verursachten Läsionen sind weniger problematisch, sie führen deshalb seltener zu einer Fehlbeurteilung. Ameisen, Ohrwürmer, Küchenschaben setzen kleine, manchmal halbmondförmige Epidermisverletzungen und zwar vorwiegend in der Umgebung von Mund- und Nasenöffnungen, am Halse und auch an den Innenflächen der Oberschenkel in der Umgebung der weiblichen Geschlechtsteile.

In Unkenntnis dieser postmortalen Erscheinungen wird Verdacht auf Würgeakt oder Lustmord etc. geäußert. Nekrophagen greifen die Haut nicht nur mit ihren Beißwerkzeugen an, sondern lösen die Epidermis mittels Fermenten selbst über ihre Exkremente. Spuren, die vertrocknen, bleiben zurück. Ein Vater wurde wegen Vergiftung seines Kindes lebenslänglich verurteilt. Man hatte „Verätzungen" im Bereich des Mundes nicht als Folgen von Einwirkung durch Nekrophagen erkannt. Die Veränderungen lokalisieren sich vorwiegend im Bereich der Haarfollikel, mehr noch in der Umgebung der Talgdrüsenausführungsgänge. Hierdurch entstehen, besonders im Bereich des Halses, jene verdächtigen Marken.

10. Identitätsfeststellung über die Haut in der frühen Leichenzeit

Statur, Körpergröße, Gewicht, gleichfalls Eigenschaften der Haut und der Hautanhangsgebilde, spiegeln Persönlichkeitsmerkmale wider. Man spricht von Farbe, Konsistenz der Haut, von Länge und Farbe der Kopfhaare, von individuellen Merkmalen wie Muttermalen, Narben, Tätowierungen etc.

Der Mensch „lebt" so lange, wie sein Erscheinungsbild in der menschlichen Gesellschaft gegenwärtig bleibt. Beispiele: Religiöser Kult, Unsterblichkeitsglaube, Herstellung von Totenmasken, von Statuen, Porträtmalerei; selbst Konservierung des Körpers: Einbalsamierung, Mumifizierung. Die Haut ist ein individuelles Bauelement des menschlichen Körpers. In der gerichtlichen Medizin spielen Eigenschaften der Haut bei der Identifizierung unbekannter Leichen eine entscheidende Rolle. Agnoszierung ist problemlos, solange der Körper noch nicht durch Fäulnis oder Verwesung verändert ist oder die Leiche zerstückelt wurde.

Aber bereits in der ersten Leichenzeit ergeben sich Schwierigkeiten: Bei Tieflagerung des Kopfes wird das Gesicht infolge der Hypostase anschwellen, sich bläulich-rot verfärben.

Nach Hochlagerung des Kopfes und Durchtrennen der Halsvenen verschwinden Totenflecke und Dunsung weitgehend. Selbst Diffusionstotenflecke mit der auffälligen Imbibition der Haut bilden sich nach mehrstündiger Lagerung des Kopfes in fließendem Wasser zurück.

Die Bestimmung des Geschlechtes — abgesehen von Hermaphroditen — verursacht keine Schwierigkeit.

Zur Altersbestimmung bieten Haarfarbe, Hautfalten und spezielle Altersveränderungen der Haut, wie Atrophie oder Pigmentflecke, gute Hinweise. Selbst Tätowierungen können auf Geburtsdatum, Militärdienstzeit, Beruf hinweisen. Berufsangaben sind aus der Verteilung und Verfärbung von Hautschwielen ablesbar.

Über Tätowierungen haben in jüngster Zeit SCHÖNFELD und über Berufsmerkmale, speziell der Hände, F. RONCHESE publiziert.

Das Papillarlinienmuster der Fingerbeere dient zur Identifikation, ist aber nur dann einsetzbar, wenn die Person früher bereits einmal registriert wurde, oder in jenen Staaten, z.B. den USA, wo Fingerabdrücke der gesamten Bevölkerung (Personalausweise etc.) vorhanden sind.

Die Identifikation ist in der frühen Leichenzeit schon dann erschwert, wenn der Körper zerstückelt oder einer Hitzeeinwirkung unterworfen wurde.

An einzelnen Hautstücken wird man folgende Testungen durchführen:

Abstammung: Mit Hilfe (von) der Uhlenhuthschen Präcipitation bzw. der Immunoelektrophorese wird festgestellt, ob die Haut vom Menschen oder Tier stammt. Ein Versuch, Blutgruppeneigenschaften aus Haut und Geweben nachzuweisen, wird durchgeführt werden müssen.

Mikroskopische Untersuchung des Geschlechtschromatins nach BARR und BERTRAM wird auch an der Leichenhaut eingesetzt. HOLZER und MARBERGER sowie SCHLEYER, PIOCH halten die cytologische Geschlechtsbestimmung für einsatzfähig, solange die Zellkernfärbung noch gelingt, also auch an nicht mehr ganz frischen Leichen und Leichenteilen!

Nicht nur an der Haut, sondern auch an relativ fäulnisresistenten Haarwurzeln, werden Geschlechtsbestimmungen vorgenommen (TOVO und DE BERNARDI sowie PIOCH, FREY-SULZER). SCHLEYER meint, daß bei über 25% chromatinpositiver Zellkerne die Diagnose absolut berechtigt sei, CASTAGNOLI und FREYSULZER gehen von 4% aus.

Bezüglich des histologischen Verhaltens der Haut soll zwischen Männern und Frauen eine Differenz insofern bestehen, als bei Männern die Papillen kurz und breit, bei Frauen schmal und hoch seien. Nach LUGER und SCHULHOF soll dies bei 70% der Menschen zutreffen. Exakte Messungen und Zählungen sind aber erforderlich.

Bestimmte Hautpartien können über Anhangsgebilde Geschlechtshinweise geben: Barthaare, Brustwarzen, Striae, Behaarungstyp, Linea fusca.

B. MUELLER faßte eine Reihe von Merkmalen zusammen; die Angaben könnten tabellarisch wiedergegeben werden. Ein sicherer Hinweis jedoch fehlt, da z.B. Falten in der Leichenhaut in Ausbildung und Erkennbarkeit vom Unterhautfettgewebepolster sowie von zu unterschiedlichen Zeiten einsetzenden Degenerationserscheinungen an elastischen Fasern abhängen.

Senil-atrophische Haut, Pigmentflecken, geben Altershinweise, ebenfalls schüttere Achsel- bzw. Schambehaarung. Unsicher sind Folgerungen aus dem Ergrauen der Kopfhaare. Markante Persönlichkeitsmerkmale wie Atherome, Tätowierungen, Narben, Pigmentanomalien in der Haut von zerstückelten Körperteilen deuten auf das Alter.

Bei Skalpierung sind nicht nur die eigentliche Haarfarbe, sondern Tönung oder Färbung, die Länge nachgewachsener, d.h. nicht gefärbter Haare, bedeutsam. Sobald ein behaartes Hautstück gefunden wird, kann man zu 57,3% folgern, daß Kopf- wie Körperhaare gleichfarben sind; in 36,3% ist die Körperbehaarung heller, in 6,3% dunkler (SIMON).

Über die Schwielenverteilung und Verfärbung, selbst über die Tönung der Kopfhaare, lassen sich Einwirkungen von Berufsstaub oder Dämpfen erkennen. Vitale Verfärbungen, z.B. über Anilin-Derivate (Gelbtönung von Haut und Haaren) oder braunrote Verfärbungen der Haut und Haare, teils auch gelbliche Nageltönungen, können auf Nitrokörper weisen. Met-Hämoglobin ? Hauthaar ist bei Pikrinsäure intensiv gelblich verfärbt (MOESCHLIN, RONCHESE). Sind sichtbare Schleimhäute bei den zerstückelten Leichenteilen zu erkennen, ist speziell die Zahnschleimhaut zu beachten.

II. Die Haut und Anhangsgebilde in der späteren Leichenzeit
1. Putrifikation

Fäulnis setzt Bakterien voraus. HÄUSSLER versteht unter Fäulnis den chemischen Vorgang einer Zersetzung des Gewebes durch Spaltpilze, der, über Zwischenstufen, zu einfachen chemischen Verbindungen führt. Bei der Fäulnis handelt es sich meist um reduktive oder oxydo-reduktive, bei der Verwesung um rein oxydative Prozesse. Spaltpilze spielen bei der Verwesung eine geringere Rolle als Schimmelpilze. Da Abläufe und Bedingungen, beginnend mit Autolyse über Fäulnis bis zur Verwesung, nicht streng voneinander zu trennen sind, beeinflussen sich die Vorgänge gegenseitig oder sie wechseln sich ab.

Die Fäulnisvorgänge sind von folgenden Voraussetzungen abhängig:

1. Sie setzen nur in Gegenwart von Flüssigkeit ein, deshalb wird eine blutreiche Haut die Autolyse, später auch die Fäulnis fördern.

2. Ernährungszustand des Gesamtorganismus. Bei ausgeprägtem *Unterhautfettgewebe* setzt die Fäulnis früher ein als z.B. bei flüssigkeitsarmer, senil-atrophischer Haut eines Kachektischen.

3. *Todesursache*. Sepsis oder Peritonitis lassen die Fäulnis explosivartig beginnen — im Gegensatz zu aseptischen Todesursachen bzw. nach intensiver Behandlung mit Sulfonamiden oder Antibiotica (sulfonamidbehandelte Haut, Penicillin-Puder) (s. hierzu die Arbeiten von H. J. WAGNER).

Wurde ein Körper *zerstückelt*, sind Fäulniserscheinungen stärker als vergleichsweise bei unversehrter Leiche. Deshalb faulen *sezierte* Leichen schneller, weil die bakterielle Kontamination groß ist.

ORFILA und LESEUR haben schon 1831 über Fäulnisvorgänge an der Leichenhaut unter Berücksichtigung der Milieueinflüsse publiziert. Sie wollten aufgrund eines von ihnen angegebenen Farbspieles Leichenfäulnisvorgänge beschreiben, sie chronologisch einordnen.

Der erste Fäulnishinweis für das bloße Auge ist die grünliche Verfärbung der Haut, die zumeist am Unterleib, rechts vorzeitiger als links, einsetzt.

SCHWERD zitiert in seiner Monographie die Arbeiten von ISHIBASHI u. FALLANI, von PALMIERI u. ROMANO, die zeigen, daß gesicherte Erkenntnisse darüber nicht vorliegen. Dies gilt für viele nekrochemische Prozesse.

LAVES und O. SCHMIDT widmeten eine Reihe von Experimenten der Frage des Vorkommens von Sulf.-Hb in der Leiche.

Man sollte daran erinnern, daß Verdoglobin nicht nur in der Leiche, sondern auch am Lebenden auftritt. Der physiologische Gehalt beträgt nach KIESE etwa 0,4% (Verdoglobin A). Verdoglobin S wird sich bei chronischem Arzneimittelmißbrauch oder autotoxisch in den Erythrocyten bilden.

O. SCHMIDT untersuchte drei Leichen, die in schwefelwasserstoffhaltigem Brunnenwasser ertrunken waren und nach einer Stunde geborgen wurden. Die unbedeckten Körperpartien waren dunkelgrün verfärbt als die Sektion 24 Std später vorgenommen wurde.

Die Grünfärbung an der Haut des Unterleibs wird bei warmer Außentemperatur, bei Bettleichen, nach 1 bis 2 Tagen zu sehen sein.

Sauerstoff muß an die Haut gelangen können: O. SCHMIDT ließ den Leichnam eines Neugeborenen 3 Wochen im Sommer halbseitig in Öl liegen, nur die unbedeckte Haut war grün bis schwarzgrün verfärbt, nach Herausnahme aus dem Öl vergingen 30 min, bis die ganze Körperhaut grünfarben war.

Auch die Sulf.-Hb-Bildung in der Flüssigkeit der Fäulnisblasen beruht auf Sauerstoffpermeation. Die Differenzierung gegenüber Met-Hb ist nicht leicht.

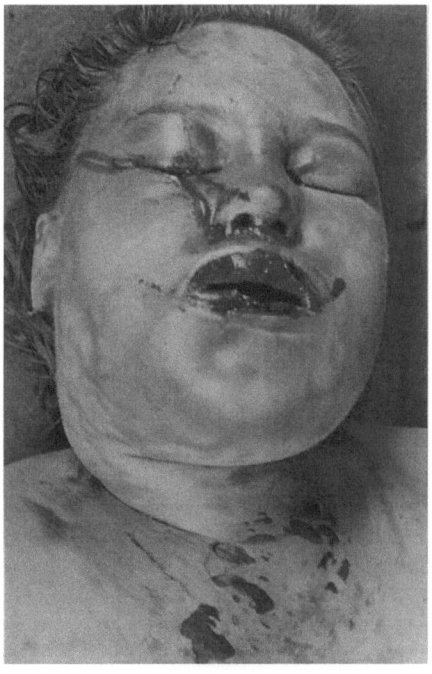

Abb. 7. Fäulnisdunsung. Abfließen der Fäulnisflüssigkeit, Verlust der Epidermis bei geplatzten Fäulnisblasen mit nachfolgender Vertrocknung

Als Folge der Autolyse, des Zusammenbruchs der Schrankenfunktionen, der physikalischen Gesetzen folgenden Flüssigkeitsverteilung, werden tieferliegende Hautanteile eine deutliche *Kolliquation* aufweisen.

Nach postmortaler Hämolyse tritt Hämoglobin durch die Gefäßwandungen; Hautvenennetze stellen sich bis zur Fingerbreite deutlichst dar, dies nicht nur im Bereich der Livores, sondern z.T. auch außerhalb. Die „durchgeschlagenen" Gefäße sind schmutzig-rot bis violett-braun verfärbt.

In der nächsten Phase kommt es zu einer Lockerung zwischen Oberhaut und Cutis. Auf leichten Druck verschiebt sich die Oberhaut. Bei Fehlen mechanischer äußerer Gewalteinwirkung wird sich infolge der Fäulnistranssudation eine Blase bilden, die anfangs, sofern sie nicht im Bereich der Totenflecke liegt, einen hellfarbenen Inhalt hat. Erst in der späteren Fäulnisperiode wird dieser schmutzig-rot-violett, bräunlich-rot oder grünlich. Neben der Oberhaut beginnen sich auch Nägel und Behaarung zu lockern.

Bei bakterieller Zersetzung entstehen Fäulnisgase. Man tastet ein Knistern, ähnlich wie wir es von dem posttraumatischen Hautemphysem des Lebenden kennen. Neben dem eigentlichen Fäulnisemphysem der Haut wird die Fäulnisgasblähung innerer Organe, speziell der Bauchhöhle, dazu führen, daß die Bauchhaut trommelhart wird. Bei mechanischer Einwirkung oder evtl. auch ohne dieselbe, platzt die Bauchhaut, weil der Gasüberdruck im Innern zu groß geworden ist. Es handelt sich um jene Phasen, in denen sich der Uterus handschuhartig ausstülpt und bei vorliegender Schwangerschaft der Gasüberdruck im Leib zu einer Sarggeburt führt.

Experimentelle Autolyse-Versuche (BRAUN-FALCO und WINTER) führten in der IV. und V. Phase von der abakteriellen Autolyse in die Fäulnis über:

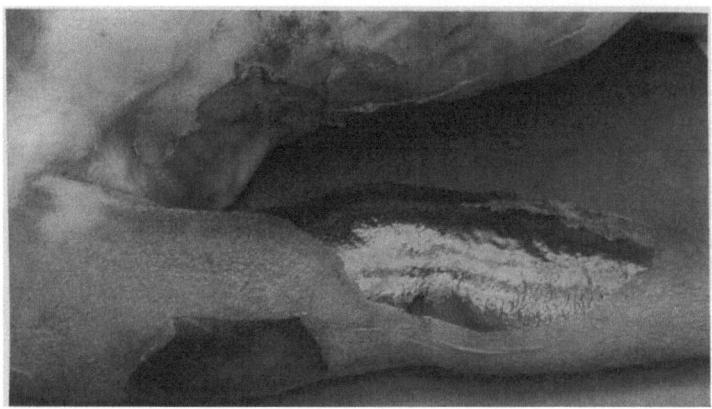

Abb. 8. Epidermablösung mit frischer Freilegung der Cutis — Diffusionstotenflecke —, „durchgeschlagene" Gefäße

Normale Haut — steril entnommen, feuchte Kammer, 37° — war im *epidermisnahen Corium* nach 48—120 Std bakteriendurchsetzt. Das Kollagen wirkte ödematisiert unter Verlust der Faserstruktur.

Elastische Fasern blieben erhalten. Wegen der schwachen Darstellung bzw. Anfärbbarkeit wird von einer *Schattenepidermis* gesprochen. Nur im völlig verwaschenen *Stratum granulosum* stellen sich einzelne basophile Kernreste dar. Auflösung der Keratohyalinkörnchen. Trennung der Epidermis vom Corium mit erkennbaren Wurzelfüßchen in den basalen Teilen der Basalzellen. Strukturverlust der Hornschicht und Quellung. Beginnende Desintegration aller subcornealen Epidermisschichten durch *Acantholyse*. — Pyknose und Karyolyse der Kerne der *Follikel*. Auflösungsvorgänge an *Talg- wie ekkrinen Schweißdrüsen*. Die Membrana propria der Endstücke bleibt erhalten, in dieser Hülle ein nicht zu differenzierendes, nekrotisches Material. Schweißdrüsenausführungsgänge sind längere Zeit gut zu differenzieren. — In der V.-Phase sind epitheliale Strukturen aufgelöst. Die Epidermis zeigt zwischen Hornschicht und Bindegewebe große, mit Bakterienhaufen angefüllte Hohlräume (Fäulnisgas!). Histochemische Untersuchungen gaben für die Beantwortung der Frage einer fäulnisbedingten Kontinuitätstrennung von Epidermis und Cutis keine sicheren Hinweise. Der PAS-positive Grenzstreifen (Basalmembran) ist auch nach Kontinuitätstrennung vielfach am oberen Corium gut zu finden. Soweit der Ausfall HALE-PAS-Reaktion eine Erklärung zuläßt, scheint es während der Autolyse nicht zu Entmischungsvorgängen mit phanerosesaurer Mucopolysaccharide zu kommen, wie sie unter pathologischen Bedingungen vielfach typisch sind, sondern lediglich zu Depolymerisationsvorgängen (BRAUN-FALCO) (Abb.7 und 8).

2. Dekomposition

Haut wie Weichteile werden in der Fäulnis durch enzymatische wie bakterielle Verdauung der Eiweiße, Kohlenhydratgärung und Fettspaltung erweicht, verflüssigt. Dieser Prozeß wird durch Nekrophagen beschleunigt; Ergebnis: eine Skeletierung.

Die Fäulnis kann auf jeder Stufe, besonders im trockenen Erdgrab oder in nicht luftdicht verschlossenem Sarge, unterbrochen werden. Sie entwickelt sich nur im flüssigen Milieu. Der Wassergehalt der Organe beträgt 70—90%. Erinnern wir uns, daß die Hornschicht nur 2%, dagegen das Corium 69—74% Wasser enthält, so wird auch hier deutlich, daß sich erste Fäulnisvorgänge im Corium bilden müssen.

Unter der Fäulnis werden die Organe flüssigkeitsärmer, sofern sie nicht sehr tief liegen bzw. sich die Haut in der Fäulnisbrühe befindet. Zwischencelluläres, aber auch zellgebundenes, Wasser wird zu Verlust gehen. Eine rasch ablaufende Fäulnis trocknet das Gewebe und damit auch die Haut aus. Die Lebensbedingungen der Fäulnisbakterien werden schlechter, sofern nicht Flüssigkeit aus der Umgebung wiederum der Haut zugeführt wird.

Die Fäulnis verändert zudem das chemische Milieu. Proteolytische Enzyme sind in der ersten Leichenzeit, d.h. bei saurer Reaktion des Gewebes, wirksam. In der späteren Phase hemmen Zersetzungsprodukte die Fäulnis. Es kommt zu einer Umkehr chemischer Vorgänge. Aus den reduktiven werden oxydative Prozesse, das bedeutet: sobald mehr Sauerstoff als Wasser im Gewebe vorhanden bzw. angeboten wird. Diese Umkehr von der vorwiegend reduktiven in die langsame, oxydative Zersetzung nennt man *Verwesung* oder *Vermoderung*. Die Oberfläche des Körpers wird wegen des Flüssigkeitsverlustes schrumpfen, bräunlichfarben, der Körper ist leichtgewichtig; die Oberfläche tastet sich torfartig und es entströmt ihr ein eigenartig ranziger oder modriger Geruch. In diesem Zustande werden niedrige Vertreter der Leichenzehrer tätig, wie Arthropoden, Crustaceen, Arachnoiden, Pseudoskorpioniden usw.

Nach etwa 2jähriger Lagerung werden die Sargleichen im Erdgrab von Milben befallen; diese entnehmen die restliche Feuchtigkeit und trocknen damit das Gewebe vollends aus.

Im 3. Jahr p.m. werden die trockenen Gewebsreste wie Haare von Anthrenus, Dermestes aufgenommen. Von den allerletzten Leichenresten und den Exkrementen der Leichenzehrer sowie den Puppenhüllen leben weitere Käferarten.

3. Nekrophagen

Gleichgültig, ob eine Leiche in der Wohnung, im Freien, in einer Leichenkammer, im Erdgrab, im Wasser usw. liegt, Aasfresser werden sich als Leichenzehrer immer einstellen. Die intakte Leichenhaut erfährt Verletzungen von so eigenartiger Form, daß sie Folgen einer zu Lebzeiten gesetzten Gewalteinwirkung vortäuschen können. Leichenzehrer schädigen die Haut sowohl von der Außenfläche als auch vom Innern des Körpers her. Jede Läsion des Integuments erschwert die *Identifikation*.

Nicht zuletzt sollte man sich die Frage vorlegen, ob aus den durch Nekrophagen gesetzten Veränderungen ein Rückschluß auf *Todes- oder Liegezeit* einer Leiche möglich ist.

Jeder Leichenfundort besitzt in Abhängigkeit von Wetterlage, dem Tag-Nacht-Rhythmus, der Jahreszeit und Organismengemeinschaft eine andere Nekrophagenzusammensetzung.

a) Fauna

In Mitteleuropa werden Fraßverletzungen durch Haus- wie Wildtiere, selbst durch Vögel, gesetzt. Zumeist handelt es sich um Nagetiere, weiter aber auch um Katze, Hund, Haus- wie Wildschwein, Fuchs und Dachs. Bei den Vögeln werden Eule und Bussard zu nennen sein. Vielfach gehen die Tiere nur bei äußerster Not an Aas: deshalb sind zur Winterszeit Leichenzehrer häufiger tätig. Andere gehen, unabhängig von Hungerzeiten, die menschliche Haut an: Ratten, Mäuse, Schweine. Auch die Haut des Hilflosen, des Betrunkenen etc., kann zu Lebzeiten angenagt werden. Betätigen sich Nagetiere, entstehen durch differente Zahnbreiten und den Zahnabstand typische Nagespuren. Nicht das Zentrum, sondern die Peripherie wird untersucht. An den Wundrändern sind Nage- bzw. Kerbspuren deutlich auszumachen. Häufig aber erschwert die Elastizität der Haut eine einwandfrei verwertbare Messung. Neben Nagespuren setzen Reißzähne schlitz- oder stichartige Verletzungen. Auch die Krallen hinterlassen strichförmige Excoriationen, selbst schlitzförmige Hautdurchtrennungen, je nach Art. Dicht nebeneinander liegen Hackwunden durch Raubvogelschnäbel (Abb. 9).

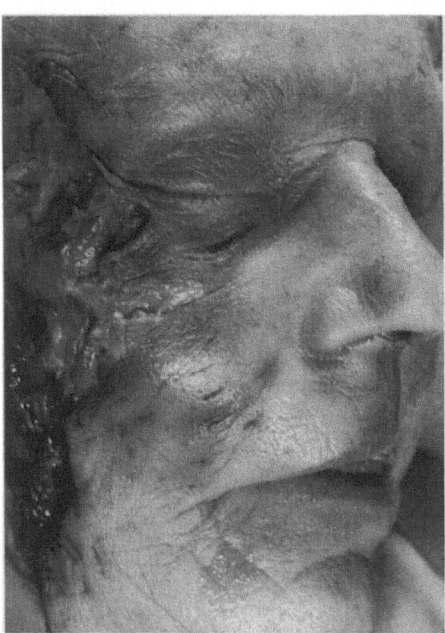

Abb. 9. Postmortaler Tierfraß — Katze

Unbekleidete Körperpartien, das weiche Gewebe, werden bevorzugt: Ohrmuscheln, Nasenspitze, Lippen, Augenlider. Die Wangengegend (Bichat'scher Pfropf) und selbstverständlich auch die Hände sind Prädilektionsstellen.

Von größter Bedeutung sind jedoch die Fliegen. Der Bakteriengeruch lockt Fliegen an (HENNIG). In der Agonie oder sofort nach dem Tode legen Stubenfliegen oder Brummer ihre Eier. Die grünschillernde Goldfliege setzt erst am faulen Gewebe, zudem bei warmer Außentemperatur, ab. Die blaue Fleischfliege legt keine Eier, sie bringt lebende Junge zur Welt.

10—24 Std nach der Eiablage der Zimmerfliegen schlüpfen die Maden. Bei günstigen Bedingungen ist die gesamte Leiche nach 2—3 Tagen von Maden bedeckt. Sie kriechen in Körperöffnungen oder -verletzungen, zerstören mit ihren proteolytischen Fermenten besonders das weiche Gewebe. Die Haut vermögen sie oberflächlich anzudauen. — Bei ihrem Weg über das Innere des Körpers greifen sie später das Unterhautfettgewebe an und setzen loch- oder siebartige Verletzungen der Haut. Vertrocknet die Haut in dieser Phase, sieht sie wie von Schrotkörnern durchlöchert aus.

In der Regel verpuppen sich Fliegenmaden nach 10—14 Tagen.

12—14 Tage später finden sich nur noch leere Puppenhülsen, nachdem die Fliegen geschlüpft sind.

Zeitliche Angaben über die Metamorphose der Fliege sind derartig von der Umgebung abhängig, daß große Verschiebungen möglich sind. Bei warmem und schwülem Wetter verläuft der Generationswechsel wesentlich rascher. In großer Schnelligkeit kann bei günstigen Umgebungstemperaturen eine Leiche mittels Fliegenmaden beseitigt werden. ,,Tres muscae consumunt cadaver equi aeque ac leo" (LINNÉ).

Allein aus dem Entwicklungszustand von Maden, dem Auffinden von Puppen, eine Liegezeitangabe zu geben, wäre ein Unterfangen — denn auch den Nekrophagen, speziell den Fliegenmaden, stellen Biophagen nach.

Zu jeder Zeit kann ein Leichnam von Insekten angegangen werden, gleich, ob sich der Körper im Zustand der Fäulnis, der Verwesung, der Mumifikation oder der Saponifikation befindet. Ausnahmsweise finden sich Fliegenmaden im Erdgrab. Sind die Eier vor der Beerdigung oder unter Benützung von Gängen der Regenwürmer abgelegt worden? Bei Exhumierung schwirren kleinste Fliegen von 2—4 mm Länge mit verstümmelten Flügeln, z.T. auch springend, über den Leichnam. Immer wieder ist man überrascht, viele Monate nach einer Beerdigung lebende Fliegen oder Käfer zu sehen.

Die Maden der Köcherfliege fressen kanalähnliche Löcher in die Haut einer Wasserleiche unter Bevorzugung nicht behaarter Körperstellen. Sie nehmen ihre Tätigkeit unabhängig vom Fäulniszustand auf und bevorzugen bereits verletzte Gewebe, wobei auch hier bekleidete Körperteile ausgespart werden (HOLZER).

Aaskäfer, insbesondere verschiedene Arten der Totengräber, üben ihre leichenzerstörende Tätigkeit ebenso aus wie Tausendfüßler, Asseln, selbst Regenwürmer und Schnecken. Nematoden der Gattung Potodea verzehren in feuchter Erde faulendes Gewebe.

Käfer, besonders auch Küchenschaben oder Ameisen, setzen oberflächliche Hautverletzungen, die bestimmte Muster wiedergeben und in der anschließenden Vertrocknung auffällig sind, ähnlich den Wanderspuren der Maden unter oberflächlicher Hautandauung. Gerade diese Defekte sind an der frischen Leiche höchst verdächtig für Säureeinwirkung, Würge- bzw. Strangulationsmerkmale etc.

Eine Wasserleiche unterliegt nicht nur Treib- oder Schiffsschraubenverletzungen, sondern Wasserratten, Wasserkäfer, Krebse, Schnecken, Flohkrebse, Seesterne, Hummer, gehen an den Leichnam. Die Ansicht über die Tätigkeit der Fische ist nicht einheitlich, zumeist werden Aale oder Neunaugen als Leichenzehrer betrachtet.

Blutegel können sich ansaugen und typische sternchenförmige Verletzungen von 3—4 mm Größe beibringen. Egel saugen sich um so rascher an, je wärmer die Leiche ist und bevorzugen blutreiche Partien, z.B. die Zone der Hypostase.

b) Flora

Stirbt der Mensch im Wasser, wird die von Kleidern unbedeckte Haut nach gewisser Zeit wie von Schlamm überzogen aussehen. Es handelt sich um einen zumeist schmutzig-graugrünen oder braun-grünen Algenrasen, der evtl. zusätzlich noch mit Schlamm bedeckt sein kann. Ein dichter geschlossener Filz von Algen ist nach HABERDA innerhalb von 2—3 Wochen bei Donauleichen ausgebildet. In der stärker verschmutzten Mur vergingen nach WERKGARTNER mindestens 8 Tage; MARESCH sah in manchen Gewässern sogar schon nach 3—4 Tagen einen kompletten Algenrasen. Die Zeit hat sich gegenüber früher wesentlich verkürzt. WEYRICH fand schon nach 4 Tagen bei Rheinleichen Algenbewuchs. Wir, in Köln, beobachteten ebenfalls frühestens nach 4 Tagen einen flächigen, 2 cm dicken Algenansatz an Beinen und Leib. Nach 5 Tagen war der gesamte Körper mit Algen überzogen (Juni), im Winter frühestens nach 17 Tagen. Die Algen bedecken die Epidermis, falls diese abgegangen ist, besiedeln sie die Cutis.

Tabelle 2. *Tierfraßspuren an der menschlichen Leiche nach* H. Suckow

Tierart	Typische Fraßspuren	Bevorzugung bestimmter Leichenteile	Vortäuschung von falschen Verletzungsspuren
Vögel, Krähen, Raben, Möwen, Eulen, Mäusebussard	messerstichähnliche Hautwunden		Messerstichwunden (scharfe Verletzungen)
Hauskatzen	Fraßstelle zeigt glatte Trennungsflächen; in deren Nähe verlaufen stichwundenähnliche Hautverletzungen, durch die Eckzähne entstanden und für Ketzenfraß beweisend, oberflächliche Vertrocknungen durch Belecken zarter Hautstellen		
Hunde	stellenweise in bogenförmiger Reihe stehende Hautabschürfungen und kleine Trennungen der Haut. Zahnabdrücke deutlich erkennbar. Manche Wunden weisen rundliche Eingangsöffnungen und einige kurze, kegelförmige Kanäle auf		Verwechslung mit Stichwunden möglich
Fliegenmaden der Musca carnaria oder Fleischfliege	Zerstörung besteht in Depilation, Erweichung und Verflüssigung der Haut. Eröffnung der Bauchwand und Beseitigung der Gewebe, auch feste Gewebe, wie Uterus. Auf Hautstellen, die einige Zeit von Maden bedeckt waren, ist eine schmutzigdunkelgrau verfärbte Stelle zu erkennen	besonders Wunden, unbedeckte Hautstellen, Mundwinkel, Lidspalten, Genitalöffnungen, unabhängig von vorausgegangener Bakterienfäulnis, denn Maden können selbstlytisch wirksam durch Absonderung bestimmter Fermente sein	
Larven der Köcherfliege (Wassermotte oder Trichoptera)	ausgedehnte oberflächliche Zerstörungen, aber auch große Löcher und Höhlen in Leichenteilen. Zahlreiche rundliche Lücken bis tief ins Gewebe hinein. Die Innenwand der Höhlen ist ganz fein zernagt	besonders unbekleidete Leichenteile von Wasserleichen	
Nagetiere: Waldwühlmaus, Wühlmaus	am Rande von Schädelknochen unregelmäßige, manchmal auch glattrandige, parallel verlaufende Dellen, immer je 2 Dellen, die durch eine Leiste getrennt sind	Knochen zum Abwetzen der Nagezähne	Verletzungen durch fremde äußere Gewalteinwirkung
Wanderratten, selten Hausratte, wenig Haus- und Feldmäuse	unregelmäßige, manchmal glattrandige Hautdefekte, paarweise, stichähnliche Wunden von den Nagezähnen und schlitzförmige, strichähnliche Bißwunden	Substanzverluste an den Händen	wurden für vital entstandene Verletzungen gehalten

Tabelle 2. (Fortsetzung)

art	Typische Fraßspuren	Bevorzugung bestimmter Leichenteile	Vortäuschung von falschen Verletzungsspuren
usschwein, ldtiere, hse, Dachse, dschweine, mster, Eichnchen, Hasen	verschleppen Leichenteile	z. B. Ohrmuscheln	
igel	beißt ein rundes Loch in die Haut, durch Saugen kommt es zu Blutungen	besonders Wasserleichen	postmortale Blutungen
sterne	ähnliche Verletzungen	besonders Wasserleichen	
necken	oberflächliche Vertrocknungen	besonders Wasserleichen	
bse	kleine Bißwunden und Hautvertrocknungen	besonders Wasserleichen	
renwürmer	ausgedehnte hellbräunliche, derblederartig anzufühlende Hautstellen, die scharf begrenzt und unregelmäßig gestaltet sind	an keine besondere Körpergegend gebunden	z. B. von Verätzungen, Verbrühungen und Verbrennungen 2. Grades, also solche, die mit Verlust der Epidermis einhergehen
chenschaben	gelbe bis braune Hautvertrocknungen	keine besondere Körpergegend bevorzugend	Schwefelsäureverätzung, wenn Veränderungen an geeigneter Stelle sitzen
eisen	teils rundliche, teils streifige (oft landkartenähnliche), pergamentartige Vertrocknungen durch oberflächliche Benagung der Haut oder durch Auflockerung chemisch wirkender Sekrete, schwärzliche, sauer reagierende Exkoriationen	keine besondere Körpergegend bevorzugend	wenn Spuren an entsprechenden Stellen (Kinn, Hals) sitzen, können Verätzungen oder Würgespuren vorgetäuscht werden
llerasseln, eisen, rwürmer	oberflächliche Hautvertrocknungen	keine besondere Körpergegend bevorzugend	Säureverätzung

Fundstelle: O. PROKOP, Forensische Medizin. Berlin: Verlag Volk und Gesundheit 1967.

Der pelzartige Überzug erschwert die Identifizierung. Persönlichkeitsmerkmale wie Narben, Tätowierungen, Verletzungen sind nicht zu erkennen. Der Algenrasen ist abzuheben; dies ist mühsam. Die Epidermis geht dabei meist zu Verlust. Verletzungen sind zu vermeiden.

Neben den Algen siedeln Schleimpilze auf der Haut; die Bezirke sind klein, rot bis violett getönt. Werden sie größer, denkt man sehr leicht an Folgen einer Gewalteinwirkung (Blutung). Beim Liegen im feuchten Keller oder im lockeren Erdreich siedeln sich Schimmelpilze auf der unbedeckten Haut an, zunächst kleinflächig, später zusammenfließend; sie bedecken das Gesicht wie eine Maske, sind grau, schneeweiß, violett-rot, gelegentlich auch gelb getönt. Die verschiedenen Farben können auch nebeneinander gesehen werden. Im Erdgrab kann man sie bereits nach 14 Tagen entdecken. Bei einem Leichenfund in einer Gartenlaube waren $3^1/_2$ Monate, nachdem der Betreffende zuletzt lebend gesehen worden war, Gesicht und Hände von Pilzen überzogen. Nach Aufenthalt im Erdgrab von 100 Tagen war der gesamte Körper von Schimmelpilzen bedeckt (Abb. 10).

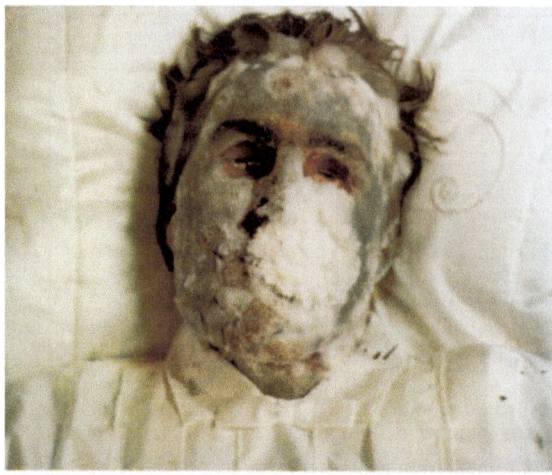
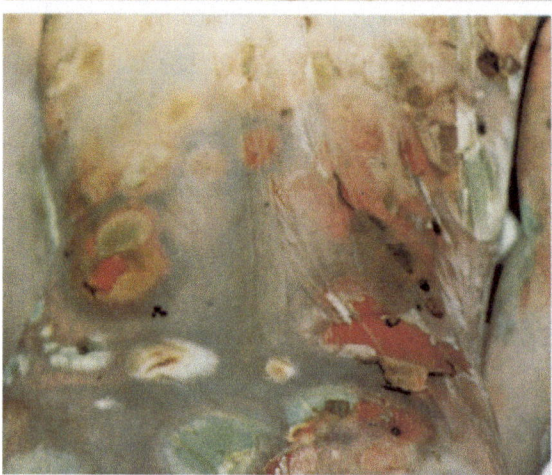

Abb. 10. Rote, weiße und grünliche Pilzrasen-Kolonien am Gesicht und Rücken; Verdoglobin-farbene Totenflecke

Dozsa stellte die das Wachstum der Pilze beeinflussenden Faktoren heraus und führte auf:
Pilzflora der Sterbenden,
Pilzflora der Kleidung, des Bahrtuches, des Sarges,
Pilzflora der Friedhofsoberfläche, des Friedhofsbodens,
Vitalität der Pilze,
Klimatische Faktoren.
Zusammensetzung des Erdreiches mit denen sich daraus ergebenden physikalischen Einwirkungen.
Die Wasserstoffionenkonzentration des Leichnams, des Erdreiches.
Lebensalter, Ernährungszustand, Krankheitsbefund nach Vergiftungen, antibiotische Behandlung usw. sind von Einfluß und stehen in enger Beziehung zur herrschenden Bakterienflora.
Jahreszeit, Sauerstoffgehalt im Sarge, in der Gruft, im lockeren Erdreich etc. regulieren die Spanne zwischen Tod und Beerdigung und nicht zuletzt die Zeit zwischen Beerdigung und Exhumierung.

Schimmelpilze siedeln sich bereits in der frühen Leichenzeit an, in der späteren überziehen sie besonders das Gesicht maskenartig. Nach 2—3 Jahren verkleinern sich die Herde. Abgestorbene Pilze sind schwärzlich. Cutis wie anliegende Kleidung sehen wie gescheckt aus. HUNZINGER unterschied drei Gruppen:

Pilze auf Fäulnisleichen,
Pilze auf trockenen oder fettig zerfallenen Leichen bis 1 Jahr p.m. und
Pilze auf Knochen.

4. Mumifikation

Ein Körper wird nach dem Tode, wie GÜNTZ bereits 1828 feststellte, infolge der Wasserverdunstung leichter. DUPONT konstatierte 1889, daß das Gewicht der Leiche pro Tag und pro Kilo um 7,7 g unter gewöhnlichen Verhältnissen abnimmt. Andere Meßserien stammen von IPSEN, der systematisch den *postmortalen Gewichtsverlust* von Früchten, wie Neugeborenen, bestimmte. Früchte verlieren, je unreifer sie sind, um so mehr an Gewicht. Im VI. Schwangerschaftsmonat täglich etwa 48 g, im VII. 34,7 g, im VIII. 21 g. Diese Differenz erklärt sich aus dem höheren Wassergehalt der unreifen Frucht. Letztere hat ferner im Verhältnis zum Körpergewicht eine relativ große, d.h. für die Verdunstung günstige Oberfläche. Drittens: Die Abdeckung der Körperoberfläche mit Vernix caseosa ist, je nach Reifegrad der Frucht, unterschiedlich.

In der ersten Leichenzeit treten Verdunstungen und Vertrocknungen nur an bevorzugten Körperpartien auf. Dieser Prozeß wird durch die Fäulnis unterbrochen. Wird diese gestört, ändern sich Umwelteinflüsse, fördern letztere einen raschen Wasserverlust, trocknet die Oberfläche, später der gesamte Körper, aus. Dieser Endzustand wird als Mumie bezeichnet, der Vorgang selbst Mumifizierung oder Mumifikation.

Wir differenzieren zwischen *natürlicher* und *artefizieller* Mumifizierung. Letztere wird z.B. in Spanien bei der Einbalsamierung — neben Desinfizientien — über wasserentziehende Substanzen künstlich herbeigeführt.

Bei der *natürlichen* Mumifikation unterscheiden wir zwei Arten:

Primäre Mumifikation. Dieser Zustand wurde unter Vertrocknung (I, 9) beschrieben. Innerhalb von etwa 2 Tagen verfärbt sich die Haut der Acren gelblich, später bräunlich bis braun-schwarz. Die Körperoberfläche wird trocken, ist gerunzelt, schrumpft, wird lederähnlich fest bzw. zäh. Bei der primären Mumifikation wird, in Abhängigkeit von äußeren Bedingungen, die Haut zunächst rasch an Wasser verlieren, dies im Gegensatz zu dem protrahierteren Wasserverlust während der Fäulnis. Die primäre Mumifikation schließt eine spätere Verwesung nicht aus.

Sekundäre Mumifikation. Diese entsteht während der Fäulnis. Ändern sich dann Umwelteinflüsse, trocknet die Haut aus. Unter Umständen hatte der Körper bereits sehr viel Wasser verloren: Fäulnisblasen waren geplatzt und hatten ihren flüssigen Inhalt entleert bzw. oberflächliche Körperanteile waren unter der Hypostase flüssigkeitsärmer geworden. Sofern diese Fäulnisbrühe von der Umgebung (Sargauskleidung, Erdboden etc.) aufgesogen wurde, wird den Fäulnisbakterien die biologische Existenz entzogen, die Fäulnis sistiert vor Erweichung bzw. Verflüssigung der Organe; der Austrocknungsprozeß setzt ein.

Zu den Einflüssen, die die Haut einer Leiche mumifizieren lassen, gehören:

a) Trockene, bewegte Luft bei einer Temperatur, die keinesfalls auffällig hoch zu sein braucht. Selbst in unseren Breiten kann im Sommer, selbst in kühlerer Jahreszeit, eine Mumifikation auftreten.

b) Liegt die Leiche in einem Sarkophag, in einem Raum mit stark hygroskopischen Wänden oder auf dem Boden, tritt die Vertrocknung wesentlich schneller und auch intensiver ein.

Makroskopischer Befund. Die Mumienhaut ist rotbraun, dunkelbraun, fast schwärzlich. Wenn die Körperoberfläche schneeweiß aussieht, haben sich auf ihr Schimmelpilze angesiedelt (BORN). Die Oberfläche sieht welk aus, tastet sich leder- bis pergamentartig. Beim Beklopfen hört man einen hölzernen Laut. Dieses Geräusch wird, sofern ausgedehntere Fäulnisvorgänge innere Organe bereits erweicht und verflüssigt haben oder wenn Leichenzehrer (z.B. Maden) die Weichteile aufgelöst haben, im Bereich des Brustkorbes trommelähnlich sein. Die Haut geht bei der reinen Mumifikation nicht zu Verlust, lediglich bei jener sekundären — nach fortgeschrittener Fäulnis.

Später werden Leichenzehrer, z.B. Dipteren oder Insekten, das Integument eigenartig durchlöchern, wie durch Schrotschüsse. Diese Leichenzehrer werden die Mumienhaut vorwiegend von innen her zerstören.

Bei der primären Mumifikation sind die Haare völlig erhalten, im Gegensatz zu der sekundären mit der vorangehenden Fäulnisauslösung der Haare.

Bei dunkelbrauner bis schwarzer Vertrocknung der Fingerbeeren ist das Nagelbett entsprechend getönt, der Nagelfalz ist geschrumpft. Demgegenüber fällt die schneeige Weiße der distalen Nagelabschnitte, die dem Nagelbett nicht anliegen, auf.

Während der vorangegangenen Fäulnis sind die Nägel bereits zu Verlust gegangen, dann wird sich das Nagelbett intensiv mumifizieren.

Mikroskopische Befunde. Nach vorangegangener Fäulnis mit Oberhautverlust stellt sich lediglich die Cutis dar. Die Kerne färben sich nicht mehr an. Bei einer noch nicht intensiven Mumifikation kommt es zur Metachromasie der Kerne und Bindegewebsfasern. Eine weitergehende Differenzierung ist bei Mumien mit hinreichender Sicherheit nicht mehr möglich.

Auch sind Talg- und Schweißdrüsen nicht mehr erkennbar.

Gewichtsverlust. POUSSANT hat das Gewicht von erwachsenen Mumien mit 5—6 kg angegeben. Da aber das Trockengewicht einer menschlichen Leiche 14 kg beträgt, weist die Differenz aus, daß nicht nur ein Wasserverlust für die Gewichtsreduzierung verantwortlich ist, sondern daß vorangehende Fäulnisvorgänge mit einem Abbau von Organgeweben, von Körpersubstanzen, diese Differenz erklärt. Leichenzehrer haben innere Organe, das Unterhautfettgewebe, die Muskulatur usw. aufgelöst.

STRAUCH fand eine 179 cm lange Mumie mit einem Gewicht von 8,9 kg.

Zeitdauer bis zur Ausbildung einer Mumifikation

a) Partielle Mumifikation. Die vorwiegend auf die Acren begrenzte Vertrocknung und spätere Mumifizierung der Haut tritt im trockenen Sommer oder in trockenem Milieu schon innerhalb von wenigen Tagen auf, bei Kleinstkindern evtl. schon innerhalb eines Tages. Die Veränderungen können protrahiert verlaufen, bei Wechsel der Umgebungsbedingungen in Schüben. Ein Mensch erhängt sich in einem zunächst geheizten Zimmer, der Ofen geht aus, erste Fäulnisvorgänge stellen sich ein. Bei entsprechender Luftbewegung wird der Körper mumifiziert: Leiche im freien Hang auf Dachboden oder in zugigem Schuppen.

b) Totale Mumifikation. Auch hier spielen verschiedenste Faktoren eine Rolle. Bei Neugeborenen sind Mumien bereits innerhalb von 2 Wochen nach dem Tode gesehen worden, die geringste Zeitspanne bei Erwachsenen beträgt $2^1/_2$ Monate. HOLZER berichtete über eine totale Mumifizierung nach 4 Monaten. Die Gesamtmumifikation der Haut in heißen Ländern mit trockener, bewegter Luft wird etwa nach einer Minimalzeit von 3—4 Wochen gesehen.

Die Annahme, daß nach Vergiftungen (Arsen, Antimon, Wismut etc.) eine beschleunigte Mumifikation eintreten kann, wurde an anderer Stelle besprochen (III). KRATTER ist dieser Meinung entgegengetreten, er verwies auf Untersuchungen in der Steiermark, wo Arsen in verhältnismäßig großen Mengen eingenommen wird. Beschleunigte Mumifikationen traten nicht auf. Auch die von SCHRETZMANN behauptete, beschleunigte Mumifikation nach CO-Einwirkung ist nicht zu bestätigen.

Forensisch-kriminalistische Bedeutung

Die konservierenden Eigenschaften einer primären Mumifikation werden vitale Hautverletzungen noch längere Zeit als Stich-, Schuß- oder Strangulationsmarken erkennen lassen. Bei bestimmter Körperlagerung, Kinn gegen die Brust gesenkt etc., oder durch Kleidungsstücke, entstehen strangulationsähnliche Marken. Liegt die Halshaut in Falten oder: um den Hals schließt sich eng anliegend ein Kleidungsstück, ist nicht mehr zu differenzieren, ob es sich um vitale oder postmortale Strangulationen oder um ein Kunstprodukt handelt (s. EVANS und TANTS, die in jüngster Zeit über einen Fall von Mumifikation und Strangulation berichtet haben). Ein Mensch hat Halsschmerzen, schlingt sich um den Hals einen Strumpf; er stirbt. Der Tod wird nicht bemerkt, die Fäulnis setzt ein. Die durch den Strumpf komprimierte Halshaut bildet eine Drosselfurche gegenüber der Fäulnisdunsung der übrigen Halshaut. Nach Vertrocknung bleibt die Furche zurück.

Histologisch sind vitale Reaktionen oder Zeichen bei Mumifizierung nicht mehr nachzuweisen. Der Gutachter ist deshalb mit bestimmten Fragestellungen über intravitale, supravitale oder postmortale Verletzungen überfordert.

Auch hier sei darauf verwiesen, daß Leichenzehrer verschiedenster Art erhebliche Verletzungen des Integuments hervorrufen können, so daß bei einer mumifizierten Leiche eine exakte, beweisfähige Aussage kaum zu erbringen ist.

5. Saponifikation (Fettwachsbildung)

Die Annahme, Adipozire oder Leichenwachs wären Folgen einer längeren Liegezeit der Leiche im Wasser, ist nur bedingt richtig.

Für die Dekomposition der Körpergewebe durch Fäulnis ist eine gewisse Feuchtigkeit Voraussetzung, diese Feuchtigkeit andererseits — entsprechend den dialektischen Gesetzen der Natur — unterbricht die Fäulnis unter bestimmten Bedingungen. Es kommt zu einer Adipozirebildung, die letztlich konservierend wirkt. Man könnte auch von einer feuchten Mumifikation sprechen. Denken wir an die Mumifikationen bei der spanischen Einbalsamierungsmethode oder fragen wir uns, ob nicht die Ägypter Leichen in einem Salzbad konservierten?

Adipozire tritt nicht nur im Wasser, sondern in jeder feuchten Umgebung, z.B. damit auch bei Erdleichen, auf. Sie ist nicht etwa eine spezifische, nur im Wasser sich einstellende Erscheinung, sondern eine der späten Leichenzeit, gleichgültig, ob es sich um begrabene oder nicht begrabene Erd- oder um Wasserleichen handelt. Didaktisch erscheint es zweckmäßig, bei der Abhandlung der Fettwachsbildung gleichzeitig auch die Hautveränderungen der Wasserleichen anzusprechen.

Die Veränderungen der Leichenhaut sind als *direkte* Folgen des Aufenthaltes im Wasser und nicht extra als *indirekte* zu differenzieren. Letztere betreffen mechanische Läsionen (Treibverletzungen, Leichenzehrer etc.).

a) Die Haut in feuchtem Milieu

Bei Arbeiten im Wasser oder nach Stehen in ihm, runzelt und verfärbt sich die Haut der Finger- bzw. Zehenbeeren. Die Waschhautbildung beruht auf einer wäßrigen Quellung des Stratum corneum. In ihrem Ausmaß hängt sie von der Expositionszeit, dem regionalen Aufbau der Haut bzw. der Dicke des Stratum corneum ab. DROSDOFF hat die Hornhautdicke der Zehenbeeren mit 1010 μ gemessen, die Hornhaut der Fingerbeeren wird mit 706 μ, die der Fußsohle mit 562 μ, und die des Handtellers mit 462 μ angegeben. Die Dicke der Hornschicht ist weiter abhängig vom Alter, Geschlecht und Beruf. In diesem Zusammenhang ist die Tabelle DROSDOFFs über das Verhältnis der Dicke des Stratum corneum zum Stratum germinativum von Bedeutung (Tabelle 3).

Bei Berücksichtigung dieser Tabellenwerte wird es verständlich, daß die Waschhaut im Bereich der Zehenbeeren am stärksten ist, bzw. allgemein dort, wo die Verhornung äußerste Stärke erreicht.

Normal beginnt die Waschhautbildung an dem Nagelfalz, an Zehen- wie Fingerbeeren. Die Haut verfärbt sich weißlich, runzelt, quillt. Weiße Verfärbung beruht auf Trübung und Quellung des Stratum corneum. Die normale Hautfarbe hängt von der Durchblutung der Haut ab. Blutgefüllte Capillaren schimmern durch das Stratum corneum. Quillt letzteres und trübt sich, hebt es sich ab, sehen wir lediglich seine Eigenfarbe.

Der Fettmantel schützt die Haut vor einer Wasserpenetration. Waschhaut bildet sich deshalb in warmem Wasser oder in einer mit fettlösenden Mitteln versetzten Flüssigkeit schneller aus. Im warmen Wasser sind nicht nur die chemischen, sondern auch die physikalischen Bedingungen für die Permeation günstiger. Die Poren werden weiter und erleichtern eine Wasserdurchlässigkeit.

Tabelle 3. *Verhältnis der Dicke des Stratum corneum zum Stratum germinativum* (DROSDOFF, 1879)

	Verhältnis in µ	Reduziertes Verhältnis
Stirn	22: 51	0,4 :1
Wange	35: 57	0,6 :1
v. Hals	32: 40	0,75:1
Gesäß	33:122	0,25:1
Palma	462:107	4 :1
Fingerbeere, 2. Finger	706:112	6 :1
Planta	562:100	5,6 :1
Zehenbeere	1010:100	10 :1

b) Haut im feuchten Milieu nach dem Tode

In jedem feuchten Milieu wird nicht nur die Haut des Lebenden, sondern auch die der Leiche physikalische Folgen der Wässerung zeigen. Dabei ist es gleich, ob es sich um Wasser, Urin oder andere Flüssigkeiten handelt, sofern diese nicht eine adstringierende Wirkung auf die Haut ausüben.

MONACELLI untersuchte über 2 Monate lang das Verhalten von Fettsubstanzen während der Autolyse. Seine Befunde werden als Produkte einer Entmischung nach hydrolytischer Spaltung von Lipoproteinverbindungen aufgefaßt (Lipophanerose). Wenn dieser Vorgang der Autolyse zugeordnet worden ist, zeigt sich die Schwierigkeit einer strengen Differenzierung zwischen Autolyse und speziellen Fäulnisvorgängen. Immerhin weisen Befunde von MONACELLI aus, daß sich im Protoplasma der Zellen des Stratum basale — Haut in physiologischer Kochsalzlösung bei $+37°$ — bereits nach 14 Tagen feine Phosphatidgranula bilden, die später auch im Stratum spinosum zu entdecken sind.

c) Wasserleiche: Direkte Einwirkung des Wassers

LEUCHTER hat 1905 beschrieben, daß eine Quellung der Fingerbeeren nach 24 Std, die der gesamten Hohlhand nach 48 Std zu sehen ist. Bei der anlaufenden Fäulnis, d.h. nach 6—8 Tagen Aufenthalts im Wasser, löse sich die Oberhaut. Nach KRATTER ist die Waschhautbildung an den Fingerbeeren nach 3—6 Std erreicht. Die Angaben der Autoren schwanken, sie stehen in Abhängigkeit nicht nur von der Wasserzeit, sondern auch von den Temperaturen des Wassers bzw. dessen Zusammensetzung.

Bei Schätzung der Wasserzeit aus der Waschhaut ist eine Aussage nur durch sofortige Untersuchung, unmittelbar nach der Ländung verwertbar. Verbleibt der Körper in nassen Kleidungsstücken, in feuchten Strümpfen und Schuhen, werden Handschuhe nicht ausgezogen, entwickelt sich die Waschhaut auch außerhalb des Wassers weiter. Hierin wird eine der Ursachen für die unterschiedliche Datenangabe der Autoren liegen.

Tabelle 4. *Waschhaut — zeitliche Verhältnisse der Entstehung*

Nagelfalz	2—3 Std	PIETRUSKY
Fingerbeeren	3—6 Std	KRATTER
	24 Std	LEUCHTER
Hohlhand	einige Stunden	CIOBAN
Fußsohle	nach 12 Std	SMITH
	nach 2 Tagen	PIETRUSKY
	nach 48 Std	LEUCHTER
	einige Tage	KRATTER
Handrücken	5—6 Tage	KOOPMANN
		PROKOP
Handgelenk-Unterarm	nach 2 Tagen	CIOBAN
Teilweise Ablösung der Haut	nach 6—8 Tagen	LEUCHTER
	nach 8—10 Tagen	KOOPMANN
Totale Ablösung ohne Nagelverlust	2—3 Tage	SCHRADER
	5—8 Tage	CIOBAN
Totale Ablösung mit Nagellösung	2—3 Wochen	SMITH, SCHRADER, PIETRUSKY
	2—3 Monate (in kaltem Wasser)	

Tabelle 5. *Anhaltspunkte für eine ungefähre Schätzung der Zeit des Aufenthaltes von Leichen im Wasser* (B. MUELLER)

Postmortale Veränderungen beim Aufenthalt einer Leiche im Wasser kommen immer wieder vor, außerdem sind die Angaben über die mikroskopischen Befunde noch nicht von verschiedenen Seiten auf ihre Zuverlässigkeit überprüft worden. *Eine schematische Verwertung der Tabelle durch den Unerfahrenen kann zu Fehlbegutachtungen führen.*

Unter 12 Std	Gänsehautbildung (nach 3—4 Std), sofern sie nicht während des Lebens vorhanden war. Beginnende Waschhautbildung nach 3—4 Std. Bißverletzungen von Garneelen an den Schleimhäuten (mindestens 4—8 Std).
12—24 Std	Befallensein der Fingerspitzen von Waschhautbildung (24 Std).
24—48 Std	Übergehen der Waschhautbildung auf die Hohlhand (28—48 Std). Ausbildung der Waschhaut an den Füßen (48 Std). Rötliche bis blaurote Verfärbung des Kopfes bei Fehlen von Fäulniserscheinungen an der Haut (ab 48 Std).
1 Woche	Verbreitung der Waschhautbildung auf die Hohlhandflächen (nach 5—8 Tagen). Beginn der Ablösung der Waschhaut von der Hohlhand (6—8 Tage). Beginnendes Ansetzen von Algenrasen (4 Tage).
7—14 Tage 1—2 Wochen	Entwicklung von dichtem Algenrasen an Stellen, denen die Kleider anliegen (8—10 Tage).
2—3 Wochen	Mikroskopisch schlechte Erkennbarkeit der elastischen Fasernetze bei Fehlen von Epithelabhebungen (2—3 Wochen). Eingehülltsein der Leiche in Algenrasen (von 14 Tagen an, sehr unsichere Merkmale).
3—4 Wochen	Abhebung der Epithelschicht im Bereich der Waschhautbildung (mikroskopisch), schlechte Färbbarkeit der elastischen Fasern der Haut (etwa 4 Wochen, sehr unsichere Merkmale).
1—2 Monate	Grünfärbung von Kopf, Hals und Brust (3—4 Wochen im Sommer). Auftreibung der ganzen Leiche, unkenntliche Gesichtszüge, Ablösung der Nägel, Nichterkennbarkeit der Augenfarbe (5—6 Wochen im Sommer). Beginnende Fettwachsbildung (frühestens nach 1—2 Monaten).
2—3 Monate	Grünfärbung von Kopf, Hals und Brust (2—3 Monate im Winter). Auftreibung der ganzen Leiche, unkenntliche Gesichtszüge, Ablösung der Nägel, Nichterkennbarkeit der Augenfarbe (12 Wochen und mehr im Winter). Erheblichere Fettwachsbildung (frühestens nach 3 Monaten).

Vom Nagelfalz und den Fingerbeeren ausgehend, greift die Waschhautbildung später auf den Handrücken und weiter auf die ulnare Fläche der Beugeseite des Unterarmes über.

Eine Waschhautbildung am Nagelfalz wird selbstverständlich dann nicht beobachtet, wenn durch kosmetische Eingriffe der Nagelfalz weitgehend entfernt wurde und somit die Quellung nicht so früh eintritt.

Erst als Folge der Fäulnis wird sich die Epidermis der Hohlhand und der Finger, mit Nägeln, abheben, bzw. handschuhartig lösen. In dieser Phase wird

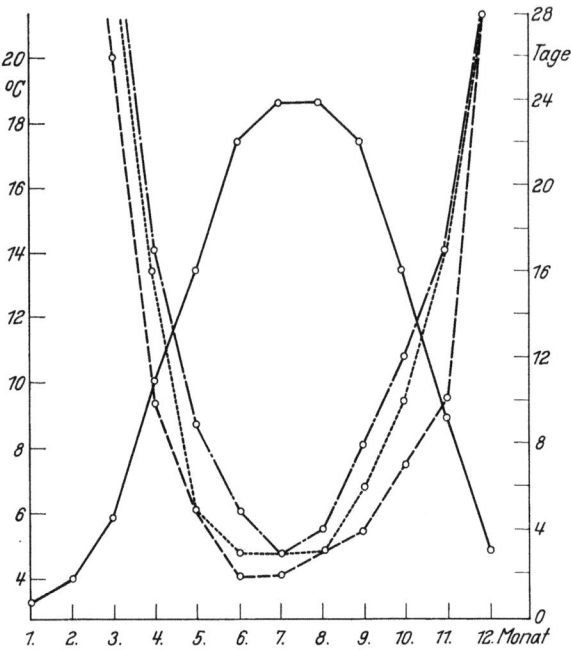

Abb. 11. Abhängigkeit der Leichenveränderungen von der Temperatur des Rheinstroms und der Liegezeit im Wasser (Reh). —— Durchschnittliche *Wassertemperatur* des Rheins in Düsseldorf, - - - - Mindestzeit für *Gasemphysem*, ... Mindestzeit für *Verflüssigung des Gehirns*, -·-·-·- Mindestzeit für *Lockerung der Fußnägel*, Lagerung der Wasserleichen im Kühlraum. Obduktion nach 2—3 Tagen

die Oberhaut kreideweiß im Bereich der verhornten Bezirke (KOLISKO). Wenn vereinzelt davon gesprochen wurde, daß die Ablösung der Haut bei Kindern rascher eintritt als bei Erwachsenen, möge man bedenken, daß hier vielleicht kein verwertbares Material vorliegt, denn der Ablösevorgang ist letztlich eine Folge der einsetzenden Fäulnis und diese kann bekanntlich unter differenten Bedingungen zu unterschiedlichen Zeiten beginnen (Abb. 12).

REH hat die Abhängigkeit der Leichenveränderungen von der Temperatur des Rheinstromes und der Liegezeit im Wasser in einem Diagramm dargestellt. Wir verweisen speziell auf das Gasemphysem der Haut sowie auf die Lockerung der Fußnägel (Abb. 11).

COLLIGNON beobachtete 1772 erstmals eine *Leichenwachsbildung*, 1789 haben die Franzosen THOURET und FOURCROY ausführlich über ihre Befunderhebungen nach Exhumierungen auf einem Pariser Friedhof in den Jahren 1786 und 1787 berichtet. Massengräber wurden wegen einer Neubelegung eröffnet. Man entdeckte nicht eine erwartete Fäulnisskelettierung, sondern die Leichen hatten ihre äußere Form behalten. Die Körperoberfläche wurde mit dem Aussehen einer gewissen Käseart verglichen, ein ranziger Käsegeruch war festzustellen. Die

Farbe wurde als grau beschrieben, besonders dort, wo das Leichenwachs noch feucht und weich war. Gelegentlich erwies sich die Oberkörperoberfläche auch als weiß. An der freien Luft trocknete das Leichenwachs, jetzt erschien die Oberfläche bröckelig, porös. Makroskopisch konnte die Oberfläche nicht als Haut angesprochen werden. Sie war nach THOURET in eine käsig-schmierige, graue Masse umgewandelt. Haare und Nägel konnten jedoch noch erkannt werden. Die Leichen rochen nicht nach Fäulnis, sondern eher etwas modrig.

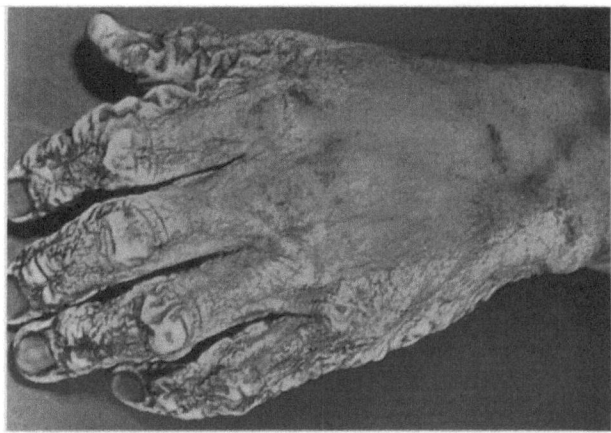

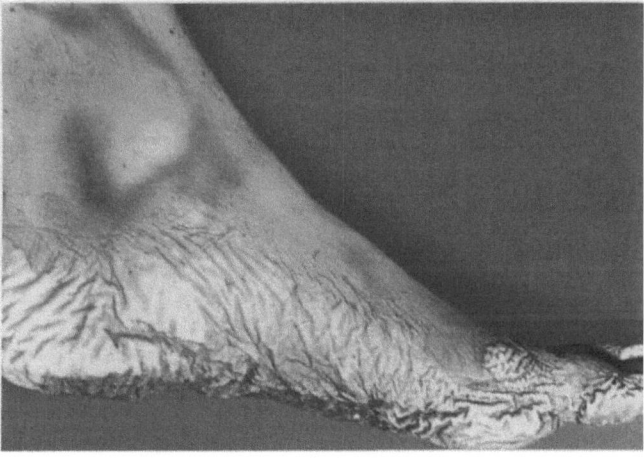

Abb. 12. Waschhaut — ,,durchgeschlagene" Gefäße

KRATTER stellte 1880 in einer Zusammenfassung die Bedingungen einer Adipozirebildung heraus. Man konnte Erklärungen vorlegen, weshalb das Unterhautfettgewebe z.B. in Fettwachs umgewandelt würde. Schwierigkeiten lagen darin, einen Grund zu erkennen, weshalb nicht nur Fettgewebe, sondern auch Muskulatur und Weichteile zu Fettwachs wurden. Viele Theorien gab es! (KRATTER, ASCARELLI, IPSEN, SCHAUENSTEIN, HOFMANN, EHRMANN, LUDWIG, EULENBERG, REUBOLD). Von ZIMMLER stammt der Begriff der sog. postmortalen Fettphanerose. REICHARDT führte chemische Untersuchungen durch und schloß sich den Ansichten der zuvor Genannten an. KRATTER, ASCARELLI und IPSEN sahen im Leichenwachs einen Umbildungsvorgang von Weichteilen in Fett. LEHMANN und VOIT unterstellten eine Neubildung von Fett aus Eiweißen (Adipo-Neogenese). Wegen bakterieller Zersetzungsprozesse des Gewebes würde es zu einer Freisetzung von Fett kommen unter Spaltung des Triglycerids in Glycerin und freie Fettsäuren; die gesättigten, höheren Fettsäuren schlagen sich nach TAMASSIA in kristalliner Form nieder und verseifen mit Kalk und Magnesia (daher der Name Saponifikation). Die erste Voraussetzung für die Entstehung von Leichenwachs wäre ein initialer Fäulnisvorgang. Nach den chemischen Untersuchungen von GOI und WENDE enthält Leichenwachs neben freien Fettsäuren Neutralfette und zu einem Achtel Kaliummagnesium — wie Ammoniakseifen. 1955 postulierten SMITH und FIDDES, daß die Fettwachsbildung als eine Fetthärtung aufzufassen sei. Es käme über eine Hydrolyse von Fett zu ungesättigten und gesättigten Fettsäuren. Bei diesem hydrolytischen Vorgang müßten als Katalysatoren im Fett Fermente wirken oder freigesetzt werden. RUTTER sowie MARSHALL nehmen an, daß diese Fermente gleichzeitig mit dem Eiweißabbau freigesetzt würden. Dadurch entstünden ammoniakalische Seifen in den frühen Stadien der Fettwachsbildung. Diese Ammoniaksaponifikation soll aber nicht die dominante Rolle spielen. MANT und FURBANK entwickelten folgende Theorie: Sie gehen von der Voraussetzung aus, daß unter sterilen Laboratoriumsbedingungen eine Fettspaltung sehr erschwert möglich ist. Deshalb würden bakterielle anaerobe Vorgänge bei der Fettwachsbildung entscheidend sein. Nach den neuesten Untersuchungen von NANIKAWA und WOITO mit der Basenverteilungschromatographie sind nur geringe Teile des Leichenwachses Seifen der Totalfettsäuren, entsprechend 2,0, 4,2 und 8,1 % der Gesamtadipoziremasse. Fettwachs stelle nur eine Verschiebung zu den stabileren, chemisch als auch katalysatorisch gesättigten Fettsäuren dar. Der Begriff Seifenbildung wäre demnach hinfällig. Die Mischung gesättigter Fettsäuren, hauptsächlich Palmitin, Stearin und Hydroxylstearinsäuren, hat schon LUKAS gefunden. Nach RUTTER und MARSHALL ist die Hydroxylstearinsäure ein wesentlicher Bestandteil der Adipozire, während Seifen und Proteine qualitativ und quantitativ variable Komponenten darstellen. Chemisch ähnliche Zusammensetzungen hat LUKAS bei den weißlichen Belägen ägyptischer Mumien gefunden. Diese Ansicht muß allerdings mit einer gewissen Vorsicht bewertet werden (Salzwasserbasen bei Mumien).

Makroskopisches Aussehen. Die Haut frisch geländeter Fettwachsleichen ist schmutzig-grau, z.T. glänzend, höckerig warzig, dazwischen sind gelegentlich rötliche, bandartige Strukturen zu erkennen. Die Oberfläche fühlt sich schmierig weich, seifig an. Eine durch Druck hervorgerufene Delle bleibt bestehen. Der Geruch ist modrig. Hautanhangsgebilde sind erhalten und zumeist dunkelgrau-braun.

Trocknet die Fettwachsleiche in der Luft, tönen sich die oberflächlichen Schichten etwas dunkler, sie werden evtl. krümelig und auf Druck konsistenter. Es lassen sich einzelne Schichten und Wachspartikel bröckelhaft ablösen. In dieser Phase ist die bedeckende Oberfläche eher spröde und zerbrechlich. Erst nach längerer Zeit von Lufttrocknung wird der überziehende Fettwachspanzer tonähnlich hart und klingt bei Beklopfen nach tönerner Masse. Haare und Nägel fallen dabei nach leichter Berührung aus.

Histologischer Befund. Die normale Schichtung der Haut ist nicht zu erkennen; anstelle der Epidermis findet sich häufig ein Pilz- und Bakterienrasen (EVANS). Die kollagenen Fasern der Dermis sind gelegentlich noch diffus darstellbar. Einzelne Haarfollikel sollen noch erkennbar sein. Das Leichenwachs stellt sich mikroskopisch in Form von sphärischen Kristallen mit radialer Strahlung dar. In der Hämatoxylin-Eosinfärbung tönt sich das Gewebe leicht bläulich. Die Kristalle sind anisotroph.

Nach Verdunstung der Feuchtigkeit zeigen sich lediglich die Folgen der Eintrocknung.

Die Entstehung von Leichenwachs ist abhängig von körpereigenen wie Umweltfaktoren. Je stärker das subcutane Fettgewebe ausgebildet ist, desto rascher entsteht Leichenwachs. Deshalb bildet sich besonders bei Säuglingen, Kleinkindern, adipösen Personen oder an Körperstellen mit reichlich vorgebildetem, subcutanen Fettgewebe schneller Leichenwachs. Dies würde der Auffassung von ZILLNER, der sog. Fettphanerose, entsprechen. Aber auch eine durch Desaminierung von Aminosäuren entstehende Fettsäurebildung könnte für das Aufkommen von Leichenwachs in diesen Gebieten herangezogen werden.

Die Umweltfaktoren spielen eine bedeutende Rolle. Bei geringerer Leichenwachsbildung der Haut kann man mit einer Wasserzeit von 3—6 Wochen rechnen. Größere flächenhafte Leichenwachsbildungen wurden nach 6—8 Wochen beobachtet. BOHNE und REIMANN sahen bei höheren Temperaturen schon Adipozire nach 14 Tagen bis 3 Wochen. REIMANN führte diese schnelle Entstehung im Sommer und im wärmeren Klimata auf relative Sauerstoffverarmung des wärmeren Wassers zurück. Ein gleicher Grund wäre bei jenen Leichen, die in tiefen Alpenseen oder in sauerstoffarmen Industriegewässern eine gewisse Zeit liegen, zu zitieren. Histologisch hat MATZDORFF bereits nach 7 Tagen Fettsäurekristalle im Unterhautfettgewebe (Talgdrüsen) gefunden. Eine vollständige Fettwachspanzerung des gesamten Körpers wird frühestens nach 12 Monaten erwartet. Die Versuche von BROCHYLA sind für diese Fragestellung von Bedeutung. Oberschenkelhaut wurde in verschiedenen Böden gleich tief vergraben. Im Sandboden war die Haut nach 52 Tagen vollständig zerstört; kein Leichenwachs. Nach Vergraben in fetter Erde zeigte sich nach 34 Tagen eine Andeutung von Leichenwachs. Die Haut und das Unterhautfettgewebe erschienen verseift.

Wenn in der Zeit nach dem 2. Weltkrieg Gräber der im Kriege Gefallenen geöffnet wurden und man selbst in trockener Erde eine typische Leichenwachsbildung feststellte, wird man sich überlegen müssen, ob hier nicht die Fäulnisflüssigkeit, die sich zwangsläufig in einem Massengrabe sammelt, nicht jene Funktionen übernimmt, die zur Adipozirebildung nötig sind. Man möge weiter berücksichtigen, daß der Wassergehalt des Erdbodens temporär sehr unterschiedlich sein kann. Es wäre eine Fehlwertung, wenn der Zustand, in dem ein Grab geöffnet wird, einzig entscheidend sein sollte. Bei der Öffnung von Massengräbern könnte man im trockenen Erdreich, in der Peripherie des Massengrabes u.U. kein Fettwachs entdecken; dieses jedoch im Zentrum des Massengrabes.

Forensisch-kriminalistische Bedeutung. Durch die Leichenwachsbildung werden Wunden bzw. Strangulationsfurchen längere Zeit postmortal erhalten (KRATTER, DANNER). Geklärt werden kann nicht, ob der sich darbietende Defekt als intravital oder postmortal entstanden angesehen werden muß.

Der Ausdruck Panzer wurde verwendet. Man sieht bei der Bergung einer Leiche gelegentlich, daß der Oberflächenpanzer geborsten ist. Unter dem Treiben wurden die Extremitäten im fließenden Wasser gegeneinander bewegt, infolgedessen kam es zu Kontinuitätstrennungen. Die Gliedmaßen können sich vom Körperstamm lösen, evtl. auch abbrechen, vorwiegend im Knie- und Ellenbogenbereich. Die geborgenen Leichenteile zeigen nach Trocknung die geborstene Oberfläche.

Bei der Ländung können Verletzungen im schmierig weichen Leichenwachs gesetzt werden.

Neben den *direkten* Einwirkungen, die von der Waschhautbildung bis zur Saponifikation führen können, stehen die *indirekten* in Gewässern. Treibverletzungen stellen sich vielfach an typischer Stelle in Gestalt von unterschiedlich tiefen Schürfungen der Haut und des Unterhautfettgewebes dar. Da die Leiche im Wasser in Bauchlage treibt, die Extremitäten zutiefst hängen, sieht man über Handrücken, den Knien und dem Fußrücken derartige Treibspuren;

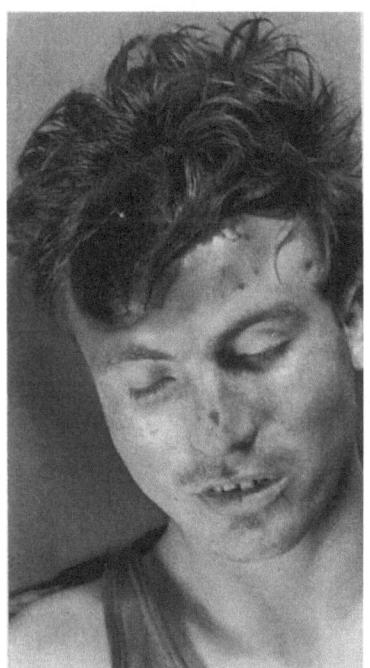

sie können sich bei Kopftieflage auch im Bereich der Stirn und des Nasenrückens ausbilden (Abb. 13).

In Abhängigkeit von der Beschaffenheit des Grundes und der Strömung können die Kopfschwarte, einschließlich der Schädelkalotte, in Stunden geschürft, abgeschliffen sein, dabei werden evtl. feinste Kieselsteinchen in, bzw. unter die verletzte Haut getrieben. Beim Treiben gegen Buhnen, Brückenpfeiler etc. entstehen Verletzungen. Man wird diese Verletzungen, die u. U. nicht an typischer Stelle sofort als Treibverletzungen zu identifizieren sind, differentialdiagnostisch jenen Läsionen gegenüberstellen, die beim Hineinspringen oder Fallen ins Wasser entstehen können.

Verletzungen durch Schiffsschrauben sind bekannt. Selbst schwerste Haut- und Körperdurchtrennungen sind möglich. Die modernen Schiffsschrauben unterscheiden sich in ihrem Verletzungsmuster von den früher üblichen.

Die *Leichenzehrer* im Wasser (Käfer, Krebschen, desgleichen aasfressende Fische) werden

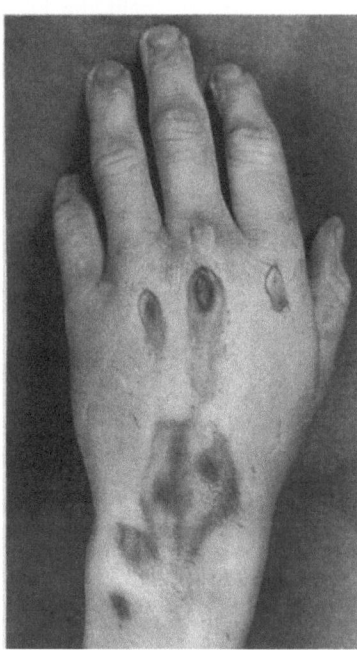 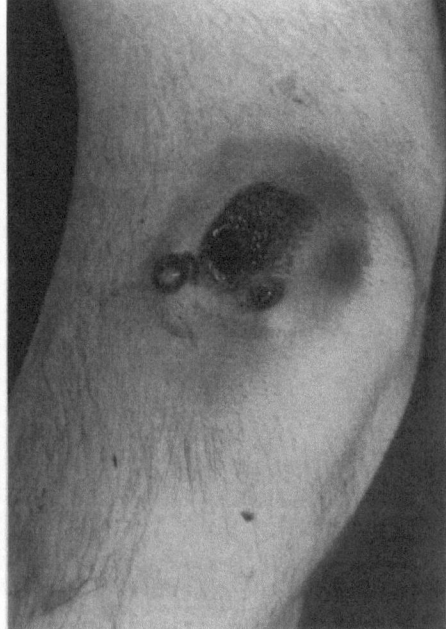

Abb. 13. Treibverletzungen einer Wasserleiche. Unten links: Hautschürfungen mit Vertrocknungen. Unten rechts: Impression eines Kieselsteines

Hautverletzungen setzen können, die differentialdiagnostisch deshalb große Schwierigkeiten bereiten, weil sie in ihrem Aussehen Ähnlichkeiten mit vital entstandenen haben können, zudem die Wundflächen selbst durch den Auswaschungsprozeß im Wasser keine vitalen Reaktionen oder Zeichen mehr erkennen lassen.

Im Wasser oder auch nach einem Antreiben können z. B. Ratten oder Vögel die freiliegenden Körperteile verletzen. Bei den Schnabelhieben der Vögel entstehen u. U. Befunde, die jenen durch stechende Werkzeuge ähneln.

6. Moormumifikation

In einer Monographie hat A. Dieck über die europäischen Moorleichenbefunde 1965 ausführlich berichtet. Welche Veränderungen stellen sich im Moor oder Anmoor, in huminsäurehaltiger Flüssigkeit ein?

Makroskopisches Aussehen und Beschaffenheit der Haut. Haut und Anhangsgebilde sind in bezug auf Farbe, Konsistenz und Erhaltungszustand von Beschaffenheit des Körpers bzw. der Leiche im Augenblick des Hineingeratens ins Moor und der Aufenthaltsdauer in ihm abhängig. Folgende Faktoren spielen eine Rolle:

1. Die Zusammensetzung des Moores bzw. Torfes.

2. Der Zustand, in dem der Körper in die Moorumgebung gebracht wird: Versinkt ein Lebender sofort im Moor oder wird ein bereits in Fäulnis begriffener Körper versenkt, nachträglich hineingeworfen oder bleibt die Leiche zunächst an der Oberfläche und versinkt dann erst.

3. Die Zeit, die vom Beginn der Bergung bis zur Besichtigung verstreicht; Temperatur außerhalb des Moores.

4. Nicht unerheblich dürfte sein, ob ein vollständig erhaltenes Integument oder nur einzelne Integumentteile einer Moorveränderung ausgesetzt werden.

5. Die Spanne zwischen Bergung und Besichtigung ist wegen der einsetzenden Vertrocknung der Körperoberfläche von Bedeutung. Farbe und Konsistenz werden sich zwischenzeitlich verändern.

6. Das Moor selbst wird sich während der Liegezeit ändern können, es kann z. T. austrocknen, seine chemische Zusammensetzung wird anders, evtl. auch der Flüssigkeitsgehalt. Primär könnte sich also eine Moorleiche entwickelt haben, die sekundär durch Veränderungen im trockengelegten Moor zu einer weiterlaufenden Fäulnis oder Verwesung geführt hat. Wie tief sank der Körper in das Moor?

7. Jahreszeitliche und damit auch Temperatur- und Flüssigkeitsschwankungen spielen eine Rolle.

8. Partiell wird die Haut verändert, sofern sich nicht der gesamte Körper im Moor befindet.

Auf differente Moorzusammensetzungen und die daraus resultierenden osmotischen Drücke wird die Leichenhaut sehr unterschiedlich reagieren. Körperflüssigkeit diffundiert aus Gewebe und Haut in die Umgebung. Entscheidend ist bei starkem und länger bestehendem Diffusionsgefälle ein Übertreten von Moorwasser. Ein regelloser Austausch ist vorstellbar, primär wird die Haut Flüssigkeit verlieren, sekundär erst dürften Moorwasserbestandteile die Haut imprägnieren. Nicht nur physikalisch-chemische Vorgänge der Diffusion und Osmose, sondern auch spezifische, nur im Moorwasser zu findende bzw. eintretende Reaktionen, spielen sich ab. Gerbstoffe wie Gerbsäuren verändern die Körperoberfläche, dringen in die Tiefe der Haut; parallel dazu jene Wassereinflüsse, wie wir sie auch bei Wasserleichen kennen. Welcher Faktor bei der Moormumifikation im Vordergrund steht, ist von Fall zu Fall sehr unterschiedlich, selbst innerhalb eines Gebietes oder gar, wenn zwei Körper dicht nebeneinander im Moor versinken, sind die Befunde unterschiedlich.

Welche konservierenden Eigenschaften wirken sich aus? SENFT hat 1862 geschrieben: Der gute Erhaltungszustand „läßt sich indessen aus dem Umstand erklären, daß sich bei den vollständigen Vertorfungsprozessen aller gerbsäure- und harzhaltigen Gewächse, z.B. der Erikazeen, laufend eine Flüssigkeit entwickelt, die aus einer, dem Holzessig ähnlichen kreosothaltigen Säure und einem dem Holzteer ähnlichen, harzigen Öl (Bitumen) besteht und die fleischigen Teile gegen Fäulnis schützt".

Nach Bergung ist die Körperoberfläche von gröberen Moorbestandteilen und Schlamm vorsichtig zu säubern. Man kann evtl. noch vorhandene Haut unzerstört vorfinden. Sie hat eine rötlich-bräunliche bis schwärzliche Farbe, ist an der Oberfläche zumeist glatt. Hautdefekte könnten erst bei der Bergung entstanden sein. Oder sind sie auf Leichenzehrer zu beziehen? Die Haut der frisch geborgenen Moorleiche ist, falls der Körper nicht vor dem Versinken im Moor faulte, erhalten. Wird sie eine gewisse Zeit der freien Luft ausgesetzt, vertrocknet sie. Jetzt erst wird sie dunkel bis schwarz. Bekannt ist z.B. die Abbildung im Lehrbuch von POLSON. Bei Beschreibung der Körperhülle hüte man sich vor Täuschungen; das Aussehen nach Lufttrocknung ist auf das der Moorgerbung nicht ohne weiteres zu übertragen. Sofortige Besichtigung ist nötig!

Unmittelbar nach Bergung ist die Haut glatt. Nach Verdunstung des Wassers wird sie etwas rauher, ja gewellt erscheinen.

Im frischem Bergungszustand ist die Haut biegsam, nicht brüchig. Ein Vergleich mit Leder ist durchaus angezeigt. Nach Vertrocknung wird die Haut härter, weniger biegsam, wirkt wie gegerbt. Die Moormumienhaut wird nie spröde oder brüchig (Abb. 14).

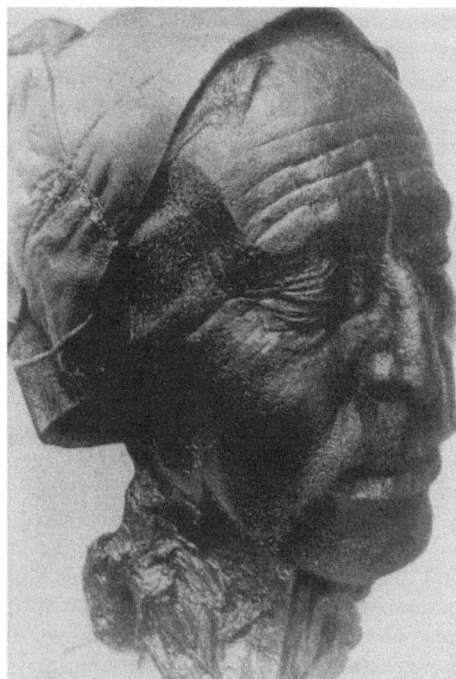

Abb. 14. Moorleiche. Heimatmuseum, Jütland

Haare bleiben erhalten, sind unmittelbar nach der Bergung fuchsig rötlich, evtl. rötlich bis dunkelbraun, biegsam. Nach Lufttrocknung und unter Feuchtigkeitsverlust dunkelt die Haarfarbe nach, gleichzeitig sind die Haare, wegen Austrocknung der Haarfollikel, leichter auszuziehen, bzw. können auf mechanischen Druck beseitigt werden.

Die Nägel sind noch gut erhalten, dunkelbraun bis schwarz. Die Lösung der Nägel aus dem Nagelfalz ist erst Folge der Lufttrocknung, es kommt unter der Verdunstung der Flüssigkeit zu einer Auflockerung am Nagelfalz.

Die experimentellen Untersuchungen von ELLERMANN (Hautstücke über ein Jahr einer Moorerde ausgesetzt) haben nicht die entsprechenden charakteristischen Veränderungen aufgewiesen, sondern jene der Adipozirebildung. Solche Versuche sind meist fehlerhaft, da sie nicht unter den physikalisch-chemischen Bedingungen vor sich gingen, wie sie das Moor anbietet.

Wurden irgendwelche Verletzungen zu Lebzeiten gesetzt, gelangte der Körper unmittelbar in das Moor, wird man unter der konservierenden Eigenschaft jene Verletzungsmarken deutlich erkennen können.

Mikroskopisch ist die Epidermis meist noch darzustellen. Nach ELLERMANN soll allerdings die Oberhaut teils fehlen, während die Lederhaut im ganzen erhalten sei. Bei länger bestehender Moormumifikation ist eine Differenzierung nicht zu erhalten. Die Lederhaut zeigt Veränderungen im Sinne einer Gerbung (s. hierzu entsprechende Lehrbücher). Die Bindegewebsfasern der Lederhaut sind noch deutlich auszumachen, zeigen aber keinerlei Kernanfärbbarkeit. Nach WALSER ist diese Darstellung nur auf kollagene Fasern beschränkt, elastische seien nicht mehr vorhanden. Das subcutane Fettgewebe zeigt lediglich bindegewebige Anteile, keine Zellmembrane. Diese mikroskopischen Befunde decken sich mit denen einer Gerbung.

Das Mark der Haare soll nicht mehr darzustellen sein, dagegen die Cuticularis. Talg- wie Schweißdrüsen stellen sich mikroskopisch nicht dar. Pigmente sind durch Moorfarbstoffe überdeckt.

7. Identitätsfeststellung über die Haut in der späteren Leichenzeit

Leichenerscheinungen, Mumifikation, Fäulnis, Wasserleichen erschweren eine Abnahme von Fingerabdrücken, machen diese sogar unmöglich. Dabei ist gerade die Daktyloskopie in vielen Fällen das einzige Mittel zur Identifizierung einer unbekannten Leiche. Deshalb muß alles unternommen werden, verwertbare Fingerabdrücke zu erhalten.

Bei den vertrockneten, geschrumpften Fingerabdrücken kann die Haut nicht durch Einspritzen von Flüssigkeit geglättet und entfaltet werden. Deswegen empfiehlt E. FRITZ, die mumifizierten Finger abzusetzen und entsprechend dem Vertrocknungsgrad 24—36 Std zu wässern. Der Erfolg ist nicht immer befriedigend. FRITZ erzielte bessere Ergebnisse nach Abtrennung der Haut der gesamten Beugefläche der Fingerkuppe und durch Wässerung für wenige Stunden nach vorheriger Abtragung des Unterhautfettgewebes. Wir haben gute Ergebnisse nach 24stündigem Einlegen in Antiformin erzielt. Danach wird das Hautstück z.B. über die Fingerkuppe des Untersuchers gespannt und entfältelt. Mit einem in Alkohol und Benzin getränkten Wattebausch wird die Oberfläche entfettet und gesäubert; dann kann ein Abdruck genommen werden.

Die Waschhaut führt zu Quellung und Fältelung der Epidermis. Die Oberfläche der Fingerbeere kann — soweit die Haut unverletzt ist — durch Unterspritzen von Flüssigkeit (Glycerin, Paraffinöl) geglättet werden (RICHTER). Punktionsstelle proximal der Fingerkuppe.

Selbst von faulen Leichen sind brauchbare Fingerabdrücke zu nehmen. Aufgabe des Untersuchers: Die Fingerbeere asservieren und sie einer erkennungsdienstlichen Bearbeitung zuleiten. Das bedeutet: Hände am Tat- oder Fundort nicht berühren, damit die Oberhaut nicht handschuhartig ab- und verlorengeht. Am Fundort fehlen zur Asservierung die richtigen Instrumente etc. Bei Bergung einer Wasserleiche z.B. sind deshalb die Hände mit einem Plastikbeutel zu umhüllen. Der Beutel ist über den Gelenken abzubinden!

Die erforderlichen, speziellen, daktyloskopischen Untersuchungen sind nur in einem kriminaltechnisch eingerichteten Laboratorium möglich.

Der Leichenschauer oder Obduzent müßte auch die Haut der Fingerbeeren konservieren, um das Untersuchungsgut einem Laboratorium zuzuleiten. Formalin oder Alkohol usw. sind nicht zu empfehlen. Der Haut wird Wasser entzogen, sie wird spröde und verliert die benötigte Elastizität. Wir trennen die Endglieder der

Finger oder nur die Haut der Fingerbeeren vom Unterhautfettgewebe. Die abgelösten einzelnen Fingerhäute werden in entsprechend dem Finger beschrifteten und mit Leitungswasser gefüllten, dickwandigen Reagenzgläsern (Plastikröhrchen) aufbewahrt. Die Haut war in Leitungswasser selbst nach 4 Wochen noch unbeschädigt, die Epidermis blieb sogar mit der Lederhaut verbunden (KOBABE).

Ist die Fäulnis so weit fortgeschritten, daß sich die Oberhaut handschuhartig gelöst hat, wird der Oberhautsack nach RICHTER mit Wachs oder Paraffin, nach REUTER mit Krukenbergschem Zinkleim ausgegossen. Es ist bekannt, daß die Innenfläche der Epidermis des Hautbalges die Papillarlinien der äußeren Oberfläche der Haut so deutlich nachzeichnet, wie man es selbst beim Lebenden selten findet. Allerdings handelt es sich hier um das Negativ der Oberfläche der Fingerbeere. Mittels der erstarrten Masse des Oberhautsackes legen wir die Papillarlinien der Fingerbeerhaut in Positivform dar.

Zur Identifizierung gibt es nunmehr zwei Möglichkeiten:
1. Fotoaufnahme der Oberfläche des „künstlichen Fingers".
2. Normaler Abdruck der Oberfläche desselben.

Liegen nur Teile der Epidermis der Fingerbeere vor — wird ein Ausguß unmöglich — fertigen wir mit Hilfe von Plastilin einen Abdruck der Innenfläche des Teilchens.

Daktyloskopische Untersuchungen können mit Erfolg trotz Verlust der Epidermis noch vorgenommen werden, weil das Stratum papillare der Lederhaut das Papillarlinienmuster der Fingerkuppe wiedergibt (REUTER).

Selbst Blutgruppen lassen sich bei gealterten oder gar in Formalin gelegenen Haaren nach YADA u.a. nachweisen, gleiches soll für die Geschlechtsbestimmungen möglich sein (MONTANARI).

III. Gewalteinwirkungen auf die Haut einer Leiche
1. Abgrenzung gegenüber agonalen wie vitalen Prozessen

Eine Fülle von Problemen stellt sich; u.a. wird die Kardinalfrage, die bei vielen Tötungsdelikten dem Sachverständigen vorgelegt wird, angesprochen. Von welch immenser Bedeutung die Problematik vitaler, agonaler, supravitaler und postmortaler Läsionen der Körperoberfläche ist, zeigen Prozesse der jüngsten Zeit. Immer sollte sich der Sachverständige darüber im klaren sein, daß er im konkreten Fall ein vitales Ereignis beweisen muß, daß nicht seine subjektive Einstellung zum Geschehnisablauf sowie Mutmaßungen oder Hypothesen Geltung haben, sondern die einfache Frage, welche sicheren Erkenntnisse aus einem morphologischen Substrat abgeleitet werden können, die den eindeutigen Schluß zulassen, daß diese Verletzung den Lebenden traf.

Bewußt werden jene Überlegungen zur Ausschlußdiagnose anderer Abläufe bzw. Todesursachen nicht angestellt, da nur über die konkrete Bewertung eines morphologischen Substrates an der Haut, nicht über weitere Organbefunde, diskutiert werden soll.

Betrachten wir unter diesen Aspekten Läsionen des Integuments, wird man sich der mikroskopischen Befunde von WALCHER über die initialen, reaktiven, entzündlichen Veränderungen einer Wunde erinnern müssen. Da die Randstellung der Leukocyten erst nach einer Überlebenszeit von ca. 30 min beginnt und dann anschließend weiße Formelemente auswandern und sich extravasal ansammeln, ist dieser Zeitraum für viele unserer Fragestellungen zu groß. Gleiches gilt für die Feststellung von RAEKALLIO, daß sich 4 Std nach einer vitalen Läsion polymorphkernige Leukocyten-Extravasate erkennen lassen und sie erst 8 Std nach einer Verletzung zahlreicher in den Randzonen von Verletzungen zu sehen sind.

Man könnte den Terminplan der Entzündung weiter verfolgen, wie es in sehr schönen Untersuchungen RAEKALLIO wie PIOCH getan haben; bezüglich der forensisch relevanten, zeitlich eingeengten Problemstellungen haben sich jedoch keine weiteren Erkenntnisse gezeigt, sofern man die Frage nach Differenzierung einer Hautverletzung mit kurzer Überlebenszeit zwischen Verletzung und Tod gegen solche der supravitalen Phase aufgreift. RAEKALLIO schreibt, daß es

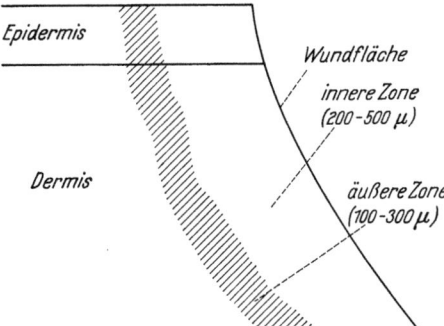

Abb. 15. Zone in der Umgebung *vitaler* Hautwunden. Innere Zone mit oft abnehmender Fermentaktivität = negative vitale Reaktion. Äußere Zone mit Zunahme der Fermentaktivität = positive vitale Reaktion. (RAEKALLIO, 1967)

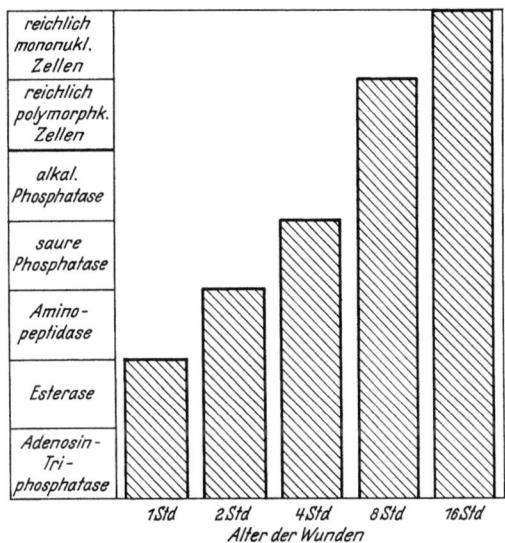

Abb. 16. *Alter der Wunden.* Bestimmung des Zeitpunktes der Läsion *vor* dem Tode. Sog. positive *vitale* Reaktion in histochemischer Darstellung. (RAEKALLIO, 1967)

noch eine Latenzperiode von mindestens 4—8 Std nach einem Trauma geben würde und daß hier fermenthistochemische Methoden weiterhelfen könnten. Nach welcher Zeit ist eine positive, vitale Reaktion zu erkennen? Tabellarisch wurden seine Ergebnisse in der 3. neubearbeiteten Auflage des Lehrbuches der Gerichtlichen Medizin von A. PONSOLD von RAEKALLIO dargestellt (Abb. 15).

Hier resümiert RAEKALLIO: ,,Wenn man keine positiven oder negativen Reaktionen bei der Darstellung der genannten Enzyme feststellen kann, ist die Wunde *entweder* nach dem Tode (postmortal) *oder* agonal, weniger als eine Stunde vor dem Tode, erzeugt worden. Erkennt man aber positive und negative vitale Reaktionen bei der Darstellung eines Enzyms oder mehrerer Fermente, so ist die Wunde bei Lebzeiten (vital) entstanden."

Sicherlich haben die fermenthistochemischen Untersuchungsmethoden Fortschritte gebracht, letzten Endes sind wir aber bei den kritischen Fragestellungen nicht wesentlich weitergekommen; wir dürfen auch nicht vergessen, daß die experimentellen Untersuchungen von RAEKALLIO an der Haut von Meerschweinchen durchgeführt wurden. RAEKALLIO meint: ,,Weil die Haut des Meerschweinchens der Haut des Menschen gleichartiger als die anderer gewöhnlicher Versuchstiere ist ..." A. FATTEH hat aber Vergleichsuntersuchungen vorgenommen. Es handelt sich dabei sowohl um Tierversuche (Meerschweinchen) als auch um menschliches Hautgewebe. Er prüfte die histochemischen Veränderungen bei Wundheilung und bei nach dem Tode gesetzten Hautverletzungen. *Beim Meerschweinchen* tritt die Zunahme der Fermentaktivitäten *wesentlich früher* ein, weil der Metabolismus der Haut der verschiedenen Species unterschiedlich ist.

	Meerschweinchen	Mensch
Ribonucleinsäure	4 Std	8 Std
Desoxyribonucleinsäure	4 Std	8 Std
Saure Phosphatase	4 Std	8 Std
Alkalische Phosphatasen	3 Std	4 Std
Nicht spezifische Esterase	10 min	30 min
Leucine Aminopeptidase	3 Std	4 Std

Man darf Ergebnisse von Tierexperimenten nicht ohne Konfrontation mit Humanmaterial für gerichtsmedizinische Zwecke verwenden.

LINDNER hat sich in den letzten Jahren speziell mit dem morphologischen Substrat der Entzündung und Wundheilung beschäftigt; seine Forschungen hierüber stellte er jüngst in einem Schema zusammen. Die Merkmale der vitalen Reaktion, der zeitliche Ablauf der Entzündung anhand des morphologisch, biochemisch und radiochemisch zur Zeit erfaßbaren Startes der wichtigsten Einzelphasen stellen sich wie folgt dar:

1—4 Std	Primäre Acidose mit Störung der Elektrolyt- und Wasserverteilung: Grundsubstanzentmischung = primäre physikalisch-chemische Zustandsänderung mit Desaggregation, Kolloiddispersion, Depolymerisierung usw. der MPS-Protein-Komplexe mit Störung der Isoionie, Isoosmie und Isotonie. Faseraufquellung (durch Beteiligung der interfibrillären Kittsubstanz am Grundsubstanzentmischungsablauf und interkristalline Quellung). Zelldemaskierung, -reizung, -aufquellung mit Beginn von Pino- und Phagocytose sowie Enzymaktivierung der ortsständigen Bindegewebszellen (Fibrocyten, Gefäßwandzellen usw.), RNS-Synthese und adaptive bzw. induktive Enzymsynthesen. Mastzellen-Degranulierung = Freisetzung von Heparin und Histamin (speciesabhängig auch von Serotonin usw.) mit Gefäß-, Zell- und Zwischensubstanzwirkungen (Permeabilitäts-, Diffusions-, Entgiftungs-, Fermenthemmungs- und weitere Einflüsse). Capillarwand-Permeabilitätsänderung durch Beteiligung an den genannten Entmischungs- und Aufquellungsvorgängen der Zwischensubstanz mit Einfluß auf die Capillarfunktion: Prästase, Stase, Hypoxie, entzündliche Hyperämie; Serum-(Fibrin-), Ery-, Leuko- usw. Austritte: Permeation, Exsudation und Emigration. ^{35}S-Sulfat-Inkorporationszunahme = Sulfatierung und Synthese von MPS (anabole und katabole Prozesse).
4—12 Std	Sekundäre Acidose: Fortsetzung der Grundsubstanzveränderung mit wechselnder Dysionie und Dysosmie, Quellung und Entquellung, Auftreten von Denaturierungs- und Degenerationsprodukten des Kollagen mit folgendem Abbau durch unspez. Proteasen, allgemeiner Zerfall der am stärksten geschädigten zelligen und zwischenzelligen Bindegewebsbestandteile des Entzündungsfeldes: Zunahme des intra- und extracellulären *Katabolismus*, von Glykolyse, Proteolyse, Lipolyse usw.: Zunahme von gefäßaktiven Abbauprodukten usw.

Schema (Fortsetzung)

12—36 Std	Zunahme der initialen, vorwiegend katabolen Prozesse, deren Intensität und Dauer vom Ort der Entzündung ebenso wie von Art, Stärke und Dauer des Entzündungsreizes abhängt; gleichzeitige Überlagerung der katabolen Vorgänge mit den genannten primären und folgenden sekundären anabolen Prozessen: Zellproliferationen (^{3}H-Thymidin- und Mitoseraten-Indices), spez. Fibroblastenproliferation.
48—72 Std	Histochemischer, autoradiographischer und radiochemischer (mit ^{35}S-Sulfat) sowie biochemischer (Uronsäuren-, Hexosamin-, MPS-) Nachweis der Grundsubstanz-Synthese (intra- und extracellulär).
3.—4. Tag	In gleicher methodischer Reihenfolge erfolgter Nachweis der Fasersynthese (mit ^{3}H-Prolin; Hydroxyprolin-Bestimmung usw.). Capillarisierung.
4.—6. Tag	Verschiebung des Zellverhältnisses mit Abnahme von Mikro- und Makrophagen zugunsten ausreifender Fibroblasten, Mastzellenneubildung.
6.—10. Tag	Abnahme des Wassergehaltes, Zunahme des Polymerisationsgrades der Grundsubstanz mit Abnahme der histochemischen Anfärbbarkeit und Zunahme des physiko-chemischen Gleichgewichtes bzw. der Eukolloidalität der Grundsubstanz; Verschiebung des Verhältnisses der Kollagenfraktionen (zugunsten der schwerer löslichen und unlöslichen) mit steigender Zahl der intramolekularen Kreuzbindungen des Kollagens. Die vollständige oder unvollständige Wiederherstellung der Ausgangssituation ist qualitativ und zeitlich abhängig von der Lokalisation des betroffenen Gewebes sowie von Art, Grad und Einwirkungsdauer der Entzündungsursache (neben dem Einfluß individueller Faktoren sowie der Reaktionslage und -eigenschaften sowie mannigfaltiger Regulationen des Gesamtorganismus).

2. Stumpfe Gewalt

Wir kennen zwar die gedeckten, d.h. subcutan gelegenen, Verletzungen innerer Organe bei intakter Haut nach Traumatisierungen. Zumeist jedoch wird die Haut ebenfalls versehrt. Die spezielle, forensische Pathologie beschäftigt sich deshalb vorwiegend mit der Untersuchung der schützenden Außenfläche des Körpers, d.h. Kleidung wie Haut, weil hier wichtige Aussagen vorliegen können.

Die Frage lautet: welche Möglichkeit habe ich, endogene von exogenen Hautveränderungen zu differenzieren bzw.
zu welcher Zeit — vital oder postmortal — wurden diese Hautläsionen gesetzt?

Der Budapester Professor PLENK schreibt schon in seinem 1781 erschienenen Buch „elementa medicinae forensis" bei der Besprechung der Strangfurche nach Erhängungstod: „an talis vivus, vel alia morte iam ante mortuus fuerit suspensus?" Es war sicherlich kein Zufall, daß PLENK den Hautverletzungen soviel Aufmerksamkeit schenkte, denn er ist einer der Begründer der wissenschaftlichen Dermatologie mit seinem Buche: Doctrina de morbis cutaneis qua hi morbi in suas classes, genera et species rediguntur (1776).

Die Problemstellung hat heute noch die gleiche Bedeutung. Sie ist keinesfalls auf Strangfurchen beschränkt, sondern auf alle Arten stumpfer Gewalteinwirkungen auf die Haut, heute speziell Betriebs- und Verkehrsverletzungen. Eine Kardinalfrage: Wurde ein Körper zu Lebzeiten oder erst nach dem Tode von einem Fahrzeug überrollt? Trotz Einsatz subtilster Untersuchungsmethoden ist diese Beantwortung nicht einfach. Die stumpfe Gewalt wird nämlich die Leichenhaut, ähnlich wie den lebenden Organismus, abhängig von der Größenform des Gegenstandes, der Kraft der Einwirkung, bezogen auf eine bestimmte Hautpartie, verletzen. Wir differenzieren:
a) Druckanämie,
b) Hautblutungen,
c) Excoriationen,
d) Platz-Quetschwunden.

a) Druckanämie

Wird die Haut zu Lebzeiten von einer großflächigen Gewalt — und nicht sehr kräftig —, z. B. durch einen Schlag mit der Hand auf die Wange, getroffen, bleibt ein blasser anämischer Bezirk zurück, der später von einer reaktiven Hyperämie umgrenzt ist. Wird ein Kind mit einem stabförmigen Gegenstand (Rohrstock) geschlagen, zeichnet sich auch hier eine blasse, streifige Zone deutlich ab, die, je nach Intensität der Gewalteinwirkung, von einer reaktiven Hyperämie umrahmt ist: sog. Doppelstreifen nach Schlagwirkung.

Nach dem Tode sind anämische Druckstellen im Bereich der Hypostase so lange zu setzen als nicht Diffusionstotenflecke vorliegen. Außerhalb der Hypostase werden sich anämische Druckstellen dort abzeichnen, wo ein relativ harter Gegenstand den Körper komprimiert. Kleidungsstücke, gewisse Dinge, die in der Kleidung stecken, der Tascheninhalt, Waffen oder Möbelstücke etc. Diese anämischen Druckstellen sind von kriminalistischer Bedeutung, besonders für die Rekonstruktion eines Tatherganges oder — besser gesagt — zur Beurteilung der Fundsituation. Sicher ist es nicht leicht, zwischen vitalen und postmortalen, anämischen Druckstellen zu differenzieren. Makroskopisch fehlt bei den postmortalen Druckeinwirkungen die reaktive Hyperämie, die aber auch nach dem Tode abblassen konnte. Im Bereich der Livores sind Entscheidungen kaum möglich. Postmortal gesetzte Druckmarken vertrocknen wegen der Flüssigkeitsverarmung des Gewebes rascher. Mikroskopisch sind die Epithelzellen abgeplattet, die Capillaren blutleer, zusammengedrückt.

b) Hautblutungen

Nach Einwirkung von stumpfer Gewalt kann die Epithelschicht zwar unversehrt bleiben, jedoch bersten Capillaren in den tiefen Hautschichten. Für die Ausbildung einer Gewebsblutung ist nicht allein die Kontinuitätstrennung der

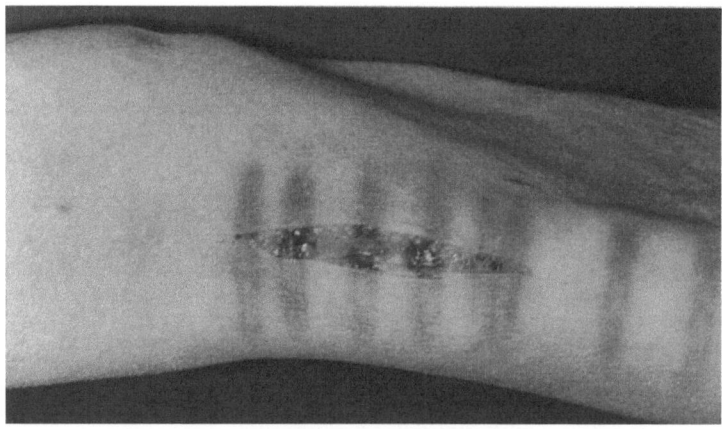

Abb. 17. Postmortale Hautblutungen in Abständen von 15—20 min ausgelöst. Doppelstreifen nach Schlag mit einem Messerrücken

Gefäßwand, sondern auch der in den Gefäßen herrschende Blutdruck entscheidend. Deshalb sind Gewebsblutungen bei nach dem Tode gesetzten Capillarverletzungen nicht zu erwarten. Sind die Capillaren, besonders auch die venösen Schenkel, in der ersten Zeit noch blutgefüllt, wird selbst *nach* dem Tode Blut ins Gewebe austreten (s. Abb. 3). Physikalische Vorgänge steuern die Blutung, deshalb sind sie auch mit dem Messer von der eingeschnittenen Gewebsfläche auszustreichen. Daß man selbst Stunden nach dem Tode noch Blutungen in der Haut hervorrufen kann, beweisen Versuche bei der Auslösung des idiomuskulären Wulstes (DOTZAUER). Damit wird deutlich, wie schwer es für den Gutachter ist, bei gewissen Problemen Stellung zu nehmen. Beim Überfahren durch Auto, Eisenbahn etc. wird z.B. ein auf Schienen liegender Toter versehrt. Es könnten in der ersten Zeit nach dem Tode noch ausgedehnte, von vitalen Blutungen schwer zu differenzierende, Gewebsveränderungen gesehen werden.

Ferner haben wir die punktförmigen, nur auf die Livores beschränkten, Hautunterblutungen zu berücksichtigen. Der Schwere nach hat die in den Capillaren absinkende Blutsäule die Gefäßwandungen zum Bersten gebracht.

Da diese Blutungen bereits wenige Stunden nach dem Tode eintreten können, werden sie bei Umlagerung der Leiche im Gegensatz zu den noch umlagerungsfähigen Livores nicht verschwinden.

Blutungen in die Haut oder in das Unterhautfettgewebe sind nicht als sichere, vitale Zeichen zu werten, besonders dann nicht, wenn die Gewalteinwirkung im Bereich der Hypostase lag.

c) Hautabschürfungen

Bei zentripetaler, erheblicher Traumatisierung werden Quetschungen, bei tangentialer Abschürfungen des Epithels bewirkt. Ob vital oder postmortal, der Epithelverlust führt später immer zu einer makroskopisch kaum voneinander zu unterscheidenden Vertrocknung der freigelegten Haut. Diese wird pergamentartig hart, rötlichbraun. Wird eine Leiche im Freien abgelegt, liegt der Körper auf Ästen, entstehen Marken, die sich für das bloße Auge von vital gesetzten kaum zu unterscheiden brauchen. Siehe hierzu die demonstrativen Versuche von PROKOP. Daß Strangfurchen erst entstehen, wenn eine Leiche erhängt wird, ist vielfach erwiesen.

Die vital gesetzte und bis in den Papillarkörper reichende Hautabschürfung läßt bei gewisser Überlebenszeit Blut, wie Gewebsflüssigkeit austreten, die je nach Intensität der Blutbeimengungen hellgelb bis braunrot gefärbt sein kann. Die Wundfläche bedeckt sich mit einer Borke als Ausdruck der vitalen Reaktion. Postmortal wird im Bereich der Livores u.U. auch Blut aussickern; die vertrocknete Excoriation ist außerhalb der Totenflecke heller getönt. Bei der mikroskopischen Untersuchung zeigt die vitale, stumpfe Hautverletzung folgendes Substrat:

Bei einer bestimmten Schwere kann es zur Sofortnekrose der Epidermis kommen. Man sieht daneben eine Trübung und Acidophilie — nach MALLORY orange-rot bis rot — des Protoplasmas als erste Phase einer Coagulationsnekrose. Bei Soforttod des Individuums werden sich Plasma- und Kernveränderungen nicht ausbilden. Eine weitere Schwierigkeit liegt darin, daß postmortale Vertrocknungen zarte, initiale, vitale Reaktionen überdecken. Wir achten deshalb mehr auf die Veränderungen des Bindegewebes im Corium. Bei frischen Hautverletzungen sieht man zwar bei der HE-Färbung im Bindegewebe keine Auffälligkeiten. Bei Einsatz empfindlicher, poli- oder metachromatischer Tingierungen, z.B. nach MALLORY, sind traumatisierte Bindegewebsbündel lebhaft carminrot, ungeschädigte kobaltblau gefärbt. Die Muskulatur, Nerven, Drüsen, Lymphknoten und Fettgewebe zeigen nach stumpfer Gewalt ähnliche Metachromasien.

Leider erzeugt nicht nur ein vitales Trauma, sondern ebenfalls eine postmortale Vertrocknung denselben Effekt. Die vitale läßt sich jedoch von der postmortalen Metachromasie differenzieren, da letztere nach Verbringen eines Hautstückes in Wasser spurlos verschwindet, während die nach vitalen Verletzungen zustande gekommenen Metachromasien, trotz des Wässerns der Haut, erhalten bleiben.

Heutzutage werden histochemische Untersuchungen eingesetzt. Wir werden im Abschnitt der thermischen, elektrischen Verletzungen näher darauf eingehen.

Vielleicht nur der Hinweis, daß die Haut infolge Pioch sofort, nach zunächst überlebter, stumpfer Gewalteinwirkung eine gesteigerte Fermentaktivität zeigt. Leider sind die schönen, experimentellen, histochemischen Befunde in praxi kaum anwendbar. Empfindliche, histochemische Veränderungen der lädierten Gewebe werden sehr rasch durch nekrochemische Einflüsse und Vertrocknungserscheinungen verändert. Im Gegensatz zu Ergebnissen bei Tierversuchen sind die Befunde anläßlich einer vielleicht Tage nach dem Tode vorgenommenen Leichenöffnung, damit auch nach einem interessierenden Ereignis, wegen der zwischenzeitlichen Veränderungen nicht optimal. Deshalb besitzen auch heute die klassischen mikro- und makroskopischen Untersuchungen ihren großen Aussagewert, z.B. das Problem der initialen Wundheilung von Epidermisverletzungen. H. Bekker sah nach 2 Std an den Schürfstellen bereits eine leukocytäre Reaktion, Emigration von Leukocyten. Dem geht eine Leukostase, die schon nach 20—30 min zu erkennen ist, voraus. Die leukocytäre Reaktion steigert sich bis zur 16. Stunde nach der Verletzung, um dann langsam abzuklingen. Die Epithelregeneration setzt nach 24 Std ein. Sie geht von den angrenzenden Epithelrändern aus, z.T. aber auch von den Ausführungsgängen der Haartalgdrüsen und von erhaltengebliebenen oder in die Haut eingepreßten Epithelinseln. Nach 36—48 Std ist die Epitheldecke wieder geschlossen, nach 4 Tagen bilden sich neue Papillen. Man könnte vorhalten, daß diese Fälle von ausgesprochenen Wundheilungen kaum kriminalistisch von Bedeutung wären. Wir benutzen jene mikroskopischen Befunde zur Abklärung der Überlebenszeit. Diese ist für die Rekonstruktion eines Tatherganges und für die Festlegung des Todeszeitpunktes (zivilrechtliche Fragen über den Todeseintritt bei gleichzeitig verunglückten Angehörigen), von Bedeutung.

Die bei der Erhängung am Halse entstehende Strangmarke ist die, durch stumpfe Gewalt bewirkte, Epithelläsion, sie setzt eine Vertrocknungszone. Es ist leicht, die Leiche eines Getöteten, z.B. nach Vergiftung nachträglich zu erhängen, um Selbstmord vorzutäuschen. Strangfurchen werden am Lebenden wie an der Leiche zu sehen sein, deshalb lautet die obligatorische Frage: welche Anhaltspunkte haben wir für den vitalen oder postmortalen Ursprung. Die Erhängungstodesfälle stehen in der Rangliste der Selbstmorde beim männlichen Geschlecht z.B. an 1. Stelle. Aus diesem Grunde werden wir bei der Abhandlung der Hautabschürfungen die Strangmarken ausführlicher besprechen.

1896 beschrieb R. Schulz folgende Unterscheidungsmerkmale vitaler bzw. postmortaler Strangulationen:

1. Durch den Strangdruck erfolgte *Formveränderung* läßt intravital oder postmortal entstandene Strangulationen nicht differenzieren.

2. Aufgrund des Druckes des Strangulationswerkzeuges auf die Haut wird diese lederartig umgewandelt.

3. Makroskopisch erkennbare (Unterhaut) Blutungen des Unterhautzellgewebes schließen eine postmortale Strangulation nicht aus.

4. Für ein vitales Geschehen spricht eine anämische Zone im Bereich der Strangmarke.

5. Größere Blutungen in der Umgebung der Strangfurche weisen häufig auf ein vitales Entstehen.

Skrzeczka unterstellt, daß eine mumifizierte Strangmarke nur nach einer *Excoriation* entstehen kann. Liegen Kleidungsstücke um den Hals, kann die Strangmarke schwerer oder kaum erkannt werden. Neben die Excoriation tritt noch die *Druckeinwirkung*, die zur Hautvertrocknung führt (Hofmann). Dittrich läßt allein den Druck als ursächlich gelten.

Letztlich sind entscheidend: Art des Strangwerkzeuges, Lage des Körpers und dessen Gewicht in der Schlinge sowie die Hangzeit.

SCHULZ hat die zwischen zwei Strangulationsfurchen eingeklemmte Haut untersucht. Dieser Zwischenkamm entsteht sowohl vital als auch postmortal. Vital soll die Blutmenge im Zwischenkamm größer sein, die Capillaren sind bis in den Papillarkörper hinein prall mit Blut gefüllt. Ferner käme es zu einer Blasenbildung an der Grenze zwischen Cutis und Epidermis. Der flüssige Blaseninhalt sei eiweißhaltig, durch Hämoglobin und Fetttröpfchen angereichert. Die Blasen seien aber nicht als vitale Zeichen beweisend. SCHULZ bekennt, daß sich die durch Strangdruck hervorgerufene Formveränderung der einzelnen Hautschichten sowohl vital als postmortal gleichen. Dagegen meinen KAPACINSKY und BESJEDKIN, über eine trübe Schwellung der Retezellen einen vitalen Befund vorlegen zu können. SCHULZ lehnt diese Bewertung ab.

Mikroskopisch ist die Cutis nach Ansicht von SCHULZ häufig verschmälert. Die Phasen sind parallel zur Oberfläche ausgerichtet. Durch Druck seien die Fettgewebszellen häufig geplatzt. ROER und KOOPMANN haben speziell die Blutungen innerhalb der Strangmarke befundet.

Die Metachromasie der Cutis mit ihren quantitativ großen Abweichungen wurde vielfach diskutiert.

LIMAN, BREMME, LESSER, HOFMANN-HABERDA halten es für unmöglich, aus dem histologischen Befund die vitalen von den postmortalen Strangmarken zu unterscheiden. *Positiv* dagegen äußern sich SCHULZ, THOMA, WALCHER, NEUGEBAUER und BLUM. Ebenfalls ANREPP und OBOLONSKY, KRATTER, ORSÓS und TIEMKE. ORSÓS hat ferner auf gewisse Veränderungen im subcutanen Fettgewebe hingewiesen. Er glaubt, in der Emulgierung des Fettes einen Hinweis für die Bewertung vorlegen zu können.

In jüngster Zeit haben die verfeinerten Methoden Fortschritte gebracht. FAZEKAS und VIRAGOS-KIS untersuchten den Histamingehalt der Haut in vitalen und postmortalen Erhängungsfurchen (40 Strangulationssuicide, 10 postmortale Erhängungen). Der Histamingehalt der Strangfurche wurde mit dem der umgebenden intakten Haut verglichen.

1. Der Gesamthistamingehalt der *vitalen Erhängungsfurche* und der intakten Halshaut derselben Leiche ist gleich groß (im Mittel 15 μg/g).

2. Der Gehalt der *vitalen Erhängungsfurche* an freiem Histamin war stets wesentlich größer (im Mittel 13,5 μg/g) als der freie Histamingehalt der intakten Halshaut derselben Leiche (im Mittel 3,6 μg/g).

3. Der freie Histamingehalt der vitalen Erhängungsfurche machte im Mittel 90% und das freie Histamin in der intakten Halshaut 24% des gesamten Histamins aus, d.h. die Erhängungsfurche enthielt um 66% mehr freies Histamin als die intakte Halshaut.

4. Wenn man das freie Histamin der intakten Halshaut als 100% betrachtet, so erwies sich der Gehalt an freiem Histamin in der Erhängungsfurche im Mittel um 275% höher.

5. Der Gesamthistamingehalt der *postmortalen Erhängungsfurche* und der intakten Haut bei ein und derselben Leiche war stets der gleiche (im Mittel 12,2 μg/g); identisch war aber auch der Gehalt an freiem Histamin in der postmortalen Erhängungsfurche der intakten Halshaut der gleichen Leiche (im Mittel 3,6 μg/g). Dies bedeutet, daß in der postmortalen Erhängungsfurche eine Histaminfreisetzung nicht stattgefunden hat.

6. Demnach kann aufgrund des wesentlich größeren Gehaltes an freiem Histamin bei der *vitalen Erhängungsfurche* — gegenüber dem in der intakten Halshaut — die im Leben vorgenommene Erhängung, von der nach dem Tode erfolgten, gut

unterschieden werden, d.h. das Plus an freiem Histamin in der durch Lebenderhängen verursachten Erhängungsfurche kann als neue vitale Reaktion betrachtet werden. So FAZEKAS 1965; 1967 kommt er aufgrund neuerer Ergebnisse zu folgendem: „In Anbetracht dessen, daß der Gehalt an freiem Histamin von der 30. postmortalen Stunde an zunimmt, kann ein Gutachten bezüglich der Frage, ob eine Erhängungsfurche in vivo entstanden ist, nur aufgrund des Vergleiches mit dem Gehalt im freien Histamin in der erwähnten Halshaut abgegeben werden." Alles ist in Fluß.

ST. BERG hat diese Untersuchungsmethode auch bei anderen Verletzungen durch stumpfe Gewalt eingesetzt und ist zu ähnlichen Ergebnissen wie FAZEKAS gekommen. Diese Befunde an *Platz- wie Quetschwunden* leiten zu dem nächsten Problem über. Im Moment des plötzlichen, natürlichen Todes kann der Körper, wie gefällt, zusammenstürzen, auf eine harte Fläche aufschlagen. Hautabschürfungen und Platz- wie Quetschwunden entstehen. Bei einem Sturz auf den Schädel werden u. U. auch Schädelbrüche gesetzt, selbst Hirnquetschungen treten ein. Wird die Ursache des Zusammensturzes, d.h. des vorangegangenen natürlichen Todes, nicht durch eine Obduktion entdeckt, ist aus den postmortalen Haut- bzw. den weiteren Verletzungen auf gewaltsamen Tod rückzuschließen.

Agonale Sturzverletzungen der Haut treten an charakteristischen Stellen auf. Man sieht sie über der Stirn, dem Nasenrücken, weniger über den Scheitelhöckern, dagegen häufiger wieder im Bereich des Hinterhauptes. Etwa 60% schlagen mit dem Gesichtsschädel, der Rest mit dem Hinterhaupt auf.

Für das Entstehen von Platzwunden und damit verbunden auch deren Größe ist nicht allein die auftreffende Gewalt entscheidend, sondern die Frage, ob Haut unmittelbar dem Knochen aufliegt bzw. ob vorspringende Knochenanteile die Entstehung einer Platzwunde auch am Lebenden wie an der Leiche begünstigen: Augenbrauen, Schienbeinkante. Das Vorkommen einer Platzwunde hängt also nicht nur von der physikalischen Beschaffenheit der Körperoberfläche ab; selbstverständlich wird man die in jüngster Zeit von WEINIG und ZINK publizierten Feststellungen über die regionalen Festigkeitsunterschiede der menschlichen Haut berücksichtigen. Ähnliche Daten waren früher schon von RAUBER-KOPSCH niedergelegt; in praxi sind sie aber wenig brauchbar, weil das Vorkommen einer Hautwunde von der Oberflächengestalt des Werkzeuges und der Gewalt, weiter vom Widerlager (Knochen oder Muskulatur) der betreffenden Hautpartie und weniger — gewiß nicht signifikant — von der Festigkeit der Haut abhängt.

Die Kopfschwarte ist derb und trotzdem sehen wir häufiger Platzwunden wegen der knöchernen Unterlage. Die Formen der Wunden, Wundrand wie Wundgrund unterscheiden sich nicht, gleich, ob kurz vor dem Tode — agonal oder postmortal — entstanden. Bei Absinken des Blutdrucks in der Agone fehlen zwar Blutungen in dieser Umgebung bzw. sie sind nur gering ausgebildet; von entscheidender Bedeutung ist jedoch das Fehlen eines kollateralen Ödems in der Wundumgebung.

3. Stich-, Schnitt- und Hiebverletzungen an der Leichenhaut

Im vorigen Jahrhundert war der Mensch bei der Todesfeststellung verunsichert. Er wollte sich davor schützen, etwa im Zustande eines Scheintodes, eingesargt oder gar begraben zu werden. Deshalb wurde in letzten Verfügungen niedergelegt, daß die Pulsadern bzw. die Herzkammern geöffnet werden sollten. Selbst in heutiger Zeit wird diese Aufgabe gelegentlich dem Arzt gestellt. Kann man solche Verletzungen von vitalen unterscheiden?

Einige Beispiele zeigen die Problematik: Eine Frau wird erwürgt, der Körper anschließend mit Stichen bedeckt, Geschlechtsteile oder Brüste verletzt. — Ein Mensch stirbt eines natürlichen Todes und fällt dann in eine den Körper zerfetzende Maschine. — Ein führerlos gewordener Pkw rast gegen eine Mauer, Gesichts- und Halshaut werden durch splitterndes Glas verletzt. — Bei einem Verkehrsopfer wird eine intrakardiale Injektion durchgeführt — beim Lebenden?

Man könnte das häufigste Beispiel nennen: Wurde eine Schnittverletzung zur Durchführung der intrathorakalen Herzmassage am Lebenden oder bereits Verstorbenen gesetzt. Es handelt sich nicht nur um ein Theoretisieren, sondern um schwerwiegende, folgenreiche Fragen. Bei einer Thorakotomie werden Herz oder Lunge verletzt, es blutet in Herzbeutel oder Pleurahöhlen; liegt im ärztlichen Eingriff letztlich die Todesursache?

Stich. Viele der zufälligen bzw. vorsätzlichen Verletzungen werden mit einem spitzen Werkzeug vorgenommen (Taschenmesser, Stilett, Mistgabel etc.). Stichverletzungen der Haut werfen schwerwiegende Fragen auf. Beispiele mögen dies erläutern:

Ein Täter berichtet, er hätte das Opfer nicht verletzt, vielmehr sei dieses während einer Rauferei in der Aufregung aus natürlicher Ursache plötzlich verstorben und nachträglich erst in das Instrument gefallen.

Oder: Vögel hacken mit ihren spitzen Schnäbeln verdächtige „Stichwunden" in die Haut der Wasserleiche.

Ein spezielles Problem wird gelegentlich angesprochen: Vitale oder postmortale Injektionsverletzung. Auf Wunsch der Angehörigen, vielfach auch routinemäßig, verabfolgen Ärzte bei einer Leichenschau Medikamente. Angehörige erheben gegen einen Arzt wegen Vernachlässigung Vorwürfe, sie meinen, der Arzt hätte wirksamere Mittel injizieren sollen, bzw. eine gehörige Wiederbelebung sei nicht vorgenommen worden. Man wird die Frage diskutieren, ob durch eine histologische Untersuchung des Injektionswundkanals die Entscheidung; ob vital oder postmortal, fällt.

Das andere Beispiel: Ein Erhängter zeigt nicht nur die typische Strangfurche, sondern auch eine Injektionsstelle. Tötung nach Verabfolgung einer Injektion, nachträgliche Erhängung zur Vortäuschung eines Selbstmordes? Handelt es sich etwa gar um eine tagelang zurückliegende Injektion?

Über die Altersbestimmung von Injektionen haben in den letzten Jahren BOLTZ wie SCHOLLMEYER gearbeitet. Tabellarisch faßte BOLTZ seine Befunde zusammen (s. Tab. 6).

SCHOLLMEYER bestätigte diese Ergebnisse.

Schnittwunden. Ein Rechtsanwalt wurde durch ein Schädeltrauma getötet, der Täter eröffnete die Pulsadern des Opfers zur Vortäuschung eines Selbstmords. Postmortale Hautschnittwunden werden bei der Leichenzerstückelung gesehen. Besonders in Großstädten werden zur Beseitigung nicht selten Körperteile in Mülltonnen, auf Schuttablageplätzen, Abwässerkanäle gelegt. Die kriminelle Leichenzerstückelung ist ein typisches Großstadtdelikt. Eine Leiche ist schwierig zu beseitigen: der Täter versucht, den Körper zu zerkleinern, um ihn unauffällig aus der Wohnung transportieren zu können. Die Teile werden in der Stadt zerstreut: Gewässer, Park, Friedhof, Acker, Feld.

Sie werden gefunden: Handelt es sich um ein anatomisches Präparat (Formalinfixierung, Zeichen von Präparationsübungen) oder um ein Operationspräparat (Spuren von Nähten, Injektionen, Desinfektionsanstriche) oder Zustand nach Tötung eines Menschen? Werden mehrere Leichenteile geborgen, versucht man, sie zusammenzufügen. Welche Verletzungen sind vital gesetzt — gehören also zur Mordausführung, welche postmortal und sind der Zerstückelung der Leiche

Tabelle 6. *Altersbestimmung*

Zeit	Stichkanal	Zellige Infiltrate	Pfropf
0—4 Std	darstellbar klaffend	—	—
4—8 Std	—	in Entwicklung	in Entwicklung
8—16 Std	schließt sich	deutlich	deutlich
16—24 Std	meist geschlossen	deutlich	die Lücke verschließend, meist im Hautniveau
24—36 Std	geschlossen	deutlich	voll ausgebildet, das Hautniveau meist überragend
36—48 Std	geschlossen	deutlich	voll ausgebildet, das Hautniveau meist überragend
48—72 Std	geschlossen	in Rückbildung	voll ausgebildet, das Hautniveau meist überragend
72—96 Std	geschlossen	spärlich	in Ablösung
5. und 6. Tag	geschlossen	meist fehlend	abgestoßen

zuzuordnen? Für die Rekonstruktion des Tatherganges ist die Altersbestimmung der postmortalen Schnittwunden — sofort nach der Tat, nach Eintritt der Totenstarre, nach beginnender Fäulnis — von entscheidender Bedeutung. Eine Differenzierung von vitalen und postmortalen Schnittwunden ist meist schwierig, besonders dann, wenn die Wunden kurz nach dem Tode gesetzt werden. Der Täter möchte nicht überrascht werden, deshalb wird er sofort nach der Tötung tätig. Die Ränder vertrocknen sowohl an den vitalen als auch an den postmortalen Schnittwunden. Es fehlen Blutungen und Begleitödeme in der Umgebung postmortal gesetzter Hautwunden, wie sie z.B. bei Thorakotomieverletzungen am Lebenden entstehen. Die Ränder der Wunde sind glatt, postmortal bleibt die Retraktion der durchtrennten Gewebe weitgehend aus.

Hiebverletzungen. Postmortale Hautverletzungen durch Axt oder Beil sind selten. Es sei denn, daß es sich um Vorgänge anläßlich einer Leichenbeseitigung handelt. Andererseits wurde einmal über einen Fall berichtet, daß ein Mensch plötzlich verstarb und auf die Schneide eines Beils stürzte. Wichtig ist das Erkennen der sog. „Pseudo-Hiebwunde" der Haut. Hierunter verstehen wir eine, durch einen gebrochenen Knochen indirekt hervorgerufene, Hautkontinuitätsunterbrechung (Sturz vom Gerüst nach Coronartod). Ein eben Verstorbener stürzt auf den Schädel mit den Folgen von Biegungs- und Berstungsbrüchen. Die Kopfhaut wird dort, wo der Schädel gar nicht direkt traumatisiert wurde, durch Knochenscherben indirekt aufgerissen. Scharfrandige Hautdurchtrennungen ohne Hautabschürfungen entstehen; typisch für Beilhiebe. Diese eigenartigen Hautwunden lassen den Verdacht einer Tötung, eines erst nachträglichen Absturzes aufkommen. Ein Selbstmord oder Unfall sollte vorgetäuscht werden! Sind Kopfhaare, die bei einer Beilverletzung scharf durchschnitten wären, überhaupt

von Injektionsstichwunden nach BOLTZ

Schüssel	Obere Epidermis	Untere Epidermis	Definitive Epidermis
—	—	—	—
erster Beginn der Zellabstoßung	—	—	—
noch unvollständig, locker	—	—	—
voll ausgebildet, dicht, breit	im Beginn der Bildung	im Beginn der Bildung	—
	Spaltung der Epidermis in 2 Anteile		
wird in den Pfropf einbezogen	ausgebildet bis zu etwa $1/3$ der Oberfläche	vorgeschritten noch nicht ganz vollständig	—
im Pfropf gelegen, aufgelockert	ausgebildet, meist nur $1/2$ der Oberfläche bedeckend	vollständig	erste Anzeichen der Neubildung
im Pfropf gelegen, aufgelockert	ausgebildet, meist nur $1/2$ der Oberfläche bedeckend	vollständig	fortschreitendes Wachstum unvollständig, eingesunken
in Ablösung	ausgebildet, meist nur $1/2$ der Oberfläche bedeckend	in Ablösung	vollständig, noch wenig differenziert, eingesunken
abgestoßen	abgestoßen	abgestoßen	im Hautniveau, differenzierter, Papillenbildung

verletzt, ist die Knochenwunde durch ein schneidendes Werkzeug entstanden oder ist sie Teil eines Biegungs- bzw. Berstungsbruchsystems?

Die Retraktion der Wundränder wird vielfach als vitale Reaktion aufgefaßt. 1896 hat R. SCHULZ als Kriterium der vitalen Reaktion die Retraktion der Gewebe bezeichnet. Vielfach wurde dieser Befund jedoch überbewertet. Nach WALCHER und auch nach B. MUELLER hat die Retraktion, im Zusammenhang mit der Frage einer vitalen oder postmortalen Entstehung, kein allzu großes Gewicht. Die Haut des Lebenden steht zwar unter erheblicher Spannung. Diese ist abhängig von der betroffenen Körperregion und nicht überall gleich. Fernerhin hängt sie von der Körperhaltung im Augenblick einer Verletzung ab. Wundränder in der Kopf- bzw. Rückenhaut retrahieren sich in der Regel nur wenig: Feste Verhaftung einer derben Haut mit der Unterlage und damit eine geringe Retraktionsfähigkeit.

Das Klaffen kann aber auch Folge eines vital entstandenen Ödems sein.

Die Fäulnisgasblähung steigert die Spannung der Haut. Wird jetzt die Haut verletzt, retrahieren sich die Wundränder. Anschließend kollabiert die vorher überspannte Haut sobald die Verletzung beispielsweise die Bauchdecke völlig durchtrennte.

Nicht nur die Haut, sondern auch die Muskulatur, greifen in die Retraktion der Hautwunde ein. Die intravital verletzte Muskulatur besitzt eine erhebliche Retraktionsfähigkeit, die aber mit dem Tode nicht erloschen ist. Eine Beobachtung, wie man sie auch auf dem Schlachthof machen kann. Die totenstarre Muskulatur läßt die Retraktion verstärken, es ist verständlich, daß postmortal gesetzte Schnittwunden der Haut, besonders dann, wenn gleichzeitig Muskulatur durchtrennt wurde, klaffen können.

4. Schußverletzung

In juristischen Lehrbüchern, wie bei BINDING oder LISZT, wird folgendes Beispiel mit einer besonderen Problematik aufgeführt: Ein Mensch schießt durch das Fenster auf seinen im Bett liegenden Feind. Die Obduktion ergab nicht nur einen „tödlichen" Brustkorbdurchschuß, sondern auch eine Apoplexia cerebri. War der Mensch etwa vor der Schußverletzung aus natürlicher Ursache verstorben, war nur auf eine Leiche geschossen worden? Auch hier die Frage nach Abgrenzung von vital und postmortal. Handelte es sich um Mord oder um Leichenschändung?

Ein anderes Beispiel: Ein Wilderer wird auf der Flucht von einem Forstbeamten niedergeschossen. Die Einschußöffnung liegt am Rücken. Eine Notwehraktion schließt sich somit aus. Die Leiche wird umgedreht und von vorne beschossen.

Oder: Leichenveränderungen können „Schußverletzungen" vortäuschen. Die Haut wird von Maden schrotschußähnlich durchlöchert. Manchmal bleiben auch nur ein oder zwei größere, regelmäßig gestaltete, rundliche Hautdefekte durch Madenfraß zurück. Ist dieser Substanzverlust an den Rändern etwas vertrocknet, sind die Maden nicht mehr vorhanden, glaubt man, eine Schußwunde zu erkennen.

Aus vielerlei Gründen wird man bei der Abhandlung der Leichenveränderung der Haut auf Formen der Schußwunden eingehen müssen und sie postmortalen Verletzungen gegenüberstellen. Verallgemeinert wäre die Aussage: Ein Nahschuß mit Pulverschmaucheinsprengung wird mit Madenfraß kaum zu verwechseln sein, eher dagegen ein absoluter Nah- oder Fernschuß.

a) Fernschuß

In Abhängigkeit von Kaliber und Munition sprechen wir bei Fehlen von Pulverschmauchniederschlägen oder Folgen eines Explosionsgasdruckes auf die Körperoberfläche von einem Fernschuß. Lediglich das Projektil, als Ausdruck einer umschriebenen, stumpfen, sich um die eigene Achse drehenden Gewalt, wirkt sich aus. Je nach Kaliber kann ein Fernschuß bereits aus 0,5 m beginnen und bis über 1000 m abgegeben werden.

Bei Beschuß der Körperoberfläche und senkrecht auf die Haut gerichteter Waffe setzt der mit Brisanz eindringende Geschoßkopf einen rundlichen Hautdefekt, einen echten Substanzverlust. Die Ränder der Wunde sind nicht miteinander zu vereinigen. Am Defektrand findet sich ein ringförmiger Beschmutzungsring und eine Epithelabschürfung. Wie entsteht beides? Das Projektil erhält beim Durchgang eines gezogenen Laufes eine Rotation um seine Längsachse. Die Flugbahn des Geschosses wird hierdurch stabilisiert, unter anderem, um bei Tangierung des Projektils mit anderen Gegenständen nicht zu kippen. Die Haut wird zwischen Projektil und der mehr oder weniger elastischen Unterlage (Muskulatur, Fettgewebe, Knochen etc.) zermalmt. Im Gegensatz zu dem damit entstehenden Substanzverlust handelt es sich beim Ausschuß um eine Kontinuitätsunterbrechung mit Aufreißen der Haut bzw. Berstung von innen. Die Einschußöffnung erscheint wie durch ein Locheisen ausgestampft. Bei nicht deformiertem, nicht gekipptem Projektil ist der Substanzverlust wegen der Elastizität der Haut kleiner als der Umfang des Geschosses. Im Augenblick des Aufpralls komprimiert der Projektilkopf die Haut, stülpt sie gegen das Unterhautfettgewebe ein, das konische Ende der Geschoßspitze durchbohrt die Haut und zermalmt sie, die Keilwirkung des eindringenden, rotierenden Projektils schürft die eingestülpte Epidermis, läßt radiäre Einrisse in der Haut entstehen. Der Nachweis von Blut- und Gewebsteilen an der Tathand oder Waffe, speziell im Laufinnern, zeigt an, daß sich zudem Druckkräfte entgegen der Schußbahn auswirken (ausführliche

Literatur H. J. WAGNER). SELLIER hat mit einer Kamera (Bildfrequenz 70 000/sec) die einzelnen Phasen beobachtet. Die durch die Rotation des Projektils der Haut mitgeteilte, radiäre Bewegung, in Verbindung mit den gegensätzlichen Druckkräften, lassen den Wundrand später nach außen stülpen. Aus dem Spalt zwischen Projektil und Schußkanal spritzen radiär komprimierte Gewebsflüssigkeit und Partikel. Physikalische Kräfte kommen zum Ansetzen; man könnte meinen, daß sich die Befunde am Lebenden oder an der Leiche gleichen.

Das Projektil reinigt sich im Bereich des Kopfes durch Abstreifen der aufgelagerten Partikelchen, der sog. Schmutzring entsteht. Das Geschoß hat während des Durchgangs durch den Lauf Reste von Schmiere, Rostpartikelchen, Pulverschmauch, Abriebteile des Geschosses mitgenommen. Durchdringt das Projektil zunächst die Kleidung, fehlt ein Schmutzring an der Haut.

Der Kliniker hat in der Differenzierung einer Ein- und Ausschußöffnung Schwierigkeiten. Weshalb? Aus Wunden blutet es. Jede Blutung stört die Übersicht.

Der Schürfsaum ist beim Lebenden zwar genauso ausgeprägt, tritt später aber an der Leiche infolge Vertrocknung für das bloße Auge erst deutlich hervor.

Man orientiert sich an folgender Regel: Der Einschuß sei im allgemeinen kleiner als der Ausschuß. Dieses ist jedoch nur bedingt richtig.

Die feingewebliche Untersuchung wurde zur Differenzierung von Ein- gegen Ausschußöffnung eingesetzt. Die Basophile ist nach KRAULAND an der Einschußwunde wesentlich deutlicher als im Bereich des Ausschusses. KRAULAND führt dies auf die Hitzewirkung über dem Projektil zurück. MUELLER behandelte die Haut mit kalten und warmen Nadelstichen. Dabei stellte sich heraus, daß die Basophile sowohl Folge von Vertrocknung als auch die einer thermischen Wirkung sein kann. Deshalb ist die Sicherheit, auf histologischem Wege einen Ausschuß zu differenzieren, nicht gegeben. Gleiches gilt für die Ringblutung und den Nachweis von CO-Hb. Die Affinität des Blutfarbstoffes für CO erlischt nicht mit dem Leben.

b) Nahschuß (relativer Nahschuß)

Werden Haut oder Haare einer Flammenwirkung oder dem Pulverschmauchniederschlag ausgesetzt bzw. Pulverplättchen in die Haut eingesprengt, handelt es sich um einen Nahschuß. Versengung von weißlicher Färbung, Kräuselung der Haare werden gesehen. In der Umgebung der Einschußöffnung hat sich ein feiner, bläulicher oder graufarbener Pulverschmauch niedergeschlagen. Wird die Haut gereinigt, sieht man, eingespießt gewissermaßen als Sekundärgeschosse, unverbrannte Pulverplättchen. Bei einem Lebenden imponieren diese Einsprengungen als feinste Blutungen. Wenn sie dichter, z.B. bei Explosionen, liegen, ist die Haut bläulich verfärbt. Beim Nahschuß entstehen am Wundrand morphologisch faßbare Veränderungen, ähnlich wie bei thermischen Läsionen, und zwar in Abhängigkeit der Pulverart und -menge (BRENKER, BAER) sowie der Entfernung der Mündung vom Körper. PUGGER hat diesen sog. Brandsaum auf den Flammenkegel bezogen, der aus der Waffe schlägt. DITTRICH sah in der Hitzecoagulation eine Thrombosierung kleiner Hautgefäße. FRAENKEL bemerkte selbst bei pulverschwachen Geschossen Brandsäume. Bis auf das Stratum basale war die Haut zu Verlust gegangen. Die Kerne waren dicht geordnet, parallel zur Oberfläche gestellt. Sofort nach Beschuß waren diese Veränderungen der gleichen Haut nicht zu sehen. Zur Hitzeeinwirkung treten Vertrocknungserscheinungen, wodurch die Verbrennungsfolgen prägnanter hervortreten (FRAENKEL).

Auch hier keine Differenzierungsmöglichkeit zwischen vital und postmortal.

Neben dem Projektil, der Mündungsflamme, des Explosionsgasdruckes entströmt der Mündung sog. Pulverschmauch. Diese Explosionsbrandrückstände hinterlassen auf der Haut, unter gewissen Bedingungen auch unter der Haut, Spuren.

Darüber hinaus entdeckte WERKGARTEN an der Schußhand Pulverschmauchniederschläge, besonders zwischen Zeigefinger und Daumen (Schwimmhaut). Für die Differenzierung von Mord oder Selbstmord ist dieser Befund ausschlaggebend. Nicht nur bei älteren Trommelrevolvern, sondern auch bei modernen Waffen, wird ein Teil der Pulverrückstände in Schußrichtung, ein anderer aus der Kammeröffnung, auch in die Gegenrichtung abgestoßen. Vergleichsuntersuchungen zwischen der rechten und linken Hand führen u. U. dann nicht zu einer Aussage, weil Selbstmörder auch beidhändig die Waffe bei Schußabgabe fassen können.

Bei Ungeübten können unter dem Zurückgleiten des Schlittens zwischen Daumen und Zeigefinger der Tathand parallel ausgerichtete, strichförmige Hautverletzungen entstehen. Sie sind bei Überlebenden schwerer zu erkennen als an der Leiche mit ihren Vertrocknungserscheinungen. Über diesen Weg kann man, indirekt gewissermaßen, rückschließen, ob eine Schußwunde vital oder postmortal beigebracht wurde, aber auch, ob es sich um einen Suicid handelt.

SCHÖNTAG konnte im Pulverschmauch Eisen, Barium, Blei und Antimon nachweisen. Nur Antimon ist als einziges Element spezifisch und daher typisch für Pulverschmauch. Die anderen aufgeführten Metalle können auch durch andere Art und Weise auf die Haut gelangen. Der Einschuß wäre hierdurch festzulegen, aber das Problem, ob der Lebende oder eine Leiche beschossen wurde, bleibt ungeklärt.

Durch den Explosionsgasdruck werden verbrannte Pulverpartikel in die Umgebung der Einschußwunde gesprengt. Da diese zudem erhitzt sind, entstehen thermische Läsionen. Die Dichte der Einsprengung — ähnlich wie beim Pulverschmauchniederschlag — steht in Abhängigkeit von der Laufentfernung zur Haut. Viele Untersuchungen betreffen den Nachweis von Metallen oder Kleidungsstücken in der Wunde, am Rand bzw. im Schußkanal (BUTZ, FRITZ, GRONZI, MEYER, STRASSMANN u.a.). Gesicherte Feststellungen über das Problem des Einschusses sind hierdurch abzuleiten, jedoch nicht, ob vital oder postmortal entstanden.

c) Einschuß bei aufgesetzter Waffe (absoluter Nahschuß)

Unter diesen Voraussetzungen kann in Abhängigkeit von Waffe, verwendeter Munition und der besonderen Körperregion die Einschußöffnung sehr unterschiedlich gestaltet sein. Bei Aufsetzen der Mündung auf die bekleidete Haut, auf den Leib oder bei einem Weichteildurchschuß von Extremitäten, wird sich das Projektil einen ähnlichen Weg durch die Haut bahnen wie beim relativen Nahschuß oder bei Fernschüssen. Der Explosionsgasdruck, damit der Pulverschmauchniederschlag und der Transport unverbrannter Pulverpartikel, dringen im Gefolge des Projektils praktisch unmittelbar in die Einschußöffnung. Je nach Unterlage wird der Explosionsgasdruck eine höhlenartige Gewebsaufreißung bewirken, in dem die Nahschußzeichen nachzuweisen sind.

Sobald unter der Haut ein flacher Knochen liegt, also nicht zunächst eine Muskelschicht, stellt sich folgender Verletzungsmechanismus ein: Die Explosionsgase dringen, während das Projektil den Plattenknochen, z.B. Stirn- oder Schläfenbein, durchschlägt, in Bruchteilen von Zeiteinheiten in das lockere Unterhautfettgewebe, wodurch die Haut gewissermaßen blasenförmig in Richtung auf die Laufmündung vorgewölbt wird.

Sobald der Gasdruck größer als die Elastizität und Dehnungsfähigkeit des Gewebes wird, reißt die Haut strahlenförmig auf. Die Kontinuitätstrennungen können mit stumpfen, ja mit scharfen Einwirkungen verwechselt werden. Im

Zentrum der mehrstrahligen Wunde wird man als Ausdruck des Einschusses, nach dem Zusammenfügen der Wundränder, stets einen Substanzverlust finden. Beim Spreizen der Wunde sind in den Taschen bzw. dem Wundkanal Pulverschmauch etc. zu entdecken. Dieser schlägt sich selbst auf die Knochenhaut nieder bzw. imprägniert den Rand der knöchernen Wunde. Bei absolutem Nahschuß ist in diesen Fällen die Einschußverletzung wesentlich größer als die des Ausschusses.

Die Explosionshöhle sollte nicht durch unnötiges Hantieren mit Instrumenten wegen Gefahr künstlicher Verletzungen und Schmutzeinschleppung sondiert werden. Die Merkmale des absoluten Nahschusses — dazu gehören auch der CO-Hb-Nachweis in Blutungen der Wundhöhle und die thermische Schädigung — lassen keine Entscheidung zu, ob dieser Schuß den toten oder lebenden Organismus traf. Unter Verwendung kleinkalibriger Waffen, bei denen das Projektil lediglich durch Treibsatz angetrieben wird, selbst bei lang gelagerter Munition oder Aufbewahren im Feuchten — eingegrabene Patronen — kann die Explosionswirkung beim aufgesetzten Schuß fehlen.

Gelegentlich geben Stanzverletzungen Hinweise auf die Haltung, mit der eine bestimmte Waffe an den Körper geführt wurde. Wenn die Haut durch den Explosionsgasdruck blasenartig vorgewölbt wird, schlägt sie gegen die Mündungsfläche, wodurch sich eine Stanzfigur, eine Schürfung, bildet. An den dann vertrockneten Epitheldefekten erkennt man das naturgetreue Abbild der Waffenmündungsfläche (WERKGARTNER, LIEBEGOTT, HUBER).

d) Ausschußverletzungen

Das austretende Projektil wird sich nicht mehr um die eigene Achse drehen. Die Haut wird somit nur ausgestülpt. Bei Größerwerden des Geschoßdruckes platzt sie auf, das Projektil hat Berührung mit der dem Unterhautfettgewebe zugewandten Fläche und nicht mit der Hornschicht. Epithelabschürfungen an den Wundrändern der Ausschußöffnung fehlen. Die Aufreißung von innen bewirkt keinen Substanzverlust, die Wundränder lassen sich gehörig adaptieren. Wurden nur Weichteile durchschlagen, wird das Projektil mit großer Brisanz bei gestreckter Bahn einen relativ kleinen, evtl. sogar rundlichen, Ausschuß bewirken. Werden festere Gewebe — evtl. auch Knochen — durchschlagen, werden diese gewissermaßen durch das Projektil als Sekundärgeschosse mitgerissen, setzen eine großstrahlige Aufreißung. Hier fehlen Pulverschmauch, Pulverpartikel, thermische Läsionen, Epithelschürfungen. Cave! Auch hier können die Wundränder vertrocknen und einen Schürfsaum vortäuschen. Man möge die Haut 24 Std in Leitungswasser wässern, die bräunliche Vertrocknungszone verschwindet dann wieder.

Neuerdings kennen wir auch beim Ausschuß den sog. Dehnungssaum. Beim Vorwölben der Haut, unmittelbar vor dem Aufreißen, löst sich das Epithel ein wenig. Wegen der anschließenden Retraktion und Schrumpfung bleibt eine schmale Zone frei von Epithel. Eine breitere Epithelschürfung, in unterschiedlicher Form, kann sich auch am Ausschuß bilden, sobald das getroffene Hautstück einem harten Gegenstand aufliegt. Der Mensch lehnt sich gegen einen Baum oder eine Mauer bzw. trägt einen metallenen Gegenstand in der Tasche. Das Projektil schlägt die Haut beim Ausdringen aus dem Körper gegen das feste Widerlager mit den Folgen von Quetschung und oberflächlicher Schürfwunde, u. U. auch mit Abdruck eines Textilmusters.

Faustregeln aufzustellen ist immer gefährlich! Sie führen zu einer Verallgemeinerung. Dies gilt besonders für das Problem der Veränderung der Haut des Lebenden oder des Toten nach Schußverletzungen.

5. Verbrennung

Durch Auftropfen von heißem Siegellack wollte man als Zeichen des Noch-Lebens Rötung oder Blasenbildung hervorrufen. Diese früher häufig geübte Lebensprobe sollte einen Scheintod ausschließen. Bei schwerer Schlafmittelvergiftung mit Koma war die Reaktion bei einer Berliner Krankenschwester jedoch negativ.

Da die Sparflamme eines Bunsenbrenners an der Leichenhaut selbst Blasen hervorruft, die für das bloße Auge den vitalen völlig gleichen, erhebt sich die konkrete Frage nach einer Differenzierungsmöglichkeit.

Nach PIOCH stellen sich der Abklärung — vital oder postmortal — zwei physiologisch bedingte Hindernisse entgegen: ,,Das Auftreten supravitaler Veränderungen und das Fehlen oder eine unterschwellige Entwicklung von reaktiven intravitalen Veränderungen bei zu kurzer Zeitspanne zwischen Trauma und Tod." PIOCH fährt fort, daß sich kurze Zeit nach lokaler Verbrennung der Haut histochemisch faßbare Veränderungen an Bausteinen und Fermentgehalt des Gewebes einstellen, die als Ausdruck vitaler Ab- und Umbauvorgänge im Bereich der Läsion zu werten sind. Den Protein-Nachweisreaktionen kommt unter den histochemischen Methoden eine besondere Bedeutung für die Erkennung vitaler Frühveränderungen nach thermischer Schädigung zu.

Mit den angewandten Methoden stellt sich regelmäßig eine positive Zone dar, die den geschädigten Bezirk demarkiert. Die Ausbildung einer zweiten und dritten Reaktionszone mit zunehmender Überlebenszeit bietet ein zusätzliches Merkmal für die Altersbestimmung der Verbrennung. Es liegt nahe, diese Befunde mit der Tätigkeit proteolytischer Enzyme in Zusammenhang zu bringen, da in dem durch die positive Reaktion hervorgehobenen Bezirk eine Grenze verläuft, bis zu der die hitzecoagulierte Dermisnekrose durch Autolyse angreifbar ist (GREUER, 1962).

Der Glykogenschwund aus den Geweben scheint uns für die Anhangsgebilde der Haut nicht verwertbar, da Glykogen bereits kürzeste Zeit nach Todeseintritt abgebaut wird.

Wenn PIOCH die nach 30—45 min einsetzende Karyolyse, d. h. das Sichtbarwerden von Feulgen-positiven Partikeln in der Dermis, der Epidermis und den Zellen der Hautanhangsgebilde, als wichtige Befunderhebung eines Vitalschadens herausstellt, so handelt es sich hier um eine Spanne, die forensisch deshalb wichtig ist, weil das interessierende Intervall zwischen Schadensetzung und Tod bzw. weitergehender Schädigung zu groß ist.

Seit alters wird zur Beseitigung einer Leiche Feuer in Anspruch genommen. Nach Zimmerbrand findet sich eine angekohlte Leiche; hat der Mensch gelebt, als das Feuer ausbrach, war er hilflos, krank, rauchte er eine Zigarette, sengte diese das Bettzeug, war die Person betrunken, stand sie unter Einwirkung von Schlafmitteln, fiel deshalb die brennende Zigarette? Aus den Befunden der Haut kann man zu diesen Problemen keine bindenden Entscheidungen liefern. Nach einem Schwelbrand wird jedoch eine COHb-Untersuchung evtl. aus dem Blut der Beckengefäße, oder die Entdeckung einer Rußaspiration, des Verschluckens von Ruß, weiterhelfen.

Bei plötzlicher Konfrontierung mit einer Hitzewelle, z. B. bei Explosion, lassen sich von der Hitzewirkung ausgesparte ,,Krähenfüße" bzw. Stirnfalten verwerten.

Der Kliniker verweist auf das *Branderythem* als vitale Reaktion. Dieses wird bei Wärmeeinwirkung von 40—50° hervorgerufen. Die Rötung beruht auf Capillarektasien. Postmortal verschwindet das vitale Erythem nach Stunden, zumindest blaßt es ab. Gelegentlich aber kann man in der Peripherie lokaler Verbrennungsbezirke noch nach Stunden, wenn nicht Tagen, deutlich das randständige Erythem mit einer Gewebsschwellung erkennen. Vielfach laufen die Capillargebiete, sofern sie nicht in hypostatischen Bezirken liegen, aus. Wurde dagegen dieses Stadium eine längere Zeit überlebt, erscheint die Haut geschwollen und gerunzelt (HOF-MANN-HABERDA).

Blasen bilden sich nach Hitzeeinwirkung von 50—70°. Die Einwirkungsdauer ist weniger von Bedeutung als der rasche Temperaturanstieg. Vital aber auch postmortal bilden sich Blasen, über die SCHJERNIG 1884 bereits schrieb.

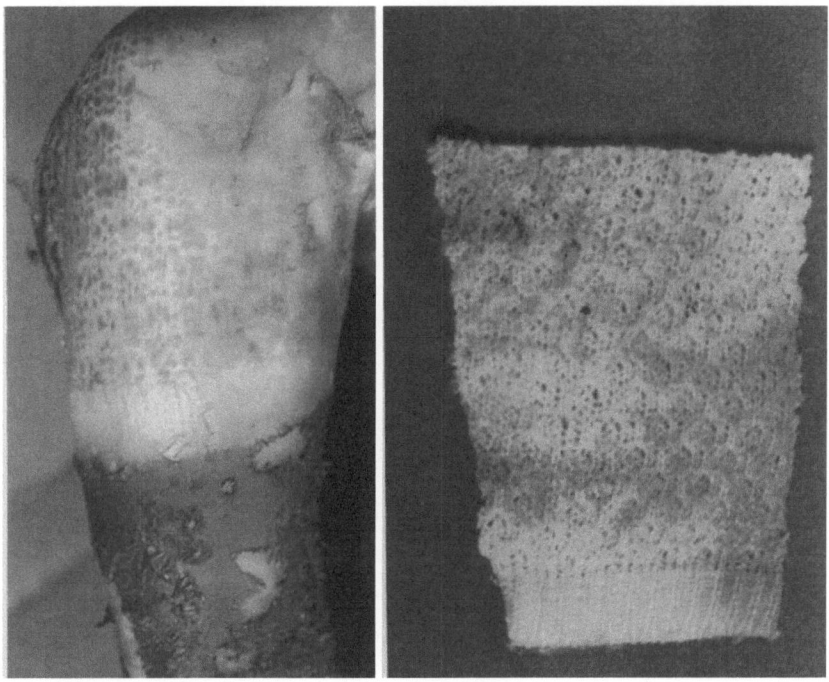

Abb. 18. Perakuter, tödlicher Verkehrsunfall. Postmortale Verbrennung der Haut durch strahlende Hitze. Die vom Kleid bedeckte Körperpartie — Oberarm — bleibt relativ unversehrt, nur Verbrennung den Maschenlöchern entsprechend (Musterung)

Bei vitalen Brandblasen ist das Exsudat eiweißreich, leukocytenhaltig, durch Fibrinabscheidung fast gelatinös. Postmortale Hautblasen enthalten nur eine seröse Flüssigkeit (SCHOLLMEYER).

Platzt die Blase z.B. auf äußeren Druck, vertrocknet die freigelegte Cutis, sie wird braun-rot, lederartig derb. Die im Corium deutlich hervortretenden Gefäße fallen durch die Vertrocknung auf. Bei postmortal entstandenen Brandblasen sollen sich injizierte Gefäße nicht so deutlich markieren. Aber auch hier ist letzten Endes die Tiefe der Läsion, eine etwaige Hitzecoagulierung des Gefäßinhaltes von Bedeutung. FALK irrt in der Annahme, das Blut schiene aus den Gefäßen verdrängt zu sein.

Liegt eine vital entstandene Brandblase später in der Zone der Livores, fällt die Entscheidung gegenüber Fäulnisblasen schwer. Da sich Fäulnisblasen selbst außerhalb von Totenflecken bilden, wird auch hier ein voreiliges Gutachten nicht abgegeben werden dürfen.

Eine Vertrocknung geplatzter Brandblasen innerhalb der Livores kann verständlicherweise ausbleiben.

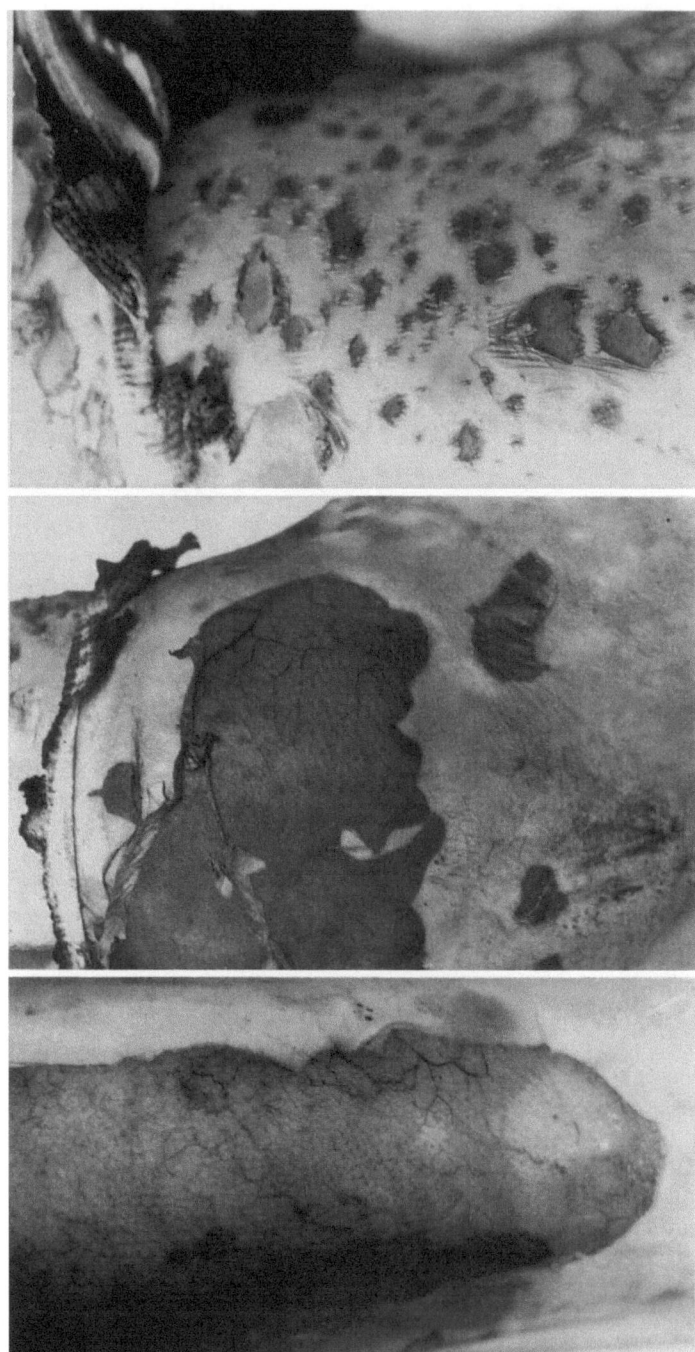

Abb. 19. Vitale Verbrennung. Oben: geplatzte Hautblasen. Mitte: ,,Thrombose'' der Hautcapillaren.
Unten: dasselbe in stärkerer Vergrößerung

SCHOLLMEYER hat vergleichende histologische Untersuchungen von Hautblasen nach Hitzeläsion bzw. nach Barbitursäurevergiftung angestellt. Bei Hitzeblasen sind die Zellen des Stratum germinativum stärker und deutlicher ausgezogen. Die roten Blutkörperchen wirken wie verklumpt. Basophile des Bindegewebes. Bei trockener stärkerer Hitze sind die Zellgrenzen kaum darstellbar. Kerne färben sich nur noch schwach an.

Bei flächenhafter Blasenbildung kann die Oberhaut handschuhförmig vom Corium gelöst werden.

Das Eiweiß der Haut wird bei Temperaturen über 65° gerinnen. Die Coagulate sehen wie gekocht aus. Die Haare sind gekräuselt, grauweißlich verfärbt,

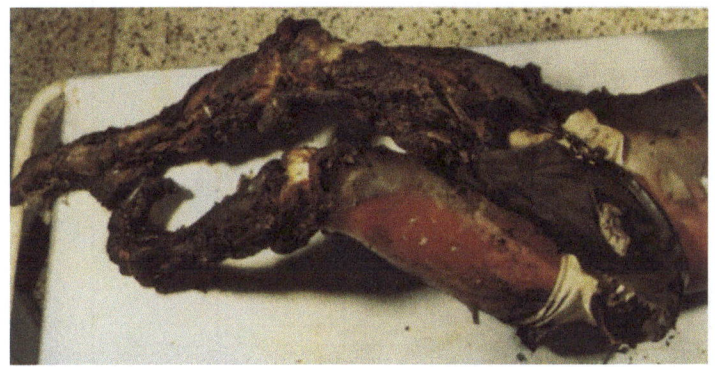

Abb. 20. Brandleiche. Einwirkung trockener Hitze zu Lebzeiten auf den linken Oberschenkel, postmortale Hitzekontraktion

die Spitzen erscheinen schwarz. Das Unterhautfettgewebe beginnt sich zu verflüssigen. Steigt die Temperatur auf etwa 140°, wird das verflüssigte Unterhautfettgewebe die Cutis zum Platzen, zum Bersten bringen, das auslaufende Fett den Brand unterhalten.

Bei ca. 400° tritt die sog. Carbonisierung ein. Ein Mitarbeiter GRÄFFs, KLAPPROTH, hat Untersuchungen zur Frage der fixierten Extremitätenversetzung bei Hitzeschrumpfleichen durchgeführt (Abb. 20). Für die Wärmekontraktur sind Hitzeeinwirkungen auf Sehnen, nicht auf die Muskeln, entscheidend; Ähnliches gilt für die sog. „Fechterstellung". Sehnen verkürzen sich unter steigender trockener Hitze durchschnittlich um maximal 61,5% ihrer ursprünglichen Länge. Die Verkürzung beginnt frühestens bei 50° C und endet spätestens bei 87° C. Die dabei freiwerdende Kraft beträgt 29 kg/cm². Letztere wiederum ist für die im Bereich der Wärmekontraktur auftretenden Platzwunden nach Verkochung des Unterhautfettgewebes verantwortlich zu machen.

In diesem Zusammenhang ist das Ergebnis jener Versuche einzufügen, das sich mit dem Problem beschäftigt, wie tief Hitze in die Haut dringt (Abb. 21).

Bei Carbonisierung der gesamten Körperoberfläche ist nicht zwischen einem evtl. kleinen vital und den sicher größeren portmortal verkohlten Hautarealen zu differenzieren. Bei einer zunächst überlebten, lokalen Carbonisierung werden Befunde vorgelegt werden können.

FÖRSTER schreibt, daß die im Grunde der Blasen noch sichtbaren Reste der Rete abgestorben und mit fädigem Fibrin durchsetzt wären. Dieses würde sich auch in den Blaseninhalt ausscheiden. Randständig wären die Zellen gequollen, Kerne noch erkennbar, aber blaß angefärbt. In den höheren Lagen sind Epithelzellen elongiert, z.T. gequollen, kernlos. Die von der Cutis abgehobenen, interpapillär gelegenen Zellen und abgeflachten Papillen sind vital, zellig infiltriert.

Aus einer Schorfbildung nach Verbrennung dritten Grades wird die Dermis-Nekrose nachzuweisen sein. Die Schorfe sind aschgrau, gelblich, braun oder mehr schwarz.

Zu einer Stase und Thrombosierung des Gefäßinhaltes kommt es beim dritten Grad der Verbrennung. Ähnliche oder gleiche Ergebnisse können wir aber auch dann erzielen, wenn die Haut in der ersten halben Stunde nach dem Tode von trockener Hitze getroffen wird. BERG sah am Rande der Läsion im ersten

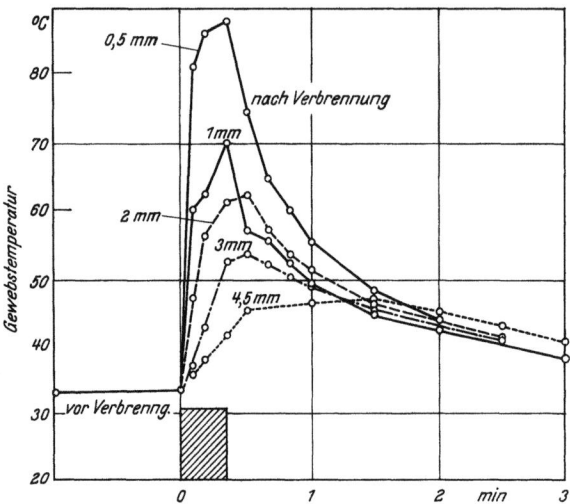

Abb. 21. Dampfapplikation von 20 sec Dauer auf rasierte Haut des Hundes, Gewebstemperaturen im Abstand von der Hautoberfläche und in Abhängigkeit von der Zeit. (PRICE, 1953)

oder zweiten Stadium nach Überlebenszeit von 3—4 Std eine Zone mit Zunahme der alkalischen wie sauren Phosphaten und der Aminopeptidasen. So interessant diese Befunde sind, sie bleiben für die meisten forensischen Problemstellungen letztlich ohne echte Aussage.

6. Verbrühung

Der Patient wurde durch einen Pfleger in eine Wanne warmen Wassers gelegt, heißes Wasser läuft nach. Er wird allein gelassen, nach einer gewissen Zeit tot, „wie gekocht" im Badewasser liegend, entdeckt. Angehörige erheben den Vorwurf einer fahrlässigen Tötung durch Verbrühung, der Angeklagte unterstellt einen natürlichen Tod mit postmortaler Verbrühung.

Aus der Klinik kennen wir das Bild der Verbrühungen, alle einzelnen Stadien. Bei feuchter Hitze werden die Haare nicht versengt. Ist der Körper bekleidet, wird er zunächst von der Flamme geschützt. Derartige Aussparungen finden wir bei der Verbrühung nicht, hier wird die Hitze durch die Kleidung gewissermaßen gespeichert, so daß bekleidete Körperpartien stärker als unbekleidete verändert sein können.

Die entscheidende Frage liegt, um auf den konkreten Fall zurückzukommen, darin, daß etwaige vitale Reaktionen durch postmortale Verbrühungen überdeckt bzw. verändert sein können. Handelt es sich zudem um einen Menschen mit schweren, seit Jahren bestehenden, organischen Erkrankungen, wird man zwar gutachtlich vorgelegte Fragen beantworten können; letzte Sicherheit ist jedoch nicht gegeben.

7. Verätzungen der Leichenhaut

Haut wie sichtbare Schleimhäute können zu Lebzeiten mit Säuren oder Laugen Kontakt bekommen. Es wird sich um Unfälle oder Suicide handeln. Wir denken aber auch an „Säurespritzen": Menschen, die aus sexueller Abartigkeit oder in einer Aggressionshandlung versuchen, anderen Säure ins Gesicht zu sprühen. Säuren z. B. gelangen direkt auf Haut und Schleimhäute oder — nach Erbrechen— indirekt auf die Körperoberfläche. — Wir stehen unter dem Eindruck, man müßte Säureeinwirkungen bei der Inspektion von Lippe, Zunge und Mundhöhle sehen; Coagulationsnekrosen sind zwar gelegentlich zu erkennen, aber nach Trinken von Säure erscheinen u. U. lediglich an den Lippen streifige Vertrocknungsbänder. Wurde erbrochen, fließt z. B. Mageninhalt über Kinn, Hals oder Brust ab, markiert sich die Abrinnstraße. In Abhängigkeit von der Länge der Überlebenszeit bilden sich oberflächliche Vertrocknungen, entstehen Nekrosen oder Säureschorfe.

Mechanische, vitale Hautläsionen oder selbst postmortale Vertrocknungen, besonders bei Neugeborenen, Säuglingen oder Kindern, an Lippen oder: das Erbrechen sauren Mageninhalts, rufen ähnliche Veränderungen hervor, wie sie bei kurzfristigen Säureeinwirkungen gesehen werden. Eine Verätzung des Lippenrotes z. B. kann vorgetäuscht werden. Es handelt sich differentialdiagnostisch um postmortale Vertrocknungen, u. U. auch um Vertrocknungen nach mechanischer Einwirkung.

Welche differentialdiagnostischen Feststellungen sind besonders bei relativ kurzer Überlebenszeit, nach Säureeinwirkung zu treffen ? Die Antwort gibt die vitale Reaktion des Gewebes. Wurde sogar bei der Sektion eine saure Erweichung des Magens gefunden, glaubte man, eine Bestätigung des Verdachtes anläßlich der Leichenschau vor sich zu haben. Entscheidend dabei bleiben die mikroskopischen und — selbstverständlich — auch ein Versuch der chemischen Untersuchungen. Vergessen wir nicht, daß ekzematöse Hautveränderungen, die später bräunlich eintrocknen, oder Insekten, besonders Ameisen-Benagungen der Leichenhaut, auch zu Fehldiagnosen führen.

Da saurer Mageninhalt gelegentlich aus den Mundwinkeln, besonders nach Wenden der Leiche oder nach Kompression des Oberleibes, vielleicht auch anläßlich eines Transportes, fließt, sich in der Umgebung des Mundes gelb-bräunliche Streifen bilden, werden diese leicht auf Salzsäure-Vergiftung bezogen.

Wenn die Oberbauchhaut in der späteren Leichenzeit handflächengroß, besonders bei kachektischen Personen, grau- bis gelb-bräunlich, fleckig verfärbt ist und man bei der Obduktion eine saure Erweichung des Magens mit Perforation findet, so daß Säure in die freie Bauchhöhle fließen konnte, werden differentialdiagnostische Überlegungen anzustellen sein.

Handelt es sich um einen eindeutig postmortalen Vorgang durch Magensäure oder um Säurevergiftung mit vitaler oder aber auch erst postmortaler Perforation ?

Da sich Säure- und Laugenwirkung in der ersten Leichenzeit deutlich markieren und bestimmte Befunde verwertbar sind, ist eine Entscheidung möglich.

Einwirkungen wie Schwefelsäure, zeichnen sich durch eine sehr rasche schmutzig-weiße, später infolge Oxydation grau-gelbliche bis grau-braune Hautnekrose aus.

Das Charakteristikum der durch Salpetersäure entstandenen Ätzschorfe liegt in ihrer gelblichen Farbe (Xanthoprotein). Nach Zusatz von Ammoniak nehmen die gelben Schorfe eine orange-rote Färbung an, letztere verschwindet nach Zusatz von Schwefel-Ammonium.

Weniger bei schwachen Lösungen als nach Anwendung konzentrierter Salzsäure zeigt die Haut Ätzschorfe; diese sind weiß bis grau-weißfarben, es bilden sich bei längerer Überlebenszeit deutliche Nekrosen und auch Geschwüre.

Auch Laugen verändern die Haut. Es entstehen zwar keine Coagulationen; deshalb sind die Laugenschorfe auch weniger fest, sie sind blaß-gelblich, vielfach transparent, weich bis zerfließlich. Säuren wie Laugen werden Anhangsgebilde der Haut verändern, vital entstehen Verschorfungen, die postmortal fehlen. In den Farbtönungen werden sich die vitalen von den postmortalen kaum differenzieren, sofern die Inspektion sehr rasch nach dem Tode vorgenommen wird.

Um eine Leiche zu beseitigen, versucht man nicht nur, sie zu zerkleinern oder zu zerstückeln, sondern legt sie in gelöschten Kalk oder in Säuren.

Nach ARNAL und MEHL ist eine völlige Zerstörung von Leichen im gelöschten Kalk nicht möglich. Im Falle WEISS wurde eine Leiche mit ungelöschtem Kalk bedeckt, die Weichteile wurden aufgelöst, die Knochen blieben jedoch erhalten. Schwefelsäure und Salzsäure bewirken eine partielle Zerstörung, speziell selbstverständlich der Haut; Salpetersäure und Königswasser sollen jedoch die Leichenteile völlig zerstören.

Experimentelle Untersuchungen liegen von OBOGLIO, CATTANEO und CARBONESCHI vor. Kaninchen sowie totgeborene, menschliche Früchte wurden in Schwefelsäure gelegt, teils nach Zerstückelung, d.h. Zerlegung der Körper. Hautstücke, Muskulatur, getrocknete oder frische Knochen, ferner ganze Gliedmaßen von Erwachsenen, wurden getestet. Um die Objekte völlig durch Schwefelsäure zu zerstören, sind different lange Einwirkungen nötig. Erhebliche Unterschiede, die vielleicht auf den Wassergehalt des Gewebes zu beziehen sind, ergeben sich. Auf die Dauer ist eine vollständige Zerstörung nur nach totaler Eintauchung der Objekte in Schwefelsäure zu erzielen.

8. Strom- und stromähnliche Veränderungen der Leichenhaut

Kann bewiesen werden, daß z.B. eine Strommarke vital oder erst postmortal entstanden ist? Dieses Problem ist, wie alle Läsionen der menschlichen Haut, nicht nur aus didaktischen Gründen anzusprechen, es handelt sich nicht um theoretische Überlegungen, sondern letztlich um Fragen des Beweiswertes bzw. der Grenze des Erkennens. Denken wir an fragliche Betriebsunfälle. Ein Arbeiter z.B. wird in der Nähe eines elektrisch betriebenen Gerätes tot aufgefunden. Arbeitskollegen halten einen Stromschlag bei ihrem Kollegen deshalb für das Nächstliegende, weil der Kollege zuvor ohne subjektive Beschwerden tätig war. Die Betriebsführung dagegen äußert Zweifel, sie vermutet einen plötzlichen Tod aus natürlicher Ursache.

Die Aufklärung dieses Todesfalles ist nicht einfach. Das Alter ist keinesfalls entscheidend. Selbst junge, scheinbar gesunde Personen, können infolge krankhafter Organveränderungen plötzlich versterben. Im Gegensatz dazu können Menschen in höherem Alter, die krank sind, effektiv wegen eines Stromschlages tot zusammenstürzen.

Gewisse Hautveränderungen werden von Arbeitskollegen bzw. Angehörigen aber auch Ärzten fälschlich als Zeichen eines Stromschlages aufgefaßt: Bläuliche Verfärbung der Gesichtshaut (Totenflecke!) oder bräunliche Eintrocknungen, z.B. an den Gliedmaßen (Hautabschürfungen).

Wir kennen Elektro-Todesfälle ohne makroskopische oder sogar mikroskopisch nachweisbare Strommarken. Das Vorkommen der Strommarke steht in Abhängigkeit zum Widerstand der Haut. Bei großflächigen Elektroden und/oder bei nasser Haut bzw. Kleidung bleiben die Strommarken aus. Andererseits ist das mikroskopische Bild einer „Strommarke", d.h. Elongation der Zellen mit Ausziehung der Zellkerne des Stratum germinativum, nicht auf Stromeinwirkungen alleine beschränkt. Früher war bereits bekannt, daß durch Hitzeeinwirkung gleiche

Veränderungen entstehen können. Es steht auch heute noch zur Diskussion, ob die Kernelongation der Strommarke eine spezifisch elektrobiologische bzw. elektromechanische oder nur die Folge einfacher Wärmeeinwirkung ist. Wie vorsichtig man urteilen muß, zeigen die Befunde von SCHÄFFNER an gefrorenen Hautstücken oder Vertrocknungen. Denn auch hier wurden Kernelongationen festgestellt. Den gleichen Effekt verursacht eine Verätzung der Haut. BÖHM versuchte mit Kongorot/Alcianblaufärbung zwischen Strom- und Wärmemarken zu unterscheiden. Zu einem tragbaren Ergebnis kam er nicht. Die an excidierten Leichenhautstücken erzeugten Strommarken mit differenter Stromfließzeit (0,5; 1,0; 1,5 sec) wiesen bei kurzer Fließzeit Marken entsprechend den Elektrodenrändern auf, diese fließen bei längerer Einwirkung zusammen.

Die Kernelongation beweist also keinesfalls die Stromeinwirkung. Man mußte andere Wege finden. Die Überlegung galt der Metallisation der Strommarke, d.h. der Inkrustation mit Metall, z.B. Kupfer, als Folge der Verdampfung des stromführenden Leiters. Positiver Metallnachweis im histologischen Präparat wurde bei einem zur Diskussion stehenden Betriebsunfall als entscheidender Beweis für die Stromeinwirkung anerkannt. Die neueren Untersuchungen von SCHÄFFNER, BÖHM, vermindern den Beweiswert der Metallisation. Minimale Spuren, z.B. von Kupfer oder Eisen, können bei irgendwelchen Tätigkeiten auf die Haut gelangen, die menschliche Körperoberfläche ist ein unterschiedlicher Metallträger. So genügt es z.B., die Haut mit einem rostigen Eisenstück zu berühren oder zu bestreichen. Dann findet sich auf der Hautoberfläche oder bei oberflächlicher Läsion, auch in der Randzone des Epitheldefektes, Metall. Solche Metallspuren bleiben tagelang in der Haut zurück. Beim Putzen eines Kupferkessels zeigt sich für eine positive Reaktion genügend Kupfer an der Hand. Durch die intakte Haut, auch durch die intakte Leichenhaut, kann Cu in das Gewebe getrieben werden.

Untersuchungen wurden mit Hilfe der von ADJUTANTIS und SKALOS benutzten Akroreaktion durchgeführt. Diese wurde durch FEIGL modifiziert. Man nimmt Filterpapierstreifen, schneidet sie spitz zu, taucht die Spitze in Rubianwasserstoffsäure und tupft damit die verdächtige Hautfläche ab. Bei Farbumschlag ins Grüne liefert diese Vorprobe den Hinweis auf Kupfer. Die Reaktion ist auch in histologischen Schnittpräparaten vorhanden. Nach SCHÄFFNER und BÖHM ist damit nicht entschieden, ob der Metallnachweis in der Haut als beweisend für eine Stromeinwirkung zu gelten hat. BOSCH ist jedoch der Meinung, daß der mit dem Lupenmikroskop sichtbare Schmelzeffekt und die Grünverfärbung der Hornschicht für Strom spezifisch seien. Es ist also nicht nur deshalb der Beweiswert einer Strommarke in Frage gestellt, weil die Kernelongationen sowie die Metallisation auch ohne Einwirkungen elektrischen Stromes entstehen können, sondern, weil nach jüngsten experimentellen Untersuchungen Strommarken auch an der Leichenhaut hervorzurufen sind. Ein Unterschied zwischen vitaler oder postmortaler Strommarke war nicht zu erkennen. Stirbt ein Mensch also plötzlich aus natürlicher Ursache und der Körper gerät nach dem Tode mit einem elektrischen Leiter in Berührung, entstehen Strommarken der Haut, aber: am untauglichen Objekt.

Wir ersehen daraus, wie problematisch die Feststellung des Elektrotodes ist, wie viele Möglichkeiten, Strommarken vorzutäuschen, existieren. Vertrocknungen an der Leichenhaut sind alltäglich. Hitzeeinwirkungen sind auch nicht selten. Abtropfendes Kerzenlicht, Verbrennungen durch einen glühenden Streichholzkopf; bei reger Reisetätigkeit und wegen der weiten Kommunikationswege ist es weiterhin durchaus vorstellbar, daß eine Leiche eingesargt wird und sich beim Verschweißen bzw. Verschließen des Sarges Hitzeeinwirkungen oder evtl. auch absprühendes Metall auf der Körperoberfläche niederschlagen. Der Sarg wird nach

Übersee gebracht, geöffnet. Man sieht jene Hautverletzungen: Kernelongation bzw. positiven Metallnachweis.

In diesem Zusammenhang sei auf eine Fehlbeurteilung aufmerksam gemacht. In histologischen Befunden von Probeexcisionen (vorwiegend der Haut, der Tonsillen oder Prostata) werden Zell- bzw. Kernveränderungen, jene „Unruhe", als Zeichen der Atypie oder der Malignität beschrieben. Es handelt sich um Veränderungen, wie man sie auch bei den Strommarken kennt. Fragt man nach, handelt es sich um Excisionen mit dem Thermokauter, einem Elektromesser. Oder: die Gewebsstücke wurden sofort in konzentrierte Fixationsflüssigkeiten, z.B. Alkohol, gegeben.

Wie wichtig die Differenzierung zwischen Strommarken und anderen Hautveränderungen ist, sei es, daß sie vital oder postmortal entstanden sind, wird ein Beispiel beleuchten: Ein Ehemann soll seine Frau mit einem Schal erdrosselt und nachträglich den toten Körper in den elektrischen Stromkreis eingeschaltet haben, um Selbstmord vorzutäuschen.

Aufgrund des Geschilderten könnte man annehmen, daß der Nachweis der Strommarke ohne jeden Beweis wäre. Das stimmt insofern nicht, als neben der Kernelongation und der Metallisation, die Wabenbildung, d.h. die wabige Auflockerung der Epidermis, von Bedeutung sein kann. Es handelt sich um die Folge von Verdampfung der Gewebsflüssigkeit. Das kommt nur bei erheblicher Hitzeeinwirkung, z.B. bei der umschriebenen Jouleschen Wärme (4000°C), vor. Bei anderen Hitzeeinwirkungen ist das unmöglich. Die klassische, histologische Untersuchung der Strommarke hat ihre Bedeutung nicht verloren.

Der Begriff Strommarke wurde von KRATTER für die pathologisch-anatomischen Veränderungen der Haut am Stromeintritts- bzw. Stromaustrittsort eingeführt. Der Begriff soll nur etwas über die Kontaktstellen der Haut mit dem elektrischen Leiter aussagen, nichts aber über Hergang und Verlauf der Verletzung.

JELLINEK, sein Schüler KAWAMURA und RIEHL, sahen in den Strommarken nur physikalisch-mechanische Auswirkungen des Stromes. Sie gaben eine büschelförmige Ausziehung der Retezellen an, wobei das Corium unverändert blieb. Mit der Frage, ob es sich bei der Strommarke um spezielle Stromwirkung oder nur um eine gewöhnliche Hitzeveränderung handelt, war im Laufe der Zeit eine große Diskussion entstanden (SCHRIDDE und BEEKMANN, MIREMENT, STRASSMANN, STRASSMANN und SCHMIDT, MUELLER wie SACHS). Mit einem glühenden Metalldraht konnten Kernelongationen erzeugt werden wie durch elektrischen Strom. Diese Reaktion wurde auf die Joulesche Wärme zurückgeführt. KOEPPEN und GERSTNER kamen nach umfangreichen Untersuchungen über die Wärmewirkungen an der Kontaktstelle des Leiters mit der Haut, in Abhängigkeit von Spannung, Zeit, Stromstärke und Wärmeversuchen mit entsprechenden Wärmemengen, zu dem Schluß, daß sich zwischen der gewöhnlichen Verbrennung und der Strommarke rein quantitative Unterschiede, nicht aber qualitative, zeigen. Die Strommarke ist daher nur eine isolierte, leichtere Form der Verbrennung durch Strom.

Makroskopische Befunde

Die Form der Strommarke steht in Abhängigkeit von der Kontaktfläche. Man kann u.U. das Abbild des stromführenden Leiters erkennen. Die Marke ist häufig grau-gelb, schmutzig- bis weißlich-grau, gelegentlich auch trübe stearinfarben. Im vielfach eingesunkenem Zentrum gelegentlich dunkelbraun verfärbt. MIREMENT weist auf die glänzende Beschaffenheit der Strommarke hin. Die lädierte Haut tastet sich häufig derb, manchmal fast pergamentartig. Die Peripherie kann leicht wallartig erhaben sein. Die Marken sind vielfach stecknadelkopfgroß und finden sich nur nach eingehender Untersuchung. Haare sind nach JELLINEK im Bereich der Strommarke nicht immer versengt. Doch sei durch Funkensprühung eine Kräuselung und Versengung möglich (STRASSMANN). Bei dicken Hornschichten soll es lediglich zur Verschiebung der Oberhaut kommen, evtl. zu Abhebungen und zur Zerstörung der Hornschicht mit Freilegung der Keimschichten des Coriums (SCHWARZ); oder es entsteht eine Verschorfung bzw. Verkohlung (STRASSMANN). Je nach Art des stromführenden Leiters kann es an den Kontaktstellen, z.B. Kupferdrahtleiter, eine grüne Verfärbung geben (JELLINEK). Jener von SCHWERDT publizierte Fall weist aus, vor welchen Schwierigkeiten ein Gutachter stehen kann.

Mikroskopische Befunde

1. *Epidermis.* Bei Schwachstromverletzungen sind Homogenisierungen und Quellungen möglich (SCHRIDDE wie SCHWARZ). Bei Haushaltsstrom- oder Starkstromeinwirkungen kommt es zur Verdampfung von Gewebsflüssigkeit und Lymphe, so daß das Bild optisch leerer Räume von wabigem oder spaltartigem Charakter entsteht. Die Hornschicht scheint aufgelockert zu sein (SCHRIDDE und BEEKMANN).

Basophilie. Das Stratum corneum kann sich vom Corium abheben (MUELLER, PIETRUSKY). Gelegentlich wird man bereits in diesem Stadium Verkohlungen der Epidermis sehen.

In den obersten Zellagen des Stratum germinativum sind die Kerne geschrumpft, die Umgebung aufgehellt (KLEIN, KOEPPEN und GERSTNER). Die Zellkerne können miteinander verklumpen und das Chromatin wie homogenisiert erscheinen (NIPPE). In den mittleren Hautschichten strecken sich Zellen und Zellkerne. Es entstehen stift- bzw. palisadenartige, z.T. regelrecht kernfadenbildende Ausziehungen (KAPLAN, PIETRUSKY, WEIMANN). In der Tiefe ordnen sich die Zellen und Kerne bürsten- oder wirbelförmig, z.T. auch haarbüschelartig (NIPPE). Nach PIETRUSKY entsteht eine spiralige Drehung. Die Kerne sind teils pyknotisch, dann auch wieder intensiver angefärbt (SCHWARZ, PIETRUSKY, KOEPPEN und GERSTNER). Nach längerer Stromeinwirkung kommt es zu blasiger Abhebung zwischen dem Stratum germinativum und der Lederhaut. Einzelne Keimzellschichten verbleiben auf der Lederhaut in Form von Inseln (STRASSMANN). Bei Starkstromeinwirkungen kann es zu totaler Zerstörung und Homogenisierung der einzelnen Zellschichten kommen. Das Gewebe zeigt eine starke Basophilie. Erwähnenswert ist, daß sich nach KLEIN wie WEIMANN die wabigen Hohlräume entlang der Schweißdrüsenausgänge gebildet haben. An den Ausziehungen und wirbelartigen Umlagerungen ist das Bindegewebe nicht beteiligt.

2. *Corium.* Das Bindegewebe unterliegt einer Schmelzung zu strukturlosen Bändern (SCHWARZ, SACHS, MUELLER, KOEPPEN). SCHRIDDE behauptet, es sähe verbacken oder verklumpt aus. Die Bindegewebsfasern lagern sich kompakt. Bei leichteren Formen kommt es zu einem ziehharmonikaartigen Zusammenschmoren der Fasern. Metachromasie sieht MIREMENT.

In letzter Zeit wurde an aus chirurgischem Material gewonnener menschlicher Haut und der Haut von weißen Ratten, mit verschiedenen histochemischen Färbemethoden, festgestellt, daß vom Rande zum Zentrum hin eine Depolymerisation der Proteine nachzuweisen ist. Ferner ergibt sich in den verlängerten Kernen abbaufähiges DNS und RNS. Eine gute Unterscheidung zwischen reaktiven und nichtreaktiven Regionen bei Strommarken hat sich ebenfalls ergeben. In einer anderen Arbeit wurde an Leichenhaut mit polarisationsoptischen Methoden die Strommarke untersucht. Dabei zeigte sich an den Strommarken bei kollagenen

Fasern intensive negative Doppelbrechung; an den unversehrten Hautstellen waren die Doppelbrechungen nicht festzustellen (G. SCHMIDT).

Über die Paralyse der Hautcapillaren, den sog. Blitzfiguren oder über das elektrische Hautödem, wurde nicht referiert, da es sich in der praktischen Fragestellung um vitale, nicht postmortale Vorgänge handelt.

9. Die postmortale percutane Resorption von Gasen

1795 wies ABERNETHY experimentell nach, daß die Haut die Fähigkeit besitzt, Kohlensäure abzugeben und Sauerstoff aus der atmosphärischen Luft aufzunehmen. FLEISCHER äußerte 1877, die Haut wäre für alle Substanzen, damit auch Gas, undurchlässig. SCHWENKENBECHER sprach sich um die Jahrhundertwende für eine Durchlässigkeit von fettlöslichen Substanzen und Gasen, jedoch nicht für Wasser und Elektrolyte, aus.

Jüngste Versuche mit radioaktiven Isotopen sicherten eine Permeabilität der menschlichen Haut auch für Wasser und Elektrolyte. Die percutane *Resorption* ist von physikalischen bzw. chemischen Eigenschaften der jeweiligen Substanzen und den strukturellen anatomischen Eigenschaften der Haut abhängig.

Ein anderer Weg führte über eine *Penetration* und zwar direkt durch die Epidermis und/oder über Haarfollikel bzw. über Schweißdrüsenausführungsgänge. Es wird angenommen, daß die Haut der Frauen leichter durchlässig als die der Männer, bzw. junger Menschen besser als die älterer, sei (BOURGET und ERNSTENE, VOLK, NADKARNI).

Bei akuten Entzündungen besteht gesteigerte, bei Sklerodermie und Myxödem eine verringerte percutane Resorption. Jeder äußere oder innere Vorgang, der den physiologischen Zustand der Haut ändert, wird sich auch auf die Permeabilität auswirken.

Die Penetration ist ein rein physikalischer Vorgang und spielt sich nicht nur an der excidierten, sondern auch an der Leichenhaut ab. Nach dem Tode kann die Haut Gase, Wasser, Elektrolyte, Halogene, Schwermetalle etc. aufnehmen.

Diese Feststellungen sind forensisch von entscheidender Bedeutung, sofern dadurch z.B. die Farbe der Totenflecke verändert bzw. chemische Befunde an excidierten Hautteilen beeinflußt wurden.

Kohlensäure. Bei Kohlensäurepartialdruck, der größer als im Gewebe ist, kann Kohlensäure von außen eindringen. Diese Bedingung wäre z.B. in einem Wein- bzw. Gärkeller erfüllt.

Sauerstoff. Nach ZUELZER wird die von der Haut aus der Luft aufgenommene Sauerstoffmenge mit 0,7 cm^3/100 cm^2 angesetzt. Innerhalb von 24 Std soll die Haut eines ruhenden Menschen bei 20°C 1,9 Liter Sauerstoff aufnehmen (GERLACH). Die in einer Sauerstoffatmosphäre percutan aufgenommene Sauerstoffmenge läßt eine Cyanose, die normalerweise nach venöser Stauung eines Armes auftritt, nicht entstehen. Diese Feststellungen der Hautphysiologen erklären die Reoxydation der zunächst dunkelblauvioletten Totenflecke (reduziertes Hämoglobin; Abb. 22). — Voraussetzung ist eine feuchte und kühle Umgebung. Die Livores nehmen als Folge einer postmortalen Sauerstoffpenetration wieder eine rötliche Farbe an. Somit kann eine Kohlenmonoxydvergiftung bei oberflächlicher Betrachtung vorgetäuscht werden. Man wird jeweils dort, wo Sauerstoff nicht an die Haut herantreten konnte, reduziertes Hämoglobin deutlich erkennen, am besten selbstverständlich im Bereich des Nagelbettes von Fingern und Zehen.

Kohlenmonoxyd. SALZMANN (1930), FLURY (1935) und BÜRGI (1942) erklärten, daß CO nicht von der Haut aufgenommen würde. Die sehr geringe Lipoidlöslichkeit wurde als Ursache genannt. Völlig anders äußert sich 1940 BREITENECKER: ,,Schließlich sei noch darauf hingewiesen, daß auch nach dem Tode CO durch die Leichenhaut in die oberflächlichen Hautblutadern aufgenommen werden kann, wodurch die Totenflecke hellrot werden. Da das Gas aber nicht tiefer als etwa 1 cm unter die Körperoberfläche eindringt, bleibt das tiefe Körperblut CO-frei."

Die Meinung wird vertreten, daß Blut in den oberflächlichen Hautgefäßen dann CO-Hb enthält, wenn der Mensch aus anderer Ursache verstarb und der Körper nachträglich in einen Schwelbrand geriet. Sicherlich spielen verschiedene Bedingungen eine Rolle; so die bekannte Temperaturabhängigkeit der Affinität,

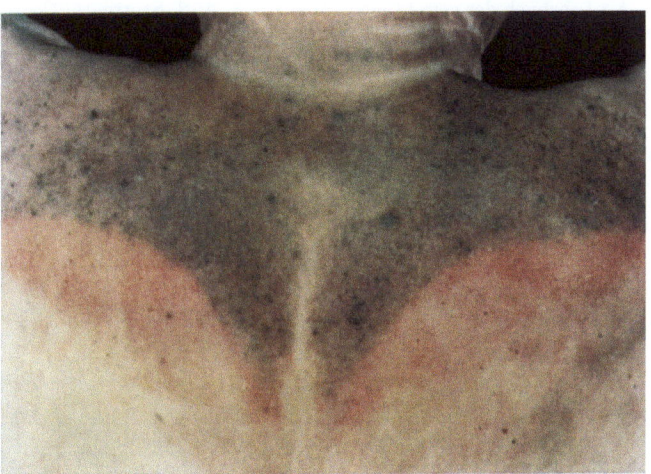

Abb. 22. Postmortale Rhexisblutungen im Bereich der Livores. *Reoxydationszone*

z. B. des Sauerstoffs oder des Kohlenmonoxydes, zum Hämoglobin. An der Leichenhaut sind Penetrationen von Gasen zu sehen, sofern der Blutfarbstoff in den Gefäßen der Leichenhaut verändert wird. Wir wissen um die Affinität des Hämoglobins, z.B. zum Sauerstoff, in Abhängigkeit von der Kälte; diese wird an der Leiche nur angesprochen, solange keine Fäulnis, keine Hämolyse besteht.

Cyan-Wasserstoff. Wird ein bestimmter Hautbezirk der Cyan-Wasserstoffkonzentration von 5—15 mg/Liter Luft ausgesetzt, sterben Meerschweinchen bereits nach 8 min, Hunde nach 47 min (WALTON und WITHERSPOON). Die Grenzkonzentrationen, innerhalb der noch keine Vergiftungserscheinungen auftraten, lagen nach SCHÜTZE bei Katzen bei 0,4% HCN in der der Haut angebotenen Luft. Bei Selbstversuchen und Angebot von 1—2% HCN an die Haut registrierte FLURY bald Intoxikationserscheinungen. Es ist nicht einzusehen, weshalb HCN nicht auch von der Leichenhaut resorbiert werden könnte; dies besonders bei Verletzungen oder an erkrankter Haut. Da der aktive Transport entfällt, handelt es sich um oberflächliche Vorgänge.

Die percutane Resorption von Schwefelwasserstoff, Tetrachlorkohlenstoff ist tierexperimentell, bzw. mit radioaktiven Substanzen, nachgewiesen. Postmortal dürften auch diese in die Haut eindringen. Ähnliches gilt für Flüssigkeiten, sofern sie lipoidlöslich sind. Wir kennen das Problem der percutanen Resorption z.B. von Benzin, Benzol, Alkohol etc. aus experimentellen Untersuchungen am Lebenden, z.B. von SCHULZ. Die percutan aufgenommenen Mengen bei medikamentöser Verabfolgung: Hautanstriche sind, bezogen auf den Gesamtkörper, unbedeutend. Früher waren diese Probleme deshalb von großer Bedeutung, weil wir z.B. Alkohol im Gewebe bzw. im Blute lediglich über das Mikrodestillationsverfahren als flüchtige, reduzierende Substanz bestimmten; heute haben wir das spezifische enzymatische Verfahren und daneben noch die Gaschromatographie. Deshalb ist z. Z. eine exakte Identifizierung, auch bei einer Blutentnahme aus oberflächlichen Hautgefäßen, möglich.

Literatur

I, 1. Algor

GRÄFF, S.: Tod im Luftangriff. Hamburg: Noelke 1955.
MUELLER, B.: Gerichtliche Medizin. Berlin-Göttingen-Heidelberg: Springer 1953.
PONSOLD, A.: Lehrbuch der gerichtlichen Medizin, 3. Aufl. Stuttgart: Georg Thieme 1967.
SEYDELER: Prag. Vjschr. 104, 138 (1869).

I, 3. Livores

BSCHOR, F.: Dtsch. Z. ges. gerichtl. Med. 55, 284 (1964).
HOFMANN-HABERDA: Lehrbuch der gerichtlichen Medizin, 11. Aufl. Wien: Urban & Schwarzenberg 1927.
MERKEL, H.: Allgemeine Pathologie, Bd. 33. München: J. F. Bergmann 1937. — MUELLER, B.: Dtsch. Z. ges. gerichtl. Med. 40, 999 (1951).
PONSOLD, A.: Lehrbuch der gerichtlichen Medizin, 3. Aufl. Stuttgart: Georg Thieme 1967.
RAUBER-KOPSCH: Lehrbuch und Atlas der Anatomie des Menschen, 14. Aufl. Stuttgart: Georg Thieme 1934—1936.
STICHNOTH, E.: Mschr. Ohrenheilk. 88, 259 (1954).
WEINIG, E., u. P. ZINK: Dtsch. Z. ges. gerichtl. Med. 60, 61—79 (1967).
ZINK, P.: Dtsch. Z. ges. gerichtl. Med. 56, 349 (1965).

I, 6. Autolyse

ALTMANN, H. W.: Handbuch der allgemeinen Pathologie, Bd. II/1. Berlin-Göttingen-Heidelberg: Springer 1955. — ANDERSON, H.: Acta path. microbiol. scand. 50, 225—227 (1960).
BLAZSO, S.: Biochem. Z. 266, 266—273 (1933). — BRACHET, B.: Arch. Biol. (Liège) 20, 7 (1942). — BRADLEY, H. C.: Autolysis and atrophy. Physiol. Rev. 2, 415—439 (1922). — BRAUN-FALCO, O.: Derm. Wschr. 134, 1341—1349 (1956). — BRAUN-FALCO, O., u. W. WINTER: Arch. klin. exp. Derm. 220, 412—442 (1964). — BÜCHNER, F.: Ärztl. Forsch. 13, 1, 307—314 (1959).
CAESAR, R.: Schweiz. Z. Path. 11, 276—282 (1948).
DIEMAIR, W., u. K. MOLLENKOPF: Z. anal. Derm. 119, 201 (1940). — DUWE, C. DE, u. L. BERTHELET: Handbuch Protoplasmaforschung, Bd. III/A, S. 4. Wien 1954.
EMDEN, G., u. F. KRAUS: Biochem. Z. 45, 1 (1912).
FRUNDER, H., u. Mitarb.: Hoppe-Seylers Z. physiol. Chem. 304, 274—283 (1956).
GOEBEL, A.: Handbuch der allgemeinen Pathologie, Bd. II/1, S. 398—418. Berlin-Göttingen-Heidelberg: Springer 1955. — GÖSSNER, W.: Virchows Arch. path. Anat. 327, 304—313 (1955). — Verh. dtsch. Ges. Path. 44. Tgg 1960, S. 204—209. — GREUER, W.: Arzneimittel-Forsch. 12. Beih. (1962).
HECHT, A.: Acta biol. med. germ. 8, 617—628 (1962). — HECHT, A., u. Mitarb.: Virchows Arch. path. Anat. 334, 267—284 (1961). — HIMES, M. B., u. Mitarb.: Arch. Path. 58, 345, 353 (1954).
JACOBI, O.: Arch. derm. Syph. (Berl.) 188, 197 (1949).
KASTEN, F. H.: J. Histochem. Cytochem. 7, 312—313 (1959). — KENT, S. P.: Arch. Path. 64, 17—22 (1957).
LAUCKER, J. L. VAN, and R. L. HOLZER: J. Path. Bakt. 35, 563—573 (1959). — Lab. Invest. 12, 102—105 (1963). — LAUER: Virchows Arch. path. Anat. 279, 618 (1931). — LEE, M. C.: J. invest. Derm. 37, 201—211 (1961). — LETTERER, H.: Naturforschung und Medizin in Deutschland 1939—1946. Tiat. Rev. 70, 1—15 (1948). — Allgemeiner und gewerblicher Tod, Allgemeine Pathologie, S. 147. — LORKE, D.: Dtsch. Z. ges. gerichtl. Med. 42, 167—172 (1953).
MÖNNIGHOFF, F. H.: Beitr. path. Anat. 102, 87—96 (1939). — MONACELLI, M.: G. ital. Derm. 69, 1093—1094 (1928). — Arch. Derm. Syph. (Berl.) 157, 31—44 (1929).; 170, 285—292 (1943). — MÜLLER, E.: Allgemeine Pathologie, Bd. II/1, S. 613—679. Berlin-Göttingen-Heidelberg: Springer 1955. — MÜLLER, R.: Frankfurt. Z. Path. 52, 433 (1938).
PASCHOUD, J. M., u. Mitarb.: Arch. klin. exp. Derm. 201, 484—494 (1955). — PIOCH, W.: Die histochemische Untersuchung thermischer Hautschäden und ihre Bedeutung für die

forensische Praxis. Lübeck: Schmidt-Römhild 1966. — PISCHINGER: Z. Zellforsch **3**, 169 (1926). — PROKOP, O.: Lehrbuch der gerichtlichen Medizin. Berlin: Volk und Gesundheit 1966.

RAEKALLIO, J.: Acta Med. leg. soc. (Liége) **18**, 1, 39—45 (1965).

SANDRITTER, W.: Z. wiss. Mikr. **62**, 283—304 (1956). — SCHAMBERG, J. FR., and H. BROWN: Arch. intern. Med. **35**, 537—545 (1925). — SCHLEYER, F.: Dtsch. Z. ges. gerichtl. Med. **46**, 1, 569 (1957). — SCHLEYER, F., e JANITZKI: Zacchia **34**, 300 (1959). — SCHMIDT, O., u. Mitarb.: Dtsch. Z. ges. gerichtl. Med. **49**, 206—212 (1959). — SCHOURUP, K.: Diss. Kopenhagen (Dansk Videnskabs Forl.) 1950. — SCHÜMMELFEDER, N.: Verh. Dtsch. Ges. Path. 33. Tgg 1949, S. 65—69. — SEVERINGHAUS, E. L., u. Mitarb.: J. biol. Chem. **57**, 163—179 (1923). — SEXMITH, E., and W. F. PETERSEN: J. exp. Med. **27**, 273—292 (1917). — STÜTTGEN, G., u. Mitarb.: Arch. klin. exp. Derm. **205**, 381—388 (1957). — SZAKALL, A.: Arb. Physiol. Lab. **13**, 49 (1943). — Arch. Derm. Syph. (Berl.) **194**, 376 (1952). — Arzneimittel-Forsch. **7**, 408 (1957).

TERBRÜGGEN, A.: Verh. Dtsch. ges. Path. 33. Tgg 1949, S. 37—57.

ZEIGER: Z. Zellforsch. **10**, 481 (1930); **20**, 1 (1935). — ZOLLINGER, H.: Schweiz. Z. Path. **11**, 276—282 (1948).

I, 7 Rigor

BARGMANN, W.: Histologie und mikroskopische Anatomie des Menschen, 6. Aufl. Stuttgart: Georg Thieme 1967.

DOTZAUER, G.: Dtsch. Z. ges. gerichtl. Med. **46**, 761 (1958).

HOFF, F.: Klinische Physiologie und Pathologie. Stuttgart: Georg Thieme 1962.

ORSOS, F.: Verh. Ges. ungar. Pathologen. Budapest: Betlen-Verlag 1940.

I, 9. Vertrocknungen

FRITZ, E.: Beitr. gerichtl. Med. **13**, 28 (1935).

GLINSKI u. HOROSZKIWICZ: Vjschr. gerichtl. Med. **25**, 243 (1903).

HERRMANN, F., u. Mitarb.: Hautarzt **11**, 8, (1960). — HOFMANN, E., u. A. HABERDA: Lehrbuch der gerichtlichen Medizin, 1. Aufl. Wien: Urban & Schwarzenberg 1927. — HOPF: Frankf. Z. Path. **63**, 1 (1952).

LARCHER: Arch. gén. Méd. **11** (1862). — LUSCHKA: Zit. bei CHIARI. In: DITTRICHs Handbuch, Bd. II. Wien u. Leipzig: Wilhelm Braumüller 1913.

MASCHKA, J. v.: Prag. med. Vjschr. **79**, 138 (1863). — MUELLER, B.: Lehrbuch der gerichtlichen Medizin. Berlin-Göttingen-Heidelberg: Springer 1953.

PIOCH, W.: Die histochemische Untersuchung thermischer Hautschäden und ihre Bedeutung für die forensische Praxis. Lübeck: Schmidt-Römhild 1966.

RAEKALLIO, J.: Enzymhistochemische Methoden bei der Untersuchung mechanisch bedingter Hautwunden. Lübeck: Schmidt-Römhild 1965.

SIEBENHAAR, D. F. J.: Encyclopädisches Handbuch der gerichtlichen Arzneikunde. Leipzig 1837—1840. — SOMMER: Med. Diss. Kopenhagen 1833. — STÜTTGEN, G.: Die normale und pathologische Physiologie der Haut. Stuttgart: Gustav Fischer 1965.

I, 10. Identifikation einer Person über die Haut in der frühen Leichenzeit

BARR, M. L.: Amer. J. hum. Genet. **12**, 118 (1960). — BARR, M. L., and E. G. BERTRAM: Nature (Lond.) **163**, 676 (1949).

CASTAGNOLI, E., u. M. FREI-SULZER: Arch. Kriminol. **140**, 1 (1967).

HOLZER, F. J.: Wien. klin. Wschr. **76**, 511 (1964).

MOESCHLIN, S.: Klinik und Therapie der Vergiftungen, 4. Aufl. Stuttgart: Georg Thieme 1964. — MUELLER, B.: Lehrbuch der gerichtlichen Medizin. Berlin-Göttingen-Heidelberg: Springer 1963.

PIOCH, W.: Über Methoden und Bedeutung feingeweblicher Untersuchungen bei der Flugunfallaufklärung. 8. Flugmed. Tgg Fürstenfeldbruck 1964. — PONSOLD, A.: Handwörterbuch der gerichtlichen Medizin und naturwissenschaftlichen Kriminalistik. Berlin: Springer 1940.

RONCHESE, F.: Occupational marks and other physical signs. New York: Grune & Stratton 1948.

SCHÖNFELD, W.: Körperbemalen, Brandmarken, Tätowieren. Heidelberg: A. Hüthig 1960. — SIMON, F.: Kenyeres-Festschrift, Budapest 1936.

II, 1. Putrifikation

BRAUN-FALCO, O., u. W. WINTER: Arch. klin. exp. Derm. **220**, 412—442 (1964).

ISHIBASHI, FALLANI, PALMIERI u. ROMANO: Zit. bei SCHWERD, Der rote Blutfarbstoff und seine wichtigsten Derivate. Lübeck: Schmidt 1962.

LAVES, W.: Dtsch. Z. ges. gerichtl. Med. **12**, 549 (1928). — LORKE, D., u. O. SCHMIDT: Dtsch. Z. ges. gerichtl. Med. **41**, 236 (1952); **42**, 164 (1952).

MERKEL, H.: Leichenerscheinungen. Aus: Ergebn. allg. Path. path. Anat. **33**, 1 (1937).
NIPPE: Dtsch. Z. ges. gerichtl. Med. **3**, 58—71 (1924).
ORFILA-LESEUR: Traité des exhumations juridiques, Paris 1831. Deutsch von GÜNTZ, Handbuch zum Gebrauch bei gerichtlichen Ausgrabungen usw. Leipzig 1832—1835.
SCHMIDT, O.: Dtsch. Z. ges. gerichtl. Med. **27**, 6 (1937); **37**, 1 (1943). — Zbl. allg. Path. path. Anat. **87**, 257 (1951). — SCHWERD, W.: Der rote Blutfarbstoff und seine wichtigsten Derivate. Lübeck: Schmidt 1962.
WALCHER, K.: Studien über die Leichenfäulnis mit besonderer Berücksichtigung der Histologie derselben. Virchows Arch. path. Anat. **268**, 17—180 (1928).

II, 3. Nekrophagen

HOFMANN-HABERDA: Lehrbuch der gerichtlichen Medizin. Wien: Urban & Schwarzenberg 1927. — HOLZER, F. J.: Dtsch. Z. ges. gerichtl. Med. **30**, 259 (1939). — HUNZIKER, H.: Z. Path. Frankfurt. **22**, 147 (1920).
MARESCH: Persönliche Mitteilung.
WERKGARTNER, A.: Persönliche Mitteilung. — WEYRICH, G.: Dtsch. Z. ges. gerichtl. Med. **19**, 118 (1932).

II, 4. Mumifikation

BORN: Zbl. allg. Path. path. Anat. **99**, 490 (1959).
CAMPS, FR. E., and E. G. EVANS: Med. Sci. law **2**, 38, 48 (1961); **2**, 155—164 (1961/62).
GÜNTZ: Der Leichnam des Neugeborenen. Leipzig 1827.
IPSEN, C.: Vjschr. gerichtl. Med. III. F. **7**, 281—315 (1894).
KRATTER: Virchows Jb. **1**, 511 (1887).
SCHRETZMANN: Dtsch. Z. ges. gerichtl. Med. **36**, 45 (1942). — STRAUCH: Dtsch. Z. ges. gerichtl. Med. **12**, 259 (1928).
TOUSSANT: Casper's Vjschr. XI. 1857.

II, 5. Saponifikation

ASCARELLI, A.: Vjschr. gerichtl. Med. **32**, 219—264 (1906).
BERG, S.: Dtsch. Z. ges. gerichtl. Med. **11**, 278—287 (1928). — BERNDT, J.: Systematisches Handbuch der gerichtlichen Arzneikunde, 4. Aufl., S. 337—338. Wien 1834. — BÖHMER, K.: Tod durch Ertrinken. In: Handwörterbuch der gerichtlichen Medizin. Berlin: Springer 1940. — BOHNE, G.: Vjschr. gerichtl. Med. **47** (Suppl. 1) 13—25 (1914). — BOSCH, K., u. F. R. KELLER: Dtsch. Z. ges. gerichtl. Med. **53**, 79—107 (1963).
CIOBAN, V.: Wien. med. Wschr. **44**, 1947—1950 (1923). — COLLIGNON: Zit. bei CHIARI, Leichenerscheinungen. In: DITTRICHs Handbuch, Bd. 2. Leipzig u. Wien: Wilhelm Braumüller 1913.
DIERKES, K.: Dtsch. Z. ges. gerichtl. Med. **30**, 262—266 (1938). — DRAPER: Vjschr. gerichtl. Med. **47**, 245—354 (1887). — DROSDOFF, V.: Arch. physiol. II, séct. **6**, 117—134 (1879).
ERMAN: Vjschr. gerichtl. Med., N. F. **37**, 51—65 (1882). — EVANS, W. E.: Med. Sci. law **3**, 145—153 (1962/63).
FÖRSTER, A.: Handwörterbuch der gerichtlichen Medizin, S. 834—836. Berlin: Springer 1940. — FOURCROY: Memoires sur les differents etats des cadavres trouves dans les fouilles de cimetive des innocents 1786 et 1787. Mém. Acad. Chir. 1789. Zit. nach MASCHKA, Handbuch der gerichtlichen Medizin 1882. — FRAENKEL, P., u. G. STRASSMANN: Vjschr. gerichtl. Med. III. F, **47**, Suppl. 4, 334—356 (1914).
GANNER: Wien med. Ztg **8** (1887). — GOLDBACH, H. J., u. H. HINÜBER: Zbl. allg. Path. path. Anat. **95**, 105—111 (1956). — GOY u. WENDE: Biochem. Z. **131**, 122 (1922).
HABERDA, A.: Vjschr. gerichtl. Med. III. F./a (1895). — HAUSBRANDT, F.: Dtsch. Z. ges. gerichtl. Med. **35—38**, 217—231 (1941—1944). — HOFMANN-HABERDA: Lehrbuch der gerichtlichen Medizin, 11. Aufl. Berlin u. Wien: Urban & Schwarzenberg 1927. — HOFMANN, E.: Lehrbuch der gerichtlichen Medizin wien S. 397—402 1878. — Wien. med. Wschr. **1879**, 5—7.
IPSEN, C.: Vjschr. gerichtl. Med. **32**, 219—264 (1906).
KOOPMANN: Abriß der gerichtlichen und sozialen Medizin. Leipzig: Georg Thieme 1939. — KRATTER, J.: Mitt. Ver. Ärzte Steiermark 1878 und Öst. ärztl. Ver. Ztg. **11** (1879). — Z. Biol. (XVI) 455—492 (1880).
LEHMANN, K. B.: Würzburger Sitzungsber. S. 19 (1888). — LESSER, A.: Vjschr. gerichtl. Med. **40**, 1—29 (1884). — LUDWIG, E.: Vortrag über Adipocire. Wien. med. Wschr. 1879. — In: Leichenfett. Aus: EULENBERG, Realencyklopädie **8**, 209 (1881). — LUKAS, A.: Forensic chemistry and scientific criminal investigation. London 1948.
MANT, A. K.: Recent work on changes after death. In: Modern trends in forensic medicine. London 1953. — MANT, A. K., and R. FURBANK: J. forens. Med. **4**, 18—35 (1957). — MATZDORFF: Dtsch. Z. ges. gerichtl. Med. **25**, 246—249 (1935). — MERLI, S.: Zacchia **35**, 10—45

(1960). Ref. Dtsch. Z. ges. gerichtl. Med. **51**, 670 (1961). — MONACELLI, M.: Arch. Derm. Syph. (Berl.), **157**, 31—44 (1929); **170**, 285—292 (1943).
NANIKAWA, R., N. TAWA u. K. SAITO: Jap. J. leg. Med. **15**, 3, 258 (1961).
ÖKRÖS, S.: Dtsch. Z. ges. gerichtl. Med. **29**, 485—500 (1938).
REH, H.: Der Tod durch Ertrinken. Habil-Schr. Düsseldorf 1966. — REICHARDT, H.: Beobachtungen über die Zersetzungsvorgänge in den Grüften und Gräbern auf den Friedhöfen. 11. Jahresbericht über das Medizinalwesen in Sachsen auf das Jahr 1880, S. 148 u. 165. — REIMANN, W.: Zur Frage der frühzeitigen Leichenwachsbildung. Wiss. Z. Univ. Halle III (1953/54). — REUBOLD: Ber. med.-phys. Ges. in Würzburg 1885. — REUTER, K., u. H. FISCHER: Dtsch. Z. ges. gerichtl. Med. **2**, 381—397 (1923). — RUTTER u. MARSHALL: Zit. in: TAYLOR's Principles and practice of medical jurispendence, vol. 1. London 1956.
SCHAUENSTEIN: Aus MASCHKA, Handbuch der gerichtlichen Medizin, Bd. 4./III. 1882. — SCHERER, H.: Diss. med. Marburg 1952. — SCHLEYER, F.: Dtsch. Z. ges. gerichtl. Med. **40**, 680—684 (1950/51). — SMITH, S., and F. S. FIDDES: Forensic medicine, 10th ed. London 1955.
TAMASSIA, A.: Rèv. sperim. di fren. e di med. leg. **9**, 161 H, 1883. — THOURET: Rapport sur les exhum. du cim. et de l'eglise des Saint-Innocents, Paris, 1789. Zit. nach MASCHKA, Handbuch der gerichtlichen Medizin 1882.
VOIT: Münch. med. Wschr. **1888**, 518.
WALCHER, K.: Virchows Arch. path. Anat. **268**, 17—180 (1928). — Ergebn. allg. Path. path. Anat. **33**, 55—137 (1937).
ZILLNER, E.: Vjschr. gerichtl. Med. **42**, N.F. 2, 1—31 (1885).

II, 6. Moormumifikation

DIECK, A.: Europ. Moorleichenfunde 1965.
ELLERMANN, W.: Vjschr. gerichtl. Med. III **54**, 181—192 (1917).
GABRIEL, M.: Dtsch. Z. ges. gerichtl. Med. **15**, 226—241 (1930).
MASDERHOFF, J.: Zit. in Handwörterbuch der gerichtlichen Medizin (v. NEUREITER, PIETRUSKY, SCHÜTT). Berlin: Springer 1940.

II, 7. Identitätsfeststellungen

FRITZ, E.: Dtsch. Z. ges. gerichtl. Med. **29**, 426 (1938).
KOBABE, A.: Kriminalistik **10**, 364 (1956).
MONTANARI, G. D., B. VITERBO, and G. R. MONTANARI: Med. Sci. and Law **7**, 208 (1967).
REUTER, K.: Arch. Kriminol. **21**, 68 (1905). — Dtsch. Z. ges. gerichtl. Med. **13**, 256 (1929). — RICHTER, M.: Arch. Kriminol. **43**, 196 (1911).
YADA, S., M. OKANE, Y. SANO, and Y. FUKUMORI: Acta Crim. Med. leg. jop. **32**, 169 (1966).

III, 1. Vitale, supravitale Hautreaktion

ABELE, G.: Dtsch. Z. ges. gerichtl. Med. **49**, 673 (1959/60).
BAHLMANN, CL.: Dtsch. Z. ges. gerichtl. Med. **32**, 133—144 (1939). — BERG, ST. P.: Dtsch. Z. ges. gerichtl. Med. **41**, 158—163 (1952). — BRAUN-FALCO, O., u. D. PETZOLDT: Arch. klin. exp. Derm. **220**, 455—473 (1964); **223**, 620—632 (1965). — Klin. Wschr. **44**, 18, 1092—1099 (1966). — BURIS, L.: Histochemical analysis of injuries. Fourth internat. meeting in forensic medicine Copenhagen, 15.—18. Aug. 1966.
DOTZAUER, G.: Dtsch. Z. ges. gerichtl. Med. **46**, 761—771 (1958).
FISCHER, J., and D. GLICK: Histochemistry: XIX Lokalisation of alkaline phosphatase in normal und path. human. skin. Proc. Soc. exp. Biol. (N.Y.) **66**, 14—18 (1947).
HOU-JENSEN, KL.: Fourth internat. meeting in forensic medicine Copenhagen, 15.—18. Aug. 1966. Histochemical demonstration of some hydrolytic enzymes in human skin wounds an their applicability as vital reactions in medico-legal practice.
KENT, S. P.: Arch. Path. **64**, 17—22 (1957). — KOPF, A.: Arch. Derm. **75**, 1—37 (1957).
LAIHO, K.: Immunohistochemical studies on fibrin in vital and postmortem subcutaneous haemorrhages. IV. intern. meeting in forensic medicine Copenhagen, 16.—18. 8. 1966. — LANSING, A. J., and D. L. ODYKE: Anat. Rec. **107**, 379—397 (1950). — LINDNER, J.: Folia Histochem. **4**, 21 (1966).
MUELLER, B.: Lehrbuch der gerichtlichen Medizin. Berlin-Göttingen-Heidelberg: Springer 1953.
ÖKRÖS, S.: Dtsch. Z. ges. gerichtl. Med. **29**, 485—500 (1938). — ORSOS, F.: Die vitalen Reaktionen u. ihre gerichtsmedizinisches Bedeutung. Gedächtnisvortrag 27. Okt. 1934, Kgl. Ärzteges. Budapest. Orvosképzés, H. 1 (1935) u. Beitr. path. Anat. **59**, 161 (1935).
PIOCH, W.: Die histochemische Untersuchung thermischer Hautschäden und ihre Bedeutung für die forensische Praxis. Lübeck: Schmidt-Römhild 1966. — PIRILÄ, V., u. O. ERÄNKO: Acta path. microbiol. scand. **27**, 650, 661 (1950). — PROKOP, O.: Lehrbuch der gerichtlichen Medizin. Berlin: Volk und Gesundheit 1966.

RAEKALLIO, J.: Histochemical studies an vital and post-mortem skin wounds. Helsinki 1961. Sonderdruck. — Acta histochem. (Jena), Suppl. **4**, 106—117 (1964). — Über die Unterscheidung vitaler und postmortaler Hautwunden mittels histochemischer Methoden. Acta med. leg. et soc. **18**, No. 1 (1965). — Exp. and molec. Path. **4**, 303—310 (1965). — J. forens. Med. **13**, 3, 85—91 (1966). — Histochemical methods in forensic medicine. Fourth internat. meeting in forensic medicine Copenhagen, 15.—18. Aug. 1966. — RASSNER, G.: Arch. klin. exp. Derm. **222**, 383—390 (1965).

SCHÜMMELFEDER, N.: Virchows Arch. path. Anat. **318**, 119 (1950). — STRUGGER: Naturwissenschaften **34**, 267 (1947).

UHER, V.: Naturwissenschaften **45**, 1, 21 (1958).

WADA, M.: Acta Med. leg. soc. (Liège) **10**, 743 (1957). — WALCHER, K.: Dtsch. Z. ges. gerichtl. Med. **15**, 16—57 (1930); — **26**, 193—211 (1936). — WERKGARTNER, A.: Dtsch. Z. ges. gerichtl. Med. **29**, 260—264 (1938).

ZIEMKE, E.: Vjschr. gerichtl. Med. **39**, Suppl. 416, 16—29 (1910). — ZINK, P.: Dtsch. Z. ges. gerichtl. Med. **56**, 349—370 (1965).

III, 2. Stumpfe Gewalt

BECKER, H.: Studien über die Abheilung von Exkoriationen unter gerichtsmedizinischen Gesichtspunkten. Med. Diss. Heidelberg 1951. — BLUM: Virchows Arch. path. Anat. **299**, 754 (1937). — BREMME: Vjschr. gerichtl. Med. **13**, 247 (1871).

CASPER-LIMAN: Praktisches Handbuch der gerichtlichen Medizin. Berlin 1889.

DOTZAUER, G.: Dtsch. Z. ges. gerichtl. Med. **46**, 761 (1958).

FAZEKAS, I. G., u. F. VIRAGOS-KIS: Dtsch. Z. ges. gerichtl. Med. **56**, 250—268 (1965); **61**, 107—116 (1967).

HOFMANN-HABERDA: Lehrbuch der gerichtlichen Medizin, 11. Aufl. Berlin u. Wien: Urban & Schwarzenberg 1927.

KALTENBACH, R.: Zbl. Gynäk. **31**, 497—498 (1888). — KLEIN, H.: Dtsch. Z. ges. gerichtl. Med. **45**, 17—20 (1956). — KOSTEN, E.: Dtsch. Z. ges. gerichtl. Med. **36**, 2, 255—258 (1942).

LESSER: Vjschr. gerichtl. Med. **32**, 219 (1880); **35**, 201 (1881).

MUELLER, B.: Dtsch. Z. ges. gerichtl. Med. **23**, 334—337 (1934).

OLBRYCHT, J. S.: Dtsch. Z. ges. gerichtl. Med. **54**, 407—423 (1963). — ORSOS, F.: Beitr. path. Anat. **95**, 163 (1935). — Dtsch. Z. ges. gerichtl. Med. **37**, 1, 33—51 (1943).

PLENK, J.: Elementa medicinæ forensis. Viena 1781.

ROER, H., u. H. KOOPMANN: Dtsch. Z. ges. gerichtl. Med. **30**, 1—8 (1938).

SCHULZ, R.: Vjschr. gerichtl. Med., N.F. **11**, 44—129 (1896).

WALCHER, K.: Dtsch. Z. ges. gerichtl. Med. **26**, 193 (1936).

ZIEMKE: Der Tod durch Erstickung. In: SCHMIDTMANNs Handbuch der gerichtlichen Medizin, II. Berlin 1907.

III, 3. Hieb, Stich, Schnitt an der Leichenhaut

BOLTZ, W.: Dtsch. Z. ges. gerichtl. Med. **40**, 181—191 (1951). — BUHTZ, G., u. EHRHARDT: Dtsch. Z. ges. gerichtl. Med. **29**, 453, 468 (1938).

FUJIWARA, K.: Dtsch. Z. ges. gerichtl. Med. **12**, 65—67 (1928).

HOUTROUW, TH.: Dtsch. Z. ges. gerichtl. Med. **15**, 417 (1930).

MUELLER, B.: Lehrbuch der gerichtlichen Medizin. Berlin-Göttingen-Heidelberg: Springer 1953.

OKAJIMA, J.: Dtsch. Z. ges. gerichtl. Med. **53**, 51—54 (1962).

SCHOLLMEYER, W.: Beitr. gerichtl. Med. **23**, 244 (1965). — SCHULZ, R.: Vjschr. gerichtl. Med., III. F., **12**, Suppl. 1, 44 (1896).

WALCHER, K.: Dtsch. Z. ges. gerichtl. Med. **26**, 193 (1936).

ZIEMKE, E.: Vjschr. gerichtl. Med. **39**, Suppl. 4, 16, 19—29 (1910); **61**, H. 2, 185—203 (1921). — Handwörterbuch der gerichtlichen Medizin. Berlin 1940. — ZUICK, K. H.: Ref. Dtsch. Z. ges. gerichtl. Med. **43**, 448 (1954).

III, 4. Schußverletzungen

BINDING: Binding Lehrbuch. Besonderer Teil, Bd. I, 2. Aufl. 1902; Bd. II, 1. Abt., 2. Aufl. 1904, 2. Abt. 1905. — BUHTZ, G.: Dtsch. Z. ges. gerichtl. Med. **18**, 609—625 (1932).

CARELIA, A.: Zacchia **33**, 73—95 (1958). Ref. Dtsch. Z. ges. gerichtl. Med. **49**, 315 (1959/60).

DITTRICH: Handbuch der ärztlichen Sachverständigentätigkeit, Bd. III. Wien u. Leipzig: W. Braumüller 1906.

ELBEL, H.: Dtsch. Z. ges. gerichtl. Med. **32**, 165—171 (1939).

FRAENKEL, P.: Vjschr. gerichtl. Med. **43**, Suppl., H 2, 154—170, 339—343 (1912). — FRITZ, E.: Dtsch. Z. ges. gerichtl. Med. **23**, 289—299 (1934).

GERLACH, WA., u. WE.: Dtsch. Z. ges. gerichtl. Med. 23, 148—151 (1934). — GORONCY, C.: Dtsch. Z. ges. gerichtl. Med. 11, 482—486 (1928). — GRÄFF, S.: Tod im Luftangriff. Hamburg: Noelke 1955. — GUARESCHI, H.: Dtsch. Z. ges. gerichtl. Med. 23, 89—96 (1934). HUBER: Dtsch. Z. ges. gerichtl. Med. 29, 249 (1938).
KRAULAND, W.: Die Basophilie des Bindegewebes als Zeichen des Einschusses. Verh. int. Kongr. gerichtl. u. soziale Medizin, Bonn 1938, S. 325—343.
LIEBEGOTT, G.: Dtsch. Z. ges. gerichtl. Med. 39, 356—363 (1948/49). — LISZT, F. v.: Lehrbuch des Deutschen Strafrechts, 23. Aufl. Berlin u. Leipzig: W. de Gruyter & Co. 1921. MEIXNER, K.: Dtsch. Z. ges. gerichtl. Med. 1, 151—153 (1922). — MEYER, W.: Vjschr. gerichtl. Med. 35, 3.F., 22—37 (1908). — MUELLER, B.: Dtsch. Z. ges. gerichtl. Med. 34, 1—3, 115—135 (1940); 35, 4, 173—179 (1941); 36, 2, 53—61 (1942).
PUPPE, G.; in: RAPMUND, O., Der beamtete Arzt und Sachverständige. Berlin: Fischer 1904.
SCHMIDT, GG: Acta Med. leg. soc. (Liège) 17, 4, 51—62 (1964). — SCHRADER, G.: Untersuchungen zur Histopathologie elektrischer Hautschädigungen. Jena: Gustav Fischer 1920. — Experimentelle Untersuchungen zur Histopathologie elektrischer Hautschädigungen durch niedergespannten Gleich- und Wechselstrom. Jena: Gustav Fischer 1932. — SCHÖNTAG, A.: Arch. Kriminol. 120, 62—66 (1957). — SELLIER: Vortrag 46. Tagg der Dtsch. Ges. für gerichtl. u. soziale Medizin 6.—9. 9. 1967 Kiel (im Druck). — STRASSMANN, G.: Beitr. gerichtl. Med. 6, 114 (1924). — Dtsch. Z. ges. gerichtl. Med. 23, 375—386 (1934).
WAGNER, H. J.: Dtsch. Z. ges. gerichtl. Med. 54, 258 (1963). — WERKGARTNER, A.: Beitr. gerichtl. Med. 6, 148 (1924). — Dtsch. Z. ges. gerichtl. Med. 11, 154—168 (1928). — WOLFF, F., u. M. LAUFER: Dtsch. Z. ges. gerichtl. Med. 56, 87—96 (1965).

III, 5. Verbrennung

BERG, ST.: Brandermittlung. Wiesbaden: Verlag Bundeskriminalamt 1962.
FALK: Der Tod durch Verbrennung und Verbrühung. In: MASCHKA, Handbuch der gerichtlichen Medizin, Bd. 1, S. 759. Tübingen: Raupp 1881. — FÖRSTER, A.: Handwörterbuch der gerichtlichen Medizin, S. 834. Berlin: Springer 1940.
GLASSTONE, S.: Die Wirkungen der Kernwaffen. Atomenergie-Kommission der Vereinigten Staaten von Amerika. Deutsche Ausgabe von H. LEUTZ. Köln-Berlin-Bonn: C. Heymanns 1960.
HENRIQUES, F., and A. R. MORITZ: Studies of thermal injury. Amer. J. Path. 23, 531, 549, 695—720, 915—942 (1947). — HOLZER, F. J.: Dtsch. Z. ges. gerichtl. Med. 34, 307—320 (1941).
JASTROWITZ, M.: Vjschr. gerichtl. Med. 32, 1—35 (1880).
MEIXNER, K.: Dtsch. Z. ges. gerichtl. Med. 18, 270—284 (1832). — MERKEL, H.: Dtsch. Z. ges. gerichtl. Med. 18, 232—249 (1932). — MORITZ, M. D., and E. D. HENRIQUES: Amer. J. Path. 23, 695—719 (1947).
MESSERSCHMIDT, O.: Auswirkungen atomarer Detonation auf den Menschen. München: K. Thiemig 1960.
PAULUS, W.: Dtsch. Z. ges. gerichtl. Med. 40, 468—471 (1951). — PIOCH, W.: Die histochemische Untersuchung thermischer Hautschäden und ihre Bedeutung für die forensische Praxis. Lübeck: Schmidt-Römhild 1966.
REH, H.: Dtsch. Z. ges. gerichtl. Med. 49, 703—709 (1959/60). — REUTER, F.: Vjschr. gerichtl. Med. 14, 28—59 (1892).
SCHILLING-SIENGALEWICZ, S.: Erkennung des Verbrennungstodes. Polska gazeta lekarska 2, 37, 675—676 (1923). Ref. Dtsch. Z. ges. gerichtl. Med. 3, 587 (1924). — SCHOLLMEYER, W.: Dtsch. Z. ges. gerichtl. Med. 51, 180—189 (1961).
TASCHEN, B.: Dtsch. Gesundh.-Wes. 36, 1142—1144 (1950). — TASCHEN, B., u. H. D. BERGEDER: Dtsch. Z. ges. gerichtl. Med. 40, 353—362 (1951).

III, 7. Verätzung der Leichenhaut

ARNAL u. MEHL: Kriminal. Rdsch. 1948.
OBOGLIO, CATTANEO et CARBONESCHI: Arch. Med. leg. 4, 407 (1934).
WEISS: Arch. Kriminol. 39, 140 (1910).

III, 8. Strom und stromähnliche Veränderungen der Leichenhaut

ADJUTANTIS, G., and G. SKALOS: J. forens. Med. 9, 1—4, 101—105 (1962).
BÖHM, E.: Dtsch. Z. ges. gerichtl. Med. 59, 22—25, 26—34 (1967); 61, 128—136 (1967). — BORNSTEIN, F.: Dtsch. Z. ges. gerichtl. Med. 56, 81—86 (1965). — BOSCH, K.: Dtsch. Z. ges. gerichtl. Med. 56, 318—323 (1965).
FRITZ, E.: Dtsch. Z. ges. gerichtl. Med. 34, 177 (1941).
GERLACH, W.: Dtsch. Z. ges. gerichtl. Med. 22, 433 (1933). — GERSTNER, H.: Virchows Arch. path. Anat. 295, 4 691—702 (1935).

HOLZER, F. J.: Dtsch. Z. ges. gerichtl. Med. 44, 418 (1955).
JELLINEK, ST.: Wien. klin. Wschr. 20, 239 (1921); 64, 501 (1952); 774—775 (1953); 41, 719—721 (1960). — Dtsch. Z. ges. gerichtl. Med. 1, 596—600 (1922); 12, 104—111 (1928). — Med. Klin. 23, 38, 1439—1442 (1922). — Elektrische Verletzungen. Leipzig: Johann Ambrosius Barth 1932. — Beitr. gerichtl. Med. 20, 56—58 (1958).
KAPLAN, A. D.: Dtsch. Z. ges. gerichtl. Med. 17, 217 (1931). — KAWAMURA, J.: Virchows Arch. path. Anat. 231, 570 (1921). — KLEIN, H.: Dtsch. Z. ges. gerichtl. Med. 47, 29—54 (1958). — KOEPPEN, S.: Dtsch. med. Wschr. 1928, 2127. — Elektromedizin 4, 215 (1961). — KOEPPEN, S. u. H. GERSTNER: Virchows Arch. path. Anat. 295, 4, 679—690 (1935). — KRATER: Tod durch Elektrizität. Wien: Franz Deuticke 1896. — KRAULAND, W.: Dtsch. Z. ges. gerichtl. Med. 40, 298—312 (1951).
MIEREMENT, C. W. G.: Klin. Wschr. 2, 1362 (1923). — MODABER, P.: Über die Metallisation, insbesondere über das Verhalten des Eisens nach elektrischen Strom. Med. Diss. Heidelberg 1965. — MUELLER, B.: Lehrbuch der gerichtlichen Medizin. Berlin-Göttingen-Heidelberg: Springer 1953. — MUNCK, W.: Dtsch. Z. ges. gerichtl. Med. 23, 97—109 (1934).
NIPPE, M.: Vjschr. gerichtl. Med. 61, 211—213 (1921).
PIETRUSKY, F.: Dtsch. Z. ges. gerichtl. Med. 29, 135—151 (1938). — PIOCH, W.: Histochemische Untersuchungen über die Darstellbarkeit früher Zell- und Gewebsalterationen nach lokaler Hitzeeinwirkung. Habil.-Schr. Bonn 1963. — Dtsch. Z. ges. gerichtl. Med. 57, 165—167 (1966). — Die histochemische Untersuchung thermischer Hautwunden und ihre Bedeutung für die forensische Praxis. Lübeck: Schmidt-Römhild 1966. — PUCCINI, G.: Minerva med. leg. 84, 4, 91—101 (1964).
RIEHL, G.: Münch. med. Wschr. 70, 1119 (1923).
SACHS: Tod durch elektrische Energie. In: PONSOLDs Lehrbuch der gerichtlichen Medizin, S. 306. Stuttgart 1950. — SCHÄFFNER, M.: Dtsch. Z. ges. gerichtl. Med. 56, 269—280 (1965). — SCHMIDT, G.: Acta Med. leg. soc. (Liège) 17, 4, 51—62 (1964). — SCHRADER, G.: Untersuchungen zur Histopathologie elektrischer Hautschädigungen. Jena: Gustav Fischer 1920. — Experimentelle Untersuchungen zur Histopathologie elektrischer Hautschädigungen durch niedergespannten Gleich- und Wechselstrom. Jena: Gustav Fischer 1932. — SCHREIBER, H.: Inaug.-Diss. München 1941. — SCHRIDDE, H.: Zbl. allg. Path. path. Anat. 32, 369 (1922). — Klin. Wschr. 4, 45, 2143—2145 (1925). — SCHRIDDE, H., u. A. BEEKMANN: Virchows Arch. path. Anat. 252, 774 (1924). — SCHWERD, W.: Dtsch. Z. ges. gerichtl. Med. 49, 218—223 (1959/60). — SCHWERD, W., u. KL. HÖCHEL: Arch. Kriminol. 138, 1—7 (1966). — SELLIER, K.: Dtsch. Z. ges. gerichtl. Med. 57, 161—165 (1966). — SOMOGYI, E.: Histochemical anaysis of electric-current marks. Fourth intern. meeting in forensic medicine Copenhagen, 15.—18. Aug. 1966. — SOMOGYI, E., P. SOTONYI u.a.: Dtsch. Z. ges. gerichtl. Med. 57, 431—438 (1966). — STRASSMANN, G., u. O. SCHMIDT: Dtsch. Z. ges. gerichtl. Med. 11, 202—210 (1928).
WAGNER, CH. E.: Untersuchungen zur Diagnostik von Stromeintrittstellen auf der menschlichen Haut. Med. Diss. Erlangen 1961. — WEINMANN, W.: Arch. Kriminol. 91, 188 (1932).

III, 9. Die postmortale percutane Resorption von Gasen

ABERNETHY: Zit. nach W. BARRAT. J. Physiol. (Lond.) 21, 192 (1897).
BOURGET: Ther. Mschr. 7, 531 (1893).
BÜRGI, E.: Die Durchlässigkeit der Haut für Arzneien und Gifte. Berlin: Springer 1942.
ERNSTENE, A. C., and M. C. VOLK: J. clin. Invest. 11, 363, 376, 383 (1932).
FLEISCHER, R.: Untersuchungen über das Resorptionsvermögen der menschlichen Haut. Habil.-Schr. 1877. — FLURY, F.: Zangger-Festschrift, Teil 2, 836 (1935).
GERLACH: Arch. Anat. Physiol. 431 (1851).
HEUBNER, W.: Zbl. Gewerbehyg. 1, 1—20 (1925/26).
NADKARNI u. Mitarb.: Arch. Derm. Syph. (Chic.) 64, 294 (1951).
SALZMANN, F.: Münch. med. Wschr. 1930 679. — SCHÜTZE, W.: Arch. Hyg. (Berl.) 98, 70 (1927). — SCHULZE, W.: Arch. Derm. Syph. (Berl.) 185, 83 (1943). — SCHWENKENBECHER, A.: Arch. Anat. Physiol. 121 (1904).
WALTON, D. C., and M. G. WITHERSPOON: J. Pharmacol. exp. Ther. 26, 315 (1926). — WILKS, S. S., and R. T. CLARK: J. appl. Physiol. 14, 313—320 (1959).
ZUELZER, G.: Z. klin. Med. 53, 403 (1904).

MIX
Papier aus verantwortungsvollen Quellen
Paper from responsible sources
FSC® C105338

If you have any concerns about our products,
you can contact us on
ProductSafety@springernature.com

In case Publisher is established outside the EU,
the EU authorized representative is:
**Springer Nature Customer Service Center GmbH
Europaplatz 3, 69115 Heidelberg, Germany**

Printed by Libri Plureos GmbH
in Hamburg, Germany

HANDBUCH DER HAUT- UND GESCHLECHTSKRANKHEITEN
J. JADASSOHN
ERGÄNZUNGSWERK

BEARBEITET VON

G. ACHTEN · J. ALKIEWICZ · R. ANDRADE · R. D. AZULAY · H.-J. BANDMANN · L. M. BECHELLI
M. BETETTO · H. H. BIBERSTEIN † · R. M. BOHNSTEDT · G. BONSE · S. BORELLI · W. BORN
O. BRAUN-FALCO · I. BRODY · S. R. BRUNAUER · W. BURCKHARDT · J. CABRÉ · F. T. CALLOMON †
C. CARRIÉ · H. CHIARI · G. B. COTTINI · H. J. CRAMER · R. DOEPFMER † · G. DOTZAUER · CHR.
EBERHARTINGER · H. EBNER · G. EHLERS · G. EHRMANN · R. A. ELLIS · A. ENGELHARDT · F.
FEGELER · E. FISCHER · H. FISCHER · H. FLEISCHHACKER · H. FRITZ-NIGGLI · H. GÄRTNER
O. GANS · M. GARZA TOBA · P. E. GEHRELS · H. GÖTZ · L. GOLDMAN · H. GOLDSCHMIDT
A. GREITHER · H. GRIMMER · P. GROSS · TH. GRÜNEBERG · J. HÄMEL · E. HAGEN · D.
HARDER · W. HAUSER · E. HEERD · E. HEINKE · H.-J. HEITE · S. HELLERSTRÖM · A. HENSCH-
LER-GREIFELT · J. J. HERZBERG · J. HEWITT · G. von der HEYDT · G. E. HEYDT · H. HILMER
H. HOBITZ · H. HOFF · K. HOLUBAR · G. HOPF · O. HORNSTEIN · L. ILLIG · W. JADASSOHN
M. JÄNNER · E. G. JUNG · R. KADEN · K. H. KÄRCHER · FR. KAIL · K. W. KALKOFF · W. D.
KEIDEL · PH. KELLER · J. KIMMIG · G. KLINGMÜLLER · N. KLÜKEN · W. KLUNKER · A. G.
KOCHS † · H. U. KOECKE · FR. KOGOJ · G. W. KORTING · E. KRÜGER-THIEMER · H. KUSKE
F. LATAPI · H. LAUSECKER † · P. LAVALLE · A. LEINBROCK · K. LENNERT · G. LEONHARDI
W. F. LEVER · W. LINDEMAYR · K. LINSER · H. LÖHE † · L. LÖHNER · L. J. A. LOEWENTHAL
A. LUGER · E. MACHER · F. D. MALKINSON · C. MARCH · J. T. McCARTHY · R. T. McCLUSKEY
K. MEINICKE · W. MEISTERERNST · N. MELCZER · A. M. MEMMESHEIMER · J. MEYER-ROHN
A. MIESCHER · G. MIESCHER † · P. A. MIESCHER · G. MORETTI · E. MÜLLER · A. MUSGER
TH. NASEMANN · FR. NEUWALD · G. NIEBAUER · H. NIERMANN · W. NIKOLOWSKI · F. NÖDL
H. OLLENDORFF-CURTH · F. PASCHER · R. PFISTER · K. PHILIPP · A. PILLAT · H. PINKUS
P. POCHI · W. POHLIT · H. PORTUGAL · M. I. QUIROGA · W. RAAB · R. V. RAJAM · B. RAJEW-
SKY · J. RAMOS E SILVA · H. REICH · R. RICHTER · G. RIEHL · H. RIETH · H. RÖCKL · N. F.
ROTHFIELD · ST. ROTHMAN † · M. RUPEC · S. RUST · T. ŠALAMON · S. A. P. SAMPAIO · R.
SANTLER · K. F. SCHALLER · E. SCHEICHER-GOTTRON · A. SCHIMPF · C. SCHIRREN · C.
G. SCHIRREN · H. SCHLIACK · W. SCHMIDT, MANNHEIM · W. SCHMIDT, MÜNCHEN · R.
SCHMITZ · W. SCHNEIDER · U. W. SCHNYDER · H. E. SCHREINER · H. SCHUERMANN † · K.-H.
SCHULZ · R. SCHUPPLI · E. SCHWARZ · J. SCHWARZ · M. SCHWARZ-SPECK · H.-P.-R. SEELIGER
R. D. G. PH. SIMONS † · J. SÖLTZ'-SZÖTS · E. SOHAR · C. E. SONCK · H. W. SPIER · R. SPITZER
D. STARCK · Z. STARY · G. K. STEIGLEDER · H. STORCK · J. S. STRAUSS · G. STÜTTGEN · M.
SULZBERGER · A. SZAKALL † · L. TAMÁSKA · A. TANAY · J. TAPPEINER · J. THEUNE · W. THIES
W. UNDEUTSCH · G. VELTMAN · J. VONKENNEL † · F. WACHSMANN · G. WAGNER · W. H. WAG-
NER · E. WALCH · G. WEBER · R. WEHRMANN · K. WEINGARTEN · G. G. WENDT · A. WIEDMANN
H. WILDE · A. WINKLER · D. WISE · A. WISKEMANN · P. WODNIANSKY · KH. WOEBER · H. WÜST
K. WULF · L. ZALA · H. ZAUN · J. ZEITLHOFER · J. ZELGER · M. ZINGSHEIM · L. ZIPRKOWSKI

HERAUSGEGEBEN GEMEINSAM MIT

R. DOEPFMER† · O. GANS · H. GÖTZ · H. A. GOTTRON · J. KIMMIG · A. LEIN-
BROCK · G. MIESCHER† · TH. NASEMANN · H. RÖCKL · C. G. SCHIRREN · U. W.
SCHNYDER · H. SCHUERMANN† · H. W. SPIER · G. K. STEIGLEDER · H. STORCK
A. WIEDMANN

VON

A. MARCHIONINI†

SCHRIFTLEITUNG: C. G. SCHIRREN

ERSTER BAND · ERSTER TEIL

SPRINGER-VERLAG BERLIN HEIDELBERG GMBH
1968

NORMALE UND PATHOLOGISCHE ANATOMIE DER HAUT I

BEARBEITET VON

G. ACHTEN · I. BRODY · O. BRAUN-FALCO · H. J. CRAMER
G. DOTZAUER · CHR. EBERHARTINGER · H. EBNER
G. EHLERS · R. A. ELLIS · E. HAGEN · H. U. KOECKE · G. MORETTI
G. NIEBAUER · H. PINKUS · P. E. POCHI · M. RUPEC
W. SCHMIDT · J. S. STRAUSS · L. TAMÁSKA · A. TANAY · H. ZAUN

HERAUSGEGEBEN VON

O. GANS UND G. K. STEIGLEDER

MIT 535 TEILS FARBIGEN ABBILDUNGEN

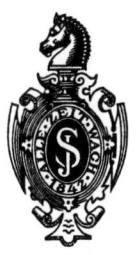

SPRINGER-VERLAG BERLIN HEIDELBERG GMBH
1968

Alle Rechte vorbehalten. Kein Teil dieses Buches darf ohne schriftliche Genehmigung des Springer-Verlages übersetzt oder in irgendeiner Form vervielfältigt werden.

© by Springer-Verlag Berlin Heidelberg 1968
Ursprünglich erschienen bei Springer-Verlag Berlin Heidelberg New York 1968
Softcover reprint of the hardcover 1st edition 1968

Library of Congress Catalog Card Number 28-17078

ISBN 978-3-662-30269-9   ISBN 978-3-662-30268-2(eBook)
DOI 10.1007/978-3-662-30268-2

Die Wiedergabe von Gebrauchsnamen, Handelsnamen, Warenbezeichnungen usw. in diesem Werk berechtigen auch ohne besondere Kennzeichnung nicht zu der Annahme, daß solche Namen im Sinn der Warenzeichen- oder Markenschutz-Gesetzgebung als frei zu betrachten wären und daher von jedermann benutzt werden dürften

Druck der Universitätsdruckerei H. Stürtz AG, Würzburg

Titel-Nr. 5518

Vorwort

Dieser Ergänzungsband über die normale Anatomie der Haut erscheint gerade ein Jahrhundert nach dem Geburtstage von Felix Pinkus (geb. am 4. April 1868), der — abgesehen von dem Beitrag über die Blutgefäße der Haut von W. Spalteholz und dem über das Pigment der Haut von B. Bloch — den ersten Band des Jadassohnschen Handbuches der Haut- und Geschlechtskrankheiten geschrieben und die normale Anatomie der Haut mit einmaliger Gründlichkeit, Weitsicht und Kritik behandelt hat. Ein wesentlicher Teil der Fakten mußte von Felix Pinkus selbst erarbeitet werden. Wenn man sich dieser Tatsache bewußt ist, kann man erst die Leistung des Autors voll würdigen.

Wir möchten den vorliegenden Band dem Gedächtnis von Felix Pinkus widmen.

Dem Buch wünschen wir, daß die Leser nach vier Jahrzehnten ebenso wie nach dem Studium des ursprünglichen Beitrages über die Anatomie der Haut sagen werden, daß er nichts von seiner Bedeutung verloren hat und ein Meilenstein der wissenschaftlichen Entwicklung geblieben ist.

O. Gans und G. K. Steigleder

Inhaltsverzeichnis

A. Histologie der normalen Haut

The Epidermis. By Ass. Professor Isser Brody, M. D., Stockholm. (With 54 Figures) . 1
    Introduction 1
A. Dermo-Epidermal Junction 2
    I. The Attachment of the Epidermis to the Dermis 2
    II. The Dermo-Epidermal Interface 4
B. Epidermal Sub-Layers 8
    I. Stratum Basale 8
    II. Transitional Cells between the Strata basale and spinosum 10
    III. Stratum spinosum 10
    IV. Stratum intermedium 11
    V. Transitional Cells or T-Cells 12
    VI. Stratum lucidum 13
        1. Plantar and Palmar Skin 13
        2. Non-Plantar and -Palmar Skin 14
    VII. Stratum corneum 14
        1. Plantar and Palmar Skin 15
        2. Non-Plantar and -Palmar Skin 15
    VIII. Transitional Zone 17
C. The Morphology of the Keratinocytes 18
    I. Cell Surface 18
        1. Cell Relief 18
        2. Plasma Membrane 20
            a) The "Horny Membrane" of Unna 20
            b) The Plasma Membrane as Revealed by Electron Microscopy 21
    II. Intercellular Space 23
    III. Attachment Zones 31
        1. Desmosomes 31
            a) The Regular Desmosome 32
            b) The Simple Desmosome 34
        2. Nexus 34
        3. The Junctional Desmosomes 35
    IV. Epidermal Fibrils 36
        1. Definitions 36
        2. General Features 37
        3. The Development of the Fibrils into Keratin Fibrils 42
            a) The Speckled Pattern 42
            b) The Keratohyalin 43
            c) The Keratin 49
    V. Mitochondria 55
    VI. The Golgi Apparatus 57
    VII. Ribosomes and alpha-Cytomembranes 57
    VIII. Other Cytoplasmic Constituents 58
    IX. Nucleus 60
    X. Cell Regeneration 61
D. The Histochemistry of the Keratinocytes 66
    I. Inorganic Substances 66

    II. Amino Acids, Proteins, Nucleic Acids and Protein-bound Sulfhydryl and Disulfide Groups 67
        1. Amino Acids and Proteins 67
        2. Nucleic Acids 68
            a) Deoxyribonucleic Acid (DNA) 68
            b) Ribonucleic Acid (RNA) 69
        3. Sulfhydryl and Disulfide Groups 70
    III. Carbohydrates 76
        1. Glycogen 76
        2. PAS-Reactive, Diastase-Resistent Polysaccharides 78
    IV. Lipids 81
        V. Enzymes 85
            1. Cytochrome Oxidase 85
            2. Monoamine Oxidase 87
            3. Succinic Dehydrogenase 87
            4. NADH- and NADPH-Tetrazolium Reductases 89
            5. Specific Coenzyme-Linked Dehydrogenases 90
            6. Phosphorylase and Amylo-1,4 → 1,6-transglucosidase 91
            7. Esterases 92
                a) Aliesterases 92
                    α) Alpha-Naphtol or Non-Specific Esterases 92
                    β) Indoxyl Acetate Esterases 95
                    γ) Tween 60 Esterases 95
                    δ) AS Esterases 95
                b) Cholinesterases 96
            8. Phosphomonoesterases 96
                a) Acid Phosphatase 96
                b) Alkaline Phosphatase 99
            9. Adenosine Triphosphatase (ATPase) 99
            10. Phosphamidase 100
            11. Nucleases 100
                a) Ribonuclease (RNase) 100
                b) Deoxyribonuclease (DNAse) 100
            12. Beta-Glucuronidase 100
            13. Proteolytic Enzymes 101
            14. Carbonic Anhydrase 102
            15. Ubiquinone 102
            16. Desulfhydrase 103
E. Dendritic Cells 103
    I. The Melanocyte 103
        1. Origin 103
        2. Demonstration, Distribution and Frequency 106
        3. Morphology 107
        4. The Transfer Process of Melanin Granules 113
        5. Enzymatic Activity 114
            a) Phenol-Oxydase 114
            b) Adenosintriphosphatase 115
    II. Langerhans Cells 116
        1. Origin 116
        2. Morphology 117
        3. Enzymatic Activity 119
References 120

Histologie, Histochemie und Wachstumsdynamik des Haarfollikels. Von Priv.-Doz. Dr. med. HANSOTTO ZAUN, Homburg a. d. Saar. (Mit 20 Abbildungen, davon 2 farbige)

Einleitung 143
    I. Die Struktur des aktiven Haarfollikels 143
        1. Die Haarzwiebel (Bulbus) 145
        2. Das Haar 147
            a) Die Haarrinde (Cortex) 148
            b) Das Haarmark (Medulla) 148
            c) Das Oberhäutchen (Epidermicula) 149

3. Die epithelialen Wurzelscheiden 150
   a) Innere Wurzelscheide 150
   b) Äußere Wurzelscheide 152
4. Die dermale Papille 153
5. Die bindegewebigen Follikelhüllen 153
   a) Glashaut 153
   b) Haarbalg 154
6. Differenzierung der Matrixzellen und Verhornung im elektronenoptischen Bild . 154
7. Der Haarfollikel in funktioneller Sicht 157
II. Die Strukturveränderungen des Follikels während des Haarcyclus 157
III. Altersveränderung des Follikels und der Kopfhaut (einschließlich sog. „Alopecia praematura") 165
IV. Histochemie des Haarfollikels 169
   1. Histotopographie anorganischer Substanzen 170
   2. Histotopographie von Kohlenhydraten 170
      a) Glykogen 170
      b) Saure Mucopolysaccharide 171
   3. Lipoide 171
   4. Histotopographie von Aminosäuren 172
   5. Sulfhydryl-(SH-) und Disulfid-(SS-)Gruppen 173
   6. Nucleinsäuren 174
   7. Histotopographie von Enzymen 175
V. Autoradiographische Befunde am Haarfollikel 175
Schluß 178
Literatur 178

Histology, Histochemistry and Electron Microscopy of Sebaceous Glands in Man. By Prof. Dr. JOHN S. STRAUSS and Dr. PETER E. POCHI, Boston. (With 22 Figures) 184

A. Distribution, Regional Variation and Gross Anatomy 184

B. Histology 192

C. Histochemistry 195
   I. Lipids 196
   II. Other Specific Substances 201
   III. Enzymes 201

D. Ultrastructure of the Human Sebaceous Gland 204
   I. Peripheral Cells 205
   II. Partially Differentiated Cells 210
   III. Fully Differentiated Cells 216

E. Sebaceous Glands in Mucous Membranes and Ectopic Sites 216
   I. Lip and Oval Mucosae 217
   II. External Genitalia 218
      1. Female 218
      2. Male 218
   III. Nipple 218
   IV. Eyelids 218
   V. Salivary Glands 218
   VI. Miscellaneous Sites 219

F. Growth and Proliferation of the Glands 219

References 220

Eccrine Sweat Glands: Elektron Microscopy; Cytochemistry and Anatomy. By Prof. Dr. RICHARD A. ELLIS, Providence. (With 23 Figures) 224

Introduction 224
   I. Development of the Eccrine Sweat Glands 225
   II. The Secretory Tubule 230
      1. Myoepithelial Cells 230
         a) Electron Microscopy 231
         b) Cytochemistry 235
         c) Function 236

    2. Clear Cells 237
        a) Electron Microscopy 237
        b) Cytochemistry 241
        c) Function 243
    3. Dark Cells 244
        a) Electron Microscopy 245
        b) Cytochemistry 247
        c) Function 248
  III. The Intradermal Sweat Duct 249
    1. Basal Cells 250
        a) Electron Microscopy 250
        b) Cytochemistry 252
        c) Function 253
    2. Superficial Cells 254
        a) Electron Microscopy 254
        b) Cytochemistry 256
        c) Function 257
  IV. The Epidermal Sweat Duct 258
        a) Electron Microscopy 258
        b) Cytochemistry 260
   V. Vascularization of the Eccrine Sweat Glands 261
  VI. Innervation of Eccrine Sweat Glands 262
References 263

Apokrine Schweißdrüsen. Von Prof. Dr. Otto Braun-Falco, München, und Dr. M. Rupec, Marburg. (Mit 46 Abbildungen, davon 1 farbig) 267
A. Historischer Überblick und Embryonalentwicklung 267
    I. Historischer Überblick 267
   II. Die Embryonalentwicklung 268
B. Die Struktur der apokrinen Schweißdrüsen 271
    I. Lokalisation und makroskopische Anatomie 271
   II. Mikroskopische Anatomie 275
    1. Der sekretorische Abschnitt 275
        a) Drüsenzellen 275
        b) Die Zellen des sog. hellen intermediären Abschnittes 279
        c) Die Myoepithelzellen 279
        d) Die Basalmembran 280
        e) Lumeninhalt 281
        f) Altersbedingte Veränderungen 282
        g) Die Innervation 284
    2. Der Ausführungsgang 284
    3. Postmortale Veränderungen 285
  III. Elektronenmikroskopische Anatomie 287
    1. Die apokrinen Drüsenzellen 287
    2. Die Myoepithelzellen 301
    3. Die Zellen des sog. hellen intermediären Abschnittes 304
    4. Ausführungsgang 304
C. Die Histochemie der apokrinen Schweißdrüsen 305
    I. Nucleinsäuren 305
   II. Proteine 305
  III. Lipide 306
   IV. Kohlenhydrate 307
    V. Eisen 309
   VI. Enzyme des energieliefernden Stoffwechsels 311
    1. Enzyme der Glykolyse 312
    2. Glycerin-1-Phosphat-Dehydrogenase (GDH) und Glycerin-1-Phosphat-
       Oxydase (GPOX) 314
    3. Malic Enzym (ME) 315
    4. Enzyme des Pentosephosphat-Cyclus 315

      5. Enzyme des Citronensäure-Cyclus 316
      6. Enzyme der Atmungskette 318
  VII. Weitere Dehydrogenasen 320
  VIII. Monoaminooxydase (MOA) 321
  IX. Hydrolytische Enzyme 321
      1. Esterasen 321
         a) Cholinesterasen 321
         b) Aliesterasen 322
      2. Phosphomonoesterasen 322
      3. Adenosintriphosphatase 324
      4. Thiaminpyrophosphatase 324
      5. β-Glucuronidase 325
      6. Leucinaminopeptidase 325
      7. Chondrosulphatase 325
D. Über den Sekretionsmodus der apokrinen Schweißdrüsen 325
E. Über hormonelle Einflüsse auf apokrine Schweißdrüsen 328
Literatur 330

Normale Histologie und Histochemie des Nagels. Von Prof. Dr. med. GEORGES ACHTEN,
  Brüssel. (Mit 34 Abbildungen) 339
Einleitung 339
A. Anatomie des Nagels 340
  I. Die Nageleinheit 340
      1. Nagelmatrix 341
      2. Nagelplatte 342
      3. Periunguiale Gewebe 342
         a) Die Nagelfurchen 342
         b) Das Eponychium 342
         c) Das Hyponychium 342
         d) Die Fingerkuppe 342
  II. Der Altersnagel 342
B. Embryologie 342
  I. Makroskopische Untersuchung 343
  II. Mikroskopische Untersuchung 344
      1. Der Nagel und seine Matrix 345
      2. Das Nagelbett (Hyponychium) 346
      3. Das Periunguiale Gewebe 346
         a) Das Eponychium 346
         b) Das Hyponychium 347
         c) Die Fingerbeere 347
         d) Lederhaut und Subcutis 348
      4. Die drei Nagelschichten 348
C. Histologie 349
  I. Der Nagel und seine Matrix 349
  II. Das Nagelbett (Hyponychium) 351
  III. Das Periunguiale Gewebe 352
      1. Eponychium 352
      2. Hyponychium 353
      3. Fingerbeere 353
      4. Lederhaut 354
      5. Gefäßversorgung 354
      6. Innervation 357
  IV. Der Altersnagel 360
D. Histochemie 361
  I. Nagelmatrix 361
  Nagelbett (Hyponychium) 361
  Periunguiale Gewebe 361
      1. Das Glykogen 361

2. Die Mucopolysaccharide 362
   a) Basalmembran und Corium 363
   b) Intercellularräume der Epidermis 363
3. Ribonucleinsäure 364
4. Die Enzyme 365
   a) Saure Phosphatasen 365
   b) Alkalische Phosphatasen 366
   c) Cholinesterasen 366
   d) Amylo-Phosphorylase 367
   Schlußfolgerungen 368
II. Der eigentliche Nagel 369
1. PAS-positive Substanzen 369
2. Basophilie 370
3. Proteine mit Sulfhydrylgruppen 370
   Schlußfolgerungen 371
4. Elektronische Mikroskopie 373
Literatur 374

Zur Innervation der Haut. Von Frau Prof. Dr. E. HAGEN, Bonn. (Mit 47 Abbildungen) . 377
Einleitung 377
Methoden 377
1. Epidermale Nerven 378
2. Das subepidermale Nervengeflecht 389
3. Gefäßnerven 398
4. Spezifisch gebaute, sensible Nervenformationen 400
   a) Der Nervenapparat des Haares 400
   b) Sensible Endkörperchen 411
Literatur 423

Die normale Histologie von Corium und Subcutis. Von Prof. Dr. W. SCHMIDT, München.
(Mit 22 Abbildungen) 430
A. Die Bauelemente des Bindegewebes von Corium und Subcutis 430
   I. Die zelligen Bestandteile des Bindegewebes 430
      1. Fibrocyten und Fibroblasten 431
      2. Histiocyten 434
      3. Gewebsmastzellen 436
      4. Plasmazellen 438
      5. Die Reticulumzelle und Fettzelle 439
   II. Die Fasern des Bindegewebes 439
       Entstehung des Kollagens und Bildung der kollagenen Fibrille 440
       1. Die argyrophile Faser 443
       2. Die kollagene Faser 445
       3. Die elastische Faser 447
   III. Die Grundsubstanz 450
B. Aggregationsweise der Bauteile und Gewebebildung 453
   Fettgewebe und Fettorgane 455
   1. Die Primitivorgane 455
   2. Das Gewebe univacuolärer Fettzellen 455
   3. Das Gewebe plurivacuolärer Fettzellen 456
   4. Cyto- und histochemische Unterschiede von weißem und braunem Fett . . 456
   5. Fettgewebe oder Fettorgane 458
   6. Die funktionelle Bedeutung des subcutanen Fettgewebes 458
   7. Vorgänge bei der Speicherung und Entspeicherung 459
C. Mikroskopische und submikroskopische Anatomie von Corium und Subcutis 461
   I. Die Basalmembran 461
   II. Das Corium 465
      1. Das Stratum papillare 465
      2. Das Stratum reticulare 470
      3. Das Corium als Ganzes 471

III. Die Subcutis 474
    Der Einbau der Gefäße in Subcutis und Corium 478
IV. Die Muskulatur der Haut 479
    1. Glatte Muskulatur 479
    2. Skeletmuskulatur 482
    3. Die myoepithelialen Zellen 482
Literatur 482

The Blood Vessels of the Skin. By Prof. Dr. GUISEPPE MORETTI, Genova. (With 165 Figures, of which are 10 in Colour) 491

A. Introduction 491
  I. General Considerations 491
  II. Historical Considerations 493
  III. Technical Considerations 495
    1. Capillaroscopic Methods 496
    2. Injection Methods 497
    3. Histological Methods 498
    4. Histochemical Methods 498
    5. Physical Methods 498
B. Notes on Comparative Anatomy, Embryology, and Prenatal and Postnatal Development of Cutaneous Blood Vessels 499
  I. General Observations 499
  II. Indications From Comparative Embryology and Comparative Anatomy in Mammals (Excluding Man) 500
    1. The Order Chioptera 503
    2. The Order Primates 505
    3. The Order Lagomorpha 506
    4. The Order Rodentia 507
    5. The Order Carnivora 507
    6. The Order Cetacea 508
    7. The Order Perissodactyla 508
    8. The Order Artiodactyla 510
  III. Embryology, Prenatal, and Postnatal Development of the Vessel Network in Man 511
C. Building Stones for the Cutaneous Blood Vessel Network 517
  I. Introductory Observations 517
  II. Arteries and Arterioles 517
    1. Artery types 517
    2. Arterioles: Types and Distributive Characteristics 519
    3. The Structure of the Arteries and Arterioles 523
    4. The Transition of the Arteries into Arterioles and of these into Capillaries . . 524
    5. The Histochemistry and Electron Microscopy of the Arterioles . . 525
  III. The Capillaries 529
    1. Definition and General Characteristics 529
    2. Papillary Loops 533
    3. Structure of the Capillaries 534
    4. Histochemistry of the Capillaries 536
    5. Electron Microscopy of the Capillaries 539
  IV. The Venules and Veins of the Skin 546
    1. Types of Venules and Veins 546
    2. The structure of the Venules and Veins 547
    3. Histochemistry and Electron Microscopy of Venules 550
  V. Arteriovenous Anastomosis (AVA) 551
    1. Types of Anastomoses 551
    2. Number and Size of Anastomoses 552
    3. Structure of the Arteriovenous Anastomoses 553
    4. Histochemistry of the Arteriovenous Anastomoses 556
  VI. Notes on the Biological Modifications of the Blood Vessels in the Skin 558
    1. Indications on the Periodic or Permanent Regeneration of Cutaneous Vessels 558
    2. Notes on the Histochemistry and Electron Microscopy of Neoformed Vessels 559
    3. Indications of Degenerative Phenomena in the Cutaneous Blood Network . . 563

VII. The Nerves of the Cutaneous Blood Vessels 564
  1. General Principles 564
  2. The Nerves of the Arteries and Arterioles, Veins and Venules and Arteriovenous Anastomoses 565
  3. The Problem of Capillary Innervation 566
D. The Architecture of the Cutaneous Blood Network 567
  I. General Observations 567
  II. The Distribution of the Arterial Vessels in the Subcutaneous and in the Dermis (apart from the Appendages) 567
    1. Networks Formed in the Subcutaneous 567
    2. Regional Aspects of the "Cutaneous" and "Fascial" Network 568
    3. Networks Formed in the Dermis 572
    4. Regional Aspects of the Dermal Networks 575
  III. The Distribution of Arterioles and Capillaries Around the Appendages 580
    1. Periglandular Networks 581
    2. Perifollicular Networks, their Static and Dynamic Aspects 583
    3. The Vascular Unit 590
    4. Smooth Muscles 594
    5. Nerve Structures 594
  IV. The Distribution of the Venous Vessels in the Dermis and Subcutaneous (Appendages Included) 595
    1. Networks Formed in the Dermis and Subcutaneous Tissue 595
    2. The Veins and Venules of the Appendages 597
    3. Regional Aspects and Factors which May Influence the Appearance of the Veins and Cutaneous Venules 598
    4. Smooth Muscles 598
    5. Nerve Structures 598
  V. Arteriovenous Anastomosis of the Dermis 598
E. An Outline of the Blood Cutaneous Network Design 599
  I. Preliminary Remarks 599
  II. How the Blood Vessel Cutaneous Network was Envisaged before Spalteholz . . 599
  III. Spalteholz's View of the Blood Network 600
  IV. The Modern Conception of the Cutaneous Blood Network 602
F. Conclusions 607
References 609

Embryologie der Haut. Von Prof. Dr. med. HERMANN PINKUS, Detroit, und Dr. med. ANTOINETTE TANAY, Detroit. (Mit 37 Abbildungen) 624
Einleitung 624
A. Entwicklung der Epidermis 625
  1. Allgemeines 625
  2. Ultrastruktur 628
  3. Histochemie 631
  4. Topographische Unterschiede 633
  5. Epidermis der Neugeborenen 636
B. Entwicklung des Coriums und des Fettgewebes 636
  1. Allgemeines 636
  2. Fasern und Zellen 638
  3. Basalmembran 639
  4. Blut- und Lymphgefäße 639
  5. Subcutanes Fettgewebe 640
  6. Histochemie 641
C. Entwicklungsmechanik der menschlichen Haut 641
D. Der Haarkomplex 644
  I. Morphologische Entwicklung 644
    1. Frühe Stadien 644
    2. Entwicklung der verschiedenen Teile 650
      a) Der Bulbus 650
      b) Unterer Follikelabschnitt 652

c) Wulst 653
d) Isthmus 653
e) Talgdrüse 653
f) Infundibulum 653
g) Haarkanal 653
h) Haar und innere Wurzelscheide 655
i) Arrector-Muskel 656
k) Apokrine Drüse 657
II. Topographische Entwicklung der Haare 658
III. Histochemie 659
IV. Quantitative Daten über fetale Haarkomplexe 660
V. Spezialisierte Drüsen 661
  1. Freie und spezialisierte Talgdrüsen 661
  2. Mammaregion 661
  3. Gehörgang und Nasenvorhof 663
E. Ekkrine Drüsen 663
  1. Allgemeines 663
  2. Ultrastruktur 665
  3. Histochemie 665
  4. Quantitative Daten und Drüsen des Neugeborenen 668
F. Nagel 669
  1. Allgemeines 669
  2. Histochemie 673
  3. Ultrastruktur 673
G. Nerven und andere Neuralleisten-Abkömmlinge 673
  1. Frühstadium 673
  2. Nerven der Finger- und Zehenbeeren 674
  3. Melanocyten und Langerhanssche Zellen 676
H. Schlußbemerkungen 677
Literatur 677

Die Altersveränderungen der Haut. Von Dozent Dr. med. H. J. Cramer, Erfurt. (Mit 7 Abbildungen) 683
Einleitung 683
1. Über Unterschiede der Altersveränderungen an bedeckter und unbedeckter Haut . 684
2. Dicke der Haut 686
3. Epidermis 686
4. Pigmentierung 691
5. Corium 691
6. Glatte Muskulatur 695
7. Talgdrüsen 695
8. Ekkrine Schweißdrüsen 696
9. Apokrine Schweißdrüsen 696
10. Die Brustdrüse 698
11. Haar und Haarfollikel 698
12. Nägel 699
13. Blutgefäße 700
14. Lymphgefäße 702
15. Nerven 702
16. Fettgewebe 703
17. Unterschiede durch Geschlecht, Konstitution und Rasse 703
Literatur 705

Hautveränderungen an Leichen. Von Prof. Dr. med. G. Dotzauer, Köln, und Dr. L. Tamáska, Köln. (Mit 22 Abbildungen, davon 5 farbig) 708
Einleitung und Problemstellung 708
I. Die Haut der frühen Leichenzeit 708
  1. Algor 708
  2. Palor 710

3. Livores 710
   a) Differentialdiagnose zwischen Cyanose und Totenflecken 714
   b) Postmortale Reoxydation der Livores 714
   c) Differentialdiagnose vitaler und postmortaler Blutungen 715
4. Postmortale Gewebswasserverschiebung 718
5. pH-Wasserstoffionenkonzentration 718
6. Autolyse 718
7. Rigor 722
8. Fettstarre 724
9. Vertrocknung der Haut 724
   a) Regulation des Wassergehaltes der intakten Haut, der sichtbaren Schleimhäute 724
      α) Vertrocknungen der intakten Haut und der sichtbaren Schleimhäute in der Agone 724
      β) Vertrocknung der intakten Haut und der Schleimhäute post mortem . . 725
   b) Vertrocknung der versehrten Haut 727
      α) Vertrocknung der Epidermis nach vitalen Verletzungen 727
      β) Vertrocknungen der Haut nach agonalen Verletzungen 727
      γ) Vertrocknungen nach postmortalen Verletzungen 728
   c) Vertrocknungen der Haut nach Einwirkung von Nekrophagen 728
10. Indentitätfeststellung über die Haut in der frühen Leichenzeit 728
II. Die Haut und Anhangsgebilde in der späteren Leichenzeit 730
1. Putrifikation 730
2. Dekomposition 733
3. Nekrophagen 733
   a) Fauna 734
   b) Flora 735
4. Mumifikation 739
5. Saponifikation (Fettwachsbildung) 741
   a) Die Haut in feuchtem Milieu 741
   b) Die Haut in feuchtem Milieu nach dem Tode 742
   c) Wasserleiche: Direkte Einwirkung des Wassers 742
6. Moormumifikation 749
7. Indentitätsfeststellung über die Haut in der späteren Leichenzeit 751
III. Gewalteinwirkungen auf die Haut einer Leiche 752
1. Abgrenzung gegenüber agonalen wie vitalen Prozessen 752
2. Stumpfe Gewalt 755
   a) Druckanämie 756
   b) Hautblutungen 756
   c) Hautabschürfungen 757
3. Stich-, Schnitt- und Hiebverletzungen an der Leichenhaut 760
4. Schußverletzung 764
   a) Fernschuß 764
   b) Nahschuß (relativer Nahschuß) 765
   c) Einschuß bei aufgesetzter Waffe (absoluter Nahschuß) 766
   d) Ausschußverletzungen 767
5. Verbrennung 768
6. Verbrühung 772
7. Verätzung der Leichenhaut 773
8. Strom- und stromähnliche Veränderungen der Leichenhaut 774
9. Die postmortale percutane Resorption von Gasen 778

Literatur 780

B. Allgemeine Pathologie

Allgemeine Pathologie des Fettgewebes. Von Priv.-Doz. Dr. GÜNTER EHLERS, Gießen.
(Mit 15 Abbildungen) 787
I. Vorbemerkungen 787
II. Anatomie des Fettgewebes 788
III. Atrophien der Haut unter besonderer Berücksichtigung des Fettgewebes . . 789
Definition und Einteilung 789
1. Primäre, physiologisch bedingte Atrophien, Atrophia cutis senilis 790

2. Sekundäre, degenerativ bedingte Atrophien 790
   a) Inanitionsatrophie 790
   b) Inaktivitätsatrophie 791
   c) Mechanisch bedingte Atrophie (Druckatrophie) 791
   d) Neurotrophisch bedingte Atrophie 792
3. Sekundäre, entzündlich bedingte Atrophien 793
   a) Atrophien nach allergischen, toxischen oder infektiösen Prozessen 793
   b) Umschriebene, entzündlich bedingte Atrophien 794
IV. Entzündliche und vorwiegend gefäßbedingte Erkrankungen des Fettgewebes . . 795
   1. Patho-Histologie der Erkrankungen des subcutanen Fettgewebes 795
      a) Erythema nodosum 796
      b) Erythema induratum Bazin 798
      c) Nodular Vasculitis 799
      d) Sarcoid Darier-Roussy 800
      e) Spontanpanniculitis Typ Pfeifer-Weber-Christian 800
      f) Spontanpanniculitis Typ Rothmann-Makai 802
      g) Panniculitis subacuta nodosa migrans 803
      h) Spontan auftretende Fettgewebsnekrosen und Fettgranulome 803
      i) Traumatogene Fettgewebsnekrose 803
      j) Fettgewebsnekrose der Brustdrüse 803
      k) Medikamentöse Lipodystrophie 804
      l) Sclerema neonatorum 805
      m) Adiponecrosis subcutanea neonatorum 806
      n) Necrosis progressiva subcutanea neonatorum 808
   2. Patho-Histologie vorwiegend gefäßbedingter Erkrankungen des subcutanen Fettgewebes 808
      a) Periarteriitis nodosa-Gruppe 809
      b) Necrobiosis lipoidica 814
      c) Necrobiosis maculosa 815
      d) Granulomatosis disciformis chronica et progressiva 815
      e) Lipogranulomatosis subcutanea hypertonica Gottron 816
      f) Pingranliquose 817
V. Tumoren des subcutanen Fettgewebes 818
   1. Gutartige Tumoren 820
      a) Lipoblastoma cutis 820
      b) Fibrolipom — Angiolipom 820
      c) Hämangioblastom 821
      d) Hibernom 821
      e) Naevus lipomatosus cutaneus superficialis Hoffmann-Zurhelle 823
   2. Bösartige Tumoren 823
      a) Liposarkom 823
      b) Hibernoma malignum 824
   3. Reticulo-histiocytäre Tumoren, systemische Erkrankungen und Metastasen des subcutanen Fettgewebes 824
VI. Experimentelle Pathologie des Fettgewebes 826
VII. Ätiologie und Pathogenese der Fettgewebserkrankungen 832
VIII. Zusammenfassende Besprechung 839
Literatur 843

Ablagerung und Speicherung in der Cutis. Von Doz. Dr. CHRISTOPH EBERHARTINGER, Wien, Dr. HERWIG EBNER, Wien, und Dr. GUSTAV NIEBAUER, Wien 862
Einleitung 862
I. Amyloide 862
II. Hyalin 868
III. Mucin 874
   1. Hyalinosis cutis et mucosae Urbach-Wiethe (Lipoidproteinose) 870
   2. Pseudomilium colloidale (Pellizari) 872
IV. Lipide 880
   1. Intracellulär 881
      a) Xanthom 881
      b) Histiocytose (Lichtenstein, Lever). Xanthogranulomatose 882
      c) Angiokeratoma corporis diffusum Fabry 884

	2. Extracellulär	884
	a) Necrobiosis lipoidica	884
	b) Extracelluläre Cholesterinose Kerl-Urbach	885
V.	Glykogen	885
VI.	Kalk	887
VII.	Urate	888
VIII.	Melanin	889
IX.	Porphyrine	892
X.	Ablagerungen von Eisen (Hämosiderin)	895
XI.	Carotinoide	897
XII.	Silber	898
XIII.	Gold	900
XIV.	Fremdkörper	900

Literatur 901

Vergleichende Histologie der Haut. Von Prof. Dr. H. U. KOECKE, Köln. (Mit 21 Abbildungen, davon 1 farbig) 920

Einleitung 920
    Die Feinstruktur des Integumentes bei den Chordata 921
  I. Grundzüge des Aufbaues der Chordatenhaut 921
 II. Die Haut der Acrania 922
III. Die Haut der Craniota (Vertebrata) 927
    1. Cyclostomata (Rundmäuler) 927
        a) Neunaugen (Petromyzonidae) 927
        b) Schleimaale (Myxinidae) 936
    2. Chondrichthyes (Knorpelfische) 941
        a) Der Bau der Haut 941
        b) Der physiologische Farbwechsel 946
        c) Das Seitenlinien-System, Funktion und Bedeutung als Fern-Tastsinnesorgan 951
    3. Teleostei (Knochenfische) 956
    4. Amphibia (Lurche) 969
        a) Der Bau der Haut und die Bildung der Basalmembran 969
        b) Die Veränderungen während der Metamorphose 986
    5. Reptilia (Kriechtiere) 987
    6. Vögel 997

Literatur 1015
    Anhang 1029
        Die Haut der Säugetiere; ausgewählte Literatur 1029

Namenverzeichnis 1034
Sachverzeichnis 1085

B. Allgemeine Pathologie
Allgemeine Pathologie des Fettgewebes
Von

G. Ehlers, Gießen

Mit 15 Abbildungen

I. Vorbemerkungen

Während seit der zusammenfassenden Publikation WERTHEIMERs und SHIPAROs aus dem Jahre 1948 der Physiologie des Fettgewebes mehr Beachtung entgegengebracht wurde, befindet sich das Gebiet der Pathologie des menschlichen Fettgewebes in seinen Anfängen. Diese Feststellung muß darauf zurückgeführt werden, daß es bisher nicht möglich war, pathogenetische Vorgänge bei krankhaften Veränderungen des Fettgewebes zu erfassen. Spezielle Untersuchungen, beispielsweise über eine Störung der Glucoseaufnahme, die Lipolyse, die Lipoprotein-Lipaseaktivität bei Glyceridaufnahme, die Bildung der Fettsäuren u.ä., sind bisher nicht bekannt geworden. Es ist jedoch zu unterstellen, daß bestimmte Stoffwechselstörungen auf genetisch bedingte Stoffwechselaberrationen des Fettgewebes selbst zurückzuführen sind. Diese Auffassung beruht auf Untersuchungen von STAUFFACHER; CROFFORD; RENAUD; RENOLD u. CAHILL; CAHILL u. RENOLD.

Bei der Durchsicht der zugängigen Literatur ist zu erkennen, daß zahlreiche Probleme im Hinblick auf die Pathologie des Fettgewebes einer weiteren Klärung bedürfen. Möglicherweise könnten Untersuchungen über die Regulation des Energiestoffwechsels von Zellen des Menschen im allgemeinen auch zu einem besseren Verständnis pathologischer Stoffwechselvorgänge im Fettgewebe beitragen.

Im vorliegenden Beitrag kann auf die Anatomie und Physiologie des Fettgewebes nicht näher eingegangen werden. Es wird von dermatologischer Seite auf entsprechende Originalien und Handbuchartikel von GANS und STEIGLEDER; SCHUPPLI; HORSTMANN; STEIGLEDER; BRAUN-FALCO u.a. aufmerksam gemacht. Das bearbeitete Kapitel wird des weiteren dadurch begrenzt, daß die akut- und chronisch-entzündlichen Erkrankungen sowie die Tumoren des Fettgewebes größtenteils in bereits erschienenen Bänden dieses Handbuches abgehandelt wurden. Das mikromorphologische Substrat von Dermatosen der genannten Krankheitsgruppen wird, vom histologischen Symptom ausgehend, besprochen oder, soweit von anderer Seite bereits erörtert, zum besseren Verständnis nochmals kurz umrissen, so daß Überschneidungen nicht zu umgehen sind. Nach Besprechung der pathologischen Veränderungen im Bereich der Subcutis soll der Versuch unternommen werden, aufgrund der in der Literatur bekannten experimentellen Untersuchungen und der Auswertung der klinischen und histologischen Morphologie der entsprechenden Krankheitszustände eine Deutung der eingeschränkten Reaktion des Fettgewebes auf Schädigungen unterschiedlicher Art vorzunehmen.

II. Anatomie des Fettgewebes

Das Unterhautfettgewebe, als sog. ,,Primitivorgan" angelegt, besteht aus einer losen Anhäufung von Fettzellen, welche sich zu Fettgewebsläppchen zusammenlagern. Im Cytoplasma der Fettzellen finden sich neben Mitochondrien zahlreiche Ribosomen. Weniger stark ausgebildet als bei anderen Zellen ist das endoplasmatische Reticulum. Durch die Fettvacuole wird der Zellkern an die Zellperipherie gedrängt. Die Zellen stehen mit einem dichten Capillarnetz in Verbindung. Zwischen der Plasma- und Basalmembran einer Fettzelle und der Basalmembran des Gefäßes findet sich der Perivascularraum, über welchen der Stoffaustausch stattfindet (SIMON; BALBONI; SHELDON; SHELDON, HOLLENBERG u. WINIGRAD; NAPOLITANO; WILLIAMSON; WASSERMANN; PLENERT; WASSERMANN u. MCDONALD). Neben den Fettzellen kommen im Fettgewebe auch Histiocyten zur Beobachtung. Höher gelegene Fettzellgruppen sind um die Hautanhangsgebilde angeordnet. Diese Zellen sollen sich färberisch (Sudan III-Färbung) von den Fettzellen der Subcutis unterscheiden (GRÜTZ).

Die Fettgewebsläppchen werden von Fettgewebssepten, einem Gerüst von Bindegewebsfasern, getragen. Des weiteren lassen sich Gitterfasern (HOFFMANN) nachweisen, die insbesondere auch in den Fettgewebsläppchen anzutreffen sind. Den Gitterfasern wird von LAUBINGER eine besondere funktionelle Bedeutung beigemessen. Die Septen lassen enge Beziehungen zur Cutis erkennen. Die Blutversorgung erfolgt durch eine retrograde Strömung vom unteren cutanen Gefäßplexus aus.

Von Bedeutung, insbesondere zum Verständnis pathologischer Veränderungen im Fettgewebe, ist die Anordnung der Blutgefäße. Neben größeren finden sich auch hier kleinere arterielle Gefäße, Arteriolen, Capillaren sowie venöse Abflußgebiete. Das capillare Strombahnnetz ist jedoch weniger dicht angeordnet als in anderen parenchymatösen Organen; die Capillarmaschen liegen weiter auseinander. Nach GOTTRON ist somit die ,,Zweiphasigkeit der physiologischen Blutdurchströmung, wie sie der Wechsel zwischen Fluxion und Ischämie darstellt, kaum gegeben".

WEISS; POPOFF u. POPOFF machten darauf aufmerksam, daß in der Subcutis vor und nach der Geburt weiße Blutkörperchen, im Frühembryonalstadium auch Erythrocyten gebildet werden können. STEIGLEDER dagegen erscheint es unsicher, ob sich Blutzellen aus differenzierten Fettzellen zu entwickeln vermögen und mißt den pericapillären Elementen eine größere Bedeutung zur Blutbildung bei (s. auch POPOFF und POPOFF; HOFFMANN).

Der Tela subcutanea muß neben rein mechanischen oder physikalischen Funktionen (Verschieblichkeit gegenüber der Muskulatur, Druckpolster, Wärmeschutz) eine wichtige Rolle im *Allgemeinstoffwechsel* zugesprochen werden (WERTHEIMER). Diese besteht sowohl in der Synthese als auch im Abbau von Fettsubstanzen. Aufgrund neuerer Untersuchungen findet der Auf- und Abbau in der Zelle über den Capillarraum statt. Der Triglycerid-Umsatz wurde besonders am Fettgewebe studiert. Freie Fettsäuren und freies Glycerin des Blutplasmas stammen überwiegend aus der Lipolyse des Fettgewebes. Der Abbau der Fette erfolgt durch Lipasen, welche die Neutralfette in Glycerin und Fettsäuren spalten. Es kann als gesichert angesehen werden, daß nicht mit Glycerin veresterte Fettsäuren frei im Blutplasma vorkommen, aber auch an bisher nicht bekannte Träger gekoppelt werden. Der Transport der Lipide im Blutplasma erfolgt nach Kopplung derselben an Proteine in Form der Lipoproteide. Chylomikronen wurden im Pericapillarraum bisher nicht nachgewiesen. Das durch Lipolyse im Fettgewebe freigesetzte Glycerin kann bei der Synthese von Glucose und Fructose Verwendung finden

(s. KIMMIG und WEHRMANN). Für die Biosynthese von Triglyceriden im Fettgewebe ist das freigesetzte Glycerin nicht wieder verwendbar; das Fettgewebe ist auf die Glykolyse angewiesen (THIELE). Die Synthese der Fettsäuren findet aufgrund von Untersuchungen mit C_{13}-markierten Vorstufen der Fettsäuren vorwiegend im Fettgewebe selbst (SHAPIRO; WERTHEIMER), weniger in der Leber statt (FAVARGER u. Mitarb.). Den Ausgangspunkt der Biosynthese von Fetten stellen die Kohlenhydrate dar. Nach der Entdeckung des Coenzyms A durch LYNEN u. Mitarb. konnte die Fettsäuresynthese geklärt werden (zur chemischen Struktur und zum Stoffwechsel der Lipide s. O. W. THIELE, 1967).

Die Fette der Subcutis bestehen vorwiegend aus Neutralfetten, den Triglyceriden der Stearin-, Palmitin- und Ölsäure. Nach CRAMER u. BRAUN sind die Myristinsäure, Laurinsäure und die ungesättigten Fettsäuren Linolen- und Arachidonsäure nur in sehr geringem Maße am Aufbau der Fette beteiligt. Die Fettsubstanzen werden als Depotfette in den Zellen abgelagert. Die Menge der Depotfette ist abhängig von der Nahrung, der Fettgewebslokalisation und dem Geschlecht (SCHAFFER; GOLDNER; MEYER u. CHAFFEE; TAYLOR u. Mitarb.; HERRMANN u. PROSE; WERTHEIMER; BALÓ; SINAPIUS).

Jedes Individuum wird wahrscheinlich nicht mit einer genetisch determinierten Anzahl von potentiellen Fettzellen geboren. Eine Zunahme der Fettreserven geht sowohl mit einer Vergrößerung als auch der zahlenmäßigen Zunahme der Fettzellen einher (RENOLD). Der unterschiedliche Fettansatz an verschiedenen Körperregionen und die ungleichmäßige Fettentspeicherung erklären sich aus den zuvor erläuterten Gesichtspunkten.

Das entspeicherte subcutane Fettgewebe wird dem ursprünglichen retikulären Gewebsverband wieder ähnlich. Bisher ist es nicht bewiesen oder wenig wahrscheinlich, daß Fettzellen die Pluripotenz ihrer Matrixzellen wieder erlangen können, so daß eine Umwandlung in Zellen des reticulo-histiocytären Systems kaum möglich erscheint (A. HOFFMANN; MICHELSON; GOTTRON, STEIGLEDER u.a.).

III. Atrophien der Haut unter besonderer Berücksichtigung des Fettgewebes

Definition und Einteilung

Unter einer Atrophie wird ein altersbedingter Hautzustand oder ein Folgezustand eines entzündlichen Prozesses verstanden. Die Atrophie des Fettgewebes kommt sowohl durch eine Volumenabnahme der Zellen als auch durch eine zahlenmäßige Verminderung derselben zustande. Die genannten Atrophieformen treten gewöhnlich kombiniert auf und werden von degenerativen Vorgängen begleitet.

Es können primär-intracelluläre den sekundär-extracellulär bedingten Atrophien gegenübergestellt werden (GANS u. STEIGLEDER). Während die erste Form der Atrophie in einer gestörten Assimilationsfähigkeit der Zelle selbst gelegen ist, entwickelt sich die zweite Form nach einer ungenügenden Zufuhr von Kohlenhydraten, Lipoiden und Eiweißkörpern bzw. nach dermal-entzündlichen Prozessen. HAUSER trennt nichtentzündliche Atrophien von solchen nach vorausgegangenen oder gleichzeitig bestehenden entzündlichen Vorgängen im Bereich der Cutis oder Subcutis ab. In Anlehnung an die genannten Autoren unterscheiden wir

1. *Primäre, physiologisch bedingte Atrophien.*
    a) Atrophia cutis senilis.

2. *Sekundäre, degenerativ bedingte Atrophien.*
a) Inanitionsatrophien.
b) Inaktivitätsatrophien.
c) Mechanisch bedingte Atrophien.
d) Neurotrophische Atrophien.
3. *Sekundäre, entzündlich bedingte Atrophien.*
a) Atrophien nach allergischen, toxischen oder infektiösen Prozessen.

Die Einteilung umfaßt ätiologische Faktoren, welche zu einer Atrophie des Fettgewebes führen können, berücksichtigt pathogenetische Vorstellungen, schließt jedoch klinische und histomorphologische Übergänge einzelner Gruppen ineinander nicht aus.

1. Primäre, physiologisch bedingte Atrophien
Atrophia cutis senilis

Die senile Atrophie des Fettgewebes ist gekennzeichnet durch einen Schwund der Fettzellen. Nach WEIDMAN sind diese Veränderungen auf eine Alterung der Zellen des subcutanen Fettgewebes zurückzuführen. Die physiologischen Alterserscheinungen sind in einem Mißverhältnis zwischen Assimilation und Dissimilation einer Zelle zu suchen, wobei deren Genese im Lebensrhythmus der Zellen selbst gelegen ist (STRÖBEL). Außer der Atrophie der Zellen selbst mißt GIERKE auch einer Veränderung der Zwischensubstanz Bedeutung bei. Neben den physiologischen und sekundären Einflüssen müssen konstitutionell-genetische Faktoren, welche ebenfalls berücksichtigt werden sollten, Beachtung finden (RENOLD).

Physiologisch bedingte Atrophien werden von solchen, die durch äußere Einflüsse bedingt sind, unterschieden. Die Abgrenzung der durch physiologisches Altern von Zellen bedingten (primäre Atrophien) von solchen durch äußere Einwirkung entstandenen Atrophien (sekundäre Atrophien) ist nicht immer durchführbar. Fließende Übergänge in pathologische Erscheinungen kommen häufiger vor.

Untersuchungen über Altersveränderungen der Haut unter Berücksichtigung verschiedener Körperregionen wurden von HILL und MONTGOMERY; EJIRI; EVANS, COWDRY und NIELSON; STRÖBEL; PERCIVAL u. Mitarb.; SAALFELD; OPPENHEIM; GOTTRON u.a. durchgeführt. Eine Beurteilung des subcutanen Fettgewebes wurde jedoch nur selten vorgenommen. Sowohl OPPENHEIM als auch STRÖBEL berichteten über einen relativ unvermittelten Übergang zwischen der altersatrophischen Cutis zur Subcutis mit Atrophie des Fettgewebes. Die bindegewebigen Septen ließen neben einer deutlichen Verschmälerung die Aufsplitterung in einzelne Fibrillen erkennen. Die in der Cutis beobachteten degenerativen Erscheinungen am Kollagen, die ,,Entartung" zu Kollazin, wurden auch in den Fettgewebssepten gefunden. Mit zunehmendem Alter war eine Abnahme der Anzahl der subcutan gelegenen Gefäße zu beobachten.

2. Sekundäre, degenerativ bedingte Atrophien
a) Inanitionsatrophie

Bei einer quantitativ oder qualitativ veränderten Ernährung kommt es zur Inanitionsatrophie des Fettgewebes (LUCIANI; ROTHMANN). Der der Hungeratrophie gleichzustellende Marasmus febrilis, der Marasmus bei chronischen Erkrankungen, z.B. der Tuberkulose, oder die Geschwulstkachexie sind ebenfalls auf eine mangelnde Zufuhr bzw. auf einen vermehrten Abbau der Fettsubstanzen zurückzuführen. Die bei der Inanitionsatrophie vorgefundenen Veränderungen der Epidermis sind sekundärer Natur und durch gleichzeitig auftretende Vitaminmangelzustände und toxische Abbauprodukte zu erklären (UNNA; LUCIANI; ROSANOW; ROTHMANN; GANS und STEIGLEDER).

Auf die Möglichkeit der Bedeutung von Inanitionsatrophien für die Entstehung von Reticulo-Endotheliosen hat GOTTRON (1952) hingewiesen. Nach der Entspeicherung von Fettzellen kommt es zur Entwicklung retikulärer Ausläufer an der Zelloberfläche. Das Auftreten einer stärkeren Reticulumfaserbildung und die Wachstumstendenz des retikulären Gewebes könnten Anhaltspunkte für die Häufung von Tumoren des reticulo-histiocytären Systems, insbesondere während der Nachkriegszeit, geben.

CZAJEWICZ und FLEMMING führten histologische Untersuchungen des Fettgewebes an hungernden Tieren durch und wiesen neben einer serösen, einfachen Atrophie eine nur geringe Wucheratrophie mit dem Nachweis mehrerer Zellkerne in der atrophischen Fettzelle nach.

In Weiterverfolgung der Versuche von FLEMMING unterscheidet SCHIDACHI histologisch drei Grade der Atrophie:

α) Seröse Atrophie mit fehlender oder geringer Wucheratrophie.

β) Volumenabnahme der Fettzellen mit seröser Atrophie und von der Peripherie der Fettläppchen zum Zentrum fortschreitende Wucheratrophie.

γ) Bindegewebsähnliche Umwandlung der Fettläppchen mit spindel- oder strangförmiger Anordnung der Zellkerne.

Diese histomorphologischen Befunde wurden von GANS in ihren Grundzügen übernommen. Wie bereits für die Einteilung der Atrophien in primäre und sekundäre Formen besprochen, können jedoch die verschiedenen histologischen Grade der Atrophie nebeneinander vorkommen oder ineinander übergehen, so daß eine Abgrenzung voneinander Schwierigkeiten bereiten kann.

Es erscheint von Interesse, daß bei sekundären Atrophien nach akuten oder chronischen Allgemeinerkrankungen, weniger bei malignen Tumoren oder im Anschluß an experimentell erzeugte Entzündungen gleichartige histomorphologische Befunde erhoben werden konnten (GANS und STEIGLEDER).

b) Inaktivitätsatrophie

Die Inaktivitätsatrophie kommt nach WEIGERT der senilen Atrophie nahe, wobei auch enge Beziehungen zur Inanitionsatrophie bestehen. Die klinische und histologische Morphologie dieser Form der Atrophie entspricht weitgehend der der Inanitionsatrophie. Charakteristische, die Inaktivitätsatrophie kennzeichnende histomorphologische Untersuchungsergebnisse liegen nicht vor (GANS und STEIGLEDER).

Nach WEIGERT ist bei der Inaktivitätsatrophie die Störung der normalen Zellfunktion auf eine Dysregulation zwischen dem Auf- und Abbau der Fettsubstanzen zurückzuführen. Als Folge dieser Störung des Gleichgewichtes von Assimilation und Dissimilation muß eine vorzeitige Alterung der Zelle angenommen werden. Durch die Inaktivität sollen die Zellen in einen Funktionszustand versetzt werden, welcher normalerweise erst im höheren Lebensalter anzutreffen ist.

c) Mechanisch bedingte Atrophie (Druckatrophie)

Mechanisch bedingte Atrophien werden nach Einwirkung von Druck und Zug von außen oder aber bei raumverdrängenden Prozessen, in der Haut durch

Tumoren oder Cysten, hervorgerufen. Pathogenetisch kommt es durch eine partielle Kompression der Blut- und Lymphgefäße zu Ernährungsstörungen des Fettgewebes. Eine nekrotische Umwandlung der den Gefäßen zugeordneten Fettgewebsareale ist nicht beobachtet worden.

Histologisch finden sich eingeengte Capillaren, Arteriolen sowie kleinere und größere arterielle Gefäße des cutanen und subcutanen Gefäßnetzes, die ebenfalls einer Druckatrophie unterliegen können. Die Fettzellen weisen einen Verlust der Fettsubstanzen auf, nehmen an Größe und Zahl ab und werden durch ein von den Indifferenzzonen der Gefäße ausgehendes Bindegewebe ersetzt. Diese Bindegewebszonen lassen zunächst einen lockeren Aufbau mit Nachweis von Histiocyten sowie fibrocytär-fibroblastischen Elementen erkennen. Später überwiegt ein zellarmes Bindegewebe mit kollagenen Fasern, die teilweise einer Hyalinisierung unterliegen und bei raumverdrängenden Prozessen in die Bindegewebskapsel gelegentlich einbezogen werden (GANS und STEIGLEDER).

d) Neurotrophisch bedingte Atrophie

Neurotrophisch bedingte Atrophien werden pathogenetisch mit Störungen des zentralen oder peripheren Nervensystems in Zusammenhang gebracht, wobei neben der Haut die Fascien, die Muskulatur und Skeletanteile in die Atrophie einbezogen werden können. Diese Form der Atrophien wird nach periphertraumatischen Nervenverletzungen, im Anschluß an eine Tabes dorsalis, Syringomyelie, Myelitis, bei Pellagra, Diabetes, Gicht oder Rheumatismus beobachtet (OPPENHEIM; BRÜNAUER; HAUSER).

Den neurotrophischen Atrophien werden hinzugerechnet (OPPENHEIM):
1. Atrophia striata neurotica.
2. Glossy skin and fingers.
3. Hemiatrophia faciei progressiva.

Über histologisch faßbare Veränderungen am Fettgewebe finden sich bei den genannten Erkrankungen nur vereinzelte, zum Teil sich widersprechende Angaben. Während BAUMANN; BRÜNAUER; KIRSCHENBERG über eine Atrophie des subcutanen Fettgewebes bis zum Schwund desselben mit Intimaveränderungen an den kleinen Arterien bei den Glossy skin and fingers sowie der Hemiatrophia faciei progressiva berichten, beschreibt SCHALTENBRAND eine Zunahme der Subcutis infolge einer Schwellung des Fettgewebes. HAUSER fand bei der Hemiatrophia faciei progressiva nur gelegentlich einen Befall des Fettgewebes in Form einer Atrophie. Bei einer eigenen Beobachtung eines Patienten mit einer Hemiatrophia faciei progressiva der rechten Gesichtshälfte (EHLERS, 1960) konnte eine normale strukturelle Ausgestaltung des Fettgewebes gefunden werden. Eine Atrophie war nicht nachweisbar. Die Fettzellen wiesen lediglich einen Verlust ihres Turgors mit gewellten Plasmamembranen auf. Die Fettgewebssepten fanden sich weder verschmälert noch verbreitert, die kollagenen Fasern zeigten bei der Hämatoxylin-Eosin-Färbung eine geringe Verwerfung mit angedeutet metachromatisch blaugrauer Tingierung. Die Wände der kleineren und größeren arteriellen Gefäße des Fettgewebes erschienen mäßig verdickt, lichtungseingeengt, hinsichtlich ihres Aufbaues aber unverändert. Entzündliche Infiltrate konnten weder in den Fettgewebsläppchen noch in den Fettgewebssepten aufgefunden werden.

Bei der Lipodystrophie dagegen läßt sich ein vollständiger Schwund der Fettzellen nachweisen. Entzündliche Zellelemente werden vermißt (GANS u. STEIGLEDER, s. dort weitere Literatur).

3. Sekundäre, entzündlich bedingte Atrophien
a) Atrophien nach allergischen, toxischen oder infektiösen Prozessen

Sekundäre Atrophien stehen am Ende vorangegangener entzündlicher Prozesse der Haut, deren Genese allergisch, toxisch oder infektiös bedingt sein kann. Diese

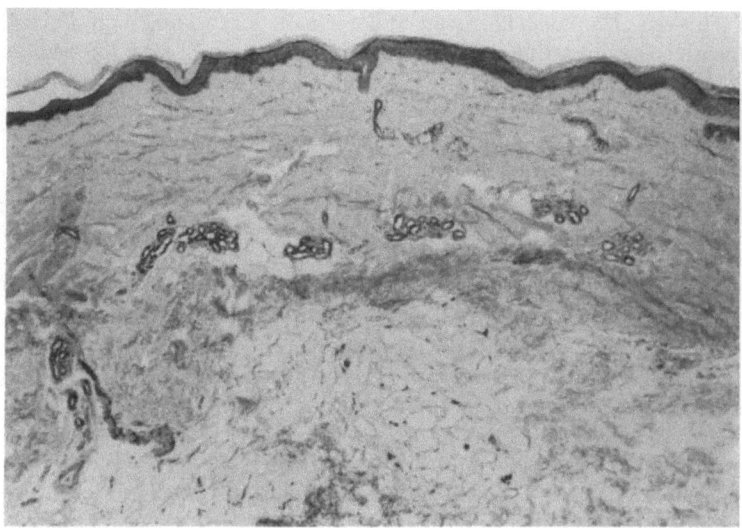

Abb. 1

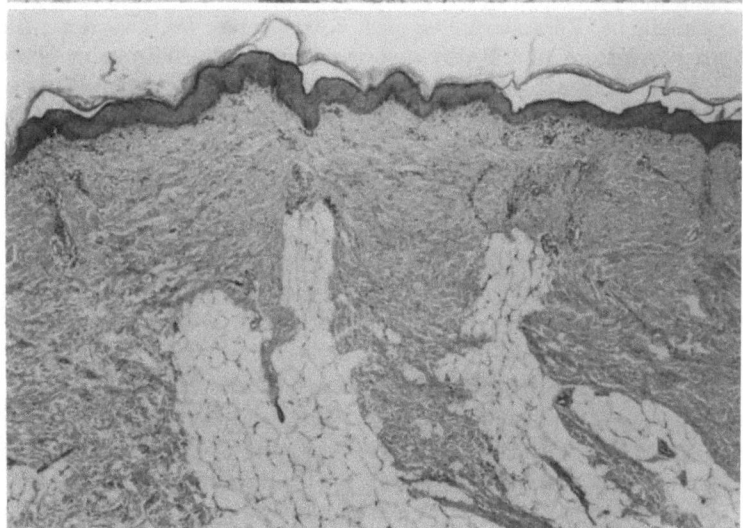

Abb. 2

Abb. 1. Werner-Syndrom. Turgorverlust der Fettzellen mit unregelmäßiger Durchsetzung des Fettgewebes von zarten, locker gefügten Bindegewebsfasern. [Aus: W. KNOTH, R. BAETHKE u. L. HOFFMANN: Hautarzt **14**, 145, 193 (1963), Abb. 11a]

Abb. 2. Rothmund-Syndrom. Vom Corium deutlich abgesetztes Fettgewebe mit gut gefüllten Fettvacuolen und breiten Fettgewebssepten. [Aus: W. KNOTH, R. BAETHKE u. L. HOFFMANN: Hautarzt **14**, 145, 193 (1963), Abb. 11b]

Form der Atrophie wird nach luischen Exanthemen, bei einem Lupus erythematodes, einer Dermatomyositis, dem Lichen ruber planus, der Acrodermatitis chronica atrophicans Pick-Herxheimer, der Anetodermia erythematosa maculosa Jadassohn (Dermatrophia chronica idiopathica maculosa), dem Lichen sclerosus et atrophicus, der sog. Kraurosis vulvae et penis sowie bei Pathothesaurismosen (GOTTRON; BLANC; STEIGER-KAZAL) beobachtet.

Histologisch kommt es zu einer unterschiedlich starken perivasalen chronischen Entzündung mit Untergang von Fettzellen und folgender Granulombildung. Nach GANS und STEIGLEDER können die Gefäßveränderungen mit Durchsetzung der Gefäßwände von Lymphocyten und Granulocyten an eine Periarteriitis nodosa erinnern. Daneben kommen außer einem Untergang von Fettzellen mit nachfolgender Granulombildung multiple disseminierte Steatonekrosen zur Beobachtung. Dies trifft insbesondere für Atrophien bei bestehender Dermatomyositis zu. Im Hinblick auf die übrigen, oben erwähnten Grunderkrankungen treten die akut- oder chronisch-entzündlichen Erscheinungen der Subcutis zurück. Die perivasal oder diffus im Corium angeordneten Rundzellinfiltrate lassen sich jedoch auch hier an zahlreichen Stellen bis in das subcutane Fettgewebe verfolgen. Die Subcutis weist ebenfalls eine deutliche Atrophie auf und nähert sich infolge der gleichzeitig bestehenden Coriumatrophie der Epidermis (BECK; BEHRING; BLANC; BREUCKMANN; DELBANCO; GANS und LANDES; GÖTZ; MONTGOMERY u. Mitarb.; GOTTRON; HAUSER; REICH; STÜHMER; WAINGER u. Mitarb.; WALTHER u.a.).

GOTTRON sah bei der Ablagerung von Amyloid an den Plasmamembranen der Fettzellen keinen Austritt von Fettsubstanzen aus der Zelle. Ölcysten und Lipogranulome wurden ebenfalls nicht gefunden. Dieser Befund steht im Gegensatz zu einer Beobachtung von BLANC, welcher über das gleichzeitige Vorkommen von Amyloid im Fettgewebe und Lipogranulomen als Folge einer Fettgewebsnekrose berichtete. LEVER beschrieb Amyloidablagerungen in Gefäßwänden der Subcutis und um Fettzellen in Mantelform.

Unterschiedliche Veränderungen des Fettgewebes bei Progerie, Akrogerie, beim Werner-Syndrom und Rothmund-Syndrom teilten GOTTRON; BASEX und DUPRÉ; KNOTH u. Mitarb. mit. GOTTRON; BASEX und DUPRÉ; WEBER fanden bei der Akrogerie und Progerie einen Schwund des Fettgewebes in Verbindung mit qualitativen und quantitativen Veränderungen der Fettzellen. Entsprechende Untersuchungen beim Werner-Syndrom durch KNOTH ließen ein turgorarmes, weniger scharf umschriebenes subcutanes Fettgewebe erkennen, welches von locker gefügten bindegewebigen Fasern unregelmäßig durchsetzt war (Abb. 1). Dagegen zeigte sich das Fettgewebe beim Rothmund-Syndrom mit gut gefüllten Fettvacuolen gegenüber dem Corium deutlich abgesetzt. Zellen der chronischen Entzündung fanden sich bei beiden Erkrankungen nur in geringem Ausmaß (Abb. 2).

b) Umschriebene, entzündlich bedingte Atrophien

Von den zuvor besprochenen, das gesamte subcutane Fettgewebe erfassenden Atrophien ist die von ROTHMANN; KRAUS; PICK; PFUHL; BLANC u. a. beschriebene *entzündlich bedingte, umschriebene Atrophie* des subcutanen Fettgewebes abzugrenzen. Diese Abgrenzung ist sowohl aus klinischen als auch aus pathogenetischen Gesichtspunkten heraus erforderlich. Die umschriebenen Atrophien sind sekundärer Natur und als Folge einer vorangegangenen, örtlich begrenzten Entzündung oder Schädigung des subcutanen Fettgewebes durch mechanische, physikalische, chemische, medikamentöse oder bakterielle Einflüsse anzusehen.

Histologisch finden sich strang- oder knotenförmige, gegenüber der Umgebung begrenzte Herde mit einer Volumen- und numerischen Abnahme der Fettzellen bis zum völligen Schwund umschriebener Fettgewebsareale. Mikromorphologisch werden alle Stadien der Atrophie angetroffen. Neben den Zellen der chronischen Entzündung fallen Riesenzellen, Ölcysten und die sog. Wucheratrophie auf. Tuberkuloide Strukturen sind seltener aufzufinden. Das untergegangene Fettgewebe wird nur teilweise durch Bindegewebe ersetzt. Von PFUHL; BLANC wurde dagegen die Wucheratrophie nicht beobachtet. Die genannten Autoren beschreiben einen Untergang der Fettzellen, gefolgt von einwandernden Histiocyten und einer bindegewebigen Sklerosierung der atrophischen Fettgewebsregionen.

IV. Entzündliche und vorwiegend gefäßbedingte Erkrankungen des Fettgewebes

Bei der Erörterung akut oder chronisch entzündlicher Krankheitszustände des subcutanen Fettgewebes müssen primär entzündliche Veränderungen der Subcutis von solchen abgegrenzt werden, welche ihren Ausgang vom Corium nehmen und sekundär auf die Tela subcutanea übergreifen.

Einer gesonderten Besprechung bedürfen solche Erkrankungen, bei denen ätiopathogenetisch die Krankheitsmanifestation an arteriellen und venösen Gefäßen des Fettgewebes im Vordergrund steht. Vorwiegend gefäßbedingte Fettgewebsentzündungen können sowohl akut- als auch chronisch-entzündlicher Natur sein. Die entzündliche Reaktion sowie die dem Trophon zugeordnete Nekrose ist abhängig von der das Gefäß treffenden Noxe, der Abwehrlage des Organismus, dem Ausmaß der Gefäßschädigung sowie der Größe des Restlumens. Bei allmählich einsetzenden, zu einem weitgehenden oder vollständigen Verschluß der Lichtung führenden, nicht entzündlichen Gefäßwandprozessen im Sinne der Endangiosis fibroblastica ist ausschließlich mit der Entwicklung einer resorptiven, granulomatös-tuberkuloiden Entzündung zu rechnen. Dennoch muß hervorgehoben werden, daß die Abgrenzung in akut- und chronisch-entzündliche Formen eine willkürliche ist, da die granulomatöse der akuten Entzündung zu folgen pflegt.

Über nomenklatorische Fragen sowie die Eingruppierung primär im Fettgewebe lokalisierter entzündlicher Veränderungen besteht bis zum gegenwärtigen Zeitpunkt keine einheitliche Auffassung. So stellen Begriffe wie Panniculitis, Lipogranulomatose, Liponekrose, mikrocystische disseminierte Steatonekrose, Dyslipoidose jeweils die gleiche Umschreibung ähnlicher oder identischer patho-histologischer Veränderungen im Bereich des subcutanen Fettgewebes dar.

Es fehlte nicht an Versuchen, die verschiedenen Formen der Fettgewebsentzündung einzuteilen (BAUMGARTNER und RIVA; KOOIJ; GOTTRON; RÖCKL und THIES; GANS und STEIGLEDER u. a.). Im folgenden werden ohne Berücksichtigung ätiologischer Faktoren oder der Erstmanifestation pathologischer Veränderungen die akut- und chronisch-entzündlichen sowie bevorzugt gefäßbedingten Erkrankungen des Fettgewebes besprochen. Die Krankheitsgruppen sind nach dem führenden histologischen Symptom geordnet und zusammengestellt. Es wird der Versuch unternommen, die für die unterschiedlichen Krankheitsbilder charakteristischen histologischen Kriterien herauszustellen, wobei spezielle pathohistologische Befunde, denen möglicherweise eine pathogenetische Bedeutung für die Entwicklung der Erkrankung zukommt, in die Besprechung einbezogen werden.

1. Patho-Histologie der Erkrankungen des subcutanen Fettgewebes

Aufgrund klinischer und histologischer Untersuchungen von 400 Patienten mit einer Vasculitis nodularis wurde von LECZINSKY auf die enge Beziehung des histologischen Befundes zwischen dem Erythema nodosum, dem Erythema induratum Bazin und allergisch bedingten Gefäßkrankheiten hingewiesen (s. auch STÜTTGEN; KNOTH und MEYHÖFER; ORBANEJA und PUCHOL; JABLONSKA;

EBERHARTINGER; FURTADO; PIERINI, ABULAFIA u. WAINFELD u. a.). Bei bestimmten Formen des Erythema nodosum kann der histologische Befund dem des Erythema induratum Bazin oder des Sarkoid Darier-Roussy ähnlich sein.

a) Erythema nodosum

Der Beginn des *Erythema nodosum* ist nach GANS; CAROL, PRACKEN und ZWIJNDREGT; MIESCHER; GOTTRON u. a. an der Cutis-Subcutis-Grenze sowie in den Randpartien der Fettgewebssepten zu suchen. Erst später greifen die entzündlichen Prozesse auf die Fettgewebsläppchen über und sind bis in tiefe Subcutisanteile zu verfolgen. Es kommt zunächst zu einer akuten Entzündung mit Gefäßerweiterung, perivasalem entzündlichem Ödem, Leukocytenemigration und Ansammlung von Lymphocyten in der Gefäßumgebung. Histiocytäre Elemente und eosinophile Leukocyten sind seltener anzutreffen, Plasmazellen fehlen. Das Infiltrat ist herdförmig angeordnet. Abscedierungen und Nekrotisierungen werden im allgemeinen vermißt. In der Umgebung pathologisch veränderter Gefäße der Subcutis kann es jedoch zur Ausbildung von Steatonekrosen, lipophagen Granulomen und epitheloidzelligen Formationen mit Riesenzellen, überwiegend vom Fremdkörpertyp, kommen (CIBILS-AGUIRRE und BRACHETTO-BRIAN; GELLERSTEDT; PICK; CAROL u. Mitarb.). Eine sog. Wucheratrophie ist wenig auffällig oder wird vollständig vermißt (CAROL u. Mitarb.; SCHUPPLI u.a.). Die Fettläppchen können gelegentlich so eingeengt werden, daß nur noch wenige Fettzellgruppen wahrnehmbar sind. Bei älteren Effloreszenzen kommt es in größeren arteriellen Gefäßen zu einer Schwellung der Endothelien mit subendothelialer Proliferation, entzündlich-hämorrhagischer Wandinfiltration, Thrombosierung des Lumens und Erythrocytenextravasation in die Umgebung der Gefäße. Entzündliche Veränderungen auch der Venen in Form einer hochgradigen Phlebitis mit Endothelschwellung, Ansammlung von polynucleären Leukocyten im Lumen sowie in der Venenwand wurden von PHILIPSON; GANS und STEIGLEDER; LEVER beschrieben. Während von vielen Autoren die pathologischen Veränderungen der Arterien und Venen stark hervorgehoben und eine Vasculitis für die Entstehung des Erythema nodosum als primär und prädominierend angesehen wird (GRZYBOWSKI; ROTNES; BERGSTRAND; MALLET; BARTÁK; SHAPOSHNIKOW u.a.), berichten MIESCHER; PAUTRIER und WORINGER sowie LÖFGREN und WAHLGREN über eine nur geringe entzündliche Beteiligung der Gefäße.

Von MIESCHER wurden Radiärknötchen beschrieben, welche für das Erythema nodosum charakteristisch sein sollen (MIESCHER; REICH; GREITHER; LÖFGREN und WAHLGREN; LEVER; DOXIADIS; NUBÉ u.a.) und in frischeren und älteren Effloreszenzen zur Beobachtung gelangen. ORBANEJA und PUCHOL sahen dagegen auch bei der Periarteriitis nodosa granulomatöse Strukturen, die mit den Miescherschen Radiärknötchen identisch waren. Die Radiärknötchen werden an der Corium-Fettgewebsgrenze, in den Bindegewebssepten der Subcutis sowie im Fettgewebe selbst gefunden (VILANOVA u. Mitarb.; VESEY u. WILKINSON; BOCK; JAMES; ITO; SHAPOSHNIKOW; GORDON; BONICELLI u. TAGLIAVINI; VANDEKERCKHOVE; BARTÁK; SCHUPPLI u.a.).

CAROL, PRACKEN und ZWIJNDREGT trennen vom typischen Erythema nodosum Sonderformen mit differierendem pathohistologischem Befund ab. Dem Erythema nodosum mit abweichendem histologischem Aufbau wird das Erythema nodosum adiponecroticans, das Erythema nodosum chronicum perilobulare, das Erythema nodosum lipogranulomatosum sowie das Erythema nodosum lipogranulomatosum bei Morbus Besnier-Boeck-Schaumann zugerechnet. Im folgenden finden lediglich die vom typischen Erythema nodosum abweichenden histomorphologischen Befunde Erwähnung.

Das *Erythema nodosum adiponecroticans* zeigt neben den für das Erythema nodosum typischen Veränderungen des Fettgewebes ausgedehnte Coagulationsnekrosen, welche dem Erythema nodosum fehlen oder lediglich in Form einer Nekrobiose angedeutet sind (ROTNES; CAROL u. Mitarb.; CIBILS-AGUIRRE u. Mitarb.; GELLERSTEDT; PICK). Daneben wurden von CAROL u. Mitarb. auffallende Gefäßveränderungen, insbesondere an den Venen, in Form der Endophlebitis obliterans nachgewiesen. Entzündliche Erscheinungen an den Arterien traten stark in den Hintergrund oder fehlten vollständig. GOTTRON hingegen hat auf eine Thrombosierung auch größerer arterieller Gefäße mit konsekutiver Gefäßwandentzündung und perivasalen entzündlichen Fettgewebsinfiltraten hingewiesen. Excisionen aus anderen, gleichzeitig entstandenen knotigen Eruptionen erbrachten ein für das Erythema nodosum typisches histologisches Substrat, so daß das Erythema nodosum adiponecroticans als Variante des Erythema nodosum aufgefaßt werden muß.

Bei dem *Erythema nodosum chronicum perilobulare* finden sich in den Fettläppchen so gut wie keine pathologischen Veränderungen. Der krankhafte Prozeß bleibt vorwiegend auf untere Anteile des Coriums sowie die Fettgewebssepten beschränkt und umschließt die Fettgewebsläppchen. Neben einem entzündlichen Ödem fallen Zellen der chronischen Entzündung, fibrocytär-fibroblastische Elemente und Riesenzellen vom Fremdkörpertyp auf. Kleinere arterielle Gefäße in den Septen zeigen eine Wandverdickung mit Lichtungseinengung. Die Gefäßwandveränderungen werden von CAROL als Endovasculitis obliterans bezeichnet.

Beim *Erythema nodosum lipogranulomatosum Carol* sind die pathohistologischen Veränderungen dagegen vorwiegend im subcutanen Fettgewebe anzutreffen. Im Corium fällt ein perivasales Infiltrat aus Histiocyten, Lymphocyten und polynucleären Leukocyten, das auf die Septen übergreift, auf. Auch fibrocytär-fibroblastische Elemente sowie Riesenzellen vom Fremdkörper- und Langhans-Typ werden vorgefunden. Auffällig sind in den Fettgewebssepten lokalisierte knötchenförmige Strukturen tuberkuloiden Aufbaues. Im Fettgewebe selbst werden neben Zellen der chronischen Entzündung Leukocyten sowie Epitheloidzellknötchen, die von Lipophagen untermischt sein können, gefunden. Abschnitte mit einer sog. Wucheratrophie kommen vor. CAROL beschreibt des weiteren histiocytäre Elemente, die sich den Fettzellen anlagern und als „Ringbänder" bezeichnet werden. Ob es sich um Lipophagen oder jugendliche Fettgewebszellen handelt, kann aus der Übersicht von CAROL, PRACKEN und ZWIJNDREGT nicht entnommen werden. In größeren Arterien fällt ein stärkeres Ödem mit subintimaler Schwellung und Durchsetzung der Gefäßwand mit Zellen der chronischen Entzündung sowie eine Periphlebitis auf.

Bei Patienten mit einem *Erythema nodosum bei Morbus Besnier-Boeck-Schaumann* (Sarkoidosis) ist das histologische Bild dem des Erythema nodosum lipogranulomatosum ähnlich. Zusätzlich werden in den Septen eosinophile Leukocyten und zahlreiche Riesenzellen vom Fremdkörper- und Langhans-Typ gefunden. Neben der Durchsetzung der Fettgewebsläppchen mit Zellen der akuten und chronischen Entzündung, die von Erythrocyten untermischt sein können, und den Zeichen einer sog. Wucheratrophie fallen zahlreiche Knötchen aus epitheloiden Zellen mit Langhansschen Riesenzellen auf. Nekrobiotische bzw. nekrotische Binde- und Fettgewebsareale mit kristalloiden Strukturen gelangen hin und wieder zur Beobachtung. Außer einer geringen Periphlebitis werden Gefäßveränderungen vermißt (CAROL, PRACKEN und ZWIJNDREGT). Die partielle tuberkuloide Ausgestaltung ist, wie auch am Beispiel des Fremdkörpergranulationsgewebes beobachtet werden kann, möglicherweise im Sinne einer besonderen Reaktionslage des Gewebes bei bestehendem Morbus Besnier-Boeck-Schaumann zu deuten.

GOTTRON fügt als weitere Variante das *Erythema nodosum nach Applikation von Jodkalium* an, bei welchem die oberen Cutisanteile besonders stark betroffen sind. Die Septen sowie die Fettgewebsläppchen lassen ähnliche Veränderungen wie das typische Erythema nodosum erkennen.

Bei dem *Erythema nodosum trichophyticum* tritt nach GOTTRON der ausgeprägte perivasale Charakter einer polymorphzelligen Entzündung in den Vordergrund. In den Septen fällt eine hochgradige knötchenförmige Infiltratdurchsetzung auf. Die Gefäßwände sind ödematös aufgelockert. Perivasal liegt ein gemischtzelliges Infiltrat. An der Zellulation beteiligen sich Histiocyten, Lymphocyten, polynucleäre und eosinophile Leukocyten, welche besonders häufig anzutreffen sind. Die Entzündung greift in Form einer retikulären Infiltration auf die Fettgewebsläppchen über. Granulome und Lipophagen wurden nicht nachgewiesen (URBACH; BALLAGI; APFFEL und BURGUN; WALTHER; FUHS u.a.).

b) Erythema induratum Bazin

Die pathologischen Veränderungen eines *Erythema induratum Bazin* nehmen nach GOTTRON ihren Ausgang von den Fettgewebssepten und finden sich in späteren Krankheitsstadien vorzugsweise in den Fettgewebsläppchen. Das Corium sowie die Fettgewebssepten weisen neben einer stärkeren ödematösen Durchtränkung im allgemeinen nur geringfügige, vorwiegend perivasal gelegene Infiltrate der chronischen Entzündung auf. Abschnittsweise kann jedoch auch ein dichtes entzündliches Infiltrat vorgefunden werden. Epitheloidzellgranulome mit Langhansschen Riesenzellen sind ebenfalls anzutreffen (GOTTRON). In den Fettgewebsläppchen findet sich ein herdförmig-multilokulär angeordnetes Infiltrat aus Histiocyten und Lymphocyten. Es kommen Knötchen mit einem typischen tuberkuloiden Aufbau zur Beobachtung. Sie weisen Langhanssche, seltener Fremdkörper-Riesenzellen auf und werden an der Peripherie von Lymphocyten und Plasmazellen begrenzt. Erythrocytenextravasate kommen vor. In der Regel sind ausgedehnte Steatonekrosen vorhanden. Eine sog. Wucheratrophie kann regionär auftreten.

Auffällig sind Gefäßabweichungen in Form der Endarteriitis obliterans sowie der Endophlebitis obliterans, die GOTTRON; CAROL u. Mitarb.; GANS und STEIGLEDER; LEVER; FISCHER; EBERHARTINGER u.a. bei einem großen Teil ihres Untersuchungsgutes nachweisen konnten und denen ätiopathogenetisch eine primäre Rolle zugestanden wird. Die Gefäße zeigen eine subintimale Proliferation, sind unter Einschluß aller Wandanteile verdickt und von Zellen der chronischen Entzündung durchsetzt. Thrombosierung mit Gefäßobliteration führen zu den bereits erwähnten Nekrosen, die das Corium und die Epidermis einschließen können. Die perivasal gelegenen Zellansammlungen sind chronisch-entzündlicher Natur. Sie können aber auch einen tuberkuloiden Bau aufweisen. Zentral wird gelegentlich eine Verkäsung oder Verflüssigung beobachtet (GANS und STEIGLEDER).

CAROL, PRACKEN und ZWIJNDREGT; GANS und STEIGLEDER beobachteten von der Norm abweichende Typen des Erythema induratum Bazin. Bei angedeuteter herdförmiger Gruppierung von Zellen der chronischen Entzündung kann ein tuberkuloider Aufbau mit Langhansschen Riesenzellen nur andeutungsweise vorhanden sein oder vollständig vermißt werden. Zentral fallen multiple kleine und größere Hohlraumbildungen auf, die ausgefallenen Fettzellen entsprechen. In den Fettgewebsläppchen finden sich neben Steatonekrosen Zeichen der sog. Wucheratrophie sowie Fibroblasten, welche von Lymphocyten untermischt sind. Die Bindegewebswucherung kann nach GANS und STEIGLEDER im Vordergrund stehen und größere Teile des Fettgewebes ersetzen.

Eine weitere Variante ist durch die Lokalisation der hauptsächlichsten krankhaften Befunde in den Fettgewebssepten gekennzeichnet. Das dichte Infiltrat setzt sich aus Histiocyten und Lymphocyten zusammen. Tuberkuloide Formationen werden gefunden. Herdförmige Coagulationsnekrosen, zahlreiche Langhanssche und Fremdkörper-Riesenzellen sowie Erythrocytenextravasate kommen vor. Die Durchsetzung der Fettgewebsläppchen mit Zellen der chronischen Entzündung sowie eine Wucheratrophie treten zurück. Auffällige Gefäßabweichungen werden vermißt. Bei ähnlichem histologischem Aufbau im Hinblick auf das Erythema nodosum gewinnen die Septumnekrosen differentialdiagnostisch an Bedeutung. CAROL u. Mitarb. betrachten diese Krankheitsform als Übergangsstadium zwischen einem Erythema induratum Bazin und Erythema nodosum und bezeichnen derartige Befunde als Erythema induratum nodosum.

Nach EBERHARTINGER stehen beim Erythema induratum Bazin die Gefäßveränderungen an den Arterien und Venen des Fettgewebes im Vordergrund, denen teils tuberkuloide, teils banal-entzündliche Gewebsreaktionen folgen. Für die Diagnose sind die im Beginn der Erkrankung an der Cutis-Subcutisgrenze oder in Septennähe anzutreffenden tuberkuloiden Knötchen charakteristisch (SPIER und RÖCKL; EBERHARTINGER). In späteren Krankheitsstadien dominieren uncharakteristische tuberkuloid-nekrotische Gewebsstrukturen mit den Zeichen einer Begleitpanniculitis (EBERHARTINGER).

c) Nodular-Vasculitis

Es ist das Verdienst von MONTGOMERY, O'LEARY und BARKER, die sog. *Nodular-Vasculitis* aus dem Formenkreis des Morbus Bazin isoliert und als Gefäßerkrankung mit nosologischer Sonderstellung herausgestellt zu haben. MONTGOMERY u. Mitarb.; MICHELSON; WOODBURNE; PHILPOTT; VILANOVA u. GRÄFLIN; D. WALTHER; TELFORD; STEIGLEDER; EBERHARTINGER; PARISH haben die tuberkulöse Genese dieser Erkrankung verneint und auf die Ähnlichkeit des histologischen Befundes mit dem des Erythema nodosum, des Erythema induratum Bazin, der Lipogranulomatosis subcutana Rothmann-Makai, der Erythrocyanose mit Fettgewebsveränderungen, der Steatonekrose der Brustdrüse sowie der Panniculitis bei Poliomyelitis hingewiesen. Der histologische Befund der angeführten Dermatosen, insbesondere des Erythema induratum Bazin, ist schwer von rein vasculären Erkrankungen des Fettgewebes abzugrenzen, da tuberkuloide Formationen bei Entzündungen im Bereich der Subcutis häufig vorkommen, andererseits in Fällen vermißt werden, welche mit großer Wahrscheinlichkeit dem Formenkreis der Tuberkulose zuzurechnen sind (MICHELSON). MICHELSON stellt die Vasculitis nodularis aufgrund ihres histologischen Befundes zwischen das Erythema nodosum und das Erythema induratum Bazin.

Nach SCHNEIDER und UNDEUTSCH beginnt die Nodular-Vasculitis ebenso wie die Lipogranulomatosis subcutanea hypertonica Gottron in ihren Frühstadien mit einer Aufquellung der Intima und sich anschließender Teile der Media. In den Quellungszonen sind metachromatisch sich anfärbende Substanzen nachweisbar, die nach SCHÜRMANN auf ein Versagen der Endothelschranke mit Plasmaimbibition, Ödem der Gefäßwand und Gewebsschädigung mit Entmischungsvorgängen in der Grundsubstanz zurückzuführen sind. Sonstige Kriterien der akuten und chronischen Entzündung werden vermißt. Dieser frühe Gefäßwandschaden kann sich einerseits zurückbilden, ohne sichtbare Schädigungen der Gefäßwandanteile hervorzurufen, andererseits bis zur fibrinoiden Nekrose mit bleibender Zerstörung der Gefäßstruktur fortschreiten.

Im weiteren Krankheitsverlauf kommt es zur Wandverdickung der Gefäße mit Einengung des Lumens bis zur Obliteration sowohl arterieller als auch venöser

Gefäße. Daneben findet sich eine subendotheliale Fibrose und mäßige Durchsetzung der Gefäßwandung mit Zellen der chronischen Entzündung. Die Nekrose kann bis zur völligen Zerstörung der Gefäßwand führen. Die elastischen Fasern bleiben weitgehend erhalten. Die sekundär entstandenen Fettgewebsnekrosen werden durch ein resorptives tuberkuloides Granulations- bzw. Resorptionsgewebe ersetzt. Ölcysten sowie fibrocytär-fibroblastische Elemente kommen zur Beobachtung. Die tuberkuloiden Granulome werden umgeben von einer retikulären Entzündung, die zwischen den einzelnen Fettzellen zur Ausbildung gelangt.

d) Sarkoid Darier-Roussy

Der histologische Aufbau des *Sarkoid Darier-Roussy* gleicht in mancher Hinsicht dem des Erythema induratum Bazin. Die Stellung des Sarkoid Darier-Roussy konnte bisher nicht eindeutig geklärt werden. Die Mehrzahl moderner Autoren, so LEITNER; COSTE; LANGCOPE und FREIMAN u.a., sehen diese Erkrankung als eine Manifestationsart des Morbus Besnier-Boeck-Schaumann an.

Die pathologischen Veränderungen sind bei nur sehr geringer Coriumbeteiligung in Form perivasaler Rundzellinfiltrate vorwiegend im Fettgewebe lokalisiert (GOTTRON; CAROL, PRACKEN und ZWIJNDREGT). Während in den Fettgewebssepten lediglich geringfügige Infiltrate aus Zellen der chronischen Entzündung nachweisbar sind, findet sich zwischen den Fettzellen eine herdförmige, an Lymphfollikel erinnernde, weniger eine diffuse Infiltratansammlung aus Histiocyten, Lymphocyten, einigen polynucleären Leukocyten und wenigen Plasmazellen. Fibrocytär-fibroblastische Elemente kommen ebenfalls zur Beobachtung. Tuberkuloide Strukturen mit Langhansschen Riesenzellen, die an einen Morbus Besnier-Boeck-Schaumann erinnern, sind in großer Zahl anzutreffen. In frischen, aktiven Herden sind nach LEVER dagegen nur wenige oder keine Langhansschen Riesenzellen aufzufinden. Lymphocyten umgeben die Epitheloidzellen oder durchmischen sie vom Rand her. Das Cytoplasma der Epitheloidzellen ist wolkig getrübt. Nekrosen werden vermißt. Nach Durchführung der Footschen Reticulumfärbung stellt sich ein Reticulumnetzwerk dar, das die Epitheloidzellknötchen umgibt oder diese durchdringt, wobei jede einzelne Epitheloidzelle von Gitterfasern umgeben sein kann (LEVER). Die herdförmigen epitheloiden Zellformationen können sich zu Konglomeraten zusammenschließen. Innerhalb der Knötchen liegen Fettzellen und kleine Ölcysten, die in der Anordnung an Fensterrosetten erinnern. Die Ausbildung sog. Fensterrosetten ist nach CAROL, PRACKEN und ZWIJNDREGT; GOTTRON; LEVER und FREIMAN für das Sarkoid Darier-Roussy typisch. Kleinere und größere Ölcysten, Fettgewebsnekrosen, eine sog. Wucheratrophie und „Ringbänder" an der Peripherie von Fettzellen sind in der Regel deutlicher ausgeprägt als beim Erythema induratum Bazin. Während GOTTRON; GANS und STEIGLEDER; FISCHER u.a. mikroskopisch faßbare Gefäßveränderungen beschrieben haben, wurden solche von CAROL, PRACKEN und ZWIJNDREGT bei einem größeren Krankengut in der Mehrzahl der Fälle nicht gefunden (NAGAHORI; IRGANG; COTTONI und SAPUPPO; JAMES; ITO; VANDEKERCKHOVE; KAMINSKY u. Mitarb.; VILANOVA u. Mitarb.; SANDBERG und ADAMS u.a.).

e) Spontanpanniculitis Typ Pfeifer-Weber-Christian

Die *Spontanpanniculitis Typ Pfeifer-Weber-Christian* (Panniculitis nodularis non suppurativa) ist eine relativ selten auftretende Erkrankung, die sich vorzugsweise im subcutanen Fettgewebe abspielt.

Histologisch finden sich sowohl in den unteren Coriumabschnitten als auch in den Fettgewebssepten nur geringfügige, perivasal gelegene Infiltrate, die sich aus Histiocyten und Lymphocyten zusammensetzen. Das gemischtzellige Infiltrat kann an der Peripherie von eosinophilen Leukocyten durchsetzt sein. Die wesentlichen pathologischen Veränderungen bleiben jedoch nahezu ausschließlich auf die Fettläppchen beschränkt.

GOTTRON und NIKOLOWSKI konnten aufgrund histologischer Untersuchungen von Knoten unterschiedlicher Bestandsdauer unter Erfassung von Frühveränderungen mehrere Stadien der Entwicklung nachweisen, auf die auch von UNGAR und LEVER hingewiesen wurde.

In Stadium I fallen zwischen den Fettzellen retikulär angeordnete, ausschließlich leukocytäre Infiltrate auf, die von wenigen Erythrocyten untermischt sein können (UNGAR; LEVER; GOTTRON und NIKOLOWSKI). Lediglich CAROL u. Mitarb. berichten von Erythrocytenextravasaten größeren Ausmaßes. Die Fettzellen selbst zeigen keine pathologischen Veränderungen. Deutliche Abweichungen finden sich hingegen am Capillarnetz. Die Capillaren sind erweitert und prall von Erythrocyten ausgefüllt. Die der terminalen Strombahn vorgeschalteten arteriellen Gefäße im Fettgewebe oder an der Cutis-Subcutisgrenze können neben einem subintimalen Ödem mit Ersatz durch jugendliches Bindegewebe eine leukocytäre Durchsetzung der Media und Adventitia aufweisen. Die elastischen Fasern sind infolge der Wandverdickung nur relativ vermindert. Auffällig ist eine Ödematisierung der Septen sowie der unteren Coriumanteile (CAROL, PRACKEN und ZWIJNDREGT; GOTTRON und NIKOLOWSKI). Die Struktur der kollagenen Fasern ist verwaschen. Dieselben sind gequollen, verbreitert und auseinandergedrängt, so daß eine retikuläre Anordnung mit Aufsplitterung des Bindegewebes resultiert. GOTTRON und NIKOLOWSKI beschreiben im Ödem liegende Infiltratzellen, die durch ein schmutzigrotes, nicht eosinophiles Cytoplasma mit exzentrisch gelegenem Zellkern charakterisiert, den Plasmazellen jedoch nicht gleichzustellen sind.

Bei länger bestehenden Efflorescenzen, die dem Stadium II entsprechen, sind die pathologischen Veränderungen ausschließlich auf die Fettläppchen beschränkt. Neben Fettzellnekrosen, untermischt von Kerntrümmern, finden sich cystisch erweiterte Hohlräume. Die nekrotischen Fettgewebsareale und Ölcysten werden von Histiocyten, Lymphocyten und Plasmazellen sowie einigen Riesenzellen vom Fremdkörpertyp umgrenzt. Das Infiltrat ist rosettenförmig angeordnet, wobei intakte Fettzellen, Nekrosen und Cysten von einem unterschiedlich breiten Infiltratsaum umgeben werden.

Das Auftreten von Zellen der chronischen Entzündung leitet über in das Stadium III der Erkrankung. Es kommt zur Entwicklung lipophager Granulome mit knötchenförmigen Infiltraten aus Histiocyten, Lymphocyten und sehr wenigen Plasmazellen, die der Entzündung einen granulomatösen Aufbau vermitteln. Insbesondere in der Umgebung der granulomatös-entzündlichen Prozesse finden sich mehrkernige, den Lipophagen entsprechende Zellen mit einem schaumigen Cytoplasma. Fettzellen und Ölcysten können randständig von Lipophagen umschlossen werden, wodurch der Eindruck drüsiger Strukturen vermittelt wird. Die Wandungen weisen jedoch auch einen endothelartigen Belag auf; die Lipophagen haben sich unter Abflachung ihrer Zellkerne eng aneinandergelagert. Eine Wucheratrophie kommt abschnittsweise zur Beobachtung. Seltener wird eine Verflüssigung der Schaumzelleninfiltrate beobachtet, so daß eine schaumige Substanz mit Kernen von Schaumzellen, Lymphocyten und polynucleären Leukocyten zur Darstellung kommt (SHAFFER; BINKLEY; LEVER). Epitheloidzellige Formationen mit Langhansschen Riesenzellen und Verkäsungen werden im allgemeinen vermißt (GOTTRON und NIKOLOWSKI). Lediglich KRINER machte auf das Vorkommen Sarkoidosis-artiger Infiltrate aufmerksam. MEYER; REYNAERS haben auf die Möglichkeit einer epitheloidzelligen Transformation von Histiocyten mit dem Nachweis von Riesenzellen in der Subcutis hingewiesen.

Die Schädigungen an größeren arteriellen Gefäßen entsprechen den unter Stadium I beschriebenen (TILDEN, GOTSHALK und AVAKIAN; NETHERTON; CUMMINS und LEVER; ALDERSON und WAY; CAROL, PRACKEN und ZWIJNDREGT; MEYER; LANGHOF; VILANOVA und AGUADÉ). Veränderungen im Sinne der Thrombangiitis obliterans kommen ebenfalls zur Beobachtung (MEYER). In seltenen Fällen kann eine Gefäßbeteiligung vermißt werden (OCANO SIERRA).

Stadium IV ist gekennzeichnet durch den reparativen Ersatz nekrotischer Fettzellen in Form eines fibrösen Gewebes, das durch den Nachweis fibrocytär-fibroblastischer Zellelemente mit Faserneubildung charakterisiert ist (BAUMGARTNER und RIVA; CAROL, PRACKEN und ZWIJNDREGT; UNGAR; LEVER; KOOIJ; HALTER; GOTTRON; GOTTRON und NIKOLOWSKI; RÖCKL und THIES; BAUMANN; GANS und STEIGLEDER; KONOPIK; KRINER; JADASSOHN; FANINGER; JAUSION u. Mitarb.; VILANOVA und AGUADÉ; DE GEORGIO; BERNDT und FRIEDRICHS; ZEUMER; SHATIN; NUNEZ-ANDRADE; WOLF; OBERLING u. Mitarb.; TENDIS; SINGH u. Mitarb.; MICHELSON; GRUPPER u. Mitarb.; HOLZEL; BINKLEY; ACKERMANN, MOSHER u. SCHWAMM u. a.).

Das Pfeifer-Weber-Christian-Syndrom spielt sich aufgrund neuerer Untersuchungen nicht nur in der Subcutis der Haut, sondern auch im Fettgewebe der inneren Organe ab. Der histologische Befund ist mit dem der Subcutis identisch (UNGAR; MOSTOFI und ENGLEMAN; SPAIN und FOLEY; MILNER u. MITCHINSON u. a.).

f) Spontanpanniculitis Typ Rothmann-Makai

Nach CAROL, PRACKEN und ZWIJNDREGT; GOTTRON und NIKOLOWSKI; RÖCKL und THIES; BAUMANN u. a. ist die *Spontanpanniculitis Typ Rothmann-Makai* (Lipogranulomatosis subcutanea Rothmann-Makai) weniger vom histologischen als vom klinischen Standpunkt aus von der Pfeifer-Weber-Christianschen Erkrankung abzugrenzen. Das histologische Substrat beider Panniculitisformen ähnelt sich weitgehend, so daß auf eine weitere Erörterung hinsichtlich der Gemeinsamkeiten verzichtet werden kann.

RÖCKL und THIES unterscheiden formalgenetisch drei Entwicklungsstadien, die denen der Pfeifer-Weber-Christianschen Erkrankung entsprechen: 1. Steatonekrose, 2. Lipophagie, Granulom- und Fettcystenbildung, 3. Ersatz durch fibröses Gewebe. Eine Leukocytenemigration vor der Entwicklung von Steatonekrosen wurde nicht beobachtet. Bei entsprechenden Frühveränderungen dürften jedoch auch polynucleäre Leukocyten in retikulärer Anordnung zwischen den Fettzellen anzutreffen sein. Die ödematöse Durchtränkung unterer Coriumanteile sowie der Fettgewebssepten scheint nicht in dem Ausmaß wie bei der Pfeifer-Weber-Christianschen Erkrankung vorzuliegen. Die Steatonekrosen werden von einem Infiltrat aus Histiocyten, Lymphocyten und polynucleären Leukocyten umgeben. Fremdkörperriesenzellen mit kristallinen Einschlüssen sind seltener anzutreffen. Ölcysten, lipophage Granulome mit tuberkuloiden Strukturen sowie eine Wucheratrophie des Fettgewebes kommen jedoch ebenfalls zur Beobachtung. Die Capillaren sind erweitert und prall mit Blut gefüllt. An der Peripherie anzutreffende größere arterielle oder venöse Gefäße zeigen neben einer subendothelialen Schwellung mit Lichtungseinengung eine Wandverdickung, Homogenisierung der Media sowie eine Schädigung der elastischen Fasern. An der entzündlichen Infiltration der Wandung beteiligen sich Histiocyten, Lymphocyten und einige polynucleäre Leukocyten. Auffällige Gefäßveränderungen können aber auch vermißt werden (CAROL u. Mitarb.; EYCKMANS; MEYER; RINALDI; KONOPIK; DUPERRAT; ZEUMER; RÖCKL und THIES u. a.).

g) Panniculitis subacuta nodosa migrans

Die *Panniculitis subacuta nodosa migrans Vilanova-Piñol-Aguadé* nimmt eine gewisse Sonderstellung ein (RABBIOSI; BUREAU, JARRY, BARRIERE, KERNEIS u. BRUNEAU; KERDEL-VEGAS; PERRY u. WINKELMANN u.a.). In den Fettgewebssepten läßt sich ein charakteristisches patho-histologisches Substrat nachweisen, das später auf die Fettläppchen übergreift. Anfänglich stehen Gefäßveränderungen in Form einer Capillaritis mit Einengung oder Verschluß des Lumens und perivasalen Infiltraten aus Histiocyten, Lymphocyten, Monocyten und Fibroblasten im Vordergrund. Kleinere muskuläre Arterien können ebenfalls betroffen sein. Durch Endothelproliferation und Zusammenfluß cellulärer Protoplasmaanteile werden nach VILANOVA u. PIÑOL-AGUADÉ riesenzellhaltige Gebilde vorgetäuscht. Die Fettgewebssepten sind ödematös aufgelockert und von fibrinoiden Nekrosen oder sklerosierten Bindegewebsabschnitten durchsetzt. Die kollagenen Fasern weisen arealweise eine Fragmentation auf. Nach Rückbildung der entzündlichen Infiltrate hinterbleiben die oben erwähnten riesenzellhaltigen Strukturen.

h) Spontan auftretende Fettgewebsnekrosen und Fettgranulome

Spontan auftretende Fettgewebsnekrosen und Fettgranulome, die sich ohne vorangegangenes Trauma oder vorangehende Entzündung entwickeln und beispielsweise Wochen oder Monate nach Abklingen eines Fleckfiebers zur Beobachtung gelangen, gehören offenbar in die Gruppe der Spontanpanniculitis Typ ROTHMANN-MAKAI (s. auch BAUMGARTNER u. RIVA). In frischen Efflorescenzen finden sich Fettgewebsnekrosen mit nachfolgender Verseifung der Fettsäuren. Erythrocytenextravasate bzw. Zellen der akuten und chronischen Entzündung werden vermißt. Erst im weiteren Krankheitsverlauf kommt es zur Hyperämie mit perivasalen Infiltraten aus Histiocyten, Lymphocyten und polynucleären Leukocyten. ABRIKOSSOFF beobachtete an den Grenzen nekrobiotischer Fettzellen die Bildung freier Tropfen verseiften Fettes von unterschiedlicher Größe. Diese werden von einem Granulationsgewebe mit Fetttropfen enthaltenden Riesenzellen umgeben. Später unterliegt das Granulationsgewebe einer fibrösen Umwandlung. Fibrocytär-fibroblastische Elemente umschließen kleine oder größere Hohlräume, die nur wenig Fett, dagegen mehr seröse Flüssigkeit enthalten (ABRIKOSSOFF; GOTTRON; BAUMGARTNER u. RIVA; PIERINI, ABULAFIA u. WAINFELD u.a.).

i) Traumatogene Fettgewebsnekrose

Die *traumatogene Fettgewebsnekrose* ist durch die Entwicklung von Lipogranulomen gekennzeichnet, die nach Einwirkung von Traumen mechanischer, chemischer oder thermischer Art entstehen. Offenbar spielt das Trauma für den Untergang von Fettzellen nur eine mittelbare Rolle. GOTTRON; KÜTTNER und BARUCH; LERICHE u.a. haben darauf aufmerksam gemacht, daß ein traumatisch bedingter segmentärer Gefäßspasmus zur Fettgewebsnekrose und Granulombildung führt. Neben einem chronischen Granulationsgewebe typischer Ausgestaltung finden sich Ölcysten mit Anlagerung von Lipophagen, die an Drüsenhalbmonde erinnern können. Schaumzellen sowie Riesenzellen vom Fremdkörpertyp sind nachweisbar (PIROTH; GOTTRON; BAUMANN; ZAVARINI u.a.). Die Veränderungen können, wenn Ölcysten von einem Granulationsgewebe umgeben werden, von Lipogranulomen entzündlicher Genese nicht unterschieden werden (PIROTH).

j) Fettgewebsnekrose der Brustdrüse

Die *Fettgewebsnekrose der Brustdrüse* stellt ein scharf umrissenes Krankheitsbild dar, das vorzugsweise beim weiblichen, selten beim männlichen Geschlecht zur Beobachtung gelangt (GOHRBANDT; GIORDANO). Dem Trauma muß für die Entstehung der Erkrankung eine bedeutende Rolle beigemessen werden (BRANCATI; ZEITLHOFER; RAST; ADAIR u. MUNZER; BARTSCH). Nach vorausgegangenen mechanischen oder chemischen Traumen entstehen Hämorrhagien, die sich allmählich in knotenförmige Gebilde umwandeln. Histologisch fällt neben Erythrocytenextravasaten der Untergang von Fettzellen mit kleineren und größeren Ölcysten sowie eine herdförmige oder retikuläre Durchsetzung benachbarter Fettgewebsabschnitte mit Zellen der akuten und chronischen Entzündung auf. Im weiteren Krankheitsverlauf findet sich ein Granulationsgewebe, gekennzeichnet durch tuberkuloide Granulome mit Riesenzellen vom Fremdkörper- und Langhans-Typ sowie fibrocytär-fibroblastische Elemente. Arterielle und venöse Gefäße zeigen neben einer subendothelialen Schwellung und Wandnekrose eine mäßige Durchsetzung mit akut oder chronisch entzündlichen Elementen. Die Abgrenzung gegenüber der Nodular-Vasculitis kann in bestimmten Entwicklungsstadien unmöglich sein (TELFORD).

k) Medikamentöse Lipodystrophie

Bei der *medikamentösen Lipodystrophie* kann es nach der Injektion bestimmter Medikamente (subcutane Injektion öliger oder wäßriger Lösungen) ebenfalls zu einer Schädigung von Fettzellen mit nachfolgendem Untergang und daraus resultierender Atrophie des subcutanen Fettgewebes kommen (GOTTRON; SCHIRREN; DEJENARUI; SZENTMIKLOSY und DAVID; KLOSTERMANN, SÜDHOF und TISCHENDORF; COLLEN u. Mitarb.; FLECK u.a.). Die aus den zerstörten Fettzellen in das Gewebe gelangenden gespeicherten Fettsubstanzen werden zum Fremdkörper und lösen Reaktionen aus, wie diese bereits bei den vorangegangenen Erkrankungen des Fettgewebes beschrieben wurden. Nach einem anfänglichen Ödem, insbesondere im Bereich der Septen, kommt es aus den Gefäßen zu einer Emigration von Monocyten, Lymphocyten und Granulocyten. Daneben fallen Erythrocytenextravasate auf. SCHIRREN; SCHEFFLER beobachteten diffus, insbesondere aber perivasal gelegene pigmenttragende Makrophagen, die teilweise eine eisenpositive Reaktion aufwiesen. Histiocytäre Elemente lagern sich den Fettzellen mit lichtmikroskopisch intakten Cytoplasmamembranen an. Durch Fettphagocytose entstehen Lipophagen. Im weiteren Krankheitsverlauf kommt es zur Entwicklung von Lipogranulomen, bestehend aus epitheloiden Zellen und Riesenzellen vom Langhans- oder Fremkörpertyp (BOLLER; PFUHL; KELLNER; STRANSKY; GOTTRON; BAUMANN; HERRMANN u. Mitarb. u.a.). Nach HERRMANN u. Mitarb.; SCHEFFLER und HAGEN kann der histologische Aufbau dem einer Nekrobiosis lipoidica ähnlich sein.

Ein fest umrissenes Krankheitsbild stellt die *Insulinlipodystrophie* (nach AGNETA in 0,1% der Fälle im Anschluß an subcutane Insulin-Injektionen) dar. Die pathologischen Veränderungen bleiben auf das Fettgewebe beschränkt. In der Mehrzahl der Beobachtungen geht dieser Form der Lipodystrophie eine Steatonekrose voraus (GANS und STEIGLEDER; KLOSTERMANN u. Mitarb.; HERRMANN u. Mitarb.; SCHIRREN). Bei fehlender Vascularisierung wird das entzündliche Infiltrat zunächst vermißt. Die Neubildung von Capillaren kann jedoch auch verstärkt sein (ENGELBACH). Die Fettgewebsnekrosen werden durch eingewanderte Granulocyten und Lipasen aufgelöst und von Histiocyten abgebaut (PFUHL; GANS und STEIGLEDER). In 10% aller Fälle kommt es zu einem völligen Schwund des subcutanen Fettgewebes (DEPISCH; STRANSKY; WOODHOUSE-PRICE; BAUMGARTNER u. RIVA; RATHERY und SIGWALD; GEBAUER; SCHEFFLER u. Mitarb. u.a.).

Neben den soeben beschriebenen Veränderungen kann sich nach Applikation von Insulin eine *Lipohypertrophie* (SCHULZE und KUNZE; BAUMGARTNER u. RIVA), das sog. Insulinlipom, entwickeln. Lipoatrophie und Lipohypertrophie werden auch als Lipodystrophie bezeichnet (ZIERZ).

In die gleiche Krankheitsgruppe ist das *Paraffinom* einzuordnen, bei dem es ebenfalls zur Entwicklung von Ölcysten mit umgebender Lipogranulombildung kommen kann. Neben den bereits erwähnten Ölcysten, die von einer fibrösen Kapsel umgeben werden, findet sich ein knötchenförmiges Granulationsgewebe aus Epitheloidzellen, Lymphocyten, Plasmazellen und Fremdkörper-Riesenzellen, in denen Vacuolen nachweisbar sind (GOTTRON; SANTLER; ARDUINO; SCHLIENGER; LEVER). Auch lymphocytäre Mikroabscesse wurden beobachtet (SCHLIENGER). SCHLIENGER fand eine Intimawucherung in arteriellen Gefäßen. Von EISENSCHMID und ORBISON wurden im Zentrum von Nekrosen und Cysten Kalkeinlagerungen gesehen. Nach SANTLER kann der beschriebene histologische Befund dem einer Necrobiosis lipoidica oder Granulomatosis disciformis chronica et progressiva Miescher gleichen.

Bei der *Lipodystrophia progressiva Simons* handelt es sich um einen örtlich begrenzten Schwund des Fettgewebes. Die Abgrenzung von medikamentös bedingten Lipodystrophien kann schwierig sein. Histologisch fällt bei regelrechter Ausgestaltung der Epidermis, der Hautanhangsgebilde und des Coriums eine Rarefizierung des subcutanen Fettgewebes mit Verbreiterung der teilweise senkrecht verlaufenden Fettgewebssepten auf. Perivasal angeordnete lympho-histiocytäre Infiltrate treten zurück und sind bevorzugt an der Corium-Fettgewebsgrenze anzutreffen (zur Ätiopathogenese, Phänomenologie und Variationsmöglichkeit der Lipodystrophia progressiva Simons s. G. WEBER u. G. ROTH, 1967).

Sklerosierende Lipogranulome, erstmals von SMETANA und BERNHARD nach Einwirkung eines Traumas (s. auch SMETANA u. BERNHARD; SAWICKY u. KANOFF u.a.) in der Inguinal-, Genital- und Analregion beschrieben, kommen auch nach der Injektion wäßriger oder öliger Lösungen zur Beobachtung (WIGHLEY und CALNAN; NEWCOMER; HERBST; SCHLIENGER). Bei einer weiteren Anzahl von Patienten konnte die auslösende Noxe nicht eruiert werden (RITTER; NEWCOMER u. Mitarb.; REES u.a.). Sklerosierende Lipogranulome sind gekennzeichnet durch den Nachweis von Fettnekrosen und Ölcysten, die von einem Granulationsgewebe sowie fibrocytär-fibroblastischen Elementen und strukturlosem Kollagen umgeben werden (WIGHLEY und CALNAN; CALNAN und HABER; ANNING; BEST u. Mitarb.; REES; PALETTE, PALETTE u. HARRINGTON). Charakteristisch für diese Form der Lipogranulome ist demnach eine zusätzliche Sklerosierung im Bereich des Fettgewebes.

1) Sclerema neonatorum

Beim *Sclerema neonatorum*, dem im Gegensatz zu den bisher besprochenen Erkrankungen des subcutanen Fettgewebes möglicherweise Störungen in der Fettsäurebildung zugrunde liegen, wird eine ödematöse von einer adipösen Form abgegrenzt. Während MENSI bei der ödematösen Form im subcutanen Fettgewebe eine blutige Durchtränkung der im übrigen gut erhaltenen Subcutis beobachtete, fanden LUITHLEN; GANS u.a. keine pathologischen Veränderungen des Fettgewebes (s. auch KORTING; HUGHES und HAMMOND; NORMAN; GRIFFEN u. MITCHELL).

Das Sclerema adiposum dagegen weist qualitative und quantitative Veränderungen des Fettgewebes auf. Es kommt zu einer Atrophie der betroffenen subcutanen Areale, die von zahlreichen Neutralfettkristallen durchsetzt sind (GANS und STEIGLEDER; LUZZATTI u. HANSEN; SIMPSON; REICH u.a.). Obliterierende

Angiitiden, Zellen der chronischen Entzündung, Riesenzellen vom Fremdkörpertyp sowie Hämorrhagien kommen zur Beobachtung (NORMAN; HOLT u. HOWLAND; LUZZATTI u. HANSEN; GRÜTZ; BLANC; MCDONALD u. a.).

Nach GRÜTZ steht der Ab- und Umbau des Fettgewebes im Vordergrund der Erkrankung, wobei sich die Fettläppchen der Struktur des Primitivorgans wieder nähern. Die Fettgewebssepten zeigen eine Verbreiterung, ödematöse Durchtränkung sowie eine verstärkte fibrocytär-fibroblastische Reaktion mit Faserneubildung. In den Fettzellen sind Vacuolen zu erkennen. Die Fettsubstanzen färben sich mit der Sudan III-Färbung ungleichmäßig an. Neben ausgefällten Fettkristallen (s. BRAUN-FALCO) finden sich Fettgewebsnekrosen sowie ein chronisch-entzündliches Infiltrat aus Histiocyten, Lymphocyten, weniger neutrophilen Leukocyten und Riesenzellen vom Fremdkörpertyp. Makrophagen wandeln sich durch Fettphagocytose in Schaumzellen um (BLANC; WORINGER u. Mitarb.). Das Granulationsgewebe kann das gesamte Fettläppchen ersetzen. GRÜTZ beobachtete eine vom Rand des Fettläppchens einsetzende Regeneration der Fettzellen.

m) Adiponecrosis subcutanea neonatorum

Bei der *Adiponecrosis subcutanea neonatorum*, dessen histologischer Befund weitgehend dem des Sclerema neonatorum (zur Nosologie der Adiponecrosis subcutanea neonatorum, des knotenförmigen Sclerema neonatorum, des Fettsclerems

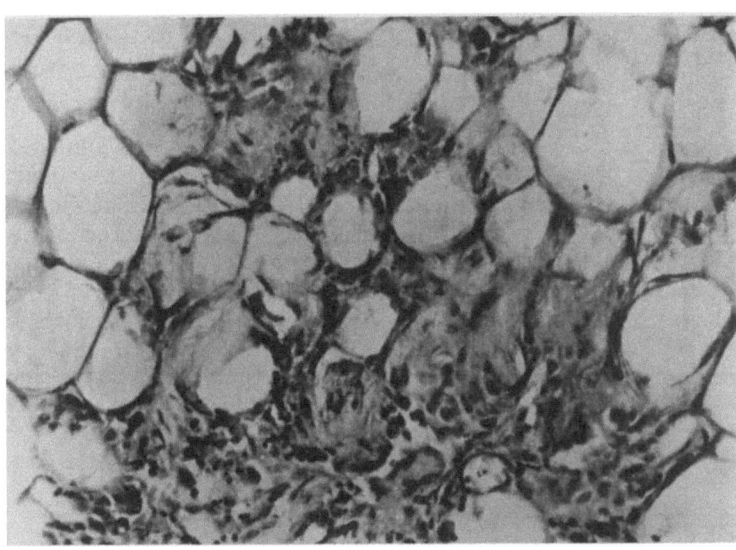

Abb. 3. Adiponecrosis subcutanea neonatorum. Umschriebene Nekrosen und Lipogranulome mit Fremdkörperriesenzellen sowie büschelförmiger Anhäufung von Fettsäurenadeln. [Aus: J. DIECKHOFF, H. C. HEMPEL u. R. KOCH: Kinderärztl. Prax. **27**, 443 (1959), Abb. 1]

sowie des generalisierten Sclerema neonatorum s. W. F. LEVER, 1958; LINDLAR u. MISGELD, 1967) gleicht (ZEEK und MADDEN; FLORY; LEVER), tritt nach LEVER die entzündliche Reaktion mit dem Nachweis von Riesenzellen stärker in den Vordergrund. ARZT fand in den Fettgewebsläppchen insbesondere perivasal gelegene Zellen der chronischen Entzündung. Abschnittsweise sieht man umschriebene Nekrosen, granulomatöse Veränderungen sowie büschelförmige Anhäufungen von Fettsäurenadeln (Abb. 3). Entsprechende mikromorphologische Untersuchungsergebnisse wurden von SCHNITLER; HOLZEL; HERING und UNDEUTSCH; DANDA und PLACHY; LANGER; MCDONALD; REYMANN; CORNBLEET und RATTNER;

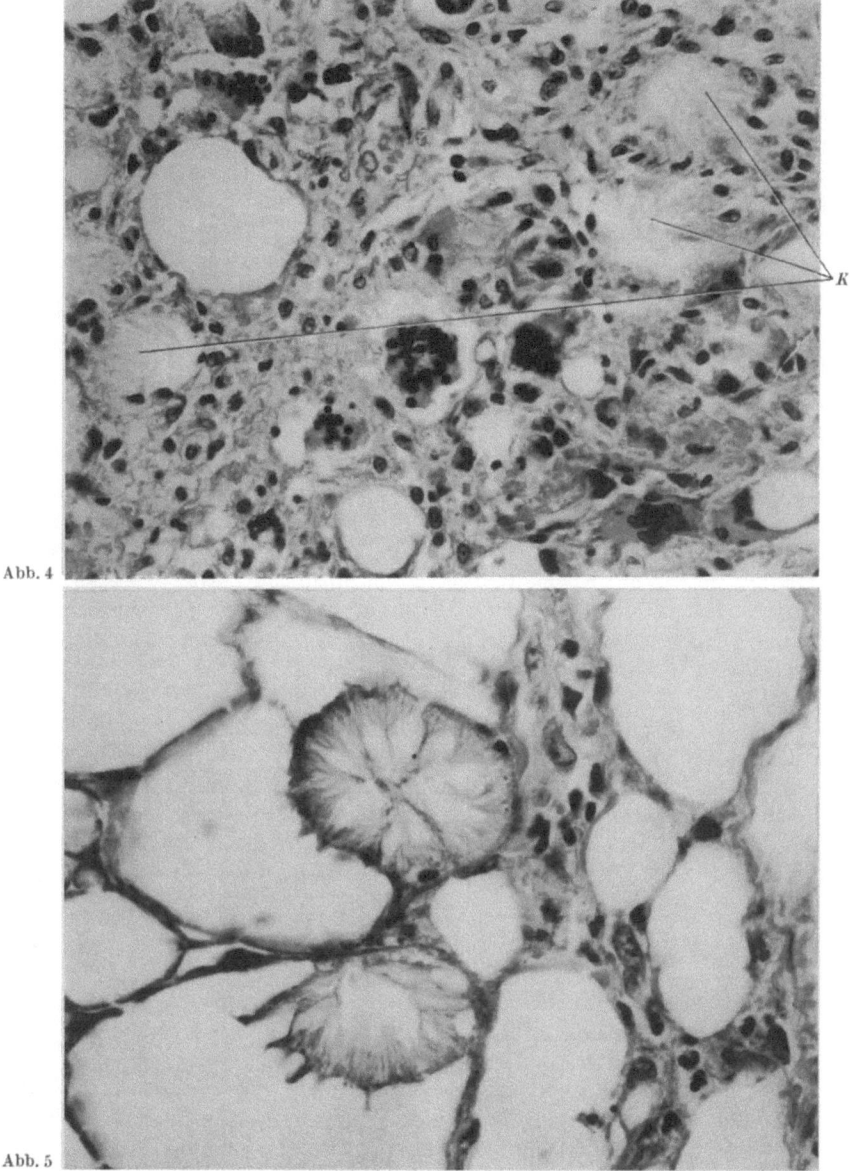

Abb. 4. Adiponecrosis subcutanea neonatorum. In den Fettzellen nadelartige Kristalle (*K*). Zwischen den Fettzellen strang- oder herdförmig angeordnetes Granulationsgewebe mit Riesenzellen. [Aus: W. OEHLERT, H. WECKE u. H. SÜTTERLE: Zbl. allg. Path. path. Anat. **107**, 499 (1965), Abb. 4]

Abb. 5. Adiponecrosis subcutanea neonatorum. Intracelluläre kristalline Fettsäureausfällungen. [Aus: W. OEHLERT, H. WECKE u. H. SÜTTERLE: Zbl. allg. Path. path. Anat. **107**, 499 (1965), Abb. 5]

FLORY; ZEEK und MADDEN; BOJLÉN und PETRY; SCHOEDD; PIAGGIO; SCRIBA; SIWE; DIECKHOFF u. Mitarb.; OEHLERT u. Mitarb.; LINDLAR u. MISGELD u. a.) mitgeteilt.

GRÜTZ hebt die Bedeutung von Fettzellvacuolen, die Umwandlung isotroper in anisotrope Fette mit Abnahme der Fettfärbbarkeit sowie die Anhäufung doppelbrechender kristalliner Substanzen hervor (s. auch HERING und UNDEUTSCH; LANGER; SIWE; DIECKHOFF u. Mitarb.). Die Kristalle sind intracellulär (Abb. 4 u. 5) gelegen (LANGER; GOTTRON; HERING und UNDEUTSCH; DIECKHOFF u. Mitarb.; OEHLERT u. Mitarb.), wurden aber auch extracellulär innerhalb der entzündlichen Infiltrate vorgefunden und bestehen aus Neutralfetten und Cholesterinestern (SIWE). BRAUN-FALCO fand aufgrund histochemischer Untersuchungen bei Beginn der Erkrankung sowohl bei der Adiponecrosis subcutanea neonatorum als auch beim Sclerema neonatorum in den mit Sudan III gut darstellbaren Fettzellen kleinste Kristalleinschlüsse. Die Neutralfette können mit der Nilblausulfatlösung sichtbar gemacht werden. Im Verlauf der Erkrankung nehmen die Kristalle auf Kosten der Neutralfette zu, bis diese das gesamte Cytoplasma ausgefüllt haben. Entsprechend der Zunahme der Kristalle nimmt die Darstellbarkeit der Neutralfette ab. NOOJIN u. Mitarb.; DIECKHOFF, HEMPEL u. KOCH konnten hingegen in den Fettnekrosen kein Cholesterin nachweisen. Freie Fettsäuren waren in geringem Umfang anzutreffen (s. auch LINDLAR u. MISGELD, 1967).

Das qualitativ veränderte Fettgewebe wird von der Peripherie der Fettläppchen her durch ein Granulationsgewebe ersetzt. Dieses kann von eosinophilen Leukocyten und Riesenzellen vom Fremdkörpertyp untermischt sein (ARZT; SCRIBA; DIECKHOFF u. Mitarb.; OEHLERT u. Mitarb. u.a.). Daneben kommen fibrocytär-fibroblastische Elemente zur Beobachtung (CAROL, PRACKEN und ZWIJNDREGT; HERING und UNDEUTSH; DIECKHOFF u. Mitarb.; OEHLERT u. Mitarb.). Nekrosen, Blutungen und Verkalkungen sind selten (ARZT; CAROL u. Mitarb.; HERING und UNDEUTSCH; LEVER; DIECKHOFF u. Mitarb.; OEHLERT u. Mitarb.; LINDLAR u. MISGELD), Gefäßveränderungen sekundärer Natur (BLANC). Der von LANGER beschriebenen positiven Esterasereaktion in Granulomen zur Abgrenzung gegenüber normalem Fettgewebe wird von KORTING keine spezifischdifferentialdiagnostische Bedeutung beigemessen. In späteren Krankheitsstadien tritt die Granulombildung zurück. Allmählich kommt es, wiederum von der Peripherie der Fettläppchen ausgehend, zu einem Ersatz des Granulationsgewebes durch Fettzellen. Schaumzellen (BLANC; WORINGER u. Mitarb.) und mehrkernige Fettzellen werden vorgefunden.

n) Necrosis progressiva subcutanea neonatorum

Die *Necrosis progressiva subcutanea neonatorum* weist ein ähnliches pathohistologisches Substrat wie die Adiponecrosis subcutanea neonatarum auf (FEHR; BUGYI; FEUERSTEIN; KORTING). Die Veränderungen sollen jedoch ihren Ausgang von der Fascie des subcutanen Fettgewebes nehmen. BUGYI weist bei der Beschreibung einer entsprechenden Beobachtung auf nekrotische Fettzellen hin, die von Histiocyten, Lymphocyten und Erythrocyten untermischt sind.

2. Patho-Histologie vorwiegend gefäßbedingter Erkrankungen des subcutanen Fettgewebes

Entzündliche Gefäßprozesse an Arteriolen, Capillaren und Venolen müssen aus klinischen und histologischen Gesichtspunkten von solchen an kleinen und mittelgroßen Arterien abgegrenzt werden (MIESCHER; RUITER; STORCK; GOUGEROT; STÜTTGEN; KORTING; ORBANEJA und PUCHOL; BOCK; SPIER; KNOTH und MEYHÖFER; JABLONSKA; EHLERS; SCHNEIDER und UNDEUTSCH u.a.).

Wir unterscheiden zwischen einer Arteriolitis-Capillaritis-Gruppe und der Periarteritis nodosa-Gruppe. Der Arteriolitis-Capillaritis-Gruppe rechnen wir die

Arteriolitis allergica (RUITER), die Papulose atrophiante maligne (DEGOS), das leukoklastische Mikrobid (MIESCHER-STORCK), das hämorrhagische Mikrobid (STORCK) sowie das Trisymptom von GOUGEROT zu. Der Purpura rheumatica Schoenlein-Henoch, obwohl histologisch häufig der Arteriolitis allergica Ruiter zugehörig, sollte aus klinischen und historischen Gesichtspunkten eine Sonderstellung zugestanden werden.

Die Hypersensitivitätsangiitis (ZEEK), die generalisierte Arteriitis (BERBLINGER), die nekrotisierende Arteriitis (MÜLLER-HOPPE), die allergische, granulomatöse, riesenzellhaltige Angiitis (CHURG-STRAUSS), die Vascular Allergy (HARKAVY) werden als Sonderform der Periarteriitis nodosa vom Typ Kussmaul-Maier-Gruber aufgefaßt (s. auch ALLEN; STÜTTGEN; BOCK; KNOTH und MEYHÖFER; ORBANEJA und PUCHOL; CERUTTI; SPIER u.a.). Im Gegensatz zur Periarteriitis nodosa cutanea handelt es sich bei den eben genannten Gefäßkrankheiten um systematisierte allergische Vasculitiden mit fakultativer Hautbeteiligung. Riesenzellhaltige, granulomatöse Befunde (HAMPERL; ALKIEWICZ) rechtfertigen nicht die Sonderstellung bestimmter Gefäßkrankheiten, wie KNOTH und MEYHÖFER nachweisen konnten. Der rhino-pharyngo-bronchialen Granulomatose Wegener kann sowohl vom klinischen als auch vom histologischen Standpunkt aus eine Sonderstellung eingeräumt werden. Die allergische Genese der Arteriitis temporalis Horton-Magath-Brown (senile, riesenzellhaltige Angiitis Erbslöh) wird von verschiedenen Autoren abgelehnt (ERBSLÖH; RANDERATH). Die Periarteriitis nodosa cutanea „benigna" stellt eine Sonderform der Periarteriitis nodosa vom Typ Kussmaul-Maier-Gruber dar, die, vorübergehend auf die Haut beschränkt, jederzeit in eine generalisierte Form mit Manifestation an den inneren Organen übergehen kann.

a) Periarteriitis nodosa-Gruppe

Veränderungen im Bereich des subcutanen Fettgewebes werden bei allergischen Gefäßkrankheiten der *Periarteriitis nodosa-Gruppe* gefunden, so daß die histologischen Befunde im Hinblick auf ihre Gemeinsamkeiten zusammenfassend besprochen werden können. Aufgrund der in der Literatur niedergelegten Befunde (RUITER; BRANDSMA u. Mitarb.; TEILUM; MIESCHER; ALLEN; GANS und STEIGLEDER; ORBANEJA und PUCHOL; DUPERRAT und MONFORT; McCOMBS; SZODORAY und VEZEKÉNY; PORTWICH; KNOTH und MEYHÖFER; EHLERS; TORO-GENKEL; LECZINSKY; INGRAM; JABLONSKA; CERUTTI; CSERMELY; TÉMINE u. Mitarb.; MOSKOWITZ u. Mitarb.; KULAGA; FISHER u. ORKIN u.a.), sowie eigener histologischer Untersuchungen an 28 Patienten mit einer *Periarteriitis nodosa cutanea* können folgende Besonderheiten festgestellt werden:

Der auffälligste krankhafte Prozeß findet sich an der Grenze von Corium und Fettgewebe sowie im Fettgewebe selbst. Im Bereich größerer Krankheitsbezirke liegen mittelgroße arterielle Gefäße, deren Lichtung nahezu vollständig verschlossen ist. Ein subintimales Ödem, Bindegewebswucherungen sowie eine entzündliche Infiltration führen zu einer stern- oder spaltförmigen Einengung des Lumens. An der Zellulation beteiligen sich vorwiegend polynucleäre Leukocyten, weniger Histiocyten, Lymphocyten und Plasmazellen. Partielle Thromben oder das Restlumen vollständig ausfüllende Blutgerinnsel mit einer später einsetzenden Rekanalisation kommen zur Beobachtung (MIESCHER; KETRON und BERNSTEIN; KNOTH u. MEYHÖFER u.a.). Die Muskellamellen der Media sind teilweise nekrobiotisch verändert. An Stellen, wo die Muskelfasern erhalten geblieben sind, sind dieselben verbreitert, fibrinoid verquollen oder frakturiert. Die Medianekrosen, nach MIESCHER für Erkrankungen der Periarteriitis nodosa-Gruppe charakteristisch, können konzentrisch angeordnet zwischen Intima und Media bzw.

zwischen Media und Adventitia gelegen (ORBANEJA und PUCHOL; STÜTTGEN u.a.) und von Epitheloidzellgranulomen umgeben sein (STÜTTGEN). Die nekrotischen Abschnitte werden durch ein zartfaseriges, zellreiches jugendliches Bindegewebe ersetzt. Die betroffenen Arterien können jedoch auch eine mehrschichtige, verdickte Muscularis aufweisen, wobei die Muskellamellen durch ein entzündliches Ödem bzw. durch ein entzündliches Infiltrat auseinandergedrängt werden. Mediaabscesse mit beginnender Aneurysmabildung kommen vor (MACAIGNE und NICAUD; KAZMEIER). Im Gegensatz zu anderen akuten Entzündungen der Gefäße sind eosinophile Leukocyten selten anzutreffen; dieselben können auch vollständig

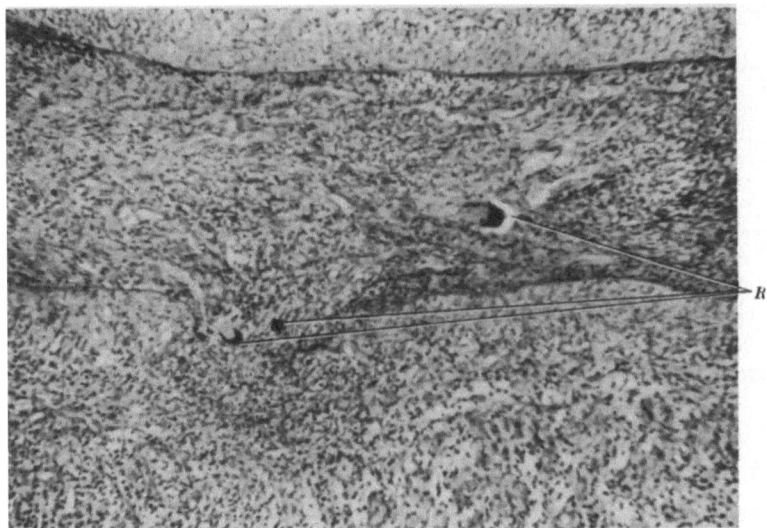

Abb. 6. Periarteriitis nodosa cutanea. Einengung des Gefäßlumens durch fibroblastisches Füllmaterial. Mediadefekt mit Aufbruch der Lamina elastica interna. Anlagerung hufeisenförmig gestalteter Riesenzellen (R) an die Elasticaabbruchstellen. [Aus: W. KNOTH u. W. MEYHÖFER: Dermatologica (Basel) 119, 1 (1959), Abb. 7]

vermißt werden. Charakteristisch dagegen ist eine Leukocytoklasie (MIESCHER; ORBANEJA und PUCHOL). Häufig wird ein unterschiedlich starker oder einseitiger Befall der Arterie mit Ausbildung von Adventitiagranulomen beobachtet. Es ist beachtenswert, daß akute oder subakut-entzündliche Gefäßwandveränderungen neben Ausheilungsstadien mit reparativem Ersatz nekrotischer Gefäßwandabschnitte vorkommen.

Die Lamina elastica interna kann abschnittsweise eine Zerstörung der Fasern mit Mediaaufbruch aufweisen. An den Abbruchstellen liegen vermehrt Zellen der chronischen Entzündung, untermischt von polynucleären Leukocyten. Besonders hervorzuheben ist der Nachweis von Riesenzellen, die mit ihrem hufeisenförmigen Kernkranz auf den Elasticaschaden gerichtet sind (KNOTH und MEYHÖFER). Obgleich in den Riesenzellen keine Elastica-Teilstücke gefunden wurden, wird die Beziehung durch die Anordnung der Riesenzellen zu den Bruchenden der elastischen Lamellen deutlich (Abb. 6).

KNOTH und MEYHÖFER haben bei einem Patienten mit nachweisbarer Hypertonie am gleichen Gefäß neben den für eine Periarteriitis nodosa typischen Gefäßveränderungen eine deutlich ausgeprägte Lamina elastica interna, die Einlagerung neugebildeter elastischer Fasern zwischen den einzelnen Muskellamellen sowie eine mehrfaserige Lamina elastica externa (sog. Hypertonie-Arterie) vorgefunden. Die Lamina elastica externa wurde durch ein mehr einseitig angelagertes granulomatöses Infiltrat begrenzt. Die betroffenen Arterien waren von Zellen der akuten und chronischen Entzündung umgeben. Eosinophile Leukocyten waren nur abschnittsweise anzutreffen. Diese Beobachtung von KNOTH und MEYHÖFER ist in pathogenetischer Hinsicht bemerkenswert.

Die Veränderungen an den arteriellen Gefäßen können in unterschiedlichem Ausmaß mit solchen an den Venen in Form der Thrombangiitis obliterans kombiniert sein. Eine subintimale Proliferation, Gefäßwandnekrosen sowie eine granulomatöse Entzündung führen zu einer Einengung der Lichtung mit Ausfüllung durch Thromben (RUITER u. Mitarb.; KORTING; MATRAS; ORBANEJA und PUCHOL; KNOTH und MEYHÖFER; BOCK; JABLONSKA; SANNICANDRO u.a.).

In der Umgebung der pathologisch veränderten Gefäße fallen Fettgewebsnekrosen, kleine Ölcysten sowie eine sog. Wucheratrophie mit Neubildung von Fettzellen auf, die durch einen zentral gelegenen Kern charakterisiert sind. Tuberkuloide und lipophage Granulome mit Riesenzellen vom Langhans- oder Fremdkörpertyp werden beobachtet (TÉMINE u. Mitarb.; CSERMELY u.a.). Zwischen den Fettzellen sind des weiteren fibrocytär-fibroblastische Elemente mit Faserneubildung zu erkennen. ORBANEJA und PUCHOL fanden Strukturen, welche den von MIESCHER für das Erythema nodosum beschriebenen Radiärknötchen gleichen. Die kollagenen Fasern der Fettgewebssepten sind arealweise homogenisiert und verschwielt.

Die *Hypersensitivitätsangiitis Zeek*, die *generalisierte Angiitis Berblinger*, die *nekrotisierende Arteriitis Müller-Hoppe* weisen akut-entzündliche Gefäßwandveränderungen und Umgebungsreaktionen auf, nehmen aber sowohl in pathogenetischer als auch in pathohistologischer Hinsicht eine gewisse Sonderstellung in der Periarteriitis nodosa-Gruppe ein.

Bei der *allergischen, riesenzellhaltigen, granulomatösen Angiitis Churg-Strauss*, der *Vascular Allergy Harkavy*, der *Arteriitis temporalis Horton-Magath-Brown* tritt bei gleichen pathologischen Veränderungen der Gefäßwände und des Fettgewebes die Ausbildung von granulomatösen Infiltraten und Riesenzellen in den Vordergrund. Die Riesenzellen können in der Langhans- oder Fremdkörperform auftreten (CHURG u. STRAUSS; HAMPERL; CARDELL u. HANLEY; KRAHULIK u. Mitarb.; FRANKENHEIM; HARRISON; REIN; RUITER; TEILUM; GANS und STEIGLEDER; RANDERATH; KNOTH und MEYHÖFER; BOCK; ERBSLÖH; EHLERS; WILLIAMS; AUFDERMAUER; SANNICANDRO u.a.). Die Unterscheidung der genannten Gefäßerkrankungen unter sich sowie deren Abgrenzung von der Periarteriitis nodosa ist nach ORBANEJA und PUCHOL nur im Anfang der nekrotischen Gefäßwandzerstörung und granulomatösen Entzündung und durch das Ausmaß der Beteiligung venöser Gefäße möglich, die bei der Periarteriitis nodosa zurücktritt. Die Art und Weise der Gefäßreaktion hängt sowohl vom auslösenden Agens als auch von der immunologischen Reaktionslage des Organismus ab. So können bei einer hyperergischen Reaktionslage exsudativ-leukocytäre Entzündungsvorgänge vom Typ des Arthus-Phänomens neben solchen vom Tuberkulintyp mit einer vorwiegend histiocytären Reaktion vorkommen. Bei einem hohen Grad der Immunität kommt es zur Ausbildung riesenzellhaltiger Granulome (LETTERER; STÜTTGEN; SANNICANDRO; AROUTUNOV u.a.).

Hautveränderungen bei der *Wegenerschen Granulomatose* sind selten und finden lediglich in Publikationen von APPAIX, PECH und CADACCIONI; REICH; JENSEN Erwähnung. Eingehende histologische Untersuchungen bei der rhino-pharyngobronchialen Granulomatose im Bereich der Haut wurden von KNOTH, BENEKE und KUNTZ (1965); KUNTZ, BENEKE und KNOTH (1967); PFEIFER u. JOCHEMS (1967); WEGENER (1967) durchgeführt.

Bei der Granulomatosis Wegener (rhino-pharyngo-bronchiale Granulomatose), der vom Klinischen und Histologischen her gesehen eine nosologische Sonderstellung zugestanden werden sollte, fallen neben Veränderungen an der Epidermis und dem Corium insbesondere solche im Fettgewebe auf. Mittelgroße Arterien muskulären Typs sind hochgradig pathologisch verändert. Die betroffenen Gefäße lassen lediglich noch eine spaltförmige Lichtung erkennen. Das Lumen ist abschnittsweise durch Fibrinmassen, verdämmernde Erythrocyten sowie histiocytär-fibrocytär-fibroblastische Elemente ausgefüllt. Rekanalisierungseffekte kommen vor. Subintimal findet sich eine Proliferation mehrfach aufeinandergereihter Zellelemente. Die Lamina elastica interna zeigt ausgedehnte Defekte und die Muscularis ist nur noch andeutungsweise zu erkennen. Zwischen den

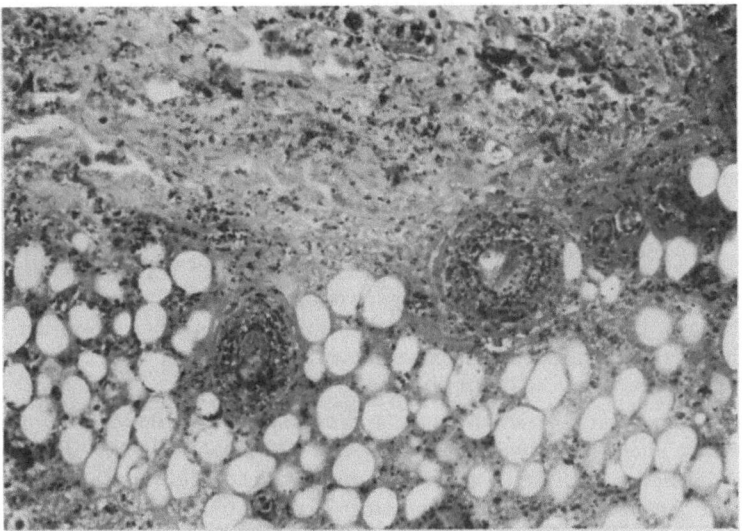

Abb. 7. Granulomatosis Wegener. Nekrotisierende Angiitis kleinerer Arterien im Fettgewebe und an der Corium-Fettgewebsgrenze. Nekrobiose und zellige Infiltration des umgebenden Fettgewebes. [Aus: W. KNOTH, G. BENEKE u. E. KUNTZ: Hautarzt 16, 289 (1965), Abb. 9]

Muskelfasern liegen Histiocyten, Lymphocyten und polynucleäre Leukocyten. Im Bereich anderer arterieller Gefäße kann das entzündliche Infiltrat zurücktreten. Die Muskelfasern sind infolge der ödematösen Durchtränkung der Gefäßwand auseinandergedrängt und unterschiedlich stark verquollen. Auch kleinere Arterien an der Corium-Fettgewebs-Grenze sind in den Krankheitsprozeß einbezogen. Diese weisen neben Intimadefekten eine partielle Thrombosierung der Lichtung, eine fibrinoide Verquellung der Media, Wandnekrosen sowie eine Durchmischung der Gefäßwand mit Zellen der chronisch-eitrigen Entzündung auf (Abb. 7). Während mittelgroße, muskuläre Arterien neben akuten subakute und chronisch-proliferierende Veränderungen erkennen lassen, sind in kleinen Arterien im allgemeinen ausschließlich Zellen der akuten Entzündung anzutreffen.

Periarteriell findet sich eine ödematöse Auflockerung des Gewebes mit begrenzendem mantelförmigem Infiltrat in Form eines chronisch bzw. chronisch-eitrigen Granulationsgewebes. Das umgebende Fettgewebe unterliegt einer Nekrose. Neben Zellen der chronisch-eitrigen Entzündung mit Karyorhexis und hyperchromatischen Kerntrümmern gelangen Fibrinabscheidungen, kleine Ölcysten sowie eine sog. Wucheratrophie zur Beobachtung (Abb. 8). Eine netzige, großzellig-granulomatöse Entzündung nach Art sog. Retothelknötchen kommt vorwiegend im Corium vor. Dieser Befund gestattet nach KNOTH trotz ähnlicher histomorphologischer Befunde an den Gefäßen eine Abgrenzung gegenüber der Periarteriitis nodosa cutanea vom Typ Kussmaul-Maier-Gruber.

Ob die *Lipatrophia anularis*, über die FERREIRA-MARQUES (1953) berichtet hat, in die Periarteriitis nodosa-Gruppe eingeordnet werden kann, ist schwer zu entscheiden. FERREIRA-MARQUES fand eine exzessive Atrophie des Fettgewebes sowie einen Ersatz bzw. eine Durchsetzung der Fettgewebsläppchen durch neugebildete kollagene und elastische Fasern. Die kollagenen Fasern zeigten eine parallele, wirbel- oder wellenförmige Anlagerung zu Bündeln. Die elastischen Fasern waren verdickt, aufgewunden und regellos angeordnet. In dem Gebiet der Neofibrillogenese konnten Histiocyten und Fibroblasten nachgewiesen werden.

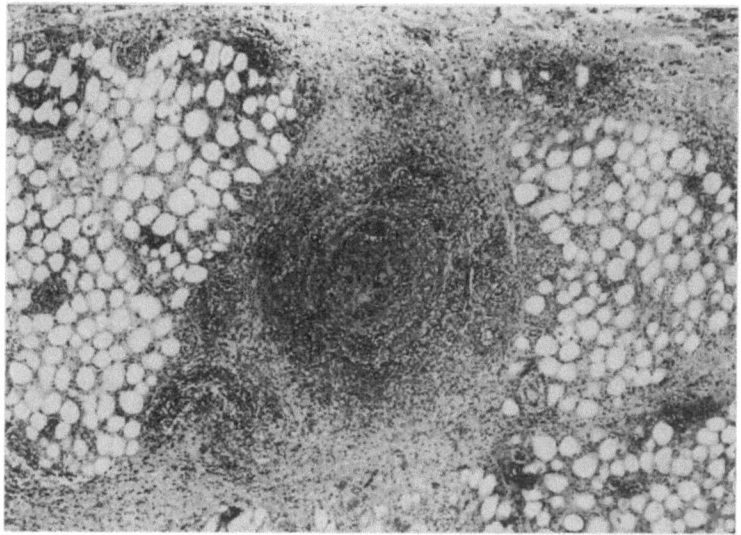

Abb. 8. Granulomatosis Wegener. Nekrotisierende Angiitis einer septalen Arterie. Periarterielle chronisch-eitrige Infiltration. Nekrobiose der Fettgewebssepten und Fettgewebsläppchen mit netzförmiger Durchsetzung von Zellen der akuten und chronischen Entzündung. [Aus: W. KNOTH, G. BENEKE u. E. KUNTZ: Hautarzt **16**, 289 (1965), Abb. 4]

Reticulumfasern wurden vermißt. In den Kollagenmassen waren rhombische Fettsäurekristalle anzutreffen. Die erhaltenen Fettzellen weisen eine gewellte oder rupturierte Cytoplasmamembran auf. Eine Fusion von Fettzellen zu Cysten, welche von Lipophagen umgeben waren, wurde beobachtet. Nekrotisches Fettgewebe selbst war nur noch in geringem Umfang nachweisbar.

Auffällig waren Gefäßveränderungen im Sinne einer Panarteriitis und Panphlebitis mit Wandverdickung, parietal angelagerten oder das Lumen verschließenden, partiell in Organisation befindlichen Schichtungsthromben, Wandruptur und Blutung. Perivasal fand sich neben der Ansammlung von Erythrocyten ein Infiltrat aus Lymphocyten und Fibroblasten mit Eindringen derselben in die Gefäßwand. An mehreren Stellen konnte eisenhaltiges Pigment aufgefunden werden.

Die Ätiologie der Lipatrophia anularis ist bisher nicht bekannt. Mechanische, chemische oder physikalische Traumen sowie Injektionen von Arzneimitteln wurden ausgeschlossen. Möglicherweise stehen vasculär-allergische Prozesse im Vordergrund der Erkrankung. Pathogenetisch gesehen könnten die Gefäßveränderungen für die Fettgewebsatrophie verantwortlich gemacht werden.

BRUINSMA hat 1967 über zwei weitere Beobachtungen mit zirkulär-bandförmiger Fettgewebsatrophie berichtet. Histologisch standen Gefäßveränderungen mit Endothelproliferation und Lichtungseinengung, Erythrocytenextravasate, eine Sklerosierung des subcutanen Fettgewebes mit Atrophie der Fettzellen sowie eine Myopathie mit ungewöhnlichen histochemischen Befunden im Vordergrund.

b) Necrobiosis lipoidica

Die *Necrobiosis lipoidica* wurde 1929 von OPPENHEIM beschrieben und 1932 von URBACH als Krankheit mit nosologischer Sonderstellung bestätigt. Auf dieses Krankheitsbild ist jedoch auch von GOLDSTEIN und HARRIS (1927) sowie von MCCORMAC (1930) aufmerksam gemacht worden (HARE).

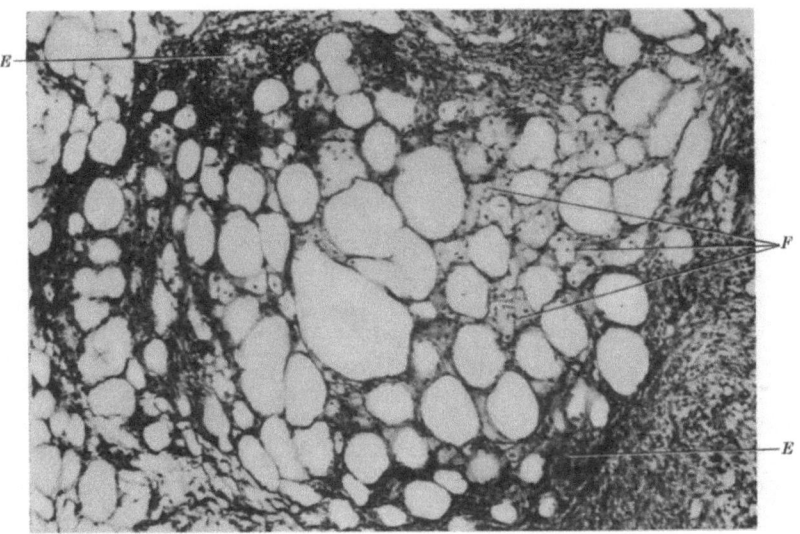

Abb. 9. Nekrobiosis lipoidica „diabeticorum". Lipogranulom mit Membranzerstörung, Zusammenfließen der Fettzellen und reaktiv-reparativer „Entzündung" (*E*). Im Zentrum Wucherung jugendlicher Fettzellen (*F*).
[Aus: W. KNOTH u. H. FÜLLER: Arch. Derm. Syph. (Berl.) **199**, 109 (1955), Abb. 8]

Eingehende histologische Untersuchungen führten KNOTH und FÜLLER (1955) durch (zur Necrosis lipoidica s. KORTING u. NÜRNBERGER, 1966). Auf die Darstellung des pathohistologischen Befundes des Coriums wird verzichtet. Es sollen lediglich solche Veränderungen Erwähnung finden, die das Fettgewebe betreffen. Vorwiegend sind obere Anteile des subcutanen Fettgewebes in das pathische Geschehen des Coriums einbezogen. An der Cutis-Subcutis-Grenze liegen Infiltrate aus Histiocyten, Lymphocyten und Plasmazellen, die jedoch seltener anzutreffen sind. BOLDT sah reichlich eosinophile Leukocyten. Daneben fallen vacuoläre Hohlräume auf, die über die normale Dimension von Fettzellen hinausreichen. Zwischen den Ölcysten unterschiedlicher Größe (SPRAFKE; KNOTH und FÜLLER) ist eine Wucherung jugendlicher Fettzellen zu erkennen, die durch einen noch zentral oder bereits exzentrisch liegenden Kern gekennzeichnet sind und nach KNOTH den Schaumzellen in Lipogranulomen gleichen. Zweikernigkeit dieser Zellen und feinwabiges Cytoplasma können demnach zur Beobachtung kommen. Außerdem finden sich Fettgewebsabschnitte, in denen neben Lymphocyten Monocyten und Epitheloidzellen sowie fibrocytär-fibroblastische Elemente anzutreffen sind (Abb. 9). Mehrkernige Riesenzellen vom Langhans- oder Fremdkörpertyp (BOLDT; HJORTH) kommen vor.

Von besonderer Bedeutung sind Veränderungen an kleineren und größeren arteriellen Gefäßen der Subcutis (s. KNOTH und FÜLLER; GÖTZ; TAPPEINER und WODNIANSKY; MULLER und WINKELMANN u. a.), die lediglich von PUCHOL vermißt wurden. Neben einer subendothelialen Wucherung, bestehend aus einem zellreichen, lockeren Bindegewebe, findet sich eine Hyperplasie der Lamina elastica interna. Die Media ist außer einer geringen Auflockerung der Muskelfasern unverändert. ENGEL und HAMMACK konnten diastaseresistente PAS-positive Substanzen nachweisen. Entzündliche Infiltrate, fibrinoide Verquellungen oder Nekrosen werden in der Gefäßwand nicht beobachtet. Die Gefäßlichtung selbst ist erheblich eingeengt, eine Thrombosierung kann vorkommen (HEILESEN; GÖTZ; BREZHENKO; GRIMMER). GRIMMER weist neben den beschriebenen Veränderungen an den Arterien auf eine subendotheliale Proliferation auch in größeren Venen mit Aufsplitterung und Unterbrechung der Fasern der Lamina elastica interna, Einengung der Lichtung und periadventitieller Wucherung des Bindegewebes hin.

Nach KNOTH ist die vorliegende Angiopathie als Endarteriitis productiva fibrosa mit geringer elastisch-fibröser Intimahyperplasie zu bezeichnen. Die mikromorphologisch faßbaren Gefäßveränderungen, die Histo- und Pathogenese der beschriebenen Angiopathien fanden bei der Erörterung der Necrobiosis lipoidica im allgemeinen nur wenig Berücksichtigung (URBACH; OPPENHEIM; BALBI; GROSS u. Mitarb.; RÖDERER; WORINGER und BURGUN; CONNOR u. a.). Seit den Mitteilungen von BOLDT; GOTTRON; SCHUERMANN; WINER; KNOTH und FÜLLER; GÖTZ; LEVER wird den Gefäßveränderungen jedoch zunehmend mehr Bedeutung beigemessen (FORMAN; PEZZAROSSA; SMITH; WORINGER und WEILL; ENGEL und HAMMACK; RINGROSE; HJORTH; BREZHENKO; GROTS, STRAUSS u. MESCON; DIMITRESCU und BĂLUS; KALDOR und NEKAM; GRIMMER u. a.).

Zusammenfassend sind bei der Necrobiosis lipoidica neben den pathologischen Gefäßveränderungen Fettzellgruppen mit zerstörten Protoplasmamembranen und Ausbildung zu unterschiedlich großen Ölcysten, Gewebsareale mit gewucherten jugendlichen Fettzellen, granulomatöse Abschnitte mit Epitheloidzellformationen sowie reaktiv-reparative Entzündungsvorgänge anzutreffen.

c) Necrobiosis maculosa

Bei der *Necrobiosis maculosa* entsprechen die histomorphologischen Veränderungen weitgehend denen der Necrobiosis lipoidica (MIESCHER), so daß auf eine weitere Erörterung verzichtet werden kann. Gefäßveränderungen wurden von MIESCHER nicht gefunden, von GERTLER; GARTMANN und KIESSLING beschrieben. Die Gefäßwände, insbesondere an der Cutis-Subcutis-Grenze, sind verdickt; abschnittsweise fällt eine Obliteration des Lumens auf. Hämorrhagien kommen zur Beobachtung. Neben den bereits erwähnten nekrobiotischen Fettgewebsarealen ist eine granulomatöse Entzündung aus Histiocyten, Lymphocyten und Riesenzellen vom Langhans- oder Fremdkörpertyp nachweisbar, welche die Nekrobiose begrenzt. In frischeren Efflorescenzen findet sich gelegentlich eine Radiärstellung der Histiocyten. Die angeführten Infiltrate können von fibrocytär-fibroblastischen Elementen sowie von eosinophilen Leukocyten und Plasmazellen untermischt sein (JONES; LEIFER; LESLIE; FORMAN; DEGOS; WORINGER).

d) Granulomatosis disciformis chronica et progressiva Miescher

Über die *Granulomatosis disciformis chronica et progressiva*, von GOTTRON (1934) als Granulomatosis tuberculoides pseudosclerodermiformis chronica beschrieben, haben 1935 MIESCHER, 1948 MIESCHER und LEDER berichtet. Nach

Hare wurden vergleichbare Fälle von Stowers (1921), McCormac (1921), Goldsmith (1928: morphoea with tuberculoid histology), Volk (1931), Vero (1934), Traub (1934) und Wise (1934) mitgeteilt.

Diese Erkrankung unterscheidet sich von der Necrobiosis lipoidica histologisch durch den Nachweis tuberkuloider Formationen um sklerosierte und hyalinisierte Bindegewebsabschnitte (Gottron; Miescher und Leder; Hare; Götz; Dorn; Reich; Knoth; Lever; Hjorth u. a.). Das histologische Bild kann an ein Sarkoid Darier-Roussy oder an einen Morbus Besnier-Boeck-Schaumann erinnern.

Gartmann; Arzt; Kogoj u. Mitarb.; Tappeiner berichten über pathologische Veränderungen auch im Fettgewebe. Kogoj fand in der Subcutis neben Stellen der Wucheratrophie perivasale Infiltrate, welche die Fettgewebsläppchen teilweise ersetzen können. Außer den Zellen der chronischen Entzündung fielen vereinzelt polynucleäre und eosinophile Leukocyten auf. Riesenzellen vom Langhans- und Fremdkörpertyp waren nachweisbar (s. auch Gartmann; Keining und Braun-Falco; Arzt u. a.). Nirgends waren dagegen Strukturen typischen tuberkuloiden Aufbaues oder Nekrosen aufzufinden. Lediglich Arzt beobachtete neben den beschriebenen Rundzellinfiltraten die Zusammenlagerung histiocytärer Elemente zu tuberkuloiden Knötchen. Tappeiner machte darauf aufmerksam, daß die Epitheloidzellkomplexe von einem schmalen Lymphocytensaum umgeben sein können. Die Blutgefäße zeigten eine Durchsetzung mit Histiocyten, Lymphocyten sowie wenigen polynucleären Leukocyten.

Bei mehreren Fällen mit Granulomatosis disciformis chronica et progressiva fanden wir histologisch faßbare Veränderungen auch im Bereich der Fettgewebssepten. Hier lassen sich runde, ovale oder bizarr konfigurierte sklerosierte Abschnitte nachweisen, die von einem granulomatösen Randwall begrenzt werden. Histiocytäre und knötchenförmig-epitheloidzellige Formationen, untermischt von Lymphocyten und wenigen Plasmazellen, umgeben die sklerosierten und hyalinisierten Bindegewebsareale. Riesenzellen vom Langhans- oder Fremdkörpertyp kommen häufiger zur Beobachtung. Die Zellen der chronischen Entzündung greifen in retikulärer Anordnung auf die Peripherie der Fettläppchen über.

Von besonderer Bedeutung sind Gefäßabweichungen, auf die Fleck; Goldsmith; Götz; Mali; Miescher und Burckhardt; K. Linser; Santler; Knoth; Hjorth; Ringrose u. a. aufmerksam machten und lediglich von Tappeiner verneint, von Keining und Braun-Falco als unwesentlich bezeichnet wurden. Kleinere und mittelgroße arterielle Gefäße in den Fettgewebsläppchen sind wandverdickt, lichtungseingeengt, hyalinisiert und zeigen eine subendotheliale Schwellung mit Neubildung zarter Bindegewebsfasern. Thrombosierungen kommen vor (Götz). Die pathologischen Gefäßveränderungen entsprechen in mehrfacher Hinsicht den bei der Necrobiosis lipoidica beschriebenen und werden von Santler der Endangiitis productiva zugerechnet. Gottron spricht von einer Endarteriopathia chronica deformans, da entzündliche Gefäßwandveränderungen nicht vorliegen. Perivasal sind ringförmig angeordnet Rundzellinfiltrate aus Histiocyten und Lymphocyten nachzuweisen, welche nur sehr selten in der Gefäßwand selbst angetroffen werden können.

e) Lipogranulomatosis subcutanea hypertonica Gottron

Auf die *Lipogranulomatosis subcutanea hypertonica* hat Gottron (1952) aufmerksam gemacht. Die Besonderheit des histologischen Befundes im Bereich des subcutanen Fettgewebes ist in den zu Lipogranulomen führenden Kreislaufstörungen zu suchen. Bei Patienten mit einem latenten oder fixierten Hypertonus kommt es zu endarteriitischen Gefäßveränderungen, die Gottron als Endarteriopathia chronica deformans bezeichnet wissen möchte, da entzündliche Zellelemente in der Gefäßwand vermißt werden. Die Blutgefäße weisen eine subendotheliale Proliferation mit Wandverdickung und Lichtungseinengung auf. Von besonderem Interesse ist der Nachweis neu gebildeter elastischer Fasern zwischen den einzelnen Muskellamellen sowie eine mehrlamelläre Lamina elastica externa. Die Mediaelastose ist für sog. Hypertoniearterien charakteristisch. Das gleichzeitige Vorkommen einer Hypertoniearterie mit Periarteriitis nodosa bei fixiertem Bluthochdruck wurde von KNOTH und MEYHÖFER beobachtet. Sekundär kommt es im Versorgungsgebiet der betroffenen Gefäße zu Gewebsnekrosen und insbesondere an der Cutis-Subcutis-Grenze zur Ausbildung einer granulomatös-retikulären Entzündung mit Lipophagen und Riesenzellen vom Fremdkörpertyp.

Bei eigenen histologischen Untersuchungen entsprechender Beobachtungen fanden sich neben den bereits beschriebenen obliterierenden, nicht entzündlichen Gefäßveränderungen Epitheloidzellen sowie Schaum- und Riesenzellen enthaltende Granulome, die in der Umgebung nekrotischer Fettgewebsareale anzutreffen waren (s. auch Fall GOTTRON; LANGHOF).

GOTTRON betrachtet aufgrund des pathohistologischen Befundes die Lipogranulomatosis subcutanea hypertonica als tiefgelegene Dermatitis lipoides atrophicans (Necrobiosis lipoidica), da primär auch hier Gefäßwandveränderungen nicht entzündlicher Art vorliegen.

f) Pingranliquose

Durch primäre Gefäßveränderungen mit begrenzten Ernährungsstörungen des Fettgewebes kann im überdimensionierten Fettpolster älterer Menschen die sog. *Pingranliquose* (WASSNER, 1962) entstehen. Histologisch findet sich eine zentrale Hohlraumbildung, welche von einer kernreichen Wandung umgeben wird. Diese zeigt eine lamelläre Schichtung. Im Anschluß an das präexistente Fettgewebe sind zusammengedrängte ovaläre Fettzellen, deren Membranen von Histiocyten umschlossen werden, zu erkennen. Eine völlige Verschmelzung der Fettzellen fällt an der Membraninnenseite auf. Ältere Wandungen sind durch einen Verlust des Kernreichtums sowie den Ersatz der Fettzellen durch ein Granulationsgewebe gekennzeichnet. Kalkeinlagerungen an der Innenwand kommen vor (Abb. 10). Auffällig sind Gefäßveränderungen in der Umgebung der Fettgewebsnekrosen. Bei größeren arteriellen Gefäßen kommen neben einer Lichtungseinengung infolge einer subendothelialen Schwellung und Proliferation Lipideinlagerungen, Hyalinisierung von Mediaabschnitten sowie nekrobiotische Gefäßwandabschnitte zur Beobachtung (Abb. 11). Gefäße kleineren Kalibers weisen lediglich eine subintimale polsterförmige Schwellung und Proliferation jugendlicher Bindegewebszellen mit Lichtungseinengung oder Verschluß des Lumens auf. Nach WASSNER lassen sich die pathologischen Gefäßveränderungen einerseits der Arteriosklerose, andererseits der Endangiitis obliterans zuordnen.

Pathogenetisch stehen bei der Pingranliquose die Gefäßveränderungen im Vordergrund. Es kommt nicht zur Nekrose einzelner Fettzellen, sondern zum Untergang von Fettläppchen. Die zum Fremdkörper gewordenen, aus der Zelle entlassenen Fettsubstanzen führen zur membranartigen Kompression angrenzender Fettgewebsbezirke. Die Einwanderung von Zellen der akuten und chronischen Entzündung mit Ausbildung eines Granulationsgewebes, die bindegewebige Umwandlung der Kapsel sowie die Kalkeinlagerungen gehören späteren Phasen an.

MÜLLER u. KRAUL (1967) haben die nosologische Sonderstellung der Pingranliquose bestätigt. Bis auf eine Hyalinisierung oder beginnende Nekrobiose zentraler Lipogranulomabschnitte konnten alle von WASSNER beschriebenen histologischen

Kriterien nachgewiesen werden. Die Erhöhung der Serum-Gesamtlipide mit obliterierender Arteriosklerose der Gefäße des subcutanen Fettgewebes wird pathogenetisch in den Vordergrund gestellt.

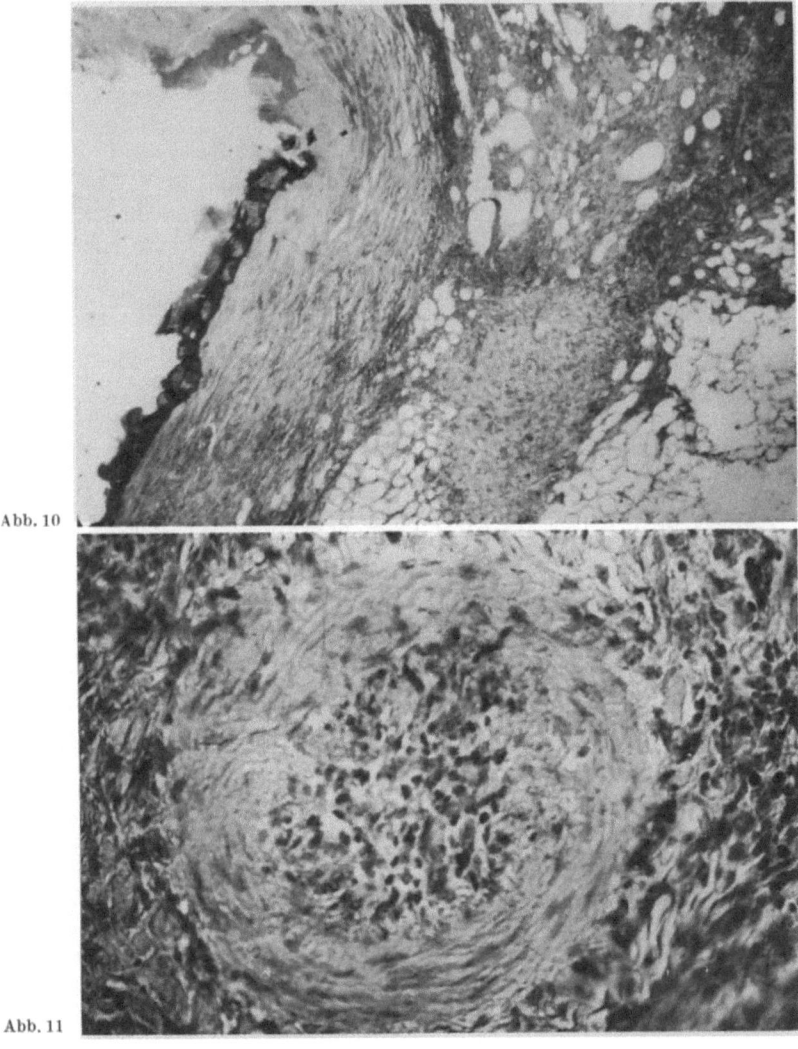

Abb. 10. Sog. Pingranliquose. Nekrotisierende Fettgewebsentzündung mit multiplen Ölcysten und Ausbildung eines großen Hohlraumes. An der Innenseite der lamellär geschichteten Cystenwand Kalkablagerungen. (Aus: U. J. WASSNER: Med. Welt 1962, 1, Abb. 5)

Abb. 11. Sog. Pingranliquose. Arterielles Gefäß in der Umgebung der Hohlraumbildung. Hyalinisierung der Gefäßwand und Verschluß des Lumens durch fibroblastisches Füllmaterial. (Aus: U. J. WASSNER: Med. Welt 1962, 1, Abb. 7)

V. Tumoren des subcutanen Fettgewebes

Tumoren des Fettgewebes sind bis auf die verhältnismäßig häufig vorkommenden Lipoblastome relativ selten anzutreffen. Die Geschwülste nehmen ihren Ausgang sowohl von den Fettzellen als auch von den Bindegewebszellen, wobei gut- und bösartige Formen unterschieden werden können.

Von besonderem Interesse sind Tumoren des braunen Fettgewebes, die als Hibernome (GERY) oder proliferierende Lipome (GLOGGENGIESSER) bezeichnet werden. Die Zellen des braunen Fettgewebes verdanken ihre Farbe dem hohen Gehalt an Atmungsfermenten (JOEL und BALL) und sind durch den Nachweis zahlreicher kleiner Fettvacuolen gekennzeichnet. Aufgrund experimenteller Untersuchungen konnte sichergestellt werden, daß dem braunen Fettgewebe die Funktion der Wärmebildung zukommt (DAWKINS und HULL; HULL und SEGALL). Die Zellen weisen einen hohen Sauerstoffverbrauch auf (DAWKINS und HULL). Bei den der Kälte ausgesetzten Tieren steigt die Hydrolyse der Triglyceride zu Fettsäuren und Glycerin an. Die Fettsäuren werden jedoch im Gegensatz zum weißen Fettgewebe nicht an das Blut abgegeben, sondern intracellulär erneut zu Triglyceriden resynthetisiert oder zu Kohlendioxyd und Wasser oxydiert, wobei chemische Energie in Wärme umgesetzt wird (BALL und JUNGAS). AHERNE und HULL fanden auch bei unreifen und reifen Neugeborenen sowie den Erwachsenen reichlich braunes Fettgewebe. Nach HULL und SEGALL enthält braunes Fettgewebe von Säuglingen nach Unterkühlung keine Fettvacuolen mehr. Das Cytoplasmaglycerin nimmt zu, ohne daß die freien Fettsäuren ansteigen. Die Untersuchungsbefunde von DAWKINS und SCOPES deuten darauf hin, daß die Fettoxydation in den Zellen des braunen Fettgewebes selbst erfolgen muß (s. auch MENSCHIK; SIDMAN und FAWCETT; ARONSON u. Mitarb.; PÖHL; SIDMAN; MELICOW; BOERNER-PATZELT; LEVER; RÉMILLARD; LANGER und LANGER-SCHIERER; NAPOLITANO und FAWCETT; BALBONI; PLENERT; HELMAN und HELLERSTRÖM; GIESEKING; LINDBERG, DE PIERRE, RYLANDER u. AFZELIUS; IKEMOTO u. a.).

Für die Entwicklung einer Anzahl von Geschwülsten des Fettgewebes könnte die prospektive Potenz der Fettzellen von Bedeutung sein. Wie bereits an anderer Stelle ausgeführt, besteht das als Primitivorgan angelegte Fettgewebe aus „reticulo-endothelialen" Zellen (WASSERMANN). GOLDNER spricht von einer histiocytären Abstammung der Fettzellen. Neben den Fettzellen konnten im Fettgewebe auch Histiocyten und silberimprägnierbare Fasern nachgewiesen werden (LAUBINGER; STEIGLEDER). Den Bindegewebszellen der Adventitialzone muß möglicherweise, insbesondere aufgrund neuer elektronenmikroskopischer Befunde (GIESEKING), eine besondere Bedeutung beigemessen werden. v. ALBERTINI betont den Reticulumzellcharakter der Pericyten, wobei die Reticulumfasern durch Silberimprägnation darstellbar sind. Auf die Bedeutung der pluripotenten Adventitialzellen haben vor allem MAXIMOW; MARCHAND sowie HERZOG hingewiesen. Experimentelle Untersuchungen veranlaßten HERZOG zu dem Rückschluß, daß diesen in der Indifferenzzone der Gefäße liegenden Zellen eine Vielzahl möglicher Differenzierungsformen innewohnt, wobei die Bildung von Lymphoblasten, Lymphocyten, Myeloblasten, neutrophilen und eosinophilen Leukocyten sowie von histiocytären Elementen möglich ist (s. auch W. KNOTH, 1958).

Nach STEIGLEDER sind die Potenzen des Fettgewebes unterschätzt, aber auch überschätzt worden. Die relativ einförmige Fettgewebsreaktion bei nicht-entzündlichen, entzündlichen, vorwiegend gefäß- oder degenerativ bedingten Prozessen ist beispielsweise weniger auf die eingeschränkte Reizantwort als auf den das Fettgewebe treffenden gleichen Reiz, die Auseinandersetzung des Gewebes mit freien Fettsäuren, zurückzuführen (STEIGLEDER). Die Vorstellungen über die Entstehung der Fettgewebsgeschwülste hängen eng mit der Entwicklung des Fettgewebes selbst zusammen. Eine allgemeingültige Deutung im Hinblick auf die Entwicklung dieser Tumoren läßt sich bisher nicht geben; diese kann nur im Zusammenhang mit pathogenetischen Vorstellungen über die Manifestation von Geschwülsten im allgemeinen gesehen werden. Wie für das Insulinlipom nachgewiesen, scheinen entzündliche Vorgänge im subcutanen Fettgewebe pathogenetisch ebenfalls eine Rolle zu spielen (HELD und DELLA SANTA; BAUMGARTNER und RIVA u. a.).

1. Gutartige Tumoren
a) Lipoblastoma cutis

Das *Lipoblastoma cutis* tritt in der Einzahl oder multipel (Lipomatosis cutis) im Bereich der Subcutis auf. Seltener werden diese Geschwülste auch subfascial, intermuskulär, in den Muskellogen oder parostal angetroffen (MADELUNG; POWER; KENIN; LEVINE und SPINNER u. a.).

Bei der histologischen Untersuchung findet sich in runder oder ovaler Anordnung ein Tumor, welcher von einer schmalen Bindegewebskapsel umgeben wird und aus verschieden großen Fettläppchen besteht. Bei tiefer gelegenen Lipomen kann die Kapsel weniger gut ausgebildet sein (WARD-HENDRICK). Die Fettzellen weisen eine unterschiedliche Größe und Entwicklungsreife auf, die Zellmembran ist gewellt. Es kommen runde, ovale, spindelige, polygonale und übergroße Formen zur Beobachtung (MATHIS). In der Regel handelt es sich um univacuolär mit Fett gefüllte Zellen, bei einem kleineren Teil sind die cytoplasmatischen Fettsubstanzen in feindisperser Form abgelagert. Der sichelförmige Zellkern liegt an der Peripherie der Fettzelle. Kerngrößenvariationen werden nicht vorgefunden, Mitosen vermißt. An den Außenzonen wachsender Geschwülste können Wachstumskerne mit jugendlichen Fettzellen nachgewiesen werden. Die runden oder ovalen Lipoblasten enthalten einen, seltener mehrere Zellkerne, welche zentral gelegen sind. Die Fettsubstanzen sind feinkörnig abgelagert. Fettzelltypen von besonderer Größe mit granuliertem Cytoplasma und zentraler Lokalisation des Zellkerns deuten nach THOMA auf ein schnelleres Wachstum der Geschwulst hin. Erst in späteren Wachstumsstadien konfluieren die Fettgranula zu unterschiedlich großen Fettvacuolen, wobei der Zellkern allmählich an die Peripherie gedrängt wird. Die Lipoblastenzonen sind von zahlreichen Capillaren durchsetzt. Die Lipome enthalten Neutralfett und stimmen hinsichtlich ihrer Zusammensetzung mit der des subcutanen Fettgewebes überein (SHANKS, PARANCHYCH und TUBA).

Nach HORNSTEIN lassen sich bei sorgfältiger Durchmusterung der Lipome neben kleinfleckigen atrophischen Arealen Bezirke mit einer sog. Wucheratrophie, lymphocytoide Knötchen und regelrechte Blutbildungsherde, insbesondere im frühkindlichen Alter, nachweisen. Daneben kommen initiale Capillarwucherungen zur Beobachtung. Diese Befunde können aufgrund eigener Untersuchungen bestätigt werden.

Die Fettläppchen selbst werden von unterschiedlich breiten Bindegewebssepten begrenzt. Die Fettgewebssepten bestehen aus schmalen kollagenen Fasern und lassen perivasal nur wenige Zellen der chronischen Entzündung erkennen. Jedes Tumorläppchen ist im Besitz einer zuführenden Arterie sowie einer abführenden Vene, denen reichlich Capillaren zwischengeschaltet sind (SHANKS, PARANCHYCH und TUBA; GRIMAUD und BEAU; HORNSTEIN; GANS und STEIGLEDER; KUSKE, PASCHOUD und SOLTERMANN; MÖBIUS, NÖDL; HERRMANN; MÜLLER u.a.).

b) Fibrolipom — Angiolipom

Unter pathologischen Zuständen können sich die Lipoblasten offenbar in andere mesenchymale Zellen differenzieren (STOUT; WILLIS; MÖBIUS u.a.). Bei *Fibrolipomen* steht die Neubildung fibrösen Bindegewebes, bei *Angiolipomen* die Ausbildung von Gefäßen im Vordergrund. Die Fettzellen dieser Geschwülste unterscheiden sich nicht von denen typischer Lipome. Myxomatöse, verkalkende oder verknöchernde Lipomabschnitte kommen vor (MERKEL; ROSER; MARCHAND; REHN; TEDESCH; LEVER; HELD und DELLA SANTA; NÖDL u.a.).

c) Hämangioblastom

Capilläre und kavernöse *Hämangioblastome* können nicht nur auf das Fettgewebe übergreifen, sondern selbst im subcutanen Fettgewebe gelegen sein.

Das *Haemangioma capillare* setzt sich unter Verdrängung der umgebenden Fettgewebsläppchen aus gruppen- oder strangförmig angeordneten, undifferenzierten Zellkomplexen zusammen. Die runden, ovalen oder spindelförmigen Zellkerne sind im allgemeinen chromatinreich, können jedoch auch ein deutlich aufgelockertes Chromatingerüst aufweisen. Die Kernpolymorphie ist gering, Teilungsfiguren gelangen selten zur Darstellung. Innerhalb der Zellgruppen kommt es zur Ausbildung kleinerer Hohlräume, die von endothelartigen Zellen mit flachen länglichen oder längsovalen Kernen begrenzt werden. Die Lichtungen enthalten verschieden große Erythrocytenaggregate.

Runde oder ovale Hohlräume unterschiedlicher Größe werden beim *Haemangioma cavernosum* bandförmig von 2—5 Zellreihen umgeben. Cytomorphologisch unterscheiden sich die angioblastischen Elemente nicht von denen der capillären Hämangiome. Der Endothelbelag kann teilweise verlorengehen, so daß die in der Lichtung nachweisbaren Blutmassen scheinbar frei im Gewebe liegen. Kavernöse Hohlräume sind in wechselndem Maße von Thromben ausgefüllt, die einer partiellen Organisation unterliegen. Abschnittsweise ragen klappen- oder septenartige Gebilde, die als Reste benachbarter, konfluierter, cystisch erweiterter Hohlräume aufzufassen sind, in die Lichtung. Die angiomatösen Komplexe werden von normal ausgestalteten Fettzellgruppen oder Fettgewebsläppchen umgeben. Die Fettzellen sind unterschiedlich groß, die Cytoplasmamembran ist gewellt. Daneben findet sich ein lockeres Bindegewebe, das den Fettgewebssepten zugeordnet werden kann. Die kollagenen Fasern sind schmal, abschnittsweise rupturiert und weisen dann eine blaugraue Tingierung auf.

d) Hibernom

Hibernome sind klinisch von Lipomen nicht abzugrenzen. Die Geschwulst besteht aus relativ kleinen Fettläppchen, wird von einem dichten Capillarnetz durchzogen (NOVY und WILSON) und ist gekennzeichnet durch den Nachweis mehrkammeriger, maulbeerartiger Fettzellen. Cytoplasmatisch diffus granulierte Zellen kommen seltener zur Beobachtung. Die Fettzellen sind rund, oval oder polygonal ausgestaltet und lassen einen zentral gelegenen Kern erkennen. Die Zellkerne zeigen ein ausgeprägtes Chromatinnetz mit 1—3 gut abgrenzbaren Nucleoli. Die Fettsubstanzen sind in Form kleiner, granulär angeordneter oder größerer Fetttropfen abgelagert. Durch Zusammenfluß der Granula zu kleineren Fettvacuolen, welche von einem schmalen Cytoplasmasaum umgeben werden, entsteht die oben beschriebene Kammerung, wobei der Kern allmählich an die Zellperipherie gedrängt wird. Die Plasmatröpfchen können auch randständig angeordnet sein. Nach GENESI zeigt das eingelagerte Fett eine unterschiedliche Anfärbbarkeit, die von der Zellentwicklung abhängig ist. Im Gegensatz zu Fettsubstanzen der Lipome sollen die der Hibernome im polarisierten Licht doppelbrechend sein (SUTHERLAND u. Mitarb.). PUTZMANN dagegen konnte doppelbrechende Lipoide nicht nachweisen. Eine Kernpolymorphie und Mitosen kommen bei Hibernomen nicht zur Beobachtung (SUTHERLAND u. Mitarb.; COX; BRINES und JOHNSON; GANS und STEIGLEDER; LEVER; GROSS und WOOD; NOVY u. WILSON; PUTZMANN u.a.).

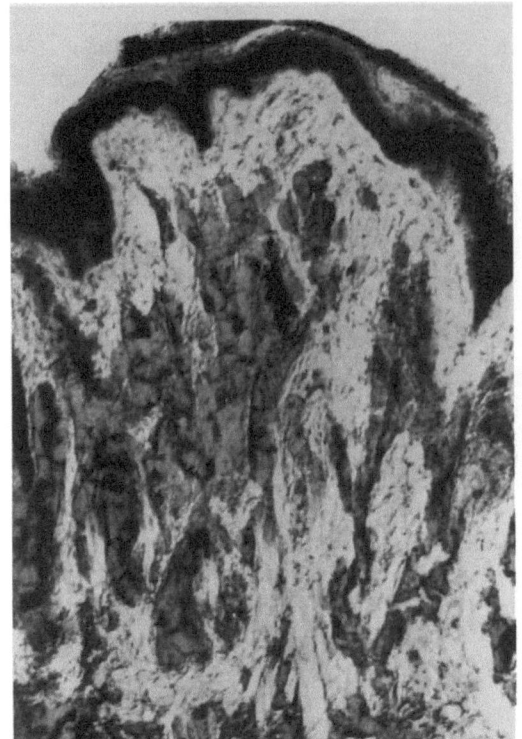
Abb. 12

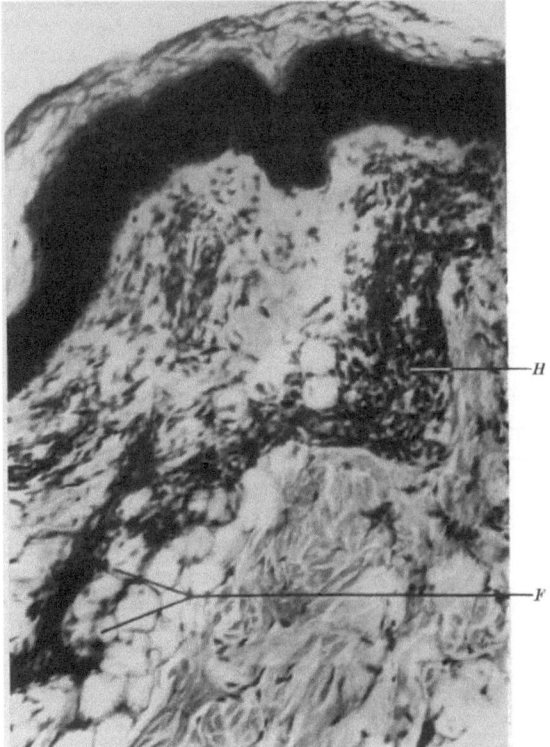
Abb. 13
(Legenden s. S. 823)

e) Naevus lipomatosus cutaneus superficialis Hoffmann-Zurhelle

Der *Naevus lipomatosus cutaneus superficialis Hoffmann-Zurhelle* (NIKOLOWSKI; THÖNE; KÚTA; HERING; GANS und STEIGLEDER; NÖDL; CRAMER; HOLTZ u.a.) ist charakterisiert durch den Nachweis dystopisch gelegener Fettzellen im Corium (zur Nomenklatur s. W. KNOTH, 1962). Die länglich angeordneten Fettzellgruppen orientieren sich ebenso wie zwischengeschaltete kollagenfaserige Anteile in vertikaler Richtung auf die Epidermis (Abb. 12). Die Fettzellen können jedoch auch isoliert liegen oder zu Läppchen angeordnet sein. Ein Zusammenhang mit dem subcutanen Fettgewebe besteht nicht. Die Fettzellgruppen entwickeln sich besonders häufig in der Nachbarschaft von Gefäßen (HOLTZ; NIKOLOWSKI; KNOTH). Dieser Befund kommt in Epidermisnähe besonders deutlich zum Ausdruck (Abb. 13). Die großvacuolären, ausgereiften Elemente zeigen wie diejenigen des Fettgewebes eine positive Fettfärbung. Die Zellkerne sind nur noch selten im Zentrum, in der Mehrzahl an der Peripherie der Fettzellen anzutreffen. Die kollagenen Fasern sind schmaler als gewöhnlich und färben sich arealweise mit polychromem Methylenblau metachromatisch an (BROCQ; RIST; GANS und STEIGLEDER; NIKOLOWSKI). Die Bindegewebsveränderungen können jedoch auch vermißt werden (ROBINSON und ELLIS; THÖNE).

2. Bösartige Tumoren

a) Liposarkom

Liposarkome entstehen nach STERNBERG als solche, können sich jedoch auch aus einem Lipom entwickeln (WILLIS; BOYD u.a.). Typische Lipome verlassen hinsichtlich ihrer biologischen Wertigkeit nach HERRMANN sehr selten ihren benignen Wachstumscharakter. Auch histologisch undifferenziert erscheinende Liposarkome, insbesondere bei Kindern, verhalten sich relativ benigne (KAUFFMANN und STOUT). Bei den Beobachtungen von KAUFFMANN und STOUT führte nur ein Liposarkom zur Metastasierung. Dagegen neigen Mischgeschwülste mit lipomatösen Anteilen eher zur malignen Entartung (HERRMANN).

Im Gegensatz zu den typischen Lipomen tritt bei den Liposarkomen die Läppchenstruktur zurück. Je nach dem Malignitätsgrad finden sich neben normalen mäßig atypische und unreife Fettzellen, die den Lipoblasten entsprechen. Reife Fettzellen können aber auch vermißt werden (GANS und STEIGLEDER). Im Cytoplasma sind unterschiedlich große Fetttropfen abgelagert. Der Zellkern ist spindel- oder sternförmig ausgestaltet und zeigt Größenunterschiede sowie Mitosen. Wabige Fettzellen und mehrkernige Fettriesenzellen mit pyknotischen Zellkernen kommen vor (WALLER). Die Riesenzellen weisen Neutralfetteinschlüsse und myxoide Strukturen auf, die sich mit Mucicarmin nicht anfärben (SCARPELLI und GREIDER). Bemerkenswert ist die zahlreichen Liposarkomen innewohnende Tendenz der Schleimbildung in Form einer partiellen Differenzierung zum Myxosarkom oder aber der schleimigen Degeneration liposarkomatöser Geschwulstanteile (ENTERLINE, CULBERSON, ROCHLIN und BRADY). Zwischen den Fettzellen findet sich in lockerer Anordnung ein Netzwerk kollagener Fasern, die der mucoiden Umwandlung unterliegen können (STOUT). Bei stärkerer Entdifferenzierung nehmen die atypischen Lipoblasten mit entsprechender Kernpolymorphie und mitotischer Aktivität zu. Die cytoplasmatischen Fettsubstanzen

---

Abb. 12. Naevus lipomatosus cutaneus superficialis Hoffmann-Zurhelle. Atopische Lagerung des Fettgewebes mit länglich, vertikal ausgerichteten Fettläppchen. [Aus: W. KNOTH: Dermatologica (Basel) **125**, 161 (1962), Abb. 2]

Abb. 13. Naevus lipomatosus cutaneus superficialis Hoffmann-Zurhelle. Perivasal angeordnete histiocytäre Elemente (*H*) mit Fettzelldifferenzierung (*F*). [Aus: W. KNOTH: Dermatologica (Basel) **125**, 161 (1962), Abb. 3]

hingegen nehmen ab und sind nur noch mit Spezialfärbungen nachweisbar, so daß nach LEVER die Differentialdiagnose gegenüber einem Fibrosarkom schwierig werden kann (STOUT; LENNERT; BLATTGERSTE; KEIL; GOTTRON und NIKOLOWSKI; ENTERLINE u. Mitarb.; MÖBIUS; WALLER; SCARPELLI u. GREIDER u.a.).

In Liposarkomen kommen nach STOUT Zellkomplexe vor, die ein Hibernom nachahmen. STOUT führt die an ein Hibernom erinnernden Strukturen auf eine gemeinsame, vom primitiven Mesenchym bereits abweichende Stammzelle zurück.

Bei Fibrolipomen ist eine maligne Entartung der mesenchymalen Bestandteile in Fibrosarkome oder Liposarkome möglich.

b) Hibernoma malignum

Das *Hibernoma malignum* ist gekennzeichnet durch unterschiedlich große runde Zellen mit zentral gelegenen Kernen. Auch Geschwulstriesenzellen kommen vor. Die Zellkerne zeigen Größenvariationen und sind relativ häufig in Mitose fixiert. Im Cytoplasma finden sich mehrere Fettvacuolen, die von Cytoplasmasäumen umschlossen und als sog. Maulbeerzellen bezeichnet werden. Die Geschwulstzellen liegen eng beieinander. Nach STOUT ist ein Geschwulststroma nur geringfügig ausgebildet, es kann auch vollständig vermißt werden. Neben den beschriebenen Geschwulstformationen können solche beobachtet werden, die dem Aufbau eines Liposarkoms (STOUT; LEVER) ähnlich sind (LENNERT; BRINES und JOHNSON; SUTHERLAND u. Mitarb.; CALLAHAHN u. CAMPBELL; GROSS und WOOD; KAUFFMANN und STOUT; ENTERLINE, CULBERSON, ROCHLIN und BRADY; STEIGLEDER u.a.).

3. Reticulo-histiocytäre Tumoren, systemische Erkrankungen und Metastasen des subcutanen Fettgewebes

Es sei darauf hingewiesen, daß bei der lymphoretikulären Hyperplasie, der Retikulose (GOTTRON: Lipophage Granulome bei chronisch-knotiger Retikulose), der *Reticulosarkomatose* (sog. Reticulosarkomatose Gottron), den *Granulomatosen* (Mycosis fungoides, Lymphogranulomatosis maligna Paltauf-Sternberg), beim sog. Plasmocytom der kleinen Reticulumzellen mit Makroglobulinämie WALDENSTRÖM (GOTTRON: „Infiltratives" Wachstum im Fettgewebe) sowie der lymphatischen und myeloischen *Leukämie* Tumor- oder Infiltratzellen auch im Fettgewebe zur Beobachtung gelangen. Die gefäßwandbezogenen, mehrherdigen blastomatösen oder granulomatösen Zellkomplexe besitzen die Neigung zur Konfluation und Infiltration (s. GOTTRON, 1960; GOTTRON und NIKOLOWSKI 1960; W. KNOTH, 1956, 1958, 1963). Aufgrund cytophotometrischer Untersuchungen durch KNOTH und SANDRITTER (1965) ist die Abgrenzung der Retikulose von einer Reticulosarkomatose und einem Hodgkin-Sarkom möglich.

Von Interesse ist der Befall ausgedehnter Gewebsbezirke coriumnaher Anteile des Fettgewebes und der Fettgewebssepten bei der chronisch-lymphatischen und myeloischen *Leukämie*, auf den TOYAMA u. NAGASHIMA; KNOTH u. BETTGE; TRUBOWITZ u. SIMS; SZYMANSKI u. BLUEFARB aufmerksam gemacht haben. Die Fettgewebssepten sind verbreitert und von Blutungen sowie leukämischen Infiltraten durchsetzt (Abb. 14). Daneben finden sich hämosiderotisches Pigment sowie nekrotische Bindegewebsabschnitte. Größere arterielle Gefäße im Fettgewebe können neben einer Wandverdickung eine erhebliche Lichtungseinengung im Sinne der Endangiosis fibroblastica aufweisen. Außer einer subendothelialen Proliferation in Form eines zellreichen fibroblastischen Füllgewebes mit Zunahme der Muskellamellen kann eine Mediaelastose gefunden werden. Auch Venen zeigen eine subendotheliale Schwellung mit zelliger Thrombosierung des Lumens. Es handelt sich um Zellen der lymphatischen oder myeloischen Reihe, die auch in

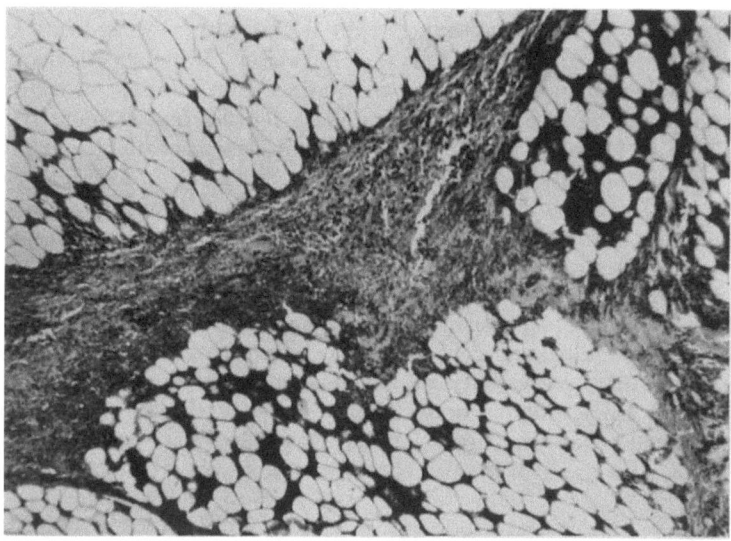

Abb. 14. Chronisch-myeloische Leukämie. In den verbreiterten und nekrobiotisch veränderten Fettgewebssepten sowie zwischen den Fettzellen myeloisch-leukämische Infiltrate. [Aus: W. Knoth u. S. Bettge: Derm. Wschr. **137**, 561 (1958), Abb. 6]

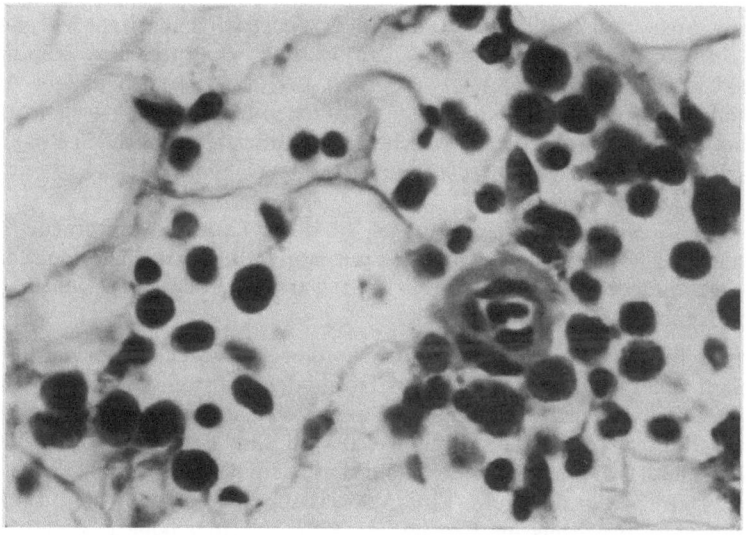

Abb. 15. Chronisch-myeloische Leukämie. Ausschnitt aus Abb. 14. Pericapillär und zwischen den Fettzellen gelegene myeloisch-leukämische Zellansammlungen aus Myelocyten, eosinophilen Myelocyten und Myeloblasten. [Aus: W. Knoth u. S. Bettge: Derm. Wschr. **137**, 561 (1958), Abb. 8]

der Wandung oder mantelförmig in der Umgebung der Gefäße anzutreffen sind. Gleichartige Zellelemente sind pericapillär oder in retikulärer Anordnung zwischen den Fettzellen anzutreffen (Abb. 15). Die Kerngröße variiert geringgradig, Mitosen kommen zur Beobachtung (Knoth und Bettge).

Eine Metastasierung maligner Tumoren der Haut, insbesondere des malignen Melanoms, sowie der inneren Organe kann nicht nur in das Corium, sondern auch in die Subcutis erfolgen. Insbesondere scheinen Pankreascarcinome in das Fettgewebe der Haut metastasieren zu können, worauf Beobachtungen von Hegler

u. WOHLWILL; JACKSON, SAVIDGE, STEIN u. VARLEY; VALENTINO; OSBORNE; HUGER; TITONE; HEGLER; BERNER u. a. hinweisen. Daneben können Veränderungen des subcutanen Fettgewebes vorkommen, die klinisch an ein Erythema nodosum oder an eine Panniculitis nodularis febrilis non suppurativa Pfeifer-Weber-Christian erinnern. Offenbar bewirken die Zellen sowohl des Primärtumors als auch die der Metastasen eine verstärkte Produktion von Lipase, welche über die Blut- und Lymphbahnen fernab von der Geschwulst zu Fettgewebsnekrosen mit umgebender chronisch-granulomatöser Entzündung führen. Auch intramurale Gefäßwandnekrosen und Venenthrombosen kommen zur Beobachtung (OSBORNE; JACKSON u. Mitarb. u. a.). Nicht immer kann entschieden werden, ob der Fettgewebsnekrose eine Metastasierung vorausgegangen ist, wobei die Fettzellen infolge des erhöhten Serumlipasespiegels einer Selbstverdauung unterliegen, oder ob die erhöhte Serumlipase pathogenetisch gesehen erst nach Vorschädigung des Fettgewebes durch Mikrotraumen und Gefäßthromben wirksam werden kann. Möglicherweise stellen venöse Thromben und vasculäre Nekrosen sowie Traumen einen Cofaktor für die Fettgewebsnekrose bei Pankreascarcinomen dar.

VI. Experimentelle Pathologie des Fettgewebes

Sowohl im dermatologischen als auch im pathologisch-anatomischen Schrifttum wurden relativ wenige Mitteilungen bekannt, die sich mit experimentellen Untersuchungen des Fettgewebes befaßt haben. Diese Feststellung findet ihre Erklärung darin, daß es bisher kaum möglich war, pathogenetische Vorgänge und Stoffwechselveränderungen bei einem Teil der uns bekannten Erkrankungen des Fettgewebes zu erfassen. So blieb es bisher bei dem Versuch einiger Autoren, durch verschiedenartige experimentelle Untersuchungen am Menschen und Tier Aufschluß über Zusammenhänge zwischen der einförmig-monotonen Reaktion des subcutanen Fettgewebes und der Einwirkung unterschiedlicher Schädigungen auf die Subcutis zu gewinnen.

Im folgenden Abschnitt werden die in der zugängigen Literatur bekannt gewordenen experimentellen Untersuchungsergebnisse nach ätiologischen Gesichtspunkten geordnet und, soweit von pathogenetischer Bedeutung, einer näheren Besprechung unterzogen.

Untersuchungen am Menschen und Tier haben es unter Berücksichtigung der Möglichkeit einer Reindarstellung von Hormonen wahrscheinlich gemacht, daß im Hypophysenvorderlappen eine von den bisher bekannten Wirkstoffen abgrenzbare Substanz gebildet wird, welche in den Fettstoffwechsel eingreift. ANSELMINO und HOFFMANN bezeichneten diesen lipotropen Faktor als lipotropes — oder Fettstoffwechselhormon. Eine Auswertung der Versuche über die Regulation des Fettstoffwechsels im Hunger bei Fettbelastung oder Diabetes mellitus hat ergeben, daß das Lipotropin zu einer Erhöhung der ungesättigten Fettsäuren im Blut, zu einem Anstieg der Blutketonkörper sowie zu einem gesteigerten Fetttransport zur Leber mit Zunahme des Leberfettgehaltes führt. Bei Tieren fällt gleichzeitig eine Steigerung des Blutzuckers sowie eine Abnahme des Leberglykogens auf. Im Nüchternblut von Diabetikern konnten stets erhöhte Mengen des Stoffwechselhormons gefunden werden, welches bei entsprechenden Kontrollpersonen fehlte. Die lipotrope Substanz wird im Serum Gesunder vermißt, läßt sich jedoch nach anschließender Fettbelastung bei Hunger nachweisen.

In diesem Zusammenhang ist die Mitteilung von BANDMANN, ROMITI u. STEHR beachtenswert, die über Fettstoffwechselstörungen bei Acanthosis nigricans „benigna" berichteten. Neben einer Atrophie des subcutanen Fettgewebes konnten

Regulationsstörungen im Zuckerstoffwechsel, ein erhöhter Grundumsatz, ein negativer Thorntest sowie eine Fettspeicherung in Leber, Knochenmark und Milz nachgewiesen werden. Hypophysäre Dysfunktionen sowie die Existenz lipotroper Hormone werden ätiopathogenetisch für die Entwicklung dieses Symptomenkomplexes diskutiert (zur Syntropie von Intelligenzdefekten, Acanthosis nigricans, Diabetes mellitus und hormonellen sowie Fettstoffwechsel-Störungen s. HEITE u. v. DER HEYDT, 1963).

KOVACEV u. SCOW haben den Einfluß von Hormonen auf die Fettsäure-Mobilisierung am subcutanen Fettgewebe der Ratte überprüft. In Fortsetzung der Versuche von ANSELMINO und HOFFMANN ist neuerdings BIRK und LI; FRIESEN sowie TRYGSTAD die Isolierung einer lipotropen Fraktion aus der tierischen Hypophyse bzw. nach Dialyse humanen Wachstumshormons gelungen. Somit finden die Untersuchungen GOODMANS u.a. über den Effekt der Wachstumshormone auf die Lipogenese des Fettgewebes von Ratten mit verstärkter Produktion freier Fettsäuren ihre Erklärung.

MOSINGER, KUHN und KUJALOVÁ untersuchten die Wirkung des lipid-mobilisierenden Hormons Epinephrin (Adrenalin) auf das menschliche Fettgewebe in vitro. Nach Ausschluß von Patienten mit abnormem Körpergewicht oder endokrinologischen Störungen konnte kein Unterschied zwischen dem Alter der Patienten und dem hormonalen Effekt gefunden werden. Die Wirkung des Epinephrins auf das subcutane Fettgewebe war weniger eindrucksvoll als auf Zellen des mesenterialen Fettgewebes. Norepinephrin zeigte eine stärkere adipokinetische Wirkung als Epinephrin. Glucagon, ACTH und TSH wiesen einen deutlich reduzierten oder keinen Wirkungseffekt auf das menschliche Fettgewebe auf. BERKOWITZ beobachtete nach Verabfolgung von Epinephrin bei der Hälfte der untersuchten Patienten mit Obesitas eine verminderte Fettmobilisierung, die jedoch bei Gewichtsreduktion wieder deutlich nachzuweisen war.

Experimentelle Untersuchungen über die Differenzierung der weißen Fettzellen am epididymalen Fettgewebe der neugeborenen Ratte durch NAPOLITANO haben ergeben, daß der Ursprung der Fettzellen in den Fibroblasten zu suchen ist. Dabei wird auf die multivalenten Potenzen der Fibrocyten und Fibroblasten hingewiesen. Die Möglichkeit anderer cytogenetischer Differenzierungen wird unter Hinweis auf die Differenzierungsmöglichkeit auch des reticulo-histiocytären Systems nicht abgelehnt (s. auch GOTTRON; RENOLD; WASSERMANN; SIMON; WILLIAMSON und LACY u.a.). Eine Umwandlung entspeicherten subcutanen Fettgewebes in die Matrixzellen scheint nach HOFFMANN; MICHELSON; STEIGLEDER u.a. wenig wahrscheinlich. Nach HOFF spricht für die hohe Differenzierung der Fettzellen, daß auf andere Lokalisationen übertragenes Fettgewebe die Eigenschaft der Standortentnahme beibehält und bis auf wenige Ausnahmen die der Gastregion nicht annimmt (LIEBELT und KIRSCHBAUM). CAMERON u. SENEVIVATNE sind der Frage nachgegangen, ob das Fettgewebe unter dem Reiz einer teilweisen Entfernung regenerationsfähig ist. Die am netzähnlichen Scrotalgewebe der Ratte vorgenommenen Versuche ließen erkennen, daß die partielle Fettgewebsentnahme keinen Wachstumsreiz darstellt. Dagegen fand sich ein reparativer Ersatz durch Granulations- und Bindegewebe. Eine Fettgewebsproliferation wurde niemals beobachtet. Die Untersuchungsergebnisse weisen ebenfalls darauf hin, daß es sich bei den Fettzellen um ein stark differenziertes Gewebe handelt.

DEMURA u. UCHIDA haben mittels der Warburgschen Apparatur die Respiration des normalen und pathologisch veränderten Fettgewebes untersucht. Der Sauerstoffverbrauch axillaren und thorakalen Fettgewebes betrug $3-4 \times 10^{-3}$ mg O_2 pro Stunde. Während nach Zusatz von Glucose eine Zunahme des Sauerstoffverbrauchs beobachtet wurde, führte 1%iges Natriumlinolenat zu einer Hemmung der Respiration normalen subcutanen Fettgewebes. Bei Entzündungen im Bereich der Subcutis war der Sauerstoffverbrauch gesteigert.

LASZLO bestimmte die freien Fettsäuren im Serum von adipösen Patienten und gesunden Kontrollpersonen während des Hungers sowie nach Glucosebelastung. Daneben wurde der Stoffwechsel des Fettgewebes in der Warburgschen Apparatur beobachtet. Die freien Fettsäuren zeigten auch während des Hungers einen hohen Spiegel, der nach Glucosebelastung gesenkt werden konnte. Die Freisetzung der Fettsäuren war abhängig von dem Ausmaß des Fettdepots. Bei Stoffwechseluntersuchungen excidierten Fettgewebes adipöser Patienten in vitro war dagegen die Mobilisierung von Fettsäuren abnorm niedrig. Eine Zunahme der Fettmobilisation erfolgte jedoch nach längerem Hungern. DOLE konnte ebenfalls zeigen, daß adipöse Menschen gegenüber gesunden Kontrollpersonen bei Hunger einen höheren Fettsäurespiegel aufweisen und daß beide Gruppen eine Depression nach Glucose zeigen. GORDON fand bei einem Teil der untersuchten Patienten mit Fettsucht, obwohl der Fettsäurespiegel in Ruhe ein hohes Plateau aufwies, keine Erhöhung der freien Plasmafettsäuren während des Hungers (s. auch BJÖRNTORP, HOOD, MARTINSSON u. PERSSON). Weitere Ergebnisse experimenteller Untersuchungen über den Lipoidstoffwechsel der Haut wurden von HSIA, GAILSOFER u. BARRY-LANE; HSIA, DREIZE u. MARQUEZ (Lipogenese in der Haut von Diabetikern); GALTON u. BRAY; HÄGGENDAL, STEEN u. SVANBORG (Durchblutung des subcutanen Fettgewebes nach Injektion von radioaktivem Xenon); GUTMAN, SCHRAMM u. SHAFRIR; BENOIT; GRIESEMER u. THOMAS (s. dort weitere Literatur) mitgeteilt.

SCAFFIDI führte Untersuchungen an Hunden über den Fettstoffwechsel von Zellen der Haut und Muskulatur nach Änderung der lokalen Temperatur durch. Analysen entsprechender Gewebsareale nach einer auf 20° C erniedrigten Körpertemperatur haben ergeben, daß die Temperaturerniedrigung keinen deutlichen Einfluß auf den Wasser- und Fettgehalt der Zellen nimmt. Eine direkte Erwärmung des Gewebes bewirkt dagegen eine Vermehrung der Hydrophilie der Fettzellen mit folgender Wasser- und Salzretention sowie eine Verminderung des intracellulären Gehalts an Fettsubstanzen, von Glykogen und Milchsäure (D'AVANZO).

Auf die Abhängigkeit der Fettsäurezusammensetzung menschlicher Fettzellen vom Alter, dem Geschlecht und der Rasse haben INSULL u. BARTSCH aufmerksam gemacht. Untersuchungsergebnisse über die Lipolyse sowie über morphologische Veränderungen der Fettzellen während der Fetteinlagerung und -mobilisation wurden von GALTON u. BRAY; GOLDRICK veröffentlicht. Die Größe der Fettzellen ist nach REH vom Ernährungszustand des Untersuchungsobjektes abhängig. Bei entsprechenden Messungen von Fettzellen des Menschen betrug der Durchmesser im Mittel zwischen 70 und 120 µ. Bei Fettgewebsatrophien lag der Durchmesser unter 70 µ, bei Adipösen oder Lipomen über 120 µ. Die obere Grenze betrug 170 µ. Für die Einlagerung von Neutralfetten steht dem Organismus neben der Vergrößerung der Fetttropfen in präexistenten Fettzellen die Möglichkeit einer Neubildung derselben zur Verfügung.

Es gibt klinische und experimentelle Hinweise dafür, daß die Fettzellen im Hinblick auf die Assimilation und Dissimilation dem vegetativen Nervensystem unterliegen (GÖERING; MÜLLER; MANSFELD u. MÜLLER; LORTAT u. VITRY; HAUSBERGER u. a.). HAUSBERGER konnte bereits 10 Std nach der Durchtrennung von Nerven mit sympathischen Faseranteilen bei Mäusen und Kaninchen einen intracellulären Glykogeneinstrom sowie eine Fettvermehrung infolge Zunahme und Vergrößerung der Fettvacuolen feststellen. An hungernden Tieren ließ sich bei identischer Versuchsanordnung der gleiche Effekt erzielen. KURÉ, OI u. OKINAKA untersuchten an Hunden den Einfluß des vegetativen Nervensystems auf das Fettgewebe. Während es nach Durchtrennung der Vorderwurzeln mit Faseranteilen des N. sympathicus oder Entfernung des Bauchgrenzstranges zu einer Vermehrung des Fettgewebes auf der operierten Seite kam, konnte nach mechanischer oder chemischer Reizung der Vorderwurzeln eine deutliche Fettgewebsatrophie beobachtet werden. Bei der Durchschneidung der Hinterwurzeln mit parasympathischen Faseranteilen wurde dagegen eine Größenabnahme der Fettzellen nachgewiesen. Die Durchtrennung des N. ischiadicus führte zu einer Verlangsamung des Fettstoffwechsels. Aufgrund der vorliegenden Befunde konnten die Angaben anderer Autoren bestätigt werden, daß der Sympathicus hemmend, der Parasympathicus fördernd in den Fettstoffwechsel eingreift.

RECHT wies auf einen lokalisierten halbseitigen Wangenfettschwund, insbesondere die Atrophie der Bichatschen Fettkörper, nach Lues oder Encephalitis hin. Ätiopathogenetisch wird der Befall des in den Basalganglien am Boden des 3. Ventrikels gelegenen trophischen Zentrums für das Fettgewebe verantwortlich gemacht, von welchem durch Vermittlung sympathischer Nervenfasern dem peripheren Fettdepot Impulse zugeleitet werden sollen.

SIDMAN u. FAWCETT beobachteten den Effekt der Durchschneidung peripherer Nerven auf einige Stoffwechselvorgänge im braunen Fettgewebe der Maus. Auffällig war die große Anzahl von Nervenfasern, die vielfach frei an den Fettzellen endeten. Die Autoren beschrieben an der denervierten Seite eine Konsistenzzunahme des braunen Fettgewebes mit Erhöhung des Glykogengehaltes sowie ätherlöslicher Lipoide. ARONSON, TEODORU, ADLER und SCHWARTZMAN fanden nach Anwendung von Cortison bei Hamstern und Mäusen eine Hypertrophie des braunen Fettgewebes, wobei der Effekt mit zunehmendem Alter der Tiere abnahm.

Autoradiographische Untersuchungen mit ^{3}H-Thymidin am weißen und braunen Fettgewebe der Ratte wurden von HELLMANN und HELLERSTRÖM durchgeführt. Aufgrund einer deutlichen Einbaurate von ^{3}H-Thymidin in die Zellkerne mit entsprechender Zellkernschwärzung wurde von den Autoren auf eine hohe mitotische Aktivität und Zellerneuerung auch des Fettgewebes geschlossen.

Von besonderem Interesse sind experimentelle Untersuchungen überwiegend am Tier, welche Hinweise auf ätiologische und pathogenetische Faktoren im Hinblick auf entzündliche Veränderungen des Fettgewebes geben können. Die Versuche entsprechen klinischen Erfahrungen, daß mechanische, chemische und thermische Traumen sowie ionisierende Strahlen eine Panniculitis auslösen können.

UMBREIT untersuchte die Wirkung von Druck und Zug auf das Fettpolster und einzelne Fettzellen des Menschen. Die Auswertungen haben ergeben, daß körperwarme empfindlicher als erkaltete Fettzellen auf Druck und Zug reagieren, daß dieselben im Hinblick auf mechanische Einflüsse jedoch sehr widerstandsfähig sind. Die erkaltete Fettzelle ist in der Lage, die entstandene Gestaltsänderung schneller auszugleichen. Zunächst verschiebt sich die Fettzelle gegen ihre Nachbarzelle ohne Deformation. Bei stärkerer Belastung durch Druck fällt eine gleichmäßige Abflachung, bei Zug hingegen eine ungleichmäßige Beanspruchung der Fettzellen auf. Nach dem Erreichen der Elastizitätsgrenze kommt es zur Membranruptur.

SLOBOSIANO, GEORGESCO und HERSCOVICI fanden nach künstlicher Quetschung der Haut in 40% der untersuchten Fälle zwischen den Fettzellen retikulär angeordnete chronisch entzündliche Infiltrate, in 2% nach vorangegangener Läsion eine Induration der geschädigten Fettgewebsareale. Ähnliche Versuche an Hunden und Katzen ließen histologische Veränderungen erkennen, die denen der Adiponecrosis subcutanea neonatorum ähnlich waren (BERNER u. HEYDE).

PROSERPIO führte mittels Klemmen in der Inguinalregion männlicher Meerschweinchen Quetschversuche über einen Zeitraum von 10 min durch und nahm 3—4 Monate später histologische Untersuchungen des Fettgewebes vor. In einer zweiten Versuchsreihe wurde nach vorheriger Kastration der Einfluß der inneren Sekretion auf die Fettgewebsnekrose untersucht. Im Hinblick auf die Nekrosen konnte kein wesentlicher Unterschied in beiden Versuchsreihen gefunden werden. Nur in fortgeschrittenen Stadien trat bei nichtoperierten Tieren eine schnellere und stärkere Reaktion mit Reparation der Nekrosen durch ein Granulationsgewebe auf. Eine Verseifung wurde niemals beobachtet. Fast ausschließlich ließen sich Neutralfette, hingegen nur wenig saure Fette nachweisen. Im Endstadium erfolgte ein Ersatz der nekrotischen Gewebsareale durch Binde- oder Fettgewebe.

WORINGER sah nach Traumen in Form einfacher Schnittwunden, die nach unterschiedlichen Zeitspannen im Anschluß an operative Eingriffe untersucht wurden, eine Wucheratrophie des Fettgewebes. Mit der Nilblausulfatfärbung ließ sich feststellen, daß resorbiertes Fett acidophil wird. An der Fettresorption beteiligten sich neben den Fettzellen selbst Histiocyten, Lymphocyten und polynucleäre Leukocyten.

Injektionen wäßriger oder öliger Substanzen können zu einem histologischen Befund führen, der ebenfalls einer Adiponecrosis subcutanea neonetorum auffallend ähnlich ist. Nach Applikation von Palmitinsäure (SIWE), Lipoiden (SAWICKY und KANOFF), Carmin, Glucose oder physiologischer Kochsalzlösung (SCHWARZMANN) in das Fettgewebe von Meerschweinchen fanden sich neben Steatonekrosen Zellen der akuten und chronischen Entzündung sowie fibrocytär-fibroblastische Elemente. Auch nach der Injektion von Cholesterin (MOSTO), Glycerol (CAMPBELL) oder öliger Lösungen (MOSTO) kam es bei Meerschweinchen, Ratten und Kaninchen an der Injektionsstelle zur Entwicklung von Fettgewebsnekrosen, die im Früh- und Spätstadium den pathohistologischen Veränderungen der menschlichen Subcutis weitgehend entsprachen. Zu ähnlichen Untersuchungsergebnissen nach intracutaner Injektion von menschlichem Oberflächenfett, Squalen, freien Fettsäuren des Talges und Resttalg (Glyceride, Wachse, Sterole usw.) in die Rückenhaut des Menschen oder in Meerschweinchenhaut kamen STRAUSS und KLIGMAN; SPIER und KLASCHKA; STRAUSS und POCHI. SPIER und KLASCHKA haben insbesondere auf die granulotaktische Wirkung des Talges mit folgender Leukocytoklasie aufmerksam gemacht. ARIMORI, HAMAMATSU und KUROKOWA beobachteten nach intradermaler Injektion von Linolsäure dem Erythema nodosum oder Erythema induratum Bazin ähnliche Reaktionen. STORCK konnte durch Olivenölinjektionen bei einem Menschen eine Panniculitis mehrfach provozieren, wobei die histologischen Veränderungen abschnittsweise an ein Shwartzmann-Sanarelli-Phänomen erinnerten. Versuche an der Ratte haben gezeigt, daß nicht nur subcutane Injektionen, sondern auch ein hoher Gehalt der Nahrung zugesetzter gesättigter Fettsäuren zu Fettgewebsgranulomen führen können (HERTING u. CRAIN).

Eine Lipogranulombildung mit und ohne Sklerosierung konnte auch nach Anwendung bestimmter Medikamente in öliger oder wäßriger Lösung (Paraffinöl, Campher u. ä.) gefunden werden (NEWCOMER; WIGLEY und CALNAN; BLANC; BAUMGARTNER u. RIVA; HERBST; SCHLIENGER u. a.). Bereits eine einmalige Injektion von 5 ml Paraffinum liqu. löste bei der Ratte im Peritoneum eine fortschreitende lipogranulomatöse Reaktion aus, die histologisch dem Paraffinom des Menschen ähnlich war (EISENSCHMID u. ORBISON). Charakteristisch waren

Fettgewebsnekrosen, ein Fremdkörpergranulationsgewebe mit Riesenzellen, Verkalkungen sowie unterschiedlich große Ölcysten, umgeben von einer fibrösen Kapsel. ÖSTERREICHER u. WATSON versuchten, aufgrund detaillierter Untersuchungen an Ratten mit Alloxan-Diabetes die zur Insulin-Lipodystrophie führende Substanz zu ermitteln. Weder nach Anwendung von handelsüblichem oder kristallisiertem Zink-Insulin, noch nach Injektion von physiologischer Kochsalzlösung, Lipaseextrakt oder Trikresol (Präservator im Handelsinsulin) konnte bei entsprechenden Versuchsgruppen eine Fettgewebsatrophie gefunden werden. JABLONSKA, HAUSMANOWA-PETRUSEWICZ u. PIWOWARCZYK (1967) konnten dagegen die pathogenetische Bedeutung postinjektioneller Traumen sowie die des Insulins selbst für die Auslösung einer Lipodystrophie an diabetischen Kaninchen nachweisen. Die Frage, warum es nur bei einem Teil der Diabetiker zur Insulindystrophie kommt, kann bisher nicht eindeutig beantwortet werden. WAIL führte mikrochemische Untersuchungen von Fettnekrosen und Fettgranulomen nach Campherölinjektion durch und fand, daß es sich bei den nachgewiesenen Lipoiden nicht um die künstlich eingeführten, resorbierten und vom Gewebe zurückgehaltenen Fettsubstanzen, sondern um Veränderungen des Eigenfettes selbst handelt.

Auch nach Einwirkung von Kälte fallen im Fettgewebe histologische Veränderungen auf, die einer Adiponecrosis subcutanea neonatorum nahekommen (BLAKE, GOYETTE, LYTER u. SWAN; FLECK). SLOBOSIANO, GEORGESCO u. HERSCOVICI verfolgten das histologische Substrat des Fettgewebes Neugeborener nach Einwirkung von Äthylchlorid und sahen in 71% der untersuchten Fälle eine deutliche entzündliche Infiltration mit nekrotischen Abschnitten, indurierten Arealen sowie eine Fettgewebsatrophie. CAMERON u. MALLIK beobachteten bei Albinoratten nach kurzdauernder Erfrierung ebenfalls Fettgewebsnekrosen mit der menschlichen Pathologie vergleichbaren Befunden und fibrosierender Endphase. HAXTHAUSEN fand bei mehreren Kindern nach Kälteeinwirkung Infiltrate im Fettgewebe des Gesichtes, welche klinisch und histologisch der Adiponecrosis subcutanea neonatorum entsprachen. Ähnliche Beobachtungen wurden von SOLOMON u. BEERMAN (Provokation der Panniculitis durch den Eiswürfeltest); ROTMAN; DUNCAN, FREEMAN u. HEATON (unauffällige immunelektrophoretische Befunde) mitgeteilt. CRACIUN u. FAGARASANO beschrieben dagegen Lipogranulome der Bauchhaut, die sich nach einer über einen größeren Zeitraum fortgesetzten Diathermiebehandlung entwickelten.

SABRAZÈS u. BIDEAU erzeugten bei jungen Meerschweinchen nach Einwirkung von Röntgenstrahlen eine Verminderung, teilweise oder völlige Atrophie des Fettgewebes. Der Grad des Fettgewebsschwundes war abhängig von der Bestrahlungsintensität sowie dem Zeitpunkt der Untersuchung. Histologisch wurde neben einem Ödem eine Ungleichmäßigkeit in Form und Größe der Fettzellen, eine Zellzerstörung mit chronischer Entzündung, die Ausbildung von Cysten und Neigung zu substitutiver Sklerosierung beobachtet. Etwa einen Monat nach Abschluß der Bestrahlungsserie konnte die Neubildung von Fettzellen nachgewiesen werden.

Von besonderem Interesse sind experimentelle Untersuchungen von PANABOKKÉ, welcher neutrale, saure und alkalische Pankreasextrakte von verschiedenen Tierarten herstellte und jeweils in das Scrotalgekröse sowie in das perineale Fettpolster weißer Ratten injizierte. Die Tiere wurden 24—72 Std nach der Injektion getötet. Aufgrund der histologischen und histochemischen Aufarbeitung des Untersuchungsmaterials kommt PANABOKKÉ zu der Feststellung, daß die Nekrose der Fettzellen nicht durch Lipase, Trypsin, Hyaluronidase oder Elastase hervorgerufen, sondern wahrscheinlich durch Amylase und Lecithinase ausgelöst wird. Es wird darauf hingewiesen, daß die Membran der Fettzelle stellenweise neben Proteinen Kohlenhydrate und Lecithin enthält, die von der Amylase und Lecithinase angegriffen werden können. Erst wenn diese Stellen der Zellmembran geöffnet sind, kann die Zellzerstörung und Fettgewebsnekrose unter Einwirkung von Lipase einsetzen.

Auf die Erörterung experimenteller Untersuchungen im Hinblick auf Erkrankungen der Periarteriitis nodosa-Gruppe muß im Rahmen dieses Beitrags verzichtet und auf entsprechende Handbuchartikel verwiesen werden. Das Reaktionsorgan wird überwiegend vom Gefäßsystem gebildet, wobei die Schädigung des Fettgewebes sekundärer Natur ist.

VII. Ätiologie und Pathogenese der Fettgewebserkrankungen

Über ätiologische Faktoren der Fettgewebserkrankungen finden sich im Schrifttum zahlreiche Hinweise, welche unter Berücksichtigung von Einzelpublikationen teilweise hypothetischen Charakters oder rein spekulativer Natur sind. Entsprechende Aussagen gelten auch für pathogenetische Vorstellungen. Es bedarf nicht der weiteren Erläuterung, daß Rückschlüsse aus dem jeweils vorliegenden histologischen Befund insbesondere auf die Pathogenese der Fettgewebserkrankungen nur unter Vorbehalt und mit gewissen Einschränkungen gezogen werden dürfen. Aus den dargelegten Gründen sollen unter Hinweis auf die Fülle von Literaturangaben nur diejenigen Berücksichtigung finden, deren Ergebnisse auf einem größeren Krankengut basieren oder welche durch bereits aufgeführte experimentelle Untersuchungen gestützt zu sein scheinen.

Wie bereits darauf hingewiesen, spielen bei der Auslösung von Erkrankungen des Fettgewebes mechanische, chemische und thermische Traumen eine nicht unerhebliche Rolle. Die im vorangegangenen Kapitel erwähnten experimentellen Untersuchungen unterstützen entsprechende klinische Beobachtungen. SCHWARZMANN; ZAVARINI führen die *traumatisch bedingten Lipogranulome* auf den Untergang von Fettzellen zurück. Die freigesetzten gespaltenen Fettsubstanzen sollen zu einer Reizung des reticulo-histiocytären Systems des Fettgewebes mit folgender resorptiver Entzündung und anschließender Sklerosierung der Fettgewebsgranulome führen. Die auslösende Noxe kann unterschiedlicher Art sein. Der eben angedeutete pathogenetische Reaktionsablauf kann nach CISTJAKOV im Anschluß an ein Trauma, eine Injektion, als Nachbarschaftsreaktion, infolge einer Störung des vegetativen Nervensystems oder nach Veränderungen der lokalen Blutversorgung bei Infektionskrankheiten, z. B. Fleckfieber, beobachtet werden. SCHLIENGER führt die *medikamentös bedingten Fettgewebsnekrosen* primär auf durch das Trauma freiwerdende Gewebslipasen zurück. Diese bewirken eine Fettzellzerstörung und Fettzersetzung mit nachfolgender Granulombildung. Nach PIROTH können entzündliche von traumatisch bedingten Lipogranulomen histologisch nicht abgegrenzt werden. Diese Beobachtung deutet darauf hin, daß weniger der auslösende Faktor als bestimmte pathogenetische Vorgänge im Fettgewebe selbst zu einem ähnlichen oder identischen histomorphologischen Bild führen.

Die Pathogenese der *Insulinlipodystrophie* ist weitgehend ungeklärt. Nach AVERY; BAUMGARTNER u. RIVA; JABLONSKA u. Mitarb. u. a. führt das durch die Injektion ausgelöste Trauma zu einer lokalen entzündlichen Reaktion im Fettgewebe, womit die Lipodystrophie in die Gruppe der traumatischen Panniculitis einzuordnen wäre. Des weiteren wird das Insulin als antiglykämische Substanz, eine Zellschädigung durch zu hohe Insulinkonzentration, ein einseitig übersteigerter Ablauf des Stoffwechsels (SCHULZE), die Existenz lipolytischer Fermente oder eine Vasoconstriction (GOTTRON) für die Auslösung der Lipodystrophie verantwortlich gemacht. Beachtenswert sind tierexperimentelle Untersuchungen von

Jablonska, Hausmanowa-Petrusewicz u. Piwowarczyk über den Einfluß des Insulins auf Muskelfasern und Fettzellen der Subcutis bei diabetischen Kaninchen. Demnach müssen die injektionsbedingten Traumen und das Insulin selbst für die Auslösung der Lipodystrophie verantwortlich gemacht werden. Gottron mißt außerdem postinjektionellen, örtlich begrenzten Durchblutungsstörungen eine besondere pathogenetische Bedeutung bei. Jablonska u. Hintz berichteten ebenfalls über inflammatorische Gefäßveränderungen; eine Degeneration oder Nekrose der Gefäßwände wurde vermißt. Die ursächliche Wirkung des Trikresol oder eine Verunreinigung der Präparate durch Pankreaslipase konnte experimentell ausgeschlossen werden. Dagegen scheint eine individuelle Reaktionsbereitschaft des Fettgewebes erforderlich zu sein, da nur bei einem gewissen Prozentsatz von Diabetikern eine Lipodystrophie nach Insulininjektion zur Entwicklung gelangt (s. dazu auch Baumgartner u. Riva).

Für die Entstehung des *Insulinlipoms* könnten chronisch-traumatische oder entzündliche Reize eine Rolle spielen. Die Möglichkeit der Fettgewebswucherung auf entzündlicher Basis wird untermauert durch das gemeinsame Vorkommen tumoröser Abschnitte und solcher Areale, die Zellen der chronischen Entzündung aufweisen. Baumgartner u. Riva halten für die Entwicklung der Lipome die Disposition des Fettgewebes zur Wucherung für erforderlich, da Lipome häufig bei Jugendlichen und Dystrophikern zur Beobachtung kommen. Nach Gottron sollte die Bedeutung des Strombahnnetzes im Fettgewebe nicht übersehen werden, da die besondere Reizbarkeit des Gefäßnervensystems bei Diabetikern bekannt ist (s. auch Schuermann). Das Auftreten einer Fettgewebsnekrose, eines Fettgewebsschwundes oder eines Lipoms nach Applikation von Insulin ist nach Gottron abhängig von der Stärke des an der peripheren Strombahn ansetzenden Reizes. Während starke Reize zur Vasoconstriction und Histolyse führen, kommt es nach schwächerer Reizung zum Fettgewebsschwund mit Ausbildung einer Fibrose, bei weiterer Reizabschwächung hingegen zum Zellwachstum und somit zur Lipomentstehung.

Bei der Entwicklung von *Fettgewebsgranulomen nach Diathermie* oder Starkstrom (Gross; Heilmann u. Sonneck; Makai; Calmann) weist die Symmetrie in der Anordnung der Knoten möglicherweise auf eine neuro-endokrine Genese hin (Fleck). Heilmann u. Sonneck denken dabei an eine unmittelbare Störung im Hypophysen-Zwischenhirn-System. Daß die Störung vegetativer Zentren bei der Auslösung der Panniculitis eine Rolle spielen könnte, gewinnt durch tierexperimentelle Untersuchungen (Luftinfusion in die Hirnventrikel führt zu einer Erniedrigung des Blutfettes, der Phosphatide und des Gesamt-Cholesterins) an Bedeutung (s. Fleck).

In diesem Zusammenhang müssen Untersuchungen über die *Adiponecrosis subcutanea neonatorum* Erwähnung finden, für deren Auslösung überwiegend Traumen bei einer erschwerten Geburt (Newcomer, Graham, Schaffert u. Kaplan; Schoedd; Zocchi; Reymann; Cruse; Cornbleet u. Rattner; McDonald; Dieckhoff, Hempel u. Koch u. a.), eine Asphyxie mit Anoxie (Zocchi; Holzel u. a.) sowie Kälteeinwirkungen (Newcomer u. Mitarb.; Slobosiano, Georgesco u. Herscovici u. a.) verantwortlich gemacht werden. Ausschlaggebend für die Entstehung der Adiponecrosis subcutanea neonatorum scheint jedoch die abnorme Beschaffenheit des Neugeborenenfettes zu sein. Mikrochemische Untersuchungen des Serums und nekrotischen Fettgewebes durch Siwe; Unshelm; Scriba; Noojin, Pace u. Davis; Dieckhoff, Hempel u. Koch zeigten gegenüber gesunden Neugeborenen einen um das Doppelte erhöhten Fettsäuregehalt im Serum bei deutlicher Herabsetzung der ungesättigten Serumlipoide. Die mittlere Jodzahl war erheblich vermindert, das mittlere Molekulargewicht der Fettsäuren zeigte bei beiden Untersuchungsgruppen gleiche Werte. Diese Befunde sprechen für einen niedrigen Gehalt an ungesättigten Fettsäuren im Serum der Kranken und schließen einen hohen Ölsäureanteil aus. Abweichungen des Cholesterinspiegels, des anorganischen Phosphors sowie der Phosphatide waren nicht zu erkennen. Aufgrund von Fermentbestimmungen konnten Veränderungen der Pankreas- und Leberlipase im Serum nicht nachgewiesen werden. Die Gesamtlipase war ebenfalls unauffällig. Im Gegensatz zu den Untersuchungen von SIWE konnten DIECKHOFF u. Mitarb. in den Fettgewebsnekrosen wenig freie Fettsäuren und kein Cholesterin nachweisen. STEIGLEDER u. Mitarb. stellten in den Fettgewebsgranulomen eine deutliche Esterasereaktion fest, die dem normalen Fettgewebe fehlt. Dieser Befund könnte auf einer verstärkten Fettspaltung oder aber auf einer Einwanderung esteraseaktiver Histiocyten beruhen.

Bemerkenswert sind vergleichende dünnschichtchromatographische Untersuchungen der Lipoide aus Excisaten normalen und pathologisch veränderten Gewebes, die von LINDLAR und MISGELD 1967 an Säuglingen mit Adiponecrosis subcutanea neonatorum durchgeführt wurden. Im Gegensatz zu Triglyceriden konnten Diglyceride nur in geringem Umfang nachgewiesen werden. Freie Fettsäuren und Cholesterin, das nur zur Hälfte in veresterter Form vorlag, erschienen im Bereich der Adiponekrose deutlich vermehrt. Gegenüber normaler Haut waren die Gesamtlipoide erheblich herabgesetzt, das Cholesterin um das Vierfache vermehrt. In der Zusammensetzung der Fettsäuren ergaben sich beachtenswerte Unterschiede: Die Palmitolinsäure war stark, die Myristinsäure deutlich verringert, die Palmitinsäure dagegen vermehrt. Die differierenden Werte in der Bestimmung der Palmitin- und Linolsäure bei verschiedenen Proben werden auf die unterschiedliche Ernährung der Kinder zurückgeführt. Die Ölsäure lag mit Werten um 30% deutlich niedriger als in der Haut Erwachsener. LINDLAR u. MISGELD fassen die nachweisbaren Lipoidveränderungen nicht als Ursache, sondern als Folge traumatischer oder zirkulatorischer Schäden auf. Dem riesenzellhaltigen Granulationsgewebe wird beim Abbau der Lipoide eine besondere Funktion beigemessen. In diesem Zusammenhang kommt dem Fermentreichtum des Granulationsgewebes, insbesondere auch dem der Riesenzellen (LINDLAR u. MISGELD: Zunahme der Lipase-Aktivität; GÖSSNER: Erhöhung der Esterase-Aktivität; GEDIGK u. BONTKE: Verstärkte Aktivität saurer Phosphatasen und unspezifischer Esterasen, geringe Lipase-Aktivität in C_{20}- und C_{22}-Polyenfettsäure-Granulomen) besondere Bedeutung zu. Die im Bereich nekrotischen Fettgewebes auftretenden Lipoide, insbesondere die freiwerdenden Fettsäuren, unterliegen der enzymatischen Einwirkung, wobei es möglicherweise auch zu einer Hydrierung der ungesättigten C_{16}-Fettsäure (LINDLAR u. MISGELD) kommt. Über ähnliche Ergebnisse aufgrund autoradiographischer und histochemischer Untersuchungen an Mycolsäuregranulomen berichten KRACHT u. GUSEK. Die verstärkte Fermentaktivität in Lipogranulomen mit dem Ziel, Fremdkörpermaterial zu beseitigen, wird von GEDIGK eher auf die adaptive Neubildung, weniger auf eine Aktivierung bereits vorhandener Fermente zurückgeführt. Die Untersuchungen unterstreichen die bisher bezweifelte hohe strukturelle und enzymatische Differenzierung der Riesenzellen vom Fremdkörper- und Langhans-Typ und bestätigen die bereits früher publizierten Befunde von STEIGLEDER und LÖFFLER (1956), STEIGLEDER und SCHULTIS (1957).

SIWE; UNSHELM fanden im Fettgewebe von gesunden Säuglingen mehr Palmitin- und weniger Ölsäure als bei älteren Kindern, ein Befund, der auf eine generell andersartige Zusammensetzung des Fettgewebes Neugeborener von dem Erwachsener (GOTTRON) hinweist. Auch PIAGGIO hat auf die Modifikation des Neutralfettes aufmerksam gemacht. Die Ansicht, daß möglicherweise die Nahrungsumstellung pathogenetisch eine Rolle spielen könnte, wird durch bereits aufgeführte experimentelle Untersuchungen gestützt.

GOTTRON hat insbesondere auf die pathogenetische Bedeutung traumatogener Reize für die Reaktion des Gefäßnervensystems mit folgender Durchblutungsstörung aufmerksam gemacht. Nach GOTTRON; HERING und UNDEUTSCH u. a. führt die erhöhte Reizbarkeit des peripheren Strombahnnervensystems beim Säugling zu einer Änderung der Durchströmung, wobei die verstärkte Gefäßreagibilität zur Stase und gefäßbezogenen Coagulationsnekrose führt. Diese Auffassung wird gestützt durch eine Mitteilung von DANDA u. PLACHY, die bei mehreren Kindern mit Adiponecrosis subcutanea neonatorum eine gestörte Blutversorgung der Subcutis nachweisen konnten. Da die Erkrankung jedoch nur relativ selten zur Beobachtung gelangt, sollen endogen-konstitutionelle Faktoren für die Auslösung der Veränderung zusätzlich von Bedeutung sein (BAUMGARTNER u. RIVA).

Primär scheinen die Störung der Fettsäurebildung, der Umbau bzw. die andersartige Zusammensetzung des embryonalen Fettgewebes pathogenetisch die bedeutendste Rolle zu spielen (CRUSE; HERING und UNDEUTSCH; NOOJIN u. Mitarb.; SCRIBA). Diese Annahme wird gestützt durch Autopsiebefunde, nach denen Nekrosen auch am visceralen Fettgewebe gefunden wurden (NOOJIN, PACE u. DAVIS; GRÜTZ u. a.). Traumen, Kälteeinwirkungen bzw. postpartaler Temperaturwechsel sind als auslösende und Lokalisationsfaktoren anzusehen und führen über das Strombahnnervensystem zum Capillarkrampf und zur Stase (Kälteischämie), welche die intracelluläre Ausfällung von Fettsäurekristallen sowie die Zerstörung der Fettzellmembranen zur Folge hat. Bei den ausgefallenen, doppelbrechenden Kristallen handelt es sich nach SCRIBA um Palmitin- und Stearinsäure. Die nunmehr extracellulär gelegenen Fettsubstanzen stellen für das Gewebe Fremdkörper dar, welche die Bildung von Granulomen zur Folge haben (GRAY; MCDONALD; GOTTRON; FLECK u. a.). In ähnlichem Sinne ist die Mitteilung von MILNER und MITCHINSON zu deuten, die autoallergische oder andere hyperergische Phänomene für die Entstehung der Adiponecrosis subcutanea neonatorum verantwortlich machen. Die Hypersensitivität mit Angriffspunkt an den Gefäßen richtet sich dabei vorwiegend gegen Bakterien. Daneben wurden aber auch Auto-Antikörper gegen Schilddrüsenkolloid und Cytoplasma von Zellen der Glandula thyreoidea (RICCI, MICHELETTI u. COSCIA) gefunden. Von Interesse sind Beobachtungen von Kindern mit Adiponecrosis subcutanea neonatorum, bei deren Mutter während der Gravidität ein Diabetes mellitus nachweisbar war (S. STEINESS; OEHLERT, WECKE u. SUTTERLE).

Für das *Sclerema neonatorum* gelten hinsichtlich der Ablagerung von Palmitin- oder Stearinsäure sowie anderer Glyceride höherer Fettsäuren ähnliche Beziehungen (GRAY). MCDONALD zieht zusätzlich Schock- oder Stresswirkungen in Betracht, wobei wiederum das Gefäßsystem die primäre Rolle bei der Auslösung der Dermatose übernimmt.

Bei dem *Pfeifer-Weber-Christian-Syndrom* sowie der *Lipogranulomatosis subcutanea Rothmann-Makai* spielt das Trauma lediglich eine provozierende Rolle (STUHLERT). Pathogenetisch kommen infektiöse Reize verschiedenster Art in Betracht (KONOPIK; MEYER; BINKLEY; SANFORD, EUBANK u. STENN; GOTTRON u. NIKOLOWSKI). BAUMGARTNER u. RIVA weisen auf die Existenz von Foci hin, obgleich kulturelle Untersuchungen von Blut und Gewebe im Hinblick auf eine bakterielle Streuung nicht überzeugend waren. Auffallend bei der Spontanpannikulitis Typ Rothmann-Makai ist eine Koinzidenz mit rheumatischen Beschwerden, so daß die Zuordnung der Erkrankung an den rheumatischen Formenkreis erwogen wurde (BAUMGARTNER und RIVA). Die Beeinflussung des Gefäßnervensystems mit folgender Durchblutungsstörung verdient offenbar insbesondere bei der Lipogranulomatosis subcutanea Rothmann-Makai Beachtung, zumal diese Erkrankung bei Kindern und Jugendlichen vorzugsweise symmetrisch vorkommt und mit einer erhöhten Reizbarkeit des peripheren Nervensystems einhergeht. Die Durchströmungsänderung führt über die Stase zur örtlichen Ischämie mit folgender Nekrose der dem betreffenden Gefäßgebiet zugeordneten Fettgewebsareale. Die gelegentliche Kombination mit einer Phlebitis oder Thrombangitis obliterans veranlaßte MEIER zur Einordnung der Erkrankung in die Periarteriitis nodosa-Gruppe oder die Bürgersche Krankheit. Die Möglichkeit, daß eine allergische Reaktionslage des Fettgewebes zu metabolischen Veränderungen führen kann oder Zwischenhirnfunktionsstörungen für die Entwicklung dieser Panniculitisformen pathogenetische Bedeutung besitzen, ist bisher experimentell nicht bewiesen (KELLNER; LOSSIE und VOEGT; zur Frage der Polyätiologie des Pfeifer-Weber-Christian-Syndroms unter Berücksichtigung endokriner Störungen sowie medikamentös bedingter Formen s. B. ALBRECTSEN, 1960).

Beachtenswert erscheint die Kombination zwischen Pfeifer-Weber-Christian-Syndrom, Pankreas-Schäden sowie einem Diabetes mellitus (BOHNSTEDT; ALBRECTSEN; MACHACEK; DE GRACIANSKY, LIÈVRE u. PARAF; DE GRACIANSKY; PAVLIK; HEUSER, LIEBERMAN, DONNWELL u. LANDING u.a.). Sowohl bei Pankreas-Carcinomen als auch bei Pankreatitis (ZELLER u. HETZ; PAVLIK; HEUSER u. Mitarb.: akute Pankreatitis, chronische Pankreatitis, exkretorische Pankreas-Insuffizienz, traumatische Pankreatitis, Pankreas-Cysten) können neben einer Hyperlipasämie (DE GRACIANSKY; COMFORT u. OSTERBERG) disseminierte Fettgewebsnekrosen gefunden werden, die möglicherweise auf komplexe enzymatische Vorgänge zurückzuführen sind. In einer Anzahl von Beobachtungen fand sich eine deutliche Zunahme der Lipaseaktivität (DE GRACIANSKY; LIÈVRE) sowie eine Vermehrung von Amylase (COHEN) und Trypsin (LEGER). PANABOKKÉ konnte durch den Nachweis mehrerer Pankreasfermente in Fettgewebsnekrosen die klinischen Befunde durch experimentelle Untersuchungen stützen.

Beim *Erythema nodosum*, dem *Erythema induratum Bazin* sowie dem *Sarkoid Darier-Roussy* spielen Gefäßveränderungen im Sinne der Panarteriitis oder Panphlebitis eine primäre Rolle für die Auslösung der Erkrankung. Die veränderte allergische Reaktionslage des Organismus gegenüber Tuberkelbakterien ist von Bedeutung. Das pathogenetische Geschehen leitet jedoch in allgemeine, nicht streng mit der Tuberkulose verknüpfte Vorgänge immunologischer und immunbiologischer Art über. So kommt die Tuberkulose für das Erythema nodosum nicht als auslösendes Moment, sondern lediglich als Schrittmacher in Betracht, wobei zahlreiche Erreger, vorzugsweise β-hämolysierende Streptokokken mit Erhöhung des Antistreptolysin-Titers, zur Krankheitsmanifestation führen (MOLLARET; VANDEKERCKHOVE; SANDBERG u. ADAMS; MEYERS u.a.). Das Erythema nodosum wird außerdem bei Lepra, Morbus Besnier-Boeck-Schaumann, Lues, Lymphogranuloma inguinale, Trichophytie, Histoplasmose, Coccidioidomykose und nach Verabfolgung verschiedener Medikamente (Sulfathiazol, Supronal, Oestrogen, Seren) beobachtet (FINUCANE; GORDON; JAMES; GUGGENHEIM; DAVISON; RODRIGUEZ; MUNTEANU; CSERVENKA; BOCK; LITTLE u. STEIGMAN; FORD; OTTO u. HOBUSCH; VESEY u. WILKINSON; HOCHLEITNER; GREITHER; BOHNSTEDT; PIERINI, ABULAFIA u. WAINFELD u.a.). Bei einem medikamentös ausgelösten Erythema nodosum stellt das Infektionsgeschehen den Realisationsfaktor erster Ordnung, das Medikament den Realisationsfaktor zweiter Ordnung dar. Die Entwicklung eines Erythema nodosum als Primärsymptom bei akuter Monocytenleukämie, chronisch lymphatischer oder myeloischer Leukämie wird nur gelegentlich gefunden (PINSKI u. STANSIFER).

Aber auch dispositionelle Faktoren, und dies trifft insbesondere für die Erythema induratum-Gruppe zu, sind für die Krankheitsmanifestation von ausschlaggebender Bedeutung. Nach EBERHARTINGER wird nur ein bestimmter Personenkreis mit adipösen Unterschenkeln, Fettverteilungsanomalien und starker Kälteempfindlichkeit von der Erkrankung betroffen. Die bei diesen Patienten während hormoneller Krisen mit allgemeiner endokriner Dysregulation gehäuft vorzufindende Erythrocyanose ist ebenfalls hier einzuordnen. Ein Zusammenhang zwischen den genannten Faktoren und der sekundären Fettgewebsreaktion wird insbesondere im Rahmen der infektions-allergischen Genese durch die von GOTTRON inaugurierte relationspathologische Konzeption verständlich, nach der eine verlangsamte Durchströmung im Bereich des terminalen Strombahnnetzes der Absiedlung von Bakterien, Toxinen und anderen Antigenen Vorschub leistet. Der Kälteeinwirkung kommt möglicherweise nur eine auslösende oder verstärkende Wirkung zu. Der Ausgangspunkt des pathogenetischen Geschehens ist aufgrund der Untersuchungen EBERHARTINGERs demnach im Gefäßsystem, zumeist an den Arterien der Cutis-Subcutis-Grenze zu suchen.

Den Erkrankungen der *Periarteriitis nodosa-Gruppe* liegt eine allergische Genese zugrunde. Die Art und Weise der Gefäßreaktion hängt vom auslösenden Agens sowie der immunologischen Reaktionslage des Organismus ab. Bei einer hyperergischen Reaktionslage können exsudativ-leukocytäre Entzündungsvorgänge vom Typ des Arthus-Phänomens neben solchen vom Tuberkulintyp mit einer vorwiegend histiocytären Reaktion vorkommen. Neuere Einteilungen der Periarteriitis nodosa-Gruppe unterscheiden zwischen allergischen und nicht-allergische Formen (RANDERATH: anoxämisch, dysorotisch, toxisch, hormonal und pressorisch bedingte Arteriitiden — s. W. KNOTH u. W. MEYHÖFER, 1959). Gemeinsam ist beiden Krankheitsgruppen jedoch der primäre Gefäßbefall mit sekundärer Schädigung des dem Gefäßgebiet zugeordneten Binde- und Fettgewebes. Im Hinblick auf weitere Einzelheiten über die Ätiologie und Pathogenese allergischer Gefäßkrankheiten muß auf entsprechende Kapitel dieses Handbuches verwiesen werden.

Bei der *Necrobiosis lipoidica, Necrobiosis maculosa* und *Granulomatosis disciformis chronica et progressiva Miescher* sind pathogenetisch hochgradige Veränderungen an den Gefäßen von primärer Bedeutung (BREZHENKO; GROTS u. Mitarb.; RINGROSE; WORINGER u. WEILL; BAZEX u. DUPRÉ; PEZZAROSSA; DIMITRESCU u. BĂLUS; FORMAN; HEILESEN; KALKOFF; LINSER; GRIMMER; KNOTH u. FÜLLER; KNOTH; SANTLER; MULLER u. WINKELMANN u.a.). GOTTRON hat für die Necrobiosis lipoidica erstmals auf Zusammenhänge zwischen abartigen Kreislaufsituationen in Form der latenten und manifesten Hypertonie, der Hypotonie sowie einer konstitutionellen Vasolabilität und pathologischen Gefäßveränderungen hingewiesen. Von Interesse ist die Möglichkeit einer Kombination der Necrobiosis lipoidica mit weiteren Gefäßerkrankungen, beispielsweise einer vasculären Purpura (GOTTRON; STÜTTGEN). Hinzu kommt die Lokalisation der Hautveränderungen im Bereich der Unterschenkel; hier sind die Kreislaufverhältnisse besonders ungünstig. Nach KNOTH steht die arterielle Angiopathie in Form der Endarteriitis productiva fibrosa mit mäßig elastisch-fibröser Intima-Hyperplasie im Vordergrund des Krankheitsgeschehens. Es ist bekannt, daß bei einem Diabetes mellitus die Gefäße frühzeitig und schwer betroffen werden. Dabei sind sowohl Hypertonie, Hypotonie, Vasolabilität als auch eine orthostatische Hypotension bei der klinischen Untersuchung von Diabetikern nachweisbar. Nach ROTTER; MEESEN u.a. sind die Gefäßveränderungen funktionell und morphologisch faßbar. Die Ernährung der Gefäße erfolgt bis zur Media durch erythrocytenfreie Blutflüssigkeit, die der Adventitia durch die Vasa vasorum. ROTTER mißt im Hinblick auf Beginn und Manifestwerden pathologischer Gefäßveränderungen der Dysorie die bedeutendste Rolle zu. Bei der Hypertension kommt es zur Spannung des Bindegewebsschwammes und somit zur Behinderung des Einstroms der Blutflüssigkeit. Andererseits führen das perivasale Ödem sowie eine intra- bzw. perivasale Entzündung zur Blockierung der Vasa vasorum. Die so bedingte Hypoxydose stellt nach ROTTER den Beginn der Gefäßveränderungen dar. Auch hypotonische oder orthostatische Dysregulationen sowie Kälteeinwirkungen (SIEGMUND) führen zu Ernährungsstörungen im Gefäßwandbereich, wobei der Säftestrom von der Gefäßlichtung zur Adventitia hin verlangsamt ist. Als Folge der Dysorie mit Ernährungsstörung der Gefäßwand stellen sich intramurale Nekrosen ein. Demzufolge könnte es sich bei den aufgeführten Erkrankungen möglicherweise um Kreislaufdysregulationen in übererregbaren terminalen Strombahngebieten handeln, wobei die orthostatischen Regulationsstörungen zur Endangiitis productiva fibrosa mittelgroßer Hautarterien führen. Eine Folge der Oligämie und Hypoxydose sind unvollständige Gewebsinfarzierungen mit sekundärer Fetteinlagerung oder Fettphanerose (GOTTRON; GANS und STEIGLEDER; KNOTH; KNOTH und FÜLLER; GÖTZ u.a.). Die bei den zuletzt aufgeführten Erkrankungen klinisch und histologisch faßbaren Befunde bedürfen jedoch einer weiteren Stützung durch experimentell-physiologische Studien, die insbesondere im Hinblick auf eine Fundierung der angedeuteten pathogenetischen Vorstellungen von wesentlicher Bedeutung wären.

Über die Pathogenese der *Fettgewebstumoren* findet sich in der Literatur eine Anzahl von Hinweisen, die jeweils der vorherrschenden Lehrmeinung Rechnung tragen. Wie bereits früher erwähnt, hängen die Vorstellungen über die Entstehung der Fettgewebsgeschwülste eng mit der Entwicklung des Fettgewebes selbst zusammen. Eine allgemeingültige pathogenetische Deutung, besonders für die Entstehung maligner Fettgewebstumoren, ist bisher nicht möglich, da die Forschung über die Genese der Tumoren im allgemeinen noch nicht abgeschlossen und in vollem Fluß ist. Aus diesem Grund sollen lediglich die Beobachtungen Erwähnung finden, die histologisch einen Hinweis auf die Entwicklung von Fettgewebstumoren geben könnten.

Neben der genetischen Bedeutung für die Manifestation von Lipomen (familiäre Häufung) finden konstitutionelle, traumatische und entzündliche Faktoren (HANHARDT; BAUMGARTNER u. RIVA; GANS u. STEIGLEDER; GOTTRON; HELD u. DELLA SANTA) sowie trophische Störungen Erwähnung. BAUMGARTNER u. RIVA sahen in eindrucksvoller Weise bei einer Panniculitis Rothmann-Makai neben entzündlichen Erscheinungen Lipome. Auf die Mitwirkung des Endocriniums sowie auf eine mesencephale Genese haben DERCUM; TOURAINE u. RENAULT; FALTA; SCHIMPF u.a. hingewiesen (s. FLECK).

Besonders beachtenswert scheinen jedoch neurogene und vasculäre Einflüsse zu sein. HORNSTEIN beobachtete bei der histologischen Untersuchung lipomatöser Tumoren von Patienten mit Neurofibromatosis generalisata eigenartige zellige Wucherungen des neurovasculären Endnetzes, d.h. der Überschneidungszone des vegetativen nervösen Endnetzes mit der terminalen Strombahn. Durch diese Untersuchungsergebnisse findet die Auffassung der nerval induzierten Entwicklung lipomatöser Tumoren eine gewisse morphologische Stütze. Für eine neurogene Genese wird des weiteren die segmentäre, ein- oder beidseitige Anordnung der Tumoren, die Schmerzhaftigkeit sowie die Entwicklung von Lipomen im Verlauf einer Polyneuritis, segmentalen Myelitis, Syringomyelie, nach einem apoplektischen Insult oder einer traumatischen Schädigung des zentralen Nervensystems herangezogen (BUSCHKE u. MATTHISSOHN; s. dazu auch BAUMGARTNER u. RIVA sowie FLECK).

GOTTRON stellte nachdrücklich die Bedeutung eines besonderen Reizes auf das terminale Strombahnnetz für die Entstehung umschriebener Fettgewebstumoren heraus, worauf bereits bei der Besprechung der Insulinlipome eingegangen wurde. Für diese Auffassung spricht das auffällige Zusammentreffen von Lipomen bei Patienten mit petechialer Blutungsneigung infolge einer erhöhten Capillarfragilität, M. Werlhof oder labilem Hypertonus (GOTTRON). Auch GERTLER weist auf die Bedeutung der Irritation des Gefäßnervensystems hin. Von Interesse sind in diesem Zusammenhang die Befunde von HORNSTEIN, der pathologische Gefäßveränderungen im Sinne der Arteriosklerose am Rand der Lipome fand, wonach weniger ausgeprägte Gefäßveränderungen gegebenenfalls zur lipomatösen Wucherung, stärkere vasculäre Schäden zu regressiven Veränderungen führen können (s. dazu H. A. GOTTRON).

VIII. Zusammenfassende Besprechung

Bei einem Vergleich der Erkrankungen des Fettgewebes fällt eine deutliche Diskrepanz zwischen der klinischen Morphologie, dem Allgemeinbefinden sowie den unterschiedlichen ätiologischen Faktoren einerseits und der Einförmigkeit des pathohistologischen Befundes andererseits auf. Es scheint eine Eigenart des Fettgewebes zu sein, auf verschiedenartige Noxen und Reize mit typischen und sich immer wiederholenden Reaktionsformen zu antworten. Experimentelle Untersuchungen über die Pathologie des Fettgewebes haben gezeigt, daß in der Regel zu Beginn der Veränderungen die Cytosteatonekrosen mit verschiedenen Erscheinungsformen im Vordergrund stehen, gleichgültig welche auslösende Noxe der Erkrankung zugrunde liegt, wobei erst im weiteren Krankheitsverlauf die Lipogranulombildung folgt. So können bei der Spontanpanniculitis, nach Traumen, bei pathologischen Gefäßveränderungen, im Fettgewebe oder in der Nachbarschaft lokalisierten entzündlichen oder tumorösen Prozessen sowie in Reorganisation befindlichen Fettgewebstransplantaten histologisch identische lipophage Granulome beobachtet werden. Die Fettgewebsgranulome lassen sich als Ausdruck einer resorptiven Entzündung oder als Fremdkörperreaktion auf geschädigte körpereigene Fettzellen deuten. Den verschiedenen Panniculitisformen gemeinsam ist die histologische Ähnlichkeit der Lipogranulome mit Fremdkörpergranulomen. Lediglich bei Fettgewebserkrankungen tuberkulöser Genese finden sich neben unspezifisch-granulomatösen Reaktionen solche charakteristischer Art, die nicht nur im Fettgewebe, sondern auch im Corium anzutreffen sind. Unregelmäßigkeiten im histologischen Aufbau der Lipogranulome sind lediglich graduellen, nicht prinzipiellen Unterschieds und von der Intensität der einwirkenden Noxe sowie der Krankheitsdauer abhängig.

Unsere Kenntnisse über den Mechanismus der Reaktionsprozesse im Fettgewebe sind bis zum gegenwärtigen Zeitpunkt mangelhaft. Es soll jedoch mit gewissem Vorbehalt versucht werden, aus dem histologischen Befund sowie den verschiedenen klinischen und experimentellen Untersuchungsergebnissen eine Deutung im Hinblick auf die eigenartige Reaktionsweise des Fettgewebes zu geben.

Die Begründung für die granulomatöse Reaktion der Subcutis auf unterschiedliche Schädigungen ist im Fettgewebe selbst zu suchen. Das Fettgewebe stellt ein Organ sui generis dar (BAUMGARTNER und RIVA; FLECK; GOTTRON u.a.), das ursprünglich aus Gefäßen und einem pluripotenten retikulären Gewebsverband (extramedulläre Blutbildung, Phagocytose, reaktive Wucherung) bestand. Die Pluripotenz der Zellen des reticulo-histiocytären Systems ist auch nach

Ablauf des Embryonalstadiums von Bedeutung und spielt bei der Abwehrreaktion des Organismus auf schädliche Einflüsse eine bedeutende Rolle. Dabei werden die Adventitialzellen, die in der Indifferenzzone der Gefäße liegen und denen ebenfalls eine Vielzahl von Differenzierungsmöglichkeiten innewohnt, dem erweiterten reticulo-histiocytären System zugeordnet. Unter diesem Gesichtspunkt gesehen müssen verschiedene Reize, welche außer den Fettzellen die pluripotenten, sich aus der jungen indifferenten Mesenchymzelle ableitenden Adventitialzellen treffen, zu einer ähnlichen oder gleichen Reaktion führen. Allerdings kann je nach Reizqualität und -quantität körpereigener oder -fremder Substanzen die Zellbildung mehr in die eine oder andere Richtung gelenkt werden; die lipogranulomatöse Reaktion des Fettgewebes bleibt jedoch erhalten.

Die ätiologischen Faktoren sind unterschiedlicher Art, zum Teil noch unbekannt. So führen mechanische, chemische, thermische und bakterielle sowie infektions- oder arzneimittelallergisch bzw. toxisch bedingte Reize zur Auslösung gleicher patho-histogenetischer Vorgänge. Die Ursache der spontanen herdförmigen Panniculitis ist bisher unbekannt. Möglicherweise liegt der entzündlichen Reaktion des Fettgewebes gegenüber äußeren Einflüssen eine dauernde oder vorübergehende Disposition, eine verstärkte Reaktionsbereitschaft und Vulnerabilität der Subcutis zugrunde. Diese Annahme verbindet nach BAUMGARTNER u. RIVA die artefizielle, entzündliche und spontane Panniculitis und bietet somit Übergangsformen. Die besondere konstitutionelle angeborene (BAUMGARTNER u. RIVA: Neuropathische oder arthritische Konstitution bei Lipogranulomatosis subcutanea Rothmann-Makai) oder erworbene und dementsprechend ständige oder vorübergehende Disposition des Fettgewebes zur entzündlich-granulomatösen Reaktion (s. auch EBERHARTINGER) scheint insbesondere bei der artefiziellen Panniculitis vorzuliegen, da es nur bei wenigen Patienten zur Lipogranulombildung kommt.

Hormonelle Störungen könnten bei der Auslösung der Panniculitis eine Rolle spielen, worauf zahlreiche experimentelle Untersuchungen hinweisen. MAKAI vermutet Beziehungen zur Schilddrüse. LEINATI konnte diese Annahme durch experimentelle Untersuchungen stützen und fand nach Thyreoidektomie oder Ovariektomie häufiger eine Lipogranulombildung als bei nicht operierten Kontrolltieren. Es wäre jedoch auch an eine Allergisierung zu denken, wobei das Fettgewebe selbst oder die Gefäße arealweise zum Schockorgan werden könnten (BAUMGARTNER u. RIVA).

Ein weiterer Faktor für die Entwicklung von Lipogranulomen ist von grundlegender Bedeutung. Gemeint sind die in den Fettzellen gespeicherten Fettsubstanzen. Wie bereits mehrfach zum Ausdruck gebracht wurde, kann es sich bei den Lipogranulomen um eine resorptive Entzündung oder um eine Fremdkörper-Reaktion handeln. Ähnlich wie nach der Injektion öliger Lösungen könnten im Hinblick auf die Fremdkörper-Reaktion freiwerdende Fettsubstanzen für die artefiziell-, entzündlich-, allergisch-, toxisch-, hyp- oder anoxämisch bedingte Panniculitis sowie die Spontanpanniculitis eine bedeutende oder sogar ausschlaggebende pathogenetische Rolle spielen. Zunächst muß die cytoplasmatische Membran, die das Abfließen der Fettsubstanzen verhindert, von Makrophagen durchbrochen werden. Diese wandeln sich nach Aufnahme der Fettsubstanzen in Epitheloid- und Schaumzellen um. Nach PFUHL ist der Mitbefall der Gefäße von Bedeutung. Unterliegen diese ebenfalls einer Nekrose, müssen erst Granulocyten die Nekrose auflösen, bevor die Makrophagen in Tätigkeit treten können. Der Fremdkörper kann in Form nekrotischen Fettgewebes oder der aus der Zelle entlassenen Fettsubstanzen und deren Umwandlungsprodukten (hydrolytische Spaltung der Fette, Verseifung der Fettsäuren) vorliegen (s. auch PFUHL; FEIJOO; PIROTH; BRAUN-FALCO; STEIGLEDER). Grenzen zwischen nekrotischen Fettzellen und die Bildung freier Tröpfchen verseiften Fettes verschiedener Größe wurden von ABRIKOSSOFF beobachtet. Die Spaltung des frei im Gewebe liegenden Fettes soll von besonderer Bedeutung sein (s. auch E. PETRI; LECÈNE u. MOULONGUET; ABRIKOSSOFF). Die intracellulären Fettsubstanzen können jedoch unter gewissen Bedingungen (Inanition, Entzündung, Ischämie) auch primär einer chemischen Umwandlung mit Fremdkörperwirkung unterliegen und somit eine lipophage Reaktion auslösen (s. dazu auch BAUMGARTNER u. RIVA; FLECK u.a.). Inwieweit eine diabetische Stoffwechsellage oder andere Stoffwechselstörungen bei bestimmten Fällen pathogenetisch wirksam sind (OEHLERT u. Mitarb.; STEINESS), ist unbekannt. Dagegen könnte die Ernährung oder Nahrungsumstellung (BAUMGARTNER u. RIVA; GOTTRON; STEIGLEDER u.a.) für intracelluläre Stoffwechselstörungen eine Rolle spielen, wobei die unterschiedliche Zusammensetzung des Depotfettes von der Art der mit der Nahrung aufgenommenen Fettsubstanzen abhängig wäre. Der Mangel von Lipasen stellt eine weitere Möglichkeit für die Störung im Umbau von Nahrungsfett zu Depotfett dar (BAUMGARTNER u. RIVA). Es scheint dabei nicht ausgeschlossen, daß verschiedene Fettarten unterschiedlich auf freiwerdende Fermente reagieren und somit mehr oder weniger dazu in der Lage sind, als Mikrofremdkörper entsprechende Gewebsreaktionen auszulösen (BAUMGARTNER u. RIVA). Daß das Fettgewebe von Säuglingen eine andere Zusammensetzung als das Erwachsener aufweist, ist bewiesen (s. dazu SIWE; UNSHELM; SCRIBA; CRUSE; NOOJIN u. Mitarb.; HERING u. UNDEUTSCH; PIAGGIO; GOTTRON; GOTTRON u. NIKOLOWSKI; GRÜTZ; STEIGLEDER; HERTING u. CRAIN u.a.). Die zu beobachtende Verseifung würde auch hier als sekundärer Vorgang anzusehen sein, welcher möglicherweise bei der Resorption des modifizierten Fettes unter Einwirkung von Gewebslipasen auftritt (WORINGER).

Nach STEIGLEDER ist die Lipogranulombildung nicht in der Morphe des Fettgewebes, sondern in der biochemischen Besonderheit der Fettzellen begründet. Die Fettsubstanzen werden durch ein „kompliziertes biologisches System von Antioxydantien davor bewahrt, ranzig zu werden (HICKMAN), welches sofort versagt, wenn das Fett seinen Kontakt mit dem Organismus verliert". Es ist nicht auszuschließen, daß unterschiedliche ätiologische Faktoren intracellulär-oxydative Vorgänge veranlassen, die zu identischen pathologischen Stoffwechselprodukten führen und dementsprechend durch einen gleichen Reiz auf das Fettgewebe die gleichförmige Reaktion desselben (WORINGER; PFUHL; BLANC; GOTTRON; FEIJOO; MICHELSON; STEIGLEDER u.a.) auslösen. Die Frage, ob und inwieweit das extracellulär gelegene Fett bereits als Fremdkörper wirkt oder ob die ausgetretenen Fettsubstanzen erst nach physikalischer oder chemischer Umwandlung reizend oder stärker reizend wirken, ist bisher nicht zu beantworten.

Aus zahlreichen Arbeiten ist zu entnehmen, daß dem Gefäß-Nervensystem bei der Auslösung der verschiedenen Pannuculitisformen ebenfalls eine bedeutende Rolle beigemessen werden muß. GOTTRON hat 1952 versucht, die Pathogenese der Fettgewebserkrankungen aus relationspathogenetischer Sicht zu klären. Dabei werden den Untersuchungen die Struktureigenheiten des Fettgewebes zugrunde gelegt, wobei den Durchströmungsverhältnissen besondere Beachtung entgegengebracht wird. Der Entzündungsbegriff wird im Hinblick auf eine bessere Deutung des stufenweise ablaufenden, veränderten Gefäßgeschehens an der Endstrombahn bewußt ausgeschaltet. Das capillare Strombahnnetz ist nach den Ausführungen GOTTRONs weniger dicht als in anderen parenchymatösen Organen angeordnet, wodurch die capillaren Maschen weiter auseinander liegen. Hierdurch ist die Zweiphasigkeit der physiologischen Blutströmung in Form des Wechsels von Fluxion und Ischämie kaum gegeben. Unter dieser Voraussetzung findet sich die Blutströmung im Fettgewebe in einem ständigen, mäßig ausgeprägten peristatischen Strömungszustand. Durch die Einwirkung eines Reizes kann der peristatische verhältnismäßig leicht in einen prästatischen Folgezustand übergehen. Für diesen Strömungswechsel spielt weniger die Reizqualität als die Reizquantität eine Rolle. Somit ist das Fettgewebe eher als andere Gewebe zum statischen Zustand der peripheren Durchströmung mit seinen Folgezuständen prädisponiert.

RÖCKL und THIES konnten aufgrund klinischer und histomorphologischer Untersuchungen an mehreren Patienten mit knotig rezidivierenden, spontan auftretenden Veränderungen der Subcutis in Form der Spontanpanniculitis Typ Rothmann-Makai die relationspathogenetische Vorstellung GOTTRONs im Hinblick auf besondere Durchströmungsverhältnisse der Gefäße des Fettgewebes untermauern. Übereinstimmend fanden sich Durchblutungsstörungen der unteren Extremitäten infolge Erfrierung, Varicose oder Thrombophlebitis mit länger bestehenden Ödemen. Der peristatische Strömungszustand mit Erhöhung der Gefäßlabilität fand seinen sichtbaren Ausdruck in der nachzuweisenden Ödembildung, in deren Folge Reize nicht näher bekannter Natur in einem umschriebenen Gewebsbezirk bis zur Stase mit Herabsetzung der Sauerstoffzufuhr und den sich daraus ergebenden Folgezuständen führen können. Der Grad der Strömungsänderung ist jedoch nicht nur von der Stärke und Dauer des einwirkenden Reizes, sondern auch von der Stärke der Reizbarkeit des vegetativen Nervensystems abhängig, die als individuell-konstitutionelle Reaktion aufzufassen ist. Daneben können andere schädliche Einflüsse, beispielsweise eine Inanition, zur weiteren Erhöhung der Reizbarkeit des Gefäßnervensystems führen (GRUBER; GOTTRON; GOTTRON u. NIKOLOWSKI). Bei langsam einsetzender Stase mit allmählich aufsteigenden Reaktionsstufen tritt zunächst eine Strömungsverlangsamung mit plasmogener und cellulärer Diapedese auf. Ein stärkerer Reiz kann unter Umgehung der Prästase unmittelbar zur Stase und Gewebsnekrose mit Histolyse der Fettzellen führen. Unter diesem Gesichtspunkt wird ABRIKOSSOFFs Beobachtung von Nekrosen in primären Efflorescenzen bei Spontanpanniculitis verständlich. Die paracellulär gelegenen, intra- oder extracellulär veränderten Fettsubstanzen werden zum Fremdkörper und veranlassen die Ausbildung lipophager Granulome. Welche Rolle die nach der primären Gewebsschädigung freiwerdende Lipase, die Blutlipase bei Hämorrhagien, die Lipasen der Leukocyten und Lymphocyten, allergische, hormonelle, zentralnervöse oder konstitutionelle Faktoren für die Auslösung der Erkrankung, die Umwandlung der Fettsubstanzen bzw. die Lipogranulombildung zusätzlich spielen, ist bisher unbekannt.

Die Ausführungen lassen erkennen, daß die lipophagen Granulome entweder Ausdruck einer resorptiven Entzündung sind oder aber als Fremdkörperreaktion gedeutet werden können. Pathogenetisch gehen nach Einwirkung unterschiedlicher ätiologischer Faktoren den Fettgewebsveränderungen Gefäßstörungen am terminalen Strombahnnetz bzw. Gefäßveränderungen entzündlicher oder nichtentzündlicher Genese voraus. Sind in den Septen verlaufende größere Gefäße betroffen, kommt es zunächst zu einer septalen Bindegewebsnekrose, später erst zu einer Nekrose des Fettgewebes selbst. Die zwischen den Fettzellen liegenden Arterien veranlassen dagegen eine primäre Fettgewebsnekrose. Aber auch Gefäßschäden im Bereich der Cutis können sich im Hinblick auf die Besonderheit der Blutversorgung rückläufig auf die Subcutis auswirken. Die Schädigungen an den körpereigenen Fettzellen in Form der Histolyse sowie deren Folgezustände sind demnach auf die besonderen Durchströmungsverhältnisse der Subcutis zurückzuführen, unter Umständen jedoch Ausdruck einer besonderen Reizbarkeit des terminalen Gefäßnervensystems. Der intracelluläre Fettstoffwechsel kann aber auch primär gestört sein und zur Fehlbildung von Fettsubstanzen führen. Voraussetzung für die dem Fettgewebe eigene Gewebsreaktion ist die hydrolytische Spaltung der Fette sowie die Verseifung der Fettsäuren. Die Lipogranulombildung, welche das tragende Moment der Fettgewebserkrankungen darstellt, ist als eine typische Reaktionsart auf unspezifische Schädigungen aufzufassen. Die Steatonekrosen können im Gegensatz zu den Verhältnissen an anderen Organen am Beginn einer Reihe pathologischer Veränderungen stehen, womit insbesondere auch im Hinblick auf die Granulombildung den Erkrankungen des subcutanen Fettgewebes ein besonderes Gepräge gegeben wird. Es muß weiteren histo- und biochemischen Untersuchungen des normalen und pathologischen Fettgewebes vorbehalten bleiben, tieferen Einblick in die Vorgänge der granulomatösen Entzündung der Subcutis zu gewinnen.

Literatur

Gesamtübersichten

ALBERTINI, A. V.: Histologische Geschwulstdiagnostik. Stuttgart: Georg Thieme 1955. — ALLEN, A. C.: The skin. St. Louis: C. V. Mosby Co. 1954. — ASCHOFF, L.: Lehrbuch der Pathologie und pathologischen Anatomie, 5. Aufl. Jena: Gustav Fischer 1921.

BAUMGARTNER, W., u. G. RIVA: Panniculitis, die herdförmige Fettgewebsentzündung. Helv. med. Acta, 12, Suppl. XIV (1945). — BLANC, W. A.: Neue Syndrome der Fettgewebspathologie. Pseudotumoröse Fettgewebsnekrosen, disseminierte Fettgewebsnekrosen, dysproteinämische Liposklerosen. Paris: Masson & Cie. 1951. — Syndroms nouveaux de pathologie adipeuse. Paris: Masson & Cie. 1959. — BOHNSTEDT, R. M.: Krankheitssymptome an der Haut in Beziehungen zu Störungen anderer Organe. Stuttgart: Georg Thieme 1963.

FEHR, E.: Diagnostik der Kinderkrankheiten. Wien: Springer 1951.

GANS, O.: Histologie der Hautkrankheiten, Bd. I/II. Berlin: Springer 1925. — GANS, O., u. G. K. STEIGLEDER: Histologie der Hautkrankheiten, Bd. I/II. Berlin-Göttingen-Heidelberg: Springer 1957.

KLOSTERMANN, G. F., H. SÜDHOF u. W. TISCHENDORF: Der diagnostische Blick. Stuttgart: Schattauer 1964. — KYRLE, J.: Vorlesungen über Histo-Biologie der menschlichen Haut und ihrer Erkrankungen, Bd. I/II. Wien u. Berlin: Springer 1925.

LEVER, W. F.: Histopathologie der Haut. Stuttgart: Gustav Fischer 1958. — LUTZ, W.: Lehrbuch der Haut- und Geschlechtskrankheiten. Basel: S. Karger 1957.

MÜLLER, L. R.: Lebensnerven und Lebenstriebe, S. 766. Berlin: Springer 1931.

SANDRITTER, W., u. J. SCHORN: Histopathologie. Stuttgart: Schattauer 1965.

THOMA, K. H.: Oral surgery. London 1952. — Oral pathology. St. Louis 1954.

VOSS, H.: Grundriß der normalen Histologie und mikroskopischen Anatomie. Leipzig: Georg Thieme 1949.

WARD-HENDRICK, A.: Diagnosis and treatment of tumors of the head and neck. Baltimore 1950. — WEIDMAN, F. D.: Ageing of the skin. Problems of ageing, 2. ed., p. 391. New York 1942. — WILLIS, R. A.: Pathology of tumors. London 1953.

Vorbemerkungen

BRAUN-FALCO, O.: Die Histochemie der Haut. In: Dermatologie und Venerologie von H. A. GOTTRON u. W. SCHÖNFELD, Bd. I/1, S. 366. Stuttgart: Georg Thieme 1961.

CAHILL jr., G. F., and A. E. RENOLD: Regulation of adipose tissue metabolism within the intact organism: a summary. In: Handbook of physiology. Sect. 5, Adipose tissue, p. 681, ed. by A. E. RENOLD and G. F. CAHILL. Baltimore: Williams & Wilkins Co. 1965. — CROFFORD: Zit. nach A. E. RENOLD 1965.

HORSTMANN, E.: Anatomie der Haut und ihrer Anhangsorgane. In: Dermatologie und Venerologie, von H. A. GOTTRON u. W. SCHÖNFELD, Bd. I/1, S. 42. Stuttgart: Georg Thieme 1961.

RENOLD, A. E.: Das Fettgewebe. Med. Prisma 6, 5 (1965). — RENOLD, A. E., and G. F. CAHILL jr.: Metabolism of isolated adipose tissue: a summary. In: Handbook of physiology. Sect. 5, Adipose tissue. Baltimore: Williams & Wilkins Co. 1965.

SCHUPPLI, R.: Erythema nodosum. — Periarteriitis nodosa. — Panniculitis. — Granuloma anulare. — Necrobiosis lipoidica diabeticorum. — Granulomatosis disciformis. — Necrobiosis maculosa. In: Handbuch der Haut- und Geschlechtskrankheiten, von J. JADASSOHN, Erg.-Werk Bd. II/2, S. 78, 105, 122, 141. Berlin-Göttingen-Heidelberg: Springer 1965. — SHAPIRO, B.: Triglyceride metabolism. In: Handbook of physiology. Sect. 5, Adipose tissue, p. 217, ed. by A. E. RENOLD and G. F. CAHILL. Baltimore: Williams & Wilkins Co. 1965. —

Stauffacher, W.: Comparative studies of muscle and adipose tissue metabolism and obese mice. Ann. N.Y. Acad. Sci. **131**, 528 (1965). — Steigleder, G. K.: Allgemeine Pathologie der Haut. In: Dermatologie und Venerologie, von H. A. Gottron u. W. Schönfeld, Bd. I/1, S. 253. Stuttgart: Georg Thieme 1961. — Neoplastisch wuchernde Zellen der Cutis und Subcutis. In: Handbuch der Haut- und Geschlechtskrankheiten, von J. Jadassohn, Erg.-Werk Bd. I/2, S. 687. Berlin-Göttingen-Heidelberg: Springer 1961.
Wertheimer, H. E.: Introduction — a perspective. In: Handbook of physiology. Sect. 5, Adipose tissue, p. 5, ed. by A. E. Renold and G. F. Cahill. Baltimore: Williams & Wilkins Co. 1965.

Anatomie des Fettgewebes

Balboni, G.: Die Ultrastruktur der Fettzelle. Arch. ital. Anat. Embriol. **68**, 67 (1963). — Baló, J.: Zur Frage der Fettmobilisierung. Acta morph. Acad. Sci. hung. **10**, 313 (1961).
Cramer, D. L.: The component fatty acid of human depot fat. J. biol. Chem. **151**, 427 (1943).
Dabelow, A.: Reaktionsweisen des Lymphknotens beim Fetttransport. Z. Zellforsch. **12**, 207 (1931).
Favarger, P.: Relative importance of different tissues in the synthesis of fatty acids. In: Handbook of physiology. Sect. 5, Adipose tissue, p. 19, ed. by A. E. Renold and G. F. Cahill. Baltimore: Williams & Wilkins Co. 1965. — Favarger, P., et H. Bodur: Recherches sur la synthèse de graisses à partier d'acetate ou de glucose. Helv. physiol. pharmacol. Acta **15**, 345 (1957).
Goldner, J.: Histiocytäre Abstammung der Fettzellen. Z. Zellforsch. **24**, 312 (1936). — Gottron, H. A.: Krankheitszustände des subkutanen Fettgewebes. Medizinische **1952**, 912. — Grütz, O.: Beiträge zur Histologie und Pathogenese der Adiponekrosis subcutanea neonatorum. Arch. Kinderheilk. **113**, 199 (1938).
Herrmann, F., P. H. Prose, L. Mandol, and G. Medoff: Investigations into the pharmacology of skin fats and oilments. I. The collection and determination of lipids on the skin. J. invest. Derm. **16**, 217 (1951). — Hoffmann, A.: Die Entwicklung des Fettgewebes beim Menschen. Z. mikr.-anat. Forsch. **56**, 415 (1950/51).
Kimmig, J., u. R. Wehrmann: Biochemie der Haut. In: Dermatologie und Venerologie, von H. A. Gottron u. W. Schönfeld, Bd. II/1, S. 1178. Stuttgart: Georg Thieme 1962.
Laubinger, W.: Über den systemartigen Zusammenhang der Gitterfasern in den Fettorganen und seine funktionelle Bedeutung. J. Morph. mikr. Anat. **81**, 230 (1938). — Lynen, F., B. Agranoff, U. Hennig u. E. Möslein: Die Bildung freier Acetessigsäure in der Leber. Angew. Chem. **70**, 716 (1958). — Lynen, F., H. Eggerer, U. Hennig u. J. Kessel: Farnesylpyrophosphat und 3-Methyl-Δ^3 butenyl-1-pyrophosphat, die biologischen Vorstufen des Squalens. Angew. Chem. **70**, 738 (1958). — Lynen, F., U. Hennig, C. Bublitz, B. Sörbo u. L. Kröplin-Rueff: Der chemische Mechanismus der Acetessigsäurebildung in der Leber. Biochem. Z. **330**, 269 (1958).
Meyer, K., and E. Chaffee: Mucopolysaccharide acid of cornea and possible relation to "spreading factor". Proc. Soc. exp. Biol. (N.Y.) **43**, 487 (1940). — Mucopolysaccharids of the skin. J. biol. Chem. **138**, 491 (1941). — Michelson, H. E.: A consideration of some diseases of the subcutaneous fat. Arch. Derm. **75**, 633 (1957).
Napolitano, L.: Die Differenzierung der weißen Fettzellen. J. Cell Biol. **18**, 663 (1963). — The fine structure of adipose tissues. In: Handbook of physiology. Sect. 5, Adipose tissue, p. 109, ed. by A. E. Renold and G. F. Cahill. Baltimore: Williams & Wilkins Co. 1965.
Plenert, W.: Der Baker-Test bei der Untersuchung des subcutanen Fettgewebes im Kindesalter. Acta histochem. (Jena) **8**, 311 (1959). — Popoff, L., et N. Popoff: L'hemopoese cutanée au cours de la vie intra-utérine. Ann. Derm. Syph. (Paris) **85**, 157 (1958).
Renold, A. E.: Das Fettgewebe. Med. Prisma **6**, 5 (1965). — Renold, A. E., and G. F. Cahill jr.: Metabolism of isolated adipose tissue: a summary. In: Handbook of physiology. Sect. 5, Adipose tissue. Baltimore: Williams & Wilkins Co. 1965.
Schaffer, J.: Das Fettgewebe. In: Handbuch der mikroskopischen Anatomie des Menschen von W. v. Möllendorf, Bd. II/2, S. 70. Berlin: Springer 1930. Z. mikr.-anat. Forsch. **22**, 579 (1930). — Shapiro, B.: Triglyceride metabolism. In: Handbook of physiology. Sect. 5, Adipose tissue, p. 217, ed. by A. E. Renold and G. F. Cahill. Baltimore: Williams & Wilkins Co. 1965. — Shapiro, B., and E. Wertheimer: The metabolic activity of adipose tissue. Metabolism **5**, 79 (1956). — Sheldon, H.: Morphology of adipose tissue: A microscopic anatomy of fat. In: Handbook of physiology. Sect. 5, Adipose tissue, p. 125, ed. by A. E. Renold and G. F. Cahill. Baltimore: Williams & Wilkins Co. 1965. — Sheldon, H., C. H. Hollenberg u. A. J. Winigrad: Beobachtungen zur Morphologie des Fettgewebes. Diabetes **11**, 378 (1962). — Simon, G.: Histogenesis. In: Handbook of physiology. Sect. 5, Adipose tissue, p. 101, ed. by A. E. Renold and G. F. Cahill. Baltimore: Williams & Wilkins Co. 1965. — Sinapius, D.: Zur Histochemie des Fettgewebes. Beitr. path. Anat. **121**, 1 (1959). —

STEIGLEDER, G. K.: Allgemeine Pathologie der Haut. In: Dermatologie und Venerologie von H. A. GOTTRON u. W. SCHÖNFELD, Bd. I/1, S. 253. Stuttgart: Georg Thieme 1961.
TAYLOR, A. C.: Survial of rat skin and changes in hair pigmentation following freezing. Exp. Zool. 110, 77 (1949). — TAYLOR, J. D., H. E. PAUL, and M. F. PAUL: Biochemistry of wound-healing. Arch. Biochem. 17, 421 (1948).
WASSERMANN, F.: The development of adipose tissue. In: Handbook of physiology. Sect. 5, Adipose tissue, p. 87, ed. by A. E. RENOLD and G. F. CAHILL. Baltimore: Williams & Wilkins Co. 1965. — WASSERMANN, F., u. McDONALD: Elektronenmikroskopische Untersuchungen über die äußeren Membranstrukturen der Fettzelle und über deren Veränderungen bei der Entspeicherung der Zelle. Z. Zellforsch. 52, 778 (1960). — WASSERMANN, H.: Die Fettorgane des Menschen. Z. Zellforsch. 3, 235 (1926). — WEISS, F.: Histologische Untersuchungen an der Haut von debilen Neugeborenen, eutrophischen und ernährungsgestörten Säuglingen unter besonderer Berücksichtigung ihres bindegewebigen und fettspeichernden Anteils sowie der klinischen Zusammenhänge. Jb. Kinderheilk. 135, 184, 272 (1932). — WERTHEIMER, H. E.: Fettspeicherung und Fettmobilisierung. Münch. med. Wschr. 31, 1153 (1958). — Introduction — a perspective. In: Handbook of physiology. Sect. 5, Adipose tissue, p. 5, ed. by A. E. RENOLD and G. F. CAHILL. Baltimore: Williams & Wilkins Co. 1965. — WILLIAMSON, J. R.: Fine structural alterations in adipose tissue in diabetic rats. Anat. Rec. 142, 291 (1962). — Adipose tissue. Morphological changes associated with lipid mobilization. J. Cell Biol. 20, 57 (1964). — WILLIAMSON, J. R., and P. E. LACY: Structurell aspects of adipose tissue: A summary attempting to synthesize the information contained in the preceding chapters. In: Handbook of physiology. Sect. 5, Adipose tissue, p. 201, ed. by A. E. RENOLD and G. F. CAHILL. Baltimore: Williams & Wilkins Co. 1965.

Atrophien der Haut

BAUMANN: Zit. nach S. R. BRÜNAUER 1935. — BAZEX, A., and A. DUPRÉ: Acrogerie (GOTTRON). A propos d'une observation. Ann. Derm. Syph. (Paris) 82, 604 (1955). — BECK, S. C.: Beitrag zur Lehre von der idiopathischen Hautatrophie. Arch. Derm. Syph. (Berl.) 100, 117 (1910). — BERING, FR.: Über Dermatitis atrophicans chronica idiopathica. Arch. Derm. Syph. (Berl.) 113, 73 (1912). — BERNSTEIN, E.: Hemiatrophia alternans facialis progressiva. Zbl. Haut- u. Geschl.-Kr. 25, 68 (1928). — BREUCKMANN, H.: Über ein der Akrodermatitis chronica atrophicans ähnliches Krankheitsbild bei Winzern mit Arsenschädigung. Arch. Derm. Syph. (Berl.) 179, 695 (1939). — BRÜNAUER, ST. R.: Atrophien. In: Haut- und Geschlechtskrankheiten von L. ARZT u. C. ZIELER, Bd. II, S. 407. Berlin u. Wien: Urban & Schwarzenberg 1935.
CZAJEWICZ: Zit. nach O. GANS u. G. K. STEIGLEDER 1955.
DELBANCO, E.: Kraurosis glandis et praeputii. Verh. Dtsch. Derm. Ges. 1908, Frankfurt a. M.
EHLERS, G.: Hemiatrophia faciei progressiva nach Hirntrauma. Derm. Wschr. 114, 958 (1961). — EJIRI, I.: Studien über die Histologie der menschlichen Haut, 1.—5. Mitt. Jap. J. Derm. 40, 173, 216 (1936); 41, 8, 64, 95 (1937). — EVANS, COWDRY u. NIELSON: Zit. nach F. PINKUS u. H. PINKUS, Anatomie. In: Fortschritte der Dermatologie 1943—1946, hrsg. v. W. LUTZ, S. 1. Basel 1948.
FLEMMING: Zit. nach O. GANS u. G. K. STEIGLEDER 1955.
GANS, O., u. E. LANDES: Akrodermatitis atrophicans arthropathica. Hautarzt 3, 151 (1952). — GIERKE: Zit. nach O. GANS u. G. K. STEIGLEDER 1955. — GÖTZ, H.: Die Akrodermatitis chronica atrophicans Herxheimer als Infektionskrankheit. Hautarzt 5, 491 GONDESEN, H.: Hemiatrophia et hypertrophia faciei sinistra. Arch. Derm. Syph. (Berl.) 189, 472 (1949); Derm. Wschr. 122, 848 (1950). — GOTTRON, H. A.: Familiäre Akrogerie. Arch. Derm. Syph. (Berl.) 181, 571 (1940). — Krankheitszustände des subcutanen Fettgewebes. Medizinische 1952, 912. — Veränderungen der Haut im Alter. Neue med. Welt 1950 I, 13, 54. (1954).
HAUSER, W.: Atrophien. In: Dermatologie und Venerologie von H. A. GOTTRON u. W. SCHÖNFELD, Bd. II/2, S. 833. Stuttgart: Georg Thieme 1958. — HEUSS: Zit. nach O. GANS u. G. K. STEIGLEDER 1955. — HILL, W. R., and H. MONTGOMERY: Regional changes and changes caused by age in the normal skin. J. invest. Derm. 3, 231 (1940). — HOFF, F.: Haut und vegetative Steuerung. Arch. Derm. Syph. (Berl.) 184, 234 (1943).
KIRSCHENBERG, E.: Zur Frage der Hemiatrophia faciei progressiva mit zentraler Genese. Ref. Zbl. Haut- u. Geschl.-Kr. 21, 299 (1927). — KNOTH, W., R. BAETHKE u. L. HOFFMANN: Über das Werner-Syndrom. Ein Beitrag zur Kenntnis der Schilddrüsenfunktion nach Radiojodstudium, der Symptomatologie der Schrifttumsfälle und der histologischen Differentialdiagnose zum Rothmund-Syndrom. Hautarzt 14, 145, 193 (1963). — KRAUS: Zit. nach O. GANS u. G. K. STEIGLEDER 1955.
LANDES, E.: Angeborene Hemiatrophia faciei dextra. Derm. Wschr. 126, 1219 (1952). — LUCIANI: Zit. nach O. GANS u. G. K. STEIGLEDER 1955.

MONTGOMERY, H., and R. R. SULLIVAN: Arodermatitis atrophicans. Arch. Derm **51**, 32. (1945). — OPPENHEIM, M.: Atrophien. In: Handbuch der Haut- und Geschlechtskrankheiten von J. JADASSOHN, Bd. VII/2, S. 500. Berlin: Springer 1931. — PERCIVAL, G. H., W. HANNEY, and D. H. DUTHIE: Fibrous changes in the dermis with special reference to senile elastosis. Brit. J. Derm. **61**, 269 (1946). — PFUHL: Zit. nach O. GANS u. G. K. STEIGLEDER 1955. — PICK, F. J.: Über Erythromelie. Ein kasuistischer Beitrag. Arch. Derm. Syph. (Berl.) (Erg.-Bd.) **113**, 915 (1900). — REICH, H.: Histologische Untersuchungen bei diffuser Sklerodermie. Arch. Derm. Syph. (Berl.) **191**, 505 (1950). — RENOLD, A. E.: Das Fettgewebe. Med. Prisma **6**, 5 (1965). — ROSANOW: Zit. nach O. GANS u. G. K. STEIGLEDER 1955. — ROTHMANN: Zit. nach O. GANS u. G. K. STEIGLEDER 1955. — SAALFELD, E.: Zur pathologischen Anatomie der Haut im Alter. Arch. Derm. Syph. (Berl.) **132**, 1 (1921). — SCHALTENBRAND, G.: Die Beziehungen zwischen Hauterkrankungen und Nervenerkrankungen. Arch. Derm. Syph. (Berl.) **187**, 506 (1949). — SCHIDACHI, J.: Über die Atrophie des subcutanen Fettgewebes. Arch. Derm. Syph. (Berl.) **90**, 97 (1908). — STEIGER-KAZAL, D.: Xanthoma molluciforme et generalisatum bei einem Kleinkinde, mit Ausgang in Anetoderma. Derm. Wschr. **112**, 125 (1941). — STRÖBEL, H.: Die Gewebsveränderungen der Haut im Verlaufe des Lebens. Arch. Derm. Syph. (Berl.) **186**, 636 (1948). — STÜHMER, A.: Balanitis xerotica obliterans und ihre Beziehungen zur Kraurosis glandis et praeputii penis. Arch. Derm. Syph. (Berl.) **156**, 613 (1928). — UNNA, P. G.: Basophiles Kollagen, Kollagen und Kollastin. Mh. prakt. Derm. **19**, 1 (1894). — Zit. nach O. GANS u. G. K. STEIGLEDER 1955. — WAINGER, C. K., and W. F. LEVER: Dermatomyositis. Arch. Derm. **59**, 196 (1949). — WALTHER, D.: Über den Lupus erythematodes profundus. Arch. klin. exp. Derm. **204**, 182 (1957). — WEBER, G.: Fehlbildungen. In: Dermatologie und Venerologie von H. A. GOTTRON u. W. SCHÖNFELD, Bd. IV, S. 156. Stuttgart: Georg Thieme 1960. — WEIGERT: Zit. nach O. GANS u. G. K. STEIGLEDER 1955.

Patho-Histologie der Erkrankungen des subcutanen Fettgewebes

ABRIKOSSOFF, A.: Über die spontan auftretenden Fettgewebsnekrosen und Fettgranulome. Zbl. Path. **38**, 542 (1926). — ADAIR, F. E., u. J. TH. MUNZER: Fettnekrose der weiblichen Brustdrüse. Amer. J. Surg. **74**, 117 (1947). — AGNETA, J. O.: Lipatrofia sclerosa insulinica. Rev. argent. Dermatosif. **39**, 156 (1955). — ALDERSON, H. E., and S. C. WAY: Relapsing febrile nonsuppurative panniculitis (Weber). Arch. Derm. **27**, 440 (1933). — ANNING, S. T.: Sklerosierendes Lipogranulom. Proc. roy. Soc. Med. **45**, 101 (1952). — APFFEL, K., u. F. BURGUN: Zur Frage des nicht tuberkulösen Erythema nodosum beim Kinde. Kinderärztl. Prax. **13**, 57 (1942). — ARDUINO, J. L.: Sklerosierendes Lipogranulom (Paraffinom) des männlichen Genitale. J. Urol. (Baltimore) **82**, 155 (1959). — ARNDT: Zit. nach F. FUNK, 1958. — ARZT, L.: Adiponekrosis subcutanea. Zbl. Haut- u. Geschl.-Kr. **49**, 584 (1935). — BALLAGI, ST.: Ein Fall von Erythema nodosum trichophyticum bei Trichophytia profunda des Kopfes. Zbl. Haut- u. Geschl.-Kr. **68**, 361 (1942). — BARTÁK, P.: Zur Kenntnis der histologischen Bilder des Erythema nodosum. Derm. Wschr. **149**, 619 (1964). — BAUMANN, R.: Die Panniculitisformen unter besonderer Berücksichtigung der Spontanpanniculitis Rothmann-Makai. Ärztl. Wschr. **8**, 609 (1953). — BERGSTRAND, H.: Is erythema nodosum a hypersensibility reaction of anaphylactic type ? Acta derm.-venereol. (Stockh.) **29**, 539 (1949). — BERNDT, H., u. W. FRIEDRICHS: Beitrag zur Klinik der Panniculitis Weber-Christian. Z. ges. inn. Med. **15**, 67 (1960). — BEST, E. W., H. L. MASON, J. W. DE WEERD u. D. C. DAHLIN: Sklerosierendes Lipogranulom des männlichen Genitale, hervorgerufen durch Mineralöl. Proc. Mayo Clin. **28**, 623 (1953). — BINKLEY, J. S.: Relapsing febrile nodular nonsuppurative panniculitis. J. Amer. med. Ass. **109**, 1419 (1937). — BOCK, H. E.: Zur Allergielage bei Erythema nodosum im Rahmen des Löfgren-Syndroms. Allergie u. Asthma **6**, 121 (1960). — BOJLÉN, K., u. S. PETRY: Necrosis adiposa neonatorum. Acta paediat. (Uppsala) **19**, 123 (1936). — BOLLER, R.: Behandlung der Insulinlipodystrophie. Klin. Wschr. **1930**, 2433. — BONICELLI, U., u. R. TAGLIAVINI: Noduläre Vasculitis und Erythema induratum. G. ital. Derm. **102**, 69 (1961). — BRANCATI, R.: Die Fettnekrose der Brustdrüse. Arch. ital. Chir. **26**, 585 (1930). — BRAUN-FALCO, O.: Die Histochemie der Haut. In: Dermatologie und Venerologie von H. A. GOTTRON u. W. SCHÖNFELD, Bd. I/1, S. 366. Stuttgart: Georg Thieme 1961. — BUGYI, G.: Heilung in zwei Fällen von Necrosis progressiva subcutanea neonatorum. Derm. Wschr. **133**, 497 (1956). — CALNAN, C. D., u. H. HABER: Sklerosierendes Lipogranulom. Proc. roy. Soc. Med. **45**, 716 (1952). — CAROL, W. L. L., J. R. PRACKEN u. H. A. v. ZWIJNDREGT: Erythema nodosum und „Relapsing febrile nodular nonsuppurative panniculitis". Arch. Derm. Syph. (Berl.) **182**, 329 (1942). — CIBILS AGUIRRE, R., u. D. BRACHETTO-BRIAN: Über die pathologische Anatomie des Erythema nodosum. Sem. méd. **1932 I**, 253. Zit. Zbl. Haut- u. Geschl.-Kr. **41**, 339

(1932). — COLLEN, W. S., L. C. BOAS, J. D. ZILINSKY u. J. J. GREENWALD: Fettschwund infolge der Insulininjektion. Eine Gegenmaßnahme. New Engl. J. Med. 241, 610 (1949). — CORNBLEET, TH., and H. RATTNER: Adiponecrosis subcutanea neonatorum. Arch. Derm. 40, 829 (1939). — COSTE: Zit. nach FR. FUNK 1958. — COTTONI, G. B., u. A. SAPUPPO: Handelt es sich bei der disseminierten symmetrischen Steatonekrose um ein Sarkoid Darier-Roussy oder eine Lipogranulomatosis subcutanea Rothmann-Makai? Hautarzt 11, 249 (1960). — CUMMINS, L. J., and W. F. LEVER: Relapsing febrile nodular nonsuppurative panniculitis (Weber-Christian-disease). Arch. Derm. 38, 415 (1938).

DANDA, J., u. V. PLACHY: Adiponecrosis subcutanea neonatorum. Čs. Derm. 31, 190 (1956). Ref. Zbl. Haut- u. Geschl.-Kr. 97, 60 (1957). — DEJENARUI, I., A. SZENTMIKLOSY u. T. DAVID: Über einen Fall von diabetischer Nekrobiose. Derm.-Vener. (Buc.) 3, 171 (1958). — DEPISCH, F.: Weiterer Beitrag zur Frage der lokalen Lipodystrophie bei Dauerinsulinbehandlung. Wien. med. Wschr. 1930 I, 168. — DIECKHOFF, J., H. C. HEMPEL u. R. KOCH: Die traumatisch bedingte Fettgewebsnekrose des Neugeborenen. Kinderärztl. Prax. 27, 443 (1959). — DOXIADIS, S. A.: Aetiologie des Erythema nodosum bei Kindern. Brit. med. J. 1949 II, 844. — DUPERRAT, B.: Panniculitis de Rothmann-Makai. Med. infant. 67, 5 (1960).

EBERHARTINGER, CHR.: Das Problem des Erythema induratum Bazin. Arch. klin. exp. Derm. 217, 196 (1963). — EISENSCHMID, J. A., u. J. L. ORBISON: Experimentelle Erzeugung peritonealer Lipogranulome bei der Ratte. Arch. Path. 66, 154 (1958). — ENGELBACH, F.: Lokalisierter Schwund des subcutanen Fettgewebes infolge von wiederholten Insulininjektionen. Ann. intern. Med. 6, 1322 (1933). — EYCKMANS, R.: Panniculite nodulaire de Rothmann-Makai. Arch. belges Derm. 10, 363 (1954).

FANINGER, A., u. M. IŠVANESKI: Ein Beitrag zur Kenntnis der spontanen, chronisch-recidivierenden Panniculitis. Hautarzt 9, 372 (1958). — FEUERSTEIN: Homoiotransplantation bei ausgehender Necrosis progressiva neonatorum. Hautarzt 8, 375 (1957). — FISCHER, H.: Beziehungen zwischen Haut und Lungen. In: Dermatologie und Venerologie von H. A. GOTTRON u. W. SCHÖNFELD, Bd. V/1, S. 247. Stuttgart: Georg Thieme 1963. — FLORY, C. M.: Fat necrosis of the newborn. Arch. Path. 45, 278 (1948). — FUHS, H.: Ein Fall von Trichophyton gypseum kerium und Erythema nodosum trichophyticum, das histologisch typisch war. Zbl. Haut- u. Geschl.-Kr. 68, 411 (1942). — FUNK, FR.: Die Sarkoidose. In: Dermatologie und Venerologie von H. A. GOTTRON u. W. SCHÖNFELD, Bd. II/2, S. 1227. Stuttgart: Georg Thieme 1958.

GANS, O.: Die Histopathologie polymorpher exsudativer Dermatosen in ihrer Beziehung zur speziellen Aetiologie. Arch. Derm. Syph. (Berl.) 130, 15 (1921). — Über Lupus pernio und seine Beziehungen zum Sarkoid Boeck. Derm. Z. 33, 64 (1921). — GEBAUER, H.: Fettgewebsdellen bei Depot-Insulin-Spritzen. Münch. med. Wschr. 1942, 350. — GELLERSTEDT: Zit. nach O. GANS u. G. K. STEIGLEDER 1955. — GEORGIO, A. DE: Su un caso di panniculite nodulare. Sindrome di Weber-Christian. Minerva derm. 34, 151 (1959). — GIORDANO: Zit. nach R. BRANCATI 1930. — GOHRBANDT: Zit. nach R. BRANCATI 1930. — GORDON, H.: Erythema nodosum. A review of one hundred and fifteen cases. Brit. J. Derm. 73, 393 (1961). — GOTTRON, H. A.: Hauttuberkulose. In: DEIST u. KRAUS, Die Tuberkulose, ihre Erkennung und Behandlung. Stuttgart: Ferdinand Enke 1950. — Krankheitszustände des subcutanen Fettgewebes. Medizinische 1952, 912. — GOTTRON, H. A., u. W. NIKOLOWSKI: Pfeifer-Christian-Webersche Krankheit in ihrer Nosologie und Pathogenese. Hautarzt 3, 530 (1952). — GREITHER, A.: Erythema nodosum und Erythema exsudativum multiforme. In: Dermatologie und Venerologie von H. A. GOTTRON u. W. SCHÖNFELD, Bd. II/1, S. 445. Stuttgart: Georg Thieme 1958. — GRUPPER, CH., M. HEBERT et J. HEWITT: Panniculite atrophiante fébrile de Weber-Christian. Bull. Soc. franç. Derm. Syph. 61, 344 (1954). — GRÜTZ, O.: Beiträge zur Histologie und Pathogenese der Adiponekrosis subcutanea neonatorum. Arch. Kinderheilk. 113, 199 (1938). — GRZYBOWSKI, M.: Sur l'anatomie pathologique de l'érythème noueux. Bull. Soc. franç. Derm. Syph. 45, 1073 (1938).

HALTER, K.: Lipogranulomatosis subcutanea Makai. Z. Haut- u. Geschl.-Kr. 1952, 305. — HERBST: Lipogranulom. Zbl. Haut- u. Geschl.-Kr. 84, 242 (1953). — HERING, H., u. W. UNDEUTSCH: Zur Klinik und Pathogenese der Adiponekrosis subcutanea neonatorum. Derm. Wschr. 134, 917 (1956). — HERRMANN, W. P., K. H. SCHULZ u. R. WEHRMANN: Zur Pathogenese der Insulin-Allergie. Derm. Wschr. 139, 73 (1959). — HOLT u. HOWLAND: Zit. nach G. W. KORTING 1958. — HOLZEL, A.: Subcutaneous fat necrosis of the newborn. Arch. Dis. Childh. 26, 89 (1951). — HUGHES u. HAMMOND: Zit. nach G. W. KORTING 1958.

IRGANG, S.: Sarkoid Darier-Roussy. Report of a case and a discussion of the histologic features. Dermatologica (Basel) 118, 145 (1959). — ITO, K.: Reconsidering the classical entity of erythema induratum in the age of modern therapy. Bull. pharm. Res. Inst. 34, 24 (1961).

JABLONSKA, S.: Hyperergische Gefäßkrankheiten in der Dermatologie. Z. Haut- u. Gschl.-Kr. 33, 37 (1962). — JADASSOHN, W.: Panniculite de Weber-Christian. Dermatologica (Basel) 116, 346 (1958). — JAMES, D. G.: Erythema nodosum. Brit. J. Med. 1961, 853. — JAUSION, H., P. BÉNARD, R. SYLVESTRE et J. P. MENANTEAU: Un cas particulier de pannicu-

litis nodulaire fébrile multirecidivante de Weber-Christian. Bull. Soc. franç. Derm. Syph. **65**, 463 (1958).
KAMINSKY, A., L. JAIMOVICH, P. VIGLIOGLIA, M. KORDON y H. ROSALES: Sarkoides de Darier-Roussy. Rev. argent. Dermatosif. **46**, 209 (1962). — KELLNER, H.: Zur Frage der Zusammenhänge zwischen lipophager Granulombildung und Erythema induratum, Sarkoid Darier-Roussy und Panniculitis non suppurativa nodularis recidivans. Hautarzt **2**, 299 (1951). — KNOTH, W., u. W. MEYHÖFER: Beitrag zum Formenkreis der Periarteriitis nodosa und zur Bewertung der Riesenzellen bei Gefäßerkrankungen. Dermatologica (Basel) **119**, 1 (1959). — KONOPIK, J.: On the pathogenesis and aetiology of panniculitis. Čs. Derm. **30**, 259 (1955). — KOOIJ, R.: Das Weber-Christiansche Syndrom als Variante der Panniculitis. Dermatologica (Basel) **101**, 322 (1950). — KORTING, G. W.: Sklerodermie und sklerodermieähnliche Erkrankungen. In: Dermatologie und Venerologie von H. A. GOTTRON u. W. SCHÖNFELD, Bd. II/2, S. 942. Stuttgart: Georg Thieme 1958. — KRINER, J.: Panniculitis de Weber-Christian con sectores de estructura sarcoidal. Arch. argent. Dermatosif. **7**, 125 (1957). — KÜTTNER, H., u. M. BARUCH: Der traumatische segmentäre Gefäßkrampf. Bruns' Beitr. klin. Chir. **120**, 7 (1920).
LACOMME, M., et FL. KREIS DE MAYO: Sur l'induration cutanée curable du nouveauné dite d'origine obstétricale. Bull. méd. (Paris) **1936**, 509. Ref. Zbl. Haut- u. Geschl.-Kr. **55**, 639 (1937). — LANGCOPE, W. T., u. D. G. FREIMAN: Zit. nach FR. FUNK 1958. — LANGER, E.: Adiponekrosis subcutanea neonatorum. Derm. Wschr. **133**, 647 (1956). — LANGHOF, H.: Panniculitis nodosa (allergica?). Zbl. Haut- u. Geschl.-Kr. **104**, 348 (1959). — LECZINSKY, C. G.: Nodular vasculitis, clinical and histological studies, based on some 400 cases. Proc. 11. Internat. Congr. Dermat. Stockh. 1957, vol. 2, p. 185 (1960). — LEITNER, ST.: Der Morbus Besnier-Boeck-Schaumann. Basel: Benno Schwabe & Co. 1949. — LERICHE: Zit. nach H. A. GOTTRON 1952. — LEVER, W. F.: Nodular nonsuppurative panniculitis (Weber-Christian disease). Arch. Derm. **59**, 31 (1949). — LEVER, W. F., and D. G. FREIMAN: Sarkoidosis. Arch. Derm. **57**, 639 (1948). — LEWANDOWSKY, F.: Zur Kenntnis der Boeck'schen Sarkoide. Arch. Derm. Syph. (Berl.) **135**, 287 (1921). — LÖFGREN, S., and F. WAHLGREN: On the histopathology of erythema nodosum. Acta derm.-venereol. (Stockh.) **29**, 1 (1949). — LUITHLEN: Zit. nach O. GANS u. G. K. STEIGLEDER 1955. — LUZZATTI u. HANSEN: Zit. nach G. W. KORTING 1958.
MALLET, M.: Etude histologique des lésions cutanées de l'érythème noueux. Bull. Soc. franç. Derm. Syph. **45**, 1064 (1938). — MCDONALD, R.: Subcutaneous fat necrosis and sclerema neonatorum. S. Afr. med. J. **1955**, 1007. — MENSI, E.: Sulle alterazioni cutanee dello sclerema. G. ital. Derm. **1912**, 209. — MEYER, A.: Die herdförmige unspezifische Entzündung der Subcutis (Panniculitis). Praxis **1955**, 201. — MICHELSON, H. E.: A consideration of some diseases of subcutaneous fat. Arch. Derm. **75**, 633 (1957). — MIESCHER, G.: Zur Histologie des Erythema nodosum. Acta derm.-venereol. (Helsingfors) **27**, 448 (1947). — Zur Frage der Radiärknötchen beim Erythema nodosum. Arch. Derm. Syph. (Berl.) **193**, 251 (1951). — MILNER, R. D. G., and M. J. MITCHINSON: Systemic Weber-Christian disease. J. clin. Path. **18**, 150 (1965). — MOSTOFI, F. K., and E. ENGLEMAN: Fatal relapsing febrile nonsuppurative panniculitis. Arch. Path. **43**, 417 (1947). — MULLER, S. A., and R. K. WINKELMANN: Necrobiosis lipoidica diabeticorum. Arch. Derm. **93**, 272 (1966).
NAGAHORI, T.: Supplementary findings in erythema induratum Bazin. Jap. J. Derm. **69**, 147 (1959). Ref. Zbl. Haut- u. Geschl.-Kr. **104**, 38 (1959). — NETHERTON, E. W.: Relapsing nodular nonsuppurative panniculitis. Arch. Derm. **28**, 258 (1933). — NEWCOMER, V. D.: Sklerosierendes Lipogranulom oder Fremdkörpergranulom nach Ölinjektion. Arch. Derm. **69**, 383 (1954). — NEWCOMER, V. D., J. H. GRAHAM, R. R. SCHAFFERT, and L. KAPLAN: Vernarbendes Lipogranulom in Beziehung zu exogenen Lipoidsubstanzen. Arch. Derm. **73**, 361 (1956). — NOOJIN, R. O., B. F. PACE, and H. G. DAVIS: Subcutaneous fat necrosis of the newborn: certain etiologic considerations. J. invest. Derm. **12**, 331 (1949). — NORMAN, GRIFFEN u. MITCHELL: Zit. nach G. W. KORTING 1958. — NUBÉ, M. J.: Miescher's granulomas in erythema nodosum. Dermatologica (Basel) **101**, 80 (1950). — NUNEZ ANDRADE, R.: Panniculitis nodular no suppurada. Sindrome de Pfeifer-Weber-Christian. Medicina (Mex.) **42**, 1 (1962).
OBERLING, FR., M. IMLER u. A. BATZENSCHLAGER: Idiopathische disseminierte Panniculitiden. Anatomisch-pathologische Daten. Bull. Soc. franç. Derm. Syph. **70**, 239 (1963). — OCANO SIERRA, J.: Panniculitis nodular febril recidivante no suppurada de Pfeifer-Weber-Christian. Acta dermo-sifiliogr. (Madr.) **53**, 19 (1962). — OEHLERT, W., H. WECKE u. H. SÜTTERLE: Die Fettgewebsnekrose des Neugeborenen bei Diabetes mellitus der Mutter. Zbl. allg. Path. path. Anat. **107**, 499 (1965). — ORBANEJA, J. G., u. J. R. PUCHOL: Über die Systematik der kutanen nekrotisierenden Gefäßerkrankungen. Hautarzt **11**, 453 (1960).
PAUTRIER, L. M.: La Maladie de Besnier-Boeck-Schaumann. Paris: Masson & Cie. 1940. — PAUTRIER, L. M., et F. WORINGER: Contribution à l'étude histologique de l'érythème noueux. Bull. Soc. franç. Derm. Syph. **45**, 1068 (1938). — PFUHL, W.: Die Aufräumung zugrunde

gegangener Fettzellen durch Histiocyten im Trypanblauentzündungsherd. Arch. Anat. Entwickl.-Gesch. 110, 533 (1940). — PIAGGIO, W.: Heilbare Hautinduration der Neugeborenen. Zbl. Haut- u. Geschl.-Kr. 42, 360 (1932). — PICK, W.: Über die persistierende Form des Erythema nodosum. Arch. Derm. Syph. (Berl.) 72, 361 (1904). — PIROTH, M.: Zur Morphologie des Lipogranuloms. Zbl. allg. Path. path. Anat. 93, 293 (1955).
RAST, J. P.: Einige morphologische Merkmale der Fettgewebssklerose. Ihre Bedeutung bei der Fibrosis mammae. Presse méd. 1956, 139. — RATHERY, F., u. J. SIGWALD: Örtlich begrenzter Fettschwund durch Insulin. Bull. Soc. méd. Hôp. Paris 46, 951 (1930). — REES, H. A.: Sclerosing lipogranuloma. Arch. Derm. 89, 277 (1964). — REICH, H.: Zur Kenntnis der Radiärknötchen (Miescher) beim Erythema nodosum. Hautarzt 3, 503 (1952). — REICH, N. E.: Sclerema subcutanea neonatorum. Arch. Derm. Syph. (Chic.) 45, 342 (1942). — REYMANN, FL.: Necrosis adiposa neonatorum. Acta derm.-venereol. (Stockh.) 35, 220 (1955). — REYNAERS, H.: Panniculite nodulaire chronique. Arch. belges. Derm. 8, 78 (1952). — RINALDI, V. G.: Pannicolite nodulare cronica progressiva tipo Rothmann-Makai. Ann. ital. Derm. Sif. 10, 44 (1955). — RITTER, E.: Sclerosing lipogranuloma. Brit. J. Derm. 68, 419 (1956). — RÖCKL, H., u. W. THIES: Herdförmige, chronisch-recidivierende Krankheitszustände des subcutanen Fettgewebes. Hautarzt 8, 58 (1957). — ROTNES, P. L.: Untersuchungen über Erythema nodosum im erwachsenen Alter. Acta dermat.-venereol. (Stockh.) 17, 117 (1936).
SANDBERG, D. H., u. J. M. ADAMS: Erythema induratum und Streptokokkeninfektion. J. Pediat. 61, 880 (1962). — SANTLER, R.: Paraffinom. Zbl. Haut- u. Geschl.-Kr. 84, 242 (1953). — SAWICKY, H. H., and N. B. KANOFF: Sclerosing lipogranuloma. Arch. Derm. 73, 264 (1956). — SCHEFFLER, H.: Lokalisierte, allergische Hautreaktionen mit Pigmentablagerung nach Insulininjektion. Medizinische 1955, 1409, 1414. — SCHEFFLER, H., u. H. HAGEN: Allergische Hautreaktionen nach Insulin in Form der Necrobiosis lipoidica. Med. Klin. 1956, 2128. — SCHIRREN, C.: Necrobiosis lipoidica diabeticorum, Lipodystrophie. Derm. Wschr. 138, 1120 (1958). — SCHIRREN sen., C. G.: Ein ungewöhnlicher Fall von lokaler Insulin-Anaphylaxie. Hautarzt 4, 531 (1953). — SCHLIENGER, F.: Zur Kenntnis der medikamentösen Lipogranulome. Dermatologica (Basel) 98, 289 (1949). — SCHNITLER, K.: Über einen Fall von multiplen Lipogranulomen bei einem Säugling. Acta derm.-venereol. (Stockh.) 19, 395 (1938). — SCHOEDD, J.: Adiponecrosis subcutanea neonatorum. Mschr. Kinderheilk. 63, 241 (1935). — SCHULZE, W., u. E. KUNZE: Über die Lipodystrophie. Z. Haut- u. Geschl.-Kr. 22, 193 (1957). — SCHUPPLI, R.: Erythema nodosum. In: Handbuch der Haut- und Geschlechtskrankheiten von J. JADASSOHN, Erg.-Werk Bd. II/2, S. 78. Berlin-Göttingen-Heidelberg: Springer 1965. — SCRIBA, K.: Subkutane Fettgewebsnekrosen bei Neugeborenen. Zbl. allg. Path. path. Anat. 93, 460 (1955). — SHAFFER, B.: Liquefying nodular panniculitis. Arch. Derm. Syph. (Chic.) 38, 535 (1938). — SHAPOSHNIKOW, O. K.: Chronic erythema nodosum. Vestn. Derm. Vener. 36, 21 (1962). — SHATIN, H.: Relapsing febrile nodular nonsuppurative panniculitis (Weber-Christian disease). Arch. Derm. 83, 1053 (1961). — SIMPSON, K.: Sclerema neonatorum (adiposum). Guy's Hosp. Rep. 84, 307 (1934). — SINGH, G., P. K. SRIVASTAVA, and K. N. GOUR: Weber-Christian syndrome in a child. Indian J. Derm. Venereol. 31, 162 (1940). — SIWE, ST. A.: Zur Pathogenese der Adiposis subcutanea (Sklerodermia neonatorum). Acta path. microbiol. scand., Suppl. 16, 438 (1933). Ref. Zbl. Haut- u. Geschl.-Kr. 48, 298 (1934). — SMETANA, H., and W. BERNHARD: Sclerosing lipogranuloma. Arch. Path. 50, 296 (1950). — SPAIN, D. M., and J. M. FOLEY: Nonsuppurative panniculitis (Weber-Christian's disease). Amer. J. Path. 20, 783 (1944). — SPIER, H. W., u. H. RÖCKL: In: Fortschritte der praktischen Dermatologie, Bd. III, S. 98. Berlin-Göttingen-Heidelberg: Springer 1960. — STRANSKY, E.: Lipodystrophie um die und fernab von den Injektionsstellen nach Insulinbehandlung bei Diabetes mellitus. Wien. med. Wschr. 1930 I, 133. — STÜTTGEN, G.: Arteriitis und Gangrän der Haut. Hautarzt 7, 353 (1956).
TELFORD, E. D.: Lesions of the skin and subcutaneous tissue in diseases of the peripheral circulation. Arch. Derm. Syph. (Chic.) 36, 952 (1937). — TENDIS, N.: Panniculitis nodosa nonsuppurativa. Dtsch. Gesundh.-Wes. 17, 1478 (1962). — TILDEN, J. L., H. C. GOTSHALK, and E. V. AVAKIAN: Relapsing febrile nonsuppurative panniculitis. Arch. Derm. Syph. (Chic.) 41, 681 (1940).
UNGAR, H.: Relapsing febrile nodular inflammation of adipose tissue (Weber-Christian syndrome): report of a case with autopsy. J. Path. Bact. 58, 175 (1946). — URBACH, E.: Pilznachweis in einem Erythema nodosum trichophyticum. Zbl. Haut- u. Geschl.-Kr. 50, 552 (1935).
VANDEKERCKHOVE, M.: Erythema induratum Bazin, Hypodermitis nodularis chronica und Nodular-Vasculitis. Arch. belges Derm. 18, 193 (1962). — VESEY, C. M. L., and D. S. WILKINSON: Erythema nodosum. A study of seventy cases. Brit. J. Derm. 71, 139 (1959). — VILANOVA, X., u. J. PIÑOL AGUADÉ: Noduläre Aphthose, Aphthose en plaques und Pfeifer-Christian-Webersche Panniculitis. Hautarzt 9, 389 (1958). — VILANOVA, X., J. PIÑOL AGUADÉ u. J. M. MORAGAS: Vasculitis nodularis und Erythema induratum Bazin. Statistische und diagnostische Studie. Bull. Soc. franç. Derm. Syph. 65, 418 (1958).

Walther, H.: Beitrag zum Erythema nodosum mycoticum. Z. Haut- u. Geschl.-Kr. 19, 203 (1955). — Wighley, J. E. M., u. C. D. Calnan: Sklerosierendes Lipogranulom. Proc. 10th Internat. Congr. of Derm. London 1952, p. 465. — Wolf, M.: Weber-Christian disease: Nonfebrile, nonsuppurative, relapsing, nodular panniculitis. Arch. Derm. 86, 802 (1962). — Woodhouse-Price, L. R.: Lokalabsorption von Fett infolge von Insulininjektion. Lancet 1930 I, 1015. — Woringer, F.: Les granulomes à corps étrangers de la peau. Thèse de Strasbourgh 1929. — Woringer, F., et G. Weiner: Le cytostéatonécrose du tissu sous-cutanée chez le nouveau né. Rev. franç. Pédiat. 4, 57 (1928).

Zavarini, G.: Atypische chronische mikronoduläre Fettgewebsentzündung. Rass. Derm. Sif. 8, 245 (1955). — Zeek, P., and E. M. Madden: Sclerema adiposum neonatorum of both, internal and external adipose tissues. Arch. Path. 41, 166 (1946). — Zeitlhofer, J.: Über Fettgranulome der Brustdrüse. Langenbecks Arch. klin. Chir. 277, 385 (1953). — Zeumer, G.: Über die herdförmigen Entzündungen im subcutanen Fettgewebe unter besonderer Berücksichtigung der Panniculitisformen. Zbl. Chir. 85, 2003 (1960). — Zieler: Zit. nach F. Funk 1958. — Zierz, P.: Haut—Leber—Pankreas. In: Dermatologie und Venerologie von H. A. Gottron u. W. Schönfeld, Bd. III/2, S. 1016. Stuttgart: Georg Thieme 1959.

Patho-Histologie vorwiegend gefäßbedingter Erkrankungen des subcutanen Fettgewebes

Alkiewicz, J.: Die subkutanen Veränderungen bei einem Fall von Periarteriitis nodosa. Przegl. Derm. vener. 28, 630 (1933). — Appaix, A., A. Pech u. J. M. Codaccioni: Maligne Granulomatose nach Wegener. J. franç. Oto-rhino-laryng. 8, 737 (1959). — Arzt, L.: Zur Differentialdiagnose granulomatöser Prozesse (Granulomatosis disciformis chronica progressiva, Necrobiosis lipoidica diabeticorum, atypisches Tbc-Granulom). Hautarzt 3, 488 (1952). — Aufdermauer, M.: Die granulomatöse Riesenzell-Arteriitis. Schweiz. med. Wschr. 89, 843 (1959).

Balbi, E.: Untersuchungen über die Pathogenese der Necrobiosis lipoidica diabeticorum Urbach-Oppenheim. G. ital. Derm. 74, 14 (1953). Ref. Zbl. Haut- u. Geschl.-Kr. 45, 467 (1953). — Bock, H. E.: Allergische Erkrankung des Herzens und Gefäßsystems. In: K. Hansen, Allergie, S. 532. Stuttgart: Georg Thieme 1957. — Die hyperergischen Gefäßerkrankungen. In: Angiologie von M. Ratschow. Stuttgart: Georg Thieme 1959. — Boldt, A.: Zur Kenntnis der Necrobiosis lipoidica („diabeticorum"). Arch. Derm. Syph. (Berl.) 179, 74 (1939). — Necrobiosis lipoidica diabeticorum. Zbl. Haut- u. Geschl.-Kr. 62, 338, 613 (1939). — Beitrag zur Klinik und Ätiologie des Granuloma anulare. Arch. Derm. Syph. (Berl.) 179, 603 (1939). — Brandsma, C. H.: Arteriolitis allergica. Dermatologica (Basel) 97, 265 (1948). — Brandsma, C. H., A. W. M. Pompen u. H. J. Weyers: Granulomatöse Panvasculitiden mit anschließender kutan-subkutaner Lokalisierung. Dermatologica (Basel) 97, 257 (1948). — Brezhenko, A. I.: On lipoid necrobiosis. Vestn. Derm. Vener. 37, 17 (1963). Ref. Zbl. Haut- u. Geschl.-Kr. 114, 292 (1963).

Cardell, M. W., and E. H. Hanley: Fatal case of giantcell or temporal arteriitis. J. Path. Bact. 63, 587 (1951). — Cerutti, P.: Periarteriitis nodosa der Haut. Minerva derm. 36, 187 (1961). — Cerutti, P., u. G. Santoianni: Über die Polyarteriitis cutanea benigna. Hautarzt 8, 109 (1957). — Churg, J., and L. Strauss: Allergic granulomatosis, allergic angiitis and periarteriitis nodosa. Amer. J. Path. 27, 277 (1951). — Connor, W. H.: Necrobiosis lipoidica diabeticorum. Arch. Derm. 34, 705 (1936). — Csermely, E.: Beitrag zur Kenntnis der Periarteriitis nodosa cutanea. G. ital. Derm. 103, 327 (1962).

Degos, R.: Dyslipoidoses cutanées du type Oppenheim-Urbach. Sem. Hôp. Paris 25, 2137 (1949). — Dyslipoidoses cutanées du type Oppenheim-Urbach. Ann. Derm. Syph. (Paris) 78, 579 (1951). — Dimitrescu, A., u. L. Bălus: Necrobiosis lipoidica bei einer Zuckerkranken. Derm.-Vener. (Buc.) 1, 262 (1956). — Dorn, A.: Zur Einordnung der Granulomatosis disciformis chronica et progressiva Miescher. Inaug.-Diss. Frankfurt a. M. 1956. — Duperrat, B., et J. Monfort: Les allergides vasculaires hypodermiques. Ann. Derm. Syph. (Paris) 85, 385 (1958). — Les vascularites nodulaires dans le cadre des hypodermites subaigues des membres inférieures. Bull. franç. Derm. Syph. 65, 441 (1958).

Eberhartinger, Chr.: Das Problem des Erythema induratum Bazin. Arch. klin. exp. Derm. 217, 196 (1963). — Ehlers, G.: Vasculäres Mikrobid beim Kleinkind unter dem Bilde einer papulösen Arteriolitis allergica. Hautarzt 12, 111 (1961). — Über allergische Hautgefäßkrankheiten. Med. Welt 1965, 1720. — Engel, M. F., and W. J. Hammack: Necrobiosis lipoidica diabeticorum. A biochemical, histochemical and electrophoretic study. Arch. Derm. 78, 73 (1958). — Erbslöh, F.: Nosologische und klinische Besonderheiten der sog. Arteriitis temporalis. Verh. dtsch. Ges. inn. Med. 60, 702 (1954).

Ferreira-Marques, F.: Lipatrophia annularis. Ein Fall einer bisher nicht beschriebenen Krankheit der Haut (des Panniculus adiposus). Arch. Derm. Syph. (Berl.) 195, 479 (1953). — Fleck, F.: Zum Problem der Granulomatosis disciformis chronica et progressiva. Derm. Wschr. 127, 541 (1953). — Über kutane Dyslipoidosen, Steatonekrosen und verschiedene Einzelformen abnorm-regionaler Fettverteilung. Z. Haut- u. Geschl.-Kr. 24, 1 (1958). —

Forman, L.: Necrobiosis lipoidica diabeticorum of the scalp. Proc. roy. Soc. Med. 47, 658 (1954). — Frangenheim, H.: Zur Frage der Riesenzellarteriitis. Zbl. allg. Path. path. Anat. 88, 81 (1952).
Gans, O.: Diskussionsbeitrag. Zbl. Haut- u. Geschl.-Kr. 78, 408 (1952). — Gartmann, H.: Drei Fälle von Granulomatosis disciformis chronica et progressiva Miescher. Derm. Wschr. 128, 676 (1953). — Gartmann, H., u. W. Kiessling: Necrobiosis maculosa Miescher. Arch. klin. exp. Derm. 218, 21 (1963). — Gertler, W.: Necrobiosis maculosa. Derm. Wschr. 138, 823 (1958). — Necrobiosis maculosa bei Altersdiabetes. Derm. Wschr. 139, 276 (1959). — Götz, H.: Zur Frage der Beziehungen zwischen der Granulomatosis disciformis chronica et progressiva (Miescher) und der Necrobiosis lipoidica diabeticorum. Hautarzt 7, 156 (1956). — Goldsmith, W. N.: Granuloma of ears (chronic). Proc. X. Internat. Congr. Derm., London 1952, p. 239. — Morphoea or tuberculosis cutis? Proc. roy. Soc. Med. 21, 1768 (1928). — Goldstein, E., and J. Harris: Xanthoma diabeticorum; unusual process of involution. Amer. J. med. Sci. 173, 195 (1927). — Gottron, H. A.: Erythema induratum Bazin und Sarkoid Darier-Roussy. Arch. Derm. Syph. (Berl.) 172, 143 (1935). — Krankheitszustände des subcutanen Fettgewebes. Medizinische 1952, 912. — Lipogranulomatosis subcutanea hypertonica. Derm. Wschr. 144, 1112 (1961). — Granuloma anulare. In: Dermatologie und Venerologie von H. A. Gottron u. W. Schönfeld, Bd. V/1, S. 241. Stuttgart: Georg Thieme 1963. — Grimmer, H.: Necrobiosis lipoidica (sine diabete). Z. Haut- u. Geschl.-Kr. 37, 1 (1964). — Gross, P., and G. F. Machaceck: Necrobiosis lipoidica diabeticorum. Arch. Derm. 32, 491 (1935). — Grots, J. A., J. S. Strauss, and H. Mescon: Necrobiosis lipoidica diabeticorum of the abdomen. Arch. Derm. 83, 505 (1961). — Gougerot, H., et B. Duperrat: Allergides nodulaires dermiques de H. Gougerot. Brit. J. Derm. 66, 283 (1954).
Hamperl, A.: Elastische Fasern als Fremdkörper. Bemerkungen zur sog. Arteriitis temporalis. Virchows Arch. path. Anat. 323, 591 (1959). — Hare, P. J.: Necrobiosis lipoidica. Brit. J. Derm. 67, 365 (1955). — Harrison, C. V.: Giant cell or temporal arteriitis, a review. J. clin. Path. 1, 197 (1948). — Heilesen, B.: Necrobiosis lipoidica diabeticorum — diabetes mellitus. Acta derm.-venereol. (Stockh.) 36, 234 (1956). — Hjorth, N.: Necrobiosis lipoidica. Granulomatosis disciformis chronica et progressiva Miescher. Acta derm.-venereol. (Stockh.) 39, 140 (1959).
Ingram, J. T.: Allergic vasculitis. Proc. 11. Internat. Congr. Derm. Stockh. 1957, vol. 2, 170 (1960).
Jablonska, S.: Hyperergische Gefäßkrankheiten in der Dermatologie. Z. Haut- u. Geschl.-Kr. 33, 37 (1962). — Jones, D. B.: Zit. nach P. J. Hare 1955.
Kaldor, I., u. L. Nekam: Immunologische Veränderungen bei Necrobiosis lipoidica. Ann. Derm. Syph. (Paris) 91, 147 (1964). — Kazmeier, F.: Symptomatologie und Differentialdiagnose der Periarteriitis nodosa. Med. Welt 1951, 774. — Keining, E., u. O. Braun-Falco: Zur Aetiologie der Granulomatosis disciformis chronica et progressiva (Miescher). Derm. Wschr. 131, 1 (1955). — Kétron, L. W., and J. C. Bernstein: Cutaneous manifestations of periarteriitis nodosa. Arch. Derm. Syph. (Chic.) 40, 929 (1939). — Knoth, W.: Die Begutachtung eines Granulomatosis disciformis chronica et progressiva-Kranken mit abgeheilter Tuberculosis cutis fistulosa. Berufsdermatosen 7, 136 (1959). — Knoth, W., G. Beneke u. E. Kuntz: Zur Kenntnis der Wegenerschen Granulomatose. Hautarzt 16, 289 (1965). — Knoth, W., u. H. Füller: Zur Patho- und Histogenese der Necrobiosis lipoidica „diabeticorum". Arch. Derm. Syph. (Berl.) 199, 109 (1955). — Knoth, W. ,u. W. Meyhöfer: Beitrag zum Formenkreis der Periarteriitis nodosa und zur Bewertung der Riesenzellen bei Gefäßerkrankungen. Dermatologica (Basel) 119, 1 (1959). — Kogoj, F., u. St. Puretić: Zur Frage der Granulomatosis disciformis chronica et progressiva Miescher. Hautarzt 4, 305 (1953). — Korting, G. W.: Über cutane Periarteriitis nodosa unter besonderer Berücksichtigung begleitender Leberstörungen und der sog. Thrombophlebitis migrans. Arch. Derm. Syph. (Berl.) 199, 332 (1955). — Korting, G. W., u. F. Nürnberger: Necrosis lipoidica. Arch. klin. exp. Derm. 225, 113 (1966). — Krahulik, L., M. Rosenthal, and E. H. Loughlin: Periarteriitis nodosa in childhood with meningeal involvement. Report of a case with study of pathologic findings. Amer. J. med. Sci. 190, 308 (1935). — Kulaga, U. v.: Cutaneous form periarteriitis nodosa. Vestn. Derm. Vener. 38, 45 (1964). Ref. Zbl. Haut- u. Geschl.-Kr. 117, 205 (1964). — Kuntz, E., G. Beneke u. W. Knoth: Die Wegenersche Granulomatose. Med. Welt 18, 295 (1967).
Langhof, H.: Lipogranulomatosis subcutanea partim exulcerans hypertonica Gottron. Zbl. Haut- u. Geschl.-Kr. 104, 348 (1959). — Leczinsky, C. G.: Nodular vasculitis; clinical and histological studies, based on some 400 cases. Proc. 11. Internat. Congr. Derm. Stockh. 1957, vol. 2, p. 185 (1960). — Leifer, W.: Zit. nach P. J. Hare 1955. — Leslie, G.: Zit. nach P. J. Hare 1955. — Letterer, E.: Morphische Manifestationen allergisch-hyperergischer Vorgänge im Verlaufe von Infektionskrankheiten. Acta allerg. (Kbh.), Suppl. 3, 6, 79 (1953). — Linser, K.: Granulomatosis tuberculoides pseudo-sclerodermiformis symmetrica chronica. Zbl. Haut- u. Geschl.-Kr. 88, 193 (1954).

MACAIGNE, N., et P. NICAUD: Les lésions de la périartérite noueuse à forme chronique. Ann. Anat. path. **11**, 235 (1934). — MALI, J. W. H.: Granulomatosis disciformis chronica et progressiva. A form of tuberculosis? Dermatologica (Basel) **101**, 84 (1950). — MATRAS, A.: Hyperergische Panvasculitis unter dem Bilde der multiplen symmetrischen Haut- und Knochengangrän. Arch. klin. exp. Derm. **207**, 521 (1958). — MCCOMBS, R. P.: Die klinische Unterscheidung zwischen der allergischen Gefäßentzündung und der Periarteriitis nodosa. Int. Arch. Allergy **12**, 98 (1958). — MCCORMAC, H.: Case for diagnosis. Proc. roy. Soc. Med. **15**, 7 (1921). Zit. nach P. J. HARE 1955. — MICHELSON, H. E.: Inflammatory nodose lesions of lower leg. Arch. Derm. **66**, 327 (1952). — MIESCHER, G.: Über kutane Formen der Periarteriitis nodosa. Dermatologica (Basel) **92**, 225 (1946). — Necrobiosis maculosa. Dermatologica (Basel) **98**, 199 (1949). — Akut-entzündliche Gefäßkrankheiten und deren Auswirkung auf die Haut. Arch. klin. exp. Derm. **206**, 135 (1957). — MIESCHER, G., u. W. BURCKHARDT: Zit. nach W. KNOTH 1959. — MIESCHER, G., u. M. LEDER: Granulomatosis disciformis chronica et progressiva (atypische Tuberkulose). Dermatologica (Basel) **97**, 25 (1948). — Granulomatosis disciformis chronica et progressiva. Schweiz. med. Wschr. **1948**, 1182. — MONTGOMERY, H., P. A. O'LEARY, and N. W. BARKER: Nodular vascular diseases of the legs: erythema induratum and allied conditions. J. Amer. med. Ass. **128**, 335 (1945). — MOSKOWITZ, R. W., A. H. BAGGENSTOSS, and C. H. SLOCUMB: Histopathologic classification of periarteriitis nodosa. A study of 56 cases confirmed at necropsy. Proc. Mayo Clin. **38**, 345 (1963). — MULLER, S. A., and R. K. WINKELMANN: Necrobiosis lipoidica diabeticorum. Arch. Derm. **93**, 272 (1966).

OPPENHEIM, M.: Über eine bisher nicht beschriebene, mit eigentümlicher lipoider Degeneration der Elastica und des Bindegewebes einhergehende chronische Dermatose bei Diabetes mellitus. Arch. Derm. Syph. (Berl.) **166**, 576 (1932). — ORBANEJA, J. G., u. J. R. PUCHOL: Über die Systematik der kutanen nekrotisierenden Gefäßerkrankungen. Hautarzt **11**, 453 (1960).

PEZZAROSSA, G.: Über die Necrobiosis lipoidica und deren Zusammenhänge mit dem Granuloma anulare. G. ital. Derm. **98**, 129 (1957). — PORTWICH, F.: Periarteriitis nodosa. Ergebn. inn. Med. Kinderheilk. **12**, 428 (1959). — PUCHOL, J. R.: Ein Fall von Necrobiosis lipoidica diabeticorum. Acta dermo-sifiliogr. (Madr.) **46**, 587 (1955).

RANDERATH, E.: Die Bedeutung der allergischen Pathogenese bei der Arteriitis. Verh. dtsch. Ges. inn. Med. **60**, 359 (1954). — REICH, H.: Die pseudosklerodermiforme tuberkuloide Granulomatose der Schienbeingegend. Derm. Wschr. **138**, 900 (1938). — Cuto-lympho-viscerale Granulomatose. Arch. klin. exp. Derm. **213**, 479 (1961). — REIN, G.: Über Riesenzellarteriitis, besonders der Aorta. Z. Kreisl.-Forsch. **44**, 393 (1955). — RINGROSE, E. J.: Smoking, necrobiosis lipoidica, granulomatosis disciformis chronica et progressiva. Arch. Derm. **79**, 635 (1959). — ROEDERER, J., F. WORINGER u. R. BURGUN: Betrachtungen über einen Fall von Necrobiosis lipoidica. Dermatologica (Basel) **99**, 131 (1949). — RUITER, M.: Allergic cutaneous vasculitis. Acta derm.-venereol. (Stockh.) **32**, 274 (1952). — Über die sogenannte Arteriolitis (Vasculitis) allergica cutis. Hautarzt **8**, 293 (1957). — Die sog. cutane Form der Periarteriitis nodosa. Brit. J. Derm. **70**, 102 (1958).

SANNICANDRO, F.: Noduläre, granulomatöse Riesenzellen-Arteriitis der Haut, vergesellschaftet mit Akrosklroedem. Dermatologica (Basel) **127**, 467 (1963). — SANTLER, R.: Zwei Fälle von Granulomatosis disciformis chronica et progressiva (Miescher). Hautarzt **5**, 14 (1954). — SCHNEIDER, W., u. W. UNDEUTSCH: Vasculitiden des subcutanen Fettgewebes. Arch. klin. exp. Derm. **221**, 600 (1965). — SCHUERMANN, H.: Necrobiosis lipoidica diabeticorum ohne Diabetes. Zbl. Haut- u. Geschl.-Kr. **59**, 250 (1938). — Necrobiosis lipoidica (diabeticorum) bei latentem Diabetes und Hypertonie. Zbl. Haut- u. Geschl.-Kr. **62**, 339 (1939). — SCHÜRMANN, P., u. H. E. MCMAHON: Die maligne Nephrosklerose, zugleich ein Beitrag zur Frage der Blutgewebsschranke. Virchows Arch. path. Anat. **291**, 47 (1933). — SMITH, J. G.: Necrobiosis lipoidica. A disease of changing concept. Arch. Derm. **74**, 280 (1956). — SPIER, H. W.: Allergie der Haut. In: Dermatologie und Venerologie von H. A. GOTTRON u. W. SCHÖNFELD, Bd. I/1, S. 613, 678. Stuttgart: Georg Thieme 1961. — SPRAFKE, H.: Beitrag zur Frage der Diabetes-Bedingtheit der Necrobiosis lipoidica diabeticorum. Derm. Wschr. **112**, 185 (1941). — STEIGLEDER, G. K.: Diskussionsbemerkung zum Vortrag J. J. HERZBERG, 23. Tagg Dtsch. Derm. Ges. Wien 1956. Arch. klin. exp. Derm. **206**, 204 (1957). — Allgemeine Pathologie der Haut. In: Dermatologie und Venerologie von H. A. GOTTRON u. W. SCHÖNFELD, Bd. I/1, S. 295, 311. Stuttgart: Georg Thieme 1961. — STORCK, H.: Über haemorrhagische Phänomene in der Dermatologie. Dermatologica (Basel) **102**, 197 (1951). — STOWERS, J. H.: Case for diagnosis. Proc. roy. Soc. Med. **15**, 7 (1921). — SZODORAY, L., u. K. N. VEZEKÉNY: Über die an Unterschenkeln junger Frauen auftretende Periarteriitis nodosa cutanea seu vasculitis nodularis. Hautarzt **10**, 263 (1959).

TAPPEINER, J., u. P. WODNIANSKY: Hauterkrankungen durch Einlagerung körpereigener Stoffe. In: Dermatologie und Venerologie von H. A. GOTTRON u. W. SCHÖNFELD, Bd. III/2, S. 1148. Stuttgart: Georg Thieme 1959. — Necrobiosis maculosa. (Ihre Beziehungen zu verwandten granulomatösen Erkrankungen.) Derm. Wschr. 146, 569 (1962). — TAPPEINER, S.: Zur Klinik und Histologie der Granulomatosis disciformis chronica et progressiva (Miescher). Arch. Derm. Syph. (Berl.) 194, 341 (1952). — TEILUM: Zit. nach ORBANEJA u. PUCHOL 1960. — TELFORD, E. D.: Veränderungen der Haut und Subcutis bei Krankheiten des peripheren Kreislaufs. Arch. Derm. 36, 952 (1937). — TORO-GENKEL, L.: Vasculitis nodular. Rev. méd. chile 87, 870 (1959). — TRAUB, E. F.: Zit. nach P. J. HARE 1955.

URBACH, E.: Beiträge zu einer physiologischen und pathologischen Chemie der Haut. X. Eine neue diabetische Stoffwechseldermatose. Necrobiosis lipoidica diabeticorum. Arch. Derm. Syph. (Berl.) 166, 273 (1932).

VERO, F.: Zit. nach P. J. HARE 1955. — VOLK, R.: Tuberkulose der Haut. In: Handbuch der Haut- und Geschlechtskrankheiten von J. JADASSOHN, Bd. X/1. Berlin: Springer 1931.

WALTHER, D.: Diskussionsbemerkung zum Vortrag J. J. HERZBERG, 23. Tagg Dtsch. Derm. Ges. Wien 1956. Arch. klin. exp. Derm. 206, 204 (1957). — WINER, L. H.: Histopathologie knotiger Veränderungen. Arch. Derm. 63, 347 (1951). — WISE, F.: Zit. nach P. J. HARE 1955. — WOODBURNE, PHILPOTT, VILANOVA u. GRAFLIN: Zit. nach F. FLECK 1958. — WORINGER, F.: Zit. nach P. J. HARE 1955. — WORINGER, FR., u. J. P. WEILL: Vergleich zwischen einer frischen und einer lang bestehenden Läsion bei Necrobiosis lipoidica diabeticorum. Bull. Soc. franç. Derm. Syph. 66, 226 (1959).

Tumoren des subcutanen Fettgewebes

AHERNE, W., and D. HULL: The site of heat production in the newborn infant. Proc. roy. Soc. Med. 57, 1172 (1964). — ARONSON, ST. A., C. V. TEODORU, M. ADLER u. G. SCHWARTZMAN: Der Einfluß von Cortison auf das braune Fettgewebe von Hamstern und Mäusen. Proc. Soc. exp. Biol. (N.Y.) 85, 115 (1954).

BALBONI, G.: Die Ultrastruktur der Fettzelle. Arch. ital. Anat. Embriol. 68, 67 (1963). — BALL, E. G., and R. L. JUNGAS: On the action of hormones which accelerate the rate of oxygen consumption and fatty acid release in rat adipose tissue in vitro. Proc. nat. Acad. Sci. (Wash.) 47, 932 (1961). — BLATTGERSTE, H.: Über einen Fall von lipoblastischem Sarkom. Zbl. Chir. 80, 1797 (1955). — BOERNER-PATZELT, D.: Das braune Fettgewebe der sog. Winterschlafdrüse des Igels. Z. mikr.-anat. Forsch. 63, 5 (1957). — BOYD: Zit. nach W. MÖBIUS. — BRINES, O. A., and M. H. JOHNSON: Hibernoma, a special fatty tumor. Report of a case. Amer. J. Path. 25, 467 (1949). — BROCQ, L.: Zit. nach E. HOFFMANN u. E. ZURHELLE. — BRUNCK, J.: Über einen metastasierenden, aber klinisch gutartig verlaufenden Naevus mit blasig entarteten Naevuszellen und deren Genese. Arch. Derm. Syph. (Berl.) 196, 170 (1953).

CALLAHAN, u. CAMPBELL: Zit. nach G. K. STEIGLEDER. — COX, R.W.: Hibernom, das Lipom des unreifen Fettgewebes. J. Path. 68, 511 (1954). — CRAMER, H. J.: Zur nosologischen Stellung des Naevus lipomatodes cutaneus superficialis (HOFFMANN-ZURHELLE). Derm. Wschr. 142, 1218 (1960).

DAWKINS, M. J. R., and D. HULL: Brown fat and the response of the new-born rabbit to cold. J. Physiol. (Lond.) 169, 101 (1963). — Brown adipose tissue and the response of new born rabbits to cold. J. Physiol. (Lond.) 172, 216 (1964). — DAWKINS, M. J. R., and J. SCOPES: Non-shivering thermogenesis and brown adipose tissue in the human newborn infant. Nature (Lond.) 206, 201 (1965).

ENTERLINE, H. T., J. D. CULBERSON, D. B. ROCHLIN, and L. W. BRADY: Liposarkoma, a clinical and pathological study of 53 cases. Cancer (Philad.) 13, 932 (1960).

FEYRTER, F.: Über den Naevus. Virchows Arch. path. Anat. 301, 417 (1938). — Blasige Umwandlung Meissnerscher Tastkörperchen der Zunge. Zugleich ein Beitrag zur Naevusfrage. Virchows Arch. path. Anat. 301, 470 (1938).

GARTMANN, H.: Über blasige Zellen im Naevus-Zellnaevus. Z. Haut- u. Geschl.-Kr. 28, 148 (1960). — GENESI, M.: Ibernoma (lipoblastoma bruno adenomorfo). Tumori 41, 430 (1955). — GERY: Zit. nach O. GANS u. G. K. STEIGLEDER 1957. — GIESEKING, R.: Der Stoffwechsel des braunen Fettgewebes im elektronenmikroskopischen Bild. Beitr. path. Anat. 125, 457 (1961). — Mesenchymales Gewebe und ihre Reaktionsformen im elektronenoptischen Bild. Stuttgart: Gustav Fischer 1966. — GLOGGENGIESSER: Zit. nach O. GANS u. G. K. STEIGLEDER 1957. — GOTTRON, H. A.: Retikulosen der Haut. In: Dermatologie und Venerologie von H. A. GOTTRON u. W. SCHÖNFELD, Bd. IV, S. 501. Stuttgart: Georg Thieme 1960. — GOTTRON, H. A., u. W. NIKOLOWSKI: Bösartige Neubildungen. In: Dermatologie und Venerologie von H. A. GOTTRON u. W. SCHÖNFELD, Bd. V, S. 488. Stuttgart: Georg Thieme 1960. — GRIMAUD, R., et A. BEAU: Un nouveau cas de lipome de la langue. J. franç. Oto-rhino-laryng. 5, 118 (1958). — GROSS, S., and C. WOOD: Hibernoma. Cancer (N.Y.) 6, 159 (1953).

HEGLER, C., u. FR. WOHLWILL: Fettgewebsnekrosen in Subcutis und Knochenmark durch Metastasen eines Carcinoms des Pankreasschwanzes. Virchows Arch. path. Anat. 274, 784 (1930). — HELD, D., u. R. DELLA SANTA: Multiple Fettgewebsverhärtung, hervorgerufen durch Thrombose der venösen Capillaren des Fettgewebes. Dermatologica (Basel) 120, 145

(1960). — HELMAN, B., u. C. HELLERSTRÖM: Zellerneuerung im weißen und braunen Fettgewebe der Ratte. Acta path. microbiol. scand. 51, 347 (1961). — HERING, H.: Kasuistischer Beitrag zum Naevus lipomatosus cutaneus superficialis (HOFFMANN-ZURHELLE). Z. Haut- u. Geschl.-Kr. 21, 123 (1956). — HERRMANN, L.: Einige bemerkenswerte Befunde bei Lipomen. Z. ärztl. Fortbild. 55, 1396 (1961). — HERZOG, GG.: Über adventitielle Zellen und über die Entstehung von granulierten Elementen. Verh. dtsch. Ges. Path. 25, 562 (1914). — Referat über die Bedeutung der Gewebezüchtung für die Pathologie. Verh. dtsch. Ges. Path. 52, 9 (1931). — Über die Bedeutung der Gefäßwandzellen in der Pathologie. Klin. Wschr. 1923, 684, 730. — Experimentelle Zoologie und Pathologie. Ergebn. allg. Path. path. Anat. 21, 182 (1925). — HOFFMANN, E., u. E. ZURHELLE: Über einen Naevus lipomatodes cutaneus superficialis der linken Glutäalgegend. Arch. Derm. Syph. (Berl.) 130, 327 (1921). — HOLTZ, K. H.: Beitrag zur Histologie des Naevus lipomatodes cutaneus superficialis (HOFFMANN-ZURHELLE). Arch. Derm. Syph. (Berl.) 199, 275 (1955). — HORNSTEIN, O.: Histologischer Beitrag zur Pathogenese subcutaner Lipome. Arch. klin. exp. Derm. 204, 397 (1957). — HUGER, TITONE, HEGLER u. BERNER: Zit. nach S. H. JACKSON, R. S. SAVIDGE, L. STEIN u. H. VARLEY 1952. — HULL, D., and M. M. SEGALL: The effects of sympathetic denervation and stimulation on brown adipose tissue in the new born rabbit. J. Physiol. (Lond.) 177, 63 (1964). — The effect of removing brown adipose tissue on heat production in the newborn rabbit. J. Physiol. (Lond.) 175, 58 (1964).

JACKSON, S. H., R. S. SAVIDGE, L. STEIN u. H. VARLEY: Pancreascarcinom in Verbindung mit Fettnekrosen. Lancet 1952 II, 962. — JOEL, C. D., and E. G. BALL: Electron transmitter system in adipose tissue. Fed. Proc. 19, 32 (1960).

KAUFFMANN, S. L., and A. P. STOUT: Lipoblastic tumors in children. Cancer (Philad.) 12, 912 (1959). — KEIL, W.: Multiple recidivierende Lipome mit lokaler sarkomatöser Entartung. Virchows Arch. path. Anat. 315, 207 (1948). — KENIN, A., J. LEVINE, and M. SPINNER: Paraostal lipoma. J. Bone Jt Surg. Ed. Vol. A 41, 1122. — KNOTH, W.: Die diagnostische Bedeutung des Gitterfasernachweises bei Dermatosen. Arch. klin. exp. Derm. 206, 744 (1956). — Klinische und histopathologische Probleme bei der Reticulosarkomatosis cutis. Verh. dtsch. Ges. Path. 41, 403 (1958). — Erkrankungen des reticulohistiocytären Systems der Haut. Habil.-Schrift Gießen 1958. — Über Naevus lipomatosus cutaneus superficialis Hoffmann-Zurhelle und über Naevus naevocellularis partim lipomatodes. Dermatologica (Basel) 125, 161 (1962). — Zur Histotopographie der Reticulosen, Reticulosarkomatosen und Granulomatosen. Arch. klin. exp. Derm. 219, 138 (1963). — KNOTH, W., u. S. BETTGE: Über besondere Veränderungen der Hautgefäße bei lymphatischer und myeloischer Leukämie. Derm. Wschr. 137, 561 (1958). — KUSKE, H., J. M. PASCHOUD u. W. SOLTERMANN: Lipomatosis der Zunge. Dermatologica (Basel) 114, 305 (1957). — KÚTA, A.: Naevus lipomatosus superficialis seu subepidermalis. Dermatologica (Basel) 103, 42 (1951).

LANGER, H., u. H. LANGER-SCHIERER: Zum chemischen Aufbau des braunen Fettgewebes von Wanderratten und europäischen Hamster. Hoppe-Seylers Z. physiol. Chem. 314, 50 (1959). — LENNERT, K.: Über ein lipoblastisches Sarkom des Mediastinums, zugleich ein Beitrag zur Kenntnis der bösartigen Fettgewebsgeschwülste. Frankfurt. Z. Path. 61, 78 (1949). — LEVER, J. D.: Die Feinstruktur des braunen Fettgewebes der Ratte mit Beobachtungen über die cytologischen Veränderungen nach Hunger und Adrenalektomie. Anat. Rec. 128, 361 (1957).

MADELUNG: Zit. nach O. GANS u. G. K. STEIGLEDER 1957. — MARCHAND, F.: Über die Herkunft der Lymphocyten und ihre Schicksale bei der Entzündung. Verh. dtsch. Ges. Path. 24, 5 (1913). Zit. nach O. GANS u. G. K. STEIGLEDER 1957. — MATHIS, H.: Die gutartigen Gewächse der Mundhöhle. Zahnärztl. Fortbild. 1953, 10. — MAXIMOW, A.: Experimentelle Untersuchungen über entzündliche Neubildung von Bindegewebe. Beitr. path. Anat., Suppl. 5, 1 (1902). — Über die Zellformen des lockeren Bindegewebes. Arch. mikr. Anat. 67, 680 (1906). — Über undifferenzierte Blutzellen und mesenchymale Keimlager im erwachsenen Organismus. Klin. Wschr. 5, 2193 (1926). — Bindegewebe und blutbildende Gewebe. In: Handbuch der mikroskopischen Anatomie des Menschen, Bd. II/1 von W. v. MÖLLENDORFF. Berlin: Springer 1927. — Über die Histogenese der entzündlichen Reaktion mit Nachprüfung der v. Möllendorffschen Trypanblauversuche. Beitr. path. Anat. 82, 1 (1929). — MELICOW, M. M.: Braunes Fettgewebe und Phäochromocytom. Arch. Path. 63, 367 (1957). — MENSCHIK, Z.: Histochemischer Vergleich vom braunen und weißem Fettgewebe. Anat. Rec. 116, 439 (1953). — MERKEL: Zit. nach O. GANS u. G. K. STEIGLEDER 1957. — MÖBIUS, W.: Über Lipome im Mundhöhlenbereich. Zahnärztl. Welt 61, 267 (1960). — MÜLLER, W.: Multiple zirkumskripte Lipome. Derm. Wschr. 151, 1406 (1965).

NAPOLITANO, L.: Die Differenzierung der weißen Fettzellen. J. Cell Biol. 18, 663 (1963). — NAPOLITANO, L., u. D. FAWCETT: Die Feinstruktur des braunen Fettgewebes bei neugeborenen Mäusen und Ratten. J. biophys. biochem. Cytol. 4, 685 (1958). — NIKOLOWSKI, W.: Über den Naevus lipomatodes cutaneus superficialis (HOFFMANN-ZURHELLE). Derm. Wschr. 122, 735 (1950). — NÖDL, F.: Gutartige Tumoren der Haut. In: Dermatologie und Venerologie von

H. A. GOTTRON u. W. SCHÖNFELD, Bd. IV, S. 214, 218, 221. Stuttgart: Georg Thieme 1960. — NOVY, F. G., and J. W. WILSON: Hibernomas, brown fat tumors. Arch. Derm. **73**, 149 (1956). — OSBORNE, R. R.: Acinöses Carcinom des Pankreas mit Funktion, begleitet von verbreiterten, herdförmigen Fettgewebsnekrosen. Arch. intern. Med. **85**, 933 (1950). — PAUTRIER, L. M., u. FR. WORINGER: Zit. nach W. KNOTH 1962. — PLENERT, W.: Der Baker-Test bei der Untersuchung des subcutanen Fettgewebes im Kindesalter. Acta histochem. (Jena) **8**, 311 (1959). — PÖHL, A.: Zur Pathologie des braunen Fettgewebes im Säuglingsalter. Öst. Z. Kinderheilk. **11**, 12 (1955). — POWER, D. A.: A parostal lipoma. Transact. path. Soc. Lond. **39**, 270 (1888). — PUTZMANN, G.: Über ein braunes Lipom. Zbl. allg. Path. path. Anat. **96**, 25 (1957).

REHN, E.: Die Fetttransplantation. Langenbecks Arch. klin. Chir. **98**, 1 (1912). — RÉMILLARD, G. L.: Histochemie und mikrochemische Beobachtungen über die Lipide des interscapularen Fettgewebes weiblicher Fledermäuse. Ann. N.Y. Acad. Sci. **72**, 1 (1958). — RIST, M.: Zit. nach E. HOFFMANN u. E. ZURHELLE. — ROBINSON, H. M., and F. A. ELLIS: Naevus lipomatosus subepidermalis seu superficialis cutis. Arch. Derm. **35**, 485 (1937). — ROSER: Zit. nach O. GANS u. G. K. STEIGLEDER 1957.

SCARPELLI, D. G., and M. H. GREIDER: A correlative cytochemical and electron microscopic study of liposarcoma. Cancer (Philad.) **15**, 776 (1962). — SHANKS, J. A., W. PARANCHYCH, and J. TUBA: Familial multiple lipomatosis. Canad. med. Ass. **77**, 881 (1957). — SIDMAN, R. L.: Histogenese des braunen Fettgewebes in vivo und in der Gewebekultur. Anat. Rec. **124**, 581 (1956). — SIDMAN, R. L., u. D. W. FAWCETT: Der Effekt der Durchschneidung peripherer Nerven auf einige Stoffwechselvorgänge im braunen Fettgewebe der Maus. Anat. Rec. **118**, 487 (1954). — STEIGLEDER, G. K.: Neoplastisch wuchernde Zellen der Cutis und Subcutis. In: Handbuch der Haut- und Geschlechtskrankheiten von J. JADASSOHN, Erg.-Werk Bd. I/2, S. 724. Berlin-Göttingen-Heidelberg: Springer 1964. — STERNBERG, S. S.: Liposarcoma arising within a subcutaneous lipoma. Cancer (Philad.) **5**, 975 (1952). — STOUT, A. P.: Liposarcoma — the malignant tumor of lipoblasts. Ann. Surg. **119**, 86 (1944). — SUTHERLAND, J. C., W. P. CALAHAN, and G. L. CAMPBELL: Hibernoma, a tumor of brown fat. Cancer (Philad.) **5**, 364 (1952). — SZYMANSKI, F. J., and S. M. BLUEFARB: Nodular fat necrosis and pancreatic diseases. Arch. Derm. **83**, 224 (1961).

TEDESCH, C. G.: Systemic multicentric lipoblastosis. Arch. Path. **42**, 320 (1946). — THÖNE, A. W.: Ein Fall von Naevus lipomatodes. Hautarzt **2**, 512 (1951). — TOYAMA, I., u. T. NAGASHIMA: Über die subkutanen Fettgewebsnekrosen, insbesondere bei Systemerkrankung des hämatopoetischen Apparates. Jap. J. Derm. **32**, 485 (1932). Ref. Zbl. Haut- u. Geschl.-Kr. **43**, 46 (1933). — TRUBOWITZ, S., and CH. F. SIMS: Subcutaneous fat in leukemia and lymphoma. Arch. Derm. **86**, 520 (1962).

VALENTINO, A.: Ein einzigartiger Fall von multiplen, subcutanen Fettgewebsnekrosen. Arch. ital. Chir. **76**, 49 (1963).

WALLER, J. I.: Liposarcoma of the scrotum. J. Urol. (Baltimore) **87**, 139 (1962).

Experimentelle Pathologie des Fettgewebes

ABRIKOSSOFF, A.: Über die spontan auftretenden Fettgewebsnekrosen und Fettgranulome. Zbl. allg. Path. path. Anat. **38**, 542 (1926). — ANSELMINO, K. J., u. F. HOFFMANN: Über das Fettstoffwechselhormon des Hypophysenvorderlappens (Lipotropin) und seine Bedeutung für die Fettumsetzung unter physiologischen und pathologischen Bedingungen. Dtsch. med. Wschr. **90**, 1697 (1965). — ARIMORI, M., T. HAMAMATSU, and S. KUROKOWA: The effect of injected fatty acids on the skin of patients with various dermatoses and with leprosy. Proc. R. internat. Congr. Derm. **2**, 1257 (1962). — ARONSON, ST. A., C. V. TEODORU, M. ADLER u. G. SCHWARTZMAN: Der Einfluß von Cortison auf das braune Fettgewebe von Hamstern und Mäusen. Proc. Soc. exp. Biol. (N.Y.) **85**, 214 (1954).

BERKOWITZ, D.: Metabolic changes associated with obesety before and after weight reduction. J. Amer. med. Ass. **187**, 399 (1964). — BERNER u. HEYDE: Zit. nach H. HERING u. W. UNDEUTSCH 1956. — BIRK, Y., and C. H. LI: Isolation and properties of a new, biologically active peptide from sheep pituitary glands. J. biol. Chem. **239**, 1048 (1964). — BLAKE, H. A., E. M. GOYETTE, C. S. LYTER, and H. SWAN: Subcutaneous fat necrosis complicating hypothermia. J. Pediat. **46**, 78 (1955).

CAMERON, G. R., u. K. C. B. MALLIK: Ausheilung im Fettgewebe nach lokaler Erfrierung. J. Path. **68**, 525 (1954). — CAMERON, G. R., u. R. D. SENEVIVATNE: Wachstum und Wiederherstellung von Fettgewebe. J. Path. **59**, 665 (1947). — CAMPBELL, J. A. A.: Subcutane Fettgewebsnekrosen, Hämolyse ohne Siderose und Tubulusatrophie der Niere nach wiederholten Glyzerolinjektionen. J. Path. Bact. **76**, 473 (1958). — CRACIUN, E. C., et J. FAGARASANO: Sur le lipogranulome bénin sous cutané par diathermie, traumatisme ou injections médicamenteuses. Ann. Anat. path. **12**, 1909 (1935).

D'AVANZO, A.: Untersuchungen über die Veränderung des Stoffwechsels der lokalen Temperatur der Gewebe. Die Fermente der Haut unter dem Einfluß lokaler Erwärmung.

Riv. Pat. sper. **4**, 301 (1929). — DEMURA, K., u. T. UCHIDA: Über die Respiration des subcutanen Fettgewebes. Jap. J. Derm. **71**, 724 (1961). — DOLE, V. P.: Relation between nonesterified fatty acids in plasma and metabolism of glucose. J. clin. Invest. **35**, 150 (1956).
EISENSCHMID, J. H., u. J. L. ORBISON: Experimentelle Erzeugung peritonealer Lipogranulome bei der Ratte. Arch. Path. **66**, 154 (1958).
FRIESEN, H.: Pituitary peptides and fat mobilization. Metabolism **13**, 1214 (1964).
GOERING, D.: Über den Einfluß des Nervensystems auf das Fettgewebe. Z. Anat. Entwickl.-Gesch. **2**, 312 (1921/22). — GOODMAN, H. M.: Der Einfluß mehrfacher Behandlung mit Wachstumshormon auf die Lipogenese im Fettgewebe der Ratte. Endocrinology **72**, 95 (1963). — GORDON, E. S.: Non-esterified fatty acids in blood of obese and lean subjects. Amer. J. clin. Nutr. **8**, 740 (1960). — GOTTRON, H. A.: Krankheitszustände des subcutanen Fettgewebes. Medizinische **1952**, 912.
HAUSBERGER, F.: Über die nervöse Regulation des Fettstoffwechsels. Klin. Wschr. **1935**, 77. — HAXTHAUSEN, H.: Fettgewebsnekrosen durch Kälteschaden. Eigentümliche, namentlich bei Kindern auftretende Nekrosen und Infiltrate im subcutanen Fettgewebe des Gesichts nach Kälteeinwirkung. Nord. Med. **1940**, 1174. — HELLMAN, B., u. C. HELLERSTRÖM: Zellerneuerung im weißen und braunen Fettgewebe der Ratte. Acta path. microbiol. scand. **51**, 347 (1961). — HERBST: Lipogranulom. Zbl. Haut- u. Geschl.-Kr. **84**, 242 (1953). — HERING, H., u. W. UNDEUTSCH: Zur Klinik und Pathogenese der Adiponecrosis subcutanea neonatorum. Derm. Wschr. **134**, 917 (1956). — HERTING, D. C., and R. C. CRAIN: Foreign body type reaction in fat cells. Proc. Soc. exp. Biol. (N.Y.) **98**, 347 (1958). — HOFF, F.: Beobachtungen an Hauttransplantaten. Klin. Wschr. **1953**, 56. — HOFFMANN, A.: Die Entwicklung des Fettgewebes beim Menschen. Z. mikr.-anat. Forsch. **56**, 415 (1950/51).
KURÉ, K., T. OI u. S. OKINAKA: Trophische Innervation des Fettgewebes bezüglich der Beziehung des Spinalparasympathicus zu derselben. Klin. Wschr. **1937 II**, 1789.
LASZLO, J.: Changes in obese patient and his adipose tissue during prolonged starvation. Sth. med. J. (Bgham, Ala.) **58**, 1099 (1965). — LI, C. H.: Lipotropin, a new active peptide from pituitary glands. Nature (Lond.) **201**, 924 (1964). — LIEBELT, A., and A. KIRSCHBAUM: Lipogenesis in "adipose tissue" transplanted to mouses ear. Anat. Rec. **124**, 326 (1956). — LORTAT, G., u. M. VITRY: Zit. nach D. GOERING 1922.
MANSFELD, W., u. F. MÜLLER: Zit. nach D. GOERING 1922. — MICHELSON, H. E.: A consideration of some diseases of the subcutaneous fat. Arch. Derm. **75**, 633 (1957). — MOSINGER, B., E. KUHN, and V. KUJALOVÁ: Action of adipokinetic hormones on human adipose tissue in vitro. J. Lab. clin. Med. **66**, 380 (1965). — MOSTO, D.: Zum Studium der subkutanen Cytosteatonekrosen. Pren. méd. argent. **18**, 414 (1931).
NAPOLITANO, L.: Die Differenzierung der weißen Fettzellen. J. Cell Biol. **18**, 663 (1963). — NEWCOMER, V. D.: Sklerosierendes Lipogranulom oder Fremdkörpergranulom nach Ölinjektion. Arch. Derm. **69**, 383 (1954).
ÖSTERREICHER, D. L., u. E. M. WATSON: Insulin-Fettatrophie. Amer. J. med. Sci. **218**, 172 (1949).
PANABOKKÉ, R. G.: Eine experimentelle Untersuchung der Fettnekrosen. J. Path. Bakt. **75**, 319 (1958). — PROSERPIO, A.: Über die sog. Fettnekrose des subcutanen Fettgewebes. Arch. ital. Chir. **35**, 67 (1933).
RECHT, GG.: Zur Kasuistik des halbseitigen Wangenfettschwunds. Dtsch. Z. Nervenheilk. **134**, 237 (1934). — REH, H.: Die Fettzelle beim Menschen und ihre Abhängigkeit vom Ernährungszustand. Virchows Arch. path. Anat. **324**, 234 (1953). — RENOLD, A. E.: Das Fettgewebe. Med. Prisma **6**, 5 (1965).
SABRAZÈS, J., u. J. BIDEAU: Bemerkungen zur Strahlenempfindlichkeit des Fettgewebes. C. R. Soc. Biol. (Paris) **123**, 691 (1936). — SAWICKY, H. H., and N. B. KANOFF: Sclerosing lipogranuloma. Arch. Derm. **73**, 264 (1956). — SCAFFIDI, V.: Untersuchungen über den Stoffwechsel durch Änderung der lokalen Temperatur der Gewebe. Der Gehalt an Wasser und Fett in der Haut und Muskeln infolge lokaler Erkältung. Riv. Pat. sper. **5**, 31 (1930). — SCHLIENGER, F.: Zur Kenntnis der medikamentösen Lipogranulome. Dermatologica (Basel) **98**, 289 (1949).— SCHWARZMANN, J. M.: Über die cutane und subcutane traumatische experimentelle Fettgewebsnekrose. Ann. Derm. Syph. (Paris) **1**, 476 (1930). — SIDMAN, R. L., u. D. W. FAWCETT: Der Effekt der Durchschneidung peripherer Nerven auf einige Stoffwechselvorgänge im braunen Fettgewebe der Maus. Anat. Rec. **118**, 487 (1954). — SIMON, G.: Histogenesis. In: Handbook of physiology. Sect. 5, Adipose tissue, p. 101, ed. by A. E. RENOLD and G. F. CAHILL. Baltimore: Williams & Wilkins Co. 1965. — SIWE, ST. A.: Zur Pathogenese der Adiponekrosis subcutanea (sklerodermia neonatorum). Acta path. microbiol. scand., Suppl. **16**, 438 (1933). — SLOBOSIANO, H., M. GEORGESCO u. P. HERSCOVICI: Beitrag zur Kenntnis der heilbaren Hautinduration des Neugeborenen. Zbl. Haut- u. Geschl.-Kr. **43**, 431 (1933). — SPIER, H. W., u. F. KLASCHKA: Histopathologie des perifollikulären Bindegewebes bei Akne. Proc. Internat. Congr. Derm. 1962, vol. II, p. 957. — STEIGLEDER, G. K.: Die Struktur der Haut als Grundlage ihrer Leistung und Erkrankung. In: Handbuch der allgemeinen Pathologie von

F. ROULET, Bd. III/2, S. 539. Berlin-Göttingen-Heidelberg: Springer 1960. — STORCK, H.: Recidivierende Panniculitis. Dermatologica (Basel) 108, 423 (1954). — STRAUSS, J. S., and A. M. KLIGMAN: The pathologic dynamics of akne vulgaris. Arch. Derm. 82, 779 (1960). — STRAUSS, J. S., and P. E. POCHI: Intracutaneous injection of sebum and comedones. Arch. Derm. 92, 443 (1965).
TRYGSTAD: Zit. nach K. J. ANSELMINO u. F. HOFFMANN 1965.
UMBREIT, CH.: Die Wirkung von Druck und Zug auf Fettpolster und Fettzelle des Menschen. Z. Zellforsch. 13, 397 (1931).
WAIL: Zit. nach A. ABRIKOSSOFF 1926. — WASSERMANN, F.: The development of adipose tissue. In: Handbook of physiology. Sect. 5, Adipose tissue, p. 87, ed. by A. E. RENOLD and G. F. CAHILL. Baltimore: Williams & Wilkins Co. 1965. — WIGLEY, J. G. M., u. C. D. CALNAN: Sklerosierendes Lipogranulom. Proc. 10. Internat. Congr. of Derm. London 1952, 465 (1953). — WILLIAMSON, J. R., and P. E. LACY: Structurell aspects of adipose tissue: a summary attempting to synthesize the information containes in the preceding chapters. In: Handbook of physiology. Sect. 5, Adipose tissue, p. 201, ed. by A. E. RENOLD and G. F. CAHILL. Baltimore: Williams & Wilkins Co. 1965. — WORINGER, FR.: Ein Beitrag zur Histopathologie des Fettgewebes. Ann. Derm. Syph. (Paris) 2, 1089 (1931).

Ätiologie und Pathogenese der Fettgewebserkrankungen. Zusammenfassende Besprechung

ABRIKOSSOFF, A.: Über die spontan auftretenden Fettgewebsnekrosen und Fettgranulome. Zbl. allg. Path. path. Anat. 38, 542 (1926). — ALBERTAZZI, F., u. E. FERRATO: Photoplethismographische und capillaroskopische Prüfung des Fingerkreislaufs in Fällen von Necrobiosis lipoidica diabeticarum. Minerva derm. 36, 450 (1961). — AVERY, H.: Insulin fat atrophy, a traumatic atrophic panniculitis. Brit. med. J. 1929 I, 597.
BAZEX, A., u. A. DUPRÉ: Gemeinsames Vorkommen von knotiger Necrobiosis lipoidica mit diabetischer Gangrän und praetibialem Myxoedem. Bull. Soc. franç. Derm. Syph. 65, 466 (1958). — BINKLEY, J. S.: Relapsing febrile nodular nonsuppurative panniculitis. Report of a case. J. Amer. med. Ass. 113, 113 (1939). — BOCK, H. E.: Zur Allergielage bei Erythema nodosum im Rahmen des Löfgren-Syndroms. Allergie u. Asthma 6, 121 (1960). — BRAUN-FALCO, O.: Die Histochemie der Haut. In: Dermatologie und Venerologie von H. A. GOTTRON u. W. SCHÖNFELD, Bd. I/1, S. 389. Stuttgart: Georg Thieme 1961. — BREZHENKO, A. I.: On lipoid necrobiosis. Zbl. Haut- u. Geschl.-Kr. 114, 292 (1963). — BUSCHKE, A., u. A. MATTHISSOHN: Symmetrische Lipomatosis. Arch. Derm. (Berl.) 120, 537 (1914).
CALMANN, A.: Pseudotumoren im Fettgewebe nach Diathermiebehandlung. Zbl. Chir. 60, 1272 (1933). — CISTJAKOV, N.: Über die Nekrosen des subkutanen Fettgewebes (Oleogranulome). Zbl. Haut- u. Geschl.-Kr. 35, 100 (1931). — CORDERO, A. A., y R. N. CORTI: Necrobiosis lipoidica. Pren. méd. argent. 1957, 787. — CORNBLEET, TH., and H. RATTNER: Adiponekrosis subcutanea neonatorum. Arch. Derm. 40, 829 (1939). — CRUSE: Zit. nach H. HERING u. W. UNDEUTSCH 1956. — CSERVENKA, I.: Antistreptolysin-Untersuchungen bei Patienten mit Erythema nodosum. Zbl. Haut- u. Geschl.-Kr. 109, 48 (1961).
DANDA, J., u. V. PLACHY: Adiponecrosis subcutanea neonatorum. Čs. Derm. 31, 190 (1956). — DATAVO, L.: Klinisch-biologische Bemerkungen über Necrobiosis lipoidica. G. ital. Derm. 98, 654 (1957). — DAVISON, A. R.: Erythema nodosum leprosum. Leprosy Rev. 30, 112 (1959). — DERCUM: Zit. nach F. FLECK 1958. — DIECKHOFF, J., H. C. HEMPEL u. R. KOCH: Die traumatisch bedingte subkutane Fettgewebsnekrose des Neugeborenen. Kinderärztl. Prax. 1959, 443. — DIMITRESCU, A., u. L. BĂLUS: Necrobiosis lipoidica bei einer Zuckerkranken. Derm.-Vener. (Buc.) 1, 262 (1956).
EBERHARTINGER, CHR.: Das Problem des Erythema induratum Bazin. Ein Beitrag zur Kenntnis der recidivierenden, subkutanen nodösen Gefäßprozesse am Unterschenkel. Arch. klin. exp. Derm. 217, 196 (1963). — ENGEL, M. F., and W. J. HAMMACK: Necrobiosis lipoidica diabeticorum. A biochemical, histochemical and electrophoretic study. Arch. Derm. 78, 73 (1958).
FALTA: Zit. nach F. FLECK 1958. — FEIJOO, L.: Über die sog. lipophagen Granulome der Haut unter besonderer Berücksichtigung der Weber-Christianschen Krankheit. Frankfurt. Z. Path. 65, 173 (1954). — FINUCANE, B.: Erythema nodosum als Manifestation einer Sarkoidose. J. Irish med. Ass. 50, 132 (1962). — FLECK, F.: Über kutane Dyslipoidosen, Steatonekrosen und verschiedene Einzelformen abnorm-regionaler Fettverteilung. Z. Haut- u. Geschl.-Kr. 24, 1, 29 (1958). — FORD, F. D. C.: Erythema nodosum im Wochenbett nach Einspritzung eines Leberextractes. Brit. med. J. 1960 I, 400. — FORMAN, L.: Necrobiosis lipoidica of the scalp. Proc. roy. Soc. Med. 47, 658 (1954).
GERTLER, W.: Multiple Lipome des Oberkörpers bei Halsrippen. Derm. Wschr. 130, 1015 (1954). — Necrobiosis lipoidica bei Hyperlipämie. Derm. Wschr. 137, 522 (1958). — GERTLER, W., u. A. SCHIECK: Zur Häufigkeit der Necrobiosis bei Diabetikern. Derm. Wschr. 141, 456 (1960). — GÖTZ, H.: Zur Frage der Beziehungen zwischen der Granulomatosis disciformis chronica et progressiva (Miescher) und der Necrobiosis lipoidica diabeticorum. Hautarzt 7, 156

(1956). — GOLDBERG, A. L., and W. A. ROSENBERG: Necrobiosis lipoidica with intercapillary glomerulosclerosis. Arch. Derm. 71, 642 (1955). — GORDON, H.: Erythema nodosum. A review of one hundred and fifteen cases. Brit. J. Derm. 73, 393 (1961). — GOTTRON, H. A.: Krankheitszustände des subcutanen Fettgewebes. Medizinische 1952, 912. — GOTTRON, H. A., u. W. NIKOLOWSKI: Pfeifer-Christian-Weber'sche Krankheit in ihrer Nosologie und Pathogenese. Hautarzt 3, 530 (1952). — GRAY, A. M. H.: Über die Identität der Adiponekrosis subcutanea neonatorum mit dem Sclerema neonatorum. Brit. J. Derm. 45, 498 (1933). — GREITHER, A.: Erythema nodosum und Erythema exsudativum multiforme. Hautarzt 5, 1 (1954). — GRIMMER, H.: Necrobiosis lipoidica sine diabete. Z. Haut- u. Geschl.-Kr. 37, I (1964). — GROSS: Zit. nach F. FLECK 1958. — GROTS, I. A., J. S. STRAUSS, and H. MESCON: Necrobiosis lipoidica diabeticorum of the abdomen. Arch. Derm. 83, 505 (1961). — GRUBER, G. B.: Diskussionsbemerkung. Zbl. allg. Path. path. Anat. 45, 397 (1929). — GRÜTZ, O.: Beitrag zur Histologie und Pathogenese der Adiponekrosis subkutanea neonatorum. Arch. Kinderheilk. 113, 199 (1938). — GUGGENHEIM, L.: Erythema nodosum bei primärer Syphilis. Dermatologica (Basel) 118, 311 (1959).

HANHARDT, E.: Neue Sonderformen von Keratosis palmoplantaris, u. a. eine regelmäßig dominante mit systematisierten Lipomen, ferner zwei einfach-recessive mit Schwachsinn und z. T. mit Hornhautveränderungen des Auges (Ektodermalsyndrom). Dermatologica (Basel) 94, 286 (1947). — HEILESEN, B.: Necrobiosis lipoidica diabeticorum — diabetes mellitus. Acta derm.-venereol. (Stockh.) 36, 234 (1956). — HEILMANN, P., u. H. J. SONNECK: Lipomatosis symmetrica nach Elektrotrauma. Derm. Wschr. 128, 1106 (1953). — HELD, D., u. R. DELLA SANTA: Multiple Fettgewebsverhärtung, hervorgerufen durch Thrombose der venösen Kapillaren des Fettgewebes. Dermatologica (Basel) 120, 145 (1960). — HERING, H., u. W. UNDEUTSCH: Zur Klinik und Pathogenese der Adiponekrosis subcutanea neonatorum. Derm. Wschr. 134, 917 (1956). — HERTING, D. D., and R. C. CRAIN: Foreign body type reaction in fat cells. Proc. Soc. exp. Biol. (N.Y.) 98, 347 (1958). — HICKMAN, K. C. D.: In: Biological antioxydants, transact. 4. Conf., J. Macy Foundation, New York 1949. — HOCHLEITNER, H.: Zur Klinik des Erythema nodosum. Derm. Wschr. 147, 418 (1963). — HOLZEL, A.: Subcutaneous fat necrosis of the newborn. Arch. Dis. Childh. 26, 89 (1951). — HORNSTEIN, O.: Histologischer Beitrag zur Pathogenese subcutaner Lipome. Arch. klin. exp. Derm. 204, 397 (1957).

JAMES, D. G.: Erythema nodosum. Brit. med. J. 1961I, 853. — JUNCKER: Necrobiosis lipoidica und diabetische Angiopathie. Zbl. Haut- u. Geschl.-Kr. 92, 396 (1955).

KALDOR, I., u. L. NEKAM: Immunologische Veränderungen bei Necrobiosis lipoidica. Ann. Derm. Syph. (Paris) 91, 147 (1964). — KALKOFF, K. W.: Necrobiosis lipoidica diabeticorum. Zbl. Haut- u. Geschl.-Kr. 87, 292 (1954). — KELLNER, H.: Zur Frage der Zusammenhänge zwischen lipophager Granulombildung und Erythema induratum, Sarkoid Darier-Roussy und Panniculitis nonsupperativa nodularis recidivans. Hautarzt 2, 299 (1951). — KNOTH, W.: Erkrankungen des reticulo-histiocytären Systems der Haut. Habil.-Schrift Gießen 1958. — Die Begutachtung eines Granulomatosis disciformis chronica et progressiva-Kranken mit abgeheilter Tuberkulosis cutis fistulosa. Berufsdermatosen 7, 136 (1959). — KNOTH, W., u. H. FÜLLER: Zur Patho- und Histogenese der Necrobiosis lipoidica „diabeticorum". Arch. Derm. Syph. (Berl.) 199, 109 (1955). — KNOTH, W., u. W. MEYHÖFER: Beitrag zum Formenkreis der Periarteriitis nodosa und zur Bewertung der Riesenzellen bei Gefäßerkrankungen. Dermatologica (Basel) 119, 1 (1959). — KONOPIK, J.: On the pathogenesis and aetiology of panniculitis. Čs. Derm. 30, 259 (1955).

LECÈNE, P., et P. MOULONGUET: La pseudo-tuberculose du péritone secondaire aux perforations du tube digestif. Ann. Anat. path. 2, 193 (1925). — LEINATI, F.: Zit. nach W. BAUMGARTNER u. G. RIVA 1945. — LINSER, K.: Necrobiosis lipoidica. Granulomatosis disciformis chronica et progressiva (Miescher). Zbl. Haut- u. Geschl.-Kr. 88, 193 (1954). — LITTLE, J. A., and A. J. STEIGMAN: Erythema nodosum in primary histoplasmosis. J. Amer. med. Ass. 173, 875 (1960). — LOSSIE, H., u. H. VOEGT: Zur Frage der hormonalen Genese der Spontanpanniculitis Rothmann-Makai. Ärztl. Wschr. 9, 1071 (1954).

MAKAI, E.: Über Lipogranulomatosis subcutanea. Klin. Wschr. 1928II, 2343. — Lipogranulomatöse Knotenbildungen im Fettgewebe. Zbl. Chir. 60, 1267 (1933). — McDONALD, R.: Subcutaneous fat necrosis and sclerema neonatorum. S. Afr. med. J. 1955, 1007. — MEESEN, H.: Experimentelle Probleme zum Kollapsproblem. Beitr. path. Anat. 102, 191 (1939). — MEIER: Zit. nach F. FLECK, 1958. — MEYER, A.: Die herdförmige unspezifische Entzündung der Subcutis (Panniculitis). Praxis 1955, 201. — MEYERS: Erythema nodosum, Arthritis. Zbl. Haut- u. Geschl.-Kr. 114, 256 (1963). — MICHELSON, A. E.: A consideration of some diseases of the subcutaneous fat. Arch. Derm. 75, 633 (1957). — MILNER, R. D. G., and M. J. MITCHINSON: Systemic Weber-Christian-disease. J. clin. Path. 18, 150 (1965). — MOLLARET, H. H.: Eine neue mögliche Ursache des Erythema induratum. Presse méd. 70, 1923 (1962). — MUNTEANU, M.: Aetiologische Betrachtungen anhand von einigen Fällen von Erythema nodosum. Derm.-Vener. (Buc.) 4, 233 (1959).

NEWCOMER, V. D., J. H. GRAHAM, R. R. SCHAFFERT u. L. KAPLAN: Vernarbendes Lipogranulom in Beziehung zu exogenen Lipoidsubstanzen. Arch. Derm. 73, 264 (1956). — NOOJIN, R. O., B. F. PACE, and H. G. DAVIS: Subcutaneous fat necrosis of newborn: Certain etiologic considerations. J. invest. Derm. 12, 331 (1949).
OEHLERT, W., H. WECKE u. H. SUTTERLE: Die Fettgewebsnekrose des Neugeborenen bei Diabetes mellitus der Mutter. Zbl. allg. Path. path. Anat. 107, 499 (1965). — OTTO, H., u. K. H. HOBUSCH: Ein Kurzbeitrag zur Aetiologie des Erythema nodosum. Z. ges. inn. Med. 14, 452 (1959).
PETRI, E.: Über extramedulläre Blutbildung bei Polycythaemia vera. Zbl. allg. Path. path. Anat. 35, 245 (1924). — PEZZAROSSA, G.: Über die Necrobiosis lipoidica und deren Zusammenhänge mit dem Granuloma anulare. G. ital. Derm. 98, 129 (1957). — PFUHL, W.: Die Aufräumung zugrunde gegangener Fettzellen durch Histiocyten im Trypanblauentzündungsherd. Z. Anat. Entwickl.-Gesch. 110, 533 (1940). — PIAGGIO, W.: Heilbare Hautinduration der Neugeborenen. Zbl. Haut- u. Geschl.-Kr. 42, 360 (1932). — PINSKI, J. B., u. PH. D. STANSIFER: Erythema nodosum als Primärsymptome der Leukämie. Arch. Derm. 89, 339 (1964). — PIROTH, M.: Zur Morphologie des Lipogranuloms. Zbl. allg. Path. path. Anat. 93, 292 (1955).
RANDERATH, E.: Die Bedeutung der allergischen Pathogenese bei der Arteriitis. Verh. Dtsch. Ges. inn. Med., 60. Kongr. 1954, S. 359. — REYMANN, FL.: Necrosis adiposa neonatorum. Acta derm.-venereol. (Stockh.) 35, 220 (1955). — RICCI, MICHELETTI u. COSCIA: Zit. nach R. D. G. MILNER u. M. J. MITCHINSON 1965. — RINGROSE, E. J.: Smoking, Necrobiosis lipoidica, granulomatosis disciformis chronica et progressiva. Arch. Derm. 79, 635 (1959). — RODRIGUEZ, J. N.: Erythema nodosum leprosum, a deep nodular form of reaction in lepromatous leprosy. Int. J. Leprosy 25, 313 (1957). — RÖCKL, H., u. W. THIES: Herdförmige chronisch recidivierende Krankheitszustände des subkutanen Fettgewebes. Hautarzt 8, 58 (1957). — ROLLINS, T. G., and R. K. WINKELMANN: Necrobiosis lipoidica-granulomatosis. Arch. Derm. 82, 537 (1960). — ROTTER, W.: Über die Bedeutung der Ernährungsstörung, insbesondere des Sauerstoffmangels, für die Pathogenese der Gefäßveränderungen mit besonderer Berücksichtigung der Endangiitis obliterans und der Arteriosklerose. Beitr. path. Anat. 110, 46 (1949). — RUTISHÄUSER, E., u. D. HELD: Capilläre Fibrinthromben in den intercytären Spalträumen des Fettgewebes. Ber. allg. spez. Path. 47, 171 (1961).
SANDBERG, D. H., and J. M. ADAMS: Erythema induratum und Streptokokkeninfektion. J. Pediat. 61, 880 (1962). — SANFORD, H. N., D. F. EUBANK u. F. STENN: Chronische Panniculitis mit Leukopenie (Pfeifer-Weber-Christian-Syndrom). Amer. J. Dis. Child. 83, 156 (1952). — SANTLER, R.: Zwei Fälle von Granulomatosis disciformis chronica et progressiva (Miescher). Hautarzt 5, 14 (1954). — SCHIMPF, A.: Familiäre supramalleoläre Lipomatosis. Derm. Wschr. 130, 1117 (1954). — SCHLIENGER, F.: Zur Kenntnis der medikamentösen Lipogranulome. Dermatologica (Basel) 98, 289 (1949). — SCHOEDD, J.: Adiponekrosis subkutanea neonatorum. Mschr. Kinderheilk. 63, 241 (1935). — SCHUERMANN, H.: Zur Klinik und Pathogenese der Dermatomyositis. Arch. Derm. Syph. (Berl.) 178, 414 (1939). — SCHULZE: Zit. nach F. FLECK 1958. — SCHWARZMANN, J. M.: Über die cutane und subcutane traumatische experimentelle Fettgewebsnekrose. Ann. Derm. Syph. (Paris) 1, 476 (1930). — SCRIBA, K.: Subcutane Fettgewebsnekrosen bei Neugeborenen. Zbl. allg. Path. path. Anat. 93, 460 (1955). SEVASTINOS, E., M. M. JALLAD, and K. YAMATO: Necrobiosis lipoidica diabeticorum, diabetes mellitus. Arch. Derm. 82, 834 (1960). — SIEGMUND, H.: Diskussionsbemerkung. Verh. Dtsch. Ges. Path., 29. Tagg 1936, S. 104. — SIWE, ST. A.: Zur Pathogenese der Adiponekrosis subkutanea (Sklerodermia neonatorum). Acta path. microbiol. scand., Suppl. 16, 438 (1933). — SLOBOSIANO, H., M. GEORGESCO u. P. HERSCOVICI: Beitrag zur Kenntnis der heilbaren Hautinduration der Neugeborenen. Zbl. Haut- u. Geschl.-Kr. 43, 431 (1933). — SMITH, J. G.: Necrobiosis lipoidica. A disease of changing concepts. Arch. Derm. 74, 280 (1956). — SPAGNOLI, U.: Necrobiosis lipoidica diabeticorum. Rass. Derm. Sif. 11, 237 (1958). — STEIGLEDER, G. K.: Die Struktur der Haut als Grundlage ihrer Leistung und Erkrankung. In: Handbuch der allgemeinen Pathologie von F. ROULET, Bd. III/2, S. 539. Berlin-Göttingen-Heidelberg: Springer 1960. — Allgemeine Pathologie der Haut. In: Dermatologie und Venerologie von H. A. GOTTRON u. W. SCHÖNFELD, Bd. I/1, S. 310. Stuttgart: Georg Thieme 1961. — Neoplastisch wuchernde Zellen der Cutis und Subcutis. In: Handbuch der Haut- und Geschlechtskrankheiten von J. JADASSOHN, Erg.-Bd. I/2, S. 724. Berlin-Göttingen-Heidelberg: Springer 1964. — STEIGLEDER, G. K., u. H. LÖFFLER: Zum histochemischen Nachweis unspezifischer Esterasen und Lipasen. Arch. klin. exp. Derm. 203, 41 (1956). — STEIGLEDER, G. K., u. K. SCHULTIS: Die Bedeutung des Nachweises unspezifischer Esterasen in Bindegewebszellen der Haut. Arch. klin. exp. Derm. 204, 448 (1957). — STEINESS, J.: Subkutane Fettgewebsnekrosen beim Neugeborenen und mütterlicher Diabetes mellitus. Acta med. scand. 170, 411 (1961). — STUHLERT, H.: Pfeifer-Christian-Webersche Krankheit und Panniculitis traumatica. Z. Haut- u. Geschl.-Kr. 16, 321 (1954). — STÜTTGEN, G.: Arteriitis und Gangrän der Haut. Ein Beitrag zur Abgrenzung der Periarteriitis nodosa cutanea. Hautarzt 7, 354 (1956).

TOURAINE, A., et P. RENAULT: Lipomatose segmentaire du tronc. Bull. Soc. franç. Derm. Syph. **45**, 924 (1938).
UNSHELM, E.: Beitrag zur Aetiologie der subcutanen Fettgewebsnekrose der Säuglinge. Mschr. Kinderheilk. **52**, 321 (1932).
VANDEKERCKHOVE, M.: Erythema induratum Bazin, Hypodermitis nodularis chronica und Nodularvasculitis. Arch. belges Derm. **18**, 193 (1962). — VESEY, C. M. R., and D. S. WILKINSON: Erythema nodosum. A study of seventy cases. Brit. J. Derm. **71**, 139 (1959).
WORINGER, F.: Contribution à l'histologie du tissu adipeux. Ann. Derm. Syph. (Paris) **2**, 1089 (1931). — WORINGER, FR., et J. P. WEILL: Necrobiosis lipoidica diabeticorum. Bull. Soc. franç. Derm. Syph. **66**, 226 (1959).
ZAVARINI, G.: Atypische, chronische, mikronoduläre Fettgewebsentzündung. Rass. Derm. Sif. **8**, 245 (1955). — ZOCCHI, S.: Über die heilbare Hautverhärtung der Neugeborenen durch geburtshilfliches Trauma. Riv. Ostet. Ginec. **14**, 335 (1932).

Literaturnachtrag (bei Korrektur, November 1967)

ACKERMANN, A. B., D. T. MOSHER, and H. A. SCHWAMM: Factitial Weber-Christian-syndrome. J. Amer. med. Ass. **198**, 731 (1966). — ALBRECTSEN, B.: Zit. nach P. DE GRACIANSKY 1967. — AROUTUNOV, V.: Nekrotisierende allergische Pan-Angiitis. Ann. Derm. Syph. (Paris) **92**, 489 (1965).
BANDMANN, H. J., N. ROMITI u. K. STEHR: Beitrag zur Klinik und zur Klassifizierung der Acanthosis nigricans. Hautarzt **16**, 492 (1965). — BENOIT, F. L.: The inhibitory effect of chloroquine on rat adipose tissue metabolism in vitro. Metabolism **16**, 557 (1967). — BJÖRNTORP, P., B. HOOD, A. MARTINSSON, and B. PERSSON: The composition of human subcutaneous adipose tissue in obesity. Acta med. scand. **180**, 117 (1966). — BRUINSMA, W.: Lipo-atrophia annularis, an abnormal vulnerability of the fatty tissue. Dermatologica (Basel) **134**, 107 (1967). — BUREAU, Y., A. JARRY, H. BARRIERE, J. P. KERNEIS et P. BRUNEAU: Les hypodermites nodulaires subaigues des membres inferieurs. Bull. Soc. franç. Derm. Syph. **65**, 401 (1958).
COHEN: Zit. nach P. DE GRACIANSKY 1967.— COMFORT u. OSTERBERG: Zit. nach P. DE GRACIANSKY 1967.
DE GRACIANSKY, P.: Panniculite de WEBER-CHRISTIAN. Diskussion d'une étiologie pancréatique. Bull. Soc. franç. Derm. Syph. **73**, 925 (1967). — Weber-Christian-syndrome of pancreatic origin. Brit. J. Derm. **79**, 278 (1967). — DE GRACIANSKY, LIÈVRE u. PARAF: Zit. nach P. DE GRACIANSKY 1967. — DUNCAN, W. C., R. G. FREEMAN, and CH. L. HEATON: Cold panniculitis. Arch. Derm. **94**, 722 (1966).
FISHER, I., u. M. ORKIN: Die kutane Form der Periarteriitis nodosa. Arch. Derm. **89**, 180 (1964). — FURTADO, T. A.: Histopatologia das hipodermites. Med. Cut. **1**, 597 (1967).
GALTON, D. J., and G. A. BRAY: Studies on lipolysis in human adipose cells. J. clin. Invest. **46**, 621 (1967). — GOLDRICK, R. B.: Morphological changes in the adipocyte during fat deposition and mobilization. Amer. J. Physiol. **212**, 277 (1967). — GRIESEMER, R. D., and R. W. THOMAS: Lipogenesis in human skin. IV. In vitro rate studies. J. invest. Derm. **47**, 432 (1966). — GUTMAN, A., H. SCHRAMM, and E. SHAFRIR: Adipose tissue glycogen. Israel J. med. Sci. **3**, 427 (1967).
HÄGGENDAL, E., B. STEEN, and A. SVANBORG: Measurement of blood flow through human abdominal subcutaneous fat tissue by local injection of radiactive xenon. Preliminary report. Acta med. scand. **181**, 215 (1967). — HEITE, H. J., u. G. VON DER HEYDT: Pigmentierte papilläre Dystrophien. In: Handbuch der Haut- und Geschlechtskrankheiten von J. JADASSOHN. Erg.-Werk Bd. III/1. Berlin-Göttingen-Heidelberg: Springer 1963. — HEUSER, E., E. LIEBERMAN, G. N. DONNELL, and B. H. LANDING: Subcutaneous fat necrosis with acute hemorrhagic pancreatitis — a case in a child with steroid-resistant nephrosis treated with 6-mercaptopurine. Calif. Med. **106**, 58 (1967). — HSIA, S. L., M. A. DREIZE, and M. C. MARQUEZ: Lipid metabolism in human skin. II. A study of lipogenesis in skin of diabetic patients. J. invest. Derm. **47**, 443 (1966). — HSIA, S. L., M. S. GAIL-SOFER, and BARRY LANE: Lipid metabolism in human skin. I. Lipogenesis from acetate-1-^{14}C. J. invest. Derm. **47**, 437 (1966).
IKEMOTO, H.: Role of brown adipose tissue in cold acclimation. Jap. J. vet. Res. **15**, 106 (1967). — INSULL jr., W., and G. E. BARTSCH: Fatty acid composition of human adipose tissue related to age, sex and race. Amer. J. clin. Nutr. **20**, 13 (1967).
JABLONSKA, ST., I. HAUSMANOWA-PETRUSEWICZ u. I. PIWOWARCZYK: Der Einfluß auf Muskeln und Subkutis bei diabetischen Kaninchen. Derm. Wschr. **153**, 497 (1967). — JABLONSKA, ST., u. R. HINTZ: Im Druck. Zit. nach JABLONSKA, ST., I. HAUSMANOVA-PETRUSEWICZ u. I. PIWOWARCZYK 1967.
KERDEL-VEGAS, FR.: Subacute Panniculitis nodosa migrans (Vilanova und Piñol-Aguadé). Hautarzt **17**, 116 (1966). — KOVACEV, V. P., and R. O. SCOW: Effect of hormones on fatty acid release by rat adipose tissue in vivo. Amer. J. Physiol. **210**, 1199 (1966).

LINDBERG, O., J. DE PIERRE, E. RYLANDER, and B. A. AFZELIUS: Studies on the mitochondrial energytransfer system of brown adipose tissue. J. Cell Biol. **34**, 295 (1967). — LINDLAR, F., u. V. MISGELD: Die Adiponecrosis subcutanea neonatorum unter lipoidchemischem Aspekt. Hautarzt **18**, 115 (1967). — LEGER: Zit. nach P. DE GRACIANSKY 1967. — LIÈVRE: Zit. nach P. DE GRACIANSKY 1967.

MACHACEK: Zit. nach P. DE GRACIANSKY 1967. — MÜLLER, H., u. U. KRAUL: Die Pingranliquose. Derm. Wschr. **153**, 583 (1967).

PALETTE, E. M., E. C. PALETTE, and R. W. HARRINGTON: Sclerosing lipogranulomatosis: its several abdominal syndromes. Arch. Surg. **94**, 803 (1967). — PANABOKKÉ, R. G.: Zit. nach P. DE GRACIANSKY 1967. — PARISH, W. E.: Bacterial antigens in nodular vasculitis. Brit. J. Derm. **79**, 643 (1967). — PAVLIK, F.: Pfeifer-Weber-Christiansche Krankheit bei exokriner Pankreasinsuffizienz. Derm. Wschr. **153**, 649 (1967). — PERRY, H. O., u. R. K. WINKELMANN: Subacute noduläre migrierende Panniculitis. Arch. Derm. **89**, 170 (1964). — PFEIFER, U., u. R. JOCHEMS: Wegenersche Granulomatose: Klinischer Verlauf und pathologisch-anatomische Befunde unter Corticosteroidbehandlung. Klin. Wschr. **45**, 839 (1967). — PIERINI, L. E., J. ABULAFIA y S. WAINFELD: Las hipodermitis. Arch. argent. Derm. **15**, 1, 105 (1965). — Hipodermitis lipogranulomatosas idiopathicas. G. ital. Derm. **107**, 1079 (1966).

RABBIOSI, G.: Ipodermite nodulare subacuta migrante: considerazioni sopra due case. Minerva derm. **33**, 55 (1958). — ROTMAN, H.: Cold panniculitis in children. Adiponecrosis e frigore of Haxthausen. Arch. Derm. **94**, 720 (1966).

SOLOMON, L. M., and H. BEERMAN: Cold Panniculitis. Arch. Derm. **88**, 897 (1963).

THIELE, O. W.: Chemie und Stoffwechsel der Lipide. Eine kurze Übersicht. Hippokrates (Stuttg.) **38**, 829 (1967).

VILANOVA, X.: Subacute, nodular, migrans hypodermites, abstract. Arch. Derm. **87**, 536 (1963). — VILANOVA, X., et J. P. PIÑOL-AGUADÉ: Hypodermite nodulaire subaigue migratrice. Ann. Derm. Syph. (Paris) **83**, 369 (1956). — Subacute nodular migratory panniculitis. Brit. J. Derm. **71**, 45 (1959). — Paniculitis necrotica. Evolucion mortal. Acta derm. sifilogr. **55**, 1 (1964).

WEBER, G., u. G. ROTH: Lipodystrophia progressiva, eine Sklerodermie en coup de sabre simulierend. Arch. klin. exp. Derm. **229**, 194 (1967). — WEGENER, F.: Die Wegenersche Granulomatose. In: Lehrbuch der speziellen und pathologischen Anatomie v. E. KAUFMANN u. M. STAEMMLER, Bd. I/1. Berlin: W. de Gruyter 1967.

ZELLER u. HETZ: Zit. nach P. DE GRACIANSKY 1967.

Ablagerung und Speicherung in der Cutis

Von

Christoph Eberhartinger, Wien,
Herwig Ebner, Wien und **Gustav Niebauer**, Wien

Einleitung

Zahlreiche Stoffe, teils im Körper selbst gebildet, teils von außen dem Körper zugeführt, werden in der Cutis abgelagert und gespeichert. Einige Substanzen sind schon physiologisch vorhanden, sie treten unter besonderen Umständen nur vermehrt, andere treten nur unter pathologischen Bedingungen auf. Oft führen diese Ablagerungen oder Speicherungen eines Stoffes in der Cutis zu einem dermatologisch wohl definierten Krankheitsbild.

Diese Ablagerungskrankheiten körpereigener Stoffwechselprodukte wurden hinsichtlich klinischer und histologischer Morphologie sowie Pathogenese von W. F. LEVER in Band III/1 dieses Handbuches ausführlich behandelt. Des weiteren stehen Speicherungen von Substanzen, die physiologischerweise in der Cutis vorhanden sind, eng mit pathologischen Veränderungen an Grundsubstanz, Kollagen und Elastica in Zusammenhang. Dieses Kapitel wurde in Band I/2 von O. BRAUN-FALCO behandelt.

Im Folgenden soll deshalb, um Überschneidungen und Wiederholungen zu vermeiden — auch der knappe, zur Verfügung stehende Raum zwingt dazu — nur überblicksmäßig diesen Problemen nachgegangen werden. Da in den genannten Handbuchbeiträgen reichlich Bildmaterial veröffentlicht wurde, wurde in diesen Kapiteln von einer Bebilderung Abstand genommen. Nur bei einzelnen Kapiteln erschien es uns notwendig etwas ausführlicher zu werden. Auf alle Fälle empfiehlt es sich, bei Fragestellungen über Speicherungen und Ablagerungen der Cutis auch die oben genannten Handbuchbeiträge zu berücksichtigen.

I. Amyloide

Amyloidose ist eine Krankheit unbekannter Ursache, charakterisiert durch die Akkumulation eines amorphen, proteinhaltigen Materials in verschiedenen Organen und Geweben (BRIGGS, 1961). Es wird allgemein angenommen, daß Amyloid unter physiologischen Bedingungen nicht vorkommt. Im Gegensatz dazu vertritt allerdings McMANUS (1950) die Ansicht, daß amyloide Substanz in sehr geringer Konzentration ein normaler Bestandteil der Grundsubstanz ist und daß es bei der Amyloidose nicht zu einer qualitativen, sondern zu einer quantitativen Veränderung in der Zusammensetzung des Bindegewebes komme.

Amyloid ist ein chemisch nicht einheitlich aufgebauter Protein-Polysaccharidkomplex (SPRAFKE, 1952; SAGHER und SHANON, 1953; LETTERER, 1959; MUSGER, 1962). Das Ergebnis biochemischer und histochemischer Untersuchungen dieser Substanz ist daher nicht einheitlich. Der positive Ausfall der Jod- und Jodschwefelsäure-Reaktion hat VIRCHOW (1854) im Amyloid eine celluloseähnliche Substanz vermuten lassen. Wenige Jahre später bezeichneten FRIEDREICH und KEKULÉ (1859) das Amyloid bereits als Eiweiß. Neben dem Eiweißanteil konnten in der Folgezeit noch Glykoproteid- und Polysaccharidkomponenten nachgewiesen werden (HASS, 1942; WAGNER, 1955). Das erklärt die histochemische Darstellbarkeit des Amyloids mit der PAS-Reaktion und bei richtiger Vorbehandlung des Gewebes auch mit der Hale- oder einer ähnlichen Reaktion (MCMANUS, 1948; JONES und FRAZIER, 1950; PALITZ und PECK, 1952; RUSZCZAK und WOZNIAK, 1961). Die gebundene Menge saurer Mucopolysaccharide scheint sehr wechselnd zu sein.

Wahrscheinlich ist die *Rot-Metachromasie* bei Färbung des Amyloids mit Methylviolett oder Kresylviolett auf die Anwesenheit dieser sauren Mucopolysaccharide zurückzuführen, obgleich mit Toluidinblau nur selten echte Metachromasie beobachtet wird. Diese Metachromasie ist bei den klassischen Amyloidfärbungen das einzige sichere differentialdiagnostische Kriterium gegenüber anderen hyalinen Proteinen (PEARSE, 1960). Die Vorbehandlung des Gewebes ist für den Ausfall der Metachromasie-Reaktionen von großer Bedeutung (PEARSE, 1960). Allerdings lassen Vergleichsuntersuchungen mit der Metachromotropie des Knorpels überhaupt daran zweifeln, ob die Metachromasie des Amyloids auf die Anwesenheit saurer Mucopolysaccharide bezogen werden darf. Es ist jedenfalls unwahrscheinlich, daß die metachromatische Reaktion des Amyloids auf der Anwesenheit von Chondroitinsulfat beruht (CARNES und FORKER, 1954, 1956). Unterschiede im färberischen Verhalten und in den histochemischen Reaktionen sind ganz besonders beim Paramyloid zu beobachten, dessen chemische Zusammensetzung mehr als beim echten Amyloid variiert (LETTERER, 1950).

Wenig ist über die chemische oder physikalische Bindung des Kongorot an das Amyloid bekannt. Bei Gewebsschnitten, die mit *Kongorot* in wäßriger oder alkoholischer Lösung ohne Differenzierung gefärbt werden, färben sich alle Strukturen rot an. Aber nur das Amyloid zeigt in selektiver Weise einen Dichroismus. Das weist darauf hin, daß die Bindung des Farbstoffes an das Amyloid von anderer Art ist als die Bindung an andere Strukturen des Gewebes (COHEN, CALKINS und LEVENE, 1959; EHRLICH und RATNER, 1961; MISSMAHL und HARTWIG, 1953, FREY, 1925; PUCHTLER, SWEAT und LEVINE, 1962). Voraussetzung des Dichroismus ist eine lineare und parallel gerichtete Anordnung von Substrat und Farbstoff. Schon das polarisationsmikroskopische Bild und der Nachweis einer positiven Doppelbrechung weisen auf die „gerichtete" submikroskopische Struktur des Amyloids hin (DIVRY und FLORKIN, 1927; MISSMAHL und HARTWIG, 1953; COHEN, CALKINS und LEVENE, 1959). Die in den letzten Jahren durchgeführten elektronenoptischen Untersuchungen der amyloiden Substanz konnten auch tatsächlich eine fibrilläre Ultrastruktur des Amyloids nachweisen (s. später). In diese wird das Kongorot *gerichtet* eingelagert. Bei polarisationsmikroskopischer Betrachtung der kongorotgefärbten Schnitte zeigt das Amyloid somit positive Doppelbrechung und einen Dichroismus; d.h., die Doppelbrechung leuchtet zwischen gekreuzten Polars in einer für Amyloid typischen grünen Farbe auf (MISSMAHL und HARTWIG, 1953; WOLMAN und BUBIS, 1965). Da dieses Phänomen selektiv nur bei Amyloid beobachtet wird, sollte in allen Zweifelsfällen eine polarisationsoptische Untersuchung der Schnitte durchgeführt werden. Der Vorteil dieser Methode ist nicht nur die Spezifität, sondern auch die Möglichkeit, schon kleinste Mengen von Amyloid nachzuweisen, so daß schon Anfangsstadien der Amyloidablagerungen histologisch sichtbar werden. Weiter ermöglicht die polarisationsoptische Untersuchung kongorotgefärbter histologischer Schnitte die Unterscheidung einer periretikulären Amyloidose von einer perikollagenen (MISSMAHL, 1965).

Wie schon oben angeführt, ist die *chemische Zusammensetzung* des Amyloids nicht konstant, so daß die histochemischen Reaktionen durchaus unterschiedlich ausfallen können. Nach HARMS (1964) sollte von *den* Amyloiden gesprochen werden. Nach GÖSSNER (1964) wird der wechselhafte Ausfall der verschiedenen Amyloidfärbungen und -reaktionen am besten verständlich, wenn man das Amyloid mit einem Schwamm vergleicht, der sich mit verschiedenen Flüssigkeiten vollsaugen kann. Mit den Färbungen und histochemischen Tests erfaßt man im wesentlichen den Schwamminhalt, der durch das Milieu bestimmt wird, in das der Schwamm eintaucht. Aufklärung über den Bau des Schwammgerüstes bringen eher die elektronen- und polarisationsmikroskopischen Befunde.

Bemerkenswert ist der regelmäßig stark positive Ausfall des histochemischen Tryptophantests an allen bisher untersuchten Amyloidformen, während sich Kollagen und bindegewebiges Hyalin bei dieser Reaktion negativ verhalten (GÖSSNER, 1961). Die Herkunft des tryptophanreichen Proteins ist nicht geklärt; die Inkorporation tryptophanreicher Serum-Eiweißkörper wird als wahrscheinlich diskutiert. Was den Einbau sulfathaltiger Mucopolysaccharide in das Amyloid betrifft, so hat KENNEDY (1962) den autoradiographischen Beweis erbracht, daß bei experimenteller Amyloidose eine vermehrte S^{35}-Sulfat-Inkorporation in die proliferierten retikulären Elemente und in die neugebildeten Amyloidsubstanzen stattfindet. Von diesem Gesichtspunkt aus müssen heute auch die Befunde von TEILUM (1956) interpretiert werden, der angenommen hat, daß Amyloid vom RES sezerniert wird. Denn auf Grund der elektronenmikroskopischen Befunde ist es wahrscheinlich, daß das aktivierte Reticulum nur die Vorstufen des Amyloids sezerniert und daß sich das eigentliche Amyloid extracellulär bildet (CAESAR, 1960). Diese Befunde ergänzend haben LINDNER und FREYTAG (1964) darauf hingewiesen, daß auch die Capillarendothelien und die Gefäßwandzellen bei einer Permeabilitätsstörung — und diese liegt bei einer Amyloidose vor — saure Mucopolysaccharide gesteigert synthetisieren. Amyloid kann auch Fettstoffe (Neutralfett und Cholesterin) absorbieren, was unter Umständen zu einer Sudanophilie, besonders im Zentrum der Schollen, führt (KREIBICH, 1913).

Die verschiedenen *klassischen Färbemethoden* für Amyloid sind bei KÖNIGSTEIN (1932) und LEVER (1963) ausführlich besprochen worden. Hier soll nur nochmals darauf hingewiesen werden, daß in der Routinehistologie die Färbung nach VAN GIESON von großer Hilfe ist, da sich Amyloid dabei hellgelb anfärbt (MIESCHER, 1945). Jedoch ein selektiver Nachweis, der schon kleinste Herde erfaßt, gelingt nur bei Betrachtung kongorotgefärbter histologischer Schnitte im Polarisationsmikroskop zwischen gekreuzten Polars. Das Amyloid leuchtet hierbei in einer grünen, anomalen Polarisationsfarbe auf (MISSMAHL, 1965). Der fluorescenzoptische Nachweis des Amyloids mit Thioflavin T dürfte wohl ebenso empfindlich sein (VASSAR und CULLING, 1959; MALAK und SMITH, 1962), ist jedoch nicht im gleichen Maße spezifisch.

Elektronenmikroskopische Untersuchungen von Amyloid wurden bei experimenteller Amyloidose, sekundärer Amyloidose (Niere), primärer Amyloidose (Haut) und bei hereditärer Amyloidose im Rahmen des familiären Mittelmeerfiebers (Niere) von COHEN und CALKINS (1959, 1960), CAESAR (1960), LETTERER, CAESAR und VOGT (1960), HASHIMOTO, GROSS und LEVER (1965) durchgeführt. Amyloid ist im elektronenoptischen Bild eine fibrilläre Substanz, somit kein amorpher, sondern ein kristalliner Körper mit „gerichteter" submikroskopischer Struktur, der mit anderen extracellulären Substanzen keinerlei Ähnlichkeit hat. Im Gegensatz zur wechselnden chemischen Zusammensetzung des Amyloids ist das elektronenoptische Bild durchaus konstant. Zwischen primärer und sekundärer Amyloidose besteht kein Unterschied. Charakteristisch sind die Elementarfibrillen und die Bündelung der Fibrillen. Die für Amyloid typische Ultrastruktur wurde intracellulär *niemals* nachgewiesen. Damit scheint heute die Theorie der intracellulären Amyloidbildung, wie sie von TEILUM (1956) angenommen wird, unwahrscheinlich. Vielmehr ist eine *extracelluläre* Entstehung des Amyloids anzunehmen. Die Amyloidfibrille unterscheidet sich in ihrer Ultrastruktur signifikant vom Kollagen, sie ist auch kollagenaseresistent und enthält kein Hydroxyprolin (CALKINS und COHEN, 1960; COHEN und CALKINS, 1964).

Das *Einteilungsschema der Amyloidosen* ist nicht einheitlich (s. LEVER, 1963). Aber fast alle Autoren unterscheiden zwei Hauptgruppen, nämlich die primäre Amyloidose (= Paramyloidose) und die sekundäre Amyloidose (= typische, klassische oder echte Amyloidose). Während erstere ohne Begleiterkrankung auftritt, ist die klassische Amyloidose Folge einer chronischen Krankheit. Die Ablagerungen bei sekundärer Amyloidose finden sich hauptsächlich in Milz, Leber, Niere und Nebenniere, während bei Paramyloidose Herzmuskel, quergestreifte Muskulatur, periphere Nerven und Haut ergriffen sein können. Alle bisher versuchten Einteilungen der Amyloidosen nach Gewebeverteilung und färberischen Eigenschaften sind artefiziell, da zu viele Überschneidungen bestehen. Nach CALKINS und COHEN (1960) sollte die Unterscheidung zwischen primärer und sekundärer Amyloidose nur davon abhängen, ob prädisponierende und assoziierte Krankheiten vorhanden sind oder nicht. Das histologische Einteilungsprinzip von MISSMAHL (1964) bietet in dieser Hinsicht neue Möglichkeiten, erfordert allerdings noch weitere Prüfungen (s. Tabelle 1).

Nach LEVER (1963) befällt die klassische, sekundäre Amyloidose in der Regel die Haut nicht. Aber auch darüber sind die Literaturangaben nicht einheitlich (s. GANS und STEIGLEDER, 1955; FREUDENTHAL, 1930; MALAK und SMITH, 1962). Das hängt eben wieder damit zusammen, daß Amyloid, bzw. *die* Amyloide chemisch nicht genau definiert sind und daß sich mit den klassischen histologischen und histochemischen Methoden Amyloid und Paramyloid nicht sicher unterscheiden lassen. Da auch elektronenmikroskopisch zwischen Amyloid und Paramyloid kein Unterschied besteht, ist es notwendig, die Frage des Vorkommens einer sekundären Amyloidose in der Haut mit der polarisationsoptischen Technik von MISSMAHL (1965) nachzuprüfen.

Polarisationsmikroskopische Untersuchungen wurden in den letzten Jahren von SCHOTT und HOLZMANN (1965) und von SCHNEIDER und MISSMAHL (1966) durchgeführt. Nach den Angaben dieser Autoren scheint es in der Haut nur zur Ablagerung von perikollagenem Amyloid zu kommen. SCHOTT und HOLZMANN (1965) konnten auch mit Hilfe polarisationsmikroskopischer Untersuchungen eine Ablagerung von Amyloid bei Mycosis fungoides nachweisen.

Die *Herkunft* des primären Amyloids ist noch nicht endgültig geklärt, doch machen einerseits elektronenmikroskopische Untersuchungen, andererseits der Nachweis einer Amyloidbildung in Fibroblastenkulturen es sehr wahrscheinlich, daß es im Gewebe an Ort und Stelle zur Entstehung des Amyloids kommt (SCHNEIDER und MISSMAHL, 1966), wobei Fibroblasten anstatt Tropokollagenmolekülen Amyloid bzw. Vorstufen des Amyloids synthetisieren (HASHIMOTO, GROSS und LEVER, 1965).

Für die Herkunft des weitaus häufiger auftretenden und auch experimentell leicht erzeugbaren sekundären Amyloids werden zahlreiche Möglichkeiten diskutiert. Schon frühzeitig wurde auf die Möglichkeit eines immunologischen Geschehens hingewiesen (LETTERER, 1940; LOESCHCKE, 1927). Mit der von KLEIN und BURKHOLDER (1959) angegebenen histoimmunologischen Fluorescenzmethode gelang VOGT und KOCHEM (1960) bei experimenteller Amyloidose, bei Amyloidablagerungen von spontan erkrankten Tieren und bei einem Fall von sekundärer Amyloidose des Menschen der Nachweis eines Antigen-Antikörperpräcipitats im

Amyloid. Diese Befunde und der Nachweis von Gammaglobulin im Bereich der Amyloidablagerungen (VAZQUES, DIXON und NEIL, 1957) machen einen immunologischen Entstehungsmechanismus wenigstens für das experimentelle Amyloid wahrscheinlich. Doch hat erst vor kurzem LETTERER (1964) darauf hingewiesen, daß keineswegs bei jeder Amyloidose eine Immunopathie vorliegt. So spielen Antikörper bei Amyloidose als Folge der multiplen Myelome, bei hereditärer Amyloidose und bei Altersamyloidose sicher keine Rolle.

Nach MISSMAHL (1965) ermöglicht die *polarisationsoptische Untersuchung kongorotgefärbter histologischer Schnitte* nicht nur den sicheren Nachweis einer Amyloidose, sondern auch die Unterscheidung einer periretikulären Form von einer perikollagenen. Auf Grund der Untersuchung von Autopsiefällen mit Amyloidose verschiedenster Genese haben Fälle, die einer klinisch und pathologisch-anatomisch gemeinsamen Gruppe angehören, immer entweder periretikuläres oder perikollagenes Amyloid. Dabei ermöglicht die Rectumbiopsie und polarisationsoptische Untersuchung des kongorotgefärbten Gewebes bereits am Krankenbett den Nachweis der Amyloidose und die Zuordnung zu einer von beiden Formen.

In Tabelle 1 ist das von MISSMAHL (1964) aufgestellte Einteilungsprinzip der Amyloidosen wiedergegeben. Daraus ist zu ersehen, daß die perikollagene Form im wesentlichen der primären Amyloidose entspricht.

Tabelle 1. *Einteilung der Amyloidosen nach* MISSMAHL (1964)

	periretikuläres Amyloid	perikollagenes Amyloid
hereditär	Amyloidose bei familiärem Mittelmeerfieber [a] Amyloidose, mit Urticaria und Taubheit einhergehend [b]	neuropathische familiäre Amyloidosen [d-f] kardiopathische familiäre Amyloidose [g]
erworben	Amyloidose als Folge einer entsprechenden Grundkrankheit	Amyloidose als Folge des multiplen Myeloms
idiopathisch	Amyloidose ohne nachweisbare Grundkrankheit [c]	Amyloidose ohne nachweisbare Grundkrankheit („primäres Amyloid")

[a] MISSMAHL, H. P., J. GAFNI u. E. SOHAR: Harefuah 64, 223 (1963).
[b] MUCKLE, T. J., and M. WELLS: Quart. J. Med. 31, 235 (1962).
[c] BLUM, A., J. GAFNI, E. SOHAR, S. SHIBOLET, and H. HELLER: Ann. intern. Med. 57, 795 (1962).
[d] ANDRADE, C.: Brain 75, 408 (1952).
[e] RUKAVINA, J. G., W. D. BOLCK, C. E. JACKSON, H. J. FALK, J. H. CUREY, and A. C. CURTIS: Medicine (Baltimore) 35, 151 (1958).
[f] SOHAR, E., J. GAFNI, A. BLUM, M. PRAS, and H. HELLER: Quart. J. Med. 32, 211 (1963).
[g] FREDERIKSEN, T., H. GØTZSCHE, H. HARBOE, N. KIAER, and K. MELLEMGARD: Amer. J. Med. 33, 328 (1962).

Die polarisationsoptischen Merkmale der periretikulären und perikollagenen Amyloidose sind von MISSMAHL (1964) ausführlich beschrieben worden: „Bei der *periretikulären Form* der Amyloidose werden die Arteriolen und Capillaren am stärksten befallen. Kleine Venen enthalten in der Regel nur geringe Amyloidablagerungen. In allen diesen Gefäßen erscheinen die ersten, bei Kongorotfärbung polarisationsoptisch erkennbaren Amyloidablagerungen zwischen gekreuzten Polars als feine, grün aufleuchtende Striche unter der Intima bzw. in Organen mit Sinusoiden in den Sinusoidwänden. Das perivasculäre, kollagene Bindegewebe bleibt auch beim Fortschreiten der Erkrankung vom Amyloid frei. Wird in der Leber, der Milz, den Nebennieren und den Glomerula der Nieren Amyloid außerhalb capillärer Strukturen abgelagert, so geschieht dies zunächst entlang präexistenter retikulärer Fasern und dann, das Parenchym verdrängend, auch außerhalb derselben. Bei der *perikollagenen Form* der Amyloidose werden vorwiegend größere Blutgefäße und insbesondere Venen von Amyloid ergriffen. Die ersten Veränderungen sind polarisationsoptisch bei Kongorotfärbung wiederum als feine grüne Striche zu sehen. Das Amyloid liegt nun aber entlang der kollagenen Fasern, welche die Muscularis der Gefäße umgeben. Von hier schreitet die Amyloidose nach innen zu entlang den Sarkolemmen, der Muscularis, nach außen zu teilweise tumorartig entlang dem perivasculären kollagenen Gewebe fort. An der quergestreiften und glatten Muskulatur sowie der Muskulatur des Herzens beginnt diese Form der Amyloidablagerung in den Sarkolemmen, an den Nerven in den Neurilemmen...".

Für die Beschreibung der *Histologie von Amyloidablagerungen* in der Haut des Menschen müssen wir uns hier allerdings auf solche Literaturangaben beschränken, bei denen die Untersuchungen mit den klassischen Färbemethoden durchgeführt wurden.

Im wesentlichen beschränkt sich die Ablagerung des Amyloids auf die obere Cutis. Seltener findet es sich, hauptsächlich an Gefäße gebunden, in den unteren Coriumschichten und in den Fettläppchen der Subcutis.

Die Epidermis zeigt fast immer zumeist sekundär bedingte Veränderungen. Es kommt häufig zur Hyperkeratose, wobei die völlig kernlose Hornschicht das restliche Epithel an Dicke übertreffen kann (GUTMANN, 1928; WINER, 1931). Durch diese starke Verhornung kann die oft beim Lichen amyloidosus klinisch imponierende Transparenz der Knötchen verschwinden. Die Basalzellschichte kann in einzelnen Bezirken eine stärkere Pigmentation zeigen (MARCHIONINI und JOHN, 1935). Bei stark ausgeprägten Fällen kommt es meist zu einer Druckatrophie der Epidermis. Über mächtigen Amyloidschollen kann es auch ganz zum Verlust des Epithels kommen.

Zu Beginn der Infiltration findet sich das Amyloid etwa in Leukocytengröße im Bereich der Papillen, besonders um Capillaren angeordnet. Teilweise wurde auch das Auftreten in Gebilden beschrieben, die eventuell der Form und Größe nach als Zellen angesprochen werden könnten und an manchen Stellen sogar Kernreste und Zellmembran erkennen ließen (NOMLAND, 1936). Besonders beim Lichen amyloidosus bleibt die Ablagerung auf den oberen Teil der Papille beschränkt (FREUDENTHAL, 1930; MARCHIONINI und JOHN, 1935; WINER, 1931). Bei anderen klinischen Manifestationen ist das Amyloid wieder in Form eines schmalen, bandförmigen Streifens eingelagert bzw. kann es überhaupt zu einer diffusen Infiltration des Coriums kommen (GABRIEL u. LINDEMAYR, 1957; STREITMANN, 1965).

Am deutlichsten ist das Amyloid in der stark verdickten Media der Arteriolen zu erkennen. Zumeist ist es in gleicher Stärke fortlaufend eingelagert und nur in manchen Fällen wechselt die Intensität der Einlagerung, wodurch rosenkranzartige Auftreibungen entstehen. Ähnliche Verhältnisse finden sich auch bei den venösen Gefäßen. Auf jeden Fall wird das Amyloid in die glatten Muskelzellen eingelagert, die elastischen Fasern der Gefäßwand bleiben jedoch unverändert. So kann man auch bei gänzlichem Verschluß eines Gefäßes den Ring der Elastica sehen (KÖNIGSTEIN, 1932). Bei den Capillaren ist das Amyloid direkt an das Endothelrohr angelagert (GOTTRON, 1932). Die Intima der Gefäße wird nur in seltenen Fällen ergriffen (IVERSON und MORRISON, 1948), doch findet sich manchmal eine auffällige Vorwölbung des Amyloids gegen das Gefäßlumen. Oft sieht man zahlreiche, weit klaffende Gefäße mit hohem Endothel, wobei nicht zu unterscheiden ist, ob es sich hier um eine vermehrte Schlängelung oder eine echte Gefäßvermehrung handelt (WEYHBRECHT, 1952). Manchmal ist auch eine Proliferation von perithelialen Zellen zu sehen, wodurch es zur Bildung zahlreicher Gefäßknäuel kommt, die an umschriebene angiomatöse Bildungen erinnern. Hin und wieder, meist unmittelbar unter dem Epithel, finden sich perivasculär Rundzellinfiltrate mit Fremdkörperriesenzellen (PEARSON, RICE und DICKENS, 1941; KONRAD, 1936; LAWLESS, 1936). In der Umgebung der Gefäße und auch um die abgelagerten Amyloidschollen sind die Mastzellen deutlich vermehrt (GOTTRON, 1932; DEGOS, DELORT und HEWITT, 1951; WEYHBRECHT, 1952). Gleichzeitig sieht man zahlreiche extravasale Erythrocytenansammlungen, die klinisch als Purpuraherde imponieren.

Von SCHILDER (1909) wurde eine Ablagerung des Amyloids im Bereiche der Talg- und Schweißdrüsen der Kopfhaut und Achselhöhlen beschrieben. Dabei ist wieder eine gewisse Beziehung zu den die Drüsen umgebenden elastischen Fasern auffällig. Es kommt nämlich zu einer Ablagerung zwischen dem Epithel der Haarbälge und Talgdrüsen und den angrenzenden elastischen Fasern. Ähnliches findet man auch bei den Schweißdrüsen. Erst bei starker Zunahme der amyloiden Infiltration kommt es zu einer Druckatrophie der elastischen Elemente, so daß schließlich die sezernierenden Drüsenendstücke von einem dicken Amyloidmantel umgeben sind. Die Drüsenepithelien werden aber dadurch nicht verändert.

Eine auffallende und regelmäßig wiederkehrende Lagebeziehung besteht zwischen den Amyloidablagerungen und den Haarfollikeln. Als spindelförmige bis zylindrische Hüllen von wechselnder Dicke liegen sie der äußeren Wurzelscheide an, von der sie nur durch die Glashaut getrennt sind. Diese Einscheidungen reichen meist von der Haarpapille bis in die Höhe der Talgdrüseneinmündung, mitunter auch höher (NÖDL und ZAUN, 1964). Durch den Druck der hyperkeratotischen Epidermis einerseits und der eingelagerten Amyloidsubstanz andererseits kann es auch zur Zerstörung des Follikels kommen. Um das Haarüberbleibsel kann sich dann ein Fremdkörperriesenzellgranulom entwickeln (MASCHKILLEISSON, 1930). Stellenweise sind jedoch überhaupt nur mehr Reste einer bindegewebigen Umhüllung zu sehen und lediglich der M. arrector sowie eine Anhäufung bizarr geformter elastischer Fasern zeigen im Verein mit den vertikalen Amyloidstreifen die einstige Lage des Follikels an (NÖDL und ZAUN, 1964).

In der Gitterfaserdarstellung nach PAP tritt im Bereiche der Ablagerung ein dichtes Fasergeflecht hervor, dessen Schwärzung oft schwächer als normal ist. Nicht nur innerhalb, auch in der unmittelbaren Umgebung der Amyloidablagerung trifft man diese Fasern, die gestaltlich und färberisch Übergänge zum kollagenen Bindegewebe aufweisen, in ungewöhnlicher Dichte und Reichhaltigkeit an (NÖDL und ZAUN, 1964).

Die kollagenen Fasern sind verbreitert, gequollen und wenig gewellt (GOTTRON, 1932). Die elastischen Fasern sind besonders im Stratum papillare knäuelförmig zusammengeballt, sonst sind sie teilweise zerstückelt und zeigen einen körnigen Zerfall. Es handelt sich dabei um druckatrophische Veränderungen.

In der Subcutis kann man neben den Amyloidablagerungen in den Wänden von Blutgefäßen auch sog. Amyloidringe finden, die durch die Ablagerung von Amyloid um einzelne Fettzellen herum entstehen (LEVER, 1958). Innerhalb der einzelnen Fettläppchen nimmt die Intensität der Ablagerung vom Rande gegen das Zentrum zu ab (GANS und STEIGLEDER, 1955).

Eine genauere Nachprüfung mit modernen Hilfsmitteln (Elektronenmikroskopie und Polarisationsmikroskopie) erfordern die Angaben über eine sekundäre Hautamyloidose (FREUDENTHAL, 1930; MALAK und SMITH, 1962). Letztere Autoren fanden bei 10,9% der untersuchten Hautepitheliome im Tumorstroma Amyloidablagerungen. Sie vermuten, daß eine Antigenwirkung des Tumors zur Amyloidablagerung im Stroma führt.

II. Hyalin

Von v. RECKLINGHAUSEN wird unter Hyalin eine Gruppe von Substanzen verstanden, deren wichtigste Gemeinsamkeit die gleichen optischen Eigenschaften und die Neigung, sich mit sauren Farbstoffen anzufärben, ist. Das starke Lichtbrechungsvermögen des Hyalins gleicht dem Amyloid, es gibt aber im Gegensatz zu diesem keine Jodreaktion, keine Metachromasiereaktion usw. (s. Amyloid).

Unter pathologischen Verhältnissen tritt Hyalin vor allem in Form von Kugeln oder verästelten Bälkchen auf; es ist undurchsichtig, stark glänzend und löst sich nicht in Wasser, Alkohol, schwachen Säuren und Basen, ist jedoch löslich in starker Kalilauge, Salzsäure und Pepsin. Hyalin färbt sich mit allen sauren Anilinfarben, nimmt aber auch Kernfarbstoffe mehr oder minder gut an (SCHMORL, 1925).

Was im Schrifttum von verschiedener Seite als Hyalin bezeichnet wird, ist allerdings durchaus nicht einheitlich. Nach ROULET (1948) wird Hyalin als eine besondere Bindegewebsumwandlung definiert, die einerseits durch Quellung der Bindegewebsfasern und wahrscheinlich andererseits durch gleichzeitige Durchtränkung mit Plasmaeiweiß entsteht. LUBARSCH (1882) unterscheidet ein epitheliales, sekretorisch entstandenes und ein bindegewebiges Hyalin; letzteres wird auch als Hyalinisierung, also als eine Zustandsänderung des Bindegewebes, bezeichnet. Wie die Untersuchungen von MÜLLER (1936) ergaben, lassen sich beim bindegewebigen Hyalin zwei Komponenten unterscheiden: eine hauptsächlichere mit Fasereigenschaften wie Kollagen, die allerdings trypsinresistent ist, und eine weitere Komponente, die durch Trypsin gespalten wird und sich wahrscheinlich aus globulären Serumeiweißkomponenten aufbaut. Auch neuere, elektronenoptische Untersuchungen sprechen dafür (RATZENHOFER und SCHAUENSTEIN, 1951; SCHAUENSTEIN und RUMPF, 1952; PROBST, 1956, 1957).

RATZENHOFER und PROBST (1953, 1957) fanden, daß die Hyalinisierung einen sehr eingreifenden Prozeß des Bindegewebes darstellt. Es gelingt mit den gewöhnlichen Methoden nicht, die Fibrillen aus den hyalinen Massen zu isolieren. Erst wenn man die sehr widerstandsfähige Grundsubstanz durch langdauernde Trypsinverdauung entfernt hat, sieht man Fibrillen, welche in sehr großer Menge im Hyalin vorhanden sind. Sie verhalten sich wie normale Kollagenfibrillen und zeigen die typische Struktur.

Die beigefügte Tabelle 2 gibt einen Überblick über das histochemische Verhalten von Hyalin, gleichzeitig die Unterscheidung zwischen bindegewebigem Hyalin und Gefäßhyalin sowie Gefäßfibrinoid, bindegewebigem Fibrinoid und Fibrin (Tabelle 2). Diese Untersuchung ist schon deshalb interessant, da sich Gefäßfibrinoid und Gefäßhyalin tinktoriell und histochemisch sehr ähnlich verhalten. Alle diese Substanzen färben sich eosinophil mit Hämatoxylin-Eosin und zeigen eine negative Reaktion mit Mucicarmin und nach FEULGEN (MONTGOMERY und MUIRHEAD, 1957).

Für eine dermatologische Histologie ist noch ein weiteres Faktum zu berücksichtigen. In der allgemeinen Pathologie werden alle transparenten, strukturlosen, homogenen Eiweißsubstanzen, die epithelialer Herkunft sind, als epitheliales Hyalin oder Kolloid bezeichnet. Als Hyalin im engeren Sinne (conjunctivales Hyalin) werden Gebilde bezeichnet, die aus dem Bindegewebe entstehen. Chemisch gesehen sind beide keine einheitlichen Körper. Ihr färberischer Unterschied liegt z.B. darin, daß sich bindegewebiges Hyalin bei van Gieson-Färbung leuchtend rot anfärbt, während sich das weniger acidophile Kolloid meist gelb darstellt. Im Hinblick auf die grundlegenden Arbeiten von UNNA werden derartige Umwandlungsprodukte der Bindegewebsfasern als Kolloid bezeichnet, da sie ja vor allen Dingen aus den kollagenen Fasern entstehen. Nach GANS (1957) sollte diese Terminologie — auf Grund der Unnaschen Ansicht, daß Kolloid vornehmlich aus dem leimgebenden Gewebe entsteht — beibehalten werden.

Nach derzeitiger Ansicht ist also diese bindegewebige Hyalinbildung als eine pathologische Neukombination von Inhalt des Bindegewebes und von Serumbestandteilen anzusehen. Dementsprechend kann nicht von einer „Ablagerung" dieser Substanz im eigentlichen Sinne gesprochen werden. Im Bereiche der Cutis kommt es bei den verschiedensten krankhaften Zuständen zur bindegewebigen Hyalinbildung. Dies ist im Rahmen dieses Handbuches im Kapitel über pathologische Veränderungen an Grundsubstanz, Kollagen und Elastica (Band I/2) von BRAUN-FALCO abgehandelt worden.

Tabelle 2. *Histochemische Reaktionen*

Material	Färbungen und						
	Mallory's Bindegewebsfärbung	Masson's Trichromfärbung	Ölrot 0	Nilblau-Sulfat	Sudan Schwarz B	Schultzsche Färbung	Kongorot
Fibrin	rot	rot	0	0	0	±	+
Bindegewebiges Fibrinoid	rot	rot	0	0	0	0	0
Gefäßfibrinoid	rot	rot	++++	++++ Blau	++++	+++	++
Gefäßhyalin	rot	rot	++++	++++ Blau	++++	+++	++
Bindegwebiges Hyalin	blau	grün	0	0	0	0	0

(Entnommen der Arbeit von MONTGOMERY und MUIRHEAD)

Im folgenden sollen zwei Krankheiten, die durch das Auftreten hyalinähnlicher Substanzen in der Cutis ihren Namen haben, ausführlicher besprochen werden, insbesondere da bei diesen Erkrankungen auch die Möglichkeit der Ablagerungen von Eiweißkörpern aus dem Serum diskutiert wird.

1. Hyalinosis cutis et mucosae Urbach-Wiethe (Lipoidproteinose)

Man versteht darunter eine seltene, wahrscheinlich recessiv vererbbare Dermatose, die sich *klinisch* in papulösen und hyperkeratotischen, auch albopapuloiden (LEINBROCK, 1960) Veränderungen an Haut und Schleimhaut äußert. Über das anatomische Substrat besteht nach den bisherigen Publikationen keine einheitliche Auffassung. Gerade nach den zuletzt erschienenen Arbeiten, die zum Großteil klinisch und histologisch sehr genau untersuchte Fälle betreffen, hat man den Eindruck, daß größere Verschiedenheiten besonders in Hinblick auf das färberische Verhalten der veränderten Gewebe vorkommen können.

Das drückt sich auch in der bisher noch nicht einheitlichen Nomenklatur dieser Erkrankung aus. WIETHE (1924) faßt die abgelagerten Massen als Hyalin auf und prägte daher den Begriff „Hyalinose". URBACH (1929), der als erster genaue histochemische Untersuchungen angestellt hat, fand reichlich Lipide in den abgelagerten Substanzen, reihte sie in die Gruppe der Lipoidosen ein und bezeichnete sie als „Lipoidproteinose". Die Bezeichnung Lipoidproteinose ist allerdings später wieder zugunsten der ersteren Bezeichnung Hyalinose fallen gelassen worden (LUNDT, 1949). Andere glaubten jedoch, den Lipoidreichtum der Veränderungen nicht ganz außer acht lassen zu dürfen und kehrten wieder zum Begriff der Lipoidproteinose zurück (EBERHARTINGER und NIEBAUER, 1959; McCUSKER und CAPLAN, 1962; MARAGNANI, 1961) bzw. haben den Namen Lipoglykoproteinose vorgeschlagen.

Bei diesem Leiden kommt es zur Ablagerung homogener, schwach eosinophiler Massen vor allem im Bereiche um die Gefäße und Schweißdrüsen der Cutis. In der Hämalaun-Eosin-Färbung erscheinen die Einlagerungen blaßrosa, in der Färbung nach VAN GIESON intensiv gelb, in der nach MALLORY rot, mit Elastica-Farbstoffen können sie nicht angefärbt werden. Typische Amyloidreaktionen werden nicht gesehen. Metachromasie wird nicht oder nur in geringem Maße beobachtet. Auch der Ausfall der Proteinreaktionen wird nicht einheitlich angegeben, so daß auf einen unterschiedlichen Proteingehalt der abgelagerten Massen geschlossen werden kann. Großes Interesse fand seit URBACH (1929) das Verhalten der Fettfärbungen. Auch hier ist offenbar eine große Variabilität anzunehmen,

für Fibrin, Fibrinoid und Hyalin

Reaktionen								
Xantho-protein-reaktion	Indol-reaktion	Reaktion auf freie Carbonyl-gruppen nach ASHBEL u. SELIGMAN	Millon-Reaktion	Nachweis von Calcium	PAS am Gefrier-Schnitt	PAS am Paraffin-Schnitt	Nachweis von eiweißgebundenen SH-Gruppen nach BARRNETT u. SELIGMAN	Kalium-Nachweis
+++	+++	0	+++	++++	+++	+	+	+
+++	+++	0	+++	++++	+++	±	0	±
0	0	+++	±	±	+++	+	++	+++
0	0	+++	±	±	+++	±	++	+++
0	0	0	0	±	±	0	±	0

denn neben massiven Fettablagerungen werden in manchen Fällen nur wenige oder gar keine Lipide gefunden. Freies Cholesterin scheint nicht vorzukommen, jedoch wurden bei einigen Fällen Cholesterinesterverbindungen gefunden. Allerdings muß in diesem Zusammenhang noch bedacht werden, ob das Auftreten von Lipiden nicht bloß sekundärer Natur ist. Ähnlich verhält es sich mit den Kohlenhydraten, deren histochemischer Nachweis verschieden stark ausfällt. Zur richtigen Interpretation der histochemischen und biochemischen Befunde muß allerdings berücksichtigt werden, daß sich auch bei gleichen Patienten die hyalinen Massen je nach Art und Alter der Läsionen chemisch und färberisch variabel verhalten (BAZEX, 1939; GROSFELD und SPAAS, 1964; IZAKI HORIUCHI und HOZAKI, 1954; LANDI und NEGRI, 1962; RASIEWICZ, RUBISZ-BRZEZINSKA und KONECKI, 1965; WEYHBRECHT und KORTING, 1954; WILE und SNOW, 1941; WISE und REIN, 1930; WOLMAN, 1964; WOOD, URBACH und BEERMANN, 1956). In dieser Beziehung sind vor allen Dingen die Nachuntersuchung eines Urbachschen Falles von KATZENELLENBOGEN und UNGAR (1957) interessant. Wohl sicher kommt es in den abgelagerten Massen im Laufe der Zeit (die Krankheit verläuft durch Jahrzehnte) zu chemischen Veränderungen und Umwandlungen. Vielleicht lassen sich dadurch die widersprechenden Resultate in der Literatur erklären.

Chemische Analysen excidierter Gewebsstücke der Veränderungen wurden verschiedentlich angestellt. Auch hier konnten nur sehr unterschiedliche Befunde erhoben werden. Dies könnte allerdings auch durch die technische Schwierigkeit derartiger Methoden zu erklären sein (POTTER und WEINSTEIN, 1959; RAMOS e SILVA, 1947; HOLTZ und SCHULZE, 1950/51; MONTGOMERY und HAVENS, 1939; WILE und SNOW, 1941).

Hinsichtlich der *Pathogenese* und der *Herkunft der hyalinen Massen*, die sich bei diesem Leiden in der Cutis finden, besteht keine einheitliche Ansicht. Eine Reihe von Autoren stellt das lokale Geschehen in den Vordergrund. Sie meinen, daß es sich primär um einen degenerativen Prozeß des Bindegewebes handelt und daß Veränderungen des Serumeiweißes erst sekundär auftreten (BAZEX und DUPRE, 1964; J. CALVET u. Mitarb., 1962; EBERHARTINGER und NIEBAUER, 1959; HEYL und DE KOCK, 1964; MIEDZINSKI und KOZAKIEWICZ, 1957; SZODORAY, 1941; KATZENELLENBOGEN und UNGAR, 1957). Andere jedoch sind der Ansicht, daß die abgelagerten Substanzen aus dem Blutstrom stammen, wofür vor allem das Auftreten der hyalinen Massen um die Gefäße und eine gewisse Ähnlichkeit mit der Amyloidose, bzw. Paramyloidose sprechen würde (BRAUN und WEYHBRECHT, 1952; HÄNIG und KREMER, 1955; KATAOKA, YAMAGATA und UEDA, 1954; LAYMON und HILL, 1957; WEYHBRECHT und KORTING, 1954; HOLTZ und SCHULZE, 1950/51). Neure Publikationen weisen darauf hin, daß sich die Lipoidproteinose und die erythropoetische Porphyrie im klinischen Bild überschneiden können. Die Lokalisation der Hautveränderungen ist allerdings etwas verschieden, insofern bei letzterer Erkrankung vor allem die lichtexponierten Hautstellen befallen sind (HORNSTEIN u. KLINGMÜLLER, 1961; FINDLAY, SCOTT und CRIPPS, 1964).

2. Pseudomilium colloidale (Pellizari)

Diese als selbständige Hauterkrankung anzusehende Veränderung wird auch als „Colloidmilium" (WAGNER), „Colloidome miliaire "(BESNIER), „Hyalom" (VIDAL-LELOIR), „Dégénérescence colloid du derme" (BESNIER und BALZER), „Conjunctivom mit hyaliner Degeneration" (MILIAN), „Elastosis colloidalis conglomerata" (FERREIRA-MARQUES und VAN UDEN, 1950) bezeichnet. Sie ist gekennzeichnet durch Auftreten kleiner, gelblicher bis bräunlicher, durchsichtiger Knötchen vor allem im Gesicht, besonders an der Stirne, aber auch an anderen chronisch aktinisch belasteten Regionen. Wenn sich statt Knötchen größere Herde bilden, so werden diese von REUTER und BECKER (1942) als „kolloide Degeneration der Haut" bezeichnet. Verschiedentlich wird eine seltenere, juvenile, und eine häufigere, im Erwachsenenalter erworbene Form unterschieden (ANDREWS, BOSELLINI). PERCIVAL und DUTHIE (1948) unterscheiden zwischen: 1. Juveniler Form mit familiärem Vorkommen, 2. Auftreten bei Erwachsenen ohne familiäres Vorkommen, gewöhnlich kombiniert mit seniler Elastose, 3. seniler Elastose und kolloidaler Degeneration, wobei eine zweifelhafte direkte ätiologische Beziehung zueinander besteht und 4. anderen Dermatosen mit sekundären kolloiden Veränderungen.

Das pathologische Substrat dieser Erkrankung sind umschriebene, kolloide Massen im oberen Corium, die sich mit Hämatoxylin-Eosin gewöhnlich eosinophil anfärben, allerdings meist schwächer als das eigentliche Kollagen. PRAKKEN (1951) beobachtete, daß der Bildung des Kolloidmiliums eine basophile Degeneration des Kollagens vorausgeht, so daß in den Anfangsstadien die kolloide Masse auch schwach basophil sein kann. Von der Epidermis ist das homogen erscheinende Kolloid durch eine schmale Zone normalen Kollagens getrennt. Das Kolloid enthält eine mäßige Zahl von Kernen. Elastische Fasern sind in der Kolloidmasse vorhanden, jedoch aufgesplittert und gegenüber dem normalen Bindegewebe rarefiziert. Die großen Spalträume sind zum Teil Fixierungsartefakte. Nach VAN GIESON färben sich die kolloidalen Massen gelb; eine spezifische histologische Nachweismethode gibt es allerdings nicht (weitere histochemische Befunde s. den Handbuchbeitrag von BRAUN-FALCO, 1964).

Die Frage, ob es sich beim Pseudomilium colloidale um ein Degenerationsprodukt der kollagenen (PRAKKEN, 1951) oder der elastischen Fasern handelt (letztere Meinung wird vor allem von FERREIRA-MARQUES und VAN UDEN, 1950, vertreten), ist allerdings nicht entschieden. Nach GANS und STEIGLEDER ist es wohl am wahrscheinlichsten, daß dieses Kolloid keine völlig einheitliche Substanz ist und daß es sowohl vom Kollagen als auch vom Elastin stammen kann.

Im Gegensatz zur herkömmlichen Auffassung, daß die kolloiden Massen nur von ortsständigen Materialien stammen, steht die von ZOON, JANSEN und HOVENKAMP (1955) geäußerte Ansicht. Diese Autoren vermuten, daß das „Kolloid" weder aus der Elastica noch aus dem Kollagen entsteht, sondern daß es durch pathologisch veränderte Blutgefäße aus dem Serum ausgeschieden wird. In diesem Sinne spricht das Ergebnis der Papierchromatographie eines derartigen Gewebeextraktes. Es fanden sich Aminosäuren, die weder in der Elastica, noch im Kollagen vorkommen. Auch BECKER und WILSON (1956) konnten eine Identität der Aminosäurezusammensetzung der kolloiden Hautveränderungen und des Serums finden, während wesentliche Unterschiede gegenüber dem Kollagen und dem Material der elastischen Fasern bestehen. Daß hier in der Hauptsache eine

Ablagerung und nicht ein Degenerationsprodukt vorliegt, wurde schon vorher von PERCIVAL und DUTHIE (1948), sowie von TOSTI (1953) angenommen. Doch konnte ZAUN (1966) bei dem von ihm beschriebenen Fall keine Dysproteinämie feststellen, weshalb er folgert, daß zumindest bei einem Teil der Pseudomilium colloidale-Fälle die kolloide Substanz nicht von Serumproteinen hergeleitet sein kann. Aber die Frage der Herkunft der kolloiden Substanz ist derzeit noch offen, zumal die Methoden derartiger Analysen technisch nicht völlig ausreichend sind. Zweifellos sind für die Pathogenese dieser Erkrankung sowohl die familiäre Disposition als auch die chronisch aktinische Hautschädigung von großer Bedeutung (PRAKKEN, 1951; ARRIGHI, 1955; ALLISON-ALLISON, 1957; TORRES, RADICE, VILLAFANE und VACCARO, 1957; GUIN und SEALE, 1959; COSTE, PIGUET und DELBARRE, 1960; HOLZBERGER, 1960; BECK und WIFLING, 1960; HELM, 1962).

Auch elektronenoptische Untersuchungen haben bisher die Frage nach der Herkunft des kolloiden Materials nicht klären können (PIREDDA, 1958). Hingegen haben historöntgenographische (mikroradiographische) Untersuchungen den eindeutigen Beweis erbracht, daß zwischen der sog. „hyalinen Homogenisierung" bei aktinischer (seniler) Elastose und dem Substrat der Kolloidmilien ein grundsätzlicher Unterschied besteht. Bei seniler Elastose ist die Röntgenstrahlenabsorption in der Zone der Homogenisierung im Vergleich zum normalen cutanen Bindegewebe stark reduziert (TOSTI und FAZZINI, 1962; NIEBAUER und STOCKINGER, 1965), es nimmt also in diesem Bereich die Gewebsdichte ab. Hingegen ist die kolloide Substanz der Kolloidmilien von außerordentlich starker Röntgenstrahlenabsorption; sie liegt sogar über der Absorption durch Hornsubstanz (TOSTI und FAZZINI, 1962; TOSTI, 1964). Somit ist das Kolloidmilium durch eine Zunahme der Gewebsdichte charakterisiert, die am wahrscheinlichsten durch Ablagerung proteinhaltigen Materials erklärt wird, während bei „aktinischer Elastose" die Gewebsdichte abnimmt, obgleich das färberisch-histologische Bild derartige Vorgänge und Unterschiede nicht vermuten ließe.

Diese sog. *„aktinische Elastose"* wird auch als Altersdegeneration der Haut („Elastosis senilis") bezeichnet. Aber nicht das Altern an sich, sondern die chronische Lichtschädigung der Haut führt zu diesem Zustand (LUND und SOMMERVILLE, 1957; SMITH und LANSING, 1959; SMITH jr., 1963; NIEBAUER, 1965). Die aktinische Elastose entwickelt sich im Laufe des Lebens nur an den freigetragenen Körperstellen, und zwar um so stärker und früher, je mehr diese Menschen der Einwirkung des Lichtes ausgesetzt waren und je pigmentärmer sie sind (ELLER und ELLER, 1951).

Von der meist atrophischen Epidermis durch einen dünnen Streifen elasticafreien Gewebes getrennt liegt im oberen Drittel des Coriums ein Gewirr von plumpen, vielfach gewundenen Fasern, das in einem späteren Stadium über verklumpte und fragmentierte Formen zu einem scholligen und schließlich amorphen Material zusammensintert. Bei Färbung mit Hämatoxylin-Eosin nehmen die beschriebenen Strukturen das Hämatoxylin an, sie färben sich bläulich (basophil) durch ihre Affinität zum basischen Farbstoff. Bei Färbung mit Resorcin-Fuchsin oder Orcein färben sie sich „wie elastisches Gewebe", d.h., sie verhalten sich fuchselinophil bzw. orceinophil. Bei Färbung nach VAN GIESON sind die gleichen Bezirke gelb. Die Orceinophilie und Fuchselinophilie der aktinischen Elastose wird durch Hyaluronidase nicht verändert, sie wird aber durch Vorbehandlung der Schnitte mit Elastase verhindert (SAMS und SMITH, 1961). Dieser Befund ist für das Substrat Elastin allerdings nicht beweisend, da das Enzym Elastase auch Mucoproteine angreift (sog. „Mucinase") (HALL, REED und TUNBRIDGE, 1952). Auch die sog. Elastica-Farbstoffe sind nicht spezifisch für das Protein Elastin. Vielmehr färben sie das interfibrilläre Kittmaterial der elastischen Fasern (BAHR und HUHN, 1952; SCHWARZ und DETTMER, 1953; LANSING, 1954).

Letztlich muß aber doch aus diesen und zahlreichen anderen histochemischen und physikalischen Befunden (s. BRAUN-FALCO, 1964; NIEBAUER und STOCKINGER, 1965) gefolgert werden, daß die elastotischen Bezirke aus chemisch ähnlichen Bausteinen zusammengesetzt sind wie das elastische Gewebe der normalen Haut. Die Basophilie spricht für die Anwesenheit saurer Gruppen in diesem Bereich. Das elastotische Gewebe verhält sich PAS-positiv (Montgomery, 1955; Winer, 1955; Braun-Falco, 1956; Steiner, 1957), wobei mit Zunahme der Degeneration die Reaktion auch stärker ausfällt. Gleichsinnig färben sich diese Zonen mit Toluidinblau intensiv orthochromatisch und mit Alcianblau, Hale oder Astrablau stark positiv (Percival, Hannay und Duthie, 1949; Braun-Falco, 1956; Sams jr. und Smith, 1961; Sams jr. und Davidson, 1962). Demnach enthalten diese Zonen vermehrt neutrale und saure Mucopolysaccharide, die im Rahmen des aktinisch bedingten Degenerationsprozesses aus der Kittsubstanz freigesetzt werden. Diese Annahme von Mucopolysacchariden in der Zone der aktinischen Elastose hat sich durch Messen des Hexosamingehaltes auch biochemisch bestätigen lassen (Smith jr., Davidson, Tindall und Sams, 1961). Somit besteht chemisch und physikalisch eine sehr große Ähnlichkeit zwischen normalem Elastin und dem Substrat der aktinischen Elastose. Auf Grund lichtoptischer Befunde besteht kein Zweifel darüber, daß die pathischen Strukturen der degenerativen „senilen" Atrophie der Haut eindeutige Übergänge in die normal geformten elastischen Fasern erkennen lassen (Feyrter u. Niebauer, 1966).

Da es aber kaum vorstellbar ist, daß im Rahmen einer degenerativen Atrophie das biologisch nur wenig aktive elastische Gewebe durch Proliferation derart an Masse zunimmt, wird von einigen Autoren für das Zustandekommen der aktinischen Elastose eine Degeneration und Umwandlung des kollagenen Gewebes verantwortlich gemacht (Percival, Hannay und Duthie, 1949; Tunbridge, Tattersall, Hall, Astbury und Reed, 1952; Gillman, Penn, Bronks und Roux, 1955; Montgomery, 1955; Winer, 1955; Steiner, 1957). In diesem Sinne sprechen auch die Befunde der Historöntgenographie (Niebauer und Stockinger, 1965); sie demonstrieren, daß bei der aktinischen Elastose die Gewebsdichte abnimmt, eine Beobachtung, die nur durch eine Abnahme des Totalgehaltes an Bindegewebe zu erklären ist. Weiters zeigen die elektronenoptischen Ergebnisse von Niebauer u. Mitarb., daß bei aktinischer Elastose *primär* eine Schädigung des kollagenen Fasermaterials vorliegt, die zum Abbau und zur Auflösung der Fasern führt.

III. Mucin

Allgemein wird heute die lichtoptisch homogene Komponente der Intercellularsubstanz als „Grundsubstanz" bezeichnet (Maximow, 1927). Sie füllt als Kontinuum die Räume zwischen Zellfasern und Gefäßen, ist normalerweise eine hochviscöse Flüssigkeit und stellt ein weitgehend unorientiertes System von Mucopolysacchariden und Skleroproteinen in wechselndem Polymerisationsgrad dar (Robb-Smith, 1954). Zellen, Fasern und Grundsubstanz bilden eine funktionelle Einheit (Horstmann, 1957). In den letzten Jahrzehnten war diese Bindegewebsgrundsubstanz Gegenstand zahlreicher Untersuchungen und wurde so von einem „abstrakten" Begriff zu einer Realität (Graumann, 1964). Entscheidende Schritte auf diesem Wege waren die Entdeckung der „spreading factors" (Duran-Reynals, McLean), die fortschreitende Aufklärung der chemischen Zusammensetzung von Bindegewebsbausteinen, insbesondere der Mucopolysaccharide (Meyer), die Isolierung der Hyaluronidase (Meyer), die Identifizierung der Hyaluronidaseaktivität mit den spreading factors (Chain und Duthie) und die Einführung der Perjodat-Leukofuchsinmethode in die histologische Technik (McManus, Lillie, Hotchkiss).

Allgemein gelten als wesentliche *Bausteine* die sog. Mucoproteide (Mucopolysaccharid-Proteinkomplexe). Ihre chemische Ähnlichkeit mit den „Schleimstoffen" ist seit langem bekannt (VIRCHOW, 1852; ROLLET, 1871; MAXIMOW, 1927). Nach LETTERER (1932) empfiehlt es sich jedoch, die Bezeichnung „Schleim mesenchymaler Herkunft" zu vermeiden und vom Schleim nur bei Produkten epithelialer Genese zu sprechen (SYLVÉN, 1945; GRAUMANN, 1964). Immerhin wird gerade im dermatologischen Schrifttum gelegentlich der Begriff „Schleimablagerung" für das vermehrte Auftreten von Mucoproteiden („Mucin") verwendet. Während über die Proteinfraktion noch wenig bekannt ist, konnte durch histochemische und biochemische Untersuchungen die Polysaccharidkomponente genauer definiert werden. Ihre Bausteine sind vor allem Hyaluronsäure und Chondroitinsulfate. Beide sind hochpolymer und enthalten Hexosamin und Glucuronsäure. Hyaluronsäure enthält äquimolekular N-Acetyl-Glucosamin und d-Glucuronsäure, die Chondroitin-Schwefelsäure hingegen N-Acetyl-d-Galaktosamin, d-Glucuronsäure und Schwefelsäure (WATSON und PEARCE, 1947a, b, 1949; BRAUN-FALCO, 1954). Da die Hyaluronsäure stark hygroskopisch ist, ist sie vor allem für den Flüssigkeitsgehalt der amorphen Grundsubstanz verantwortlich und verleiht ihr den gelartigen Charakter. Besonders das junge, undifferenzierte Bindegewebe hat einen hohen Wassergehalt (BENSLEY, 1934). Das Wasser selbst liegt in gebundener, nicht in freier Form vor, so daß bei den sog. Mucinosen (Krankheiten, bei denen das Mucin in der Haut besonders vermehrt ist) in der Regel keine „eindrückbaren Ödeme" bestehen.

Woher die Mucopolysaccharide stammen, ist nicht sicher. Es werden mehrere Möglichkeiten diskutiert. Sicher ist jedenfalls, daß die Haut selbst zur Synthese von Hexosamin, dem allen Mucopolysacchariden gemeinsamen Baustein, fähig ist (WEBER, 1958). Die meisten Autoren nehmen an, daß Mucopolysaccharide genauso wie das Kollagen von den Fibroblasten sezerniert werden (Fibroblastentheorie). Dafür spricht schon die Beobachtung, daß vor allem junges, fetales Bindegewebe reichlich Mucopolysaccharide enthält und daß die Fibroblastenaktivität mit einer Anreicherung von Schleimsubstanzen einhergeht. Auch experimentell erhobene Befunde in der Gewebekultur von Fibroblasten sprechen dafür (TRYB, 1923; KREIBICH, 1927; GERSH und CATCHPOLE, 1949; BOLLET, BOAS und BONIN, 1954; CURRAN und KENNEDY, 1955; GROSSFELD u. Mitarb., 1955, 1957; NODA, 1965).

Eine spezialisiertere Meinung hinsichtlich der Bildung von Mucopolysacchariden stammt unter anderem von ASBOE-HANSEN. Er vermutet, daß die Gewebsmastzellen außer Heparin und Histamin auch Hyaluronsäure produzieren. Diese Annahme beruht auf der nachgewiesenen Vermehrung von Mastzellen bei myxödematösen Veränderungen der Haut, wobei sich die Zahl der Mastzellen proportional dem Grad der Metachromasie verhält. Der Autor nimmt an, daß die Mastzellen Vorstufen sowohl des gerinnungshemmenden Schwefelpolysaccharids Heparin als auch der nicht gerinnungshemmenden Hyaluronsäure sezernieren (ASBOE-HANSEN, 1950a u. b, 1954, 1956). Diese Meinungen blieben jedoch nicht unwidersprochen, teils aus prinzipiellen Überlegungen (BURKL, 1952; WEISSMANN und MEYER, 1952, 1954; TAYLOR und SAUNDERS, 1957; MEYER, 1960; NIEBAUER, 1960), teilweise auf Grund von Befunden bei Mucinosen, bei denen eine Mastzellvermehrung nicht nachgewiesen wurde (MONTGOMERY und UNDERWOOD, 1953; TAPPEINER, 1955; KEINING und BRAUN-FALCO, 1956; BRAUN-FALCO, 1957a; WODNIANSKY, 1957). Sicher besteht jedoch die Ansicht zu Recht, daß eine gewisse Beziehung zwischen Mastzellen und Bindegewebsstoffwechsel besteht, jedoch mehr im Sinne einer regulierenden als einer produzierenden Funktion (z.B. Beeinflussung des Bindegewebsstoffwechsels mit dem Mastzellenprodukt Heparin, NIEBAUER, 1960) (s. auch Schema 3).

Schließlich wird die Möglichkeit des humoralen Antransportes saurer Mucopolysaccharide diskutiert (RENAUT, 1903, 1903/04; HIERONYMI, 1954; SCHALLOCK und LINDNER, 1957). Blut enthält ja sicher saure Mucopolysaccharide (WINZLER, 1957), die bei verschiedenen Mucinosen erheblich vermehrt sein können.

Solche Erhöhungen fanden beim Lichen myxoedematosus TAPPEINER (1955), EBERHARTINGER und EBNER (1965), beim prätibialen Myxödem WODNIANSKY (1957), beim Skleromyxödem KEINING und BRAUN-FALCO (1956) sowie MONTGOMERY und UNDERWOOD (1953). Es ist aber noch nicht gesichert, ob die Vermehrung saurer Mucopolysaccharide im Serum die Mucinosen im Sinne einer Ablagerung verursacht, oder ob die Vermehrung im Serum nur sekundär durch das lokale Geschehen zustande kommt.

Die *Regulierung der Mucinmenge* mesenchymaler Grundsubstanz erfolgt auf verschiedenen Wegen, wovon der zentral-hormonale und der lokal-enzymatische Mechanismus wohl am wichtigsten sein dürfte (Schema 1). Es ist seit langem bekannt, daß es bei endokrinen Störungen zu einer Mucinanreicherung in der Haut kommt. Es scheinen hier vor allem die Funktion der Thyreoidea und Hypophyse eine besondere Bedeutung zu haben, wobei ein Gleichgewichtszustand zwischen der Funktion der Schilddrüse und der Hypophyse anzunehmen ist (RAWSON, STERNE und AUB, 1942). Bei Störung einer dieser Funktionen, so speziell beim Ausfall der Thyreoidea, werden größere Mengen des thyreotropen Hypophysenhormons gebildet (GRAUMANN, 1964; KINT und CANDAELE, 1963;

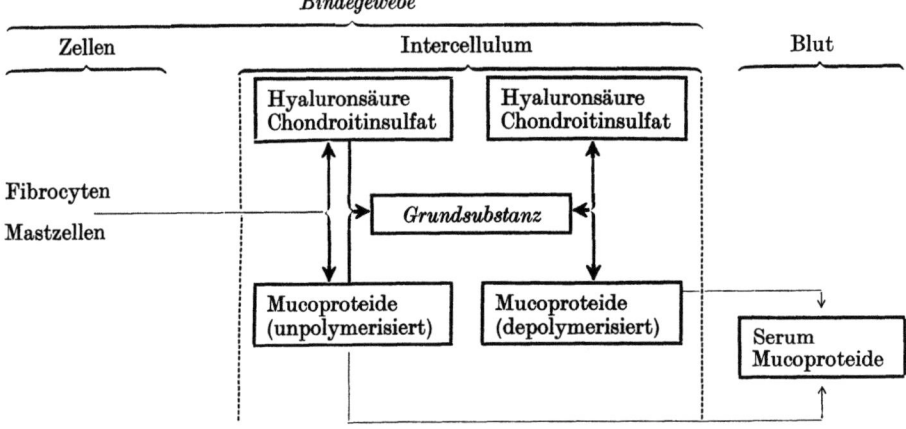

Schema 1. Beziehungen der Bindegewebsgrundsubstanz zu den Zellen des Bindegewebes und zum Blut. (Nach PERNIS, entnommen aus W. GRAUMANN, Handbuch der Histochemie, Bd. II/2)

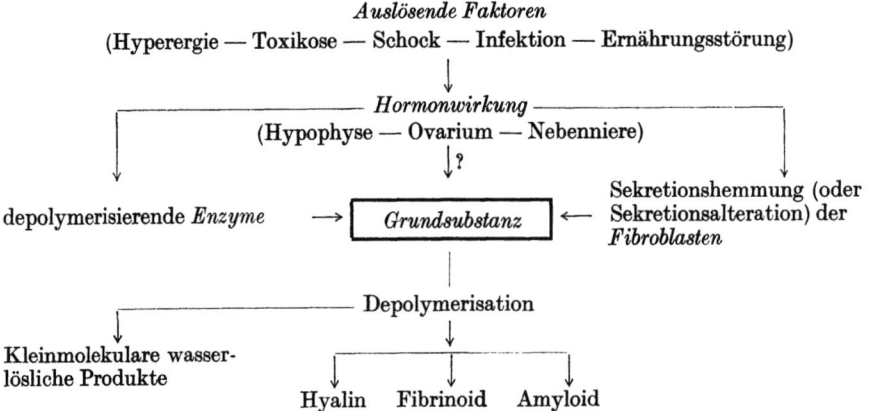

Schema 2. Schematische Darstellung der Degradation der Bindegewebsgrundsubstanz. (Nach DE BRUX, entnommen aus W. GRAUMANN, Handbuch der Histochemie, Bd. II/2)

BEIERWALTES, 1962). Von diesem werden wiederum mehrere Faktoren angenommen, so unter anderem ein hypothetischer histotroper Faktor, der die Mucinanreicherung beim prätibialen, lokalisierten Myxödem bei Hyperthyreose bewirken soll (WODNIANSKY, 1957). Allerdings wird bei Komplikationen der Hyperthyreose wie Exophthalmus und prätibiales Myxödem das thyreotrope Hormon nicht vermehrt gefunden, eine Tatsache, die obigen Ansichten etwas widerspricht (UTIGER u. Mitarb., 1965). Inwieweit LATS (long acting thyroid stimulator) hier von Bedeutung ist, sei noch dahingestellt (BONNYNS, 1967).

Beim hypothyreotischen, diffusen Myxödem liegt die Ursache der Störung vor allem im Ausfall des Schilddrüsenhormons selbst und nicht primär in den Störungen der Hypophyse. WINER u.a. meinen hierzu, daß beim hypothyreotischen Myxödem der Abbau der Schleimsubstanzen gestört, aber die Bildung derselben nicht verändert ist. Offenbar ist das Schilddrüsenhormon für die Depolymerisierung der Mucoproteide von Bedeutung. Neben den genannten Hormonen scheinen auch noch andere und schließlich auch noch Vitamine für den Mucingehalt der Haut von Bedeutung zu sein (WINER, BIERMAN und STERNBERG, 1963; Übersicht bei BRAUN-FALCO, 1964).

Die enzymatische Regulierung des Gehaltes an Mucopolysacchariden der Haut erfolgt vor allem über das sich normalerweise im Gleichgewicht befindende System Hyaluronsäure-Hyaluronidase (TROTTER und EDEN, 1942; KEINING und BRAUN-FALCO, 1952). Die depolymerisierende Wirkung des Ferments Hyaluronidase und der auf diesen Wegen bedingte Abbau der Kittsubstanz des Bindegewebes ist bekannt. Damit wird auch die „spreading"-Wirkung der Hyaluronidase erklärt, obwohl beim Zustandekommen dieses Effektes auch andere Enzymsysteme mitwirken dürften (WELLS, 1954). (Über andere Fermente mit mucolytischer Wirkung s. bei BRAUN-FALCO, 1964). Bei einigen Mucinosen scheint nun das Enzymsystem entweder indirekt durch die bei Schilddrüsenerkrankungen bestehende Hormonstörung oder direkt durch eine lokale Behinderung der Hyaluronidasefreisetzung gestört zu sein.

Bei der *histochemischen Darstellung* der sog. Schleimstoffe ist vor allem die Frage der Fixierung zu beachten, da sich diese Substanzen hinsichtlich ihrer Löslichkeit recht unterschiedlich verhalten (Das gilt schon für die Grundsubstanz des normalen Hautbindegewebes, NIEBAUER und RAAB, 1961.) Nach GRAUMANN (1964) empfiehlt sich neben den üblichen Methoden insbesondere die Fixation mit Bleiacetat und die Gefriertrocknung. Im letzteren Falle müssen die Polysaccharid-Protein-Komplexe durch Alkohol-Denaturierung wasserunlöslich gemacht werden.

Zwei histochemische Methoden sind in diesem Zusammenhang von besonderem Interesse: die PAS-Färbung und der Nachweis echter Metachromasie. Ihre Ergebnisse sind in der Regel nicht gleichsinnig, sondern eher gegenläufig (s. BRAUN-FALCO, dieses Handbuch, Band I/2). Die Untersuchungen von SYLVÉN (1938) über

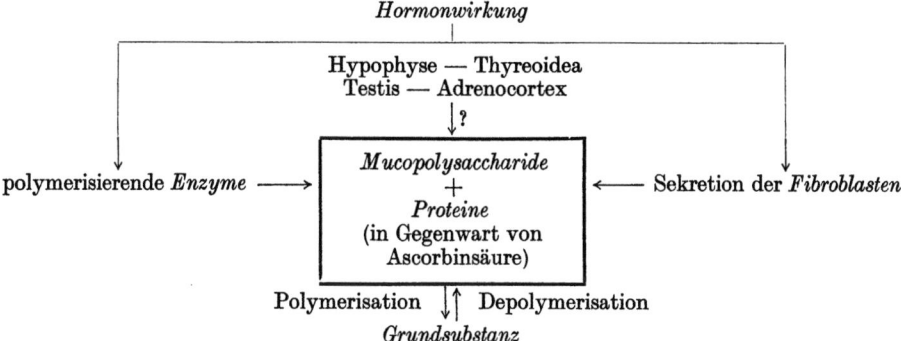

Schema 3. Schematische Darstellung der Aggregation der Bindegewebsgrundsubstanz.
(Nach DE BRUX, entnommen aus W. GRAUMANN, Handbuch der Histochemie, Bd. II/2)

die Elektivität und die Fehlerquellen der Schleimfärbung mit *Mucicarmin* im Vergleich zu Metachromasie-Reaktionen zeigen die weitgehende Unspezifität der Mucicarminreaktion. Nach SYLVÉN läßt ihr positiver Ausfall keinesfalls auf das Vorhandensein von „Schleim" im Bindegewebe und auch nicht auf Degeneration schließen. SYLVÉN (1938a, 1939, 1941, 1945) hat in einer Reihe von Arbeiten Zustände der „mesodermalen Verschleimung" nicht als degenerative Vorgänge, sondern einfach als eine „Zustandsänderung der bindegewebigen Grundsubstanz" definiert, wobei die Ursache der Metachromasie in einer Änderung der Polysaccharid-Protein-Bindung und dem Freiwerden elektronegativer Gruppen zu suchen sei. Nach EHRICH (1952) kommt möglicherweise noch eine gesteigerte sekretorische Aktivität der Fibroblasten hinzu (GRAUMANN, 1964). Nach SYLVÉN ist der Nachweis einer diffusen Gewebsmetachromasie ein Symptom besonderer Gewebsaktivität und nicht ein Degenerationszeichen!

Durch histoenzymatische Verfahren — vor allem durch Vorbehandlung des Gewebes mit Hyaluronidase — kann z.B. die Metachromasie partiell zum Verschwinden gebracht werden. Diese Methode ist zur Kontrolle anderer Untersuchungsmethoden von einigem Wert; es muß jedoch berücksichtigt werden, daß alle Hyaluronidasepräparate auch proteolytische Aktivität zeigen.

Einen guten Überblick über den derzeitigen Stand der histochemischen Methoden zum Nachweis von Mucopolysaccharidkomplexen in der Grundsubstanz gibt der Verhandlungsbericht des Kolloquiums der Gesellschaft für Histochemie im Jahre 1962 (LINDNER).

Mannigfache Zustände können zur *„Anreicherung"* saurer Mucopolysaccharide in der Cutis führen. BRAUN-FALCO (1964) gibt im Kapitel: „Pathologische Veränderungen der mesenchymalen Grundsubstanz der Haut" dieses Handbuches dafür folgende Möglichkeiten an:

1. Eine vermehrte Bildung von Grundsubstanzen, bzw Grundsubstanzbausteinen oder eine Störung im Aufbau-Abbau-Verhältnis der interfibrillären Grundsubstanz.

2. Entmischungszustände in den interfibrillären Grundsubstanzen mit Phanerose vor allem saurer Mucopolysaccharide.

3. Anreicherung saurer, mucopolysaccharidreicher mukoider Ödeme im Hautbindegewebe.

Eine besondere Bedeutung im Sinne pathologischer Ablagerungsspeicherungen von Mucin in der Cutis haben in diesem Zusammenhang jene Erkrankungen, die als Mucinosen, Myxodermien bzw. Myxödem im Sinne der Dermatologie (SCHÜRMANN, 1938) bezeichnet werden. Auf diese soll hier speziell eingegangen werden.

Wie schon gesagt, ist es seit langem bekannt, daß Schleimablagerungen in der Haut im Zusammenhang mit Störungen der inneren Sekretion, sei es Hypo- oder Hyperthyreose, vorkommen. Auf dieser Erkenntnis basierend, wurde entsprechend den Auffassungen von SCHUERMANN, MONTGOMERY und UNDERWOOD, BRAUN-FALCO und LEVER, folgende Einteilung der *Mucinosen* getroffen:

1. Myxoedema diffusum bei Hypothyreose,
2. Myxoedema circumscriptum praetibiale bei Hyperthyreose,
3. Lichen myxoedematosus, Skleromyxödem und
4. Skleroedema adultorum bei Euthyreose.

Während bei den hypo- und hyperthyreotischen Mucinosen die pathogenetische Bedeutung der Schilddrüse außer Zweifel steht, wird Ätiologie und Pathogenese der euthyreotischen Myxodermien noch diskutiert.

Für die histologische Beschreibung ist die vorangehende Unterteilung von geringerer Bedeutung, da sich bei allen Mucinosen im wesentlichen analoge feingewebliche Veränderungen finden. Je nach Alter des Patienten, der Lokalisation des entnommenen Gewebsstückes und dem Grade der Erkrankung kann allerdings das histologische Bild des Myxoedema diffusum Unterschiede aufweisen (GANS und STEIGLEDER).

Als charakteristisches Merkmal finden sich bei allen „schleimführenden" Erkrankungen im Cutisbereiche flächenhafte oder umschriebene Ablagerungen, die mit Hilfe der eingangs erwähnten histochemischen Nachweise als „Schleim" zu identifizieren sind. Bei Anwendung von Routinefärbungen können diese bei leichten Formen allerdings übersehen werden. Beim Skleroedema adultorum beruht die Metachromasie der Ödemsubstanz jedoch auf der Anwesenheit wasserlöslicher Hyaluronsäure (HOLUBAR u. MACH, 1967).

An der Epidermis sind nur geringe, sekundär bedingte Veränderungen zu erkennen. In der Basalzellschicht ist mitunter der Melaningehalt vermehrt (MONTGOMERY und UNDERWOOD, 1953; KEINING und BRAUN-FALCO, 1952).

Im Corium, beim Lichen myxoedematosus und beim Skleromyxödem mehr in den oberen, sonst eher in den tieferen Schichten sind reichliche Ablagerungen von Schleim zu erkennen. Entsprechend dem klinischen Bilde sind diese Ablagerungen beim Lichen myxoedematosus auf relativ kleine Areale beschränkt, während sie beim Skleromyxödem in Form eines Horizontalbandes angeordnet sind. Das Mucin kann homogen, fädig geronnen, in seltenen Fällen auch kristallin erscheinen (TAPPEINER und WODNIANSKY, 1959).

Die kollagenen Bündel sind durch die Einlagerungen auseinandergedrängt, aufgequollen und zersplittert (REUTER, 1931; SCHNITZER, 1961; CAROL, 1932). Manche dieser Bündel zeigen feinfibrilläre Büschel von basophiler Tinktion an den Enden, so daß man den Eindruck gewinnt, daß das kollagene Gewebe nicht nur rein passiv auseinandergedrängt, sondern auch in diesen Prozeß einbezogen wird (TAPPEINER, 1955). Die fragmentierten kollagenen Fasern zeigen im Gegensatz zu den noch erhaltenen im polarisierten Licht keine Doppelbrechung (KEINING und BRAUN-FALCO, 1952). Insbesondere in den oberen Cutisschichten bilden sie ein verworrenes Geflecht und erst in der Tiefe verlaufen sie allmählich wieder in parallelen Bündeln (GANS und STEIGLEDER, 1955). Auch die elastischen Fasern sind stark vermindert, fragmentiert und aufgelockert (FISCHER, 1949; EBERHARTINGER, 1956; SWEITZER und LAYMON, 1938; WODNIANSKY, 1957; NEUMANN, 1935). In älteren Efflorescenzen sind nur mehr spärliche Faserreste nachweisbar (TAPPEINER, 1955). Die Anfärbbarkeit der elastischen Fasern (Weigertsche Resorcinfärbung, Gomori, Aldehydfuchsinfärbung) ist jedoch normal (KEINING und BRAUN-FALCO, 1952). Die Gitterfasern sind deutlich vermehrt (MONTGOMERY und UNDERWOOD, 1953; KONRAD und WINKLER, 1956).

Innerhalb der Schleimablagerungen finden sich reichlich längliche Zellen mit sternförmigen Fortsätzen, die an embryonale Bindegewebszellen erinnern und als jugendliche Fibroblasten gedeutet werden (KOPF, 1956; DALTON und SEIDELL, 1953; MEYER und NISHIYAMA, 1961). Für diese Zellen ist durchwegs eine diffuse, gelegentlich auch feingranulierte, cytoplasmatische Metachromasie (Toluidinblau) kennzeichnend. Umgeben sind sie vielfach von einem metachromatischen Hof, der durch die Abscheidung metachromatischen Materials entstanden sein könnte (KEINING und BRAUN-FALCO, 1952). Daneben wird von manchen Autoren eine Vermehrung der Mastzellen beschrieben (ASBOE-HANSEN, 1956; VILLANOVA, PINOL und MORAGAS, 1960; BERNHARDT, 1931; TRYB, 1922). Teilweise findet sich auch perivasculär und am Rande der Herde ein mäßiges Rundzellinfiltrat (CEELEN, 1921; v. ZEZWITSCH, 1959; SCHUERMANN, 1938; BUTLER und LAYMON, 1937; HAMMINGA und KEINING, 1954). Die Hautanhangsgebilde sind, besonders in stark ausgeprägten Fällen, rarefiziert (MILLER und MOPPER, 1955; EBERHARTINGER, 1956). Die glatten Muskelzellen der Mm. arrectores pilorum können durch feinfädiges, mucinöses Material auseinandergedrängt sein, wodurch eine Störung der

Anordnung des Verlaufes der Muskelzellen zustande kommt. Die Zellen an und für sich sind jedoch nicht verändert (KEINING und BRAUN-FALCO, 1952).

Von GOTTRON und KORTING (1953) wurden an den Gefäßen der Cutis-Subcutisgrenze hochgradige Veränderungen beschrieben. Die Gefäßwände sind in toto, besonders aber Media und Intima, verdickt, das Lumen schlitzförmig eingeengt. Daneben finden sich sog. Sperrarterien, die zwischen Membr. elastica interna und Endothel mauerartig angeordnet eine mehrschichtige Einlagerung aus glatten Muskelzellen aufweisen. Diesen Gefäßveränderungen wird von vielen Autoren eine wichtige pathogenetische Bedeutung zugemessen, da es durch die Kreislaufverlangsamung zur Hypoxie kommt, die eine Ablagerung von Mucopolysacchariden begünstigt (GOTTRON, 1954; KORTING und WEBER, 1963; TAPPEINER, 1955).

Von PINKUS wurde 1957 als *Alopecia mucinosa* ein Krankheitsbild beschrieben, das klinisch hinsichtlich des Verlaufes und des Ausmaßes der Veränderungen eine große Divergenz zeigte. Ähnliche Fälle wurden von BRAUN-FALCO im gleichen Jahre unter der Bezeichnung Mucophanerosis intrafollicularis et seboglandularis publiziert, der gleichzeitig schon eine Unterteilung in symptomatische und idiopathische Formen dieser Erkrankung schuf. Da die Erscheinungen auch an unbehaarten Körperstellen auftreten können, wurde von anderen Autoren die Benennung Mucinosis follicularis vorgeschlagen (JABLONSKA, CHORZELSKI und LANCUCKI, 1959; TAPPEINER, PFLEGER und HOLZNER, 1962, THIES, 1964). Histologisch kommt es zu auffallenden degenerativen Veränderungen der Talgdrüsen. Die Talgdrüsenläppchen haben ihren normalen Aufbau völlig verloren. Die Mutterzellen am Rande sind meist erhalten, zeigen aber schon in ihrem Cytoplasma Vacuolenbildung oder sind ödematös aufgetrieben. Die weiter innen liegenden Zellen haben ihre Stuktur gänzlich verloren, ihr Cytoplasma ist in Auflösung begriffen. Zwischen den Zellen bilden sich Hohlräume, die mit einem homogenen, mucinösen Material, das sich mit Astra-, Toluidin- und Alcianblau anfärbt, erfüllt sind. Gleichartige Veränderungen finden sich im Bereiche des Haarfollikels mit besonderer Ausprägung in der Höhe der Einmündung der Talgdrüsenausführungsgänge. Auch hier finden sich diese mucinösen Veränderungen. In der Umgebung der derart veränderten Follikel treten stellenweise ziemlich intensive, entzündliche Infiltrate auf, die aus Lymphocyten, Histiocyten, vereinzelt Plasmazellen und Fibroblasten aufgebaut sind (KIM und WINKELMANN, 1962).

Elektronenmikroskopische Untersuchungen von ORFANOS und GAHLEN (1964) haben gezeigt, daß es bei dieser Erkrankung besonders im oberen Stratum spinosum und im Stratum granulosum zum Auftreten 150—200 mµ großer, rundlicher, osmiophiler, als „Cytosome" bezeichneter Elemente kommt. Die Autoren nehmen an, daß es sich hier um die morphologische Manifestation des entgleisten Zellstoffwechsels handelt.

Da ein Großteil der sensiblen Innervation der Haut im Haarfollikelbereich gelegen ist (NIEBAUER, 1966) kommt es relativ häufig in der erkrankten Region zu Sensibilitätsstörungen (ARNOLD, 1962; CABRÉ und KORTING, 1965). Auch eine Verminderung der Schweißsekretion in diesen Arealen wurde beschrieben (BORDA u. Mitarb., 1964).

IV. Lipide

Als Lipide werden alle natürlich vorkommenden, fettähnlichen Stoffe bezeichnet, die unlöslich in Wasser sind, aber löslich in Äther, Chloroform, Aceton und Kohlenwasserstoffen (PEARSE, 1961). Demnach handelt es sich um eine chemisch weitgehend heterogene Gruppe von Substanzen.

Die *Neutralfette* sind Ester des dreiwertigen Alkohols Glycerin mit drei höheren Fettsäuren. Mengenmäßig sind sie bei weitem die wesentlichsten fettigen Substanzen der Nahrung und der Fettdepots. Als *Lipoide* werden fettartige Substanzen bezeichnet, die entweder neben Glycerin noch andere Stoffe, meist polarer, wasserlöslicher Art enthalten (z.B. Phosphat, stickstoffhaltige Basen) oder Verbindungen anderer Alkohole (z.B. Sphingosin) sind (ZÖLLNER, 1957). Sie sind wichtige Zellbestandteile und möglicherweise eng mit den Vorgängen bei der Fettsäureoxydation verknüpft. Das *Cholesterin* ist eine cyclische Verbindung, deren Grundgerüst vom Cyclopentanoperhydrophenantrenring gebildet wird. Es ist eine Intermediärsubstanz beim Aufbau zahlreicher Verbindungen mit Sterinskelet und wahrscheinlich hat es auch eigene biologische Funktionen.

Mit entsprechend empfindlichen Methoden gelingt es auch bei normalen Zuständen in praktisch allen Zellen der Haut Lipide nachzuweisen.

In diesem Kapitel soll nur auf solche Krankheitsbilder näher eingegangen werden, bei denen es zur massiven Ablagerung von Lipiden im Hautbereich kommt und die Lipidanhäufung das führende Krankheitssymptom ist.

Für eine morphologisch-histologische Einteilung ist die Lokalisation der Lipide maßgeblich.

1. Intracellulär.
a) Xanthom.
b) Histiocytose (LICHTENSTEIN, 1953; LEVER, 1963); Xanthogranulomatose (TAPPEINER und WODNIANSKY, 1959); systematisierte Lipoidspeicherkrankheit (KEINING und BRAUN-FALCO, 1961); normocholesterinämische, disseminierte Xanthomatose (GANS und STEIGLEDER, 1955); sogenannte Lipoidose (FEYRTER, 1955).
c) Angiokeratoma corporis diffusum FABRY.
2. Extracellulär.
a) Necrobiosis lipoidica.
b) Extracelluläre Cholesterinose KERL-URBACH.

1. Intracellulär

a) Xanthom

Der feingewebliche Aufbau und die histochemische Analyse der hypercholesterinämischen und hyperlipämischen Xanthome läßt keine markanten Unterschiede erkennen (BORRIE, 1957; URBACH, 1933; MONTGOMERY und OSTERBERG, 1938), obgleich FISCHER und NIKOLOWSKI (1960) auf einige histologische Details hinwiesen, die zur Differentialdiagnose beitragen können. Eine sichere Unterscheidung ist jedoch aus dem histologischen Bild nicht möglich. Charakteristisch ist die sog. Xanthomzelle, die aus Zellen des RES, aus Histiocyten und eventuell auch aus fixen Bindegewebszellen durch Lipideinlagerung entstehen kann (SCHAANNING und NYQUIST, 1932; SIEMENS, 1921). Diese Zellen sind oval, scharf begrenzt. Das Plasma erscheint hell, anfangs homogen, erst später retikulär schaumig. Durch amitotische Zellteilung entstehen die sog. Toutonschen Riesenzellen, die oft über 50 µ groß werden (MATRAS, 1956; SIEMENS, 1921).

Die Epidermis ist zumeist unverändert, über größeren Knoten eventuell etwas verdünnt. In älteren Efflorescenzen kann man im Stratum basale sudanpositive Körnchen und Schollen nachweisen. Anfangs liegen in den oberen Coriumschichten die Schaumzellen oft ringförmig um die Gefäße. Später ist oft die gesamte Cutis von Schaumzellen durchsetzt. Die Xanthombildung wird von einer verschiedengradigen entzündlichen Reaktion begleitet. Das Infiltrat ist aus polymorphkernigen Leukocyten, Lympho- und Histiocyten aufgebaut (TAPPEINER und WODNIANSKY, 1959). Die entzündlichen Begleiterscheinungen treten mit zunehmendem Alter der Veränderungen in den Hintergrund. Es kommt im weiteren Verlauf zu einer Kompression der Gefäße, wodurch Zellkerne pyknotisch werden, bzw. die Xanthomzellen direkt zerfallen, so daß Lipide frei im Gewebe liegen. Schließlich bilden sich nadel- und wetzsteinförmige Cholesterinkristalle (BURNS,

1920; BARKER-BEESON und ALBRECHT, 1923; MOOK und WEISS, 1923; WEIDMAN und FREEMAN, 1924). Zuweilen kommt es in der tiefen Cutis auch zur Ausbildung von Pseudocysten. Das sind wandlose, mit Erythrocyten und Zellresten gefüllte Höhlen, die wahrscheinlich ebenfalls durch Zerfallsvorgänge der Xanthomzellen entstehen (JORGE und BRACHETTO-BRIAN, 1932).

Im Rahmen der Regression treten vermehrt kollagene Fasern auf, so daß endlich ein zellarmes, fibröses Narbengewebe resultiert (PFLEGER und TIRSCHEK, 1956). Eventuell kann es auch zu einer Restitutio ad integrum kommen.

Verschiedene histochemische Untersuchungsmethoden zeigen an, daß die in Xanthomzellen abgelagerten Lipide in ihrer Zusammensetzung schwanken können (WOLMAN, 1964). In jungen Efflorescenzen findet sich reichlich Neutralfett und verestertes Cholesterin, während mit zunehmendem Alter die Neutralfette abnehmen und vermehrt freies Cholesterin auftritt.

Im polarisierten Licht erweisen sich die kristallinen und kleineren Teile der Einlagerung als anisotrop (FRANZ, 1936; WIEDMANN, 1937). Die Doppelbrechung verschwindet bei Erwärmung und tritt bei Erkalten des Schnittes zum größten Teile wieder auf (NÖDL, 1951). Wie SECKFORT und BRAUN-FALCO (1957) nachgewiesen haben, geben die Lipide der Xanthomzellen auch eine intensive Plasmalreaktion. Elektronenmikroskopische Untersuchungen der Xanthomzelle wurden von IMAEDA (1960) durchgeführt.

b) Histiocytose (Lichtenstein, Lever); Xanthogranulomatose

Wie auch LEVER (1963) in seinem Handbuchbeitrag hinweist, stellen die Abt-Letterer-Siwesche, die Hand-Schüller-Christiansche Erkrankung und das eosinophile Granulom nur Varianten eines einzigen Krankheitsbildes dar (FARBER, 1941, 1944; WEINSTEIN, FRANCIS und SPROFKIN, 1947; LAYMON und SEVENANTS, 1948; PINKUS, COPPS, CUSTER und EPSTEIN, 1949; LICHTENSTEIN, 1953; VESLOT, DUPERRAT, BROWAES, GARNIER und PLEY, 1951; FEYRTER, 1955; GANS und STEIGLEDER, 1955; DUMMERMUTH, 1958; MACH, 1962; ausführliche Literaturangaben bei RÖCKL und VOGT, 1960). Im Vordergrund steht bei allen die Proliferation von histiocytären Elementen (JAEGER und DELACRETAZ, 1954), während die Lipideinlagerungen erst sekundär auftreten (CEELEN, 1933; GOTTRON, 1942) und in Einzelfällen gänzlich fehlen können (GROSS und JACOX, 1942; DENNIS und ROSAHN, 1951). Als Ursache der intracellulären Lipideinlagerungen wird eine Störung des Zellstoffwechsels angenommen (CHIARI, 1931). Möglicherweise ist dieses Phänomen Ausdruck eines Rückfalles der Zelle in embryonale Potenzen (ZÖLLNER, 1957). Von SIWE (1949) wird das Vorliegen einer intracellulären Fermentstörung der Histiocyten, die eine Digestierung des phagocytierten Lipids verhindert, angenommen. Das Naevoxanthoendotheliom ist als monosymptomatische Variante einer generalisierten Histiocytose zu betrachten (LAMB und LAIN, 1937; THANNHAUSER, 1958). Auch das feingewebliche Bild stimmt weitgehend überein.

Histologisch können verschiedene, ineinander übergehende Stadien der Entwicklung vorliegen. Beim klassischen Verlauf des Morbus Hand-Schüller-Christian kommt es nach dem proliferativen Stadium, in dem sich eine Anhäufung von Histiocyten und Eosinophilen findet, zum granulomatösen Stadium, welches sich durch intracelluläre Ansammlung von Cholesterin zum xanthomatösen Stadium weiterentwickelt. Letztlich kommt es zu einem fibrotischen Endstadium. In keiner Phase der Erkrankung läßt sich extracelluläres Cholesterin nachweisen. Nach LEVER (1955) tritt der Morbus Hand-Schüller-Christian relativ selten an der Haut auf. In seinem Handbuchbeitrag (1963) gibt er eine Mitbeteiligung der

Haut bei 30% der Gesamtfälle an. In einer erst vor kurzem erschienenen Zusammenstellung von 180 Fällen fanden AVIOLI, LASERSOHN und LOPRESTI (1963) bei 25% der Fälle Hautveränderungen beschrieben. Es kommt primär zu einem Ödem des Papillarkörpers, zu einer Dilatation der Capillaren und zum Austritt von Erythrocyten (GOTTRON, 1942; LEVER und LEEPER, 1950). Auch das Epithel zeigt abschnittsweise eine ödematöse Aufquellung. In der weiteren Folge kommt es im Corium zu umschriebenen Ansammlungen von Histiocyten. Diese haben ein helles, homogenes, leicht eosinophiles Protoplasma und große, unregelmäßige Kerne. An manchen Stellen fließt das Cytoplasma der Histiocyten ineinander über; vereinzelt dringen sie destruierend in die Epidermis ein. Besonders im Genital-, Axillar- und Kopfbereich kommt es zur Ausbildung von Granulomen. Hier finden sich daneben noch unregelmäßig gelagerte Riesenzellen vom Fremdkörpertyp, Lymphocyten, vereinzelt Plasmazellen und Eosinophile (BERNUTH, 1933; FARBER, 1941; WALLACE, 1950; BOJOWA und DZIEDZIUSZKO, 1950). Gelegentlich besitzen hier die Histiocyten ein vacuolisiertes Cytoplasma und weisen bei Fettfärbung kleine Mengen phagocytierten Lipids auf (WALLACE, 1950).

Erst im weiteren Verlaufe kommt es zum Auftreten von Schaumzellen, eventuell auch von Toutonschen Riesenzellen (BERNUTH, 1933; BOJOWA und DZIEDZIUSZKO, 1952). In älteren Herden kommt es zur Gefäßneubildung, Fibrose, während die Schaumzellen wieder schwinden.

Histochemisch wurde die Entwicklung der xanthomatösen Veränderungen von PFENNINGS und SCHÜMMELFEDER (1952) an inneren Organen genauer studiert. Es zeigte sich, daß die Lipideinlagerung in der Peripherie der Granulome beginnt und zentralwärts fortschreitet, ferner, daß nicht sichtbar stapelnde Granulome und Granulomabschnitte mit der Plasmalreaktion faßbare Aldehyde enthalten. Das Fortschreiten der Lipideinlagerung wurde von den Autoren als dem Vorgange einer pathologischen Verfettung anderer Art ähnlich gedeutet.

Unter gekreuzten Polars sieht man eine Anreicherung doppelbrechender Fettsubstanz, teilweise typische Kristalle in Form von Malteserkreuzen. Auch die Prüfung im polarisierten Licht nach Umkristallisation bei 60° weist auf das Vorhandensein von Cholesterin und Cholesterinverbindungen hin. Auffällig ist die enorm stark positive Plasmalreaktion nach FEULGEN und VOIT, welche auf einen großen Gehalt der Zellen an Acetalphosphatiden hinweist. Daneben zeigt die Blaufärbung der Fettsubstanz mit Nilblausulfat und auch der positive Reaktionsausfall mit der Fischlerschen Methode das Vorhandensein von Fettsäuren mit einer Kettenlänge von über 6 C-Atomen an. Die positive Bakersche Reaktion spricht für das Vorhandensein von Phospholipoiden (KUTSCHER und VRLA, 1949; BRAUN-FALCO und BRAUN-FALCO, 1957). FEYRTER (1955) weist besonders auf das Ergebnis der Thionin-Weinsteinsäure-Einschlußfärbung hin, mit der rhodiochrome Lipoproteide, in denen kryptacide Komplexe salzartig an die Aminogruppen der Aminosäuren gebunden erscheinen, eine rosenrote Farbe geben.

Auf Grund elektronenoptischer Befunde berichteten BASSET und TURIAF (1965) erstmals über das Vorkommen tubulärer, stäbchen- oder tennisschlägerartiger Strukturen in den pathologischen Histiocyten einer pulmonalen Histiocytosis X. Im folgenden Jahr konnten die gleichen Autoren auch in weiteren Fällen dieser Erkrankung ihre elektronenoptischen Befunde bestätigen. Sie nahmen anfangs an, daß es sich bei diesen Organellen um virale Zelleinschlüsse handle und diskutierten daher ihre mögliche ätiologische Rolle. Weitere Untersuchungen zeigten jedoch, daß die von BASSET und TURIAF (1965) sowie von BASSET und NÉZELOF (1966) beschriebenen intracytoplasmatischen Einschlüsse proliferativer Histiocyten die gleiche Struktur, Form und Anordnung aufweisen wie die erstmals von BIRBECK u. Mitarb. (1961) beschriebenen sog. „Langerhanszell-Organellen".

c) Angiokeratoma corporis diffusum Fabry

Untersuchungen der letzten Jahre haben gezeigt, daß es sich bei den von FABRY (1898) erstmals beschriebenen Hautveränderungen um die cutanen Manifestationen einer generalisierten Lipoidspeichererkrankung handelt, in deren Rahmen auch Herzmuskel, Nierenglomerula, Kerne des Hirnstammes, autonome Ganglien etc. ergriffen werden. Weiter wurde eine Erblichkeit der Erkrankung festgestellt. Aus diesem Grunde wurde von DE GROOT (1964) die Bezeichnung *Thesaurismosis lipoidica hereditaria* für diese Erkrankung vorgeschlagen.

Über die Zusammensetzung der abgelagerten Lipide sind die Meinungen noch geteilt. RUITER und DE GROOT (1967) nehmen an, daß es sich um inosithaltige Aminophosphatide handelt, während SWEELEY und KLIONSKY (1963) diese pathologischen Stoffwechselprodukte eher für neutrale Glykolipide (Sphingosintrihexosid) halten.

Histologisch findet man im Corium, besonders unmittelbar unter der Epidermis kleine, capilläre Angiome. Das darüberliegende Epithel zeigt Zeichen einer Hyperkeratose (KENDALL, DAVIDSON und PFAFF jr., 1962). Es soll sich hier um Aneurysmata und Erweiterungen präexistenter Blutgefäße handeln (RUITER, 1958). Gelegentlich sieht man schon in der HE-Färbung die charakteristischen Veränderungen, und zwar zeigen die glatten Muskelzellen der Media kleinster Arterien eine Schwellung und wabig-vacuoläre Aufhellung des Protoplasmas. Viel besser werden diese Veränderungen bei Betrachtung formalinfixierter, ungefärbter Gefrierschnitte im polarisierten Lichte sichtbar (HORNBOSTEL und SCRIBA, 1953). Man sieht dabei, daß sowohl die glatten Muskelzellen als auch die Endothelzellen der Gefäße doppelbrechende Substanz enthalten.

Für die histochemische Darstellung der Lipide beim Angiokeratoma corporis diffusum ist eine besondere Fixierung notwendig (PITTELKOW, KIERLAND und MONTGOMERY, 1957; LEVER, 1963). Von RUITER (1954) wurde erstmals eine Sudanschwarz-Scharlachrotfärbung am formolfixierten und chromierten Paraffinschnitt zur Darstellung der Lipidablagerung angegeben. Diese sind hierbei lichtmikroskopisch als schwarze oder rote Körperchen wechselnder Größe zu erkennen. Weiters eignet sich die 3:4 Benzpyren-Fluorescenzmethode (BERG, 1951) zur Darstellung der Lipide. Elektronenmikroskopisch sind die Lipideinlagerungen in Form osmiophiler, lamellärer Körper nachweisbar, wobei ein elektronenoptisch helles Zentrum von einem System konzentrisch angeordneter abwechselnd dichter und heller Linien umgeben ist (RUITER und DE GROOT, 1967).

Mit diesen Methoden ist es nach RUITER und DE GROOT (1967) möglich auch in unveränderter Haut kranker Personen, ja sogar in Fällen, bei denen keine klinischen Hautveränderungen bestehen, den Nachweis der charakteristischen Lipideinlagerung zu erbringen.

2. Extracellulär

Wie schon einleitend erwähnt, kommt es bei der Necrobiosis lipoidica und der extracellulären Cholesterinose zu einer vorwiegend extracellulären Ablagerung der Lipide. Diese erfolgt durchwegs in pathologisch verändertes Gewebe.

a) Necrobiosis lipoidica

Charakteristischerweise sieht man bei dieser Erkrankung in den mittleren und tiefen Cutisschichten ausgedehnte, unscharf begrenzte Areale, in deren Bereich das Bindegewebe, besonders um zentrale Gefäße angeordnet, schollig-nekrobiotisch umgewandelt ist. Die Wand der Gefäße ist verdickt, es findet sich eine subendotheliale

Gewebswucherung und eine Proliferation der Intima. Sicher stellen diese Gefäßveränderungen die ersten histologisch faßbaren Veränderungen der Nekrobiosis dar (ROEDERER, WORINGER und BURGUN, 1949). Es kommt zu einer zunehmenden Einengung des Lumens und zum Verschluß kleinster Gefäße (ZEISLER und CARO, 1934; BOLDT, 1939; LAYMON und FISHER, 1949; WOLFF, 1964).

Die nekrobiotischen Bezirke sind von einem aus Lymphocyten, Histiocyten und Monocyten aufgebauten, entzündlichen Infiltrat umgeben, das stellenweise zungenförmig in die Herde vordringt (LAYMON und FISHER, 1949). Gelegentlich sind hier auch Riesenzellen, hämosiderinhaltige Makrophagen, vereinzelt auch lipoidbeladene Histiocyten zu sehen (CONNOR, 1936; URBACH, 1933; BRUCE-JONES, 1937; HITCH, 1937; MICHELSON und LAYMON, 1937).

In den meisten Fällen — sie können allerdings gelegentlich auch fehlen (LEIFER, 1941) — sind Lipideinlagerungen, die sich mit Sudan III braunrot anfärben, vorwiegend perivaskulär im Interstitium zu beobachten. Im polarisierten Licht ist gewöhnlich keine Doppelbrechung zu sehen. Chemisch dürfte es sich hauptsächlich um freies Cholesterin, Neutralfett und Phospholipoide handeln (USHER und RABINOWITSCH, 1937; BELOTE und WELTON, 1939).

b) Extracelluläre Cholesterinose Kerl-Urbach

Vielleicht handelt es sich bei dieser Dermatose um kein selbständiges Krankheitsbild, sondern um eine Sonderform des Erythema elevatum et diutinum, bei dem es sekundär zu einer reichlichen Einlagerung von Lipiden kommen kann (HERZBERG, 1958). Die feingeweblichen Veränderungen entsprechen auch weitgehend dem beim Erythema elevatum beschriebenen Bild. Das gänzliche Fehlen von Schaum- und Riesenzellen wird als typisch für die Erkrankung angesehen (LAYMON, 1937; SOBEL und POLLOCK, 1948). Daneben findet sich in der Färbung nach Sudan III in frischen Efflorescenzen staubförmig um die Gefäße angeordnet, bräunlich rote Substanz, die extracellulär gelagert ist und keine Doppelbrechung erkennen läßt (LAYMON, 1937; FROST und ANDERSON, 1939). In älteren und größeren Knoten sind diese Einlagerungen mehr diffus und doppelbrechend. Bei Digitoninzusatz entstehen zahlreiche Cholesterinnadeln, die bei Chloralzusatz wieder verschwinden (URBACH, 1933). Der Cholesteringehalt ist in den betreffenden Hautstellen auf das fünffache erhöht. Drei Viertel des Cholesterins liegt dabei in freier Form vor, im Gegensatz zum Xanthom, bei dem drei Viertel bis fünf Sechstel des Cholesterins verestert ist (WOLMAN, 1964).

V. Glykogen

Glykogen ist eine im tierischen Organismus sehr häufig anzutreffende Substanz. Es kommt in Zellen aller Gewebearten — zumindest unter gewissen Bedingungen — vor. Wahrscheinlich besitzen alle Zellen die Möglichkeit, Glykogen zu bilden, wobei die Gründe zur Glykogenbildung durchaus nicht einheitlich sind. Auch die funktionelle Bedeutung der Glykogenvorkommen ist sehr unterschiedlich. Jedenfalls ist der Glykogengehalt Kennzeichen einer speziellen Stoffwechselsituation, nicht aber das Charakteristikum einer speziellen Zellart.

Sicherlich ist das Vorhandensein von Glykogen nicht, wie früher angenommen wurde, ein Degenerationszeichen, sondern vielmehr ein Anzeichen aktiver Zellleistungen (GRAUMANN, 1964). Die biologische Bedeutung des Glykogens liegt in seiner Wichtigkeit als Baustein im strukturellen Gefüge bestimmter Zellen, als Nährstoff für glykogenhaltige, aber auch andere Zellen, als Nebenprodukt des Proteinabbaues und als notwendige Stufe der Blutzuckerbildung aus Nichtkohlenhydraten.

Besonders eingehend ist die funktionelle Bedeutung des Glykogenvorkommens im Cytoplasma an embryonalem Gewebe und in Tumoren studiert worden, sowie unter speziellen physiologischen Bedingungen, so im Zusammenhang mit der Vascularisation und anaeroben Stoffwechsellage. Befunde, die aber hier nicht diskutiert werden können (GRAUMANN, 1964).

Die Erforschung des Glykogenvorkommens in der Haut ist gerade in letzter Zeit eingehend studiert worden (STEIGLEDER, 1961). Stehen doch für die Routinehistochemie die PAS-Reaktion und ihre Modifikationen als einfache und erprobte Methoden zur Darstellung des Glykogens (nach Vorbehandlung des Gewebes mit Diastase oder Speichel) zur Verfügung. Neben diesen gibt es noch die älteren Methoden wie mit Lugolscher Lösung, nach BAUER-FEULGEN, nach CASELLA und die Best-Carmin-Reaktion (s. PEARSE, 1961).

Im Integument findet sich normalerweise histochemisch nachweisbares Glykogen speziell in der Epidermis und in den Hautanhangsgebilden. Unter den verschiedensten pathologischen Bedingungen kann dieser Stoff vermehrt vorkommen, wobei letztlich der Grund dieser Glykogenanreicherung noch nicht geklärt ist (STEIGLEDER, 1961). Zahlreiche Arbeiten behandeln vor allem das Vorkommen von Glykogen im Zusammenhang mit epithelialen Tumoren (STEIGLEDER, 1961). Veränderungen der Glykogenverteilung in epithelialen Hautanhangsgebilden wurden weniger ausführlich studiert. Im Vergleich zum epithelialen Glykogenvorkommen liegen nur Einzelbefunde über Glykogenanreicherungen bei Veränderungen im Hautbindegewebe vor. Hier ist vor allem die Beobachtung von HARE (1955) zu nennen, der reichlich Glykogen bei Necrobiosis lipoidica cum et sine diabete, aber auch bei Necrobiosis maculosa, Granulomatosis disciformis, in geringerem Ausmaß auch bei Granuloma anulare fand. Glykogen liegt hierbei frei und in Histiocyten phagocytiert in den peripheren Partien der nekrobiotischen Herde und im unmittelbar benachbarten Corium. Die Ablagerungen von Glykogen und Fett sind unabhängig voneinander. Die Menge des abgelagerten Glykogens war in diesen Fällen unabhängig von der Tatsache, ob es sich um ein diabetisches oder nichtdiabetisches Individuum handelt. Letzlich ist die Bedeutung der Glykogenablagerungen bei diesen Erkrankungen noch unbekannt, ihr diagnostischer Wert wird jedoch diskutiert. Allerdings scheint das Glykogenvorkommen bei diesen Leiden nicht regelmäßig zu sein (WOLFF, 1964; GRAY, GRAHAM und JOHNSON, 1965). Im geringeren Maße fand HARE (1955) überdies Glykogen in Knoten von rheumatischer Arthritis und bei Gefäßkrankheiten wie Arteriosklerose, Morbus Raynaud, hypostatisches Ulcus. BAZEX und DUPRÉ (1952) beschrieben Glykogen im erkrankten Bindegewebe bei Skleromyxödem. BANGLE (1952) untersuchte das Glykogenvorkommen bei Tumoren (Dermatofibroma protuberans, Hämangiopericytom, Sarcoma idiopathicum Kaposi) und konnte Glykogen vor allem in Endothelzellen und der glatten Muskulatur nachweisen.

Auch im Rahmen der von GIERKE (1929) erstmals beschriebenen Glykogenspeicherkrankheit kann es neben den massiven Glykogenablagerungen in den inneren Organen in manchen Fällen zur Einlagerung von Glykogen in die Haut kommen. Es besteht dadurch die Möglichkeit, mit Hilfe des histochemischen Glykogennachweises in Hautbiopsien die Diagnose zu verifizieren. Die Ablagerung findet sich dabei hauptsächlich im Schweißdrüsenepithel und in den Fibrocyten (SELBERG, 1952). Weiters kommen auch an der Haut noch uncharakteristische Veränderungen der Behaarung und im Rahmen der Lipämie Xanthome zur Beobachtung (GRAFE, 1955). Bei der „Glykogenose" dürfte es sich um eine spezifische Abbauhemmung des Glykogens handeln, wobei verschiedene Typen unterschieden werden können, denen unterschiedliche Enzymdefekte zugrunde liegen (RECANT, 1955; MASON und ANDERSEN, 1941; DI SANT'AGNESE, ANDERSON und MASON, 1950;

DI SANT-AGNESE, ANDERSON, MASON und BAUMAN, 1950). Es wird jedoch auch das Vorliegen einer abnormen chemischen Glykogenkonstitution und einer abartigen, besonders innigen Proteinbindung als Ursache der Erkrankung diskutiert (GRAUMANN, 1964).

VI. Kalk

Zu Kalkablagerungen in der Haut kann es im Rahmen sehr unterschiedlicher Krankheitsbilder kommen (LEVER, 1963). Hier sollen, ungeachtet der vorliegenden Grundkrankheit und des daraus resultierenden klinischen Bildes, die gemeinsamen histologischen Charakteristika besprochen werden.

Der chemische Aufbau der in die Haut eingelagerten Kalkmassen ist einfach. Sie bestehen größtenteils aus kohlen- bzw. phosphorsaurem Kalk, gelegentlich finden sich Spuren von Magnesiaverbindungen (GANS und STEIGLEDER, 1955).

Zum Kalknachweis im Gewebe gibt es verschiedene Methoden. Nach ERÖS färbt sich kalkhaltiges Gewebe auch nach Entkalkung lebhaft rot, während Binde- und Muskelgewebe blaßrot erscheinen. Für die folgenden Kalknachweise ist die Tatsache wichtig, daß alle Fixierungsflüssigkeiten mit Ausnahme des Alkohols entkalkend wirken. Bei Anwendung der Färbemethode nach KOSSA werden die kalkhaltigen Stellen schwarz gefärbt. Damit sollen besonders die phosphorsauren Kalke zur Darstellung gebracht werden. Auch in der Färbung nach GÖMÖRI erscheinen die Kalksalze schwarz, wobei besonders die Randzone deutlich gefärbt wird.

Sicher wird das Calcium nur in pathologisch verändertes Gewebe eingelagert (KERL, 1919; JESSERER, 1960). Daneben sind aber für die Lokalisation der Ablagerung auch noch andere Faktoren von Bedeutung. Ähnlich wie bei der Calcinose der inneren Organe dürfte auch in der Haut das alkalische Milieu bevorzugt werden. Daher erfolgt die Kalkablagerung oft an Hautstellen mit niedriger metabolischer Aktivität und daher niedrigem Kohlensäuregehalt (BRODY und BELLIN, 1937). Weiters werden noch örtliche Zirkulationsstörungen mit der Kalkablagerung in Verbindung gebracht.

Die Kalkansammlungen finden sich in den tiefen Coriumschichten und in der Subcutis (NAEGELI, 1932; SCHIFF und KERN, 1953; WISKEMANN, 1955; TAPPEINER und WODNIANSKY, 1959). Nur an manchen Stellen drängen die Kalkmassen gegen die Epidermis vor. Diese ist im wesentlichen unverändert und erscheint nur an diesen Stellen verschmälert. Eventuell kann es auch zum Einreißen und zur Fistelbildung kommen (GANS und STEIGLEDER, 1955). In seltenen Fällen wurden auch Kalkablagerungen innerhalb der Epidermis beschrieben (WEIDMANN und SHAFFER, 1926).

Die Kalkmassen sind großteils von einer Kapsel aus kernarmen, dichtfaserigem und meist völlig hyalin entartetem Bindegewebe umgeben. Vielfach wird auch ein heller Hof erwähnt, der aus kristallinischen Kalkkörperchen besteht (NAEGELI, 1932). An Zellen findet man reichlich Fremdkörperriesenzellen und in geringerem Ausmaße Fibroblasten, Lymphoid- und Plasmazellen (BRODY und BELLIN, 1937; PONHOLD, 1941; WISKEMANN, 1955). Teilweise sieht man in den kernreichen Riesenzellen als Zeichen einer Phagocytose kleine Kalkpartikel eingeschlossen. Sie sind nicht nur unmittelbar am Kalkherd zu finden, sondern auch in der Umgebung. Auffallend sind degenerative Veränderungen der elastischen Fasern, die verquollen und fragmentiert erscheinen. Gerade diese pathologisch veränderten elastischen Elemente haben eine große Affinität zum Calcium (WINER, 1952). Häufig findet man im Zentrum von Kalkablagerungen Aufhellungen, die bei einer Elasticafärbung intensiv Farbstoff annehmen (PONHOLD, 1941). Ähnliche degenerative Veränderungen der elastischen Fasern, zumeist verbunden mit einer Aufhellung der kollagenen Bündel, sieht man auch weit von den Kalkablagerungen entfernt. Auch fallen Riesenzellen auf, die sich den morphologisch nur gering veränderten elastischen Fasern anlagern. Beim *Pseudoxanthoma elasticum* ist die Kalkablagerung an den elastischen Fasern das am frühesten nachweisbare histologische Symptom (FINNERUD und NOMLAND, 1937; GRONBLAD, 1948; GOODMAN u. Mitarb., 1963). Diese Ablagerung läßt sich auch historöntgenographisch gut darstellen (NIEBAUER u. Mitarb., 1965). Ähnlich wie die anderen Bindegewebsfasern bestehen auch die elastischen Fasern aus Fibrillen und Kittsubstanz. Elektronenmikroskopisch wurde nachgewiesen, daß Kalksalze nur in die Kittsubstanz der elastischen Faser eingelagert werden (SCHMITT-ROHDE und WEICHHARDT, 1955).

An den Gefäßen sind auch weit von den Kalkherden entfernt Veränderungen festzustellen. Die Elastica erscheint aufgelockert, verdünnt und gleichzeitig kommt es zu einer kompensatorischen Wucherung der Intima mit einer Neubildung zarter elastischer Fasern, wodurch stellenweise das Lumen eingeengt wird (PONHOLD, 1941). Die Hautanhangsgebilde bleiben unverändert.

In manchen Fällen kann es nach vorangegangener Verkalkung auch zur Bildung von Knochengewebe kommen. Durch die Riesenzellen kommt es zur lacunären Resorption des Kalkgewebes und auf den Resten der verkalkten Grundlage wird durch Osteoblasten osteoides Gewebe gebildet (MUSGER, 1935; BÄFVERSTEDT, 1941).

VII. Urate

Durch die Desaminierung und Oxydation von Nahrungspurinen einerseits und durch den physiologischen Abbau körpereigener Purine andererseits entsteht im menschlichen Organismus Harnsäure. Eine „Harnsäuresynthese", wie sie in großem Maße bei den urikotelen Tieren (Vögeln, Reptilien) stattfindet, spielt beim Menschen keine Rolle. Ausgeschieden wird die Harnsäure zum überwiegenden Teil über die Nieren, in geringerem Maße über Magensaft, Galle und Schweißdrüsen (NIINO, 1939; FREUDENTHAL und GESEROWA, 1929; ZÖLLNER, 1957).

Zu einer *Ablagerung von Uraten im Hautbereich* kommt es nun beim Ansteigen des Harnsäurespiegels im Blut. Die Urate dialysieren in vivo in alle extracellulären Flüssigkeitsräume und finden sich dort in der gleichen Konzentration wie im Plasma. Steigt der Harnsäurespiegel, so kommt es zu einer Übersättigung der Lösung. Im Blut bleibt sie infolge des hohen Eiweißgehaltes stabil, im Interstitium fallen die Urate jedoch aus. Zumeist tritt dieses Ereignis ziemlich plötzlich ein. Klinisch resultiert der akute Gichtanfall. Relativ selten kommt es dazu ohne diese akuten Erscheinungen (KAISER, 1920; EBNER und RAAB, 1964). Die auslösende Ursache für das Ausfallen der Urate im interstitiellen Gewebe ist letztlich ungeklärt (TAPPEINER und WODNIANSKY, 1959). Bedeutungsvoll sind hierbei nur die bei neutraler Reaktion entstehenden primären, monobasischen Salze der Harnsäure.

Die Stelle, an der es zur Ausbildung der Tophi kommt, also der Ort des Niederschlages der Urate, ist sicherlich durch lokale Faktoren bestimmt. THANNHAUSER (1956) hat darauf hingewiesen, daß gerade in den Gewebsspalten des Knorpels die interstitielle Flüssigkeit besonders schlecht zirkuliert. Auch GOTTRON und KORTING (1957) unterstrichen die Bedeutung der örtlichen Durchblutungsverhältnisse für die Ablagerung von Uraten im Bindegewebe. Histologisch wurden am Rande der Uratablagerungen wandverdickte Gefäße beobachtet (NIINO, 1940). Vielleicht gibt es neben einer zirkulatorischen noch eine zusätzliche histochemische Disposition von kollagen- und mucopolysaccharidreichem Gewebe für das Ausfallen der Urate.

Die Ablagerung der Uratkristalle erfolgt in unverändertes Gewebe. Die nach Herauslösung der Kristalle nachweisbaren Gewebsveränderungen sind sekundären Charakters.

Als einfachstes Mittel zum *Nachweis der Urate* im Inhalt der Tophi ist das Nativpräparat zu erwähnen. Es finden sich zahlreiche, zumeist büschelförmig zusammenliegende, wechselnd große Kristallnadeln. Daneben sieht man noch kleine Mengen uneinheitlicher Salzgemische und charakteristische Cholesterintafeln. Mit dem entnommenen Untersuchungsmaterial macht man am besten gleichzeitig die Murexidprobe (LEVER, 1963). Zur Fixierung des histologischen Präparates verwendet man am zweckmäßigsten Alkohol, da durch Formalin die Kristalle zerstört werden. Weitere histochemische Nachweise s. bei LEVER (1963).

Die *Histologie* zeigt eine stellenweise leicht hyperkeratotische, in anderen Abschnitten mäßiggradig atrophische Epidermis. Auf weite Strecken erweist sich die Epidermis jedoch als unverändert. In den mittleren und tiefen Coriumschichten, teilweise auch in der Subcutis, finden sich rund oder ovalär konfigurierte Bezirke, die sich mit Eosin zartrosa anfärben und eine schollige, wolkige Strukturierung erkennen lassen. Diese Areale sind von einem dichten, fortlaufenden Infiltratsaum umgeben, der vorwiegend aus Lymphocyten, Histiocyten und vielkernigen Fremdkörperriesenzellen aufgebaut ist. Bei vielen epidermisnahe gelegenen Knoten stellt diese Zone der bindegewebigen Reaktion die einzige Trennschicht gegen die Epidermis dar. An manchen Stellen können die Uratablagerungen die Epidermis fistelartig durchbrechen (GOTTRON und KORTING, 1957). Besonders deutlich erkennt man die oben beschriebenen Veränderungen bei Durchführung der kombinierten Alcianblau-PAS-Färbung. Die Knoten färben sich dabei hellblau wolkig an, im bindegewebigen Randsaum sind in vermehrtem Maße PAS-positive Strukturen zu erkennen. Bei Anwendung der Silberimprägnationsmethode nach GOMORI findet sich ein zartes Netzwerk versilberbarer Fasern innerhalb der Knoten. Nach GRÜN (1926) soll es sich hierbei nicht um Fasern im eigentlichen Sinne, sondern um Eiweißstrukturen handeln.

VIII. Melanin

Die enzymatische Synthese des Pigments Melanin und die Reifung der Melanosomen zu vollmelanisierten Granula innerhalb spezialisierter Zellen der Epidermis (Melanocyten), die Abgabe der Granula in Form eines cytokrinen Vorganges, die phagocytäre Speicherung des Pigments in Malpighizellen oder Histiocyten und schließlich der Abtransport des Pigments sind physiologische Vorgänge. Das quantitative Ausmaß der Melaninsynthese und Pigmentspeicherung in den Zellen sind bestimmend für die Hautfarbe und genetisch fixiert. Abweichungen von der Norm manifestieren sich als Hyper- und Depigmentierungen. Der Hauptort der Melaninbildung und -speicherung ist intraepidermal gelegen; über die Physiologie und Pathologie der intraepidermalen Pigmentstoffwechselvorgänge muß auf die entsprechenden Kapitel des Handbuches verwiesen werden.

Nur in Ausnahmefällen (z.B. bei Mongolenfleck oder bei bestimmten pathologischen Zuständen) kommt es auch zu einer dermalen Melaninablagerung, die über das physiologische Ausmaß hinausgeht.

Zum besseren Verständnis sollen die biochemischen und morphologischen *Grundlagen des Melaninstoffwechsels* hier kurz referiert werden:

Auf Grund bisheriger Untersuchungen ist beim Menschen *L-Tyrosin* dasjenige Substrat aus dem die Melanocyten Pigment bilden (RAPER, 1928; EVANS u. RAPER, 1937). Im nichtaktivierten Melanocyten scheint die Umwandlung des Tyrosins nur langsam vor sich zu gehen. Sobald sich jedoch in Gegenwart des Ferments *Tyrosinase* (FITZPATRICK u. Mitarb., 1950 bis

1963; MASON u. Mitarb., 1948—1956) und molekularen Sauerstoffs kleine Mengen Dopa gebildet haben, läuft die Reaktion schneller ab. Der nächste Schritt ist die Umwandlung des Dopa zum entsprechenden Chinon. Auch diese Reaktion erfordert die Gegenwart einer Phenoloxydase; sie wird entsprechend dem Substrat als Dopaoxydase bezeichnet. Tyrosinase und Dopaoxydase sind ein einheitliches Enzym, dessen Wirkgruppe Kupfer ist und dessen Aktivität von der Wertigkeit des Kupfers abhängt. Das reduzierte Enzym (Cuproverbindung) ist sowohl gegenüber Tyrosin als auch gegenüber Dopa aktiv. Die oxydierte Form des Enzyms ist gegenüber Tyrosin unwirksam (aber aktivierbar) und gegenüber Dopa von vornherein aktiv. Dopachinon oxydiert im weiteren Reaktionsverlauf spontan zum roten Farbstoff Dopachrom, aus dem schließlich über 5,6-Dihydroxyindol die Melaninmuttersubstanz hervorgeht. Dieses Polymer ist mit seinem Chinon im „Melaningranulum" an die Amino- oder Sulphhydrilgruppen einer Proteinmatrix gebunden. Die endgültige chemische Struktur des proteingebundenen Melaninmoleküls ist allerdings nicht bekannt (MASON, 1959; HEMPEL, 1966).

Über die *Lokalisation der Tyrosinaseaktivität* in Suspensionen von Zellteilchen wurde schon von HERRMANN u. BOSS (1945) und dann von LERNER, FITZPATRICK u. Mitarb. (1949) berichtet. Kombinierte elektronenoptische und biochemische Studien haben zu der Erkenntnis geführt, daß die Tyrosinaseaktivität an distinkte cytoplasmatische Teilchen gebunden ist, die *nicht* mit modifizierten Mitochondrien identisch sind. Diese tyrosinaseaktiven Körperchen werden heute als „Prämelanosomen" bezeichnet (FITZPATRICK, QUEVEDO u. Mitarb., 1966), während nur die reifen, d. h. vollmelanisierten Granula als „Melanosomen" beschrieben werden. Diese Organellen entstammen der Golgiregion dem endoplasmatischen Reticulum (HIRSCH, 1937; BARNICOT u. BIRBECK, 1958; SEIJI u. Mitarb., 1961, 1963 und HIRSCH u. Mitarb., 1965). Die Synthese der Melaningranula erfolgt gewissermaßen in drei Stufen: zuerst kommt es zur Bildung der „Protyrosinase" aus Polypeptiden (Ribosome), dann folgt ein Zwischenstadium, in dem sich diese Protyrosinasemoleküle zu „Prämelanosomen" ordnen und schließlich folgt das Stadium, in dem die Biosynthese des Melanin beginnt und sich das Pigment innerhalb der Prämelanosomen anreichert. In dieser Phase enthält das Granulum aktive Tyrosinase. Diese Organellen finden sich nur im Cytoplasma der Melanocyten. Das Endprodukt dieses Vorganges ist das „Melanosom", in dem die Pigmentbildung zu Ende geführt ist; daher enthält diese Organelle auch keine aktive Tyrosinase mehr. Als „*Melaningranulum*" wird heute nur das lichtoptisch wahrnehmbare Produkt der Melaninsynthese bezeichnet, es kann innerhalb und außerhalb der Melanocyten liegen.

Die *histochemischen Eigenschaften des Melanins* sind im Lehrbuch von PEARSE ausführlich dargestellt; insbesondere seine Differentialdiagnose gegenüber Hämosiderin, argentaffine Granula anderer Art, chromaffine Granula, Pseudomelanin und verschiedene Lipopigmente. Bei einem Pigment, das völlig unlöslich ist in Lösungsmitteln, die das Gewebe nicht zerstören, aber löslich ist in N NaOH, das gebleicht wird durch starke Oxydationsmittel in weniger als 48 Std und das ammoniakalisches Silbernitrat reduziert, handelt es sich nach PEARSE fast immer um Melanin. Nach diesem Autor ist die *Ferri-Ferricyanidreaktion* (SCHMORLS Reaktion) entschieden empfindlicher als die Technik der Melanindarstellung mit ammoniakalischem Silber. Allerdings ist die Schmorl-Reaktion unspezifischer, denn es reagieren überhaupt die Diphenole, auch chromaffines Gewebe, SH-Gruppen usw. (ADAMS, 1956). Von LILLIE wurde 1957 eine Modifikation dieser Methode angegeben, die nach Art der Turnbull-Blaumethode abläuft und für Melanin sehr spezifisch sein soll.

Zum *enzymhistochemischen Nachweis der melaninbildenden Phenolasen* eignen sich die Tyrosinase- bzw. Dopaoxydasereaktion (FITZPATRICK u. KUKITA, 1959) und ihre empfindlicheren Modifikationen, wie z.B. die kombinierte Dopa-ammoniakalische-Silbernitratmethode von MISHIMA (1960) oder die Anwendung markierten Tyrosins für Autoradiographien (FITZPATRICK u. KUKITA, 1956).

Nur gröbere Melaningranula geben eine positive, diastaseresistente *PAS-Reaktion*. Daher verhalten sich die Granula in den Melanophagen und Melanomzellen meist PAS-positiv und die kleineren intraepidermalen Granula meist PAS-negativ (LANGER u. STÜTTGEN, 1960; MONTAGNA, CHASE u. Mitarb., 1951).

Nur die Melanocyten sind in der Lage Melanosomen zu synthetisieren. Die Vorstufen dieser Zellen, die sog. Melanoblasten stammen aus der *Neuralleiste* (RAWLES, 1947, 1948; ZIMMERMANN, 1950, 1954; ZIMMERMANN u. Mitarb., 1948, 1959), aus der sie während des neonatalen Lebens in drei Richtungen wandern: in die Haut und Übergangsschleimhaut, in das Auge (Uveatractus und Retina) und in das Zentralnervensystem (Leptomeninx). Nach dem 6. Embryonalmonat haben die epidermalen Melanocyten ihre endgültige Position an der Epidermis-Cutisgrenze eingenommen (MISHIMA u. Mitarb., 1966). Die *dermalen Melanoblasten* scheinen zu diesem Zeitpunkt „aufgebraucht" zu sein. Nur bei bestimmten Rassen (Asiaten, Inder, Neger) bleiben sie oft über diese Zeit hinaus in der Region des caudalen Endes der Neuralleiste und des Neuralrohres liegen, wandeln sich schon intradermal in Melanocyten um und bilden dann den sog. „*Mongolenfleck*", der als ein Restlager des embryonalen Be-standes an dermalen Melanocyten aufgefaßt wird (STARCK, 1964). Auch im späteren Leben bleibt diese Beziehung der Hautmelanocyten zu den neuralen Strukturen erkennbar (NIEBAUER u. WIEDMANN). Während die Melanocyten der Haut die Fähigkeit der Melaninbildung zumindest intraepithelial ihr ganzes Leben behalten (positive Dopaoxydasereaktion), sind die Melanocyten des Auges und der Leptomeninx nur eine begrenzte embryonale Zeitspanne zur Melaninbildung fähig.

Die *Terminologie der melaninenthaltenden Zellen* wurde den modernen Erfordernissen entsprechend bei der 6. Internationalen Pigmentzellkonferenz in Sofia 1965 festgelegt und von FITZPATRICK, QUEVEDO jr., LEVENE u. Mitarb. (1966) publiziert. Als „*Melanocyt*" wird nur die reife, zur enzymatischen Melaninsynthese fähige Zelle bezeichnet. Der Definition von BLOCH entsprechend wird diese Zelle auch heute noch im europäischen Schrifttum häufig als „*Melanoblast*" bezeichnet. Doch wurde international festgelegt, daß als Melanoblast nur jene unreifen Zellen zu bezeichnen sind, die von der Neuralleiste entstammend zur Pigmentbildung noch nicht fähig sind. Grundsätzlich zu unterscheiden sind die pigmenttragenden Zellen des Bindegewebes, die sog. „*Melanophagen*". Hingegen ist der Ausdruck „*Melanophoren*" den Pigmentzellen bei Fischen, Amphibien usw. vorbehalten, die contractile Eigenschaften haben.

Die *elektronenmikroskopischen Eigenschaften der Melanocyten* wurden eingehend von BIRBECK u. Mitarb. (1957—1963), BREATHNACH u. Mitarb. (1963—1965) und ZELICKSON u. Mitarb. (1962—1965) beschrieben. Diese Befunde bestätigen die Eigenschaft des Melanocyten als „Drüsenzelle", worauf schon MASSON auf Grund der Ergebnisse lichtoptischer Befunde hingewiesen hat. Das Produkt dieser Zellen, die Melanosomen, hat charakteristische ultrastrukturelle Eigenschaften, die abhängig vom Zelltyp verschieden sind. Das heißt, epidermale Melanocyten, dermale Melanocyten, Naevuszellen, Melanomzellen usw. synthetisieren strukturell verschieden aussehende Melanosomen, so daß eine Zelldifferenzierung schon auf Grund der ultrastrukturellen Eigenschaften der Melanosome möglich ist. Besonders MISHIMA (1966) hat auf diesen „*Melanosome-Polymorphismus*" hingewiesen; ein Befund, der besonders für das Studium dermaler Pigmentablagerungen von großer Bedeutung ist.

Die Melanocyten sind sog. „*Dendritenzellen*" (BILLINGHAM u. Mitarb., 1948—1953; NIEBAUER u. Mitarb., 1953—1965). Der Abtransport des Pigments erfolgt über die Dendriten durch Abgabe an die Epidermiszellen in Form einer „cytokrinen Sekretion" (MASSON). An diesem Vorgang beteiligen sich die Malpighizellen aktiv im Sinne von Phagocytose der Melaningranula, die sich sodann vor allem im apikalen Teil der Zellen in Form sog. „Kernkappen" anreichern (RAPPAPORT, 1956; DROCHMANS, 1966).

Unter *physiologischen* Bedingungen finden sich *in der Derma intracytoplasmatische Melanineinlagerungen* in zwei grundsätzlich verschiedenen Zellarten: 1. In Zellen, die das Melaninpigment autochthon gebildet haben; sog. „dermale Melanocyten" (auch „Cutis-Melanoblasten" genannt) und 2. in Bindegewebszellen, die das Pigment phagocytiert haben („Melanophagen"). Nur unter pathologischen Bedingungen kommt es auch in anderen Zelltypen zum Auftreten von Melanin wie in Naevuszellen, Melanomzellen usw. (s. dazu den Handbuchbeitrag von COTTINI, Bd. II/1).

Das Auftreten *dermaler Melanocyten* ist am ehesten mit der Einwanderung der Melanoblasten aus der Neuralleiste in die Cutis erklärbar, in dem Sinne, daß sich diese Zellen schon vor ihrem Eintritt in den epithelialen Verband in aktive Melanocyten umwandeln. Eine abschließende Beweisführung dieser Vorstellung ist allerdings noch nicht gelungen und es bleibt nach wie vor die Frage offen, ob nicht in dem einen oder anderen Falle dermale Melanocyten *sekundär* aus der Epidermis oder aus dem Haarfollikel in das Corium gelangen (SZABO, 1959—1963; KINOSHITA, 1960). Klinisch manifestieren sich Ansammlungen dermaler Melanocyten als Mongolenfleck, Naevus Ota oder Blauer Naevus (ausführliche Beschreibung im Handbuchbeitrag von COTTINI, Bd. II/1).

Die Mehrzahl der Autoren stimmt heute darin überein, daß das Melanin der *Melanophagen* aus den epidermalen Melanocyten stammt und daß es durch Phagocytose aufgenommen wird. Wie allerdings der Transport des Melanins vor sich geht, ist noch weitgehend unbekannt. MIESCHERs Vorstellung, daß die Aufnahme über ein gelöstes Pigment erfolgt, ist nicht bewiesen. Für diese Theorie ist auch die Studie von BECKER (1927), daß die Pigmentzellen der Dermis identisch sind mit den perivasculären Histiocyten, also den gleichen Zellen, die Fett und Hämosiderin speichern, kein ausreichender Beweis. Vom histochemischen Standpunkt aus ist MIESCHERs Theorie schwer vorstellbar, da sich das Melanin nur in stark alkalischen Medien löst. Ebenso ist die Hypothese von MEIROWSKY u. Mitarb. (1951) einer Kondensation gelösten epithelialen Pigments zu Coriumpigment nicht bewiesen.

Elektronenmikroskopische Untersuchungen ermöglichen es ohne weiteres, zwischen melaninbildenden dermalen Melanocyten und pigmentspeichernden Melanophagen zu unterscheiden (CHARLES u. INGRAM, 1959; DROCHMANS, 1963; MISHIMA, 1966). Letztere speichern die Melaningranula in Organellen, deren ultrastrukturelle Charakteristika identisch sind mit den Lysosomen (sog. „lysosomale Speicherung", NOVIKOFF, 1961). Da diese Organellen reich an saurer Phosphatase sind, lassen sich die Melanophagen auch histochemisch von den phosphatasenegativen Melanocyten unterscheiden.

Besonders MEIROWSKY hat auf die Anordnung dermaler Pigmentzellen um Blut- und Lymphgefäße hingewiesen. Nach seiner Auffassung bilden die dermalen Pigmentzellen ein von der Epidermis unabhängiges System, wobei das Melanin der Zellen ein metabolisches Produkt des Zellkernes ist. Neben dieser hauptsächlich perivasculären Anordnung der Melanophagen ist auch eine perineurale Anordnung erkennbar, die als „subepidermale *perineurale Pigmenthülle*" von KAWAMURA (1954) besonders herausgestellt wurde. Dieser Autor erblickt in den Melanocyten der Epidermis und in der nervösen Peripherie der Haut mit ihrer perineuralen Pigmenthülle einen zusammengehörigen Komplex.

Der *Abtransport des dermalen Pigments* erfolgt über die Lymphgefäße. Dafür sprechen pathologisch-anatomische Befunde, die sich bei bestimmten Hauterkrankungen und Neoplasien im Lymphbahnbereich erheben lassen (PAUTRIER u. Mitarb., 1927; PATTERSON, 1959; GAIL, 1957).

Wie vorhin ausgeführt findet unter physiologischen Bedingungen die Melaninsynthese in der Haut des Menschen nur in den Melanocyten statt. Das gilt auch z.B. für den Naevus coeruleus, den Mongolenfleck usw. Es gibt jedoch Ausnahmefälle, bei denen in der Haut eine autochthone Melaninbildung zustande kommt, ohne daß Tyrosinase oder Dopaoxydase an der Ablagerungsstelle des Pigments nachweisbar wäre. Das ist der Fall bei den *universellen Melanodermien* im Rahmen von weit fortgeschrittenen Melanomen (FITZPATRICK u. Mitarb., 1954). Bei diesen kommt es zu einer abnormen Melaninablagerung in der Cutis, während die epidermalen Melanocyten unverändert sind. Im Rahmen dieser Erkrankungen gelangen die Vorstufen des Melanins (Dopa, 5,6-Dihydroxyindol) aus den Blutgefäßen in das Corium und werden dort durch unspezifische oxydierende Fermentsysteme in den Histiocyten und in der extracellulären Flüssigkeit in Melanin umgewandelt (LEONHARDI, 1955).

IX. Porphyrine

Die Einbeziehung der Porphyrien in das Kapitel über Ablagerungen und Speicherungen in der Cutis geht von der einfachen Vorstellung aus, daß bei diesen Erkrankungen tatsächlich Porphyrine in der Haut abgelagert und dann als Fotosensibilisatoren wirksam werden. Für die Ablagerung oder Speicherung photodynamisch wirksamer Porphyrine in der Haut des Menschen sprechen allerdings nur Einzelbefunde.

Während bei der klassischen Porphyria congenita Günther und bei den hepatischen Porphrieformen das Uroporphyrin als wesentliche photosensibilisierende Substanz bezeichnet wird, scheint für die Photosensibilisierung bei der zweiten erythropoetischen Porphyrieform, nämlich der protoporphyrinämischen Lichturticaria, das Protoporphyrin verantwortlich zu sein. Die Voraussetzung dafür ist gegeben, denn im Gegensatz zu älteren Befunden (FISCHER u. SCHNELLER, 1920) ist neuerdings auch bei dieser Substanz eine photosensibilisierende Wirkung nachgewiesen worden (WEGNER, 1948; SCHENK u. WIRTH, 1953).

Nur einige wenige fluorescenzmikroskopische Befunde über eine Ablagerung der Porphyrine in der Haut bei Porphyrien liegen vor.

Der fluorescenzmikroskopische Nachweis von Porphyrinen im Gewebe erfordert allerdings eine einwandfreie Technik, da schon die ungeeignete Vorbehandlung des Gewebes zum Herauslösen des rotfluorescierenden Stoffes und damit zu einer falsch negativen Reaktion führt. Über eine optimale histologische Technik für Biopsiematerial der Tarda-Leber zum Zwecke des fluorescenzmikroskopischen Porphyrinnachweises haben HOLZNER u. NIEBAUER (1963) berichtet.

Eine weitere Fehlerquelle bei der Beurteilung von Schnitten ist die Eigenfluorescenz des Gewebes (ausführlich darüber in den Arbeiten von BOMMER, 1929 und bei NIEBAUER, 1961). Auch sie ist unter anderem von der Vorbehandlung des Gewebes abhängig, weshalb die Untersuchung nativer Gefrierschnitte am geeignetsten ist. Zum Beispiel wird nach Fixieren des Materials in Formol die „Eigenfluorescenz" zahlreicher Strukturen intensiver, es fluorescieren dann auch die Kollagenbündel und einige epitheliale Elemente, weshalb im strengen Sinne von einer Sekundärfluorescenz nach Formolfixierung zu sprechen wäre. Im unfixierten, nativen Gewebe der normalen Haut fluorescieren bläulich-weiß die elastischen Fasern, die Drüsenmembranen und die Hornsubstanz. Goldgelb fluorescierende Granula finden sich im Schweißdrüsenepithel, in der Wand größerer Arterien und in bestimmten Zellen (NIEBAUER, 1961). Weiter beschrieben BOMMER u. HAMPERL eine streifenförmige Zone an der Grenze zwischen dem Stratum granulosum und dem Stratum lucidum mit stark ausgeprägter Fluorescenz, die wegen ihres ziegelroten Farbtones der Fluorescenz rings um die Haarpapillen ähnlich ist (DE LERMA, 1958). Allerdings hat NIEBAUER in unfixierten Kryostatschnitten der normalen Haut diese Rotfluorescenz nicht nachweisen können. BOMMER (1929) beschreibt auch eine rotfluorescierende Substanz in Follikeltrichtern der Gesichtshaut, während die Talgdrüsen selbst keine rote Fluorescenz zeigen und vermutet, ein durch Bakterien gebildetes Porphyrin nachgewiesen zu haben. Auch MONTAGNA (1956) beschreibt das gelegentliche Vorkommen einer roten Fluorescenz in Comedonen und vermutet Porphyrin.

Bei der Güntherschen Krankheit fanden BORST u. KÖNIGSDORFER (1929) im obersten Corium, direkt unter der Epidermis, sowie auch im Stratum corneum feine Porphyringranula (Nachweis erst nach Alkalisieren der Schnitte deutlich). LANGHOF, MÜLLER u. RIETSCHEL (1961) beobachteten bei *familiärer, protoporphyrinämischer Lichturticaria* eine intensive rotbraune, fleckige Fluorescenz der gesamten Epidermis, die im Stratum corneum am stärksten war. Daneben fielen im Corium und in der unteren Epidermis gelb bis orange fluorescierende Körnchen auf. Nach 30 sec Belichtung verschwand die Rotfluorescenz in der für das Porphyrin typischen Weise. Untersucht wurden trocken eingebettete Gefrierschnitte. Die Natur dieses fluorescierenden Stoffes konnte nicht genauer analysiert werden. Es wird nur *vermutet*, daß es sich dabei um Protoporphyrin handelt.

Bei dem von LANGHOF, MÜLLER u. RIETSCHEL (1962) als Dermatitis solaris subita recidivans beschriebenen Fall wurde ebenfalls in einem Hautexzisat eine diffuse rosarote Fluorescenz im Stratum corneum, weniger intensiv in den darunter liegenden Epidermisschichten, nachgewiesen. Diese Fluorescenz zeigte allerdings kein Löschphänomen, weshalb es sich nicht um Porphyrinfluorescenz handeln kann. Da die Patientin große Mengen phenolphthaleinhaltiger Abführmittel eingenommen hatte, wird von den Autoren die Möglichkeit des Nachweises einer derartigen Substanz oder eines Indolabkömmlings diskutiert. Bei solchen Untersuchungen muß also auch an die Möglichkeit der Ablagerung medikamentöser rotfluorescierender Substanzen gedacht werden!

LANGHOF u. RIETSCHEL (1962) haben auch bei einem Patienten mit cutaner Porphyrie an einer bedeckt getragenen Hautstelle (Leistenbeuge) eine fleckförmige Rotfluorescenz, die das Löschphänomen nach 20 sec. zeigte, nachgewiesen, während der fluorescenzmikroskopische Befund an der freigetragenen Haut (Handrücken) negativ war. Weitere Untersuchungen in dieser Richtung sind allerdings erforderlich, um zu einem abschließenden Urteil zu kommen. Denn sowohl MAGNUS, JARRETT u. Mitarb. (1961), als auch SUUROMOND (1965) haben in den unfixierten Kryostatschnitten der Hautbiopsien von Fällen mit protoporphyrinämischer Lichtdermatose *keine* pathologische Fluorescenz nachweisen können.

Anders ist allerdings die Situation vom Standpunkt biochemischer Untersuchungen: Schon in der normalen Haut des Menschen haben PATHAK und BURNETT (1964) weit schwankende Werte zwischen 0,09 µg/g und 0,48 µg/g Uroporphyrin nachgewiesen. Ein signifikanter Anstieg der Gewebskonzentration bei Porphyrien wurde nicht festgestellt, doch müßten Untersuchungen dieser Art an einem größeren Material wiederholt werden.

Auch in der sehr umfangreichen Literatur über *Porphyria cutanea tarda*, der weitaus häufigsten Porphyrinkrankheit, finden sich keine sicheren histologischen Angaben über eine Ablagerung rotfluorescierender Substanzen in der Cutis, obgleich das Ergebnis von Belichtungsversuchen für Porphyrinablagerungen in der Haut sprechen würde. WISKEMANN und WULF (1959) haben bei Porphyria cutanea tarda regelmäßig pathologische Erytheme durch langwelliges UV- und sichtbares Licht entsprechend dem Absorptionsspektrum der ausgeschiedenen Porphyrine nachweisen können. Diese Befunde lassen das direkte Mitwirken der Porphyrine als Fotosensibilisatoren, zumindest bei der erythematösen Reaktion, vermuten. Auch bei protoporphyrinämischen Lichtdermatosen fanden MAGNUS (1964) und WISKEMANN u. WEHRMANN (1965) eine abnormale Maximal-Lichtempfindlichkeit bei Wellenlängen um 400 µm. Bei starker Empfindlichkeit kann sich das auslösende Spektralbereich bis zu 600 µm im sichtbaren Spektrum erstrecken. Nach diesen Autoren bekräftigen derartige Befunde die Ansicht, daß bei Porphyrie das Licht spezifisch von den Porphyrinmolekülen der Haut aufgenommen wird und so zu einer photobiologischen Wirkung führt.

FORMANEK und NIEBAUER (1966) haben bei einigen Tardapatienten Hautbiopsien fluorescenzmikroskopisch untersucht, und zwar sowohl von bedeckten als auch von frei getragenen Körperstellen. Diese Untersuchungen wurden unter den gleichen methodischen Voraussetzungen durchgeführt wie der Porphyrinnachweis in Leberbiopsien (HOLZNER und NIEBAUER). In keinem Hautschnitt ließen sich auf diese Weise rotfluorescierende Substanzen in der Epidermis oder im Corium nachweisen.

Mit diesen Befunden ist allerdings die Vorstellung der Porphyria cutanea tarda als einfache, photodynamisch ausgelöste Lichtdermatose nicht ohne weiteres vereinbar. Die Blasenbildung ist bei dieser Erkrankung immer subepidermal und unilokulär. Sie tritt nur in Zonen einer weit fortgeschrittenen Schädigung des Hautbindegewebes auf. Im Vordergrund steht eine basophile Degeneration des Bindegewebes und eine hochgradige pathologische Veränderung der Elastica im Sinne einer aktinischen (senilen) Elastose des oberen und mittleren Coriums, während im subepidermalen Bereich die elastischen Fasern nicht angefärbt sind. (Ausführlich über die Histologie der akuten und chronischen Hautschädigungen als Folge der aktinischen oder traumatischen Noxe bei Porphyrien s. LEVERs Handbuchbeitrag in Vol. III/1). Vor allem letzterer Befund wird von KLOSTERMANN und RITZENFELD (1963) für den „Festigkeitsverlust der dermoepidermalen Verbindung" verantwortlich gemacht. Die Wände der kleinen Gefäße sind oft auffallend verdickt und färben sich stark PAS-positiv an; ein entzündliches Infiltrat des Coriums fehlt fast völlig. Es scheint also so zu sein, daß im Rahmen der Porphyrie an den belichteten Hautstellen frühzeitig und hochgradig eine degenerative Schädigung des Bindegewebes einsetzt. Es ist durchaus möglich, daß diese Terrainschädigung ein wesentlicher Faktor für die aktinisch-traumatisch bedingte Blasenbildung ist.

X. Ablagerungen von Eisen (Hämosiderin)

Mit der Kost gelangen täglich etwa 10—20 mg Eisen in den Darm, wovon normalerweise weniger als 1 mg resorbiert wird. Etwa in der gleichen Größenordnung liegt die tägliche Eisenausscheidung in Harn, Stuhl, Schweiß und durch den Haarausfall. Sie ändert sich auch nicht bei erhöhtem Eisenangebot (AUFDERHEIDE, HORNS u. Mitarb, 1953; LEIPERT, 1964). Somit hat der Körper nur eine sehr beschränkte Fähigkeit, einmal aufgenommenes Eisen wieder abzugeben. Auf diesem Wege kommt es bei bestimmten Formen schwerer chronischer Anämie, bei Malaria, Blutstauung, parenteraler Eisenzufuhr, Bluttransfusionen usw. zur *Hämosiderose*. Mit *Hämochromatose* bezeichnet man das pathologisch-anatomische Syndrom einer Eisenthesaurismose, Hämosiderose bzw. Siderose verbunden mit fibrotischen Organveränderungen. Die idiopathische Hämochromatose ist charakterisiert durch vermehrte Eisenresorption, exzessive Eisenablagerung und Fibrose in sämtlichen Geweben. Klinisch ist sie beim Vollbild durch die Trias *braunes Hautkolorit, Lebercirrhose* und *Diabetes mellitus* gekennzeichnet. Es gilt heute als gesichert, daß ihr eine angeborene Stoffwechselstörung zugrunde liegt. Von der idiopathischen Hämochromatose sind die anderen Formen der Eisenthesaurismosen abzutrennen (s. Tabelle). Diese Siderosen zeigen neben der Eisenspeicherung keine Gewebsläsion. Morphologisch und klinisch ist die Differenzierung der Lebercirrhose mit ausgedehnter Siderose von einer idiopathischen Hämochromatose meist unmöglich. Diese Formen können nur durch die Untersuchungen des Eisenstoffwechsels und der Erythrocytenkinetik mit Fe^{59} und Cr^{51} auseinander gehalten werden (BRUNNER, 1965).

Klassifikation des Hämochromatosesyndroms (BRUNNER, 1965)

---

1. Idiopathische Hämachromatose
2. Siderosen:
    a) Eisenverwertungsstörungen:
       idiopathische refraktäre Anämie
       sideroachrestische Anämie
    b) Eisenüberangebot:
       endogen: Hämolyse
       exogen: Transfusionen bzw. i.v. Eisentherapie
       Nahrung: perorale Eisentherapie, Cytosiderose der Bantu-Neger
       Trinkwasser: Kaschin-Beck-Krankheit (Mongolei)
    c) Lebercirrhose mit Siderose (sekundäre Hämochromatose)

Als ein besonderes, aber nicht spezifisches Charakteristikum der Hämochromatose wird die Bronzefärbung der Haut bezeichnet. Sie wird kaum durch die Eisenablagerungen, sondern vor allem durch Melaninablagerungen hervorgerufen. Diese Hyperpigmentation der Haut ist nur beim voll entwickelten Krankheitsbild mit großer Häufigkeit vorhanden, Prozentangaben schwanken zwischen 84—97% der Fälle. Als Initialsymptom wurde sie von verschiedenen Autoren in 26% (SHELDON, 1935), 32% (FINCH und FINCH, 1955) bzw. 40% (BUTT und WILDER, 1938) angegeben.

Die *histologische Untersuchung der Haut* hat die Aufgabe, die Erhöhung des Eisengehaltes nachzuweisen, um so die Differentialdiagnose gegenüber anderen mit Hyperpigmentierung des Integuments einhergehenden Dermatosen zu erleichtern. Die Hautprobeexcision ist heute allerdings nicht mehr das wichtigste diagnostische Hilfsmittel, vielmehr nur eine von mehreren Laboratoriumsmethoden zum Nachweis einer Hämochromatose. Für die Diagnose wesentlich ist besonders die histologische Untersuchung des Leberpunktats, die Bestimmung des Plasmaeisens und der Eisenbindungskapazität.

Mit der Berliner Blau-Reaktion wird meist nur ein recht bescheidener Teil des vorhandenen Eisens dargestellt, weshalb diese Methode von SOLTERMANN (1956) für den Nachweis von Hämochromatose als völlig ungeeignet bezeichnet wird, während mit der Turnbullblau-Methode eine sehr gute Darstellung des Hämosiderins gelingt.

Das Depoteisen kommt als wasserlösliches, kristallines Protein vor, *Ferritin*, und als wasserunlösliches, größeres Eiweiß-Eisenaggregat, *Hämosiderin*. Letzteres entsteht immer dann, wenn Eisen über den zur Hämsynthese erforderlichen Bedarf angenommen wird, oder wenn Eisen bei Störungen der Hämsynthese nicht verwertet werden kann. Der Unterschied beider eisenhaltigen Proteine scheint mehr in ihrer physikalischen Form zu liegen als in ihrem chemischen Aufbau (LEIPERT, 1964). GÖSSNER (1953) sowie GEDIGK und STRAUSS (1953) bewiesen histochemisch, bzw. fluorescenzmikroskopisch, daß der eisenfreie Restkörper des Hämosiderins außer Eiweiß saure Mucopolysaccharide und einen mit dem Ceroid verwandten Lipoidkörper enthält. Allgemein wird angenommen, daß mikroskopisch als braungelbes, körnig-scholliges Pigment sichtbar und histochemisch nachweisbar nur das Hämosiderin ist. Neuerdings bevorzugt man im internationalen Schrifttum dafür die Bezeichnung „Siderinpigment" (VOLLAND und PRIBILLA, 1955), da die moderne Eisenforschung im Gegensatz zu der noch von LUBARSCH vertretenen Auffassung lehrt, daß es sich hierbei keineswegs ausschließlich um Blutabbauprodukte im Sinne hämatogener bzw. hämoglobinogener Pigmente zu handeln braucht. Übrigens scheint Eisen auch dann mit den üblichen histochemischen Methoden (d. h. ohne vorherige Demaskierung) nachweisbar zu werden, wenn der Ferritingehalt einer Zelle ein gewisses Maß übersteigt. Es ergibt sich dann eine diffuse Blaufärbung des Cytoplasmas (THALER, 1964).

Grundsätzlich ist nicht alles „Hämosiderin" einfach als pathologisch zu bewerten. Das gilt nicht nur für Milz, Leber und Knochenmark. Auch in der Peripherie findet sich schon physiologisch Hämosiderin, z. B. in den Tonsillen, Lymphfollikeln des Wurmfortsatzes, des Zungengrundes usw. Im Bereich der Haut hat RICHTER (1933) auf das unter physiologischen Bedingungen vorkommende eisenpositive Pigment im Epithel der apokrinen Schweißdrüsen und in den diesen Drüsen benachbarten histiocytären Elementen sowie in Myoepithelien hingewiesen.

Bei der *Hämochromatose* liegt das Hämosiderin in dichtester Anordnung in dem die großen Gefäße und besonders auch die gewöhnlichen und apokrinen Schweißdrüsen umgebenden Bindegewebe und auch in den Schweißdrüsen selbst. Manchmal liegt es auch in der Nachbarschaft von Talgdrüsen (HEDINGER, 1953). Die Granula liegen teils fein verteilt, teils in Klumpen in den fixen Bindegewebszellen. Nur bei einem Teil der beschriebenen Fälle wurde Hämosiderin in der Basalschicht nachgewiesen (MONTGOMERY und O'LEARY, 1950; MAGNUSON und RAULSTON, 1942; HEDINGER, 1953). ALTHAUSEN u. Mitarb. (1951) haben z. B. bei keinem ihrer Fälle Eisen in der Basalschicht gefunden. MONTGOMERY, HAMILTON u. Mitarb. (1930) fanden bei 4 von 16 Hämochromatosefällen das Hämosiderin besonders in den Dendritenzellen der Epidermis, wohin es nach Ansicht der Autoren aus der Umgebung der cutanen Gefäße durch Vermittlung der fixen Bindegewebszellen gelangt ist. Dies wäre eine Bestätigung der Theorie von PAUTRIER über die Transportfunktion der Langerhansschen Zellen im Sinne einer Stoffwechselvermittlung. Auch LOEWENTHAL (1929) und TORNABUONI (1929) fanden bei Schambergscher Dermatose in den Langerhanszellen eisenpositives Pigment. MONTGOMERY, HAMILTON u. Mitarb. fanden bei 2 der Hämochromatosefälle das Hämosiderin besonders auch in der Membrana propria der Schweißdrüsen.

SOLTERMANN fand mit der Turnbullblau-Methode bei lebenswarm fixiertem Material schon normalerweise in allen axillären Hautexcisionen Hämosiderin im Epithel der a-Drüsen und bei Leichenmaterial in 86% der untersuchten Fälle. Häufig sind auch Myoepithelien und Zellen der Membrana propria eisenhaltig. Auch die Epithelien der e-Drüsen können mitunter Hämosiderin enthalten. Aber auch interstitiell, perivasculär und diffus in der Cutis sowie in den Basalzellen der Epidermis wurde Eisen in granulärer Form auch bei Normalpersonen gefunden. Daher sollte nach SOLTERMANN der histochemisch positive Eisenbefund in der Haut nur sehr vorsichtig beurteilt werden. Er ist allein nicht ausreichend, um die Diagnose einer Hämochromatose als gesichert anzusehen. Insbesondere wird betont, daß der Hämosiderinnachweis in der Axillarhaut denkbar ungeeignet ist, da gerade dort physiologischerweise immer Eisen gefunden wird. Dieser Hinweis ist wichtig, da die Biopsie aus der Axillargegend wegen des Reichtums an Schweißdrüsen von mehreren Autoren für den Hämochromatosenachweis empfohlen wird (HEDINGER, 1953). Man soll auch nicht die Haut der Beine zur Probeexcision wählen, da dort häufiger Hämosiderinablagerungen, z. B. im Rahmen des varicösen Symptomenkomplexes, vorkommen (SCHWARZMANN, 1930).

Aber auch der negative Eisenbefund ist im Sinne einer Ausschlußdiagnose nicht beweisend, da nicht jeder Fall von Hämochromatose in der Haut mikroskopisch darstellbares Eisen enthält.

Zahlreiche Erkrankungen führen im Rahmen einer hämorrhagischen Diathese zur sekundären Hämosiderose der Haut. Diese Krankheitsbilder im Detail zu besprechen geht über den Rahmen des Kapitels. Charakteristisch für die sekundäre Hauthämosiderose ist die positive Eisenreaktion des Pigments, das sich meist nicht in der Epidermis, sondern nur in der Cutis findet, das resorptionsfähig ist, aber lange unverändert liegen bleiben kann und besonders bei den lokalisierten Formen nur langsam verschwindet (SELLEI, 1929). Auch die Hämosiderose bei Dermatosis pigmentaria progressiva Schamberg, bei Purpura anularis teleangiectodes Majocchi und Dermatitis lichenoides purpurica pigmentosa Gougerot und Blum ist sekundärer Natur. Diese Krankheitsbilder kommen durch eine verschiedenartig auftretende Capillaritis zustande.

XI. Carotinoide

Carotinoide sind Pigmentstoffe pflanzlichen Ursprunges, die auf Grund ihrer chemischen Konstitution in *Carotine* und *Xanthophylle* unterteilt werden können. Die Carotine sind stark ungesättigte Kohlenwasserstoffe, während die Xanthophylle Hydroxylderivate dieser Verbindungen darstellen. Sie sind lipoidlöslich und werden im Darm bei Anwesenheit von Nahrungsfett und Gallensäuren resorbiert. Im Blut sind sie an Lipoproteine, besonders an das β-Lipoprotein, gebunden. Die Carotine sind leicht löslich in Petroläther, schwer löslich in Methylalkohol, während sich die Xanthophylle genau umgekehrt verhalten. Diese beiden Stoffe sind nicht immer im gleichen Verhältnis vorhanden. Sie haben nur einen geringen Farbunterschied, so daß sie durch direkte colorimetrische Analysen nicht ganz genau getrennt werden können. Weiter sind sie sehr lichtempfindlich, besonders gegenüber ultravioletten Strahlen und unterliegen leicht einer Autooxydation mit rapidem Farbverlust (THOMSON, 1934). In reiner Form haben die Carotinoide einen intensiv gelbroten Farbton und sind geschmack- und geruchlos (SEQUEIRA, 1937). Zum Unterschied vom sog. Lipofuscin oder Abnützungspigment werden die Carotinoide auch als „echte" Lipochrome bezeichnet (THOMSON, 1934). Es unterliegt keinem Zweifel mehr, daß die gelbe Farbe der tierischen Fette und Lipoide hauptsächlich auf diese Pflanzenfarbstoffe, die mit der Nahrung in den Körper gelangen, zurückzuführen ist.

Der Carotinoidblutspiegel wird durch drei Faktoren reguliert (LEVER, 1963): 1. Zufuhr mit der Nahrung, 2. Resorption vom Darm aus, 3. Löslichkeit im Serum. Diese ist, da die Carotinoide an Lipoproteine gebunden sind, dem Lipidspiegel im Serum proportional (MARCHIONINI und PATEL, 1937). Bei der Entstehung einer Carotinämie mit folgender Ablagerung lipochromen Pigmentes in der Haut spielt in erster Linie die stark erhöhte Zufuhr durch einseitige Ernährung eine Rolle (BUSMAN und WOODBURNE, 1931; LEVIN und SILVERS, 1931; RATTNER und GINSBERG, 1932; SEZARY und VERNE, 1939; REISCH, 1960), doch kann es auch im Rahmen eines Diabetes mellitus, Myxödems oder eines nephrotischen Syndroms durch die Erhöhung des Lipoidspiegels zum gleichen Bilde kommen. Zum Teil wird das Auftreten einer Carotinosis auch mit einer Störung des Umbaues der Carotine zu Vitamin A in Zusammenhang gebracht (LUTZ, 1957).

Die Haut nimmt bei übermäßiger Einlagerung von Carotinoiden typischerweise einen kanariengelben bis orangen Farbton an. Als Prädilektionsstellen sind Handteller, Fußsohlen, Gesicht und Hals zu bezeichnen (BLUEFARB, RODIN und HOIT, 1954). Bei stark ausgeprägten Fällen kann es allerdings auch zu einer universellen Verfärbung der Haut kommen, wobei aber typischerweise Skleren und Schleimhäute frei bleiben (KOTELNIKOW, 1936; MATSUDA, 1937; AYRES, 1940).

Zum histologischen Nachweis der Pigmentablagerung eignet sich der Gefrierschnitt am besten, da außer mit Fettlösungsmitteln auch mit Wasser der Farbstoff teilweise entfernt wird (KAUFMANN, 1933). Mit den gewöhnlichen Färbemethoden färben sich die Carotinoide nicht. Exakt kann ihre Anwesenheit und Konzentration nur durch chemische oder spektroskopische Methoden nachgewiesen werden (KAUFMANN, 1933).

Im feingeweblichen Schnitt imponiert eine deutliche Gelbfärbung des Stratum corneum (LUTZ, 1957). Die übrigen Epidermisschichten sind zwar ähnlich, aber wesentlich schwächer gefärbt. Die Hornschicht zeigt infolge ihres Lipoidreichtums eine besondere Affinität zu den Carotinoiden. Eine Steigerung weist die Gelbfärbung der Hornschichte um die Schweißdrüsenausführungsgänge auf. In dem Protoplasma der Basalzellen finden sich hin und wieder grobe, intensiv-gelbe Granula eingestreut (GANS und STEIGLEDER, 1957). Papillarkörper, Cutisbindegewebe und Schweißdrüsenepithel sind ebenfalls, doch in geringerem Maße als die Epidermis, diffus gelb gefärbt. Für die Entstehung und Lokalisation der Carotinosis dürften die Schweißdrüsen eine wesentliche Rolle spielen (ČAJKOVAC, 1938; MORO, 1932). Wenigstens konnte bei Tieren, die keine Schweißdrüsen besitzen, wie z. B. Kaninchen, Meerschweinchen, Ziegen, experimentell keine Carotinosis erzeugt werden. Bei anderen Versuchstieren wieder wurde die Pigmentablagerung durch Pilocarpin gesteigert und durch Atropin gehemmt, so daß ein Zusammenhang mit der Schweißdrüsenfunktion wahrscheinlich erscheint (ANZAI, 1931). Das subcutane Fettgewebe bleibt gewöhnlich frei, bzw. tritt hier die Verfärbung wesentlich langsamer und später auf als in der Epidermis; erst postmortal soll das Fettgewebe den Farbstoff stark annehmen (GANS und STEIGLEDER, 1957).

XII. Silber

Seit langem ist die Tatsache bekannt, daß nach längerem Gebrauch silberhaltiger Arzneimittel schiefergraue Verfärbungen der Haut auftreten können. Je nach Entstehung und Ausdehnung der Silbereinlagerungen sind verschiedene Formen der Argyrose zu unterscheiden (KANITZ, 1909): 1. Die lokale, gewerblich bedingte Argyrose der Silberarbeiter. 2. Die lokale Imbibitions-Argyrose. 3. Die universelle Argyrose.

Bei der *lokalen, gewerblich bedingten Argyrose* der Silberarbeiter kommt es im Verlaufe kleiner Verletzungen zum Eindringen von Silbersplittern in die Haut. Histologisch finden sich hier gewisse, durch die Art der Entstehung verständliche, Besonderheiten (OPPENHEIM, 1934; HARKER und HUNTER, 1935). Gleiches kann auch nach Einbringung von Silberdrähten bei kosmetischen Operationen gesehen werden (KESSEL, 1941). In der Cutis finden sich, umgeben von einer bindegewebigen Kapsel, größere Silberteilchen. In der Umgebung liegen zumeist noch mehrere kleinere Silberpartikel. Die elastischen Fasern des umgebenden Gewebes sind mit Silber imprägniert (GANS und STEIGLEDER, 1957).

Die *lokale Imbibitionsargyrose* kann im Anschluß an eine lang dauernde lokale Verwendung silberhaltiger Präparate im Schleimhautbereich am Ort der Verwendung auftreten.

Eine *universelle Argyrose* kann einerseits durch Resorption nach langdauernder lokaler (CRIADO, 1930; ZACKS, 1933; WISE, 1934; FOX, 1937; BERNSTEIN, 1938; MØLLER, 1955), peroraler (GOTTRON, 1933; KERL, 1933; MADDEN, 1933; HERRMANN, 1934; CURSCHMANN, 1937; HADLEY, 1941; BRODTHAGEN, 1955; BIEBER, 1957) oder parenteraler (MATRAS, 1930; HABERMANN, 1940) Gabe von Silberpräparaten, andererseits aber natürlich auch durch intensiven beruflichen Kontakt entstehen (WEYHBRECHT, 1953). Die zu einer universellen Argyrose führende Silbermenge schwankt in weiten Grenzen. GANS wies schon 1933 darauf hin, daß viele Menschen trotz Einnahme großer Silbermengen keine Argyrose bekommen, während andere Personen schon nach wesentlich geringeren Mengen dieses Krankheitsbild zeigen. Diese Tatsache macht wahrscheinlich, daß beim Entstehen der universellen Argyrose eine individuelle Disposition eine Rolle spielt (KWIATKOWSKI, 1935; GOLDSCHLAG, 1936; CHANIAL, 1955). Die makroskopisch sichtbare Verfärbung der Haut und die feingewebliche Silberablagerung bleiben durch Jahre und Jahrzehnte bestehen. GOTTRON (1933) beobachtete allerdings nach Jahrzehnten eine spontane Aufhellung. AMITRANO (1938) sah beim Säugling sogar ein Verschwinden innerhalb von Wochen.

Die exakte Diagnosestellung erfolgt durch den Nachweis des metallischen Silbers im Gewebe. Einfach gelingt dies mit Hilfe der sog. Leuchtbildmethode von HOFFMANN, die von HABERMANN (1940) erstmals zu diesem Zwecke herangezogen wurde (MATRAS, 1930; MADDEN, 1933; SOTGIU und DE GIORGO, 1937; ZOON, 1934). Im Dunkelfeld werden die Silberkörnchen durch ihre hellen Lichtreflexe viel besser als im Hellfeld sichtbar. Nach Behandlung der Schnitte mit einer 1%igen KCN-Lösung verschwindet das Aufleuchtphänomen der Silberkörnchen (ZOON, 1934). Absolut beweisend für die Diagnose ist der spektralanalytische Silbernachweis im Gewebe (ROYSTER, 1932; GAGER und ELLISON, 1935; MØLLER, 1955).

Die lokale Imbibitionsargyrie und die universelle Argyrose zeigen das gleiche feingewebliche Bild, über welches im allgemeinen eine einheitliche Meinung herrscht. Das metallische Silber findet sich in Form feiner, runder, braunschwarzer Körnchen mehr oder minder diffus über die Cutis verstreut. Bevorzugte Lokalisationsstellen sind die Basalmembran der Schweißdrüsen, die bindegewebige Grenzschichte der Haarfollikel und Talgdrüsen. Außerdem sind die Silberkörnchen auch noch subepidermal, angelagert an die feinen, senkrecht zum Stratum basale verlaufenden elastischen Fasern, zu sehen (Elastophilie) (STILLIANS, 1937; BOERSMA und BARKER, 1948; WEYHBRECHT, 1953). In gleicher Weise ist auch die Elastica der Gefäße imprägniert (ZOON, 1934; CASCOS, 1936).

Uneinheitlich ist die Ansicht über die Lokalisation der Silberkörnchen hinsichtlich der Bindegewebszellen. Während von manchen Autoren nur ein extracelluläres Vorkommen der Silberpartikel beschrieben wurde, sahen andere Silber auch in Endothelzellen und perivasculären Phagocyten (ZOON, 1934; LANGERON, DELATTRE und PAGET, 1933; CASCOS, 1936; BERNSTEIN, 1938; HILL und MONTGOMERY, 1941). Hier besteht ein Unterschied zur experimentell erzeugten Argyrose der Tiere, bei denen nach Angaben von LENARTOWICZ und JALOWY (1938) das Silber hauptsächlich in den Zellen des RES abgelagert wird.

Über eine Fremdkörperreaktion des Gewebes bei der lokalisierten und universellen Argyrose finden sich nur vereinzelt Angaben (EBERHARTINGER, EBNER und NIEBAUER, 1965).

XIII. Gold

Ähnlich wie zur Argyrose kann es auch nach Verabreichung von Goldpräparaten zur *Chrysiasis cutis* (Chrysocyanose, Auriasis) kommen. Erstmals wurde dieses Phänomen von HANSBORG (1928) beschrieben. Auffällig ist im klinischen Bild, daß sich die schiefergraue bis lividbläuliche Verfärbung der Haut besonders an den lichtexponierten Stellen findet (REYNAERS, 1952; CARDIS und CONTE, 1936; GOUGEROT und CAETEAUD, 1931; LOPEZ, 1931; CASCOS, 1936; NOVÉ-JOSSERAND, GATÉ, CHARPY, JOSSERAND und CUILLERET, 1931; HOCHLEITNER, 1959). Das Auftreten der Hautveränderungen soll weitgehend von der zugeführten Menge abhängig sein (SCHMIDT, 1941; LORENZEN, 1931; CARDIS et CONTE, 1936). Allerdings sollen Nierenfunktionsstörungen nach Meinung von WIGLEY (1932) als dispositioneller Faktor eine Rolle spielen.

Ähnlich wie bei der Argyrose kann das Gold mittels der Leuchtbildmethode von HOFFMANN, aber auch mikrochemisch und spektralanalytisch nachgewiesen werden. Im Gewebe scheint das Gold teilweise als Metall, teilweise in noch unbekannten Verbindungen vorzuliegen (GANS und STEIGLEDER, 1957).

In der Haut findet man die Goldkörnchen, die meist größer und ungleichmäßiger als die Silberkörnchen sind, vor allem in der Cutis und um die Hautanhangsgebilde (Haarwurzelscheide, bindegewebiger Haarbalg, Schweißdrüsen, aber auch in Talgdrüsen und Haarpapillen). Man findet es ferner als subepithelialen Metallsaum. Nach einigen Beobachtungen soll das Gold eher intracellulär in phagocytierende Bindegewebszellen abgelagert werden (RATHERY, DEROT, DOUBROW und JAMMET, 1934; ZIMMERLI und LUTZ, 1929; CASCOS, 1936). Andere Autoren fanden die Goldpartikelchen frei im Gewebe. Entzündliche Reaktionen sollen nach KOCHS (1938) nicht vorkommen. Von Bedeutung ist ferner, daß Goldteilchen auch in der Epidermis zu erkennen sind. Die Basalzellschicht ist voll von glänzenden Körnchen (KOCHS, 1938). In den höheren Epidermislagen ist das Gold mehr diffus verteilt (GANS und STEIGLEDER, 1957). Goldablagerungen in der Subcutis und der Rinden- und Marksubstanz der Haare wurden nicht beschrieben.

XIV. Fremdkörper

In die Cutis eingebrachte Fremdkörper können, wenn sie mehr oder weniger lange dort liegenbleiben, eine Reaktion der Umgebung zur Folge haben. Diese wird im allgemeinen unter dem Begriff *Fremdkörpergranulom* zusammengefaßt (NIMPFER, 1933). Wie GAHLEN und KLÜKEN (1952) darauf hinwiesen, ist jedoch die Häufigkeit der Ausbildung eines Fremdkörpergranuloms gemessen an der Häufigkeit der Fremdkörpereinsprengung an sich sehr selten. Sie hängt jedoch zu nicht geringem Teil von der chemischen Zusammensetzung des eingebrachten Fremdkörpers ab. So kommt es bei Berylliumeinsprengungen fast obligat zur Granulombildung. In letzter Zeit wurde mehrfach über das Auftreten von Granulomen nach Anwendung zirkoniumhaltiger Externa berichtet (BALER, 1965). Wahrscheinlich spielt daneben noch eine besondere, abartige Reaktionslage des Organismus eine Rolle (FLECK, 1954).

Die Zeit, die von der Einbringung des Fremdkörpers bis zur Ausbildung des Granuloms verstreichen kann, ist verschieden und kann Wochen bis Jahrzehnte ausmachen. Für diese Tatsache werden physikalische Faktoren verantwortlich gemacht, da es primär zu einer langsamen Auflösung und Verteilung des eingesprengten Fremdkörpers in die Umgebung kommt, wodurch entzündliche Veränderungen im Gewebe ausgelöst werden (EPSTEIN, GERSTL, BERK und BELBER, 1955). Erst später kommt es dann zur eigentlichen Granulombildung. Bekannter-maßen findet man in solchen Fällen in der Cutis, an manchen Stellen bis zum Epithel vordringend, dicht gedrängte, rundliche Granulome von typisch tuberkuloidem Bau, die aus Epitheloid- und Riesenzellen — teilweise vom Langhans-, teilweise vom Fremdkörpertyp — aufgebaut sind.

Im Zentrum können auch Einschmelzungsherde gesehen werden (DUTRA, 1949). Innerhalb der Granulome breitet sich ein Netz von argentaffinen Fasern kleinsten Kalibers aus (GAHLEN und KLÜKEN, 1952; FLECK, 1954).

Größte Schwierigkeiten kann allerdings der histologische Nachweis der Fremdkörper bereiten (CIVATTE, 1955). Oft findet man schon bei Routinefärbung in den meist reichlich vorhandenen Riesenzellen stark lichtbrechende, nadel- oder plättchenförmige Kristalle (LÖHE, 1950; MACHER, 1955). Manchmal scheint von den Fremdkörperriesenzellen nur mehr ein schmaler Cytoplasmasaum übriggeblieben zu sein, während durch dichtgedrängte Kristalle ein Hohlraum vorgetäuscht wird (MACHER, 1953). Am besten gelingt der Nachweis der Fremdkörper im polarisierten Licht, in dem innerhalb der Riesenzellen hellscheinende Partikelchen zur Darstellung kommen (MACHER, 1953; GINSBERG und BECKER, 1951; BULEY und KULWIN, 1954; LAPIERE, 1955; DUPERRAT, 1955; BOLGERT und AMADO, 1956). Weitere kompliziertere Methoden zum Fremdkörpernachweis sind die chemische Untersuchung nach Veraschung, die spektrographische Analyse, die Röntgenabsorptionsspektrographie (CROSSLAND, 1955) und die Historöntgenographie (BREITENECKER und NIEBAUER, 1960).

Es darf allerdings nicht verwundern, wenn nicht selten der Fremdkörper überhaupt nicht nachzuweisen ist, da die Granulome auch nach der Resorption des Fremdkörpers bestehen bleiben (GAHLEN und KLÜKEN, 1952).

Besondere Erwähnung sollen noch jene Fremdkörperreaktionen finden, die nach Injektion von Mineralölen entstehen können (Paraffinome, Vaselinome) (ARZT, 1919; BAZIN, 1929; SPITZMÜLLER, 1929). Neben dem typischen Fremdkörpergranulationsgewebe finden sich charakteristischerweise Vacuolen der Riesenzellen, die durch Phagocytose erklärt werden (SCHLIENGER, 1949). Daneben sieht man noch teils einzelstehende, teils gruppierte und von einer fibrösen Kapsel umgebene Cystenbildungen mit sudanophilem Inhalt. Auch chemisch gelingt der Nachweis des Mineralöles (GIOIA, 1929). Bemerkenswert ist vielleicht noch die Veränderung der färberischen Affinität des umgebenden Bindegewebes, das sich nach VAN GIESON gelb und nach MALLORY braunrot anfärbt (GANS und STEIGLEDER, 1957).

Literatur

Amyloide

BRIGGS, G. W.: Amyloidosis. Ann. intern. Med. 55, 943 (1961).
CAESAR, R.: Die Feinstruktur von Milz und Leber bei der experimentellen Amyloidose. Z. Zellforsch. 52, 653—673 (1960). — Elektronenmikroskopische Untersuchungen an menschlichem Amyloid bei verschiedenen Grundkrankheiten. Path. et Microbiol. (Basel) 24, 387—396 (1961). — Elektronenmikroskopische Beobachtungen bei Nierenamyloidose des Goldhamsters. Frankfurt. Z. Path. 72, 506—516 (1963). — CALKINS, E., and A. S. COHEN: Diagnosis of amyloidosis. Bull. rheum. Dis. 10, 215 (1960). — CARNES, W. H., and B. R. FORKER: The metachromasy of amyloid. J. Histochem. Cytochem. 2, 469—470 (1954). — Metachromasy of amyloid. Lab. Invest. 5, 21—43 (1956). — COHEN, A. S., and E. H. CALKINS: Electron microscopic observations on a fibrous component in amyloid of diverse origin. Nature (Lond.) 183, 1202 (1959). — The isolation of amyloid fibrils and a study of the effect of collagenase and hyaluronidase. J. Cell Biol. 21, 481 (1964). — COHEN, A. S., H. CALKINS and C. I. LEVENE: Studies on experimental amyloidosis. I. Analysis of histology and staining reactions of casein induced amyloidosis in the rabbit. Ann. J. Path. 35, 971 (1959).
DEGOS, R., J. DELORT et J. HEWITT: Amyloidose cutanée (Amyloidosis der Haut). Bull. Soc. franç. Dermat. Syph. 58, 534 (1951). — DELANK, H.-W., G. KOCH, G. KÖNN, H.-P. MISSMAHL u. K. SUWELACK: Familiäre Amyloid-Polyneuropathie Typus Wohlwill-Corino Andrade. Ärztl. Forsch. 19, 401 (1965). — DIVRY, P., et M. FLORKIN: C. R. Soc. biol. (Paris) 97, 1808 (1927). Zit. nach COHEN u. CALKINS 1964.
EHRLICH, J. C., and I. M. RATNER: Amyloidosis of the isles of Langerhans. Amer. J. Path. 38, 49—59 (1961).

FREUDENTHAL, W.: Amyloid in der Haut. Arch. Derm. Syph. (Berl.) 162, 40—94 (1930). — FREY, A.: Zur Frage nach der Ursache des Bichroismus gefärbter Fasern. Naturwissenschaften 13, 403—406 (1925). — FRIEDREICH, N., u. A. KEKULÉ: Zur Amyloidfrage. Virchows Arch. path. Anat. 16, 50 (1859).

GABRIEL, H., and W. LINDEMAYR: Amyloidosis cutis nodularis atrophicans. Dermatologica (Basel) 115, 508—515 (1957). — GANS, O., u. G. K. STEIGLEDER: Histologie der Hautkrankheiten, I. Bd. Berlin-Göttingen-Heidelberg: Springer 1955. — GÖSSNER, W.: Vergleichende histochemische Untersuchungen über die Proteinkomponente von Amyloid, Hyalin und Kollagen. Histochemie 2, 199 (1961). — Diskussionsbeitrag beim Kolloquium „Fortschritte der Amyloidforschung" in Halle 1964. — GOTTRON, H.: Systematisierte Haut-Muskel-Amyloidose unter dem Bilde eines Sclerodema amyloidosum. Arch. Derm. 166, 584 (1932). — GUTMANN, C.: Weiteres über Amyloid der Haut. Derm. Z. 53, 235 (1928).

HARMS, H.: Diskussionsbeitrag beim Colloquium über „Fortschritte der Amyloidforschung" in Halle 1964. — HASHIMOTO, K., B. G. GROSS, and W. F. LEVER: Lichen amyloidosus. Histochemical and electron microscopic studies. J. invest. Derm. 45, 204—219 (1965). — HASS, G.: Studies of amyloid. II. The isolation of a polysaccharide from amyloid-bearing tissues. Arch. Path. 34, 92 (1942). — HELLER, H., H. P. MISSMAHL, E. SOHAR, and J. GAFNI: Amyloidosis. Its differentiation into perireticulin and pericollagen types. J. Path. Bact. 88, 15 (1964).

IVERSON, L., and A. B. MORRISON: Primary systemic amyloidosis. Arch. Path. 45, 1—20 (1948).

JONES, R. S., and D. B. FRAZIER: Primary cardiovascular amyloidosis. Arch. Path. 50, 366—384 (1950).

KENNEDY, J. S.: Sulphur-35 in experimental amyloidosis. J. Path. Bact. 83, 165—181 (1962). — KLEIN, P., u. P. BURKHOLDER: Ein Verfahren zur fluorescenzoptischen Darstellung der Komplementbindung und seine Anwendung zur histo-immunologischen Untersuchung der experimentellen Nierenanaphylaxie. Dtsch. med. Wschr. 84, 2001 (1959). — KÖNIGSTEIN, H.: Amyloid der Haut. In: Handbuch der Haut- und Geschlechtskrankheiten, IV, 3. Teil. Berlin: Springer 1932. — KONRAD, J.: Amyloidosis des rechten Unterschenkels. Zbl. Haut- u. Geschl.-Kr. 53, 148 (1936). — KREIBICH, C.: Über Amyloiddegeneration der Haut. Arch. Derm. Syph. 116, 385 (1913).

LAWLESS, T. K.: Primary amyloidosis of the skin. Arch. Derm. 33, 932 (1936). — LETTERER, E.: Die Amyloidosen im Lichte neuer Forschungsmethoden. Dtsch. med. Wschr. 75, 15 (1950). — Über die geweblichen und humoralen Störungen des Eiweiß-Stoffwechsels. IV. Franz Volhard-Gedächtnisvorlesung. Stuttgart: Friedr.-Karl Schattauer 1958. — Allgemeine Pathologie. Stuttgart: Georg Thieme 1959. — Fortschritte der Amyloidforschung. Jena 1940. — LETTERER, E., R. CAESAR u. A. VOGT: Studien zur elektronenoptischen und immunmorphologischen Struktur des Amyloids. Dtsch. med. Wschr. 85, 1909 (1960). — LEVER, W. F.: Ablagerungskrankheiten körpereigener Stoffwechselprodukte. In: Handbuch der Hautkrankheiten, hrsg. von J. JADASSOHN, Erg.-Werk Bd. III/1. Berlin-Göttingen-Heidelberg: Springer 1963. — Histopathologie der Haut. Stuttgart: Gustav Fischer 1958. — LINDNER, J., u. G. FREYTAG: Ein Beitrag zur Amyloidentstehung. In: Fortschritte der Amyloidforschung, Symp. in Halle 1964. — LOESCHCKE, H.: Vorstellungen über das Wesen von Myelin und Amyloid aufgrund von serologischen Versuchen. Beitr. path. Anat. 77, 231 (1927).

MALAK, J. A., and E. W. SMITH: Secondary localized cutaneous amyloidosis. Arch. Dermat. 86, 465 (1962). — MARCHIONINI, A., u. F. JOHN: Über lichenoide und poikilodermieartige Hautamyloidose. Arch. Derm. Syph. 173, 545 (1935). — MASCHKILLEISSON, L. N.: Über Amyloidose der Haut. Acta derm. venereol. (Stockh.) 11, 77—119 (1930). — McMANUS, J. F. A.: Diskussionsbemerkung. Ann. N.Y. Acad. Sci. 52, 987 (1950). — The periodic acid routine applied to the kidney. Ann. J. Path. 24, 643—653 (1948). — MIESCHER, G.: Beitrag zur Klinik der Paramyloidose (Pseudomyxoedema paramyloidosum). Dermatologica (Basel) 91, 177 (1945). — MISSMAHL, H. P.: Rectumbiopsie zum Nachweis der Amyloidose. Dtsch. med. Wschr. 88, 1783 (1963). — Diagnose einer primären, perikollagenen Amyloidose mit Hilfe der Rectumbiopsie. Dtsch. med. Wschr. 89, 122 (1964). — Erbbedingte generalisierte Amyloidosen. Dtsch. med. Wschr. 89, 709 (1964). — Diagnose der generalisierten Amyloidosen. Dtsch. med. Wschr. 90, 394 (1965). — MISSMAHL, H. P., u. M. HARTWIG: Polarisationsoptische Untersuchungen an der Amyloidsubstanz. Virchows Arch. path. Anat. 34, 489—508 (1953). — MUSGER, A.: Stoffwechsel- und Ablagerungskrankheiten der Haut. In: Lehrbuch der Haut- und Geschlechts-Krankheiten, hrsg. von E. RIECKE, H. G. BODE u. G. W. KORTING. Stuttgart: Gustav Fischer 1962.

NÖDL, F., u. H. ZAUN: Zur Klinik und Histologie der systematisierten Haut-Muskel-Paramyloidose. Arch. klin. exp. Derm. 220, 393 (1964). — NOMLAND, R.: Localized amyloidosis of the skin. Arch. Derm. Syph. (Chic.) 33, 85 (1936).

PALITZ, L. L., and S. PECK: Amyloidosis cutis: a macular variant. Arch. Derm. Syph. 65, 451 (1952). — PEARSE, A. G. E.: Histochemistry, theoretical and applied, 2nd ed. London: Churchill 1960. — PEARSON, B., H. M. RICE, and K. L. DICKENS: Primary systemic amyloidosis. Arch. Path. 32, 1—10 (1941). — PUCHTLER, H., F. SWEAT, and M. LEVINE: On the binding of Congo red by amyloid. J. Histochem. Cytochem. 10, 355 (1962).

RUSZCZAK, Z., u. L. WOZNIAK: Amyloidosis cutis localisata nodosa cum anetodermia. Hautarzt 12, 254 (1961).

SAGHER, F., and J. SHANON: Amyloidosis cutis. Familial occurrence in three generations. Arch. Derm. 87, 171 (1953). — SCHILDER, P.: Über die amyloide Entartung der Haut. Frankfurt. Z. Path. 3 (1909). Zit. nach GANS u. STEIGLEDER. — SCHNEIDER, G.: Über die Pathogenese der Amyloidose. Immunologische, histochemische und morphologische Untersuchungen. Ergebn. allg. Path. path. Anat. 44, 1 (1964). — SCHNEIDER, W., u. H. P. MISSMAHL: Lichen amyloidosus als Beispiel der perikollagenen, primären, hautbeschränkten und vorwiegend umschriebenen Amyloidose. Arch. klin. exp. Derm. 224, 235—247 (1966). — SCHOTT, H. J., u. H. HOLZMANN: Polarisationsoptischer Nachweis von Amyloid-Ablagerung bei Mycosis fungoides. Arch. klin. exp. Derm. 222, 632—641 (1965). — SPRAFKE, H.: Über Amyloidosen. Derm. Wschr. 126, 1017 (1952). — STREITMANN, B.: Amyloidosis cutis nodularis atrophicans. Z. Haut- u. Geschl.-Kr. 38, 115—123 (1965).

TEILUM, G.: Periodic acid-schiff-positive reticulo-endothelial cells producing glycoprotein. Functional significance during formation of amyloid. Amer. J. Path. 32, 945 (1956).

VASSAR, P. S., and F. C. CULLING: Fluorescent stains. With special reference to amyloid and connective tissue. Arch. Path. 68, 487 (1959). — VAZQUES, T. T., F. J. DIXON, and A. L. NEIL: Demonstration of specific antigen and antibody in experimentally produced amyloid. 54th Annual Meeting of the Amer. Assoc. of Pathologists, Washington, D. C., April 11th—13th, 1957. Ref. in: Amer. J. Path. 33, 614 (1957). — VIRCHOW, R.: Weitere Mitteilungen über das Vorkommen der pflanzlichen Zellulose beim Menschen. Virchows Arch. path. Anat. 6, 268 (1854). — VOGT, A., u. H. G. KOCHEM: Histo-serologische Untersuchungen mit fluorescin-markiertem Antikomplement. Nachweis komplementbindender Substanzen im Amyloid. Z. Zellforsch. 52, 640—652 (1960).

WAGNER, B. M.: Histochemical studies of fibrinoid substances and other abnormal tissue proteins. Arch. Path. 60, 221 (1955). — WEYHBRECHT, H.: Lichen amyloidosus unter dem klinischen Bild eines verrukösen Lichen chronicus Vidal. Derm. Wschr. 125, 460 (1952). — WINER, L. H.: Local amyloidosis of the skin. Arch. Derm. 23, 866—871 (1931). — WOLMAN, H., and J. J. BUBIS: The cause of the green polarization color of amyloid stained with Congo red. Histochemie 4, 351 (1965).

Hyalin

ALLISON, J. R., and J. ALLISON jr.: Colloid milium. Arch. Derm. 76, 218—220 (1957). — ANDREWS, G. C.: Diseases of the skin, ed. 4. Philadelphia: W. B. Saunders Co. 1954. — ARRIGHI, F.: Pseudo-milium colloide. Bull. Soc. franç. Derm. Syph. 62, 440—445 (1955).

BAHR, G. F., u. K. H. HUHN: Über den Einfluß der Kittsubstanzen bei der Färbung des kollagenen und elastischen Gewebes. Arch. Derm. Syph. (Berl.) 194, 400—404 (1952). — BAZEX, A.: Un cas de lipoido-proteinose (maladie de Urbach-Wiethe). Bull. Soc. franç. Derm. Syph. 46, 136—142 (1939). — BAZEX, A., et A. DUPRÉ: La lipoido-protéinose est elle une dégénérescence du système musculaire lisse de la peau ? Ann. Derm. Syph. (Paris) 91, 5—22 (1964). — BECK, F., u. L. WIFLING: Ein Beitrag von 5 Fällen von Pseudomilium colloidale Pellizari in Nordbayern. Z. Haut- u. Geschl.-Kr. 28, 113 (1960). — BECKER, J. F., and H. T. H. WILSON: Colloid milium. Brit. J. Derm. 68, 345—349 (1956). — BESNIER, E.: Zit. nach L. ARZT, Zur Kenntnis des „Pseudo-Milium colloidale". Arch. Derm. 118, 785 (1913). — BESNIER, E., u. F. BALZER: Zit. nach L. ARZT, Zur Kenntnis des „Pseudo-Milium colloidale". Arch. Derm. 118, 785 (1913). — BOSELLINI, J. L.: Zit. nach L. ARZT, Zur Kenntnis des „Pseudo-Milium colloidale". Arch. Derm. 118, 785 (1913). — BRAUN, W., u. H. WEYHBRECHT: Beitrag zur Klinik und Pathogenese der Hyalinosis cutis et mucosae (Lipoid-Proteinose [Wiethe-Urbach]). Arch. Derm. 194, 538—554 (1952). — BRAUN-FALCO, O.: Über das Wesen der senilen Elastosis. Derm. Wschr. 134, 1021—1042 (1956). — Pathologische Veränderungen an Grundsubstanz, Kollagen und Elastica. In: Handbuch der Haut- u. Geschlechtskrankheiten, Erg.-Werk Bd. I/2, S. 519ff. Berlin-Göttingen-Heidelberg: Springer 1964. — BREITENECKER, L., u. G. NIEBAUER: Historöntgenographische Untersuchungen. Acta histochem. (Jena), Suppl. 2, 124 (1960).

CALVET, J., A. BAZEX, A. DUPRÉ, A. RIBET et G. HEMOUS: Lipoide-protéinose de la peau et des muqueuses. Maladie d'Urbach-Wiethe on hyalinose cutanéo-muqueuse. Presse méd. 70, 973—975 (1962). — COSTE, F., B. PIGUET et F. DELBARRE: Milium colloide et manifestations ostéo-articulaires. A propos de deux cas. Ann. Derm. Syph. (Paris) 87, 149—162 (1960).

Eberhartinger, Chr., u. G. Niebauer: Beitrag zur Kenntnis der Lipoidproteinose (Urbach-Wiethe). (Hyalinosis cutis et mucosae). Hautarzt 10, 54—65 (1959). — Eller, J. G., and W. D. Eller: Tumors of the skin. London: Henry Kimpton 1951.
Ferreira-Marques, J., u. N. van Uden: Die Elastosis conglomerata. Beitrag zur Kenntnis des Kolloidmiliums im allgemeinen, seiner Histogenese im besonderen und zugleich zur Pathologie des elastischen Gewebes. Arch. Derm. 192, 2—60 (1950). — Feyrter, F., u. G. Niebauer: Zur Frage der degenerativen senilen Atrophie der Haut. Derm. Wschr. 152, 1176 (1966). — Über elastische Fasern und Elastose. Med. Welt 1966, 2097. — Über Unnas Kollastin, Kollacin und Elacin. Z. Haut- u. Geschl.-Kr. 40, 218 (1966). — Findlay, G. H., F. P. Scott, and D. J. Cripps: Porphyria and lipid-proteinosis. A clinical, histological and biochemical comparison of 19 South-African cases. Brit. J. Derm. 78, 69—80 (1966).
Gans, O., u. G. K. Steigleder: Histologie der Hautkrankheiten. Berlin-Göttingen-Heidelberg: Springer 1957. — Gillman, Th., J. Penn, D. Bronks, and M. Roux: Abnormal elastic fibers. Arch. Path. 59, 733—751 (1955). — Grosfeld, J. C. M., J. Spaas, and J. Auping: Hyalinosis cutis et mucosae. Ned. T. Geneesk. 108, 1025—1032 (1964). — Guin, J. D., and E. R. Seale: Colloid degeneration of the skin (colloid milium). A report of seven cases. Arch. Derm. 80, 533—537 (1959).
Hänig, E., u. H. Kremer: Bericht über 2 Fälle von familiärer Hyalinosis cutis et mucosae (Lipoid-Proteinose). Hautarzt 6, 491—494 (1955). — Hall, D. A., R. Reed, and R. E. Tunbridge: Structure of elastic tissue. Nature (Lond.) 170, 264—266 (1952). — Helm, F.: Ein Beitrag zum Favre-Racouchotschen Syndrom. Hautarzt 12, 265 (1962). — Heyl, R., and D. H. de Kock: A chromatographic study of skin lipids in lipoid-proteinosis. J. invest. Derm. 42, 333—336 (1964). — Holtz, K. H., u. W. Schulze: Beitrag zur Klinik und Pathogenese der Hyalinosis cutis et mucosae (Lipoid-Proteinose Urbach-Wiethe). Arch. Derm. Syph. (Berl.) 192, 206 (1950/51). — Holzberger, P. C.: Concerning adult colloid milium. Arch. Derm. 82, 711—716 (1960). — Hornstein, O., u. G. Klingmüller: Sogenannte Hyalinosis cutis (Urbach-Wiethe) unter dem Bild einer Lichtdermatose (Hidroa vacciniformis ähnlich). Derm. Wschr. 141, 1007 (1961).
Izaki, M., T. Horiuchi, and H. Hozaki: Lipoidosis cutis et mucosae (Lipoidproteinose Urbach-Wiethe): report of a case. Keio J. Med. 3, 163—177 (1954).
Kataoka, H., S. Yamagata, and Y. Ueda: Hyalinosis cutis et mucosae. Jap. J. Derm. 64, 29—37 (1954). — Katzenellenbogen, I., and H. Ungar: Lipoid proteinosis. (Reinvestigation of a case previously reported by Urbach and Wiethe in 1929). Dermatologica (Basel) 115, 23—35 (1957). — Klingmüller, G., u. O. Hornstein: Plotoporphyrinämische Lichtdermatose mit eigentümlicher Hyalinosis cutis. Hautarzt 16, 115 (1965).
Landi, G., e P. L. Negri: Lipoproteinosi di Urbach-Wiethe: Osservazioni chimiche et istochimiche su di un caso. Rass. Derm. Sif. 15, 80—90 (1962). — Lansing, A. J.: Ageing of elastic tissue and the systemic effect of elastase. In: Ciba Foundation Colloquia on Ageing vol. 1, p. 88—108, ed. by G. E. Wolstenhome. London: J. & A. Churchill, Ltd. 1954. — Laymon, C. W., and E. M. Hill: An appraisal of hyalinosis cutis et mucosae. Arch. Derm. 75, 55—65 (1957). — Leinbrock, A.: Albopapuloide Veränderungen bei Hyalinosis cutis et mucosae. Arch. Derm. 211, 341 (1960). — Lubarsch, O.: Ergebnisse der Pathologie, Bd. 4, S. 449. Wiesbaden: J. F. Bergmann 1892. Zit. nach E. Müller. — Lund, H. Z., and R. L. Sommerville: Basophilic degeneration of the cutis. Amer. J. clin. Path. 27, 183—190 (1957). — Lundt, U.: Beitrag zur Kenntnis der Hyalinosis cutis et mucosae. Arch. Derm. Syph. (Berl.) 188, 128 (1949).
Maragnani, U.: Su due casi familiari di lipoproteinosi di Urbach-Wiethe. Minerva Derm. 36, 166—177 (1961). — Marchionini, A., u. K. S. Aygün: Untersuchungen über das Kolloidmilium in Anatolien. Derm. Wschr. 1941/II, 897—909. — McCusker, J. J., and R. M. Caplan: Lipoidproteinosis (Lipoglycoproteinosis). Amer. J. Path. 40, 599—613 (1962). Miedziński, F., u. J. Kozakiewicz: Zur Kenntnis der Hyalinosis cutis et mucosae. Dermatologica (Basel) 114, 106—112 (1957). — Milian, G.: Zit. nach O. Gans u. G. K. Steigleder, Histologie der Hautkrankheiten. Berlin-Göttingen-Heidelberg- Springer 1957. — Montgomery, H., and F. Z. Havens: Xanthomatosis. IV. Lipoidproteinosis (phosphatide lipoidosis). Arch. Otolaryng. 29, 650 (1939). — Montgomery, P. O. B.: A characterization of basophilic degeneration of collagen by histochemical and microspectroscopic procedures. J. invest. Derm. 24, 107—110 (1955). — Montgomery, P. O. B., and E. E. Muirhead: A differentiation of certain types of fibrinoid and hyalin. Amer. J. Path. 33, 286 (1957). — Müller, E.: Untersuchungen über Wesen und Entstehungsbedingungen bindegewebigen Hyalins. Beitr. path. Anat. 97, 41 (1936).
Niebauer, G.: Aktinische Elastose und Cancerogenese. Ann. ital. Derm. Clin. Sper. 19, 115 (1965). — Niebauer, G., u. L. Stockinger: Über die senile Elastosis. Arch. klin. exp. Derm. 221, 122—143 (1965).
Pellizari, C.: Zit. nach L. Arzt, Zur Kenntnis des „Pseudo-Milium colloidale". Arch. Derm. 118, 785 (1913). — Percival, G. H., and D. A. Duthie: Notes on a case of colloid

pseudomilium. Brit. J. Derm. 60, 399 (1948). — PERCIVAL, G. H., P. W. HANNAY, and D. A DUTHIE: Fibrous changes in the dermis, with special reference to senile elastosis. Brit. J. Derm. 61, 269—276 (1949). — PIREDDA, A.: Le alterazioni altoastrutturali nella pseudo milio colloide. G. ital. Derm. 99, 496 (1958). — POTTER, B., and P. WEINMANN: Lipoidproteinosis. Arch. Derm. 80, 111—112 (1959). — PRAKKEN, J. R.: Colloid and senile degeneration of the skin. Acta derm.-venereol. (Stockh.) 31, 713—721 (1951). — PROBST, A.: Zur Pathologie des Bindegewebes. Münch. med. Wschr. 98, 70 (1956). — Zur Pathologie der Fasern und der Grundsubstanz des Bindegewebes. Wien. klin. Wschr. 1957, 787. — PROBST, A., u. M. RATZENHOFER: Elektronenmikroskopische Fibrillenstudien bei tuberkulösen Nekrosen. Beitr. path. Anat. 118, 228 (1957).

RAMOS e SILVA, S.: Lipid proteinosis (Urbach Wiethe). Arch. Derm. 55, 42 (1947). — RASIEWICZ, W., J. RUBISZ-BRZEZINSKA, and J. KONECKI: Hyalinosis cutis et mucosae Urbach-Wiethe. Dermatologica (Basel) 130, 145—157 (1965). — RATZENHOFER, M., u. A. PROBST: Zur Morphologie des Hyalins. Verh. Dtsch. Ges. Path. 37. Tagg 1953, S. 247. — RATZENHOFER, M., u. E. SCHAUENSTEIN: Zur Struktur von Piehollagen, Kollagen und Hyalin nebst Bemerkungen über die Hyalinentstehung in verschiedenen Organen und Karzinomen. Verh. Dtsch. Ges. Path. 35. Tagg 1951, S. 233. — REUTER, M. J., and S. W. BECKER: Colloid degeneration (collagen degeneration) of the skin. Arch. Derm. Syph. 46, 695 (1942). — ROULET, F.: Methoden der pathologischen Histologie. Wien: Springer 1948.

SAMS jr., W. M., and J. G. SMITH jr.: The histochemistry of chronically sun damaged skin. J. invest. Derm. 37, 447—453 (1961). — SAMS jr., W. M., J. G. SMITH jr., and E. A. DAVIDSON: The connective tissue histochemistry of normal and some pathologic skin. J. Histochem. Cytochem. 10, 710—718 (1962). — SCHAUENSTEIN, E., u. G. RUMPF: Physikochemische Befunde am bindegewebigen Hyalin. Z. Biol. 105, 117 (1952). — SCHMORL, G.: Die pathologisch-histologischen Untersuchungsmethoden. Leipzig: F. C. W. Vogel 1925. — SMITH jr., J. G.: The dermal elastoses. Arch. Derm. 88, 382—392 (1963). — SMITH jr., J. G., E. A. DAVIDSON, J. P. TINDALL, and W. M. SAMS: Hexosamine and hydroxyproline alterations in chronically sun damaged skin. Proc. Soc. exp. Biol. (N.Y.) 108, 533—535 (1961). — SMITH jr., J. G., and A. J. LANSING: The distribution of solar elastosis (senile elastosis) in the skin. J. Geront. 14, 496 (1959). — SCHWARZ, W. E., u. N. DETTMER: Elektronenmikroskopische Untersuchungen des elastischen Gewebes in der Media der menschlichen Aorta. Virchows Arch. path. Anat. 323, 243—268 (1953). — STEINER, K.: Mucid substances and cutaneous connective tissue in dermatoses. J. invest. Derm. 28, 403—418 (1953). — SZODORAY, L.: Über die Lipoidproteinose (Lipoidosis cutis et mucosae) Urbach-Wiethe. Dermatologica (Basel) 83, 375—386 (1941).

TOMPKINS, J., and I. M. WEINSTEIN: Lipoidproteinosis: Two cases reports including liver biopsies, special blood analyses and treatment with e lipotropic agent. Ann. intern. Med. 41, 162 (1954). — TORRES, E. A., J. C. RADICÉ, N. U. VILLAFANE u. S. VACCARO: Pseudomilium coloide. Pren. med. argent. 44, 566—570 (1957). Zit. nach HOLZBERGER. — TOSTI, A.: Pseudo milio colloide familiare. Ann. ital. Derm. Sif. 8, 161 (1953). — Microradiografia da contatto della cute umana. Monografia di Ann. ital. derm. clin. sperim. industria grafica nationale, Palermo (1964). — TOSTI, A., e L. FAZZINI: Indagini foto-e Roentgen. Ann. ital. derm. clin. sperim. 16, 185—192 (1962). — TUNBRIDGE, R. E., R. N. TATTERSALL, D. A. HALL, W. T. ASTBURY, and R. REED: The fibrous structure of normal and abnormal human skin. Clin. Sci. 11, 315—331 (1952).

URBACH, E., u. C. WIETHE: Lipoidosis cutis et mucosae. Virchows Arch. path. Anat. 273, 285—319 (1929).

VIDAL-LELOIR: Zit. nach O. GANS u. K. G. STEIGLEDER, Histologie der Hautkrankheiten. Berlin-Göttingen-Heidelberg: Springer 1957.

WAGNER: Zit. nach L. ARZT, Zur Kenntnis des „Pseudo-Milium colloidale". Arch. Derm. 118, 785 (1913). — WEYHBRECHT, H., u. G. W. KORTING: Zur Pathogenese der Hyalinosis cutis et mucosae. Arch. Derm. 197, 459—478 (1954). — WIETHE, C.: Über lokale Hyalinablagerungen in den oberen Luftwegen. Z. Hals-, Nas.-Ohrenheilk. 10, 359 (1924). — WILE, U. J., and J. S. SNOW: Lipoid proteinosis. Report of a case. Arch. Derm. 43, 134—144 (1941). — WINER, L. H.: Elastic fibers in unusual dermatoses. Arch. Derm. Syph. (Chic.) 71, 338—348 (1955). — WISE, F., and CH. R. REIN: Lipoidosis cutis et mucosae (lipoid proteinosis of Urbach). Report of the disease in two sisters, with a histologic and histochemical investigation in one case. Arch. Derm. 37, 201—218 (1938). — WOLMAN, M.: Lipids. In: Handbuch der Histochemie von W. G. GRAUMANN u. K. H. NEUMANN, Bd. V, S. 273. Stuttgart: Gustav Fischer 1964. — WOOD, M. G., F. URBACH, and H. BEERMAN: Histochemical study of a case of lipoid proteinosis. J. invest. Derm. 26, 263—274 (1956).

ZAUN, H.: Pseudomilium colloidale. Kolloidmilium. Elastosis colloidalis conglomerata. Arch. klin. exp. Derm. 224, 408 (1966). — ZOON, J. J., L. H. JANSEN, and A. HOVENKAMP: The nature of colloid milium. Brit. J. Derm. 67, 212—217 (1955).

Mucin

ARNOLD, H. L.: Dysesthesia in alopecia mucinosa. Arch. Derm. **85**, 409 (1962). — ASBOE-HANSEN, G.: The origin of synovial mucin, Ehrlichs mast cell-a secretory element of the connective tissue. Ann. rheum. Dis. **9**, 149 (1950a). — A survey of the normal and pathological occurence of mucinous substances and mast cells in the dermal connective tissue in man. Acta derm.-venereol. (Stockh.) **30**, 338 (1950b). — The mast cell. Int. Rev. Cytol. **3**, 399 (1954). — Two cases of circumscribed myxoedema following of thyreotoxicosis with radioactive iodine. Acta derm.-venereol. (Stockh.) **36**, 225 (1956). — ASBOE-HANSEN, G., and O. WEGELIUS: Histamine and mastcells. Acta physiol. scand. **37**, 350 (1956). BEIERWALTES, W. H.: Acid mucopolysaccharide studies in localized myxoedema. Proc. 12. internat. Congr. Derm. vol. **1**, p. 771—776, 1962. — BENSLEY, S. H.: On the presence, properties and distribution of the intercellular ground substance of close connective tissue. Anat. Rec. **60**, 93 (1934). — BERNHARDT, R.: Myxoedema papulatum et tuberosum. (Zur Frage des Lichen ruber moniliformis Kaposi.) Arch. Derm. Syph. (Berl.) **164**, 689 (1931). — BOLLET, A. J., N. F. BOAS, and J. J. BONIN: Synthesis of hexosamine by connective tissue (in vitro). Science **120**, 348 (1954). — BONNYNS, M.: 1st Meeting europ. Thyreoid Ass. 1967. — BORDA, J. M., J. ABULAFIA, and F. CARDENAS: Alopecia mucinosa con alteraciones sudorales. Arch. argent. Derm. **14**, 287 (1964). — BRAUN-FALCO, O.: Histochemische und morphologische Studien an normaler und pathologisch veränderter Haut. Arch. Derm. Syph. (Berl.) **198**, 111 (1954). — Zum Formenkreis der Myxodermien. Derm. Wschr. **133**, 540 (1956). — L'Histochimie des myxodermies. Bull. Soc. franç. Derm. Syph. **64**, 600 (1957a). — Mucophanerosis intrafollicularis et seboglandularis. Derm. Wschr. **136**, 1289 (1957b). — In: Pathologische Veränderungen an Grundsubstanz, Kollagen und Elastica. Handbuch der Haut- und Geschlechtskrankheiten (Hrsg. J. JADASSOHN), Erg.-Werk Bd. I/2. Berlin-Göttingen-Heidelberg New York: Springer 1964. — BURKL, W.: Über Mastzellen und ihre Aufgaben. Wien. klin. Wschr. **64**, 411 (1952). — BUTLER, J., and C. W. LAYMON: Nodular diffuse scleroderma. Arch. Derm. Syph. (Chic.) **35**, 919 (1937).

CABRÉ, J., u. G. W. KORTING: Zum symptomatischen Charakter der „Mucinosis follicularis"; ihr Vorkommen beim Lupus erythematodes chronicus. Derm. Wschr. **149**, 513 (1964). — CAROL, W. L. L.: Über atypisches Myxödem. Acta derm.-venereol. (Stockh.) **13**, 127 (1932). — CEELEN, W.: Über Myxödem. Beitr. path. Anat. **69** (1921). — CHAIN u. DUTHIE: Zit. nach W. GRAUMANN, Handbuch der Histochemie. Stuttgart: Gustav Fischer 1964. — CURRAN, R. C., and J. S. KENNEDY: Utilization of sulphate by fibroblasts in the quartz focus. Nature (Lond.) **175**, 435 (1955).

DALTON, J. E., and M. A. SEIDELL: Studies on lichen myxedematouss (papular mucinosis). Arch. Derm. **67**, 194 (1953). — DURAN-REYNALS, F.: Zit. nach W. GRAUMANN, Handbuch der Histochemie. Stuttgart: Gustav Fischer 1964.

EBERHARTINGER, CHR.: Ein Fall von Myxoedema circumscriptum symmetricum crurum. Wien. med. Wschr. **1956**, 449. — EBERHARTINGER, CHR., u. H. EBNER: Zur Kenntnis des Lichen myxoedematosus. Z. Haut- u. Geschl.-Kr. **19**, 108 (1965). — EHRICH, W. E.: Nature of collagen diseases. Amer. Heart J. **43**, 121 (1952).

FERREIRA-MARQUES, J.: Sensory imbalance in alopecia mucinosa. Arch. Derm. **84**, 302 (1961). — FISCHER, F. v.: Beitrag zur Klinik und Pathogenese des Myxoedema tuberosum. Dermatologica (Basel) **98**, 270 (1949).

GANS, O., u. G. K. STEIGLEDER: Histologie der Hautkrankheiten, I. Bd. Berlin-Göttingen-Heidelberg: Springer 1955. — GERSH, J., and H. R. CATCHPOLE: The organization of ground substance and basement membrane and its significance in tissue injury, disease and growth. Amer. J. Anat. **85**, 457 (1949). — GOTTRON, H. A.: Skleromyxödem. (Eine eigenartige Erscheinungsform von Myxothesaurodermie.) Arch. Derm. Syph. (Berl.) **199**, 71 (1954). — GOTTRON, H. A., u. G. W. KORTING: Zur Pathogenese des Myxoedema circumscriptum tuberosum. Arch. Derm. Syph. (Berl.) **195**, 625 (1953). — GRAUMANN, W. G.: In: W. G. GRAUMANN u. K. H. NEUMANN, Handbuch der Histochemie, Bd. II/2, Polysaccharide. Stuttgart: Gustav Fischer 1964. — GROSSFELD, H., L. MEYER, and G. GODMAN: Differentiation of fibroblastes in tissue culture as determined by mucopolysaccharide production. Proc. soc. exp. Biol. (N.Y.) **88**, 31 (1955). — Mucopolysaccharide production in tissue culture. J. biophys. biochem. Cytol. **3**, 391 (1957).

HAMMINGA, H., u. F. J. KEUNING: Lichen myxoedematosus (mucinosis papulosa cutis). Dermatologica (Basel) **109**, 86 (1954). — HIERONYMI, G.: Über Vorkommen und Verteilung saurer Mucopolysaccharide in Geschwülsten. Frankfurt. Z. Path. **65**, 409 (1954). — HOLUBAR, K., u. K. W. MACH: Scleredema (Bäschke). Acta derm.-venereol. (Stockh.) **47**, 102 (1967). — HORSTMANN, E.: In: Handbuch der mikroskopischen Anatomie des Menschen. Die Haut, Bd. III/3. Berlin-Göttingen-Heidelberg: Springer 1957. — HOTCHKISS, R. D.: A microchemical reaction resulting in the staining of polysaccharide structures in fixed tissue preparations. Arch. Biochem. **16**, 131 (1948).

JABLONSKA, ST., T. CHORZELSKI u. J. LANCUCKI: Mucinosis follicularis. Hautarzt 10, 27 (1959). — KEINING, E., u. O. BRAUN-FALCO: Vergleichende Betrachtungen über das Keloid, Sklerödem und myxomatöse Hautveränderungen. Derm. Wschr. 126, 633 (1952). — Zur Klinik und Pathogenese des Skleromyxoedems (gleichzeitig ein histochemischer Beitrag zur Natur der mucinösen Einlagerungen). Acta derm.-venereol. (Stockh.) 36, 37 (1956). — KIM, R., and R. K. WINKELMANN: Follicular mucinosis -(Alopecia mucinosa). Arch. Derm. 85, 490 (1962). — KINT, A., et D. CANDAELE: Arch. belges Derm. 19, 25 (1963). — KONRAD, J., u. A. WINKLER: Skleromyxoedem (Arndt-Gottron). Arch. Derm. Syph. (Berl.) 202, 254 (1956). — KOPF, A. W.: Lichen myxedematosus (skleromyxedema). Arch. Derm. 73, 623 (1956). — KORTING, G. W., u. G. WEBER: Bericht über eine solitäre tuberöse Myxodermie des linken Handrückens. Arch. klin. exp. Derm. 216, 354 (1963). — KREIBICH, C.: Mucin bei Hauterkrankung. Arch. Derm. Syph. (Berl.) 153, 799 (1927). — LETTERER, E.: Zit. nach W. GRAUMANN, Handbuch der Histochemie. Stuttgart: Gustav Fischer 1964. — LEVER, W. F.: Ablagerungskrankheiten körpereigener Stoffwechselprodukte. In: Jadassohnsches Handbuch der Haut- und Geschletskrankheiten, Erg.-Werk Bd. III/1. Berlin-Göttingen-Heidelberg: Springer 1963. — LILLIE, R. D.: Zit. nach W. GRAUMANN, Handbuch der Histochemie. Stuttgart: Gustav Fischer 1964. — LINDNER, J.: Weitere Befunde zur Enzymhistochemie der Bindegewebszellen. Acta histochem. (Jena), Suppl. IV, 128 (1964). — LOEVEN, W. A.: The binding collagen-mucopolysaccharide in connective tissue. Acta anat. (Basel) 24, 217 (1955).

MAXIMOW, A.: Bindegewebe und blutbildende Gewebe. In: W. v. MÖLLENDORFF, Handbuch der mikroskopischen Anatomie des Menschen, Bd. II/1. Berlin: Springer 1927. — McLEAN, F.: Zit. nach W. GRAUMANN, Handbuch der Histochemie. Stuttgart: Gustav Fischer 1964. — McMANUS, J. F. A.: Histological demonstrations of mucin after periodic acid. Nature (Lond.) 158, 202 (1946). — MEYER, H., u. S. NISHIYAMA: Zur Klinik und Histologie des Lichen myxoedematosus. Derm. Wschr. 144, 1237 (1961). — MEYER, K.: The chemistry of the ground substances of connective tissue. In: Connective tissue in health and disease, ed. by G. ASBOE-HANSEN, p. 54. Copenhagen: E. Munksgaard 1954. — Struktur und Biologie der Polysaccharidsulfate im Bindegewebe. Symp. über Struktur und Stoffwechsel des Bindegewebes, 16. und 17. 10. 1959, Münster, S. 12, hrsg. v. W. H. HAUSS u. H. LOSSE. Stuttgart: Georg Thieme 1960. — Zit. nach W. GRAUMANN, Handbuch der Histochemie. Stuttgart: Gustav Fischer 1964. — MILLER, TH. H., and C. MOPPER: Lichen myxoedematosus. Arch. Derm. 71, 542 (1955). — MONTGOMERY, H., and L. J. UNDERWOOD: Lichen myxoedematosus. (Differentiation from cutaneous myxoedema or mucid states.) J. invest. Derm. 20, 213—235 (1953).

NEUMANN, H.: Die Schleimpapel-Krankheit (Lichen myxoedematosus). Derm. Wschr. 1935/II, 1263—1294. — NIEBAUER, G.: Der gegenwärtige Stand der Mastzell-Forschung. Klin. Wschr. 38, 673 (1960). — Morphologie und Funktion der Mastzellen bei allergischen Reaktionen. Wien. klin. Wschr. 75, 174 (1963). — NIEBAUER, G., u. W. RAAB: Histochemische Untersuchungen des Hautbindegewebes nativer Gefrierschnitte. (Der Einfluß der Vorbehandlung.) Acta histochem. (Jena) 12, 26 (1961). — NODA, M.: Studies on fractional determination of the acid mucopolysaccharides in cutaneous tissues. Jap. J. Derm. 75, Ser. B 396—406 (1965).

ORFANOS, C., u. W. GAHLEN: Elektronenmikroskopische Befunde bei der Mucinosis follicularis. Arch. klin. exp. Derm. 218, 435 (1964).

PINKUS, H.: Alopecia mucinosa. Arch. Derm. 76, 419 (1957).

RAWSON, R. W., G. D. STERNE, and J. C. AUB: Physiological reactions of the thyreoid stimulating hormone of the pituitary. Endocrinology 30, 240 (1942). — RENAUT, J.: Zit. nach O. BRAUN-FALCO, Handbuch für Haut- und Geschlechtskrankheiten, Erg.-Werk Bd. I/2, Pathologische Veränderungen an Grundsubstanz, Kollagen und Elastica. Berlin-Göttingen-Heidelberg-New York: Springer 1964. — REUTER, M. J.: Histopathology of the skin in myxedema. Arch. Derm. Syph. (Chic.) 24, 55 (1931). — ROBB-SMITH, A. H. D.: Normal morphology and morphogenesis of connective tissue. In: G. ASBOE-HANSEN, Connective tissue in health and disease. Kopenhagen: Munksgaard 1954. — ROLLET, A.: Von den Bindesubstanzen. In: Strickers Handbuch der Lehre von den Geweben des Menschen und der Tiere, Bd. I. Leipzig 1871.

SCHALLOCK, G., u. H. LINDNER: Beitrag zur Frage der Entmischungszustände in der Grundsubstanz des Bindegewebes. Medizinische 1957, 12. — SCHNITZER, A.: Über zwei Fälle von Skleroedema adultorum. Dermatologica (Basel) 84, 215 (1941). — SCHUERMANN, H.: Über Hauterscheinungen mit Beziehungen zum Myxoedem und Basedow'scher Krankheit. Arch. Derm. Syph. (Berl.) 176, 544 (1938). — SWEITZER, S. E., and C. W. LAYMON: Scleredema adultorum (Buschke). Arch. Derm. Syph. (Chic.) 37, 420 (1938). — SYLVÉN, B.: Über das Vorkommen von metachromatischen Substanzen in wachsenden Geweben und ihre Bedeutung. Klin. Wschr. 1938a, 1545. — Experimentelle Beiträge zur Kenntnis der

Färbung mit Mucicarmin nach P. MAYER. Z. wiss. Mikr. 55, 462 (1938b). — Über die Elektivität und die Fehlerquellen der Schleimfärbung mit Mucicarmin im Vergleich mit metachromatischer Färbung. Virchows Arch. path. Anat. 303, 280 (1938c). — Über das Vorkommen von hochmolekularen Esterschwefelsäuren im Granulationsgewebe und bei der Epithelregeneration. Acta clin. scand. 86, Suppl. 66, 5 (1941). — Ester sulphuric acids of high molecular weight and mast cells in mesenchymal tumors. Acta radiol. (Stockh.) Suppl. 59 (1945). — SZIRAI, J. A.: Zit. nach W. GRAUMANN, Handbuch der Histochemie. Stuttgart: Gustav Fischer 1964.

TAPPEINER, J.: Zur Pathogenese des Lichen myxoedematosus (Mucinosis papulosa cutis). Arch. klin. exp. Derm. 201, 160 (1955). — TAPPEINER, J., L. PFLEGER u. H. HOLZNER: Zur Mucinosis follicularis (Alopecia mucinosa Pinkus). Arch. klin. exp. Derm. 215, 209 (1962). — TAPPEINER, J., u. P. WODNIANSKY: Hautveränderungen durch Einlagerung körpereigener Substanzen. In: Dermatologie und Venerologie, Bd. III/2, hrsg. v. H. A. GOTTRON u. W. SCHÖNFELD. Stuttgart: Georg Thieme 1959. — TAYLOR, H. E., and A. M. SAUNDERS: The association of metachromatic ground substance with fibroblastic activity in granulation tissue. Amer. J. Path. 33, 525 (1957). — THIES, W.: Mucinosis follicularis (Alopecia mucinosa Pinkus). Hautarzt 15, 422 (1964). — TROTTER, W. R., and K. C. EDEN: Localized pretibial myxoedema in association with toxic goitre. Quart. J. Med. 11, 229 (1942). — TRYB, H. A.: Über eine seltene Erkrankung der Haut mit Schleimanhäufung. Arch. Derm. Syph. (Berl.) 143, 428 (1922).

UTIGER, R. D., TH. LEMARCHAND-BERAUD, and A. VANNOTTI: Current topics in thyreoid research. New York and London: Academic Press 1965.

VILANOVA, X., J. PINOL et J. M. DE MORAGAS: Lichen myxoedematosus. Bull. Soc. franç. Derm. Syph. 67, 382 (1960). — VIRCHOW, R.: Die Identität von Knochen-, Knorpel- und Bindegewebs-Körperchen sowie über Schleimgewebe. Verh. phys.-med. Ges. Würzb. 2, 150 (1852).

WATSON, E. M., and R. H. PEARCE: The mucopolysaccharide content of the skin in localized (pretibial) myxedema. Amer. J. clin. Path. 17, 507 (1947a). — The biochemistry of the skin: a review with particular reference to the mucopolysaccharides. Brit. J. Derm. 59, 327 (1947b). — The mucopolysaccharide content of the skin in localized (pretibial) myxedema. Amer. J. clin. Path. 19, 442 (1949). — WEBER, G.: Vergleichende Untersuchungen über das quantitative Verhalten proteingebundener Kohlehydrate im Blutserum bei Dermatosen. Acta derm.-venereol. (Stockh.), Suppl. 38, 1—52 (1958). — WEISSMANN, B., and K. MEYER: Structure of hyaluronic acid: the glucuronic linkage. J. Amer. chem. Soc. 74, 4729 (1952). — The structure of hyalobiuronic acid and hyaluronic acid from umbilical cord. J. Amer. chem. Soc. 76, 1753 (1954). — WELLS, G. C.: Connective tissue ground substance in ST. ROTHMANN, Physiology and histochemistry of the skin. Chicago: Chicago University Press 1954. — WIENER, R., A. IANNACCONE, J. EISENBERG, S. I. GRIBOFF, A. W. LUDWIG, and L. J. SOFFER: Influence of hormone therapy on body fluids, electrolyte balance and mucopolysaccharides in myxedema. J. clin. Endocr. 15, 1131 (1955). — WINER, L. H., S. M. BIERMAN, and TH. STERNBERG: Observations of acid mucopolysaccharide and mastcells in the skin of hairless mice following the topical application of estrone and pregnenolone. J. invest. Derm. 41, 141—146 (1963). — WINZLER, R. J.: Zit. nach O. BRAUN-FALCO, Handbuch für Haut- und Geschlechtskrankheiten, Erg.-Werk Bd. I/2, Pathologische Veränderungen an Grundsubstanz, Kollagen und Elastica. Berlin-Göttingen-Heidelberg-New York: Springer 1964. — WODNIANSKY, P.: Über die Ätiologie und Pathogenese des Myxoedema circumscriptum praetibiale symmetricum. Arch. klin. exp. Derm. 205, 22 (1957).

ZEZSCHWITZ, K. A. v.: Beitrag zum Problem des Lichen myxoedematosus. Arch. klin. exp. Derm. 208, 301 (1959).

Lipide

AVIOLI, L., J. T. LASERSOHN, and J. H. LOPRESTI: Histiocytosis X (Schüller-Christian disease). Medicine (Baltimore) 42, 119 (1963).

BARKER-BEESON, B., and P. G. ALBRECHT: A contribution to the study of xanthoma tuberosum, with report of a case. Arch. Derm. Syph. (Chic.) 8, 695 (1923). — BASSET, F., et C. NÉZELOF: Presence en microscopie électronique des structures filamenteuses originales dans les lésions pulmonaires et osseuses de l'histiocytose X. Etat actuel de la question. Soc. Méd. Hôpitaux de Paris 117, 413—426 (1966). — BASSET, F., et J. TURIAF: Identification par la microscopie électronique de particules de nature probablement virale dans les lésions granulomateuses d'une histiocytose "X" pulmonaire. C. R. Acad. Sci. (Paris) 261, 3701—3703 (1965). — BELOTE, G. H., and D. G. WELTON: Necrobiosis without diabetes. Arch. Derm. Syph. (Chic.) 40, 887 (1939). — BERNUTH, F. v.: Über einen Fall von allgemeiner granulomatöser Xanthomatose (Schüller-Christiansche Krankheit). Arch. Kinderheilk. 100, 115 (1933). — BIRBECK, M. S. C., A. S. BREATHNACH, and J. D. EVERALL: An electron microscope study of basal melanocytes and high-level clear cells (Langerhans cells) in vitiligo. J. invest. Derm. 37, 51—64 (1961). — BOJOWA, E., and A. DZIEDZIUSZKO: Lipogranulomatosis. Zit nach Zbl. Haut- u. Geschl.-Kr. 78, 155 (1952). — BOLDT, A.: Zur Kenntnis der Necrobiosis lipoidica ("diabeticorum"). Arch. Derm. Syph. (Berl.) 179, 74 (1939). — BORRIE, P.: Essential hyperlipaemia and idiopathic hypercholesterolaemic xanthomatosis. Brit. med. J. 1957, No 5050, 911. — BRAUN-FALCO, O., u. BRAUN-FALCO, F.: Zum Syndrom „Diabetes insipidus und disseminierte Xanthome". Z. Laryng. Rhinol. 36, 378 (1957). — BRUCE-JONES, D. B. S.: A case clinically resembling morphea with a tuberculosis background and indeterminate histology suggestive of necrobiosis lipoidica. Brit. J. Derm. 49, 328 (1937). — BURNS, F. S.: A contribution to the study of the etiology of xanthoma multiplex. Arch. Derm. Syph. (Chic.) 2, 415 (1920).

CEELEN, W.: Über die Lipoidgranulomatose (Hand-Schüller-Christiansche Krankheit). Dtsch. med. Wschr. 1933 I, 680. — CHIARI, H.: Die generalisierten Xanthomatosen vom Typus Schüller-Christian. Ergebn. allg. Path. path. Anat. 24, 396 (1931). — CONNOR, W. H.: Necrobiosis lipoidica diabeticorum. Arch. Derm. 34, 705 (1936).

DENNIS, J. W., and P. D. ROSAHN: The primary reticulo-endothelial granulomas. Amer. J. Path. 27, 627 (1951). — DUMMERMUTH, G.: Reticulogranulomatose. Helv. paediat. Acta 13, 15 (1958).

FABRY, J.: Ein Beitrag zur Kenntnis der Purpura haemorrhagica nodularis (Purpura papulosa haemorrhagica Hebrae). Arch. Derm. Syph. (Berl.) 43, 187 (1898); — Zur Klinik und Ätiologie des Angiokeratoma. Arch. Derm. Syph. (Berl.) 123, 294 (1916). — FARBER, L.: The nature of "solitary or eosinophilic granuloma" of bone. Amer J. Path. 17, 625 (1941); — The nature of some diseases ascribed to disorders of lipid metabolism. Amer. J. Dis. Child. 68, 350 (1944). — FEYRTER, F.: Zur Frage der sog. Lipoidosen. Virchows Arch. path. Anat. 327, 643 (1955). — FISCHER, H., u. W. NIKOLOWSKI: Zur formalen Genese der hyperlipidämischen Xanthome. Arch. klin. exp. Derm. 210, 141 (1960). — FRANZ, G.: Über Xanthomatose mit besonderer Beteiligung des Gefäßsystems. Zugleich ein Beitrag zur Frage der Arteriosklerose. Frankfurt. Z. Path. 49, 431 (1936). — FROST, R., and C. R. ANDERSON: Extracellular cholesterosis of URBACH. Arch. Derm. Syph. (Chic.) 39, 1061 (1939).

GANS, O., u. G. K. STEIGLEDER: Histologie der Hautkrankheiten, I. Bd. II. Aufl. Berlin-Göttingen-Heidelberg: Springer 1955. — GOTTRON, H. A.: Aussprache. Derm. Z. 62, 287 (1931). — Schüller-Christiansche Krankheit unter besonderer Berücksichtigung der Hautveränderungen. Arch. Derm. Syph. (Berl.) 182, 691 (1942). — GROOT, W. P. DE: Genetic aspects of the thesaurismosis lipoidica hereditaria Ruiter-Pompen-Wyers (Angiokeratoma corporis diffusum). Dermatologica (Basel) 129, 281—283 (1964). — GROSS, P., and H. W. JACOX: Eosinophilic granuloma of bone and certain other reticuloendothelial hyperplasia of bone. Amer. J. med. Sci. 203, 673 (1942).

HERZBERG, J. J.: Die extracelluläre Cholesterinose (Kerl-Urbach), eine Variante des Erythema elevatum diutinum. Arch. klin. exp. Derm. 205, 477 (1958). — HITCH, J. M.: Necrobiosis lipoidica diabeticorum (Urbach and Oppenheim). Arch. Derm. Syph. (Chic.) 36, 536 (1937). — HORNBOSTEL, H., and K. SCRIBA: Zur Diagnostik des Angiokeratoma Fabry mit cardiovascorenalem Symptomenkomplex als Phosphatidspeicherungskrankheit durch Probeexcision der Haut. Klin. Wschr. 31, 68 (1953).

IMAEDA, T.: Electron microscopic study of xanthoma cells. J. invest. Derm. 34, 331 (1960).

JAEGER, H., et J. DELACRETAZ: Maladie de Hand-Schüller-Christian. Dermatologica (Basel) 108, 426 (1954). — JORGE, J. K., u. D. BRACHETTO-BRIAN: Der histologische Bau des solitären angeborenen Xanthoms. Prensa med. argent. 18, 1129 (1932).

KEINING, E., u. O. BRAUN-FALCO: Dermatologie und Venerologie. München: J. F. Lehmann 1961. — KENDALL, R. F., R. C. DAVIDSON, and J. PFAFF jr.: Angiokeratoma corporis diffusum. Arch. Derm. Syph. (Chic.) 86, 328 (1962). — KERL, W.: Multiple Knotenbildungen, reichlich Lipoid enthaltend. Zbl. Haut- u. Geschl.-Kr. 37, 36 (1931). — KNOTH, W., u. H. FÜLLER: Zur Patho- und Histogenese der Necrobiosis lipoidica „diabeticorum". Arch. Derm. Syph. (Berl.) 199, 109 (1954/55). — KUTSCHER, W., u. V. VRLA: Über einen Fall von Hand-Schüller-Christianscher Krankheit (Cholesteringranulomatose). Klin. Wschr. 1949, 369.

LAMB, J. H., and E. S. LAIN: Naevo-xantho-endothelioma. Its relation to the juvenile Xanthoma. Sth. med. J. (Bghm, Ala.) 30, 585 (1937). — LAYMON, C. W.: Extracellular cholesterosis. Arch. Derm. 35, 269 (1937). — LAYMON, C. W., and I. FISHER: Necrobiosis lipoidica (diabeticorum?). Arch. Derm. Syph. (Chic.) 59, 150 (1949). — LAYMON, C. W., and J. J. SEVENANTS: Systemic reticuloendothelial granuloma. A comparison of Letterer-Siwe disease, Schüller-Christian disease and eosinophilic granuloma. Arch. Derm. 57, 873 (1948). — LEIFER, W.: Necrobiosis lipoidica diabeticorum in a nondiabetic person. Arch. Derm. Syph. (Chic.) 44, 717 (1941). — LEVER, W. F.: Hauterscheinungen bei Lipoidosen. Derm. Wschr. 132, 1086 (1955); — Ablagerungskrankheiten körpereigener Stoffwechselprodukte. In: Jadassohnschen Handbuch der Haut- und Geschlechtskrankheiten, Bd. III/1. Berlin-Göttingen-Heidelberg: Springer 1963. — LEVER, W. F., and R. W. LEEPER: Eosinophilic granuloma of the skin. Report of cases representing the two different diseases described as eosinophilic granuloma of the skin. Arch. Derm. Syph. (Chic.) **62**, 85 (1950). — LICHTENSTEIN, L.: Histiocytosis X. Integration of eosinophilic granuloma of bone "Letterer-Siwe disease" and "Schüller-Christian disease" or related manifestations of a single nosologic entity. Arch. Path. **56**, 84 (1953).

MACH, K.: Pathologische Zustände des retothelialen Systems der Haut. Hautarzt **13**, 390 (1962). — MATRAS, A.: Beitrag zu den Xanthomatosen der Haut und deren Behandlung. Wien. klin. Wschr. **1956**, 777. — MICHELSON, H. E., and C. W. LAYMON: Necrobiosis lipoidica diabeticorum. Arch. Derm. Syph. (Chic.) **35**, 1130 (1937). — MONTGOMERY, H., and A. E. OSTERBERG: Xanthomatosis. Correlation of clinical, histopathologic and chemical studies of cutaneous xanthoma. Arch. Derm. **37**, 373 (1938). — MOOK, W. H., and R. S. WEISS: Xanthoma and hypercholesterinemia. Arch. Derm. Syph. (Chic.) 8, 19 (1923). — MÜLLER, D.: Die intrazerebrale Form der Lipoidgranulomatose. Fortschr. Neurol. Psychiat. **31**, 225—267 (1963).

NÖDL, F.: Zur Histo-Pathogenese der Xanthomatose. Arch. Derm. **193**, 176 (1951).

PEARSE, E. A. G.: Histochemistry — Theoretical and applied, 2nd ed. London: J. & A. Churchill Ltd. 1961. — PFENNINGS, K. B., u. N. SCHÜMMELFEDER: Histochemische Untersuchungen an Granulomen einer Lipoidgranulomatose (Hand-Schüller-Christiansche Krankheit). Zbl. allg. Path. path. Anat. **88**, 95 (1952). — PFLEGER, L., u. H. TIRSCHEK: Xanthomatose bei idiopathischer Hyperlipämie und Pankreatitis. Wien. klin. Wschr. **1956 I**, 435—438. — PINKUS, H., L. A. COPPS, S. CUSTER, and S. EPSTEIN: Reticulogranuloma. Report of a case of eosinophilic granuloma of bone associated with nonlipid reticulosis of skin and oral mucosa under the clinical picture of Hand-Schüller-Christian disease. Amer. J. Dis. Child. **77**, 503 (1949). — PITTELKOW, R. B., R. R. KIERLAND, and H. MONTGOMERY: Polariscopic and histochemical studies in angiokeratoma corporis diffusum. Arch. Derm. **76**, 59 (1957).

RÖCKL, H., u. D. VOGT: Spontan abgeheilter Fall einer Lipoidgranulomatose vom Typus der Hand-Schüller-Christianschen Krankheit mit Manifestationen an Haut, Schleimhaut und Dura mater (Pachymeningosis haemorrhagica). Hautarzt **11**, 500 (1960). — ROEDERER, J., F. WORINGER et R. BURGUN: Considerations sur un cas de necrobiose lipoidique. Dermatologica (Basel) **99**, 131 (1949). — RUITER, M.: Angiokeratoma corporis diffusum. Arch. Derm. Syph. **68**, 21 (1953). — Histological investigation of the skin in angiokeratoma corporis diffusum in particular with regard to the associated disturbance of phosphatid metabolism. Dermatologica (Basel) **109**, 273 (1954). — Some further observations on angiokeratoma corporis diffusum. Brit. J. Derm. **69**, 137 (1957). — Das Angiokeratoma corporis diffusum Syndrom und seine Hauterscheinungen. Hautarzt **9**, 15 (1958). — RUITER, M., and W. P. DE GROOT: Methods of demonstration of lipid deposits in angiokeratoma corporis diffusum. Dermatologica (Basel) **135**, 75—83 (1967).

SCHAANNING, CHR. K., u. B. NYQUIST: Über Xanthom und Xanthomatose. Med. Rev. **49**, 433 (1932). — SCRIBA, K.: Zur Pathogenese des Angiokeratoma corporis diffusum Fabry mit cardio-vasorenalem Symptomenkomplex. Verh. dtsch. Ges. Path. **34**, 221 (1950). — SECKFORT, H., u. O. BRAUN-FALCO: Acetalphosphatide bei xanthomatösen Erkrankungen. Klin. Wschr. **35**, 866 (1957). — SIEMENS, H. W.: Zur Kenntnis der Xanthome. Arch. Derm. Syph. (Berl.) **136**, 159 (1921). — SIWE, S. A.: The reticulo-endothelioses in children. Advanc. Pediat. **4**, 117 (1949). — SOBEL, N., and J. H. POLLOCK: Extracellular cholesterosis with pulmonary involvement. Arch. Derm. Syph. (Chic.) **58**, 206 (1948). — SWEELEY, C. C., and B. KLIONSKY: Fabry's disease: Classification as sphingolipidosis and partial characterization of novel glycolipid. J. biol. Chem. **238**, 3148 (1963).

TAPPEINER, J., u. P. WODNIANSKY: Hauterkrankungen durch Einlagerung körpereigener Substanzen. In: Handbuch der Dermatologie und Venerologie, hrsgg. von H. A. GOTTRON u. W. SCHÖNFELD, Bd. III/2. Stuttgart: Georg Thieme 1959. — THANNHAUSER, S. J.: Lipidosis, 3. Aufl. New York: Grune & Stratton 1958. — TURIAF, J., u. F. BASSET: Deux nouveaux cas d'histiocytose "X" a localisations pulmonaires et osseuses avec présence dans les lésions granulomateuses de particules tubulaires intracytoplasmiques suggérant une structure virale. Soc. Méd. Hôpitaux de Paris **117**, 373—383 (1966).

URBACH, E.: Cutane Lipoidosen. Derm. Z. **66**, 371 (1933). — URBACH, E., E. EPSTEIN u. K. LORENZ: Extrazelluläre Cholesterinose. Arch. Derm. Syph. (Berl.) **166**, 243 (1932). — USHER, B., and I. M. RABINOWITSCH: Necrobiosis lipoidica diabeticorum. Report of a case with clinical, pathologic and histochemical observations. Arch. Derm. Syph. (Chic.) **35**, 180 (1937).

VESLOT, DUPERRAT, BROWAES, GARNIER et PLEY: La maladie de Letterer-Siwe: sa place dans le cadre des reticulo-endothelioses. Étude d'une forme icterique de cette affection. Arch. franç. Pediat. **8**, 225 (1951).

WALLACE, W. S.: Reticulo-endotheliosis. Hand-Schüller-Christian disease and the rarer manifestations. Amer. J. Roentgenol. **62**, 189 (1950). — WEIDMAN, F. D., and W. FREEMAN: Xanthoma tuberosum. Two necropsies disclosing lesions of the central nervous system and other tissues. Arch. Derm. Syph. (Chic.) 9, 149 (1924). — WEINSTEIN, A., H. C. FRANCIS, and B. F. SPROFKIN: Eosinophilic granuloma of bone. Report of a case with multiple lesions of bone and pulmonary infiltration. Arch. intern. Med. 79, 176 (1947). — WIEDMANN, A.: Untersuchungen der Frage der Ätiologie des Xanthoma tuberosum. Arch. Derm. 175, 71 (1937). — WOLFF, K.: Über eine generalisierte Necrobiosis lipoidica. Z. Haut- u. Geschl.-Kr. 37, 97 (1964). — WOLMAN, M.: Lipide. In: Handbuch der Histochemie, hrsgg. von W. GRAUMANN u. K. H. NEUMANN, Bd. V. Stuttgart: Gustav Fischer 1964.

ZEISLER, E. P., and M. R. CARO: Necrobiosis lipoidica diabeticorum. Arch. Derm. Syph. (Chic.) 30, 796 (1934). — ZÖLLNER, N.: Lipoidstoffwechsel in THANNHAUSERs Lehrbuch des Stoffwechsels und der Stoffwechselkrankheiten. Stuttgart: Georg Thieme 1957.

Glykogen

BANGLE, R.: Amer. J. Path. 28, 1027 (1952). — BAZEX, A., et A. DUPRÉ: Mucinose papuleuse du type scléromixoedème de ARNDT-GOTTRON. Minerva derm. 34, 85 (1959).

GANS, O., u. G. K. STEIGLEDER: Histologie der Hautkrankheiten, II. Aufl. Berlin-Göttingen-Heidelberg: Springer 1957. — GIERKE, E.: Hepato-Nephromegalia glykogenica. Beitr. path. Anat. 82, 497 (1929). — GRAFE, E.: Die Glykogenspeicherkrankheit. In: Handbuch der inneren Medizin, hrsgg. von BERGMANN, W. FREY u. H. SCHWIECK, IV. Aufl., Bd. VII/2. Berlin-Göttingen-Heidelberg: Springer 1955. — GRAUMANN, W.: Polysaccharide. Handbuch der Histochemie, Bd. II/2. Stuttgart: Gustav Fischer 1964. — GRAY, H. R., J. H. GRAHAM, and W. C. JOHNSON: Necrobiosis lipoidica: a histopathological and histochemical study. J. invest. Derm. 44, 369 (1965).

HARE, P. J.: Necrobiosis lipoidica. Brit. J. Derm. 67, 365 (1955).

MASON, H. H., and D. H. ANDERSEN: Glykogen disease. Amer. J. Dis. Child. 61, 795 (1941).

PEARSE, A. G. E.: Histochemistry. London: J. & A. Churchill ltd. 1961.

RECANT, L.: Recent development in the field of glykogen metabolism and the diseases of glykogen storage. Amer. J. Med. 19, 610 (1955).

SANT'AGNESE, DI P. A., D. H. ANDERSEN, and H. H. MASON: Glykogen storage disease of the heart. II. Critical review of the literature. Pediatrics 6, 607 (1950). — SANT'AGNESE, DI P. A., D. H. ANDERSEN, H. H. MASON, and W. A. BAUMAN: Glykogen storage disease of the heart. I. Report of two cases in siblings with chemical an pathologic studies. Pediatrics 6, 402 (1950). — SELBERG, W.: Zur Klinik und Pathologie der Glykogenspeicherkrankheit. Dtsch. med. Wschr. 77, 1020 (1952). — STEIGLEDER, G. K.: Allgemeine Pathologie der Haut. In: Dermatologie und Venerologie, hrsgg. von H. A. GOTTRON u. W. SCHÖNFELD. Stuttgart: Georg Thieme 1961.

WOLFF, K.: Über eine generalisierte Necrobiosis lipoidica. Z. Haut- u. Geschl.-Kr. 37, 97 (1964).

Kalk

BAFVERSTEDT, B.: Über Calcinosis cutis. Acta derm.-venereol. (Stockh.) 22, 213 (1941). — BRODY, J., and D. E. BELLIN: Calcinosis with scleroderma. Arch. Derm. 36, 85 (1937).

FINNERUD, C. W., and R. NOMLAND: Pseudoxanthoma elasticum. Proof of calcification of elastic tissue; occurence with and without angioid streaks in the retina. Arch. Derm. 35, 653 (1937).

GANS, O., u. G. K. STEIGLEDER: Histologie der Hautkrankheiten, Bd. I. Berlin-Göttingen-Heidelberg: Springer 1955. — GOODMAN, R. M., E. W. SMITH, D. PATON, R. A. BERGMAN, CH. L. SIEGEL, O. E. OTTESEN, W. M. SHELLEY, A. L. PUSCH, V. A. McKUSICK: Pseudoxanthoma elasticum: A clinical and histopathological study. Medicine (Baltimore) 42, 297 (1963). — GRONBLAD, E.: Calcinosis cutis in Pseudoxanthoma elasticum. Acta derm.-venereol. (Helsinki) 28, 270 (1948).

JESSERER, H.: Calcinosis interstitialis (Kalkgicht). Med. Klin. 55, 2229 (1960).

KERL, W.: Beiträge zur Kenntnis der Verkalkungen der Haut. Arch. Derm. Syph. 126, 172 (1919).

LEVER, W. F.: Ablagerungskrankheiten körpereigener Stoffwechselprodukte. In: Handbuch der Haut- und Geschlechtskrankheiten, hrsg. von J. JADASSOHN, Erg.-Werk, Bd. III/1. Berlin-Göttingen-Heidelberg: Springer 1963.

MUSGER, A.: Knochenbildung in der Haut. Acta derm.-venereol. (Stockh.) 16, 1 (1935).

NAEGELI, O.: Kalkablagerungen. In: Handbuch der Haut- und Geschlechtskrankheiten, hrsg. von J. JADASSOHN, Bd. IV/3. Berlin: Springer 1932. — NIEBAUER, G., u. L. STOCKINGER: Über die Elastosis senilis. Arch. exp. Derm. 221, 122 (1965).

PONHOLD, J.: Zur Histologie der Kalkgicht. Arch. Derm. 182, 412 (1941).

SCHIFF, B. L., and A. B. KERN: Metabolic calcinosis in the newborn. Arch. Derm. 68, 672 (1953). — SCHMITT-RHODE, J. M., u. E. WEICHHARDT: Das Thibierge-Weissenbach-Syndrom (Sklerodermie mit Calcinosis) an Hand eines Falles. Dtsch. med. J. 1955, 577.

TAPPEINER, J., u. P. WODNIANSKY: Hautveränderungen durch Ablagerung von Kalk. In: Handbuch der Dermatologie und Venerologie, hrsg. von H. A. GOTTRON u. W. SCHÖNFELD, Bd. III/2. Stuttgart: Georg Thieme 1959.
WEIDMAN, F. D., and L. W. SHAFFER: Calcification of the skin, including the epiderm, in connection with extensive bone resorption. Arch. Derm. 14, 503 (1926). — WINER, L. H.: Solitary congenital nodular calcification of the skin. Arch. Derm. 66, 204 (1952). — WISKEMANN, A.: Calcinosis cutis universalis und Poikilodermie. Arch. Derm. 199, 507 (1955).

Urate

EBNER, H., u. W. RAAB: Chronische Hautgicht. Hautarzt 15, 429 (1964).
FREUDENTHAL, W., u. Z. GESEROWA: Harnsäurekristalle in Hydrocystomen. Arch. Derm. 158, 724 (1929).
GOTTRON, H. A., u. G. W. KORTING: Chronische Hautgicht. Arch. klin. exp. Derm. 204, 483 (1957). — GRÜN, E.: Zur Histologie der Gichtknoten. Arch. Derm. Syph. (Berl.) 152, 3 (1926).
KAISER, S.: Primäre Hautgicht. Arch. Derm. (Berl.) 151, 386 (1926).
LEVER, W. F.: Ablagerungskrankheiten körpereigener Stoffwechselprodukte. In: Handbuch der Haut- und Geschlechtskrankheiten von J. JADASSOHN, Erg.-Werk, Bd. III/1. Berlin-Göttingen-Heidelberg: Springer 1963.
NIINO, S.: Ein Beitrag zur Histogenese der Gichtknoten. Jap. J. Derm. 46, Nr 1 (1939). Zit. nach Zbl. Haut- u. Geschl.-Kr. 64, 334 (1940).
TAPPEINER, J., u. P. WODNIANSKY: Hauterkrankungen durch Einlagerung körpereigener Substanzen. In: Dermatologie und Venerologie, hrsg. von H. A. GOTTRON u. W. SCHÖNFELD, Bd. III/Teil 2. Stuttgart: Georg Thieme 1959. — THANNHAUSER, L. J.: Über die Pathogenese der Gicht. Dtsch. med. Wschr. 81, 492 (1956).
ZÖLLNER, N.: Nukleinstoffwechsel in THANNHAUSERs Lehrbuch des Stoffwechsels und der Stoffwechselkrankheiten. Stuttgart: Georg Thieme 1957.

Melanin

ADAMS, C. W. M.: A stricter interpretation of the ferric ferricyanide reaction with particular reference to the demonstration of protein-bound sulphhydril and di-sulphide groups. J. Histochem. Cytochem. 4, 23—35 (1956).
BARNICOT, N. A., and M. S. C. BIRBECK: The electron microscopy of human melanocytes and melanin granules, in the biology of hair growth (ed. MONTAGNA and ELLIS), p. 239—254. New York: Academic Press. Inc. 1958. — BECKER, S. W.: Melanin pigmentation; systematic study of pigment of human skin and the upper mucous membranes with special consideration of pigment dendritic cells. Arch. Derm. 16, 259—290 (1927). — Dermatological investigations of melanin pigmentation. Special Publ. N.Y. Acad. Sci. 4, 82—125 (1948). — Historical background of research on pigmentary diseases of the skin. J. invest. Derm. 32, 185—196 (1959). — BECKER, S. W., and A. A. ZIMMERMANN: Further studies on melanocytes and melanogenesis in the human fetus and newborn. J. invest. Derm. 25, 103—112 (1955). — BECKER jr., W. S., T. B. FITZPATRICK, and H. MONTGOMERY: Human melanogenesis: Cytology and histology of pigment cells (Melanodendrocytes). Arch. Derm. Syph. (Chic.) 65, 511—523 (1952). — BILLINGHAM, R. E.: Dendritic cells. J. Anat. (Lond.) 82, 93—109 (1948). — Dendritic cells in pigmented human skin. J. Anat. (Lond.) 83, 109—115 (1949). — BILLINGHAM, R. E., and P. B. MEDAWAR: A study of the branched cells of the mammalian epidermis with special reference to the fate of their division products. Phil. Trans B 237, 151—171 (1953). — BILLINGHAM, R. E., and W. K. SILVERS: The melanocytes of mammals. Quart. Rev Biol. 35, 1—40 (1960). — BIRBECK, M. S. C.: Electron microscopy of melanocytes: The fine structure of hair bulb premelanosomes. Ann. N.Y. Acad. Sci. 100, 540—547 (1963). — BIRBECK, M. S. C., and N. A. BARNICOT: Electron microscopic studies on pigment formation in human hair follicles. In: Pigment cell biology, ed. by M. GORDON, 647 p., p. 549—561. New York: Academic Press 1959. — BIRBECK, M. S. C., A. S. BREATHNACH, and J. D. EVERALL: An electron microscope study of basal melanocytes and high-level clear cells (Langerhans cells) in vitiligo. J. invest. Derm. 37, 51—64 (1961). — BIRBECK, M. S. C., and E. H. MERCER: The electron microscopy of the human hair follicle. Part 1. Introduction and the hair cortex. J. biophys. biochem. Cytol. 3, 203 (1957). — BLOCH, N.: Das Problem der Pigmentbildung in der Haut. Arch. Derm. Syph. (Berl.) 124, 129—208 (1917). — BLOCH, B., u. P. RYHINER: Histochemische Studien in überlebendem Gewebe über fermentative Oxydation und Pigmentbildung. Z. ges. exp. Med. 5, 179—263 (1916/17). — BREATHNACH, A. S.: Electron microscopy of a small pigmented cutaneous lesion. J. invest. Derm. 42, 21—25 (1964). — BREATHNACH, A. S., M. S. BIRBECK, and J. D. EVERALL: Observations bearing on the relationship between Langerhans cells and melanocytes. Ann. N.Y. Acad. Sci. 100, 223 (1963). — BREATHNACH,

A. S., T. B. FITZPATRICK, and L.-M.-A. WYLLIE: Electron microscopy of melanocytes in human piebaldism. J. invest. Derm. **45**, 28—37 (1965). — BREATHNACH, A. S., and D. P. GOODWIN: Electron microscopy of nonkeratinocytes in the basal layer of white epidermis of the recessively spotted guinea pig. J. Anat. (Lond.) **99**, 377—387 (1965). — BREATHNACH, A. S., and L. M. WYLLIE: Electron microscopy of melanocytes and melanosomes in freckled human epidermis. J. invest. Derm. **42**, 388—394 (1964). — Electron microscopy of melanocytes and Langerhans cells in human fetal epidermis at fourteen weeks. J. invest. Derm. **44**, 51—60 (1965).

CHARLES, A., and J. T. INGRAM: Electron microscope observations of the melanocyte of the human epidermis. J. biophys. biochem. Cytol. **6**, 41—44 (1959). — COTTINI, G. B.: Die Hautmelanome. In: Handbuch der Haut- u. Geschlechtskrankheiten, Erg.-Werk Bd. II/1, S. 568—675. Berlin-Göttingen-Heidelberg: Springer 1963.

DROCHMANS, P.: Electron microscope studies of epidermal melanocytes and the fine structure of melanin granules. J. biophys. biochem. Cytol. **8**, 165—180 (1960). — Melanin granules: Their fine structure, formation and degradation in normal and pathological tissues. Int. Red. exp. Path. **2**, 357—422 (1963). — The fine structure of melanin granules (the early, mature and compounds forms). In: Structure and control of the melanocytes, ed. by G. DELLA PORTA and O. MÜHLBOCK. Berlin-Heidelberg-New York: Springer 1966. — DUVE, C. DE: The lysosome concept, in lysosomes, ed. by A. V. S. REUCK and M. P. CAMERON, p. 1—35. Boston: Little Brown & Co. 1963. — DUSHANE, G. P.: An experimental study of the origin of pigment cells in amphibia. J. exp. Zool. **72**, 1 (1935). — The development of pigment cells in vertebrates. The biology of melanomas. New York: Publ. Acad. Sci. 1948.

EVANS, W. C., and H. S. RAPER: The accumulation of 1—3:4-dihydroxyphenylalanine in the tyrosinase-tyrosine reaction. Biochem. J. **31**, 2162—2170 (1937).

FITZPATRICK, T. B.: Human melanogenesis; the tyrosinase reaction in pigment cell neoplasm, with particular reference to malignant melanoma. Arch. Derm. Syph. (Chic.) **65**, 379—391 (1952). — Zur Rolle der Tyrosinase bei der Säugetier-Melanogenese. Hautarzt **10**, 520 (1959). — FITZPATRICK, T. B., W. S. BECKER jr., B. A. LERNER, and H. MONTGOMERY: Tyrosinase in human skin: demonstration of its presence and of its role in human melanin formation. Science **112**, 223—225 (1950). — FITZPATRICK, T. B., and A. S. BREATHNACH: Das epidermale Melanin- Einheit-System. Derm. Wschr. **147**, 481—489 (1963). — FITZPATRICK, F. B., T. B. BRUNET, and A. KUKITA: The nature of hair pigment. In: The biology of hair growth, p. 255—303 (ed. MONTAGNA and R. ELLIS). New York: Academic Press 1958. — FITZPATRICK, T. B., and A. KUKITA: A histochemical autoradiographic method for demonstration of tyrosinase in human melanocytes, nevi, and malignant melanoma. J. invest. Derm. **26**, 173—183 (1956). — Tyrosinase activity in vertebrate melanocytes. In: Pigment cell biology, ed. by M. GORDON, 647 p., p. 489—524. New York: Academic Press 1959. — FITZPATRIK, T. B., and A. B. LERNER: Biochemical basis of human melanin pigmentation. Arch. Derm. (Chic.) **69**, 133—149 (1954). — FITZPATRICK, T. B., H. MONTGOMERY, and A. B. LERNER: Pathogenesis of generalized dermal pigmentation secondary to malignant melanoma and melanuria. J. invest. Derm. **22**, 163 (1954). — FITZPATRICK, T. B., W. C. QUEVEDO jr., A. L. LEVENE, J. V. McGOVERN, Y. MISHIMA, and A. G. OETTLE: Terminology of vertebrate melanin containing cells. Science **152**, 88—89 (1966). — FITZPATRICK, T. B., M. SEIJI, and D. McGUGAN: Melanin pigmentation. New Engl. J. Med. **265**, 328, 374, 430 (1961).

GAIL, D.: Über das Vorkommen von Melanin und Hämosiderin im peripheren Lymphknoten. Frankfurt. Z. Path. **68**, 64 (1957).

HEMPEL, K.: Investigation on the structure of melanin in malignant melanoma with ^{3}H- and ^{14}C-Dopa labelled at different positions. In: Structure and control of the melanocytes, ed. by G. D. PORTA and O. MÜHLBOCK. Berlin-Heidelberg-New York: Springer 1966. — HERRMANN, H., and M. B. BOSS: Dopa oxydase activity in extracts from ciliary body and in isolated pigment granules. J. cell. comp. Physiol. **26**, 131 (1945). — HERZBERG, J. J.: Zur Diagnostik und Therapie der Melanocytoblastome. Arch. klin. exp. Derm. **203**, 142—202 (1956). — HIRSCH, G. C.: Theorie der Golgikörper. Proc. kon. med. Akad. Wet. **40**, 614—623 (1937). — HIRSCH, H. M., A. S. ZELICKSON, and J. F. HARTMANN: Localization of melanin synthesis within the pigment cell. Determination by a combination of electron microscopic autoradiography and topographic planimetry. Z. Zellforsch. **65**, 409 (1965). — HORSTMANN, E.: Die Haut. In: Handbuch der mikroskopischen Anatomie des Menschen, Bd. III/3, S. 1—276 (W. BARGMANN ed.). Berlin-Göttingen-Heidelberg: Springer 1957.

KAWAMURA, T.: Über die menschliche Haarscheide, unter besonderer Berücksichtigung ihrer Innervation und subepidermalen perineuralen Pigmenthülle. Hautarzt **5**, 106—109 (1954). — Über die Herkunft der Naevuszellen und die genetische Verwandtschaft zwischen Pigmentzellnaevus, blauem Naevus und Recklinghausenscher Phakomatose. Hautarzt **7**, 7—14 (1956). — KINOSHITA, R.: Studies on unitary construction of pigmented nevus. Jap. J. Derm. **70**, 178 (1960).

LANGER, E., u. G. STÜTTGEN: Histochemische Befunde mit dem Schiffschen Reagens (PAS) am Melaninpigment menschlicher Gewebe und Blastome. Arch. klin. exp. Derm. **210**, 466—471 (1960). — LEONHARDI, G.: Über Harnchromatogenese bei Melanommetastasen in der Leber. Arch. Derm. Syph. (Berl.) **200**, 255 (1955). — LERNER, A. B., and T. B. FITZPATRICK: Biochemistry of melanin formation. Physiol. Rev. **30**, 91—126 (1950). — LERNER, A. B., T. B. FITZPATRICK, E. CALKINS, and W. H. SUMMERSON: Mammalian tyrosinase: preparation and properties. J. biol. Chem. **178**, 185—195 (1949). — Mammalian tyrosinase: the relationship of copper to enzymatic activity. J. biol. Chem. **187**, 793—802 (1950). — LILLIE, R. D.: Metal reduction reactions of the melanins: Histochemical studies. J. Histochem. Cytochem. **5**, 325—333 (1957). — Ferrous jon uptake. Arch. Path. **64**, 100—103 (1957).

MASON, H. S.: The chemistry of melanin. III. Mechanism of the oxidation of dihydroxyphenylalanine by tyrosinase. J. biol. Chem. **172**, 83—90 (1948). — Pigment cells in man. In: Biology of melanomas (R. W. MINE, ed.). N.Y. Acad. Sci. Spec. Publ. **4**, 15—51 (1948). — Structures and functions of the phenolase complex. Nature (Lond.) **177**, 79—81 (1956). — Structure of melanins. In: Pigment cell biology, ed. by M. GORDON, 647 p., p. 563—582. New York: Academic Press 1959. — MASON, H. S., W. L. FOWLKS, and E. PETERSON: Oxygen transfer and electron transport by the phenolase complex. J. Amer. chem. Soc. **77**, 2914—2915 (1955). — MASSON, P.: Pigment cells in man. In: Biology of melanomas, ed. by M. GORDON et al. N.Y. Acad. Sci. spec. Publ. **6**, 15—51 (1948). — My conception of cellular nevi. Cancer (Philad.) **4**, 9—38 (1951). — MEIROWSKY, E.: Über den Ursprung des melanotischen Pigments der Haut und des Auges. Leipzig 1908. — MEIROWSKY, E., and L. W. FREEMAN: Chromatin-melanin relationship in malignant melanoma. J. invest. Derm. **16**, 257 (1951). — MIESCHER, G.: Die Chromatophoren in der Haut des Menschen, ihr Wesen und die Herkunft ihres Pigments. Ein Beitrag zur Phagocytose der Bindegewebszellen. Arch. Derm. Syph. (Berl.) **131**, 313—425 (1922). — MISHIMA, Y.: New technique for comprehensive demonstration of melanin premelanin and tyrosinase sites. J. invest. Derm. **34**, 355—360 (1960). — Cellular and subcellular differentiation of melanin phagocytosis and synthesis by lyso-somal and melanosomal activity. J. invest. Derm. **46**, 70—75 (1966). — Macromolecular characterizations in neoplastic and dysfunctional human melanocytes. In: Structure and control of the melanocyte, ed. by G. D. DELLA PORTA and O. MÜHLBOCK). Berlin-Heidelberg-New York: Springer 1966. — MISHIMA, Y., and A. V. LOUD: Ultrastructure of unmelanized pigment cells in induced melanogenesis. Ann. N.Y. Acad. Sci. **100**, 607—617 (1963). — Electron microscopic studies on the process of melanization of pigment cells in vivo and in vitro. Proc. of XII. Internat. Congr. of Dermatology. Excerpta Med. **55**, 1217—1222 (1963). — MISHIMA, Y., A. V. LOUD, and F. F. SCHAUB jr.: Electron microscopy of premelanin. J. invest. Derm. **39**, 55—62 (1962). — MISHIMA, Y., and F. F. SCHAUB jr.: Origin of the nevus cell. Electron microscopic and induced melanin formation. Proc. of the XII. Internat. Congr. of Dermatology. Excerpta Med. **55**, 1588—1592 (1963). — MISHIMA, Y., and S. WIDLAN: Embryonic development of melanocytes in human hair and epidermis. Their cellular differentiation and melanogenic activity. J. invest. Derm. **46**, 263—277 (1966). — MONTAGNA, W., H. B. CHASE, and W. C. LOBITZ jr.: Histology and cytochemistry of human skin. II. The distribution of glycogen in the epidermis, hair follicles, sebaceous glands and eccrine sweat glands. Anat. Rec. **114**, 231—248 (1952). — MUSGER, A.: Melano-Phakomatose. Hautarzt **14**, 106—110 (1963).

NIEBAUER, G.: Der Aufbau des peripheren neurovegetativen Systems im Epidermal-Dermalbereich. Acta neuroveg. (Wien) **15**, 109—123 (1956). — Das Verhalten der Pigmentzellen in bestrahlter und unbestrahlter Haut. Ann. ital. Derm. clin. speriment. **16**, 93—103 (1961/62). — Theorie und Praxis der Pigmentstoffwechsel-Erkrankungen. Hautarzt **15**, 258—265 (1964). — Über die Dendritenzellen bei Vitiligo. Dermatologica (Basel) **130**, 317—324 (1965). — NIEBAUER, G., u. N. SEKIDO: Über die Dendritenzellen der Epidermis. (Eine Studie über die Langerhans-Zellen in der normalen und ekzematösen Haut des Meerschweinchens). Arch. klin. exp. Derm. **222**, 23—42 (1965). — NIEBAUER, G., u. A. WIEDMANN: Zur Histochemie des neurovegetativen Systems der Haut. Acta neuroveg. (Wien) **18**, 280—296 (1958). — NOVIKOFF, A. B.: Lysosomes and related particles. In: The cell (BRACHET-MIRSKY, ed.), vol. II, p. 423—488. New York: Academic Press 1961.

PATTERSON, T. J. S.: Enlarged lymphatic glands in a case of multiple pigmented naevi. Brit. J. Surg. **46**, 418 (1959). — PAUTRIER, L. M., et J. LEVY: Contribution a l'étude de l'histo-physiologie cutanée. Les echanges dermo-epidermiques et le reseau tropho-melanique. Ann. Derm. Syph. (Paris) **8**, 700 (1927). — PEARSE, A. G. E.: Histochemistry, theoretical and applied. London: Churchill Ltd. 1961.

RAPER, H. S.: Aerobic oxidases. Physiol. Rev. **8**, 245—282 (1928). — RAPPAPORT, B.: Studies on atopic dermatitis: III. The effect of corticotropine, cortisone and hydrocortisone on storage of melanin in basal cells and on dopaoxidase reaction. Arch. Path. **61**, 395—400 (1956). — RAWLES, M. E.: Origin of pigment cells from the neural crest in the mouse embryo. Physiol. Zool. **20**, 248—266 (1947). — Origin of melanophores in development of color patterns

in vertebrates. Physiol. Rev. **28**, 382—408 (1948). — Origin of the mammalian pigment cell and its role in the pigmentation of hair. In: Pigment cell growth (M. GORDON, ed.). New York: Academic Press Inc. 1953.
SEIJI, M.: Formation of mammalian melanin. Jap. J. Derm. **73**, 4—6 (1963). — SEIJI, M., and T. B. FITZPATRICK: The reciprocal relationship between melanization and tyrosinase activity in melanosomes (melanin granules). J. Biochem. **49**, 700—706 (1961). — SEIJI, M., T. B. FITZPATRICK, and M. S. C. BIRBECK: The melanosome: distinctive subcellular particle of mammalian melanocytes and the site of melanogenesis. J. invest. Derm. **36**, 243—252 (1961). — SEIJI, M., T. B. FITZPATRICK, R. T. SIMPSON, and M. S. C. BIRBECK: Chemical composition and terminology of specialized organelles (melanosomes and melanin granules in mammalian melanocytes). Nature (Lond.) **197**, 1082—1084 (1963). — SEIJI, M., and S. IWASHITA: On the site of melanin formation in melanocytes. J. Biochem. **54**, 465—467 (1963). — Intracellular localization of tyrosinase and site of melanin formation in melanocyte. J. invest. Derm. **45**, 305—314 (1965). — SEIJI, M., K. SHIMAO, M. S. C. BIRBECK, and T. B. FITZPATRICK: Subcellular localization of melanin biosynthesis. Ann. N.Y. Acad. Sci. **100**, 497—533 (1963). — SNELL, R. S.: An electron microscopic study of the dendritic cells in the basal layer of guinea pig epidermis. Z. Zellforsch. **66**, 457—470 (1965). — STARCK, D.: Herkunft und Entwicklung der Pigmentzellen. Handbuch der Haut- und Geschlechtskrankheiten, Erg.-Werk, Bd. I/2, S. 138—175. Berlin-Göttingen-Heidelberg: Springer 1964. — STARICCO, R. G.: The melanocytes and the hair follicle. J. invest. Derm. **35**, 185—194 (1960). STRONG, R. M.: Color of the skin and corium pigmentation. Arch. Path. Lab. Med. **3**, 938 (1927). — SZABO, G.: Tyrosinase in the epidermal melanocytes of white human skin. Arch. Derm. **76**, 324—329 (1957). — Quantitative histological investigations on the melanocyte system of the human epidermis. In: Pigment cell biology, ed. by M. GORDON, p. 99—125. New York: Academic Press 1959. — Studies on mammalian pigmentation. II. The displacement of hair melanocytes during experimental carcinogenesis. Anat. Rec. **137**, 170 (1960). — The effect of carcinogens on melanocytes. Ann. N.Y. Acad. Sci. **100**, 269—278 (1963).
WEIDENREICH, F.: Die Lokalisation des Pigments und ihre Bedeutung in Ontogenesis und Phylogenesis der Wirbeltiere. Z. Morph. Anthrop., Suppl. **2**, 59 (1912). — WEISSENFELS, N.: Licht-phasenkontrast- und elektronenmikroskopische Untersuchungen über die Entstehung des Propigment. Granula in Melanoblastenkulturen. Z. Zellforsch. **45**, 60—73 (1956). WELLINGS, S. R., and B. V. SIEGEL: Electron microscopic studies on the subcellular origin and ultra-structure of melanin granules in mammalian melanomes. In: The pigment cell. Biological and clinical aspects (ed. RILEY and FORTNER). Ann. N.Y. Acad. Sci. **100**, 548—568 (1963). — WIEDMANN, A.: Studien über das neurohormonale System der menschlichen Haut. Acta neuroveg. (Wien) **3**, 354—372 (1951). — Zur Frage der sog. Langerhans-Zellen der Haut. Hautarzt **3**, 249—252 (1952). — Neuere Untersuchungen über das neuro-vegetative System der Haut. Hautarzt **4**, 125—129 (1953). — Über das neurovegetative System der Haut. Hautarzt **14**, 60—64 (1963). — Über die Struktur des neurovegetativen Systems. Hautarzt **15**, 13—16 (1964).
YOSHIDA, Y., and Y. TOGASHI: Studies on tyrosinase reaction. I. A new method of activating the tyrosinase reaction. J. invest. Derm. **24**, 573—574 (1955). II. Studies on the new method of tyrosinase reaction. J. invest. Derm. **25**, 363—364 (1955).
ZELICKSON, A. S.: The fine structure of the human melanotic and amelanotic malignant melanoma. J. invest. Derm. **39**, 605—613 (1962). — The melanocyte and the melanin granule. Electron microscopy of skin and mucous membrane, p. 96. Springfield (Ill.) Ch. C. Thomas 1963. — ZELICKSON, A. S., and J. F. HARTMANN: The fine structure of the melanocyte and melanin granule. J. invest. Derm. **36**, 23—27 (1961). — ZELICKSON, A. S., M. M. HIRSCH, and F. J. HARTMANN: Melanogenesis: A autoradiographic study at the ultrastructural level. J. invest. Derm. **43**, 327—332 (1964). — Localization of melanin synthesis. J. invest. Derm. **45**, 458—463 (1965). — ZIMMERMANN, A. A.: Die Entwicklung der Hautfarbe beim Neger vor der Geburt. Mitt. Thurgauischen Naturforsch. Ges. **37**, 34—71 (1953). — ZIMMERMANN, A. A., and S. W. BECKER jr.: Melanoblasts and melanocytes in fetal negro skin. In: Illinois monographs in medical sciences, vol. VI. Urbana: University of Illinois Press 1959. — ZIMMERMANN, A. A., and TH. CORNBLEET: The development of epidermal pigmentation in the negro fetus. J. invest. Derm. **11**, 383—392 (1948).

Porphyrine

BOMMER, S.: Weitere Untersuchungen über sichtbare Fluoreszenz beim Menschen. Acta derm.-venereol. (Stockh.) **10**, 391 (1929). — BORST, M., u. H. KÖNIGSDÖRFFER: Untersuchungen über Porphyrie mit besonderer Berücksichtigung der Porphyria congenita. Leipzig: S. Hirzel 1929.
DE LERMA, B.: Die Anwendung von Fluoreszenzlicht in der Histochemie. Handbuch der Histochemie, Bd. I/1, S. 78—159. Stuttgart: Gustav Fischer 1958.

FISCHER, H., u. K. SCHNELLER: Zur Kenntnis der natürlichen Porphyrine. III. Über exogene Porphyrinbildung und Ausscheidung. Hoppe-Seylers Z. physiol. Chem. **130**, 302 (1920). — FORMANEK, J., u. G. NIEBAUER: Ergebnisse klinischer und chemischer Untersuchungen bei Porphyria cutanea tarda, Wien. Z. inn. Med. **47**, 438 (1966).
HAMPERL, H.: Die Fluoreszenzmikroskopie menschlicher Gewebe. Virchows Arch. path. Anat. **292**, 1 (1934). — HOLZNER, J. H., u. G. NIEBAUER: Fluoreszenzmikroskopischer Nachweis von Porphyrin in der Leber. Acta hepato-splenol. (Stuttg.) **10**, 110 (1963).
KLOSTERMANN, G. F., u. P. RITZENFELD: Über Porphyria cutanea tarda. Versuch einer pathogenetischen Betrachtungsweise auf Grund neuer histologischer Befunde. Arch. klin. exp. Derm. **216**, 373 (1963).
LANGHOF, H., H. MÜLLER u. L. RIETSCHEL: Untersuchungen zur familiären, protoporphyrinämischen Lichturticaria. Arch. klin. exp. Derm. **212**, 506 (1961). — LANGHOF, H., H. MÜLLER u. L. RIETSCHEL: Dermatitis solaris subita recidivans. Arch. klin. exp. Derm. **214**, 549 (1962). — LANGHOF, H., u. L. RIETSCHEL: Zur Frage der Lichtsensibilisation durch Porphyrine. Arch. klin. exp. Derm. **214**, 230 (1962). — LERMA, B. DE: Die Anwendung von Fluoreszenzlicht in der Histochemie. Handbuch der Histochemie. Bd. I, Allgemeine Methodik, 1. Teil, S. 78—159. Stuttgart: Gustav Fischer 1958.
MAGNUS, J. A.: Photobiologische Wirkungen bei protoporphyrinämischen Lichtdermatosen. Arch. klin. exp. Derm. **219**, 724 (1964). — MAGNUS, J. A., A. JARRETT, T. A. J. PANKERD, and C. RIMINGTON: Erythropoietic protoporphyria. A new porphyria syndrome with solar urticaria due to protoporphyrinaemia. Lancet (Lond.) **1961 II**, 448. — MONTAGNA, W.: The structure and function of skin. New York: Academic Press 1956.
NIEBAUER, G.: Über Zellen mit eigenfluoreszierenden Granula in der Haut des Menschen. Derm. Wschr. **144**, 773 (1961).
PATHAK, M. A., and J. W. BURNETT: The porphyrin content of skin. J. invest. Derm. **43**, 119 (1964).
SCHENK, G. P., u. H. WIRTH: Photo-oxidation von Thioharnstoff zu Aminoimino-methansulfinsäure. Naturwissenschaften **40**, 141 (1953). — SUUROMOND, D.: Erythropoetic protoporphyria. Dermatologica (Basel) **131**, 276 (1965).
WEGNER, A. J.: Untersuchungen über die Lichtsensibilisierung weißer Mäuse durch Porphyrin. Z. ges. inn. Med. **3**, 123 (1948). — WISKEMANN, A., u. R. WEHRMANN: Protoporphyrinämische Lichtdermatosen. Klinik, Biochemie, Hämatologie, Lichtprovokation und Erbgang der elf Patienten aus fünf Familien. Arch. klin. exp. Derm. **223**, 347 (1965). — WISKEMANN, A., u. K. WULF: Zur Lichtprovokation der Porphyrin-Dermatosen. Arch. klin. exp. Derm. **209**, 454 (1959). — Belichtungsversuche bei kongenitaler Porphyrie und cutaner Spätporphyrie. Dermat. Wschr. **144**, 1007 (1961).

Eisenablagerung

ALTHAUSEN, T. L., R. K. DOIG, S. WEIDEN, R. MOTTERAM, C. N. TURNER u. A. MOORE: Hemochromatosis. Arch. intern. Med. **88**, 553 (1951). — AUFDERHEIDE, A. C., H. L. HORNS, and R. J. GOLDISH: Secondary hemochromatosis. I. Transfusion (exogenous) hemochromatosis. Blood **8**, 824 (1953).
BRUNNER, H. E.: Die Differentialdiagnose hämatologischer Erkrankungen mit Isotopenmethoden. Schweiz. med. Wschr. **95**, 285 (1965). — BUTT, H. R., and R. M. WILDER: Hemochromatosis. Arch. Path. **26**, 262 (1938).
FINCH, S. C., and C. A. FINCH: Idiopathic hemochromatosis, an iron storage disease. Medicine (Baltimore) **34**, 381 (1955).
GEDIGK, P., u. G. STRAUSS: Zur Histochemie des Hämosiderins. Verh. Dtsch. Ges. Path. 37. Tagg Marburg 1953. — GÖSSNER, W.: Histochemischer Nachweis einer organischen Trägersubstanz im Hämosiderinpigment. Virchows Arch. path. Anat. **323**, 685 (1953).
HEDINGER, C.: Zur Pathologie der Hämochromatose. Hämochromatose als Syndrom. Helv. med. Acta **20**, Suppl. 32 (1953).
LEIPERT, TH.: Zur Biochemie des Eisenstoffwechsels. Wien. Z. inn. Med. **45**, 393 (1964). — LOEWENTHAL, L.: A case of progressive pigmentary dermatosis (Schamberg), with reference to the blood cholesterol and epidermal siderosis. Brit. J. Derm. **41**, 473 (1929).
MAGNUSON, H. J., and B. O. RAULSTON: The iron content of the skin in hemochromatosis. Ann. intern. Med. **16**, 687 (1942). — MONTGOMERY, H., and P. A. O'LEARY: Pigmentation of the skin in Addison's disease, acanthosis nigricans and hemochromatosis. Arch. Derm. **21**, 970 (1930).
RICHTER, W.: Beiträge zur normalen und pathologischen Anatomie der apokrinen Hautdrüsen des Menschen mit besonderer Berücksichtigung des Achselhöhlenorgans. Virchows Arch. path. Anat. **287**, 277 (1933).
SCHWARZMANN, J. M.: Sur la dermatose pigmentee et purpurique de membres inferieurs et la pigment hemosiderique dans la peau. Donnee cliniques, histologiques et experimentales.

Acta derm.-venereol. (Stockh.) **11**, 1 (1930). — SHELDON, J. H.: Haemochromatosis. London and Oxford: University Press 1935. — SELLEI, J.: Die lokalisierten und progredienten Hämosiderosen. Arch. Derm. **157**, 517 (1929). — SOLTERMANN, W.: Die Bedeutung des Eisennachweises in der Haut für die Diagnose einer Hämochromatose unter besonderer Berücksichtigung der Axillargegend und der apokrinen Schweißdrüsen. Dermatologica (Basel) **112**, 335 (1956).

THALER, H.: Die Histologie der Eisenspeicherung in der Leber. Wien. Z. inn. Med. **45**, 447 (1964). — TORNABUONI, G.: Dermatosi di Schamberg. G. ital. Derm. **70**, 1217 (1929).

VOLLAND, W., u. W. PRIBILLA: Über die Siderinpigmente (unter besonderer Berücksichtigung ihrer Genese). Klin. Wschr. **33**, 145 (1955).

WEWALKA, F.: Eisenstoffwechselprobleme bei Leberkrankheiten. Wien. Z. inn. Med. **45**, 433 (1964).

Carotine

ANZAI, M.: Studies on the pathogenesis of carotinosis. Jap. J. med. Sci., Trans. V Path. **1**, 175—190 (1931). — AYRES jr., S.: Carotinemia. (Los Angeles Derm. Soc. 9. 1. 1940.) Arch. Derm. **42**, 366—367 (1940).

BLUEFARB, S. M., H. H. RODIN, and L. HOIT: Carotinemia. (Chicago Derm. Soc. 26. 4. 1954.) Arch. Derm. **70**, 827—828 (1954). — BUSMAN, G. J., and A. R. WOODBURNE: Carotinemia. Arch. Derm. **24**, 901 (1931).

ČAJKOVAC, Š.: Zur Frage der Carotinodermie der Haut. Liječn. Vjesn. **60**, 750—753 (engl. Zusammenfassung 779—780) (1938).

GANS, O., u. G. K. STEIGLEDER: In: Histologie der Hautkrankheiten, 2. Aufl., Bd. II. Berlin-Göttingen-Heidelberg: Springer 1957.

KAUFMANN, E.: Aurantiasis cutis (BAELZ). In: Handbuch der Haut- und Geschlechtskrankheiten, hrsg. von J. JADASSOHN, Bd. IV/2. Berlin: Springer 1933. — KOTELNIKOW, W.: Fall von exogener Xanthodermie bei einer Schwangeren. Ginek. **1**, 91 (1935). Zit. in Zbl. Haut- u. Geschl.-Kr. **51**, 123 (1935).

LEVER, W. F.: Carotinosis. In: Handbuch der Haut- und Geschlechtskrankheiten, hrsg. von J. JADASSOHN, Erg.-Werk, Bd. III/1. Berlin-Göttingen-Heidelberg: Springer 1963. — LEVIN, O. L., and S. H. SILVERS: Carotinemia resulting from restricted diet as observed in dermatologic practice. J. Amer. med. Ass. **96**, 2190—2193 (1931). — LUTZ, W.: In: Lehrbuch der Haut- und Geschlechtskrankheiten, 2. Aufl. Basel: S. Karger 1957.

MARCHIONINI, A., u. C. PATEL: Klinische und experimentelle Untersuchungen über den Vitamin A- und Carotingehalt des menschlichen Blutserums bei Hautkrankheiten. Arch. Derm. Syph. (Berl.) **175**, 419 (1937). — MATSUDA, S.: Über die Aurantiasis cutis (Bälz) s. Carotinosis (Minura) infolge übermäßigen Genusses von japanischem Meerlattich (Ama-Nori, Porphyra tenera Kjellmann, Bangiales). Jap. J. Derm. **41**, 105—106 (1937). — MORO, E.: Über das Wesen der gelben Hautfärbung nach carotinoidreicher Kost. Acta paediat. (Stockh.) **13**, 364—368 (1932).

RATTNER, H., and J. E. GINSBERG: Carotinosis and alcohol-petroleumbenzine extract, demonstration of carotene. Arch. Derm. **40**, 831—832 (1932). — REISCH, M.: Localized carotenoid pigmentation (Aurantiasis). Arch. Derm. (Chic.) **82**, 820 (1960).

SEQUEIRA, J. H.: Carotinaemia in Europeans in the tropics. Brit. J. Derm. **49**, 69—74 (1937). — SÉZARY, A., et J.-P. VERNE: Xanthochromie cutanée caroténique. Bull. Soc. franç. Derm. Syph. **46**, 1331—1335 (1939).

THOMSON, J. G.: Über Lipochrome im menschlichen Körper, Z. ges. exp. Med. **92**, 692 (1934).

Silber

AMITRANO, L.: Alcuni casi di argirosi in neonati in seguito a trattamento delle oftalmie con preparato di argento. Rinasc. med. **15**, 724 (1938).

BERNSTEIN, E. T.: Argyria (generalized), resulting from intranasal use of mild protein silver. Arch. Derm. **37**, 1089 (1938). — BIEBER, PH.: Argyrie cutanée. Bull. Soc. franç. Derm. **64**, 210 (1957). — BOERSMA, D., and B. L. BARKER: Sites of disposition of silver in argyria. With special reference to the axillary glands. Arch. Derm. **57**, 1009 (1948). — BRODTHAGEN, A.: Argyria. Acta derm.-venereol. **35**, 234 (1955).

CASCOS, A.: Étude comparative des pigmentations metalliques. Argyrose et chrysose. Ann. Derm. Syph. (Paris) **7**, 751 (1936). — CHANIAL, G.: Un curieux cas d'argyrie cutanée. Bull. Soc. franç. Derm. Syph. **62**, 345 (1955). — CRIADO, M. F.: Merkwürdige Pigmentierungen der Nägel. Act. dermo-sifilogr. (Madr.) **22**, 738 (1930). — CURSCHMANN, H.: Über Argyrie nach langdauernder Adsorganmedikation. Med. Klin. **1937**/II, 1158.

EBERHARTINGER, CHR., H. EBNER u. G. NIEBAUER: Argyrose und lymphoreticuläre Reaktion (Bericht über 2 Fälle von universeller Argyrose). Z. Haut- u. Geschl.-Kr. **38**, 161 (1965).

Fox, H.: Argyrie due to mild protein silver. Arch. Derm. **35**, 1193 (1937).
Gager, L. T., and E. M. Ellison: Generalized (therapeutic) argyria. Case report with necropsy and notes on diagnosis and prevention. Int. Clin. **4**, 118 (1935). — Gans, O.: Diskussion. Zbl. Haut- u. Geschl.-Kr. **43**, 13 (1933). — Gans, O., u. K. G. Steigleder: Histologie der Hautkrankheiten, II. Bd. Berlin-Göttingen-Heidelberg: Springer 1957. — Goldschlag, F.: Argyrosis. Zbl. Haut- u. Geschl.-Kr. **53**, 595 (1936). — Gottron, H. A.: Argyrie. Zbl. Haut- u. Geschl.-Kr. **43**, 612 (1933).
Habermann, R.: Über Argyria cutis nach Silbersalvarsan. Derm. Z. **40**, 65 (1940). — Hadley, H. G.: Argyria. Acta derm.-venereol. (Stockh.) **22**, 197 (1941). — Harker, J. M., and D. Hunter: Occupational argyria. Brit. J. Derm. **47**, 441 (1935). — Herrmann, F.: Argyrosis. Zbl. Haut- u. Geschl.-Kr. **48**, 104 (1934). — Hill, W. R., and H. Montgomery: Argyria. Arch. Derm. **44**, 588 (1941).
Kanitz, H.: Über Argyrie der Haut. Arch. Derm. **94**, 49 (1909). — Kerl, W.: Argyrie. Zbl. Haut- u. Geschl.-Kr. **45**, 300 (1933). — Kessel, O.: Argyrosis der Ohrmuschel und einige praktische Bemerkungen. Hals-, Nas.- u. Ohrenarzt, 1. Teil **31**, 250 (1941). — Kwiatkowski, St. L.: Diskussion. Zbl. Haut- u. Geschl.-Kr. **51**, 163 (1935).
Langeron, L., A. Delattre et M. Paget: Modifications histologiques et chimiques au cours de l'argyrie. C.R. Soc. Biol. (Paris) **114**, 132 (1933). — Lenartowicz, J., et B. Jalowy: Essais de production d'argyrie artificielle chez les animaux. Ann. Derm. Syph. (Paris) **9**, 483 (1938).
Madden, J. F.: Argyria. Arch. Derm. **28**, 264 (1933). — Matras, A.: Argyrie. Zbl. Haut- u. Geschl.-Kr. **32**, 181 (1930). — Møller, P.: Argyria caused by application of silver nitrate to the fauces for several years. Acta derm.-venereol. (Stockh.) **35**, 180 (1955).
Oppenheim, M.: Argyria localis bei einem Silberschmied. Zbl. Haut- u. Geschl.-Kr. **48**, 2 (1934).
Royster, L. T.: Argyria. Report of a case in a patient aged five and a half years. J. Pediat. **1**, 736 (1932).
Sotgiu, G., et A. de Giorgo: Argirosi. G. ital. Derm. **72**, 813 (1937). — Stillians, A. W.: Argyria. Arch. Derm. **35**, 67 (1937).
Weyhbrecht, H.: Allgemeine Argyrose bei gleichzeitiger Hepatopathie (Trichloräthylen-Intoxikation?) und die Beziehungen der beiden Krankheitszustände zueinander. Derm. Wschr. **127**, 494 (1953). — Wise, F.: Argyrosis (?) of the nail beds. Arch. Derm. **29**, 624 (1934).
Zacks, M. A.: Argyria in a child following intranasal use of argyrol. Laryngoscope (St. Louis) **43**, 680 (1933). — Zoon, J. J.: Über histologische Befunde bei Argyria cutis. Derm. Z. **70**, 125 (1934).

Gold

Cardis, F., et M. Conte: La chrysocyanose. Ann. Derm. Syph. (Paris) **7**, 229 (1936). — Cascos, A.: Étude comparative des pigmentations metalliques. Argyrose et chrysose. Ann. Derm. Syph. (Paris) **7**, 751 (1936).
Gans, O., u. G. K. Steigleder: Argyrie und Chrysiasis. In: Histologie der Hautkrankheiten, II. Bd. Berlin-Göttingen-Heidelberg: Springer 1957. — Gougerot, H., et A. Caeteaud: Pigmentation reticulée survenue après une erythrodermie aurique. Bull. Soc. franç. Derm. Syph. **38**, 47 (1931).
Hansborg, H.: Zit. nach Kochs. Acta tuberc. scand. **4** (1928). — Hochleitner, H.: Fremdkörpereinlagerungen. In: Dermatologie und Venerologie von H. A. Gottron u. W. Schönfeld, Bd. III/1. Stuttgart: Georg Thieme 1959.
Kochs, A. G.: Zur Kenntnis der Chrysiasis. Arch. Derm. **178**, 323 (1938).
Lopez, P.: Hautaurosis im Verlauf einer Sanocrysinbehandlung. Progr. Clinica **39**, 402 (1931). — Lorenzen, J. N.: Über das Auftreten von Chrysiasis bei früher mit Natriumaurothiosulfat behandelten Lungentuberculösen. Beitr. Klin. Tuberk. **76**, 686 (1931).
Nové-Josserand, L., Gaté, Charpy, Josserand et P. Cuilleret: Pigmentation aurique de la peau, chez trois enfants tuberculeux soumis à un traitement prolongé par les sels d'or: chrysocyanose. Bull. Soc. franç. Derm. Syph. **38**, 117 (1931).
Rathery, Fr., M. Dérot, S. Doubrow et Jammet: Chrysopexie et chrysocyanose. (Étude anatomoclinique). Bull. Soc. med. Hôp. Paris **3**, 1217 (1934). — Reynaers, H.: Chrysocyanose des parties découvertes. Arch. belges Derm. **8**, 75 (1952).
Schmidt, O. E. L.: Chrysiasis. Arch. Derm. **44**, 446 (1941).
Wigley, J. E.: Some observations on the deposition of gold in the skin. Brit. J. Derm. **44**, 69 (1932).
Zimmerli, E., u. W. Lutz: Eine eigenartige Form von Pigmentierung nach Goldbehandlung. Arch. Derm. **172**, 523 (1929).

Fremdkörper

ARZT, L.: Demonstration eines Falles. Arch. Derm. **133**, 67 (1919).
BALER, G. R.: Zirkoniumgranulomes caused by topical therapy. Arch. Derm. **91**, 145 (1965). — BAZIN, A. T.: Two cases of paraffinoma. Brit. med. J. **1929** No 3597, 1101. — BOLGERT et R. AMADO: Granulome silicotique avec histologie atypique. Bull. Soc. franç. Derm. Syph. **63**, 356 (1956). — BREITENECKER, L., u. G. NIEBAUER: Historöntgenographische Untersuchungen. Acta histochem. (Jena), Suppl. II, 124 (1960). — BULEY, H. M., and M. H. KULWIN: Sarcoid-like silica granuloma. Arch. Derm. **70**, 828 (1954).
CIVATTE, J.: Quelques problèmes posés par les granulomes silicotiques et les granulomes béryllliques cutanés. Sem. Hôp. Paris **1955**, 3757. — CROSSLAND, P. M.: Silicon granuloma of the skin. Arch. Derm. **71**, 457 (1955).
DUPERRAT, A.: Les granulomes silicotiques cutanés. Minerva derm. **29**, 150 (1954). — DUTRA, F. R.: Beryllium granulomas of the skin. Arch. Derm. **60**, 1140 (1949).
EPSTEIN, E.,'B. GERSTL, M. BERK, and J. P. BELBER: Silica pregranuloma. Arch. Derm. **71**, 645 (1955).
FLECK, E. F.: Zur Differentialdiagnose und Behandlung des Berylliumgranuloms der Haut. Derm. Wschr. **129**, 649 (1955).
GAHLEN, W., u. N. KLÜKEN: Über Fremdkörpergranulome und M. Besnier-Boeck. Arch. Derm. **194**, 121 (1952). — GANS, O., u. G. K. STEIGLEDER: Fremdkörper-Paraffinome, Vaselinome. In: Histologie der Hautkrankheiten, Bd. II. Berlin-Göttingen-Heidelberg: Springer 1957. — GINSBERG, J. E., and L. A. BECKER: Silicon granuloma of skin due to traumatics and inoculation. J. Amer. med. Ass. **147**, 751 (1951). — GIOIA, E.: Elaiomi e liponecrosi (nuovi fatti e nuove ipotesi patogeniche). Arch. Soc. ital. Chir. 698 (1929).
LAPIERE, S.: Granulomes silicotiques. Cas 2. Arch. belges Derm. **11**, 70 (1955). — LÖHE, H.: Ungewöhnlicher Fall von Fremdkörperschädigung. Derm. Wschr. **121**, 82 (1950).
MACHER, E.: Talcumgranulome als vermeintliche Lupusknötchen. Z. Haut- u. Geschl.-Kr. **18**, 192 (1955). — Die Bedeutung des Talcumgranuloms in der Dermatologie. Hautarzt **4**, 529 (1953).
NIMPFER, TH.: Fremdkörpereinsprengungen in die Haut als berufliche Schädigung bei Installateuren. Derm. Z. **66**, 313 (1933).
SCHLIENGER, F.: Zur Kenntnis der medikamentösen Lipogranulome. Dermatologica (Basel) **98**, 289 (1949). — SPITZMÜLLER, W.: Zur Klinik der Fremkörpertumoren nach Paraffininjektionen. Wien. klin. Wschr. **1929 I**, 866.

Vergleichende Histologie der Haut

Von

H. U. Koecke, Köln*

Mit 21 Abbildungen, davon 1 farbig

Einleitung

Die Haut (Integument) stellt die äußere Begrenzung eines Tieres dar; die Gewebe der Haut bilden daher eine Schranke gegenüber den Umwelteinflüssen, müssen aber gleichzeitig einen Kontakt zur Außenwelt aufrechterhalten, so daß die großen Sinnesorgane eine wesentliche Unterstützung und Ergänzung erfahren. Die Haut besitzt durch ihre große Flächenausdehnung in den Körperregionen eine regionale Gliederung (Regionalspezifität), die sich in unterschiedlicher Feinstruktur und der Verschiedenartigkeit ihrer Derivate zeigt und so im Grunde schon eine vergleichende Histologie am Individuum notwendig macht. Im wesentlichen wird darüber hinaus der makroskopische und mikroskopische Aufbau der Haut durch drei Gruppen von Faktoren bestimmt:

a) durch die Zugehörigkeit zu einer der Klassen der Wirbeltiere, grob gesprochen also durch die genetischen Faktoren;

b) durch die Lebensweise der Tiere, d. h. ihre Physiologie und Ökologie;

c) durch die Faktoren der Außenwelt: Makro- und Mikroklima, wobei aquatische und terrestrische Umgebung von entscheidender formender Bedeutung sind.

PINKUS (1964) stellt daher mit Recht fest: „die Haut als Begriff ist eine Abstraktion". Zugleich ergibt sich auch, daß eine vergleichende Histologie der Haut, auf engem Raum zusammengedrängt, nur eine sehr unvollständige und auswählende Betrachtung sein kann. Seit den großen Zusammenfassungen von BIEDERMANN (1926, 1928a—c), v. KAMPEN (1927), sowie RABL, LANGE, SCHUMACHER, BALLOWITZ, BOAS, DE MEIJERE, v. EGGELING, PENNERS und PEYER (1931) ist eine ausführliche vergleichende Betrachtung der Haut nicht mehr vorgenommen worden. Und heute, in einer Zeit, in der vor allem die experimentelle Analyse und funktionelle Betrachtung im Mittelpunkt des Interesses steht, muß in einer Darstellung der Histologie auch die Funktion stärker als früher Berücksichtigung finden, wenn sie für den experimentell arbeitenden Forscher eine Erleichterung bei seiner Arbeit bringen soll. Neuere zusammenfassende Darstellungen über den Feinbau des Integumentes liegen nur für einzelne Wirbeltierklassen im Rahmen von Monographien vor (BLACKSTAD, 1963; v. OSTEN, 1957; RAUTHER, 1940; RAWLES, 1960). Es ist auch der Versuch unternommen worden, die biologischen und medizinischen Probleme der Wirbeltierhaut einem größeren Leserkreis zugänglich zu machen (ADAM, 1964a und b; FIEDLER, 1964; HAGEN, 1964; KOECKE, 1964; LÜDICKE, 1964). Entsprechend der medizinischen Bedeutung ist die Haut der Säugetiere und des Menschen besonders intensiv ein Gegenstand der Forschung; unter den verschiedenen Gesichtspunkten sind daher die neueren Erkenntnisse mehrfach dargestellt worden (BIEGERT, 1961; HERXHEIMER, 1960; HORSTMANN, 1957; MEDAWAR, 1953; MONTAGNA, 1961, 1963;

---

* Jetzt Marburg/Lahn.

PINKUS, 1954; ROTHMAN, 1954; STÜTTGEN et al., 1965; WEDDELL, 1960; WELLS, 1954; WINKELMANN, 1960; GABE, 1967). Wir glauben zweckentsprechend auszuwählen, wenn wir im Rahmen dieses Handbuches zunächst eine Übersicht über den Feinbau der Haut bei den Wirbeltierklassen mit Ausnahme der Säugetieer geben, wobei vor allem neuere Ergebnisse im Vordergrund stehen sollen. Bestimmte Teilgebiete können kurz behandelt werden, da sie an anderen Stellen dieses Handbuches eine ausführliche Darstellung erfahren (PINKUS: Anatomie, 1964; RICHTER: Haare, 1963; STARCK: Pigmentzellen, 1964; STARY: Chemie der Cutis, 1963; MALKINSON und ROTHMAN: Stoffaufnahme durch die Haut, 1963). Darüber hinaus sollen Vorgänge an der Haut gesondert betrachtet werden, die für den Aufbau und die Erhaltung der Hautstruktur besonders wichtig sind; die Kenntnisse über solche Vorgänge haben z. T. in der letzten Zeit durch intensive Bearbeitung eine wesentliche Erweiterung erfahren.

Die Feinstruktur des Integumentes bei den Chordata

Einige Bemerkungen über die Systematik der Chordaten seien hier vorausgeschickt. Nach der heutigen Ansicht sind die echten Wirbeltiere aus einer hypothetischen Tiergruppe hervorgegangen, deren heute lebende Formen als Acrania (= Leptocardia, früher Cephalochordata) einen eigenen Tierstamm bilden (STENSIÖ, 1964). Die Hoffnung, eine aus Schichten des Silurs geborgene fossile Form (Jamoytius kerwoodi White) stelle einen Vorfahren der Acrania dar, hat sich leider nicht bestätigt (RITCHIE, 1960). Die rezenten Acrania leben nur noch in wenigen Gattungen, zu denen u. a. das bekannte Lanzettfischchen (Branchiostoma lanceolatum) gehört. Der 2. Stamm der Chordaten sind die Vertebrata (Craniota), unter denen die Kieferlosen = Agnatha in der Stammesgeschichte sehr frühzeitig einen eigenen Entwicklungsgang begonnen haben und heute allein durch die Cyclostomata (Rundmäuler mit Schleimfischen und Neunaugen) vertreten sind. Die mit Kiefern versehenen Wirbeltiere (Gnathostomata) bilden die dem Beschauer geläufigen großen Klassen: die Knorpelfische (Chondrichthyes mit Rochen, Haien u.a.), die Knochenfische (Osteichthyes), zu denen der weitaus größte Teil der etwa 40000 bekannten Arten gehört. Alle bisher erwähnten Gruppen umfassen nur Tiere, deren Lebensraum ausschließlich das Wasser war und ist. Erst in der Klasse der Amphibia (Lurche) sind nach einer langen Übergangszeit die physiologischen Möglichkeiten verwirklicht worden, die ein Leben auf dem Lande möglich machen. Die Klassen der Reptilien (Kriechtiere) und Vögel (Aves) werden oft wegen ihrer engen stammesgeschichtlichen Verwandtschaft und gewisser anatomischer Ähnlichkeiten als Sauropsida zusammengefaßt. Schließlich stellen die Säugetiere mit den Primaten und dem Menschen die als letzte in der Phylogenese entstandene Klasse der Wirbeltiere dar.

I. Grundzüge des Aufbaues der Chordatenhaut

Die Haut aller Chordaten besteht aus zwei verschiedenen Gewebetypen, die deutlich voneinander abgegrenzte Hautschichten aufbauen. Das zusammenhängende Oberflächengewebe ist die *Epidermis;* sie entsteht bei der Embryonalentwicklung aus dem Ektoderm des Keimes. Die Zellen der Epidermis bilden einen Gewebsverband ohne Blutgefäße, sie sind bei ihrer Ernährung auf Stoffe angewiesen, die aus den tieferen Gewebeschichten und durch die Intercellularspalten transportiert werden. Diese Spalten sind von einer Grundsubstanz erfüllt, auf deren Entstehung noch zurückzukommen ist. Bei allen erwachsenen Chordaten sind die Epidermiszellen in mehreren Schichten übereinander angeordnet, eine Ausnahme bildet nur die Epidermis der Acranier. Dagegen sind bei den Larvenformen oder Jugendstadien ein- oder zweischichtige Epithelverbände vorhanden. Die Epidermis erfährt also wesentliche Umbauten im Verlaufe der Individualentwicklung. Ist die Epidermis in Form eines mehrschichtigen Epithels aufgebaut, so sind die Zellen der Schichten keineswegs untereinander mehr gleichwertig. Über einer basalen Zellschicht mit der Fähigkeit zur Vermehrung beginnen die Zellen mit Differentierungsprozessen, die je nach Tierart sehr verschieden sind. So können Hautdrüsen, zusammenhängende oberflächliche Hornschichten, Hornschuppen, Federn, Haare, Klauen, Nägel etc. entstehen.

Unter der Epidermis folgen die Gewebe des *Corium* (Dermis oder Cutis); sie entstammen dem Mesoderm des Keimes, enthalten aber auch Zellen der Neuralleiste (Ektomesenchym) und der Plakoden. Das Corium baut sich aus den cellulären, geformten und ungeformten Elementen des Bindegewebes auf und ist Träger von Blutgefäßen, Nerven und Muskeln. Die Grenzschicht gegen die Epidermis besitzt eine besondere Textur aus Fasern, eingebettet in die Grundsubstanz des Corium, und unterlagert die Epidermis als Basalmembran. Den Anschluß an die tiefer gelegenen Muskeln oder anderen Gewebe des Körpers übernimmt eine bindegewebige Schicht: die *Subcutis*, deren Abgrenzung fließend ist.

Beide Gewebsschichten der Haut: Epidermis und Corium stehen in engen Wechselbeziehungen zueinander, die während des ganzen Lebens eines Tieres andauern und mit der Embryonalentwicklung begonnen haben. Nur der ungestörte Ablauf der gegenseitigen Beeinflussung im Verlauf der Morphogenese macht die Entstehung einer so komplizierten großflächigen Gewebshülle mit ihren Derivaten und regionalen Gliederungen möglich. Die Wechselbeziehungen werden besonders deutlich (und experimentell zugänglich), wenn die Haut entsteht oder tiefgreifenden Veränderungen unterworfen wird; das ist bei intensivem Wachstum der Fall, beim Übergang von Larven- in Jugendstadien (Metamorphose), bei Häutungsprozessen und bei Verwundungen. Wir werden versuchen, die wesentlichen Ergebnisse, die eine Untersuchung der genannten Vorgänge sichtbar gemacht hat, für das Verständnis einer vergleichenden Histologie der Haut heranzuziehen.

II. Die Haut der Acrania

Die Haut der Acranier besitzt eine Eigenschaft, die am Integument der adulten Chordaten nicht noch einmal verwirklicht ist: auch bei adulten Acraniern ist die bedeckende *Epidermis* wie bei wirbellosen Tieren ein nur einschichtiges Epithel. Im Aufbau der gesamten Haut dagegen ist bereits die komplexe Zusammensetzung aller Wirbeltierhäute verwirklicht: das Integument ist gegliedert in Epidermis, Corium mit Basalmembran, Subcutis und enthält Sinneszellen, Nerven, Gefäße. Im einzelnen liegen folgende Verhältnisse vor (Abb. 1).

Das *einschichtige Epithel* besteht aus prismatischen Zellen (FRANZ, 1923; OLSSON, 1961), von denen im dorsalen Bereich etwa 140 eine Fläche von ca. 0,67 mm^2 bedecken (LELE, PALMER und WEDDELL, 1958). Die Oberfläche wird von einer dünnen Schicht bedeckt, die früher als Cuticula, aber bereits von FRANZ (1923) auf Grund seiner Versuche als eine Schleimlage angesehen wurde. Tatsächlich handelt es sich um eine Mucoproteinschicht (OLSSON, 1961), die Zellen sind also von einer „Glykocalyx" im Sinne von BENNETT (1963) überzogen. In diese Schleimschicht strecken die Epithelzellen grobe Mikrovilli hinein (Länge 2600—3300 Å, Dicke 900—1400 Å, OLSSON, 1961). Die obere Zone des Cytoplasmas der Epithelzellen wird ferner von großen Blasen eingenommen, deren feinfädiger Inhalt nach außen zwischen die Mikrovilli entleert zu werden scheint. Die früheren Beschreibungen der Haut des Lanzettfischchens kannten diese Vesikel als eine Art „Stäbchensaum" am apikalen Zellpol und geben recht zutreffende Abbildungen; die Vesikel können bis zu 1 μ lang sein. Der übrige Zellkörper enthält neben Mitochondrien zahlreiche Vesikel und ein ausgedehntes Feld von Golgi-Membranen, während ein ausgeprägtes endoplasmatisches Reticulum nicht beobachtet wurde (OLSSON, 1961). An der Basis enthalten die Zellen Tonofilamente und zahlreiche Vacuolen, in denen Glykogen gespeichert ist, wodurch lichtmikroskopisch das Bild eines kurzen basalen Stäbchensaumes hervorgerufen wird. Die seitlichen Plasmamembranen der Epithelzellen sind vielfältig gefaltet und bilden Zellfortsätze, so daß die benachbarten Zellen miteinander verzahnt sind. Merkwürdigerweise finden sich aber keine Desmosomen. Der große Zellkern liegt basal. Obwohl die Lanzettfischchen fleckig gefärbt sind, kommen keine besonderen Pigmentzellen vor. Das Pigment, wahrscheinlich Melanin, ist in den Epithelzellen selbst enthalten (FRANZ, 1923; OLSSON, 1961) und bildet dort Granula, die von einer Membran umgeben sind; ihre Feinstruktur ist bisher nicht untersucht worden.

Die Epithelzellen ruhen auf einer *Basalmembran* des Hautbindegewebes. Die Schichten dieses Bindegewebes sind in den früheren Beschreibungen verschieden interpretiert worden. Doch glauben wir, daß man nach der Aufklärung der Feinstruktur insbesondere der oberen Faserschichten durch OLSSON (1961) die Einteilung von RABL (1931) beibehalten sollte. Danach ist die eigentliche Basalmembran eine sehr dünne Schicht, die in Kontakt mit den Epithelzellen steht. Sie ist etwa 1100 Å dick (OLSSON, 1961) und zeigt die Charakteristika der Vertebratenbasalmembran: eine den Epithelzellen zugekehrte Schicht besteht aus dichtem Material, das der adepidermalen Membran entspricht. Eine zweite tiefer gelegene Schicht ist weniger dicht und wird von eindringenden Kollagenfibrillen sehr geringen Durchmessers durchsetzt, die senkrecht aus den tieferen Faserschichten emporsteigen; ihre Verteilung in der Basalmembran ist durch die Maskierung nicht zu verfolgen.

Die in der Körpertiefe folgende Faserschicht stellt das *Corium* dar (vgl. Abb. 1 a). Es besteht aus zahlreichen Lagen von Kollagenfasern, die sich schichtweise im Winkel von 90° überlagern und deren Verlaufsrichtungen etwa einen Winkel von 45° zur Längsachse des Körpers bilden. Die Fasern sind etwa 750 Å dick und zeigen die typische Querstreifung. Die Zahl der Faserlagen unterliegt regionalen Unterschieden und beträgt 16—40. Aus dieser Faserschicht kommen die sehr viel dünneren Fibrillen, die in die Basalmembran einstrahlen. Die untere (innere) Grenze wird von den Zellfortsätzen eingenommen, die weitverzweigte Fibrocyten der Subcutis gegen die Faserschicht ausstrecken.

Die *Subcutis* ist sehr unterschiedlich dick, heftet die Haut an die Myotome an und geht in die Myosepten über; im rostralen Bereich fehlt sie ganz. Die Subcutis wird von gallertiger Grundsubstanz gebildet, die Schleimreaktion zeigt. Eingebettet in die Grundsubstanz sind absteigende Faserbündel aus dem Corium und Fibrocyten, deren Fortsätze oft die Faserbündel begleiten. Man muß diese Schicht als Subcutis betrachten, da sie den Anschluß an die Faserschichten der Muskelfascien vermittelt, in bestimmten Körperregionen fehlt und im Gegensatz zum Corium sehr verschieden dick ist. Offenbar fehlt den Acraniern die Möglichkeit, Fett in Fettzellen zu speichern und so eine celluläre Subcutis aufzubauen. So wird durch die Vermehrung der Bindegewebsgrundsubstanz eine turgeszente und druckfeste Schicht aufgebaut, die vielleicht auch eine Ernährungsreserve darstellt. Denn die Grundsubstanz wird von einem ausgeprägten System von Hohlräumen durchzogen (FRANZ, 1927), deren Lumina von Zellen ausgekleidet sind. Obwohl FRANZ sagt, daß in den Hohlräumen keine Zirkulation stattfindet, da sie blind geschlossen sind und keine Verbindungen zu den Blutgefäßen vorhanden sind, wird ein Flüssigkeitsaustausch mit der umgebenden Grundsubstanz und eine gewisse Fluktuation der umschlossenen Flüssigkeit anzunehmen sein. Man kann die cutanen Hohlräume wohl mit Lymphgefäßen vergleichen.

Die *Innervation* des Integumentes ist keinswegs einfach, sondern sehr engmaschig ausgebildet und zeigt erhebliche regionale Unterschiede. Es kommen

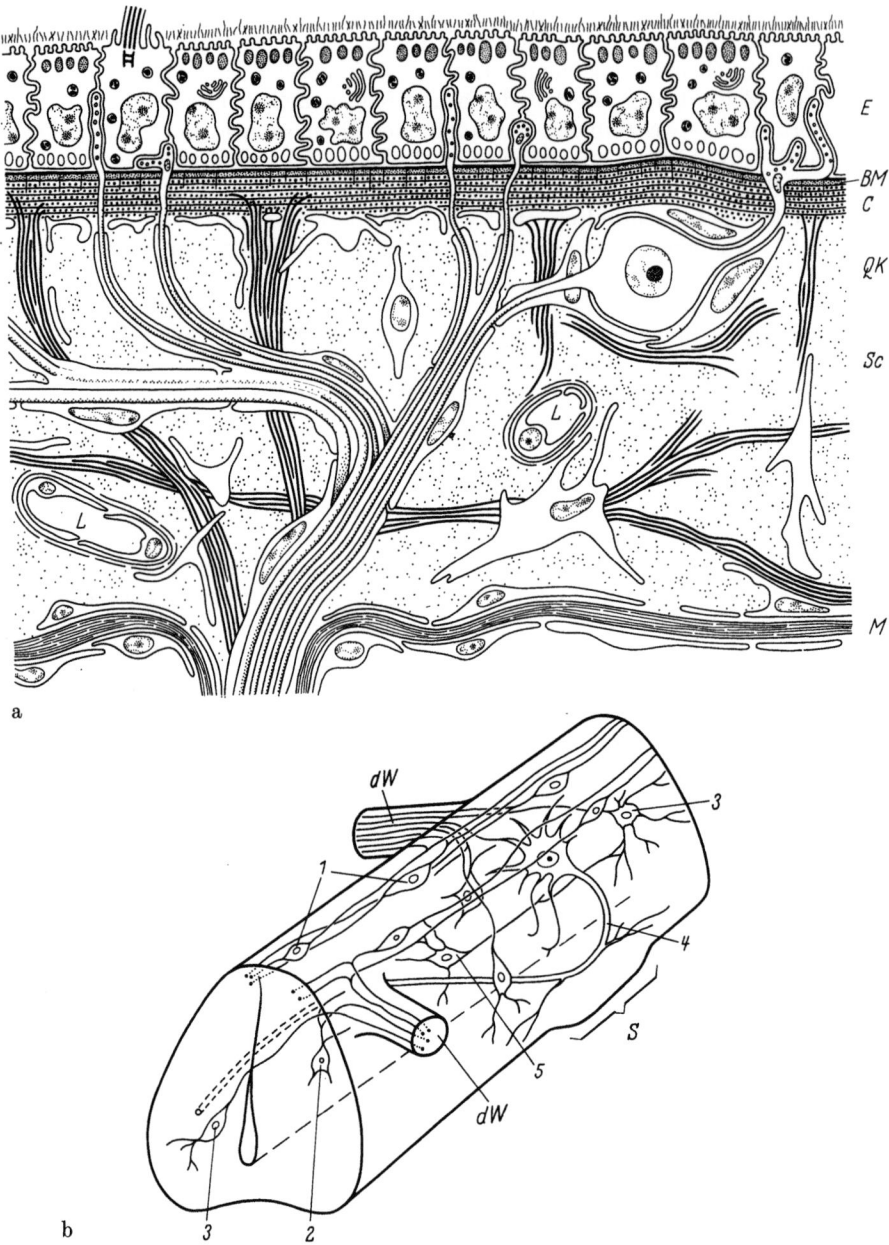

Abb. 1a u. b. Haut und Zentralnervensystem des Lanzettfischchens (Branchiostoma lanceolatum). a Die Haut mit ihren Schichten an der ventro-lateralen Körperseite; an der Subcutis ist der Übergang in ein Myoseptum dargestellt. *E* Epidermis, *BM* Basalmembran, *C* Corium, *M* Muskelfascie, *Sc* Subcutis, *QK* Quatrefagessche Körperchen. Im Epithel sind eine Sinneszelle mit Geißel sowie freie Axonendigungen gezeichnet. Unter dem Corium liegt ein Quatrefagessches Körperchen, dessen Ganglienzelle mit mehreren Dendriten an eine Epithelzelle heranreicht. Durch das Myoseptum tritt ein Nervenstämmchen mit 6 Axonen verschiedenen Durchmessers in die Haut ein, alle Axone sind von Schwannschen Zellen (ohne Myelinscheidenbildung, entsprechend wie bei Cyclostomen) begleitet. Bei *L* zwei der Lymphspalten, von Endothel ausgekleidet. Die dargestellten Verhältnisse sind wegen der besseren Übersicht nicht in allen Teilen maßstabgerecht und beruhen z.T. auf Analogieschlüssen, da im einzelnen keine genauen Feinstrukturuntersuchungen vorliegen. (Unter Benutzung der Abbildungen von BONE; FRANZ; KRAUSE; LELE, PALMER und WEDDELL; OLSSON.) b Ausschnitt aus dem „Rückenmark" mit den für die Hautinnervation wichtigen Neuronen (somato-sensorisch). Es werden 2 dorsale Wurzeln (*dw*) und die synaptische ventrale Zone (*S*) für die motorische Muskelinnervation (sog. „ventrale Wurzel") gezeigt. *1* bipolare A-Zelle des dorsalen Tractus, *2* segmentales Einzelneuron, *3* Neuron jenseits des Zentralkanals, *4* Rohde-Neuron, *5* longitudinales Verbindungsneuron

vier verschiedene Typen von sensorischen Elementen vor: a) freie Nervenendigungen; b) mit Kapseln versehene Nervenendigungen; c) sekundäre Sinneszellen; d) die Quatrefagessche Körperchen. Bei den Larven ist die Entfaltung des nervösen Apparates noch keineswegs so ausgedehnt wie bei den adulten Tieren. Der einfachere Bau des Zentralnervensystems macht es dabei möglich, bestimmte Neurone im sog. Rückenmark des Lanzettfischchens den sensorischen Elementen zuzuordnen (BONE, 1959, 1960).

a) Die freien Nervenendigungen sind Axone, die das Zentralnervensystem durch die dorsalen Wurzeln verlassen. Die gebündelten Axone treten in die intermuskulären Bindegewebssepten (Myosepten) ein, wo sie sich in einen Ramus dorsalis und einen stärkeren Ramus ventralis teilen (FRANZ, 1923). Auch diese Rami verteilen noch einmal die in ihnen zusammen verlaufenden Axone auf zwei Abzweigungen. Die Axone sind nicht alle gleichwertig, sondern zeigen verschiedene Durchmesser, eine Eigenart, die schon an der dorsalen Wurzel sichtbar ist (LELE, PALMER und WEDDELL, 1958): neben sehr dünnen Axonen (unter 1 μ Durchmesser) ist die Mehrzahl der Fasern zwischen 1—2 μ dick und besonders große Axone haben 4 μ Durchmesser. Beim Eintritt in die Subcutis verzweigen sich die Nervenstämmchen in Bündeln von 3—8 Axone, die schräg durch die Grundsubstanz und zwischen die locker angeordneten kollagenen Fasern zur Cutis verlaufen. Dabei sind die Axone von Schwannschen Zellen begleitet, denn eine Auszählung der Kerne zeigt eindeutig, daß es sich nicht um Nervenzellkerne handelt. Die Axone treten senkrecht durch das Fasernetz der Cutis, wobei sichtbare kreuzförmige Spalten in der Faserlage den Weg freigeben. Die Axone dieser kleinen Bündel sind von verschiedenem Durchmesser. Unmittelbar unter der Epidermis verteilen sich die Axone in verschiedene Richtungen und senden zahlreiche Kollateralen an die Epithelzellen. Es entsteht ein außerordentlich dichter subepithelialer Plexus. Die terminalen Verzweigungen der Axone scheinen zwischen die Epithelzellen vorzudringen, und es wird angenommen, daß sie als freie Axone zwischen den Zellen in Intercellularlücken ähnlich den Verhältnissen in der Cornea enden. Außerordentlich wichtig scheint ein Befund zu sein, der durch Auszählung der Verteilung von Epithelzellen im dorsalen Hautbereich auf die terminalen Axonkollateralen gewonnen wurde (LELE, PALMER und WEDDELL, 1958): ein Axon versorgt das Areal von sieben Epithelzellen, jede Epithelzelle erhält mindestens zwei Nervenendigungen, die außerdem von verschiedenen Axonen aus verschiedenen Richtungen an die Zelle herantreten. Diese Befunde werden deshalb so wichtig sein, weil der Ursprung der sensorischen Axone im Zentralnervensystem (BONE, 1959, 1960) von verschiedenen Zelltypen ausgeht (Abb. 1b). Denn in der Larve sind die ebenfalls durch die dorsalen Wurzeln eintretenden visceralen sensorischen Axone des Atriumsystems noch nicht vorhanden, so daß die Hautinnervation erkennbar wird. Die Masse der Axone wird von bipolaren, sog. A-Zellen in die dorsalen Wurzeln entsandt; diese Zellen bilden zwei dorsale Stränge im Zentralnervensystem und sind seit RETZIUS bekannt. Sie geben aber nur einen Ast in die Wurzel ab, die andere Kollaterale verläuft von der T-förmigen Verzweigungsstelle weiter im dorsalen Tractus dieser Zellen. Der zweite Zelltyp liegt in der Nähe des Zentralkanals und kreuzt mit dem Zellfortsatz für die dorsale Wurzel von seiner Seite auf die andere über. Diese Zellen sind wie die A-Zellen in der ganzen Länge des Zentralnervensystems gleichmäßig vorhanden. Ein dritter Zelltyp liegt schließlich als Einzelneuron an jeder dorsalen Wurzel, ist stark verzeigt und entsendet nur einen Fortsatz in die Wurzel. Als letzter Typ von Zellen ist das große Rohde-Neuron zu nennen, das auf der jeweils anderen Seite des Zentralkanals liegt, als Kolossalfaser seine langen Neuriten durch das „Rückenmark" sendet und der dorsalen Wurzel einen großen Fortsatz mit zahlreichen Ausläufern zuwendet.

Von diesen Endungen tritt einer durch die dorsale Wurzel zum Integument aus. Leider ist man noch weit entfernt davon, allen diesen Neuronen bestimmte physiologische Funktionen zuzuordnen, denn trotz der relativ einfachen Organisation bieten die Acranier für den Physiologen recht schwierige Bedingungen. Die Rohde-Zellen nehmen eine besondere Stellung ein; sie sind nicht gleichmäßig verteilt, sondern fehlen beim Lanzettfischchen in den Körpersegmenten 12—39. Da sie mit den Schwimmbewegungen zu tun haben, sind sie bereits frühzeitig im Zentralnervensystem der Larven vorhanden. Die Rohde-Zellen stehen durch ihre Dendriten mit den drei im „Rückenmark" vorhandenen Tractus in Verbindung und sind so angeordnet, daß jeweils eine Rohde-Zelle zu einer dorsalen Wurzel, und zwar der gegenüberliegenden Seite gehört (FRANZ, 1923).

b) Wesentlich weniger ist über die mit Kapseln versehenen Nervenendigungen bekannt. Im Integument der Metapleuralfalten, unter der äußeren Oberfläche, enden die Axone der dorsalen Wurzeln (ventraler Ast) in Kapseln, die von Gruppen von Bindegewebszellen gebildet werden (BONE, 1960). Die terminalen Axonkollateralen scheinen zwischen den Bindegewebszellen zu liegen, doch sind Einzelheiten nicht bekannt. Durchschneidung der sensorischen Wurzeln bewirkt die Degeneration der Axone, nicht aber der Kapseln. Eine Kapsel wird in der Regel von Axonen aus mehreren verschiedenen dorsalen Wurzeln versorgt. Jedoch nicht alle Axone der sensorischen Wurzeln des Metapleuralfaltenbereichs enden in diesen Organen. Ein kleiner Teil zieht zum Epithel der Innenseite der Metapleuralfalten und bildet dort das bereits beschriebene terminale Geflecht.

c) Über den ganzen Körper verstreut, aber gehäuft am Rostrum und am Schwanz auftretend finden sich Sinneszellen im Epithel (FRANZ, 1923; BONE, 1960). Ihre Darstellung ist schwierig, da sie sehr stark von der Methodik abhängig ist. Im wesentlichen werden die alten Befunde von DOGIEL bestätigt. Es handelt sich um gestreckte Zellen mit einem oder mehreren haarförmigen Fortsätzen an der Oberfläche, die an der Basis mit breitem Zellfuß der Basalmembran aufsitzen. BONE (1960) konnte an Methylenblau-Präparaten die Sinneszellen mit den ableitenden Axonen vor allem im Bereich des Mundes und des Rostrums nachweisen. Es kann kein Zweifel bestehen, daß es sich um sekundäre Sinneszellen handelt, die von den gleichen sensorischen Fasern erfaßt werden, die in der Umgebung die freien Nervenendigungen bilden. An den Präoraltentakeln oder dem Velarapparat treten die Sinneszellen zu echten Sinnesknospen zusammen; ihre Innervation erfolgt von den sensorischen Wurzeln der III.—VII. „Spinalnerven", allerdings mit bestimmten Besonderheiten (FRANZ, 1923).

d) Als besondere Sinnesorgane des Integumentes müssen die de Quatrefagesschen Körperchen in den Rostralflossen bewertet werden (FRANZ, 1923; BONE, 1959). Sie bestehen aus einer oder mehreren großen bipolaren Ganglienzellen, die umgeben sind von einer dünnen Kapsel von „Nebenzellen", die der Nervenscheide entsprechen sollen, also vielleicht Schwannsche Zellen sind (Abb. 1a). Das Neuron entsendet einen langen Fortsatz aus der Kapsel in die Subcutis, einen kurzen Fortsatz mit Verzweigungen durch die Cutis und zwischen die Epithelzellen; die Körperchen liegen nämlich einzeln oder zu vielen zusammen an der Grenze von Cutis und Subcutis im Hautbindegewebe und können die sehr dünne Cutis des Rostrums vorwölben. Sie sind bereits in der Ontogenese frühzeitig vorhanden, ihre Entstehung ist daher noch unbekannt. Die Innervation der Körperchen erfolgt von den sensorischen I. und II. „Spinalnerven" (FRANZ, 1923). Diese Spinalnerven erhalten ihre Axone aber von besonderen Neuronen am vorderen Ende des „Rückenmarkes" unmittelbar hinter dem Gehirnbläschen mit dem Pigmentfleck und dem Rest des Neuroporus. Es sind die B-Zellen, bipolare Neurone, die eine dorsale Gruppe bilden und deren einer Fortsatz durch die genannten Wurzeln zum

Rostrum zieht, während der andere Fortsatz durch das Zentralnervensystem bis zum caudalen Ende zu verfolgen ist. Es scheint sich um modifizierte A-Zellen zu handeln. Die Synapsen zu den Neuronen der de Quatrefagesschen Körperchen sind noch nicht bekannt, aber aus der Zahl der B-Zellen, Körperchen und Axone in den zugehörigen „Spinalnerven" muß eine solche synaptische direkte Verbindung erschlossen werden (BONE, 1959). Ebenfalls unbekannt sind die Verbindungen des im ZNS verbleibenden Axons der B-Zellen mit anderen Neuronen. Doch darf man wohl soweit gehen zu sagen, daß diese Körperchen Sinnesreize am Rostrum aufnehmen; diese werden von den B-Zellen durch die ganze Länge des ZNS weiter vermittelt und haben wesentlichen Effekt auf die Fortbewegung (Schwimmbewegung) der Larven und des adulten Tieres. In der Funktion dürfte dieser Komplex dem Koordinationssystem des Mauthnerschen Apparates von Cyclostomen, Fischen und aquatischen Amphibien analog sein.

Überblickt man die Verhältnisse der Haut bei den Acraniern, so ergibt sich, daß eine regionale Gliederung vor allem durch die nervösen Elemente gegeben ist. Das Unvermögen, ein mehrschichtiges Epithel aufzubauen, läßt bei den primitiven Chordaten die Entstehung von Epithelderivaten nicht zu. Darüber hinaus ist auch das Corium uniform ausgebildet, allerdings in der Art und Weise, die nun für alle Chordaten charakteristisch sein wird. Das Fehlen der Fettzellen schließlich unterbindet die Variationsmöglichkeiten der Subcutis, die als ein Gallertpolster an die unbekannten aquatischen Vorfahren erinnert.

III. Die Haut der Craniota (Vertebrata)

1. Cyclostomata

Die Haut der Rundmäuler zeigt eine Reihe von Merkmalen, die charakteristisch für die Vertebratenhaut sind, oder doch für die Haut einiger Klassen: die Vielschichtigkeit der Epidermis, die Differenzierung von Epidermiszellen in verschiedene Drüsenzelltypen, ein besonderes System von Hautsinnesorganen: die Seitenlinie, und schließlich der Unterschied zwischen der Haut von Larven und der erwachsenen Form. Der Feinbau ist bei den durch ihre Lebensweise und Anatomie unterschiedenen Neunaugen (Petromyzonidae) und Schleimaalen (Myxinidae) im einzelnen recht verschieden.

a) Neunaugen (Petromyzonidae)

Bei den Neunaugen liegen nur wenige neuere Arbeiten über die Haut vor, obwohl seit einigen Jahren die neurosekretorischen Verhältnisse, die Hypophyse, die Umwandlung der Leber bei der Metamorphose und der Chorda starkes Interesse gefunden haben.

Die *Epidermis* baut sich aus mehreren Zellschichten auf, wobei die Art des Tieres und sein Alter erhebliche Unterschiede in der Dicke der Epidermisschichten bedingen. So ist z. B. das einheimische Bachneunauge nur ca. 15—17 cm lang, das Meerneunauge der europäischen Küstengewässer wird dagegen 1 m lang und wiegt bis zu 1200 g oder mehr. Da die Neunaugen mehrere Jahre als Larven verbringen (sog. Ammocoetes) und in den ersten beiden Jahren ein starkes Wachstum während der sommerlichen Futterperiode durchlaufen (vgl. HARDISTY, 1951), so verändert sich auch die Haut. Bei den 1 cm großen Larven bedeckt ein kubisches einschichtiges Epithel die Hautoberfläche; an der Basis sind einzelne Ersatzzellen eingeschoben. Dieses Oberflächenepithel zeigt bereits den charakteristischen Belag einer „Deckplatte" (s. u.). Ist die Larve 3—4 cm lang, so sind bereits

3—4 Epithelzellschichten vorhanden und die Differenzierung in verschiedene Drüsenzelltypen ist abgeschlossen. Bei einer Größe von 10 cm sind die Verhältnisse schon dem des erwachsenen Fluß- oder Bachneunauges sehr ähnlich: eine geschlossene oberflächliche Epithelzellschicht deckt die mittleren Zellschichten ab, die Regeneration erfolgt im Bereich einer geschlossenen basalen Zellschicht.

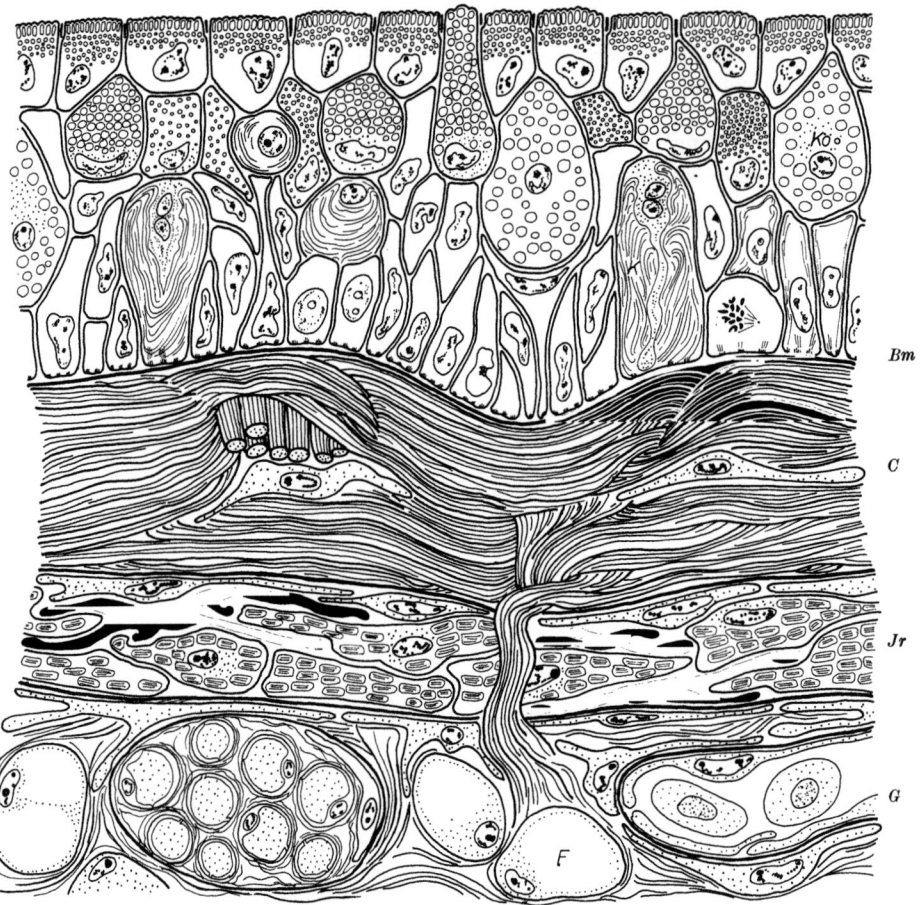

Abb. 2. Bachneunauge (Petromyzon planeri), Haut. Das Epithel zeigt die Zellen des Stratum cuticulare mit Schleimvacuolen, Körnerzellen mit basaler Begleitzelle und die Entstehung einer Körnerzelle; Schleimzellen in verschiedenen Reifungsphasen und Kolbenzellen. Das straffe Corium wird von einer Pigmentzellschicht unterlagert; in die Subcutis ist ein Gefäß und ein Nerv eingezeichnet (vgl. Text). *Bm* Basalmembran, *C* Corium, *G* Gefäß, *F* Fettzelle, *Ir* Iridocyt, *K* Kolbenzelle, *Kö* Körnerzelle, *Sc* Stratum cuticulare

Im einzelnen sind bei den mittelgroßen Arten folgende Epithelverhältnisse vorhanden. Drei ziemlich scharf getrennte Epithelzellzonen sind ausgeprägt (FICALBI, 1924) (Abb. 2). Auf der Basalmembran sitzen die Zellen des *Stratum basale* in einschichtiger Lage; nur diese Zellen zeigen Mitosen. Nach NIAZI (1963) handelt es sich um die Zellschicht, die bei größeren Verletzungen und der darauf folgenden Regeneration durch Zellteilungen den Zellverlust ausgleichen. Das Stratum basale entspricht demnach dem Stratum germinativum der höheren Wirbeltiere. Allerdings sind die Epithelzellen bei den Cyclostomen nicht kubisch oder hochprismatisch, sondern verjüngen sich spindelförmig in ihrem oberen Teil, weil die folgenden Zellen der oberflächlicheren Schichten ebenfalls unregelmäßige Spindelformen aufweisen.

Eine histophotometrische Messung des DNS-Gehaltes (nach Feulgen-Färbung, MANFREDI ROMANINI, 1956, 1957) und eine karyometrische Messung zeigt, daß die Kerne des Stratum basale den größten Inhalt besitzen und auch am meisten DNS enthalten sollen. Man muß nach den heutigen Kenntnissen über die S-Phase und die DNS-Synthese im Interphasekern bezweifeln, ob den gemessenen Werten von MANFREDI ROMANINI in der vorliegenden Form noch viel Bedeutung zukommt. Denn angeregt waren diese Messungen aus phylogenetischen Erwägungen, die von MIRSKY und RIS (1951) über den DNS-Gehalt in Kernen von Petromyzon, von Teleostiern und anderen Wirbeltieren angestellt wurden.

Zur Oberfläche hin folgen die Schichten des *Stratum intermedium*, die beim Bachneunauge 3—4, beim Flußneunauge 6—10 und beim Meeresneunauge 10 und mehr Zellagen umfassen. Die überwiegende Menge bilden spindelförmige Epithelzellen, deren Zellkerne und Cytoplasma recht ähnlich den Basalzellen sind. In den vielschichtigen Epithelien kommt die Spindelform der Zellen dadurch zustande, daß viele Epithelzellen auch der höheren Schichten noch mit einem langen Fortsatz wie bei einem mehrreihigen Epithel auf der Basalmembran haften. An einem älteren Regenerat des Schwanzes beim Flußneunauge konnte STUDNICKA (1912) durch die Vielschichtigkeit des Regenerates die weiten Intercellularspalten zwischen den Epithelzellen der mittleren Schicht sehen und bildet die Zellen mit zahlreichen Zellbrücken vom Typ der Bizzozeroschen Noduli ab. Der Autor spricht von ,,Stachelzellen". Man darf also annehmen, obwohl keine elektronenmikroskopischen Untersuchungen vorliegen, daß die Epithelzellen der mittleren Schicht den Zellen des Stratum spinosum der höheren Wirbeltiere entsprechen und durch zahlreiche Desmosomen aneinander haften. Die Spindelform vieler Epithelzellen kommt auch durch die große Zahl von Drüsenzellen zustande, die mit ihren Zellkörpern die einfachen Epithelzellen zur Seite drängen. *Drei Typen von Drüsenzellen* sind vorhanden: 1. Einfache Schleimzellen; sie liegen zahlreich unter der oberflächlichen Zellschicht und strecken z.T. ihre mit Schleim erfüllten Protoplasten zwischen die oberen Epithelzellen zur Oberfläche, wo der Schleim entleert wird. Diese den Becherzellen ähnliche Drüsenzellen degenerieren unter vacuoliger Aufquellung und werden aus dem Zellverband ausgestoßen. In den vielschichtigen Epithelien der größeren Arten kann ihre Differenzierung und die allmähliche Anhäufung der Schleimsubstanz beobachtet werden. 2. Große Körnerzellen mit zentral gelegenem Kern; das Plasma ist erfüllt mit zahlreichen runden Granula. Das Zellvolumen beträgt ein Vielfaches des Volumens der einfachen Epithelzellen und auch der Schleimzellen. Nach FICALBI (1924) messen Körnerzellen bei Larven 10—30 μ im Durchmesser, bei Bachneunaugen 20—40 μ und bei Meeresneunaugen bis zu 40 μ im Durchmesser. Da diese Drüsenzellen sehr zahlreich sind, pressen sie die benachbarten Epithelzellen zusammen, so daß flache Hüllzellen die Drüsenzellen zu umgeben scheinen. MANFREDI ROMANINI (1957) findet kleine ,,überzählige Kerne" mit DNS zwischen den Granula, als sei bei der Differenzierung eine Zerklüftung des Kernes vorausgegangen. Auch die Entwicklung dieses Drüsenzelltypes läßt sich im Epithel verfolgen. Aus den Regenerationsversuchen von NIAZI (1963) läßt sich schließen, daß bei den Larven etwa 26 d verstreichen, bis im Epithel des Regenerates wieder neue Körnerzellen vorhanden sind. Wichtig scheint zu sein, daß STUDNICKA (1912) bei seinen Untersuchungen über das Regenerat (ebenfalls die Schwanzspitze) des ausgewachsenen Tieres nur wenige Körnerzellen findet. Nach unseren Beobachtungen bei Lampetra planeri entstehen die Körnerzellen nach der Teilung einer Basalzelle, wobei die obere Tochterzelle sich abrundet, aber noch durch eine Plasmabrücke mit der Basalzelle in Verbindung bleibt. Das Cytoplasma läßt lichtmikroskopisch eine Schichtung (konzentrisch) erkennen, so daß in diesen jungen Körnerzellen ein stark entwickeltes endoplasmatisches Reticulum vermutet werden kann. Bei den großen Neunaugenarten mit vielschichtigem Epithel bleiben lange Fortsätze bestehen, die bis zur Basalmembran reichen und vielleicht aus der beobachteten Teilungsform der Zellen zu erklären sind. Nach eigenen phasenkontrastmikroskopischen Beobachtungen sitzen aber ein oder zwei Epithelzellen wie ein Kelchstiel an der Basis der großen Körnerzellen und halten sie mit dem größten Teil ihres Zelleibes basal umfaßt. Dabei sitzen die „Stielzellen" mit einem Ausläufer auf der Basalmembran. Auch die alten Abbildungen der frühen Untersucher lassen eine solche Interpretation zu. Demnach haben die Körnerzellen dauernd Kontakt mit der basalen Epithelzelle, die bei der letzten Zellteilung gemeinsam mit der Körnerzelle entstanden ist. Die Zahl der Granula im Plasma nimmt zu, wenn die Zelle größer wird. Sehr häufig strecken die Körnerzellen, ähnlich den Schleimzellen, lange flaschenhalsförmige Zellfortsätze zwischen die oberen Epithelzellen, so daß eine Sekretion ins Außenmedium bzw. in den der Haut anhaftenden Schleim sehr wahrscheinlich ist, vielleicht aber nur auf besondere Reize erfolgt. 3. Ein ganz merkwürdiger Zelltyp sind schließlich die sehr großen Kolbenzellen, die in gewisser Hinsicht den Kolbenzellen vieler Knochenfische ähnlich sind. Über ihre Funktionen ist nichts bekannt, auch PFEIFFER (1960, 1963) rechnet sie nicht zu den Zellen, die sog. „Schreckstoffe" produzieren. Seine Ansicht, es handele sich bei Kolben- und Körnerzellen nicht um verschiedene Zelltypen, sondern um verschiedene Entwicklungsstufen eines Zelltyps, kann aber nach Entstehung und Feinbau der Kolbenzellen nicht zutreffen. Die Kolbenzellen sind stets zweikernig und erreichen eine Länge von 35 µ (Flußneunauge). Sie sind in der Haut der gesamten Körperoberfläche mit Ausnahme der Flossensäume und der Mundregion vorhanden und erreichen im vielschichtigen Epithel der großen Arten erhebliche Größen. Nach FICALBI (1924) finden sich in der Seitenhaut 500 dieser Zellen pro 1 mm^2. Sie beginnen ihre Differenzierung in der Basalzellenschicht als zweikernige Zellen, nach den Regenerationsversuchen von NIAZI dauert es ca. 35 d, bis neue Kolbenzellen im Regenerationsepithel vorhanden sind, und etwa 90 d nach der Abtrennung der Schwanzspitze ist das Epithel des Regenerates in seinem Aufbau wieder weitgehend normal. Die Zellen wachsen in die Länge, dabei bleiben die Kerne am apikalen Pol, umgeben von Cytoplasma, das eine zentrale Zone in der Zelle einnimmt. Denn bereits in den frühen Phasen nehmen die Zellprodukte: lange dichte Fäden, die peripheren Zellteile ein. Die ausdifferenzierte Zelle bleibt mit breitem Zellfuß auf der Basalmembran und reicht bis in die Zone der Körnerzellen, oft bis zur oberen Epithelzellenschicht. Eine Entleerung des Inhaltes wurde bisher nicht beobachtet. Die peripheren, dicht gepackten Fibrillen bilden aus spiralig verlaufenden Bündeln in der Zelle eine kompakte Hülle, so daß Plasma und Kerne auf eine zentrale Zone wie in einer Röhre beschränkt sind. Die Fibrillen sind doppelbrechend, ihre Molekularstruktur muß also eine hohe Ordnung aufweisen, wie es zu erwarten ist. Wir stellen eine positive Doppelbrechung (unter Gips, 551 nm) an den längsorientierten Fibrillen fest, wie sie an Querschnitten schon von M. SCHULTZE (loc. cit. bei BIEDERMANN, 1926) 1861 ermittelt wurde.

Zwischen diesen Zelltypen müssen noch besondere Epithelzellen verborgen sein, die ein photolabiles Pigment enthalten (STEVEN, 1951). Diese Epithelzellen sind nicht mit Lipophoren zu verwechseln, die nur in den Bindegewebsschichten der Haut vorhanden sind. Es sind vielmehr rundliche Epithelzellen der mittleren Schicht von ca. 10 µ Durchmesser (Larven des Bachneunauges), die in Gruppen beisammenliegen und besonders häufig in der Haut des Schwanzes vorkommen. Das Pigment bleicht am Licht aus und zeigt eine maximale Absorption des Lichtes bei 490—520 nm. Es ist seit langem bekannt, daß die Larven in der Haut Lichtreceptoren besitzen müssen (vgl. STEVEN, 1950) und besonders in der Schwanz-region eine erhöhte Lichtempfindlichkeit aufweisen. Die stärkste Empfindlichkeit findet STEVEN (1950) bei einer Wellenlänge des auf die Haut einfallenden Lichtes am Schwanz bei 530 nm. Zwei Befunde ergeben, daß die genannten Epithelzellen als Lichtreceptoren arbeiten. STEVEN (1951) kann nämlich nachweisen, daß die Gruppen von Epithelzellen von kleinen Nervenstämmen des Lateralissystems (Lateralis posterior des Accessorius) innerviert werden; einzelne Axone treten durch die Epidermis und nach Verzweigung mit Endknöpfchen an die pigmentführenden Epithelien heran. Ferner ist bekannt, daß in der Haut von Fischen und Amphibienlarven ein blau fluorescierendes Pterin als photolabiler Farbstoff vorkommt (HAMA, 1953, 1959, 1963; KAUFFMANN, 1959; ZIEGLER-GÜNDER, 1954, 1956; ZIEGLER, 1960, 1961, 1963; Zusammenfassung über Pterine bei ZIEGLER, 1965). Zwar ist bisher eine Lokalisation dieser Farbstoffe nur in den Chromatophoren gelungen, bei der kurzen Zeit aber, in der Genaueres über die Pterine und ihren Stoffwechsel bekannt geworden ist, bedeutet diese Einschränkung kein Hindernis beim Vergleich. Außerdem ist bekannt, daß Riboflavin und Pterine fast stets zusammen vorkommen, da die Flavinenzyme Elektronen bei Dehydrierung von Pterin aufnehmen können (vgl. ZIEGLER, 1965), und japanische Untersucher finden in der Haut einer japanischen Lamprete einen hohen Gehalt an Riboflavin und anderen B-Vitaminen. Die Dehydrierung der lichtempfindlichen Pterine durch Licht und die dabei frei werdenden Elektronen ergeben in mehrfacher Hinsicht Möglichkeiten, Membranpotentiale der betreffenden Zellen zu verändern, auf Umwegen oder direkt, oder Stoffe freizusetzen, die als Transmitter für die durch Synapsen angeschlossenen Nervenzellen wirken. Wenn auch noch im einzelnen überhaupt keine Vorstellung darüber besteht, wie die Vorgänge einer Lichtreizung vor sich gehen, darf man wohl die genannten Epithelzellen aus den dargelegten Gründen als spezielle Sinneszellen ansehen.

Die oberflächlichen Epithelzellen bilden das *Stratum superficiale oder Stratum cuticulare*, bestehend aus einer Zellschicht. An der Oberfläche haben die Zellen eine Differenzierung ausgebildet, die als „Deckplatte" seit langem bezeichnet wird; bereits frühere Autoren (vgl. RABL, 1931) sahen in der senkrechten Streifung der „Deckplatte" feinste Lamellen, die eingesenkte Alveolen an der Zelloberfläche gegeneinander abgrenzen. Unsere eigenen phasenkontrastoptischen Beobachtungen zeigen, daß die einzelnen Zellen durch Schlußleisten gegeneinander abgegrenzt sind und auch die „Deckplatten" nichts anderes darstellen als eine differenzierte Zelloberfläche, da die Schlußleisten die „Deckplatten" durchsetzen. Es handelt sich um eine Schicht eingesenkter Schleimvacuolen, die durch Öffnungen mit dem Außenmedium in Verbindung stehen. Die Ähnlichkeit mit den entsprechenden Differenzierungen beim Amphioxusepithel und das Vorkommen entsprechend gebauter Schleimvacuolen in der Oberfläche von Epithelien bei Amphibienlarven (eigene elektronenmikroskopische Beobachtungen, vgl. Amphibien; SCHULZ und DE PAOLA, 1958; PFLUGFELDER und SCHUBERT, 1965; KELLY, 1966) läßt den Schluß zu, daß es sich um gleichartige schleimerfüllte Einsenkungen der Zelloberfläche handelt. Unter „Schleim" wird dabei ganz allgemein eine Substanz verstanden, die feinfädiger Natur ist und im färberischen Verhalten (ohne Anwendung spezifischer Nachweise) den Substanzen in Becherzellen gleicht. Diese Oberflächendifferenzierung ist schon bei den Epithelzellen der einschichtigen Epidermis der Larven vorhanden. Die Zellen des Stratum cuticulare sind nicht spindelförmig, sondern kubisch, mit wechselnder Form des basalen Zellpoles; der Kern ist groß und rundlich. In älteren Zellen findet sich Schleimsubstanz in zunehmendem Maße auch im Innern des Zellkörpers, dicht unter den Alveolen der Oberflächenzone. Unterbrochen wird die Schicht des Oberflächenepithels durch die schon erwähnten flaschenförmigen Fortsätze von Schleim- und Körnerzellen, die Schlußleisten bleiben an solchen Durchtrittsstellen erhalten. Das Stratum cuticulare überzieht mit seinen typischen Zellen auch die Cornea.

Trotz des vielschichtigen Aufbaues ihres Epithels ist die Haut der Neunaugen keine osmotische Barriere (HARDISTY, 1954). Abgesehen von den verschiedenen Möglichkeiten einer Osmoregulation (HARDISTY, 1956; MORRIS, 1958) durch Kiemen und Nieren ist die Haut eine sehr empfindliche Austauschzone beim Wechsel vom Süßwasser zum Seewasser und umgekehrt. Dabei ist das Bachneunauge mit seiner dünneren Haut empfindlicher als das Flußneunauge, das ja auch eine Laichwanderung aus Brack- oder Meerwasser in die Flüsse unternimmt und dabei eine irreversible Umstellung seiner Osmoregulation erfährt (MORRIS, 1958). Die weiten Intercellularspalten zwischen den Epithelzellen und die zahlreichen Drüsenzellen werden wohl den geringen osmotischen Widerstand der Haut verursachen.

Unterlagert ist die Epidermis von einer *Basalmembran,* die in den frühen Larvenstadien vom Corium nicht unterschieden werden kann (RABL, 1931). Die Basalmembran baut sich als dünne Schicht aus Kollagenfasern auf, die als Geflecht in einer dichten Grundsubstanz zusammengekittet sind. Nach den Beschreibungen von FICALBI (1924) kann man annehmen, daß die basalen Zellen mit Füßchen und Desmosomen an der Grundsubstanz verankert sind, elektronenmikroskopische Befunde liegen nicht vor. Dennoch sind die Befunde von FICALBI so eindeutig, daß sie in dieser Hinsicht interpretiert werden dürfen: er zeigt feine Knöpfchen mit Tonofibrillen an der Basis der Epithelzellen, und schon ältere Autoren hatten den festen Zusammenhang der Knöpfchen mit der Basalmembran beim Ablösen der Epidermis erkannt. Eine Bildung von Epidermisleisten oder zapfenförmigen Einsenkungen kommt nicht vor, die Grenze Epithel–Bindegewebe ist glatt.

Das *Corium* ist ein straffes Bindegewebe und setzt sich aus zahlreichen Lagen von kollagenen Faserbündeln zusammen, die parallel der Oberfläche verlaufen. Die breiten Bündel sind geordnet: jede Lage nimmt zur folgenden in ihrer Verlaufsrichtung etwa einen Winkel von 90° ein, wobei (nach RABL) zur Körperachse auf dem Rücken ein Winkel von 45° gebildet wird. Zwischen den Faserbündeln liegen flach ausgebreitete Fibrocyten und einzelne Melanophoren; durchbrochen werden die Schichten von aufsteigenden kleinen Faserbündeln und elastischen Elementen. Die Dicke des Corium nimmt natürlich mit dem Alter der Larven zu, und man darf sich dieses Dickenwachstum wohl so vorstellen, wie es von KEMP (1959) für Amphibienlarven beschrieben wurde, d.h. die Dickenzunahme geschieht durch Vermehrung der Faserlagen, die auf der Unterseite des Corium abgelagert werden. Beim adulten Flußneunauge mißt RABL eine Dicke des Corium (Rücken) von 90 μ, beim Meeresneunauge von 300 μ; bei Larven von 9 cm Länge ist das Corium nur 9 μ dick. Beim Bachneunauge kann man z.B. 15—20 Faserlagen in der Rückenhaut und am Kopf unterscheiden.

Die Verbindung des straffen Coriumbindegewebes mit dem Körper wird durch eine *Subcutis* hergestellt. Sie ist in den verschiedenen Körperregionen unterschiedlich dick und besteht hauptsächlich aus Fettzellen, zwischen denen Faserbündel aus dem Corium zur Muskelfascie ziehen. In der Subcutis liegen auch die Blutgefäße für die Hautversorgung, Lymphspalten und Nervenstämmchen. An der Grenze zwischen Corium und Subcutis breiten sich zahlreiche *Melanophoren und Chromatophoren* aus, die eine vielzellige geschlossene Schicht von Farbzellen bilden können und die gefleckte oder dunkle oder marmorierte Färbung der Neunaugen bedingen. Die Melanophoren gleichen denen der Fische und lassen durch Verlagerung der Pigmentgranula im Zellkörper einen Farbwechsel entstehen; die Tiere sind im Licht dunkel und in der Nacht heller (YOUNG, 1935), passen sich aber nicht wie manche Fische der Untergrundfärbung an. Eine nervöse Beeinflussung der Melanophoren scheint nicht vorzuliegen, sondern nur eine hormonelle Steuerung durch Hypophyse und Pinealorgan (YOUNG, 1935; YOUNG und BELLERBY, 1935; LANZING, 1954), obwohl die Verhältnisse wegen der technischen Schwierigkeiten keineswegs geklärt sind. Die Entfernung der beiden, noch sehr augenähnlich entwickelten Pinealorgane stört den Ablauf des Hell-Dunkelrhythmus der Melanophoren, die Tiere bleiben dunkel, d. h. das Melanin ist in den Melanophoren ausgebreitet. Die Entfernung der Hypophyse dagegen führt zur Aufhellung der Tiere, d. h. die Melaningranula in den Melanophoren werden im Zentrum des Zellkörpers gesammelt. LANZING (1954) konnte durch Extrakte aus Neunaugen-Hypophysen beim Frosch eine Dunkelfärbung durch die Verteilung der Melaningranula in den Melanophoren bewirken (MDH = melanin dispersing hormone). Im gleichen Sinne sprechen die Befunde von YOUNG (1935): Wurde Extrakt aus Säuger-Hypophyse in die hypophysektomierten (aufgehellten) Neunaugen injiziert, so erfolgte eine Verdunkelung, d. h. Melaninausbreitung in den Melanophoren. — Außer den Melanophoren kommen noch andere Chromatophoren: Lipophoren und Iridocyten in der Farbzellenschicht vor; beide Zelltypen sind besonders reichlich in der Bauchhaut vorhanden. Die Lipophoren der Larven des Bachneunauges enthalten ein Carotin, das nach den Untersuchungen von STEVEN (1951) identisch ist mit Lutein. Diese Zellen können aber ihr Pigment nicht verlagern, im Gegensatz zu den entsprechenden Farbzellen bei echten Fischen. Die Iridocyten enthalten Guaninkristalle, welche das Licht reflektieren, Einzelheiten darüber sind bei den Cyclostomen nicht bekannt.

Die *Innervation der Haut* steht im engsten Zusammenhang mit der Anordnung der Sinneszellen (TRETJAKOFF, 1927; STEFANELLI, 1932; BOEKE, 1934; FAHRENHOLZ, 1936; STEVEN, 1951). Sowohl durch Silberimprägnation als auch durch Vitalfärbung mit Methylenblau läßt sich zeigen, daß die Nervenstämmchen das Corium durchstoßen und dann noch eine weite Strecke parallel unter der Basalmembran verlaufen, ehe sie sich in einzelne Axone aufteilen und in die Epidermis vordringen. „Freie Nervenendigungen" werden bis unter das Stratum cuticulare nachgewiesen, und aus den Untersuchungen von STEVEN (1951) geht hervor, daß sie mit Endknöpfchen, d. h. Synapsen an den speziellen, mit photolabilen Pigmenten gefüllten Epithelzellen enden. Je eine Gruppe von Epithelzellen wird von einem Axon mit verschiedenen Kollateralen versorgt. Diese Zellen sind also der erste Typ von Sinneszellen in der Epidermis. Die Axone gehören dem Seitenliniennerven an (s. u., am Rumpf: N. lateralis posterior), aus dessen Hauptstamm sie in einzelnen Bündeln durch das Corium treten. Ob außerdem Axone frei zwischen den Epithelzellen ohne zugehörige Sinneszellen enden, konnte bisher nicht festgestellt werden. Die peripheren Nerven zeigen bei den Cyclostomen eine besondere Feinstruktur (PETERS, 1960). Wie sich an den ventralen und dorsalen Wurzeln der Spinalnerven zeigen läßt, besitzen die Axone keine Myelinscheide, sondern sind nur von Schwannschen Zellen umkleidet. Je größer der Axondurchmesser ist, um so mehr Schwannsche Zellen bedecken den Zellfortsatz. Dünne (ca. 1 μ) Axone werden im Querschnitt nur von einer Schwannschen Zelle umfaßt, dickere Axone (Durchmesser 4—8 μ) zeigen 4—6 Schwannsche Zellen im Querschnitt. Da für die Schleimaale (s. dort) auch für Hirnnerven entsprechende Verhältnisse nachgewiesen wurden (PETERS, 1963), so kann angenommen werden, daß die aus dem Lateralissystem in die Haut eintretenden Nervenbündel in ihrer Feinstruktur ebenfalls „marklose" Nerven darstellen. Die Schwannschen Zellen werden von einer Basalmembran aus kollagenen Fibrillen (Endoneurium) umgeben. Der zweite Typ von Sinneszellen ist auf bestimmte kleine epitheliale *Hautsinnesorgane* beschränkt, deren Gesamtheit das schon genannte *Seitenliniensystem* darstellt. Die eng umgrenzten Sinnesorgane sind runde oder ovale Gruben im Epithel (Abb. 3a und b). Im Gegensatz zu den Organen des Seitenliniensystems bei Fischen und Amphibien sind sie also nicht in ein Kanalsystem unter die Oberfläche versenkt worden, sondern bleiben als offene Sinnesgruben in einer primitiven Form erhalten. Die Sinnesgruben, auch Neuromasten genannt, sind in Reihen angeordnet; auf dem Rumpf verlaufen auf jeder Körperseite drei solcher Seitenlinien, eine dorsale Reihe dicht unter dem Flossensaum, eine laterale und eine ventrale Reihe. Am Kopf ist die reihenförmige Anordnung komplizierter; an der Mundregion sind kurze Reihen von Sinnesgruben, ebenso an den Kiemenöffnungen. Im Bereich des Auges liegt eine gebogene supraorbitale und eine suborbitale Reihe, und schließlich ist eine rostrale Reihe im Bereich der Oberlippe zu lokalisieren. Entsprechend ist die Innervation durch Hautäste der Hirnnerven recht kompliziert. Sowohl Rami des Trigeminus wie des Facialis stehen mit den Sinnesgruben der Kopfseitenlinien in Verbindung (vgl. TRETJAKOFF, 1927); die Rumpfseitenlinie wird durch den sog. N. lateralis posterior versorgt, der Teilen des Accessorius entspricht. Die verschiedenen Anteile dieses Lateraliskomplexes der Hirnnerven sind durch Ganglien und Commissuren untereinander verknüpft und müssen physiologisch wohl als eine Einheit betrachtet werden. Das gilt vor allem für die Anteile aus dem Facialis (sog. N. lateralis anterior) und den Accessorius (sog. N. lat. posterior), deren Neurone z.T. im gleichen Kerngebiet der Medulla liegen (Nucleus medialis), z.T. in benachbarten Kernen, oder aber mit Fasern ins Cerebellum reichen, in den Nucleus medialis und in den Kern des VIII. Hirnnerven (Nucleus octavo-motorius posterior, vgl. ARIENS-KAPPERS et al., 1960). — Die einzelne Sinnesgrube liegt in einer Einsenkung der Epidermis, da das vielschichtige Epithel der Umgebung in das einschichtige Sinnesepithel übergeht. FAHRENHOLZ (1936) beschreibt die Neuromasten als rinnenförmige Einsenkungen, so daß die Sinnesorgane wie Rinnen zwischen zwei Epithelhügeln liegen; daraus leitet er eine besondere Funktion ab, die vor allem den beiden seitlichen Epidermiswülsten zukommt (s.u.). Außerdem liegt die Sinnesgrube über einer vorgewölbten Bindegewebspapille, in der ein kleiner Nervenast des jeweils zugehörenden Lateralisnerven zur Oberfläche verläuft. Das Epithel der Grube setzt sich aus hohen Stützzellen zusammen, zwischen denen birnenförmige große Sinneszellen eingeschlossen sind. Die Befunde früherer Untersucher wurden von TRETJAKOFF mit Vitalfärbung durch Methylenblau bestätigt. Die Sinneszellen werden von den Axonen, die unter der Epidermis ein dichtes Geflecht bilden und in die Epidermis vordringen, mit typischen „Endplatten", also wohl becherförmigen Synapsenzonen umfaßt. Es dürfte sich demnach um sekundäre Sinneszellen handeln, wie sie in ihrem Feinbau und der nervösen Versorgung von den Seitenlinienorganen der Fische bekannt sind (s. dort). An der Oberfläche sind zwischen Stütz- und Sinneszellen Schlußleisten ausgebildet, die gesamte Oberfläche ist mit einer dünnen Schicht schleimigen Sekretes bedeckt.

Schließlich sind Sinneszellen auch in *Hautsinnesknospen* vorhanden, die verstreut im Epithel vorkommen (BOEKE, 1932; FAHRENHOLZ, 1936a und b) (Abb. 3b). Die Sinneszellen ragen zwischen den normalen Epithelzellen des Stratum cuticulare mit ihrem apikalen Zellpol und feinen Sinneshaaren ins Außenmedium. Die ganze Knospe wird von Stützzellen unterhalb des Stratum cuticulare pyramidenförmig aufgebaut, so daß die Sinneszellen völlig isoliert vom umgebenden normalen Epithel mit den Kolbenzellen und Schleimzellen sind. Die Stützzellen erreichen die Basalmembran, durch die ein Bündel von Axonen in die Sinnesknospe eintritt; die Axone verteilen sich in der Knospe auf die Sinneszellen, die wie in den Neuromasten sekundäre Sinneszellen sind. Das Axonbündel steigt aus der Subcutis senkrecht durch das Corium zur Sinnesknospe auf. Ob außerhalb der beiden

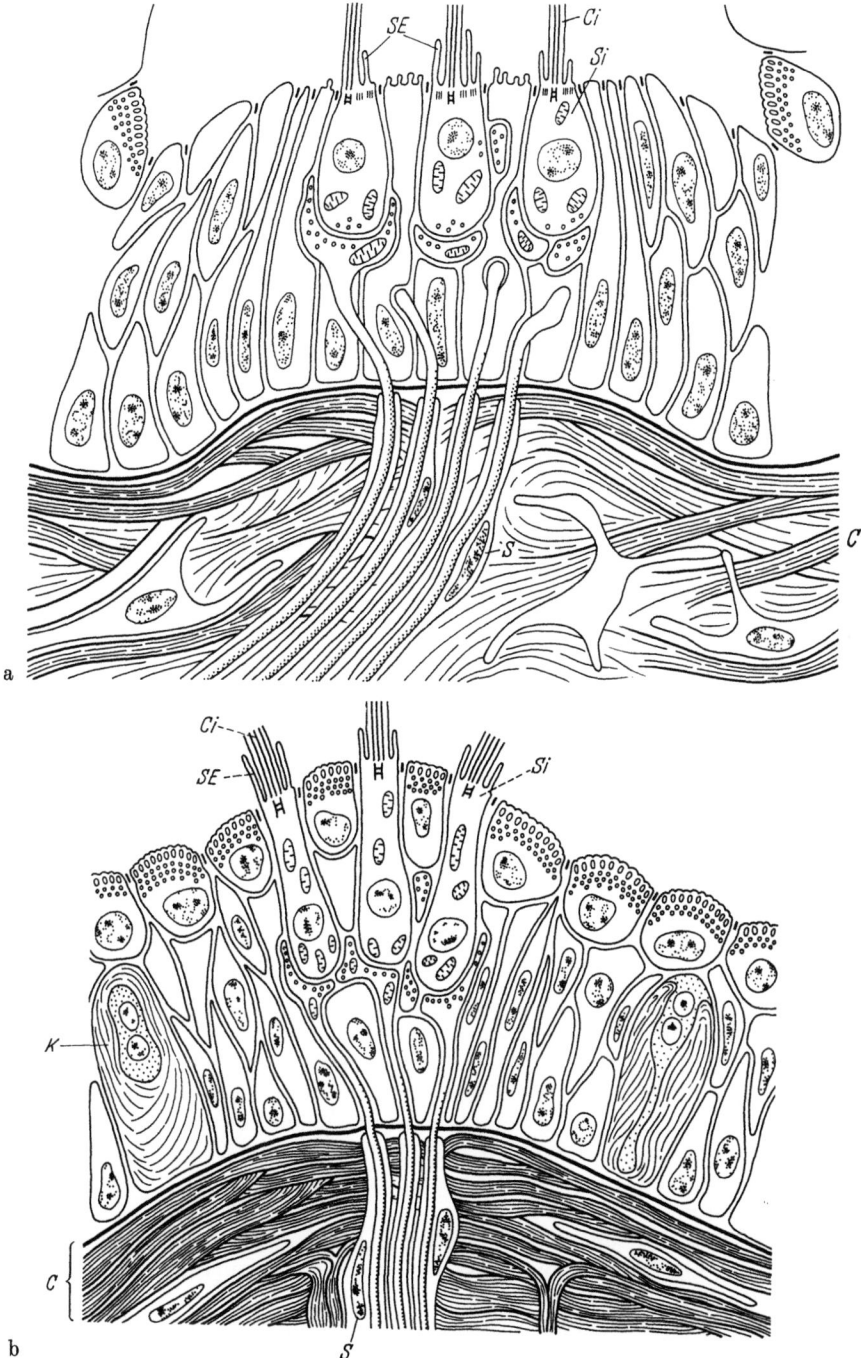

Abb. 3a u. b. Neunauge, Sinnesknospen der Haut. Die Sinneszellen sind in ihrer Struktur den Verhältnissen bei Fischen entlehnt (FLOCK und WERSÄLL, 1962); die Axone und die mutmaßliche Begleitung durch Schwannsche Zellen entsprechen den peripheren Nerven von Cyclostomen (PETERS, 1960). (In Anlehnung an FAHRENHOLZ, 1936.) a Sinnesknospe der Seitenlinie; in einer rinnenförmigen Epitheleinsenkung liegt über einer Auflockerung des Coriums eine Gruppe von Sinneszellen, die durch große Stützzellen umgeben werden. Die seitliche Begrenzung der Knospe wird durch gestreckte Epithelzellen = Mantelzellen vorgenommen. Erst seitlich der Sinnesknospen sind Zellen des Stratum cuticulare vorhanden, die das vielschichtige Epithel der Rinnen überkleiden. Aus dem Corium steigen die Axone auf, die Schwannschen Zellen reichen wahrscheinlich nur bis zur Basalmembran. b Freie Sinnesknospe in der Haut. Eine Gruppe von Sinneszellen ist in das Epithel eingeschoben, besondere Stützzellen sind nicht ausgebildet, die oberflächlichen Epithelzellen gehören dem Stratum cuticulare an, jedoch sind keine Schleimzellen in der unmittelbaren Umgebung vorhanden. *C* Corium, *S* Schwannsche Zellen, *K* Kolbenzellen, *Si* Sinneszellen, *Ci* Kinocilium, *SE* Stereocilium oder Microvilli

Typen von Sinnesknospen noch verstreute Sinneszellen im Epithel (außer den pigmentführenden!) vorkommen, ist umstritten. Während STEVEN (1951) keine weiteren Sinneszellen findet, bildet TRETJAKOFF (1927) zahlreiche einzelstehende Sinneszellen mit zugehörigen Axonen im Epithel der Lippen ab. FAHRENHOLZ (1936a und b) bestätigt die älteren Untersuchungen und beschreibt, allerdings mit einer unspezifischen Molybdänhämatoxylinmethode (nach HELD), eine Reihe von Sinneszellen mit Sinneshaaren an ihrer Oberfläche. Nach den Abbildungen zu urteilen scheint aber eine Verwechslung mit Schleimzellen sehr wohl möglich zu sein. Eine runde Zelle, die früher als Leukocyt im Epithel angesehen wurde und die wir nach unseren Präparaten für eine Entwicklungsstufe des Zelltyps der Körnerzellen halten, beschreibt FAHRENHOLZ als Tastzelle („Merkelsche Tastzelle"). Sie soll besonders zahlreich in den Epithelwülsten seitlich der Neuromast-Sinnesknospen vorhanden sein, so daß diese Epithelverdickungen besondere Tastfunktionen besitzen sollen. Auch Axone an solchen Tastzellen werden beschrieben. Da aber die Epithelwülste keine Körnerzellen enthalten, sondern erst seitlich im Epithel die normale Verteilung der Zelltypen im vielschichtigen Epithel vorhanden ist, liegt gerade die Möglichkeit nahe, daß von den Epithelwülsten als kleinen Regenerationszentren ein steter Zellstrom zu den Seiten hin besteht und darum besonders viele undifferenzierte Körnerzellen vorhanden sein müssen. Hier wird die Elektronenmikroskopie noch manche Klärung bringen müssen.

b) Schleimaale (Myxinidae)

Die Haut der Schleimaale besitzt eine besondere Differenzierung, die bei den Neunaugen noch nicht vorhanden ist: eingesenkte *alveoläre Schleimdrüsen*. Sie sind vom Kopf bis zum Schwanz segmental angeordnet und liegen auf jeder Seite ventrolateral, an der unteren Grenze der Myomeren (NEWBY, 1946). Es sind also in jedem Körpersegment zwei Schleimdrüsen vorhanden. Der Durchmesser einer Drüse beträgt bei der pazifischen Form Polistrotrema (Bdellostoma) stouti ca. 1,3 mm, der sehr kurze Ausführungsgang ist nur 0,5 mm lang. Die Feinstruktur der Drüsen wird weiter unten berücksichtigt. Diese Drüsen sind neben den verschiedenartigen Schleimzellen der vielschichtigen Epidermis hauptsächlich an der Produktion der überraschend großen Schleimmengen beteiligt, die von den Myxiniden ausgeschieden werden können.

Die *Epidermis* ist mehrschichtig und setzt sich aus fünf Zelltypen zusammen. RABL gibt an, daß bis zu 20 Zellschichten übereinander liegen können, und bei erwachsenen Exemplaren von Myxine besteht die Epidermis auf dem Rücken aus 6—8 Zellschichten (130 μ dick), auf dem Bauch aus 4—5 Zellschichten. Eine deutliche Trennung in verschiedene Epidermiszonen, etwa ein Stratum basale und ein Stratum mucosum, ist wegen der sehr großen Schleim- und Fadenzellen nur sehr unvollständig, der Aufbau weicht daher von dem der Neunaugenepidermis erheblich ab. Die Zusammenfassung von BLACKSTAD (1963), ergänzt durch elektronenmikroskopische und histochemische Untersuchungen, macht die Berücksichtigung älterer Arbeiten überflüssig. Die Befunde lassen auch einige der umstrittenen Erscheinungen in der Neunaugen-Epidermis klarer werden. Die basale Zellschicht setzt sich aus undifferenzierten Epithelzellen zusammen, die fast alle die Basalmembran berühren und etwa die Hälfte der Epidermisdicke ausmachen. Ähnlich wie bei den Neunaugen sind die apikalen Zellteile spindelförmig ausgezogen. Eine deutliche, ca. 0,5 μ dicke Ektoplasmaschicht der Epithelzellen besteht aus einer Lage dicht gepackter Tonofibrillen, die weitgehend parallel verlaufen, aber Bündel von Fibrillen auch ins Endoplasma abgeben. Diese periphere Lage von Tonofibrillen ist bei den Myxiniden früher als eine Kondensation der

Grundsubstanz des Plasmas betrachtet worden und wurde bei den Petromyzonten als Mantel von Epithelfasern an der Außenfläche der Zellen beschrieben; diese Fasern sollten in den Intercellularen von Zelle zu Zelle ziehen und sind besonders in der Abbildung von KRAUSE (1923) hervorgehoben. Der Tonofibrillenmantel der undifferenzierten Epithelzellen ist jedoch noch bedeckt von einer dünnen Schicht Cytoplasma mit zahlreichen Vesikeln. Die Plasmamembran ist sehr stark gefaltet, so daß benachbarte Zellen in ihren Grenzen zueinander ein kompliziertes Bild von Verzahnungen bieten. Desmosomen mit Tonofibrillen sind in der üblichen Weise vorhanden. Der Kern der Epithelzellen zeigt oft tiefe Einbuchtungen, in denen Mitochondrien liegen können. Im Endoplasma liegen die typischen Zellorganellen, die keine Besonderheiten aufweisen. Daneben sind aber zahlreiche größere oder kleinere Blasen vorhanden, in denen fibrilläres Material eingeschlossen ist und die als Vorstufen der Schleimbildung gedeutet werden. Denn aus den undifferenzierten Epithelzellen entwickeln sich alle hochdifferenzierten Zelltypen der Epidermis. Die Basis der Epithelzellen ist von zahlreichen Halbdesmosomen und kleinen Pinocytoseblasen besetzt, so daß die dort vorhandenen Tonofibrillenbündel, die in den Zellkörper aufsteigen, ziemlich parallel verlaufen und eine basale Streifung der Zellbasis im lichtmikroskopischen Bild hervorrufen.

Aus den indifferenten Epithelzellen gehen *drei Drüsenzelltypen* hervor: a) die kleinen Schleimzellen, b) die großen Schleimzellen (sog. Spinnenzellen) und c) die Fadenzellen. Die Drüsenzellen liegen in den oberen Epidermisschichten. An der Grenze zu den indifferenten Epithelzellen sind die basalen Teile der Zellen spindelförmig, da die apikalen Teile der indifferenten Epithelzellen eine ähnliche Form haben. Es liegen also ähnliche Verhältnisse wie bei den Neunaugen hinsichtlich der Zellgestalt vor.

a) *Die kleinen Schleimzellen* färben sich intensiv mit Mucicarmin (NEWBY, 1946), ihr Inhalt ist PAS-positiv (BLACKSTAD, 1963). Die tiefer gelegenen, also noch nicht voll ausdifferenzierten Schleimzellen enthalten zahlreiche Granula verschiedener Art, von denen ein Teil mit Sudanschwarz B angefärbt wird. Bei den reifen Schleimzellen ist der Kern in charakteristischer Weise flach gegen die Zellbasis verlagert worden, das Cytoplasma ist erfüllt von Granula, die elektronenmikroskopisch teils typische homogene Mucigengranula unterschiedlicher Dichte sind, wie sie in allen Schleimzellen vorkommen, teils aber komplexe und lamellär geschichtete Körper darstellen; außerdem kommen Lipoidtropfen vor. Zwischen den Granula sind Mitochondrien und Golgi-Lamellen vorhanden, eine Umwandlung von Mitochondrien in Granula kann nicht beobachtet werden. Die Schleimzellen bilden schließlich die oberen Zellschichten. Die an der Oberfläche der Epidermis liegenden Schleimzellen weisen einen ganz ähnlichen „Cuticularsaum" auf wie bei den Neunaugen; es kommt offenbar nicht zu einer massierten Schleimabgabe wie bei echten Becherzellen. Für Myxine liegen die elektronenmikroskopischen Befunde vor, die unsere Annahme über das Vorhandensein von Alveolen an der Zelloberfläche und den Vergleich mit Epithelzellen von Amphibienlarven stützen. An der Oberfläche befinden sich nämlich etwa 0,85 μ tiefe Einsenkungen, die mit Reihen von Granula in Verbindung stehen und durch dichtes Plasma voneinander getrennt sind. Mikrovilli und lappige Zellausläufer ragen zwischen den Einsenkungen hervor.

b) *Große Schleimzellen* (ca. 45 μ Durchmesser) werden wegen der zentralen Lage des Kernes und der radiären Ausstrahlung von Plasmasträngen vom Perikaryon durch die Schleimsekrete des Zellinnern auch „Spinnenzellen" genannt. Sie liegen in den basalen Epidermisschichten. Ähnlich wie bei den Körnerzellen der Neunaugen legen die Abbildungen älterer Autoren nahe, daß eine Art Stielzelle die große Schleimzelle trägt. Die großen Schleimvacuolen enthalten einen homogenen Inhalt, der sich mit Mucicarmin färbt, aber im Gegensatz zu den kleinen Schleimzellen PAS-negativ ist. Die Plasmastränge bestehen aus Membranen, welche die Schleimvacuolen voneinander trennen; kleinere Granula sind in den reifen Zellen nicht mehr vorhanden. OLSSON (1959) findet die großen Schleimzellen auch im Ductus nasopharyngicus und nimmt aufgrund der histochemischen Reaktionen und des Sekretmodus an, daß die β-Zellen der Adenohypophyse modifizierte „Spinnenzellen" sind. In den alveolären Schleimdrüsen liefern die großen Schleimzellen eine dünnflüssige Schleimsubstanz (NEWBY, 1946).

c) Eine besondere Differenzierung weisen die merkwürdigen *Fadenzellen* auf; sie sind keine Schleimzellen üblicher Art und können in gewisser Hinsicht den Kolbenzellen der Neunaugen verglichen werden, doch ist ihre Funktion besser bekannt. Es sind große, birnförmige oder gestreckte Zellen (Länge bis 150 μ, Dicke ca. 60 μ; NEWBY, 1946) in den mittleren Schichten der Epidermis; ihr apikaler Zellteil ragt zwischen den kleinen Schleimzellen bis an die Epidermisoberfläche, so daß ihr Inhalt dort entleert werden kann. Dieser Inhalt ist im lebenden Zustand der Zellen undurchsichtig, an fixierten und gefärbten Zellen zeigen sich spiralig gewundene Fäden verschiedener Dicke, die Doppelbrechung zeigen. Daneben enthalten die Zellen Granula. Beide, Fäden und Granula sind PAS-negativ, beide enthalten Tyrosin. Das Protein der Fäden ist nach seinem Gehalt an Aminosäuren und seinem Röntgendiagramm weder mit Kollagen, Keratin oder Myosin zu vergleichen (FERRY, 1941). In reifen Fadenzellen liegt der Kern im apikalen Teil des Cytoplasmas, umgeben von homogenen Granula. Dort beginnt auch der Faden mit einfachen Schlingen in etwa 25—35 zirkulär angeordneten Schleifen. Die folgenden Schleifen wenden sich aber an der Peripherie des Zellkörpers basal und laufen im Innern des Plasmas zum apikalen Teil zurück, so daß eine komplizierte Anordnung des aufgewickelten Fadens entsteht (NEWBY, 1946). Bei der Differenzierung und Größenzunahme sich entwickelnder Fadenzellen zeigt sich ein enger Zusammenhang zwischen den Granula und Teilstücken des Fadens, der offenbar aus den einzelnen Schlingen erst zusammengesetzt wird zu einem durchgehenden Faden. Ebenso ist eine Dickenzunahme des Fadens bei der Bildung zu erkennen. Wird eine reife Fadenzelle eröffnet, so tritt der zusammengerollte Faden als ein ca. 110 μ mal 60 μ großes oval geformtes Körperchen aus. Am apikalen Ende beginnt der Faden sich zu entspiralisieren und liegt dann als mehrere Zentimeter langer etwa 1,3 μ dicker „Sekretfaden" im dünnflüssigen Schleim. Im Wasser ändert dieser Schleim sehr bald seine Konsistenz und wird zu einer fadenziehenden Gallerte, in der ein Schleimaal völlig eingebettet sein kann. Die Feinstruktur des Fadens in der Zelle (BLACKSTAD, 1963) zeigt eine Zusammensetzung aus 60—80 Filamenten pro Faden, jedes 100—120 Å dick und durch eine Grundsubstanz zusammengekittet. Die Doppelbrechung ist durch eine solche Anordnung des Materials erklärt. Jedes Filament scheint eine periodische Querstreifung im Abstand von 30—40 Å zu besitzen. Die Vorgänge bei der Aufquellung im Wasser und die nachfolgenden Veränderungen an der schleimigen Gallerte sind leider bisher nicht erneut untersucht worden; die älteren Befunde (vgl. BIEDERMANN, 1930) sind entsprechend der Methodik zu primitiv, um Aufschlüsse zu ergeben. Nach einiger Zeit zieht sich nämlich die Schleimgallerte unter Abgabe von Wasser wieder zusammen.

Der fünfte Zelltyp: die Sinneszellen werden bei der Innervation der Haut berücksichtigt.

Unterlagert ist die Epidermis von einer *Basalmembran* und den daran anschließenden Schichten des *Corium*, beide in der Feinstruktur bei Myxine durch die Untersuchungen von BLACKSTAD (1963) bekannt. Die *Basalmembran* (PAS-positiv, 0,3—0,5 μ dick) ist eine fast homogen erscheinende Schicht, aus der sehr feine Fibrillen gegen die Halbdesmosomen der basalen Epithelzellen durch einen schmalen Spaltraum unter den Zellen aufsteigen. Aus dem Corium strahlen feinste Fibrillen aus dem Maschenwerk dicker, 200—700 Å messender Kollagenfibrillen in die Basalmembran ein, dort sind sie dann aber nicht mehr zu erkennen, sondern offenbar durch die kittende Grundsubstanz maskiert. *Das Corium* ist deutlich aus drei Schichten aufgebaut. Unmittelbar unter der Basalmembran sind in einer 2—3 µ dicken Schicht die kollagenen Fibrillen sehr unregelmäßig als Maschenwerk angeordnet, diese Zone ist daher nur schwach doppelbrechend im polarisierten Licht und außerdem PAS-negativ. Es folgt dann eine Zone (ca. 9 µ Dicke), die als Stratum compactum bezeichnet werden könnte und schon seit langem bekannt ist. In ihr liegen mehrere (bis 5) dichte Schichten kollagener Faserbündel, die alle parallel zur Basalmembran verlaufen, in ihren Verlaufsrichtungen sich aber in der bekannten Weise um ca. 90° überkreuzen. Diese obere Coriumschicht wird von Melanophoren unterlagert und damit deutlich vom tieferen Coriumbindegewebe abgegrenzt. Letzteres ist eine etwa 80 µ dicke Lage aus verschiedenen Schichten kollagener Fasern, die aber nicht so dicht gepackt sind wie im oberflächlicheren Stratum compactum, jedoch einen entsprechenden Verlauf zeigen. Die Fibrillen zeigen die typische Querstreifung des Kollagens und messen zwischen 450—700 Å im Durchmesser. Außerdem sind feine Fibrillen ohne erkennbare Querstreifung vorhanden. Zwischen den Lagen der Fibrillen liegen langgestreckte Zellen, die z.T. PAS-positive Granula enthalten und Fibroblasten sein dürften. Aufsteigende Faserbündel durchsetzen beide Schichten des Coriums in ähnlicher Weise, wie es für die Haut der Neunaugen beschrieben wurde. Capillaren sind zwischen den Bündeln vor allem im Stratum compactum vorhanden, wo ein engmaschiges Capillarnetz dicht unter der Epidermis ausgebildet ist (MARINELLI und STRENGER, 1956). Da die Melanophoren tiefer liegen, hat die Haut besonders auf der Bauchseite der Tiere durch das Blut einen rötlichen Farbton. Ein vergleichbares Capillarnetz fehlt bei den Neunaugen.

Die *Subcutis* ist stark ausgebildet und enthält hauptsächlich große Fettzellen, zwischen denen Bindegewebsstränge die Nerven und Blutgefäße zum Corium führen. Die Subcutis stellt aber keine feste Verbindung mit den Muskelsegmenten her, sondern wird von weiten *Lymphräumen* unterlagert, so daß die gesamte Haut schlaff auf dem Körper befestigt ist (COLE, 1926). Teils sind diese Sinus mit Blut gefüllt und stellen eine Verbindung zwischen Arterien- und Venensystem dar, teils enthalten sie echte Lymphe und stehen mit Venen in Verbindung, nehmen also am Blutkreislauf nicht teil. Alle Lymphräume sind von einem dünnen Endothel umkleidet. Im Kopfgebiet gliedern sich die Lymphräume in verschiedene Systeme, im gesamten Rumpfgebiet sind drei subcutane Lymphsinus vorhanden, in denen Blut zirkuliert. Zwei laterale Räume sind durch ein dorsales mittleres Septum getrennt, sowie durch Septen in Höhe der Schleimdrüsen seitlich gegen einen unpaaren ventralen Lymphsinus abgegrenzt. Das Caudalherz des Venensystems steht mit dem Lymphsinus im Schwanzgebiet in direkter Verbindung. Die Nerven und Gefäße der Haut treten allein durch die genannten Septen in die Subcutis ein. MARINELLI kleidet den Tatbestand in folgende anschauliche Worte: „Überblicken wir die Gesamtlage, so könnten wir sagen, daß das Tier in einem mit Blut gefüllten Sack schwimmt, in dem es mit einigen zarten Bindegewebsbändern in Lage gehalten wird."

Die tief eingesenkten *Schleimdrüsen* sind echte alveoläre Drüsen, wie sie sonst bei Cyclostomen und Fischen (mit Ausnahmen, z.B. Leuchtorgane, Giftdrüsen) nicht vorkommen. Der epitheliale Teil ist tief in die Subcutis vorgewölbt und wird von den segmental angeordneten Platten der Musculi decussati der rechten bzw. linken Körperseite überdeckt (MARINELLI und STRENGER, 1956). Wegen ihrer auffallenden Morphologie und Funktion sind sie mehrfach genau untersucht worden, zuletzt von SCHAFFER (1925), NEWBY (1946), MARINELLI und STRENGER (1956), BLACKSTAD (1963). Bei einer Reizung der Tiere wird der Drüseninhalt ausgepreßt, und zwar in Nachbarschaft der Reizquelle stärker als an anderen Körperzonen. Daher befinden sich die Drüsen nicht alle in gleichen Sekretionszuständen. Das Drüsenepithel besteht aus den Zellen der Epidermis: indifferenten Zellen, großen und kleinen Schleimzellen und mehreren tausend Fadenzellen. Der Inhalt einer Alveole ist aus Schleim und zerfallenden Fadenzellen zusammengesetzt, die ihre Fäden z.T. schon abgewickelt haben; es liegt holokrine Sekretion vor. Die abgestoßenen Zellen werden von den indifferenten Epithelzellen ersetzt. Das Epithel des kurzen Ausführungsganges baut sich aus undifferenzierten Epithelzellen, großen und kleinen Schleimzellen auf; Fadenzellen fehlen. Es geht ohne scharfe Grenze in das Körperepithel über. In der Drüse ist der Schichtenbau durch die Anhäufung reifer Schleim- und Fadenzellen verlorengegangen, und eine geschlossene Basalzellenschicht in regelmäßiger Anordnung ist nicht vorhanden; vielmehr sind die basalen indifferenten Zellen flach auf die Basalmembran gedrückt, so daß zu vermuten ist, der Zellnachschub vollziehe sich vom Epithel des Ausführungsganges her. Das Coriumbindegewebe umgibt die Drüse in Form einer Kapsel, die zwar noch die Faserschichten des Corium enthält, aber unterhalb des Ausführungsganges sehr stark abgewandelt ist: die Kapsel enthält ein sehr enges capillares Gefäßnetz und zahlreiche quergestreifte Muskelbündel. Die Herkunft dieser Muskelzüge ist ebenso wie ihr genauer Verlauf nicht geklärt, doch darf angenommen werden, daß es sich um Teile der erwähnten Mm. decussati handelt. Sie pressen bei Reizung des Tieres die Drüsen zusammen, so daß der schleimige Inhalt entleert wird. Das Kapselbindegewebe mit den Capillaren springt ins Innere der Drüsen in Form von Trabekeln vor, auf diese Weise die sezernierende Oberfläche vergrößernd.

Die *Innervation und die Anordnung der Sinneszellen* der Haut ist wesentlich anders als bei den Neunaugen. Die Sinnesgruben des Seitenliniensystems sind bis auf wenige Reste am Kopf reduziert oder fehlen ganz. Sinneszellen kommen als einzeln stehende sekundäre Sinneszellen und zu mehreren vereinigt in Sinnesknospen vor. Sie sehen ganz ähnlich aus wie bei Neunaugen; allerdings fehlen neuere Untersuchungen. Die Haut der Schleimaale ist lichtempfindlich (NEWTH und Ross, 1955; STEVEN, 1955), denn obwohl die Augen der Myxiniden stark reduziert sind, reagieren die Tiere bei Belichtung der Haut mit Licht der Wellenlängen zwischen 500 und 520 nm. Die bisher nicht bekannten Photoreceptoren der Haut müssen am vorderen und hinteren Ende des Tieres besonders gehäuft vorhanden sein. Doch dürften ähnliche Verhältnisse wie bei den Neunaugen vorliegen (s. dort), wo die Frage des photolabilen Pigmentes und die nervöse Versorgung besonderer pigmenthaltiger Epithelzellen ausführlich diskutiert wurde. Die Epidermis ist von zahlreichen freien Nervenendigungen durchsetzt, die auch an die Sinneszellen herantreten. Da ein Lateralissystem fehlt, bilden Neurone (uni- oder bipolar) einen besonderen subcutanen Plexus (BONE, 1963); ein Teil der Neurone liegt an den kleinen subcutanen Gefäßen und reguliert wahrscheinlich die Blutfüllung und die Durchströmung der großen subcutanen Lymphräume. Im Bereich der Schleimdrüsen treten die Neurone zu einem ausgedehnten Plexus zusammen. Die Nervenzellen des subcutanen Plexus, einschließlich der an den Gefäßen liegenden Teile und der in den Drüsenkapseln, stehen mit Neuronen der ventralen Spinalnerven in synaptischer Verbindung, sind also nicht, wie es bei Neunaugen der Fall ist, direkte Vermittler von Impulsen zum ZNS durch das Lateralissystem. NEWTH und Ross (1955) konnten zeigen, daß die Lichtreaktion der Haut tatsächlich Impulse auslöst, die durch das Rückenmark von Myxine zum Gehirn weitergeleitet werden. Die Autoren heben hervor, wie ungewöhnlich und einzigartig dieser spinale Weg der Impulse von einem Photoreceptor zum Gehirn für Wirbeltiere ist. Das Fehlen des Lateralissystems macht sich natürlich auch in der Gliederung der zentralen Trigeminus-, Vagus- und Glossopharyngicus-Ganglien morphologisch bemerkbar. Die peripheren Nerven gleichen in der Feinstruktur denen der Neunaugen (PETERS, 1963): die Axone besitzen keine Myelinscheiden und werden nur von Schwannschen Zellen umschlossen, die von einer Basalmembran aus locker verflochtenen kollagenen Fibrillen mit Fibroblasten als einem Endoneurium umlagert sind. Je nach Axondurchmesser bilden eine oder mehrere Schwannsche Zellen im Querschnitt die Hülle des Axons. Sowohl Hirn- als Spinalnerven zeigen übereinstimmend diese Verhältnisse.

2. Chondrichthyes (Knorpelfische)
a) Der Bau der Haut

Die Haut der Selachier (Haie und Rochen) ist durch besondere Derivate ausgezeichnet: *die Hautzähnchen, sog. Placoidschuppen* (s. Abb. 4). Es sind keine echten Schuppen, sondern nach caudal gekrümmte Hohlzähnchen, die den gleichen Aufbau besitzen wie die Kieferzähne der Selachier und diesen auch entsprechen. Bei den Haien sind die Placoidschuppen in regelmäßigen Reihen in der Haut angeordnet; bei den Rochen sind sie unregelmäßig verteilt, einzelne Körperzonen sind sogar frei von Zähnchen. Im fertigen Zustand überragen die oberen Teile der Placoidschuppen die Epidermis, an der Basis sind sie im Bindegewebe des Corium verankert; epidermale und mesenchymale Zellen sind am Aufbau dieser Hartgebilde beteiligt, obwohl bis heute der Anteil der Gewebe bei der Entwicklung der Zähnchen nicht erkannt werden konnte (BARGMANN, 1938; LISON, 1949; W. J. SCHMIDT, 1951; POOLE, 1956). Der Aufbau der Placoidschuppen wird weiter unten beschrieben.

Die *Epidermis* der Selachier ist vielschichtig, meistens sind 4—8 Zellschichten vorhanden (KRAUSE, 1923; RABL, 1931). Jedoch zeigt ein Vergleich verschiedener Körperzonen, daß z. B. beim schwarzen Dornhai (Spinax niger), einem kleinen, ca. $1/2$ m messenden nordatlantischen und auch in der Nordsee heimischen Hai auf der Bauchseite, der Unterseite des Kopfes, in der Umgebung der Flossenansätze und der Kiemenöffnungen bis zu 19 Epithelzellschichten übereinander liegen (JOHANN, 1899). Eine *erhebliche Variation* der Epidermisdicke ist auch zwischen den verschiedenen Arten von Haien und Rochen ausgeprägt (DANIEL, 1928); die verschiedenen Lebensbedingungen, das Vorhandensein der Placoidschuppen und ihre Verteilung, die erheblichen Größenunterschiede zwischen den Arten wirken sich nun in zunehmendem Maße auf den Feinbau der Haut aus. Die relative Gleichförmigkeit der Haut bei den niederen Chordaten (sieht man von den Zuständen während der Larvenentwicklung ab) kann bei der Mannigfaltigkeit der Formen und der Erweiterung der Lebensräume nicht mehr beibehalten werden.

Ein Stratum basale aus prismatischen teilungsfähigen Epithelzellen bildet die untere Zellschicht der Epidermis. Eine mittlere Lage aus polyedrischen Zellen wird Stratum spinosum genannt. Diese Zellen sind durch „Intercellularbrücken", also Desmosomen miteinander verbunden und weisen Tonofibrillen auf. An der Oberfläche ordnen sich die Zellen zu einer Schicht an, deren Zellen abgeflacht sind und entsprechend den Verhältnissen bei Cyclostomen als Stratum cuticulare bezeichnet werden. Denn diese oberflächlichen Zellen zeigen wieder einen „Cuticularsaum", über dessen Beschaffenheit aber keine neueren Untersuchungen vorliegen. Wir verweisen auf die Befunde bei Cyclostomen. In diesem Zusammenhang ist von Interesse, daß bei Haifischembryonen von einer Größe über 40 mm

(Mustelus laevis) die Epidermis zweischichtig ist: eine niedrige unregelmäßig geformte Basalzellenschicht wird von hochprismatischen Zellen überlagert, in der sich zwei Zelltypen differenziert haben: Wimperepithelzellen mit Cilien und mehrkernige Drüsenzellen, die offenbar Schleimstoffe produzieren. Über das genaue Schicksal im Verlaufe der Entwicklung ist nichts bekannt. RAUTHER (1927) bestätigt das Vorhandensein der Cilien bei embryonalen Epithelien von Acanthias und Mustelus, findet außerdem eine „Deckplatte' aus eingesenkten Alveolen zwischen den Cilien. Diese Verhältnisse erinnern an Epithelien von Amphibienlaren; die Potenzen zur Bildung von Cilien und von Schleim sind in Epithelzellen also vorhanden. Es bleibt die Frage offen, welche Art der Oberflächendifferenzierung bei den erwachsenen Tieren schließlich verwirklicht ist. Für Rochen wird eine Schleimbildung in der gesamten oberen Epithelzellenschicht des Kopfes angegeben.

Zwischen den mit Tonofibrillen versehenen Epithelzellen kommen zwei *Typen von Drüsenzellen* vor: *Becherzellen* (Schleimzellen) und *„seröse"* *Drüsenzellen*. Die Becherzellen finden sich vor allem in der Haut der Rochen, da dort die Placoidschuppen reduziert sind; aber auch seröse Drüsenzellen kommen vor. In der Regel finden sich seröse Drüsenzellen aber nur bei Haien, denen dafür die Schleimzellen fehlen. Auf die Schleimzellen in der Haut der Embryonen wurde schon hingewiesen. Die Becherzellen differenzieren sich aus den Basalzellen, indem Tochterzellen an Größe zunehmen und durch die Zellschichten in die distale Zone wandern. Dort wird die Schleimsubstanz produziert, der Kern bleibt im basalen Zellteil, und die stark vergrößerte Zelle gleicht einer typischen Becherzelle; sie öffnet sich an der Oberfläche und entleert dort ihr Sekret. Die „serösen" Drüsenzellen erreichen erhebliche Größen und liegen im Stratum spinosum, reichen aber auch von der Basalzellenschicht bis zur Oberfläche. Sie sind von Sekretgranula erfüllt, die sich je nach Differentierungszustand mit Orange G oder Säurefuchsin anfärben oder zu einer homogenen Sekretmasse zusammengeflossen sind. Der Zellkern ist in die Cytoplasmareste an der Peripherie der Zelle gedrängt worden.

Das Epithel wird von zahlreichen *Leukocyten* (besonders eosinophilen) durchwandert; sie stammen aus dem dichten Capillarnetz unter der Basalmembran. Zahlreiche *Melanophoren* können zwischen den Zellen des Stratum spinosum ihre Ausläufer erstrecken; die Epithelzellen selbst nehmen aber kein Pigment auf. Teils liegen die Melanophoren in der Epidermis, teils sitzen sie im Corium und lassen ihre Ausläufer nur in das Epithel aufsteigen. Für den Farbwechsel sind aber vor allem die tiefer gelegenen Pigmentzellen im Corium wesentlich.

Eine Einsenkung des Epithels in Form echter *Drüsen* kommt im allgemeinen nicht vor. Jedoch sind an den zu Begattungsorganen umgestalteten Teilen der Bauchflossen bei männlichen Tieren Epithelfalten in wechselnder Ausbildung vorhanden, die besonders zahlreiche große Becherzellen enthalten. Sie fungieren als echte Schleimdrüsen (DANIEL, 1928) und können z. B. bei der bekannten Rochengattung Raja sogar eine komplexe Form mit zwei Lappen ausbilden, wobei das Sekret durch eine Papille austritt. Nach BOLOGNANI FANTIN (1963) handelt es sich um tubulöse Drüsen von serösem Typ, da eine Prüfung auf saure Mucopolysaccharide negativ ausfällt; das Sekret in Form feiner Granula ist PAS-positiv. Epithelfalten an Flossenstacheln, die umgebildete oder verschmolzene Hautzähne darstellen, sind als Giftdrüsen seit langem bekannt. Die Stacheln auf der Schwanzflosse der Stechrochen sind rinnenförmig und enthalten in der Furche ein von Drüsenzellen durchsetztes Epithel, deren Sekret als Gift gefürchtet ist und bei Verletzungen durch die Stacheln in die Wunde gelangt (FLEURY, 1950; HALSTEAD und MODGLIN, 1950; Zusammenfassung bei HALSTEAD und MITCHELL, 1963). Die Stechrochen dürften unter den Selachiern als „giftige Tiere" die bekanntesten sein. Das Gift wirkt auf den Kreislauf und beeinflußt den Herzmuskel, der gelähmt wird. Im Tierversuch (FLEURY, 1950; RUSSEL und VAN HARREVELD, 1954; RUSSEL, BARRITT und FAIRCHILD, 1957) wirkt das Gift in Form eines rohen Extraktes tödlich. Die zuletzt genannten Autorengruppen haben sorgfältige physiologische Untersuchungen bei verschiedenen Tierarten und auch beim Menschen durchgeführt. Da es sich aber bei den beiden Drüsenarten um spezialisierte Organe in Beziehung zu bestimmten Funktionen wie Begattung und Abwehr handelt, kann hier nicht näher auf sie eingegangen werden.

Eine *Basalmembran* unterlagert die Epidermis. RABL (1931) erkennt zwischen eigentlicher Basalmembran und der unteren Grenze der basalen Epithelzellen eine feine Kittschicht, so daß wohl vergleichbare Verhältnisse wie bei der Haut der Schleimaale vorliegen (s. dort). Das *Corium* ist in zwei deutlich getrennte Schichten gegliedert: die obere, an die Basalmembran grenzende Schicht ist locker aus einem Maschenwerk von Fasern aufgebaut und durch eine Lage flach ausgebreiteter Fibrocyten von der Basalmembran getrennt. Die lockere Schicht kann als Stratum laxum (RABL) oder Str. spongiosum gekennzeichnet werden. In ihren Bindegewebsmaschen verlaufen Capillaren, die ein dichtes Netz bilden und umgeben sind von zahlreichen Melanophoren und wenigen Xanthophoren. Daneben sind Fibroblasten vorhanden. Auch elastische Fasern durchziehen das Maschenwerk. Im einzelnen kann Ausdehnung und Dichte dieser Schicht sehr wechselnd sein. Die Bedeutung der Pigmentzellen für den Farbwechsel wird weiter unten betrachtet. — Eine elastische „Grenzmembran" aus dicht verflochtenen, sehr feinen elastischen Fasern trennt die obere Schicht des Corium von einer straffen tiefen Schicht: dem Stratum compactum. Hier liegen kollagene Faserbündel eng gepackt in Lagen; der Verlauf der Faserrichtung geht parallel zur Körperoberfläche, etwa 45° im Winkel zur Körperlängsachse, wobei sich Bündel der einzelnen aufeinanderfolgenden Schichten fast rechtwinklig in ihrem Verlauf kreuzen. Dadurch kommt eine charakteristische Textur zustande, welche zusammen mit den Placoidschuppen die Straffheit und Widerstandsfähigkeit der Selachierhaut bedingen. Die Zahl der Schichten des Stratum compactum schwankt zwischen 8 und 40; demzufolge sind die Integumente sehr verschieden dick. Auch die gröberen Faserbündel, zwischen denen elastische Netze liegen, wechseln in ihrer Dicke sehr von Art zu Art. Wie schon mehrfach bei der Struktur des Corium beschrieben, sind vertikale Faserbündel von der Tiefe bis zum Stratum spongiosum als verflechtende Elemente überall eingelagert; ihre feineren Fasern verlieren sich in dem Maschenwerk des Str. spongiosum und der Basalmembran. Die Gesamtdicke der Haut wird also weniger durch die Epidermis als durch die Ausbildung des Corium bedingt. Die Festigkeit der Haut ermöglicht eine Verarbeitung zu Leder, dem bekannten Chagrinleder oder „Galuchat". Im Fernen Osten wurden Waffen und Lackkästen schon im Mittelalter mit Selachierhaut überzogen, die eingefärbt und deren Zähne angeschliffen wurden. Später wurde ein ähnlich bearbeitetes Leder als Schmuckleder auch für Handtaschen, Uhren, Necessaires, Kästchen etc. in Europa und Amerika modern (BRÜHL, 1933). Je nach dem verwendeten Rohmaterial hat dieses Leder sehr verschiedene Namen erhalten.

Die *Subcutis* verbindet das Corium mit der Muskelfascie und ist in den Körperregionen sehr unterschiedlich gebaut. So kann es ein Gallertgewebe aus retikulären Bindegewebsbündeln mit viel Grundsubstanz sein, es kann Fettzellen enthalten, kann aber auch wie ein straffes Sehnengewebe aus kollagenen Fasern in Fortsetzung der Gewebe von Muskelfascien gebaut sein.

In der Haut verankert sind die *Placoidschuppen (Hautzähne)* (Abb. 4a), die im einzelnen durch die Form und durch zusätzliche Spitzen des über die Epidermis hervorragenden Teiles sehr verschieden aussehen können. Sie erreichen bei einzelnen Arten auf dem Rücken eine erhebliche Größe (Durchmesser 4 cm bei Trygoniden). Sie überdecken sich jedoch nicht, sondern sind durch Hautgewebe voneinander getrennt, auch wenn sie in dichten regelmäßig angeordneten Reihen stehen. Diese Anordnung hängt mit dem Faserverlauf des straffen Corium zusammen, in dessen Faserbündeln die Verankerung der Zähne hineinreicht. Die Grundform der Placoidschuppen besteht aus einer unregelmäßig rhombisch geformten Basalplatte, auf der ein kurzer Stiel mit dem distalen gekrümmten Zahnteil sitzt. Da ein steter Ersatz für abgestoßene Zähnchen und ein Abbau alter Zähne vorhanden ist, sind benachbarte Placoidschuppen oft von ungleicher Größe. Basalplatte und Zahnteil sind hohl und öffnen sich an der Basis, so daß eine Pulpahöhle mit besonderen Bindegewebszellen vorhanden ist und deren Inneres mit dem Bindegewebe, den Blutgefäßen und Nerven des Corium in Verbindung steht (GNADEBERG, 1926). Die

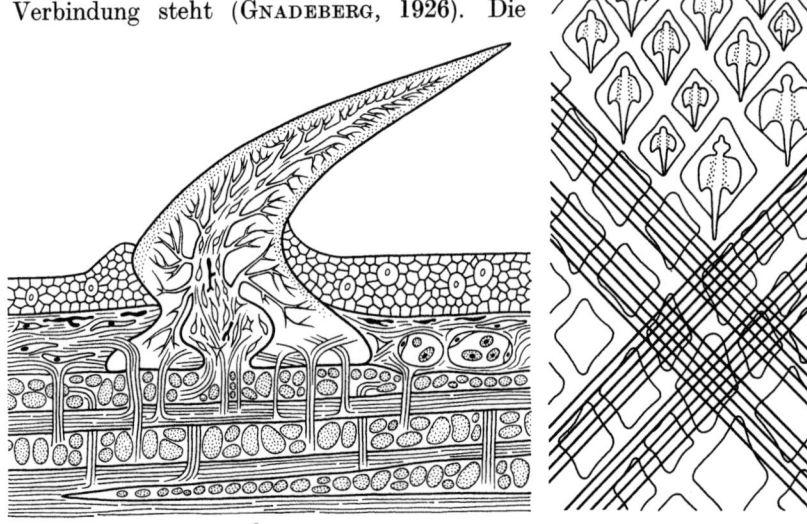

Abb. 4a u. b. Haut und Placoidschuppen eines Haies. a Schnitt durch die Haut und die Medianebene einer Placoidschuppe; daneben die Schuppen in Aufsicht in ihrer Beziehung zum Verlauf der Fasern des Coriums. Die Schuppe durchbricht das Epithel und ist mit Faserbündeln verankert. (Nach KLAATSCH und GNADEBERG.) b Entwicklungsreihe von Placoidschuppen beim Katzenhai (Embryo). Links oben Anlage aus Epithelplatte und dermaler Papille, daneben ist die Schuppenform durch die Epithelanlage bereits ausgeprägt. Unten fortgeschrittenes Stadium mit Gefäß in der Pulpaanlage. Die Schichtung des Coriums in Stratum laxum und Stratum compactum ist vorhanden, sehr gut sichtbar wird die Verflechtung der Faserbündel in Stratum compactum. Azan 350/1

Pulpahöhle kann sehr weit und mit großer Öffnung ausgebildet sein oder bis auf geringe Reste durch die Hartsubstanz verdrängt werden. Der Zahn selbst wird bei der Entwicklung durch das Zusammenwirken einer Zellschicht der Epidermis: den Ganoblasten (früher auch Schmelzorgan oder Ameloblasten genannt) und den Zellen einer bindegewebigen Papille: den Odontoblasten gebildet. Diese Zahnanlage, deren Entwicklung aus Abb. 4b ohne weitere Erläuterung ersichtlich ist, gleicht in sehr auffallender Weise den Anlagen von Reptilienschuppen und von Federn; die Entwicklung der Hautzähne wurde zuletzt von W. J. SCHMIDT (1951) analysiert. Nach der Feinstruktur des Zahnes wird die Bildung der Hartsubstanz nur von den Odontoblasten vorgenommen, und SCHMIDT vermutet, daß die Schicht der epidermalen Ganoblasten die Form des Zahnes bestimmt, ohne am Aufbau direkt beteiligt zu sein. Die Kenntnisse über die frühe Entwicklung von Federanlagen können diese Auffassungen heute stützen, wenn auch dort gerade umgekehrt allein die epidermalen Teile der Anlage die Feder aufbauen. Aber zunächst ist in den Stadien, die morphologisch den Hautzahn-Anlagen ähnlich sehen, eine zeitlich abgestufte Wechselwirkung zwischen den Zellen der bindegewebigen Papille und den epidermalen Teilen der

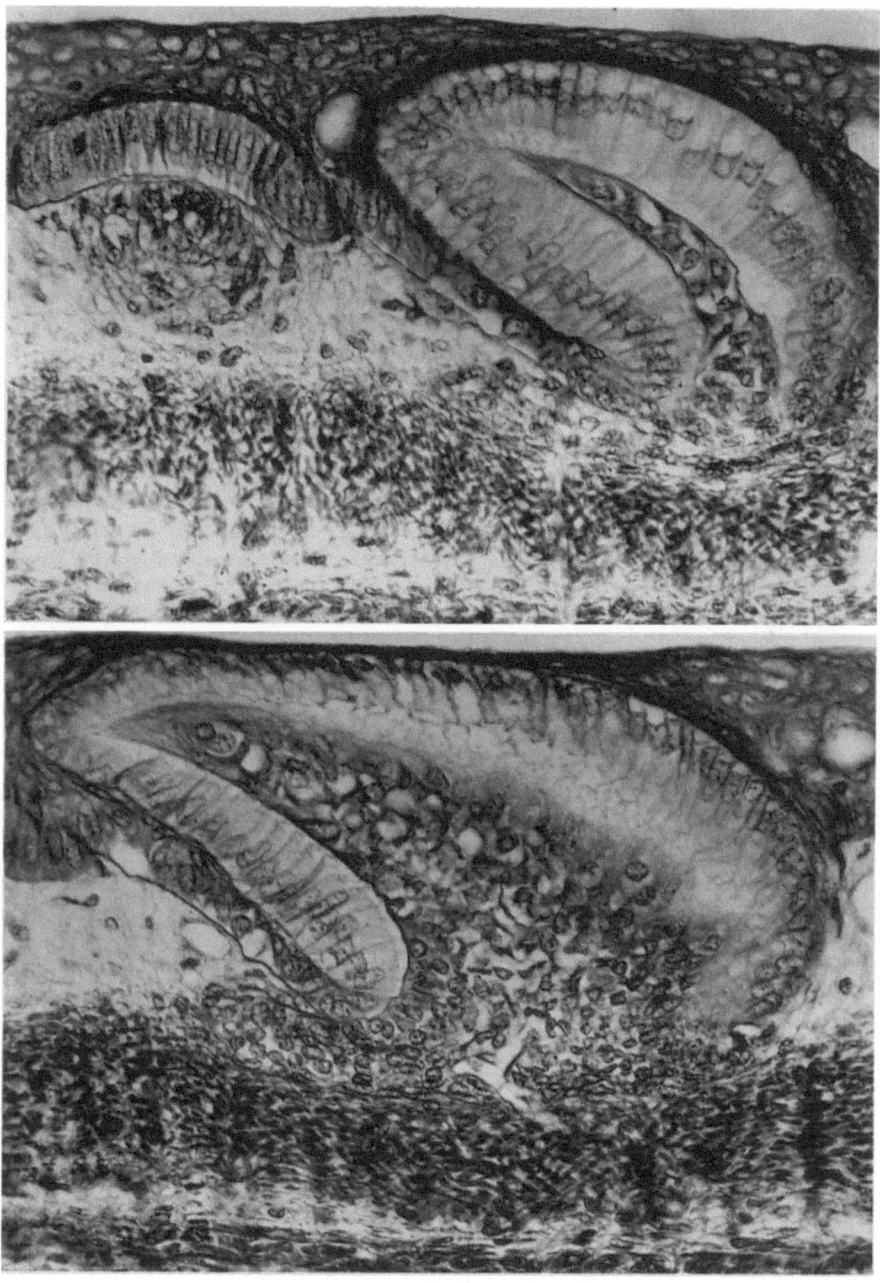

Abb. 4b

Anlage unbedingt notwendig. Der Zahn besteht aus Dentin, das von der Pulpa her von zahlreichen feinen Kanälen (ähnlich den Tomesschen Fasern) durchsetzt wird; in dieses System feiner Röhren entsenden die bei der Bildung der Hartsubstanz allmählich auf die Pulpahöhle zurückgedrängten Odontoblasten feine Zellausläufer (LISON, 1949; W. J. SCHMIDT, 1951; POOLE, 1956). An der

Oberfläche wird im distalen Teil des Zahnes das Dentin von einer abgewandelten, besonders harten Dentinschicht, dem Durodentin überzogen; diese Schicht wurde früher vielfach als „Schmelz" angesehen. Echter Schmelz kommt aber bei den Fischen nicht vor, und wie sich aus zahlreichen Untersuchungen (BARGMANN, 1938; W. J. SCHMIDT, 1938, 1940, 1949; GROSS-LERNER, 1957; POOLE, 1956) ergibt, auch nicht auf den Mundzähnen, die ja den Placoidschuppen homolog sind. Die fossilen Zähne von Knochenfischen aus dem Devon zeigen bereits den jetzt von rezenten Formen bekannten Feinbau (W. J. SCHMIDT, 1959), so daß es sich um ursprüngliche Verhältnisse handelt und nicht um eine Abwandlung des Zahntyps im Verlaufe der Phylogenese. Die Basalplatte besteht nur aus Dentin der einfachen Form. Die Feinstruktur der Placoidschuppen (SCHMIDT, 1951; POOLE, 1956) im Bereich des Durodentins besteht aus Kristallen von Hydroxyapatit ($Ca_{10}(PO_4)_6(OH)_2$), zwischen denen nur wenig organisches Material verblieben ist. Die Oberfläche wird von einer dünnen Grenzlamelle gebildet, in der die Achsen der Kristalle tangential zur gekrümmten Oberfläche angeordnet sind; die Grenzlamelle wird sehr früh in der Anlage sichtbar und liegt unmittelbar den Zellgrenzen der Ganoblasten an. Sie ist wohl identisch mit der Basalmembran und wird bei der Verkalkung als erste mit Hartsubstanz imprägniert. Es folgt eine Schicht, in der die Kristallachsen vertikal zur Oberfläche stehen, der Rest an organischem Material ist gering. Die Mineralsalze werden bei der Entstehung der Schuppen in dieser Schicht entsprechend dem Verlauf der feinen Kollagenfibrillen abgelagert, und diese Fibrillen werden von den Odontoblasten in vertikaler Richtung zur Basalmembran aufgebaut. Nach einer sehr dünnen Übergangszone beginnt die Region des typischen Dentins: tangential zur Oberfläche verlaufende Kollagenfasern mit eingelagerten Kristallen, deren Achsen parallel zu den Faserbündeln ausgerichtet sind. Die Dentinschicht stellt die Masse des Zahnes dar und wird vom System der Kanälchen in vertikaler Richtung durchsetzt. Die Durodentinschicht der Oberfläche unterscheidet sich daher optisch vom Dentin, da im Durodentin das Kollagen fast restlos durch Mineralsalze ersetzt worden ist und die Achsen der Kristalle entsprechend der ehemaligen vorgeformten Unterlage senkrecht zu den Kristallachsen im Dentin verlaufen. Im Dentin und unter der Grenzlamelle können Melaningranula eingeschlossen sein, die aus den Pigmentzellen des Corium stammen und bei der Anlage im Bereich der Pulpa gelegen haben. Die Basalplatte der Schuppen ist von unregelmäßigerem Feinbau, hier fehlen die Kanälchen. Statt dessen sind Faserbündel des Corium in die Hartsubstanz eingeschlossen worden, so daß die Platte an zahlreichen Stellen wie mit Sharpeyschen Fasern im Stratum compactum verankert ist. Neben mechanischem Verlust von Schuppen kommt es in der normalen Haut auch zum Abbau der Hautzähnchen (BUDKER, 1936, 1938; PETIT und BUDKER, 1936), zuerst wird die Basalplatte von großen vielkernigen Zellen, sog. Odontoklasten aufgelöst, dann von der Pulpa her das Dentin und die harte Oberschicht, dabei wird eine Demineralisierung vorgenommen, und eine gelatinöse Konsistenz ist zeitweilig die Folge.

b) Der physiologische Farbwechsel

Die *Pigmentzellen* der Epidermis und des Corium sind die Grundlage für die Zeichnungen der Selachier und ihren physiologischen Farbwechsel. Obwohl auch Xanthophoren vorkommen (DANIEL, 1928; HOGBEN, 1936; WARING, 1936), fehlen den Knorpelfischen die brillanten roten, gelben, blauen und grünen Farben der Knochenfische. Im allgemeinen weisen Selachier graue und braune Farben der Haut auf, die auf der Oberseite dunkler und an der Bauchseite heller sind. Dort sind die mit Guaninkristallen gefüllten Leukophoren (Iridocyten) im Corium vorhanden und geben der Haut einen hellen, oftmals silbrigen Glanz. Es kommen aber auch Fleckenzeichnungen und Marmorierungen vor wie beim Leopardhai oder manchen Katzenhaien sowie bei Rochen z. B. Zitterrochen. Einige wenige Rochenarten tragen auffällige sog. Augenflecke, die im Zentrum blaue Farben zeigen und von einem braun-schwarzen und gelben Farbring umgeben sind (Texas-Rochen, gefleckter Zitterrochen). Einige Haie (Walhai, Stierkopfhai, die kleineren Stierkopfhaie) besitzen goldgelbe oder orange Fleckungen aus Xanthophoren, die mit den braunen oder rötlichen Melanophoren zusammen auffallende Zeichnungen der Haut ergeben. Die Farben können aber auch verändert werden, je nach dem Untergrund der Umgebung und den Lichtverhältnissen. Die Selachier sind in unserem Zusammenhang die erste Tiergruppe, bei denen ein Farbwechsel genauer untersucht ist; wir haben bei den Cyclostomen bereits auf die Beeinflussung der Pigmentzellen hingewiesen. Es ist daher zweckmäßig, kurz einige allgemeine Erscheinungen beim *physiologischen Farbwechsel* zu beschreiben. Ein solcher Farbwechsel geht in einer relativ kurzen Zeit vor sich und ist nicht durch eine quantitative Zunahme der Pigmente bedingt, d. h. die Zahl der Pigmentzellen und die in den Zellen enthaltene Menge des Pigmentes bleiben trotz des Farbwechsels gleich. Es wird vielmehr das Pigment in den Zellen verschoben, so daß in der Aufsicht auf die Haut die im einzelnen vom Pigment überdeckten Flächen sich verändern. Früher wurde von einer Kontraktion bzw. Expansion der Pigmentzellen gesprochen, in Verkennung der tatsächlich ablaufenden Vorgänge. In Wirklichkeit liegt aber Aggregation bzw. Dispersion der Pigmentgranula im Zelleib der Pigmentzellen vor. Ist in einem Hautabschnitt in allen Melanophoren das Pigment (in Form der festen Granula) bis in die feinen Zellausläufer verteilt, so wird eine absolut größere Fläche der Haut von Pigment überdeckt als wenn die Zellen ihre Pigmente in der Nähe des Zellkernes zusammenballen und der übrige Zellkörper mit seinen weit verzweigten Ausläufern durchscheinend ist. Die Pigmentzellen sind also ein Effektorsystem. Der physiologische Farbwechsel beruht auf einem einfachen Vorgang in Hunderttausenden von Pigmentzellen. Liegen solche verschiedenfarbigen Zellen in mehreren Schichten übereinander, so können durch Verdecken oder Freigeben der einen oder anderen Schicht ganz unterschiedliche und brillante Farbwechsel hervorgerufen werden. Für die Effektoren = Pigmentzellen kann man nun, unabhängig von dem gesamten Effekt am Tier, einen objektiven Index zur Beurteilung des Farbwechsels aufstellen, indem man das Maß der Pigmentverlagerung in den Zellen berücksichtigt: von der völligen Zusammenballung im Zentrum der Zelle bis zur völligen Ausbreitung der Granula bis in die feinsten Zellausläufer. Gute Zusammenfassungen, die sich mit den Fragen des physiologischen Farbwechsels befassen, finden sich bei FINGERMAN (1963) und WARING (1963). Die Ursachen zu einer Beeinflussung der Pigmentzellen in Richtung auf einen Farbwechsel können in Wahrnehmungen mit den Augen liegen und sind für gewöhnlich als Untergrund-Effekte bekannt: ein Tier dunkelt auf dunklem Untergrund in der Farbe nach, d. h. Melanophoren verteilen das Pigment im Zellkörper; auf hellem Untergrund wird die Haut heller, es kommt zu einer Zusammenballung des Pigmentes in den Melanophoren. Auch unter Ausschaltung der Augen kann noch ein Farbwechsel bei verschiedenen Lichtverhältnissen durchgeführt werden; man sagt dann, die Pigmentzellen seien ihre eigenen Receptoren und damit „unabhängige Effektoren". Wie lückenhaft eine solche Betrachtung ist, zeigt unsere Kenntnis von den photolabilen Pigmenten der Haut heute, auf die bei den Neunaugen ausführlicher eingegangen worden ist. Bei der direkten Lichteinwirkung ist der Effekt gerade umgekehrt wie bei dem Untergrundeffekt: Dunkelheit bewirkt eine Aufhellung der Tiere, Licht eine stärkere Dunkelfärbung. Schließlich gibt es Ursachen, die mit Licht überhaupt nichts zu tun haben, nämlich innere Erregungszustände der Tiere wie z. B. bei

Verletzungen, in der Brunstzeit usw.; sie können sehr rasche Farbwechsel bewirken. Die Verlagerung der Pigmentgranula in den Zellen ist an isolierten Fischschuppen (MATTHEWS, 1931; VERNE und VILTER, 1935; KINOSITA, 1963), in Gewebekultur an Amphibien-Melanophoren (KULEMANN, 1960; NOVALES und NOVALES, 1966) und bei Pigmentzellen des Guppy (Lebistes reticulatus) auch elektronenmikroskopisch (FALK und RHODIN, 1957) untersucht worden, so daß ein genauer Einblick in die Vorgänge gewonnen wurde. MATTHEWS gibt in seinen Beobachtungen und schönen Zeichnungen eine unmißverständliche Vorstellung von der Verlagerung des Pigmentes in den Melanophoren (Fundulus heteroclitus). Übereinstimmend läßt sich zeigen, daß die Pigmentzellen keine Flächenveränderungen erfahren, wenn die Pigmentgranula verlagert werden. Läßt man bestimmte Hormone auf die Melanophoren einwirken, so wandern die Granula in die Ausläufer der Zellen, und bald ist die Zelle von gleichmäßig verteilten Pigmentkörnern erfüllt. Auch direkte Belichtung erzielt einen Effekt: bei Pigmentzellen des Krallenfrosches (KULEMANN, 1960), des Grasfrosches (ZETTNER, 1956), des blinden mexikanischen Höhlenfisches (BURGERS, BENNINK und VAN OORDT, 1963), sowie der Eidechse Anolis (HADLEY, 1931) werden in der Gewebekultur oder an isolierten Hautstücken bzw. Schuppen die Pigmentgranula in den Zellen bis in die Ausläufer transportiert. Der Bewegungsvorgang hängt von der Anwesenheit von ATP ab. Da FALK und RHODIN (1957) ein besonderes Endoplasma in den Melanophoren nachweisen konnten, in dem fibrilläre Elemente eingebettet sind, besonders zahlreich an der Grenze Ekto-Endoplasma, so ist an der Abhängigkeit der Pigmentbewegungen von Plasmabewegungen nicht zu zweifeln. Vor allem deshalb nicht, weil in jüngster Zeit für Amöben mit einer verbesserten Technik ganz ähnliche Fibrillen, ebenfalls an der Grenze Ekto-Endoplasma gehäuft, elektronenmikroskopisch nachgewiesen und ihre Abhängigkeit der Funktion von ATP wahrscheinlich gemacht werden konnte (S. DANNEEL, 1965; BHOWMICK, 1966). Wir dürfen also sagen: im Grunde beruht der physiologische Farbwechsel der Tiere darauf, daß die Farbzellen mittels fibrillärer Differenzierungen ihres Cytoplasmas die Granula in der Zelle transportieren, entweder durch echte Verkürzung der Fibrillen nach dem Gleitmechanismus der Fibrillen quergestreifter Muskeln (S. DANNEEL, 1965), oder durch Erzeugung lokaler Plasmaströmungen nach dem Muster amöboider Bewegungen. Damit wird das Effektorsystem der Pigmentzellen aber noch interessanter, als es ohnehin schon ist, denn die Frage der direkten Hormoneinwirkung bekommt dadurch eine außerordentliche Bedeutung für den physiologischen Farbwechsel. KINOSITA (1963) nimmt allerdings an, daß bei der Einwirkung der Hormone Zellpotentiale verändert werden, so daß die Granula elektrophoretisch entlang von elektrischen Potentialgradienten wandern sollen.

Welche Hormone regulieren nun im Körper das Verhalten der Pigmentzellen? Die Ausbreitung des Pigmentes in den Melanophoren, Xantho- und Erythrophoren wird durch eine Gruppe von Hormonen bewirkt, die in der Pars intermedia der Hypophyse synthetisiert und als MSH (melanocyte-stimulating-hormone), MDH (melanin-dispersing-hormone) oder auch Intermedin bezeichnet werden. Seit der Extraktion aus Hypophysen (LERNER und LEE, 1956; LEE und LERNER, 1956) ist eine große Zahl von Untersuchungen über Natur und Struktur dieser Hormone gemacht worden (Zusammenfassungen bei KARKUN und LANDGREBE, 1963; WARING, 1963; GESCHWIND, 1966; SCHWYZER, 1966). Es sind Polypeptide von geringem Molekulargewicht, deren Zusammensetzung aus Aminosäuren bekannt und deren Synthese im Laboratorium für mehrere Hormone gelungen ist. Die Hypophyse macht zwei Gruppen von MSH: α-MSH und β-MSH, die sich in der Reihenfolge der Aminosäuren und der Molekülgröße unterscheiden. Während aber α-MSH von allen Tierarten, die bisher untersucht wurden, immer in gleicher Form aufgebaut wird, ist β-MSH bei den verschiedenen Tierarten etwas unterschiedlich zusammengesetzt. Sowohl α-MSH (vgl. BOISSONAS, 1962; HOFMANN, WOOLNER, SPÜHLER und SCHWARTZ, 1958; HOFMANN, WOOLNER, YAJIMA, SPÜHLER, THOMPSON, SCHWARTZ, 1958; HOFMANN, 1960; SCHWYZER und LI, 1958; SCHWYLER, COSTOPANAGIOTES und SIEBER, 1963) als auch ein β-MSH, das dem aus Rinderhypophysen gewonnenen entspricht (SCHWYZER, KAPPELER, ISELIN, RITTEL und ZUBER, 1959; SCHWYZER, ISELIN, KAPPELER, RIMIKER, RITTEL und ZUBER, 1963), konnten bisher synthetisiert werden. Um den Wirkungsmechanismus der Hormone zu klären, sind in verschiedenen Laboratorien auch analoge Verbindungen aufgebaut und auf ihre Melanophoren-stimulierende Wirkung geprüft worden (z. B. GUTTMANN und BOISSONAS, 1961; LEE, LERNER und BUETTNER-JANUSCH, 1963). Ein weiteres Hypophysenhormon, das auf die Nebenniere wirkt (ACTH), ist in seinem Aufbau aus Aminosäuren dem MSH ähnlich, so daß es ebenfalls auf die Pigmentzellen wirkt, wenn auch nicht in der intensiven Weise wie MSH. Auch ACTH ist inzwischen in mehreren Laboratorien synthetisiert worden, da es für die Klinik und die Dermatologie das wichtigste der Melanophorenhormone ist (HOFMANN, YAJIMA, YANAIHARA, LIU, LANDE, 1961; HOFMANN, YAJIMA, LIU und YANAIHARA, 1962; LI, MEIENHOFER, SCHNABEL, CHUNG, LO und RAMACHANDRAN, 1961; RABEN, LANDOLT, SMITH, HOFMANN, YAJIMA, 1961; SCHWYZER und SIEBER, 1963). Eine gegenteilige Wirkung übt ein Hormon der Epiphyse aus, das Melatonin (LERNER, CASE, TAKAKASHI, LEE, MORI, 1958; LERNER, CASE, HEINZELMAN, 1959). Nach seiner Extraktion konnte die Struktur ebenfalls aufgeklärt werden. Es bewirkt eine Zusammenballung des Pigmentes in den Melanophoren und läßt damit die Tiere hell werden. Geringe Abwandlungen beim Aufbau seines Moleküls haben zur Folge, daß die Intensität seiner Wirkung stark absinkt (LERNER und LEE, 1962). Die hochwirksame, d. h. natürliche Form des Melatonins kann als ein Antagonist zum MSH betrachtet werden, da es ebenso wirksam wie dieses ist und in Melanocyten, die unter MSH-Wirkung die Pigmentausbreitung vorgenommen haben, eine Konzentration der Granula hervorruft. Der Antagonismus Hypophyse-Epiphyse konnte für Amphibien von BAGNARA (1964) sehr klar gezeigt werden. Nun reagieren aber bei einer direkten Belichtung die Pigmentzellen des bekannten Krallenfrosches unterschiedlich; Xenopus scheint eine Ausnahme zu dem für Amphibien festgestellten Sachverhalt zu sein, daß die Melanophoren bei Belichtung ihr Pigment ausbreiten, bei Dunkelheit im Zentrum aggregieren. Im Schwanz, auch im Falle einer Isolierung, erfolgt im Licht bei Krallenfroschlarven eine Zusammenballung des Pigmentes, so daß die Gewebe hell und durchsichtig sind. Bei Dunkelheit breitet sich das Pigment aus. Im übrigen Körper dagegen zeigen die Melanophoren das umgekehrte Verhalten und folgen damit der allgemeinen Regel: Licht bewirkt eine Ausbreitung des Pigments, Dunkelheit die Zusammenballung. BAGNARA (1960) hat diese Widersprüche durch eine interessante Hypothese zu klären versucht. Aus der Zeitdauer, die jeweils bei der Pigmentverlagerung im Bereich des Körpers und im Schwanz notwendig ist, schließt er auf die Synthese einer photochemischen Substanz in der Schwanzhaut, die im Licht in kurzer Zeit verändert wird. Diese Substanz bewirkt die Ausbreitung des Pigmentes in den Schwanzmelanophoren. Wenn wir an die photolabilen Pterine denken, die bereits bei den Neunaugen erwähnt und in der Haut von Amphibienlarven ebenfalls vorhanden sind, so erhält diese Annahme eine sehr große Wahrscheinlichkeit. Auf der anderen Seite ist die Epiphyse der niederen Wirbeltiere lichtempfindlich, da sie einem der beiden Augen des phylogenetisch alten zweiten Augenpaares entspricht und Zellelemente enthält, die den Stäbchen und Zapfen der Retina vergleichbar sind (KELLY und

v. d. Kamer, 1960; Eakin, 1961; Eakin und Westfall, 1961, Oksche und Vaupel-v. Harnack, 1965). Bei Dunkelheit schüttet die Epiphyse Melatonin aus, eine Aufhellung der Tiere erfolgt. Offensichtlich müssen diese Vorgänge dadurch unterstützt werden, daß der Schwellenwert für Melatonin bei den Schwanzmelanophoren höher liegt als bei den Körpermelanophoren.

Um aber den Farbwechsel vollständig zu verstehen muß man wissen, daß auch Adrenalin und Noradrenalin eine Zusammenballung des Pigmentes und damit eine Aufhellung der Tiere bewirkt. Das ist für Fische, Amphibien und Reptilien bekannt (Wright, 1955; Wright und Lerner, 1960; Burgers, Bennink und van Oordt, 1963; Zimmerman und Dalton, 1961; Kleinholz, 1938). Allerdings ist Melatonin 100000fach wirksamer als Adrenalin (Lerner, Case und Takahashi, 1960); bereits 1 µg/ml Aquarienwasser läßt bei Krallenfroschlarven für lange Zeit die Pigmentaggregation in den Melanophoren vor sich gehen. Damit wird die Frage einer nervösen Beeinflussung des Farbwechsels erneut zu stellen sein. Von Fischen und Reptilien ist der direkte nervöse Einfluß auf Pigmentzellen bekannt, z. T. sogar mit einer Doppelinnervation. Bei Amphibien ist der nervöse Einfluß nicht direkt zu erkennen, aber auch nicht auszuschließen. Noradrenalin ist eine der Transmittersubstanzen an Synapsen, und da außerdem adrenergische Systeme im Zentralnervensystem bekannt geworden sind und für Amphibien sogar in der Pars intermedia der Hypophyse nachgewiesen werden konnten (Enemar und Falck, 1965), ist eine zweifache Möglichkeit zur nervösen Beeinflussung der Pigmentzellen gegeben. Im Gegensatz dazu geht der Einfluß durch das Auge beim Untergrundeffekt über eine Steuerung der Ausschüttung von MSH vor sich (Dierst und Ralph, 1962). Beim Frosch ist nachgewiesen worden, daß eine Zerstörung des Hypothalamus eine starke Herabsetzung der Ausschüttung von MSH zur Folge hat (Kastin und Ross, 1965). Die mögliche Einwirkung des Hypothalamus auf die Pars intermedia der Hypophyse sieht Etkin (1962) in der nervösen Verbindung zwischen diesen beiden Teilen und zieht aus seinen morphologischen und experimentellen Befunden den Schluß, daß eine neurosekretorische Bahn vom Hypothalamus den Zwischenlappen kontrolliert. Durch die zahlreichen bekannt gewordenen Faktoren beim Zustandekommen des physiologischen Farbwechsels ist heute keineswegs eine allgemein verbindliche und gültige Theorie über den Mechanismus und seine Gliederung aufzustellen. Sowohl eine „Ein- Hormontheorie" als eine „Zwei-Hormontheorie" und schließlich die nervöse Kontrolle sind als Erklärungen herangezogen worden. Ohne Zweifel ist der Mechanismus bei der Vielfalt der Tiere keineswegs einheitlich.

Der *Farbwechsel bei den Selachiern* zeigt einen sehr deutlichen Untergrund-Effekt: Haie und Rochen auf dunklem Boden eines Aquariums werden dunkler gefärbt; über hellem Boden verblassen die Farben. Dieser Effekt ist zeitabhängig und braucht mehrere Tage bis zum Maximum seiner Ausprägung, außerdem spielt die Belichtung eine wichtige Rolle. Von der Pigmentausbreitung bzw. Aggregation sind epidermale und dermale Melanocyten betroffen. Die Abhängigkeit dieses Effektes von der Hypophyse ist seit langem bekannt (Hogben, 1936; Parker, 1936, 1938; Vilter, 1937; Waring, 1936, 1938). Entfernung des Hypophysenhinterlappens mit der Pars intermedia führt zu einer Aufhellung der Tiere, d. h. Zusammenballung des Pigmentes in den Melanophoren. Wird danach aber Hypophysenextrakt injiziert, so färbt sich die Haut wieder dunkel. Dieser Effekt kann aber schon dadurch erzielt werden, indem Blut von dunklen Tieren in helle Tiere übertragen wird. Waring (1942) konnte außerdem zeigen, daß in der Dunkelheit (d. h. bei der langsamen Aufhellung) in den Hypophysen der Tiere mehr MSH gespeichert ist als bei Tieren im Licht. Die Beteiligung des Nervensystems beim Untergrund-Effekt ist nicht geklärt. Durch Reizung im Rückenmark läßt sich eine Aufhellung der zugehörigen Hautsegmente erreichen (VILTER, 1937) und auch die Durchschneidung der Flossennerven verursacht auf dunklen Flossen helle Bänder (PARKER, 1936; WARING, 1938). Dagegen zeigt die Zerstörung des ganzen Brachialplexus (ABRAMOWITZ, 1939) an den Brustflossen und der Umgebung in der Haut keine Aufhellung. Da der Effekt der Aufhellung bei Durchtrennung der Nerven aber in wenigen Minuten vor sich geht, muß an die Wirkung von Adrenalin gedacht werden, da auch die Injektion von Adrenalin eine Zusammenballung des Pigmentes und damit die Aufhellung von Haien und Rochen verursacht. ABRAMOWITZ gibt außerdem zu bedenken, daß bei den Operationen im Gehirn auch die Hypophyse beschädigt worden sein könnte. Neuere Untersuchungen liegen darüber nicht vor. Es muß noch besonders vermerkt werden, daß junge Tiere den Untergrund-Effekt schneller zeigen, und daß ferner die Individuen recht unterschiedlich reagieren können und der Nagelrochen überhaupt keinen Effekt zeigt. — Die Beteiligung des Auges an der Beeinflussung der Hautfärbung läßt sich durch „geblendete" Tiere zeigen, denn sie nehmen eine mittlere Färbung an, die aber von der Belichtung abhängig ist (HOGBEN, 1936); auf belichtetem weißen Untergrund werden die Tiere etwas dunkler als auf belichtetem dunklen Untergrund. Es ist zu erwarten, daß heute weitere Untersuchungen folgen werden, denn inzwischen lassen sich an betäubten Haien in den großen marinen Versuchslaboratorien dunkle Plastikschalen auf die Augen setzen, so daß die gleichen Tiere unter verschiedenen Bedingungen geprüft werden können und damit individuelle und jahreszeitliche Schwankungen auszuschalten sind.

c) Das Seitenlinien-System, Funktion und Bedeutung als Fern-Tastsinnesorgan

Bei den Knorpelfischen ist das System der Seitenlinien-Sinnesorgane in typischer Form und vollem Umfang entwickelt. Die Neunaugen besaßen, wie wir festgestellt hatten, nur flache Sinnesgruben, die phylogenetisch als Vorläufer eines Seitenlinien-Systems bewertet werden. Die Bedeutung, die das voll ausgebildete Seitenlinien-System bei Knorpel- und Knochenfischen und den Amphibienlarven und in einigen Fällen auch noch für erwachsene aquatische Amphibien (z. B. Krallenfrosch) besitzt, besteht in der Möglichkeit einer Wahrnehmung selbst sehr geringer Wasserbewegungen und Wasserströmungen, so daß die Fähigkeit der Seitenlinien-Organe mit Recht als „Ferntastsinn" (DIJKGRAAF, 1934) bezeichnet wird. Im inkompressiblen Medium Wasser ist dieser Ferntastsinn für die Orientierung, das Auffinden von Beute, für die Stellung des Körpers zur Strömung (in Flüssen, bei Gezeiten, bei stärkeren Meeresströmungen usw.) notwendig. Je nach der Durchsichtigkeit des Wassers ist ja der Gesichtssinn für größere Entfernungen nur sehr beschränkt wirksam. Die Haut übernimmt damit in Anpassung an die aquatische Lebensweise die Aufgabe der Kommunikation mit der Umwelt, auf die einleitend hingewiesen wurde, obwohl sie andererseits in zunehmendem Maße eine osmotische Barriere sein muß. LOWENSTEIN (1957) bezeichnet die Wirkungsweise der Seitenlinie sogar als die eines Echolotes, indem die Wasserwellen bei der Bewegung des Fisches von nahen Objekten reflektiert werden und so ihre Anwesenheit verraten. Sehr gute Zusammenfassungen über Funktion und Struktur der Seitenlinien-Organe sind von WRIGHT (1951), DIJKGRAAF (1952, 1963) und LOWENSTEIN (1957) geschrieben worden.

Das sog. *Seitenlinien-System* besteht aus einer sehr großen Zahl von einzelnen Sinnesknospen, den Neuromasten, wie sie in der Grundstruktur schon bei den Neunaugen vorhanden sind. Diese Sinnesknospen sind reihenartig angeordnet, und von den Knorpelfischen ab wird ein Teil von ihnen in Hautkanäle versenkt.

Die übrigen Sinnesknospen bleiben als oberflächliche, freie Neuromasten im Körperepithel eingeschaltet. Alle Sinnesknospen in der äußeren Bedeckung eines Tieres gehören also zum System der „Seitenlinie", die ihren Namen von dem besonders auffälligen Teil an der Körperseite der Fische hat; die „Seitenlinie" tritt oft durch starke Pigmentierung hervor und verläuft von der Kiemenregion etwa in der Mitte der Körperseite bis zum Schwanz. Am Kopf sind mehrere Reihen (auf dem Unterkiefer, an den Augen, am Oberkopf) in wechselnder Ausbildung vorhanden; und eine weitere Reihe von Sinnesknospen ist als Rückenlinie bis zur Rückenflosse angeordnet. In der Regel werden bei allen Fischen die Sinnes-

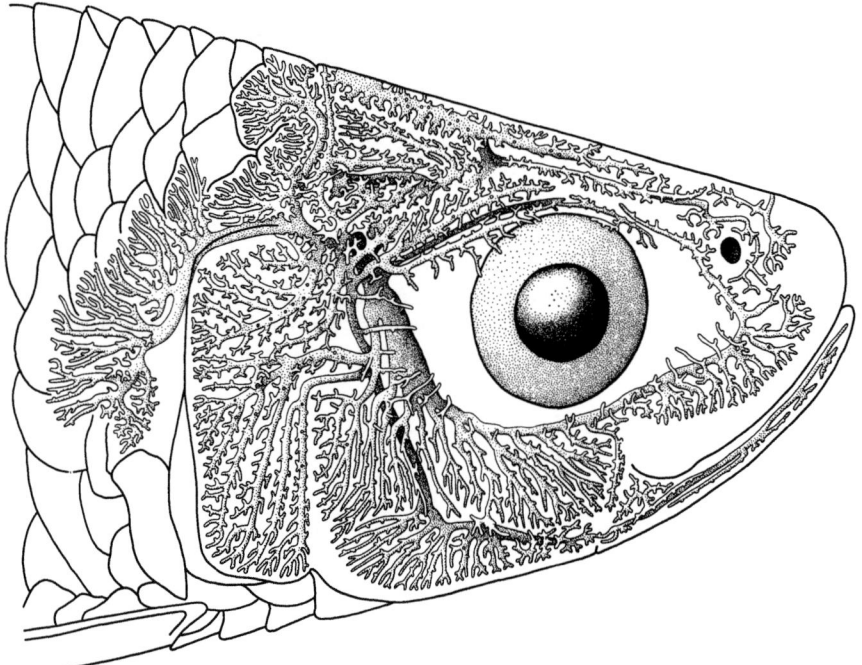

Abb. 5. Kopf der Sardine (Clupea pilchardus Walb.) mit den Kanälen der Seitenlinienorgane. Von den ursprünglichen Längskanälen zweigen zahlreiche Nebenkanälchen ab, so daß bis hinter den Kiemendeckel das gesamte Kopfgebiet vom Lateralisorgan erfaßt wird. (Verändert nach WOHLFAHRT, 1938)

knospenreihen am Kopf und auf der Seite bei der Entwicklung in Kanäle der Haut versenkt, die Rückenlinie und weitere Sinnesknospen am Kopf bleiben als oberflächliche Sinnesgruben oder -hügel bestehen. Bei den Amphibien wird der ursprüngliche Zustand beibehalten, so daß keine Kanalsysteme entstehen; außerdem kommen häufig drei parallele Reihen an der Körperseite vor, eine Anordnung, die an die primitiveren Verhältnisse der Cyclostomen erinnert. Die verschiedene morphologische Ausbildung der Seitenlinien und der Seitenlinienkanäle kann hier nicht berücksichtigt werden. Abb. 5 zeigt nur einen sehr instruktiven Fall: Bei der bekannten Sardine des Mittelmeeres fehlen am Rumpf die Seitenlinien (WOHLFAHRT, 1937). Dafür sind die Kanäle am Kopf ganz besonders verzweigt angelegt und mit zahlreichen kleinen Ästen ausgestattet. — Die durchgehenden Kanäle mit den Sinnesknospen am Kopf und am Rumpf stehen durch segmental angeordnete dünne Röhrchen mit der Oberfläche in Verbindung (Abb. 6a). Bei den beschuppten Fischen münden die Öffnungen der Röhrchen entsprechend ihrer Entstehung aus oberflächlichen Epitheleinsenkungen über den Schuppen, so daß die Schuppen um diese Röhrchen herum aufgebaut werden; die Schuppen werden also von den zuführenden Kanälchen „durchsetzt". Das System dieser zahlreichen Röhrchen ermöglicht es, an jeder Stelle des versenkten Seitenlinienkanals Wasserströmungen auch kleinsten, d. h. eng begrenzten Umfanges (feine Wasserstrahlen z. B. im Experiment) aufzunehmen und die Flüssigkeit im System in Bewegung zu setzen.

Die *Innervation* der Sinnesknospen erfolgt durch Hirnnerven, und zwar durch besondere Äste des V., VII., X. und XI. Am Kopf sind Äste des Trigeminus und der sog. Lateralis anterior als Teil des Facialis vorhanden, am Rumpf der sog. Lateralis posterior des Vagus und evtl. des Glossopharyngicus. Die Ursprungskerne in der Medulla liegen nahe beieinander und stehen mit der Ursprungsregion des Stato-Acusticus in Verbindung. Man faßt daher das Lateralissystem mit dem Statoacusticussystem zusammen als eine physiologische und durch die phylogenetische Entstehung auch morphologische Einheit auf, zumal der Sinnesapparat im Vestibularorgan dem der Sinnesknospen im Seitenliniensystem in vielen Einzelheiten ähnlich ist. Auch bei Tieren, die ein Cerebellum entwickelt haben, bleiben die Wurzeln der Lateralisnerven in der Medulla. Schließlich müssen noch die ungewöhnlich großen Mauthnerschen Neurone in der Medulla erwähnt werden, deren Axone als Riesenfasern durch das Rückenmark bis zum Schwanz ziehen. Die Mauthnerschen Neurone sind von den Cyclostomen bis zu den Amphibien vorhanden und koordinieren die Schwimmbewegungen des Schwanzes und der Körpermuskulatur (STEFFANNELLI, 1951; WILSON, 1959). Jedes der beiden Neurone besitzt außerordentlich zahlreiche Dendriten, mit denen u.a. Verbindungen zu den Kernen des Vestibularapparates und des Lateralissystems aufgenommen werden. Außerdem sind Zellkörper und Dendriten mit vielen Synapsen bedeckt (ROBERTSON, BODENHEIMER und STAGE, 1963), die von Neuronen der genannten Kerne und aus dem Tectum opticum, dem sensorischen Ganglion des Trigeminus und vom Nucleus motorius tegmenti stammen. Die zentrale Verknüpfung des Lateralissystems mit den Gleichgewichts- und Bewegungszentren zeigt die große Bedeutung, die bei den wasserlebenden Formen den Seitenlinienorganen zukommt.

Der *Aufbau der Sinnesknospen* ist im Prinzip bei allen Tieren gleich und sehr gut bekannt (DIJKGRAAF, 1952; FLOCK und WERSÄLL, 1962; FLOCK und DUVALL, 1965; GÖRNER, 1962, 1963; HAMA, 1962, 1965; MURRAY, 1955; TRUJILLO-CENÓZ, 1961). Das normale Körperepithel wird in einer platten- oder birnenförmigen Sinnesknospe durch hohe Zellen ersetzt: Stützzellen, die von der Basalmembran bis an die Oberfläche reichen; vielfach ist an der seitlichen Begrenzung der Knospe ein Mantel besonders dünner und langgestreckter Stützzellen vorhanden, welche die Knospe schalenförmig umgeben können und manchmal als besondere Zellen: sog. Mantelzellen angesehen worden sind (vgl. Abb. 3a). An der Basalmembran liegen flache, indifferente Epithelzellen, die entweder eine geschlossene basale Zellschicht bilden können oder als einzelne Zellen zwischen Stützzellen eingeschlossen werden. Bei einer Verletzung von Sinnesknospen, etwa durch mechanische Einwirkung oder durch Parasitenbefall, und beim Absterben alternder Zellen werden von den basalen indifferenten Epithelzellen neue Stützzellen und neue Sinneszellen geliefert (GRONER, 1940). Eingeschlossen von den Stützzellen werden im Zentrum der Knospe die eigentlichen Sinneselemente: sekundäre, kurze Sinneszellen, deren Zellkörper die Basalmembran nicht erreichen und auf der basalen Seite verbreitert sind. An der Apex tragen die Sinneszellen feine Sinneshaare: ein echtes Kinocilium mit den typischen Innenstrukturen aller Cilien und Geißeln, und etwa 50 Stereocilien, die einfachen Mikrovilli gleichen. Die Cilien ragen in eine gelatinöse Masse hinein, welche als Cupula auf der Sinnesknospe sitzt und etwa 0,1 mm lang ist. Bei den freien Sinnesknospen ist die Cupula lang und schmal (vgl. Abb. 16), bei den versenkten Knospen dagegen ist sie dem Lumen des Kanals angepaßt und breiter, so daß sie den Kanal wie eine kegelförmige Scheibe an dieser Stelle verschließt.

Eine Reizung der Sinneszellen erfolgt also nicht durch unmittelbaren Zugang des Außenmediums zu den „Sinneshaaren", sondern durch die Verbiegung der Cupula und damit die Bewegung aller Cilien aller Sinneszellen einer Knospe unter der Cupula. Wie FLOCK und WERSÄLL (1963) sowie FLOCK und DUVAL (1965) zeigen konnten,

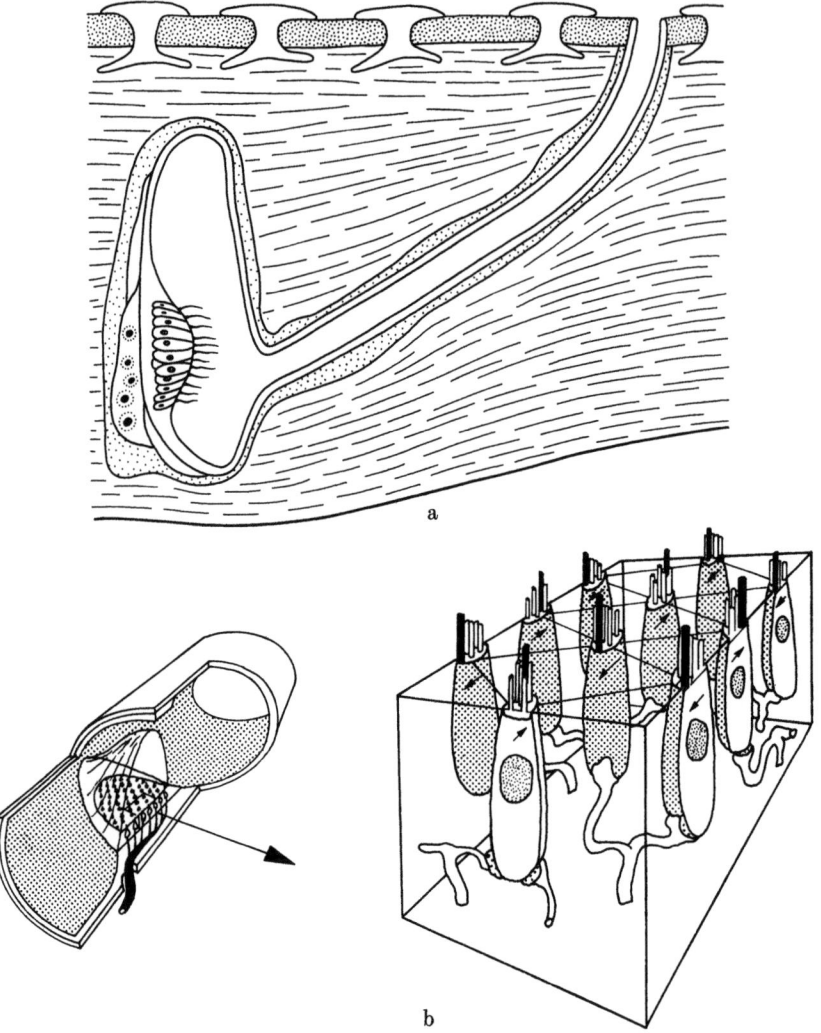

Abb. 6a u. b. System der Seitenlinie. a Schematischer Schnitt durch einen Seitenlinienkanal beim Hai. Es ist ein zuführender Kanal gezeigt, der von der Oberfläche in den quer geschnittenen eigentlichen Seitenlinienkanal reicht; dort liegt eine Sinnesknospe (Neuromast), die Cupula ist nicht dargestellt; die darunter liegenden Nervenfasern des Lateralisnerven sind im Querschnitt zu denken. Das Kanalsystem ist von einem Fasermantel umhüllt. (Schematisch, nach GILBERT, 1962.) b Die Lage der Cilien auf den Sinneszellen eines Neuromasten und die Axone in einem schematischen Blockdiagramm (von FLOCK und WERSÄLL, 1962); links die Lage des Neuromasten mit der Cupula im Seitenlinienkanal, rechts die Sinneszellen: schwarz die Kinocilien, die Pfeile geben die Richtung an, in der die Cupula abgebogen werden muß, um eine Erhöhung der Frequenz der Impulse zu erzeugen

sind die Sinneszellen in einer Knospe verschieden; abwechselnd sitzt das Kinocilium entweder auf der zum Kopf gerichteten Seite der Zelle oder auf der zum Schwanz gerichteten Seite (Abb. 6b). Die benachbarten Zellen einer in der Achse des Kanals ausgerichteten Reihe haben also die Kinocilien jeweils auf der entgegengesetzten Seite stehen. Außerdem ist am Basalkörper des Kinociliums nur an der von den Stereocilien abgewendeten Seite eine besondere Differenzierung vorhanden. Diese Befunde sind für die Erklärung der Funktion der Sinneszellen von größter Bedeutung. Es ist bekannt, daß ein Wasserstrom vom Schwanz zum Kopf, der also die Cupula einer Sinnesknospe zum Kopf hin beugt, in den ableitenden Nervenfasern einer Sinnesknospe zwei Effekte erzeugt: Ein Teil der Axone zeigt eine erhöhte Frequenz der Impulse, ein anderer Teil dagegen eine Hemmung im Sinne einer Abnahme der Impulsfrequenz (SAND, 1937; DIJKGRAAF, 1965; GÖRNER, 1961). Wird der Wasserstrom umgekehrt, so zeigen die vorher gehemmten Axone eine Erhöhung der Impulsfrequenz und die vorher stärker erregten Fasern eine Hemmung und Frequenzverminderung. Da im Gleichgewichtsorgan des Stachelrochens die gleichen Verhältnisse hinsichtlich des Aufbaues und der Anordnung der Sinneszellen und der Erregung der Axone vorliegen, kann an der tatsächlichen Bedeutung der Befunde nicht gezweifelt werden (LOWENSTEIN und WERSÄLL, 1959; LOWENSTEIN, OSBORNE und WERSÄLL, 1964; FLOCK, 1964). Das bedeutet also, daß die Abbiegung der Cupula in einer Richtung bei den Sinneszellen, an deren Kinocilium die Differenzierung des Basalkörpers in der Richtung des verbiegenden Wasserstromes liegt, den ableitenden Axonen eine exzitatorische Erregung vermittelt, und bei den Sinneszellen, deren Basalkörper gegen den Wasserstrom stehen, die hemmende Erregung auf die Axone übertragen wird. Damit ist im Grunde die Funktion der Seitenlinienorgane geklärt. Ergänzend muß gesagt werden, daß von den Sinnesknospen auch in Ruhe ständig Impulse weitergeleitet werden (Dauerentladung). Aus dieser Form der Funktion geht auch hervor, daß die Seitenlinien nicht dem Hören dienen können, wie DIJKGRAAF immer wieder betont hat, um der irrigen Ansicht vom Hören der Fische mit der Haut entgegenzutreten. — Entsprechend der Funktion ist die Innervation der Sinnesknospen nicht einfach gestaltet. Alle Sinneszellen besitzen an ihrem breiten basalen Zellpol eine Synapsenzone, an der freie Axone mit becherförmigen, knopfartigen oder tief in Einbuchtungen der Sinneszellen vorspringenden Fortsätzen angeschlossen sind; synaptische Vesikel sind vorhanden. Die vom Ast des Lateralisnerven kommenden Axonbündel verlaufen in der Haut zunächst parallel der Oberfläche und geben kleinere Bündel an Gruppen von Sinnesknospen ab. Die Axone treten durch die Basalmembran und liegen zwischen den Stützzellen. Dort hört die Myelinscheide auf und die freien Axone kommen mit den Sinneszellen in Verbindung. Die Axone haben aber keineswegs alle den gleichen Durchmesser. HAMA (1962) bestätigt die Befunde anderer Autoren (KATSUKI, YOSHINO und CHEN, 1951) über die Anwesenheit von zwei Typen von Axonen, indem er auch zwei Typen von Axonenden an den Sinneszellen beim japanischen Aal elektronenmikroskopisch nachweist. Die gröbere Morphologie der Innervation bei Sinnesknospen des Krallenfrosches (MURRAY, 1955) könnte ein Anhalt für physiologisch verschiedenartige Axone sein. Beim Krallenfrosch wird jede Knospe von zwei etwa gleichen Ästen des Lateralisnerven versorgt; sie verlaufen im Stratum spongiosum eine Strecke weit parallel zueinander. Vor dem Eintritt in die Sinnesknospe verzweigen sich die Bündel und lösen sich dann in der Knospe in die Axone auf. Diese Anordnung ist erstaunlich regelmäßig ausgebildet. Eine zweite Innervation erfolgt aber noch durch ein unregelmäßig ausgebildetes Bündel dünner Axone, das getrennt von den „Zwillingsbündeln" in die Knospe eintritt und dort ebenfalls dann seine Axone an Sinneszellen verteilt. Es besteht also die Möglichkeit, daß neben der Richtung des Wasserstromes auch die Intensität der Abbiegung der Cupula wahrgenommen wird. Denn beim japanischen Aal zeigen die dünnen Axone eine Dauerentladung und einen niedrigen Schwellenwert für die Veränderungen der Lage der Cupula, die dickeren Axone dagegen machen keine Dauerentladung und sprechen erst auf stärkere Reize an, haben also einen höheren Schwellenwert (KATSUKI, YOSHINO und CHEN, 1951; KATSUKI und YOSHINO, 1952).

Die *Cupula* wird von den Sinneszellen gebildet. Merkwürdigerweise sezernieren die Sinneszellen in Form feiner Tröpfchen ein Material, das auf der Oberfläche der Sinnesknospe zur Cupula zusammenfließt (GRONER, 1940) und zwischen den „Sinneshaaren", also Stereo- und Kinocilien eine „Sekretstreifung" zeigt. Beim Krallenfrosch sind die Sekretgranula in den Sinneszellen PAS-negativ (MURRAY, 1955) und färben sich mit Toluidinblau und Nilblausulfat metachromatisch rot. Die oben angeführten elektronenmikroskopischen Arbeiten zeigen Sekretgranula in verschiedener Dichte im apikalen Teil der Sinneszellen, so daß an der Sekretbildung kein Zweifel bestehen kann.

Das *Seitenliniensystem der Selachier* folgt im wesentlichen dem dargestellten typischen Verlauf. In einigen Formen aber, z.B. den Haien Heptanchus und Chlamydoselache sind primitive Verhältnisse beibehalten worden, indem die Sinnesknospen nicht in Kanäle versenkt wurden, sondern nur in flachen Epithelrinnen angeordnet sind. Besonders spezialisierte Teile des Seitenliniensystems sind die tief eingesenkten Lorenzinischen Ampullen, die mit langen, gallertgefüllten Kanälen an der Außenfläche der vorderen Körperteile münden; sie sind bei Haien und Rochen ausgebildet (über Aufbau und Funktkon vgl. MURRAY, 1962; DIJKGRAAF, 1963). Beim Zitterrochen (Torpedo) liegen etwa 100 völlig geschlossene blasenförmige, versenkte Sinnesknospen auf jeder Seite der elektrischen Organe und in der Umgebung der Nasengruben. Auch sie gehören zum Seitenliniensystem (SZABO, 1958). Schließlich gibt es sog. Grubenorgane bei Haien und Rochen, die den Geschmacksknospen ähnlich sind. Es handelt sich aber nach der Innervation um Sinnesknospen der Seitenlinie, die durch eine Auffaltung des Corium und des Epithels in kleine enge Gruben versenkt sind (vgl. BUDKER, 1958).

Die *Innervation der Haut der Selachier* erfolgt außer vom Lateralissystem der Hirnnerven auch von sensorischen Fasern der Spinalnerven (WUNDERER, 1908; WEDELL, 1941; LOWENSTEIN, 1956). Aus einem doppelt angelegten Plexus im Corium steigen Faserbündel zur Epidermis, wo Axone zwischen die Epithelzellen vordringen und ein Geflecht freier Nervenendigungen bilden. Besonders dicht sind diese Nervenplexus im Epithel der Flossen. Beim Übertritt in die Epidermis verlieren die Axone ihre Myelinscheide. Zwischen den Stützelementen der Flossensäume, den sog. Flossenstrahlen: hornige Stäbe dermalen Ursprungs, liegen besondere Tastkörperchen, sog. Terminalkörperchen nach WUNDERER. Es sind rundlich-ovale Gebilde aus Bindegewebszellen, ähnlich einem Meißnerschen Körperchen; aus dem Plexus an der Basis der Flossen ziehen Nerven in die Flossen und geben Äste an die Terminalkörperchen ab. Dort dringen die Axone zwischen die Polsterzellen des Körperchens vor und bilden ein Geflecht; die Myelinscheide hört am Rande des Gebildes auf. LOWENSTEIN (1956) konnte diese alten Befunde bestätigen und in elektrophysiologischen Versuchen zeigen, daß es sich um echte Pressoreceptoren handelt; sie sind gewissermaßen Proprioceptoren, da sie durch ihre Reizung die Verformung der Flossen angeben. Es wäre interessant zu wissen, in welcher Weise sie mit dem Lateralissystem und den Mauthnerschen Neuronen verknüpft sind, da die Flossen bei den Schwimmbewegungen und vor allem bei den Haien beim Angriff auf eine Beute (Brustflossen!) eine wesentliche Funktion haben. Interessanterweise haben sich bisher ähnliche Terminalkörperchen bei Knochenfischen nicht nachweisen lassen.

3. Teleostei (Knochenfische)

Die Haut der Knochenfische ist im allgemeinen gekennzeichnet durch ihre Schuppen. Sie sind, anders als die Hautzähnchen der Selachier, im Bindegewebe des Corium eingebettet und stets von der Haut überdeckt. Bei der außerordentlich großen Zahl von Arten (über 20000) und den verschiedensten Lebensräumen des Wassers, die von Fischen bewohnt werden, ist eine Abwandlung dieses allgemeinen Grundtyps eines Hautskeletes selbstverständlich. Einmal existieren verschiedene Schuppenformen, deren Ausbildung bei den Fischen durch die Verwandtschaft der Gruppen untereinander bestimmt wird. Zweitens kann durch eine weitgehende Reduktion der Schuppen eine lederartige oder weiche Haut entstehen (z. B. Welse, Aale). Drittens können große Skeletplatten der Haut den Körper in einen starren Panzer einschließen (Seepferdchen, Mondfisch, Kofferfisch). Die Vielfalt der Hautstruktur bei Fischen wird in den großen Zusammenfassungen von RAUTHER (1927), RABL (1931), SCHNAKENBECK (1955), VAN OOSTEN (1957) und BERTIN (1958) beschrieben.

Das *Epithel* ist bei allen Fischen vielschichtig, die Dicke und die Zahl der Zellschichten sind aber bei den Arten sehr verschieden. So können über Knochenplatten nur zwei Epithelschichten auf der Haut vorhanden sein, in der Regel bedecken aber 10—30 Schichten die Haut (Abb. 7). Auch die Körperteile zeigen eine sehr regionalspezifische Differenzierung im Aufbau der Haut. Am Kopf fehlen häufig die Schuppen, und die Epidermis ist dicker als am übrigen Körper; ebenfalls ist die Bauchseite anders beschaffen als Seiten und Rücken usw. Eine 7 cm lange Elritze hat ungefähr eine Epidermisdicke von 100 µ, beim erwachsenen Hecht ist die durchschnittliche Dicke 100—150 µ (PFEIFFER, 1960; KRAUSE, 1923). Die Größe des Fisches ist also nicht von sehr wesentlicher Bedeutung. Eine Zusammenfassung von Meßergebnissen geben HARDER (1964), PFEIFFER (1960), RABL (1931). Die Schichten von Epithelzellen sind nur sehr unregelmäßig übereinandergelagert. Auf der Basalmembran sitzen hochprismatische indifferente Epithelzellen als Stratum basale (Str. germinativum). Mitosen sind in diesen Zellen häufig. Zahlreiche Lymphocyten können in den Intercellularspalten vorhanden sein. Die nach außen folgenden Zellen sind unregelmäßig spindelförmig gestaltet, ähnlich wie es bereits für Neunaugen und Selachier beschrieben wurde. Die oberen Epithelschichten setzen sich aus polygonalen Zellen zusammen und werden von stark abgeflachten Zellen gegen die Außenfläche abgedeckt. Oberflächliche Differenzierungen auf der Deckzellenschicht, die gewissermaßen ein Stratum cuticulare bilden, sind als Cuticularräume, Deckplatten oder Schleimüberzüge in mannigfacher Form beschrieben worden. Auf die möglichen Oberflächendifferenzierungen wurde bereits mehrfach hingewiesen. Die Epithelzellen aller Schichten enthalten Tonofibrillen und überspannen die breiten Intercellularspalten mit Zellbrücken. Die Verzahnung der Zellen untereinander und die Ausbildung von Desmosomen an den Kontaktstellen sind ebenso wie die Tonofibrillen elektronenmikroskopisch nachzuseisen (MULLINGER, 1964). Eine Verhornung der Zellen kommt nur in bestimmten Familien vor (Cypriniden, Catastomiden), indem zur Laichzeit beim Männchen und in einigen Arten auch beim Weibchen sog. Perlorgane ausgebildet werden. Am Kopf, auf dem Rücken, an den Seiten und auf den Brustflossen entstehen kleine Hornwarzen, meist über dem Rande der Schuppen und oft in regelmäßiger Anordnung. Es können sogar längere stachelartige Gebilde sich entwickeln; nach Beendigung der Laichperiode fallen Warzen und Stacheln wieder ab. An der Stelle der Perlorgane sind große Epithelzellen mit Granula als eine Art Keimlager dauernd vorhanden. Sie vermehren sich mit Beginn der Laichzeit sehr stark, so daß ein kleiner Zellkegel sich über die benachbarte Epidermis erhebt. In den oberflächlichen Zellschichten setzt eine Verhornung ein, so daß feste Lagen von zusammenhängenden Hornschuppen eine feste Spitze bilden. Leider ist über die hormonelle Steuerung dieses Vorganges und die Herkunft der Perlorgane nichts bekannt. Sinnesknospen fehlen im Bereich der Wucherungen, so daß ihre Homologie mit dem Epithel der Sinnesknospen vermutet wurde.

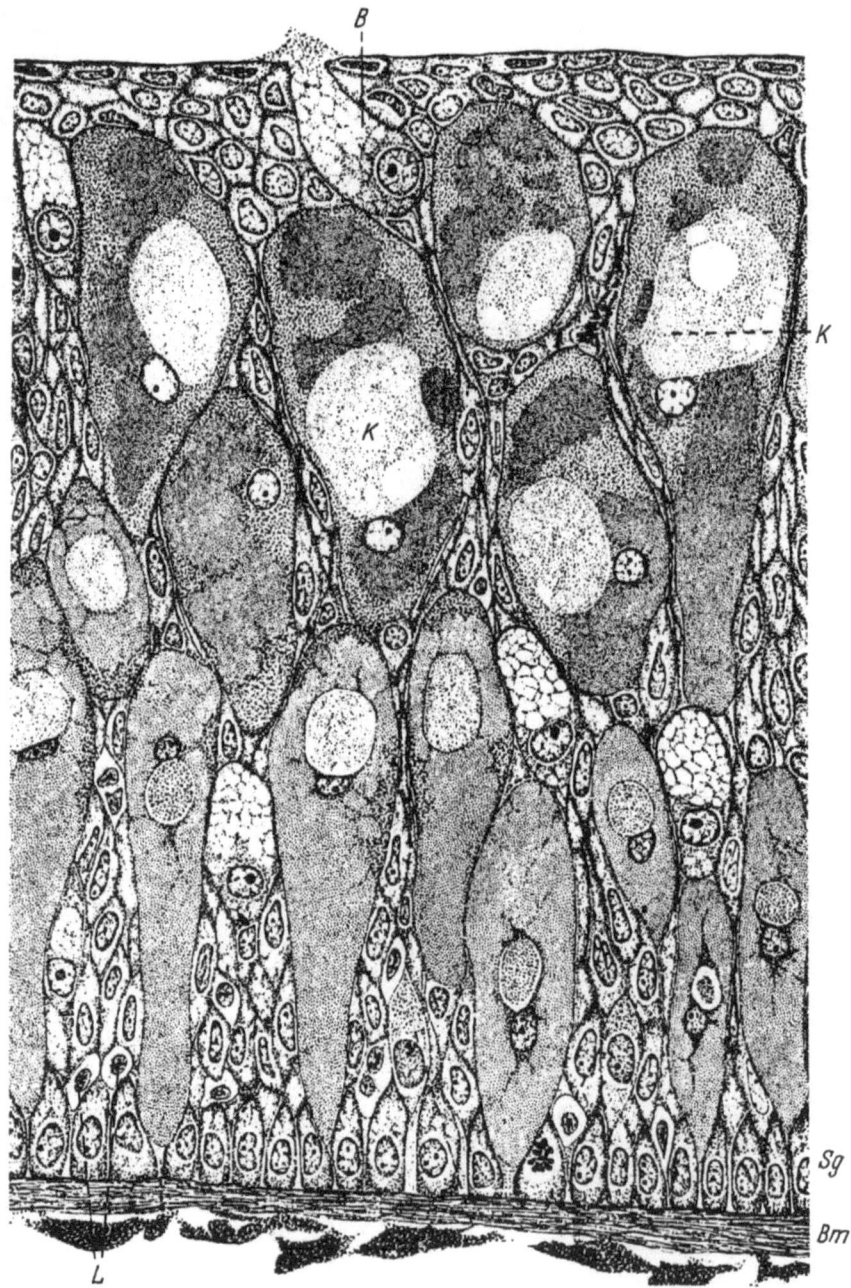

Abb. 7. Hautepithel von der Körperseite eines erwachsenen Aals. (Nach AUST, 1936.) Neben den Becherzellen (Schleimzellen) sind sehr zahlreiche Kolbenzellen im vielschichtigen Epithel vorhanden. Über dem klar abgegrenzten Stratum germinativum liegen eingewanderte Lymphocyten. Bezeichnungen: *B* Becherzellen, *Bm* Basalmembran, *K* Kolbenzellen, *L* Lymphocyten, *Sg* Stratum germinativum

Drüsenzellen sind in der Fischhaut sehr zahlreich vorhanden. Einfache *Becherzellen* von typischem Aufbau sind in allen Differenzierungsstadien in den mittleren Schichten zu finden und entleeren an der Oberfläche ihr schleimiges Sekret. Bei manchen Arten sind außerdem seröse Drüsenzellen vom Typ der *Körnerzellen* vorhanden, wie wir sie bei den Selachiern und Neunaugen genannt haben (Panzerwelse, dem im Holothuriendarm lebenden Fierasfer, ,,Himmelsgucker" Uranoscopus, Seepferdchen, Petermännchen u.a.) und erhebliche Größen erreichen können und in den mittleren Zellschichten liegen. Ebenfalls nur bei bestimmten Gruppen vorhanden sind die *Kolbenzellen*, der dritte Typ von Drüsenzellen bei Fischen. Es sind große Zellen von gestreckter Gestalt, z.B. bei der Elritze 40 μ hoch und 17 μ im Durchmesser; ähnliche Größen werden von verschiedensten Fischen berichtet. Es gibt aber auch kleinere und abgerundete Kolbenzellen. Meist sitzen sie mit der Zellbasis auf der Basalmembran auf und strecken ihren verdickten Zellkörper in die oberen Epidermisschichten; dadurch bekommen sie ein kolbenförmiges Aussehen. Der dichte homogene Zellinhalt läßt in der Nähe des Zellkernes (manchmal auch zwei Zellkerne) eine Vacuole erkennen. Durch ihre Morphologie erinnern sie an die Kolbenzellen der Neunaugen, aber der Zellinhalt scheint doch sehr wesentlich verschieden davon zu sein. Bei manchen Arten enthält die Epidermis sehr viele Kolbenzellen, so daß nur dünne Stränge von Epithelzellen zwischen den Zellen übrigbleiben. Bei anderen Arten sind nur wenige Kolbenzellen vorhanden; außerdem können Kolbenzellen gar nicht mit der Basalmembran in Verbindung stehen. PFEIFFER (1960, 1962) ist der Meinung, daß ganz verschiedene Zellen als ,,Kolbenzellen" beschrieben worden sind und nimmt an, daß ,,echte" Kolbenzellen nur auf bestimmte Gruppen von Fischen beschränkt sind. Sie sollen einen sog. Schreckstoff produzieren, der bei einer Verletzung der Haut frei wird und eine Schreckreaktion bei den anderen Tieren hervorruft. Dabei ist es wichtig, daß viele dieser Arten Fischschwärme bilden. Da aber noch keine neueren Untersuchungen über die Feinstruktur und die Entwicklung der verschiedenen Kolbenzellen vorliegen, muß abgewartet werden, ob solche ,,echten Kolbenzellen" besondere Alarmsubstanzen produzieren und welche Funktionen die übrigen großen Drüsenzellen der Haut haben. Ähnlich wie bei den Selachiern kommt es bei bestimmten Formen zur Einsenkung der Epithelalveolen, in denen gehäuft Drüsenzellen im Epithel ausdifferenziert sind. Echte Drüsen kann man diese Komplexe aber nicht nennen. Sie werden als *Giftdrüsen* an der Basis von Stacheln (Petermännchen, Skorpionfische, Froschfische u.a.) oder der Brustflossen (Welse, BAILEY und TAYLOR, 1950) vor allem von bodenbewohnenden Fischen benutzt. Wie bei den Selachiern sind es auch hier nur wenige moderne Untersuchungen, die Aufschluß über die tatsächliche Giftwirkung und ihre Physiologie geben. Beim Rotfeuerfisch (Familie der Skorpionfische), einem in Zoo-Aquarien wegen seiner Farben und seines bizarren Aussehens häufig gehaltenen Fisch, sind in den großen Stacheln der Flossen ähnlich wie bei den Stacheln der Selachier tiefe Einsenkungen, in denen das Epithel besondere Drüsenzellen enthält (HALSTEAD, CHITWOOD und MODGLIN, 1955). Sie sind groß, von polygonaler Form und enthalten feine Granula. Dieses Gift und das von verwandten Skorpionfischen (Steinfische) läßt sich aus den Drüsensäckchen als eine helle Flüssigkeit gewinnen, analysieren und auf seine physiologische Wirkung prüfen (SAUNDERS, 1959, 1960). Das Gift verursacht bei geringer Dosierung im Experiment beim Kaninchen einen starken Abfall des Blutdruckes, der nicht durch Beeinflussung des Sympathicus hervorgerufen wird. Die Wirkung beruht auf einer bestimmten Fraktion des Sekretes, die aus Protein oder einer Mischung von Proteinen besteht und in geringen Mengen Mäuse bereits tötet. Am Kaninchen ließ sich neben dem Abfall des Blutdruckes eine verstärkte Atmung und bei höheren Dosen schließlich Atmungsstillstand bei sehr geringem Blutdruck feststellen. Im EKG ist Tachykardie, Vorhofflimmern und eine nicht näher in der Ursache definierte Schädigung des Myokards zu sehen. Außer den unangenehmen und schmerzhaften lokalen

Folgen bei einer Verletzung durch Stacheln der Skorpionfische sind also tatsächlich erhebliche Vergiftungserscheinungen möglich. Beim großen und kleinen Petermännchen, die beide auch in der Nordsee vorkommen, sind die scharfen Stacheln der Rückenflossen eine häufige Verletzungsursache und besitzen ebenfalls Giftdrüsen; die starken Schmerzen nach dem Stich können beim Schwimmen eine Gefährdung der betroffenen Person darstellen. Die sorgfältigen Untersuchungen von HALSTEAD und MODGLIN (1958) sowie RUSSEL und EMERY (1960) lassen eine große Ähnlichkeit der Giftwirkung mit der von Stechrochen erkennen. Der Blutdruck fällt rapide ab, es kommt zu unregelmäßigem Herzschlag und ischämischen Schäden im Herzmuskel. Die Atmung wird unregelmäßig, wahrscheinlich durch den geringen Blutdurchfluß in der Pulmonalis. Dagegen zeigt sich keine Beeinflussung der neuromuskulären Synapsen, wie oft angenommen wurde. 3—8 ml des rohen Drüsenextraktes wirken bei Katzen und Hunden letal.

Das Epithel wird, besonders in den basalen Schichten, oft von zahlreichen *Wanderzellen*, vor allem *Lymphocyten* durchsetzt.

Eine deutlich abgegrenzte *Basalmembran* unterlagert das Epithel. An besonders günstigen Objekten mit dicker Basalmembran konnte RABL (1931) zeigen, daß die basalen Epithelzellen mit feinen Fortsätzen in einer dünnen Schicht der Grundsubstanz verankert sind und dann erst auf eine dichte Schicht feinster, maskierter Fasern treffen. An der Haut der Rückenflosse des japanischen Fisches Chasmichthys konnte FUJII (1966) elektronenmikroskopisch zeigen, daß die Basalmembran unter den Epithelzellen mit einer homogen erscheinenden Schicht beginnt und dann etwa 18 Lagen kollagener Fibrillen folgen, die in regelmäßiger Weise parallel verlaufen und deren Verlaufsrichtung von Lage zu Lage um 90° wechselt, also den gleichen Aufbau bedingen wie bei allen bisher bekannt gewordenen Basalmembranen in Haut und Cornea von Wirbeltieren. Flach ausgebreitete Fibrocyten liegen der Unterseite der Basalmembran an, doch auch Melanophoren können diese Lage einnehmen. Beim Goldfisch ist die Basalmembran der beschuppten Haut 7000—8000 Å dick und von entsprechendem Aufbau (LOUD und MISHIMA, 1963). Aus der Basalmembran strahlen feine Fasern senkrecht in das *Corium* ein, welches in seinem oberen Teil locker aufgebaut ist und daher als Stratum laxum bezeichnet wird. Die Entstehung von Basalmembran und Corium ist bei Embryonen verschiedentlich untersucht worden, wir verweisen auf die Verhältnisse bei Amphibienlarven, wo vor allem elektronenmikroskopische Studien die Vorgänge um den Aufbau der Bindegewebsschichten aufgehellt haben. Der innere Teil des Corium ist durch parallel gelagerte Faserbündel, die sich schichtweise überkreuzen, besonders dicht und zugfest und wird wegen seines Aufbaues Stratum compactum genannt. Seine innere Struktur wird besonders gut sichtbar, wenn durch Trypsinverdauung die Epidermis und das lockere Bindegewebe entfernt werden und dünne Schichten des Corium in Flächenpräparaten unter polarisiertem Licht photographiert werden (FAURE-FREMIET, 1938) (Abb. 8). Die Überkreuzung der Schichten in Winkeln zwischen 60—90° tritt als schachbrettartiges Muster mit unregelmäßig großen Feldern hervor. Durchsetzt werden diese Schichten von elastischen Fasernetzen und vertikalen Bündeln kollagener Fasern. Entsprechend der Körperform sind Dicke des Stratum compactum und die Winkel, in denen sich die Schichten überlagern, sehr unterschiedlich. Bis zu 50 Schichten kollagener Fasern können das Stratum compactum aufbauen, wodurch natürlich eine sehr feste, lederartige Beschaffenheit der Fischhaut zustande kommt. Beim Stör ist z.B. das Stratum compactum 5 mm dick; in der Regel ist die Dicke in der Rückenhaut 200—600 μ (HARDER, 1964). Die Schichten der Haut, vor allem die Epidermis, werden während des Wachstums vom geschlüpften Jungfisch zum erwachsenen Individuum z.T. erheblich in ihrem Aufbau verändert. Besonders weitgehende Abwandlungen der Epidermis erfolgen bei solchen Arten, die eine Metamorphose durchmachen, wie z.B. der Aal bei seiner Wanderung aus dem Meer in die Flüsse. Nicht nur die Größe der Larven, sondern auch die verschiedenen osmotischen Bedingungen beim Wechsel von Salz- in Süßwasser wirken sich aus. Beim Aal nimmt mit dem Wachstum der Larven auch die Zahl der Epithelzellenschichten zu, während der Übergang ins Süßwasser vor allem die Ausdifferenzie-

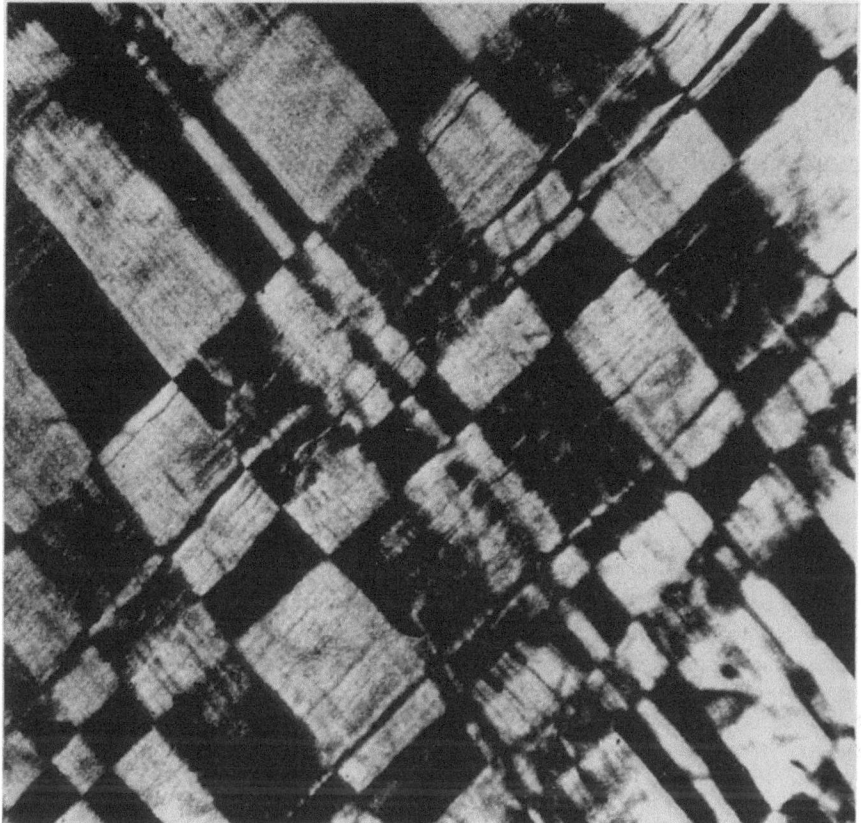

Abb. 8. Fischhaut; Aufsicht auf die frei präparierte Faserbündelschicht des Corium im Bereich des Stratum compactum, polarisiertes Licht. Die Überkreuzung der doppelbrechenden Kollagenfaserbündel wird als Muster durch Auslöschen bzw. Aufleuchten des Materials sichtbar (FAURÉ-FRÉMIET, 1938)

rung von Drüsenzellen (besonders der großen Kolbenzellen) bewirkt (AUST, 1936). Bei der Abwanderung der laichreifen Aale ins Meer erfolgt ein erneuter Umbau unter Zerfall von Epithelzellen.

Durch eine meist dünne *Subcutis* wird die Verbindung zur Muskelfascie hergestellt. Das Gewicht der frischen Haut kann 6—10% des Körpergewichts ausmachen (VAN OOSTEN, 1957) und der hohe Gehalt an kollagenen Fasern des Corium bedingt die industrielle Verwertung zur Bereitung von Fischleim. Doch unterscheidet sich das Kollagen der Haut verschiedener Fischarten. Durch Erwärmung läßt sich eine Denaturierung des Kollagens erreichen, die sich durch sog. thermische Schrumpfung zeigt: die Fasern schrumpfen bei einer bestimmten Temperatur irreversibel. Diese Temperatur ist spezifisch für bestimmte Kollagene (GUSTAVSON, 1955) und hängt mit der Lebensweise der Fische zusammen: bei Tiefsee- und Kaltwasserfischen liegt die kritische Temperatur je nach Art bei

37—45° C, bei Warmwasserfischen oder Fischen aus Oberflächenwasser dagegen bei 50—57°. Diese auffallende Übereinstimmung konnte bei einer großen Zahl europäischer und japanischer Fische nachgewiesen werden. Die Analyse der beteiligten Kollagene zeigt, daß die kritische Temperatur um so tiefer liegt, je weniger Hydroxyprolin im Kollagenmolekül vorhanden ist, d.h. mit steigendem prozentualen Anteil des Hydroxyprolin steigt auch die Temperatur für die thermische Schrumpfung. Diese für die Untersuchung der Kollagene sehr wichtigen Befunde haben dazu geführt, daß Kollagene der Fischhaut weiter analysiert wurden, um die molekulare Organisation zu klären (PIEZ und GROSS, 1960). Die intramolekulare Stabilität des Kollagens könnte durch Wasserstoffbrücken des Hydroxyprolins bewirkt werden, so daß weniger Hydroxyprolin auch eine geringere Stabilität bewirken würde. PIEZ und GROSS (1960) zeigen aber, daß es die Pyrrolidinringe des Prolins und Hydroxyprolins sind, welche die intramolekulare Stabilität bedingen; die Wasserstoffbrücken dienen dem intermolekularen Verband und bleiben in der Zahl immer gleich; denn bei sinkender Beteiligung von Prolin und Hydroxyprolin werden die fehlenden Hydroxybindungen durch andere Aminosäuren (Serin und Threonin) ersetzt. So führt eine biologische Eigentümlichkeit im Aufbau des Corium-Kollagens der Fischhaut zu wesentlichen Ergebnissen über den Zusammenhalt molekularer Strukturen. Daß eine für die Fischarten wesentliche biologische Bedeutung im speziellen Kollagenaufbau verborgen sein muß, ist demnach zwingend anzunehmen.

Das Stratum laxum (auch Str. spongiosum oder Str. vasculare genannt) des Corium muß noch genauer betrachtet werden. In dieser Schicht liegen die charakteristischen Bestandteile der beschuppten Fischhaut: die *Schuppen*. Ferner sind die zahlreichen *Farbzellen* dort vorhanden, welche die z.T. intensiven Farbmuster und den physiologischen Farbwechsel hervorrufen. Und schließlich ist das Stratum laxum reich an *Nerven und Capillaren*, so daß eine besondere Hautatmungsfunktion bei vielen Fischen ausgebildet ist.

Die *Schuppen* sind integumentale Skeletbildungen, plattenförmig und so im Stratum laxum eingelagert, daß ihr innerer Teil dem Stratum compactum aufliegt und der periphere Teil mit einer faserigen Schicht unter der Epidermis verankert ist. Die Schuppen durchbrechen also im Gegensatz zu den Placoidschuppen der Selachier nicht die Epidermis, sondern werden stets davon verdeckt. Zumeist liegen die Schuppen dachziegelartig übereinander angeordnet, doch sind die Unterseite: der Schuppenboden und die Oberseite: das Schuppendach von einer faserigen Schuppentasche umschlossen. Zwischen diese Schuppentaschen kann Basalmembran und Epidermis in flachen Furchen eingesenkt sein. Es gibt ihrer Form nach zwei Typen von Schuppen bei den heute lebenden Knochenfischen: Rundschuppen (Cycloidschuppen) und Kammschuppen (Ctenoidschuppen). Erstere sind rundlich mit glattem Rand, Kammschuppen besitzen eine gerade hintere (körpernahe) Kante mit feinen Zähnchen: dem Kamm. Im einzelnen ist die Form der Schuppen sehr stark von der Körperregion und dem Alter der Tiere abhängig und erheblichen Veränderungen unterworfen, doch sind Cycloidschuppen bzw. Ctenoidschuppen Gruppenmerkmale, die aber über die „Primitivität" einer Fischgruppe keine Auskunft geben können. Beide Schuppentypen leiten sich phylogenetisch von den altertümlichen Ganoid- und Cosmoidschuppen her. Jede Schuppe trägt auf ihrer Oberseite radiäre Einkerbungen, die von einem Zentralfeld zur Peripherie verlaufen. Auffälliger dagegen sind die konzentrisch angeordneten Furchen, die sich um das Zentralfeld anordnen. Form und Oberflächenstruktur einer Schuppe kann als Klassifikationsmerkmal dienen, wenn die Schuppe ausgewachsen ist (VAN OOSTEN, 1957). Jede Schuppe besteht aus einer fibrillären Platte (NEAVE, 1940; WALLIN, 1956), die sich aus dünnen Schichten parallel gelagerter kollagener Fibrillen zusammensetzt. Darauf ist eine Knochenschicht aufgelagert, deren Oberfläche von den genannten Reliefstrukturen geprägt wird. Im Bereich der radiären Furchen fehlt die Knochenschicht, so daß die fibrilläre Platte am Grunde der Furchen auch von der Oberseite zugänglich ist. Die Struktur der Schuppen kommt durch ihre Entwicklung zustande. Bereits bei sehr kleinen Tieren (12—50 mm Körperlänge) werden Ansammlungen von Fibroblasten in der Cutis gebildet, die eine dermale Papille darstellen. Besondere Verhältnisse abweichender Art kommen vor, wenn zunächst eine Larvenform entwickelt und dann eine Metamorphose durchgemacht wird (z.B. die Glasaale des Aales). Die Anordnung der Papillen bleibt regelmäßig und reihenförmig, so daß die Schuppen später ebenfalls in regelmäßigen Reihen, von der Seitenlinie beginnend, über den Körper ventral und dorsal angeordnet sind. Beim Wachstum der Tiere werden neue Reihen zwischengeschaltet, so daß gewisse Unregelmäßigkeiten in Form scheinbar verzweigter Reihen entstehen. Zwischen den Zellen der dermalen Papille tritt sehr bald Bindegewebsgrundsubstanz auf, in der Fibrillen sichtbar werden. Durch die sich in die Länge streckende zentrale Fasermasse werden die Zellen in eine obere und eine untere Schicht auseinandergedrängt und sitzen nun der sich erweiternden Faserplatte als Skleroblasten auf. In der oberen Schicht der Faserplatte setzt dann die Einlagerung von Mineralsalzen [überwiegend $Ca_3(PO_4)_2$, $Mg_3(PO_4)_2$, $CaCO_3$] in großen Kristallen ein. Dabei werden aber keine Zellen eingeschlossen, und auch keine Kanälchen bleiben ausgespart, so daß eine homogen erscheinende Knochenschicht (sog. Hyalodentin) entsteht. Ist der Prozeß abgeschlossen, so verschwinden die Skleroblasten auf der Unter- und Oberseite der entstandenen Platte. Das weitere Wachstum der Schuppen erfolgt nur am Rande der Platten, wodurch die konzentrischen Ringe entstehen. Auch die älteren Schuppen herangewachsener Tiere zeigen daher kein Dickenwachstum, sondern nur ein Flächenwachstum. In einigen Fischarten, z.B. beim Goldfisch erfolgt jedoch noch eine dünne Auflagerung weiterer Mineralsalze auf die Schuppenoberseite. Da sich beim Wachstum der Tiere auch die Körperoberfläche vergrößert und neue Schuppen nicht mehr angelegt werden können, muß durch Flächenwachstum der Schuppen gewährleistet werden, daß eine lückenlose Bedeckung des Körpers durch Schuppen erhalten bleibt. Dieser Vorgang ist die Grundlage für eine Altersbestimmung von Fischen. In den gemäßigten Klimazonen erfolgt entsprechend dem Nahrungsangebot ein rhythmisches Wachstum der Tiere, das im Herbst allmählich zum Stillstand kommt (vgl. BROWN, 1957) und außer vom Nahrungsangebot von sehr verschiedenen Faktoren abhängt. Das Flächenwachstum der Schuppen ist während der Wachstumsperiode ebenfalls gesteigert und erlischt dann, so daß einer der konzentrischen Ringe entsteht, die oben als Relief der Schuppen genannt wurden. Starke Wachstumsphasen zeigen sich als breite Ringe der Schuppen, ähnlich wie die Jahresringe am Baumholz. In wärmeren Gewässern verwischen sich aber die rhythmischen Wachstumsvorgänge. Die Bestimmung der Wachstumsvorgänge hat für die Fischerei sehr große Bedeutung; aus genauen Untersuchungen lassen sich Vorhersagen über zu erwartende Fangergebnisse der kommenden Jahre machen oder geben bei Fischkulturen über notwendige Fütterungsmaßnahmen Aufschluß.

Bei Verletzungen der Fischhaut erfolgt eine *Regeneration der Schuppen* (NEAVE, 1940). Wird die einzelne Schuppe verletzt, was z.B. bei den wenigen großen Schuppen eines Spiegelkarpfens der Fall sein kann, so wandern die am Rande der Schuppen liegenden Skleroblasten in das verletzte Gebiet und bauen ähnlich wie bei der Entwicklung eine neue Schuppenplatte auf. Sind bei einer Verletzung zwar die Schuppen verlorengegangen, aber die bindegewebigen Umhüllungen (Schuppentasche) noch erhalten geblieben, so wird in kurzer Zeit eine neue

Schuppe gebildet, die sich kaum von der alten Schuppe unterscheidet. Vor allem von der Randzone, die ja Wachstumszone ist, wandern Skleroblasten in die Schuppentasche, bilden zuerst auf der unteren Bindegewebsfläche eine Zellschicht und füllen die Tasche mit Grundsubstanz und kollagenen Fibrillen. Die Mineralisierung beginnt dann im Zentrum und breitet sich zu den wachsenden Rändern der Platte aus. Dabei ist auch die Oberseite der sich bildenden Schuppe von Zellen bedeckt, die aber nicht wie bei echten Osteoblasten in die entstehende Hartsubstanz eingeschlossen werden. Ist bei der Verletzung das Corium so weit in Mitleidenschaft gezogen worden, daß Schuppentaschen zerstört wurden oder verlorengegangen sind, so dauert es Monate, bis neue Schuppen entstanden sind. Ihre Anordnung und Form weicht meist erheblich von den ursprünglichen Verhältnissen ab. In der verheilten Haut erfolgt eine Neubildung von dermalen Schuppenpapillen, und zwar in Anlehnung an die Schuppen des Wundrandes. Offenbar müssen Skleroblasten von anderen Schuppentaschen in das Hautregenerat einwandern, damit Papillen entstehen. Es gibt zahlreiche Fälle, in denen das Regenerat völlig ohne Schuppen bleibt. Entstehen aber Schuppen, so lehnt sich die Anordnung in gewisser Weise an die am Wundrand verbliebenen alten Schuppen an.

Die *Farbzellen* der Fischhaut enthalten entweder braune oder schwarze Melanine (Melanophoren), rote Farbstoffe (Erythrophoren), gelbe Farbstoffe (Xanthophoren) oder kristalline Plättchen von Guanin (Guanophoren oder Iridocyten), welche Licht reflektieren. Die leuchtenden Farben, z. B. der bekannten Korallenfische, des Neonfisches und vieler anderer Arten kommen durch Kombination der verschiedenen Farbzelltypen im durchscheinenden Stratum laxum zustande. Die Iridocyten unterlagern die übrigen Farbzellen in einer dichten Lage, so daß einfallendes Licht von den plattenförmigen Kristallen reflektiert wird, den Silberglanz der Fische bewirkt oder die Leuchtkraft der darüber angeordneten anderen Farbzellen erhöht. Die Kombination der Farbzellen ist in den prächtigen Farbtafeln von BALLOWITZ (1917) erstmals dargestellt worden. Die Feinstruktur aller Farbzelltypen ist aus elektronenmikroskopischen Untersuchungen gut bekannt (FUJII, 1966; BIKLE, TILNEY und PORTER, 1966; LOUD und MISHIMA, 1963; MATSUMOTO, 1965; MISHIMA und LOUD, 1963; FALK und RHODIN, 1957). Obwohl im differenzierten Zustand die Chromatophoren ganz verschiedene Farbstoffe enthalten, stammen sie aber alle vom gleichen Zellstamm ab: sie sind Derivate von Neuralleistenzellen (ORTON, 1953; HAMA und OBIKA, 1960; HAMA, 1963). Charakteristisch für alle Farbzellen sind die Pigmente, die in Form spezifischer Granula im Cytoplasma der Zellen vorkommen. Die Melanophoren sind weit verzweigte Zellen, in deren perinucleärem Zellkörper und den Zellausläufern Melanosomen liegen, die (in besonderer Struktur zusammengelagert) Melanine enthalten. Eben durch die corpusculäre Form der Pigmentorganelle ist überhaupt ein physiologischer Farbwechsel durch Transport der Pigmente in den Zellen möglich. Neben den schon beim Abschnitt Farbwechsel erwähnten Untersuchungen von FALK und RHODIN (1957) über den Mechanismus des Transportes der Granula sind erneute elektronenmikroskopische Befunde und Beobachtungen an isolierten Schuppen mit Melanophoren durch BIKLE, TILNEY und PORTER (1966) bekannt geworden. Diese Autoren finden Mikrotubuli (225 Å Durchmesser) von gestrecktem unverzweigtem Verlauf in den Melanophoren, die sich bei Aggregation und Dispersion der Granula in der Zelle nicht verändern. Die Granula scheinen auf festen Bahnen bewegt zu werden, so daß jedes Pigmentkörperchen wieder zu seinem Ausgangsort in der Zelle zurückkehrt. Die Bedeutung der Mikrotubuli wird so gedeutet, daß sie als Gleitbahnen dienen und den Weg der Granula bestimmen. Die Erythrophoren enthalten rote oder orange Pterine in runden Körperchen, den Pterinosomen, die eine geschichtete Innenstruktur besitzen (MATSUMOTO, 1965). Außerdem sind Carotinoide in den Zellen vorhanden, die in Lipoide gelöst sind und in dieser Form als Tropfen ebenfalls von einer Membran umschlossen werden (LOUD und MISHIMA, 1963). Die Xanthophoren besitzen gelbe und farblose, fluorescierende Pterine, eingeschlossen in Pterinosomen, sowie ebenfalls Carotinoide in gleicher Form gespeichert wie in Erythrophoren. Wegen ihres Lipoidgehaltes werden beide Zelltypen oft als Lipophoren bezeichnet; sie sind sternförmig verzweigt. Da die roten und gelben Pterine sowie die farblosen Verbindungen enge chemische Verwandtschaft aufweisen und ineinander übergeführt werden können, ist die Bezeichnung „Pterinophoren" (ZIEGLER, 1963) korrekter, da mit der Umwandlung der Pterine auch der Farbton wechselt, ein Xanthophor also zum Erythrophor wird. Als „Lipophoren" sollen nur Zellen bezeichnet werden, in denen der Pteringehalt ganz oder fast ganz reduziert worden ist und die Carotinoide die überwiegende Menge an Farbstoff bilden. Bereits früher wurde darauf hingewiesen, daß ein großer Teil der Pterine photolabil ist, und KAUFFMANN (1959) konnte zeigen, daß bei Zierfischen (Warmwasser) ein sehr hoher Anteil der Pterine in der Haut farblos ist. Dabei unterscheiden sich jedoch Xanthophoren und Erythrophoren im Gehalt an farblosen Pterinen, die fest an die Membranen der Pterinosomen gebunden sind (MATSUMOTO, 1965). Auf die mögliche Bedeutung der lichtempfindlichen Pterine als Quelle für eine Lichtrezeption der Haut wurde bereits hingewiesen. Die Iridocyten (Guanocyten) schließlich enthalten verschieden große Kristallplättchen, die sich isolieren lassen und deren Vergleich mit reinem Guanin zeigt, daß es sich um Kristallaggregate oder Einkristalle von Guanin handelt (NECKEL, 1954). Es ist zu vermuten, daß die Kristalle beim Farbwechsel ebenso wie die Farbstoffe der übrigen Farbzellen in den Zellen verlagert werden, da die Amphibieniridocyten auf Melanocyten-stimulierendes Hormon ansprechen (BAGNARA, 1958, 1964).

Der *physiologische Farbwechsel* der Fische kann sehr rasch vor sich gehen, wenn Tiere in Erregung versetzt werden. Seit den klassischen Untersuchungen durch v. FRISCH (1911) an der Elritze sind die Fische immer wieder wegen dieser schnellen Farbveränderungen, die sich z.T. in veränderten Zeichnungen der Haut äußern, untersucht worden. Es ist aber auch der langsamer verlaufende Untergrundeffekt, der bei den Selachiern im einzelnen erörtert wurde, festzustellen: auf dunklem Untergrunde werden die Tiere langsam dunkler in der Hautfarbe, auf hellem Untergrund blassen die Farben ab (Zusammenfassung bei WARING, 1963). Diese Veränderungen betreffen vor allem die Melanophoren, die bei der Dispersion des Pigmentes die Iridocyten abdecken und neben der Vergrößerung der einzelnen dunklen Farbflecke zugleich die Reflexion des „Silberglanzes" vermindern. Die Untergrundeffekte sind von der Hypophyse abhängig, die Einzelheiten wurden im Abschnitt über den physiologischen Farbwechsel beschrieben. Bei den Knochenfischen tritt aber ein neuer, komplizierender Faktor hinzu: es erfolgt eine nervöse Beeinflussung der Farbzellen. Der phylogenetisch ältere Zustand der Selachier und Cyclostomen, bei denen nur Hormone den Farbwechsel regulieren, wird also erweitert. Diese Komplikation ergibt bei den verschiedenen Knochenfischarten eine sehr unterschiedliche Reaktion unter experimentellen Bedingungen (vgl. WARING, 1963), so daß eine allgemeine, für alle Fische zutreffende Betrachtung der Faktoren beim Farbwechsel noch nicht möglich ist. Klar ist jedoch, daß Hypophysektomie bei Fischen ein Erblassen der Farben erzeugt; ferner, daß trotz Hypophysektomie ein langsamer Untergrundeffekt stattfindet. Schließlich erfolgt nach Injektion von Hypophysenextrakt eine Dunkelfärbung der Fische. Der Hormonwirkung steht die Beeinflussung durch Neurone entgegen. Bereits von FRISCH (1911) konnte die Beteiligung von Neuronen am Farbwechsel der Elritze zeigen; die Ganglienzellen sind durch Spinalnerven und sympathischen Ganglien mit den Farbzellen verbunden und bewirken eine Aggregation der Farbstoffe in den Zellen, also eine Aufhellung der Tiere. Die Axone der zentralen Ganglienzellen verlassen bei der Elritze das Rückenmark durch die spinalen Wurzeln in Höhe des 15. Wirbels, bei anderen Fischen durch Wurzeln mehrer Segmente des ZNS und verlaufen im Truncus sympathicus nach rostral und caudal; in den sympathischen Ganglien bilden sie Synapsen mit sympathischen Neuronen, und diese treten in der Haut mit ihren Axonen an die Farbzellen heran. Eine Durchtrennung der Axone führt zu einer Ausbreitung des Pigmentes in den betroffenen, d.h. von den durchtrennten Axonen innervierten Melanophoren (vgl. GRAY, 1956), wenn die Tiere auf hellen Untergrund eingestellt, also aufgehellt waren. Bereits sehr frühzeitig war die Innervation der Farbzellen nachgewiesen (BALLOWITZ, 1893) und von den Autoren z.T. als Doppelinnervation aufgefaßt worden (z.B. ABRAMOWITZ, 1935, 1936; PARKER und ROSENBLUETH, 1941; PARKER, 1942, 1945). Mit Sicherheit hat sich aber eine doppelte Wirkung, also Ausbreitung und Zusammenballung der Farbstoffe durch nervöse Kontrolle bisher nicht nachweisen lassen. Denn diese Kontrolle wird offenbar durch den Schwellenwert der Farbzellen für Farbwechselhormone kompliziert. Schon ABRAMOWITZ (1936) erkannte, daß Farbzellen in einem Tier verschieden reagieren können; Xanthophoren folgten anderen Reizen als Melanophoren (bei Fundulus). Außerdem kann trotz Injektion von Hypophysenextrakt eine Ausbreitung der Farbgranula in Melanophoren nicht erzielt werden, es sei denn, die zugehörenden Nerven sind durchschnitten worden. Es ergibt sich also, daß in manchen Arten die nervöse Kontrolle (zur Aggregation der Farbstoffe) die hormonale Wirkung der Hypophyse (zur Ausbreitung der Farbstoffe durch MSH) überwiegt. In anderen Arten dagegen ist ein Antagonismus vorhanden, dessen Gleichgewicht nur bei besonderen Zuständen zur einen oder anderen Seite verändert wird. Die Aufklärung der Struktur von Farbwechselhormonen und ihre chemische Darstellung (vgl. Abschnitt Farbwechsel) läßt erwarten, daß auch die noch ungeklärten Mechanismen des Farbwechsels bei Knochenfischen besser analysiert werden können. Für die Histologie ist wichtig, daß die alten Befunde von BALLOWITZ elektronenmikroskopisch ihre volle Bestätigung gefunden haben. In der Tat finden sich im Stratum laxum des Coriums zahlreiche marklose Axonbündel (WHITEAR, 1952; FUJII, 1966), von denen manche die Plasmamembranen der Melanophoren berühren und synaptische Vesikel enthalten (FUJII, 1966; BIKLE, TILNEY und PORTER, 1966). In diesen Regionen liegen im Plasma der Farbzellen zahlreiche pinocytotische Blasen. FUJII spricht die Axone als adrenergische Nervenendigungen an. Es ist bekannt, daß die Melanophoren isolierter Schuppen auf Adrenalin mit der Aggregation des Pigmentes antworten. Eine weitere Form der Synapse findet sich manchmal an den Ausläufern der Farbzellen, wo Axone zahlreiche synaptische Bläschen von 500 Å Durchmesser enthalten, wie sie typisch für cholinergische Neurone sind. Damit vertritt FUJII wieder eine doppelte Innervation der Melanophoren. Jedenfalls kann der Kontakt zwischen freien Axonen und Melanophoren gezeigt werden, und dieser Befund ist bereits von großer Bedeutung für die Diskussion des Farbwechsels. Außerdem wird den Pinocytoseblasen an der Oberfläche der Farbzellen eine Bedeutung bei der Aufnahme von Transmittern oder Hormonen zugeschrieben.

Das Stratum laxum wird wegen seines *Gefäßreichtums* oft auch Str. vasculosum genannt. Durch die Gefäßversorgung übernimmt dieser Teil der Cutis die Funktion der Hautatmung bei sehr vielen Fischen. Besonders in der Haut mit reduzierten Schuppen kann ein sehr großer Anteil der Atmung durch die Capillaren der Haut erfolgen; bekannte Beispiele sind Aal, Welse, Schlammspringer. Doch auch in der beschuppten Haut sind die Hautgefäße zahlreich. Bei der Quappe (Lota lota), einem im Süßwasser vorkommenden Dorschfisch, haben die Blutgefäße in einem mm² der Haut eine Oberfläche von 0,59 mm² und zusammen eine Länge von 20 mm (zit.nach HARDER aufgrund verschiedener Autoren, 1964). Bei der Haut mit reduzierten oder fehlenden Schuppen bekommt die Hautatmung die Bedeutung einer Ersatzatmung; vor allem schlammbewohnende Fische, Fische von warmen Flachwasser- und Gezeitenzonen können die Kiemenatmung durch Hautatmung wirksam unterstützen (vgl. LEINER, 1937; CARTER, 1957). Ein Aal kann pro Std 12 cm³ CO_2/g Körpergewicht bei 12° C ausscheiden. Werden die Kiemen ausgeschaltet, so steigt die CO_2-Abgabe auf 15 cm³. Die CO_2-Ausscheidung spielt eine größere Rolle beim

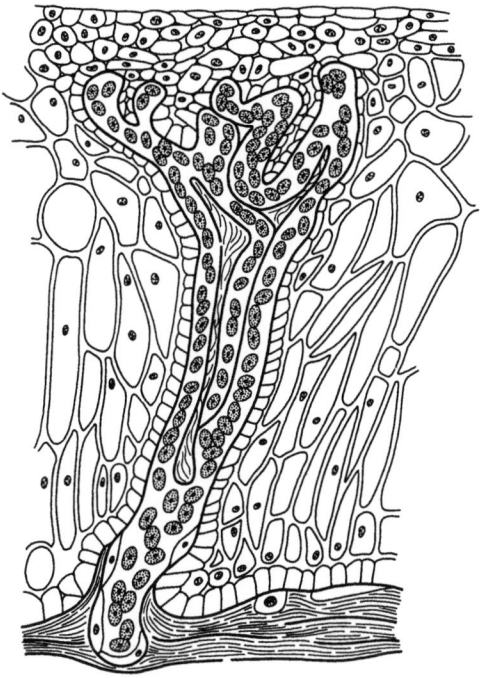

Abb. 9. Hautatmung eines Gobiiden (Trypanchen aus Sumatra, Mangrovezone); Ausschnitt aus der Haut der Kopfoberseite. In das vielschichtige Epithel wird ein Gefäß aus dem Corium vorgetrieben, das sich in der oberflächlichen Schicht in mehrere Capillarschlingen aufteilt. (Nach SCHÖTTLE, 1932)

Aufenthalt in Luft als im Wasser, wo die Kiemen als CO_2-Abscheider fungieren. Die Länge der Capillaren in 1 mm² der Haut entspricht mit 17,7 mm bei einer Oberfläche von 0,45 mm² etwa den Verhältnissen bei der Quappe (JAKUBOWSKI, 1961), aber die Lage der Capillaren in den oberen Schichten begünstigt den Gasaustausch. Die Gefäße werden unter das Epithel verlagert und können sogar als emporsteigende Schlingen mit kleinen Bindegewebspapillen bis dicht unter die Epitheloberfläche vordringen (Abb. 9). Bei den im tropischen Flachwasser lebenden Schlammspringern (Gobiidae), die für längere Zeit das Wasser zu verlassen pflegen, sind die Gefäßverhältnisse am stärksten auf den Gasaustausch eingerichtet (SCHÖTTLE, 1932). Da die Körperhaut Schuppen besitzt, sind die speziellen Bezirke in der Haut des sehr großen Kopfbereiches mit den Kiemendeckeln zu finden. Bei einzelnen Arten ist auch die Oberseite des Rumpfes mit besonderen Capillaren versehen; stets ist aber die Ventralseite des Körpers, die ja im Schlamm eingebettet liegt, frei von respiratorischen Bezirken. Solche besonderen Capillaren können die etwa 200 μ dicke Epidermis als aufsteigende Gefäßschlingen durchsetzen; oder es werden breite Coriumpapillen aufgewölbt, über denen die Epidermis nur 1—2schichtig ist, so daß die Capillarwände gleichzeitig Basalmembran der respiratorischen Epithelzone darstellen. In anderen Fällen dringen Capillarschlingen mit dem Bindegewebe der Basalmembran in die Epidermis vor, so daß ein Netz von „intraepidermalen" Capillaren nur noch von einer dünnen Epithelzellenschicht auf der Oberfläche bedeckt wird. Hier sind fast die histologischen Strukturen der Kiemen erreicht worden. Die Gefäße werden z.T. von der Arteria subclavia, z.T. aus Ästen der Kiemenbögen und der Carotis externa versorgt.

Die *Innervation* der Fischhaut erfolgt durch zwei Systeme: somatosensible spinale Nerven bilden einen cutanen Plexus; die Lateraliskomponenten der Hirnnerven stellen den nervösen Teil des Seitenliniensystems dar. Im Bereich der Lippen, Kiemen und an besonderen, modifizierten Flossenteilen sowie Körperanhängen (Barteln) kommen noch Geschmacksknospen hinzu, deren Innervation von den Hirnnerven VII, IX und X erfolgt; sie können hier nicht berücksichtigt werden. — Der *cutane Nervenplexus* aus segmentalen spinalen Fasern (SCHARRER, 1935; SCHARRER, SMITH und PALAY, 1947; WHITEAR, 1952) wird aus größeren Nerven zusammengesetzt, die an der unteren Grenze des Stratum laxum im Bereich der zahlreichen Farbzellen verlaufen und die segmentale Anordnung noch deutlich erkennen lassen. Von diesen Nerven steigen kleinere Äste senkrecht bis unter die Basalmembran hoch. Da die Schuppen einen Teil des Corium einnehmen, müssen die Nerven um die Schuppenränder herum zur Oberfläche verlaufen. Durch das Wachstum der Schuppen während des individuellen Lebens der Tiere wird also auch die gröbere Anatomie des cutanen Nervenplexus ständig verändert, vor allem bei Jungfischen. Unter der Basalmembran verzweigen sich die kleinen Nervenfasern, zumeist über der Schuppe, an der sie emporgewachsen sind und über die caudal folgende Schuppe. Das bedeutet immerhin, daß ein recht großes Gebiet vom gleichen Nervenästchen innerviert wird und keineswegs der Bereich einer Schuppe auch sinnesphysiologisch eine Einheit darstellt. Unter der Basalmembran verlaufen kleine Bündel von Axonen, ohne in der Verteilung irgendeine Gesetzmäßigkeit der Anordnung erkennen zu lassen. Der Durchmesser der einzelnen Axone ist im Bündel unterschiedlich und beträgt 5,5 µ—1 µ. Die Axone verlassen das Bündel an beliebigen Stellen und treten durch die Basalmembran in die Epidermis ein, wo sie unter Verzweigung zwischen die Epidermiszellen bis dicht unter die Epitheloberfläche vordringen. Beim Durchdringen der Basalmembran hört die Myelinscheide auf, so daß wahrscheinlich freie Axonenden in den Intercellularen der Epithelzellen liegen. WHITEAR (1952) kommt nach den physiologischen Versuchen vieler Untersucher zu dem Schluß, daß diese Nervenendigungen für den Tastsinn verantwortlich sind. Auch die Flossen enthalten ein entsprechendes Nervennetz (SCHARRER, 1935), aber bei bestimmten Fischen konnten SCHARRER, SMITH und PALAY (1947) nachweisen, daß die freien Nervenendigungen im Flossenepithel auch eine chemische Sensibilität aufweisen, obwohl sie spinaler Herkunft sind und Äste des Facialis bzw. Geschmacksknospen in den Flossen nicht vorhanden sind.

Das *Seitenliniensystem* (Morphologie vgl. DEVILLERS, 1958) wird von den Lateralisanteilen der Hirnnerven versorgt, wie bereits früher beschrieben wurde. Ebenfalls wurden die Funktionen und der Feinbau dieser Sinnesorgane bereits geschildert. Bei den Knochenfischen sind die Schuppen über den Seitenlinienkanälen durchbohrt, da sie in den Schuppentaschen um die bereits vorhandenen kanalförmigen Einsenkungen der Epidermis aufgebaut werden. Meist überlappen sich die Schuppen über den Seitenlinien nicht, und außerdem können sie den von ihnen erfaßten Teil des Kanalsystems als eine knöcherne Röhre umgeben. Über die Anordnung der Seitenlinienkanäle wurde bei den Selachiern ausführlich berichtet. Der Nervenstamm der Lateralisäste liegt in der Nähe der Muskelfascie und gibt Seitenäste ab, die in das Corium eintreten; jede dieser Verzweigungen versorgt zahlreiche Sinnesknospen der Seitenlinie (v. WOELL-WARTH, 1934; SCHWARTZ, 1965). Die zu den Sinnesknospen führenden Äste verlassen die größeren Stämmchen und treten in die Faserbündel des Stratum compactum ein, wo sie über längere Strecken parallel zu den Fasern verlaufen. Erst kurz vor den von ihnen versorgten Endorganen durchstoßen sie das Stratum compactum und vermischen sich mit den Nervenfasern des cutanen Plexus, wo sie oft nur noch sehr schwer von den spinalen Nerven unterschieden werden können (WHITEAR, 1952). Im Stratum laxum verzweigen sich dann diese kleinen Lateralisäste an der Basis der Schuppen, die zu den Seitenlinienkanälen in Beziehung stehen, und die Axone durchdringen die Basalmembran unter den Sinnesknospen. Dort bilden sie die synaptischen Verbindungen mit den Receptorzellen, auf die im einzelnen bereits bei den Selachiern eingegangen wurde. Ein Teil der Sinnesknospen (Neuromasten) des Lateralissystems liegt außerhalb der Seitenlinienkanäle und läßt bei verschiedensten Fischgruppen den charakteristischen Bau (mit einer Cupula) vermissen. Oft sind solche Sinnesknospen als Tast- oder Geschmacksknospen mißdeutet worden. In neuerer Zeit sind solche offenbar spezialisierten und bestimmten physiologischen Aufgaben zugeordneten Seitenlinienknospen sorgfältig untersucht worden. Bei den Katzenwelsen z.B. sind die in einzelne Gruben versenkten Sinnesknospen in der Körperhaut verstreut vorhanden und am Kopf besonders dicht angeordnet. Jedes Organ besteht aus einem engen Kanal in der Epidermis, dessen Oberfläche von besonders geformten Epithelzellen bedeckt ist. Der Kanal ist von einer gallertigen Substanz erfüllt. Am Grunde liegt eine Zellplatte, die von der Basalmembran der angrenzenden Epidermis unterlagert ist. Das ganze Organ: Kanal und Zellplatte ist in seiner Ausdehnung nicht tiefer als die umgebende Epidermis und wölbt sich also auch nicht ins Corium vor. Die basale Zellplatte besteht aus Receptorzellen (Sinneszellen) und Stützzellen (MULLINGER, 1964). Die Sinneszellen werden von den Stützzellen getragen und berühren die Basalmembran nicht, erhalten aber von Axonen zahlreiche Synapsen. An der Zelloberfläche ragen zahlreiche Mikrovilli ins Lumen des Kanals, doch besitzen die Sinneszellen keine Cilien. Die Stützzellen liegen der Basalmembran auf, so daß der Zelleib in der Hauptsache unter den Sinneszellen liegt und dort auch den Zellkern enthält. An der Oberfläche liegen die schmalen, zusammengedrängten Fortsätze der Stützzellen zwischen den breiten Sinneszellen und zeigen unregelmäßig geformte, oft breite Mikrovilli. Die zugehörigen Nervenfasern der ,,Sinnesknospen" entstammen dem Lateralissystem. In dieser Form der Seitenlinienorgane fehlen die typischen Bestandteile, die für die Perception von mechanischen Reizen notwendig sind: Cilium und Cupula. Im Augenblick wird die Möglichkeit diskutiert, daß diese sog. ,,kleinen Grubenorgane" als Receptoren für elektrische Reize funktionieren.

4. Amphibia (Lurche)

a) Der Bau der Haut und die Bildung der Basalmembran

Die Amphibien durchlaufen bei ihrer Entwicklung mit wenigen Ausnahmen eine *Metamorphose*. Die Larven sind wasserlebend oder werden bei einigen Arten im Uterus behalten. Durch die Metamorphose wird die Struktur der Haut stark verändert, denn fast immer verlassen die metamorphosierten Tiere das Wasser und gehen zum Landleben über, obwohl sie an die Nähe des Wassers oder an eine sehr feuchte Umgebung gebunden bleiben. Die Haut muß dem Umgebungswechsel angepaßt werden. Eine kleine Gruppe von Amphibien, die Blindwühlen (Gymnophiona) leben im Erdreich und haben eine geringelte Haut, in der als Rest des phylogenetisch alten Panzers ausgestorbener Amphibien (Stegocephala) Kalkplatten eingelagert sind. Doch auch ihre Larven sind wasserlebend oder bleiben im Uterus.

Die Haut der Larven ist (neben der geringeren Zahl der Epithelzellenschichten) durch Drüsenzellen ausgezeichnet; bei den metamorphosierten Tieren werden versenkte extraepitheliale Drüsen gebildet, und die Epithelzellen der oberflächlichen Zellschichten verhornen (vgl. Abb. 14). Große zusammenhängende Teile dieser verhornenden Schicht werden von Zeit zu Zeit abgestoßen.

Die großen Zellen der Amphibien haben ein günstiges Objekt seit Beginn der Mikroskopie dargestellt, und so sind zahlreiche ältere Untersuchungen an der

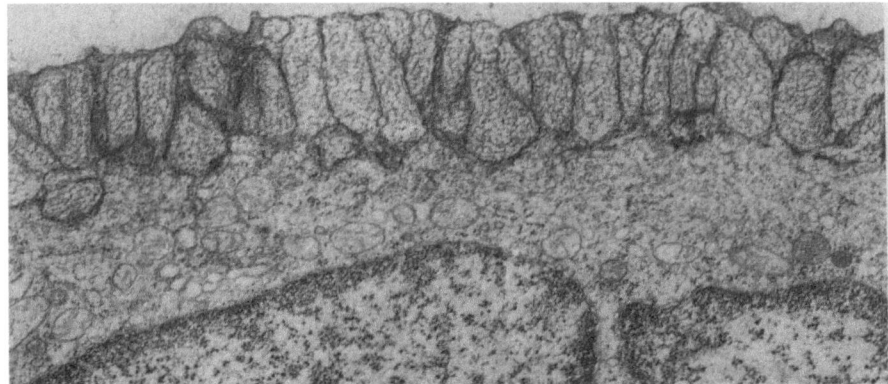

Abb. 10. Oberfläche des ,,Stratum cuticulare" im Epithel einer Salamander-Larve (5 cm Länge). Ausschnitt aus der Oberfläche einer Epithelzelle, zahlreiche ,,Schleim"-Vacuolen liegen dichtgedrängt in der apikalen Plasmaschicht und werden durch dichte Plasmahüllen voneinander getrennt; darunter ein Teil des Zellkernes. 13 500/1

Amphibienhaut gemacht worden. Die Zusammenfassungen von BIEDERMANN (1926, 1930) und von RABL (1931) geben eine gedrängte Übersicht. Hier dagegen sollen vor allem die elektronenmikroskopischen Befunde der letzten Jahre in der Hauptsache Berücksichtigung finden, da sie wesentlich zum Verständnis der Kontroversen über einzelne Zelltypen und Zelleinschlüsse bei den Autoren früherer Jahrzehnte beitragen.

Die *Epidermis der Larvenhaut* ist zwei- oder dreischichtig. Bei den Larven der Urodelen (Molch, Salamander, Axolotl) sind sechs Zelltypen im Epithel zu unterscheiden. Auf der Basalmembran liegen die indifferenten Epithelzellen, die dichte Bündel von Tonofibrillen enthalten und mit Halbdesmosomen an der basalen Zellmembran versehen sind (WEISS und FERRIS, 1954; PORTER, 1954; KELLY, 1966). Mitosen sind zahlreich. Die Epithelzellen an der Oberfläche haben besondere Differenzierungen ausgebildet. Ein Zelltyp trägt Cilien in großer Zahl, so daß die noch sehr kleinen Larven langsame Bewegungen durch den Cilienbesatz der Oberfläche ausführen. Diese Zellen sind offenbar einem raschen Abnutzungsprozeß unterworfen und werden in großer Zahl abgestoßen und durch neue Zellen der mittleren Schicht ersetzt (KOECKE, unveröffentliche Beobachtungen). Die Cilien haben den typischen Aufbau, ein Basalkörper ist vorhanden und trägt lange Verankerungsfibrillen (quergestreift), die in den Zellkörper einstrahlen. Zwischen den Wimperzellen stehen Drüsenzellen, deren Oberfläche von zahlreichen eingesenkten Schleimvacuolen eingenommen wird (Abb. 10). Zwischen den Vacuolen ragen Mikrovilli empor (KELLY, 1966). Zumeist aber sind die Vacuolen nach unseren Beobachtungen durch hyaline Schichten des Cytoplasmas voneinander getrennt, die sich an der Oberfläche fortsetzen und so unregelmäßig wabenförmige Wände bilden. Die Schicht der Vacuolen und Oberflächendifferenzierungen wurde in den alten Arbeiten als ,,Deckplatte" bezeichnet und ihre Struktur vielfach diskutiert. Wir haben schon beim Lanzettfischchen und bei den Neunaugen auf diese Verhältnisse hingewiesen. Die schleimbildenden Epithelzellen können auch einzelne Cilien tragen, oft finden sich nahe der Oberfläche zahlreiche Centriole, so daß eine Cilienbildung unterdrückt worden sein muß. Über die Faktoren, die bei den indifferenten Epithelzellen eine Entwicklung in Richtung auf Schleimsekretion oder Cilienbildung lenken, ist nichts bekannt. Entsprechend der sekretorischen Tätigkeit finden sich in den Zellen mit Schleimvacuolen große und zahlreiche Golgi-Felder. Ein dritter Zelltyp in der oberflächlichen Schicht ist nicht häufig und scheint ebenfalls sekretorisch tätig zu sein (KELLY, 1966). An der Oberfläche liegen dichte Granula, von einer Membran umgeben; im Plasma sind ausgedehnte Golgi-Felder und stark entwickelte Kanäle des endoplasmatischen Reticulums vorhanden. Die Funktion dieser Zellen ist nicht bekannt. Nach eigenen Beobachtungen halten wir es nicht für ausgeschlossen, daß es sich um einzelne ,,alte" Epithelzellen handelt, die noch embryonales Pigment enthalten. Zwischen allen Zellen sind weite Intercellularlücken, die von Zellfortsätzen überspannt werden; Desmosomen sind groß und zahlreich ausgebildet, ihre Feinstruktur wurde von KELLY (1966) ausführlich untersucht. An der Oberfläche liegen die Zellmembranen zum Verschluß der Intercellularen dicht aneinander und bilden die ,,Schlußleisten". Schleimzellen in Form von großen Becherzellen kommen nur in der Kopfhaut und der Kiemenregion vor, sie zeigen die von zahlreichen Geweben bekannte Feinstruktur. Charakteristisch für das Larvenepithel der Urodelen sind die in der mittleren Schicht gelegenen großen Leydigschen Zellen; sie bilden oft eine geschlossene mittlere Zellschicht und verschwinden bei der Metamorphose. Ihre besondere Feinstruktur und ihr Drüsencharakter ist in der Funktion noch nicht gedeutet. Die Zellen sind größer als die umgebenden Epithelzellen und die Becherzellen, sie haben einen Durchmesser von ca. 25 µ. Etwa 2 µ große Granula erfüllen das Cytoplasma in der Umgebung des Kernes. Der Inhalt der Granula ist PAS-positiv und von einer Membran umschlossen. Das periphere Cytoplasma der Zellen ist sehr dünnflüssig und enthält nur wenig differenzierte Bestandteile. Jedoch finden sich Bündel von Tonofibrillen unter der Plasmamembran, die das seit langem bekannte ,,Langerhanssche Netz" bilden (HAY, 1961; KELLY, 1966). Leydigsche Zellen teilen sich. Es wird vermutet, daß ihr Sekret in die Intercellularen abgegeben wird, da sie nicht an die Oberfläche kommen und sich auch nicht öffnen, etwa vergleichbar den Becherzellen. Neben der Beschränkung der Becherzellen auf die Kopfhaut zeigt sich eine regionale Gliederung im Feinbau auch noch an den Extremitäten (HAY, 1960). Dort ist eine dicke Epidermis aus 3—5 Schichten vorhanden, in der Drüsenzellen fehlen. Bei einigen Larvenformen kommen Schreckstoffe in der Haut wie bei schwarmbildenden Fischen vor (KULZER, 1954; PFEIFFER, 1966), die in besonderen ,,Riesenzellen" gebildet werden sollen. PFEIFFER gibt für Kaulquappen von Bufo 100—400 solcher Zellen pro mm^2 an.

Die Larvenhaut der Anuren (Kröten, Frösche) enthält nur in wenigen Fällen Leydigsche Zellen (z.B. beim Krallenfrosch, PFLUGFELDER und SCHUBERT, 1965). Die oberflächlichen Zellen sind Wimperepithelzellen oder mit Schleimvacuolen gefüllte Zellen wie bei den Urodelen. Jedoch zeigen die basalen Epithelzellen fädige Einschlüsse, die bei Urodelen nicht vorkommen: sog. Eberthsche Figuren; sie sind wie die Langerhansschen Netze lange Zeit hindurch Gegenstand von Diskussionen gewesen. Es handelt sich um relativ dicke Bündel aus Tonofibrillen, die parallel oder gewunden zusammengelagert und als basal gelegene Stränge

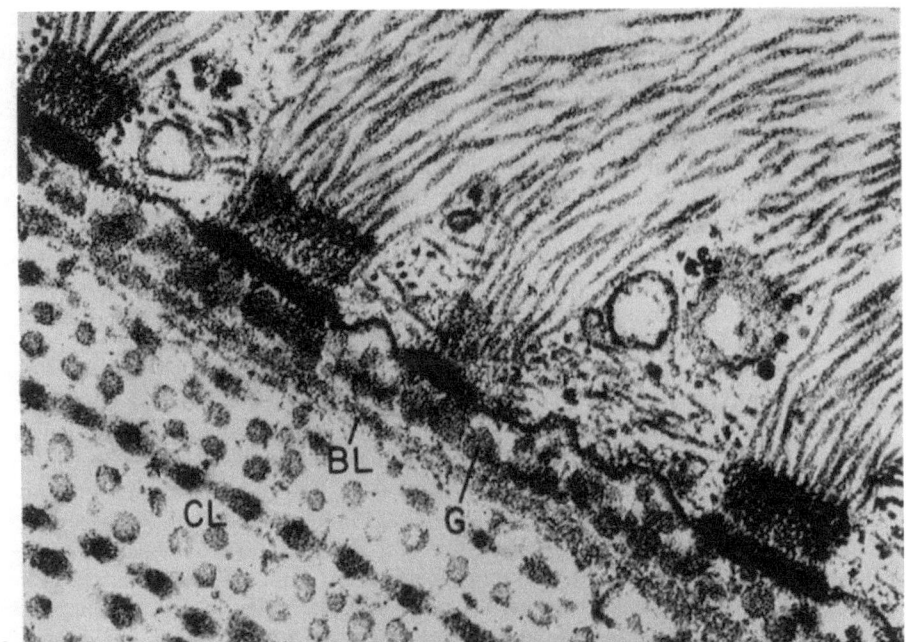

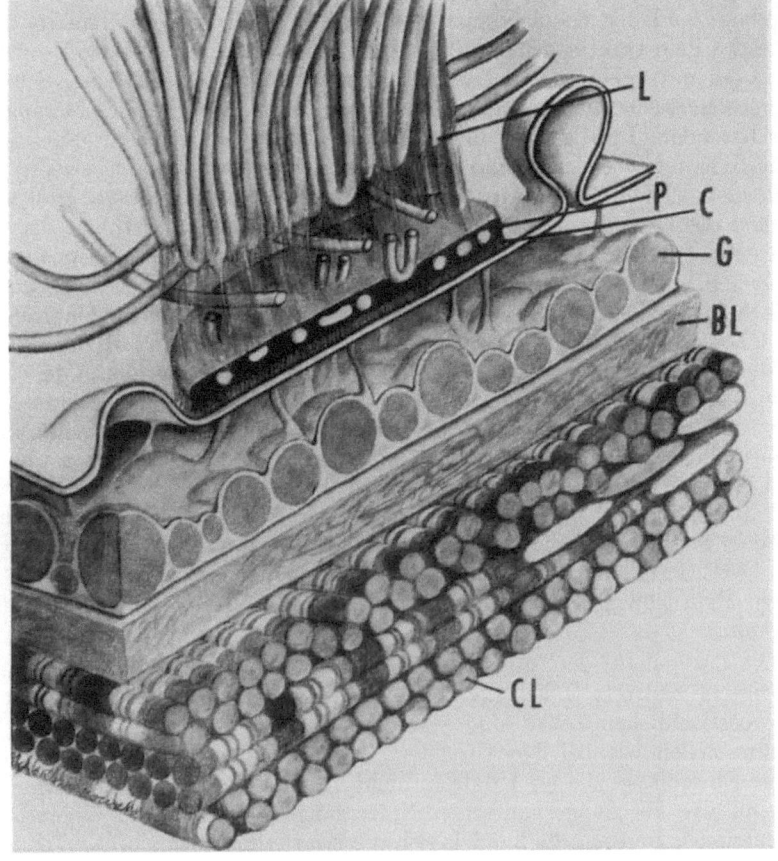

Abb. 11 a u. b. (Legende s. S. 973)

auch lichtmikroskopisch erkennbar sind (CHAPMAN und DAWSON, 1961; SINGER und SALPETER, 1961). Die Tonofibrillen liegen den Halbdesmosomen eng an und strahlen von dort in die Bündel ein. Wie im Bereich von Desmosomen bilden die Fibrillen enge Schleifen (SINGER und SALPETER, 1961; KELLY, 1966), enden also nicht an der Zone der Halbdesmosomen, sondern laufen zurück in das große Bündel (Abb. 11). Eine befriedigende Erklärung für die Funktion der Tonofilamentbündel kann bisher nicht gegeben werden, denn mit der Verhornung der Zellen haben sie offenbar nichts zu tun (KEMP, 1959).

Die *Grenze der basalen Epithelzellen* gegen das Bindegewebe und die *Basalmembran* sind bei den Amphibien besonders gut untersucht worden. Die einer Analyse so günstigen Verhältnisse des Feinbaues und das zu beeinflussende Wachstum der Larven und ihre Metamorphose haben dabei außerordentlich wichtige Ergebnisse gewinnen lassen. Seit die grundlegenden Untersuchungen von ROSIN (1946) gezeigt haben, daß die Basalmembran den Körper der Amphibien als ein Netz von überkreuzten Fasern in enger Anlehnung an die Form und Beanspruchung der Haut umschließen, sind zahlreiche weitere Einzelheiten durch die elektronenmikroskopische Technik aufgeklärt worden. Unmittelbar unter den Epithelzellen liegt eine sehr dünne Schicht, 250—400 Å dick, zwischen den Plasmamembranen der Epithelzellen und den körperwärts folgenden kollagenen Fibrillen der eigentlichen Basalmembran. Diese Schicht wurde von SALPETER und SINGER (1959) als „adepidermale Membran" charakterisiert und beschrieben. Sie besteht aus sehr feinem fibrillären Material, in das kleine runde Körperchen (200—600 Å) eingebettet sind (WEISS und FERRIS, 1954; SALPETER und SINGER, 1959; HAY, 1964; KELLY, 1966). Von den hier genannten Autoren wird angenommen, daß es sich um Lipoidtröpfchen handelt, die aber so fest mit den Mucopolysacchariden der Grundsubstanz verbunden sind, daß sie bei einer mechanischen Entfernung des Epithels auf der Oberfläche des Bindegewebes verbleiben (KELLY, 1966). In sehr überzeugender Weise kann KELLY die feste Verhaftung der Tröpfchen mit der Unterlage demonstrieren und zugleich nachweisen, daß jedes Tröpfchen von einer Hülle aus Mucopolysacchariden umschlossen ist, so daß es für Lipasen von der Oberfläche aus nicht angreifbar ist. Während der Veränderungen der Haut in der Metamorphase verschwinden die Tröpfchen innerhalb weniger Tage.

Die eigentliche *Basalmembran* ist ca. 4 µ dick und setzt sich aus 20—22 Lagen von Kollagenfibrillen zusammen (bei Larven von ca. 25 mm Länge), kann aber bei älteren Larven (75 mm, Frosch) bis zu 40 Fibrillenschichten enthalten (Abb. 12). Diese Basalmembran, so muß besonders betont werden, ist aber nur bei Larven eine echte Basalmembran. In der Metamorphose wird sie von der Epidermis gelöst, umgebaut und durch einwandernde Zellen durchsetzt und stellt schließlich die straffe Lage des Corium, das Stratum compactum dar. Eine jede Lage der larvalen Basalmembran ist etwa 500 Å dick und besteht aus Grundsubstanz und fünf Schichten von kollagenen Fibrillen, die alle parallel verlaufen. Eine entsprechende Struktur wurde bereits beim Lanzettfischchen, den Neunaugen und Fischen beschrieben. Jede Lage der Fibrillenschichten kreuzt die angrenzende Lage mit etwa 90° in der Verlaufsrichtung der Fibrillen; dabei ist im einzelnen die Lage am Körper, in der Umgebung der Kiemen und an den Gliedmaßen für die Winkelverhältnisse maßgebend (ROSIN, 1946). Es wird aber eine sehr regelmäßige orthogonale Struktur stets beibehalten. Die einzelnen Lagen von Fibrillen werden durch senkrechte Bündel aus gleichartigen Fibrillen durchstoßen, so daß eine Verklam-

Abb. 11 a u. b. Struktur der Desmosomen in der Haut des Molches (Taricha torosa) (KELLY, 1966). a Hemidesmosomen an der Basis larvaler Epithelzellen; Bündel von Tonofibrillen sind am Desmosom befestigt, in der adepidermalen Membran liegen zahlreiche Substanztropfen (G), die Basallamelle (BL) grenzt die „Membran" gegen die Lagen kollagener Fasern ab (CL). b Schema eines Hemidesmosoms an der Basalmembran; C Kittschicht aus dichter Substanz unter der Platte (P) des Desmosoms, L Schlingen der Tonofilamente

merung der Schichten (außer durch die Grundsubstanzverkittung) besteht. Aus den senkrechten Bündeln treten einzelne Fibrillen in die parallel zur Oberfläche verlaufenden Lagen ein, so daß insgesamt ein außerordentlich stark verflochtenes Gewebe aus Fibrillen besteht (WEISS und FERRIS, 1954, 1956; KEMP, 1959; SALPETER und SINGER, 1959; EDDS und SWEENY, 1962).

Die *Entstehung der Basalmembran* während der Entwicklung ist in zweifacher Hinsicht wichtig. Einmal müssen die morphologischen Vorgänge beim Aufbau der Fibrillen und ihre Zusammenlagerung zu geordneten Schichten verfolgt werden.

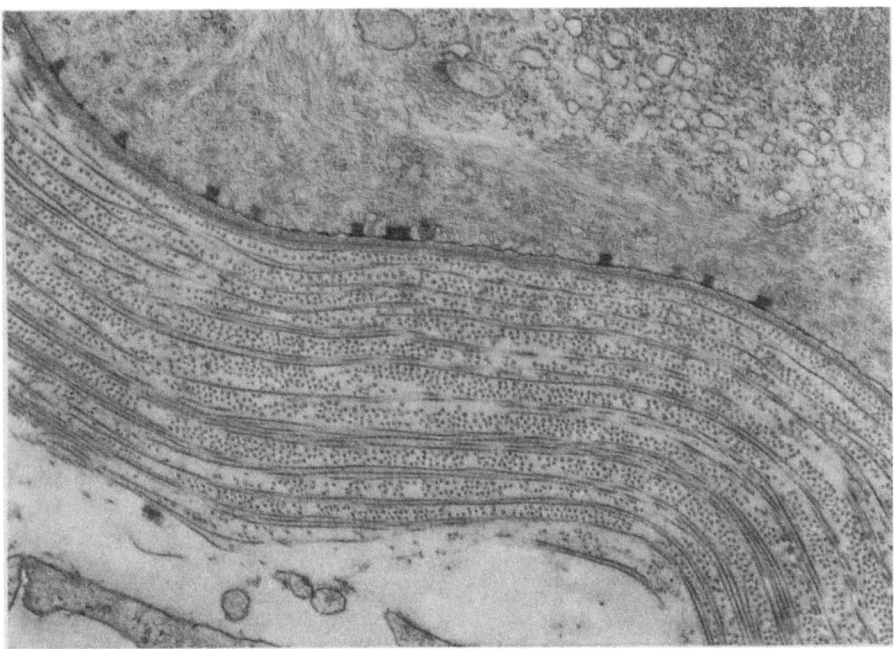

Abb. 12. Basalmembran des Körperepithels einer Salamanderlarve (5 cm Länge); unter den Epithelzellen mit Tonofibrillen und Halbdesmosomen folgt eine breite Zone: adepidermale Membran; daran schließen sich 20 Schichten kollagener Fasern an, die teils längs oder schräg angeschnitten sind, teils im Querschnitt in sich überkreuzenden Lagen getroffen sind. 14 500/1

Zum anderen muß die stoffliche Zusammensetzung und die Herkunft der Substanzen geklärt werden. Bei Froschlarven beginnt der Aufbau der Basalmembran zwischen Ektoderm und Mesoderm noch vor dem Einsetzen des Herzschlages (sog. Stadium 18 nach SHUMWAY). Zunächst entsteht eine adepidermale Membran aus Grundsubstanz mit rundlichen Körpern, wie sie für Larven charakteristisch ist; ihre Dicke beträgt 0,1—0,5 µ. An der Innenseite sind erste Kollagenfibrillen von 150 Å Durchmesser in ungeordneter Lage vorhanden (KEMP, 1959; EDDS und SWEENY, 1962). Die Ektodermzellen bilden zu diesem Zeitpunkt noch eine einschichtige geschlossene Zellschicht, in den Zellen sind die embryonalen Dottereinschlüsse zahlreich vorhanden, später werden sie immer weiter abgebaut und fehlen dann in den Zellen älterer Larven. Im Stadium 20 werden dann die entstandenen kollagenen Fibrillen zu geordneten Schichten zusammengelagert, so daß in den inneren Lagen die orthogonale Struktur sichtbar wird. Der entstandenen Basalmembran liegen Mesenchymzellen dicht an, offenbar gibt es zwei funktionell verschiedene Formen (EDDS und SWEENY, 1962), so daß die Bezeichnung Fibroblast nicht ohne weiteres angewendet werden sollte. Mit zunehmendem Alter der

Larven (eine durchgehende Blutzirkulation besteht noch nicht in allen Körperteilen) werden zwischen die schon geordneten Fibrillen weitere Fibrillen eingelagert, eine zunehmende Dichte der Fibrillenschichten wird sichtbar. Zugleich differenzieren die Epithelzellen die Halbdesmosomen aus. Im Stadium 23, wenn die Zirkulation vollständig ist und die äußeren Kiemen der Larven von einem Operculum überdeckt werden, also die typische Form der „Kaulquappe" ausgebildet wird, sind 6—8 Lagen von Fibrillen vorhanden. Mit dem Beginn der Nahrungsaufnahme durch den Mund und Darmtractus (vorher wurde der Dotter des Entoderms abgebaut) im Stadium 25 besteht die Basalmembran aus 14—18 Schichten. Der Durchmesser der Fibrillen ist auf 350 Å angewachsen. Bei Larven von 2,5 cm Länge sind 20 Schichten und bei Larven von 3,2 cm Länge 32 Schichten festzustellen. Die Basalmembran wird von typischen Fibroblasten unterlagert. Das Epithel ist zweischichtig und hat die Wimper- und Drüsenzellen an der Oberfläche ausdifferenziert. Die Kräfte, die zur Orientierung der Fibrillen und zum Aufbau der orthogonalen Struktur der Lagen zueinander führen, sind völlig unbekannt. Durch Versuche mit Verletzungen und Amputationen wurde mehrfach die Neubildung der Basalmembran verfolgt, um diese Faktoren zu analysieren. Entsprechende Mechanismen liegen ja beim Aufbau des Corneabindegewebes vor, wo ebenfalls Regenerationsversuche gemacht wurden. Die erneute Bildung einer Basalmembran im Bereich einer Hautwunde (WEISS und FERRIS, 1956; SALPETER und SINGER, 1960) beginnt damit, daß die Epithelzellen die Wunde oberflächlich verschlossen haben; dann erscheint zuerst wieder die typische adepidermale Membran mit den globulären Körperchen. Später lagern sich zahlreiche Fibrocyten an das Wundcoagulum an und nach ca. einer Woche erscheinen die ersten kollagenen Fibrillen, unregelmäßig gelagert und von 150—200 Å Durchmesser. Der bei der Wundsetzung entstandene Rand der Basalmembran bleibt unverändert. Zwischen die alten Fibrillen von 500 Å Durchmesser legen sich die neugebildeten Fibrillen. Während der 2. Woche formen die Epithelzellen Halbdesmosomen an der Kontaktfläche mit der adepidermalen Membran, zugleich beginnt eine Lagerung der epidermisnahen Kollagenfibrillen in regelmäßigen Schichten unter Aufbau der orthogonalen Anordnung. Die im Bereich der Fibrocyten abgelagerten Fibrillen dagegen werden noch regellos in der Grundsubstanz sichtbar. Der Prozeß der Ausrichtung der Fibrillen schreitet von der epidermalen Seite zum inneren Teil der Basalmembran während der 3. Woche fort, so daß 9 Fibrillenschichten gezählt werden können, außerdem erreichen jetzt die Fibrillen ihre endgültige Dicke von 500 Å im Durchmesser. Der Ordnungsprozeß verläuft also offenbar unter Wirkung der Epidermis, wobei die Anordnung in Fibrillenschichten und der Aufbau der orthogonalen Struktur miteinander gekoppelt sind. In den folgenden Wochen wird allmählich eine Basalmembran mit der ursprünglichen Schichtenzahl aufgebaut, die mit der alten Membran verflochten ist.

Die *Herkunft der Substanzen* zum Aufbau der Membran deutet gleichfalls auf eine besondere Wirkung des Epithels bei der Organisation der Fibrillenschichten hin. Als charakteristischer Bestandteil von Kollagen läßt sich Hydroxyprolin schon bei Embryonen und Larven nachweisen (EDDS, 1958; EDDS und SWEENY 1961). Der Gehalt an Hydroxyprolin in der Basalmembran nimmt vom Stad. 20 bis 25 auf das fünffache zu. Nur sehr wenig Tyrosin ist nachzuweisen, jedoch immer vorhanden und mit der Zunahme der Ausdehnung der Basalmembran auch proportional ansteigend. Es sind also am Aufbau der Membran neben den Mucopolysacchariden, von denen Hexosamin als Hydrolyseprodukt ebenfalls nachgewiesen wurde, auch noch andere Proteine außer Kollagen in bestimmten Mengen beteiligt. Außerdem kommt eine Regionalspezifität dadurch zum Ausdruck, daß sich Basalmembran von Körper und Schwanz in der chemischen Zusammensetzung unterscheiden. Die Anwendung autoradiographischer Methoden bei der Regeneration zum Studium der wachsenden Basalmembran (HAY und REVEL, 1963; HAY, 1964) des Axolotls und von Salamanderlarven lassen den Ort des Einbaues radioaktiver Aminosäuren erkennen. H^3-Prolin findet sich bereits 30 min nach der Injektion in die Tiere in den Fibroblasten unter der Basalmembran und in Knorpelzellen des Gliedmaßenknorpels. Nach 2—4 h sind radioaktive Produkte in der Nachbarschaft der Zellen vorhanden. Doch auch die Epidermiszellen zeigen schon nach 15 min einen Einbau des markierten Prolins. Später sammelt sich das aktive Produkt an der Basis der Epithelzellen an und erscheint nach 2—4 h in großen Mengen in der Basalmembran und in den Intercellularen zwischen den Epithelzellen. Doch auch andere Gewebselemente sind nach diesem Zeitraum, wenn auch schwach, markiert, z. B. Muskeln. Von den Autoren werden diese Befunde so gedeutet, daß neben den Fibroblasten auch die Epithelzellen einen Teil von Substanzen für die Basalmembran synthetisieren und dort ablagern. Nun ist aber Prolin keineswegs charakteristisch für Kollagen, und auch die Epithelzellen können Prolin in Eiweißstoffe einbauen, die gar nichts mit der Basalmembran zu tun haben. Daß aktives Material in den Intercellularen erscheint, ist nach der intensiven Produktion durch Fibroblasten und der allgemeinen Ausbreitung des injizierten Prolins zu erwarten. Aus ihren elektronenmikroskopischen Bildern über den Schichtenbau der Larvenhaut beim Frosch schließen LEESON und THREADGOLD (1961) auf eine Beteiligung der Epithelzellen bei der Bildung der kollagenen Fibrillen. KALLMAN und GROBSTEIN (1965) haben nun eine Technik entwickelt, die eine einwandfreie Beurteilung der Beteiligung von Epithel und Mesenchym am Aufbau der Basalmembran erlaubt. Wenn auch embryonales Drüsenmaterial der Maus als Objekt genommen wurde, so sind seine Ergebnisse doch gerade im Hinblick auf die Versuche bei Amphibien diskutiert worden. Durch die Trennung des Epithels vom Mesenchym können die Gewebe einzeln mit H^3-Prolin markiert werden. In der Gewebekultur werden beide Komponenten zwar zusammengefügt, bleiben aber durch ein Millipore-Filter (Porengröße 0,45 µ) stets vom direkten Kontakt getrennt. Tatsächlich wird Prolin in beide Zelltypen eingebaut. Aber das Produkt der Mesenchymzellen ist eine lösliche Form und wird durch das Filter transportiert und unter den Epithelzellen abgelagert. Die Auflösung durch Kollagenase beweist den Kollagencharakter der entstehenden Schicht, während sich die eingebauten Substanzen im Epithel nicht durch Kollagenase oder auch nicht durch Hyaluronidase abbauen lassen. Aus diesen Befunden und dem morphologischen Ablauf der Basalmembranentwicklung läßt sich eindeutig schließen, daß die Fibroblasten die Substanzen für die Basalmembran aufbauen und die Epithelzellen die Polymerisation zu geformten Fibrillen bewirken, wahrscheinlich durch Abgabe eines Stoffes, der als Mucopolysaccharidkomplex angenommen wird. Der Polymerisations-Katalysator könnte durchaus auch Prolin enthalten, so daß der Einbau von Prolin in den Epithelzellen und die Anhäufung des Produktes an der Zellbasis die Ergebnisse von HAY und REVEL bedingen.

In der Larvenhaut folgt auf die Basalmembran, die dem Stratum compactum des adulten Corium homolog ist, nur noch eine *Subcutis* aus lockeren Fasern, Fibrocyten und Wanderzellen, in der die Grundsubstanz das Übergewicht hat. Zahlreiche *capillare Gefäße* bilden ein dichtes Netz, so daß z. B. beim Axolotl die Hautgefäße 40% der Atmung übernehmen (CZOPEK, 1957). Die breiten Flossensäume der Schwänze dienen als zusätzliche respiratorische Organe. Mit dem zunehmenden Alter der Larven kann das Netz der Capillaren noch verdichtet werden (STRAWINSKI, 1956; CZOPEK, 1955, 1957, 1959). Die wechselnden Bedingungen der Außenwelt werden durch Erweiterung und Verengung der

Capillaren kompensiert (SZARSKI, 1958), und auch die jahreszeitlichen Schwankungen scheinen sich entsprechend der Aktivität der Tiere in der Capillardurchströmung und Oberflächenveränderung der Gefäße zu zeigen. So können bei erhöhtem CO_2-Gehalt der umgebenden Luft mehr Capillaren in der Haut geöffnet und durchblutet werden (bis zu 60%) als unter „Normalbedingungen". Eine ähnliche zusätzliche Öffnung von Capillaren erfolgt bei Verschluß der Lunge. Es ist seit langem bekannt, daß bestimmte Arten in einem für den Gasstoffwechsel ungünstigen Lebensraum der Larven eine besonders starke Gefäßversorgung der Haut entwickeln oder sogar Hautlappen und lange Papillen auf der Haut ausbilden, in denen die Gefäße, ähnlich wie bei den Schlammspringern nur von einem dünnen Epithel überdeckt werden (NOBLE, 1925).

Unter der Basalmembran liegen die dermalen *Farbzellen*, unter denen bei den Larven die Melanophoren überwiegen. Einzelne Melanophoren kommen auch zwischen den Epidermiszellen vor (MEYER und LOETZKE, 1954), aber der *physiologische Farbwechsel* wird von den dermalen Farbzellen ausgeführt. Die zweite Gruppe von Farbzellen, die in der Larvenhaut häufig vorkommen, sind „Pterinophoren" (vgl. vorher), also gelbe Zellen mit Pterinen. Der Einfluß des Melanocyten-stimulierenden Hormons scheint bei der Entwicklung von entscheidender Bedeutung zu sein; es ist das erste Hormon (MSH), das in der Entwicklung gebildet und wirksam wird (PEHLEMANN, 1962). Die Melanophoren teilen sich nur unter dem Einfluß dieses Hormons (PEHLEMANN, 1966), so daß nach Hypophysektomie die Larven weiter wachsen und die Hautoberfläche sich vergrößert, aber die Population der Pigmentzellen bleibt unverändert: die Larven bleiben hell. Das Auftreten der Pterine hängt von der Ausdifferenzierung von „Pterinophoren" in den Larven ab (HAMA, 1963; OBIKA, 1963; GOTO, 1963), die sich wie die Melanophoren aus Zellen der embryonalen Neuralleiste entwickeln (HAMA und OBIKA, 1960; OBIKA, 1963; BAGNARA und RICHARDS, 1965); die Synthese erfolgt in den larvalen Pterinophoren. Auch ihr Verhalten wird wahrscheinlich durch die Farbwechselhormone schon bei der Entwicklung gesteuert. Die Beobachtungen v. FRISCHs (1920) über die Farben des Feuersalamanders zeigen, daß der Untergrund einen Einfluß auf die Ausbreitung der gelben, d. h. durch „Pterinophoren" gefärbten Hautpartien hat. Tatsächlich wird die Menge der Pterine bei den auf hellem Untergrund lebenden Larven erheblich gesteigert (ZIEGLER-GÜNDER, 1959), doch ist nicht bekannt, ob die Zahl der „Pterinophoren" oder die Syntheseleistung der einzelnen Farbzellen gestiegen ist. Die Experimente von BAGNARA (1961) zeigen aber, daß bei hypophysektomierten Larven die Menge der Pterine gegenüber normalen Larven stark zurückbleibt; die Injektion von MSH bewirkt eine Vermehrung der Pterine in hypophysektomierten Larven. Diese Verhältnisse deuten doch sehr auf eine vergleichbare Entwicklungskontrolle wie bei den Melanophoren hin. Ein Teil der „Pterinophoren" beginnt im Lauf des Larvenlebens auch Carotinoide einzulagern und wird so zu rot-gelben Xanthophoren. Es muß noch darauf hingewiesen werden, daß die Veränderung der Hautfärbung durch Vermehrung der Pigmentzellen oder Pigmente natürlich nicht einen raschen physiologischen Farbwechsel darstellt, sondern einen gewissen Dauerzustand und damit einen sog. morphologischen Farbwechsel bedingt. An den Pigmentzellen können selbstverständlich dann auch die Vorgänge des physiologischen Farbwechsels stattfinden. Schließlich sind auch Iridocyten (mit Guaninkristallen) in der Schicht der Farbzellen vorhanden (ZIEGLER-GÜNDER, 1954, 1955). Auch bei ihnen wird durch die Einwirkung von MSH die Einlagerung des Guanins beeinflußt (BAGNARA und NEIDLEMAN, 1958). Der physiologische Farbwechsel wird bei larvalen und adulten Amphibien hormonal gesteuert; es kann hier auf die Ausführungen des Abschnittes Farbwechsel hingewiesen werden. Melanophoren und „Pterinophoren" bzw. Xanthophoren reagieren auch in der Larvenhaut auf MSH mit Ausbreitung der Pigmentgranula (vgl. u. a. BAGNARA, 1964); Melatonin verursacht Aggregation der Farbstoffe (vgl. BAGNARA, 1960, 1963). Dagegen verhalten sich Iridocyten (Guanophoren) anders: sie reagieren auf Melatonin gar nicht (BAGNARA, 1964) und auf MSH mit einer Aggregation der Kristalle (BAGNARA, 1958, 1964). Das ist für die Effekte der Hautfärbung zwar sehr sinnvoll, aber schwer zu erklären. Vielleicht sind die alten Beobachtungen von COLLIN (1936) und TUSQUES (1939) doch von Bedeutung: mit Methylenblaufärbung läßt

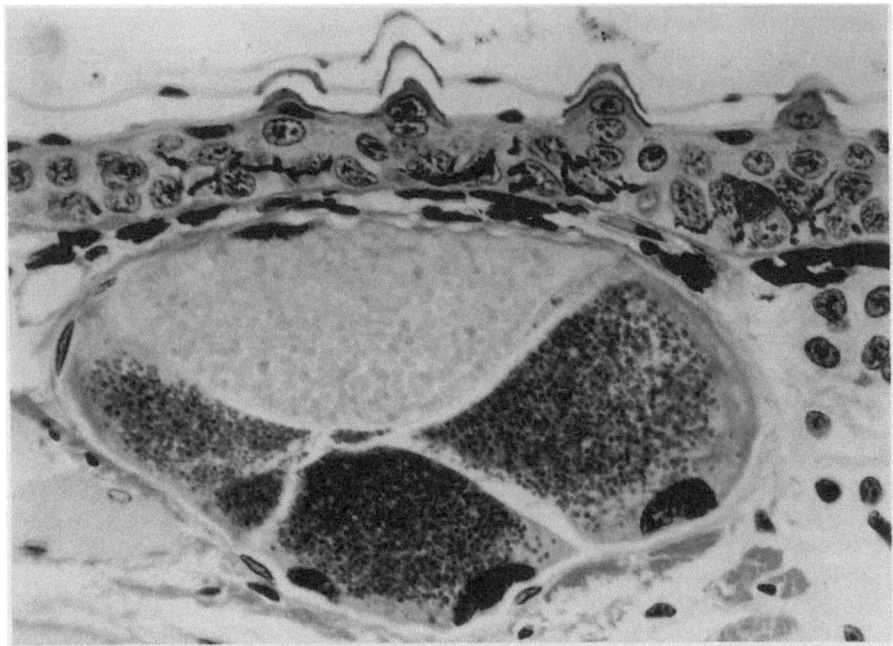

Abb. 13. Feuersalamander, junges Tier; Haut des Schwanzes mit Giftdrüse. Das Epithel läßt durch übereinandergeschichtete Zellgruppen kleine Höcker entstehen; die oberflächlichen Zellen sind verhornt und heben sich als zusammenhängende Schicht ab, 4 solcher Schichten sind zu erkennen. Pigmentzellen unterlagern die Basalmembran, einzelne Melanophoren liegen auch im Epithel. In der Giftdrüse sind die 4 sichtbaren Zellen in verschiedenen Sekretionszuständen. Azan, 500/1

sich bei Kaulquappen erkennen, daß an einem Teil der Melanophoren und auch der Guanophoren Nervenendigungen vorkommen. Der Untergrundeffekt ist ausgeprägt vorhanden: bei Belichtung werden die Larven dunkel, bei Dunkelheit blassen die Farben ab, d. h. Melanin wird in den Farbzellen zusammengeballt (BOGENSCHÜTZ, 1965). Die Augen spielen zwar eine Rolle, bei der Wahrnehmung des Lichtes müssen aber noch andere Receptoren vorhanden sein. Auf die besonderen Farbwechselverhältnisse bei hellem und dunklem Untergrund bzw. bei Licht und Dunkelheit der Krallenfroschlarven wurde bereits hingewiesen.

Innervation und Seitenlinienorgane werden weiter unten erläutert.

Die *Haut der adulten Amphibien* ist von einer mehrschichtigen Epidermis bedeckt, deren obere Zellschichten verhornen (Abb. 13). 3—5 oder mehr Epithelzellschichten mit einer Gesamtdicke von ca. 30 µ (bis 150 µ) bilden eine osmotische Barriere, die als physiologisches Musterbeispiel eine sehr genaue Untersuchung erfahren hat (vgl. USSING, 1960; FARQUHAR und PALADE, 1966). Die Zahl der Zellschichten hängt sehr stark von den Lebensbedingungen der einzelnen Arten ab und kann bis auf 10 und mehr gesteigert sein (Zusammenstellungen bei NOBLE, 1925;

Rabl, 1931). Die Basalzellenschicht (Stratum germinativum) besteht aus kubischen Epithelzellen, die durch Teilungen für Zellersatz sorgen. Aber durch die periodische Häutung in Form des Abwerfens der verhornten Oberflächenzellen findet nur eine rhythmische Teilungsaktivität statt, die unter hormonaler Kontrolle steht. Die Häutung erfolgt in unregelmäßigen Abständen von Wochen oder Monaten und ist früher mit dem Wachstum der Tiere in Verbindung gebracht worden. Es hat sich aber gezeigt, daß Thyroxin die Häutung bei den meisten Amphibien auslöst, bei einigen Arten dagegen (Kröte, Krallenfrosch) wirken Steroide der Nebennierenrinde anstatt Thyroxin (Adams, Richards und Kuder, 1930; Adams, Kuder und Richards, 1932; Jørgensen und Larsen, 1960, 1961, 1964; Stefano und A. Donoso, 1964; Jørgensen, Larsen und Rosenkilde, 1965; Kaltenbach und Clark, 1965). Der Mechanismus der Häutung ist keineswegs klar, denn durch die Hormone werden nicht etwa die basalen Zellen in ihrer Teilungsaktivität so stark beeinflußt, daß allein ihr Wachstumsrhythmus entscheidend für die Häutung ist. Bei fehlendem Thyroxin (nach Entfernung der Schilddrüse) geht ein langsames Dickenwachstum der Epidermis mit oberflächlicher Verhornung ohne Häutungen weiter. Die Basalzellen haben zahlreiche Halbdesmosomen gegen das Bindegewebe ausgebildet und entsenden Zellausläufer in die Basalmembran, so daß diese keine glatte Schicht an ihrer Oberseite mehr besitzt, sondern ein feines Relief entstanden ist. Die Epithelzellen sind von zahlreichen Tonofilamenten in Bündeln durchzogen (Pillai, 1962; Voute, 1963; Parakkal und Matoltsy, 1964; Farquhar und Palade, 1964, 1965). Die Zellen der mittleren Schicht können undeutlich gegeneinander als Stratum spinosum und als Stratum granulosum im distalen Teil der Epidermis hinsichtlich ihres Differenzierungsgrades unterschieden sein. Die unregelmäßig geformten Zellen des Stratum spinosum enthalten Tonofilamente, aber außerdem entwickelt sich das endoplasmatische Reticulum stärker, ebenso die Golgi-Felder. Lysosomen sind vorhanden und enthalten alkalische Phosphatasen. Mit der weiteren Differenzierung entstehen im Zusammenhang mit den Golgi-Vesikeln große Sekretgranula, die lichtmikroskopisch PAS-positiv sind und an den Zelloberflächen in die Zwischenzellspalten abgegeben werden. Dort bleiben sie als geformte, von einer Membran umgebene Körperchen noch einige Zeit erhalten. Die Zellen des Stratum granulosum sezernieren also Mucopolysaccharid-haltiges Material in den Intercellularraum. Da die Zwischenzellspalten bis unter die verhornten, oberflächlichen Epithelzellen reichen und ein zusammenhängendes Spaltensystem bilden (Farquhar und Palade, 1966), werden die Substanzen sich dort ausbreiten. Die Intercellularen öffnen sich an der Basalmembran zum Bindegewebe, so daß die Gewebsflüssigkeit mit den in ihr enthaltenen Stoffen ungehindert einfließen kann. Vielleicht ist die Aufgabe der sezernierten Mucopolysaccharide darin zu sehen, daß durch ihre große Wasserbindungsfähigkeit Flüssigkeiten im Intercellularraum festgehalten werden (vgl. unten; Parakkal und Matoltsy, 1964). Überdeckt werden die Zellen des Stratum granulosum von den stark abgeflachten, verhornten 1—2 Zellschichten des Stratum corneum. Seine Zellen haben alle Granula abgegeben, nur Reste der Lysosomen sind manchmal zu erkennen. Der Kern ist geschrumpft und das Plasma durch dichte Filamente ersetzt worden, zwischen denen noch einzelne Zellorganellen liegen können. Von großer Bedeutung ist, daß nun die Zellfortsätze eingezogen worden sind, mit denen in allen anderen Schichten die Intercellularspalten überbrückt werden. Dort sind bei einem Teil der Zellfortsätze typische Desmosomen ausgebildet (Millonig, 1958; Dewey und Barr, 1964; Farquhar und Palade, 1964, 1965, 1966), an denen die Zellmembranen durch einen Spalt von ca. 200 Å getrennt bleiben. An anderen Stellen dagegen verschmelzen die äußeren Schichten der Zellmembranen und bilden eine

„macula occludens" (FARQUHAR und PALADE, 1965). Im Stratum corneum dagegen sind die Intercellularspalten bis auf wenige Reste verschwunden, die Zellen liegen dicht beieinander und zeigen verschiedene Stadien von Desmosomen-Abwandlungen; stellenweise verschmelzen die Zellmembranen. Bereits an den Zellkontakten des Stratum granulosum sind die Veränderungen von Desmosomen zu Membranverschmelzungen im Gange. An der Oberfläche nun sind die Membranen der angrenzenden verhornten Zellen überall verschmolzen (Dicke des Membrankomplexes ca. 170 Å), so daß eine vollständige Abdichtung der Intercellularen gegen das Außenmedium gewährleistet wird. Diese weitreichende Verschmelzung: Zonula occludens ist auch weitgehend an tiefer gelegenen Zell-

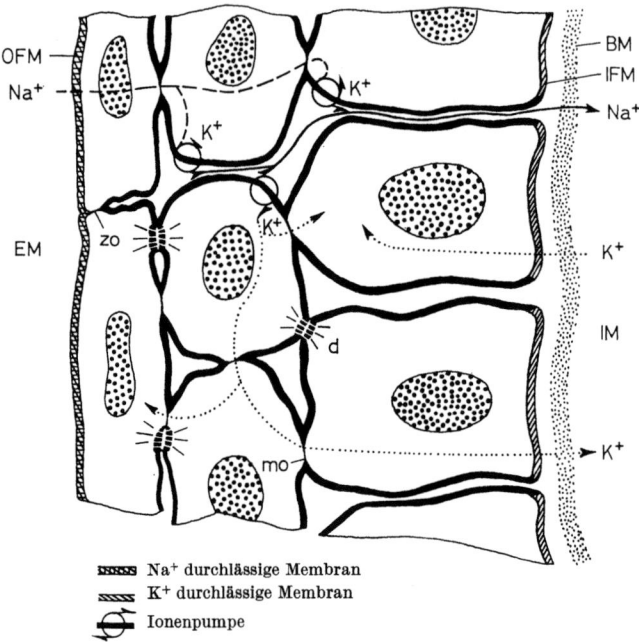

Abb. 14. Schema der Amphibienepidermis (FARQUHAR und PALADE, 1966). Es werden die Wege von Na+-Ionen, K+-Ionen und die Austauschmöglichkeiten durch die Zellmembranen in die Grundsubstanz der Intercellularen gezeigt; vgl. Text. *BM* Basalmembran, *EM* äußeres Medium, *IFM* innere Zellmembran, *IM* inneres Medium, *OFM* äußere Zellmembran, *zo* Zonula occludens

membranen der verhornten Zellen eingetreten. Der Nachweis von ATPase (FARQUHAR und PALADE, 1966) zeigt, daß in allen Zellmembranen der Epithelzellen dieses Ferment vorhanden ist, mit Ausnahme an der oberflächlichen Membran der Zellen des Stratum corneum, im Bereich der Desmosomen und Zellmembranverschmelzungen und der basalen Membran der Zellen des Stratum germinativum. Mit anderen Worten: überall an den Intercellularspalten können Epithelzellen aktive Stofftransporte durchführen (Abb. 14). Diese morphologischen und enzymhistochemischen Befunde sind für das Verständnis der Physiologie des Hautepithels von größter Wichtigkeit. Die dünne Haut der Amphibien wird von großen Lymphräumen unterlagert. In der Luft geht daher sehr viel Wasser verloren, während im Wasser ein erheblicher Einstrom von Wasser in die Gewebsflüssigkeit erfolgt. Dieses letztere osmotische Problem wurde bereits bei den Neunaugen und ihren Laichwanderungen erörtert. Der Wasseraustausch wird wie der Gasaustausch von der Umgebungstemperatur, dem Häutungszustand der Haut, der Körperregion beeinflußt. Es ist unmöglich, hier auf die Einzelheiten der Osmoregulierung einzugehen, die unter der Kontrolle von Hypophysenhormonen steht und z. T. durch den Füllungszustand der Gefäße bedingt ist. Darüber hinaus findet außerdem eine aktive Ionenaufnahme durch die Epithelien aus dem umgebenden Medium statt, vor allem von Na^+-Ionen, so daß eine sog. Natriumpumpe vorliegt. Die Larvenhaut hat die Fähigkeit zur aktiven Stoffaufnahme noch nicht (TAYLOR und BARER, 1965), erst bei der Metamorphose wird sehr rasch ein elektrisches Potential der Haut aufgebaut, das Voraussetzung für die Ionenpumpe ist (KOEFOED-JOHNSEN und USSING, 1958; USSING, 1960; INAMURA, TAKEDA und SASAKI, 1965). Erst mit dem Umbau der Haut in der Metamorphose beginnt der aktive Transport von Na^+-Ionen ins Innere. Dieser Vorgang wird durch den Nachweis der ATPase (FARQUHAR und PALADE, 1966) verständlich: durch die Oberflächenmembran der verhornten Zellen können Na^+-Ionen frei hindurchtreten, die gleiche Membran ist aber impermeabel für K^+-Ionen; andere kleine Ionen wie Li^+ oder Cl^- können ebenfalls durch die Membran hindurch, nicht dagegen größere Ionen wie SO_4^--Ionen. Durch die spezialisierte Membran an der Basis der Epithelzellen des Stratum germinativum werden K^+-Ionen aus der Gewebsflüssigkeit aufgenommen und von Zelle zu Zelle weitergegeben, indem sie die Verschmelzungszonen der Zellmembranen (maculae occludentes) passieren. Dadurch sind die mit ATPase versehenen freien Membranen aller Epithelzellen an den Intercellularspalten in der Lage, durch die Ionenpumpe Na^+- gegen K^+-Ionen auszutauschen und die von der Oberfläche eingedrungenen Na^+-Ionen in die Intercellularspalten abzugeben. Damit fließen die Na^+-Ionen ins Innere durch die Gewebsflüssigkeiten, die freien Zugang zum Intercellularsystem haben. Voraussetzung ist die Abdichtung der Spalten gegen die Oberfläche, wie sie durch die Zellen des Stratum corneum vorgenommen wurde. Es ist damit auch verständlich, warum dieser Prozeß bei den Larven noch nicht einsetzen kann, da hier ganz anders differenzierte Zellen die Oberfläche bilden. Tatsächlich zeigen die physiologischen Untersuchungen, daß die eigentliche Barriere in der Oberflächenmembran zu suchen ist (CEREIJIDO und CURRAN, 1965), deren Permeabilität durch die Anwesenheit von Ca und antidiuretischem Hormon (ADH) in der Haut beeinflußt wird: Ca setzt die Aufnahme von Na^+-Ionen herab, ADH fördert die Na^+-Aufnahme. Beide Faktoren wirken unabhängig voneinander und beeinflussen den aktiven Transport an den Membranen des Intercellularsystems nicht (CURRAN und GILL, 1962; HERRERA und CURRAN, 1963; CURRAN, HERRERA und FLANIGAN, 1963). Der Einstrom von K^+-Ionen auf der Innenseite ist abhängig von der Anwesenheit von Na^+-Ionen (CURRAN und CEREIJIDO, 1965). Die Beeinflussung der Vorgänge durch den Organismus ist also nicht nur durch hormonelle Faktoren möglich, sondern auch durch die Mobilisierung von Ca; und tatsächlich finden sich sehr alte Befunde bestätigt, nach denen kristalline Körperchen im Corium der Anuren vorhanden sind (TAYLOR, TAYLOR und BARKER, 1966). Es liegen an der Grenze von Stratum spongiosum zum Str. compactum erhebliche Mengen von Ca-phosphat in Form von kristallinen Aggregaten gespeichert, die mit der Verknöcherung des Skeletes nicht verändert werden und offenbar bei anderer Gelegenheit mobilisiert werden können.

Aus den Gefäßen im Corium stammen die *Wanderzellen* (Lymphocyten und Leukocyten bzw. Makrophagen), die in die Epidermis einwandern und zwischen den Epithelzellen liegen können.

Unterlagert wird die Epidermis von einer dünnen *Basalmembran*, deren obere Schicht aus regellos angeordneten kollagenen Fibrillen mit einem Saum aus sehr feinem granulären Material an die basalen Epithelzellen grenzt und durch die starke Faltung der Zellmembranen und die Zellausläufer ein unregelmäßiges Oberflächenrelief erhält. Eine kompaktere Lage aus kollagenen Fibrillenbündeln, die körperwärts folgt, ist keineswegs so regelmäßig aufgebaut wie bei den Larven: die Bündel bilden keine Schichten, sondern sind mit wechselnder Verlaufsrichtung ineinander verflochten (KEMP, 1961; A. J. SCHMIDT, 1962). Es folgt das Stratum spongiosum des Corium; ein lockeres Netzwerk kollagener und auch elastischer Fasern durchzieht die Grundsubstanz. Zahlreiche Fibrocyten, Wanderzellen und Farbzellen sind in dieser Schicht vorhanden und bilden ein sehr stark verzweigtes System von Zellausläufern in der Masse der Grundsubstanz. Die Basalmembran wird von flach ausgebreiteten Fibrocyten unterlagert. Die Farbzellen des Stratum spongiosum sind am physiologischen Farbwechsel beteiligt, ihr Verhalten und die Charakteristika wurden bei den Larven bereits beschrieben. Die Verlagerung von Pigmentgranula in den Zellen wird außer durch Hormone auch durch verschiedene Stoffe hervorgerufen (WRIGHT und LERNER, 1960). Ein Teil der ,,Pterinophoren" enthält bei den adulten Tieren mehr Carotinoide, so daß sehr satte rote Farbtöne in den Zeichnungen der Amphibien vorkommen. Doch sind auch Pterine weiter vorhanden (HAMA, 1953, 1959; GOTO, 1963; OBIKA und BAGNARA, 1964). Die Grundsubstanz, so wenig sie in morphologischer Hinsicht besondere Strukturen erkennen läßt, ist einem langfristigen Umbau unterworfen (GEDEVANISHVILI, 1964). So ist eine jahreszeitliche Veränderung der histochemischen Färbbarkeit der Mucopolysaccharide festzustellen, und auch die Zahl der Fibrocyten soll abnehmen. Bereits frühzeitig war aufgefallen, daß der Wassergehalt und damit die Gesamtdicke der Haut jahreszeitliche Schwankungen durchmacht, da während der Winterruhe eine Einschränkung des Stoffwechsels erfolgt. Eingelagert ins Stratum spongiosum sind die zahlreichen capillaren Gefäße, Lymphgefäße und kleinen Nervenstämmchen, welche die Haut versorgen. Sowohl Blut- als auch Lymphcapillaren bilden zwei Netze aus, ein subepidermales in der Nähe des Epithels, dem auch die Gefäße bei der Hautatmung angehören, und ein tiefer gelegenes subcutanes Netz. Aus der Subcutis steigen Bündel glatter Muskelzellen in das Stratum spongiosum auf, meist zusammen mit Netzen elastischer Fasern; sie gelangen durch Lücken der kollagenen Faserschichten des Stratum compactum in die obere lockere Gewebszone. Die innere Lage des Corium: das Stratum compactum ist durch eine Schicht von Melanophoren und kristallinen Körperchen vom Stratum spongiosum abgegrenzt. Es handelt sich um die schon diskutierten Einlagerungen von Ca-phosphat (TAYLOR, TAYLOR und BARKER, 1966), die bereits im vorigen Jahrhundert beschrieben wurden, aber in ihrer Bedeutung sehr unklar waren. Die Schicht wurde auch von VOUTE (1963) elektronenmikroskopisch gesehen. Vielleicht lassen sich die gespeicherten Substanzen als ein Rest der Schuppen deuten, die als phylogenetisches Relikt eine völlig andere Funktion bekommen haben, während sie bei den Gymnophionen noch Skeletplatten aufbauen. Die Faserbündel des Stratum compactum sind schichtenweise angeordnet und kreuzen sich in ihrer Verlaufsrichtung, so daß die bekannte orthogonale Struktur der larvalen Basalmembran beibehalten wurde (KEMP, 1961; A. J. SCHMIDT, 1962; VOUTE, 1963; PFLUGFELDER und SCHUBERT, 1965). Denn die Fasermassen sind tatsächlich die in die Tiefe verlagerten Teile der larvalen Basalmembran (vgl. unten). Eine faserige *Subcutis* verbindet das Corium mit der Muskelfascie; Fettgewebe ist selten. In der Subcutis liegen die größeren Gefäße und Nerven, die Äste in die obere Hautschicht abgeben. Die großen, bereits erwähnten Lymphsäcke und -gefäße sind ebenfalls in der Subcutis gelegen, so daß sie durch diese Sinus in eine der Haut und eine der Fascie anliegende Faserschicht geteilt wird. Die Subcutis trägt auch die Flossensäume oder Hautfalten, da dort das Corium sehr dünn ist.

Eingesenkt in das Stratum spongiosum sind die für die adulte Amphibienhaut charakteristischen *Drüsen*. Die Größe der Drüsenalveolen oder -acini bestimmt regional die Dicke des Stratum spongiosum. Es handelt sich um Giftdrüsen (Körnerdrüsen) mit flüssigem Sekret, Schleimdrüsen und Duftdrüsen. Die Sekrete sind seit langem als Gifte bekannt und rufen Schleimhautreizungen hervor. Es handelt sich um Substanzen verschiedener Stoffklassen, die in ihrer chemischen Struktur und pharmakologischen Wirkung im Gegensatz zu den Fischgiften schon frühzeitig genau untersucht wurden. Die Krötengifte sind Herzgifte von Glykosidcharakter, die der Salamander Alkaloide und biogene Amine (z.B. 5-Hydroxytryptamin). Ihre pharmakologisch gut bekannten Eigenschaften erübrigen hier eine weitere Darstellung. Die Zahl der Drüsen ist sehr groß; so kommen z.B. beim Grasfrosch pro mm^2 Hautfläche auf dem Rücken 30—45 Drüsen vor, davon sind 8—10 Giftdrüsen; beim Laubfrosch sind die entsprechenden Zahlen sogar 120—130, davon 75% Giftdrüsen.

Die Schleimdrüsen besitzen einen kurzen Ausführungsgang, da sie unmittelbar unter dem Epithel im Corium liegen; abgeflachte Epithelzellen grenzen das Ganglumen gegen die übrige Epidermis ab. Das sezernierende Epithel besteht aus großen Zellen mit zahlreichen Vacuolen, deren Inhalt PAS-positiv ist und mit zunehmender Sekretion große wäßrige Blasen im Plasma bildet (SPANNHOF, 1954; VOUTE, 1963; PFLUGFELDER und SCHUBERT, 1965). An der Oberfläche besitzen die Schleimzellen unregelmäßig geformte Mikrovilli, die Reste der Zellorganelle werden mit dem Kern in das basale Plasma gedrängt. Der ganze Vorgang wird als holokrine Sekretion gedeutet. Das Sekret ist flüssig, zeigt eine schwach positive PAS-Reaktion und erfüllt das Drüsenlumen. Der Sekretionsvorgang scheint cyclisch zu verlaufen, da zahlreiche Drüsen entleert zu sein pflegen. In solchen Drüsenalveolen tritt dann deutlich eine basale Zellschicht hervor, die als Ersatzzellen die sezernierenden Zellen unterlagert haben; sie bilden in der Sekretionsphase eine dünne, aber geschlossene Lage flacher Epithelzellen und differenzieren sich zu Drüsenzellen aus. Eine dünne Basalmembran (in Fortsetzung der Basalmembran des Körperepithels) umkleidet die Drüsenepithelien. Darunter liegen glatte Muskelzellen, die z.T. eine dicke muskuläre Schicht bilden können, z.T. aber auch fehlen (z.B. Krallenfrosch). Die Muskelzellen werden von Nervenstämmchen des sympathischen Systems innerviert, so daß bei bestimmten Reizen das Sekret ausgepreßt oder sogar ausgespritzt werden kann. Capillaren treten an die Drüsen heran. Zumeist liegen zahlreiche Fibrocyten und Farbzellen in der Nähe der Drüsen.

Die *Giftdrüsen („Körnerdrüsen")* fallen durch ihre Größe und die Sekretgranula auf, die sich bei der Azanfärbung in Abstufungen von bläulich, orange bis rot anfärben. Der Ausführungsgang wird von flachen Epithelzellen ausgekleidet, die in das Drüsenepithel überleiten. Die Drüsenzellen befinden sich in verschiedenen Phasen der Sekretproduktion. Nur wenige Zellen haben ihre volle Aktivität erreicht und erfüllen das Lumen fast ganz (SPANNHOF, 1954; PFLUGFELDER und SCHUBERT, 1965; ältere Angaben bei BIEDERMANN, 1930). Andere Zellen bilden eine Lage von Ersatzzellen oder eine seitlich an der Drüsenwandung liegende Epithelzellgruppe, in der einzelne Zellen schon kleine Sekretgranula enthalten. Die aktiven Drüsenzellen enthalten eine große Anzahl verschiedenartiger Sekretgranula im apikalen Plasma, so daß Zellkern und Zellorganelle auf das basale Plasma zurückgedrängt werden. Letzteres ist durch ein sehr stark ausgebildetes endoplasmatisches Reticulum mit sehr weiten Zisternenräumen gekennzeichnet. Die Granula sind teils aus dichter, homogen erscheinender Substanz aufgebaut; andere Granula sind spindelförmig („Navicellen") und haben eine komplizierte Innenstruktur. Werden die Drüsen entleert, etwa auf Reizung durch Chemikalien, so füllen sich aus der Ersatzzellengruppe neue Drüsenzellen mit Sekret. Umhüllt sind die Alveolen von Basalmembran, glatten Muskelzellen, Fibrocyten und

Melanophoren. Capillaren und Nerven treten an die Drüsen heran. Die glatten Muskelzellen bewirken die Entleerung des Sekretes. Es kommen auch gemischte Drüsen vor, in denen außer den Körnerzellen auch Schleimzellen vorhanden sind. Duftdrüsen sind modifizierte „Körnerdrüsen". An den Flanken und Gliedmaßen können während der Brunstzeit besondere Hautverdickungen als Warzen auftreten, die eine Umklammerung des Weibchens erleichtern. In diesen Bereichen sind dann die Schleimdrüsen vergrößert und bilden ein zähklebriges Sekret.

Die *Innervation der Haut* erfolgt durch einen subcutanen Nervenplexus, der sehr verschiedene Axone enthält: spinale afferente Fasern für Epidermis und Cutis, Fasern des Lateralissystems für die Sinnesknospen der Seitenlinienorgane, sympathische efferente postganglionäre Fasern von den sympathischen Ganglien, die zur glatten Muskulatur und zu den Gefäßen in Beziehung treten. Die Nervenstämmchen treten mit den Bündeln glatter Muskelzellen durch die Lücken des Stratum compactum, verzweigen sich sehr stark und bilden einen Plexus nahe der Epidermisgrenze und einen im Stratum spongiosum (WHITEAR, 1955). Aus 8—15 μ dicken markhaltigen Fasern dringen verzweigte Enden in die Epidermis vor, wo sie ein Netz von marklosen Axonenden bilden. Ihre Reizung erfolgt durch leichten Druck oder durch Berührung mit einer haarfeinen Spitze (ADRIAN, MCKEEN, CATTELL und HOAGLAND, 1931; MARUHASHI, MIZIGUCHI und TASAKI, 1952) oder mittels eines eng begrenzten Luftstrahls. Sie gelten als die Receptoren für Berührungsreize. Beim Krallenfrosch treten die Nerven in besondere Epidermispapillen ein (FAHRENHOLZ, 1929; MURRAY, 1955), die durch regelmäßig aufgeschichtete Epithelzellen als kleine spitze Höcker gebildet werden (Abb. 15). Auch beim Frosch sind kleine Warzen besonders berührungsempfindlich, während dicht danebengelegene Teile der Epidermis nicht gereizt werden können. Man wird sich die Lage der freien Axonteile in der Epidermis wohl so vorzustellen haben, wie es MUNGER (1965) für das Schnauzenepithel beim Opossum beschreibt: Zwar enden die Schwannschen Zellen an der Basalmembran, aber die Epithelzellen umgreifen die Axone in ähnlicher Weise, so daß sie keineswegs in den Intercellularspalten ungeschützt verlaufen. Weitere markhaltige dicke Fasern teilen sich im Stratum spongiosum auf und lassen markarme sehr stark verzweigte Endigungen mit varicösen Verdickungen entstehen (WHITEAR, 1955). Diese varicösen Endnetze können an die Drüsen herantreten oder ohne sichtbare Beziehung zu Strukturen im Stratum spongiosum verteilt sein. Eine Beziehung zu den 6—9 μ dicken Fasern, die auf Druckreize reagieren und ein ovales Areal von 3×4 oder 5×6 mm versorgen (MARUHASHI, MIZIGUCHI und TASAKI, 1952) läßt sich mit Sicherheit noch nicht herstellen. Andere Fasern verlaufen zu Papillen des Corium, wo sie in einer Anhäufung von großen Zellen (Merkelschen Zellen) sich aufzweigen. Schließlich sind noch markarme sehr dünne Nervenfasern vorhanden, die bereits in dieser Form in die Haut eintreten und auf alle möglichen Reize mit anhaltenden Impulsfolgen antworten. Alle diese erwähnten Nerven entstammen dem spinalen System und treten zum größten Teil durch die dorsalen Wurzeln und zum kleineren Teil durch die ventralen Wurzeln in die Haut ein. Die aus den sympathischen Ganglien stammenden Axone sind teils mit Markscheiden versehen, teils markarm; sie legen sich den glatten Muskelzellen der Drüsen an, so daß die Drüsenalveolen ein doppeltes dichtes Nervennetz umgibt.

Das *Seitenliniensystem* erhält seine Nervenversorgung aus den Lateralisästen der V., VII. und VIII. Hirnnerven. Die Larven besitzen ein gut entwickeltes System von Sinnesknospen, die in Reihen am Kopf und am Rumpf angeordnet sind (vgl. WRIGHT, 1951). Über die Funktion war bereits gesprochen worden. Nur ein Teil der adulten Amphibien behält nach der Metamorphose die Seitenlinienorgane, Die Sinnesknospen bleiben im Epithel an der Oberfläche (Abb. 15) und werden nicht wie bei den Fischen in die Tiefe der Haut verlagert. Eine solche Sinnesknospe setzt sich bei den Larven aus 5—10 großen Sinneszellen (Receptorzellen) zusammen, die von Stützzellen umschlossen werden. An der Oberfläche der Receptorzellen sind Mikrovilli und dickere Stereocilien vorhanden sowie pro Zelle ein echtes Cilium (vgl. Fische); an der Basis reichen die Receptorzellen nicht bis zur Basalmembran, sondern werden von den Stützzellen umschlossen (JAUDE, 1966). Die Stützzellen sind zahlreicher und langgestreckt, reichen von der Basalmembran bis zur Ober-

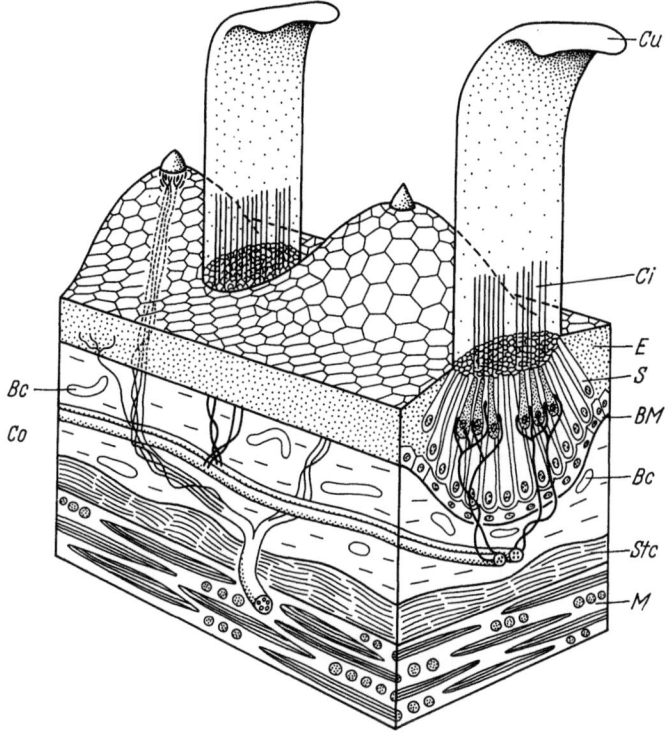

Abb. 15. Tasthügel und Seitenlinien-Sinnesknospen vom Krallenfrosch; schematisiertes Blockdiagramm. Es sind 2 Tasthügel mit der empfindlichen Spitze und Neuromasten mit Cupula der Seitenlinie dargestellt. Die Sinnesknospe enthält 2 Gruppen von je ca. 17 Sinneszellen (Schwankungen von 7—33 Sinneszellen sind möglich) und wird von 2 getrennten afferenten Fasern des Lateralissystems innerviert. Die Tasthügel erhalten einen davon unabhängigen cutanen afferenten Nerven. (Kombiniert nach GÖRNER, 1961, und MURRAY, 1955). *Co* Corium, *C* Cilien, *Cu* Cupula, *Bc* Blutcapillare, *Bm* Basalmembran, *E* Epithel, *M* Muskelschicht, *S* Stützzellen, *Stc* Stratum compactum

fläche; am Rande gegen das Körperepithel sind sie als besonders flache Mantelzellen ausgebildet. An der Oberfläche ist eine Cupula aus gallertigem Material von den Stützzellen ausgeschieden worden, welche die Cilien umschließt. Durch die unterlagernde Basalmembran treten Axone an die Receptorzellen heran; typische Synapsen sind dort ausgebildet. Bei erwachsenen Tieren, z. B. dem Krallenfrosch, sind die Knospen wesentlich zellreicher (GÖRNER, 1962), so werden 7—33 Sinneszellen pro Knospe gezählt; das Prinzip des Feinbaues wird aber nicht verändert. Die Innervation scheint eine Doppelinnervation zu sein (MURRAY, 1955), denn nach dem Verlassen des großen Lateralisnerven in der Subcutis oder nach dem Aufsteigen in das Stratum spongiosum teilen sich die Fasern in zwei parallel verlaufende Stränge, die in der Nähe der Sinnesknospen wieder jeder einen Ast abteilen; jede Sinnesknospe erhält also zwei (parallel verlaufende) kleine Axonbündel. Außerdem tritt ein weiterer Ast aus dünneren Fasern, meist ebenfalls doppelt, an die Knospe heran. Alle Fasern treten durch die Basalmembran, und die Axone verzweigen sich in der Knospe, wobei sie an die zentral gelegenen Sinneszellen gelangen. Jede Receptorzelle erhält damit Synapsen von verschiedenen Axonen. Die mögliche funktionelle Bedeutung war bereits diskutiert worden.

b) Die Veränderungen während der Metamorphose

Bei dem weitgehenden Umbau des larvalen Körpers in der Metamorphose werden neben den Organen vor allem die Bindegewebe ausgedehnter Körperzonen betroffen, u.a. die der Haut. Die Umstellung des Epithels auf die neuen Bedingungen ist relativ einfach: Die oberen Schichten und die Drüsenzellen gehen allmählich verloren und werden vom Stratum germinativum durch eine neue Population von Epithelzellen ersetzt, deren Differenzierung einen anderen Weg einschlägt als bei der Larve. Drüsenknospen werden gebildet (VANABLE, 1964), die sich zu den typischen extraepithelialen Drüsen entwickeln und bei ihrer Anlage und Ausgestaltung gegenüber anderen Drüsen keine Abweichungen zeigen. Damit ist uns hinsichtlich des Epithels zunächst das Verständnis der Vorgänge erschwert, da die entscheidenden Faktoren das Reaktionssystem selbst, d.h. die Epithelzellen betreffen und das Grundproblem das der Differenzierung ist. Das Bindegewebe dagegen wird z.T. in der Metamorphose aufgelöst, wie z.B. bei der Einschmelzung des Schwanzes und der Kiemen der Larven, um in anderer Form erneut aufgebaut zu werden, von den gleichen Zellen, die schon in der Larve vorhanden sind. Beim Abbau des larvalen Bindegewebes sind zwei Enzyme tätig, die bereits isoliert werden konnten: eine Hyaluronidase (SILBERT, NAGAI und GROSS, 1965), die der Hodenhyaluronidase der Säuger ähnlich ist, und eine Kollagenase (GROSS und LAPIERE, 1962; GROSS, LAPIERE und TANZER, 1963). Die Hyaluronidase baut die Mucopolysaccharide der Grundsubstanz ab und ist eine β-endo-N-acetylhexosaminidase. Bereits R. WEBER (1957) hatte die Aufmerksamkeit auf die Fermentaktivität in den Geweben bei der Metamorphose gelenkt und konnte Kathepsin nachweisen. Doch wird durch Kathepsin das dauerhafte Gerüst des Bindegewebes: das Kollagen nicht abgebaut (GROSS, LAPIERE und TANZER, 1963). Der Umbau der Haut beginnt damit, daß die larvale Basalmembran von der Epidermis gelöst wird und unter dem Stratum germinativum ein schmaler flüssigkeitsgefüllter Spaltraum entsteht (KEMP, 1961, 1963; USUKU und GROSS, 1965). Zugleich werden zahlreiche Vacuolen in den basalen Epithelzellen sichtbar, denn diese Zellen synthetisieren eine Kollagenase (GROSS und LAPIERE, 1962; GROSS, 1964; EISEN und GROSS, 1965), die eine Auflösung und Auflockerung der oberen Schicht der Basalmembran bewirkt. Wird die Proteinsynthese in den Epithelzellen durch Puromycin gehemmt, so unterbleibt die Synthese des Fermentes. Mit dem Einsetzen der Metamorphose, die auch experimentell durch Injektion von Thyroxin oder lokal durch Thyroxindepots eingeleitet werden kann, beginnen die Epithelzellen mit dem Aufbau und der Sekretion des kollagenolytischen Fermentes. Aus dem Bindegewebe dringen dann Fibrocyten entlang der vertikalen Fibrillenbündel in die larvale Basalmembran vor. Zunächst schieben sie nur lange Zellausläufer vor, aber bald lockert sich die dichte Basalmembran (Dicke 2—6 μ in der Larve) erheblich auf (bis zu 17 μ in einigen Tagen). Die Fibrocyten dringen zwischen die Fibrillenschichten vor und auch bis in den Spalt unter der Epidermis. Neben den Fibrocyten kommt ein zweiter Zelltyp vor, dessen Plasma von zahlreichen Vacuolen durchsetzt ist; die Bedeutung dieser Zellen läßt sich noch nicht nachweisen. Bei der Auflockerung der Basalmembran werden die kollagenen Fibrillen auseinandergedrängt und zahlreiche feine, neue Fibrillen werden sichtbar. Die Auflockerung kommt durch die Auflösung der Grundsubstanz zustande, denn die Bindegewebszellen sondern die obengenannte Hyaluronidase ab. Da sich diese Aktivität durch Puromycin nicht hemmen läßt und eine Zerstörung der Zellen (Frieren und Auftauen) die Ausbeute an Hyaluronidase erhöht, kann als sicher gelten, daß die Bindegewebszellen dieses Ferment bereits vor der Metamorphose gespeichert haben. In den einzuschmelzenden Gewebspartien des Körpers werden die kollagenen Fasern immer dünner, der Wassergehalt sinkt rapide. In der übrigen Haut dagegen bauen die eingedrungenen Fibrocyten große Mengen neuer Fibrillen auf, die Zellen sind sehr verzweigt und liegen den Fibrillenbündeln eng an. Unter dem Epithel befinden sich zahlreiche Bindegewebszellen, auch die Farbzellen wandern dort ein. Die Aktivität der Fibrocyten baut eine dicke Schicht aus Grundsubstanz und regellos angeordneten dünnen Kollagenfibrillen auf: Das Stratum spongiosum entsteht. Eine neue, dünne Basalmembran grenzt die relativ ungeordnete Zone gegen das Epithel ab. Die weiter an Dicke zunehmende „larvale Basalmembran" ist in die Tiefe gerückt und zum Stratum compactum der Haut geworden. Sicher sind beim Aufbau der neuen Haut zahlreiche Fermente notwendig (GROSS, LAPIERE und TANZER, 1963); die Bestimmungen der Kathepsinaktivität im Schwanz von Krallenfroschlarven ergibt die höchste Aktivität in den Geweben bei Beginn der Metamorphose (R. WEBER, 1957), mit zunehmendem Abbau des Schwanzes sinkt auch die Aktivität ab.

5. Reptilia (Kriechtiere)

Die Haut der Reptilien ist durch das Fehlen von Hautdrüsen und die starke Verhornung der oberen Epithelschichten gekennzeichnet. Die Verhornung erzwingt zwei neue Vorgänge, die bisher für die Funktionsfähigkeit der Haut nicht notwendig waren: a) eine mit dem Wachstum der Tiere gekoppelte periodische Verhornung und Häutung; b) eine Gliederung der dicken Hornschichten an der Oberfläche in Schuppen, um die Beweglichkeit der Haut zu erhalten. Obwohl viele Reptilien, durch ihre Haut geschützt, Bewohner von sehr trockenen Gebieten sind, darf man sich die Haut nicht als undurchlässig vorstellen. Beim Kaiman ist der Wasserverlust durch die Haut immerhin noch so stark, daß er dem von Amphibien vergleichbar wird und etwa 30—50% des Verlustes bei Amphibien ausmacht. Und selbst bei Wüstenreptilien ist der Wasserverlust bei der Atmung geringer als der durch die Haut (BENTLEY und SCHMIDT-NIELSEN, 1965, 1966), wobei noch etwa 5% des Wasserverlustes vom Kaiman erreicht wird. Die phylogenetisch sehr heterogenen Reptilien sind außerdem in vielen Einzelheiten außerordentlich voneinander verschieden. Für die Haut gilt das ebenso wie für andere Organe. Der Häutungsvorgang ist nur bei den Schlangen und Eidechsen periodisch ausgebildet; Krokodile verlieren die Hornschichten in kleinen Stücken und ohne Periodizität. Die Schildkröten schließlich tragen einen Knochenpanzer, auf dem die epitheliale Horndecke nur eine geringe Bedeutung hat. Auch andere Formen bilden echte Knochenschuppen, welche die Hornschuppen unterlagern. Wie bei den Fischen müssen wir uns auf wenige Formen beschränken. Bei *Krokodilen und Schildkröten* ist die Haut, vor allem die Epidermis relativ einfach gebaut, ein vielschichtiges Epithel bildet durch Verhornung zahlreicher oberflächlicher Zellschichten eine feste Körperbedeckung, die in Schuppen gegliedert ist (vgl. SPEARMAN, 1966). Da aber keine regelmäßige Häutung stattfindet, wachsen die Schuppen an ihrem Rande weiter, um dem Wachstum des Tiers zu folgen. Das Corium besteht aus kollagenen Faserzügen, die eine besondere Lage zueinander einnehmen und so die mechanischen Beanspruchungen aufnehmen, die durch die Schuppen- oder Panzerbedeckung entstehen.

Besonderes Interesse hat aber die Haut der *Schlangen und Eidechsen (sog. Squamaten)* gefunden, da ihre periodischen Häutungsvorgänge einen komplizierten

Epithelaufbau bedingen, die Schuppengliederung konstant und also genetisch bedingt ist und bei den Schlangen ein Teil der Schuppen der Fortbewegung dient. Die Schuppen werden von Epidermis, Corium und Subcutis gebildet und überdecken sich dachziegelartig (Abb. 16). Die starke Verhornung und komplizierte Epithelschichtung erfolgt nur auf der Schuppenoberfläche. In den Rinnen zwischen den Schuppen ist das Epithel sehr viel dünner und macht den cyclischen Proliferations- und Verhornungsprozeß der Häutung nur in sehr begrenztem Umfang mit.

Die *Epidermis der Schuppenoberseite* bietet je nach der Häutungsphase ein sehr verschiedenes Bild (vgl. BECHTEL, 1957; GOSLAR, 1958, 1964; MADERSON, 1965). Kurz nach der Häutung besteht die Epidermis aus zwei getrennten Schichten:

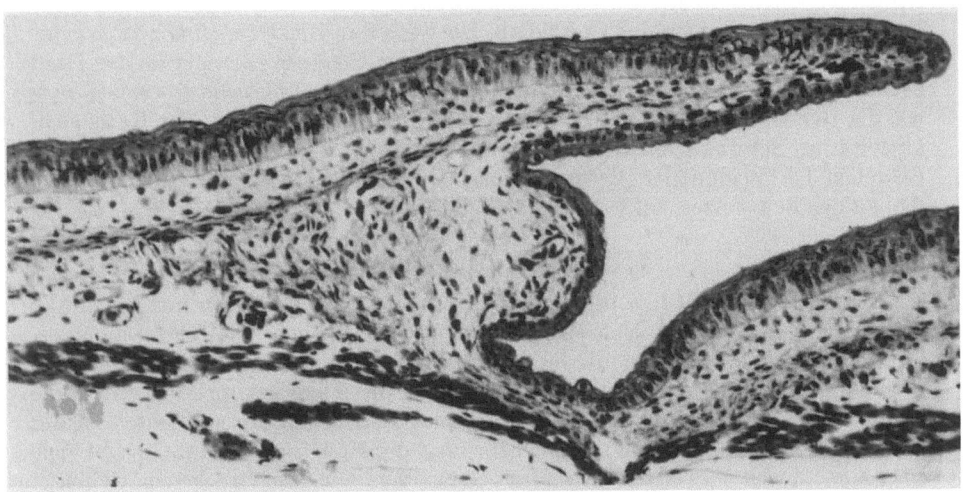

Abb. 16. Schuppenanlage eines Embryo der Kreuzotter; die Anlage trägt auf der Oberseite ein vielschichtiges Epithel und geht in die elastische Falte zwischen den Schuppen über, sie überdeckt bereits einen Teil der folgenden Schuppenanlage. Im Bindegewebe sind die entstehenden charakteristischen Faserzüge zu erkennen, abgeschlossen wird das Hautmesenchym durch eine Muskelplatte. (Häm. nach HEIDENHAIN, 200/1)

dem Stratum germinativum als einfacher Lage kubischer Zellen auf der Basalmembran (früher Stratum profundum) sowie einem aus vielen Zellagen aufgebauten Stratum corneum. Eine Übergangszone sich differenzierender Zellen wie im Stratum granulosum oder Stratum spinosum der Säuger fehlt zunächst. Die indifferenten Epithelzellen des Stratum germinativum enthalten Tonofibrillen und sind untereinander mit Desmosomen verbunden (HORSTMANN, 1964). An der Basis dringen die Epithelzellen mit Fortsätzen gegen die Basalmembran vor, so daß eine „Verzahnung" der Zellen zu bestehen scheint. In Wirklichkeit handelt es sich aber um regelmäßige Leisten, deren Verlaufsrichtung parallel und in Richtung der Schuppenachsen liegt (SCHMIDT, 1917; POCKRANDT, 1936/37). Es entsteht also hier zum erstenmal ein gesetzmäßiges Reliefbild des Unterhautbindegewebes, wie es für die Haut der Säugetiere so charakteristisch ist (HORSTMANN, 1957, 1962). Zwar beruht dieses Relief im wesentlichen auf der basalen Verformung der Zellen, jedoch sind auch regelrechte Coriumleisten durch Epithelwälle bekannt, also völlig homolog den Erscheinungen bei Säugetieren. Das Stratum corneum kann 10 oder mehr Zellschichten umfassen und wird von einer zunächst unvollständigen Lage flacher, heller Zellen unterlagert: die spätere Häutungsschicht. Ihr Cytoplasma zeichnet sich durch Vacuolen und osmiophile Einschlüsse aus. Die zur Oberfläche folgenden, flachgestreckten Zellen bilden in mehreren Lagen die innere Hornschicht. In diesen Zellen lassen sich feine Granula und Keratinfibrillen nachweisen

(HORSTMANN, 1964), jedoch keine Keratohyalintropfen. Darüber liegen weitere Zellschichten, deren völlig verhornte Epithelzellen entweder stark abgeflacht oder im Gegensatz dazu gerade blasig aufgetrieben sind und ihre Hornsubstanz vor allem im Bereich der Zellperipherie abgelagert haben. Man faßt diese Schichten als harte Hornschicht zusammen. Es handelt sich um abgestorbene Zellen, obwohl zwischen den Bündeln der Keratinfilamente noch Mitochondrien eingeschlossen sind; doch fallen alle histochemischen Fermentreaktionen negativ aus (G. WEBER, 1961; GOSLAR, 1964). In der weichen Hornschicht dagegen zeigen die Zellen noch eine Aktivität von Phosphatasen, Esterasen und auch von ATPase. Die scharfe Abgrenzung zwischen den toten und den noch nicht gänzlich verhornten Zellschichten kommt dadurch zustande, daß die Endphase der Verhornung bei den Reptilien erst kurz vor der Häutung einsetzt und unter Kontrolle von Geschlechtshormonen steht (GOSLAR, 1958). An der Oberfläche wird die harte Keratinschicht durch eine zusammenhängende Zellschicht bedeckt, das sog. Oberhäutchen. Es handelt sich um ganz flache Zellen, deren Zellgrenzen in der Aufsicht sich noch deutlich abheben und deren Oberfläche entweder ein besonders Relief bildet oder sogar haarförmige feine und dickere Fortsätze besitzt (SCHMIDT, 1912, 1913; HORSTMANN, 1964; MADERSON, 1964). Im Falle der Geckos dienen solche haarfeinen Fortsätze an der Oberfläche zur Unterstützung der Kletterbewegung an senkrechten Wänden oder Gegenständen, indem sie einen hohen Reibungswiderstand mit den Unebenheiten der Oberfläche erzeugen und so das Abgleiten verhindern. Eine besonders interessante Funktion der Oberfläche ist bei einer Wüstenechse (Moloch horridus) festgestellt worden (BENTLEY und BLUMER, 1962). Die feinen Fortsätze des „Oberhäutchens" wirken als capillares Netz, wenn die Tiere mit dem Tau oder mit Wasser auf dem Boden in Berührung kommen. Die Haut saugt sich auf der Oberfläche mit einem Wassernetz voll, das bis in die Mundregion sich vorschiebt und dort vom Tier mit Hilfe großer Schleimdrüsen eingeschluckt wird. Auf diese Weise können die Tiere lange Zeit ohne echtes Trinken in der Wüste überleben. — Neben dem mikroskopisch sichtbaren Oberflächenrelief ist außerdem die Zelloberfläche (bei glattem Oberhäutchen) von einer nur mit dem Elektronenmikroskop sichtbaren Feinstruktur von Leisten und Wabenmustern überzogen (HOGE und SANTOS, 1953), dessen Ausbildung artspezifisch ist und somit eine besondere Konstanz zeigt.

Nach der Häutung wird in etwa 3—4 Wochen eine neue, aus 12—16 Zellschichten bestehende Epithelzone unter dem Stratum corneum durch Proliferation der basalen Epithelzellen aufgebaut. Die Tochterzellen schieben sich aus dem Stratum germinativum in die höher gelegenen Zellschichten und breiten sich dort parallel zur Oberfläche aus, ihre Form wird also beim Verlassen der Keimschicht völlig verändert. So entsteht eine dicke sog. „intermediäre Schicht" von Zellen zwischen den Hornlagen des Stratum corneum und den indifferenten Zellen des Stratum germinativum. In den zur Grenze des alten Stratum corneum gelegenen Zellen findet dann sehr rasch eine Verhornung statt (SCHMIDT, 1913; BREYER, 1929; MADERSON, 1965), wobei die Aktivität der meisten histochemisch nachweisbaren Fermente ebenfalls schnell abnimmt (GOSLAR, 1964). Die obere Zellschicht, die also direkt unter den größeren und mit Vacuolen durchsetzten Häutungszellen des vorhergehenden Proliferationsschubes liegt, differenziert sich zu einem „Oberhäutchen" aus, indem die feinen Haarfortsätze und Zähnchen entstehen (HORSTMANN, 1964). Die verhornten Fortsätze greifen in Einstülpungen der Häutungszellen, so daß eine Verzahnung der beiden Zellschichten entsteht, die lichtmikroskopisch als eine deutliche, gestreifte Trennzone zwischen alter und neuer Epidermis der Schuppe seit langem bekannt ist. Die rasch verhornten Zellen bilden schließlich die obere, harte Keratinzone. Die tiefer gelegenen Zellen der neuen, „intermediären" Epidermis verhornen langsamer, zeigen noch zahlreiche Fermentaktivitäten und werden zur weichen Hornschicht, unterlagert von den basalen Epithelzellen. Damit ist der Prozeß der Proliferation und der Differenzierung als Vorbedingung für eine Häutung abgeschlossen. Eine Schuppe besteht aus zwei einander entsprechenden übereinander gelagerten Schichtenfolgen. Bei der Häutung wird durch einen nicht näher bekannten Prozeß in der Schicht der Häutungszellen ein Abbau vorgenommen; die Anwesenheit von Aminopeptidasen und freien Aminosäuren scheint die beginnende Auflösung der Zellen zu bewirken (GOSLAR, 1964). Dadurch wird am neuen Oberhäutchen ein Spalt zwischen den alten und neuen Epithelschichten erzeugt, der die kurz vor der Häutung einsetzende makroskopische Trübung der Haut zur Folge hat. 2—3 Wochen vor der Häutung ist die Trennung vollständig und die Haut wird wieder farbkräftig und glänzend. Schließlich erfolgt die Häutung, die gesamte Oberhaut wird als das bekannte „Natternhemd" abgestreift. In dieser alten Epidermishülle sind noch alle Zellschichten erkennbar (SCHMIDT, 1959) und verschiedene Stoffe nachzuweisen, z.B. Sphärite aus Lipoiden, Purine u.a. kristalline Ausfüllungen. Die Häutung wird hormonal gesteuert, aber es ist noch unklar, in welcher Weise. Thyroxin unterdrückt die Häutung, fördert aber die Verhornung (HALBERKANN, 1953, 1954), erst einige Zeit nach Thyroxingabe kommt es zur Häutung; den gleichen Effekt kann man auch durch Zuführen von thyreotropem Hypophysenhormon erzielen. Merkwürdig ist dagegen, daß nach Entfernung der Schilddrüse (NOBLE und BRADLEY, 1933) ebenso wie nach Hypophysektomie nicht der Ablauf der Häutung, wohl aber die Periode zwischen den Häutungen verändert wird, indem sie eine Verlängerung erfährt. Bei Zufuhr von Thyroxin wird der Häutungscyclus dann wieder normal. Nur der Hypophysenvorderlappen hat Einfluß, Entfernung von Zwischen- und Hinterlappen bleibt wirkungslos. Trotzdem ist durch Sexualhormone die Häutung ebenfalls zu beeinflussen (GOSLAR, 1958). Die jahreszeitlichen Veränderungen in der Hypophyse im Zusammenhang mit der Fortpflanzungsaktivität und Entfaltung der Gonaden sind ebenso wie die der Schilddrüse gut bekannt. Auch ACTH hemmt das Einsetzen der Häutung. Ist also der Mechanismus der Beeinflussung sehr unklar, so zeigt die Blockierung der Schilddrüse durch Thiouracil noch weniger aufschlußreiche Ergebnisse. RATZERSDORFER, GORDON und CHARIPPER (1949) finden, daß unter Thiouracil nicht die Periode zwischen den Häutungen verändert wird, wohl aber verlängert sich die Häutung selbst. Das ließe sich mit der langsameren Verhornung der Epithelien erklären. Dagegen stellt HALBERKANN (1954) bei einem Teil der Versuchstiere überhaupt keine Veränderung des Häutungscyclus fest, bei anderen wird die einsetzende Häutungsphase rückgängig gemacht. Wird das Methylthiouracil 9 Tage nach der letzten Häutung gegeben (Ringelnatter), so erfolgt die Häutung zum normalen, allerdings sehr frühen Zeitpunkt. Den direkten Einfluß des Thyroxins sieht GOSLAR (1964) in der Wirkung auf die Häutungszellen; MADERSON (1965) dagegen beschreibt die Einwanderung eosinophiler Granulocyten in das Epithel und ihre Ansammlung in der Häutungsschicht, wo sie die Auflösung bewirken sollen.

Die *Epithelien in den Rinnen zwischen den Schuppen* folgen dem Häutungscyclus nicht, sie bestehen aus wenigen Zellschichten, die an der Oberfläche eine normale Verhornung zeigen. Diese dünne Schicht verhornter Zellen wird bei der Häutung mit den Schuppenteilen abgegeben, so daß die dicken Schuppenfelder durch eine dünne Membran zusammenhängen; es ist dies ja die Vorbedingung für ein geschlossenes Abstreifen der alten Epidermis in Form des „Natternhemdes".

Im Epithel sind *Melanophoren* vorhanden, die bereits während der Embryonalentwicklung eingewandert sind und den Bereich des Stratum germinativum nicht verlassen (FIORONI, 1961). Sie entsenden Zellausläufer zwischen die oberen Epithelschichten und lagern zwischen und in den Epithelzellen ihr Melaninpigment ab. Entsprechend der Häutung werden sie rhythmisch tätig, spielen aber für die Ausfärbung der Haut keine Rolle. Wenn die Verhornung einer neuen Epithelgeneration (intermediäre Schicht) beginnt, ziehen die Melanophoren ihre Ausläufer zurück (FIORONI, 1961). Es bestehen also analoge Verhältnisse wie beim Haarwachstum und Haarwechsel der Säuger (vgl. DANNEEL und WEISSENFELS, 1953). Es gibt aber auch Fälle (z.B. Chamäleon), wo sehr große Melanophoren in tieferen Lagen des Coriumbindegewebes lange Fortsätze bis ins Epithel senden und dort Melanin ablagern.

Unterlagert wird die Epidermis von der *Basalmembran*, die den üblichen Aufbau hat (HORSTMANN, 1964). Darunter liegt das *Corium*, das sich wie bei den Amphibien in zwei strukturmäßig und funktionell sehr verschiedene Zonen gliedert: das oberflächliche *Stratum laxum* und darunter das *Stratum compactum*. Das Stratum laxum ist die Schicht der Pigmentzellen, Gefäße und Nerven und kann geradezu als Pigmentschicht bezeichnet werden (FIORONI, 1961). Denn die zahllosen verschiedenen Farbzellen des Stratum laxum bilden die Grundlage für das Erscheinungsbild der Reptilien mit ihren sehr auffälligen Mustern, die bei Schlangen, Eidechsen und Schmuckschildkröten ihren Höhepunkt der Ausbildung erreichen. Durch die Erweiterung von Hautfalten am Nacken, an der Kehle können in der Erregung besonders auffällige Muster als Drohgebärde sichtbar gemacht werden (Kobra, Kragenechse, Anolis u.a.). Die Farbzellen sind wie bisher besprochen Melanophoren, Guanophoren (Iridocyten), Xantho- und Erythrophoren. Sie brauchen im einzelnen nicht mehr betrachtet zu werden und wurden von SCHMIDT (1917) sehr sorgfältig beschrieben. Inzwischen konnten auch Pterine in den Xantho- und Erythrophoren nachgewiesen werden (GÜNDER, 1954; ORTIZ und WILLIAMS-ASHMAN, 1963; ORTIZ, BÄCHLI und WILLIAMS-ASHMAN, 1963). Die Guanophoren bilden in der Regel eine sehr dicke Schicht, so daß reflektiertes bläuliches Licht mit den gelben oder roten Farbstoffen wie bei den Fischen und Amphibien Mischfarben (z.B. blau) ergeben kann oder den irisierenden Glanz der Farben unterstützt. Der *physiologische Farbwechsel* der Reptilien ist einer Analyse nicht so gut zugänglich wie bei den niederen Wirbeltieren, denn nur in wenigen Arten sind die Farbzellen der mikroskopischen Beobachtung zugänglich, so daß der Farbwechsel nicht nach dem Verhalten des Pigmentes in den Zellen, sondern nur durch mikroskopische Betrachtung des Farbzustandes des Tieres beurteilt werden kann (vgl. WARING, 1963). Obwohl eine nervöse Kontrolle wahrscheinlich ist, konnte ein direkter Beweis bisher dafür nicht erbracht werden. In den wenigen günstigen Fällen dagegen, bei denen man die Melanophoren direkt beobachten kann, zeigt sich die hormonale Kontrolle und Beeinflussung durch MSH, Adrenalin, Hypophysektomie. In den Schwimmhäuten einer Wasserschildkröte sind die Melanophoren gut sichtbar. Die Verlagerung des Pigmentes erfolgt nach Injektion von MSH (Hypophysenextrakt) im Sinne der Ausbreitung der Granula in den Melanophoren, unter Adrenalin erfolgt die Aggregation (WOOLLEY, 1956). Auch der Untergrundeffekt ist deutlich ausgeprägt. Auch bei der Gattung Anolis, die zu den Leguanen gehört, sind die Melanophoren in der isolierten, durchsichtigen Haut sehr gut sichtbar, da die Schuppen klein und dünn sind (HOROWITZ, 1957, 1958). Schon früher waren mit der Haut von Anolis Versuche durchgeführt worden (HADLEY, 1931; KLEINHOLZ, 1938). Hypophysektomie und Adrenalin hellen die Haut durch Aggregation der Granula in den Melanophoren auf; MSH bringt die dunkle Färbung zustande. Wie im einzelnen die Erregungszustände der Tiere bei Kämpfen mit Artgenossen, sonstige Reizung (Chamäleon, Krötenechse) und der Untergrund via Augen auf den Farbwechsel Einfluß nimmt, ist nicht bekannt.

Das Bindegewebe des Stratum laxum bildet die Grundlage für die Vorwölbung der Schuppen und stellt eine Verschiebeschicht dar; zugleich bilden die Faserzüge auch eine Verankerung der Schuppen (SCHMIDT, 1912, 1913; POCKRANDT, 1936). In der feineren Architektur zeigt sich eine Anpassung an die Beanspruchung der Schuppen (Abb. 17), so daß a) die Schuppen verschiedener Körperregionen nicht gleichartig vom Bindegewebe unterlagert werden, b) jede Schuppe in ihrem vorderen Teil anders gestützt wird als im hinteren Abschnitt, der die nächste Schuppe überdeckt und so einen vorstehenden Rand besitzt. Daher finden sich in den großen Bauchschuppen der Schlange besonders übersichtliche Verhältnisse, da sie zur Fortbewegung benutzt werden (vgl. unten). In den starren Schuppen der Krokodile bzw. unter den Panzern der Schildkröte stellt das Stratum laxum nur ein dichtes Fasernetz aus kollagenen Fibrillen dar, das durch aufsteigende Faserbündel gefestigt wird und allmählich in die regelmäßig angeordneten Faserlagen des Stratum compactum übergeht (vgl. SCHMIDT, 1921; LANGE, 1931). In den großen Schuppen der Squamaten steigen einzelne Faserschichten aus den oberflächlichen Lagen des Stratum compactum in das lockere Bindegewebe des Stratum laxum auf und breiten sich bis in den hinteren Rand der Schuppe aus, wo sie in der Basalmembran verankert sind. Am vorderen Teil der Schuppe verlaufen Faserbündel vertikal zur Oberfläche, durchsetzen das Stratum laxum und strahlen ebenfalls mit Faserbündeln in die Basalmembran ein. In der Mitte der Schuppe besteht ein Geflecht aus sich kreuzenden Bündeln kollagener Fasern. Das Bindegewebe in der Furche zur nächsten Schuppe wird durch unregelmäßig angeordnete Fasern aufgebaut, zwischen denen große turgescente Bindegewebszellen oder Fettzellen ein Druckpolster bilden. Die großen Faserzüge sind durchsetzt von einem dichten Netz elastischer Fasern, die hier zum erstenmal in größeren Mengen in der Haut vorhanden sind und z. T. durchbrochene Membranen bilden. Unter der gesamten Schuppenfläche durchsetzen sie als aufsteigende vertikale elastische Netze das kollagene Fasergerüst. POCKRANDT (1936) zeigt, daß ein längs verlaufendes und ein quer zur Körperachse verlaufendes elastisches System vorliegt; verbunden sind diese Netze durch lange Faserstränge (elastisch), die in parallelen Zügen die Schuppen mit den seitlichen Nachbarschuppen verbinden; sie ziehen quer durch das Schuppenbindegewebe und geben in den Nachbarschuppen aufsteigende Fasern bis in die Nähe der Basalmembran ab. Diese elastischen Querverbindungen sind bei der starken Dehnung der Haut beim Ver-

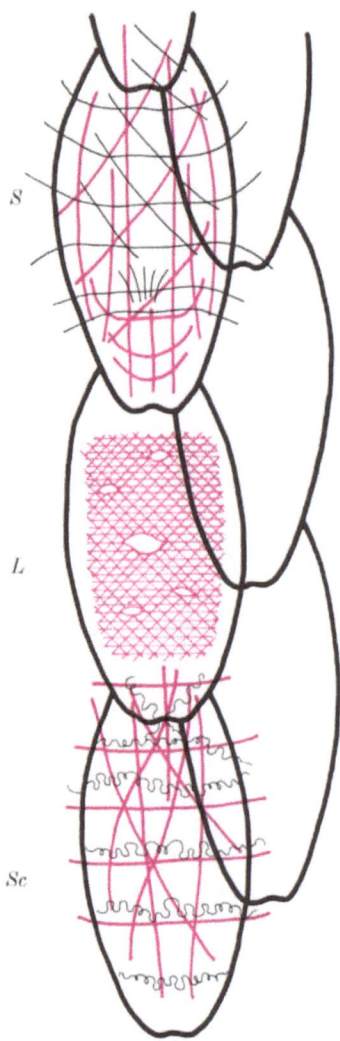

Abb. 17. Funktionelle Anpassung der Coriumstruktur unter den Rückenschuppen einer Ringelnatter (Tropidonotus natrix). Darstellung elastischer Fasern in verschiedenen Schichten: Im Schuppenkörper S, in der elastischen Lamelle L und in der Subcutis Sc. Rot = Fasern des Längssystems, schwarz = Fasern des Quersystems. (Nach POCKRANDT, 1936)

schlingen von Beute von Bedeutung. Es ist bedauerlich, daß die so deutlich sichtbare „funktionelle Struktur" des Reptilienbindegewebes in der nachfolgenden Zeit keine genaue Bearbeitung und tiefere Analyse mehr erfahren hat.

Im Zusammenhang mit dem Bindegewebe muß die *Muskulatur* betrachtet werden, die bei den Schlangen an den Bauchschuppen ansetzt und eine Fortbewegung der Tiere ohne die „schlängelnde" Körperbewegung ermöglicht; bei der durch Körperbiegungen bewirkten Bewegungsweise dienen die Bauchschuppen der Abstützung an Unebenheiten des Untergrundes (vgl. BELLAIRS und UNDERWOOD, 1951; LISSMANN, 1950; LÜDICKE, 1962/64). Die cutane Muskulatur entstammt der Skeletmuskulatur und ist entweder modifizierte Rippenmuskulatur (M. costocutaneus-Gruppe) oder besteht aus Teilen des verlagerten M. rectus und M. obliquus subcutaneus (ventraler Hautmuskel in seiner Gesamtheit, vgl. HOFFMANN, 1890; WIEDEMANN, 1931/32; eine gute Zusammenfassung der anatomischen Verhältnisse gibt LÜDICKE, 1962/64). Die Muskelpartien sind segmental und sehr kompliziert angeordnet, da auch die Schuppen untereinander mit Muskeln verbunden sind. Die Hautmuskeln liegen unter dem Stratum compactum und benutzen die Faserbündel, die in die Haut aufsteigen, als Sehnen. Durch eine Kontraktionswelle von hinten nach vorne werden die Schuppen gehoben und gesenkt, wobei die Rippen aber gegenüber der Wirbelsäule keine Bewegung erfahren, also als starres Widerlager der Haut-Rippenmuskeln dienen (LISSMANN, 1950). HESS (1963, 1965) konnte bei der Hautmuskulatur zwei verschiedene Fasertypen nachweisen, die langsamen und die schnellen Fasern. Sie unterscheiden sich dadurch, daß die schnelle Faser einen sehr regelmäßigen Aufbau der elektronenmikroskopisch sichtbaren Fibrillen und nur eine typische motorische Endplatte von einem Axon besitzt. Die langsamen Fasern dagegen zeigen nicht die sonst als Leitbahnen ausgebildeten Tubuli des endoplasmatischen Reticulums und haben multiple Synapsenendigungen von abweichendem Aufbau; so fehlt die starke Faltung der postsynaptischen Zellmembran, die bei schnellen Fasern an der motorischen Endplatte charakteristisch ist. Durch diese Feststellungen wird sich sicher eine erneute Überarbeitung der Erkenntnisse über die Bewegung der Schlangen anschließen müssen. Zu ergänzen bleibt noch, daß die stärkste Hautmuskulatur bei großen Schlangen, z.B. der Boa zu finden ist; daß ferner ein sehr unterschiedlich großer Anteil der Rumpffläche von Hautmuskeln bedeckt sein kann (zwischen 50—80%) und die im Erdreich lebenden wühlenden Schlangen alle ihre Rumpfschuppen abspreizen können und daher in der gesamten Rumpfhaut eine starke Muskulatur besitzen.

Die *Blutgefäße des Stratum laxum* sind in ihrer Anordnung von der Ausbildung der Schuppen abhängig (SCHMIDT, 1910; POCKRANDT, 1936/37; LÜDICKE, 1940). Aus dem regelmäßigen Netz der subcutanen Arterien und Venen steigen kleine Äste durch Lücken des Stratum compactum in das Bindegewebe der oberen Coriumschicht auf und bilden dort ein engmaschiges Capillarnetz (Abb. 18), das die Papille der Schuppe durchsetzt. Die Sprossung der Gefäße ist von FIORONI (1961) in den Schuppenanlagen verfolgt worden. LÜDICKE (1940) konnte zeigen, daß Anastomosen den Kurzschluß der Capillarnetze ermöglichen, und daß ferner die Arteriole ähnlich wie in den Darmzotten zunächst ungeteilt im medianen Teil der Schuppenpapille aufsteigt und sich erst in der Schuppenspitze in Capillaren teilt. POCKRANDT (1936/37) vermutet eine Beteiligung an einer Hautatmung bei Wasserschlangen, da die Capillarnetze ungewöhnlich dicht ausgebildet und z.T. die Gefäße in die Epidermis vorgeschoben sind. Auch im flachen Ruderschwanz sind die Capillaren unmittelbar unter der Epidermis gelegen. Hier werden also Verhältnisse der Hautdurchblutung erreicht wie bei den Amphibienlarven oder den Fischen der Gezeitenzone (Gobiiden, s. vorher). Wir erwähnen die Befunde deshalb, weil die Art des arteriellen Zuflusses und die Anastomosen eine Regulation der Hautzirkulation doch sehr wahrscheinlich machen. Die Reptilien sind als wechselwarme Tiere auf die Zufuhr von Wärme angewiesen, die sie durch direkte Sonnenbestrahlung, aus der Luft bzw. dem Wasser und als Untergrundabstrahlung aufnehmen. Durch ihr Verhalten stellen sie sich auf die Bedingungen zur Erwärmung sehr genau ein. Es ist aber weiter sehr gut bekannt, daß die einmal erreichte optimale Körpertemperatur (ca. 32—39° C, die Arten verhalten sich verschieden) sehr genau eingehalten wird, es erfolgt also eine

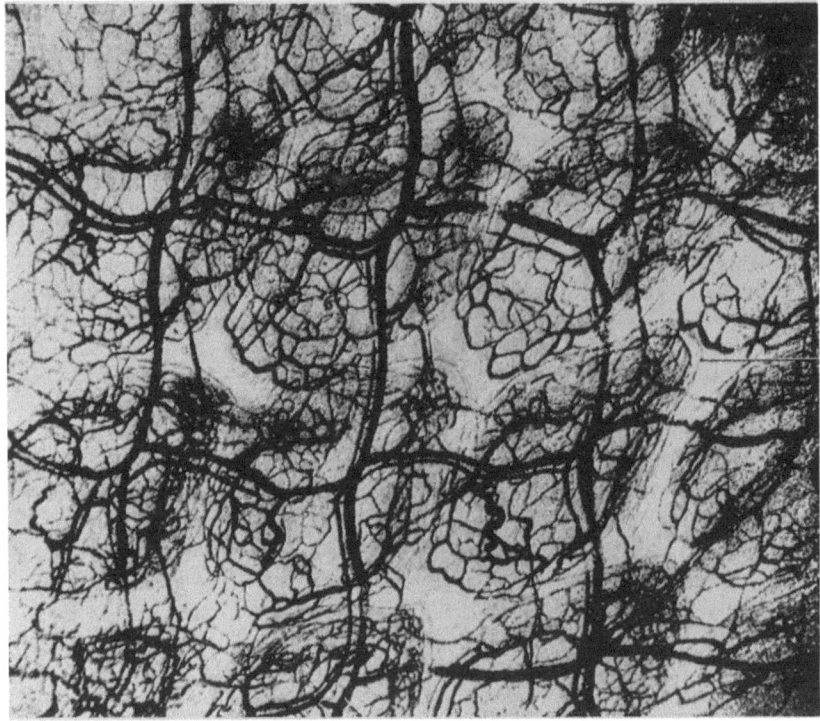

Abb. 18. Anordnung der Blutgefäße unter den dorsalen Halsschuppen der Schlanknatter (Zamenis dahli Fitz.). Die gleichförmige doppelte Gefäßanordnung und die aufsteigenden Capillarnetze der Schuppen sind durch Tuscheinjektion sehr deutlich zu erkennen (LÜDICKE, 1940). 25/1

Thermoregulation. Die capillaren Hautgefäße stellen ein besonders günstiges System dar, durch das sowohl Wärme mit der Körperoberfläche aufgenommen und abgeleitet werden kann, wie auch eine Drosselung der Wärmeaufnahme bzw. Wärmeabgabe bei kühlerer Umgebung vorgenommen werden muß. Schließlich wird auch der physiologische Farbwechsel beeinflußt: stark erwärmte Tiere werden heller, kühle Tiere (z. B. beim Beginn der morgendlichen Erwärmung) sind dunkler. Werden verschieden große Tiere der gleichen Art unter gleichen Bedingungen einer Wärmebestrahlung ausgesetzt, so werden die kleineren Individuen eher heller als die großen. Denn die Melanophoren absorbieren Wärme, die Guanophoren reflektieren vor allem im infraroten Wellenbereich (BOGERT, 1959). Die direkte Beteiligung der Blutgefäße kann beim texanischen Taubleguan (Holbrookia) nachgewiesen werden. Diese Tiere graben sich ein, um der nächtlichen Abkühlung entgegenzuwirken. Am Morgen lassen sie zuerst nur den Kopf von der Sonne bescheinen, den sie hervorstrecken. In einem großen Blutsinus des Kopfes wird auf diese Weise das Blut vorgewärmt, bis die Tiere schon sehr aktiv sind, wenn sie die Erde vollständig abschütteln. Über die Thermoreceptoren der Haut ist (mit Ausnahme der Grubenorgane bei den Grubenottern) wenig bekannt. Nur BULLOCK und DIECKE (1956) berichten bei ihren Untersuchungen über das Grubenorgan, daß Nervenableitungen auch von der Bauchseite von Schlangen gemacht wurden. Bei Temperaturerhöhungen waren keine Reaktionen zu verzeichnen, nur bei der Abkühlung um mehrere Grad kam es zu einer vorübergehenden Frequenzerhöhung. Eine zentrale Steuerung durch den hypothalamischen Bereich des Gehirns am 3. Ventrikel ist nach den Untersuchungen von RODBARD, SAMSON und FERGUSON (1950) immerhin wahrscheinlich. Bei einer größeren Anzahl von Schildkröten konnte nämlich durch Einpflanzen von Silberdraht in Gehirnteile gezeigt werden, daß bei Erwärmung der genannten Region ein Blutdruckanstieg innerhalb von 20 sec. erfolgt, der sein Maximum einige Minuten nach Beginn der Erwärmung erreicht. Das bedeutet natürlich auch eine verstärkte Durchblutung der Haut. Eine Abkühlung des Hirngebietes mit dem Silberdraht senkte den Blutdruck. Eine periphere Erwärmung bzw. Abkühlung des Tieres wirkt offenbar zunächst nicht über den Stoffwechsel des Herzmuskels auf den Blutdruck, sondern über ein zentral-nervöses Kontrollzentrum. Die starke Steigerung der Atmungsfrequenz bei erhöhten Körpertemperaturen (ca. 40° C) dient nicht der Wärmeregulierung, sondern ist nur durch den erhöhten O_2-Verbrauch bei erhöhtem Stoffwechsel bedingt (NIELSEN, 1961). Dagegen kann die erst kürzlich bekannt gewordene Wasserabgabe durch die Haut (vgl. oben) durchaus einer Temperaturregulation dienen.

Das *Stratum compactum* im Corium setzt sich aus Faserschichten zusammen, ähnlich wie die entsprechende Schicht bei adulten Amphibien. In jeder Schicht liegen dicht gepackte Faserbündel parallel zueinander; dagegen wechselt die Verlaufsrichtung der Fasern von Schicht zu Schicht. Die Fasern übereinander liegender Schichten überschneiden sich also in gewissen Winkeln. Die Schuppen prägen dabei die Winkelverhältnisse: da sie mit Fasern des Stratum compactum verankert und selbst in schräg über den Körper verlaufenden Reihen angeordnet sind, so folgen die Fasern den Schrägzeilen der Schuppen. Eingeschlossen in die Faserschichten sind vertikale Bündel sowie die aus der Subcutis aufsteigenden Blutgefäße und Nerven. Auf die Komplikation der Architektur beim Vorhandensein von echten Knochenschuppen in der Haut können wir hier nicht eingehen.

Die *Subcutis* ist die aus lockerem Bindegewebe, Faserbündeln und z. T. auch aus Fettpolstern bestehende Verbindungsschicht, in der die Hautmuskulatur eingelagert ist (s. oben). Die Subcutis enthält ein charakteristisches Maschenwerk von Gefäßen und Nerven, die wieder in ihrer Verteilung durch die Anordnung der Schuppen bestimmt werden. Ein sehr gleichmäßiges Geflecht von nahezu quadratischen oder sechseckigen Maschen ist so angeordnet, daß die Knotenpunkte der Verzweigungen etwa in der Mitte unter den Schuppen liegen (Abb. 18). Und zwar ist ein Doppelstrang aus Arterie und Vene vorhanden, meist begleitet von einem Nerven. Dickere Gefäße versorgen an verschiedenen Stellen dieses System, indem sie durch die Muskulatur stoßen und besonders in den Hautmuskeln einen sehr gewundenen Verlauf (zur Verschiebung des Gefäßes bei der Bewegung) nehmen können. Fettzellen können die Verzweigungsstellen stützen. Aus diesem Netz treten die kleinen Gefäße zur Bildung der Capillaren in der Schuppenpapille aus.

Die *Innervation und die Hautsinnesorgane* der Reptilien sind nur sehr ungenügend bekannt. Die somatischen afferenten Neurone liegen in den Spinalganglien, und die davon ausgehenden Rami dorsales bedingen eine segmentale Innervation der Haut. Dort sind die Axone als freie Nervenendigungen in der Epidermis verbreitet, oder sie enden an besonderen Sinnesorganen, die als Tastorgane angesehen werden. Über eine Beteiligung des sympathischen Systems bei der Hautinnervation ist nichts bekannt. Die segmentale Innervation der Körperoberfläche läßt sich als Dermatome bei Eidechsen (VAN TRIGT, 1917) und Schlangen (TEN CATE, 1936) zeigen. Das einem Spinalnerven zugeordnete Hautsegment hat am Rumpf etwa die Form eines Rechtecks, dessen Länge ca. $3^1/_2$ Wirbelkörperlängen entspricht; an und auf den Extremitäten sind die Grenzen natürlich verschoben. Die gegenseitige Überlappung der Dermatome ist erheblich; so beträgt die Überdeckung der benachbarten Areale bei der Eidechse $^2/_3$, bei der Natter $^1/_2$ der Dermatombreite. Da die Bauchseite der Reptilien bei der Wärmewahrnehmung und Wärmeaufnahme vom Untergrund im Verhalten der Tiere eine zentrale Rolle spielt, so ist nicht verwunderlich, daß die Dermatome auf der Ventralseite breiter als auf der Dorsalseite sind, also sich ventral noch stärker überschneiden. Diese Anordnung ist unter den höheren Wirbeltieren nur bei den Reptilien ausgebildet. Die Nervenstämmchen der spinalen Rami, die in die Subcutis eingetreten sind, enthalten markhaltige Axone verschiedenen Durchmessers (SCHMIDT, 1910, dort auch die älteren Befunde). Aus dem regelmäßig den Gefäßen folgenden Nervenplexus steigen kleine Stämmchen ins Stratum laxum empor, wo eine starke Verzweigung der Fasern stattfindet. Ein großer Teil der Fasern gelangt an die Basalmembran; dort dringen die Axone ins Epithel vor, wobei die Markscheiden an der Epithelgrenze aufhören. Im Epithel bilden die Axone ein Geflecht, das besondere und auffällige varicöse Verdickungen zeigt, die nach Silberimprägnation und Methylenblaufärbung sichtbar sind und als Endkolben bezeichnet wurden (SCHMIDT, 1910; JABUREK, 1927; SCHARTAU, 1936). Die segmentale Überschneidung, die ja die Überlappung der Dermatome bedingt, wird auch im histologischen Bild sichtbar (SCHARTAU, 1936). Daß die alte Annahme, die Endverzweigungen der Axone würden in die Epithelzellen vordringen, nicht den wirklichen Verhältnissen entspricht, kann nach den bisher bekannt gewordenen elektronenmikroskopischen Befunden an anderen Tierklassen wohl mit Sicherheit angenommen werden. Die als Tastorgane angesprochenen *Sinnesorgane* sind in der Haut des Kopfes und des Rumpfes sehr zahlreich vorhanden. Jede Schuppe enthält eines oder, vor allem am Kopf, mehrere dieser Organe. BREYER (1929) zählt an einem Tier der Mauereidechse 5810 Tastorgane, bei der Zauneidechse sind es 4964; SCHMIDT (1910) findet auf bestimmten Kopfschildern 70 bzw. 100 Tastflecke. Sie können sehr klein im Durchmesser sein (8 μ), oder als deutliche große helle Flecken auf den Schuppen erscheinen, da das Pigment in ihrer Umgebung reduziert ist. Die Unstimmigkeiten, die hinsichtlich des Feinbaues dieser „Tastflecke" bestehen, machen es schwer, zu einer Beurteilung der Organe zu gelangen. Offenbar bestehen im einzelnen recht erhebliche Unterschiede im Aufbau, und neuere Untersuchungen fehlen darüber. Als sicher kann gelten, daß der am meisten ausgebildete Typ der Organe keine Sinnesknospe des Epithels darstellt, sondern ein Polster von Zellen in einer Coriumpapille (SCHMIDT, 1910, 1912, 1913, 1914, 1917/18; JABUREK, 1927; BREYER, 1929). Die Organe bestehen aus einer Gruppe von großen Zellen unter der Basalmembran und sind von dünnen Faserkapseln umschlossen (Abb. 19). Der Komplex liegt in einer papillenförmigen Vorwölbung des Corium gegen die Epidermis und wird von einem Nervenast versorgt, dessen Axone zwischen die großen Zellen vordringen sollen. Es wäre also eine Art von Meissnerschen Tastkörperchen entstanden, und die großen Zellen dürften mit den „Merkelschen Tastzellen" zu identifizieren sein. Über dem Komplex ist die Epidermis in verschiedener Weise modifiziert. So können bei Eidechsen und Geckos im Stratum basale über der Coriumpapille einige große Epithelzellen liegen, die von flachen Mantelzellen an den Seiten gegen das übrige Epithel abgegrenzt sind. Das Oberhäutchen ist jedoch geschlossen darüber ausgebildet und trägt besonders lange haarfeine Fortsätze, die in einzelnen Arten zu einem langen Haar verschmolzen sind. Beide Haartypen nehmen natürlich Berührungen unter Verbiegung auf, die Verformung überträgt sich durch die besonders geformten Epithelzellen auf das Coriumpolster. Es ist daher nicht wahrscheinlich, daß die großen Epithelzellen über der Papille Sinneszellen sind, wie SCHMIDT (1913, 1924) annimmt. In anderen Fällen liegen nämlich über den vorgewölbten Coriumpapillen im Epithel Reihen von großen Epithelzellen bis zur harten Hornschicht regelmäßig übereinander geschichtet, oder ein flächiger Komplex modifizierter verhornter Zellen ermöglicht als Polster die Druckübertragung auf die Coriumpapille, dabei fehlt das harte Oberhäutchen der Epidermis. Es muß aber gesagt werden, daß die Beurteilung erschwert wird durch die ungenaue Kenntnis

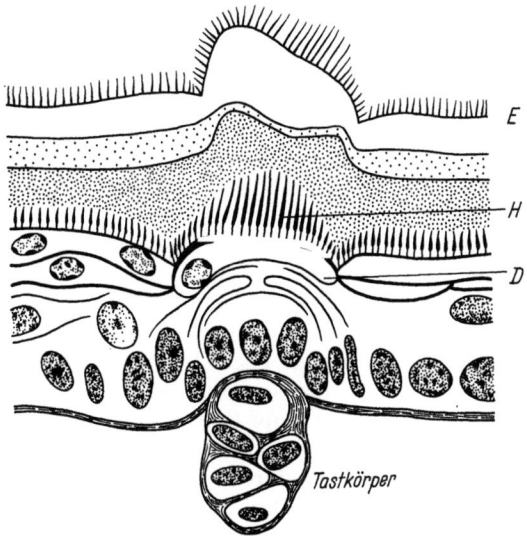

Abb. 19. Tastorgan am Schwanz einer Eidechse (Blattschwanzgecko, Uroplatus fimbriatus); in einer Bindegewebskapsel liegen große Zellen eingeschlossen, das Epithel darüber wird von schalenförmig angeordneten Zellen gebildet, die als Abschluß eine Deckplatte (D) bilden. Darüber sind die Hornfortsätze der neuen Oberfläche ausgebildet (H); überlagert wird die neue Epidermis von der alten, stark verhornten Epithelschicht E, an deren Oberfläche die alten Hornfortsätze stehen. (Nach W. J. SCHMIDT, 1913)

der tatsächlichen Innervierung im Bereich der Tastflecke. Es ist durchaus möglich, daß Axone zwischen die säulenförmig aufgeschichteten Epithelzellen vordringen, wie JABUREK (1927) angibt. Dann müßten die in der Coriumpapille gelegenen Zellkerne den Schwannschen Zellen der Nerven angehören. — Weitere Sinnesorgane sollen als eingesenkte epitheliale Sinnesknospen vorkommen, und schließlich sind Pacinische Körperchen von MERKEL im Corium beschrieben worden (zit. nach SCHMIDT, 1917/18), doch sind diese Befunde nie wieder bestätigt worden. Zwar sind die Schwierigkeiten bei der histologischen und vor allem physiologischen Untersuchung der Reptilienhaut unvergleichlich größer als bei Amphibien- und Säugerhäuten. Dennoch ist es sehr bedauerlich, daß bei den phylogenetisch so wichtigen Gruppen der Reptilien keine modernen Untersuchungen vorliegen, da ihr Verhalten bei der Thermoregulation und die unbezweifelbare Homologie zwischen Reptilienschuppe, Vogelfeder und Säugerhaar sehr aufschlußreiche Ergebnisse erwarten lassen.

6. Vögel

Die Haut der Vögel wird durch die Entwicklung von Federn gekennzeichnet, die als Derivate der Epidermis ein Klassenmerkmal darstellen. Die starke Verankerung der Federn in der Haut bedingt, ähnlich wie bei den Schuppen der

Reptilien, daß die Gliederung und der feinere Aufbau der Haut von der Anordnung der Federn geprägt ist. Die Federn sind nicht überall gleichmäßig in der gesamten Haut vorhanden, sondern stehen in festgelegten Reihen, die während der Embryonalentwicklung in artspezifischer Weise auftreten (embryonale Pterylose). Die federtragenden Partien der Haut (sog. Federfluren) werden von Zonen ohne Federn in ihrer Ausdehnung abgegrenzt, so daß schmale Hautstreifen ohne Federn (sog. Federraine) die befiederten Hautpartien umgeben und eine bestimmte Symmetrie erzeugen. An den Extremitäten schließlich sind in der Regel anstatt der Federn echte Hornschuppen vorhanden, die aber den Federn homolog sind und bei bestimmten Rassen domestizierter Vögel (Hühner, Tauben u. a.) oder auch bei spezialisierten Arten durch Federn ersetzt werden (vgl. unten). Bis auf einige große Drüsen (Salzdrüsen, Bürzeldrüse) mit ganz spezialisierten Aufgaben fehlen der Vogelhaut jegliche Drüsen oder Drüsenzellen in der Epidermis (Zusammenfassungen bei LANGE, 1931; STRESEMANN, 1934). Die einfache Beschaffung von Tiermaterial und die ungewöhnlich günstigen Bedingungen bei den Embryonen für experimentelle Eingriffe haben die Haut der Vögel zu einem bevorzugten Objekt für die Kausalanalyse der Morphogenese gemacht. Fast alles, was heute über die Wechselwirkungen der Gewebe in der Haut bei der Embryonalentwicklung und die Entstehung von Epithelderivaten, von Regionalspezifität u. a. bekannt ist, wurde an der Vogelhaut erschlossen.

Die *Epidermis* ist nur aus wenigen Zellschichten (2—4) aufgebaut, da die Haut von den Federn bedeckt wird und mechanischer Schutz durch die Epidermis nicht mehr notwendig ist. Nur die frei zutage liegenden Hautpartien am Kopf, an besonderen Hautlappen, am Kamm machen eine Ausnahme. Die Oberfläche der Haut ist aber überall an Rumpf und Kopf (hintere Extremitäten ausgenommen) nicht glatt, sondern durch Falten des Unterhautbindegewebes in Felder und Furchen unregelmäßig zerklüftet, wodurch eine starke Verschieblichkeit der oberen Hautschichten bewirkt wird. Das Stratum germinativum besteht aus kubischen oder stark abgeflachten Zellen, je nach der Dicke der oberflächlichen Epithelzellschichten; Mitosen sind häufig. Die oberen Zellen der Epidermis sind wechselnd geformt und verhornen, ohne daß in der Regel Keratohyalingranula sichtbar werden. Die Zellen flachen sich ab, der Kern bleibt noch erhalten, doch lagert sich die Hornsubstanz nur an der Peripherie der Zellen ab. Die so entstehenden hohlen Hornzellen des Stratum corneum erinnern also an die Verhältnisse der lockeren Hornschicht der Reptilien (SPEARMAN, 1966). Und ähnlich wie bei diesen lassen sich Phosphatasen und Esterasen vor der endgültigen Verhornung nachweisen. Das Stratum corneum besteht an der Oberfläche aus mehreren Schichten sehr flacher, zusammenhängender Hornzellen, die in Lagen abschilfern. Eine Mitosekontrolle scheint in manchen Stellen der Epidermis zu bestehen: nach eigenen Beobachtungen (unveröffentlicht, Taube adult und Nestling) werden regelmäßige Säulen aus Epidermiszellen (4—5 Lagen) gebildet, die an der Oberfläche verhornen und so eine gewellte Hornlage entstehen lassen. Einzelne Hautfalten zeichnen sich durch eine vielschichtige Epidermis aus, die an der Basis mit Leisten im Corium verankert ist, also doch wohl eine gewisse Konstanz haben dürften, während die benachbarten Faltungen keine Abweichungen vom üblichen Epidermisaufbau zeigen. Die Abhängigkeit der Epidermisdifferenzierung von Wirkstoffen wie Cortison, Vitamin A konnte bei Vögeln klar gezeigt werden (Zusammenfassung bei FELL, 1964). Die elektronenmikroskopische Untersuchung der sich differenzierenden Epidermis erfolgte am Schnabel, den Extremitäten und der Rückenhaut (FITTON-JACKSON und FELL, 1963; FELL, 1964). Durch die Gewebekultur werden Verhältnisse erzielt, die dem bereits geschlüpften Tier gleichen, da die Oberflächenschichten das embryonale Periderm (eine besondere Epithelschicht) verlieren und eine reguläre Verhornung durchmachen. Es zeigt sich, daß die Basalzellen mit feinen Fortsätzen in einer dünnen Basalmembran von typischem Aufbau verankert sind; sie enthalten außer den Zellorganellen noch Bündel aus sehr feinen Fibrillen. Die nach oben folgenden „Stachelzellen" liegen in zwei bis drei Schichten und sind abgeflacht und durch Desmosomen verbunden wie auch die Basalzellen. In den „Stachelzellen" sind ebenfalls Tonofilamente vorhanden, die an die Desmosomen heranreichen. Aus dem Einbau radioaktiv markierter Substanzen läßt sich vielleicht schließen, daß ähnlich wie bei den Amphibien die Epithelzellen dieser beiden Schichten sulfatierte Mucopolysaccharide aufbauen (PELC und FELL, 1960). Durch die Verhornung wird diese Synthese blockiert, unter Vitamin A dagegen so stark gefördert, daß große oberflächliche Schleimvacuolen entstehen, die sehr an die im Oberflächenepithel von Amphibienlarven erinnern. In solchen Fällen unterbleibt die Keratinisierung der Zellen; ein Stratum corneum entsteht also nicht und die schleimbildenden Zellen bilden eine Oberflächenschicht. — Die verhornenden Zellen der zwei oberflächlichen Schichten schließlich enthalten große Vacuolen mit Flüssigkeit und unter der Zellmembran wird ein sehr dichtes, aus Fibrillen bestehendes Material in Schichten abgelagert, die doppelbrechend in polarisiertem Licht sind. Die einzelne verhornende Zelle verliert ihre Zellorganelle, wird aber nicht zu einer festen Masse, sondern ist ein Hohlkörper. Die Befunde von SPEARMAN (1966) sind durchaus richtig, und das Stratum corneum der Vögel kann nicht mit dem der Säuger ohne weiteres verglichen werden.

Die Abwandlungen der Haut bei den verschiedenen Arten betreffen aber nicht die Epidermis, sondern den Aufbau von *Corium und Subcutis*. Bei den Reptilien ist das Corium zwar von der Art der Schuppen und Panzer in seiner faserigen Struktur weitgehend abhängig, aber ein Stratum laxum und Stratum compactum war abgegrenzt; die artspezifische Größe des Tieres zeigte sich in der Dickenausdehnung dieser Schichten. Bei den Vögeln ist diese relative Einheitlichkeit nicht mehr gegeben. Es zeigt sich ein großer Unterschied, der nicht auf der bloßen Größenzunahme des Körpers beruht, wenn die Haut eines großen Laufvogels (z. B. Emu, Strauß) und die eines kleinen Singvogels miteinander verglichen werden. Die Wasservögel benötigen einen sehr starken Schutz gegen Wärmeverlust und besitzen starke Fettpolster der Haut. Und so lassen sich viele „Typen" des Hautbindegewebes aufstellen, die nicht alle direkt mit deutlich erkennbaren Funktionen zusammenhängen (vgl. LANGE, 1931; LÜDICKE, 1964). Die Einlagerung der Federn und ihrer Muskeln komplizieren außerdem die Struktur der Schichten. LANGE (1928, 1929) findet bei seinen vergleichenden Untersuchungen bei großen Laufvögeln den Typ ausgebildet, bei dem unter einem lockeren Stratum laxum noch das Stratum compactum ähnlich wie bei den Reptilien vorhanden ist und von starken aufsteigenden Faserbündeln durchsetzt wird. Mit der Abnahme der Größe der Tiere (Singvögel, Tauben) fällt die tiefere Schicht im Corium fort. Zwischen diesen klaren Bautypen kommen aber fließende Übergänge vor; die Vogelhaut hat also Tendenzen, sich in Anpassung an die Größe der Tiere und die Funktionen der Oberflächengewebe unterschiedliche Schichten von Geweben zu schaffen, die nicht immer homologisiert werden können. Die Dicke des Corium bei mittelgroßen Vögeln (Huhn, Raubvögel, Taucher) beträgt am Rumpf 100 bis 200 µ, bei großen Laufvögeln (Kasuar) ist die dünnere Oberschicht 50—60 µ, die straffe Unterschicht 400—500 µ dick.

Die Epidermis wird von einer dünnen *Basalmembran* unterlagert, die in die kollagenen Fasern des Corium übergeht und als eigene Grenzschicht des Bindegewebes manchmal kaum zu erkennen ist. Eine sehr engmaschige Papillenbildung der oberen Bindegewebszone kommt auch in der Rumpfhaut offenbar öfters vor, als die bisherigen Beschreibungen vermuten lassen. LANGE (1929) hat solche Epithelleisten bei den großen Laufvögeln eingehend dargestellt, nach unseren Beobachtungen kommen sie aber auch in der Haut von kleinen Vögeln wie z. der Taube vor. Ein Zusammenhang mit den Hautgefäßen scheint zu bestehen. Das Corium setzt sich aus verflochtenen Faserbündeln zusammen, die zwar in der Hauptsache parallel zur Oberfläche verlaufen, aber sich nach allen Richtungen kreuzen und durchflechten. So kommt ein relativ straffes Bindegewebe zustande, in das zahlreiche capillare Blutgefäße bis dicht unter die Epidermis vordringen. Netze aus elastischen Fasern durchsetzen die kollagenen Bündel. Eine regelmäßige Schichtung wie bei den Reptilien ist nur in seltenen Fällen anzutreffen und in den Häuten der großen Laufvögel mit reduzierter Befiederung deutlich entwickelt (LANGE, 1928). In der Regel sind aber keine getrennten Zonen im Corium in Form eines Stratum laxum und Stratum compactum vorhanden. Es ist sogar schwierig, Corium und Subcutis voneinander zu scheiden, da Fetteinlagerungen, Federn und Muskeln die Schichtung völlig verwischen und verändern. An der inneren Grenze des straffen Coriumbindegewebes liegt ein Gefäßplexus aus kleinen Arterien, Venen und Capillaren; von hier dringen die Capillargefäße bis zur Epidermis vor (LANGE, 1928). In vielen Fällen kann die Zone der Gefäße als ein Stratum vasculosum (nach FREUND, 1926) außerordentlich gut ausgebildet sein. Die Versorgung des Stratum vasculosum erfolgt aus einem grobmaschigen Gefäßnetz größerer Arterien und Venen in der Subcutis; diese entspringen den Hauptstämmen der Arterien bzw. führen in die großen Venen des Körpers. Aus dem unteren Plexus der Subcutis steigen kleinere Äste schräg aufwärts, zerteilen sich zur Versorgung der Fettläppchen und bilden in der oberen Subcutis ein Gefäßnetz 2. Ordnung (LANGE, 1928). Von einem Plexus aus wird das flache Gefäßnetz unter dem Corium (Stratum vasculosum) in Form aufsteigender kleiner Gefäße gebildet, und von diesen dringen ausschließlich Capillaren in die Fasermasse des Corium vor. Im Gegensatz zur Hautdurchblutung bei den Säugetieren spielt aber die Vasomotorik bei der Thermoregulation in der Rumpfhaut der Vögel keine Rolle; das Gefieder stellt mit der eingeschlossenen Lufthülle eine Isolierschicht dar, so daß die Hauttemperatur weitgehend konstant gehalten wird (Zusammenfassung bei KING und FARNER, 1961). Die physiologische Thermoregulation im Bereich der Rumpfhaut wird durch die Stellung der Federn, also durch eine Veränderung der Durchlässigkeit der Isolierschicht erreicht. Die beiden Muskelsysteme (vgl. unten), welche die Federn bewegen, müssen daher einer zentralen Kontrolle im Zusammenhang mit der Körpertemperatur unterliegen, wobei auch die Stellung der Federn durch nervöse Bahnen ins ZNS zurückgemeldet wird. Die Vasomotorik der Hautgefäße ist durch eine Motorik der Federn, deren Wirkung außerhalb des Körpers liegt, ersetzt worden. Ob es sich um einen eigenen Weg in der Phylogenese zur Erreichung der Homoiothermie handelt oder ob die Säugetiere eine Weiterbildung der ursprünglichen Form der physikalischen Thermoregulation vorgenommen haben, muß dahingestellt bleiben. Beide Klassen leiten sich von den Reptilien her, und in beiden Klassen gehen die charakteristischen Hautderivate: Federn und Haare auf die Schuppen zurück. Und auch die Säugetiere besitzen Muskeln an den Haaren, so daß diese aufgerichtet werden können. Aber das Haarkleid bietet weniger Schutz gegen die Umgebungstemperatur, so daß die „Schale" durch verminderte oder vermehrte Durchblutung der oberflächlichen Gefäße in der Thermoregulation einbezogen werden muß (vgl. SCHOLANDER, WALTERS, HOCK und IRVING, 1950). Die physiologischen Gesichtspunkte im Vergleich einer phylogenetischen Entstehung beider Hauttypen sind daher außerordentlich fesselnd, aber noch ungenügend analysiert. Denn auch für die Vögel gilt hinsichtlich der Thermoregulation, was für die Säuger von THAUER (1964) ausdrücklich hervorgehoben wird: auch außerhalb des ZNS müssen in der Tiefe des Körpers („Kern") Kältereceptoren vorhanden sein, und die efferente Innervation der visceralen und somatischen Organe ist in hohem Grade an die Entstehung der Homoiothermie angepaßt worden. Auch bei Vögeln läßt sich durch Abkühlung der Haut ein reflektorisches Kältezittern erzeugen. In den Füßen und den mit Schuppen bedeckten Teilen des Mittelfußes und des Unterschenkels dagegen sind die Gefäße für die Thermoregulation die wichtigste Einrichtung; hier sind besondere Gefäßnetze und andere Spezialisierungen anzutreffen, die besonders gut für arktische Vögel untersucht sind, deren Besprechung aber hier nicht erfolgen kann (vgl. CHATFIELD, LYMAN und IRVING, 1953; BARTHOLOMEW und DAWSON, 1954; IRVING und KROG, 1955; HOWELL und BARTHOLOMEW, 1961; KAHL, 1963).

Eine *besondere Vascularisierung* erhalten bei sehr vielen Vogelgruppen (z.B. Hühnervögel, Enten, Tauben, Möven, Raubvögel, Singvögel u.a.) bestimmte Areale der Haut auf Bauch und Brust, die als „Brutflecke" bekannt sind (LANGE, 1928; BAILEY, 1952; SELANDER und KUICH, 1963). Das Stratum vasculosum dieser Zonen wird während der Brutzeit durch vermehrte Capillarschichten verdickt, das umgebende Bindegewebe wird auffallend zellreich und bei einigen Arten kommt es zum Umbau der Fasermassen im Corium (Falkenvögel). Rundzellinfiltrate sind häufig, und die unterlagernde Subcutis verliert ihre Fettschicht. Diese Hautpartien dienen ohne Zweifel der erhöhten Wärmeabgabe des Körpers, die auf die zu bebrütenden Eier übertragen wird; in der Regel fehlen Federn in diesem Bereich. Die starke Gefäßversorgung des Stratum vasculosum wird von großen Arterien übernommen, die als besondere „Arteriae incubatoriae" in die Haut von der Achselhöhle her einstrahlen und Äste der A. thoracica externa sind.

Unter dem Corium beginnt ein unregelmäßig ausgebildetes Fettpolster, dessen Läppchen von straffen kollagenen Faserbündeln durchzogen wird und das Lager für die größeren Gefäße und Nervenstämme der Haut bildet. Nach LANGE (1928) kann diese Schicht als *Subcutis* angesehen werden, da sie auf der Unterseite durch kollagenes Bindegewebe abgeschlossen wird und die *Federbälge* mit den Federn ähnlich wie die Haarwurzeln der Säugetiere tief in die Fettpolster eingesenkt sind. Durch die Muskelplatten der Federn wird die Subcutis unregelmäßig in eine obere und eine untere Schicht zerteilt; die mit kollagenen Fasern und starken elastischen Netzen versehenen Muskelbündel bilden zusammen das sog. Stratum musculoelasticum. Die Federbälge sind röhrenförmige Einsenkungen der Epidermis und mit einem mehrschichtigen Epithel ausgekleidet, das an der Oberfläche verhornte Zellschichten trägt. Auch das straffe Bindegewebe der oberen Coriumschicht wird mit in die Tiefe genommen und umschließt das Epithelrohr mit einem festen Mantel. An der Basis geht das Epithel des Federbalges in die Keimzone des Federepithels über (vgl. unten). Die Federbälge sind schräg in die Haut eingelassen und stehen in gleichmäßigen Reihen im Bereich der Federfluren, so daß in der Haut eine regelmäßige Reihenfolge von Federbälgen vorhanden ist, entsprechend der embryonalen Entwicklung der Federanlagen (embryonale Pterylose). Die Federbälge sind mit Bündeln glatter Muskelzellen verbunden, die im Stratum musculoelasticum liegen und mit elastischen Sehnen an den festen Bindegewebsscheiden der Federbälge ansetzen. Die Muskelbündel bilden anatomische Einheiten und verbinden bestimmte Federbälge miteinander. Im Prinzip sieht das so aus, daß je 7 Federbälge eine Einheit bilden: um einen zentral gelegenen Balg sind 6 benachbarte angeordnet. Diese Federbälge sind durch breitflächige Bündel gekoppelt: sog. Retraktoren, die eine Annäherung der Einheiten bewirken und damit eine lokale Zusammenziehung der Haut. Andere Muskelbündel verbinden den distalen Teil der Federbälge mit den basalen Teilen der in einer Reihe benachbarten Federbälge: Erektoren (Arrectores plumarum), ihre Kontraktion richtet

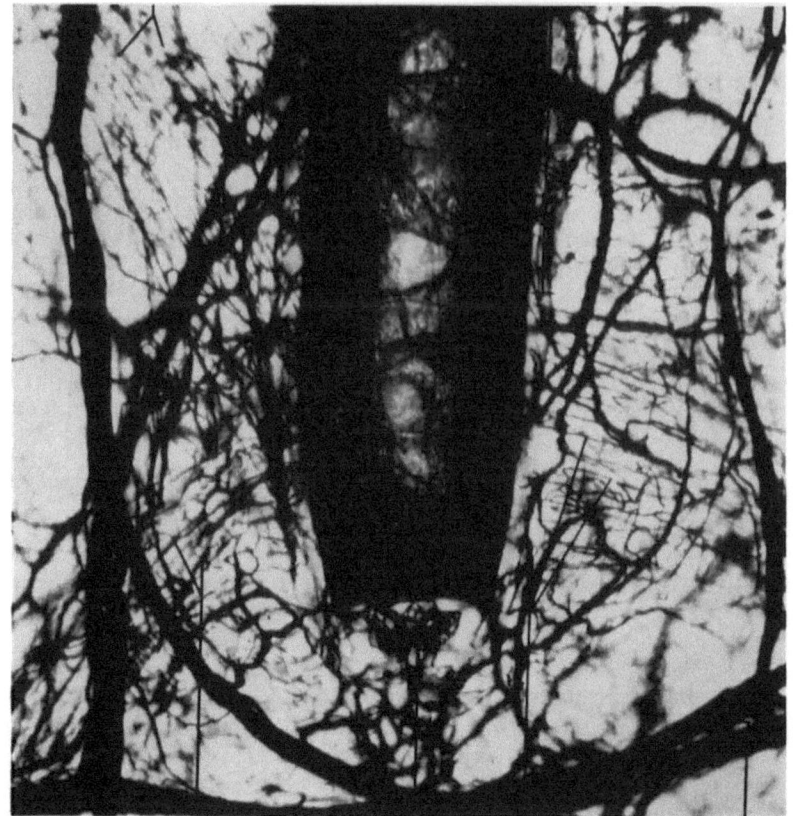
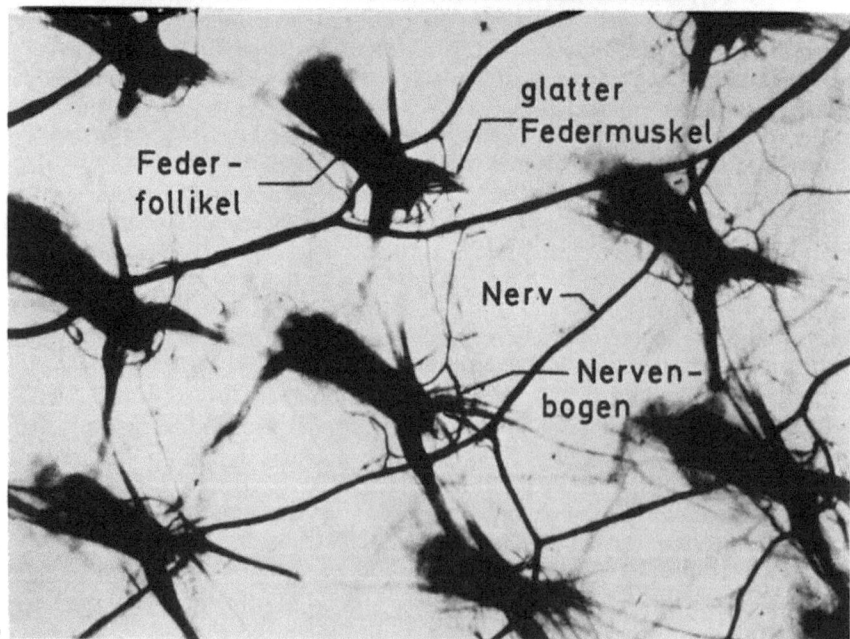

Abb. 20a u. b. (Legende s. S. 1003)

die in den Federbälgen steckenden Federn auf: das Gefieder wird gesträubt. Eine dritte Gruppe verbindet die distalen Teile der Federbälge von benachbarten Reihen: Depressoren; ihre Kontraktion hält die Federn dicht an die Haut gepreßt; das gesträubte Gefieder kann wieder glatt angelegt werden (STETTENHEIM, LUCAS, DENNINGTON und JAMROZ, 1962). Diese Bewegungen sind die Grundlagen der Veränderung der Isolierschicht bei der Thermoregulation. Die glatten Muskelbündel werden von sympathischen Neuronen innerviert, die in den sympathischen Ganglien liegen und ausschließlich postganglionär sein sollen. Diese alten Befunde sind aber nicht mehr nachgeprüft worden, und es muß nach den Erfahrungen über glatte Muskelzellinnervation bei Säugetieren bezweifelt werden, ob tatsächlich ausschließlich postganglionäre adrenergische Fasern dort enden. Da bei den Säugern auch cholinergische und präganglionäre Fasern in glatten Muskelbündeln enden, und bei den Vögeln die sympathischen Nerven zusammen mit den Spinalnerven die Haut erreichen, dürfte eine Nachprüfung wohl angebracht sein. Die Stellung der Federn wird durch zahlreiche Lamellenkörperchen am Federbalg kontrolliert (vgl. unten). Die großen Konturfedern (Schwanz, Schwungfedern) sind geradezu mit einer Scheide aus Lamellenkörperchen am Federbalg versehen. Eine weitere Möglichkeit zur Bewegung der Federn ist durch quergestreifte Hautmuskeln gegeben. Sie werden als Hautrumpfmuskulatur an Kopf, Hals, Brust, Bauch und Rücken von den großen Muskelpartien des M. trapezius, M. serratus superficialis, M. sternohyoideus, M. pectoralis, M. latissiumus dorsi und M. deltoides abgegeben. Die Faserschichten oder einzelne zerstreute Muskelfasern (Hals, Kopf) steigen vom Ursprungsmuskel in die Subcutis, so daß dort Muskelplatten vorhanden sind. Ihre Ansatzflächen sind aber in den Bindegewebszügen der Subcutis verankert, es erfolgt dadurch nur eine willkürliche Bewegung ganzer Federfluren zusammen, einzelne Federn sind also hierbei nicht erfaßt (vgl. BERGER, 1960). Damit wird diese Hautmuskulatur als Mittel des Ausdrucks wie Kampfstellung, Balzerregung usw. benutzt. Bekannt sind die Kopfhauben des Kakadus oder die Schmuckfedern der Paradiesvögel; beide Federgruppen werden durch bestimmte Teile der quergestreiften Hautrumpfmuskulatur bewegt. Diese Muskulatur wird naturgemäß von spinalen efferenten Neuronen innerviert bzw. im Bereich des M. sternohyoideus vom N. hypoglossus. Doch erfolgt eine übergeordnete Kontrolle durch Zentren im Stammhirn. Für das Huhn bzw. den Hahn konnten v. HOLST u. Mitarb. (vgl. JECHOREK und v. HOLST, 1956; v. HOLST, 1957; v. HOLST und ST. PAUL, 1960) zeigen, daß die elektrische Reizung bestimmter eng begrenzter Zonen des Stammhirnes das Verhalten angeborener Instinkthandlungen zustande bringt; in dem uns interessierenden Rahmen werden die mit Federbewegungen verknüpften Balz- und Imponiergehaben auf Reizung durchgeführt, Angriffsstellung und Angriff ebenso wie Furchtreaktionen. — Die *Gefäßversorgung* im Bereich der Federbälge ist sehr gut ausgebildet (Abb. 20a). Dem bereits genannten subcutanen Gefäßplexus entstammen Gefäßschlingen, welche die Basis der Federbälge umgeben und zahlreiche kleinere Gefäße an die glatten Muskelbündel, in das Bindegewebe und an die Lamellenkörperchen abgeben; in den Erfolgsorganen zerteilen sich die Gefäße in zahlreiche capillare Netze (PETERSON, RINGER, TETZLAFF und LUCAS, 1965). An der Basis des Balges dringen die Gefäße auch in das Bindegewebe der wachsenden Feder ein (s. unten).

Abb. 20a u. b. Gefäße und Nerven in Beziehung zu Federn. a Ausschnitt aus dem Gefäßplexus an der Basis einer Schenkelfeder des Huhnes. Der Federbalg wird von einem doppelten Gefäßbogen umgeben, von dort erfolgt die Versorgung des Capillarplexus der Federpapille, der Muskeln und des Federbalges. Tuscheinjektion. b Aufsicht auf einen Teil des Schenkelbezirkes beim Huhn. Die in Reihen stehenden Federbälge werden von einem regelmäßigen Nervennetz versorgt, jeder Nerv gibt an die Muskeln und den Federbalg mehrere kleine Äste ab, die als Bögen um die Federbasis angeordnet sind. Leukofuchsin-Färbung, Totalpräparat. (a und b: PETERSON, RINGER und TETZLAFF, 1965)

Die *Innervation der Haut* ist segmental: Die Neurone der afferenten Hautfasern liegen in den Spinalganglien; ihre Axone versorgen die Haut, so daß trapezförmige Dermatome in der Haut festzustellen sind (KAISER, 1924). Diese Dermatomzonen überlappen sich ähnlich denen der Reptilien sehr erheblich ($1/2$—$1/1$ ihrer Breite) und sind in den Extremitäten in der Ausbreitung abgewandelt; insgesamt sind 32 Dermatome vorhanden. Mit den segmentalen Spinalnerven verlaufen aber auch die postganglionären sympathischen Fasern, deren Erfolgsorgane z.T. die glatten Federmuskeln sind. Die Schwierigkeit einer Trennung der peripheren Axone hinsichtlich ihrer Zugehörigkeit zum spinalen oder sympathischen System wird durch den gemeinsamen Verlauf sehr vergrößert, und es fehlen neuere Untersuchungen. Das subcutane Nervennetz (Abb. 20b) ist ziemlich gleichmäßig ausgebreitet (TETZLAFF, PETERSON und RINGER, 1965) und besteht aus Fasern verschiedenen Durchmessers. An den Federbälgen treten kleine Bündel von Axonen aus der Faser an die glatten Muskelbündel heran, andere gelangen in die Lamellenkörperchen. An der Basis enes jeden Federbalges ist ein charakteristischer Nervenfaserbogen vorhanden, der seine Fasern von benachbarten Stämmchen des großmaschigen Nervenplexus erhält. Diese komplizierte Mischung von Axonen ist aber noch nicht weiter untersucht worden. Aus dem subcutanen Plexus steigen Nervenäste ins Corium auf, wo sich ein engmaschiges Netz dünner Fasern ausbreitet (SCHARTAU, 1938). Ein Teil der Axone dringt in die Epidermis vor, wo sie sich als freie Nervenendigungen oder mit Endknöpfchen zwischen die Epithelzellen verteilen. SCHARTAU findet Ganglienzellen im Coriumnetz und nimmt an, daß ein Teil der Axone im Epithel dem sympathichen System angehört. Von den subepidermalen Ganglienzellen werden ebenfalls zahlreiche Ausläufer in die Epidermis vorgeschickt. Der Aufbau des Rückenmarkes läßt ARIËNS KAPPERS (ARIËNS KAPPERS, HUBER und CROSBY, 1960) vermuten, daß die Empfindlichkeit der Vogelhaut hinsichtlich des spinalen Systems sehr viel geringer ist als die bei Reptilien und Amphibien; die Haut wird durch die Federn abgeschirmt. Die weitaus geringere Zahl der dorsalen Wurzelfasern und die geringere Zahl der somatischen sensorischen Neurone läßt dies vermuten. Das würde aber auch bedeuten, daß tatsächlich ein Teil der peripheren Nerven dem sympathischen System zugehören würde. Neben den Nervennetzen und freien Verzweigungen in der Epidermis sind im Corium und der Subcutis zahlreiche Sinneskörperchen vorhanden; es wurden bereits die an den Federn gehäuft vorkommenden Lamellenkörperchen genannt. Diese Körperchen entsprechen im Aufbau den Vater-Pacini-Körperchen der Säugetiere (WINKELMANN und MYERS III, 1961), sind in der Größe und Form ein wenig davon abweichend und heißen bei den Vögeln „Herbstsche Körperchen". Die etwa eiförmig gestalteten Körperchen enthalten ein (oder mehrere?) Axon, das ohne Markscheide im Innern des Zapfens endet. Umgeben wird der Axonzapfen von zahlreichen Zellen, die einen Innenkolben bilden. Die Untersuchungen von CLARA (1925) und SCHILDMACHER (1931) zeigen, daß dieser Teil des Körperchens bilateralsymmetrisch gebaut ist. Ohne Zweifel treffen damit die Befunde von PEASE und QUILLIAM (1957) über die Feinstruktur der Pacinischen Körperchen bei Säugern auf die „Herbstschen Körperchen" der Vögel zu, denn eine so weitgehende Übereinstimmung hinsichtlich des Schalenbaues und der Symmetrie ist wohl kaum anders zu deuten. Wir können daher die celluläre Innenzone mit den zahlreichen Zellkernen und dem Längsspalt als die Wachstumszone der „Herbstschen Körperchen" betrachten. Nach außen folgen zahlreiche konzentrische Lagen des Außenkolbens, die aus schalenförmig zusammengelegten flachen Zellen bestehen, zwischen denen Flüssigkeit, kollagene Fasern und Blutcapillaren eingeschlossen sind. Jedoch unterscheiden sich die Lamellenkörperchen der Vögel in der histochemisch erfaßbaren Substanzzusammensetzung (WINKELMANN und MYERS III,

1961). Die Flüssigkeit zwischen den Lamellenschalen enthält saure Mucopolysaccharide, die sich mit der PAS-Reaktion rot und auch mit Alcianblau anfärben sowie gegen die Einwirkung von Hyaluronidase unempfindlich sind. Der Achsenzylinder wird umgeben von einer Schicht mit starker Aktivität spezifischer Acetylcholinesterase, während das Axon selbst keine Aktivität dieser Esterase erkennen läßt. Hinsichtlich der Funktion darf man wohl die alte Auffassung verwerfen, die Lamellenkörperchen der Vögel würden den Blutdruck registrieren (CLARA, 1925). Nach den genauen elektrophysiologischen Untersuchungen an Lamellenkörperchen der Säugetiere (vgl. LOEWENSTEIN und SHALAK, 1966) und den Befunden von SCHWARTZKOPFF (1948) dürfen die „Herbstschen Körperchen" der Vögel als Druckreceptoren bei Verformungen des Bindegewebes angesehen werden. Denn die im Lauf des Vogels sitzenden zahlreichen Lamellenkörperchen übernehmen die Stöße des Untergrundes, auf dem der Vogel sitzt („Vibrationssinn"), da durch die anatomische Anordnung des Knochen-Bindegewebsapparates die Vibration sich in einer Verformung der Körperchen überträgt. In der nicht von Federn bedeckten Haut (Hals und Kopf vieler Arten) sowie in der Haut des Schnabels finden sich neben den Herbstschen Körperchen noch Merkelsche Tastkörperchen im Bindegewebe sowie spezialisierte Sinneskörperchen, da der Schnabel vielfach als besonders Tast- oder Temperatursinnesorgan im Leben bestimmter Vogelarten dient. Wir können hier nicht weiter darauf eingehen (vgl. BOTEZAT, 1906; CLARA, 1925; KROGIS, 1931; DIJKSTRA, 1933).

Pigmente kommen in der Haut der Vögel nur in besonderen Fällen vor; vor allem ist die mit Federn bedeckte Haut fast immer frei von Pigmentzellen. Bei bestimmten Rassen, z. B. Seidenhuhn oder bei Tauben (vgl. LUBNOW, 1957; KUHN und KOECKE, 1956), sind Pigmentzellen in der Haut vorhanden, dringen aber nicht in die wachsenden Federn ein, so daß ein weißes Gefieder entsteht. In der Regel ist es aber umgekehrt: die Haut bleibt ohne Pigment und alle Farben sind in die Federn eingelagert worden. Nur bei nackten Hautregionen (Kopf, Kämme, Halslappen) unterlagern zahlreiche Melanophoren und Xanthophoren die Epidermis, so daß farbige Hautpartien entstehen, wie es bereits für Reptilien, Amphibien und Fische besprochen wurde. Die Farbstoffe sind Carotinoide und entsprechen den roten und gelben Federfarbstoffen (vgl. VÖLKER, 1962, 1963).

Das charakteristische Hautderivat der Vögel ist die *Feder*. Im fertigen Zustand besteht sie nur aus verhornten Epithelzellen, ist also allein ein Epidermisprodukt, beim Wachstum sind dagegen Bindegewebe und Gefäße der Cutis von wesentlicher Bedeutung. Die Feder ist das komplizierteste Epidermisderivat der Haut bei den Wirbeltieren. Entstehung und Wachstum der Feder haben daher eine besonders eingehende Untersuchung erfahren, deren Ergebnisse hier nur gestreift werden können. Zusammenfassungen finden sich bei LILLIE (1942), RAWLES (1960), COHEN und 'ESPINASSE (1961). Eine Feder besteht aus einem durchgehenden Schaft, von dem an beiden Seiten Federäste (Rami) entspringen. Jeder Federast trägt wieder auf jeder Seite eine Reihe dünner Federstrahlen (Radii). Dieses Verzweigungssystem bildet eine flache, mehr oder weniger bilateral-symmetrische Federfahne, deren Achse vom Schaft dargestellt wird. An der Basis fehlen dem Schaft die Seitenäste, er ist nackt und steckt als Spule (Calamus) im Federbalg. Der feste Zusammenhalt der Federfahne wird durch besondere Randstrukturen der Federstrahlen bewirkt, wo kleine Haken des einen Strahles in krempenförmige Abbiegungen des folgenden Strahles eingreifen. Die Abhängigkeit des feineren Aufbaues von der Funktion, z. B. Zusammenhalt der Fahnen bei Schwungfedern bei Belastung durch den Flug, sind ausführlich von SICK (1937), die Abhängigkeit der Struktur von der Körperregion von HEMPEL (1931) und die bei Wasservögeln durch RUTSCHKE (1960) untersucht worden. Die Veränderungen in der Federstruktur bei der Bildung besonders auffallender Schmuckfedern wurde durch BRINCKMANN (1958) und beim Wechsel vom Jugendgefieder zum Gefieder des adulten Vogels durch GÖHRINGER (1951) analysiert, um nur einige grundlegende Arbeiten zu nennen. Die Federn eines Vogels sind in Form, Größe und Struktur keineswegs gleichartig; das geschilderte Bild gilt für die großen und auffälligen sog. Konturfedern. Sie bedecken als äußere Schicht den Körper und prägen in der Regel durch ihre Färbungen den typischen Habitus eines Vogels. Die großen Konturfedern des Flügels sind als Schwungfedern, die des Schwanzes als Steuerfedern bekannt. Als Abwandlungen dieses komplizierten Typs sind die Pelzdunen anzusehen; sie liegen unter den Konturfedern und ihre Strahlen sind nicht verhakt, sondern bilden eine luftige Isolierschicht. Besonders Wasservögel sind mit solchen Dunen ausgerüstet. Daneben kommen noch Fadenfedern vor (v. PFEFFER, 1952) und sog. Afterfedern, die als Doppelbildungen der Konturfedern aus der gleichen Anlage entstehen und deshalb für die Morphogenese der Federn von Interesse sind (vgl. LILLIE und JUHN, 1938; STEINER, 1943; ZISWILER, 1962). Zusammenfassungen über die Formen der Federn sind bei BIEDERMANN (1928) und STRESEMANN (1927/1934) sowie MAYAUD (1950) nachzulesen.

Das Wachstum einer Feder geht beim adulten Vogel folgendermaßen vor sich. An der Basis des tief eingesenkten Federbalges liegt eine neue Federanlage. Dort schlägt das mehrschichtige Epithel des Federbalges in einen dicken Epithelring um, dessen Zellen das Stratum germinativum für die neue Feder darstellen und wegen seiner Form als Ringwulst, Hals oder einfach als Matrix bezeichnet wird. Das Epithel des Ringwulstes geht an der Spitze des Federkeimes in eine flache Epithelkappe über, so daß eine knopfförmige Vorwölbung in das Lumen des Federbalges vorragt. Das Coriumbindegewebe setzt sich in Form einer Papille mit Gefäßen in den Epithelconus fort: die Pulpa. Dieses zellreiche Mesenchym ist für die entstehende Feder außerordentlich wichtig, denn es bestimmt während der Embryonalentwicklung und auch später den regional-spezifischen Charakter der Feder, z.B. Rückenfeder, Schwungfeder etc. Da bei der Federerneuerung gewissermaßen jeder Federkeim wieder in einem embryonalen Zustand sich befindet, erfolgt also auch die spezifische Differenzierung der Feder unter dem Einfluß des Pulpamesenchyms. Durch die mitotische Aktivität der Epithelzellen des Ringwulstes schiebt sich ein dicker Epithelzylinder vor, dessen Zellen in drei Schichten gesondert sind und das Pulpamesenchym umschließen. Eine äußere Epithellage aus wenigen Zellschichten (sog. Stratum corneum) wird zur Federscheide; die Zellen verhornen und umschließen die Feder bis zu ihrer vollständigen Ausdifferenzierung und Entfaltung. Eine dicke mittlere Lage aus Epithelzellen (sog. Stratum intermedium) stellt das eigentliche federbildende Gewebe dar; eine dünne innere Schicht aus wenigen Lagen von Zellen (sog. Stratum cylindricum) schließt das Mesenchym der wachsenden Feder von den Federzellen ab: die Pulpascheide. Ein solcher Abschluß ist besonders in den Spitzenteilen der Feder wichtig, denn während die basalen Teile noch wachsen und in der mittleren Zone eine Differenzierung zu Federzellen einsetzt, sind die oberen Teile der Feder bereits fertig und abgestorben. Daher wird unter der inneren Epithelschicht das Pulpamesenchym allmählich aus den oberen Zonen der Feder zurückgezogen und muß von der Epithelkappe im Hohlzylinder geschützt werden. Die Gefäßversorgung ist wegen des intensiven Wachstums der Federgewebe außerordentlich reich ausgebildet (LILLIE, 1940; GOFF, 1949): Von einer zentralen Arterie, die aus dem allgemeinen Plexus der subcutanen Gefäße stammt, verzweigt sich ein enges Capillarnetz im Mesenchym unter dem Epithel; an der Spitze der Pulpa zerteilt sich die Arterie in einen Gefäßbaum. Am Ringwulst ist das Capillarnetz besonders engmaschig ausgebildet. Große Sinus nehmen das Blut aus den Capillaren wieder auf; erstere vereinigen sich in der Nähe der Pulpabasis zu mehreren venösen Gefäßen, die in das allgemeine subcutane Gefäßnetz münden. Das Wachstum vollzieht sich aber nicht gleichmäßig, sondern in rhythmischen Aktivitätsphasen. Sie lassen sich durch den Einbau von markierten Substanzen (^{35}S-Natriumsulfat, ^{35}S-Methionin, ^{35}S-DL-Cystin) darstellen und genau erfassen (LÜDICKE, 1961, 1963, 1965, 1966; LÜDICKE und GEIERHAAS, 1963; LÜDICKE und TEICHERT, 1963); es entstehen sog. Zuwachsstreifen, die manchmal schon bei der ausgewachsenen Feder ohne jede Vorbehandlung als Querbänder in der Federstruktur (nicht in der Färbung!) sichtbar sind. Das federbildende Epithel der mittleren Schicht (Stratum intermedium) erfährt eine komplizierte Differenzierung (GREITE, 1934) und zeigt außerdem eine besondere chemische Eigenart. Während Federscheide und inneres Epithel an der Pulpa α-Keratin aufbauen, aus dem auch die Säugetierhaare bestehen, machen die Federzellen das charakteristische β-Keratin (RUDALL, 1947; MERCER, 1961). Bei der embryonalen Federentwicklung wird die Synthese von β-Keratin erst nach einer Anlaufzeit erreicht, beim Hühnchen erscheint das adulte β-Keratin in der wachsenden Dune erst am 14. Bebrütungstage, und die Disulfidbindungen scheinen erst am 13. und 14. Tage aufgebaut zu werden (BELL und THATHACHARI, 1963). Die endgültige Form des Keratins wird über eine Reihe von Vorstufen erreicht, die sich auch isolieren lassen (MALT, SPEAKMAN und BELL, 1964). Die Feinstruktur des β-Keratins ist gut bekannt (FRASER und MCRAE, 1959; SCHOR und KRIMM, 1961) und läßt sich wahrscheinlich elektronenmikroskopisch als 12 Å dicke Fibrillen isolieren (BELL, MALT und STEWART, 1964), ist aber in der stark wachsenden Feder zu größeren Einheiten zusammengelagert (FILSHIE und ROGERS, 1962; KOECKE, unveröffentlicht). Unter welchem Einfluß die Sonderung der Epithelschichten und die Synthese von α- bzw. β-Keratin vor sich geht, ist nicht bekannt. Denn auch im Ringwulst des Federkeimes bei erwachsenen Tieren ist keine morphologische Sonderung der zahlreichen Epithelzellen in Keimschichten zu erkennen; die Gliederung setzt erst etwas höher im wachsenden Federkeim in einer Differenzierungszone ein. Es ist ferner bekannt, daß die Hornschuppen an Lauf und Fuß der Vögel aus α-Keratin bestehen (RUDALL, 1947; SPEARMAN, 1966), und daß während der Embryonalentwicklung Epithelien von Federanlagen und Schuppenanlagen noch gegeneinander ausgetauscht werden können. Das führt selbst dann zu normalen Federn bzw. Schuppen, wenn die ausgetauschten Epithelien mit der histologischen Differenzierung begonnen hatten (SENGEL, 1958; RAWLES, 1963). MERCER (1961) schließlich konnte elektronenmikroskopisch im Ringwulst der wachsenden Feder keine Unterschiede zwischen den Epithelzellen dieser Keimzone feststellen. Das für die definitive Feder allein wichtige Epithel ist das des Stratum intermedium, also diejenige Schicht, deren Zellen charakteristisches Federkeratin vom β-Typ produzieren. In der Differenzierungszone der wachsenden Feder wird dieses Epithel in Leisten gegliedert (Primärleisten), die von der dorsalen Seite des Epithelzylinders schräg distalwärts nach ventral verlaufen; an der dorsalen Seite entsteht ein breiter Epithelstreifen: die Schaftanlage, die als gerade Leiste von der Spitze bis zur Basis des Federkeimes sich erstreckt. Alle Primärleisten enden also an dieser Schaftanlage und stehen in ihrer Orientierung in einem bestimmten Winkel dazu. Das Epithel innerhalb der Primärleisten differenziert sich zu verschiedenen Zelltypen, die besondere Verbände bilden: einen mittleren säulenförmigen Teil für den Federast (Ramus), und zwei am Ramus ansetzende plattenförmige Verbände: Federstrahlen (Radii). Die Epithelsäule des zukünftigen Ramus reicht durchgehend von der Schaftanlage bis zur ventralen Spitze der Primärleiste und trägt auf jeder Seite eine große Zahl von Epithelzellplatten als Anlagen der Federstrahlen. Andere Epithelzellen der Primärleisten bilden noch Hilfsstrukturen, die hier nicht weiter erläutert werden sollen. In unserem Rahmen sind nur zwei Vorgänge wichtig: a) die Sonderung und Verhornung der Epithelien in der Differenzierungszone; b) die Farbeinlagerung in die wachsenden Epithelien.

Zu a). Sobald die Gliederung der Epithelzellen zu den genannten Zellverbänden erfolgt ist, setzt in den Zellen die Verhornung ein. Die in der Nähe des Pulpamesenchyms gelegenen Zellen (Zellen der Federäste und angrenzende Teile der Federstrahlen) beginnen die Hornproduktion. Doch läßt sich im Gegensatz zum Haar der Säugetiere keine eng abgegrenzte Verhornungszone erkennen, denn während der Verhornung wachsen die Zellen weiter: d.h., es werden Proteine synthetisiert und RNS ist reichlich vorhanden (KONING, 1957). Elektronenmikroskopisch unterscheiden sich die verhornenden Federzellen von den Zellen im Haar; in den Federzellen treten nur Keratinfibrillen und keine granulären Elemente auf, ihre Ribosomen bleiben intakt (FILSHIE und ROGERS, 1962) und der Gehalt an RNS bleibt bis zur vollständigen Verhornung erhalten (SPEARMAN, 1966). Die in den verschiedenen Federteilen aufgebauten Proteine unterscheiden sich in der Aminosäure-Zusammensetzung (SCHROEDER und KAY, 1955), ist aber für alle Typen von Federn einer Art in den entsprechenden Federabschnitten gleich. Die Zellen der Pulpa enthalten Phosphatasen in relativ hohen Mengen (KONING, 1957; HINSCH, 1960), deren Aktivität mit dem Transport der Nachschubsubstanzen für die rapide wachsenden Epithelien in Zusammenhang gebracht werden. Die enge Beziehung zur Schuppe kommt in der gleichen Verteilung: hoher RNS-Gehalt im basalen Epithel der Schuppenanlagen und hoher Gehalt an Phosphatasen in den Mesenchymzellen dieser Anlagen zum Ausdruck (THOMSON, 1964). Die unmittelbare Bedeutung dieser Substanzen für die Morphogenese der Federn läßt sich dadurch zeigen, indem die Phosphatasen abgeblockt werden (HAMILTON und KONING, 1956): die Entwicklung der Feder wird stark gestört. Die Verwandtschaft der Feder mit der Reptilienschuppe wird durch das Keratin deutlich. Die geschilderte harte Hornschicht bei Eidechsen und Schlangen und auch die oberflächlichen Lagen der Schildkrötenpanzer enthalten typisches β-Keratin, also „Federkeratin" (RUDALL, 1947; SPEARMAN, 1966); die weiche Hornschicht dagegen ist aus α-Keratin aufgebaut. Während des cyclischen Aufbaues der Schuppen bei Schlangen und Eidechsen (s. dort) erfolgt also ebenfalls eine Sonderung in Epithelzellen mit der Produktion von α- bzw. β-Keratin. Die Schuppen der Krokodile enthalten gemischt beide Keratintypen. Auf der anderen Seite wird die (indirekte) Verwandtschaft der Feder mit dem Haar während des Federwechsels sichtbar. Die Zellen in den Epithelsäulen für die Federäste bilden ein zentrales Mark (Medulla) aus großen Zellen, die starke periphere Hornmäntel ausgebildet haben und in denen nach dem Austrocknen Luft eingeschlossen ist (SCHMIDT und RUSKA, 1961, 1962). Die äußeren Zellschichten gliedern sich in abgeflachte Rindenzellen (Cortex) und eine bedeckende Zellschicht, die Cuticula. Die flachen Zellen der Cuticula gleichen denen der Haarcuticula (AUBER und APPLEYARD, 1951) und auch die Rindenschicht ist mit der des Haares (abgesehen vom Typ des Keratins) vergleichbar (AUBER, 1955). Die Rindenzellen sind von längsverlaufenden Fibrillen erfüllt, die zu Strängen in dem lufterfüllten Hohlraum der abgestorbenen Zellen zusammengeschlossen sind und evtl. Melaninpigment umschließen (SCHMIDT und RUSKA, 1963). Die Zellgrenzen sind stark verzahnt und unterstützen so den Zusammenhalt. Schließlich ist die Gesamtgliederung der Federleiste und auch des Schaftes in diese drei distinkten Zellschichten wie beim Haar vollzogen worden. Nur die Medullazellen sind anders als die entsprechenden Medullazellen des Haares, vor allem wegen der eingeschlossenen Luft. Die Reptilienschuppe als das phylogenetisch älteste Epidermisderivat hat eine Sonderung in zwei Richtungen erfahren: Entwicklung zur Feder oder zum Haar. Die ersteren haben die Bildung von β-Keratin übernommen und spezialisiert, die letzteren die Bildung von α-Keratin. Beide sind in ihrer Struktur trotz der grob-morphologischen Unterschiede in vieler Hinsicht einander ähnlich geblieben. Vielleicht darf man überspitzt sagen, daß die Feder ein verzweigtes altertümliches Haar ist. Leider kennen wir die Entstehungsformen der Feder nicht, denn Archaeopteryx, der Urvogel, besitzt schon voll ausgebildete typische Federn.

Die feinere Ausformung der Federstrukturen wird durch zahlreiche genetische Faktoren bestimmt, deren Veränderungen infolge von Mutationen bestimmte Strukturabwandlungen beim Federwachstum erzeugen. Besonders aufschlußreich sind solche Mutanten, die in die Morphogenese der Federn oder Schuppen eingreifen (ABBOTT und ASMUNDSON, 1957; GOETINCK und ABBOTT, 1963; SENGEL und ABBOTT, 1963). Die Epidermis ist bei der Mutante „scaleless" nicht in der Lage, mit dem unterlagernden Mesenchym zu reagieren und Federn oder Schuppen zu bilden. Die Mesenchymzellen sind von dieser Mutation in ihrer Fähigkeit zur Federpulpabildung bzw. Schuppenunterlage aber nicht eingeschränkt, wenn man gesunde Epidermis anbietet, etwa in Kombinationskulturen. Von gleicher Bedeutung sind solche Mutationen, welche die Bildung der Federn und ihr Wachstum nicht beeinflussen, wohl aber die Struktur der sich ausdifferenzierenden Federzellen. Es gibt mindestens 7 solcher Mutanten beim Huhn und bei der Taube. Bei der Mutante „frizzle" (Strupphuhn) wird der Aufbau der Proteinkette des β-Keratins verändert (KRIMM, 1960); es entsteht ein abartiges β-Keratin, in dem der Mengenanteil einiger Aminosäuren und die Textur der Fibrillen durch eine abgeänderte Lage von Prolin in der Sequenz abgewandelt ist. Die Folge ist eine defekte Federstruktur; häufig fallen dadurch die Federn rasch aus, und die nackten Hühner sterben, weil ihre Thermoregulation den Wärmeverlust durch die Haut nicht kompensieren kann. Ähnliche Defekte der Federstruktur liegen bei der Wollfedrigkeit bzw. der Seidenfedrigkeit vor; hier fehlen die festen Zusammenhalte in der Federfahne durch mangelnde Verhakung der Federstrahlen untereinander (JONES und MORGAN, 1956; MILLER, 1956). Auch durch Hormone (vor allem Thyroxin, JUHN und BATES, 1960) wird auf dem Umweg über das Wachstum und die Wachstumsgeschwindigkeit die Federstruktur beeinflußt.

Zu b). Während des Federwachstums werden die leuchtenden oder dunklen Farben eingelagert, die in der toten ausgewachsenen Feder die Muster und Zeichnungen des Vogelgefieders bedingen. Nur während der kurzen Wachstumsspanne kann also eine Farbgebung bzw. Farbänderung vorgenommen werden. Daraus ergibt sich, daß bei Vögeln kein nennenswerter physiologischer Farbwechsel wie bei den bisher besprochenen Wirbeltierklassen vorkommt, obwohl Farbwechselhormone bei Vögeln ebenfalls nachgewiesen wurden. Farbeffekte müssen dadurch hervorgerufen werden, daß durch Federbewegungen verdeckte Musterteile plötzlich aufgedeckt und durch die Körperhaltung besonders deutlich gezeigt werden (vgl. MORRIS, 1956). Die Farbstoffe sind sehr verschiedenartig und können entweder im Körper synthetisiert oder aber mit der Nahrung aufgenommen und an die Federzellen weitergegeben werden. Die schwarzen, braunen, braunroten oder gelblichen Melanine werden in Melanocyten aufgebaut und in die Federepithelzellen übertragen. Oder es handelt sich um grüne oder gelbe, z. T. fluorescierende Pigmente, die im Körper der Vögel, vor allem Papageien und Sittichen aufgebaut und in Federzellen gespeichert werden. Andere Pigmente sind kupferhaltige Porphyrine (Turaco), die in alkalischen Medien löslich sind, so daß Turaco-Federn im Trinkwasser von Vogelgehegen wegen der alkalischen Verunreinigung mit Exkrementen Farbe abgeben: „abfärben". Sehr viele Farbstoffe werden aber mit der Nahrung als Carotinoide aufgenommen und unverändert in den Federzellen (sog. Lipochrome) gespeichert oder vorher geringfügig abgeändert, so daß ein hellerer oder dunklerer Farbton entsteht (Zusammenfassung bei VÖLKER, 1960, dort die ältere Literatur; neuere wesentliche Arbeiten: VÖLKER, 1962, 1963, 1964). Die Einlagerung in die Federzellen erfolgt auf recht verschiedene Weise. Die Carotinoide bilden mit Lipoiden und Keratin kleine Grana, die z.T. ausgerichtet in die Keratinbündel im Innern der Federzellen eingebaut sind (MATTERN, 1956; SCHMIDT, 1956). Je nach ihren physikalischen Eigenschaften, z.B. dem gebundenen Hydratationswasser, können sich verschiedene Farbtöne ergeben, so daß durch bloßes Erhitzen oder Quetschen der Federn ein Farbumschlag von rot nach violett oder orange erzeugt wird. Die Ablagerung der Lipoidtröpfchen mit den Farbstoffen ist schon im Epithel der Primärleisten vorhanden, und das Pulpamesenchym enthält als Überträger die Tröpfchen ebenfalls. Das Lipoid wirkt als Träger für die Carotinoide (DRIESEN, 1953). Da die endgültige Form der Pigmentablagerung aber vom Einbau in die Hornfibrillen der Federzellen abhängt, so folgt die Anreicherung des Pigmentes in den Federzellen der Keratinisierungszone: die älteren Federzellen an den (peripheren) Spitzen der Säulen für Federstrahlen und Federäste zeigen die intensivste Einlagerung. Die fluorescierenden Papageienfarbstoffe werden auf gleiche Weise durch Lipoidtropfen in die Federzellen gebracht (DRIESEN, 1953), sind aber später offenbar stark verteilt zwischen den Keratinfibrillen orientiert eingelagert, ohne erkennbare Aggregate zu bilden (SCHMIDT, 1961). Die roten Porphyrinfarbstoffe der Turacos und der Trappe liegen wieder als sehr kleine Grana (Turaco, SCHMIDT und RUSKA, 1963) oder molekular verteilt (Trappe, SCHMIDT und RUSKA, 1965) in den Hornmänteln oder Hornsträngen der Federzellen vor. Komplizierte Verhältnisse liegen bei der Ablagerung der Melaninpigmente in Federzellen vor. Wie bei allen Wirbeltieren werden Melanine in Form von Granula mit bestimmter Feinstruktur auch bei den Vögeln nur in Melanocyten aufgebaut. Diese Farbzellen wandern in die Epithelien der Primärleisten ein, beginnen mit der Synthese des Pigmentes und übertragen mit langen Zellausläufern die Pigmentgranula in die Federzellen (vgl. KOECKE und SCHITTENHELM, 1961) (Abb. 21). Im einzelnen ist dieser Vorgang noch nicht geklärt, aber der Mechanismus setzt voraus, daß beide Zelltypen einem aufeinander abgestimmten Rhythmus von Produktion bzw. Abgabe sowie Aufnahme des Pigmentes folgen müssen. Die hierbei wesentlichen Vorgänge der Morphogenese von Farbmustern können nicht berücksichtigt werden (vgl. KUHN, 1956; RAWLES, 1960; DANNEEL und SCHUMANN, 1963). Die eingelagerten Melaningranula werden in die Keratinmäntel der Federzellen oder die Keratinstränge im Innern der Zellen eingeschlossen und färben auf diese Weise Federstrahlen und Federäste. Durch eine rhythmische oder zeitlich begrenzte Einlagerung werden in den Federn Querstreifen („Sperberung") oder Flecken erzeugt. Die Farben entsprechen den Farbtönen des Melanins. In sehr vielen Fällen erfolgt aber ein geordneter Einbau der Granula in die Federzellen, so daß eine oder mehrere gleichmäßig ausgerichtete Lagen von Pigmentkörnern in den flachen Federzellen aufgeschichtet sind. Durch eine solche Lagerung wird der Effekt des Schillerns von Federn bewirkt, indem die Granula als dünne Blättchen Interferenzfarben entstehen lassen und durch ihre geordnete Lage eine Summation des Effektes eintritt (SCHMIDT, 1948, 1952). Die Federn der Kolibris (GREENWALT, BRANDT und FRIEL, 1960; SCHMIDT und RUSKA, 1962), von Tauben (SCHMIDT und RUSKA, 1961), der Nektarvögel (DURRER und VILLIGER, 1962) verdanken ihren vielfarbigen Glanz dieser „Strukturfarbe". Vielfach sind die Pigmentgranula im fertigen Zustand lufterfüllt, in Form kleiner Röhren oder mit wabenförmigem Aufbau (SCHMIDT und RUSKA, 1962; DURRER und VILLIGER, 1966). Es kann als sicher gelten, daß alle schillernden Federn nach dem gleichen Schema aufgebaut sind. Das echte Pigment wird in solchen Federzellen also kaum in seiner ursprünglichen Farbgebung benutzt, sondern bildet ein

Substrat für einen optischen Effekt. Besonders interessant ist dabei, daß auffallende Muster aus verschiedenartigen Schillerfarben gebildet werden, wie z.B. die Augen auf den Schwanzfedern beim Pfau (DURRER, 1962). Hier werden Farben von grünrot über gelb und türkis bis zum Dunkelblau im Zentrum des Augenfleckes sichtbar. Ihre Entstehung geht darauf zurück, daß während des Federwachstums die Melaningranula nicht nur in paralleler Lage und in Schichten eingebaut werden, sondern Raumgitter mit verschiedenen Abständen zwischen den stäbchenförmigen Pigmentkörperchen und mit verschiedener Tiefe, d.h. Zahl der Schichten geschaffen werden (Abb. 21 c). Die einzelnen Federzonen unterscheiden sich durch die Art dieser Melaningitter. Die schmalen Spalten zwischen den als Gitterstäbchen wirkenden Pigmentkörperchen lassen nur beschränkte Einfalls- und Reflexionswinkel des Lichtes zu; dadurch entsteht in einer bestimmten Federzone durch das Beugungsgitter eine bestimmte Farbe, die anders als beim einfachen Schiller unabhängig vom Standpunkt des Betrachters ist und eine ziemliche Konstanz zeigt.

Eine weitere „Strukturfarbe" muß noch erwähnt werden, die häufig in Federn vorkommt: blau. Echte blaue Federfarbstoffe sind sehr selten. Vielmehr entsteht das Strukturblau als Tyndalleffekt, weil Licht durch ein trübes Medium fällt. Dieses Medium wird von den Federzellen geschaffen, indem eine andere Art der Verhornung durchgeführt wird; statt der dicken peripheren Hornmäntel wird die Zelle von einem engen Wabenwerk von Keratin durchzogen, in dessen Kämmerchen beim Austrocknen der Federn Luft eindringt (AUBER, 1957; SCHMIDT und RUSKA, 1962, 1965). Die Kammern sind etwa 0,2 μ im Durchmesser. Die erfolgende Lichtstreuung ist für kurzwelliges (blaues) Licht etwa 16mal stärker als für rotes Licht, so daß vor allem blaues Licht zurückgeworfen wird. Das Blau der Eichelhäherfedern wird auf diese Weise erzeugt. Um die Farbe aber sichtbar zu machen, muß ein dunkler Untergrund vorhanden sein. Die „Blauzellen" werden daher von Melaninpigment unterlagert. Diese Kombination von echtem Pigment mit „Strukturfarbe" ist schon lange bekannt und ausführlich für viele Vögel beschrieben worden (FRANK, 1939), aber erst durch die Elektronenmikroskopie richtig verständlich gemacht worden. Durch die Kombination des Strukturblau mit gelben Lipochromen entstehen grüne Mischfarben, bei Kombination mit roten Lipochromen violette Farbtönungen.

Die Federn werden zumeist periodisch gewechselt: *Mauser*. Es erfolgt also ähnlich wie bei den Haaren eine Erneuerung des Federkleides. Vielfach ist ein Jahresrhythmus des Federwechsels ausgebildet, so daß nach der Fortpflanzungsperiode das Federkleid gewechselt wird. Manche Arten machen aber 2 oder 3 Mausercyclen durch. Werden alle Federn abgeworfen und durch neue ersetzt, so spricht man von einer Vollmauser. Es können aber auch nur bestimmte Federgruppen wie Schwungfedern etc. ersetzt werden; es liegt dann eine Teilmauser vor. In den gemäßigten Klimazonen und in Trockengebieten mit ihrer ausgeprägten Periodik von Temperatur- und Feuchtigkeitsschwankungen wird auch die periodische Mauser eingehalten. Sind die Klimaschwankungen weniger einschneidend, so verwischt sich die cyclische Mauseraktivität. Denn ein Beginn zur Neubildung von Federn wird von äußeren Faktoren: Temperatur, Nahrungsangebot, Tageslänge (d.h. Licht) u.a. beeinflußt. Der endogene Rhythmus des Federwechsels, zu dem die äußeren Bedingungen als „Zeitgeber" oder „Schlüsselreize" koordiniert sein müssen, wird durch Hormone hervorgerufen. In der Regel setzt die Mauser nach einer Fortpflanzungsperiode ein, und bei Vögeln, die größere Wanderungen durchführen, darf die Mauser nicht gerade während des Vogelzuges im Gange sein. In ihrer ausführlichen Zusammenfassung geben STRESEMANN und STRESEMANN (1966) einen Überblick über die zahlreichen Befunde des Zeitpunktes und der Reihenfolge des Federwechsels und den allgemeinen Bedingungen.

Weitere Literatur findet sich bei WAGNER und MÜLLER (1963). Die Grundlage für die Mauser bildet der Federkeim, dessen Epithel (des Ringwulstes) eine Ruheperiode einschaltet und bei Beginn des Federwechsels wieder aktiviert wird. Das Wachstum des Epithels und die Veränderungen im Mesenchym der Pulpa des Federkeimes leiten die Bildung einer neuen Feder ein, wie es vorher geschildert

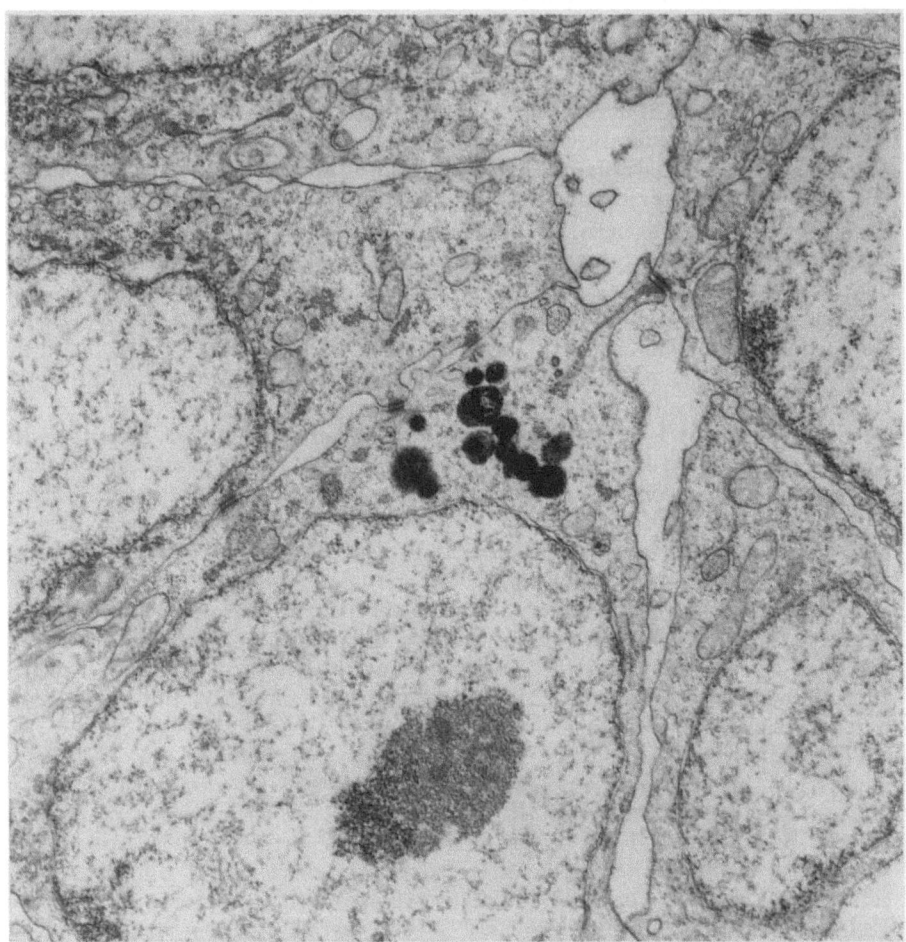

Abb. 21 a—c. Vogelfeder und Melanin; Einlagerung des Pigmentes in die Federepithelzellen. a Federzellen einer Rückendune der Ente (Embryo, 16 d). Die Federzellen sind durch Desmosomen verbunden und lassen große Intercellularlücken entstehen, durch die Fortsätze der Pigmentzelle vorgeschoben werden können. In der mittleren Federzelle ist bereits Melanin in Form großer Granula eingelagert. 20000/1. b Ausschnitt aus stark verzahnten Federzellen (Differenzierungszone) der Schwanzdune eines 20 d alten Entenkükens. Der Ausläufer einer Pigmentzelle wird so eng von der Federzelle umschlossen, daß die Zellmembranen stellenweise zusammenfließen (wie bei einer Zona occludens); später werden die Membranen fragmentiert, so daß die Melaningranula und der Inhalt des Zellausläufers von den Epithelzellen aufgenommen werden. 50000/1. c Schematische Darstellung der Lage von Melaninkörperchen in Federzellen vom Pfau (Schwanz). Die verhornenden und austrocknenden Federzellen lassen lufterfüllte Hohlräume entstehen, die Melaninstäbchen bilden ein Interferenzgitter. (Nach DURRER, 1965)

wurde. Durch den sich vergrößernden Federkeim werden die Hornschichten an der Spule der alten Feder von denen des Federbalges gelöst: die alte Feder fällt aus (sog. Ecdysis) oder wird beim „Putzen" vom Vogel losgerupft. Man muß sich dabei vor Augen halten, daß der feste Halt der Spule im Federbalg allein durch die zusammenhängenden Hornschichten gewährleistet ist; er kann durch Ausrupfen der Feder gelöst werden, wobei meist der oberflächliche Teil des Feder-

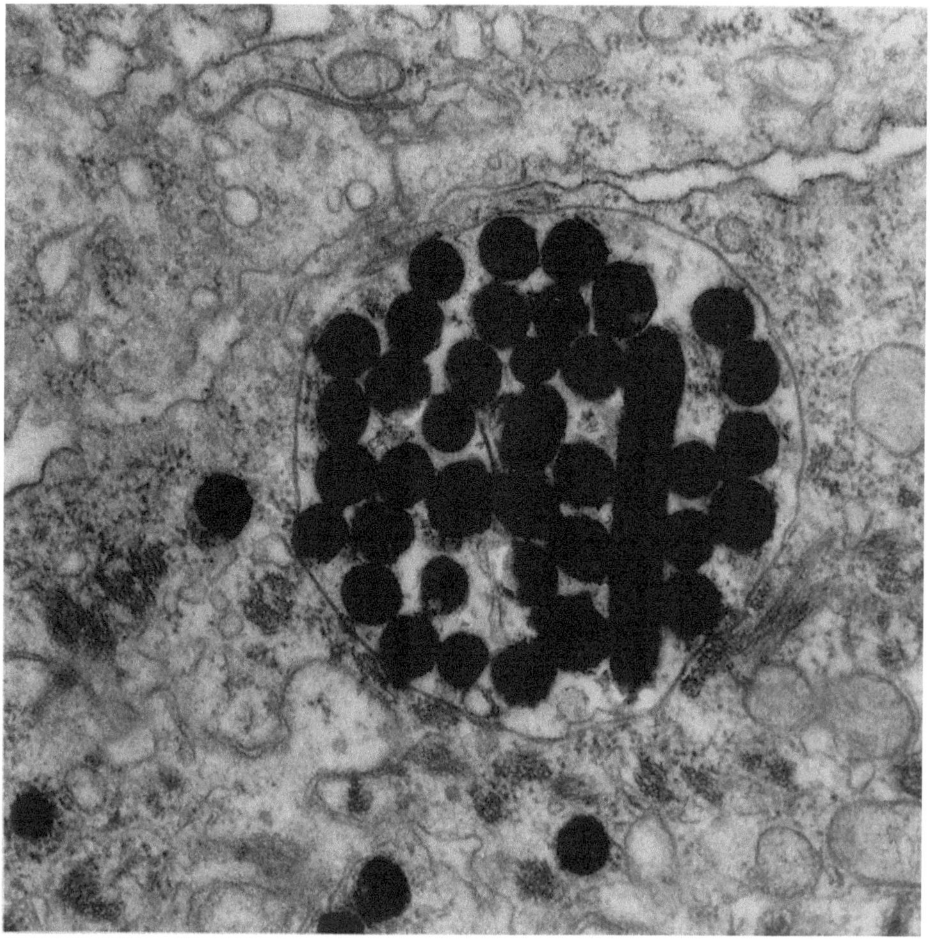

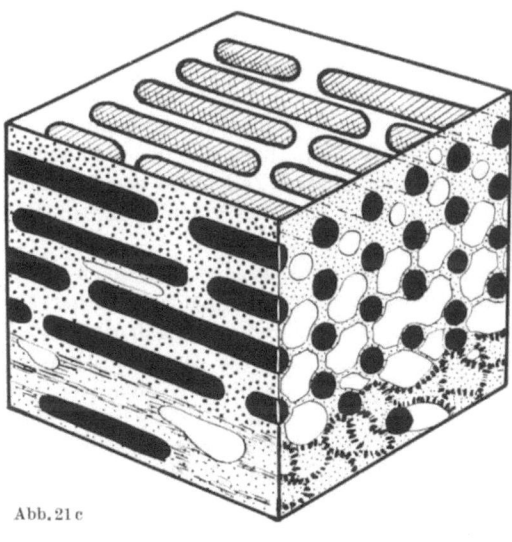

Abb. 21 c

keimepithels mit abgerissen wird. Es ist also nicht, wie seit langem angenommen wurde, der Federausfall die primäre Erscheinung, sondern das einsetzende Wachstum der neuen Feder (BECKER, 1959; WATSON, 1963). Dadurch werden auch die hormonellen Einflüsse auf die Mauser verständlich (vgl. HÖHN, 1961; JÖCHLE, 1961; TIXIER-VIDAL, 1963). Das Schilddrüsenhormon bewirkt die Mauser, seine Ausschüttung und sein jahreszeitlich schwankender Spiegel wird durch das thyreotrope Hormon der Adenohypophyse gesteuert; diese wiederum wird vom Hypothalamus korrigiert. Die mannigfachen Einwirkungen der äußeren Bedingungen, vor allem auch der Geschlechtsorgane auf die Mauser, greifen über das hypothalamisch-hypophysäre System in den Federwechsel ein. Die Photoperiode, also der Tag-Nacht-Rhythmus und die dabei auftretende Lichtmenge beeinflussen durch das zentrale System die Gonadenentfaltung und auch die Mauser (vgl. FOLLET und FARNER, 1966; FARNER, OKSCHE und LORENZEN, 1962; KOBAYASHI und OBUKO, 1955; KOBAYASHI, BERN, NISHIOKA und HYODO, 1961). Wie beim Haarwechsel der Säugetiere ist also eine komplizierte Regulation der Wachstumsaktivität des federbildenden Epithels ausgebildet worden, die mit der Kontrolle der mitotischen Aktivität im Hautepithel verglichen werden sollte (vgl. BULLOUGH und LAURENCE, 1960, 1961; BULLOUGH, 1962; EBLING und HERVEY, 1964; COHEN, 1965; FINEGOLD, 1965). Durch besondere Situationen, in denen die Tiere einem plötzlichen Schock ausgesetzt sind, kann eine ,,Schreckmauser" hervorgerufen werden (DATHE, 1955), die einem Stress gleichzusetzen ist. Hier dürfte die starke Kontraktion der Federmuskulatur das Abwerfen der Federn bewirken, obwohl auch eine Schreckmauser durch Hyperthyreose einige Zeit nach dem Stress auftreten kann (JÖCHLE, 1961). Hinsichtlich der normalen periodischen Mauser war schon lange bekannt, daß die Schilddrüse jahrescyclische Veränderungen durchmacht (KÜCHLER, 1935; HÖHN, 1949).

Die Gemeinsamkeiten zwischen Federn und Haaren werden noch durch zwei Befunde hervorgehoben. a) Die Stellung der Federn in den gleichmäßig angeordneten Reihen der Federfluren kann durch Wirbelbildungen gestört sein (GOESSLER, 1937). b) Bei männlichen Vögeln kommt eine Glatzenbildung vor, die der vom Menschen bekannten Alopecie sehr gleicht (beim Kampfläufer, v. OORDT und JUNGE, 1936; beim Lappenstar, HAMILTON, 1959); in beiden Formen zeigen die Männchen während der Balzzeit kahle Kopfhautpartien. Nach der Brutperiode wachsen wieder Federn nach. Wurden die Männchen kastriert, so unterbleibt die Glatzenbildung. Die genauere Untersuchung zeigt, daß durch die Verabreichung von Testosteron die Federlosigkeit für viele Monate aufrechterhalten werden kann und auch außerhalb der Brutperiode erzeugt wird. Nur bestimmte Hautbezirke sind aber ansprechbar. Die Ursache der Glatzenbildung liegt in einer Hemmung der Federkeime, deren Wachstum gestoppt wird. Die alten Federn gehen allmählich verloren, es werden aber keine neuen nachgeschoben (HAMILTON, 1959). Einzelne Federn können längere Zeit in der sonst kahlen Haut noch stehenbleiben; werden sie gerupft, so wachsen auch in diesen Follikeln keine neuen Federn nach.

Abschließend muß noch erwähnt werden, daß nach einer Mauser das nachwachsende Gefieder in Struktur oder Färbung vom vorhergegangenen abweichen kann. Während der Entwicklung der Vögel nach dem Schlüpfen werden verschiedene Altersphasen durchgemacht, die durch bestimmte Gefiedertypen gekennzeichnet sein können. Das eben geschlüpfte junge Tier besitzt ein Dunenkleid, das nach einer gewissen Zeit durch ein Jugendgefieder ersetzt wird. Auch die Federkleider von Jungtieren können noch mit zunehmendem Alter verschieden voneinander sein. Der adulte Vogel schließlich hat das typische Erwachsenengefieder; aber dessen Aussehen hängt davon ab, in welcher Periode des Sexual-cyclus oder der Jahreszeit sich der Vogel befindet. So entwickeln viele Arten für die Fortpflanzungsperiode unter dem Einfluß der Geschlechtshormone ein bestimmtes Hochzeits- oder Prachtkleid, das in den beiden Geschlechtern verschieden ist (vgl. WITSCHI, 1961). Von den afrikanischen Webervögeln ist bekannt, daß die Entstehung von Pigmentmustern auf den Federn vom Luteinisierungshormon der Hypophyse beeinflußt wird (HALL, RALPH und GRINWICH, 1965). Das Epithel des Federkeimes wird also während seines Wachstums zu sehr verschiedenen Leistungen gedrängt, je nach hormonalem Einfluß; ebenso wird die Pigmentbildung und -einlagerung modifiziert. Wegen des auffallenden Effektes dieser Beeinflussung hat die Untersuchung des Gefieders in der Hormonforschung frühzeitig große Bedeutung erlangt. Die Ausprägungen verschiedener Gefiedertypen sind unter den Bezeichnungen Geschlechtsdimorphismus, Saisondimorphismus, Altersdimorphismus seit langem in vielen Fällen beschrieben und diskutiert worden.

Literatur

ABBOTT, U. K., and V. S. ASMUNDSON: Scaleless, an inherited ectodermal defect in the domestic fowl. J. Hered. 48, 63—70 (1957). — ABRAMOWITZ, A. A.: Regeneration of chromatophore nerves. Proc. nat. Acad. Sci. (Wash.) 21, 137—141 (1935). — The double innervation of caudal melanophores in fundulus. Proc. nat. Acad. Sci. (Wash.) 22, 233—238 (1936). — The non-identity of the neurohumors for the melanophores and xanthophores of fundulus. Amer. Naturalist 70, 372—378 (1936). — The pituitary control of chromatophores in the dogfish. Amer. Naturalist. 73, 208—240 (1939). — ADAMS, A. E., A. KUDER, and L. RICHARDS: The endocrine glands and molting in Triturus viridescens. J. exp. Zool. 63, 1—55 (1932). — ADAMS, A. E., L. RICHARDS, and A. KUDER: The relations to the thyroid and pituitary glands to moulting in Triturus viridescens. Science 72, 323—324 (1930). — ADRIAN, E. D., K. MCKEEN CATTELL, and H. HOAGLAND: Sensory discharges in single cutaneous nerve fibres. J. Physiol. (Lond.) 72, 377—391 (1931). — ARIËNS KAPPERS, C. U.: Anatomie comparée du système nerveux. Paris: Masson & Cie. 1947. — ARIËNS KAPPERS, C. U., G. C. HUBER, and E. C. CROSBY: The comparative anatomy of the nervous system of vertebrates, including man, vol. I. New York: Hafner Publ. Co. 1960. — AUBER, L.: Cortex and medulla of bird feathers. Nature (Lond.) 176, 1218—1219 (1955). — The structures producing "non-iridescent" blue color in bird feathers. Proc. Zool. Soc. Lond. 129, 455—486 (1957). — AUBER, L., and H. M. APPLEYARD: Surface cells of feather barbs. Nature (Lond.) 168, 736—737 (1951). — AUST, S.: Die Epidermis von Anguilla vulgaris F. während seiner Entwicklung. Zool. Jb., Abt. Anat. 62, 1—44 (1936/37).

BAGNARA, J. T.: Hypophyseal control of guanophores in anuran larvae. J. exp. Zool. 137, 265—284 (1958). — Pineal regulation of the body lightening reaction in amphibian larvae. Science 132, 1481—1483 (1960). — Chromatotrophic hormone, pteridines, and amphibian pigmentation. Gen. comp. Endocr. 1, 124—133 (1961). — The pineal and the body lightening reaction of larval amphibians. Gen. comp. Endocr. 3, 86—100 (1963). — Stimulation of melanophores and guanophores by melanophore-stimulating hormone peptides. Gen. comp. Endocr. 4, 290—294 (1964). — Independent actions of pineal and hypophysis in the regulation of chromatophores of anuran larvae. Gen. comp. Endocr. 4, 299—303 (1964). — BAGNARA, J. T., and S. NEIDLEMAN: Effect of chromatotrophic hormone on pigments of anuran skin. Proc. Soc. exp. Biol. (N.Y.) 97, 671—673 (1958). — BAGNARA, J. T., and C. M. RICHARDS: Expression of specific pteridines in amphibian xenoplastic neural crest transplants. Amer. Zool. 5, 664 (1965). — BAILEY, R. E.: The incubation patch of passerine birds. Condor 54, 121—136 (1952). — BAILEY, R. M., and W. R. TAYLOR: Schilboëdes hildebrandi, a new ameiruid catfish from Mississippi. Copeia (Ann. Abor) 1 (1950). — BALLOWITZ, E.: Die Nervenendigungen der Pigmentzellen, ein Beitrag zur Kenntnis des Zusammenhanges der Endverzweigungen der Nerven mit dem Protoplasma der Zellen. Z. wiss. Zool. 56, 673—706 (1893). — Über die Erythrophoren und ihre Vereinigung mit Iridocyten und Melanophoren bei Hemichromis bimaculatus Gill. Vierter Beitrag zur Kenntnis der Chromatophoren und der Chromatophoren-Vereinigungen bei Knochenfischen. Arch. Zellforsch. 14, 193—219 (1917). — BARGMANN, W.: Zur Frage der Homologisierung von Schmelz und Vitrodentin. Z. Zellforsch. 27, 492—499 (1938). — BARTHOLOMEW, G. A., and W. R. DAWSON: Temperature regulation in young pelicans, herons and gulls. Ecology 35, 466—472 (1954). — BECHTEL, H. B.: Microscopical aspects of ecdysis in snakes. Herpetologica 13, 171—181 (1957). — BECKER, R.: Die Strukturanalyse der Gefiederfolgen von Megapodius freyc. reinw. und ihre Beziehungen zu der Nestlingsdune der Hühnervögel. Revue suisse Zool. 66, 411—527 (1959). —

BELL, E., and Y. T. THATHACHARI: Development of feather keratin during embryogenesis of the chick. J. Cell Biol. 16, 215—223 (1963). — BELLAIRS, A. d'A., and G. UNDERWOOD: The origin of snakes. Biol. Rev. 26, 193—237 (1951). — BENNETT, H. S.: Morphological aspects of ectracellular polysaccharides. J. Histochem. Cytochem. 11, 14—23 (1963). — BENTLEY, P. J., and W. F. C. BLUMER: Uptake of water by the lizard, Moloch horridus. Nature (Lond.) 194, 699—700 (1962). — BENTLEY, P. J., and K. SCHMIDT-NIELSEN: Permeability to water and sodium of the crocodilian, Caiman sclerops. J. cell. comp. Physiol. 66, 303—309 (1965). — Cutaneous water loss in reptiles. Science 150, 1547—1549 (1966). — BERGER, A. J.: The musculature. In: Biology and comp. physiol. of birds, vol. 1, p. 301—344 (ed. A. J. MARSHALL). New York and London: Academic Press 1960. — BIEDERMANN, W.: Vergleichende Physiologie des Integumentes der Wirbeltiere. Ergebn. Biol. 1, 1—342 (1926). — Vergleichende Physiologie des Integumentes der Wirbeltiere, 3. Teil. Ergebn. Biol. 3, 354—541 (1928). — BIKLE, D., L. G. TILNEY, and K. R. PORTER: Microtubules and pigment migration in the melanophores of Fundulus heteroclitus L. Protoplasma (Wien) 61, 322—345 (1966). — BLACKSTAD, TH. W.: The skin and slime glands. In: The biology of myxine, p. 195—230 (ed. A. BRODAL and R. FÄNGE). Oslo: Oslo Universitetsforlaget 1963. — BOAS, J. E. V.: Federn. In: Handbuch der vergleichenden Physiologie der Wirbeltiere, Bd. I, S. 271—374 (Hrsg. L. BOLK, E. GÖPPERT, E. KALLIUS u. W. LUBOSCH). Berlin u. Wien: Urban & Schwarzenberg 1931. — BOEKE, J.: II. Niedere Sinnesorgane. In: Handbuch der vergleichenden Anatomie der Wirbeltiere, Bd. II/2, S. 855—878 (Hrsg. L. BOLK, E. GÖPPERT, E. KALLIUS u. W. LUBOSCH). Berlin u. Wien: Urban & Schwarzenberg 1934. — BOGENSCHÜTZ, H.: Untersuchungen über den lichtbedingten Farbwechsel der Kaulquappen. Z. vergl. Physiol. 50, 598—614 (1965). — BOGERT, C. M.: How reptiles regulate their body temperature. Sci. Amer. 200, 105—120 (1959). — BOISSONAS, R. A.: Die chemische Forschung auf dem Gebiet des MSH. In: Gewebs- und Neurohormone. Physiologie des Melanophorenhormons, S. 195—204 (8. Symp. Dtsch. Ges. Endokrinol.). Berlin-Göttingen-Heidelberg: Springer 1962. — BOLOGNANI FANTIN, A. M.: Contributo alla conoscenza istochimica della ghiandola dell'apparato copulatore di Raja clavata. Monit. zool. ital. 70/71, 301—312 (1963). — BONE, Q.: The central nervous system in larvae Acraniates. Quart. J. micr. Sci. 100, 509—527 (1959). — A note on the innervation of the integument in Amphioxus, and its bearing on the mechanism of cutaneous sensibility. Quart. J. micr. Sci. 101, 371—379 (1960). — Some observations upon the peripheral nervous system of the hagfish, Myxine glutinosa. J. marine biol. Ass. 43, 31—47 (1963). — BOTEZAT, E.: Die Nervenendapparate in den Mundteilen der Vögel und die einheitliche Endigungsweise der peripheren Nerven bei den Wirbeltieren. Z. wiss. Zool. 84, 205—360 (1906). — BREYER, H.: Über Hautsinnesorgane und Häutung bei Lacertilien. Zool. Jb. Abt. Anat. 51, 549—580 (1929). — BRINCKMANN, A.: Die Morphologie der Schmuckfedern von Aix galericulata L. Revue suisse Zool. 65, 485—608 (1958). — BROWN, M. E.: Experimental studies on growth. In: The physiology of fishes, vol. I, p. 361—400 (ed. M. E. BROWN). New York: Academic Press 1957. — BRÜHL, L.: Fischhaut. In: Die Rohstoffe des Tierreiches, Bd. I, S. 228—260 (Hrsg. F. PAX u. W. AHRNDT). Berlin: Gebrüder Borntraeger 1933. — BUDKER, P.: Sur la destruction et la chute des dents mandibulaires des Sqales. C. R. Acad. Sci. (Paris) 203, 386—387 (1936). — Les cryptes sensorielles et les denticules cutanés des plagiostomes. Ann. Inst. océanogr. Monaco 18, 207—288 (1938). — Les organes sensoriels cutanés de Sélaciens. In: Traité de Zoologie, vol. XIII/2, p. 1033—1062 (ed. P. GRASSÉ). Paris: Masson & Cie. 1958. — BULLOCK, T. H., and F. P. J. DIECKE: Properties of an infra-red receptor. J. Physiol. (Lond.) 134, 47—87 (1956). — BULLOUGH, W. S.: The control of mitotic activity in adult mammalian tissue. Biol. Rev. 37, 307—342 (1962). — BULLOUGH, W. S., and E. B. LAURENCE: The control of epidermal mitotic activity in the mouse. Proc. roy. Soc. B 151, 517—536 (1960). — The control of mitotic activity in mouse skin. Dermis and hypodermis. Exp. Cell Res. 21, 394—405 (1960). — Stress and adrenaline in relation to the diurnal cycle of epidermal mitotic activity in adult male mice. Proc. roy. Soc. B 154, 540—556 (1961). — BURGERS, A. C. J., P. J. H. BENNINK, and G. J. VAN OORDT: Investigations into the regulation of the pigmentary system of the blind mexican cave fish, Anoptichthys jordani. Proc. kon. ned. Akad. Wet. C 66, 189—195 (1963). — BURGESS, G. H. O.: Absence of keratin in teleost epidermis. Nature (Lond.) 178, 93—94 (1956).

CARTER, G. S.: Air breathing. In: Physiology of fishes, vol. I, p. 65—79 (ed. M. E. BROWN). New York: Academic Press 1957. — CATE, J. TEN: La coordination des mouvements locomoteurs après la section transversale de la meelle épinière chez les couleuves. Archs. néerl. Physiol. Ser. IIIc 21, 195—201 (1936). — CEREIJIDO, M., and P. F. CURRAN: Intracellular electrical potentials in frog skin. J. gen. Physiol. 48, 543—557 (1965). — CHAPMAN, G. H., and A. B. DAWSON: Fine structure of the larval anuran epidermis, with special reference to the figures of Eberth. J. biophys. biochem. Cytol. 10, 425—435 (1961). — CHATFIELD, P. O., C. P. LYMAN, and L. IRVING: Physiological adaptation to cold of peripheral nerve in the leg of the herring gull (Larus argentatus). Amer. J. Physiol. 172, 639—644 (1953). — CLARA, M.: Über den Bau des Schnabels der Waldschnepfe. Z. mikr.-anat. Forsch. 3, 1—108 (1925). —

COHEN, J., and P. G. ESPINASSE: On the normal and abnormal development of the feather. J. Embryol. exp. Morph. **9**, 223—251 (1961). — COHEN, S.: The stimulation of epidermal proliferation by a specific protein (EGF). Develop. Biol. **12**, 394—407 (1965). — COLE, F. J.: A monograph on the general morphology of myxinoid fishes, based on a study of myxine. Part VI. The morphology of the vascular system. Trans. roy. Soc. Edinb. **54**, 309—342 (1926). — COLLIN, R.: Sur l'innervation des mélanocytes et des guaninocytes dans la queue du tétard de Rana temporaria L. C. R. Soc. Biol. (Paris) **122**, 669—671 (1936). — CURRAN, P. F., and M. CEREIJIDO: K fluxes in frog skin. J. gen. Physiol. **48**, 1011—1033 (1965). — CURRAN, P. F., and J. R. GILL jr.: The effect of calcium on sodium transport by frog skin. J. gen. Physiol. **45**, 625—641 (1962). — CURRAN, P. F., F. C. HERRERA, and W. J. FLANIGAN: The effect of Ca and antidiuretic hormone in Na transport across frog skin. II. Sites and mechanism of action. J. gen. Physiol. **46**, 1011—1027 (1963). — CZOPEK, J.: Vascularization of respiratory surfaces in Leiopelma hochstretteri Fitzinger and Xenopus laevis (DAUDIN). Acta anat. (Basel) **25**, 346—360 (1955). — The vascularisation of respiratory surfaces in Ambystoma mexicanum (Cope) in ontogeny. Zoologica Pol. **8**, 131—149 (1957). — Skin and lung capillaries in European commom newts. Copeia (Ann Arbor) **91**—96 (1959).

DANNEEL, R., u. H. SCHUMANN: Die Entstehung des Farbmusters beim Lakenfelder Huhn. Wilhelm Roux' Arch. Entwickl.-Mech. **154**, 405—416 (1963). — DANNEEL, R., u. N. WEISSENFELS: Die Herkunft der Melanoblasten in den Haaren des Menschen und ihr Verbleib beim Haarwechsel. Biol. Zbl. **72**, 630—643 (1953). — DANNEEL, S. (SCHÄFER-DANNEEL): Strukturelle und funktionelle Voraussetzungen für die Bewegung von Amoeba proteus. Z. Zellforsch. **78**, 441—462 (1967). — DATHE, H.: Über die Schreckmauser. J. Ornithol. (Leipzig) **96**, 5—14 (1955). — DEVILLERS, CH.: Le système latéral. In: Traité de Zoologie, vol. XIII/2, p. 940—1032 (ed. P. GRASSÉ). Paris: Masson & Cie. 1958. — DEWEY, M. M., and L. BARR: A study of the structure and distribution of the nexus. J. Cell Biol. **23**, 553—585 (1964). — DIERST, K. E., and C. L. RALPH: Effect of hypothalamic stimulation on melanophores in the frog. Gen. comp. Endocr. **2**, 347—353 (1962). — DIJKGRAAF, S.: Untersuchungen über die Funktion der Seitenorgane an Fischen. Z. vergl. Physiol. **20**, 162—214 (1934). — Bau und Funktion der Seitenorgane und des Ohrlabyrinths bei Fischen. Experientia (Basel) **8**, 205—244 (1952). — Elektrophysiologische Untersuchungen an der Seitenlinie von Xenopus laevis. Experientia (Basel) **12**, 276—278 (1956). — The functioning and significance of the lateral-line organs. Biol. Rev. **38**, 51—105 (1963). — DIJKSTRA, C.: Die De- und Regeneration der sensiblen Endkörperchen des Entenschnabels (Grandry- und Herbst-Körperchen) nach Durchschneidung des Nerven, nach Fortnahme der ganzen Haut und nach Transplantation des Hautstückchens. Z. mikr.-anat. Forsch. **34**, 75—185 (1933). — DRIESEN, H. H.: Untersuchungen über die Einwanderung diffuser Pigmente in die Federanlage, insbesondere beim Wellensittich [Melopsittacus undulatus (SHAW)]. Z. Zellforsch. **39**, 121—151 (1953). — DURRER, H.: Schillerfarben beim Pfau. Eine elektronenmikroskopische Untersuchung. Verh. naturforsch. Ges. Basel **73**, 204—224 (1962). — DURRER, H., u. W. VILLIGER: Schillerfarben der Nektarvögel (Nectariniidae). Eine elektronenmikroskopische Untersuchung an Nectarinia sperata brasiliana (Gm) — Sumatra und Nectarinia cuprea septentrionalis (Vincent) — Luluabourg, Kasai, Kongo. Revue suisse Zool. **69**, 801—813 (1962). — Schillerfarben der Trogoniden. Eine elektronenmikroskopische Untersuchung. J. Ornithol. (Leipzig) **107**, 1—26 (1966).

EAKIN, R. M.: Photoreceptors in the amphibian frontal organ. Proc. nat. Acad. Sci. (Wash.) **47**, 1084—1088 (1961). — EAKIN, R. M., and J. A. WESTFALL: The development of photoreceptors in the stirnorgan of the treefrog., Hyla regilla. Embryologia (Nagoya) **6**, 84—98 (1961). — EBLING, F. J., and G. R. HERVEY: The activity of hair follicles in parabiotic rats. J. Embryol. exp. Morph. **12**, 425—438 (1964). — EDDS jr., M. V.: Development of collagen in the frog embryo. Proc. nat. Acad. Sci. (Wash.) **44**, 296—305 (1958). — EDD jr., M. V., and P. R. SWEENY: Chemical an morphological differentiation of the basement lamella. In: Synthesis of molecular and cellular structure, p. 111—138. 19. Symp. of the Society for study of development and growth, 1960. New York: Ronald Press Co. 1961. — Development of the basement lamella. In: Electron microscopy, vol. II, QQ 2. 5th Intern. Congr. for Electronmicroscopy Philadelphia 1962 (ed. S. S. BREESE jr.). New Yorkand London: Academic Press 1962. — EISEN, A. Z., and J. GROSS: The role of epithelium and mesenchyme in the production of a collagenolytic enzyme and a hyaluronidase in the anuran tadpole. Develop. Biol. **12**, 408—418 (1965). — ENEMAR, A., and B. FALCK: On the presence of adrenic nerves in the pars intermedia of the frog, Rana temporaria. Gen. comp. Endocr. **5**, 577—583 (1965). — ETKIN, W.: Hypothalamic inhibition of pars intermedia activity in the frog. Gen. comp. Endocr., Suppl. **1**, 148—159 (1962). — FAHRENHOLZ, C.: Die Tastsinnesorgane in der Haut des afrikanischen Krallenfrosches (Xenopus calcaratus PETERS). Morph. Jb. **63**, 454—479 (1929). — Tastzellen und Tastorgane in der Neunaugenhaut. Z. mikr.-anat. Forsch. **39**, 116—134 (1936). — Die sensiblen Einrichtungen der Neunaugenhaut. Z. mikr.-anat. Forsch. **40**, 323—380 (1936).

FALK, S., and J. RHODIN: Mechanism of pigment migration within teleost melanophores. In: Electron microscopy. Proc. Stockholm Conference, p. 213—215. New York: Academic Press 1957. — FARNER, D. S.: Hypothalamic neurosecretion and phosphatase activity in relation to photoperiodic control of the testicular cycle of Zonotrichia leucophrys gambelii. Gen. comp. Endocr., Suppl. 1, 160—167 (1962). — FARNER, D. S., A. OKSCHE, and L. LORENZEN: Hypothalamic neurosecretion and the photoperiodic response in the white-crowned sparrow, Zonotrichia leucophrys gambelii. In: Neurosecretion (Mem. Soc., Endocr. No 12), p. 187—195 (ed. H. HELLER and R. B. CLARK). London and New York: Academic Press 1962. — FARQUHAR, M. G., and G. E. PALADE: Functional organization of amphibian skin. Proc. nat. Acad. Sci. (Wash.) 51, 569—577 (1964). — Cell junctions in amphibian skin. J. Cell Biol. 26, 263—291 (1965). — Adenosine triphosphatase localization in amphibian epidermis. J. Cell Biol. 30, 359—379 (1966). — FAURE-FREMIET, E.: Structure du derme téliforme chez les Scombridés. Archs. Anat. micr. Morph. exp. 34, 219—230 (1938). — FERRY, J. D.: A fibrons protein from the slime of the hagfish. J. biol. Chem. 138, 263—268 (1941). — FICALBI, E.: Struttura del tegumento dei Pteromyzonti. IV. Le cellule epidermiche speciali. Archo. ital. Anat. Embriol. 21, 1—54 (1924). — FIEDLER, W.: Die Haut der Säugetiere als Ausdrucksorgan. Stud. gen. Berlin 17, 362—390 (1964). — FILSHIE, B. K., and G. E. ROGERS: An electron microscope study of the fine structure of feather keratin. J. Cell Biol. 13, 1—12 (1962). — FINEGOLD, M. J.: Control of cell multiplication in epidermis. Proc. Soc. exp. Biol. (N.Y.) 119, 96—100 (1965). — FIORONI, P.: Zur Pigment- und Musterentwicklung bei squamaten Reptilien. Revue suisse Zool. 68, 727—874 (1961). — FITTON-JACKSON, S., and H. B. FELL: Epidermal fine structure in embryonic chicken skin during atypical differentiation induced by vitamin A in culture. Develop. Biol. 7, 394—419 (1963). — FLEURY, R.: L'appareil venimeux des Sélaciens Trygoniformes (anatomie, histologie, physiologie). Mém. Soc. zool. Fr. 30, 1—38 (1950). — FLOCK, Å.: Structure of the macula utriculi with special reference to directional interplay of sensory responses as revealed by morphological polarization. J. Cell Biol. 22, 413—431 (1964). — FLOCK, Å., and A. J. DUVALL: The ultrastructure of the kinocilium of the sensory cells in the inner ear and lateral line organs. J. Cell Biol. 25, 1—8 (1965). — FLOCK, Å., and J. WERSÄLL: Synaptic structure in the lateral line canal organ of the teleost fish Lota vulgaris. J. Cell Biol. 13, 337—343 (1962). — A study of the orientation of the sensory hairs of the receptor cells in the lateral line organ of fish, with special reference to the function of the receptors. J. Cell Biol. 15, 19—27 (1962). — FOLLETT, B. K., and D. S. FARNER: The effect of the daily photoperiod on gonadal growth, neurohypophyseal hormone content, and neurosecretion in the hypothalamo-hypophyseal system of the Japanese quail (Coturnix coturnix japonica). Gen. comp. Endocr. 7, 111—124 (1966). — Pituitary gonadotropins in the Japanese quail (Coturnix coturnix japonica) during photoperiodically induced gonadal growth. Gen. comp. Endocr. 7, 125—131 (1966). FORSDAHL, K. A.: Mechanism of pigment-granule movement in melanophores of the lizard anolis carolinensis. Nytt Mag. Zool. 8, 37—44 (1959). — FRANK, F.: Die Färbung der Vogelfeder durch Pigment und Struktur. J. Ornithol. (Leipzig) 87, 426—523 (1939). — FRANZ, V.: Haut, Sinnesorgane und Nervensystem der Akranier. Jena. Z. Naturwiss. 59, 401—526 (1923). — Morphologie der Akranier. Ergebn. Anat. Entwickl.-Gesch. 27, 464—692 (1927). — FRASER, R. D. B., and T. P. MCRAE: Molecular organization of feather keratin. J. molec. Biol. 1, 387—397 (1959). — FREUND, L.: Besondere Bildungen im mikroskopischen Aufbau der Vogelhaut. Zool. Anz., Suppl. 2, 153—158 (1926). — FRISCH, K. v.: Beiträge zur Physiologie der Pigmentzellen in der Fischhaut. Pflügers Arch. ges. Physiol. 138, 319—387 (1911). — Über den Einfluß der Bodenfarbe auf die Flecken bezeichnung des Feuersalamanders. Biol. Zbl. 40, 390—414 (1920). — FUJII, R.: Correlation between fine structure and activity in fish melanophore. In: Structure and control of the melanocyte, p. 114—123 (ed. G. DELLA PORTA and O. MÜHLBOCK). Berlin-Heidelberg-New York: Springer 1966.

GABE, M.: Le tégument et ses annexes. In: Traité de Zoologie, vol. XVI/1, p. 1—233 (ed. P. P. GRASSÉ). Paris: Masson & Cie. 1967. — GEDEVANISHVILI, M. D.: The seasonal variation in amounts of mucopolysaccharide constituents in the ground substance of frog dermis. In: Zweiter Int. Kongr. Histo- und Cytochemie, S. 159 (Hrsg. T. H. SCHIEBLER, A. G. E. PEARSE u. H. H. WOLFF). Berlin-Göttingen-Heidelberg: Springer 1964. — GESCHWIND, I. I.: Chemistry of the melanocyte-stimulating hormones. In: Structure and control of the melanocyte, p. 28—43 (ed. G. DELLA PORTA and O. MÜHLBOCK). Berlin-Heidelberg-New York: Springer 1966. — GNADEBERG, W.: Untersuchungen über den Bau der Placoidschuppen der Selachier. Jena. Z. Naturwiss. 62, 473—500 (1926). — GÖHRINGER, R.: Vergleichende Untersuchungen über das Juvenil- und Adultkleid bei der Amsel (Turdus merula L.) und beim Star (Sturnus vulgaris L.). Revue suisse Zool. 58, 279—358 (1951). — GÖRNER, P.: Beitrag zum Bau und zur Arbeitsweise des Seitenorgans von Xenopus laevis. Zool. Anz., Suppl. 25, 193—198 (1962). — Untersuchungen zur Morphologie und Elektrophysiologie des Seitenlinienorgans vom Krallenfrosch (Xenopus laevis Daudin). Z. vergl. Physiol. 47, 316—338 (1963). — GOESSLER, E.: Wirbelbildungen in den Federfluren der Vögel. Revue suisse Zool. **44**, 371—380 (1937). — GOETINCK, P. F., and U. K. ABBOTT: Tissue interaction in the scaleless mutant and the use of scaleless as an ectodermal marker in studies of normal limb differentiation. J. exp. Zool. **154**, 7—19 (1963). — GOFF, R. A.: Development of the mesodermal constituents of feather germs of chick embryos. J. Morph. **85**, 443—481 (1949). — GOSLAR, H. G.: Über die Wirkung verschiedener Sexualhormone auf die Häutungsvorgänge der Ringelnatter (Natrix natrix L.). Derm. Wschr. **137**, 139—146 (1958). — Beiträge zum Häutungsgeschehen der Schlangen. I. Mitteilung: Histologische und topochemische Untersuchungen an der Haut von Natrix natrix L. während der Phasen des normalen Häutungszyklus (Jena). Acta histochem. **5**, 182—212 (1958). — Beiträge zum Häutungsvorgang der Schlangen. 2. Mitteilung: Studien zur Fermenttopochemie der Keratogenese und Keratolyse am Modell der Reptilienhaut. Acta histochem. (Jena) **17**, 1—60 (1964). — GOTO, T.: Über die Veränderungen der Pterine in den Entwicklungsstadien von einem Frosch, Rhacophorus schlegelii var. arborea. Jap. J. Zool. **14**, 69—81 (1963). — Über einen blau fluoreszierenden Stoff „Bufo-chrom", seine Isolierung aus der Haut einer Kröte Bufo vulgaris und sein Verhalten in den Entwicklungsstadien. Jap. J. Zool. **14**, 83—90 (1963). — Fluoreszierender Stoff aus Bufo vulgaris. Konstitutionsaufklärung des Pteridins „Bufo-chrom". Jap. J. Zool. **14**, 91—95 (1963). — GRAY, E. G.: Control of the melanophores of the minnow (Phoxinus phoxinus (L.)). J. exp. Biol. **33**, 448—459 (1956). — GREENWALT, C. H., W. BRANDT, and D. D. FRIEL: The iridescent colors of humming bird feathers. Proc. amer. philos. Soc. **104**, 249—253 (1960). — GREITE, W.: Die Strukturbildung der Vogelfeder und ihre Pigmentierung durch Melanine. Z. wiss. Zool. **145**, 283—334 (1934). — GRONER, W.: Die Entwicklung der Crista und Cupula im statischen Apparat und in den freien Sinneshügeln der Fische. Z. wiss. Zool. **153**, 310—372 (1940). — GROSS, J.: Studies on the biology of connective tissues: remodelling of collagen in metamorphosis. Medicine (Baltimore) **43**, 291—303 (1964). — GORSS, J., and C. M. LAPIERE: Collagenolytic activity in amphibian tissues: a tissue culture assey. Proc. nat. Acad. Sci. (Wash.) **48**, 1014—1022 (1962). — GROSS, J., C. M. LAPIERE, and M. L. TANZER: Organization and disorganization of extracellular substances: the collagen system. In: Cytodifferentiation and macromolecular synthesis. (21st Symp. Soc. Study Dev. Growth, 1962) p. 175—202. New York and London: Academic Press 1963. — GROSS-LERNER, H.: Über Bau und Entwicklung der Reusenzähne von Cetorhinus maximus Gunner. Z. Zellforsch. **46**, 357—386 (1957). — GUSTAVSON, K. H.: The function of hydroxyproline in collagens. Nature (Lond.) **175**, 70—74 (1955). — GUTTMANN, S., and R. A. BOISSONAS: Influence of the structure of the N-terminal extremity of -MSH on the melanophore stimulating activity of this hormone. Experientia (Basel) **17**, 265—267 (1961).

HADLEY, C. E.: Color changes in excised and intact reptilian skin. J. exp. Zool. **58**, 321—331 (1931). — HALBERKANN, J.: Untersuchungen zur Beeinflussung des Häutungszyklus der Ringelnatter durch Thyroxin. Arch. Derm. **197**, 37—41 (1953). — Der Häutungsablauf der Ringelnatter unter Methyl-Thiouracil. Naturwissenschaften **41**, 237—238 (1954). — Zur hormonalen Beeinflussung des Häutungszyklus der Ringelnatter. Z. Naturforsch. **9b**, 77—80 (1954). — HALL, P. F., C. C. RALPH, and D. L. GRINWICH: On the locus of the action of interstitial cell-stimulating hormone (ICSH or LH) on feather pigmentation of african weaver birds. Gen. comp. Endocr. **5**, 552—557 (1965). — HALSTEAD, B. W., M. J. CHITWOOD, and F. R. MODGLIN: The anatomy of the venom apparatus of the zebrafish (Pterois volitans (Linnaeus). Anat. Rec. **122**, 317 (1955). — HALSTEAD, B. W., and L. R. MITCHELL: A review of the venomous fishes of the pacific area. In: Venomous and poisonous aninals and noxious plants of the pacific region, p. 173—202 (ed. H. L. KEEGAN and W. V. MACFORLANE). Oxford-London-New York-Paris: Pergamon Press 1963. — HALSTEAD, B. W., and F. R. MODGLIN: A preliminary report on the venom apparatus of the Bat-Ray, Holorhinus californicus. Copeia (Ann Arbor) 165—175 (1950). — Weeverfish stings and the venom apparatus of weevers. Z. Tropenmed. Parasit. **9**, 129—146 (1958). — HAMA, K.: Fine structure of the lateral line organ of the japanese sea eel. In: Electron microscopy, vol. II, N-4. 5th Intern. Congr. for Electronmicroscopy Philadelphia 1962 (ed. S. S. BREESE jr.). New York and London: Academic Press 1962. — Some observations on the fine structure of the lateral line organ of the japanese sea eel lyncozymba nystromi. J. Cell Biol. **24**, 193—210 (1965). — HAMA, T.: Substances fluorescentes du type ptérinique dans la peau on les yeux de la grenouille (Rana nigromaculata) et leurs transformation photochimiques. Experientia (Basel) **9**, 299 (1953). — Histological distribution of pterins in the skin of bull-frog. Anat. Rec. **134**. 326—327 (1959). — The relation between the chromatophores and pterin compounds. Ann. N.Y. Acad. Sci. **100**, 977—986 (1963). — HAMA, T., and M. OBIKA: Pterin synthesis in the amphibian neural crest cell. Nature (Lond.) **187**, 326—327 (1960). — HAMILTON, H. L., and A. L. KONING: Effects of a phosphatase-inhibitor on the structure of the developing down feather. Amer. J. Anat. **99**, 53—80 (1956). — HAMILTON, J. B.: A male pattern baldness in wattled starlings resembling the conditions in man. Ann. N.Y. Acad. Sci. **83**, 429—447 (1959). — HARDISTY, M. W.: Duration of the larval period in the brook lamprey lampetra planeri). Nature (Lond.) **167**, 38—39 (1951). — Permeability to water of the lamprey integument. Nature (Lond.)

174, 360—361 (1954). — Some aspects of osmotic regulation in lampreys. J. exp. Biol. **33**, 431—447 (1956). — HAY, E. D.: The fine structure of nerves in the epidermis of regenerating salamander limbs. Exp. Cell Res. **19**, 299—317 (1960). — Secretion of a connective tissue protein by developing epidermis. In: The epidermis, p. 97—116 (ed. W. MONTAGNA and W. C. LOITZ, jr.). New York and London: Academic Press 1964. — HAY, E. D., and J. P. REVEL: Autoradiographic studies of the origin of the basement lamella in Ambystoma. Develop. Biol. **7**, 152—168 (1963). — HEMPEL, M.: Die Abhängigkeit der Federstruktur von der Körperregion, untersucht an Xantholaema rubricapilla. Jena. Z. Naturwiss. **65**, 659—737 (1931). — HERRERA, F. C., and P. F. CURRAN: The effect of Ca and antidiuretic hormone on Na transport across frog skin. I. Examination of interrelationships between Ca and hormone J. gen. Physiol. **46**, 999—1010 (1963). — HESS, A.: Two kinds of extrafusal muscle fibers and their nerve ending in the garter snake. Amer. J. Anat. **113**, 347—363 (1963). — The sarcoplasmic reticulum, the T system, and the motor terminals of slow and twitch muscle fibers in the garter snake. J. Cell Biol. **26**, 467—476 (1965). — HIGASHI, H., S. HIRAO, I. YAMADA, and R. KIKUCHI: Vitamin contents in the lamprey, entosphemus japonicus Martens. J. Vitaminol. **4**, 88—99 (1958). — HINSCH, G. W.: Alkaline phosphatase of the developing down feather: substrates, activators, and inhibitors. Develop. Biol. **2**, 21—41 (1960). — HÖHN, E. O.: Seasonal changes in the thyroid gland and the effects of thyroidectomy in the mallard, in relation to molt. Amer. J. Physiol. **158**, 337—344 (1949). — Endocrine glands, thymus and pineal body. In: Biol. and comp. Physiol. of birds, vol. II, S. 87—114 (ed. A. J. MARSHALL). New York and London: Academic Press 1961. — HOFFMANN, C. K.: Reptilien. III. Schlangen und Entwicklungsgeschichte der Reptilien. In: Bronns Klassen und Ordnungen des Thier-Reichs, Bde 6/3. Leipzig: C. F. Wintersche Verl.handlg. 1890. — HOFMANN, K.: Synthesis of melanocyte-stimulating hormone derivatives. Ann. N.Y. Acad. Sci. **88**, 689—707 (1960). — HOFMANN, K.: M. E. WOOLNER, G. SPÜHLER, and E. T. SCHWARTZ: Studies on polypeptides. X. The synthesis of a pentapeptide corresponding to an amino acid sequence present in corticotropin and in the melanocyte stimulating hormones. J. Amer. chem. Soc. **80**, 1486—1488 (1958). — HOFMANN, K., M. E. WOOLNER, H. YAJIMA, G. SPÜHLER, T. A. THOMPSON, and E. T. SCHWARTZ: Studies on polypeptides. XII. The synthesis of a physiologically active blocked tridecapeptide amine possessing the amino acid sequence of -MSH. J. Amer. chem. Soc. **80**, 6458—6459 (1958). — HOFMANN, K., H. GAJIMA, T. LIU, and N. YANAIHARA: Studies on polypeptides. XXIV. Synthesis and biological evaluation of a tricosapeptide possessing essentially the full biological activity of ACTH. J. Amer. chem. Soc. **84**, 4475—4480 (1962). — HOFMANN, K., H. YAJIMA, N. YANAIHARA, T. LIU, and J. LANDE: Studies on polypeptides. XIII. The synthesis of a tricosapeptide possessing essentially the full biological activity of natural ACTH. J. Amer. chem. Soc. **83**, 487—489 (1961). — HOGBEN, L.: The pigmentary effector system. 7. The chromatic function in elasmabranch fishes. Proc. roy. Soc. B **120**, 142—158 (1936). — HOGE, A. R., and P. S. SANTOS: Spbmicroscopic structure of „stratum corneum" of snakes. Science **118**, 410—411 (1953). — HOLST, E. v.: Die Auslösung von Stimmungen bei Wirbeltieren durch „punktförmige" elektrische Erregung des Stammhirns. Naturwissenschaften **44**, 549—551 (1957). — HOLST, E. v., u. U. v. SAINT PAUL: Vom Wirkungsgefüge der Triebe. Naturwissenschaften **47**, 409—422 (1960). — HOROWITZ, S. B.: The effect of sulhydryl inhibitors and thiol compounds on pigment aggregation and dispersion in the melanophores of Anolis carolinensis. Exp. Cell Res. **13**, 400—402 (1957). — The energy requirements of melanin granula aggregation and dispersion in the melanophores of Anolis carolinensis. J. cell. comp. Physiol. **51**, 341—357 (1958). — HORSTMANN, E.: Die Morphologie der Epidermis. Excerpta Med. Congr. Ser. **55**, 362—372 (1962). — Proc. XII. Intern. Congr. Dermat. — Elektronenmikroskopische Untersuchungen an der Epidermis von Reptilien. Verh. Anat. Ges., Jena 1964. Erg.-H. Anat. Anz. **113**, 87—93 (1964). — HOWELL, T. R., and G. A. BARTHOLOMEW: Temperature regulation in laysan and black footed albatrosses. Condor **63**, 180—185 (1961). — HUNT, C. C., and P. G. NELSON: Structural and functional changes in the frog sympathetic ganglion following cutting of the presynaptic fibres. J. Physiol. (Lond.) **177**, 1—20 (1965).

INAMURA, A., H. TAKEDA, and N. SASAKI: The accumulation of sodium and calcium in a specific layer of frog skin. J. cell. comp. Physiol. **66**, 221—226 (1965). — IRVING, L., and J. KROG: Temperature of skin in the arctic as a regulator of heat. J. appl. Physiol. **7**, 355—364 (1955).

JABUREK, L.: Über Nervenendigungen in der Epidermis der Reptilien. Zugleich ein Beitrag über die feinere Struktur der Nervenendknöpfchen sowie deren Beziehung zu den Epidermiszellen. Z. mikr.-anat. Forsch. **10**, 1—49 (1927). — JAKUBOWSKI, M.: The structure and vascularization of the skin of the eel (Anguilla anguilla L.) and the viviparous blenny (Zoarces viviparus L.). Acta biol. cracov., Sér. Zool. **3**, 1—22 (1961). — JAUDE, S. S.: Fine structure of lateral-line organs of frog tadpoles. J. Ultrastruct. Res. **15**, 496—509 (1966). — JECHOREK, W., u. E v. HOLST: Fernreizung freibeweglicher Tiere. Naturwissenschaften **43**, 455 (1956). — JÖCHLE, W.: Experimentelle Untersuchungen zur neuroendokrinen Steuerung der Mauser beim Haushuhn. In: Gewebs- und Neurohormone. Physiologie des Melanophorenhormons, p. 416—421. 8. Symp. Dtsch. Ges. Endokrinologie (1961). Berlin-Göttingen-Heidelberg: Springer 1962. — JOHANN, L.: Über eigentümliche epitheliale Gebilde (Leuchtorgane) bei Spinax niger. Z. wiss. Zool. **66**, 136—160 (1899). — JONES, D. J., and W. MORGAN: Wooly feathering in the fowl. J. Hered. **47**, 137—141 (1956). — JØRGENSEN, C. B., and L. O. LARSEN: Hormonal control of moulting in amphibians. Nature (Lond.) **185**, 244—245 (1960). — Molting and its hormonal control in toads. Gen. com. Endocr. **1**, 145—153 (1961). — Further observations on molting and its hormonal control in Bufo bufo (L.). Gen. comp. Endocr. **4**, 389—400 (1964). — JØRGENSEN, C. B., L. O. LARSEN, and P. ROSENKILDE: Hormonal dependency of molting in amphibians: effect of radiothyroidectomy in the toad Bufo bufo (L.). Gen. comp. Endocr. **5**, 248—251 (1965). — JUHN, M., and R. W. BATES: Thyroid function in silky feathering. J. exp. Zool. **143**, 239—243 (1960).

KAHL, M. P.: Thermoregulation in the wood stork, with special reference to the role of the legs. Physiol. Zool. **36**, 141—151 (1963). — KAISER, L.: De segmentale innervatie van de huid bij de duif. Archs. néerl. Physiol. **9**, 299—379 (1924). — KALLMAN, F., and C. GROBSTEIN: Source of collagen at epithelio-mesenchymal interfaces during inductive interaction. Develop. Biol. **11**, 169—183 (1965). — KALTENBACH, J. C., and N. B. CLARK: Direct action of thyroxin analogues on molting in the adult newt. Gen. comp. Endocr. **5**, 74—86 (1965). — KARKUN, J. N., and F. W. LANDGREBE: Pituitary hormones affecting the chromatophores. In: Comparative endocrinology, vol. I, p. 81—110 (ed. U.S. v. EULER and H. HELLER). New York and London: Academic Press 1963. — KASTIN, A. J., and G. T. ROSS: Melanocytestimulating hormone activity in pituitaries of frogs with hypothalamic lesions. Endocrinology **77**, 45—48 (1965). — KATSUKI, Y., S. YOSHINO, and J. CHEN: Neural mechanism of the lateral-line organ of fish. (Fundamental neural mechanism of sensory organs in general. Jap. J. Physiol. **1**, 264—268 (1951). — Response of the single lateral-line fiber to the linearly rising current stimulating the endorgan. Jap. J. Physiol. **2**, 219—231 (1952). — Action current of the single lateral-line nerve fiber of fish. II. On the discharge due to stimulation. Jap. J. Physiol. **1**, 179—194 (1951). — KAUFFMANN, TH.: Untersuchungen über die fluoreszierenden Pigmente in der Haut von Zierfischen. Z. Naturforsch. **14b**, 358—363 (1959). — KELLY, D. E.: Fine structure of desmosomes, hemidesmosomes and an adepidermal globular layer in developing newt epidermis. J. Cell Biol. **28**, 51—72 (1966). — KELLY, D. E., and J. C. VAN DE KAMER: Cytological und histochemical investigations on the pineal organ of the adult frog (Rana esculenta). Z. Zellforsch. **52**, 618—639 (1960). — KEMP, N. E.: Development of the basement lamella of larval anuran skin. Develop. Biol. **1**, 459—476 (1959). — Replacement of the larval basement lamella by adult-type basement membrane in anuran skin during metamorphosis. Develop. Biol. **3**, 391—410 (1961). — Metamorphotic changes of dermis in skin of frog larvae exposed to thyroxine. Develop. Biol. **7**, 244—254 (1963). — KING, J. R., and D. S. FARNER: Energy metabolism, thermoregulation and body temperature. In: Biology and comp. physiology of birds, vol. II, p. 215—288 (ed. A. J. MARSHALL). New York and London: Academic Press 1961. — KINOSITA, H.: Electrophoretic theory of pigment migration within fish melanophore. Ann. N.Y. Acad. Sci. **100**, 992—1003 (1963). — KLEINHOLZ, L. H.: Studies in reptilian colour changes. II. The pituitary and adrenal glands in the regulation of the melanophores of Anolis carolinensis. J. exp. Biol. **15**, 474—491 (1938). — Studies in reptilian colour changes. III. Controle of the light phase and behavior of isolated skin. J. exp. Biol. **15**, 492—499 (1938). — KOBAYASHI, A., H. A. BERN, R. S. NISHIOKA, and Y. HYODO: The hypothalamo-hypophyseal neurosecretory system of the parakeet, Melopsittacus undulatus. Gen. comp. Endocr. **1**, 545—564 (1961). — KOBAYASHI, H., and K. OBUKO: Prolongation of molting period in the canary by long days. Science **121**, 338—339 (1955). — KOECKE, H. U., u. W. SCHITTENHELM: Die Entwicklung der Schillerfärbung während des Federwachstums und die Einlagerung des Melaninpigmentes in die Federzellen bei der Stockente (Anas boschas L.). Wilhelm Roux-Arch. Entwickl.-Mech. **153**, 283—313 (1961). — KOEFOED-JOHNSEN, V., and H. H. USSING: The nature of the frog skin potential. Acta physiol. scand **42**, 298—308 (1958). — KOMNICK, H., u. K. E. WOHLFARTH-BOTTERMANN: Das Grundplasma und die Plasmafilamente der Amöbe Chaos chaos nach enzymatischer Behandlung der Zellmembran. Z. Zellforsch. **66**, 434—456 (1965). — KONING, A. L.: Histochemical localization of certain constituents of developing juvenile wing feather. Amer. J. Anat. **100**, 17—50 (1957). — KRAUSE. R.: Mikroskopische Anatomie der Wirbeltiere in Einzeldarstellungen, Bd. I—IV. Berlin u. Leipzig: W. de Gruyter & Co. 1923. — KRIMM, S.: Structure of frizzle mutant feather keratin. J. molec. Biol. **2**, 247—249 (1960). — KROGIS, A.: On the topography of HERBST's and GRANDRY's corpuscles in the adult and embryonic duckbill. Acta zool., Stockholm **12**, 241—263 (1931). — La disposition des corpuscules de HERBST et de GRANDRY dans le bec des oiseaux adultes. C. R. Soc. Biol. (Paris) **108**, 742—744 (1931). — KÜCHLER, W. J.: Jahrezyklische Veränderungen im histologischen Bau der Vogelschilddrüse. J. Ornithol. (Leipzig) **83**, 414—461 (1935). — KUHN, O.: Die Färbungsmuster der Vögel, ihre morphologischen Grundlagen und entwicklungsphysiologischen Probleme. Biol. Zbl. **75**,

51—67 (1956). — KUHN, O., u. H. U. KOECKE: Das Schicksal der Melanoblasten im Integument verschiedener Traubenrassen. Z. Zellforsch. **44**, 557—584 (1956). — KULEMANN, H.: Untersuchungen der Pigmentbewegungen in embryonalen Melanophoren von Xenopus laevis in Gewebekulturen. Zool. Jb., Abt. allg. Zool. Physiol. **69**, 169—192 (1960). — KULZER, E.: Untersuchungen über die Schreckreaktion der Erdkrötenkaulquappe (Bufo bufo L.). Z. vergl. Physiol. **36**, 443—463 (1954).

LANGE, B.: Die Brutflecke der Vögel und die für sie wichtigen Hauteigentümlichkeiten. Morph. Jb. **59**, 601—712 (1928). — Über die Haut von Struthio, Rhea und Dromaeus. (Ein Beitrag zur Kenntnis der Vogelhaut. Morph. Jb. **62**, 464—506 (1929). — Integument der Sauropsiden. In: Handbuch der vergleichenden Anatomie der Wirbeltiere, Bd. I, S. 375—448 (Hrsg. L. BOLK, E. GÖPPERT, E. KALLIUS u. W. LUBOSCH). Berlin u. Wien: Urban & Schwarzenberg 1931. — LANZING, W. J. R.: The occurrence of a water-balance-, a melanophore-expanding and an oxytocic principle in the pituitary gland of the river-lamprey (Lampetra fluviatilis L.). Acta endocr. (Kbh.) **16**, 277—284 (1954). — LEE, T. H., and A. B. LERNER: Isolation of melanocyte-stimulating hormone from hog pituitary gland. J. biol. Chem. **221**, 943—959 (1956). — LEE, T. H., A. B. LERNER, and V. BUETTNER-JANUSCH: Species differencies and structural requirements for melanocyte-stimulating activity of melanocyte-stimulating hormones. Ann. N.Y. Acad. Sci. **100**, 658—667 (1963). — LEESON, R. C., and L. T. THREADGOLD: The differentiation of the epidermis in Rana pipiens. Acta anat. (Basel) **44**, 159 (1961). — LEINER, M.: Die Physiologie der Fischatmung. In: Bronns Klassen und Ordnungen des Tierreiches. Echte Fische, Bd. 1, S. 827—910. Leipzig: Akademische Verlagsgesellschaft 1937. — LELE, P. P., E. PALMER, and G. WEDDELL: Observations on the innervation of the integument of Amphioxus, Branchiostoma lanceolatum. Quart. J. micr. Sci. **99**, 421—440 (1958). — LERNER, A. B., J. D. CASE, R. V. HEINZELMAN: Structure of melatonin. J. Amer. chem. Soc. **81**, 6084—6085 (1959). — LERNER, A. B., J. D. CASE, and Y. TAKAHASHI: Isolation of melatonin and 5-methoxy-indole-3-acetic acid from bovine pineal glands. J. biol. Chem. **235**, 1992—1997 (1960). — LERNER, A. B., J. D. CASE, Y. TAKAHASHI, T. H. LEE, and W. MORI: Isolation of melatonin, the pineal gland factor that lightens melanocytes. J. Amer. chem. Soc. **80**, 2587 (1958). — LERNER, A. B., and T. H. LEE: Isolation of homogeneous melanocyte stimulating hormone from hog pituitary gland. J. Amer. chem. Soc. **77**, 1066—1067 (1955). — The melanocyte-stimulating hormones. In: Vitamins and hormones, vol. 20, p. 337—346 (ed. R. S. HARRIS and I. G. WOOL). New York and London: Academic Press 1962. — LI, C. H., J. MEIENHOFER, E. SCHNABEL, D. CHUNG, T. LO, and J. RAMACHANDRAN: The synthesis of a nonadecapeptide possessing adrenocorticotripic and melanotropic activities. J. Amer. chem. Soc. **82**, 5760—5762 (1960). — Synthesis of a biologically active nonadecapeptide corresponding to the first nineteen amino acid residues of adrenocorticotropins. J. Amer. chem. Soc. **83**, 4449—4457 (1961). — LILLIE, F. R.: Physiology of the development of the feather. III. Growth of the mesodermal constituents and blood circulation in the pulp. Physiol. Zool. **13**, 143—175 (1940). — On the development of feathers. Biol. Rev. **17**, 247—266 (1942). — LILLIE, F. R., and M. JUHN: Physiology of the development of the feather. II. General principles of development with special reference to the afterfeather. Physiol. Zool. **11**, 434—449 (1938). — LISON, L.: Recherches sur l'histogenèse de l'email dentaire chez les Sélaciens. Archs. Biol. (Paris) **60**, 111—135 (1949). — LISSMANN, H. W.: Rectilinear locomotion in a snake (Boa occidentalis. J. exp. Biol. **26**, 368—379 (1950). LOEWENSTEIN, W. R., and R. SHALAK: Mechanical transmission in a Pacinian corpuscle. An analysis and a theory. J. Physiol. (Lond.) **182**, 346—378 (1966). — LOUD, A. V., and Y. MISHIMA: The induction of melanization in goldfish scales with ACTH, in vitro. Cellular and subcellular changes. J. Cell Biol. **18**, 181—194 (1963). — LOWENSTEIN, O.: Pressure receptors in the fins of the dogfish Scylliorhinus canicula. J. exp. Biol. **33**, 417—421 (1956). — The sense organs: the acustico-lateralis system. In: The physiology of fishes, vol. II, p. 155—186 (ed. M. E. BROWN). New York: Academic Press 1957. — LOWENSTEIN, O., M. P. OSBORNE, and J. WERSÄLL: Structure and innervation of the sensory epithelia of the labyrinth in the thornback ray (Raja clavata). Proc. roy. Soc. B **160**, 1—12 (1964). — LOWENSTEIN, O., and J. WERSÄLL: A functional interpretation of the electron-microscopic structure of the sensory hairs in the cristae of the elasmabranch Rajy clavata in terms of directional sensitivy. Nature (Lond.) **184**, 1807—1808 (1959). — LUBNOW, E.: Die Pigmentierung des japanischen Seidenhuhns. Biol. Zbl. **76**, 316—342 (1957). — LÜDICKE, M.: Über die Capillargebiete des Blutgefäß-Systems im Kopf der Schlangen (Tropidonotus natrix L. and Zamenis Dahli Fitz.). Z. Morph. Ökol. Tiere **36**, 401—445 (1940). — Die Kennzeichnung der Zuwachsstreifen in der wachsenden Konturfeder mit Hilfe von radioaktivem Natriumsulfat. Z. vergl. Physiol. **44**, 133—173 (1961). — Über die Aufnahme von radioaktivem Schwefel in die wachsende Vogelfeder nach Applikation von ^{35}S-Methioninlösungen. Z. vergl. Physiol. **44**, 414—450 (1961). — 5. Ordnung der Klasse Reptilia: Serpentes. In: Handbuch der Zoologie, Bd. 7/1, S. 1—128. Berlin: W. de Gruyter & Co. 1962, 1964. — Der Schwefelgehalt der wachsenden Vogelfeder im Bereich ihrer Melaninfelder. Naturwissenschaften **49**, 189—190 (1962). —

Das Integument der Vögel. Stud. gen. **17**, 390—406 (1964). — Die Beziehungen des ventralen Coriumraumes der wachsenden Flugfeder zu den radioaktiven Querbändern nach Applikation von ^{35}S-Sulfat- und ^{35}S-DL-Cystinlösungen. Biol. Zbl. **84**, 273—297 (1965). — Die Querbänder der Flugfedern von Tauben nach der Behandlung mit Farb-, Plumbit- und Silbernitratlösungen im Vergleich zu den radioaktiven Mustern nach Applikation von ^{35}S-Natriumsulfat und ^{35}-S-DL-Cystinlösungen. J. Ornithol. (Leipzig) **107**, 205—224 (1966). — LÜDICKE, M., u. B. GEIERHAAS: Über das Ablagerungsmuster des radioaktiven Schwefels in der wachsenden Konturfeder nach Applikation von ^{35}-S-DL-Cystinlösungen. J. Ornithol. (Leipzig) **104**, 142—167 (1963). — LÜDICKE, M., u. H. TEICHERT: Über den Ort der Aufnahme des radioaktiven Schwefels in der Federanlage nach Injektion von ^{35}S-DL-Cystin- und ^{35}S-Natriumsulfatlösungen. Naturwissenschaften **50**, 737 (1963).

MADERSON, P. F. A.: Keratined epidermal derivatives as an aid to climbing in Gekkonid lizards. Nature (Lond.) **203**, 780—781 (1964). — Histological changes in the epidermis of snakes during the sloughing cycle. Proc. Zool. Soc. Lond. **146**, 98—113 (1965). — MALKINSON, F. D., and S. ROTHMAN: Percutaneous absorption. In: Handbuch der Haut- u. Geschlechtskrankheiten, Erg.-Werk, Bd. 1/3, S. 90—156. Normale und pathologische Physiologie der Haut, Bd. I (Hrsg. A. MARCHIONINI u. H. W. SPIER). Berlin-Göttingen-Heidelberg: Springer 1963. — MALT, R. A., G. J. STEWART, P. T. SPEAKMAN, and E. BELL: A fibrous polymer from embryonic feather. J. roy. micr. Soc., Ser. III, **83**, 373—375 (1964). — MANFREDI ROMANINI, M. G.: La quantità di acido deossiribonucleico nei wari tipi cellulari dell'epidermide dé Lampetra. Z. Anat. Entwickl.-Gesch. **120**, 101—114 (1957). — MARINELLI, W., u. A. STRENGER: Myxine glutinosa (L.). Vergleichende Anatomie und Morphologie der Wirbeltiere, 2. Liefg. Wien: Franz Deuticke 1956. — MARUHASHI, K. MIZIGUCHI, and I. TASAKI: Action currents in single afferent nerve fibres elicited by stimulation of the skin of the toad and the cat. J. Physiol. (Lond.) **117**, 129—151 (1952). — MATSUMOTO, J.: Studies on the fine structure and cytochemical properties of erythrophores in swordtail, Xiphophorus Helleri, with special reference to their pigment granules (Pterinosomes). J. Cell Biol. **27**, 493—504 (1965). — MATTERN, I.: Zur Histologie und Histochemie der lipochromatischen Federn einiger Cotingiden (Schmuckvögel). Z. Zellforsch. **45**, 96—136 (1936). — MATTHEWS, S. A.: Observations on the pigment migration within the fish melanophore. J. exp. Zool. **58**, 471—486 (1931). MAYAUD, N.: Téguments et phanères. In: Traité de Zoologie, vol. XV, p. 4—77 (ed. P. GRASSÉ). Paris: Masson & Cie. 1950. — MEIJERE, J. C. H. DE: Haare. In: Handbuch der vergleichenden Anatomie der Wirbeltiere, Bd. I, S. 585—632 (Hrsg. L. BOLK, E. GÖPPERT, E. KALLIUS u. W. LUBOSCH). Berlin u. Wien: Urban & Schwarzenberg 1931. — MERCER, E. H.: Keratin and keratinization. An essay in molecular biology. In: Int. series Monogr. on pure and applied biology. 12. Oxford-London-NewYork-Paris: Pergamon Press 1961. — MEYER, M., u. H. H. LOETZKE: Über melaninhaltige Zellen und die Schwarzzeichnung am Schwanzende einheimischer Anurenlarven. Z. mikr.-ant. Forsch. **65**, 443—476 (1959). — MILLER, W. J.: Silky plumage in the ring neck dove. J. Hered. **47**, 37—40 (1956). — MILLONIG, G.: L'ultrastruttura dei noduli di Bizzozero nella cute di Tritone. Boll. Soc. ital. Biol. sper. **34**, 578—582 (1958). — MIRSKY, A. E., and H. RIS: The desoxyribonucleic acid content of animal cells and its evolutionary significance. J. gen. Physiol. **34**, 451—462 (1951). — MISHIMA, Y., and A. V. LOUD: The ultrastructure of unmelanized pigment cells in induzed melanogenesis. Ann. N.Y. Acad. Sci. **100**, 607—617 (1963). — MORRIS, D.: The feather postures of birds and the problem of the origin of social signals. Behaviour **9**, 75—113 (1956). — MORRIS, R.: The mechanism of marine osmoregulation in the lampern (Lampetra fluviatilis L.) and the canses of its breakdown during the spawning migration. J. exp. Biol. **35**, 649—665 (1958). — MULLINGER, A. M.: The fine structure of ampullary electric receptors in amiurus. Proc. roy. Soc. B **160**, 345—359 (1964). — MUNGER, B. L.: The intraepidermal innervation of the snout skin of the opossum. A light and electron microscope study, with observations on the nature of MERKEL's Tastzellen. J. Cell Biol. **26**, 79—97 (1965). — MURRAY, R. W.: The lateralis organs and their innervation in Xenopus laevis. Quart. J. micr. Sci. **96**, 351—361 (1955). — Temperatur receptors. Advanc. comp. Physiol. **1**, 117—175 (1962).

NEAVE, F.: On the histology and regeneration of the teleost scale. Quart. J. micr. Sci. **81**, 541—568 (1940). — NECKEL, I.: Chemische und elektronenmikroskopische Untersuchungen über das Guanin in der Haut einiger Fische. Mikroskopie **9**, 113—119 (1954). — NEWBY, W. M.: The slime glands and thread cells of the hagfish, Polistotrema stouti. J. Morph. **78**, 397—409 (1946). — NEWTH, D. R., and D. M. Ross: On the reaction to light of myxine glutinosa L. J. exp. Biol. **32**, 4—21 (1955). — NIAZI, I. A.: The histology of tail regeneration in the Ammocoetes. Canad. J. Zool. **41**, 125—146 (1963). — NIELSEN, B.: On the regulation of the respiration in reptiles. I. The effect of temperature and CO_2 on the respiration of lizards (Lacerta). J. exp. Biol. **38**, 301—314 (1961). — NOBLE, G. K.: The integumentary, pulmonary, and cardiac modifications correlated with increased cutaneous respiration in the Amphibia: a solution of the "hairy frog" problem. J. Morph. **40**, 341—416 (1925). — NOBLE, G. K., and H. T. BRADLEY: The relation of the thyroid and hypophysis to the molting process in

the lizard, Hemidactylus brookii. Biol. Bull. **64**, 289—298 (1933). — NOVALES, R. R., and B. J. NOVALES: Cytological and ultrastructural aspects of amphibian melanophore control. In: Structure and control of the melanocyte, p. 52—59 (ed. G. DELLA PORTA and O. MÜHLBOCK). Berlin-Heidelberg-New York: Springer 1966.
OBIKA, M.: Association of pteridines with amphibian larval pigmentation and their biosynthesis in developing chromatophores. Develop. Biol. **6**, 99—112 (1963). — OBIKA, M., and J. T. BAGNARA: Pteridines as pigments in amphibians. Science **143**, 485 (1964). — OKSCHE, A., u. M. VAUPEL-V. HARNACK: Vergleichende elektronenmikriskopische Studien am Pinealorgan. Prog. Brain Res. **10**, 237—258 (1965). — OLSSON, R.: The neurosecretory hypothalamus system and the adenohypophysis of myxine. Z. Zellforsch. **51**, 97—107 (1959). — The skin of Amphioxus. Z. Zellforsch. **54**, 90—104 (1961). — OORDT, G. J. VAN, u. G. C. A. JUNGE: Die hormonale Wirkung der Gonaden auf Sommer- und Prachtkleid. III. Der Einfluß der Kastration auf männliche Kampfläufer (Philomactus pugnax). Wilhelm Roux' Arch. Entwickl.-Mech. **134**, 112—121 (1936). — OOSTEN, J. V.: The skin and the scales. In: The physiology of fishes, vol. 1, p. 207—244 (ed. M. BROWN). New York: Academic Press 1957. — ORTIZ, E., E. BÄCHLI, D. PRICE, and H. G. WILLIAMS-ASHMAN: Red pteridine pigments in the dewlaps of some Anoles. Physiol. Zool. **36**, 97—103 (1963). — ORTIZ, E., and H. G. WILLIAMS-ASHMAN: Identification of skin pteridines in the pasture lizard, Anolis pulchellus. Comp. Biochem. Physiol. **10**, 181—190 (1963). — ORTON, G. L.: Development and migration of pigment cells in some teleost fishes. J. Morph. **93**, 69—99 (1953).
PARAKKAL, P. F., and G. MALTOTSY: A study of the fine structure of the epidermis of Rana pipiens. J. Cell Biol. **20**, 85—94 (1964). — PARKER, G. H.: Color changer in elasmobranchs. Proc. nat. Acad. Sci. (Wash.) **22**, 55—60 (1936). — Melanophore response in the young of Mustelus canis. Proc. Amer. Acad. Arts Sci. **72**, 269—282 (1938). — Sensitization of melanophores by nerve cutting. Proc. nat. Acad. Sci. (Wash.) **28**, 164—170 (1942). — Melanophore activators in the common american eel Anguilla rostrata Le Seur. J. exp. Zool. **98**, 211—235 (1945). — PARKER, G. H., and A. ROSENBLUETH: The electric stimulation of the concentrating (adrenergic) and the dispersing (cholinergic) nerve-fibers in the melanophores of the catfish. Proc. nat. Acad. Sci. (Wash.) **27**, 198 (1941). — PEASE, D. C., and T. A. QUILLIAM: Electron microscopy of the Pacinian corpuscle. J. biophys. biochem. Cytol. **3**, 331—341 (1957). — PEHLEMANN, F. W.: Experimentelle Untersuchungen zur Determination und Differezierung der Hypophyse bei Anuren (Pelobates fuscus, Rana esculenta). Wilhelm Roux' Arch. Entwickl.-Mech. Org. **153**, 551—602 (1962). — Die Teilung dermaler Melanophoren von Xenopus laevis-Larven. Naturwissenschaften **53**, 207 (1966). — Der Einfluß des Melanophorenhormons auf die Farbzellverteilung. Umschau **66**, 606 (1966). — PELC, S. R., and H. B. FELL: The effect of excess Vitamin A on the uptake of labelled compounds by embryonic skin in organ culture. Exp. Cell Res. **19**, 99—113 (1960). — PETERS, A.: The structure of the peripheral nerves of the lamprey (Lampetra fluviatilis). J. Ultrastruct. Res. **4**, 349—359 (1960). — The periphal nervous system. In: The biology of myxine, p. 92—123 (ed. A. BRODAL and R. FÄNGE). Oslo: Oslo Universitetsforlaget 1963. — PETERSON, R. A., R. K. RINGER, M. J. TETZLAFF, and A. M. LUCAS: Ink perfusion for displaying capillaries in the chicken. Stain Technol. **40**, 351—356 (1965). — PETIT, G., e P. BUDKER: Contribution a l'étude de la différenciation des dents cutanèes, liée à la présence de cryptes sensorielles chez quelques espèces de Sélaciens. Bull. Inst. océanogr. **695**, 1—46 (1936). — PEYER, B.: Hartgebilde des Integumentes. In: Handbuch der vergleichenden Anatomie der Wirbeltiere, Bd. I, S. 703—752 (Hrsg. L. BOLK, E. GÖPPERT, E. KALLIUS u. W. LUBOSCH). Berlin u. Wien: Urban & Schwarzenberg 1931. — PFEFFER, K. V.: Untersuchungen zur Morphologie und Entwicklung der Fadenfedern. Zool. Jb. Abt. Anat. **72**, 67—100 (1952). — PFEIFFER, W.: Über die Schreckreaktion bei Fischen und die Herkunft des Schreckstoffes. Z. vergl. Physiol. **43**, 578—614 (1960). — The fright reaction of fish. Biol. Rev. **37**, 495—511 (1962). — Die Verbreitung der Schreckreaktion bei Kaulquappen und die Herkunft des Schreckstoffes. Z. vergl. Physiol. **52**, 79—98 (1966). — Die Schreckreaktion der Fische und Kaulquappen. Naturwissenschaften **53**, 565—570 (1966). — PFLUGFELDER, O., u. G. SCHUBERT: Elektronenmikroskopische Untersuchungen an der Haut von Larven- und Metamorphosestadien von Xenopus laevis nach Kaliumperchloratbehandlung. Z. Zellforsch. **67**, 96—112 (1965). — PIEZ, K. A., and J. GROSS: The amino acid composition of some fish collagens: The relation between composition and structure. J. biol. Chem. **235**, 995—998 (1960). — PILLAI, P. A.: Electron microscopic studies on the epidermis of newt with an enquiry into the problem of induced neoplasia. Protoplasma (Wien) **55**, 10—62 (1962). — POCKRANDT, D.: Beiträge zur Histologie der Schlangenhaut. Zool. Jb. Abt. Anat. **62**, 275—322 (1936/37). — POOLE, D. F. G.: The fine structure of the scales and teeth of Raia clavata. Quart. J. micr. Sci. **97**, 99—107 (1956). — PORTER, K. R.: Observations on the fine structure of animal epidermis. In: 3. Internat. Conf. Electr. Micros. 1054, p. 539—546. London: Roy. Microscop. Soc. 1956.
RABEN, M. S., R. LANDOLT, F. A. SMITH, K. HOFMANN, and H. YAJIMA: Adipokinetic activity of synthetic peptides related to corticotropin. Nature (Lond.) **189**, 681—682 (1961). —

Rabl, H.: Integument der Anamnier. In: Handbuch der vergleichenden Anatomie der Wirbeltiere, Bd. I, S. 271—374 (Hrsg. L. Bolk, E. Göppert, E. Kallius u. W. Lubosch). Berlin u. Wien: Urban & Schwarzenberg 1931. — Ratzersdorfer, C., A. S. Gordon, and H. A. Charipper: The effect of thiourea on the thyroid gland and molting behaviour of the lizard, Anolis carolinensis. J. exp. Zool. 112, 13—27 (1949). — Rauther, M.: Echte Fische. Teil 1 (Anatomie, Physiologie und Entwicklungsgeschichte. In: Bronns Klassen und Ordnungen des Tierreiches, 6. Bd., I. Abt. Pisces, 2. Buch: Echte Fische. Leipzig: Akademische Verlagsgesellschat 1927—1940. — Rawles, M. E.: The integumentary system. In: Biology and comparative physiology of birds, vol. I, p. 189—240 (ed. A. J. Marshall). New York and London: Academic Press 1960. — Tissue interactions in scale feather development as studied in dermal-epidermal recombinations. J. Embryol. exp. Morph. 11, 765—789 (1963). — Richter, R.: Die Haare. In- Handbuch der Haut- u. Geschlechtskrankheiten, Erg.-Werk 1/3, S. 182—576. Normale und pathologische Physiologie der Haut, Bd. I (Hrsg. A. Marchionini u. H. W. Spier). Berlin-Göttingen-Heidelberg: Springer 1963. — Ritchie, A.: A new interpretation of jamoylius kerwoodi white. Nature (Lond.) 188, 647—649 (1960). — Robertson, J. D., T. S. Bodenheimer, and D. E. Stage: The ultrastructure of Mauthner cell synapses and nodes in goldfish brains. J. Cell Biol. 19, 159—199 (1963). — Rodbard, S., F. Samson, and D. Ferguson: Thermosensitity of turtle brain as manifested by blood pressure changes. Amer. J. Physiol. 160, 402—408 (1950). — Rosin, S.: Über Bau und Wachstum der Grenzlamelle der Epidermis bei Amphibienlarven; Analyse einer orthogonalen Fibrillenstruktur. Revue suisse Zool. 53, 133—201 (1946). — Ross, D. M.: The sense organs of Myxine glutinosa L. In: The biology of myxine, p. 150—160 (ed. A. Brodal and R. Fänge). Oslo: Oslo Universitetsforlaget 1963. — Rudall, K. M.: X-ray studies of the distribution of protein chain types in the vertebrate epidermis. Biochim. biophys. Acta (Amst.) 1, 549—562 (1947). — Russel, F. E., and A. van Harreveld: Cardiovascular effects of the venom of the round stingray, "Urobatis halleri". Arch. int. Physiol. 62, 322—333 (1954). — Russel, F. E., W. C. Barritt, and M. D. Fairchild: Electrocardiographic patterns evoked by the venom of the stingray. Proc. Soc. exp. Biol. (N.Y.) 96, 634—635 (1957). — Russel, F. F., and J. A. Emery: Venom of the weevers Trachinus draco and Trachinus vipera. Ann. N.Y. Acad. Sci. 90, 805—819 (1960). — Rutschke, E.: Untersuchungen über Wasserfestigkeit und Struktur des Gefieders von Schwimmvögeln. Zool. Jb., Abt. Syst. 87, 441—506 (1960).

Salpeter, M. M., and M. Singer: The fine structure of the adepidermal reticulum in the basal membrane of the skin of the newt, Triturus. J. biophys. biochem. Cytol. 6, 35—40 (1959). — Differentiation of the submicroscopic adepidermal membrane during limb regeneration in adult triturus, including a note on the use of the term basement membrane. Anat. Rec. 136, 27—39 (1960). — Sand, A.: The mechanism of the lateral sense organs of fishes. Proc. roy. Soc. B 123, 472—495 (1937). — Saunders, P. R.: Venom of the stonefish Synanceja verrucosa. Science 129, 272—274 (1959). — Pharmacological and chemical studies of the venom of the stonefisch (Genus Synanceja) and other scorpionfishes. Ann. N.Y. Acad. Sci. 90, 798—804 (1960). — Schaffer, J.: Zur Kenntnis der Hautdrüsen bei den Säugetieren und bei Myxine. Z. Anat. Entwickl.-Gesch. 76, 320—337 (1925). — Scharrer, E.: Die Empfindlichkeit der freien Flossenstrahlen des Knurrhahns (Trigla) für chemische Reize. Z. vergl. Physiol. 22, 145—154 (1935). — Scharrer, E., S. W. Smith, and S. L. Palay: Chemical sense and taste in the fishes, prionotus and trichogaster. J. comp. Neurol. 86, 183—198 (1947). — Schartau, O.: Beiträge zur Innervation der Reptilien. I. Allgemeinere morphologische Verhältnisse des Rückenmarks; Innervation der Haut, der Unterhaut und des in der Verknöcherung befindlichen Wirbelkörpers der Blindschleiche. Z. mikr.-anat. Forsch. 39, 172—214 (1936). — Schildmacher, H.: Untersuchungen über die Funktion der Herbstschen Körperchen. J. Ornithol. (Leipzig) 79, 374—415 (1931). — Schmidt, A. J.: Architectural regularity of the subepidermal reticulum of fibers in the adult newt, Triturus viridescens (Diemictylus v.). J. Morph. 111, 275—285 (1962). — The basement membrane of the epidermis of the adult newt, Diemictylus viridescens: the collagen of the fibers of the adepidermal reticulum. Acta anat. (Basel) 50, 170—185 (1962). — Schmidt, W. J.: Das Integument von Voeltzkowia mira Bttgr. Ein Beitrag zur Morphologie und Histologie der Eidechsenhaut. Z. wiss. Zool. 94, 605—720 (1910). — Studien am Integument der Reptilien. I. Die Haut der Geckoniden. Z. wiss. Zool. 101, 139—258 (1912). — Studien am Integument der Reptilien. IV. Uroplatus fimbriatus (Schneid) und die Geckoniden. Zool. Jb., Abt. Anat. 36, 377—464 (1913). — Studien am Integument der Reptilien. V. Anguiden. Zool. Jb., Abt. Anat. 38, 1—102 (1914). — Die Chromatophoren der Reptilienhaut. Arch. mikr. Anat., Abt. I, 90, 98—259 (1917). — Studien am Integument der Reptilien. VIII. Über die Haut der Acrochordinen. Zool. Jb., Abt. Anat. 40, 155—202 (1917/18). — Die Panzerhaut der Weichschildkröte Emyda granosa und die funktionelle Bedeutung ihrer Strukturen. Arch. mikr. Anat., Abt. I, 95, 186—246 (1921). — Über die aus Tonofibrillen hervorgehenden Tastborsten der Eidechsen. Z. Zellen- u. Gewebelehre 1, 327—356 (1924). — Polarisationsoptische Untersuchung schmelzartiger Außenschichten des Zahnbeins von Fischen. I. Die emailartige

Außenlage der Schlundzähne von Cyprinoiden. Z. Zellforsch. **28**, 761—783 (1938). — Polarisationsoptische Untersuchung schmelzartiger Außenschichten des Zahnbeins von Fischen. II. Das porzellanartige Dentin (Durodentin) der Selachier. Z. Zellforsch. **30**, 235—272 (1940).— Ergebnisse einer Untersuchung über das Schillern von Federn. Z. Naturforsch. **3b**, 55—57 (1948). — Polarisationsoptische Untersuchung schmelzartiger Außenschichten des Zahnbeins von Fischen. III. Das Durodentin von Myliobatis. Z. Zellforsch. **34**, 165—178 (1949). — Polarisationsoptische Untersuchung schmelzartiger Außenschichten des Zahnbeins von Fischen. IV. Der angebliche Schmelz der Placoidschuppen. Z. Zellforsch. **36**, 198—221 1951). — Wie entstehen die Schillerfarben der Federn? Naturwissenschaften **39**, 313—318 (1952). — Polarisationsoptik und Farberscheinungen der lipochromführenden Federäste von Xipholene lamelli pennis. Z. Zellforsch. **45**, 152—175 (1956). — Durodentin bei einem devonischen Fisch (Laccognathus panderi Gross). Z. Zellforsch. **49**, 493—514 (1959). — Kristalline Einlagerungen im Natternhemd von Python reticulatus Gray. Z. Zellforsch. **50**, 766—783 (1959). — Histologische Untersuchungen an Papageienfedern mit gelbem eigenfluoreszierenden Pigment. Z. Zellforsch. **55**, 469—485 (1961). — SCHMIDT, W. J., u. H. RUSKA: Elektronenmikroskopische Untersuchung der Pigmentgranula in den schillernden Federstrahlen der Taube Columba trocaz H. Z. Zellforsch. **55**, 379—388 (1961). — Tyndallblau-Struktur von Federn im Elektronenmikroskop. Z. Zellforsch. **56**, 693—708 (1962). — Die Markzellen des Federschaftes auf Grund polarisations- und elektronenmikroskopischer Untersuchungen an Ara und Cotinga. Z. Zellforsch. **56**, 713—727 (1962). — Über das schillernde Federmelanin bei Heliangelus und Lophophorus. Z. Zellforsch. **57**, 1—36 (1962). — Rindenzellen von Federn im Elektronenmikroskop. Z. Zellforsch. **60**, 80—88 (1963). — Zur Morphologie des Porphyrinpigmentes der Turacus-Federn. Z. Zellforsch. **61**, 202—213 (1963). — Koproporphyrinführende Brustfedern der Trappe Eupodotis senegalensis im Licht-, Fluorescenz- und Elektronenmikroskop. Z. Zellforsch. **66**, 427—433 (1965). — Zusammenwirken von Strukturblau mit Phaeomelanin zur Erzeugung von violett bei Chloëbiafedern. Z. Zellforsch. **66**, 519—528 (1965). — SCHNAKENBECK, W., u. PISCES: In: Handbuch der Zoologie, Bd. VI/1, S. 551—1115 (Hrsg. J.-G. HELMCKE u. H. v. LENGERKEN). Berlin: W. de Gruyter & Co. 1955. — SCHÖTTLE, E.: Morphologie und Physiologie der Atmung bei wasser-, schlamm- und landlebenden Gobiiformes. Z. wiss. Zool. **140**, 1—114 (1932). — SCHOLANDER, P. F., V. WALTERS, R. HOCK, and L. IRVING: Body insulation of some arctic and tropical mammals and birds. Biol. Bull. **99**, 225—236 (1950). — SCHOLANDER, P. F., R. HOCK, V. WALTERS, and L. IRVING: Heat regulation in some arctic and tropical mammals and birds. Biol. Bull. **99**, 237—258 (1950). — SCHOR, R., and S. KRIMM: Studies on the structure of feather keratin. I. X-ray diffraction studies and other experimental data. Biophys. J. **1**, 467—487 (1961). — Studies on the structure of feather keratin. II. A helix model for the structure of feather keratin. Biophys. J. **1**, 489—515 (1961). — SCHRAEDER, W. A., and L. M. KAY: The amino acid composition of certain morphologically distinct parts of white turkey feathers, and of goose feather barbs and goose down. J. Amer. chem. Soc. **77**, 3901—3908 (1955). — SCHUMACHER, S.: Integument der Mammalier. In: Handbuch der vergleichenden Anatomie der Wirbeltiere, Bd. I, S. 449—504 (Hrsg. L. BOLK, E. GÖPPERT, E. KALLIUS u. W. LUBOSCH). Berlin u. Wien: Urban & Schwarzenberg 1931. — SCHWARTZ, E.: Bau und Funktion der Seitenlinie des Streifenhechtlings (Aplocheilus lineatus Cuv. u. Val.). Z. vergl. Physiol. **50**, 55—87 (1965). — SCHWARTZKOPFF, J.: Der Vibrationssinn der Vögel. Naturwissenschaften **35**, 318—319 (1948). — SCHWYZER, R.: Chemische Synthese der Melanotropine und des corticotropen Hormons der Hypophyse. Naturwissenschaften **53**, 189—197 (1966). — SCHWYZER, R., H. KAPPELER, B. ISELIN, W. RITTEL u. H. ZUBER: Synthese und biologische Aktivität von geschützten Polypeptidsequenzen des Melanophoren-stimulierenden Hormons (-MSH) des Rindes. Helv.-chim. Acta **42**, 1702—1708 (1959). — SCHWYZER, R., and C. H. LI: A new synthesis of a pentapeptide L-Histidin-L-phenylalanyl-L-arginyl-L-triptophyl-glycin and its melanocyte-stimulating activity. Nature (Lond.) **182**, 1669—1670 (1958). — SCHWYZER, R., and P. SIEBER: Total synthesis of adrenocorticotrophic hormone. Nature (Lond.) **199**, 172—174 (1963). — SELANDER, R. K., and L. L. KUICH: Hormonal control and development of the incubation patch in icterids, with notes on behaviour of cowbirds. Condor **65**, 73—90 (1963). — SENGEL, P.: Recherches expérimentales sur la différenciation des germes plumaires et du pigment de la peau de l'embryon de poulet en culture in vitro. Ann. Sci. (Zool.) natur. (Paris) **11**, 431—514 (1958). — La différenciation de la peau et des germes plumaires de l'embryon de poulet en culture in vitro. Ann. biol. Sér. 3 **43**, 29—52 (1958). — Le développement de la peau et des phanères chez l'embryon de poulet. Rev. suisse Zool. **72**, 569—577 (1965). — SENGEL, P., and U. K. ABBOTT: In vitro studies with the scaleless mutant. J. Hered. **54**, 255—262 (1963). — SICK, H.: Morphologisch-funktionelle Untersuchungen über die Feinstruktur der Vogelfeder. J. Ornithol. (Leipzig) **85**, 206—372 (1937). — SILBERT, J. E., Y. NAGAI, and J. GROSS: Hyaluronidase from tadpole tissue. J. biol. Chem. **240**, 1509—1511 (1965). — SINGER, M., and M. M. SALPETER: The bodies of Eberth and associated structures in the skin of the frog tadpole. J. exp. Zool. **147**, 1—19 (1961). — SPANNHOF, L.: Zur Genese, Morphologie und Physiologie der Hautdrüsen bei Xenopus laevis Daudin. Wiss. Z. Humboldt-

Univ. Berl., Math.nat. Reihe **3**, 295—305 (1954). — SPEARMAN, R. I. C.: The keratinization of epidermal scales, feathers and hairs. Biol. Rev. **41**, 59—96 (1966). — STARCK, D.: Herkunft und Entwicklung der Pigmentzellen. In: Handbuch der Haut- u. Geschlechtskrankheiten, Erg.-Werk Bd. 1/2, S. 139—175. Normale und pathologische Anatomie der Haut. II. (Hrsg. O. GANS u. G. K. STEIGLEDER). Berlin-Göttingen-Heidelberg-New York: Springer 1964. — STARY, Z.: Mucosaccharides and glycoproteins. Chemistry and physiopathology. Ergebn. Physiol. **50**, 174—408 (1959). — Chemistry of the cutis. In: Handbuch der Haut- u. Geschlechtskrankheiten, Erg.-Werk Bd. 1/3, S. 577—706. Normale und pathologische Physiologie der Haut. I. (Hrsg. A. MARCHIONINI u. H. W. SPIER). Berlin-Göttingen-Heidelberg: Springer 1963. — STEFANELLI, A.: Terminazioni nervose di moto e di senso nei Petramizonti. Arch. zool. ital. **17**, 85—101 (1932). — The Mauthnerian apparatus in the ichthyopsida; its nature and function and correlated problems of neurohistogenesis. Quart. Rev. Biol. **26**, 17—34 (1951). — STEFANO, F. J. E., and A. O. DONOSO: Hypophysoadrenal regulation of moulting in the toad. Gen. comp. Endocr. **4**, 473—480 (1964). — STEINER, H.: Der strukturelle Aufbau der Kasuarfeder, ein Beitrag zum Afterschaftproblem. Rev. suisse Zool. **50**, 287—294 (1943). — STENSIÖ, E.: Les cyclostomes fossiles on Ostracodermes. In: Traité de Palaeontologie, vol. IV/1, p. 96—382 (ed. J. PIVETEAU). Paris: Masson & Cie. 1964. — STETTENHEIM, P., A. M. LUCAS, E. M. DENINGTON, and C. JAMROZ: The arrangement and action of the feather muscles in chickens. Proc. XIII. Int. Orn. Congr. Ithaca 1962, p. 918—924. — STEVEN, D. M.: Some properties of the photoreceptors of the brook lamprey. J. exp. Biol. **27**, 350—364 (1950). — Sensory cells and pigment distribution in the tail of the Ammocoete. Quart. J. micr. Sci. **92**, 233—247 (1951). — Experiments on the light sense of the hag, Myxine glutinosa L. J. exp. Biol. **32**, 22—38 (1955). — STRAWINSKI, S.: Vascularization of respiratory surfaces in ontogeny of the edible frog, Rana esculenta L. Zoologica Pol. **7**, 327—365 (1956). — STRESEMANN, E.: Sauropsida: Aves. In: Handbuch der Zoologie, Bd. VII/2 (Hrsg. W. KÜKENTHAL u. T. KRUMBACH). Berlin u. Leipzig: W. de Gruyter & Co. 1927/34. — STRESEMANN, E., u. V. STRESEMANN: Die Mauser der Vögel. J. Ornithol. (Leipzig) **107** (Sonderh.), 3—445 (1966). — STUDNIČKA, F. K.: Über Regenerationserscheinungen im caudalen Ende des Körpers von Petromyzon fluviatilis. Arch. Entwickl.-Mech. Org. **34**, 187—238 (1912). — STÜTTGEN, G., H. IPPEN, G. MORETTI, H. BRÜSTER, G. GOERZ u. B. KINKELIN: Die normale und pathologische Physiologie der Haut. Stuttgart: G. Fischer 1965. — SZABO, T.: Quelques précisions sur la morphologie de l'appareil sensoriel de Savi dans Torpedo marmorata. Z. Zellforsch. **48**, 536—537 (1958). — SZARSKI, H.: Some reactions of skin capillaries of the frog. In: Proc. XV. Int. Congr. Zool. London 1958, p. 531—533 (ed. H. R. HEWER and N. D. RILEY). London 1959.

TAYLOR jr., R. E., and S. B. BARKER: Transepidermal potential difference: development in anuran larvae. Science **148**, 1612—1613 (1965). — TAYLOR jr., R. E., H. C. TAYLOR, and S. B. BARKER: Chemical and morphological studies on inorganic phosphate deposits in Rana catesbeiana skin. J. exp. Zool. **161**, 271—286 (1966). — TETZLAFF, M. J., R. A. PETERSON, and R. K. RINGER: A phenylhydrazine-leucofuchsin sequence for staining nerves and nerve endings in the integument poultry. Stain Technol. **40**, 313—316 (1965). — THAUER, R.: Der nervöse Mechanismus der chemischen Temperaturregulation des Warmblüters. Naturwissenschaften **51**, 73—80 (1964). — THOMSON, J. L.: Morphogenesis and histochemistry of scales in the chick. J. Morph. **115**, 207—233 (1964). — TIXIER-VIDAL, A.: Histophysiologie de l'adénohypophyse des oiseaux. In: Cytologie de l'adénohypophyse, p. 255—273 (ed. J. BENOIT, C. DA LAGE). Colloq. Intern. Centre Nat. Rech. Sci. Paris, vol. 128, 1963. — TRETJAKOFF, D.: Das periphere Nervensystem des Flußneunauges. Z. wiss. Zool. **129**, 359—452 (1927). — TRIGHT, H. VAN: La dermatomerie du léard. Arch. néerl. Physiol. Ser. III **2**, 51—176 (1917/18). — TRUJILLO-CENÓZ, O.: Electron microscope observations on chemo- and mechanoreceptor cells of fishes. Z. Zellforsch. **54**, 654—676 (1961). — TUSQUES, J.: L'innervation des chromatophores. C. R. Soc. Biol. (Paris) **130**, 56—58 (1939).

USSING, H. H.: The frog skin potential. J. gen. Physiol. **43**, Suppl. 1, 135—147 (1960). — USUKU, G., and J. GROSS: Morphologic studies of connective tissue resorption in the tail fin of metamorphosing bullfrog tadpole. Develop. Biol. **11**, 352—370 (1965).

VANABLE, J. W.: Granular gland development during Xenopus laevis metamorphosis. Develop. Biol. **10**, 331—357 (1964). — VERNE, J., and V. VILTER: Réactions pharmaco dynamiques des mélanocytes de l'ecaille isolée de Carassius. C. R. Soc. Biol. (Paris) **119**, 1312—1314 (1935). — VILTER, V.: Recherches histologiques et physiologiques sur la fonction pigmentaire des Sélaciens. Bull. Stn. biol. Arcachon **34**, 63—136 (1937). — VÖLKER, O.: Die Farbstoffe im Gefieder der Vögel. Fortschr. Chem. org. Naturstoffe **18**, 177—222 (1960). — Die chemische Charakterisierung roter Lipochrome im Gefieder der Vögel. J. Ornithol. (Leipzig) **102**, 430—438 (1961). — Experimentelle Untersuchungen zur Frage der Entstehung roter Lipochrome in Vogelfedern. J. Ornithol. (Leipzig) **103**, 276—286 (1962). — Gefiederfarben der Vögel und Carotinoide. Natur u. Museum **93**, 39—53 (1963). — Die gelben Mutanten des Rotbauchwürgers (Laniarius atrococcineus) und der Gouldamadine (Chloebia gouldiae) in biochemischer Sicht. J. Ornithol. (Leipzig) **105**, 186—189 (1964). — Federn, die am Licht ausbleichen. Natur u. Museum **94**, 10—14 (1964). — VOUTE, C. L.: An electron microscopic study of the skin of the frog (Rana pipiens). J. Ultrastruct. Res. **9**, 497—510 (1963).

WAGNER, H. O., u. C. MÜLLER: Die Mauser und die den Federausfall fördernden und hemmenden Faktoren. Z. Morph. Ökol. Tiere **53**, 107—151 (1963). — WALLIN, O.: Mucopolysaccharides and the calcification of the scale of the roach (Leuciscus rutilus). Quart. J. micr. Sci. **97**, 329—332 (1956). — WARING, H.: A preliminary study of the melanophore-expanding potency of the pituitary gland in the frog and dogfish. Proc. Trans. (Liverpool) biol. Soc. **49**, 65—90 (1936). — Colour change in the dogfish (Scyllium canicula). Proc. Trans. (Liverpool) biol. Soc. **49**, 17—64 (1936). — Chromatic behaviour of elasmobranchs. Proc. roy. Soc. B **125**, 264—282 (1938). — The co-ordination of vertebrate melanophore responses. Biol. Rev. **17**, 120—150 (1942). — Color change mechanisms of cold-blooded vertebrates. New York and London: Academic Press 1963. — WATSON, G. G.: Feather replacement in birds. Science **139**, 50—51 (1963). — WEBER, G.: Vergleichende bioenzymatische Untersuchungen in der Hornschicht von Mensch und Schuppentieren (Squamaten). Naturwissenschaften **48**, 83 (1961). — WEBER, R.: On the biological function of cathepsin in tail tissue of Xenopus larvae. Experientia (Basel) **13**, 153—155 (1957). — Die Kathepsinaktivität im Schwanz von Xenopuslarven während Wachstum und Metamorphose. Rev. suisse Zool. **64**, 326—336 (1957). — WEDELL, G.: The pattern of cutaneous innervation in relation to cutaneous sensibility. J. Anat. (Lond.) **75**, 346—367 (1941). — WEISS, P. A., and W. FERRIS: Electromicrograms of larval amphibian epidermis. Exp. Cell Res. **6**, 546—549 (1954). — Electronmicroscopic study of the texture of the basement membrane of larval amphinian skin. Proc. nat. Acad. Sci. (Wash.) **40**, 528—540 (1954). — The basement lamella of amphibian skin. Its reconstruction after wounding. J. biophys. biochem. Cytol. **2**, Suppl., 275—281 (1956). — WHITEAR, M.: The innervation of the skin of teleost fishes. Quart. J. micr. Sci. **93**, 289—305 (1952). — Dermal nerve-endings in Rana and Bufo. Quart. J. micr. Sci. **96**, 343—349 (1955). — WIEDEMANN, E.: Zur Ortsbewegung der Schlangen und Schleichen. Zool. Jb., Abt. Physiol. **50**, 557—596 (1931/32). — WILSON, D. M.: Function of giant MAUTHNER's neurons in the lungfish. Science **129**, 841—842 (1959). — WINKELMANN, R. K., and T. T. MYERS. III. The histochemistry and morphology of the cutaneous sensory end-organs of the chicken. J. comp. Neurol. **117**, 27—36 (1961). — WITSCHI, E.: Sex and secondary sexual characters. In: Biology and comp. physiology of birds, vol. II, p. 115—168 (ed. A. J. MARSHALL). New York and London: Academic Press 1961. — WOELLWARTH, C. v.: Über die Beziehungen der Seitensinnesorgane der Fische zum Nervensystem. Z. vergl. Physiol. **20**, 215—250 (1934). — WOHLFAHRT, T. A.: Anatomische Untersuchungen über die Seitenkanäle der Sardine (Clupea pilchardus Walb.). Z. Morph. Ökol. Tiere **33**, 381—412 (1937). — WOOLLEY, P.: Colour change in a Chelonian. Nature (Lond.) **179**, 1255—1256 (1957). — WRIGHT, M. R.: The lateral line system of sense organs. Quart. Rev. Biol. **26**, 264—280 (1951). — WRIGHT, M. R., and A. B. LERNER: On the movement of pigment granules in frog melanocytes. Endocrinology **66**, 599—609 (1960). — WRIGHT, P. A.: Physiological response of frog melanophores in vitro. Physiol. Zool. **28**, 204—218 (1955). — WUNDERER, H.: Über Terminalkörperchen der Anamnier. Arch. mikr. Anat. Entwickl.-Gesch. **71**, 504—569 (1908).

YOUNG, J. Z.: The photoreceptors of lampreys. I. Light-sensitive fibres in the lateral line nerves. J. exp. Biol. **12**, 229—238 (1935). — The photoreceptors of lampreys. II. The function of the pineal complex. J. exp. Biol. **12**, 254—269 (1935). — YOUNG, J. Z., and C. W. BELLERBY: The response of the lamprey to injection of anterior lobe pituitary extract. J. exp. Biol. **12**, 246—253 (1935).

ZETTNER, A.: Über die Lichtreaktion der Froschhautchromatophoren. Z. Biol. **108**, 210—216 (1956). — ZIEGLER, I.: Tetrahydropterin-Derivat als lichtempfindliche Verbindung bei Amphibien und Insekten. Z. Naturforsch. **15b**, 460—465 (1960). — Quantitative Bestimmung von gelbem Pterin und Riboflavin in der Haut des Feuersalamanders (Salamandra salamandra). Biochem. Z. **334**, 425—430 (1961). — Tetrahydropterin und Melanophoren-Differenzierung bei Fischen. Z. Naturforsch. **18b**, 551—556 (1963). — Pterine als Wirkstoffe und Pigmente. In: Erg. Physiologie **56**, p. 1—66. Berlin-Heidelberg-New York: Springer 1965. — ZIEGLER-GÜNDER, I.: Nachweis und Lokalisation von Pterinen und Riboflavin in der Haut von Amphibien und Reptilien. Z. vergl. Physiol. **36**, 78—114 (1954). — Histologische Lokalisation von Ribonucleoproteiden als Substrat von Pterin in der Haut der Amphibien. Zool. Anz., Suppl., **18**, 447—452 (1955). — Untersuchungen über die Purin- und Pterinpigmente in der Haut und in den Augen der Weißfische. Z. vergl. Physiol. **39**, 163—189 (1956). — Zur Konstitution und physiologischen Bedeutung der photolabilen Haut- und Augenpterine. Zool. Anz., Suppl., **20**, 97—101 (1957). — Die Pterine in der Haut und in den Augen von Salamandra salamandra nach Aufzucht auf verschiedenfarbigem Untergrund. Experientia (Basel) **15**, 429—430 (1959). — ZIMMERMANN, S. B., and H. C. DALTON: Physiological responses of amphibian melanophores. Physiol. Zool. **34**, 21—33 (1961). — ZISWILER, V.: Die Afterfeder der Vögel. Untersuchungen zur Morphogenese und Phylogenese des sog. Afterschaftes. Zool. Jb., Abt. Anat. **80**, 245—308 (1962).

Anhang

Die Haut der Säugetiere; ausgewählte Literatur

In der Einleitung wurde kurz erwähnt, daß die Haut der Säugetiere bei der Besprechung im Rahmen dieses Abschnittes ausgeklammert werden sollte. Die Überschneidungen mit anderen Abschnitten dieses Handbuches wären sehr zahlreich und wenig nützlich gewesen. Die medizinische Forschung an der Haut ist vielfach auf Versuchstiere angewiesen, so daß über aktuelle und wichtige Fragen, über Bau und Physiologie der Säugetierhaut in den entsprechenden Publikationen medizinischer Fachzeitschriften zahlreiche Befunde vorgetragen werden.

Aus diesem Grunde erscheint es zweckmäßig, für den an bestimmten Problemen interessierten Leser eine Auswahl von Literatur über Säugetierhaut zu geben, die im wesentlichen nicht in medizinischen Journalen veröffentlicht wurde, sondern in Zeitschriften biologischen oder zoologischen Inhalts. Anhand dieser aufgeführten Literatur ist es dann leicht möglich, bei Bedarf weitere Publikationen zu finden. Das nachfolgende Literaturverzeichnis ist daher nach Sachgruppen geordnet; die Zitate sind nicht im allgemeinen Literaturverzeichnis aufgeführt.

a) Primatenhaut

BIEGERT, J.: Volarhaut der Hände und Füße sowie entsprechende Bildungen auf Nase und Schwanz. In: Primatologia, Handbuch der Primatenkunde, Bd. II/1/3, S. 3/1—3/326 (Hrsg. A. HOFER, A. H. SCHULTZ u. D. STARCK). Basel u. New York: S. Karger 1961.

ELLIS, R. A., and W. MONTAGNA: The skin of primates. VI. The skin of the gorilla (Gorilla gorilla). Amer. J. physic. Anthrop. 20, 79—93 (1962).

MONTAGNA, W.: The skin of lemurs. Ann. N.Y. Acad. Sci. 102, 190—209 (1962). — MONTAGNA, W., and R. A. ELLIS: The skin of primates. I. The skin of the potto (Perodicticus potto). Amer. J. physic. Anthrop. 17, 137—161 (1959). — The skin of primates. II. The skin of the slender loris (Loris tardigradus). Amer. J. physic. Anthrop. 18, 19—43 (1960). — MONTAGNA, W., K. YASUDA, and R. A. ELLIS: The skin of primates. III. The skin of the slow loris (Nycticebus coucang). Amer. J. physic. Antrop. 18, 19—43 (1960). — The skin of primates. V. The skin of the black lemur (Lemus macao). Amer. J. physic. Anthrop. 19, 115—123 (1961). — MONTAGNA, W., and J. S. YUN: The skin of primates. VIII. The skin of the Anubis baboon (Papio doguera). Amer. J. physic. Anthrop. 20, 131—141 (1962). — The skin of primates. XV. The skin of the chimpanze Pan satyrus. Amer. J. physic. Anthrop. 21, 189—203 (1963).

PARAKKAL, P. F., W. MONTAGNA, and R. A. ELLIS: The skin of primates. XI. The skin of the white browed gibbon (Hylobates hoolock). Anat. Rec. 5, 169—178 (1962).

YASUDA, K., T. AOKI, and W. MONTAGNA: The skin of primates. IV. The skin of the lesser bushbaby (Galago senegalensis). Amer. J. physic. Anthrop. 19, 23—33 (1961).

b) Feinbau der Haut

BARGEN, G. V.: Elektronenmikriskopische Untersuchung der Kaninchenhaut. Z. Zellforsch. 50, 459—471 (1959).

CUMMINS, H.: Dermatoglyphics: a brief review. In: The epidermis, p. 375—386 (ed. W. MONTAGNA and W. C. LOBITZ jr.). New York and London: Academic Press 1964.

DOWNES, A. M., L. F. SHARRY, and G. E. ROGERS: Separate synthesis of fibrillar and matrix proteins in the formation of keratin. Nature (Lond.) 199, 1059—1061 (1963).

ELLIS, R. A.: Vascular patterns of the skin. In: Advances biology of skin, vol. II. Blood vessels and circulation, p. 20—37 (ed. W. MONTAGNA and R. A. ELLIS). Oxford-London-New York-Paris: Pergamon Press 1961.

FARQUHAR, M. G., and G. E. PALADE: Junctional complexes in various epithelia. J. Cell Biol. 17, 375—412 (1963). — FORSLIND, B., and G. SWANBECK: Keratin formation in the hair follicle. I. An ultrastructural investigation. Exp. Cell Res. 43, 191—209 (1966).

HERTZMANN, A. B.: Effects of heat on the cutaneous blood flow. In: Advances biology of skin, vol. II. Blood vessels and circulation, p. 98—116 (ed. W. MONTAGNA and R. A. ELLIS). Oxford-London-New York-Paris: Pergamon Press 1961.

KALLMAN, F., and N. K. WESSELLS: Periodic repeat units of epithelial cell tonofilaments. J. Cell Biol. 32, 227—231 (1967).

Marchmann, A., and R. Brunish: Acid mucopolysaccharides in rat skin. An electrophoretic study of dermal and subcutaneous tissue. Proc. Soc. exp. Biol. (N.Y.) **119**, 1064—1968 (1965). — Matoltsy, A. G., and P. Parakkal: Membrane-coating granules of keratinizing epithelia. J. Cell Biol. **24**, 297—307 (1965). — Medawar, P. B.: The micro-anatomy of the mammalian epidermis. Quart. J. micr. Sci. **94**, 481—506 (1953).

Nakai, T.: A study of the ultrastructural localization of hair keratin synthesis utilizing electron microscopic autoradiography in a magnetic field. J. Cell Biol. **21**, 63—74 (1964).

Odland, G. F.: The fine structure of cutaneous capillaries. In: Advances biology of skin, vol. II. Blood vessels and circulation, p. 57—70 (ed. W. Montagna and R. A. Ellis). Oxford-London-New York-Paris: Pergamon Press 1961.

Pease, D. C., and W. Pallie: Electron microscopy of the digital tactile corpuscles and small cutaneous nerves. J. Ultrastruct. Res. **2**, 352—365 (1959).

Rogers, G. E.: Structural and biochemical features of the hair follicle. In: The epidermis, p. 179—236 (ed. W. Montagna and W. C. Lobitz jr.). New York and London: Academic Press 1964. — Roth, S. I., and W. H. Clark jr.: Ultrastructural evidence related to the mechanism of keratin synthesis. In: The epidermis, p. 303—337 (ed. W. Montagna and W. C. Lobitz jr.). New York and London: Academic Press 1964.

Snell, R. S.: An electron microscopic study of keratinization in the epidermal cells of the guinea-pig. Z. Zellforsch. **65**, 829—846 (1965). — The fate of epidermal desmosomes in mammalian skin. Z. Zellforsch. **66**, 471—487 (1965). — Spearman, R. I. C.: The evolution of mammalian keratinized structures. In: The mammalian epidermis and its derivatives. Symp. Zool. Soc. Lond. **12**, 67—81 (1964).

Weiner, J. S., and K. Hellmann: The sweat glands. Biol. Rev. **35**, 141—186 (1960). — Winkelmann, R. K., S. R. Scheen jr., R. A. Pyka, and M. Coventry: Cutaneous vascular patterns in studies with injection preparation and alkaline phosphatase reaction. In: Adances biology of skin. Vol. II. Blood vessels and circulation, p. 1—19 (ed. W. Montagna and R. A. Ellis). Oxford-London-New York-Paris: Pergamon Press 1961.

c) Haare und Haarwechsel

Billingham, R. E., R. Mangold, and W. K. Silvers: The neogenesis of skin in the antlers of deer. Ann. N.Y. Acad. Sci. **83**, 491—498 (1959). — Boardman, W.: The hair pattern developed on disorientated skin grafted in 1-day-old-rats. Aust. J. biol. Sci. **15**, 674—682 (1962). — Borodach, G. N., and W. Montagna: Fat in skin of the mouse during cycles of hair growth. J. invest. Derm. **26**, 229 (1956). — Braun-Falco, O.: Über die mitotische Aktivität in der Haarmatrix bei der Albinomaus während eines künstlich induziertes Haarcyclus. Arch. klin. exp. Derm. **215**, 63 (1962). — Braun-Falco, O., u. H. Frenz: Über Veränderungen des Wassergehaltes der Haut während des Haarwachstumscyclus bei der Ratte. Arch. klin. exp. Derm. **212**, 64 (1960). — Braun-Falco, O., u. H. Theisen: Über Veränderungen im Hautbindegewebe während des Haar-Wachstumscyclus bei der Maus. Arch. klin. exp. Derm. **209**, 426 (1959). — Butcher, E. O.: Restitutive growth in the hair follicle of the rat. Ann. N.Y. Acad. Sci. **83**, 369—377 (1959).

Charles, A.: The ultrastructure of the epidermis. In: The mammalian epidermis and its derivatives. Symp. Zool. Soc. Lond. **12**, 39—54 (1964). — Chase, H. B., and G. J. Eaton: The growth of hair follicles in waves. Ann. N.Y. Acad. Sci. **83**, 365—368 (1959). — Cohen, J.: The transplantation of individual rat and guinea-pig whisker papillae. J. Embryol. exp. Morph. **9**, 117—127 (1961). — Transplantation of hair papillae. In: The mammalian epidermis and its derivatives. Symp. Zool. Soc. Lond. **12**, 83—96 (1964).

Ebling, F. J., and E. Johnson: The control of hair growth. In: The mammalian epidermis and its derivatives. Symp. Zool. Soc. Lond. **12**, 97—130 (1964).

Jarrett, A., and R. I. Spearman: The keratin defect and hair-cycle of a new mutant (matted) in the house mouse. J. Embryol. exp. Morph. **5**, 103—110 (1957). — Johnson, E., and F. J. Ebling: The effect of plucking hairs during different phases of the follicular cycle. J. Embryol. exp. Morph. **12**, 465—474 (1964).

Lyne, A. G.: The systemic and adaptive significance of vibrissae in marsupials. Proc. Zool. Soc. Lond. **133**, 97—133 (1959).

Oliver, R. F.: Whisker growth after removal of the dermal papilla and lengths of follicle in the hooded rat. J. Embryol. exp. Morph. **15**, 331—347 (1966). — Histological studies of whisker regeneration in the hooded rat. J. Embryol. exp. Morph. **16**, 231—244 (1966). — Ectopic regeneration of whiskers in the hooded rat from implanted lengths of vibrissa follicle wall J. Embryol. exp. Morph. **17**, 27—34 (1967).

Parakkal, P. F.: The fine structure of the dermal papilla of the guinea pig hair follicle. J. Ultrastruct. Res. **14**, 133—142 (1966).

Rogers, G. E.: Electron microscope studies of hair and wool. Ann. N.Y. Acad. Sci. **83**, 378—399 (1959). — Newer findings on the enzymes and proteins of hair follicles. Ann. N.Y.

Acad. Sci. 83, 408—428 (1959). — ROTH, S. I., and E. B. HELWIG: The cytology of the dermal papilla, the bulb, and the root sheaths of the mouse hair. J. Ultrastruct. Res. 11, 33—51 (1964). — The cytology of the cuticle of the cortex, the cortex, and the medulla of the mouse hair. J. Ultrastruct. Res. 11, 52—67 (1964). — RYDER, M. L.: Follicle arrangement in skin from wild sheep, primitive domestic sheep and in parchment. Nature (Lond.) 182, 781—783 1958).

SEARLE, A. G., and R. I. SPEARMAN: "Matted", a new hair-mutant in the house-mouse: genetics and morphology. J. Embryol. exp. Morph. 5, 93—102 (1957). — SLEE, J.: Developmental morphology of the skin and hair follicles in normal and in "ragged" mice. J. Embryol. exp. Morph. 10, 507—529 (1962). — SPEARMAN, R. I.: The skin abnormatity of "ichthyosis", a mutant of the house mouse. J. Embryol. exp. Morph. 8, 387—395 (1960). — STRAILE, W. E.: A study on the neoformation of mammalian hair follicles. Ann. N.Y. Acad. Sci. 83, 499—506 (1959). — Possible functions of the external root sheath during growth of the hair follicle. J. exp. Zool. 150, 207—223 (1962). — STRAILE, W. E., H. B. CHASE ,and C. ARSENAULT: Growth and differentiation of hair follicles between periods of activity and quiescence. J. exp. Zool. 148, 205—221 (1961).

WESSELLS, N. K., and K. D. ROESSNER: Nonproliferation in dermal condensations of mouse vibrissae and pelage hairs. Develop. Biol. 12, 419—433 (1965).

d) Abgewandelte Haarformen

MOHR, E.: Die Körperbedeckung der Stachelschweine. Z. Säugetierkd. 29, 17—33 (1964).
RYDER, M. L.: Structure of rhinoceros horn. Nature (Lond.) 193, 1199—1201 (1962).

e) Nervenversorgung der Haut

DIAMOND, J., J. A. B. GRAY, and D. R. INMAN: The relation between receptor potentials and the concentration of sodium ions. J. Physiol. (Lond.) 142, 382—394 (1958).

FALK, B., and H. RORSMAN: Observation on the adrenergic innervation of the skin. Experientia 19, 205—206 (1963).

HENSEL, H.: Allgemeine Sinnesphysiologie, Hautsinne, Geschmack, Geruch. Berlin-Heidelberg-New York: Springer 1966. — HERXHEIMER, A.: The anatomic innervation of the skin. In: Advances biology of skin, vol. I. Cutaneous innervations, p. 63—73 (ed. W. MONTAGNA and R. A. ELLIS). Oxford-London-Mew York-Paris: Pergamon Press 1960.

IGGO, A.: An electrophysiological analysis of afferent fibres in primate skin. Acta neuroveg. (Wien) 24, 225—240 (1963). — The periphal mechanism of cutaneous sensation. In: Studies in physiology, p. 92—100 (ed. D. R. CURTIS and A. K. McINTYRE). Berlin-Heidelberg-New York: Springer 1965. — INMAN, D. R.: The electrophysiology of single mammalian mechano-receptors. Symp. Soc. exp. Biol. 16, 317—344 (1962). — ISHIKO, N., and W. R. LOEWENSTEIN: Effects of temperature on the generator and action potentials of a sense organ. J. gen. Physiol. 45, 105—124 (1961).

LINDBLOM, U.: Properties of touch receptors in distal glabrous skin of the monkey. J. Neurophysiol. 28, 966—985 (1965). — LOEWENSTEIN, W. R.: Excitation and inactivation in a receptor membrane. Ann. N.Y. Acad. Sci. 94, 510—534 (1961). — LOEWENSTEIN, W. R., and M. MENDELSON: Components of receptor adaptation in a Pacinian corpuscle. J. Physiol. (Lond.) 177, 377—397 (1965).

MILLER, S., and G. WEDDELL: Mechanoreceptors in rabbit ear skin innervated by myelinated nerve fibres. J. Physiol. (Lond.) 187, 291—305 (1966). — MUNGER, B. L.: The intraepidermal innervation of the snout skin of the opossum. A light and electron microscope study, with observations on the nature of MERKEL's Tastzellen. J. Cell Biol. 26, 79—97 (1965).

OSEKI, M., and M. SATO: Initiation of impulses at non-myelinated nerve terminal in Pacinian corpuscles. J. Physiol. (Lond.) 170, 167—185 (1964).

SHANTHAVEERAPPA, T. R., and G. H. BOURNE: New observations on the structure of the Pacinian corpuscle and its relation to the perineural epithelium of peripheral nerves. Amer. J. Anat. 112, 97—109 (1963).

WALL, P. D.: Two transmission systems for skin sensations. In: Sensory communication, p. 475—496 (ed. W. A. ROSENBLATT). New York and London: M.I.T. Press and John Wiley & Sons 1961. — WALTER, P.: Die sensible Innervation des Lippen-Nasenbereiches von Rind, Schaf, Ziege, Schwein, Hund und Katze. Z. Zellforsch. 53, 394—410 (1961). — WEDDELL, G.: Studies related to the mechanism of common sensibility. In: Advances biology of skin, vol. I. Cutaneous innervation, p. 112—160 (ed. W. MONTAGNA). Oxford-London-New York-Paris: Pergamon Press 1960. — The innervation of cutaneous blood vessels. In: Advances biology of skin, vol. II. Blood vessels and circulation, p. 71—78 (ed. W. MONTAGNA and R. A. ELLIS). Oxford-London-New York-Paris: Pergamin Press 1961. — WEDDELL, G., W. PALLIE, and E. PALMER: The morphology of peripheral nerve termination in the skin. Quart. J. micr.

Sci. **95**, 483—501 (1954). — WEDDELL, G., E. PALMER, and W. PALLIE: Nerve endings in mammalian skin. Biol. Rev. **30**, 159—195 (1955). — WINKELMANN, R. K.: The innervation of hair follicle. Ann. N.Y. Acad. Sci. **83**, 400—407 (1959). — Similarities in cutaneous nerve end-organ. In: Advances biology of skin, vol I. Cutaneous Innervation, p. 48—62 (ed. W. MONTAGNA). Oxford-London-New York-Paris: Pergamon Press 1960.

f) Besondere Anpassungen

α) An Wasserleben

LUCK, C. P., and P. G. WRIGTH: Acpects of the anatomy of the skin of the hippopotamus Hippopotamus amphibius. Quart. J. exp. Physiol. **49**, 1—14 (1964).
MONTAGNA, W., and R. A. ELLIS: Sweat glands in the skin of Ornithorhynchus paradoxus. Anat. Rec. **137**, 271—277 (1960). — MONTAGNA, W., and R. J. HARRISON: Specialisations in the skin of the seal Phoca vitulina. Amer. J. Anat. **100**, 81—114 (1957).
PARRY, D. A.: The structure of whale blubber and a discussion of its thermal properties. Quart. J. micr. Sci. **90**, 13—25 (1949).
SCHEFFER, V. B.: Hair patterns in seals, Pinnipedia. J. Morph. **115**, 291—303 (1964). — Estimating abandance of pelage fibres on fur of seal skin. Proc. Zool. Soc. Lond. **143**, 37—41 (1964). — SOKOLOV, W. E.: Adaptations of the skin in marine mammal fauna of the U.S.S.R. to some conditions of aquatic life. Proc. 15th Int. Congr. Zool. Lond. **1959**, p. 277—280. — Some similarities and dissimilarities in the structure of the skin among the members of the suborders odontoceti and mystacocety (Cetacea). Nature (Lond.) **185**, 745—747 (1960). — Adaptations of the mammalian skin of the aquatic mode of life. Nature (Lond.) **195**, 464—466 (1962).

β) An Wüstenleben

MARGOLENA, L. A.: Sudoriferous glands of sheep and goats. Z. mikr.-anat. Forsch. **69**, 217—225 (1962).
SOKOLOV, W.: Skin adaptations of some rodents to life in the desert. Nature (Lond.) **193**, 823—825 (1962).

g) Kontrolle von Mitosen

BULLOUGH, W. S., C. L. HEWETT, and E. B. LAURENCE: The epidermal chalone: a preliminary attempt at isolation. Exp. Cell Res. **36**, 192—200 (1964). — BULLOUGH, W. S., and E. B. LAURENCE: The control of epidermal mitotic activity in the mouse. Proc. roy. Soc. B **151**, 517—536 (1959—1960). — The production of the epidermal cells. In: The mammalian epidermis and its derivatives. Symp. Zool. Soc. Lond. **12**, 1—23 (1964).
CHU, C. H. U.: A study of the subcutaneous connective tissue of the mouse, with special reference to nuclear type, nuclear division and mitotic rhythm. Anat. Rec. **138**, 11—25 (1960).
DODSON, J. W.: On the nature of tissue interactions in embryonic skin. Exp. Cell Res. **31**, 233—235 (1963).
GELFANT, S.: Patterns of epidermal cell division. I. Genetic behavior of the G_1-cell population. Exp. Cell Res. **32**, 521—528 (1963).
HELL, E. A., and C. N. D. CRUICKSHANK: The effect of injury upon the uptake of ^{3}H-thymidine by guinea pig epidermis. Exp. Cell Res. **31**, 128—139 (1963).
WESSELLS, N. K.: Effects of extra-epithelial factors in the incorporation of thymidine by embryonic epidermis. Exp. Cell Res. **30**, 36—55 (1963).

h) Wundheilung

ARGYRIS, T. S.: The growth-promoting effects of wounds on hair follicles already stimulated by plucking. Anat. Rec. **143**, 183—188 (1962). — Wound healing and the control of gowth of the skin. In: Advances biology of skin, vol. V. Wound healing, p. 231—249 (ed. W. MONTAGNA and R. E. BILLINGHAM). Oxford-London-Endinburgh-New York-Paris-Frankfurt: Pergamon Press 1964. — ARGYRIS, T. S., and B. F. ARGYRIS: Factors affecting the stimulation of hair growth during wound healing. Anat. Rec. **142**, 139—145 (1962). — ARGYRIS, T. S., and M. E. TRIMBLE: On the mechanism of hair growth stimulation in the wound healing. Develop. Biol. **9**, 230—254 (1964).
BLOCK, P., I. SEITER, and W. OEHLERT: Autoradiographic studies of the initial cellular response to injury. Exp. Cell Res. **30**, 311—321 (1963).
CABRINI, R. L., and F. A. CARRANZA jr.: Histochemical localization of β-glucoronidase in healing wounds. Naturwissenschaften **48**, 131 (1961). — CARRANZA jr., F. A., and R. L. CABRINI: Histochemical distribution of acid phosphatase in healing wounds. Science **135**, 672 (1962). — CHU, C. H. U.: A study of the subcutaneous connective tissue of the mouse,

with special reference to nuclear type, nuclear division and mitotic rhythm. Anat. Rec. **138**, 11—25 (1960).

GLÜCKSMANN, A.: Cell turnover in the dermis. In: Advances biology of skin, vol. V. Wound healing, p. 76—94 (ed. W. MONTAGNA and R. R. BILLINGHAM). Oxford-London-Edinburgh-New York-Paris-Frankfurt: Pergamon Press 1964.

HANKE, W.: Die Beeinflussung der Wundheilung bei Säugetieren durch histostatische und morphogenetische Substanzen. Wilhelm Roux' Arch. Entwickl.-Mech. **153**, 669—702 (1962).

JACKSON, D. S.: The healing wound as an experimental model for biochemical studies of connective tissue. In: Advances biology of skin, vol. V. Wound healing, p. 30—38 (ed. W. MONTAGNA and R. E. BILLINGHAM). Oxford-London-Edinburgh-New York-Paris-Frankfurt: Pergamon Press 1964.

JOHNSON, F. R., and R. M. H. MCMINN: The cytology of wound healing of body surfaces in mammals. Biol. Rev. **35**, 364—412 (1960).

LEBLOND, C. P.: Relationship of cell formation and cell migration in the renewal of stratified squamous epithelia. In: Advances biology of skin, vol. V. Wound healing, p. 39—67. (ed. W. MONTAGNA, and R. E. BILLINGHAM). Oxford-London-Edinburgh-New York-Paris-Frankfurt: Pergamon Press 1964.

MILLER, L., and H. W. WHITTING: Mast cells and wound healing of the skin in the rat. Z. Zellforsch. **65**, 597—606 (1965).

PUGATCH, E. M. J.: The growth of endothelium and pseusoendothelium on the healing surface of rabbit ear chambers. Proc. roy. Soc. B **160**, 412—422 (1964).

ROSS, R.: Studies of collagen formation in healing wounds. In: Advances biology of skin, vol. V. Wound healing, p. 144—164 (ed. W. MONTAGNA, and R. E. BILLINGHAM). Oxford-London-Edinburgh-New York-Paris-Frankfurt: Pergamin Press 1964. — ROSS, R., and E. P. BENDITT: Wound healing and collagen formation. I. Sequential changes in components of guinea pig skin wounds observed in the electron microscope. J. biophys. biochem. Cytol. **11**, 677—700 (1961). — Wound healing and collagen formation. III. A quantitative radiographic study of the utilization of proline-H^3 in wounds from normal and scorbutic guinea pigs. J. Cell Biol. **15**, 99—108 (1962). — Wound healing and collagen formation. V. Quantitative electron microscope radioautographic observations of proline-H^3 utilization by fibroblasts. J. Cell Biol. **27**, 83—106 (1965).

SCHOEFL, G. I., and G. MAJNO: Regeneration of blood vessels in wound healing. In: Advances biology of skin, vol. V, Wound healing, p. 173—193 (ed. W. MONTAGNA and R. E. BILLINGHAM). Oxford-London-Edinburgh-New York-Paris-Frankfurt: Pergamon Press 1964.

STRAILE, W. E.: The composition of mammalian skin expanding near contracting wounds. J. exp. Zool. **140**, 405—414 (1959). — The expansion and shrinkage of mammalian skin near contracting wounds. J. exp. Zool. **141**, 119—132 (1959).

WINTER, G. D.: Movement of epidermal cells over the wound surface. In: Advances biology of skin, vol. V. Wound healing, p. 113—127 (ed. W. MONTAGNA and R. E. BILLINGHAM). Oxford-London-Edinburgh-New York-Paris-Frankfurt: Pergamon Press 1964.

Namenverzeichnis

Die *kursiv* gesetzten Seitenzahlen beziehen sich auf die Literatur

Aavik, O. R.   96, *120*, 284, *330*
Abbott, U. K., u. V. S. Asmundson   1008, *1015*
— s. Goetinck, P. F.   *1019*
— s. Sengel, P.   *1026*
Abel, J. H., s. Ellis, R. A.   *264*
Abele, D. C., s. Dobson, R. L.   *264*
Abele, G.   *783*
Abernethy   778, *786*
Abramowitz, A. A.   951, 966, *1015*
Abrikossoff, A.   803, 841, 842, *846, 855, 857*
— s. Wail   *857*
Abulafia, J., s. Borda, J. M.   *906*
— s. Pierini, L. E.   796, *861*
Achs, R., R. G. Harper u. M. Siegel   636, *677*
Achten, G.   342, 344, 345, 346, 348, 349, 362, 364, 365, 366, 370, *374*, 627, 632, 636, 654, 669, *677*
— u. J. M. Simonart   699, *705*
Ackermann, A.   253, *263*
Ackermann, A. B., D. T. Mosher u. H. A. Schwamm   802, *860*
Adachi, K., u. W. Montagna   101, 102, *120*, 176, *178*, 202, *220*, 325, *330*, 431, *482*, 696, *705*
Adachi, N. K., s. Moretti, G., u. R. A. Ellis   *133*
— s. Moretti, G., N. Mescon u. P. Pochi   *133*
Adair, F. E., u. J. Th. Munzer   804, *846*
Adam, H.   271, *330*
Adams, A. E., A. Kuder u. L. Richards   920, 979, *1015*
— L. Richards u. Kuder   920, 979, *1015*
Adams, C. W. M.   890, *912*
Adams, E. C., s. McKay, D. G.   *680*
Adams, J. M., s. Sandberg, D. H.   *849, 859*
Adams-Ray, J., G. Bloom u. M. Ritzén   436, *482*
— u. H. Nordenstam   436, *482. 487*
— s. Rhodin, J.   *488*

Adjutantis, G., u. G. Skalos   775, *785*
Adler, E., H. v. Euler u. G. Günther   89, *120*
Adler, M., s. Avonson, St. A.   *853, 855*
Adolph, W. E., R. F. Baker u. G. M. Leiby   37, *120*
Adrian, E. D., K. McKeen Cattell u. H. Hoagland   984, *1015*
— u. K. Umrath   412, *423*
Afzelius, B. A.   300, *330*
— s. Lindberg, O.   *861*
Agneta, J. O.   804, *846*
Agranoff, B., s. Lynen, F.   *844*
Aherne, W., u. D. Hull   677, 819, *853*
Ahrndt, W., u. F. Pax, s. Brühl, L.   *1016*
Aiba, K.   413, *423*
Akkeringa, L. I.   406, *423*
Albertazzi, F., u. E. Ferrato   *857*
— s. Ormea, F.   *619*
Albertini, A. v.   37, *120*, 819, *843*
Albrecht, P. G., s. Barker-Beeson, B.   *908*
Albrectsen, B.   836, *860*
Albright, J. T., s. Sognnaes, R. F.   *138*
Alderson, H. E., u. S. C. Way   802, *846*
Alex, M., s. Lansing, A. I.   *486*
Alexander, P., u. R. F. Hudson   74, *120*
Alfert, M., s. Bern, H. A.   *121*
Algire, G. H.   558, *615*
Alkiewicz, J.   669, *677*, 809, *850*
— u. W. Gorny   699, *705*
Allegra   585
Allegra, F.   631, *677*
— u. W. Marcheselli   177, *178*
Allen   531
Allen, A. C.   104, *120*, 809, *843*
Allen, E. V., N. W. Barker u. E. A. Hynes   497, *609, 615*
Allen, J. M., u. J. J. Slater   324, *330*
Allen, N., u. J. G. Nichols   382, *423*
Allenby, C. F., E. Palmer u. G. Weddell   384, *423*

Allgower, M.   558, *615*
Allison, J. R., u. J. Allison jr.   873, *903*
Allison jr., J., s. Allison, J. R.   873, *903*
Althausen, T. L., R. K. Doig, S. Weiden, R. Motteram, C. N. Turner u. A. Moore   896, *916*
Altmann, H. W.   720, *780*
Alverdes, K.   268, 269, 270, 273, 274, 275, 284, *330*, 663, *677*
Amado, R., s. Bolgert   *919*
Amante, L., s. Bairati, A.   *483*
Amitrano, L.   899, *917*
Amoretti, A. R.   387, *423*
Andersen, D. H., s. Mason, H. H.   *911*
— s. Sant'Agnese, P. A. di   *911*
Andersen, H.   362, 363, 364, *374*
Anderson, C. R., s. Frost, R.   *909*
Anderson, H.   *780*
Anderson, J. P., s. Barka, T.   *330*
Andersson-Cedergren, E., s. Sjöstrand, F. S.   *138*
Andrade   695
Andrade, C.   *866*
André, P.   289, *330*
Andreasen, E.   62, *120*, 163, *178*
Andres, K. H.   406, *423*
Andrew, N. V., s. Andrew, W.   *120*
Andrew, W.   62, *120*
— u. N. V. Andrew   62, *120*
Andrews, G. C.   872, *903*
Andrews, T., s. Daniel, C.   *424*
Anning, S. T.   805, *846*
Anrepp u. Obolonsky   759
Anselmino, K. J., u. F. Hoffmann   826, 827, *855*
— u. F. Hoffmann, s. Trygstad   *857*
Anzai, M.   898, *917*
Aoki, T.   284, *330*
— s. Yasuda, K.   *1029*
Apffel, K., u. F. Burgun   798, *846*
Appaix, A., A. Pech u. J. M. Codaccioni   811, *850*

Appelmans, F., R. Wattiaux u. C. de Duve 97, *120*
— s. Duve, C. de *126*
Appleyard, H. M., u. C. M. Greville 149, *178*
— s. Auber, L. *1015*
Araki, Y., u. S. Ondo 253, *263*
Arase, M., s. Benditt, E. P. *483*
Archer, V. E., s. Luell, E. *181*
Arduino, J. L. 805, *846*
Arey, L. B. 499, 500, 511, *613*, 630, *677*
— W. Burrows, J. P. Greenhill u. R. M. Hewitt *613*
Argyris, B. F., s. Argyris, T. S. *1032*
Argyris, F. S. 88, 92, 95, *120*
Argyris, T. S. *1032*
— u. B. F. Argyris *1032*
— u. M. E. Trimble *1032*
Ariëns Kappers, C. U. 934, 1004, *1015*
— G. C. Huber u. E. C. Crosby 1004, *1015*
Arimori, M., T. Hamamatsu u. S. Kurokowa 830, *855*
Armen, D., s. Laden, E. L. *131*
Armstrong, J., s. Freeman, R. G. *705*
Arnal u. Mehl 774, *785*
Arndt *846*
Arndt, K. A., s. Eisen, A. Z. *126*
Arnold, H. L. 880, *906*
Arnold, J. 493, *609*
Aronson, St. A., C. V. Teodoru, M. Adler u. G. Schwartzman 819, 829, *853*, *855*
Arootunov 811
Aroutunov, V. *860*
Arrighi, F. 873, *903*
Arsenault, C., s. Straile, W. E. *1031*
Arthur, R. P., u. W. B. Shelley 384, *423*
Arzt, L. 806, 808, 816, *846*, *850*, 901, *919*
— u. K. Zieler *681*
— s. Besnier, E. *903*
— s. Besnier, E., u. F. Balzer *903*
— s. Bosellini, J. L. *903*
— u. C. Zieler, s. Brünauer, St. R. *845*
— s. Pellizari, C. *904*
— s. Wagner *905*
Asboe-Hansen *487, 705*
Asboe-Hansen, G. 438, 451, 453, *482, 483*, 875, 879, *906*
— u. O. Wegelius 875, *906*
— s. Meyer, K. *907*
Ascarelli, A. 745, *782*
Aschoff, L. *843*

Ashmore, H., u. M. Uttley 178, *178*
Asmundson, V. S., s. Abbott, U. K. *1015*
Astbury, W. 371, *374*
Astbury, W. T. 49, 50, *120*, 448, *483*
— u. S. Dickinson 18, *120*
— u. A. Street 18, 49, *120*
— u. H. J. Woods 18, 49, 50, 74, *120*
— s. Bailey, K. *120*
— s. Turnbridge, R. E. *489*, *905*
Astore, I., s. Barman, J. M. *178*
Atikinson, S., F. Cormia u. S. A. Unrau 165, *178*
Ato, N. 277, *330*
Atusi, N. 272, *330*
Aub, J. C., s. Rawson, R. W. *907*
Auber, L. 145, 147, 177, *178*, 652, *677*, 1008, 1011, *1015*
— u. H. M. Appleyard 1008, *1015*
Auerbach 536, *615*
Auerbach, R., s. Scott, E. J. van, u. T. M. Ekel *183*
Aufderheide, A. C., H. L. Horns u. R. J. Goldish 895, *916*
Aufdermauer, M. 811, *850*
Aufhammer 43, *120*
Auping, J., s. Grosfeld, J. C. M. *904*
Aurell, G. 664, *677*
Aust, S. 958, 961, *1015*
Avakian, E. V., s. Tilden, J. L. *849*
Avery, H. 832, *857*
Avioli, L., J. T. Lasersohn u. J. H. Lopresti 883, *908*
Aygün, K. S., s. Marchionini, A. *904*
Ayres jr., S. 898, *917*

Bacarini, E., s. Mancini *680*
Baccaredda-Boy, A., u. G. Moretti 537, *615*
— G. Moretti u. G. Farris 530, 575, 576, 580, 592, 608, *615*, *621, 623*
— G. Moretti u. B. Filippi 530, 575, 576, 580, 592, 608, *615, 621*
— G. Moretti u. A. Rebora 529, 531, 533, 575, *615, 621*
— G. Moretti, S. Zocchi u. F. Crovato 537, *615*
Bächli, E., s. Ortiz, E. *1024*
Baelz, s. Kaufmann, E. *917*
Baer 765
Baethke, R., s. Knoth, W. *845*
Bafverstedt, B. 888, *911*

Baggenstoß, A. H., s. Moskowitz, R. W. *852*
Bagnara, J. T. 949, 965, 977, *978, 1015*
— u. S. Neidleman 977, *1015*
— u. C. M. Richards 977, *1015*
— s. Obika, M. *1024*
Bahlmann, Cl. *783*
Bahr, F. G. 440, 448, 449, *483*
Bahr, G. F., u. K. H. Huhn 873, *903*
Bailey, K., W. T. Astbury u. K. M. Rudall 18, 49, 50, *120*
Bailey, R. E. 1001, *1015*
Bailey, R. M., u. W. R. Taylor 959, *1015*
Baillie, A. H., K. C. Calman u. J. A. Milne 202, *220*
Bairati, A. 564, *615*
Bairati, A., L. Amante, St. de Petris u. B. Pernis 439, 444, *483*
Baker 81, 85
Baker u. Curtis 704
Baker, B. L., s. Montes, L. F. 334, *706*
Baker, J. R., s. Fishman, W. H. *127*
Baker, R. F., s. Adolph, W. E. *120*
Baker, R. V., M. S. C. Birbeck, H. Blaschko, T. B. Fitzpatrick u. M. Seiji 110, *120*
Balbi, E. *850*
Balboni, G. 788, 819, *844, 853*
Baldes, E. J., s. Gilje, O., u. O'Leary *610, 617*
Baldes, F. J., s. Gilje, O., u. R. Kierland *610*
Baldino, N., s. Gualdi, A. *264*
Baler, G. R. 900, *919*
Ball, E. G., u. R. L. Jungas 819, *853*
— s. Barrnett, R. J. *483*
— s. Joel, C. D. *854*
Ballagi, St. 798, *846*
Ballantyne jr., D. L., u. J. M. Converse 559, *615*
Ballantyne, D. L., s. Converse, J. M. *616*
Ballowitz, E. 920, 964, 966, *1015*
Baló, J. 789, *844*
— u. J. Banga 450, *483*
Balogh, K. 526, *615*
Balsamo, C. A., s. Matoltsy, A. G. *132*
Bălus, L., s. Dimitrescu *850, 857*
Balzer, F., s. Besnier, E. *903*
Bammer, H. G. 477, *483*

Bandmann, H.-J., u. K. Bosse 144, 145, 146, 149, 150, 164, *178*
— N. Romiti u. K. Stehr 826, *860*
— u. H. W. Spier 481, *483*
Banfield, W. G. 693, *705*
Banfield, W. S. 638, *677*
Banga, J. 450, *483*
— s. Baló, J. *483*
Bangle, R. 886, *911*
Banks, B. M., s. Monis, B., u. A. M. Rutenburg *133*
Bannister, R. G., s. Romanul, F. C. A. *619*
Bargen, G. v. 2, 3, 19, 21, 37, 38, 43, 44, 55, 57, 60, 61, *120, 1029*
Bargmann, W. 148, 150, *178*, 279, 327, *330*, 379, *423*, 445, 447, 459, 480, *483*, 534, 536, 539, 547, 548, 550, 551, *615*, 724, *781*, 941, 946, *1015*
— K. Fleischhauer u. A. Knoop 268, 326, *330*
— u. A. Knoop 301, 304, *330*
— s. Möllendorff, W. v. *705*
Barka, T., u. J. P. Anderson 306, *330*
Barker, B. L., s. Boersma, D. *917*
Barker, N. W., s. Allen, E. V. 609, *615*
— s. Montgomery, H. *852*
Barker, S. B., s. Taylor jr., R. E. *1027*
— s. Taylor jr., R. E., u. H. C. Taylor *1027*
Barker-Beeson, B., u. P. G. Albrecht 882, *908*
Barman, J. M., I. Astore u. V. Pecoraro 162, *178*
— V. Pecoraro u. I. Astore 162, *178*
Barnett, R., u. A. Seligman 370, 372, *374*
Barnett, R. J., u. A. M. Seligman 526, 536, 556, *615*
Barnicot, N. A., u. M. S. Birbeck 104, 108, 109, 110, 111, 112, 114, 117, *120*, 890, *912*
— M. S. C. Birbeck u. F. W. Cuckow 104, 111, 112, *120, 121*
— s. Birbeck, M. S. C. *121, 122, 912*
— s. Birbeck, M. S. C., u. Mercer *179*
Barr, L., s. Dewey, M. M. *125, 126, 1017*
Barr, M. L. *781*
— u. E. G. Bertram 729, *781*
Barrat, W. *786*

Barriere, H., s. Bureau, Y. *860*
Barritt, W. C., s. Russel, F. E. *1025*
Barrnett, R. J. 44, 70, 71, 72, 73, 74, 92, *121*
— u. E. G. Ball 459, 460, *483*
— u. A. M. Seligman 70, 71, 72, 73, 80, 81, 92, *121, 173, 178*
Barron, E. S. G. 71, 72, 76, 89, *121*
— u. G. Kalnitzky 89, *121*
Barry Lane s. Hsia, S. L. *860*
Barták, P. 796, *846*
Bartholomew, G. A., u. W. R. Dawson 1001, *1015*
— s. Howell, T. R. *1020*
Bartsch 804
Bartsch, G. E., s. Insull jr., W. *860*
Baruch, M., s. Küttner, H. *848*
Basset, F., R. Mallet u. J. Turiaf 117, *121*
— u. C. Nézelof 117, *121*, 883, *908*
— u. J. Turiaf 117, *121*, 883, *908*
— s. Turiaf, J. 140, *910*
Bates, R. W., s. Juhn, M. *1021*
Batzenschlager, A., u. Oberling, Fr. *848*
Bauer-Feulgen 886
Baumann 792, *845*
Baumann, R. 802, 803, 804, *846*
Bauman, W. A., s. Sant'Agnese, P. A. di *911*
Baumberger, J. P., V. Suntzeff u. E. V. Cowdry 5, *121*
Baumgartner, W., u. G. Riva 795, 802, 803, 804, 805, 820, 830, 832, 833, 835, 838, 839, 840, 841, *843*
— u. G. Riva, s. Leinati, F. *858*
Bazex, A. 871, *903*
— u. A. Dupré 794, 837, 845, 857, 871, 886, *903, 911*
— s. Calvet, J. *903*
Bazin, A. T. 901, *919*
Bear, R., u. H. Rugo 371, *374*
Bear, R. S. 440, 448, *483*
Beau, A., s. Grimaud, R. *853*
Beaufay, H., s. Duve, C. de *126*
— s. Novikoff, A. B. *134*
Bechtel, H. B. 988, *1015*
Beck, F., u. L. Wifling 873, *903*
Beck, S. C. 794, *845*
Becker, H. 758, *784*
Becker, J. 455, 458, 459, *483*
Becker, J. F., u. H. T. H. Wilson 872, *903*

Becker, L. A., s. Ginsberg, J. E. *919*
Becker, R. 1014, *1015*
Becker, S. K., T. G. Fitzpatrick u. H. Montgomery 691, *705*
Becker, S. W. 104, 106, *121*, 892, *912*
— s. Reuter, M. J. *905*
Becker jr., S. W., T. B. Fitzpatrick u. H. Montgomery 5, 104, 105, 106, 107, 114, *121, 912*
— u. A. A. Zimmermann 387, *423*, 639, *677, 912*
— s. Fitzpatrick, T. B. *127, 913*
— s. Zimmermann, A. A. 142, 429, 682, *915*
Becker, V. 283, *330*
— u. J. Reitinger 286, *330*
— s. Fitzpatrick, T. B. *913*
Beckett, E. B., G. H. Bourne u. W. Montagna 226, 262, 263, 365, 367, *374*, 513, 613, 664, 676, *677*
— s. Montagna, W. *133*
Beckmann, A., s. Schridde, H. *786*
Beerman, H., s. Solomon, L. M. *861*
— s. Wood, M. G. *338. 905*
Behnke, O. 303, *330*
Behrens, M., s. Feulgen, R. *127*
Behring, Fr. 794, *845*
Behrmann, H. T. *178*
Beierwaltes, W. H. 877, *906*
Bejdl, W. 435, *483*
Bélanger, L. F. 177, *179*
Belber, J. P., s. Epstein, E. *919*
Bell, Malt u. Stewart 1007
Bell, E., u. Y. T. Thathachari 1007, *1016*
— s. Malt, R. A. *1023*
Bellairs, A. d'A., u. G. Underwood *1016*
Bellerby, C. W., s. Young, J. Z. *1028*
Bellin, D. E., s. Brody, J. *911*
Bellmann, S. B., u. E. Vercander *615*
Bellocq, Ph. 494, 497, 515, 563, 569, 570, 571, 572, 575, 576, 580, 590, 602, 609, 613, *615*, 621, 622
Belote, G. H., u. D. G. Welton 885, *908*
Bénard, P., s. Jausion, H. *847*
Benditt, E. P., R. L. Wong, M. Arase u. E. Roeper 437, *483*
— s. Combs, J. W. *484*
— s. Ross, R. 488, *1033*

Benefenati, A., s. Brillanti, F. 705
Beneke, G., s. Knoth, W. 851
— s. Kuntz, E. 851
Benett, s. Robertis, de 382
Benett, H. S., s. De Robertis, E. 424
Benfenfenati, A., u. F. Brillanti 184, 185, 191, 220
Bengoechea, M. E., s. Jabonero, V., u. A. Perez-Casas 425
Bennett, H. S. 70, 72, 121, 541, 615, 955, 1016
— J. H. Luft u. J. C. Hampton 529, 539, 615
Benninghoff, A. 454, 471, 479, 483, 499, 523, 524, 534, 535, 536, 548, 550, 554, 558, 613, 615
— A. Hartmann u. T. Hellman 615
Bennink, P. J. H., s. Burgers, A. C. J. 1016
Benoit, C. da Lage, s. Texier-Vidal, A. 1027
Benoit, F. L. 828, 860
Bensch, K. G., s. Gerald, G. B. 484
— s. Gordon, G. B. 485
Bensley, S. H. 450, 451, 452, 453, 483, 875, 906
Bentley, J. P., s. Jackson, D. S. 486
— u. W. F. C. Blumer 989, 1016
— u. K. Schmidt-Nielsen 987, 1016
Berblinger 809
Berg 884
Berg, S. 772, 782
Berg, St. 785
Berg, St. P. 783
Bergeder, H. D., s. Taschen, B. 785
Bergen, F. v. 278, 330
Berger, A. J. 1003, 1016
Bergman, R. A., s. Goodman, R. M. 911
Bergstrand, H. 796, 846
Berk, M., s. Epstein, E. 919
Berkowitz, D. 827, 855
Berlin, L. B., u. I. G. Pridvizhkin 631, 638, 659, 677
— s. Pridvizhkin, I. G. 681
Bern, Ellias, Powers u. Harkness 44
Bern, H. A. 177, 179
— M. Alfert u. S. M. Blair 69, 121
— J. J. Ellias, P. B. Pickett, T. R. Powers u. M. N. Harkness 71, 121
— D. R. Harkness u. S. M. Blair 179

Bern, H. A., s. Harkness, D. R. 180
— s. Kobayashi, A. 1021
Bernard, C. 76, 121
Bernardi, de, s. Tovo 729
Berndt, H., u. W. Friedrichs 802, 846
Berndt, J. 782
Berner, s. Huger 854
Berner u. Heyde 830, 855
Bernhard, W., s. Smetana, H. F. 849
Bernhardt, R. 879, 906
Bernstein, E. 845
Bernstein, E. T. 899, 917
Bernstein, I. A. 47, 63, 67, 68, 69, 70, 121
— s. Fukuyama, K. 127, 128
Bernstein, J. C., s. Kétron 851
Bernuth, F. v. 883, 908
Berres, H. H. 563, 615, 684, 685, 686, 691, 693, 696, 705
Bersaques, J. de., u. S. Rothman 121
Bertamino, R., E. Rampini u. C. Ruffini 581, 621
Berthelet, L., s. Duwe, C. de 780
Berthet, J. 294, 330
— u. C. de Duve 97, 121
Bertin 957
Bertram, E. G., s. Barr, M. L. 781
Besjedkin, s. Kapacinsky 759
Besnier, E. 872, 903
— u. F. Balzer 872, 903
Best, E. W., H. L. Mason, J. W. de Weerd u. D. C. Dahlin 805, 846
Bettge, S., s. Knoth, W. 854
Bettmann, S. 468, 483, 494, 496, 497, 530, 609, 610, 615
Bevelander, G., s. Johnson, P. L. 181
Bhattacharyya, B., s. Chowdhuri, S. 179
Bhowmick 948
Bianchi, L. 491, 553, 610, 615
Bideau, J., s. Sabrazés, J. 856
Bieber, Ph. 899, 917
Biedermann, W. 920, 930, 938, 970, 983, 1006, 1016
Biegert, J. 920, 1029
Biempica, L., u. L. F. Montes 268, 277, 287, 294, 296, 299, 300, 318, 323, 324, 326, 327, 330
Bierman, S. M., s. Winer, L. H. 908
Bikle, D., L. G. Tilney u. K. R. Porter 964, 966, 1016
Billingham, R. E. 104, 105, 106, 107, 113, 121, 912
— R. Mangold u. W. K. Silvers 1030

Billingham, R. E. u. P. B. Medawar 5, 104, 105, 106, 107, 110, 116, 121, 642, 677, 891, 912
— u. J. Reynolds 5, 121
— u. W. K. Silvers 5, 104, 105, 106, 113, 116, 121, 677, 678, 912
— s. Haller jr., A. J. 617
Bimts, K. N. 581, 597, 621
Binding 764, 784
Binkley, J. S. 801, 802, 835, 846, 857
Birbeck, H., s. Baker, R. V. 120
Birbeck, M. S. C. 31, 38, 44, 107, 109, 110, 113, 115, 121, 146, 147, 179, 912
— u. N. A. Barnicot 104, 110, 112, 113, 121, 891, 912
— A. S. Breathnach u. J. D. Everall 107, 108, 109, 116, 117, 118, 119, 121, 883, 891, 908, 909, 912
— u. E. H. Mercer 51, 75, 121, 122, 146, 149, 150, 152, 154, 155, 156, 179, 891, 912
— — u. N. A. Barnicot 104, 122, 147, 179
— s. Barnicot, N. A. 120, 121, 912
— s. Breathnach, A. S. 220, 912
— s. Seiji, M. 137
— s. Seiji, M., u. T. B. Fitzpatrick 915
— s. Seiji, M., T. B. Fitzpatrick u. R. T. Simpson 915
— s. Seiji, M., K. Shimao u. T. B. Fitzpatrick 915
Birk, Y., u. C. H. Li 827, 855
Bittar, E. O., s. Ferreira-Marques, J. 610
Bizzozero, E., u. M. Dogliotti 690, 705
Björntorp, P., B. Hood, A. Martinsson u. B. Persson 828, 860
Black, M. M., s. Zweifach, B. W. 142
Blackberg, S. N., s. Laidlaw, G. F. 131
Blackstad, Th. W. 920, 936, 937, 938, 940, 1016
Blair, S. M., s. Bern, H. A. 121, 179
Blair s. Horkness 177
Blake, H. A., E. M. Goyette, C. S. Lyter u. H. Swan 831, 855
Blanc 794, 795, 841
Blanc, W. A. 806, 808, 830, 843

Bland, E. F., s. Grant, R. T. 610, 617
Blaschko, A. 5, 43, 46, *122*, 465, *483*
Blaschko, H., s. Baker, R. V. *120*
Blattgerste, H. 824, *853*
Blazso, S. *780*
Blechschmidt, E. 474, 475, 476, *483*, 642, 643, 644, 661, *678*
Blinzinger, K., u. N. Matussek 446, 451, *483*
Bloch, Br. 1, 74, 103, 104, 105, 106, *122*
Bloch, B., u. P. Ryhiner *912*
Bloch, N. 891, *912*
Block, P., I. Seiter u. W. Oehlert *1032*
Block, R. J. *122*
Block, W. D., s. Rukavina, J. G. *866*
Blocker jr., T. G., s. Washburn jr., W. W. *141*
Bloom, G., u. J. W. Kelly 437, *483*
— s. Adams-Ray, J. *482*
Bloomberg, R., s. Hambrick jr., G. W. *679*
Bluefarb, S. M., s. Szymanski, F. J. *855*
— H. H. Rodin u. L. Hoit 898, *917*
Blum 759, *784*
Blum, A., J. Gafni, E. Sohar, S. Shibolet u. H. Heller *866*
— s. Sohar, E. *866*
Blumer, W. F. C., s. Bentley, P. J. *1016*
Boardman, W. *1030*
Boas, J. 339, *374*
Boas, J. E. V. 920, *1016*
Boas, L. C., s. Collen, W. S. *847*
Boas, N. F., s. Bollet, A. J. *906*
Bochud, J. M. 474, 475, 476, 478, *483*
Bock, H. E. 796, 808, 809, 811, 836, *846*, *850*, *857*
Bode, H. G., s. Riecke, E. *903*
Bodenheimer, T. S., s. Robertson, J. D. *1025*
Bodur, H., s. Favarger, P. *844*
Böhm, E. 775, *785*
Böhmer, K. *782*
Boeke, J. 383, 398, 406, 413, *423*, 564, *615*, 933, 934, *1016*
Boerner-Patzelt, D. 819, *853*
Boersma, D., u. B. L. Barker 896, *917*
Bogenschütz, H. 978, *1016*
Bogert, C. M. 994, *1016*
Bohne, G. 747, *782*

Bohnstedt, R. M. 836, *843*
Boido, V., s. Moretti, G. *182*
Bois, I., s. Sylvén, B. *140*
Boissonas, R. A. 949, *1016*
— s. Guttmann, S. *1019*
Bojlén, K., u. S. Petry 807, *846*
Bojowa, E., u. A. Dziedziuszko 883, *909*
Boldt, A. 814, 815, 885, *850*, *909*
Bolgert u. R. Amado 901, *919*
Bolk, L., E. Göppert, E. Kallius, W. Lubosch s. Boas, J. E. V. *1016*
Boller, R. 804, *846*
Bollet, A. J., N. F. Boas u. J. J. Bonin 875, *906*
Bolognani Fantin, A. M. 942, *1016*
Boltz, W. 761, *784*
Boman, K. 411, *423*
Bommer, S. 893, *915*
Bond, V. P., s. Cronkite, F. P. *125*
Bone, Q. 924, 925, 926, 927, 940, *1016*
Bonicelli, U., u. R. Tagliavini 796, *846*
Bonin, J. J., s. Bollet, A. J. *906*
Bonnet, R. 378, 401, *423*
Bonneville, M. A. 628, *678*
Bonnyns, M. 877, *906*
Bontke, E., s. Gedigk, P. *332*
Borcea, M. E. 387, *423*
Borda, J. M., J. Abulafia u. F. Cardenas 880, *906*
Bordley *494*
Bordley, J., M. H. Grow u. W. B. Sherman 494, 531, 610, *615*
Borello, P. *610*
Borges, P. R. F., s. Fishman, W. H. *127*
Born 740, *782*
Born, S., s. Herxheimer *127*
Bornstein, F. *785*
Borodach, G. N., u. W. Montagna 163, *179*, *1030*
Borrie, P. 881, *909*
Borsetto, P. L. 267, *330*, 657, 664, *678*
Borst, M., u. H. Königsdörffer 893, *915*
Bosch, K. 775, *785*
— u. F. R. Keller *782*
Bosellini, J. L. 872, *903*
Boss, M. B., s. Herrmann, H. *913*
Bosse, K., s. Bandmann, H.-J. *178*
Boström, H., E. Odeblad u. U. Friberg 79, *122*

Botezat, E. 378, *423*, 1005, *1016*
Bourget 778, *786*
Bourlond, A. 357, 358, 360, 374, 378, *423*
— u. R. K. Winkelmann 415, *423*
— s. Dupont, A. 375, *424*
— s. Leloup, R. 375, *426*
Bourne, E. J., s. Haworth, W. N. *129*
Bourne, G., s. Beckett, E. *374*
Bourne, G. H. *337*
— u. H. B. Tewari 55, 57, 86, 88, *122*, 277, 278, 299, *330*
— s. Beckett, E. B. *263*, 613, *677*
— s. Brandes, D. *330*
— s. Shantharcerappa *427*, *1031*
Bowen, R. H. 110, 112, *122*, 195, *220*
Bowmann, s. Tood 612, 622, *623*
Boyd 823, *853*
Boyd, E. 516, *613*
Braasch, N. K., u. M. J. Nickson 497, *610*
Brachet, B. *780*
Brachet, J. 69, 72, *122*, 364, *374*
— u. A. E. Mirsky *335*
Brachet-Mirsky, s. Novikoff, A. B. *914*
Brachetto-Brian, D., s. Cibils Aguirre, R. *846*
— s. Jorge, J. K. *909*
Brack, E. 695, *705*
Bradfield, J. R. G. 76, 78, *122*
— s. Gibbons, I. R. *128*
Bradley, H. C. *780*
Bradley, H. T., s. Noble, G. K. *1023*
Bradshaw *527*
Bradshaw, M., M. Wachstein, J. Spence u. J. M. Elias 96, 99, 115, 119, 120, *122*, 539, *615*
Brady, L. W., s. Enterline, H. T. *853*
Branca, A. 697, *705*
Branca, P. A. 273, 275, 279, *330*
Brancati, R. 804, *846*
— s. Giordano *847*
— s. Gohrbandt *847*
Brandau, H., u. D. Pette 316, *330*
— s. Pette, D. *335*
Brandes, D., u. G. H. Bourne 278, *330*
Brandsma, C. H. 809, *850*
— A. W. M. Pompen u. H. J. Weyers *850*

Brandt, P. W., s. Hackenbrock, C. R. 264
Brandt, W., s. Greenwalt, C. H. *1019*
Branson, H. R., s. Pauling, L., u. R. B. Corey 134
Branwood, A. W. 434, *483*
Braun, W., u. H. Weyhbrecht 871, *903*
Braun-Falco *183*
Braun-Falco, F., s. Braun-Falco, O. *909*
Braun-Falco, O. 2, 3, 11, 15, 17, 18, 20, 21, 23, 31, 37, 45, 51, 55, 56, 58, 66, 67, 69, 75, 76, 77, 78, 79, 81, 82, 83, 85, 86, 87, 88, 90, 91, 92, 93, 95, 96, 97, 100, 101, 102, *122*, 145, 162, 163, 169, 172, 175, 176, *179*, 201, 202, *220*, 235, 236, 241, 242, 248, 253, *263*, *264*, 307, 309, 318, 322, 325, *330*, 364, *374*, 447, 448, 449, 453, 462, 463, 474, 481, *483*, 526, 537, 538, 550, *615*, 685, 693, 720, 732, *780*, 787, 806, 808, 840, *843*, *846*, *857*, 862, 869, 872, 873, 874, 875, 877, 878, 880, *903*, *906*, *1030*
— u. F. Braun-Falco 883, *909*
— u. O. Frenz 163, *179*, *1030*
— u. A. Kint 158, 159, 163, *179*, *182*
— — u. W. Vogell 49, *122*
— A. Langner u. E. Christophers 79, 80, *122*
— u. G. Petry 3, 31, 35, 38, 40, *122*, *123*
— u. D. Petzold 56, 87, 88, 89, 90, 102, 103, *123*, 174, 176, 179, 241, *264*, 311, 318, *331*, 498, 526, 537, 550, *610*, *615*, *783*
— u. B. Rassner 163, *179*, *331*
— u. B. Rathjens 2, 66, 87, 88, 89, 90, 102, *123*, 170, 176, *179*, 235, 241, 248, *264*, 481, *483*, 526, *615*
— u. M. Rupec 98, 99, *123*
— u. K. Salfeld 437, *483*
— u. H. Theisen 163, *179*, *1030*
— u. W. Vogell 31, 38, 40, *123*
— u. G. Weber 5, 23, 78, 79, 80, 81, 84, 85, *123*, *135*
— u. W. Winter 81, *123*, 286, *331*, 720, 721, 732, *780*, *781*
— u. H. Zaun 163, *179*

Braun-Falco, O., s. Keining, E. 851, 907, 909
— s. Marghescu, S. *132*
— s. Petzoldt, D. 335
— s. Rassner, B. *182*
— s. Renaut, J. *907*
— s. Rupec, M. 137
— s. Seckfort, H. *910*
— s. Winter, W. 338
— s. Winzler, R. J. *908*
— s. Witzel, M. *183*
Braus, H. 466, 470, *483*
Braus u. Elze 478, 481
Braus, H., u. C. Elze 548, *615*, *616*
Bray, G. A., s. Galton, D. J. *860*
Breathnach, A. S. 3, 104, 105, 109, 116, 117, 118, 119, *123*, *912*
— M. S. Birbeck u. J. D. Everall 195, *220*, 891, *912*
— T. B. Fitzpatrick u. L.-M.-A. Wyllie *912*, *913*
— u. D. P. Goodwin *913*
— D. Goodwin u. L. M.-A. Wyllie 104, 108, 117, *123*
— u. L. M.-A. Wyllie 11, 25, 26, 38, 58, 104, 117, *123*
— u. L. M. Wyllie 627, 628, 676, *678*, *913*
— s. Birbeck, M. S. C. *121*, 908, 909, *912*
— s. Fitzpatrick, T. B. *127*, *913*
Breese jr., S. S., s. Edd jr., M. V., u. P. R. Sweeny *1017*
— s. Hama, K. *1019*
Breitenecker 779
Breitenecker, L., u. G. Niebauer 901, *903*, *919*
Bremme 759, *784*
Brenker 765
Breschet, G., u. A. Roussel de Vouzeme 224, *264*
Breuckmann, H. 794, *845*
Breyer, H. 989, 996, *1016*
Brezhenke, A. I. 815, 837, *850*, *857*
Briggs, G. W. 862, *901*
Brillanti, F., u. A. Benefenati 695, *705*
— s. Benfenati, A. *220*
Brim, J., s. Demis, D. J. *610*
Brinckmann, A. 1006, *1016*
Brines, O. A., u. M. H. Johnson 821, 824, *853*
Brinkman, A. 220, *220*
Brinkmann, A. 267, 268, 275, 277, *331*
Brochyla 747
Brocq, L. 823, *853*
Brodal, A., u. R. Fänge, s. Blackstad, Th. W. *1016*
— — s. Peters, A. *1024*

Brodie, A. F., u. J. S. Gots 89, *123*
Brodthagen, A. 899, *917*
Brody, I. 2, 3, 4, 8, 9, 10, 11, 12, 13, 14, 16, 17, 18, 19, 20, 21, 22, 23, 24, 25, 26, 27, 28, 29, 30, 31, 32, 33, 34, 35, 36, 37, 38, 39, 40, 41, 42, 43, 44, 45, 46, 47, 49, 51, 52, 53, 54, 55, 56, 57, 58, 59, 60, 63, 68, 75, 76, 78, 83, 84, 111, *123*, 299, *331*
— u. D. E. Bellin 887, *911*
— u. K. S. Larsson 11, 20, 31, 34, 35, 38, 40, 49, *124*, 629, *678*
Bronks, D., s. Gillman, Th. *904*
Brophy, D., s. Dobson, R. L. *264*
— s. Lobitz jr., W. C. *221*
— s. Lobitz, W. C., u. J. B. Holyoke 265
— s. Pass, F. *680*
Browases, s. Veslot *910*
Brown, G. E. 534, *616*
— u. H. Z. Giffin 533, *616*
— u. G. M. Roth 533, *616*
— u. C. Sheard 533, *616*
Brown, G. W., s. Glenner, G. G. *128*
Brown, H., s. Schamberg, J. Fr. *781*
Brown, M. E. 963, *1016*
Brown u. Danielli 22
Bruce-Jones, D. B. S. 885, *909*
Brühl, L. 943, *1016*
Brünauer, s. Baumann *845*
Brünauer, St. R. 792, *845*
Brüster, H., s. Stüttgen, G. *1027*
Bruhas, F. 339, *374*
Bruinsma, W. 814, *860*
Brun, R., K. Enderlin u. A. de Weck 187, 188, *220*
— s. Grasset, N. *221*
Brunck, J. 853
Brunet, P., s. Fitzpatrick *127*
Brunet, T. B., s. Fitzpatrick, F. B., u. A. Kukita *913*
Brunish, R., s. Marchmann, A. *1030*
Brunner, H. 76, *124*
Brunner, H. E. 895, *916*
Brusilow, S. W., s. Munger, B. L. 265, *335*
— s. Munger, B. L., u. R. E. Cooke 265
Bschor, F. 715, *780*
Btoian 384
Bubis, J. J., s. Wolman, H. *903*
Bublitz, C., s. Lynen, F. *844*

Bucciante, G., s. Gasparini, F. 613
Bucciante, L. 495, 551, *610*, *616*
Buchanan, T. J., s. Walls, E. W. *612*, *620*
Bucher, O. 445, 447, 481, *483*
Budker, P. 946, 956, *1016*
— s. Petit, G. *1024*
Bücher, Th., s. Pette, D. 335
Büchner, F. 780
Buettner-Janusch, V., s. Lee, T. H. *1022*
Bugyi, G. 808, *846*
Buhtz, G., u. Ehrhardt *784*
Buley, H. M., u. M. H. Kulwin 901, *919*
Bulliard, H., s. Giroud, A. *128*, *180*
— s. Giraud, A., u. C. P. Leblond *128*, *180*
Bullock, T. H., u. F. P. J. Diecke 995, *1016*
Bullough, W. S. 64, 65, *124*, 1014, *1016*
— C. L. Hewett u. E. B. Laurence 65, *124*, *1032*
— u. M. Johnsen 64, *124*
— u. E. B. Laurence 65, *124*, 145, 161, 162, *179*, 1014, *1016*, *1032*
— u. I. Rytömaa 64, 65, 66, *124*
Bunting, H. 469, *483*
— G. B. Wislocki u. E. W. Dempsey 230, 237, 238, 241, 261, *264*, 277, 278, 279, 310, 323, *331*, 482, *484*
— s. Wislocki, G. B. *142*, *490*, *620*
Burch, G. E., u. J. H. Phillips *483*
— s. Hibbs, R. G. *611*, *617*
Burckhardt, W., s. Miescher, G. *852*
Bureau, Y., A. Jarry, H. Barriere, J. P. Kerneis u. P. Bruneau 803, *860*
Burgers, A. C. J., P. J. H. Bennink u. G. J. van Oordt 948, 950, *1016*
Burgess, G. H. O. *1016*
Burgi, E. 778, *786*
Burgos, M. H., s. Fawcett, D. W. 332
Burgun, F., s. Apffel, K. *846*
— s. Roederer, J. *852*, *910*
Buris, L. *783*
Burk, D., s. Du Buy, H. G. *125*
Burkholder, P., s. Klein, P. *902*
Burkl, W. 875, *906*
Burne u. Tewari 98

Burneau, P., s. Bureau, Y. *860*
Burnett, J. W., s. Pathak, M. A. *916*
Burns, F. S. 881, *909*
Burrows, H. 635, *678*
Burrows, M. 349, *374*
Burrows, W., s. Arey, L. B. *613*
Burstone, M. S. 85, 87, 90, 92, 96, 100, *124*
— s. Dannenberg, A. M. *484*
Burtner, H. J., s. Glenner, G. G. *128*
Burton, A. C. 492, *610*
Burton, J. F. 556, *616*
Buschke, A., u. A. Matthissohn 838, *857*
Buschke, W. 282, *331*
Busman, G. J., u. A. R. Woodburne 898, *917*
Butcher, E. O. 162, 163, *179*, *1030*
— u. A. W. Grokoest 163, *179*
— s. Johnson, P. L. *181*
Butler, J., u. C. W. Laymon 879, *906*
Butt, H. R., u. R. M. Wilder 895, *916*
Butterworth, T., s. Shelley, W. B. *336*
Buttge, U. 466, 467, *483*, 691, *705*
Butz 766
Byon, S. *678*

Cabré, J., u. G. W. Korting 880, *906*
Cabrini, R. L., u. F. A. Carranza jr. *1032*
— s. Carranza jr., F. A. *616*, *1032*
Caesar, R. 720, *780*, 864, *901*
— s. Letterer, E. *902*
Caeteaud, A., s. Gougerot, H. *918*
Cahill jr., G. F., u. A. E. Renold 787, *843*
— s. Renold, A. E. *843*
— u. A. E. Renold, s. Wassermann, F. *857*
Cahn, M. M., u. W. B. Shelley 284, *331*
— s. Shelley, W. B. *336*
Cain, A. J. 198, *220*
Čajkovac, Š. 898, *917*
Calahan, W. P., s. Sutherland, J. C. *855*
Calkins, E., u. A. S. Cohen 865, *901*
— s. Cohen, A. S. 865, *901*
— s. Cohen, A. S., u. C. I. Levene 865, *901*
— s. Lerner *914*
Callahan, u. Campbell 824, *853*

Calman, K. C., s. Baillie, A. H. *220*
Calmann, A. 833, *857*
— u. H. Haber 805, *846*
Calnan, C. D., s. Wighley, J. E. M. *850*
— s. Wigley, J. G. M. *857*
Calvet, J., A. Bazex, A. Dupré, A. Ribet u. G. Hemous 871, *903*
Cameron, G. R., u. K. C. B. Mallik 831, *855*
— u. R. D. Senevivatne 827, *855*
Cameron, I. L., u. R. E. Smith 459, *484*
Cameron, M. P., s. Reuck, A. S. V. de *331*, *335*
Cameron, R. 289, *331*
Campbell, s. Callahan 824, *853*
Campbell, A. W., s. Goldblum, R. W. *128*, *180*
Campbell, G. L., s. Sutherland, J. C. *855*
Campbell, J. A. A. 830, *855*
Camps, Fr. E., u. E. G. Evans *782*
Candaele, D., s. Kint, A. *907*
Caneghem, P. van 272, 273, 275, *331*, 697, *705*
— s. Spier, H. W. *138*, *183*
Capanna, E., u. M. V. Civitelli *423*
Caplan, R. M., s. McCusker, J. J. *904*
Carasso, N., u. P. Favard 299, *331*
Carboneschi, s. Oboglio *785*
Cardell, M. W., u. E. H. Hanley 811, *850*
Cardell jr., R. R., s. Hu, F. *130*
Cardenas, F., s. Borda, J. M. *906*
Cardis, F., u. M. Conte 900, *918*
Carelia, A. *784*
Carnes, W. H., u. B. R. Forker 863, *901*
Caro, M. R., s. Zeisler, E. P. *911*
Carol, W. L. L. 879, *906*
— J. R. Pracken u. H. A. v. Zwijndregt 796, 797, 798, 800, 801, 802, 808, *846*
Caron, G. A., s. Sarkany, I. *266*
Carossini, G. 269, 270, *331*
Carranza, F. A., u. R. L. Cabrini 559, *616*, *1032*
— s. Cabrini, R. L. *1032*
Carrier, E. B. 530, 533, *616*
Carter, G. S. 967, *1016*
Cascos, A. 899, 900, *917*, *918*

Case, J. D., s. Lerner, A. B., u. R. V. Heinzelman 1022
Casella 886
Casper-Liman 784
Caspersson, T., u. J. Schultz 69, 124
Caspersson, T. O. 47, 124, 364, 374
Cassebohm, J. F. 493, 610
Castagnoli, E., u. M. Frei-Sulzer 729, 781
Castigli, C., u. A. Moriconi 509, 511, 613
Catchpole, H. R., s. Gersh, J. 484, 485, 617, 906
Cate, J. ten 996, 1016
Cattaneo, s. Oboglio 785
Caulfield, J. B., u. G. F. Wilgram 4, 35, 36, 124
— s. Wilgram, G. F., u. W. F. Lever 141
— s. Wilgram, G. F., u. E. B. Madgic 141
Cauna, N. 357, 365, 367, 374, 377, 400, 414, 418, 419, 423, 469, 484, 566, 516, 675, 678
— u. G. Mannan 400, 412, 423
— u. L. L. Ross 417, 418, 419, 423
Causey, G. 674, 678
Cavazzana, P. 272, 329, 331, 553, 616
Ceelen, W. 879, 882, 906, 909
Cereijido, M., u. P. F. Curran 981, 1016
— s. Curran, P. F. 1017
Ceresa, F. 636, 639, 678
Cerutti, P. 809, 850
— u. G. Santoianni 850
Chaffee, E., s. Meyer, K. 844
Chain u. Duthie 906
Chambers, R., u. G. S. Rényi 36, 124
— u. B. W. Zweifach 495, 541, 602, 610, 616, 622
Champetier, G., u. A. Litvac 18, 21, 30, 37, 50, 124
— s. Giroud, A. 128, 375
Chanial, G. 899, 917
Chapman, G. H., u. A. B. Dawson 973, 1016
Charipper, H. A., s. Ratzersdorfer, C. 1025
Charles, A. 37, 44, 49, 124, 148, 155, 156, 179, 204, 205, 220, 237, 238, 241, 264, 287, 292, 293, 299, 301, 302, 304, 325, 327, 331, 423, 1030
— u. J. T. Ingram 104, 105, 107, 109, 124, 892, 913
— u. F. G. Smiddy 35, 37, 58, 124
Charpy, s. Nové-Josserand, L. 918

Chase, H. B. 145, 162, 163, 179
— u. G. J. Eaton 179, 1030
— W. Montagna u. J. D. Malone 163, 179
— H. Rauch u. V. W. Smith 158, 179
— s. Eisen, A. Z. 126, 180
— s. Lyne, A. G. 131
— s. Montagna, W. 181, 376, 914
— s. Montagna, W., u. H. B. Chase 181
— s. Montagna, W., A. Z. Eisen u. A. H. Rademacher 133, 181, 222, 334
— s. Montagna, W., u. J. B. Hamilton 133, 181, 334
— s. Montagna, W., u. W. C. Lobitz 133, 265, 334
— s. Montagna, W., J. D. Malone u. H. P. Melaragno 181
— s. Montagna, W., u. H. P. Melaragno 181
— s. Shipman, M. 183
— s. Straile, W. E. 1031
Chase, N. 484
Chase, W. H. 323, 331, 456, 484
Chason, J. L., s. Landers, J. W. 623
Chatfield, P. O., C. P. Lyman u. L. Irving 1001, 1016
Chen, J., s. Katsuki, Y. 1021
Chèvremont, M., u. J. Frédéric 70, 71, 72, 124, 370, 372, 374
— s. Frédéric, J. 484
Chiale, C. 494, 516, 563, 610, 613, 616
Chiari 782
— s. Luschka 781
Chiari, H. 882, 909
Chiarugi, G. 499, 613
Chitwood, M. J., s. Halstead, B. W. 1019
Chlopin, N. G. 627, 678
Chorzelski, T., s. Jablonska, St. 907
Chowdhuri, S., u. B. Bhattacharyya 148, 179
Christophers, E., u. A. M. Kligman 21, 29, 125
— s. Braun-Falco, O. 122
Chu, C. H. U. 1032, 1033
Chung, D., s. Li, C. H. 1022
Churg, J., u. L. Strauss 809, 811, 850
Cibils-Aguirre, R., u. D. Brachetto-Brian 796, 797, 846
Cioban, V. 743, 782
Cistjakov, N. 832, 857
Civatte, A., s. Darier, J. 616

Civatte, J. 901, 919
Civitelli, M. V., s. Capanna, E. 423
Claessens, F. L. E., s. Cormane, R. H. 125, 180
Clara, M. 191, 220, 220, 444, 484, 495, 507, 510, 511, 513, 551, 552, 553, 554, 555, 556, 610, 613, 616, 640, 678, 1004, 1005, 1016
Clark, E. R. 500, 613
— u. E. L. Clark 511, 551, 613, 616
Clark, E. L., s. Clark, E. R. 613, 616
Clark, N. B., s. Kaltenbach, J. C. 1021
Clark, R. T., s. Wilks, S. S. 786
Clark, W., s. Hibbs, R. 375
— s. Hibbs, R. G. 129
Clark jr., W. H., u. R. G. Hibbs 104, 107, 108, 109, 110, 111, 112, 117, 125
— s. Eisen, A. Z. 126
— s. Roth, S. I. 136, 1030
Claude Bernard, M. 631, 678
Clemmesen, T. 559, 616
Cockerell, J., s. Freeman, R. G. 705
Cockett, F. B., s. Dodd, H. 616, 621
Codaccioni, J. M., s. Appaix, A. 850
Cogan, D. G. 558, 616
— s. Kuwabara, T. 623
Cohen 836, 860
Cohen, A. S., u. E. H. Calkins 864, 865, 901
— H. Calkins u. C. I. Levene 863, 901
— s. Calkins, E. 865, 901
Cohen, C. 50, 125
Cohen, D. M., s. Rony, H. R. 136
Cohen, J. 1030
— u. P. G. Expinasse 1005, 1017
Cohen, L. A., s. Glenner, G. 485
Cohen, R. B., s. Seligman, A. M. 137
Cohen, S. 1014, 1017
Cohen, S. B., s. Shelley, W. B. 138, 183, 223, 336
Cohnheim, J. 384, 424
Cole, F. J. 939, 1017
Collen, W. S., L. C. Boas, J. D. Zilinsky u. J. J. Greenwald 804, 847
Collignon 744, 782
Collin, R. 978, 1017
Combs, J. W., D. Lagunoff u. E. P. Benditt 438, 484
Comel, M. 491, 517, 529, 530, 533, 610, 616, 704, 705

Comel, M., u. E. Urian 529, 608, *616*, *623*
Comfort u. Osterberg 836, *860*
Connor, W. H. 815, *850*, 885, *909*
Conrads, H., s. Pau, H. *427*
Conte, M., s. Cardis, F. *918*
Contino 268, 273, 274, *331*
Conventry, M. B., s. Winkelmann, R. K. *623*, *1030*
Converse, J. M., u. D. L. Ballantyne 558, 559, 560, 562, *616*
— u. F. T. Rapaport 559, *616*
— s. Ballantyne jr., D. L. *615*
Conway, H. 559, *616*
— D. Joslin, T. D. Rees u. R. B. Stark 559, *616*
Cooke, R. E., s. Munger, B. L., u. S. W. Brusilow *265*
Cooper 154
Cooper, J. H. 462, *484*
Cooper, Z. K. 636, *678*, 683, 704, *705*
— s. Thuringer, J. M. *140*
Copps, L. A., s. Pinkus, H. *910*
Cordero, A. A., u. R. N. Corti *857*
Corey, R. B., u. L. Pauling *125*
— s. Pauling, L. *134*
— s. Pauling, L., u. H. R. Branson *134*
Corfield, M. C., A. Robson u. B. Skinner *125*
Cori, C. F., s. Cori, G. T. *125*
Cori, G. T., u. C. F. Cori 91, *125*
Cormane, R. H., u. F. L. E. Claessens 90, 91, *125*, *176*, *180*
Cormane, R. H. G., u. G. L. Kalsbeek 99, 119, *125*, *176*, *180*
Cormia, F. E. 165, 169, *180*, 495, 572, 575, 581, 583, 584, 586, 588, 593, 594, 606, *621*, 700, *705*
— u. A. Ernyey 498, 522, 523, 538, 550, 572, 575, 581, 583, 584, 586, 588, 589, 594, 606, *610*, *616*, *621*, *622*
— s. Atkinson, S. *178*
Cornbleet, T. 329, *331*
Cornbleet, Th., u. H. Rattner 806, 833, *847*, *857*
— s. Zimmermann, A. A. *142*, *429*, *915*
Corti, R. N., s. Cordero, A. A. *857*
Coscia, s. Ricći *859*
Cosslett, V. E., A. Engstrom u. H. H. Patteeya *622*
Coste 800, *847*

Coste, F., B. Piguet u. F. Delbarre 873, *903*
Cottini, G. B. 891, *913*
— u. A. Sapuppo 800, *847*
Coventry, M., s. Winkelmann, R. *376*
Cowdry, E. V. 5, *125*, 450, *484*
— u. H. C. Thompson jr. 62, *125*
— s. Baumberger, J. P. *121*
— s. Evans, R. 705, *845*
— s. Ma, C. K. *706*
— s. Seno, S. *333*
Cowper, W. 493, *610*
Cox, J., s. Karrer, H. E. *486*
Cox, R. W. 821, *853*
Cox jr., A. J., s. Reaven, E. P. *136*
Craciun, E. C., u. J. Fagarasano 831, *855*
Craig, K. Mc., s. Farber
Crain, R. C., s. Herting, D. C. *856*, *858*
Cramer, D. L. 789, *844*
Cramer, H. J. 172, *180*, 537, *616*, 823, *853*
Crane, F. L. s Hatefi, Y. *129*
Criado, M. F. 899, *917*
Crick, F. H. C. 50, *125*
— s. Rich, A. *488*
Crips, D. J., s. Findlay, G. H. *904*
Crofford 787, *843*
Cronkite, E. P., V. P. Bond, T. M. Fliedner u. J. R. Rubin 63, *125*
Crosby, E. C., s. Ariëns Kappers *1015*
Crossland, P. M. 901, *919*
Crounse, R. G. 75, *125*
— u. E. J. van Scott 162, *180*
— s. Rothberg *136*
Crovato, F., u. E. Rampini 498, *610*
— s. Baccaredda-Boy, A., G. Moretti u. S. Zocchi *615*
— s. Moretti, G. 611, *618*, *623*
— s. Moretti, G., A. Rebora u. C. Giacometti *621*
Cruickshank, C. N. D., u. S. A. Harcourt 114, *125*
— s. Hell, E. A. *1032*
Cruse 833, 835, *857*
Cruz-Sobral, F., s. Meireles Pinto, M. I. *132*
Csepláк, G., s. Melczer, N. *132*
Csermely, E. 809, 811, *850*
Cservenka, I. 836, *857*
Cuckow, F. W., s. Barnicot, N. A. 120, *121*
Cuilleret, P., s. Nové-Josseraud, L. *918*

Culberson, J. D., s. Enterline, H. T. *853*
Culling, F. C., s. Vassar, P. S. *903*
Cummins *1029*
Cummins, L. J., u. W. F. Lever 802, *847*
Curey, J. H., s. Rukavina, J. G. *866*
Curran, P. F., u. M. Cereijido 981, *1017*
— u. J. R. Gill jr. 981, *1017*
— F. C. Herrera u. W. J. Flanigan 981, *1017*
— s. Cereijido, M. *1016*
— s. Herrera, F. C. *1020*
Curran, R. C., u. J. S. Kennedy 875, *906*
Curschmann, H. 899, *917*
Curtis, s. Baker 704
Curtis, A. C., s. Montes, L. F. *334*, *706*
— s. Rukavina, J. G. *866*
Custer, S., s. Pinkus, H. *910*
Czajewicz 791, *845*
Czopek, J. 976, *1017*

Dabelow, A. 455, 458, 482, *484*, 634, 635, 661, 662, 663, 698, *705*, *844*, *1028*
Dähn, W. 66, *125*
Daems, W. Th. 296, *331*
— u. J. P. Persijn 294, *331*, 451, *484*
Dahlin, D. C., s. Best, E. W. *846*
Dalton, A. J. 110, *125*
— u. M. D. Felix 57, *125*, 299, *331*
— s. Kuff, E. L. *333*
Dalton, H. C., s. Zimmermann, S. B. *1028*
Dalton, J. E., u. M. A. Seidell 879, *906*
Danda, J., u. V. Plachy 806, 835, *847*, *857*
Daniel 941, 942, 946
Daniel, C., Ph. D. Pease u. T. Andrews *424*
Daniel, P., s. Pritschard, M. *619*
Danielli 22
Daniels jr., F., s. Lobitz jr., W. C. *221*
Danielson, L., s. Ernster, L. *126*
Danneel, R. *125*, 654, *678*
— u. E. Lubnow 104, 110, 112, *125*
— u. H. Schumann 1010, *1017*
— u. N. Weissenfels 991, *1017*
Danneel, S. 948, *1017*

Dannenberg, A. M., M. S. Burstone, D. D. S. Paul, G. Walter u. J. W. Kinsley 435, *484*
Danner 747
Danziger, S., s. McKay, D. G. *680*
Darian-Smith, I., P. Mutton u. R. Proctor *424*
Darier, J. 494, 550, *610*
— A. Civatte, G. Flandin u. A. Tranck *616*
Dastur, D. 357, *375*
Datavo, L. *857*
Dathe, H. 1014, *1017*
D'Avanzo, A. 828, *855*
David, s. Korb 720
David, H. 284, 289, *331*
David, L. T. *331*
David, T., s. Dejenarui, I. *847*
Davidson, E. A., s. Sams, W. M. *488*
— s. Sams jr., W. M., u. J. G. Smith jr. *905*
— s. Smith jr., J. G., J. P. Tindall u. W. M. Sams *905*
Davidson, P., u. M. M. Hardy 647, *678*
Davidson, R. C., s. Kendall, R. F. *909*
Davis, B. K. 158, *180*
Davis, E., u. J. Landau 534, *616*
Davis, H. G., s. Noojin, R. O. *848, 859*
Davis, M., u. J. Lawler 356, *375*
Davis, M. J., u. F. C. Lawler 491, 531, 533, 534, 596, 599, *610, 616, 621*
— u. A. L. Lorincz 495, 496, *610*
Davison, A. R. 836, *857*
Dawkins, M. J. R., u. D. Hull 819, *853*
— u. J. Scopes 819, *853*
Dawson, A. B., s. Chapman, G. H. *1016*
Wawson, W. R., s. Bartholomew *1015*
Day, F. D. 693, *705*
De, P., s. Moberger, G. *133*
De Bersaques u. Rothman *43*
Degos, R. 809, 815, *850*
— J. Delort u. J. Hewitt 867, *901*
De Graciansky, P. *860*
— Lièvre u. Paraf *860*
Deguchi, Y. 76, *125*
Deist u. Kraus, s. Gottron, H. A. *847*
Dejenarui, I., A. Szentmiklosy u. T. David 804, *847*
Delacretaz, J., s. Jaeger, H. *909*

Delank, H.-W., G. Koch, G. Könn, H. P. Missmahl u. K. Suwelack *901*
Delattre, A., s. Langeron, L. *918*
Delbanco, E. 794, *845*
Delbarre, F., s. Coste, F. *903*
De Lerma, B. 893, *915*
Della, R., s. Held, D. *858*
Della Porta, G., u. O. Mülhbock 105, *125*
Della Santa, R., s. Held, D. *853*
Delort, J., s. Degos, R. *901*
Deme, S., s. Melczer, N. *222*
Demis, D. J., u. J. Brim 497, *610*
— s. Zimmer, J. G. *621*
Dempsey, E. W., u. A. J. Lansing 447, 449, *484*
— u. G. B. Wislocki 85, *125*
— s. Bunting, H. *264, 331, 483*
— s. Lansing, A. I. *486*
— s. Wislocki, G. B. *142, 490, 620*
— s. Wislocki, G. B., u. D. W. Fawcett *142*
Demura, K., u. T. Uchida 827, *856*
Denington, E. M., s. Stettenheim, P. *1027*
Dennis, J. W., u. P. B. Rosahn 882, *909*
Depisch, F. 804, *847*
Dercum 838, *857*
Derksen, J. C., G. Heringa u. A. Weidinger 18, 37, 50, *125, 371, 375*
— G. C. Heringa 18, 37, 50, 54, *125*
De Robertis, E. *424*
— u. H. S. Benett *424*
Dérot, M., s. Rathery, Fr. *918*
De Sousa, A., u. S. Rodriguez 598, *621*
de-Thé, G. 303, *331*
Dettmer, N., J. Neckel u. H. Ruska 444, 451, *484*
— u. W. Schwarz 444, *446*
— s. Herrath, E. v. *485*
— s. Schwarz, W. E. *489, 905*
Deutsch, F. 533, 534, *616*
Devillers, Ch. 968, *1017*
Dewey, M. M., u. L. Barr 34, 35, *125, 126, 979, 1017*
— s. Sjöstrand, F. S. *138*
Diamond, J., J. A. B. Gray u. D. R. Inman *1031*
Di Bella, R. J., s. Hashimoto, K., B. Gross u. W. F. Lever *679*
Dick 685
Dick, J. C. 2, *125*, 462, 465, 468, 471, 472, *484*

Dickens, K. L., s. Pearse, A. G. E. *903*
Dickinson, S., s. Astbury, W. T. *120*
Dieck, A. *783*
Diecke, F. P. J., s. Bullock, T. H. *1016*
Dieckhoff, J., H. C. Hempel u. R. Koch 806, 807, 808, 833, 834, *847, 857*
Diemair, W., u. K. Mollenkopf *780*
Dierkes, K. *782*
Dierst, K. E., u. C. L. Ralph 950, *1017*
Dieter, W., u. C. Sung Sheng 580, *621*
Dieulafé u. Durand 494, 497, 517, 563, 567, *610, 616, 621*
Dijkgraaf, S. 951, 953, 955, 956, *1017*
Dijkstra, C. 1005, *1017*
Dimitrescu, A., u. L. Bălus 815, 837, *850, 857*
Dittrich 758, 765, *782, 784*
Dittrich, s. Luschka *781*
Divry, P., u. M. Florkin 863, *901*
Dixon, A. D. *424*
Dixon, F. J., s. Vazques, T. T. *903*
Dobson, R, L. 237, 243, 247, 249, 250, 253, *264*
— D. C. Abele u. D. M. Hale 243, 249, *264*
— V. Formisano, W. C. Lobitz u. D. Brophy 240, 247, *264*
— u. W. C. Lobitz 240, 247, 248, *264*
Dockerty, M. B., s. Kratzer, G. L. *680*
Dodd, H., u. F. B. Cockett 546, 597, *616, 621*
Dodson, J. W. *1032*
Doeg, K. A., S. Krueger u. D. M. Ziegler 102, *125*
Doeg, K. A., s. Green, D. E. *128*
Dogiel, A. S. 378, *424*, 564, *616*
Dogliotti, M., s. Bizzozero, E. *705*
Doig, R. K., s. Althausen *916*
Dole, V. P. 828, *856*
— s. Schwartz, I. L., u. J. H. Thaysen *266*
Donnell, G. N., s. Heuser, E. *860*
Donnelly, G. H., u. S. Navidi 218, 221
Donoso, A. O., s. Stefano, F. J. E. *1027*
Dorfman, A. 450, *484*
— s. Schiller, S. *488*

Dorfman, R. I., s. Ferchielli, E. *221*
Dorn, A. 816, *850*
Dorris, F. 105, *125*
Dotzauer u. Naeve 719
Dotzauer, G. 716, 719, 723, 757, *781, 783, 784*
Doubrow, S., s. Rathery, Fr. *918*
Downes, A. M., L. F. Sharry u. G. E. Rogers *1029*
Doxiadis, S. A. 796, *847*
Doyle, W. L. 244, *264*
Draper 782
Dreize, M. A., s. Hsia, S. L. *860*
Driesen, H. H. 1010, *1017*
Drochmans, P. 104, 107, 109, 112, 113, 114, 115, 117, *125*, 891, 892, *913*
Drosdoff 8, *125*, 741, 742, *782*
Droz, B. 407, *424*
Dry, F. W. 158, *180*
DuBuy, H. G., M. W. Woods, D. Burk u. M. D. Lackey 110, *125*
Duggins, O. H., u. M. Trotter 147, *180*
Duhring 2, *125*
Dummersmuth, G. 882, *909*
Duncan, W. C., R. G. Freeman u. Ch. L. Heaton 831, *860*
Dunlap, C. E., s. Farber, E. *126*
Duperrat, s. Veslot *910*
Duperrat, A. 901, *919*
Duperrat, B. 802, *847*
— u. J. M. Mascaro 654, *678*
— u. J. Monfort 809, *850*
— s. Gougerot, H. *851*
Dupont, A., u. A. Bourland 357, 358, 359, *375, 378, 387, 424*
Dupré, A. 23, 78, 79, 85, *125, 126*, 364, *375*
— s. Bazex, A. *845, 857, 903, 911*
— s. Calvet, J. *903*
Duran-Reynals, F. 452, *484*, 874, *906*
Durand, s. Dieulafé *610, 616, 621*
Durjee, A. W., s. Wright, I. S. *620*
Durrer, H. 1011, 1012, *1017*
— u. W. Villiger 1010, *1017*
Durward, A., u. K. M. Rudall 495, 497, 500, 501, 502, 503, 506, 507, 573, 575, 589, 590, *610, 613, 621*
Du Shane, G. P. 105, *126, 913*
Duthie s. Chain *906*
Duthie, D. A., s. Percival, G. H. *846, 904, 905*

Duthie, D. A., s. Percival, G. H., u. P. W. Hannay *905*
Dutra, F. R. 901, *919*
Duvall, A. J., s. Flock, Å. *1018*
Duve, C. de 97, 294, 325, *331*, 435, *484, 913*
— u. H. Beaufay 101, *126*
— B. C. Pressman, R. Gianetto, R. Wattiaux u. F. Appelmans 97, *126*
— u. R. Wattiaux 98, *126*
— s. Berthet, J. *121*
— s. Novikoff, A. B. *134*
— s. Wattiaux, R. *120, 141*
Duwe, C. de, u. L. Berthelet *780*
Dziallas, P. 550, *616*
Dziedziuszko, A., s. Bojowa, E. *909*

Eakin, R. M. 950, *1017*
— u. J. A. Westfall 950, *1017*
Eames, R. A., s. Gamble, H. J. *424*
Eastlick, H. L. 105, *126*
Eaton, G. J., s. Chase, H. B. *179, 1030*
Eberhartinger, Chr. 796, 798, 799, 837, 840, *847, 850*, 857, 879, *906*
— u. H. Ebner 876, *906*
— — u. G. Niebauer 899, *917*
— u. G. Niebauer 870, 871, *904*
Eberl-Rothe, G., u. P. A. Langegger 669, 673, *678*
Eberth, C. J. 536, *616*
Ebling, F. J., u. G. R. Hervey 1014, *1017*
— u. E. Johnson *1030*
— s. Johnson, E. *1030*
Ebner, H., u. W. Raab 888, *912*
— s. Eberhartinger, Chr. 906, *917*
Eckstein, H. C. 74, *126*
Edds jr., M. V. 975, *1017*
— u. P. R. Sweeny 974, 975, *1017*
Eden, K. C., s. Trotter, W. R. *908*
Eder, M. 87, *126*
Edwards, G. A., u. L. Makk 19, 37, *126*
Edwards, G. A., s. Grimley, Ph. M. *129*
Edwards, L. J. *180*
Eggeling, v. 920
Eggeling, H. v. 268, *331*, 661, *678*
Eggerer, H., s. Lynen, F. *844*
Ehlers, G. 792, 808, 809, 811, *845, 850*

Ehlers, G., s. Knoth, W. *130, 181*
Ehrhardt, s. Buhtz, G. *784*
Ehrich, W. E. 878, *906*
Ehring, F. 61, *126*
Ehrlich, J. C., u. I. M. Ratner 863, *901*
Ehrmann 745
Ehrmann, S. 103, *126*
Eichenlaub, F. J., u. R. A. Osbourn 627, *678*
Eichner, F. 261, *264*, 467, *484*, 573, *621*
Eidinger, D., s. Leblond, C. P. *618*
Eidinger, E., s. Glegg, R. E. *485*
Eisen, A. Z., K. A. Arndt u. W. H. Clark 98, 99, *126*
— u. J. Gross 986, *1017*
— J. B. Holyoke u. W. C. Lobitz jr. 218, *221*
— W. Montagna u. H. B. Chase 17, 71, 72, 88, *126, 173, 180*
— s. Montagna, W. *181, 222*
— s. Montagna, W., A. H. Rademacher u. H. B. Chase *133, 265, 334*
Eisenberg, J., s. Wiener, R. *908*
Eisenschmid, J. H., u. J. L. Orbison 805, 830, *847, 856*
Ejiri, J. 165, *180*, 685, 686, 688, 691, 695, 699, 700, 704, *705, 790, 845*
Ekel, T. M., s. Scott, E. J. van 137, *183*
— s. Scott, E. J. van, u. R. Auerbach *183*
Ekholm, R. *424*
Elbel, H. *784*
Elias, J. M., s. Bradshaw, M. *122*
Elias, S. M., s. Bradshaw, H. *615*
Eller, J. G., u. W. D. Eller 873, *904*
Eller, W. D., s. Eller, J. G. 873, *904*
Ellermann, W. 750, 751, *783*
Ellias, J. J., s. Bern, H. A. *121*
Ellis, F. A., s. Robinson, H. M. *855*
Ellis, R. 354, 355, 356, *375*
Ellis, R. A. 7, 8, 10, 77, 87, 88, 91, 92, 95, *126*, 165, *180*, 209, 210, 211, 212, 213, 214, 215, 232, 236, 237, 240, 241, 245, 247, 253, 257, 258, *264*, 301, 302, 303, 304, 312, 323, 326, *331*, 492, 495, 527, 528, 530, 563, 581, 583, 585, 606, *610, 616, 621, 622*, 665, 669, *678, 1029*

Ellis, R. A., u. J. H. Abel 244, *264*
— u. R. C. Henrikson 204, 205, 216, *221*
— u. W. Montagna 77, 91, 92, *126*, 176, *180*, 201, *221*, 236, 242, 248, 253, 254, 260, *264*, 312, *331*, 506, 517, 563, 581, 583, *613*, *616*, *1029*
— W. Montagna u. H. Fanger 204, *221*, 324, *331*, 581, 583, *621*, 700, 705
— u. G. Moretti 492, 495, 558, 563, 586, 587, 588, 589, 606, 607, *610*, *616*, *621*, *622*, *623*
— s. Montagna, W. *133*, *179*, *181*, *222*, *265*, *334*, *426*, 611, *614*, *618*, *621*, *622*, *623*, *706*, 1029, *1032*
— s. Montagna, W., u. A. F. Silver *222*
— s. Montagna, W., u. K. Yasunda *265*
— s. Moretti, G. *222*, *611*, *618*, *621*, *622*, *623*
— s. Moretti, G., u. N. K. Adachi *133*
— s. Moretti, G., u. H. Mescon *133*
— s. Parakkal, P. F. *614*, *1029*
— s. Yasuda, K. *338*
Ellison, E. M., s. Gager, L. T. *918*
Elschner, H., s. Steigleder, G. K. *139*
Elsen, Arndt, u. Clark 96
Elze, C. 468, 469, 470, 471, 477, *484*, *483*
— s. Braus, H. 478, *615*, *616*
Emden, G., u. F. Kraus 780
Emery, J. A., s. Russel, F. F. *1025*
Emery, J. L., u. M. McMillan 636, *678*
Emrich, H. M., s. Schulz, I. *266*
Enderlin, K., s. Brun, R. 220
Endo, M. 270, 271, *331*, *332*, 657, *678*
Enemar, A., u. B. Falck 950, *1017*
Engel 607, *623*
Engel, M. F., u. W. J. Hammack 815, *850*, 857
Engelbach, F. 804, *847*
Enghusen, E. 443, 444, 445, 448, *484*
Engleman, E., s. Mostofi, F. K. *848*
Engman, M. F., u. R. C. Mac Cardle 67, *126*
Engman jr., M. F., s. Mac Cardle *131*

Engman sen., M. F., s. Mac Cardle, R. C. *131*
Engström, A., u. J. B. Finean 440, 447, *484*
Engström, H., u. J. Wersäll 379, *424*
Engstrom, A., s. Cosslett, V. E. *622*
Enterline, H. T., J. D. Culberson, D. B. Rochlin u. L. W. Brady 823, 824, *853*
Epstein, E., B. Gerstl, M. Berk u. J. P. Belber 900, *919*
— s. Urbach, E. *910*
Epstein jr., E. H., u. W. L. Epstein 220, *221*
Epstein, S., s. Pinkus, H. *910*
Epstein, W. L., u. H. I. Maibach 61, *126*
— s. Epstein jr., E. H. *221*
Eränkö, O., s. Pirilä *135*, *783*
Erbslöh, F. 809, 811, *850*
Erickson, J. O., s. Laden, E. L. *131*
Ericsson, J. L. E., B. F. Trump u. J. Weibel 294, 296, *331*, 332
Erman 782
Ernstene, A. C., u. M. C. Volk 778, *786*
Ernster, L., M. Ljunggreen u. L. Danielson 96, *126*
— s. Lindberg, O. *131*
Ernyey, A., s. Cormia, F. E. *610*, *616*, *621*, *622*
Esoda, E. C. J., s. Flesch, P. *127*
— s. Flesch, P., u. D. A. Roe *127*
— s. Roe, D. A. *136*
Espinasse, P. G., s. Cohen, J. *1017*
Essner 435
— u. A. B. Novikoff 296, *332*, 435, *484*
— s. Goldfischer, S. *332*, *485*
Estborn, B., s. Reichard, P. *136*
Etkin, W. *1017*
Eubank, D. F., s. Sanford, H. N. *859*
— s. Ludwig, E. *782*
Eulenberg 745
Euler, H. v., s. Adler, E. *120*
Euler, U. S. v., u. H. Heller, s. Karkun, J. N. *1021*
Evans, Cowdry u. Nielson 790, *845*
Evans, A. M. 511, *613*
Evans, M. J., J. B. Finean u. D. L. Woolf 384, *424*
Evans, R., E. V. Cowdry u. P. E. Nielson 685, 686, 688, 690, *705*
Evans, W. C., u. H. S. Raper 889, *913*

Evans, W. E. 741, 746, *782*
Evensen, A., s. O. Heldaas 64, *126*
Everall, J. D., s. Birbeck, M. S. C. *121*, *908*, *909*, *912*
— s. Breathnach, A. S. *220*, *912*
Everett, N. B., s. Leblond, G. P. *181*
Eyckmans, R. 802, *847*
Ezell, D., s. Lewis, S. R. *131*

Fabry 881
Fabry, J. 881, 884, *909*
Fänge, R., u. A. Brodal, s. Blackstad, Th. *1016*
— s. Peters, A. *1024*
Fagarasano, J., s. Craciun, E. C. *855*
Fahrenholz, C. 933, 934, 935, 936, 984, *1017*
Fairchild, M. D., s. Russel, F. E. *1025*
Falcao, L., s. Meireles Pinto, M. I. *132*
Falchi, G. 387, *424*
Falck, B., s. Enemar, A. *1017*
Falin, L. I. 76, 78, *126*
Falk 769, *785*
Falk, B., u. H. Rorsman 526, *617*, *1031*
Falk, H. J., s. Rukavina, J. G. *866*
Falk, S., u. J. Rhodin 948, 964, *1018*
Fallani, s. Ishibashi *781*
Falta 838, *857*
Fan, J., s. Pinkus, H. *135*
Fanger, H., s. Ellis, R. A. *705*
— s. Ellis, R. A., u. W. Montagna *221*, *331*, *621*
Faninger 802
Faninger, A., u. M. Išvaneski 802, *847*
Farber, E., u. C. D. Louviere 87, *126*
— W. H. Sternberg u. C. E. Dunlap 89, *126*
Farber, E. M., E. A. Hines jr., M. Montgomery u. K. McCraig 569, *621*, 700, 701, *705*
Farber, L. 882, 883, *909*
Farbman, A. I. 22, 84, *126*
Farner, D. S. *1018*
— A. Oksche u. L. Lorenzen 1014, *1018*
— s. Follett, B. K. *1018*
— s. King, J. R. *1021*
Farquhar, M. G., u. G. E. Palade 2, 4, 19, 21, 22, 31, 32, 33, 34, 35, 36, 37, 38, 40, 49, 84, 99, 100, 116, 120, *126*, 288, *332*, 978, 979, 980, 981, *1018*, *1029*

Farquhar, M. G., s. Palade, G. E. *134*
— s. Rinehart, J. F. 619
Farris, G., s. Baccaredda-Boy, A., u. G. Moretti 615, *621*, *623*
Farris, G., s. Moretti, G. *614*, *618*, 623
Farris, M. S. W., s. Mikhail, G. R. *618*
Fasske, E., u. H. Themann 31, 56, 78, 86, *126*
Fatteh, A. 754
Faure-Fremiet, E. 960, 961, *1018*
Favard, P., s. Carasso, N. 331
Favarger, P. *844*
— u. H. Bodur 789, *844*
Fawcett, D., s. Napolitano L. 487, *854*
Fawcett, D. W. 57, 58, 59, 110, *126*, 244, 253, *264*, 457, 458, 460, 461, *484*, 529, *617*, *618*
— u. M. H. Burgos 299, *332*
— s. Sidman, R. L. *855*, *856*
— s. Wislocki, G. B., u. E. W. Dempsey *142*
Fazekas, I. G., u. F. Viragos-Kis 759, 760, *784*
Fazzini, L., s. Tosti, A. 905
Fegeler, F., u. M. Rahmann-Esser 68, 70, *126*
— s. Rahmann-Esser, M. 135
Fehr, E. 808, *843*
Feijoo, L. 840, 841, *857*
Felix, D. M., s. Dalton, A. J. *125*, *331*
Fell 998
Fell, H. B., s. Fitton-Jackson, S. *1018*
— s. Pele, S. R. *1024*
Felsher, Z. 5, *127*
Ferguson, D., s. Rodbard, S. *1025*
Ferrato, E., s. Albertazzi, F. *857*
Ferreira-Marques, J. 78, 116, *127*, 424, 813, *850*, *906*
— E. O. Bittar u. J. F. Leonforte 491, *610*
— u. C. A. Parra 12, 62, 76, 78, *127*
— u. N. van Uden 872, *904*
Ferris, W., s. Weiss, P. *141*, *376*, *1028*
Ferry, J. D. 938, *1018*
Feuerstein 808, *847*
Feulgen u. Voit 883
Feulgen, R., K. Imhäuser u. M. Behrens 84, *127*
— u. K. Voit 84, *127*
Feyrter 881
Feyrter, I. 853, 881, 882, 883, *909*
— u. G. Niebauer 874, *904*

Ficalbi, E. 928, 929, 930, 932, *1018*
Fiddes, F. S., s. Smith, S. 783
Fiedler, W. 920, *1018*
Filippi, B., s. Baccaredda-Boy, A., u. G. Moretti 615, *621*
Filshie, B. K., u. G. E. Rogers 51, 75, *127*, 155, *180*, *1007*, *1008*, *1018*
Finch, C. A., s. Finch, S. C. 895, *916*
Finch, L., s. Rogers, G. E. 136
Finch, S. C., u. C. A. Finch *916*
Findlay, G. H. 92, 93, 95, 113, *127*, 176, *180*, 202, 221
— F. P. Scott u. D. J. Cripps 872, *904*
Finean, J. B., s. Engström, A. 484
— s. Evans, M. J. 424
Finegold, M. J. 1014, *1018*
Fingermann 947
Finley, E. 499, 511, *613*
Finnerud, C. W., u. R. Nomland 888, *911*
Finucane, B. 836, *857*
Fiorni, H., s. Mancini, R. E. 487
Fioroni, P. 990, 991, 993, *1018*
Firket, A. 365, *375*
Firket, H. 78, *127*
Fischer, F. v. 879, *906*
Fischer, H. 798, 800, *847*
— u. W. Nikolowski 881, *909*
— u. K. Schneller 893, *916*
— s. Reuter, K. 783
Fischer, J., u. D. Glick 783
— s. Steigleder, G. K. *139*, *183*
Fischer, R. 80, 81, *127*
— s. Gedigk, P. 332
Fischler 81, 83
Fisher, I., u. M. Orkin 809, *860*
— s. Laymon, C. W. 909
Fishman 101
Fishman, W. H., u. J. R. Baker 100, 101, *127*
— J. R. Baker u. P. R. F. Borges 100, *127*
— s. Hayashi, M. 129
Fitton-Jackson, S., u. H. B. Fell 998, *1018*
Fitzgerald, M. J. T. 378, 387, 424
— u. S. M. Lavelle 424
Fitzpatrick, T. B. 114, *127*, *913*
— S. W. Becker jr., A. B. Lerner u. H. Montgomery 114, *127*, 889, 890, *913*
— u. A. S. Breathnach 113, 117, *127*, 889, 890, *913*

Fitzpatrick, T. B., P. Brunet u. A. Kukita *127*, 889, 890, *913*
— u. A. Kukita 889, 890, *913*
— u. A. B. Lerner 104, 114, *127*, 889, 890, *913*
— H. Montgomery u. A. B. Lerner 889, 890, 892, *913*
— W. C. Quevedo jr., A. L. Levene, J. V. McGovern, Y. Mishima u. A. G. Oettle 890, 891, *913*
— M. Seiji u. D. McGugan 890, *913*
— s. Baker, R. V. 120
— s. Becker jr., W. S. *121*, *912*
— s. Breathnach, A. S. *912*, *913*
— s. Lerner, A. B. *131*, *914*
— s. Lerner, A. B., E. Calkins u. W. H. Summerson 914
— s. Seiji, M. *137*, *915*
— s. Seiji, M., u. M. S. C. Birbeck *915*
— s. Seiji, M., K. Shimao u. M. S. C. Birbeck *915*
— s. Seiji, M., R. T. Simpson u. M. S. C. Birbeck *915*
Fitzpatrick, T. G., s. Becker, S. K. 705
Flandin, C., s. Darier, J. 616
Flanigan, W. J., s. Curran, P. F. *1017*
Flaschenträger, B., u. E. Lehnartz 30, *127*, 440, 447, 448, 456, *484*
Fleck, E. F. 900, 901, *919*
Fleck, F. 804, 816, 831, 833, 835, 838, 839, 841, *850*
— u. M. Fleck 180
— s. Dercum 857
— s. Falta 857
— s. Gross 858
— s. Meier 858
— s. Schulze 859
— s. Woodburne, Philpott, Vilanova u. Graflin 853
Fleck, M., s. Fleck, F. 180
Fleischauer, K. 5, *127*
Fleischer, R. 778, *786*
Fleischhauer, K. 268, *332*, 465, 467, *484*, 645, 658, 663, *678*
— u. E. Horstmann 354, *375*, 465, *484*, 663, 669, *678*
— s. Bargmann, W., u. Knoop 330
Flemming 791, *845*
Flesch, P. 72, 78, 80, *127*, 162, *180*, 371, *375*
— u. E. C. J. Esoda 78, 80, *127*
— D. A. Roe u. E. C. J. Esoda 78, 80, 81, *127*

Flesch, P., u. A. Satanove 72, 73, *127*
— s. Mescon, H. *132*
— s. Roe, D. A. *136*
— s. Scott, E. J. van *137*
Fleury, R. 942, 943, *1018*
Fliedner, T. M., s. Cronkite, E. P. *125*
Flock, Å. 955, *1018*
— u. A. J. Duvall 953, 954, 955, *1018*
— u. J. Wersäll 935, 953, 954, *1018*
Florey, H. W., J. C. F. Poole u. G. A. Meek 541, *617*
Florkin, M., s. Divry, P. *901*
Flory, C. M. 806, 807, *847*
Flury, F. 778, 779, *786*
Förster, A. 771, *782, 785*
Foley, J. M., s. Spain, D. M. *849*
Follett, B. K., u. D. S. Farner 1014, *1018*
Follis, R. H. 450, *484*
Foot, N. C. 445, *484*
Foraker, A. E., u. W. J. Wingo 173, 176, *180*
Foraker, A. G., u. W. J. Wingo 72, 87, 89, *127*
Forchielli, E., G. S. Rao, I. R. Sarda, N. B. Gibree, P. E. Pochi, J. S. Strauß u. R. I. Dorfman 190, *221*
Ford, F. D. C. 836, *857*
Fordyce, J. A. 217, *221*
Forker, A. S., s. Calkins, E. *901*
Forman, L. 815, 837, *851, 857*
Formanek, J., u. G. Niebauer 894, *916*
Formisano, V., u. W. C. Lobitz 247, *264*
— s. Dobson, R. L. *264*
— s. Montagna, W. *133, 181, 222, 265, 487, 618*
Formisano, V. R., u. W. Montagna 87, 88, *127*, 176, *180*
Forsdahl, K. A. *1018*
Forslind, B., u. G. Swanbeck *1029*
Fosnaugh, R. P., s. Hu, F. *130*
Fourcroy 744, *782*
Fowlks, W. L., s. Mason, H. S. *914*
Fox, H. 899, *918*
Fraenkel, P. 765, *784*
— u. G. Strassmann *782*
Francis, H. C., s. Weinstein, A. *911*
Frangenheim, H. 811, *851*
Frank, F. 1011, *1018*
Frank, L., s. Rapp, Y. *812*
Franz, G. 882, *909*
Franz, V. 922, 923, 924, 925, 926, *1018*

Franzini-Armstrong, C., u. K. Porter 235, *264*
Franzl, R. E., s. Rappaport, M. M. *135*
Fraser, R., H. Lindley u. G. Rogers 373, *375*
— u. G. Rogers 373, *375*
Fraser, R. D. B., u. T. P. Mc Rae *127*, 1007, *1018*
— T. P. MacRae u. G. E. Rogers 54, 74, 75, *127*
Frasher, W. G., s. Sobin, S. S. *612*
Frazier, D. B., s. Jones, R. S. *902*
Frazier, W. R., s. Weiß, S. *620*
Fréderic u. Chèvremont *75*
Fréderic, J., u. M. Chèvremont 434, *484*
— s. Chèvremont, M. *124, 374*
Frederiksen, T., H. Gøtzsche, H. Harboe, N. Kiaer u. K. Mellemgard *866*
Freeman, L. W., s. Meirowsky, E. *132, 914*
— s. Meirowsky, E., u. A. Wiseman *132*
Freeman, R. G., E. G. Cockerell, J. Armstrong u. J. M. Knox 686, *705*
— s. Duncan, W. C. *860*
Freeman, W., s. Weidman, F. D. *910*
Freerksen, E. 478, *484*, 548, 550, *617*
Frei, J. V. 288, *332*
— u. H. Sheldon 11, 19, 20, 25, 26, 37, 58, 59, *127*
Freiman, D. G., s. Langcope, W. T. *848*
— s. Lever, W. F. *848*
Freinkel, R. K. 76, *127*
Frei-Sulzer, M., s. Castagnoli, E. *781*
Frenz, H., s. Braun-Falco, O. *1030*
Frenz, O., s. Braun-Falco, O. *179*
Freudenthal, W. 865, 867, 868, *902*
— u. Z. Geserowa 888, *912*
Freund, L. *1018*
Frey, A. 863, *902*
Frey, M. v. 377, *424*
Frey-Sulzer 729
Freytag, G., s. Lindner, J. *902*
Friberg, U., s. Boström, H. *122*
Friboes, W. 2, 3, 20, *127*
Frick, A., s. Schulz, I. *266*
Frieboes, W. 628, *678, 679*
Friedman, I., s. Szanto, P. B. *337*

Friedreich, N., u. A. Kekulé 863, *902*
Friedrich u. Schossberger 329, *332*
Friedrichs, W., s. Berndt, H. *846*
Friel, D. D., s. Greenwalt, C. H. *1019*
Friesen, H. 827, *856*
Frisch, K. v. 965, 977, *1018*
Frithiof, L., u. J. Wersäll 25, 26, 58, 59, 84, *127*
Fritz, E. 726, 751, 766, *781, 783, 784, 785*
Fromter, E., s. Schulz, I. *266*
Frost, R., u. C. R. Anderson 885, *909*
Frunder, H. *780*
Führers, M. 643, 658, *679*
Füller, H., s. Knoth, W. *851, 858, 909*
Fuhs, H. 798, *847*
Fujii, R. 960, 964, 966, *1018*
Fujita, S., s. Kaku, H. *130*
Fujiwara, K. *784*
Fukumori, Y., s. Yada, S. *783*
Fukuyama, K., u. I. A. Bernstein 47, 63, 69, 70, *127*
— T. Nakamura u. I. A. Bernstein 63, 68, 69, *127, 128*
Fular, W. 62, *128*
Fullmer, H. M., u. R. D. Lillie 444, 448, *484*
Fulton, G. P., R. G. Jackson u. B. R. Lutz 558, *617*
Funk, F., s. Arndt *846*
— s. Zieler *850*
Funk, Fr. *847*
— s. Coste *847*
Furbank, R., s. Mant, A. K. *782*
Furtado, T. A. 796, *860*
Furusawa, H., s. Yasuda, K. *266*
— s. Yasuda, K., u. N. Ogata *338*
— s. Yasuda, K., u. O. Saeki *338*
Fusari, R. *424*
Fusaro, R. M., u. R. W. Goltz 247, 253, *264*, 309, *332*
— s. Goltz, R. W. *128, 332*

Gabe, M. 921, *1018*
Gabriel, H., u. W. Lindemayr 867, *902*
Gabriel, M. *783*
Gafni, J., s. Blum, A. *866*
— s. Heller, H. *902*
— s. Missmahl, H. P. *866*
— s. Sohar, E. *866*
Gager, L. T., u. E. M. Ellison 899, *918*
Gahlen, W., u. N. Klüken 900, 901, *919*

Gahlen, W., s. Orfanos, C. *907*
Gail, D. 892, *913*
Gail-Sofer, M. S., s. Hsia, S. L. *860*
Gairns, F. W. 106, *128*
Gajima, H., s. Hofmann, K. *1020*
Galente, L. F., s. Thies, W. *223*
Galewsky, E. 169, *180*
Galton, D. J., u. G. A. Bray 828, *860*
Gamble, H. J. *424*
— u. R. A. Eames *424*
Ganner *782*
Gans, O. 11, 17, 66, 67, *128*, 791, 795, 796, 804, 805, *843*, *847*, 851, 869, 899, *918*
— u. E. Landes 794, *845*
— u. T. Parkheiser 66, *128*
— u. G. K. Steigleder 606, 622, 684, 695, *705*, 787, 798, 791, 792, 795, 796, 798, 800, 802, 804, 805, 809, 811, 820, 821, 823, 838, *843*, *845*, *846*, 865, 868, 872, 879, 881, 882, 887, 898, 899, 900, 901, *902*, *903*, *904*, *906*, *909*, 911, *917*, *918*, *919*
— s. Steigleder G. K. *139*, *707*
— u. K. G. Steigleder, s. Vidal-Leloir *905*
Gansler, H. 303, *332*, 398, *424*
Gardner, J. H., u. H. F. Raybuck 638, *679*
Garn, S. M. 148, *180*
Garnier, s. Veslot *910*
Garrachon, J., J. Munoz u. M. Ortega 539, *617*
Garrod, M., s. Lloyd, D. *375*
Gartmann, H. 816, *851*, *853*
— u. W. Kiessling 815, *851*
Gasparini, F., u. G. Bucciante 513, *613*
Gastgeber, W. 643, *679*
Gaté, s. Nové-Josserand, L. *918*
Gay 275, *332*
Gebauer, H. 804, *847*
Gedevanishvili, M. D. 982, *1018*
Gedigk u. Bontke 834
Gedigk, P. 278, *332*
— u. E. Bontke 278, *332*
— u. R. Fischer 278, *332*
— u. G. Strauß 896, *916*
Geierhaas, B., s. Lüdicke, M. *1023*
Geiger, R. 638, *679*
Geiger, W. 704, *705*
Geipel, P. 218, *221*
Gelfant, S. 64, *128*, *1032*
Gellerstedt 796, 797, *847*

Genesi, M. 821, *853*
Genschow, G., s. Staubesand, J. *614*
Georgesco, M., s. Slobosiano, H. *856*, *859*
Georgio, A. de 802, *847*
Gerald, G. B., L. R. Miller u. K. G. Bensch *484*
Gerlach *786*
Gerlach, W. 778, *785*
Gerlach, Wa., u. We. Gerlach 778, *785*
Gerlach, We., s. Gerlach, Wa. *785*
Gerschler, H., s. Wöhlisch, E. *490*
Gersh, J., u. H. R. Catchpole 441, 444, 451, 452, 463, *484*, *485*, 539, 562, *617*, 875, *906*
Gerstl, B., s. Epstein, E. *919*
Gerstner, H. *785*
— s. Koeppen, S. *786*
Gertler, W. 815, *839*, *851*, *857*
— u. A. Schieck *857*
Gery 819, *853*
Geschwind, I. I. 948, *1018*
Geserowa, Z., s. Freudenthal, W. *912*
Gessler, A. E., C. E. Grey, M. C. Schuster u. J. J. Kelsch 37
— C. E. Grey, M. C. Schuster, J. J. Kelsch u. M. N. Richter 36, *128*
Giacometti, C., s. Moretti, G. *182*
— s. Moretti, G., A. Rebora u. F. Crovato *621*
Giacometti, L. 533, *617*
— s. Machida, H. *614*
Gianetto, R., s. Duve, C. de *126*
Gibbons, I. R., u. J. R. G. Bradfield *128*
Gibbs, H. F. 163, *180*
Gibbs, R. H., s. Williams jr. *142*
Gibree, N. B., s. Forchielli, E. *221*
Gibson u. Bradfield 40
Gierke 790, *845*
Gierke, E. 886, *911*
Gieseking, R. 440, 441, 442, 443, *485*, 819, *853*
Giffin, H. Z., s. Brown, G. E. *616*
Gilbert 954
Gilje, O. *617*
— R. Kierland u. E. J. Baldes 495, *610*
— P. A. O'Leary u. F. J. Baldes 493, 533, 534, *610*, *617*
Gill jr., J. R., s. Curran, P. F. *1017*

Gillespie, J. M. 74, *128*
— I. J. O'Donell, E. O. P. Thompson u. E. F. Woods 74, *128*
Gilman, Th., J. Penn, D. Bronks u. M. Roux 874, *904*
Gimbel, N. S., s. Mikhail, G. R. *618*
Ginsberg, J. E., u. L. A. Becker 901, *919*
— s. Rattner, H. *917*
Gioia, E. 901, *919*
Giordano 804, *847*
Giorgo, A. de, s. Sotgiu, G. *918*
Giroud, A., u. H. Bulliard 70, 71, 72, *128*, 147, *180*
— — u. C. P. Leblond *128*, 172, *180*
— u. G. Champetier 18, 37, 50, *128*, 371, *375*
— u. C. P. Leblond 70, 71, 72, *128*, *180*
Glasstone, S. *785*
Glegg, R. E., E. Eidinger u. C. P. Leblond 445, *485*
— s. Leblond, C. P. *618*
Glenner, G., u. L. A. Cohen 437, *485*
Glenner, G. G., H. S. Burtner u. G. W. Brown 87, *128*
Glick, D., s. Fischer, J. *783*
Glickman, F. S., s. Rapp, Y. *812*
Glinski u. Horoszkiwicz 726, *781*
Glodny, H., s. Rausch, L. *136*
Gloggengiesser 819, *853*
Gloor-Rutishauser, N. 272, 329, *332*, 697, 704, *705*
Glücksmann, A. *1033*
Gnadeberg, W. 944, *1018*
Goda, T. 110, *128*
Godman, G., s. Grossfeld, H. *906*
Goebel, A. *780*
Göhringer, R. 1006, *1018*
Göppert, E., s. Boas *1016*
Gördel, P. 166, *180*
Goering, D. 828, *856*
— s. Lortat, G. *856*
— s. Lortat, G., u. M. Vitry *856*
— s. Mansfeld, W., u. F. Müller *856*
Görner, P. 953, 955, 985, *1018*
Goerttler, K. 166, 167, 168, 169, *180*
Goerz, G., s. Stüttgen, G. *1027*
Goessler, E. 1014, *1018*, *1019*
Gössner 834
Gössner, W. 446, *485*, 780, 864, 896, *902*, *916*

Goetinck, P. F., u. U. K. Abbott 1009, *1019*
Götz, H. 794, 815, 816, 838, *845, 851, 857*
Goff, R. A. 1006, *1019*
Gohrbandt 804, *847*
Goi u. Wendl 746
Goldbach, H. J., u. H. Hinüber *782*
Goldberg 434, 441
Goldberg, A. L., u. W. A. Rosenberg *858*
Goldberg, B., u. H. Green 433, 440, 441, *485*
Goldblum, R. W., W. N. Piper u. A. W. Campbell 10, 70, 71, 72, 75, 81, *128*, 173, *180*
Goldhaber, L., s. Schiller, S. *488*
Goldfischer, S., E. Essner u. A. B. Novikoff 323, *332*, 436, *485*
Goldish, R. J., s. Aufderheide, A. C. *916*
Foldman, P., s. Pinkus, H. *681*
Goldmann, L., u. W. Kounker 495, *610*
Goldner, J. 789, 819, *844*
Goldrick, R. B. 828, *860*
Goldschlag, F. 899, *918*
Goldsmith, W. N. 816, *851*
Goldstein, D. J. 279, 280, 324, *332*
Goldstein, E., u. J. Harris 814, *851*
Goldstein, L. 69, *128*
Gondesen, H. *845*
Goldzieher, J. W., W. B. Rawls, I. S. Roberts u. M. A. Goldzieher 685, 686, 688, 700, *705*
Goldzieher, M. A., s. Goldzieher, J. W. *705*
Golgi 57
Golgi-Mazzoni 377
Golodetz, L., s. Unna, P. G. *141*
Goltz, R. W., R. M. Fusaro u. J. Jarvis 10, 79, *128*, 309, *332*
— s. Fusaro, R. M. 264, *332*
Gomori, G. 85, 92, 96, 97, *128, 264*, 321, *332, 617*
Gomori, M. D. 498, 556, *610*, 659
Gonzales, J. E., s. Landers, J. W. *623*
Goodall, A. M., u. S. M. Yang 497, 500, 511, *610, 613*
Goodall, H. M. *613*
Goodman, H. M. 827, *856*
Goodman, R. M., E. W. Smith, D. Paton, R. A. Bergman, Ch. L. Siegel, O. E. Ottesen,

W. M. Shelley, A. L. Pusch u. V. A. McKusick 888, *911*
Goodwin, D. P., s. Breathnach, A. S. *123, 913*
Gordis, L., u. H. M. Nitkowsky 294, *332*
Gordon, A. S., s. Ratzersdorfer, C. *1025*
Gordon, E. S. 796, 828, 836, *847, 856, 858*
Gordon, G. B., L. R. Miller u. K. G. Bensch 436, *484*
Gorny, W., s. Alkiewicz, J. *705*
Goroncy, C. *785*
Goslar, H. G. 988, 989, 990, *1019*
Gothe, J. 384, *424*
Goto, M. *424*
Goto, T. 977, 982, *1019*
— T. Kaga u. T. Oono 665, 667, *679*
— s. Kaga, T. *679*
Gots, J. S., s. Brodie, A. F. *123*
Gotshalk, H. C., s. Tilden, J. L. *849*
Gottron, H. A. 788, 789, 790, 791, 794, 795, 797, 798, 800, 802, 803, 804, 808, 815, 816, 817, 824, 827, 832, 833, 834, 835, 837, 838, 839, 841, 842, *844, 845, 847, 851, 853, 856, 858, 867, 868, 880, 882, 883*, 899, *902, 906, 909, 918*
— u. G. W. Korting 880, 888, 889, *906, 912*
— u. W. Nikolowski 796, 801, 802, 824, 835, 839, 841, 842, *847, 853, 858*
— u. W. Schönfeld 122, *707, 853, 855*
Gøtzsche, H., s. Frederiksen, T. *866*
Gougerot 808, 809
Gougerot, H., u. A. Caeteaud 900, *918*
— u. B. Duperrat *851*
Gour, K. U., s. Singh, G. *849*
Goyette, E. M., s. Blake, H. A. *855*
Graciansky, de 836
Graciansky, P. de, s. Albrectsen, B. *860*
— s. Cohen *860*
— s. Comfort u. Osterberg *860*
— s. Leger *861*
— s. Lièvre *861*
— s. Machacek *861*
— s. Panabokké, R. G. *861*
— s. Zeller u. Hetz *861*
Gräff, S. 85, *128*, 709, 771, 780, *785*

Grafe, E. 886, *911*
Graflin s. Woodburne *853*
Graham, J. H., s. Gray, H. R. *911*
— s. Newcomer, V. D. 848, *859*
Grandry 377
Grant, R. T., u. E. F. Bland 495, 553, *610, 617*
Grassé, P., s. Budker, P. *1016*
— s. Devillers, Ch. *1017*
— s. Gabe, M. *1018*
— s. Mayaud, N. *1023*
Grasset, N., u. R. Brun 187, 188, *221*
Grassmann, W. 440, 441, 442, 446, *485*
— u. I. Trupke 18, *128*
— s. Kühn, K. *486*
Graumann, W. 2, *128*, 444, 449, 450, 452, 453, 462, 478, *485*, 634, 635, 644, *679*, 698, *705*, 874, 875, 876, 877, 878, 885, 886, 887, *906, 911*
— s. Chain u. Duthie *906*
— s. Duran-Reynals, F. *906*
— s. McLean, F. *907*
— s. Letterer, E. *907*
— s. Lillie, R. D. *907*
— s. Meyer, K. *907*
— s. Szirai, J. A. *908*
— u. K. H. Neumann, s. Wolman, M. *905*
Gray, A. M. H. 835, *858*
Gray, E. G. 966, *1019*
Gray, H., u. W. H. Lewis 500, *613*
Gray, H. R., J. H. Graham u. W. C. Johnson 886, *911*
Gray, J. A. B., s. Diamond, J. *1031*
Gray, M. B., s. Perry, E. T. *335*
Grayson, J. 477, *485*
Greb, W. 5, *128*, 465, 466, 467, 468, 469, *485*
Green, D. E. *128*
— D. M. Ziegler u. K. A. Doeg 85, 86, 102, *128*
Green, H., s. Goldberg, B. *485*
Greenhill, J. P., s. Arey, L. B. *613*
Greenlee jr., T. K., s. Ross, R. *136*
Greenwald, J. J., s. Collen, W. S., L. C. Boas u. J. D. Zilinsky *847*
Greenwalt, C. H., W. Brandt u. D. D. Friel 1010, *1019*
Greider, M. H., s. Scarpelli, D. G. *855*
Greig, D. M. 278, *332*
Greite, W. 1007, *1019*
Greither, A. 796, 836, *847, 858*

Grenberg, T. F. 634, 637, 638, 639, *679*
Greuer, W. 720, 768, *780*
Greulich, R. C. 64, *129*
— s. Leblond, C. P. *131*
Greville, C. M., s. Appleyard, H. M. *178*
Grey, C. E., s. Gessler, A. E. *128*
Griboff, S. I., s. Wiener, R. *908*
Griesemer, R. D., u. R. W. Thomas 828, *860*
Griffen, s. Norman *848*
Griffin, A. C., s. Ogura, R. *134*
Griffith, J. A., s. Roberts, E. *619*
Griffith jr., J. O. 530, *617*
Grigorova, O. P. 515, *613*
Grimaud, R., u. A. Beau 820, *853*
Grimley, Ph. M., u. G. A. Edwards 31, *129*
Grimm, D., s. Oehlert, W. *182*
Grimmer, H. 815, 837, *851, 858*
Grimwade, A. E., s. Hollander, A. *617*
Grinwich, D. L., s. Hall, P. F. *1019*
Grobstein, C., s. Kallman, F. *1021*
Grokoest, A. W., s. Butcher, E. O. *179*
Gronblad, E. 888, *911*
Groner, W. 953, 956, *1019*
Gronzi 766
Groodt, A. de, u. Fr. de Groodt 151, *180*
Groodt, Fr. de, s. Groodt, A. de *180*
Groot, W. P. de 884, *909*
— s. Ruiter, M. *910*
Groote, G. de, s. Vandenbroucke, J. *337*
Gross 833, *858*
Gross, B., s. Hashimoto, K. *375*
— s. Hashimoto, K., R. J. Di Bella u. W. F. Lever *679*
Gross, B. G. 300, *332*
— s. Hashimoto, K. *264, 332, 902*
— s. Hashimoto, K., u. W. F. Lever *129, 679*
— s. Hashimoto, K., R. Nelson u. W. F. Lever *129, 679*
Gross, G., s. Hashimoto, K. *679*
Gross, J. 371, 375, 440, 441, 442, 444, 449, *485*, 986, *1019*
— J. H. Highberger u. F. O. Schmitt 440, 441, 443, *485*

Gross, J., u. C. M. Lapiere 986, *1019*
— C. M. Lapiere u. M. L. Tanzer 986, 987, *1019*
— u. F. O. Schmitt 440, 441, 443, 444, *485, 488, 489*
— s. Eisen, A. Z. *1017*
— s. Piez, K. A. *1024*
— s. Silbert, J. E. *1026*
— s. Usuku, G. *1027*
Gross, P., u. H. W. Jacox 882, *909*
— u. G. F. Machaceck 815, 816, *851*
Gross, S., u. C. Wood 821, 824, *853*
Grosser, O. 494, 503, 507, 518, 551, 553, 554, *610, 613, 617*
Grosser-Brockhoff, F., u. W. Schoedel 492, *610*
Grossfeld, H., L. Meyer u. G. Godman 906
Grossfeld, J. C. M., J. Spaas u. J. Auping 871, 875, *904*
Gross-Lerner, H. 946, *1019*
Groth, W. 274, *332*
Grots, I. A., u. S. K. Targovnik 201, *221*
— J. S. Strauss u. H. Mescon 815, 837, *851, 858*
Grow, M. H., s. Bordley, J. *610, 615*
Gruber, G. B. 842, *858*
Grün, E. 889, *912*
Grüneberg, H. 635, *679*
Grüneberg, Th., u. A. Szakall 13, 14, 50, 51, *129*
Grütz, O. 788, 806, 835, 841, 844, 847, *858*
Grupper, Ch., M. Hebert u. J. Hewitt 802, *847*
Grzybowski, M. 796, *847*
Gualdi, A., u. N. Baldino 240, *264*
Guareschi, H. *785*
Günder 991
Günther, G., s. Adler, E. *120*
Günther, H. 459, *485*
Güntz 739, *782*
— s. Orfila-Leseur *782*
Güttes, E. 110, 112, *129*
Guggenheim, H. 836, *858*
Guiducci, A. A., u. A. B. Hyman 216, *221*
— s. Hyman, A. G. *221*
Guijot, O., s. Hausberger, F. X. *485*
Guin, J. D., u. E. R. Seale 873, *904*
Gundermann, O., s. Jaensch, W. *613*
Gurins, I. G., s. Kalantaevskaya, K. G. *706*
Gurlt 265

Gusek s. Kracht 834
Gusek, W. 430, 431, 433, 434, 436, 437, 438, 439, *485*
Gusner, K. v. 698, *705*
Gustavson, K. H. 961, *1019*
Gutman, A., H. Schramm u. E. Shafrir 828, *860*
Gutmann, C. 867, *902*
Guttmann, S., u. R. A. Boissonas 949, *1019*

Haber, H., s. Calman, C. D. *846*
Haberda, A. 721, 735, *782*
— s. Hofmann, E. *781*
Habermann, R. 899, *918*
Hackenbrock, C. R., u. P. W. Brandt 251, *264*
Hadley, C. E. 948, 991, *1019*
Hadley, H. G. 899, *918*
Hadok, R., s. Szanto, P. B. *337*
Häggendal, E., B. Steen u. A. Svanborg 828, *860*
Häggqvist, G. 479, 481, *485, 627, 633, 641, 679*
Hänig, E., u. H. Kremer 871, *904*
Häussler 730
Hagedorn-Jensen 720
Hagen 920
Hagen, E. 377, 389, 390, 395, 398, 421, *424*
— u. S. Werner 379, 381, 392, 393, 409, 410, 419, 420, 421, 422, *424*
Hagen, H., s. Scheffler, H. *849*
Haguenau, F. 301, 302, *332*
Halberkann, J. 990, *1019*
Hale, D. M., s. Dobson, R. L. *264*
Hall, D. A., R. Reed u. R. E. Turnbridge 447, 449, *485, 873, 904*
— s. Turnbridge, R. E. *489, 905*
Hall, E., s. Schmitt, F. O. *489*
Hall, P. F., C. C. Ralph u. D. L. Grinwich 1015, *1019*
Haller jr., A. J., u. R. E. Billingham 559, *617*
Halperin, V., S. Kolas, K. R. Jefferis, S. O. Huddleston u. H. B. G. Robinson 217, *221*
Halstead, B. W., M. J. Chitwood u. F. R. Modglin 959, *1019*
— u. L. R. Mitchell 942, *1019*
— u. F. R. Modglin 942, 960, *1019*
Halter, K. 217, *221*, 272, *332*, 802, *847*
Hama, K. 31, *129*, 931, 953, 955, *1019*

Hama, T. 964, 977, 982, *1019*
— u. M. Obika 964, 977, *1019*
Hamamatsu, T., s. Arimori, M. *855*
Hambrick jr., G. W., u. R. Bloomberg 638, 642, *679*
Hamburger, V., s. Willer, B. *615*
Hamilton, H., s. Koning, A. *375*
Hamilton, H. B. 169, *180*
Hamilton, H. L. 105, *129*
— u. A. L. Koning 1008, *1019*
Hamilton, J. B. 187, *221*, 1014, *1019*
— u. A. E. Light 143, *180*
— s. Montagna, W. *133*, *222*, *376*
— s. Montagna, W., u. H. B. Chase *181*, *334*
Hamilton, J. W., s. Kuntz, A. *618*
Hammack, W. J., s. Engel, M. F. *850*, *857*
Hammett, F. S., u. L. Walp 72, *129*
Hamminga, H., u. F. J. Keuning 879, *906*
Hamperl, A. 809, 811, *851*
Hamperl, H. 218, *221*, 893, *916*
Hampton, J. C., s. Bennett, H. S. *615*
Hanawa, S. 76, *129*
Hanhardt, E. 838, *858*
Hanke, W. *1033*
Hanley, E. H., s. Cardell, M. W. *850*
Hannay, P. W., s. Percival, G. H., u. D. A. Duthie *905*
Hanney, W., s. Percival, G. H. *846*
Hansborg, H. 900, *918*
Hansen, s. Luzzatti *848*
Hansen, K., s. Bock, H. E. *850*
Hanson, J. 62, *129*
Hanušová, S. 58, 83, *129*
Hanzon, V., s. Sjöstrand, F. S. *138*
Happey, F., u. A. G. Johnson 151, 155, 156, *180*
Harboe, H., s. Frederiksen, T. *866*
Harcourt, S. A., s. Cruickshank, C. N. D. *125*
Harder 957, 960, 967
Hardisty, M. W. 927, 932, *1019*, *1020*
Hardy, J. A., s. Jarrett, A. *130*
Hardy, M. H. 69, *129*, 173, 174, *180*, 500, 507, 607, *613*, *621*, *623*
— s. Davidson, P. *678*

Hare, P. J. 814, 816, *851*, 886, *911*
— s. Jones, D. B. *851*
— s. Leifer, W. *851*
— s. Leslie, G. *851*
— s. Traub, E. F. *853*
— s. Vero, F. *853*
— s. Wise, F. *853*
— s. Woringer, F. *853*
Harkavy 809
Harker, J. M., u. D. Hunter 898, *918*
Harkness u. Blair 177
Harkness, D. R., u. H. A. Bern 175, 177, 178, *180*
— s. Bern, H. A. *179*
Harkness, M. N., s. Bern, H. A. *121*
Harkness, R. D., A. M. Marko, H. M. Muir u. A. Neuberger 441, *485*
Harms, H. 864, *902*
Harper, R. G., s. Achs, R. *677*
Harreveld, A. van, s. Russel, F. E. *1025*
Harrington, R. W., s. Palette, E. M. *861*
Harris, J., s. Goldstein, E. *851*
Harris, R. J. C. *333*
Harris, R. S., u. I. G. Wool, s. Lerner, A. B. *1022*
Harrison, C. V. 811, *851*
Harrison, G. A. 300, *332*
Harrison, R. G. 105, *129*
Harrison, R. J., s. Montagna, W. *181*, *613*, *614*, *1032*
Hartl, H., s. Martius, H. *334*
Hartmann, A., s. Benninghoff, A. *615*
Hartmann, J. F., s. Hirsch, H. M. *913*
— s. Zelickson, A. S. *142*, *915*
— s. Zelickson, A. S., u. H. M. Hirsch *142*, *915*
Hartwig, M., s. Missmahl, H. P. *902*
Hartz, P. H. 217, *221*
Harvey, H. 492, 493, *610*
Hasegawa, J., u. A. Siegel 101, *129*
Hashimoto, K. 666, 667, 672
— u. G. Gross 673, *679*
— B. Gross, R. J. di Bella u. W. F. Lever 628, 630, 631, 673, 676, *679*
Hashimoto, K., B. G. Gross u. W. F. Lever 38, 59, *129*, 227, 228, 229, 230, 248, 256, 257, 258, 259, 260, 261, *264*, 277, 287, 293, 294, 296, 297, 299, 300, 304, 323, 325, 326, 327, *332*, 628, 629, 665, 676, *679*, 864, 865, *902*

Hashimoto, K., B. G. Gross, R. Nelson u. W. F. Lever *129*, *373*, 628, 630, 631, *679*
— s. Gross, G. *679*
Hashimoto, T. 313, 314, 315, 316, 318, 325, *332*
Hass, G. 863, *902*
Hatefi, Y., R. L. Lester, F. L. Crane u. C. Widmer 102, *129*
Hausberger, F. X. 455, 456, 458, 459, 460, 461, *485*, 828, *856*
— u. O. Gujot 458, 459, 461, *485*
Hausbrandt, F. *782*
Hauser, W. 789, 792, 794, *845*
Hausman, L. A. 148, 150, *180*
Hausmanowa-Petrusewicz, I., s. Jablonska, St. *860*
Havens, F. Z., s. Montgomery, H. *904*
Havlicek, H. 492, *610*
Hawkins, J. 87, *129*
Haworth, W. N., S. Peat u. E. J. Bourne 91, *129*
Haxthausen, H. 831, *856*
Hay, E. D. 288, *332*, 639, *679*, 971, 973, 976, *1020*
— u. J. P. Revel 976, *1020*
Hayashi, M., u. W. H. Fishman 101, *129*
Hayashi, T. 675, *679*
Heaton, Ch. L., s. Duncan, W. C. *860*
Hebert, M., s. Grupper, Ch. *847*
Hecht, A. 720, *780*
Hecht, A., u. Mitarb. *780*
Hedinger, C. 896, 897, *916*
Hegel, U., s. Schulz, I. *266*
Hegler, s. Huger *854*
Hegler, C., u. Fr. Wohlwill 825, 826, *853*
Heidenhain 988
Heidenhain, M. 36, *129*
Heilesen, B. 815, 837, *851*, *858*
Heilman, P., u. H. J. Sonneck 833, *858*
Heimberger, H. 552, *617*
Heinzelman, R. V., s. Lerner, A. B. *1022*
Heite 827
Heite, H.-J., u. G. von der Heydt *860*
— u. H. Zaun 697, *705*
Helander, H. F. 287, 288, 293, 299, 326, 328, *332*
Held 936
Held, D., u. R. Della Santa 820, 821, 838, *853*, *858*
— s. Rutishäuser, E. *859*
Heldaas, O., s. Evensen, A. *126*

Hell, E. A., u. C. N. D. Cruickshank *1032*
Heller, H., u. Euler, U. S. v., s. Karkun, J. N. *1021*
— H. P. Missmahl, E. Sohar u. J. Gafni *902*
— s. Blum, A. 866
— s. Sohar, E. 866
Heller, J. 360, *375*
Hellerström, C., s. Hellman, B. *854*, *856*
Hellman, B., u. C. Hellerström 819, 829, *854*, *856*
Hellmann, K. 87, 92, 96, *129*, 204, *221*, 262, *264*, 284, 321, *332*
— s. Weiner, J. S. 266, *1030*
Hellman, T., s. Benninghoff, A. *615*
Hellström, B., u. H. J. Holmgren 438, 451, *485*, 638, *679*, 694, 704, *705*
Helly 450
Helm, F. 873, *904*
Helwig, E. B. 11, *129*
— s. Roth, S. I. *182*, *1031*
Hempel, H. C., s. Dieckhoff, J. *847*, *857*
Hempel, K. 890, *913*
Hempel, M. 1005, *1020*
Hemous, G., s. Calvet, J. *903*
Henle, F. 493, *611*
Hennig 734
Henning, U., s. Lynen, F., B. Agranoff u. E. Möslein *844*
— s. Lynen, F., C. Bublitz, B. Sörbo u. L. Kröplin-Rueff *844*
— s. Lynen, F., H. Eggerer u. J. Kessel *844*
Henrickson, R. C. 209, *221*
— s. Ellis, R. A. *221*
Henriques, E. D., s. Moritz, M. D. *785*
Henriques, F., u. A. R. Moritz *785*
Hensel, H. 389, *424*, *1031*
— A. Iggo u. I. Witt *424*
Herbst 805, 830, *847*, *856*
Herbst, F. S. M., s. Matoltsy, A. G. *132*
Hering 823
Hering, H. *854*
Hering, H., u. W. Undeutsch 806, 808, 835, 841, *847*, *856*, *858*
— u. W. Undeutsch, s. Berner u. Heyde *855*
— u. W. Undeutsch, s. Cruse *857*
Heringa, G. C. 413, *425*, 443, 444, 445, 453, *485*
Heringa, G., s. Derksen, J. *125*, *375*

Heringa, G., s. Derksen, J. C., u. A. Weidinger *125*
Herrath, E. v., u. N. Dettmer 444, *485*
Herrera, F. C., u. P. F. Curran 981, *1020*
— s. Curran, P. F. *1017*
Herrmann, F. 67, *129*, 724, 781, 899, *918*
— P. H. Prosa, L. Mandol u. G. Medoff 789, *844*
Herrmann, H. 702, *705*, *706*
— u. M. B. Boss 890, *913*
Herrmann, L. 820, 823, *854*
Herrmann, W. P., K. H. Schulz u. R. Wehrmann *847*
Herscovici, P., s. Slobosiano, H. *856*, *859*
Hershey, F. B. 76, 88, *129*
— Ch. Lewis, J. Murphy u. Th. Schiff 474, *485*
Hertig, A. T. 499, *613*
— s. McKay, D. G. *680*
Herting, D. C., u. R. C. Crain 830, 841, *856*, *858*
Hertzmann, A. B. 609, *623*, 1029
Hervey, G. R., s. Ebling, F. J. *1017*
Herxheimer, A. 564, 566, *617*, 920, *1031*
Herxheimer, K. 2, *125*, *129*
Herxheimer u. Born, S. *127*
Herzberg, J. J. 885, *909*, *913*
— s. Steigleder, G. K. *852*
— s. Walther, D. *853*
Herzenberg, H. 270, 277, 309, 328, 329, *332*
Herzog, Gg. 819, *854*
Herzog, s. Marchand 439
Hess, A. 993, *1020*
Hett, J. 400, *425*
Hetz, s. Zeller *861*
Heubner 786
Heuser, E., E. Lieberman, G. N. Donnell u. B. H. Landing 836, *860*
Heuss *845*
Hewer, H. R., s. Szarski, H. *1027*
Hewett, C. L., s. Bullough, W. S. *1032*
— s. Bullough, W. S., u. E. B. Laurence *124*
Hewitt, J., s. Degos, R. *901*
— s. Grupper, Ch. *847*
Hewitt, R. M., s. Arey, L. B. *613*
Heyde, s. Berner *855*
Heydt, v. der *827*
Heydt, G. von der, s. Heite, H. J. *860*
Heyl, R., u. D. H. de Kock 871, *904*

Heynold, H. 267, 275, 277, 332, 581, *621*
Hibbs 495, 534, 535, 541, 550
Hibbs, R. G. 204, 205, *221*, 237, 241, 250, 251, 256, 257, *264*, 268, 287, 289, 293, 295, 296, 297, 299, 300, 301, 302, 325, 326, 327, *332*
— G. E. Burch u. G. H. Phillipe 492, 527, 528, 529, 534, 535, 539, 541, *611*, *617*
— u. W. H. Clark 19, 24, 31, 32, 37, 38, *129*
— u. W. Clark 364, *375*
— s. Clark jr., W. H. *125*
Hickman, K. C. D. 841, *858*
Hicks, R. M. 299, *332*
Hieronymi, G. 875, *906*
Higashi, H., S. Hirao, I. Yamada u. R. Kikuchi *1020*
— s. Takeuchi, T. *140*
Highberger, J. H., s. Gross, J., u. F. O. Schmitt *485*
— s. Schmitt, F. O. *488*, *489*
Hill, C. R., s. Montagna, W. *133*, *181*
Hill, E. M., s. Laymon, C. W. *904*
Hill, W. R., u. H. Montgomery *485*, 685, 686, 688, 690, 691, 693, 695, 696, 699, 700, 703, *706*, 790, *845*, 899, *918*
Himes, M. B., u. Mitarb. 780
Himmel, J. M. 686, 690, 691, 695, 696, 699, 700, *706*
Hines, E. A., s. Farber, E. M. *621*, *705*
Hinsch, G. W. 1008, *1020*
Hintsch, R., s. Jablonska, St. *860*
Hintzsche, E. 66, *129*
Hinüber, H., s. Goldbach, H. J. *782*
Hirao, S., s. Higashi, H. *1020*
Hirsch 147, 148, 149
Hirsch, G. C. 890, *913*
Hirsch, H. M., A. S. Zelickson u. J. F. Hartmann 890, *913*
— s. Zelickson, A. S., u. J. F. Hartmann *142*
Hirsch, M. M., s. Zelickson, A. S., u. F. J. Hartmann *915*
His, W. 499, *613*
Hitch, J. M. 885, *909*
Hjorth, N. 814, 815, 816, *851*
Hoagland, H., s. Adrian, E. D. *1015*
Hobusch, K. H., s. Otto, H. *859*
Hochleitner, H. 836, *858*, 900, *918*

Hock, R., s. Scholander, P. F. *1026*
Hodge, A. J. 441, 442, *485*
— u. F. O. Schmitt 443, *485*
— s. Schmitt, F. O. *489*
Höchel, Kl., s. Schwerd, W. *786*
Höhn, E. O. 1014, *1024*
Hoepfner, Th., s. Jaensch, W. *613*
Hoepke, H. 2, 8, 10, 13, 14, 15, 20, 21, 23, 29, 62, 103, *129, 134*, 151, *180*, 411, *425*
Hörstadius, S. 674, *679*
Hoff 722, *781*
Hoff, F. 459, *485*, 827, *845, 856*
Hoffmann, A. 455, 456, 458, 461, *485*, 788, 789, 827, *844, 856*
Hoffmann, C. K. 993, *1020*
Hoffmann, E., u. E. Zurhelle *854*
— s. Brocq *853*
— s. Rist, M. *855*
Hoffmann, F., u. K. J. Anselmino, s. Trygstad *857*
— s. Anselmino, K. J. *855*
— s. Johnson, P. L. *130*
Hoffmann, L., s. Knoth, W. *845*
Hoffmann-Ostenhof, O. 72, 85, 89, *129*
Hoffmann-Zurhelle, s. Hering *854*
— s. Holtz, K. H. *854*
— s. Nikolowski *854*
Hofmann, E. 711, 726, 745, 758, *782*
— u. A. Haberda 759, 769, *781*
Hofmann, K. 900, 948, *1020*
— M. E. Woolner, G. Spühler u. E. T. Schwartz 849, *1020*
— — H. Yajima, G. Spühler, T. A. Thompson u. E. T. Schwartz 949, *1020*
— H. Yajima, T. Liu u. N. Yanaihara 949, *1020*
— — N. Yanaihara, T. Liu u. J. Lande 949, *1020*
— s. Raben, M. S. *1024*
Hofmann-Haberda 780, 782, *784*
Hofmann, U., s. Kühn, K. *486*
Hogben, L. 946, 950, 951, *1020*
Hoge, A. R., u. P. S. Santos 989, *1020*
Hohanel, M., s. Weiß, E. *612*
Hoit, L., s. Bluefarb, S. M. *917*
Holland, M., u. L. Meyer 515, *613*

Hollander, A., S. C. Sommers u. A. E. Grimwade 536, *617*
Hollenberg, C. H., s. Sheldon, H. *844*
Hollmann, K.-H. 302, *332, 333*
Holmgren, E. 273, 275, 279, 326, *333*, 697, *706*
Holmgren, H. 637, 638, *679*
— u. H. Johansson 637, 641, *679*
— s. Hellström, B. *679*
— s. Jorpes, E. *486*
Holmgren, H. J., s. Hellström, B. *485, 705*
Holner, H., s. Tappeiner, J. *908*
Holst, E. v. 1003, *1020*
— u. U. v. Saint Paul 1003, *1020*
— s. Jechorek, W. *1020*
Holt u. Howland 806, *847*
Holter, H. 304, *333*, 435, *485*
Holtz, K. H. 823, *854*
— u. W. Schulze 871, 872, *904*
Holubar, K., u. K. W. Mach 879, *906*
— s. Wolff, K., u. R. K. Winkelmann *142*
Holyoke, J. B., u. W. C. Lobitz 237, *264*
— s. Eisen, A. Z. *221*
— s. Lobitz jr., W. C. *131, 221, 621, 680*
— s. Lobitz, W. C., u. D. Brophy *265*
— s. Lobitz, W. C., u. W. Montagna *265*
Holzberger, s. Torres, E. A., J. C. Radicé, N. U. Villafane u. S. Vaccaro *905*
Holzberger, P. C. 873, *904*
Holzel, A. 802, 806, 833, *847, 858*
Holzer, F. J. 729, 735, 740, *781, 782, 785*
Holzer, R. L., s. Laucker, J. L. van *780*
Holzgrove, H., s. Schulz *266*
Holzmann, H., s. Schott, H. J. *903*
Holzner, J. H., u. G. Niebauer 893, 894, *916*
Homma, H. 272, 277, 286, 309, *333*, 462, *485*
Hood, B., s. Björntorp *828, 860*
Hopf *781*
Hoppe-Seyler, H. 559, *617*
Horio, M., u. T. Vondo 373
Horiuchi, T., s. Izaki, M. *904*
Horn, G. 664, *679*
Hornbostel, H., u. K. Scriba 884, *909*

Horner, W. E. 192, *221*, 267, *333*
Horning 67
Horns, H. L., s. Aufderheide, A. C. *916*
Hornstein, O. 820, 838, 839, *854, 858*
— u. G. Klingmüller 872, *904*
— s. Klingmüller, G. *904*
Horoszkiwicz, s. Glinski *781*
Horowitz, S. B. 991, *1020*
Horstmann, E. 2, 3, 5, 6, 7, 8, 10, 11, 12, 13, 17, 20, 21, 37, 38, 40, 44, 45, 55, 57, 60, 62, 72, 76, 80, 86, 88, 104, 105, 114, *129, 130,* 134, 147, 148, 151, 152, 153, 154, *180,* 225, *264,* 268, 270, 275, 279, 280, *330, 333,* 350, 352, 354, 356, 357, *375, 425,* 465, 466, 467, 471, 475, *485,* 511, 520, 521, 530, 550, 559, 567, 572, 573, 575, 579, 580, 581, 597, 598, 605, 609, *613, 617, 621,* 622, 623, 624, 663, 671, *679,* 693, 697, 699, *706,* 787, *843,* 874, *906, 913,* 920, 949, 988, 989, 991, *1020*
— s. Fleischhauer *375*
— s. Fleischhauer, K. *484, 678*
— u. A. Knoop 20, 21, 31, 34, 37, 38, 40, 43, 44, 45, 55, 56, 57, 60, 86, *130,* 364, *375*
Hortega 110
Hotchkiss, R. D. 874, *906*
Hou-Jensen, Kl. *783*
Houtrouw, Th. *784*
Hovenkamp, A., s. Zoon, J. J. *905*
Howell, T. R., u. G. A. Bartholomew 1001, *1020*
Howland, s. Holt *847*
Hoyer, H. 384, *425*, 493, 494, 507, 510, 552, 553, 554, 611, *613, 617*
Hozaki, H., s. Izaki, M. *904*
Hsia, S. L., M. A. Dreize u. M. C. Marquez 828, *860*
— M. S. Gail-Sofer u. Barry Lane 828, *860*
Hsu, K. C., s. Riffkind, R. A. *488*
Hu, F. *104*
— u. R. R. Cardell jr. 2, 3, 19, 21, 37, 110, 113, 115, *130*
— R. J. Starrico, H. Pinkus u. R. P. Fosnaugh 104, *130*
Hubener, L. F., s. Zeligman, I. *223*

Huber 767, *785*
Huber, G. C., s. Ariëns Kappers, C. U. *1015*
Huber, W., s. Serri, F. *376*
Huber, W. H., s. Serri, F. *223*
Huber, W. M., s. Serri, F., u. H. Mescon 336, *681*
— s. Serri, F., u. W. Montagna 336, *614, 681*
Huddleston, S. O., s. Halperin, V. *221*
Hudson, R. F., s. Alexander, P. *120*
Hübener, G., s. Mayer-List, R. *618*
Hueck, W. 44, *130*
Hueter, C. 493, *611*
Huger 826
— Titone, Hegler u. Berner 826, *854*
Hughes u. Hammond 805, *847*
Huhn, K. H., s. Bahr, G. F. *903*
Hull u. Segall 819
Hull, D., s. Aherne, W. *677, 853*
— s. Dawkins, M. J. R. *853*
— s. Huger *854*
Hultin, J. V., s. Winkelmann, R. K. 337, *707*
Hunt, C. C., u. A. K. McIntyre *425*
— u. P. G. Nelson *1020*
Hunter, D., s. Harker, J. M. *918*
Hunter, R., s. Pinkus, H. *135*
Hunziker, H. 739, *782*
Hurley, H., u. G. Koelle 367, *375*
— u. H. Mescon 365, 367, *375*
Hurley jr., H. J., u. H. Mascon *617*
— u. W. B. Shelley 268, 270, 280, 282, 284, 285, 310, 330, *333, 482, 485, 486*
— W. B. Shelley u. G. B. Koelle 96, *130*, 204, *221*, 284, *333*
— u. J. Witkowski 236, *264*, 265, *325, 333*
— s. Mescon, H. 611, *618, 621*
— s. Perry, E. T. *335*
— s. Shelley, W. B. *336*
Hutchinson, C., u. C. E. Koop 471, *486*
Huzella, T. 440, *486*
Hyman, A. B., u. A. A. Guiducci 216, *221*
— s. Guiducci, A. A. *221*
Hynes, E. A., s. Allen *609, 615*
Hynes, W. 559, *617*

Hyodo, Y., s. Kobayashi, A. *1021*
Hyrtl, J. 493, 497, 507, *611, 613*

Iannaccone, A., s. Wiener, R. *908*
Ichikawa, T., s. Yasuma, A. *142*
Ieta, T., s. Kaga, T. *679*
Igarashi, Y., s. Kaku, H. *130*
Iggo, A. 412, *425, 1031*
— s. Hensel, H. *424*
Ihjima, Sh., u. T. Oono 323, *333*
Iidaka, T. *679*
Iijima, T. 297, *333*
— s. Kurosumi, K., u. T. Kitamura *333*
Ikada, M. 657, *679*
Ikemoto, H. 819, *860*
Illig, L. 495, 496, 497, 517, 523, 524, 530, 531, 534, 566, 567, *611, 617*
Im 526
Im, M. J. C. *130*
— u. W. Montagna 506, *613*
Imaeda, T. 882, *909*
Imhäuser, K., s. Feulgen, R. *127*
Imler, M., s. Oberling, Fr. *848*
Inamura, A., H. Takeda u. N. Sasaki 981, *1020*
Ingalls, N. W. 634, *679*
Ingelmark, B. E. 443, 446, *486*
Ingram, J. T. 809, *851*
— s. Charles, A. *124, 913*
Inman, D. R. *1031*
— s. Diamond, J. *1031*
Insull jr., W., u. G. E. Bartsch 828, *860*
Ippen, H., s. Stüttgen, G. *1027*
Ipsen, C. 739, 745, *782*
Iraque 606, *622*
Irgang, S. 800, *847*
Irie, M., s. Yoshimura, F. *338*
Irving, L., u. J. Krog 1001, *1020*
— s. Chatefield, P. O. *1016*
— s. Scholander, P. F. *1026*
Išaneski, M., s. Faninger, A. *847*
Iselin, B., s. Schwyzer, R. *1026*
Ishibashi, Fallani, Palmieri u. Romano 731, *781*
Ishikawa, H., u. G. Klingmüller 539, *617*
Ishiko, N., u. W. R. Loewenstein *1031*
Ishimoto, Y. 446, *486*, 638, *679*
Ito, J., s. Yamamoto, T. *429*
Ito, K. 796, 800, *847*
Ito, S. 275, 300, *333*

Ito, T., u. K. Iwashige 697, *706*
Iverson, L., u. A. B. Morrison 867, *902*
Iwashige, K. 309, 311, *333*, 696, *706*
— s. Ito, T. *706*
Iwashita, S., s. Seiji, M. *137, 915*
Izaki, M., T. Horiuchi u. H. Hozaki 871, *904*

Jablonska, S. 795, 808, 809, 811, 831, 832, *847, 851*
Jablonska, St., T. Chorzelski u. J. Lancucki 880, *907*
— I. Hausmanowa-Petrusewicz u. I. Piwowarczyk 831, 833, *860*
— u. R. Hintz 833, *860*
Jabonero, V. 398, *425*, 566, *617*
— M. E. Bengoechea u. A. Perez-Casas 378, 404, 409, *425*
— u. A. Perez-Casas *425*
— s. Prieto, R. L. *427*
Jaburek, L. 996, 997, *1020*
Jackson, C. E., s. Rukavina, J. G. *866*
Jackson, D. S. 441, *486, 1033*
— u. J. P. Bentley 441, *486*
Jackson, R. G., s. Fulton, G. P. *617*
Jackson, S. H., R. S. Savidge, L. Stein u. H. Varley 826, *854*
— s. Huger *854*
Jacobi, O. *780*
Jacox, H. W., s. Gross, P. *909*
Jadassohn, W. 802, *847*
Jaeger, H., u. J. Delacretaz 882, *909*
Jaensch, W. 515, *613*
— W. Wittneben, Th. Hoepfner, G. Leupold u. O. Gundermann 515, *613*
Jaimovich, L., s. Kaminsky, A. *848*
Jakubowski, M. 967, *1020*
Jakus, M. A., s. Schmitt, F. O. *489*
Jallad, M. M., s. Sevastinos, E. *859*
Jalowy, B. 406, *425*, 444, 445, *486*, 674, 675, *679*
— s. Lenartowicz, J. *918*
James, D. G. 796, 800, 836, *847, 858*
Jamine, F. *611*
Janitzki, s. Schleyer, F. *781*
Jammet, s. Rathery, Fr. *918*
Jamroz, C., s. Stettenheim, P. *1027*

Jansen, L. H., s. Zoon, J. J. 905
Jarrett, Spearman, Riley u. Cane 99
Jarrett, A. 18, 21, 81, 103, 130, 190, 221, 454, 486
— u. P. A. Riley 99, 119, 120, 130
— u. R. I. C. Spearman 11, 18, 21, 26, 30, 75, 81, 96, 101, 103, 117, 130, 1030
— R. I. Spearman u. J. A. Hardy 11, 130
— s. Magnus, J. A. 916
Jarry, A., s. Bureau, Y. 860
Jarvis, J., s. Goltz, R. W. 128, 332
Jasswoin, G. W. 431, 486
Jastrowitz, M. 785
Jaude, S. S. 985, 1020
Jausion, H., P. Bénard, R. Sylvestre u. J. P. Menanteau 802, 847
Jechorek, W., u. E. v. Holst 1003, 1020
Jefferis, K. R., s. Halperin, V. 221
Jeffrey, G. M., J. Sikorski u. H. J. Woods 75, 130
Jellinek, St. 776, 777, 785
Jensen 811
Jesserer, H. 887, 911
Jirka, M., u. J. Kotas 248, 265
Jochems, s. Pfeifer 811
Jöchle, W. 1014, 1020, 1021
Joel, C. D., u. E. G. Ball 819, 854
Johann, L. 941, 1021
Johansson, H., s. Holmgren, H. 679
John, F. 397, 398, 425, 482, 486, 566, 567, 617
— s. Marchionini, A. 902
Johnson, A. G., s. Happey, F. 180
Johnson, E., u. F. J. Ebling 1030
— s. Ebling, F. J. 1030
Johnson, F. R., u. R. M. H. McMinn 1033
Johnson, M., s. Bullough, W. S. 124
Johnson, M. H., s. Brines, O. A. 853
Johnson, P. L., E. O. Butcher u. G. Bevelander 176, 181
— H. Hoffmann u. G. K. Rolle 71, 130
Johnsen, S. G., u. J. E. Kirk 185, 191, 221
Johnson, W. C., s. Gray, H. R. 911
Jones, D. B. 815, 851
Jones, D. J., u. W. Morgan 1009, 1021

Jones, R. S., u. D. B. Frazier 863, 902
Jordan, H. E. 439, 486
Jorge, J. K., u. D. Brachetto-Brian 882, 909
Jørgensen, C. B., u. L. O. Larsen 979, 1021
— L. O. Larsen u. P. Rosenkilde 979, 1021
Jorpes, E., H. Holmgren u. O. Wilander 437, 486
Joslin, D., s. Conway, H. 616
Josserand, s. Nové-Josserand, L. 918
Jostock, P. J., u. G. Klingmüller 512, 613
Juchems, R., s. Pfeifer, U. 861
Juhlin, L., u. W. B. Shelley 526, 537, 617
Juhn, M., u. R. W. Bates 1009, 1021
— s. Lillie, F. R. 1022
Juncker 858
Jungas, R. L., s. Ball, E. G. 853
Junge, G. C. A., s. Oordt, G. J. van 1024

Kadanoff, D. 378, 383, 402, 404, 411, 425
— W. Wassilev u. I. Matev 425
Kaga, T. 307, 323, 333
— T. Goto u. T. Ieta 679
— s. Goto, T. 679
Kagemoto, H., s. Yasuda, K. 338
— s. Yasuda, K., u. K. Kobayashi 338
— s. Yasui, I. 334, 338, 682
Kahl, M. P. 1001, 1021
Kaiser, L. 1004, 1021
Kaiser, S. 888, 912
Kajikawa, K. 433, 441, 486
Kaku, Igarashi, Masu u. Fujita 68, 70
Kaku, H., Y. Igarashi, S. Masu u. S. Fujita 130
Kalantaevskaya, K. G., u. I. G. Gurins 696, 706
Kaldor, I., u. L. Nekam 815, 851, 858
Kalkoff, K. W. 837, 858
Kallapravit, B. 184, 190, 221
Kallenbach, E., s. Sarkar, K. 336
Kallius, E., s. Boas, J. E. V. 1016
Kallman, F., u. C. Grobstein 976, 1021
— u. N. K. Wessells 1029
Kallmann, F. L., s. Porter, K. R. 135
Kalnitzky, G., s. Barron, E. S. G. 121

Kalsbeek, G. L., s. Cormane, R. H. 180
Kalsbeek, L., s. Cormane, R. H. G. 125
Kaltenbach, J. C., u. N. B. Clark 979, 1021
Kaltenbach, R. 784
Kamei, Y., s. Steigleder, G. K. 139, 183, 489, 612, 620
Kamer, J. C. v. de, s. Kelly, D. E. 1021
Kamide, J. 378, 425
Kamin, H., s. Williams jr., Ch. H. 142
Kaminsky, A., L. Jaimovich, P. Viglioglia, M. Kordon u. H. Rosales 800, 848
Kampen, v. 920
Kan, M. 679
Kanaizuka, Z. 481, 486
Kanitz, H. 898, 918
Kano, K. 696, 706
— s. Kurosumi, K. 221, 265
Kanoff, N. B., s. Sawicky, H. H. 849, 856
Kantner, M. 411, 425, 690, 702, 706
Kapacinsky u. Besjedkin 759
Kaplan, A. D. 777, 786
Kaplan, L., s. Newcomer, V. D. 848, 859
Kappeler, H., s. Schwyzer, R. 1026
Karkun, J. N., u. F. W. Landgrebe 948, 1021
Karlsbad, G., s. Petris, S. de 488
Karlson, P. 101, 102, 103, 114, 130, 337
Karnovsky, M. J. 40, 130
Karrenberg, C. L. 657, 679
Karrer, H. E. 31, 32, 33, 34, 130, 433, 449, 486
— u. J. Cox 432, 441, 447, 486
Kasahara, M., s. Malcolm, R. 426
— S. Miller, M. R. 375, 426, 618
Kasten, F. H. 780
Kastin, A. J., u. G. T. Ross 950, 1021
Kataoka, H., S. Yamagata u. Y. Ueda 871, 904
Kato, S. 272, 333
— u. M. Nagata 274, 333
Katsuki, Y., S. Yoshino u. J. Chen 955, 1021
Katzberg, A. A. 467, 469, 486, 634, 636, 679, 690, 706
— s. Thuringer, J. M. 682, 707
Katzenellenbogen, I., u. H. Ungar 871, 904

Kauffmann, Th. 931, 965, *1021*
Kauffmann, S. L., u. A. P. Stout 823, 824, *854*
Kaufmann, E. 898, *917*
Kawabata, I. 277, 287, 288, 289, 293, 297, 299, 301, 303, 323, 325, 326, 327, *333*
Kawahata, A. 225, *265*
Kawamura, J. 776, *786*
Kawamura, T. 384, 407, *425*, 892, *913*
— K. Nichihara u. H. Nakajima 674, *679*, *680*
Kawase, O., u. K. Sunahara 469, *486*
Kay, L. M., s. Schraeder, W. A. *1026*
Kayser, F. 329, *333*
Kazmeier, F. 810, *851*
Keddie, F., u. D. Sakai 59, *130*
Keech, M. K. 440, 441, 447, 449, *486*
— u. R. Reed 447, *486*
— — u. W. J. Wood 447, *486*
Keegan, H. L., u. W. V. Macforlane, s. Halstead, B. W. *1019*
Keibel, F., u. F. P. Mall *681*
Keil, W. 824, *854*
Keining, E., u. O. Braun-Falco 816, *851*, 874, 876, 877, 879, 880, 881, *907*, *909*
Kekulé, A., s. Friedreich, N. *902*
Keller, F. R., s. Bosch, K. *782*
Kellner, G. 412, 419, *425*
Kellner, H. 804, 836, *848*, *858*
Kelly, D. E. 31, 33, 35, *130*, 630, 631, *680*, 931, 970, 971, 973, *1021*
— u. J. C. van de Kamer 949, 950, *1021*
Kelly, J. W., s. Bloom, G. *483*
Kelsch, J. J., s. Gessler, A. E. *128*
Kemp, N. E. 932, 973, 974, 982, 986, *1021*
Kendall, R. F., R. C. Davidson u. J. Pfaff jr. 884, *909*
Kenin, A. J. Levine u. M. Spinner 820, *854*
Kennedy, J. S. 864, *902*
— s. Curran, R. C. *906*
Kent, S. P. 780, *783*
Kerdel-Vegas, Fr. 803, *860*
Kerl, W. 881, 887, 899, *909*, *911*, *918*
Kerl-Urbach 881
Kern, A. B., s. Schiff, B. L. *911*
Kerneis, J. P., Bureau, Y. *860*

Kersting, K. H., s. Staubesand, G. *337*
Kessel, J., s. Lynen, F. *844*
Kessel, O. 899, *918*
Kessel, R. G. 300, *333*
Kétron, L. W., u. J. C. Bernstein 809, *851*
Keuning, F. J., s. Hamminga, H. *906*
Kiaer, N., s. Frederiksen, T. *866*
Kierland, R. R., u. P. A. O'Leary 452, 469, *486*
Kierland, R. R., s. Pittelkow, R. B. *910*
Kierland, R., s. Gilje, O., u. E. J. Baldes *610*
Kiese 731
Kiessling, W., s. Gartmann, H. *851*
Kikuchi, R., s. Higashi, H. *1020*
Kim, R., u. R. K. Winkelmann 880, *907*
Kim, Y. S., s. Kosugi, T. *181*
Kimball, F. B., s. Sheldon, H. *489*
Kimmig, J., u. R. Wehrmann 13, 14, 76, *130*, 789, *844*
King, J. R., u. D. S. Farner 1000, *1021*
Kinkelin, B., s. Stüttgen, G. *1027*
Kinoshita, H., s. Ohno, T. *335*
Kinoshita, R. 891, *913*
Kinosita, H. 948, *1021*
Kinsley, J. W., s. Dannenberg, A. M. *484*
Kint, A., u. D. Candaele 876, *907*
— s. Braun-Falco, O. 122, *179*, *182*
Kint s. Braun-Falco *182*
Kirk, E. 187, 188, *221*
Kirk, J. E., s. Johnsen, S. G. *221*
Kirkman, H., u. A. E. Severinghaus 110, 112, *130*
Kirschbaum, A., s. Liebett, A. *856*
Kirschenberg, E. 792, *845*
Kiss, F. *425*
Kitamura, K. 674, *680*
Kitamura, T., s. Kurosumi, K. 221, *265*, *333*
— s. Kurosumi, K., u. T. Iijima *333*
Kittel, F. *425*
Klaar, J. 268, 272, 282, 286, 329, *333*
Klaatsch u. Gnadeberg 944
Klapproth 771
Klaschka, F., s. Spier, H. W. *856*
Klein, H. 777, 784, *786*

Klein, H. J., s. Rudolph, G. *488*
Klein, P., u. P. Burkholder 865, *902*
Kleinholz, L. H. 950, 991, *1021*
Klemperer, P. 451, *486*
Kligman, A. 350, *375*
Kligman, A. M. 13, 14, 21, 24, 29, *130*, 145, 158, 160, 162, *181*
— u. W. B. Shelley 185, *221*
— s. Christophers, E. *125*
— s. Maguire, H. C. *181*
— s. Pillsbury, D. M. *622*
— s. Strauß, J. S. *223*, *857*
— s. Strauß, J. S., u. P. E. Pochi *223*
Klingmüller, G. 495, 606, *611*, *622*
— u. O. Hornstein *904*
— s. Hornstein, O. *904*
— s. Ishikawa *617*
— s. Jostock, P. J. *613*
Klionsky, B., s. Sweeley, C. C. *910*
Klostermann, G. F., u. P. Ritzenfeld 894, *916*
— H. Südhof u. W. Tischendorf 804, *843*
Klüken, N., s. Gahlen, W. *919*
Kneeland, J. E. 267, 301, 303, *333*
Knese, K. H., u. A. Knoop 433, 441, *486*
Knoche, H. 169, *181*, 377, 400, *425*
Knoop, A., s. Bargmann, W. *330*
— s. Bargmann, W., u. K. Fleischhauer *330*
— s. Horstmann, E. *130*, *375*
— s. Knese, K. H. *486*
Knoth, W. 813, 814, 815, 816, 819, 823, 824, 837, 838, *851*, *854*, *858*
— R. Baethke u. L. Hoffmann 793, 794, *845*
— G. Beneke u. E. Kuntz 811, 812, 813, *851*
— u. S. Bettge 824, 825, *854*
— u. H. Füller 814, 815, 837, 838, *851*, *858*, *909*
— u. W. Meyhöfer 795, 808, 809, 810, 811, 817, 837, *848*, *851*, *858*
— M. Ruhbach u. G. Ehlers 93, 96, *130*, 176, *181*
— s. Kuntz, E. *851*
— s. Miescher, G., u. W. Burckhardt *852*
— s. Poutrier, L. M. *855*
Knox, J. M., s. Freeman, R. G. *705*
— s. Ogura, R. *134*

Kobabe, A. 752, *783*
Kobayashi, A., H. A. Bern, R. S. Nishioka u. Y. Hyodo 1014, *1021*
Kobayashi, H., u. K. Obuko 1014, *1021*
Kobayashi, K., s. Yasuda, K., u. H. Kagemoto *338*
Kobayasi, T. 288, *333*
Koch, F. 272, *333*
Koch, G., s. Delank, H.-W. *901*
Koch, R., s. Dieckhoff, J. *847, 857*
Kochem, H. G., s. Vogt, A. *903*
Kraus 794, *845*
Kraus u. Deist, s. Gottron, H. A. *847*
Kraus, F., s. Emden, G. *780*
Krause 377
Krause, C. 267, *333*
Krause, R. 924, 937, 941, 957, *1021*
Kreibich, C. 43, *130*, 864, 875, *902, 907*
Kreis de Mayo, Fl., s. Lacomme, M. *848*
Kremer, H., s. Hänig, E. *904*
Krimm, S. 1009, *1021*
— s. Schor, R. *1026*
Kriner, J. 801, 802, *848*
Krog, J., s. Irving, L. *1020*
Krogh, A. 491, 529, 530, 531, 533, 567, *611, 617*
Krogis, A. 1005, *1021*
Kromayer, F. 43, *131*
Krompecher, E. *333*
Krompecher, St. 447, *486*
Kroplin-Rueff, L., Lynen, F. *844*
Kropp, P. J., s. Pinkus, H. *135*
Krueger, S., s. Doeg, K. A. *125*
Krumbach, T., u. W. Kükenthal, s. Stresemann, E. *1027*
Kruse, M. 67, *131*
Kruszynski, J. 66, *131*
Krzystalowicz, F. 700, *706*
Kuder, A., s. Adams, A. E. *1015*
Küchler, W. J. 1014, *1021*
Kudicke, R., s. Steigleder, G. K. *139, 183, 489, 612, 620*
Kühn, K. 442, *486*
— W. Grassmann u. U. Hofmann 442, *486*
Kükenthal, W., u. T. Krumbach, s. Stresemann, E. *1027*
Külczycki, W. 493, 497, *611*
Küntzel, A. 18, *131*
Küttner, H., u. M. Baruch 803, *848*

Kuff, E. L., u. A. J. Dalton 299, *333*
— s. Schneider, W. C. *137*
Kuhlo, B., s. Staubesand, G. *337*
Kuhn, E., s. Mosinger, B. *856*
Kuhn, O. 1010, *1021*
— u. H. U. Koecke 1005, *1022*
Kuich, L. L., s. Selander, R. K. *1026*
Kujalová, V., s. Mosinger, B. *856*
Kukita, A., s. Fitzpatrick, T. B. *127, 913*
— s. Fitzpatrick, F. B., u. T. B. Brunet *913*
Kuklova-Sturova 530, *617, 618*
Kulaga, U. v. 809, *851*
Kulemann, H. 948, *1022*
Kulwin, M. H., s. Buley, H. M. *919*
Kulzer, E. 971, *1022*
Kuno, Y. 225, 226, 253, *265*
Kuntz, A., u. J. W. Hamilton 564, 566, *618*
Kuntz, E., G. Beneke u. W. Knoth 811, *851*
— s. Knoth, W. *851*
Kunze, E., s. Schulze, W. *849*
Kuré, K., T. Oi u. S. Okinaka 829, *856*
Kuriki, S. 669, *680*
Kurokowa, S., s. Arimori, M. *855*
Kurosumi 237
Kurosumi, K. 287, 297, 299, 325, 326, 327, *333*
— u. T. Kitamura 288, *333*
— — u. T. Iijima 268, 287, 288, 290, 292, 293, 296, 297, 299, 300, 301, 302, 303, 304, 325, 326, 327, *333*
— — u. K. Kano 204, 205, 221, 241, *265*
— T. Matsuzawa u. F. Saito 267, 327, *333*
— M. Yamagishi u. M. Sekine 268, 291, 297, *333, 334*
— s. Matsuzawa, T. *265, 334*
Kuske, H., J. M. Paschoud u. W. Soltermann 820, *854*
Kusnetz, M. 696, *706*
Kúta, A. 823, *854*
Kutsche, A., s. Schwarz, W., u. H. J. Werker *489*
Kutscher, W., u. V. Vrla 883, *909*
Kuwabara, T., u. D. G. Cogan *623*
Kvorning, S. A. 187, *221*
Kwiatkowski, St. L. 899, *918*
Kyrle, J. 270, *334*, 843

Kochs, A. G. 900, *918*
Kock, D. H. de, s. Heyl, R. *904*
Kock, R., s. Ritzenfeld, P. *136*
Kockel 726
Koecke 920, 970, 1007
Koecke, H. U. 115, *130, 425*
— u. W. Schittenhelm 1010, *1021*
— s. Kuhn, O. *1022*
Koefoed-Johnsen, V., u. H. H. Ussing 981, *1021*
Koelle, G. B. 556, *617*
— s. Hurley, H. J. *130, 375*
— s. Hurley, H. J., u. W. B. Shelley *333*
— s. Hurley jr., H. J. *221*
— s. Shelley, W. B. *138, 183, 223, 336*
Kölliker, A. 217, *221*, 267, 285, *333*, 342, 345, 361, *375*, 493, 494, 599, *611, 622*
Kölliker, A. V. 378, *425*
König, J. 471, *486*
Koenig, H. 294, *333*
Königsdörffer, H., s. Borst, M. *915*
Königstein, H. 864, 867, *902*
Könn, G., s. Delank, H.-W. *901*
Koeppen, S. 777, *786*
— u. H. Gerstner 776, 777, *786*
Kogoj, F. 2, 3, *130*
— u. St. Puretić 816, *851*
Kohan, A. B. 627, *680*
Koibuchi, S. 184, *221*
Kolas, S., s. Halperin, V. *221*
Kolhaus, J. C. 493, *611*
Kolisko 744
Kollmann 726
Komatsu, M., s. Niizuma, S. *426*
Kominkora, E., s. Zika, K. *622*
Komnick, H. 244, *265*
— u. K. E. Wohlfarth-Bottermann *1021*
Kondo, T., s. Horio, M. *375*
Konecki, J., s. Rasiewicz, W. *905*
Koning, A. *375*
— u. H. Hamilton 365, *375*
Koning, A. L. 1008, *1021*
— s. Hamilton, H. L. *1019*
Konopik, J. 802, 835, *848, 858*
Konrad, J. 867, *902*
— u. A. Winkler 879, *907*
Kooij, R. 795, 802, *848*
Koop, C. E., s. Hutchinson, C. *486*
Koopmann 743, 759, *782*
Koopmann, H., s. Roer, H. *784*

Kooyman, D. J.   66, 67, *130*
Kopf, A.   726, *783*
Kopf, A. W.   96, 99, *130*, 176, *181*, 322, 323, 324, *333*, 879, *907*
Kopriwa, B., s. Leblond, C. P. *131*
Kopsch, s. Rauber   717, *780*
Korb und David   720
Kordon, M., s. Kaminsky, A. *848*
Korting, G. W.   805, 808, 811, *848, 851*
— u. F. Nürnberger   814, *851*
— u. G. Weber   880, *907*
— s. Cabré, J.   *906*
— s. Gottron, H. A.   *906, 912*
— s. Holt u. Howland   *847*
— s. Hughes u. Hammond   *847*
— s. Riecke, E.   *902*
— s. Weyhbrecht, H.   *905*
Kosaka, Y.   184, *221*, 660, 668, 669, *680*
— s. Taniguchi, T.   *223*
Kosten, E.   *784*
Kosugi, T., u. Y. S. Kim   165, *181*
Kotas, J., s. Jirka, M.   *264*
Kotelnikow, W.   898, *917*
Kounker, W., s. Goldmann, L. *610*
Kovacev, V. P., u. R. O. Scow   827, *860*
Kozakiewicz, J., s. Miedzinski, F.
Kracht u. Gusek   834
Krahulik, L., M. Rosenthal u. E. H. Loughlin   811, *851*
Krantz, W.   352, *375*
Kratter   *782*
Kratter, J.   740, 742, 743, 744, 745, 747, 759, 776, *782*
Kratzer, G. L., u. M. B. Dockerty   635, *680*
Kraucher, G.   628, *680*
Kraul, U., s. Müller, H.   817, *861*
Krauland, W.   765, *785, 786*

Lackey, M. D., s. Du Buy, H. G. *125*
Lacomme, M., u. Fl. Kreis de Mayo   *848*
Lacy, P. E., s. Williamson, J. R.   *845, 857*
Laden, E. L., J. O. Erickson u. D. Armen   37, *131*
Lagunoff, D., s. Combs, J. W. *484*
Laidlaw, G. F., u. S. N. Blackberg   106, *131*
Laiho, K.   *783*
Lain, E. S., s. Lamb, J. H.   *909*

Lamb, J. H., u. E. S. Lain   882, *909*
Lambertini, G.   415, *426*
Lancucki, J., s. Jablonska, St. *907*
Landau, J., s. Davis, E.   *616*
Lande, J., s. Hofmann, K. *1020*
Landers, J. W., J. L. Chason, J. E. Gonzales u. W. Palutke   *623*
Landes, E.   *845*
— s. Gans, O.   *845*
Landgrebe, F. W., s. Karkun, J. N.   *1021*
Landi, G., u. P. L. Negri   871, *904*
Landing, B. H., s. Heuser, E. *860*
Landis, E. M.   530, 531, *618*
Landolt, A. M.   635, *680*
Landolt, R., s. Raben, M. S. *1024*
Langcope, W. T., u. D. G. Freiman   800, *848*
Lange, B.   920, 992, 998, 999, 1000, 1001, *1022*
Langegger, P. A., s. Eberl-Rothe, G.   *678*
Langer, E.   808, *848*
— u. G. Stüttgen   890, *914*
Langer, H., u. H. Langer-Schierer   819, *854*
Langerhans, P.   116, *131*
Langeron, L., A. Delattre u. M. Paget   899, *918*
Langer-Schierer, H., s. Langer, H.   *854*
Langhof, H.   802, 817, *848, 851*
— H. Müller u. L. Rietschel   893, *916*
— u. L. Rietschel   893, *916*
Langner, A., s. Braun-Falco, O. *122*
Lankau jr., C. A., s. Strain, W. H.   *183*
Lansing   449
Lansing, A. J.   705, 873, *904*
— u. D. I. Opdyke   77, *131*
— u. D. L. Odyke   *783*
— T. B. Rosenthal, M. Alex u. E. W. Dempsey   449, 450, *486*
— s. Dempsey, E. W.   *484*
— s. Smith jr., J. G.   *905*
Lanz, T. V.   478, *486*
Lanzing, W. J. R.   933, *1022*
La Pava, S. de, u. J. W. Pickren   219, *221*
Lapiere, C. M., s. Gross, J. *1019*
— s. Gross, J., u. M. L. Tanzer   *1019*
Lapiere, S.   639, *680*, 901, *919*

Larcher   725, 726, *781*
Larner, A. E., s. Lobitz jr., W. C.   *221*
Larsen, L. O., s. Jørgensen, C. B.   *1021*
— s. Jørgensen, C. B., u. P. Rosenkilde   *1021*
Larsson, K. S., s. Brody, I. *124, 678*
Lasersohn, J. T., s. Avioli, L. *908*
Laszlo, J.   828, *856*
Laterjet, R.   103, *131*
Laubinger, W.   456, 458, 475, *486*, 788, 819, *844*
Laucker, J. L. van, u. R. L. Holzer   *780*
Lauer   *780*
Laufer, M., s. Wolff, F.   *785*
Laurence, E. B., s. Bullough, W. S.   *124, 179, 1016, 1032*
— s. Bullough, W. S., u. C. L. Hewett   *124*
Lauter, S., u. A. Terhecherbrügge   703, *706*
Lavelle, S. M., s. Fitzgerald, M. J. T.   *424*
Laves, W.   731, *781*
Lawler, F. C., s. Davis, M. J. *610, 616, 621*
Lawler, J. C., u. L. R. Lumpkin   533, *618*
Lawler, J., s. Davis, M.   *375*
Lawless, T. K.   867, *902*
Laymon, C. W.   885, *909*
— u. I. Fisher   885, *909*
— u. E. M. Hill   871, 872, *904*
— u. J. J. Sevenants   882, *909*
Laymon, C. W., s. Butler, J. *906*
— s. Michelson, H. E.   *910*
Laymon, C. W., s. Sweitzer, S. E.   *907*
Leale-Leali   493, *611*
Leblond, C. P.   62, 70, 72, *131*, 177, 178, *181, 1033*
— N. B. Everett u. B. Simmons   177, *181*
— R. E. Glegg u. D. Eidinger   539, *618*
— R. C. Greulich u. J. P. M. Pereira   8, 10, 62, 63, 64, 69, *131*
— B. Messier u. B. Kopriwa   63, *131*
— u. B. E. Walker   63, *131*
— s. Giroud, A.   *128, 180*
— s. Giroud, A., u. H. Bulliard   *128*, 180
— s. Glegg, R. E.   *485*
— s. Messier, B.   *133, 334*
— s. Puchtler, H.   *619*
Lecène, P., u. P. Moulonguet   841, *858*

Leczinsky, C. G. 795, 809, 848, 851
Leder, M., s. Miescher, G. 852
Ledoux-Corbusier, M. 680
Lee 721
Lee, D. G., u. K. Schmidt-Nielsen 284, 334
Lee, J. L., s. Rothberg, S. 136
Lee, M. C. 245, 247, 248, 257, 258, 260, 261, 265
Lee, M. M. 473, 486
Lee, T. H., u. A. B. Lerner 949, 1022
— — u. V. Buettner-Janusch 949, 1022
— s. Lerner, A. B. 1022
Leeper, R. W., s. Lever, W. F. 909, 910
Leeson, C. R. 302, 334
Leeson, R. 482, 486
Leeson, R. C., u. L. T. Threadgold 976, 1022
Le Fevre, P. G. 72, 131
Leger 836, 861
Lehmann, H. J. 426
Lehmann, K. B. 745, 783
Lehnartz, E., s. Flaschenträger, B. 127, 484
Lehninger, A. L. 289, 334
Leiby, G. M., s. Adolph, W. E. 120
Leifer, W. 815, 851, 885, 909
Leinati, F. 840, 858
Leinbrock, A. 870, 904
Leiner, M. 967, 1022
Leipert, Th. 895, 896, 916
Leitan, V. P. 638, 680
Leitner, St. 800, 848
Lele, P. P., E. Palmer u. G. Weddell 922, 924, 925, 1022
— u. G. Weddell 384, 426
Leloup, R., u. A. Bourlond 357, 375, 389, 426
Lemarchand-Beraud, Th., s. Utiger, R. D. 908
Lenartowicz, J., u. B. Jalowy 899, 918
Lennert, K. 824, 854
— u. G. Weitzel 95, 131
Leonforte, J. F., s. Ferreira-Marques, J. 610
Leonhardi, G. 76, 86, 131, 892, 914
— u. G. K. Steigleder 175, 181
Leontowitsch, A. 401, 426
Leriche 803, 848
Lerma, B. de 893, 916
Lerne, u. Hull 640
Lerner, A. B. 85, 104, 114, 131
— J. D. Case u. R. V. Heinzelman 949, 1022

Lerner, A. B., J. D. Case, u. Y. Takahashi 950, 1022
— — — T. H. Lee u. W. Mori 949, 1022
— u. T. B. Fitzpatrick 114, 131, 890, 914
— — E. Calkins u. W. H. Summerson
Lerner, A. B., u. J. S. Mc Guire 131
— u. T. H. Lee 948, 949, 1022
— s. Case, J. D. 1022
— s. Fitzpatrick, T. B. 127, 913
— s. Fitzpatrick, T. B., S. W. Becker jr. u. H. Montgomery 127
— s. Fitzpatrick, T. B., u. H. Montgomery 913
— s. Lee, T. H. 1022
— s. Lee, T. H., u. V. Buettner-Janusch 1022
— s. Wright, M. R. 1028
Leslie, P. 815, 851
Lesser, A. 759, 782, 784
Lester, R. L., s. Hatefi, Y 129
Letterer, E. 811, 862, 863, 865, 866, 875, 851, 902, 907
— R. Caesar u. A. Vogt 864, 902
Letterer, H. 719, 720, 780
Leuchtenberger, C., u. H. Z. Lund 47, 68, 69, 131
Leuchter 742, 743
Leupold, G., s. Jaensch, W. 613
Levene, A. L., s. Fitzpatrick, T. B. 913
Levene, C. I., s. Cohen, A. S., u. H. Calkins 901
Lever, I. D. 456, 458, 461, 486
Lever, J. D. 819, 821, 824, 854
Lever, W. F. 2, 4, 8, 10, 11, 13, 14, 15, 21, 24, 108, 131, 796, 798, 800, 801, 802, 805, 806, 815, 816, 843, 848, 862, 864, 865, 868, 878, 881, 882, 884, 887, 897, 902, 907, 909, 911, 917
— u. D. G. Freiman 800, 848
— u. R. W. Leeper 883, 909, 910
— s. Cummins, L. J. 847
— s. Hashimoto, u. B. G. Gross 679
— s. Hashimoto, K., u. B. G. Gross 679
— s. Hashimoto, K., B. Gross u. R. J. Di Bella 679
— s. Hashimoto, K., B. G. Gross u. R. Nelson 129, 679

Lever, W. F., s. Wainger, C. K. 846
— s. Wilgram, G. F. 141
Lever, W. 607, 622
— s. Hashimoto, K. 264, 332, 375, 902
Levi, G. 529, 534, 535, 618
Levi, S. 378, 426
Levin, O. L., u. S. H. Silvers 898, 917
Levine, J., s. Kenin, A. 854
Levine, M., s. Puchtler, H. 903
Levonen, E., s. Rackallio, J. 619
Levy, J., s. Pautrier, L. M. 914
Lewandowsky, F. 848
Lewis, B. 342, 344, 345, 346, 347, 348, 349, 351, 370, 375
— u. H. Montgomery 342, 360, 375
Lewis, B. L. 669, 670, 671, 673, 680
— u. H. Montgomery 699, 706
Lewis, Ch., s. Hershey, F. B. 485
Lewis, S. R., C. M. Pomerat u. D. Ezell 37, 114, 131
Lewis, T. 491, 496, 531, 611, 618
Lewis, W. H. 491, 558, 618
— s. Gray, H. 613
Lewis, Y. S., s. Smith, D. E. 489
Li, C. H. 856
— J. Meienhofer, E. Schnabel, D. Chung, T. Lo u. J. Ramachandran 1022
— s. Birk, Y. 855
Li, C. H., s. Schwyzer, R. 1026
Liadsky, C., s. Pullar, P. 681
Liberkühn, J. N. 493, 611
Lichtenstein 881
Lichtenstein, L. 881, 882, 910
Liebegott, G. 767, 785
Liebett, A., u. A. Kirschbaum 827, 856
Lieberman, E., s. Heuser, E. 860
Lièvre 836, 861
Lièvre, s. de Graciansky 860
Light, A. E. 169, 181
— s. Hamilton, J. B. 180
Lillie 83
Lillie, F. R. 1005, 1006, 1022
— u. M. Juhn 1006, 1022
Lillie, R. D. 444, 486, 874, 890, 907, 914
— s. Fullmer, H. M. 484
Liman 759
Lindberg, O., J. de Pierre, E. Rylander u. B. A. Afzelius 819, 861
— u. L. Ernster 86, 131

Lindberg, S., S. E. Lindell u. H. Westling 638, *680*
Lindblom, U. 426, *1031*
Linde, K. W. *680*
Lindell, S. E., s. Lindberg, S. *680*
Lindemayr, W., s. Gabriel, H. *902*
Lindholm, E. 471, *486*, 704, 706
Lindlar, F., u. V. Misgeld 806, 807, 808, 834, *861*
Lindley, H., s. Fraser, R. *375*
Lindner, D. 431, 436, *486*
Lindner, H., s. Schallock, G. *907*
Lindner, J. 754, *783*, 878, *907*
— u. G. Freytag 864, *902*
Linke 638
Linke, K. W. 443, 444, 469, *486*, 693, *706*
Linné 735
Linser, K. 816, 837, *851*, *858*
Lionetti, F., s. Mager, M. *131*
Lison, L. 81, *131*, 941, 945, *1022*
Lissmann, H. W. 993, *1022*
List, C. F., u. M. M. Peet *426*
Liszt, F. v. 764, *785*
Little, J. A., u. A. J. Steigman 836, *858*
Litvac, A., s. Champetier, G. *124*
Liviere, u. Paraf 836
Livini, F. 631, *680*
Liu, T., s. Hofmann, K. *1020*
— s. Hofmann, K., H. Yajima, N. Yanaihara u. J. Lande *1020*
Ljunggreen, M., s. Ernster, L. *126*
Lloyd, D. 371, *375*
— u. M. Garrod 371, *375*
Lloyd, D. P. C. 253, *265*
Lo, T., s. Li, C. H. *1022*
Lobitz, W. C., J. B. Holyoke u. D. Brophy 253, 257, 258, *265*
— — u. W. Montagna 249, 257, 258, *265*
— J. B. Holyoke jr. u. W. Montagna 583, *621*
— u. H. L. Mason 253, *265*
— s. Dobson, R. L. *264*
— s. Dobson, R. L., V. Formisano u. D. Brophy *264*
— s. Formisano, V. *264*
— s. Holyoke, J. B. *264*
— s. Montagna, W. *265*
— s. Montagna, W., u. H. B. Chase *334*
Lobitz jr., W. C., D. Brophy, A. E. Larner u. F. Daniels jr. 201, *221*

Lobitz jr., W. C., u. J. B. Holyoke 78, *131*, 201, 221
— — u. W. Montagna 631, 664, *680*
— s. Eisen, A. Z. *221*
— s. Montagna, W. 121, *133*, *914*
— s. Montagna, W., u. H. B. Chase *181*, 222
— s. Pass, F. *680*
Lo Cascio, M. 512, 513, 516, 563, 606, 607, *613*, *618*, 622, 623
Lochte, T. 147, 148, 149, 150, 158, *181*
Locke, M. 31, *131*, 334, 336
Loeb, J. 511, *613*
Löffler, H., s. Steigleder, G. K. *139*, *183*, 223, *859*, 620
Löfgren, S., u. F. Wahlgren 796, *848*
Löhe, H. 901, *919*
Loeschke, H. 329, *334*, 865, *902*
Loetzke, H. H., s. Meyer, M. *1023*
Loeven, W. A. *907*
Loewenstein, W. R. *1031*
— u. M. Mendelson *1031*
— u. R. Shalak 1005, *1022*
— s. Ishiko, N. *1031*
Loewenthal, J., s. Mackenzie, D. C. *618*
Loewenthal, L. *916*
Loewenthal, L. J. A. 241, 248, 249, *265*
Loewi, G., u. K. Meyer 450, 452, *487*
Loftfield, R. B. 47, 58, *131*
Lombard, W. P. 494, *611*
Lombardo, C. 171, *181*
Lopez, P. 900, *918*
Lopresti, J. H., s. Avioli, L. *908*
Lorenz, K., s. Urbach, E. *910*
Lorenzen, J. N. 900, *918*
Lorenzen, L., s. Farner, D. S. *1018*
Lorincz, A. L., s. Davis, M. J. *610*
Lorke, D. 780
— u. O. Schmidt *781*
Lortat, G., u. M. Vitry 828, *856*
Lossie, H., u. H. Voegt 836, *858*
Loud, A. V., u. Y. Mishima 960, 964, 965, *1022*
— s. Mishima, Y. *914*, *1023*
— s. Mishima, Y., u. F. F. Schaub *914*
Loughlin, E. H., s. Krahulik, L. *851*
Louviere, C. D., s. Farber, E. *126*

Lovett-Doust, J. W. 530, *618*
Lowenstein, O. 951, 956, *1022*
— M. P. Osborne u. J. Wersäll 955, *1022*
— u. J. Wersäll 955, *1022*
Lubarsch, O. 869, 896, *904*
Lubnow, E. 104, 110, 112, *131*, 1005, *1022*
— s. Danneel, R. *125*
Lubosch, W., s. Boas, J. E. V. *1016*
Lubowe, I. I. *181*
Lucas, A. M., s. Peterson, R. A. *1024*
— s. Stettenheim, P. *1027*
Luciani 790, 791, *845*
Luck, C. P., u. P. G. Wrigth *1032*
Ludford, R. J. 43, *131*, 195, 201, *222*
Ludowieg, J., s. Schiller, S. *488*
Ludwig 182
Ludwig, A. W., s. Wiener, R. *908*
Ludwig, E. 169, *181*, 467, *487*, 745, *782*
Lüdicke, M. 993, 994, 999, 1007, *1022*, *1023*
— u. B. Geierhaas 1007, *1023*
— u. H. Teichert 1007, *1023*
Luell, E., u. V. E. Archer 148, *181*
Lüneburg 267, 328, *334*
Luft, J. H., s. Bennett, H. S. *615*
Luger u. Schulhof 729
Luh, W., s. Pette, D. *335*
Luithlen 805, *848*
Lukas, A. 746, *782*
Lumpkin, L. R., s. Lawler, J. C. *618*
Lund, H. Z., u. R. L. Sommerville 873, *904*
— s. Leuchtenberger, C. *131*
Lundgren, H. P., u. W. H. Ward 49, 50, 51, 52, *131*
— s. Ward, W. H. *141*
Lundt, V. 870, *904*
Lupidi, I., s. Ottaviani, G. *680*
Luschka 726, *781*
Lutz, B. R., s. Fulton, G. P. *617*
Lutz, W. 843, 898, *917*
— s. Zimmerli, E. *918*
Luzzatti, u. Hansen 805, 806, *848*
Lyman, C. P., s. Chatfield, P. O. *1016*
Lynch, F. W. 447, *487*, 511, *613*, 638, *680*
Lyne, A. G. *1030*
— u. H. B. Chase 119, *131*

Lyne, A. G., u. B. F. Short 681
Lynen, F., B. Agranoff, U. Hennig u. E. Möslein 844
— H. Eggerer, U. Hennig u. J. Kessel 789, 844
— U. Hennig, C. Bublitz, B. Sörbo u. L. Kröplin-Rueff 789, 844
Lynfield, Y. L. 162, 181
Lyter, C. S., s. Blake, H. A. 855

Ma, C. K., u. E. V. Cowdry 685, 693, 706
Macaigne, N., u. P. Nicaud 810, 852
MacCardle, R. C., M. F. Engman jr., u. M. F. Engman sen. 67, 131
— s. Engman, M. F. 126
— s. Scott, E. J. van 223
Macforlane, W. V., u. H. L. Keegan, s. Halstead, B. W. 1019
MacGregor, I. A. 559, 618
Mach, K. 882, 910
Mach, K. W., s. Holubar, K. 906
Machaceck, G. F., s. Gross, P. 851
Machacek 836, 861
Macher 430, 436
Macher, E. 901, 919
— u. W. Vogel 495, 533, 534, 535, 539, 541, 542, 543, 544, 545, 546, 611, 618
Machida, H. 633, 641, 659, 664, 665, 667, 668, 676, 680
— E. Perkins, W. Montagna u. L. Giacometti 506, 614
— s. Montagna, W. 614
— s. Yasuda, K., u. T. Suzuki 338
Mackenzie, D. G., u. J. Lowenthal 558, 618
MacManus, J. F. A., s. Miller, J. 133
MacRae, T. P., s. Fraser, R. D. B. 127
— s. Fraser, R. D. B., u. G. E. Rogers 127
Madden, E. M., s. Zeck, P. 850
Madden, J. F. 899, 918
Madelung 820, 854
Maderson, P. F. A. 988, 989, 990, 1023
Madgic, E. B., s. Wilgram, G. F. 141
Mager, M., W. McNary jr., u. F. Lionetti 66, 131
Magnan, C. 331
Magnin, P. H., u. S. Rothman 113, 131

Magnoni, A., s. Simonetta, B. 336
Magnus, J. A. 894, 916
— A. Jarrett, T. A. J. Pankerd u. C. Rimington 894, 916
Magnus, I. A., u. R. H. S. Thompson 96, 131
Magnuson, H. J., u. B. O. Raulston 896, 916
Maguire, H. C. 181
— u. A. M. Kligman 163, 181
Maibach, H. I., s. Epstein, W. L. 126
Maillet, M. 378, 387, 426
Majno, G. 492, 529, 534, 535, 536, 539, 540, 541, 558, 562, 611, 618
— s. Schoefl, G. I. 619, 1033
Makai, E. 833, 840, 858
Makai, T., s. Rappaport, H. 136
Makk, L., s. Edwards, G. A. 126
Malak, J. A., u. E. W. Smith 864, 865, 868, 902
Malcolm, R., H. J. R. Miller 378
— H. J. R. Miller III u. M. Kasahara 426
Mali, J. W. H. 816, 852
Malinovský, L. 414, 426
Malkinson, F. D., u. S. Rothman 921, 1023
Mall, F. P., s. Keibel, F. 681
Mallet, M. 796, 848
Mallet, R., s. Basset, F. 121
Mallik, K. C. B., s. Cameron, G. R. 855
Mallory 757
Malone, J. D., s. Chase, H. B. 179
— s. Montagna, W. 181
Malpighi, M. 493, 611
Malt, R. A., P. T. Speakman u. E. Bell 1007
— G. J. Stewart, P. T. Speakman u. E. Bell 1023
Maltotsy, G., s. Parakkal, P. F. 1024
Manca, P. V. 285, 286, 309, 334
Manchot, C. 493, 518, 599, 611, 618, 622
Mancini, R. E., u. E. Bacarini 637, 641, 680
— O. Vilar, E. Stein u. H. Fiorni 433, 450, 451, 452, 487
Mandol, L., s. Herrmann, F. 844
Manfredi Romanini, M. G. 929, 1023
Manganotti, G. 563, 618, 690, 693, 706

Mangold, R., s. Billingham, R. E. 1030
Mannan, G., s. Cauna, N. 423
Mansfeld, W., u. F. Müller 828, 856
Mant, A. K. 782
— u. R. Furbank 746, 782
Maragnani, U. 870, 904
Marberger 729
Marchand, u. Herzog 439
Marchand, F. 536, 618, 819, 821, 854
Marcheselli, W., s. Allegra, F. 178
Marchionini, A., u. K. S. Aygün 904
— u. F. John 867, 902
— u. C. Patel 898, 917
Marchmann, A., u. R. Brunish 1030
Maresch 735, 782
Marghescu, S., u. O. Braun-Falco 92, 132
Margolena, L. A. 1032
Margolies, A., u. F. Weidman 217, 222
Marinelli, W., u. A. Strenger 939, 940, 1023
Marko, A. M., s. Harkness, R. D. 485
Marks, P. 644, 680
Maron, H. 144, 181, 706
Marquez, M. C., s. Hsia, S. L. 860
Marshall, s. Rutter 783
Marshall, A. J., s. Höhn, E. O. 1020
— s. King, J. R. 1021
Martin, B., u. M. Platts 352, 354, 375
Martin, E. A., u. R. T. Wales 218, 222
Martin, K., s. Spier, H. W. 138, 183, 337
— s. Spier, H. W., u. G. Pascher 139
Martinez Perez, R. 357, 375, 384, 426
Martinotti, L. 43, 132
Martinsson, s. Björntorp 828, 860
Martius, H., u. H. Hartl 268, 334
Maruhashi, J., K. Mizuguchi u. I. Tasaki 426
Maruhashi, K., Miziguchi u. I. Tasaki 984, 1023
Marwah, A. S., u. Meyer, J. 706
Marzulli, F. N. 15, 132
Mascagni, P. 493, 611
Mascaro, J. M., s. Duperrat, B. 678
Maschka, s. Schauenstein 783
Maschka, s. Thouret 783

Maschka, J. v. 726, *781, 782,* 785
Maschkilleisson, L. N. 868, *902*
Masderhoff, J. *783*
Mason, H. H., u. D. H. Andersen 886, *911*
— s. Sant'Agnese, P. A. di *911*
Mason, H. L., s. Best, E. W. 846
— s. Lobitz, W. C. *265*
Mason, H. S. 114, *132,* 890, 891, *914*
— W. L. Fowlks u. E. Peterson 890, *914*
Masshoff, W. 62, *132*
Masson, P. 62, 104, 105, 106, 107, 108, 110, 113, 115, 116, *132,* 356, *375,* 387, *426,* 495, 513, 553, 554, 566, *611, 614, 618,* 640, *680,* 891, *914*
Masu, S., s. Kaku, H. *130*
Matev, I., s. Kadanoff, D. *425*
Mathews, M. B., s. Schiller, S. *488*
Mathis, H. 820, *854*
Matoltsy, A. G. 21, 31, 37, 38, 39, 44, 50, 51, 54, 71, 72, 74, 75, *132*
— u. C. A. Balsamo 21, 29, 30, 38, 50, 51, *132*
— u. F. S. M. Herbst 21, 30, *132*
— u. M. Matoltsy 21, 30, 37, 44, 76, 83, *132*
— u. P. Parakkal *1030*
Matoltsy, M., s. Matoltsy, A. G. *132*
— u. P. F. Parakkal 11, 20, 21, 22, 23, 25, 26, 29, 58, 59, *132,* 260, *265, 374, 375*
— s. Parakkal, P. F. *182*
Matras, A. 811, *852,* 881, 899, *910, 918*
Matsuda, S. 898, *917*
Matsumoto, J. 964, 965, *1023*
Matsumoto, R. 387, *426*
Matsumoto, S. 114, *132*
Matsuzawa, T., u. K. Kurosumi 236, 243, *265,* 301, 304, 324, *334*
— s. Kurosumi, K. *333*
Mattern, I. 1010, *1023*
Matthews, S. A. 948, *1023*
Matthissohn, A., s. Buschke, A. *857*
Maunsbach, A. B. 294, 299, *334*
Matussek, N., s. Blinzinger, K. *483*
Matzdorff 747, *782*
Maurici, M. de, s. Silvestri *707*
Maximow, A. 430, 434, 443, 450, *487,* 499, 558, *611, 614, 618,* 819, *854,* 874, 875, *907*

Mayaud, N. 1006, *1023*
Mayer, P., s. Sylvén, B. *907, 908*
Mayer-List, R., u. G. Hübener 530, *618*
Maynard, E. A., R. L. Schultz u. D. C. Pease 543, *618*
McCarthy, J. T., s. Steigleder, G. K. *139, 223*
McCombs, R. P. 809, *852*
McCormac, W. 814, 816, *852*
McCraig, W., s. Farber, E. M. *705*
McCusker, J. J., u. R. M. Caplan 870, *904*
McDonald, R. 806, 833, 835, *848, 858*
McDonald, s. Wassermann, F. *845*
McDonald, T. F., s. Wassermann, F. *489, 490*
McGovern, J. V., s. Fitzpatrick, T. B. *913*
McGugan, D., s. Fitzpatrick, T. B. *913*
McGuire, J. S., s. Lerner, A. B. *131*
McIntyre, A. K., s. Hunt, C. C. *425*
McKay, D. G., E. C. Adams, A. T. Hertig u. S. Danziger 631, 633, *680*
McKeen Cattell, K., s. Adrian, E. D. *1015*
McKenzie, J., s. Singh, M. *183*
McKusick, V. A., s. Goodman, R. M. *911*
McLean, F. 874, *907*
McLoughlin, C. B. 639, 642, *680*
McMahon, H. E., s. Schürmann, P. *852*
McManus, J. F. A. 463, *487,* 862, 863, 874, *902, 907*
McMillan, M., s. Emery, J. L. *678*
McMinn, R. M. H., s. Johnson, F. R. *1033*
McNary jr., W., s. Mager, M. *131*
McRae, T. P., s. Fraser, R. D. B. *1018*
McWhorter, C. A., s. Wilson, R. B. *682*
Medawar, u. Billingham 116
Medawar, P. B. 5, 62, 104, 105, 107, 116, 117, *132,* 146, *181,* 920, *1030*
— s. Billingham, R. E. *121, 677, 912*
Medoff, G., s. Herrmann, F. *844*
Meek, G. A., s. Florey, H. W. *617*

Meesen, H. 837, *858*
Mehl, u. Arnal 785
Mehregan, A. H. 273, *334*
Meienhofer, J., s. Li, C. H. *1022*
Meier 836, *858*
Meijere, J. C. H. de 920, *1023*
Meireles Pinto, M. I., L. Falcao, T. Cruz-Sobral u. M. J. X. Morato 77, *132*
Meirowsky, E. 104, 110, *132,* 892, *914*
— u. L. W. Freeman 110, *132,* 892, *914*
— u. A. Wiseman 104, *132*
Meisel, E., s. Wachstein, M. *489*
Meissner, G. 377, 413, 417, *426*
Meixner, K. *785*
Melaragno, H., s. Montagna, W. *376*
Melaragno, H. P., s. Montagna, W. *706*
— s. Montagna, W., u. H. B. Chase *181*
— s. Montagna, W., H. B. Chase u. J. D. Malone *181*
Melczer, N. 278, *330, 334*
— u. G. Cseplák 23, 37, *132*
— u. S. Deme 195, 196, *222*
Melicow, M. M. 819, *854*
Mellemgard, K., s. Frederiksen, T. *866*
Memmesheimer 310
Memmesheimer, A., s. Way, St. C. *337, 707*
Menanteau, J. P., s. Jausion, H. P. *847*
Mendelson, M., s. Loewenstein, W. R. *1031*
Menefee, M. G. 3, 40, *132*
Meneghini, N. 516, 563, 569, 575, *614, 618, 621,* 700, *706*
Menschik, Z. 457, *487,* 819, *854*
Mensi, E. 805, *848*
Mercantini, E. S. 436, *487*
Mercer, E. H. 2, 3, 24, 31, 33, 35, 36, 37, 38, 39, 40, 44, 50, 57, 62, 68, 75, 104, *132,* 147, 156, *181,* 299, *334,* 371, 373, *375,* 1007, *1023*
— B. L. Munger, G. E. Rogers u. S. I. Roth 37, *132,* 154, *181*
— s. Birbeck *122*
— s. Birbeck, M. S. C. *121, 122, 179, 912*
— s. Birbeck, M. S. C., u. N. A. Barnicot *179*
Merenmies, L., s. Setälä, K. *138*

Merkel 821, *854*
Merkel, F. 377, 384, *426*
Merkel, H. 710, *780, 782, 785*
Merker, H. J. 31, *132*, 294, *334*, 433, 441, 443, *487*
— s. Schwarz, W. *489*
— s. Schwarz, W., u. A. Kutsche *489*
Merli, S. *782, 783*
Mertschnigg 43, *132*
Mescon, H., u. P. Flesch 17, 44, 70, 71, 72, 81, *132*
— J. Hurley u. G. Moretti 495, 497, 526, 527, 552, 553, 554, 555, 556, 557, 566, 599, 611, *618, 621*
— u. J. S. Strauß 219, *222*
— s. Grots, I. A. *851, 858*
— s. Hurley, H. *375*
— s. Hurley jr., H. J. *617, 621*
— s. Moretti, G. *133, 222, 376, 611, 618, 621, 622, 623*
— s. Moretti, G., N. K. Adachi u. P. Pochi *133*
— s. Moretti, G., u. R. A. Ellis *133, 222*
— s. Pochi, P. E., u. J. S. Strauß *223*
— s. Serri, F. *376*
— s. Serri, F., u. W. M. Huber *336, 681*
— s. Serri, F., u. W. Montagna *336, 614, 681*
— s. Serri, F., u. M. L. Speranza *681*
— s. Shelly, W. B. *266*
Mesnil de Rochemont, R. du s. Wöhlisch, E. *490*
Mesirow, S. M., u. R. B. Stoughton 101, *133*
Messerschmidt, O. *785*
Messier, B., u. C. P. Leblond 62, 63, *133*
— u. C. P. Leblond 327, *334*
— s. Leblond, C. P. *131*
Metzner, R. *337*
Meyer 766
Meyer, A. 801, 802, 835, *848, 858*
Meyer, H., u. S. Nishiyama 879, *907*
Meyer, J., u. J. P. Weinmann 100, *133*
— A. S. Marwah u. J. P. Weinmann 690, *706*
Meyer, K. 450, 452, 478, *487*, 874, 875, *907*
— u. E. Chaffee 789, *844*
— u. M. M. Rapport 450, 452, 453, *487*
— s. Loewi, G. *487*
— s. Weissmann, B. *908*
Meyer, L., s. Grossfeld, H. *906*

Meyer, L., s. Holland, M. *613*
Meyer, M., u. H. H. Loetzke 977, *1023*
Meyers 836, *858*
Meyhöfer, W., s. Knoth, W. 848, *851, 858*
Meza-Chávez, L. 218, *222*
Mian, E., s. Cornel, M. *616, 623*
Miani, A., u. U. Ruberti 546, 549, 550, *618*
Micheletti, s. Ricci *859*
Michels, N. A. 105, *133*
Michelson, A. E. 841, *858*
Michelson, H. E. 789, 799, 802, 827, *844, 848, 852, 856*
— u. C. W. Laymon 885, *910*
Midgley, A. R., s. Pierce, G. B. *488*
Miedziński, F., u. J. Kozakiewicz 871, *904*
Mierement, C. W. G. 776, 777, *786*
Miescher, G. 796, 808, 809, 815, *848, 852*, 864, 892, *902, 914*
— u. W. Burckhardt 816, *852*
— u. M. Leder 815, 816, *852*
— u. A. S. Schönberg 185, *222*
Mikhail, G. R., M. S. W. Farris u. N. S. Gimbel 522, 523, *618*
— u. A. Miller-Milinska 695, *706*
Milan, G. 872, *904*
Miles, A. E. W. 216, 217, *222*
Millard, A., u. K. M. Rudall 75, *133*
Miller 358
Miller, A. M., s. Perkins, O. C. *222*
Miller, J., u. J. F. A. Mac Manus 62, *133*
Miller III, H. J. R. s. Malcolm, R. *426*
Miller, L., u. H. W. Whitting *1033*
Miller, L. R., s. Gerald, G. B. *484*
— s. Gordon, G. B. *485*
Miller, M., H. Ralston u. M. Kasahara 357, 358, *375*
Miller, M. R., H. J. Ralston III u. M. Kasahara 413, *426*
— H. J. Ralston u. M. Kasahara 564, *618*
Miller, S., u. G. Weddel *426, 1031*
— s. Weddell, G. *428*
Miller, Th. H., u. C. Mopper 879, *907*
Miller, W. J. 1009, *1023*

Miler-Milinska, A., s. Mikhail, G. R. *706*
Millonig, G. 40, *133*, 979, *1023*
Milne, J. A., s. Baillie, A. H. *220*
Milner, R. D. G., u. M. J. Mitchinson 802, 835, *848, 858*
— u. M. J. Mitchinson, s. Ricci, Micheletti u. Coscia *859*
Minamitani, K. 267, 268, 275, 277, 278, 279, *334*
Mine, R. W., s. Mason, H. S. *914*
Mine, T. 274, *334*
Mirsky, A. E., u. H. Ris 929, *1023*
— s. Brachet, J. *335*
Misgeld, V., s. Lindlar, F. *861*
Mishima, Y. 97, 98, 99, 115, 117, *133*, 676, *680*, 890, 891, 892, *914*
— u. A. V. Loud 890, *914*, 964, *1023*
— — u. F. F. Schaub jr. 890, *914*
— u. F. F. Schaub jr. 890, *914*
— u. S. Widlan 676, 677, *680*, 890, *914*
— s. Fitzpatrick, T. B. *913*
— s. Loud, A. V. *1022*
Mislawsky, A. N. 275, *334*
Missmahl, H. P. 863, 864, 865, 866, *902*
— J. Gafni u. E. Sohar *866*
— u. M. Hartwig 863, *902*
— s. Delank, H.-W. *901*
— s. Heller, H. *902*
— s. Schneider *903*
Missotten, L. 543, *618*
Mitchell, s. Norman *848*
Mitchell, L. R., s. Halstead, B. W. *1019*
Mitchinson, M. J., s. Milner, R. D. G. *848, 858*
— u. R. D. C. Milner, s. Ricci, Micheletti u. Coscia *859*
Miyake, S., s. Yamada, H. *429*
Miziguchi, s. Maruhashi, K. *1023*
Mizuguchi, K., s. Maruhashi *426*
Moberger, G., u. P. De 69, *133*
Mochizuki, D. 660, 668, 669, *680*
Modaber, P. *786*
Modglin, F. R., s. Halstead, B. W. *1019*
— s. Halstead, B. W., u. M. J. Chitwood *1019*
Möbius, W. 820, 824, *854*

Möbius, W., s. Boyd *853*
Möllendorf, W. V., u. W. Bargmann 622, 623, *705*
Möllendorff, M. V. *129*, 430, 434, *487*
— s. Maximow, A. *907*
Moeller 526
Mönnighoff, F. H. 720, *780*
Moeschlin, S. 730, *781*
Möslein, E., s. Lynen, F. *844*
Mogi, E. 268, 270, *334*, 663, *680*
Mohr, E. *1031*
Molinari, S., s. Pease, D. C. *619*
Mollaret, H. H. 836, *858*
Mollenkopf, K., s. Diemair, W. *780*
Møller, P. 899, *918*
Mollier, S., s. Ruckert, J. *614*
Monacelli, M. 494, 563, *611*, *618,*, 720, 742, *780*, *783*
Monash, S. 350, *376*
Monfort, J., s. Duperrat, B. *850*
Monis, B., B. M. Banks u. A. M. Rutenburg 101, *133*
— u. A. M. Rutenburg 101, *133*
Monroe, A. 493, *611*
Montagna *181*
Montagna, W. 2, 4, 5, 10, 11, 13, 14, 17, 18, 20, 38, 55, 57, 58, 62, 64, 66, 71, 72, 73, 74, 76, 77, 78, 81, 85, 86, 87, 90, 91, 92, 93, 95, 99, 100, 101, 102, 104, *133*, 143, 145, 148, 151, 153, 154, 157, 158, 168, 169, 171, 172, 174, 176, *181*, 193, 195, 197, 200, 202, 218, 220, *222*, 224, 227, 235, 236, 237, 238, 241, 242, 243, 248, 250, 253, 258, 260, 261, *265*, 268, 269, 270, 271, 272, 275, 277, 278, 279, 282, 283, 284, 286, 295, 306, 307, 308, 309, 310, 311, 312, 316, 318, 322, 323, 324, 325, 326, 327, 328, 329, 330, *334*, 366, 371, *376*, *426*, 430, 431, 435, 437, 456, 474, 481, 482, *487*, 493, 502, 504, 505, 506, 511, 526, 627, 538, 563, 564, 581, 583, 584, 585, 586, 587, 588, 589, 606, 609, *611*, *614*, *618*, *621*, *622*, *623*, 642, 656, 657, 659, 665, 668, *680*, 696, 697, 704, 705, *706*, 893, *916*, 920, *1029*
— u. E. B. Beckett 92, 96, *133*
— u. H. B. Chase 171, *181*
— H. B. Chase u. J. B. Hamilton 76, 77, 81, *133*, 170, 171, *181*, 201, *222*, 308, *334*, 363, *376*

Montagna, W., H. B. Chase u. W. C. Lobitz jr. 76, 77, *133*, 171, *181*, 201, *222*, 241, 245, 257, *265*, 275, 278, 279, 305, 308, 310, *334*, 890, *914*
— — J. D. Malone u. H. P. Melaragno 171, *181*
— — u. H. P. Melaragno 171, *181*, 370, 371, 372, *376*
— A. Z. Eisen, A. H. Rademacher u. H. B. Chase 17, 44, 71, 72, 74, *133*, 173, *181*, 201, *222*, 236, 257, *265*, 305, *334*
— u. R. A. Ellis 92, 93, 95, 96, *120*, *133*, 143, 171, *179*, *181*, 202, 203, 204, 218, *222*, 236, 248, 256, 260, 261, *265*, 284, 308, 310, 311, 312, 318, 321, 322, 323, *334*, *426*, 495, 503, 506, 527, 566, 583, 584, 585, 586, 588, 589, 609, *611*, *614*, *618*, *621*, *622*, *623*, 700, *706*, *1029*, *1032*
— — u. A. F. Silver 220
— u. V. R. Formisano 87, 88, 90, 92, *133*, 176, *181*, 202, *222*, 235, 236, 241, 252, *265*, 481, *487*, 526, 537, 538, 550, 581, *618*
— u. R. J. Harrison 153, *181*, 495, 508, 539, *614*, *1032*
— u. C. R. Hill 79, *133*, 177, *182*
Montagna, W., u. W. C. Lobitz jr. 121
— H. Machida u. E. Perkins 506, *614*
— u. H. P. Melaragno 695, *706*
— C. R. Noback u. F. G. Zak 76, 77, 81, *133*, 193, 195, 196, 198, 199, 200, 201, *222*, 278, 284, 307, 323, *334*
— Ch. R. Noback u. F. G. Zak 278, 284, 307, 323, *334*
— u. E. J. van Scott 144, 145, 147, 150, 152, 157, *182*, 185, 192, *222*,
— K. Yasuda u. R. A. Ellis 243, 248, *265*, *1029*
— u. S. S. Yum *426*
— u. J. S. Yun 85, 86, 90, *133*, 152, 153, *182*, 202, *222*, 243, 248, *265*, 318, *334*, 506, 510, 526, 538, 583, 588, *614*, *618*, *621*, *1029*
— s. Adachi, K. 120, *178*, 220, 330, 482, *705*
— s. Beckett, E. *374*
— s. Beckett, E. B. *263*, *613*, 677

Montagna, W., s. Borodach, G. N. *179*, *1030*
— s. Chase, H. B. *179*
— s. Eisen, A. Z. *126*, *180*
— s. Ellis, R. A. *126*, *180*, 221, *264*, *613*, *705*, *1029*
— s. Ellis, R. A. u. H. Fanger 221, *331*, *621*
— s. Formisano, V. R. *127*, *180*
— s. Harrison *613*
— s. Im, M. J. C. *613*
— s. Lobitz, W. C. *621*
— s. Lobitz jr., W. C. *680*
— s. Lobitz, W. C. u. J. B. Holyoke *265*
— s. Machida, H. *614*
— s. Moretti, G. *222*, *618*, *621*, *622*
— s. Parakkal, P. *614*, *1029*
— s. Saunders, C. H. de *612*
— s. Saunders, R. L. de C. H. *681*
— s. Serri, F. *376*
— s. Serri, F. u. W. M. Huber *336*, *614*, *681*
— s. Serri, F. u. H. Mescon *336*, *614*, *681*
— s. Shipman, M. *183*
— s. Yasuda, K. *183*, *223*, *266*, *338*, *490*, *1029*
Montanari, G. D., B. Viterbo u. G. R. Montanari 752, *783*
Montanari, G. R.,, s. Montanari, G. D. *783*
Montes, L. F., B. L. Baker u. A. C. Curtis 280, 282, 305, 307, 308, 309, 329, 330, *334*, *638*, *697*, *704*, *706*
— s. Biempica, L. *330*
Montgomery 469
Montgomery u. Hamilten 896
Montgomery, H., u. F. Z. Havens 871, *904*
— u. P. A. O'Leary 896, *916*
— — u. N. W. Barker 799, *852*
Montgomery, H., s. Becker, S. K. *705*
— s. Becker jr., S. W. *121*
— s. Becker jr., W. S. *912*
— s. Farber, E. M. *621*, *705*
— s. Fitzpatrick, T. B. *127*, *913*
— s. Fitzpatrick, T. B. u. A. B. Lerner *913*
— s. Hill, W. R. *485*, *706*, *845*, *918*
— s. Lewis, B. *375*
— s. Lewis, B. L. *706*
— s. Ormsby, O. S. *134*
— u. A. E. Österberg 881, *910*
— s. Pittelkow, R. B. *910*
— u. R. R. Sullivan 794, *846*

Montgomery, H., u. L. J. Underwood 875, 876, 878, 879, *907*
— s. Winkelmann, R. K. *337*
Montgomery, P. O. B. 874, *904*
— u. E. E. Muirhead 869, 870, *904*
Mook, W. H., u. R. S. Weiß 882, *910*
Moore, A., s. Althausen, T. L. *916*
Moore, D. M., u. H. Ruska 541, *618*
Moore, R. D., u. M. D. Schoenberg 448, *487*
Mopper, C., s. Miller, Th. H. *907*
Moragas, J. M. de, s. Vilanova, X. *908*
Moragas, J. M., s. Vilanova, X. u. J. Piñol Aguadé *849*
Morato, M. J. X., s. Meireles Pinto, M. I. *132*
Moretti, Adachi, Mescon u. Pochi 87, 88, 95
Moretti, G. 162, 163, *182*, 513, 517, *614*
— N. K. Adachi u. R. A. Ellis 92, 95, *133*
— u. F. Crovato 498, 525, 536, 537, 538, 539, 550, *611*, *618*, *623*
— R. A. Ellis u. H. Mescon 7, 8, 88, *133*, 204, *222*
— R. A. Ellis u. H. Mescon 491, 495, 529, 533, 572, 575, 576, 578, 581, 583, 590, 592, 604, 606, *611*, *618*, *621*
— u. G. Farris 503, 504, 505, 506, 520, 578, 608, *614*, *618*, *623*
— C. Giacometti, V. Boido u. R. Rebora 163, *182*
— u. H. Mescon 96, *133*, 202, *222*, 366, *376*
— u. W. Montagna 204, *222*, 495, 520, 529, 533, 572, 573, 576, 577, 581, 583, 590, 592, 604, 606, *618*, *621*, *622*
— u. E. Rampini 507, 508, *614*
— A. Rebora, C. Giacometti u. F. Crovato 575, *621*
— s. Baccaredda-Boy, A. *615*
— s. Baccaredda-Boy, A. u. A. Rebora *615*, *621*
— s. Baccaredda-Boy, A. u. G. Farris *615*, *621*, *623*
— s. Baccaredda-Boy, A. u. B. Filippi *615*, *621*
— s. Baccaredda-Boy, A., S. Zocchi u. F. Crovato *615*
— s. Ellis, R. A. *610*, *616*, *621*, *622*, *623*

Moretti, G. s. Mescon, H. *611*, *618*, *621*
— s. Pochi, P. *133*
— s. Rampini, E. *612*, *619*, *622*, *623*
— s. Stüttgen, G. *1027*
Morgan, C., s. Riffkind, R. A. *488*
Morgan, W., s. Jones, D. J. *1021*
Mori, T. *680*
Mori, W., s. Lerner, A. B. *1022*
Moriconi, A., s. Castigli, C. *613*
Morike, K. 351, 352, 354, *376*
Morioka, Y. 270, *334*
Morita, S. 481, *487*, 669, *680*
Moritz, A. R., s. Henriques, F. *785*
Moritz, M. D., u. E. D. Henriques *785*
Moriyama, G. 310, *334*
Moro, E. 898, *917*
Morris, D. 1009, *1023*
Morris, R. 932, *1023*
Morrison, A. B., s. Iverson, L. *902*
Moses, M. J. 68, *133*
Mosher, D. T., s. Ackermann, A. B. *860*
Mosinger, B., E. Kuhn u. V. Kujalová 827, *856*
Moskowitz, R. W., A. H. Baggenstoß u. C. H. Slocumb 809, *852*
Mosto, D. 830, *856*
Mostofi, F. K., u. E. Engleman 802, *848*
Motteram, R., s. Althausen, T. L. *916*
Moulé, Y. 277, *334*
Moulin, F. de 36, *133*
Moulonguet, P., s. Lecène, P. *858*
Moyer, F. 107, 110, *133*
Mraček, F. *336*
Muckle, T. J., u. M. Wells *866*
Mühlbock, O., u. G. della Porta s. Fujii, R. *1018*
— u. G. della Porta, s. Geschwind, I. I. *1018*
Mülhbock, O., s. Della Porta, G. *125*
Mueller, B. 709, 711, 712, 713, 727, 730, 743, 763, 765, 776, 777, *780*, *781*, *783*, *784*, *785*, *786*
Müller, C. 150, *182*
— s. Wagner, H. O. *1028*
Müller, D. *910*
Müller, E. 719, 720, *780*, 869, *904*
— s. Lubarsch, O. *904*
Müller, F., s. Mansfeld, W. *856*
Müller, H., u. V. Kraul *861*

Müller, H., s. Langhof, H., u. L. Rietschel *916*
Müller, L. R. *843*
Müller, O. 494, 496, 525, 536, 559, *611*, *618*
Müller, R. 719, 720, *780*
Müller, W. 820, 828, *854*
Müller-Hoppe 809
Müller-Kraul 817
Muir, H. M., s. Harkness, R. D. *485*
Muirhead, E. E., s. Montgomery, P. O. B. *904*
Muller, S. A., u. R. K. Winkelmann 815, 837, *848*, *852*
Mullinger, A. M. 957, 969, *1023*
Munck, W. *786*
Munger, B. 241, 244, 245, 247, 248, 250, *265*
Munger, B. L. 268, 287, 291, 294, 301, 310, 327, *335*, 383, *426*, 984, *1023*, *1031*
— u. S. W. Brusilow 248, 253, 257, 258, *265*, 301, 305, 326, *335*
— — u. R. E. Cooke 248, *265*
— s. Mercer, E. H. *181*, *132*
— s. Patrizi, G. *134*
Munger, B. L., s. Patrizzi, G. *427*
Munoz, J., s. Garrachon, J. *617*
Munro, D. D. 178, *182*
Munteanu, M. 836, *858*
Munzer, J. Th., s. Adair, F. E. *846*
Murphy, J., s. Hershey, F. B. *485*
Murray, R. W. 953, 955, 956, 984, 985, *1023*
Murtula, G. 685, 689, *706*
Musger, A. 862, 888, *902*, *911*, *914*
Mustakallio, K. 99, 119, 120, *134*
Musumeci, V. 563, *618*, 700, *706*
Mutton, P., s. Darian-Smith, I. *424*
Myers, T. T., s. Winkelmann, R. K. *1028*

Nachlas, M. M., u. A. M. Seligman 92, *134*
Nadkarni u. Mitarb. 778, *786*
Naegeli, O. 887, *911*
Naeslund, J. 663, *680*
Nagahori, T. 800, *848*
Nagai, Y., s. Silbert, J. E. *1026*
Nagamitsu, G. 310, *335*
Nagano, T. 299, *335*
Nagashima, T., s. Toyama, I. *855*

Nagata, U., s. Kato, S. *333*
Nagel, A. 477, 479, 480, 481, *487*
Nageotte, J. 440, *487*
Nagy-Vezekényi, K., s. Szodoray, L. *140*
Nakai, T. 175, 177, *182, 1030*
— u. P. Shubik 115, *134*
Nakajima, H., s. Kawamura, T. *679, 680*
Nakamura, J. 176, *182*
Nakamura, S. H. K. 435, 437, *487*
Nakamura, T., s. Fukuyama *127, 128*
Nakano, T., s. Taniguchi, T. *223*
Nanikawa 746
Nanikawa, R., N. Tawa u. K. Saito *783*
Napolitano, L. 455, 456, 457, 460, *487*, 788, 827, *844, 854, 856*
— u. D. Fawcett 456, *487*, 819, *854*
Nasy, A. N. 196, *222*
Nauck, E. T., s. Olivet, I. *335*
Navidi, S., s. Donnelly, G. H. *221*
Nay, T. 105, *134*
Neave, F. 962, 963, *1023*
Neckel, I. 965, *1023*
— s. Dettmer, N. *484*
Needham, D. M., u. C. F. Shoenberg 302, *335*
Negri, P. L., s. Landy, G. *904*
Neidleman, S., s. Bagnara, J. T. *1015*
Neil, A. L., s. Vazques, T. T. *903*
Nekam, L., s. Kaldor, I. *851, 858*
Nelke, A. 685, 690, 691, 695, 702, *706*
Nelson, P. G., s. Hunt, C. C. *1020*
Nelson, R., s. Hashimoto, K. *375*
— s. Hashimoto, K., B.G. Gross u. W. F. Lever *129, 679*
Nemetschek, H. 302, 303, 304, *335*
Nesterow, A. J. 494, *611*
Netherton, E. W. 802, *848*
Neuber, E. *706*
Neuberger, A., s. Harkness, R. D. *485*
Neugebauer 759
Neumann, H. 879, *907*
Neumann, J. 695, *706*
Neumann, K. H., s. Graumann, W. G. *906*
— u. W. G. Graumann, s. Wolman, M. *905*

Neureiter, s. Masderhoff, J. *783*
Newton, D. 378, *426*
Newby, W. M. 936, 937, 938, 940, *1023*
Newcomer, V. D. 805, 830, 848, *856*
— J. H. Graham, R. R. Schaffert u. L. Kaplan 805, 833, *848, 859*
Newth, D. R., u. D. M. Ross 940, *1023*
Nézelof, C., s. Basset, F. *121, 908*
Niazzi, I. A. 928, 929, 930, *1023*
Nicaud, P., s. Macaigne, N. *852*
Nichihara, K., s. Kawamura, T. *679, 680*
Nichols, J. G., s. Allen, N. *423*
Nickau, B. 494, *611*
— s. Weiß, B. *620*
Nickson, M. J., s. Braasch, N. K. *610*
Nicolaides 22
Nicolaides, N. 196, *222*
— u. T. Ray 196, *222*
— u. G. C. Wells 199, 203, 204, *222*
Nicolau, S. 81, *134*
Niebauer, G. 116, *134*, 378, 387, 402, 404, 407, *426, 487*, 873, 875, 880, 893, 904, 907, *914, 916*
— u. W. Raab 436, 450, 451, 469, *487*, 877, *907*
— u. N. Sekido 387, *426*, 891, *914*
— u. L. Stockinger 873, 874, 888, *904, 911*
— u. A. Wiedmann *426*, 436, *487*, 891, *914*
— s. Breitenbecker, L. *903, 919*
— s. Eberhartinger, Chr. *904, 917*
— s. Feyrter, F. *904*
— s. Formanek, J. *916*
— s. Holzner, J. H. *916*
Nielsen, B. 995, *1023*
Nielson, s. Evans 845
Nielson, P. E., s. Evans, R. *705*
Niessing, K., u. H. Rollhauser 539, *618*
Niggli-Stokar, U. *426*
Niino, S. 888, *912*
Niizuma, S. *426*
— K. Nozaki, M. Komatsu u. T. Numata *426*
Niklas, A., u. W. Oehlert 175, *182*
Nikolowski, W. 823, *854*
— u. R. Wittig 697, *706*

Nikolowski, W., s. Fischer, H. *909*
— s. Gottron, H. A. *847, 853, 858*
Nimpfer, Th. 900, *919*
Nippe, M. 777, 782, *786*
Nishihara, K. 387, *426*
Nishioka, R. S., s. Kobayashi, A. *1021*
Nishiyama, S., s. Meyer, H. *907*
Nitkowsky, H. M., s. Gordis, L. *332*
Nitta, H. 253, *265*
Noback, C. R. *182*
— s. Montagna, W. *133, 222*
Noback, Chr. R., s. Montagna, W., u. F. G. Zak
Nobis, A., s. Lehn, H. *182*
Noble, G. K. 977, 978, *1023*
— u. H. T. Bradley 990, *1023*
Noda, M. 875, *907*
Nödl, F. 820, 821, 823, *854, 882, 910*
— u. H. Zaun 868, *902*
Noetzel, H. 477, *487*
Nolte *780*
Nomland, R. 867, *902*
— s. Finnerud, C. W. *911*
Noojin, R. O., B. F. Pace u. H. G. Davis 808, 833, 835, *848, 859*
Nordenstam, H., u. Adams-Ray 436, *487*
— s. Adams-Ray, J. *482*
— s. Rhodin, J. *488*
Nordquist, R. E., s. Olson, R. L. *134*
Norman, Griffen u. Mitchell 805, 806, *848*
Novales, B. J., s. Novales, R. R. *1024*
Novales, R. R., u. B. J. Novales 948, *1024*
Nové-Josserand, L., Gaté, Charpy, Josserand u. P. Cuilleret 900, *918*
Novikoff 89
Novikoff, A. B. *134*, 294, 309, 326, *335*, 435, 436, *487*, 892, *914*
— H. Beaufay u. C. de Duve *134*
— s. Essner, E. *332, 484*
— s. Goldfischer, S. *332, 485*
Novikoff, Beaufay u. de Duve 97
Novy, F. G., u. J. W. Wilson 821, *855*
Nozaki, K., s. Niizuma, S. *426*
Nubé, M. J. 796, *848*
Nürnberger, F., s. Korting, G. W. *851*
Numata, T., s. Niizuma, S. *426*
Nunez Andrade, R. 802, *848*

Nurnberg, M., s. Steigleder, G. K. *139*
Nyholm, M., s. Setälä, K. *138*
Nyquist, B., s. Schaanning, Chr. K. *910*

Oberling, Fr., M. Imler und A. Batzenschlager 802, *848*
Oberste-Lehn, H. 5, *134*
— u. A. Nobis 144, 165, *182*
Obika, M. 977, *1024*
— u. J. T. Bagnara 982, *1024*
— s. Hama, T. *1019*
Oboglio, Cattaneo u. Carboneschi 774, *785*
Obolonsky, s. Anrepp 759
O'Brien, J. P. 267, *335*
Obručnik, M. 690, *706*
Obuko, K., s. Kobayashi, H. *1021*
Ocano Sierra, J. 802, *848*
Odeblad, E., s. Boström, H. *122*
Odland, G. 364, *376*
Odland, G. F. 2, 3, 17, 19, 21, 25, 31, 32, 33, 34, 35, 37, 40, 44, 45, 46, 47, 51, 57, 58, 59, 68, 75, 101, 104, 107, 108, 109, *134*, 147, 173, *182*, 462, *487*, 492, 495, 499, 540, 541, 542, 543, 545, 546, 550, 551, 567, *611*, *619*, *1030*
O'Donell, I. J., s. Gillespie, J. M. *128*
Odyke, D. L., s. Lausing, A. J. *783*
Oehl 13, 15, *134*
Oehlert, W., u. D. Grimm 178, *182*
— H. Wecke u. H. Sütterle 807, 808, 835, 841, *848*, *859*
— s. Block, P. *1032*
— s. Niklas, A. *182*
— s. Schultze, B. *137*
Ökrös, S. *783*
Österreicher, D. L., u. E. M. Watson 831, *856*
Oettle, A. G., s. Fitzpatrick, T. B. *913*
Ogata, N., s. Yasuda, K. *266*
— s. Yasuda, K., u. H. Furusawa *338*
Ogura, Knox, Griffin u. Kusuhara 71, 72
Ogura, R., J. M. Knox u. A. C. Griffin 71, *134*
Ohmura, H., u. T. Yasuda 325, *335*
Ohno, T., u. H. Kinoshita 272, *335*
— s. Yamamoto, T. *429*
Ohyama, T., s. Yamamoto, T. *429*
Oi, T., s. Kuré, K. *856*

Okajima 660, 668
Okajima, J. *784*
Okajima, K., u. K. Yamada 481, *487*
Okane, M., s. Yada, S. *783*
Okinaka, S., s. Kuré, K. *856*
Okonkwo, B., S. Rust u. G. K. Steigleder 438, *487*
Oksche, A., u. M. Vaupel-v. Harnack 950, *1024*
— s. Farner, D. S. *1018*
Okun, M. R. 105, 106, *134*
Oláh, I., u. P. Röhlich 25, 26, 59, 84, *134*
Olbrycht, J. S. *784*
O'Leary, P. A., s. Gilje, O. *610*, *617*
— s. Kierlaud, R. R. *486*
— s. Montgomery, H. 852, *916*
Olin 11, *134*
Olin, T. E. 627, 660, 661, *680*
Oliver, R. F. *1030*
Olivet, I., u. E. T. Nauck 268, *335*
Olsen, B. R. 442, *487*, *488*
Olson, R. L., u. R. E. Nordquist 98, *134*
Olsson, R. 922, 923, 924, 938, *1024*
Omoto, H., s. Yamamoto, T. *429*
Ondo, S., s. Araki, Y. *263*
Ono, S. 383, *426*
Oono, T., s. Goto, T. *679*
— s. Ihjima, Sh. *333*
Oordt, G. J. van, u. G. C. A. Junge 1014, *1024*
— s. Burgers, A. C. J. *1016*
Oorsoś u. Tiemke 759
Oosten, J. v. 957, 961, 962, *1024*
Opdyke, D. I., s. Lansing, A. I. *131*
Oppenheim, M. 790, 792, 814, 815, *846*, *852*, 898, *918*
Orbaneja, J. G., u. J. R. Puchol 795, 796, 808, 809, 810, 811, *848*, *852*
Orbaneja u. Puchol, s. Teilum *853*
Orbant 700, *706*
Orbison, J. L., s. Eisenschmid, J. H. *847*, *856*
Orentreich, N. 168, *182*
Orfanos, C. 383, 410, *426*, *427*
— u. W. Gahlen 880, *907*
Orfila-Leseur 730, *782*
Organos u. Gahlen 59,
Orkin, M., s. Fisher, I. 809, *860*
Orlovskaya, G. V. 638, *680*
Ormea, F. 272, *335*, 365, 376, *427*, 495, 566, 564, 566, 567, *611*, *615*, *619*

Ormea, F., M. Visetti u. F. Albertazzi 552, *619*
Ormsby, O. S., u. H. Montgomery 104, *134*
Orsos, F. 724, 759, *781*
Ortega, M., s. Garrachon, J. *617*
Ortiz, E., E. Bächli, D. Price u. H. G. Williams-Ashman 991, *1024*
— u. H. G. Williams-Ashman 991, *1024*
Ortiz Picon, J. M. 62, *134*
Orton, G. L. 964, *1024*
Osborne 826
Osborne, M. P., s. Lowenstein, O. *1022*
Osborne, R. R. *855*
Osbourn, R. A., s. Eichenlaub, F. J. *678*
Oseki, M., u. M. Sato *1031*
Osment, L. S., s. Winkelmann, R. H. *428*
Osserman, E. F., s. Riffkind, R. A. *488*
Osten v. 920
Osterberg, s. Comfort *860*
Osterberg, A. E., s. Montgomery, H. *910*
Ota, R. 277, 278, *335*
Ottaviani, G. 569, *621*
— u. I. Lupidi 640, *680*
Ottesen, O. E., s. Goodman, R. M. *911*
Otto, H., u. K. H. Hobusch 836, *859*
Ottoson, D., F. Sjöstrand, S. Stenström u. G. Svaetichin 2, 3, 21, 31, *134*
Overbeck, L., s. Petry, G. *135*
Overton, J. 31, *134*

Pace, B. F., s. Noojin, R. O. *848*, *859*
Padykula, H. A. 87, *134*
Pätzold, A. 468, *488*
Paget, M., s. Laugeron, L. *918*
Pahlke, G. 446, *488*
Palade, G. E. 55, *134*, 300, *335*, 418, *427*, 534, 541, *619*
— u. M. G. Farquhar 2, 3, 4, *134*
— u. K. R. Porter 58, *134*
— u. P. Siekevitz 277, *335*
— s. Farquhar, M. G. *126*, *332*, *1018*, *1029*
— s. Palay, S. L. *427*
— s. Siekevitz, P. *138*
Palay, S. L. 204, 205, 222, 382, 418, *427*
— u. G. E. Palade 382, 418, *427*
— s. Scharrer, E. *1025*

Palette, E. C., s. Palette, E. M. 861
Palette, E. M., E. C. Palette u. R. W. Harrington 805, 861
Palitz, L. L., u. S. Peck 863, 903
Pallie, W., s. Pease, D. C. 427, 1030
— s. Weddel, G. 376, 620, 1031, 1032
— s. Weddell, G. u. E. Palmer 428
Palmer, E., s. Allenby, C. F. 423
— s. Lele, P. P. 1022
— s. Weddel, G. 376, 428, 707, 1031, 1032
— s. Weddell, G. u. W. Pallie 428
Palmieri, s. Ishibashi 781
Palutke, W., s. Landers, J. W. 623
Pamuken, F., s. Szanto, P. B. 337
Paná, C. 329, 330, 335
Panabokké, R. G. 831, 836, 856, 861
Panebianco, G. 563, 619
Pankerd, T. A. J., s. Magnus, J. A. 916
Papa, C. M. 224, 265
Pappas, G. D., s. Porter, K. 488
Pappenheim, Giemsa u. Gram 83
Paraf, s. de Graciansky 860
Parakkal, P. F. 1030
— u. A. G. Matoltsy 154, 155, 156, 182
— u. G. Maltotsy 979, 1024
— W. Montagna u. R. A. Ellis 506, 614, 1029
— s. Matoltsy, A. G. 132, 265, 375, 1030
Paranchych, W., s. Shanks, J. A. 855
Pardo, O. A., s. Pardo-Castello, V. 376
Pardo-Castello, V., u. O. A. Pardo 342, 376
Parish, W. E. 799, 861
Parker, G. H. 950, 951, 966, 1024
— u. A. Rosenblueth 966, 1024
Parkheiser, T., s. Gaus, O. 128
Parkhurst, H. T., s. Smith, C. 138
Parra, C. A., s. Ferreira-Marques, J. 127
Parrisius, W. 494, 611
— u. Witterlin 611, 612
Parry, D. A. 1032
Parse, A. G. E. 135

Parshley, M. S., u. H. S. Simms 36, 134
Parvis-Preto, V., u. A. Ugo 506, 614
Pascher, G. 21, 30, 134
— s. Spier, H. W. 138
— s. Spier, H. W., u. K. Martin 139
Paschoud, J. M. u. Mitarb. 780
— s. Kuske, H. 854
Pass, F., D. Brophy, M. L. Pearson u. W. C. Lobitz jr. 631, 680
Patel, C., s. Marchionini, A. 917
Pathak, M. A., u. J. W. Burnett 894, 916
Paton, D., s. Goodman, R. M. 911
Patrizi, G., u. B. L. Munger 75, 134, 384, 427
Patteeya, H. H., s. Cosslett, V. E. 622
Patterson, T. J. S. 892, 914
Patzelt, V. 8, 20, 21, 31, 36, 38, 43, 44, 62, 76, 134
— s. Pernkopf, E. 125, 135, 681
Pau, H., u. H. Conrads 384, 427
Paul, D. D. S., s. Dannenberg, A. M. 484
Paul, H. E., s. Taylor, J. D. 845
Paul, M. F., s. Taylor, J. D. 845
Paule, W. J., s. Pease, D. C. 619
Pauling, L. 50, 134
— u. R. B. Corey 50, 134
— u. H. R. Branson 50, 134
— s. Corey, R. B. 125
Paulus, W. 785
Pautrier, L. M. 848
— u. J. Levy 892, 914
— u. Fr. Woringer 2, 135, 796, 848, 855
Pava, de la u. Pickren 218
Pavlik, F. 836, 861
Pawlowski, A. 378, 427, 680, 681
— u. G. Weddell 427
Pax, F., u. W. Ahrndt, s. Brühl, L. 1016
Peachey, L. D. 205, 222
Pearce, R. H., u. E. M. Watson 469, 488
— s. Watson, E. M. 908
Pearse 56, 76, 85, 90, 96, 99, 100, 102, 114, 880
Pearse, A. G. 247, 265
Pearse, A. G. E. 277, 278, 306, 323, 335, 863, 880, 886, 890, 903, 910, 911, 914

Pearse, A. G. E., u. D. G. Scarpelli 86, 89, 90, 135
— s. Scarpelli, D. G. 137
— s. Tranzer, J. P. 140
Pearson, B., H. M. Rice u. K. L. Dickens 867, 903
Pearson, M. L., s. Pass, F. 680
Pearson, R. W. 135
— u. B. Spargo 2, 3, 135
Pease, D. C. 20, 36, 37, 135, 288, 335, 464, 488, 539, 546, 619
— u. S. Molinari 539, 619
— u. W. Pallie 415, 418, 427, 1030
— u. W. J. Paule 539, 619
— u. T. A. Quilliam 416, 418, 427, 1004, 1024
— s. Maynard, E. A. 618
— s. Scott, B. L. 336
Pease, Ph. D., s. Daniel, C. 424
Peat, S., s. Haworth, W. N. 129
Pech, A., s. Appaix, A. 850
Peck, S. M. 104, 135
— s. Palitz, L. L. 903
Pecoraro, V., s. Barman, J. M. 178
Peet, M. M., s. List, C. F. 426
Pehlemann, F. W. 977, 1024
Pelc, S. R., u. H. B. Fell 999, 1024
Peleger, L., s. Tappeiner, J. 908
Pellizari, C. 904
Pelzer, R. H., s. Redisch, W. 622
Penn, J., s. Gillman, Th. 904
Penners 920
Percival, G. H., u. D. A. Duthie 872, 873, 904, 905
— P. W. Hannay u. D. A. Duthie 790, 846, 874, 905
— u. C. P. Stewart 103, 135
Pereira, J. P. M., s. Leblond, C. P. 131
Perez 421
Pérez, A. P. R., s. Pérez, R. M. 681
Pérez, R. M. 675, 681
— u. A. P. R. Pérez 675, 681
Perez-Casas, A., s. Jabonero, V. 425
— s. Jabonero, V. u. M. E. Bengoechea 425
Perkins, E., s. Machida, H. 614
— s. Montagna, W. 614
Perkins, O. C., u. A. M. Miller 217, 222
Pernis, B., s. Bairati, A. 483
— s. Petris, S. de 488,
Pernkopf, E., u. V. Patzelt 5, 8, 10, 13, 14, 20, 21, 23, 29, 125, 135, 624, 681

Perruccio, L. 607, *622*
Perry, E. T., H. J. Hurley, M. B. Gray u. W. B. Shelley 284, *335*
Perry, H. O., u. R. K. Winkelmann 803, *861*
Persijn, J. P., s. Daems, W. Th. *331*, *484*
Persson, B., s. Björntorp, P. *828*, *860*
Peter, K. 272, 273, 274, *335*
Peters, A. 933, 935, 941, *1024*
Petersen, H. 443, 468, 470, *488*, 521, 572, 604, *619*, *621*, *622*
Petersen, W. F., s. Sexmith, E. *781*
Peterson, E., s. Mason, H. S. *914*
Peterson, H. 261, *265*
Peterson, R. A., R. K. Ringer, M. J. Tetzlaff u. A. M. Lucas 1003, *1024*
— s. Tetzlaff, M. J. *428*, *1027*
Petit, G., u. P. Budker 946, *1024*
Petri, E. 841, *859*
Petris, S. de, G. Karlsbad u. B. Pernis 438, 439, *488*
Petris, St. de, s. Bairati, A. *483*
Petry, G. 32, 35, *135*, 447, 448, 479, *488*
— L. Overbeck u. W. Vogell 35, *135*
— s. Braun-Falco, O. *122*, *123*
Petry, S., s. Bojlén, K. *846*
Pette, D. 314, *335*
— u. H. Brandau 315, 316, *335*
— u. Th. Bücher 313, *335*
— u. W. Luh 316, *335*
— s. Brandau, H. *330*
Petzoldt, D., u. O. Braun-Falco *335*
— s. Braun-Falco, O. *123*, *179*, *264*, *331*, *610*, *615*, *783*
Peyer, B. 920, *1024*
Pezzarossa, G. 815, 837, *852*, *859*
Pfaff jr., J., s. Kendall, R. F. *909*
Pfaltz, C. R. 698, *706*
Pfeffer, K. v. 1006, *1024*
Pfeifer, U., u. R. Juchems *861*
Pfeiffer u. Jochems 811
Pfeiffer, W. 930, 957, 959, 971, *1024*
Pfennings, K. B., u. N. Schümmelfeder 883, *910*
Pfleger, L., u. H. Tirschek 882, *910*
Pflugfelder, O., u. G. Schubert 931, 971, 982, 983, *1024*

Pfuhl, W. 794, 795, 804, 840, 841, *846*, 848, *849*, *859*
Phillipe, G. H., s. Hibbs, R. G. *611*, *617*
Phillips, J. H., s. Burch, G. E. *483*
Philp, G. R., s. Wellings, S. R. *337*
Philpott 799
Philpott, s. Woodburne *853*
Piaggio, W. 807, 841, *849*, *859*
Pick, F. J. 794, *846*
Pick, W. 796, 797, *849*
Pickett, P. B., s. Bern, H. A. *121*
Pickren, J. W., s. La Pava, S. de *221*
Pierce, G. B., A. R. Midgley u. J. Sri Ram 463, *488*
Pierce jr., G. B. 639, *681*
Pierini, L. E., J. Abulafia u. S. Wainfeld 796, 803, 836, *861*
Pierre, J. de, s. Lindberg, O. *861*
Pietrusky, s. Masderhoff, J. *783*
Pietrusky, F. 743, 777, *786*
Pietrzykowska, A. 563, *619*
Piez, K. A., u. J. Gross 962, *1024*
Piguet, B., s. Coste, F. *903*
Pilate, M. 412, *427*
Pillai, P. A. 979, *1024*
Pillsbury, D. N., W. B. Shelley u. A. M. Kligmann 607, *622*
Pinkus, F. 1, 2, 3, 10, 12, 13, 14, 20, 21, 23, 62, *135*, 143, 149, 150, 154, 157, *182*, 220, 224, 227, *265*, 268, 270, 271, 272, 273, *335*, 342, 344, *376*, 384, 407, *427*, 445, 447, 467, 468, 471, *488*, 511, 614, 624, 627, 636, 638, 640, 642, 644, 645, 646, 647, 650, 652, 654, 655, 656, 657, 661, 663, 664, *681*
— u. H. Pinkus, s. Evans, Cowdry u. Nielson 845
Pinkus, H. 10, 17, 37, 62, 105, 106, *135*, 144, 147, 160, 165, *182*, 218, *223*, *335*, *427*, 627, 631, 644, *681*, 686, 696, 698, 699, *706*, 880, *907*, 920, 921
— L. A. Copps, S. Custer u. S. Epstein 882, *910*
— u. R. Hunter 63, 64, *135*
— J. R. Rogin u. P. Goldman 664, *681*
— u. Staricco, R. J. 106
— R. J. Starrico, P. J. Kropp u. J. Fan 107, 115, *135*

Pinkus, H., s. Hu, F. *130*
— s. Starrico, R. J. *139*, *707*
Pinol, J., s. Vilanova, X. *908*
Piñol-Aguadé, J. P., s. Vilanova, X. 849, *861*
— s. Vilanova, X. u. J. M. Moragas 849
Pinski, J. B., u. Ph. D. Stansifer 836, *859*
Pioch, W. 721, 727, 729, 753, 768, *780*, *781*, *783*, *785*, *786*
Piper, W. N., s. Goldblum, R. W. *128*, *180*
Piredda, A. 873, *905*
Pireteau, J., s. Stensiö, E. *1027*
Pirilä, V., u. O. Eränkö 99, *135*, *783*
Piroth, M. 803, 832, 840, *849*, *859*
Pisces, s. Schnakenbeck, W. *1026*
Pischinger *781*
Pischzek, F., u. P. Schmidt 531, *619*
Pissot, L. 278, *335*
Pittelkow, R. B., R. R. Kierland u. H. Montgomery 884, *910*
Piwowarczyk, I., s. Jablonska, St. *860*
Plachy, V., s. Danda, J. *847*, *857*
Platts, M., s. Martin, B. *375*
Plenert, W. 788, 819, *844*, *855*
Plenk, H. 2, *135*, 443, 444, 445, 456, 462, 479, *488*
Plenk, J. 755, *784*
Pley, s. Veslot *910*
Poclu, P. E., u. J. S. Strauß 185, 187, 188, 189, 217, *223*
— — u. H. Mescon 187, 190, *223*
— s. Forchielli, E. *221*
— s. Strauß, J. S. *223*, *857*
— s. Strauß, J. S. u. A. M. Kligman *223*
Pockrandt, D. 988, 992, 993, *1024*
Pöhl, A. 819, *855*
Pohl, L., s. Teller, H. *489*, *707*
Polley, E. H. *427*, 565, 566, *619*
Pollock, J. H., s. Sobel, N. *910*
Pomerat, C. M., s. Lewis, S. R. *131*
Pompen, A. W. M., s. Brandsma, C. H. *850*
Ponhold, J. 887, 888, *911*
Ponsold, A. 709, 711, 715, 753, *780*, *781*
Poole, D. F. G. 941, 945, 946, *1024*

Poole, J. C. F., s. Florey, H. W. 617
Popoff, L., u. N. Popoff 637, 638, *681*, 788, *844*
Popoff, N., s. Popoff, L. *681*, 788, *844*
Popoff, N. W.   495, 513, 553, *612, 614, 619, 706*
Pories, W. J., s. Strain, W. H. *183*
Port, E.   350, *376*
Porta, G. della, u. O. Mühlbock, s. Fujii *1018*
— u. O. Mühlbock, s. Geschwind, J. J. *1018*
Porter, K.   364, *376*
— u. G. D. Pappas   441, 442, *488*
— s. Franzini-Armstrong, C. *264*
Porter, K. R.   2, 3, 21, 31, 35, 37, 110, *135*, 444, *488, 970, 1024*
— u. F. L. Kallmann   58, *135*
— s. Bikle, D.   *1016*
— s. Palade, G. E.   *134*
Portwich, F.   809, *852*
Potter, B., u. P. Weinmann   871, *905*
Poussant   740
Power, D. A.   820, *855*
Powers, T. R., s. Bern, H. A. *121*
Pracken, J. R., s. Carol, W. L. L.   *846*
Prakken, J. R.   872, 873, *905*
Pranich, K., s. Wood, M. G. *338*
Pras, M., s. Sohar, E.   866
Pressman, B. C., s. Duve, C. de *126*
Pribilla, W., s. Volland, W. *917*
Price   772
Price, D., s. Ortiz, E.   *1024*
Pridvizhkin, I. G., u. L. B. Berlin   631, 634, 639, *681*
— s. Berlin, L. B.   *677*
Prieto, R. L., u. V. Jabonero *427*
Pritchard, M., u. P. Daniel   553, 554, *619*
Privat, Y., s. Vitry, G.   *489*
Probst, A.   869, *905*
— u. M. Ratzenhofer   *905*
— s. Ratzenhofer, M.   *905*
Proctor, R., s. Darian-Smith, I.   *424*
Prokop, O.   737, 743, *781, 783*
Prose, P. H., s. Herrmann, F. *844*
Proserpio, A.   830, *856*
Prunieras, M.   85, *135*
Puccinelli, V.   32, *135*
Puccini, G.   *786*

Puchol, J. R.   815, *852*
— s. Orbaneja, J. G.   *848, 852*
Puchol u. Orbaneja, s. Teilum   *853*
Puchtler, H., u. C. P. Leblond   539, *619*
— u. F. Sweat   444, *488*
— — u. M. Levine   863, *903*
Pugatch, E. M. J.   *1033*
Pullar, P., u. C. Liadsky   627, 633, *681*
Pumphrey, A. M., s. Redfearn, E. R.   *136*
Puppe, G.   *785*
Puretić, St., s. Kogoj, F.   *851*
Purkinje, J. E.   494, *612*
Purkinje, u. Wendt   224, *265*
Pusch, A. L., s. Goodman, R. M.   *911*
Putzmann, G.   821, *855*
Pyka, R., s. Winkelmann, R. *376*
Pyka, R. A., s. Winkelmann, R. K.   *623, 1030*

Quast, P.   480, 481, *488*
Quevedo jr., W. C., s. Fitzpatrick, T. B.   *913*
Quilliam, T. A., s. Pease, D. C. *427*
— s. Pease, D. C. *1024*
Quilliam, Z. A., u. M. Sato   418, *427*

Raab, W., s. Ebner, H.   *912*
— s. Niebauer, G.   *487, 907*
Raab, W. P., s. Steigleder, G. K.   *139, 183*
Rabbiosi, G.   803, *861*
— s. Serri, F.   *137*
Raben, M. S., R. Landolt, F. A. Smith, K. Hofmann u. H. Yajima   949, *1024*
Rabinowitsch, I. M., s. Usher, B.   *910*
Rabl, H.   18, 21, 43, 62, *135*, 267, *336*, 920, 923, 931, 932, 936, 940, 943, 957, 960, 970, 979, *1025*
Rachmatullin, Z. C.   675, *681*
Radaelli, F.   607, *622*
Rademacher, A. H., s. Montagna, W.   *181, 222*
— s. Montagna, W., A. Z. Eisen u. H. B. Chase *133, 265, 334*
Radicé, J. C., s. Torres, E. A. *905*
Raekallio, J.   559, *619*, 721, 727, 752, 753, 754, *781, 784*
— u. E. Levonen   559, *619*
Rahmann-Esser, M., u. F. Fegeler   70, *135*
— s. Fegeler, F.   *126*

Raigrotzki, J.   559, *619*
Ralph, C. C., s. Hall, P. F. *1019*
Ralph, C. L., s. Dierst, K. E. *1017*
Ralston, H., s. Miller, M.   *375*
Ralston III, H. J., s. Miller, M. R.   *426*
Ralston, H. J., s. Miller, M. R. *618*
Ramachandran, G. N.   442, *488*
Ramachandran, J., s. Li, C. H. *1022*
Ramos, u. Silva, S.   871, *905*
Rampini, E., G. Moretti u. A. Rebora   495, 520, 522, 586, 587, 588, 607, 608, *612, 619, 622, 623*
— s. Bertamino, R.   *621*
— s. Crovato, F.   *610*
— s. Moretti, G.   *614*
Randall, I. F.   *488*
Randerath, E.   809, 811, 837, *852, 859*
Ranvier, M. L.   36, 81, *135*
Rapaport, F. T., s. Converse, J. M.   *616*
Raper, H. S.   889, *914*
— s. Evans, W. C.   *913*
Rapkine, L.   72, *135*
Rapmund, O., s. Puppe, G. *785*
Rapp, Y., F. S. Glickman u. L. Frank   496, *612*
Rappaport, B.   891, *914*
Rappaport, H., T. Makai u. H. Swift   104, *136*
Rappaport, M. M., u. R. E. Franzl   84, *135*
— s. Meyer, K.   *487*
Rasiewicz, W., J. Rubisz-Brzezinska u. J. Konecki   871, *905*
Rasmussen, A. T.   458, 459, *488*
Rassner, B., H. Zaun u. O. Braun-Falco   169, *182*
— s. Braun-Falco, O.   *179*
Rassner, G.   5, *136*, 311, 316, 318, *336, 784*
— s. Braun-Falco, O.   *331*
Rast, J. P.   804, *849*
Rathery, Fr., M. Dérot, S. Doubrow u. Jammet   900, *918*
Ratherg, F., u. J. Sigwald   804, *849*
Rathjens, B., s. Braun-Falco, O.   *123, 179, 264, 483, 615*
Rattner, H., u. J. E. Ginsberg   898, *917*
— s. Cornbleet, Th.   *847, 857*
Ratner, I. M., s. Ehrlich, J. C. *901*

Ratschow, M., s. Bock, H. E. *850*
Ratzersdorfer, C., A. S. Gordon u. H. A. Charipper 990, *1025*
Ratzenhofer, M., u. A. Probst 869, *905*
— u. E. Schauenstein 869, *905*
— s. Probst, A. *905*
Rauber-Kopsch 413, *427*
Rauber u. Kopsch 717, 760, 780
Rauch, H., s. Chase, H. B. *179*
Raulston, B. O., s. Magnuson, H. J. *916*
Rausch, L., u. H. Glodny 70, 72, *136*
Rauther, M. 920, 942, 957, *1025*
Rav, I., s. Forchielli, E. *221*
Rawles 105
Rawles, M. 387, *427*
Rawles, M. E. 642, *681*, 890, *914*, *915*, 920, 1005, 1007, 1010, *1025*
Rawls, W. B., s. Goldzieher, J. W. *705*
Rawson, R. W., G. D. Sterne u. J. C. Aub 876, *907*
Ray, T., s. Nicolaides, N. *222*
Raybuck, H. F., s. Gardner, J. H. *679*
Reaven, E. P., u. A. J. Cox jr. 47, 66, 67, 68, *136*
Rebaudi, St. 285, 329, *336*
Rebora, A., s. Baccaredda-Boy, A., u. G. Moretti 615, *621*
— s. Moretti, G., C. Giacometti u. F. Crovato *621*
— s. Rampini, E. *612*, *619*, *622*, *623*
Rebora, R., s. Moretti, G. *182*
Recant, L. 886, *911*
Recht. Gg. 829, *856*
Redfearn, E. R., u. A. M. Pumphrey 102, *136*
Redisch, W., u. R. H. Pelzer 607, *622*
Reed, R., s. Hall, D. A. 485, *904*
— s. Keech, M. K. *486*
— s. Keech, M. K., u. W. J. Wood *486*
— s. Turnbridge, R. E. 489, *905*
Rees, H. A. 805, *849*
Rees, T. D., s. Conway *616*
Reh, H. 744, *783*, *785*, 828, *856*
Rehn, E. 821, *855*
Reich, H. 794, 796, 805, 811, 816, *846*, *849*, *852*
Reich, N. E. 796

Reichard, P., u. B. Estborn 63, *136*
Reichardt, H. 745, *783*
Reimann, W. 747, *783*
Rein, Ch. R., s. Wise, F. *905*
Rein, G. 811, *852*
Reinertson, R. P., s. Scott, E. J. van *183*
Reisch, M. 898, *917*
Reiser, K. A. 384, *427*, 566, 567, *619*
Reiss, H. *681*
Reitano, R. 563, *619*
Reiter, W. *427*
Reith, E. J., s. Rhodin, J. A. G. *136*
Reitinger, J., s. Becker, V. *330*
Rémillard, G. L. 819, *855*
Renaud 787
Renault, P., s. Touraine, A. *860*
Renaut, J. 494, 497, 598, 606, 607, *612*, *622*, *623*, 875, *907*
Rennagel, W. R., s. Rony, H. R. *136*
Renold, A. E. 787, 789, 790, 827, *843*, *844*, *846*, *856*
— u. G. F. Cahill jr. 787, *843*, *844*
— u. G. F. Cahill, s. Wassermann, F. *857*
— s. Cahill jr., G. F. *843*
— s. Crofford *843*
Rényi, G. S., s. Chambers, R. *124*
Reubold 745, *783*
Reuck, A. V. S. de, u. M. P. Cameron 331, *335*
Reuter, F. 752, *785*
Reuter, K. 752, *783*
— u. H. Fischer *783*
Reuter, M. J. 879, *907*
— u. S. W. Becker 872, *905*
Revel, J. P., s. Hay, E. D. *1020*
Reymann, Fl. 806, 833, *849*, *859*
Reynaer, H. 801, *849*, 900, *918*
Reynolds, E. S. 40, *136*
Reynolds, J., s. Billingham, R. E. *121*
Rhodin, J. 2, 4, 21, 31, 37, 57, 84, *136*
— J. Adams-Ray u. H. Nordenstam 436, *488*
— s. Falk, S. *1018*
— s. Sjöstrand, F. S. *138*
Rhodin, J. A. G. 304, *336*
— u. E. J. Reith 21, 37, 38, 47, *136*
Ribet, A., s. Calvet, J. *903*
Rice, H. M., s. Pearson, B. *903*

Rich, A., u. F. H. Crick 441, *488*
Richards, C. M., s. Bagnara, J. T. *1015*
Richards, L., s. Adams, A. E. *1015*
Richardson, K. C. 301, *336*, 378, *427*
Richter, M. 751, 752, *783*
Richter, M. N., s. Gessler, A. E. *128*
Richter, R. 116, *136*, 156, 173, *182*, 357, *376*, *427*, 566, *619*, 699, *706*, 921, *1025*
Richter, W. 272, 277, 283, 285, 296, 309, 310, 311, 329, *336*, 896, *916*
— u. W. Schmidt 272, *336*
Richter, W. H. *427*
Rici, Micheletti u. Coscia 835, *859*
Riecke, E., H. G. Bode u. G. W. Korting *902*
Riegel, P. 628, 630, 631, *681*
Riehl, G. 103, *136*, 776, *786*
Riemersma, J. C. 22, *136*
Rietschel, L., s. Langhof, H. *916*
— s. Langhof, H., u. H. Müller *916*
Rifkind, R. A., E. F. Osserman, K. C. Hsu u. C. Morgan 438, *488*
Riggio, T. 498, *612*
Riley, J. F., u. G. B. West 437, 474, *488*
Riley, N. D., s. Szarski, H. *1027*
Riley, P. A., s. Jarrett, A. *130*
Rimington, C., s. Magnus, J. A. *916*
Rinaldi, V. G. 802, *849*
Rinehart, J. F., u. M. G. Farquhar 539, *619*
Ringer, R. K., s. Peterson, R. A. *1024*
— s. Tetzlaff, M. J. 428, *1027*
Ringrose, E. J. 815, 816, 837, *852*, *859*
Ris, H., s. Mirsky, A. E. *1023*
Rist, M. 823, *855*
Ritchie, A. 921, *1025*
Rittel, W., s. Schwyzer, R. *1026*
Rittenberg, D., s. Schoenheimer *489*
Ritter, E. 805, *849*
Ritzén, M., s. Adams-Ray, J. *482*
Ritzenfeld, P. 2, 3, 55, 56, 87, 90, 103, *136*, *122*, *130*
— u. R. Koch 56, 87, *136*
— s. Klostermann, G. F. *916*

Riva, G., s. Baumgartner, W. 843
— u. W. Baumgartner, s. Leinati, F. 858
Rivelloni, G. 67, *136*
Robb-Smith, A. H. D. 874, *907*
Robb-Smith, A. H. T. 448, 450, 452, *488*
Robertis, de 418
— u. Benett 382, 418
Roberts, E., u. J. A. Griffith 531, *619*
Roberts, I. S., s. Goldzieher, J. W. 705
Robertson 382
Robertson, J. D. 22, 34, *136*, 288, *336*
— T. S. Bodenheimer u. D. E. Stage 953, *1025*
Robin, Ch. 267, *336*
Robinson, H. B. G., s. Halperin, V. 221
Robinson, H. M., u. F. A. Ellis 823, 855
Robson, A., s. Corfield, M. C. 125
Rochlin, D. B., s. Enterline, H. T. 853
Rodbard, S., F. Samson u. D. Ferguson 995, *1025*
Rodin, H. H., s. Bluefarb, S. M. 917
Rodriguez, J. N. 836, *859*
Rodriguez-Perez, A. P. 427
Rodriguez, S., s. De Sousa, A. 621
Roe, D. A. 37, 74, *136*, 371, 376
— P. Flesch u. E. C. J. Esoda 78, 80, 81, *136*
— s. Flesch, P., u. E. C. J. Esoda 127
Röckel, H., u. W. Thies 795, 842, *849*, *859*
— u. D. Vogt 882, *910*
— s. Spier, H. W. 849
Roederer, J., F. Woringer u. R. Burgun 815, *852*, 885, *910*
Röhlich, P., s. Oláh, I. 134
Roeper, E., s. Benditt, E. P. 483
Roer, H., u. H. Koopmann 759, 784
Roessner, K. D., s. Wessells, N. K. *1031*
Rogers, G. E. 51, 72, 74, 75, 87, 89, *136*, 154, 155, 172, 176, *182*, 204, 205, *223*, 437, *488*, *1030*
— L. Finch u. G. Youatt 74, *136*
— s. Downes, A. M. *1029*
— s. Filshie, B. K. 127, 180, *1018*

Rogers, G. E. s. Fraser, R. *375*
— s. Fraser, R. D. B., u. T. P. MacRae 127
— s. Mercer, E. H. *181*, 132
Rogers u. Filshie 52
Rogin, J. R., s. Pinkus, H. 681
Rolle, G. K., s. Johnson, P. L. 130
Rollet 875
Rollhäuser, H. 445, 447, 453, 455, 472, 473, *488*
— s. Niessing, K. 618
Rollins, T. G., u. R. K. Winkelmann 859
Romano, s. Ishibashi 781
Romanul, F. C. A., u. R. G. Bannister 527, *619*
Romiti, N., s. Bandmann, H. J. 860
Ronchese, F. 686, 688, *706*, 707, 729, 730, *781*
Ronge, H. 702, *707*
Rony, H. R., G. J. Scheff, D. M. Cohen u. W. R. Rennagel 73, *136*
— u. S. J. Zakon 187, *223*
Rook, A. 182
Rorsman, H., s. Falck, B. 617, *1031*
Rosa, C. G., u. K. C. Tsou 55, *136*
Rosahn, P. D., s. Dennis, J. W. 909
Rosales, H., s. Kaminsky, A. 848
Rosanow 791, *846*
Rosati, P. 509, *614*
Rosenberg, W. A., s. Goldberg, A. L. 858
Rosenblatt, W. A., s. Wall, P. D. *1031*
Rosenblueth, A., s. Parker, G. H. *1024*
Rosenkilde, P., s. Jørgensen *1021*
Rosenthal, M., s. Krahulik, L. 851
Rosenthal, T. B., s. Lansing, A. I. 486
Roser 821, *855*
Rosin, A. 96, *136*
Rosin, S. 973, *1025*
Ross, D. M. *1025*
— s. Newth, D. R. *1023*
Ross, G. T., s. Kastin, A. J. *1021*
Ross, J. B. 5, 7, *136*
Ross, L. L. 427
— s. Cauna, N. 423
Ross, R. *1033*
— u. E. P. Benditt 432, *488*, *1033*
— u. T. K. Greenlee jr. 31, *136*

Rossatti, B. 559, *619*
Roth, G., s. Weber, G. 805, *861*
Roth, G. M., s. Brown, G. E. 616
Roth, S. I., u. W. H. Clark jr. 2, 4, 12, 14, 21, 31, 32, 35, 36, 37, 38, 39, 40, 44, 47, 57, 58, 60, 68, 84, *1030*
— u. E. B. Helwig 145, 146, 149, 151, 152, 153, 155, 156, 171, *182*, *1031*
— s. Mercer, E. H. *132*, *181*
Rothberg, S., R. G. Crounse u. J. L. Lee 61, 68, *136*
Rothmann 790, 791, 794, *846*, 921
Rothman, S. 13, 14, 15, 17, 43, 72, 73, 76, *131*, *137*, 180
— u. Fr. Schaaf *137*
— s. Bersaques, J. de 121
— s. Magnin, P. H. *131*
— s. Malkinson, F. D. *1023*
— s. Santoianni, P. *137*
— s. Weitkamp, A. W. 223
Rothman, St. 277, 284, *336*
Rothmann-Makai 803
Rothmann, S. 566, 604, *619*, *623*
Rotman, H. 831, *861*
Rotnes, P. L. 796, 797, *849*
Rotter, W. 702, *707*, 837, 838, *859*
— u. L. Wagner 513, *614*, 640, *681*
Rouiller, Ch. 292, *336*
Roulet, F. 869, *905*
Roussel de Vouzeme, A., s. Breschet, G. 264
Roux, M., s. Gillman, Th. *904*
Royster, L. T. 899, *918*
Ruberti, U., s. Miani, A. 618
Rubin, J. R., s. Cronkite, E. P. 125
Rubisz-Brzezinska, J., s. Rasiewicz, W. *905*
Ruckert, J., u. S. Mollier 499, *614*
Rudall, K. M. 18, 37, 49, 50, 71, 74, *137*, 371, *376*, *1007*, *1008*, *1025*
— s. Bailey, K. 120
— s. Durward, A. 613, *610*, *621*
— s. Millard, A. *133*
Rudolph, G., u. H. J. Klein 435, *488*
Ruffini 377
Ruffini, A. 566, *619*, *622*
Ruffini, C., s. Bertamino 621
Rugo, H., s. Bear, R. *374*
Ruhbach, M., s. Knoth, W. 130, *181*
Ruiter, M. 808, 809, 811, *852*, 884, *910*
— u. W. P. de Groot 884, *910*

Rukavina, J. G., W. D. Bolck, C. E. Jackson, H. J. Falk, J. H. Curey u. A. C. Curtis 866
Rumpf, G., s. Schauenstein, E. 905
Rupec, M. 31, 32, 33, 34, 36, 37, *137*, 278, 288, 294, 295, 296, 297, 299, 311, 323, *336*
— u. O. Braun-Falco 11, 12, 14, 20, 21, 26, 58, 59, *123*, *137*
Ruska, C., s. Ruska, H. *427*
Ruska, H., u. C. Ruska *427*
— s. Dettmer, N. *484*
— s. Moore, D. M. *618*
— s. Schmidt, W. J. *1026*
Russel, F. E., u. A. van Harreveld 943, *1025*
— W. C. Barritt u. M. D. Fairchild 943, *1025*
Russel, F. F., u. J. A. Emery 960, *1025*
Rust, S., u. G. K. Steigleder 69, *137*
— s. Okonkwo, B. *487*
Ruszcak, Z., u. L. Wozniak 863, *903*
Rutenburg, A. M., u. A. M. Seligman 556, *619*
— s. Monis, B. *133*
— s. Monis, B., u. B. M. Bank *133*
Rutenburg, S. H., s. Seligman, A. M. *137*
Rutishäuser, E., u. D. Held *859*
Rutschke, E. 1005, *1025*
Rutter u. Marshall 746, *783*
Ruysch, F. 493, *612*
Ruyssen, R., u. L. Vandendriessche *331*
Ryder, M. L. 177, 178, *182*, 495, 497, 498, 500, 501, 503, 511, 573, 581, 589, 604, 608, *612*, *614*, *622*, *623*, *1031*
Ryhiner, P., s. Bloch, B. *912*
Rylander, E., s. Lindberg, O. *861*
Rytömaa, T., s. Bullough, W. S. *124*

Saalfeld, E. 688, 700, *707*, 790, *846*
Sabrazès, J., u. J. Bideau 831, *856*
Sacchi, S. 525, 536, 550, *619*
Sachs 776, 777, *786*
Saeki, O., s. Yasuda, K., u. H. Furusawa *338*
Sagher, F., u. J. Shanon 862, *903*
Saint Paul, U. v., s. Holst, E. v. *1020*

Saito, F., s. Kurosumi, K. *333*
Saito, K., s. Nanikawa, R. *783*
Sajner, J. 628, *681*
Sakai, D., s. Keddie, F. *130*
Salfeld, K., s. Braun-Falco, O. *483*
Saller, K. 459, *488*
Salmon 516, 563, 564, 569, 570, 571, 572, 580, 602, *614*, *619*, *622*, *623*
Salpeter, M. M., u. M. Singer 973, 974, 975, *1025*
— s. Singer, M. *1026*
Salzmann, F. 778, *786*
Samejima, T. 638, *681*
Samman, P. D. 571, *622*
Sams, W. M., J. G. Smith u. E. A. Davidson *488*
Sams jr., W. M., u. J. G. Smith jr. 873, 874, *905*
— — u. E. A. Davidson 874, *905*
Sams, W. M., s. Smith jr., J. G., E. A. Davidson u. J. P. Tindall *905*
Samson, F., s. Rodbard, S. *1025*
Sand, A. 955, *1025*
Sandberg, D. H., u. J. M. Adams 800, 836, 849, *859*
Sanderson, K. V., u. H. Thiede 144, *182*
Sandison, J. C. 558, *619*
Sandritter 824
Sandritter, W. 67, 69, *137*, *781*,
— u. J. Schorn *843*
Sanford, H. N., D. F. Eubank u. F. Stenn 835, *859*
Sannicandro, F. 811, *852*
Sannicandro, G. 536, 537, *619*
Sano, Y., s. Yada, S. *783*
Sant'Agnese, P. A. di, D. H. Andersen u. H. H. Mason 886, *911*
— D. H. Andersen, H. H. Mason u. W. A. Bauman 887, *911*
Santler, R. 169, *182*, 805, 816, 837, *849*, *852*, *859*
Santoianni, G., s. Cerutti, P. *850*
Santoianni, P., u. S. Rothman 100, *137*
Santos, P. S., s. Hoge, A. R. *1020*
Sapuppo, A., s. Cottoni, G. B. *847*
Sarda, I. R., s. Forchielli, E. *221*
Sarkany, I. 225
— u. G. A. Caron 224, 225, *266*

Sarkar, K., u. E. Kallenbach 279, *336*
Sasakawa, M. 76, *137*, *170*, *182*, 201, *223*
Sasaki, N., s. Inamura, A. *1020*
Satanove, A., s. Flesch, P. *127*
Sato, M., s. Oseki, M. *1031*
— s. Quilliam, Z. A. *427*
Saunders, A. M., s. Taylor, H. E. *908*
Saunders, C. H. de 495, 497, 499, 546, 596, 602, 603, 604, *612*, *619*, *622*, *623*
— u. W. Montagna 499, 602, *612*
Saunders, P. R. 959, *1025*
Saunders, R. L. de, C. H., u. W. Montagna 639, *681*
Savidge, R. S., s. Huger *854*
— s. Jackson, S. H. *854*
Savill, A., u. C. Warren 158, *182*
Sawicky, H. H., u. N. B. Kanoff 805, 830, *849*, *856*
Saxton, C. A., s. Swift, J. A. *337*
Scaffidi, V. 828, *856*
Scarpelli, D. G., u. A. G. E. Pearse 98, *137*
— u. M. H. Greider 823, 824, *855*
— s. Pearse, A. G. E. *135*
Schaaf, Fr., s. Rothman, S. *137*
Schaanning, Chr. K., u. B. Nyquist 881, *910*
Schäfer-Danneel, s. Dannel, S. *1017*
Schaefer, E. A. 500, *614*
Schäffner, M. 775, *786*
Schaffer, J. 2, 10, 31, *137*, 267, 268, 272, 274, 275, 279, 282, 288, *335*, *336*, *337*, 789, *844*, 940, *1025*
Schaffert, R. R., s. Newcomer, V. D. 848, *859*
Schallock, G., u. H. Lindner 875, *907*
Schallwegg *705*, *706*
Schallwegg, O. 468, 469, 472, 473, *488*, 683, 684, 685, 686, 688, 691, 695, 696, 697, 699, 702, 704, *707*
Schaltenbrand, G. 792, *846*
Schamberg, J. Fr., u. H. Brown *781*
Scharrer, E. 968, *1025*
— S. W. Smith u. S. L. Palay 968, *1025*
Schartau, O. 996, 1004, *1025*
Schaub jr., F. F., s. Mishima, Y. *914*
— s. Mishima, Y., u. A. V. Loud *914*

Schauenstein 745, *783*
Schauenstein, E., u. G. Rumpf 869, *905*
— s. Ratzenhofer, M. *905*
Schauer, A. 437, 438, 451, *488*
— u. E. Werle 437, *488*
Scheffer, V. B. *1032*
Scheffler, H. 804, *849*
— u. H. Hagen 804, *849*
Scheen, S. R., s. Winkelmann, R. K. 376, *623, 1030*
Scheff, G. J., s. Rony, H. R. *136*
Schenk, G. P., u. H. Wirth 893, *916*
Scherer, A. *783*
Schidachi, J. 791, *846*
Schiebler, T. H., A. G. E. Pearse u. H. H. Wolff, s. Gedevanishvili, M. D. *1018*
Schieck, A., s. Gertler, W. *857*
Schiefferdecker, P. 224, 253, *266*, 267, 268, 270, 271, 272, 275, 325, 327, 329, *336*, 480, 481, *488*
Schiff, B. L., u. A. B. Kern 887, *911*
Schiff, Th., s. Hershey, F. B. *485*
Schilder, P. 868, *203*
Schildmacher, H. 1004, *1025*
Schiller, S., M. B. Mathews, L. Goldfaber, J. Ludowieg u. A. Dorfman 451, *488*
Schilling-Siengalewicz *785*
Schimpf, A. 838, *859*
Schirren, C. 804, *849*
Schirren sen., C. G. 804, *849*
Schittenhelm, W., s. Koecke, H. U. *1021*
Schjernig 769
Schleyer, F. 719, 729, *781, 783*
— u. Janitzki *781*
Schlienger, F. 805, 830, *849, 856, 859,* 901, *919*
Schmidt, A. J. 982, *1025*
Schmidt, G. 778, *786*
Schmidt, Gg. *785*
Schmidt, M. B. 700, *707*
Schmidt, O. 731, *782*
— u. Mitarb. 719, *781*
— s. Lorke, D. *781*
— s. Strassmann, G. *786*
Schmidt, O. E. L. 900, *918*
Schmidt, P., s. Pischzek, F. *619*
Schmidt, S. 644, *681*
Schmidt, W. 300, *336*, 431, 434, 435, 452, *488*
— s. Richter, W. *336*
Schmidt, W. J. *137*, 147, 148, *182*, 257, *266*, 440, 448, *488*, 941, 944, 945, 946, 988, 989, 990, 991, 992, 993, 996, 997, 1010, *1025, 1026*
Schmidt, W. J., u. H. Ruska 1008, 1010, 1011, *1026*
Schmidt-Nielsen, K., s. Bentley, P. J. *1016*
— s. Lee, D. G. *334*
Schmidtmann, s. Ziemke *784*
Schmitt, F. O., J. Gross u. J. H. Highberger 440, 441, *488, 489*
— E. Hall u. M. A. Jakus 440, 441, *489*
— u. A. J. Hodge 440, 442, *489*
— s. Gross, J. *485*
— s. Gross, J., u. J. H. Highberger *485*
— s. Hodge, A. J. *485*
Schmitt-Rhode, J. M., u. E. Weichhardt 888, *911*
Schmorl, O. 869, *905*
Schnabel, E., s. Li, C. H. *1022*
Schnakenbeck 957
Schnakenbeck, W., u. Pisces 957, *1026*
Schneider u. Undeutsch 799, 808, *852*
Schneider, G. *903*
Schneider, W. C., u. E. L. Kuff 55, 84, *137*
Schneider, W., u. H. P. Missmahl 865, *903*
Schnellander, F. G., s. Wolff, K. *620*
Schneller, K., s. Fischer, H. *916*
Schnitzer, A. 879, *907*
Schnitler, K. 806, *849*
Schnitzer, K. L. 530, *619*
Schnyder, U. W., s. Weibel, E. R. *141*
Schober, B. 217, *223*
Schoedd, J. 807, 833, *849, 859*
Schoedel, W., s. Grosser-Brockhoff, F. *610*
Schoefl, G. I. 558, 559, *619*
— u. G. Majno 558, 562, *619, 1033*
Schönberg, A., s. Miescher, G. *222*
Schoenberg, M. D., s. Moore, R. D. *487*
Schönfeld, W. 496, *612*, 729, *781*
— s. Gottron, H. A. *122, 707, 853, 855*
Schoenheimer, R., u. D. Rittenberg 461, *489*
Schöntag, A. 766, *785*
Schöttle, E. 967, *1026*
Scholander, P. F., V. Walters, R. Hock u. L. Irving 1000, *1026*
Scholander, P. F., R. Hock, V. Walters u. L. Irving *1026*
Schollmeyer, W. 761, 769, 771, *784, 785*
Schor, R., u. S. Krimm 1007, *1026*
Schorn, J. 553, 554, 556, *619,* 620
— s. Sandritter, W. *843*
Schorr, E., s. Zweifach, B. W. *142*
Schossberger, s. Friedrich *332*
Schott, H. J., u. H. Holzmann 865, *903*
Schourup, K. 719, *781*
Schrader, G. 743, *785, 786*
Schramm, H., s. Gutman, A. *860*
Schreiber, H. 468, 477, *489, 786*
Schretzmann 740, *782*
Schridde, H. 776, 777, *786*
— u. A. Beekmann 776, 777, *786*
Schrodt, G. R., s. Walker, S. M. *141*
Schroeder, W. 492, *612*
Schroeder, W. A., u. L. M. Kay 1008, *1026*
Schubert, G., s. Pflugfelder, O. *1024*
Schuemmelfeder, N. 85, *137*, 720, *781, 784*
— s. Pfennings, K. B. *910*
Schürmann 799
Schuermann, H. 815, 833, *852, 859,* 878, 879, *907*
Schürmann, P., u. E. H. McMahon *852*
Schütt, s. Masderhoff, J. *783*
Schütze, W. 779, *786*
Schulhof, s. Luger 729
Schultis, K., s. Steigleder, G. K. *139, 266, 859*
Schultz, J., s. Caspersson, T. *124*
Schultz, R. L., s. Maynard, E. A. *618*
Schultze, B., u. W. Oehlert 63, 69, *137*
Schulz u. de Paola 931
Schulz u. Ullrich 243, 253
Schulz, K. H., s. Herrmann, W. P. *847*
Schulz, I., K. J. Ullrich, E. Fromter, H. M. Emrich, A. Frick, U. Hegel u. H. Holzgrove *266*
Schulz, R. 758, 759, 763, 779, *784*
Schulze 832, *859*
Schulze, W. *786*
— u. E. Kunze 805, *849*
— s. Holtz, K. *904*

Schumacher, S. 920, *1026*
Schumacher, S. V. 494, 503, 508, 511, 513, 554, *612, 614, 620*
Schumann, H., s. Danneel, R. *1017*
Schummer, A. 509, *614*
Schuppli, R. 787, 796, *843, 849*
Schuster, M. C., s. Gessler, A. E. *128*
Schwalm, H. 530, *620*
Schwamm, H. A., s. Ackermann, A. B. *860*
Schwanitz, J. 158, *182*
Schwartz, E. 969, *1026*
Schwartz, E. T., s. Hofmann, K. *1020*
Schwartz, I. L., u. J. H. Thaysen 253, *266*
— — u. V. P. Dole 253, *266*
Schwartzkopff, J. 1005, *1026*
Schwartzman, G., s. Aronson, St. A. *853, 855*
Schwarz 777
Schwarz, E. 68, 137
— u. H. W. Spier 68, *137*
Schwarz, W. 441, 447, 449, *489*, 638, *681*
— u. N. Dettmer 449, *489*, 873, 874, *905*
— u. H. J. Merker 444, *489*
— H. J. Merker u. A. Kutsche 434, 441, *489*
— s. Dettmer, N. *484*
Schwarzmann, J. M. 830, 832, *856, 859*, 897, *916*
Schwenkenbecher, A. 778, *786*
Schwerd, W. 731, *782, 786*
— u. Kl. Höchel *786*
— s. Ishibashi u. a. *781*
Schwyzer, B. Costopanagiotes u. Sieber 949
Schwyzer, R. 948, 949, *1026*
— B. Iselin, H. Kappeler, Rimikel, W. Rittel u. H. Zuber 949
— H. Kappeler, B. Iselin, W. Rittel u. H. Zuber 949, *1026*
— u. C. H. Li 949, *1026*
— u. P. Sieber 949, *1026*
Scolari, E. 494, *612*
Scolari, E. G. 691, *707*
Scopes, J., s. Dawkins, M. J. R. *853*
Scothorne, A., s. Scothorne, R. *376*
Scothorne, R., u. A. Scothorne 365, *376*
Scott 274
Scott, B. L., u. D. C. Pease 302, 304, *336*

Scott, E. J. van 5, 62, 63, 66, *137*, 145, 162, 163, 169, *182, 183*
— u. T. M. Ekel 10, *137*, 145, 153, 169, *183*
— — u. R. Auerbach 145, *183*
— u. P. Flesch 72, 73, *137*
— u. R. C. MacCardle 192, *223*
— R. P. Reinertson u. R. Steinmueller 162, 163, 164, *183*
— s. Crounse, R. G. *180*
— s. Montagna, W. *182, 222*
Scott, F. P., s. Findlay, G. H. *904*
Scott, G. H. *137*
Scott, T. G. 238, *266*
Scow, R. O., s. Kovacev, V. P. 827, *860*
Scriba, K. 807, 808, 833, *849, 859, 910*
— s. Hornbostel, H. *909*
Seale, E. R., s. Guin, J. D. *904*
Searle, A. G., u. R. I. Spearman *1031*
Seckfort, H., u. O. Braun-Falco 882, *910*
Segall, s. Hull 819
Segall, M. M., s. Huger *854*
Seibert, H. C., u. M. Steggerda 699, 704, *707*
Seidell, M. A., s. Dalton, J. E. *906*
Seifert, K. 449, *489*
Seiji, Shimao, Fitzpatrick u. Birbeck 115
Seiji, M. *915*
— u. T. B. Fitzpatrick 890, *915*
— — u. M. S. C. Birbeck 110, 115, *137, 915*
— — R. T. Simpson u. M. S. C. Birbeck *915*
— u. S. Iwashita 115, *137, 915*
— K. Shimao, M. S. C. Birbeck u. T. B. Fitzpatrick 110, *137, 915*
— s. Baker, R. V. *120*
— s. Fitzpatrick, T. B. *913*
Seino, S., s. Yamamoto, T. *429*
Seiter, I., s. Block, P. *1032*
Seitz, L. 329, *336*
Sekido, N. 387, *427*
— s. Niebauer, G. *426, 914*
Sekine, M., s. Kurosumi, K. *333*
Selander, R. K., u. L. L. Kuich 1001, *1026*
Selberg, W. 886, *911*
Selby, C. 364, *376*

Selby, C. C. 2, 3, 21, 24, 25, 35, 37, 38, 39, 40, 43, 44, 55, 56, 58, 59, 86, *137*, 463, 464, *489*, 628, *681*
Seligman, A. M., u. S. H. Rutenburg *137*
— K.-C. Tsou, S. H. Rutenburg u. R. B. Cohen 87, 101, *137*
— s. Barrnett, R. J. *121, 178, 374, 615*
— s. Nachlas, M. M. *134*
— s. Rutenburg, A. M. *619*
Sellei, J. 897, *917*
Sellier 765, *785*
Senevivatne, R. D., s. Cameron, G. R. *855*
Sengel, P. 642, *681*, 1007, 1009, *1026*
— u. U. K. Abbott 1009, *1026*
Seno, S., u. E. V. Cowdry 333
Sequeira, J. H. 897, *917*
Sergeev, K. K. 412, *427*
Sevastinos, E., M. M. Jallad u. K. Yamato 859
Serri, F. *137*, 236, 241, 248, *266*, 270, *336*, 365, *376*, 511, 512, 513, 516, 538, *614*, 639, 640, 675, 676, *681*
— u. W. H. Huber 218, *223*
— W. M. Huber u. H. Mescon 271, 322, *326*, 365, 366, *376*, 632, 633, 637, 641, 657, 658, 659, 665, 667, 669, 671, 673, 675, 676, *681*
— W. Montagna u. W. M. Huber 271, 324, *336*, 366, *376*, 511, 512, 513, 514, *614*, 632, 633, 638, 641, 659, 665, *681*
— — u. H. Mescon 271, 307, 312, *336*, 362, 365, 367, 368, *376*, 511, 512, 513, *614*, 632, 633, 636, 638, 641, 657, 658, 659, 665, 667, 669, 671, 673, *681*
— u. G. Rabbiosi 88, *137*
— M. L. Speranza u. H. Mescon 632, 633, 638, 641, 659, 665, *681*
Serri, H. 538, 539, *620*
Setälä, K., L. Merenmies, L. Stjernvall u. M. Nyholm 2, 3, 19, 37, *138*
Seto, H. 404, 415, *427*
Sevenants, J. J., s. Laymon, C. W. *909*
Severinghaus, A. E., s. Kirkman, H. *130*
Severinghaus, E. L., u. Mitarb. *781*
Sexmith, E., u. W. F. Petersen *781*
Seydeler 709, *780*

Sézary, A., u. J.-P. Verne 898, *917*
Shaffer 801
Shaffer, B. 801, *849*
Shaffer, L. W., s. Weidman, F. D. *912*
Shafrir, E., s. Gutman, A. *860*
Shalak, R., s. Loewenstein, W. R. *1022*
Shanks, J. A., W. Paranchych u. J. Tuba 820, *855*
Shanon, J., s. Sager, F. *862, 903*
Shanthaveerappa, T. R., u. G. H. Bourne *427, 1031*
Shapiro, B. 787, 789, *843, 844*
— u. E. Wertheimer 789, *844*
— s. Wertheimer, E. *490*
Shaposhnikow, O. K. 796, *849*
Sharry, L. F., s. Downes *1029*
Shatin, H. 802, *849*
Sheard, C., s. Brown, G. E. *616*
Sheldon, H. 788, *844*
— C. H. Hollenberg u. A. J. Winigrad 788, *844*
— u. F. B. Kimball 441, *489*
— u. H. Zetterqvist 56, *138*
— s. Frei, J. V. *127*
Sheldon, J. H. 895, *917*
Shelley, W. B. 268, *336*
— u. T. Butterworth 272, 329, *336*
— u. M. M. Cahn 330, *336*
— S. B. Cohen u. G. B. Koelle 87, *138*, 176, *183*, 202, *223*, 321, *336*
— u. H. J. Hurley 268, 273, 277, 278, 323, 330, *336*
— u. H. Mescon 240, 243, 247, *266*
— s. Arthur, R. P. *423*
— s. Cahn, M. M. *331*
— s. Hurley, H. J. *130*, 221, 333, *485, 486*
— s. Hurley, H. J., u. G. B. Koelle *333*
— s. Juhlin, L. *617*
— s. Kligman, A. M. *221*
— s. Perry, E. T. *335*
— s. Pillsbury, D. M. *622*
Shelley, W. M., s. Goodman, R. M. *911*
Sherman, W. B., s. Bordley, J. *610, 615*
Shibolet, S., s. Blum, A. *866*
Shimai, K., u. K. Yasuda *335, 337*
Shimao, K., s. Seiji, M. *137*
— s. Seiji, M., M. S. C. Birbeck u. T. B. Fitzpatrick *915*
Shimizu, H. 287, *336*
Shipman, M., H. B. Chase u. W. Montagna 171, *183*

Shoenberg, C. F., s. Needham, D. M. *335*
Short, B. F., s. Lyne, A. G. *681*
Shubik, P., s. Nakai, T. *134*
Shukla, R. C. 108, *138*
Shumway 974
Sick, H. *1026*
Sidman, R. L. 819, *855*
— u. D. W. Fawcett 819, 829, *855, 856*
Siebenhaar, D. F. J. 725, *781*
Sieber, P., s. Schwyzer, P. *1026*
Siebert, G. 86, 138, 175, *183*
Siegel, H., s. Hasegawa, J. *129*
Siegel, B. V., s. Wellings, S. R. *915*
Siegel, Ch. L., s. Goodman *911*
Siegel, M., s. Achs, R. *677*
Siegel, V., s. Wellings, S. R. *141*
Siegmund, H. 838, *859*
Siekevitz, P., u. G. E. Palade 47, 58, 69, *138*
— s. Palade, G. E. *335*
Siemens, H. W. 10, 11, *138*, 881, *910*
Sievers, A. 299, *336*
Sigwald, J., s. Rathery, F. *849*
Sikorski, J., s. Jeffrey, G. M. *130*
Silbert, J. E., Y. Nagai u. J. Gross 986, *1026*
Silva, S., s. Ramos *905*
Silver, A. F., s. Montagna, W., u. R. A. Ellis *222*
Silvers, S. H., s. Levin, O. L. *917*
Silvers, W. K., s. Billingham, R. E. *121*, 677, *678, 912, 1030*
Silvestri, U. 690, 694, 695, 696, 699, 702, *707*
— u. Me de Maurici 693, *707*
Simmons, B., s. Leblond, C. P. *181*
Simms, H. S., s. Parshley, M. S. *134*
Simon, F. 730, *781*
Simon, G. 788, 827, *844*, 856
Simonart, J. M., s. Achten, G. *705*
Simonetta, B., u. A. Magnoni 269, *336*
Simpson, G. G. 506, 507, *614*
Simpson, K. 805, *849*
Simpson, R. T., s. Seiji, M., T. B. Fitzpatrick u. M. S. C. Birbeck *915*
Sims, Ch. F., s. Trubowitz, S. *855*

Sims, R. T. 177, *183*
Sinapius, D. 789, *844*
Sinclair 377
Singer, M., u. M. M. Salpeter 973, *1026*
— s. Salpeter, M. M. *1025*
Singh, G., P. K. Srivastava u. K. N. Gour 802, *849*
Singh, M., u. J. McKenzie 165, 169, *183*
Sitte, P. 287, *337*
Siwe, St. A. 807, 808, 830, 833, 834, 841, *849*, 856, *859*, 882, *910*
Sjöstrand, F. S. 22, 55, 57, 58, 110, *138*, 287, 299, 300, *337*
— E. Andersson-Cedergren u. M. M. Dewey 31, 34, *138*
— u. V. Hanzon 57, *138*
— u. J. Rhodin 55, *138*
Sjöstrand, F., s. Ottoson, D. *134*
Skalos, G., s. Adjutantis, G. *785*
Skinner, B., s. Corfield, M. C. *125*
Skrzeczka 758
Slack, H. G. B. 446, *489*
Slater, J. J., s. Allen, J. M. *330*
Slee, J. *1031*
Slegers, J. F. G. 243, 253, *266*
Slobosiano, H., M. Georgesco u. P. Herscovici 829, 831, 833, *856, 859*
Slocumb, C. H., s. Moskowitz, R. W. *852*
Smetana, H. F., u. W. Bernhard 805, *849*
Smiddy u. Clark 39
Smiddy, F. G., s. Charles, A. *124*
Smiljanic, A. M., s. Weitkamp, A. W. *223*
Smith 743
Smith, C., u. H. T. Parkhurst 76, 77, *138*
Smith, D. E. 437, 438, *489*
— u. Y. S. Lewis 437, *489*
Smith, D. S. 304, *336, 337*
Smith, D. T. 114, *138*
Smith, E. W., s. Goodman, R. M. *911*
— s. Malak, J. A. *902*
Smith, F. A., s. Raben, M. S. *1024*
Smith, J. G. 815, *852, 859*, 873, *905*
— s. Sams, W. M. *488*
Smith jr., J. G. 187, 188, *223*
— E. A. Davidson, J. P. Tindall u. W. M. Sams 874, *905*
— u. A. J. Zansing 873, *905*
— s. Sams jr., W. M. *905*

Smith jr., J. G. s. Sams jr., W. M., u. E. A. Davidson 905
Smith, J. L. 197, *223*
Smith, R. E. 459, *489*
— s. Cameron, I. L. *483*
Smith, S., u. F. S. Fiddes 746, *783*
Smith, S. W., s. Scharrer, E. *1025*
Smith, V. W., s. Chase, H. B. *179*
Snell, R. S. 2, 19, 20, 21, 31, 37, 38, 49, 51, 55, 60, 114, *138*, *915*, *1030*
Snow, J. S., s. Wile, U. J. *905*
Sobel, N., u. J. H. Pollack 885, *910*
Sobin, S. S., W. G. Frasher u. H. M. Tremer 497, *612*
Sörbo, B., s. Lynen, F. *844*
Soffer, L. J., s. Wiener, R. *908*
Sognnaes, R. F., u. J. T. Albright 43, *138*
Sohar, E., J. Gafni, A. Blum, M. Pras u. H. Heller 866
— s. Blum, A. 866
— s. Heller, H. *902*
— s. Missmahl, H. P. 866
Sokolov, W. E. *1032*
Solomon, L. M., u. H. Beerman 831, *861*
Soltermann, W. 896, 897, *917*
Somers, G. F., s. Summer, J. B. *140*
Sommer 725, 726, *781*
Sommers, G. C. 693, *707*
Sommers, S. C., s. Hollander, A. *617*
Sommerville, R. L., s. Lund, H. Z. *904*
Somogyi, E. *786*
— P. Sotonyi u.a. *786*
Sonneck, H. J., s. Heilmann, P. *858*
Sotgiu, G., u. A. de Giorgo 899, *918*
Sotonyi, P., s. Somogyi, E. *786*
Sottermann, W., s. Kuske, H. *854*
Southwood, W. F. W. 685, 686, 687, 688, 690, 691, 692, 704, *707*
Spaas, J., s. Grosfeld, J. C. M. *904*
Spagnoli, U. *859*
Spain, D. M., u. J. M. Foley 802, 849
Spalteholz, W. 494, 497, 500, 501, 511, 516, 517, 518, 519, 520, 521, 522, 524, 526, 527, 530, 546, 548, 550, 552, 553, 563, 567, 568, 569, 570, 571, 572, 573, 574, 575, 581, 583, 586, 590, 592, 594, 595, 596, 597, 598, 600, 601, 602, 604, 605, 606, 607, *612*, *614*, *620*, *622*, *623*
Spannhof, L. 983, *1026*
Spargo, B., s. Pearson, R. W. *135*
Speakman, P. T., s. Malt, R. A. *1023*
Spearman, R. I. C. 987, 998, 999, 1007, 1008, *1027*, *1030*, *1031*
— s. Jarrett, A. *130*, *1030*
— s. Jarrett, A., u. J. A. Hardy *130*
— s. Searle, A. G. *1031*
Spence, J., s. Bradshaw, H. *615*
— s. Bradshaw, M. *122*
Speranza, M. L., s. Serri, F., u. H. Mescon *681*
Sperling, G., 273, 274, 284, *337*
Spieler, U. 286, *337*
Spier, H. W. 15, *138*, 808, 809, *852*
— u. P. v. Caneghem 21, 30, 47, 67, 69, 71, 75, 77, 91, 92, 100, *138*, 176, *183*
— u. K. Martin 96, 99, *138*, 176, *183*, 322, *337*
— u. F. Klaschka 830, *856*
— u. G. Pascher 51, 68, *138*, *139*
— — u. K. Martin 96, 99, *139*
— u. H. Röckl 799, *849*
— s. Bandmann, H. J. *483*
— s. Schwarz, E. *137*
Spinner, M., s. Kenin, A. *854*
Spitzmüller, W. 901, *919*
Sprafke, H. 814, *852*, 862, *903*
Sprofkin, B. F., s. Weinstein, H. *911*
Spühler, G., s. Hofmann, K. *1020*
Spuler, A. 662, *681*
Sreebny, L. M., s. Tamarin, A. *140*
Sri Ram, J., s. Pierce, B. G. *488*
Srivastava, P. K., s. Singh, G. *849*
Stafford, H. A. 86, *139*
Stage, D. E., s. Robertson, J. D. *1025*
Standeert, L. O., s. Vandenbroucke, J. *337*
Stansifer, Ph. D., s. Pinski, J. B. *859*
Starck 430
Starck, D. 105, *139*, 625, 635, 637, 674, 676, *681*, 682, 891, *915*, 921, *1027*
Staricco, R. G. 152, 153, *183*, *915*
Stark, R. B., s. Conway, H. *616*
Starrico, R. J. 104, *139*
— u. H. Pinkus 5, 104, 114, 115, *139*, 691, *707*
— s. Hu, F. *130*
— s. Pinkus *135*
Stary, Z. 921, *1027*
Staubesand, J. 529, *620*
— u. G. Genschow 507, *614*
Staubesand, G., B. Kuhlo u. K. H. Kersting 299, *337*
Staubesand, J. 435, *489*
Stauffacher, W. 787, *844*
Steen, B., s. Häggendal, E. *860*
Stefanelli, A. 406, *427*, 933, 953, *1027*
Stefano, F. J. E., u. A. O. Donoso *1027*
Stefko, W. 515, *614*
Steggerda, M., s. Seibert, H. C. *707*
Stegner 271, *337*
Stehr, K., s. Bandmann, H. J. *860*
Steiger-Kazal, D. 794, *846*
Steigleder, G. K. 11, 18, 23, 58, 67, 69, 70, 72, 73, 74, 76, 77, 78, 80, 81, 83, 85, 87, 88, 92, 93, 94, 96, 100, 101, 102, *139*, 172, 173, 174, 175, 176, *183*, 202, 204, *223*, 450, *489*, 685, 693, 700, 702, 703, *707*, 787, 788, 789, 799, 819, 824, 827, 840, 841, *844*, *845*, *852*, 855, *856*, 859, 886, *911*
— u. H. Elschner 23, 92, 93, 94, *139*
— u. I. Fischer 100, *139*, 176, *183*
— u. O. Gans 17, 18, 43, *139*, 684, 686, 693, *707*
— Y. Kamei u. R. Kudicke 101, *139*
— R. Kudicke u. Y. Kamei 101, 102, *139*, 176, *183*, 435, 474, *489*, 498, 527, 539, *612*, *620*
— u. H. Löffler 23, 92, 93, 94, 95, *139*, 176, *183*, 202, 204, *223*, 526, 538, 550, *620*, 834, *859*
— u. J. T. McCarthy 194, *223*
— — u. M. Nurnberg 14, 15, *139*
— u. W. P. Raab 100, *139*, 176, *183*
— u. K. Schultis 92, 96, *139*, 256, 260, *266*, *427*, 834, *859*

Steigleder, G. K., u. D. R. Weakley 23, 78, 79, 80, 81, 92, *139*, 364, *376*
— s. Gans, O. *622*, *705*, *843*, *902*, *904*, *906*, *909*, *911*, *917*, *918*
— s. Leonhardi, G. *181*
— s. Okonkwo, B. *487*
— s. Rust, S. *137*
Steigman, A. J., s. Little, J. A. *858*
Steigmann, F., s. Szanto, P. B. *337*
Stein, E., s. Mancini, R. E. *487*
Stein, L., s. Huger *854*
— s. Jackson, S. H. *854*
Steiner, H. 1006, *1027*
Steiner, K. 72, 73, *139*, 269, 270, *331*, *337*, 633, 634, 637, 639, 641, 642, 657, *682*, *874*, *905*
Steiness, J. 835, 841, *859*
Steinmueller, R., s. Scott, E. J. van *183*
Stenn, F., s. Sanford, H. N. *859*
Stensiö, E. 921, *1027*
Stenström, S., s. Ottoson *134*
Sternberg, H. 625, 633, 635, 636, *682*
Sternberg, S. S. *855*
Sternberg, Th., s. Winer, L. H. *908*
Sternberg, W. H., s. Farber, E. *126*
Sterne, G. D., s. Rawson, R. W. *907*
Stettenheim, P., A. M. Lucas, E. M. Denington u. C. Jamroz 1003, *1027*
Steven, D. M. 930, 931, 933, 936, 940, *1027*
Stewart, C. P., s. Percival, G. H. *135*
Stewart, G. J., s. Malt, R. A. *1023*
Stichnoth, E. 715, *780*
Stillians, A. W. 899, *918*
Stilwell, D. L. 412, *427*
Stjernvall, L., s. Setälä, K. *138*
Stockinger, L. *427*
— s. Niebauer, G. *904*, *911*
Stoeckel, W. *681*
Stoeckenius, W. 59, *139*, 437, 439, *489*
Stöhr jr., P. 564, 566, 567, *620*, 644, 646, 647, 648, 651, *682*
Stöhr jr., Ph. 377, 389, 398, 415, 421, *427*
Stoian, M. *427*
Storck, H. 808, 809, 830, *852*, *857*

Stoughton, R., u. G. Wells 450, 463, *489*
Stout, A. P. 820, 823, 824, *855*
— s. Kaufmann, S. L. *854*
Stoves, J. L. 172, *183*
Stowers, J. H. 816, *852*
Straile, W. E. 114, *139*, 140, *1031*
— H. B. Chase u. C. Arsenault *1031*
Strain, W. H., C. A. Lankau jr. u. W. J. Pories 177, *183*
Stransky, E. 804, *849*
Strassmann, G. 766, 776, 777, 785
— u. O. Schmidt 776, *786*
— s. Fraenkel, P. *782*
Strauch 740, *782*
Straus, W. 435, *489*
Straus jr., W. L. 268, *337*
Strauß, G., s. Gedigk, P. *916*
Strauß, J. S. 218, *223*
— u. A. M. Kligman 188, 218, *223*, 830, *857*
— — u. P. E. Pochi 187, 190, *223*
— u. P. E. Pochi 185, 187, 190, 191, *223*, 830, *857*
— s. Forchielli, E. *221*
— s. Grots, J. A. *851*, *858*
— s. Mescon, H. *222*
— s. Pochi, P. E. *223*
— s. Pochi, P. E., u. H. Mescon *223*
Strauß, L., s. Churg, J. *850*
Strawinski, S. 976, *1027*
Street, A., s. Astburg, W. T. *120*
Streeter, G. L. 631, *682*
Streitmann, B. 867, *903*
Strenger, A., s. Marinelli, W. *1023*
Stresemann, E. 998, 1006, *1027*
— u. V. Stresemann 1011, *1027*
Stresemann, V., s. Stresemann, E. *1027*
Ströbel, H. 683, 684, 685, 686, 688, 690, 691, 693, 707, 790, *846*
Strong, R. M. *915*
Stroughton, R. B., s. Mesirow, S. M. *133*
Strugger *784*
Studnička, F. K. 929, *1027*
Stühmer, A. 794, *846*
Stüttgen, G. 15, *140*, 321, *337*, 724, *781*, 795, 808, 809, 810, 811, 837, *849*, *859*
— H. Ippen, G. Moretti, H. Brüster, G. Goerz u. B. Kinkelin 921, *1027*
— u. Mitarb. *781*
— s. Langer, E. *914*

Stuhlert, H. 835, *859*
Sucquet, J. P. 493, 553, 599, *612*, *620*, *623*
Sucquet-Hoyer 513
Südhof, H., s. Klostermann, G. F. *843*
Sütterle, H., s. Oehlert, W. *848*, *859*
Suga, Y. 675, *682*
Sullivan, R. R., s. Montgomery, H. *846*
Sumner, J. B., u. G. F. Somers 87, *140*
Summerson, W. H., s. Lerner *914*
Sunahara, K., s. Kawase, O. *486*
Sunder-Plasmann, P. 567, *620*
Sung Sheng, C., s. Dieter, W. *621*
Suntzeff, V., s. Baumberger, J. P. *121*
Suskind, R. R. 196, 198, 200, 201, 204, *223*
Sutherland, J. C., W. P. Calahan u. G. L. Campbell 821, 824, *855*
Sutton, R. L. 607, *623*
Suuromond, D. 894, *916*
Suwelack, K., s. Delank, H.-W. *901*
Suzuki, T., s. Yasuda, K., u. H. Machida *338*
— s. Yasui, I. *338*
Svaetichin, G., s. O'Hoson, D. *134*
Švajger, A. 271, 327, *337*
Svanborg, A., s. Häggendal, E. *860*
Swammerdam, J. 493, *612*
Swan, G. A. 114, *140*
Swan, H., s. Blake, H. A. *855*
Swanbeck, G., u. N. Thyresson 83, *140*
— s. Forslind, B. *1029*
Swann, M. M. 64, *140*
Sweat, F., s. Puchtler, H. *488*, *903*
Sweeley, C. C., u. B. Klionsky *884*, *910*
Sweeny, P. R., s. Edd jr., M. V. *1017*
Sweitzer, S. E., u. C. W. Laymon 879, *907*
Swift, H., s. Rappaport, H. *136*
Swift, H. H. *140*
Swift, J. A. 63, 114, *140*, 146, *183*
— u. C. A. Saxton 288, *337*
Sylvén, B. 437, 438, 451, 453, 469, *489*, 875, 877, 878, *907*
— u. I. Bois 101, *140*

Sylvestre, R., s. Jausion, H. 847
Szabó, G. 5, 7, 104, 106, 107, 113, 114, *140, 183,* 225, *266*
Szabo, T. 956, *1027*
Szakall, A. 13, 14, *140, 781*
— s. Grüneberg, Th. *129*
Szanto, P. B., F. Steigmann, F. Pamuken, I. Friedman u. R. Hadok 293, *337*
Szarski, H. 977, *1027*
Szentmiklosy, A., s. Dejenarui, I. *847*
Szirai, J. A. *908*
Szodoray, L. 2, 18, 21, *140,* 272, *337,* 871, *905*
— u. K. Nagy-Vezekényi 3, 11, 18, 80, 81, *140*
— u. K. N. Vezekény 809, *852*
Szymanski, F. J., u. S. M. Bluefarb 824, *855*
Szymonowicz, L. *427*
Szymonowicz, M. *428*
Szymonowicz, W. 378, 402, 406, *428,* 674, 675, *682*

Tabachnik, J. 68, *140*
Tagliavini, R., s. Bonicelli, U. *846*
Takagaki, T., s. Wada, M. *266*
Takahashi, N. 301, *337*
Takahashi, Y., s. Lerner, A. B. *1022*
Takamura, K. 323, *337*
Takeda, H., s. Inamura, A. *1020*
Takeda, S. 657, 663, *682*
Takeuchi, T. 91, *140,* 201, *223*
— K. Higashi u. S. Watamuki 91, *140*
Takino, M. *428*
Tamarin, A. 302, 303, 304, *336, 337*
— u. L. M. Sreebny 31, 32, *140*
Tamassia, A. 746, *783*
Tamponi, M. 378, 387, *427*
Tanaka, K. 275, *337*
Tandler, B. 302, 303, 304, *337*
Taniguchi, T. 184, *223,* 660, 668, 669, *682*
— Y. Kosaka u. T. Nakano 184, *223*
Tants 741
Tanzer, M. L., s. Gross, J., u. C. M. Lapiere *1019*
Tappeiner, J. 875, 876, 879, 880, *908*
— L. Peleger u. H. Holzner 880, *908*
— u. P. Modniansky 815, *852, 853,* 879, 881, 887, 888, *908, 910, 912*

Tappeiner, S. 272, *337,* 816, *853*
Tapper, D. N. *428*
Targovnik, S. K., s. Grots, I. A. *221*
Tartuferi, F. 267, *337*
Tasaki, I., s. Maruhashi, J. *426*
— s. Maruhashi, K. *1023*
Taschen, B. 785
— u. H. D. Bergeder *785*
Tattersall, R. N., s. Tunbridge, R. E. *905*
— s. Turnbridge, R. E. *489*
Tawa, N., s. Nanikawa, S. *783*
Taylor, s. Ruter u. Marshall *783*
Taylor, A. C. 303, *337,* 789, *845*
Taylor, H. C., s. Taylor jr., R. E. *1027*
Taylor, H. E., u. A. M. Saunders 875, *908*
Taylor, J. D., H. E. Paul u. M. F. Paul 789, *845*
Taylor jr., R. E., u. S. B. Barker 981, *1027*
— H. C. Taylor u. S. B. Barker 981, 982, *1027*
Taylor, W. R., s. Bailey, R. M. *1015*
Tedesch, C. G. 821, *855*
Teichert, H., s. Lüdicke, M. *1023*
Teilum 809, 811, *853*
Teilum, G. 864, 865, *903*
Telford, E. D. 799, 804, *849, 853*
Teller, H., G. Vester u. L. Pohl 447, *489,* 684, 693, *707*
Témine u.a. 809, 811
Tench, E. M. 635, *682*
Tendis, N. 802, *849*
Teodoru, C. V., s. Aronson, St. A. *853, 855*
Terbrüggen, A. 720, *781*
Terhecherbrügge, A., s. Lauter, S. *706*
Terzakis, J. A. 243, 244, *266*
Tetzlaff, M. J., R. A. Peterson u. R. K. Ringer *428,* 1004, *1027*
— s. Peterson, R. A. *1024*
— s. Bourne, G. H. *122, 330*
Tewfik, H. 275, *337*
Thaler, H. 896, *917*
Thannhauser, L. J. 888, *912*
Thannhauser, S. J. 882, *910*
Thathachari, Y. T., s. Bell, E. *1016*
Thauer, R. 1000, *1027*
Thaysen, J. H., s. Schwartz, I. L. *266*
— s. Schwartz, I. L., u. V. P. Dole *266*

Theisen, H., s. Braun-Falco, O. *179, 1030*
Themann, H., s. Fasske, E. *126*
Thiede, H., s. Sanderson, K. V. *182*
Thiele, O. W. 789, *861*
Thies, W. 284, *337, 428,* 880, *908*
— u. L. F. Galente 204, *223*
— s. Röckl, H. *849, 859*
Thölen, H. 635, *682*
Thöne, A. W. 823, *855*
Thoenes, W. 293, 326, *337*
Thoma 759
Thoma, K. H. 820, *843*
Thoma, R. 511, *615*
Thomas, R. W., s. Griesemer, R. D. *860*
Thompson, N. 250, 253, *266*
Thompson, O. P., s. Gillespie, J. M. *128*
Thompson, R. H. S., s. Magnus, I. A. *131*
Thomson, J. G. 897, *917*
Thomson, J. L. 1008, *1027*
Thomson, R. H. 114, *140*
Thompson, T. A., s. Hofmann, K. *1020*
Thompson jr., H. C., s. Cowdry, E. V. *125*
Thouret 744, *783*
Threadgold, L. T., s. Leeson, R. C. *1022*
Thunberg, T. 87, 93, *140*
Thuringer, J. M. 61, 62, 63, *140*
— u. Z. K. Cooper 62, 63, *140*
— u. A. A. Katzberg 636, *682,* 690, *707*
Thyresson, N. 163, *183*
— s. Swanbeck, G. 83, *140*
Tiedemann, A. 559, *620*
Tiemke, s. Oorsoś 759
Tietze, A. 474, 475, *489*
Tilden, J. L., H. C. Gotshalk u. E. V. Avakian 802, *849*
Tilney, L. G., s. Bikle *1016*
Tindall, J. P., s. Smith jr., J. G., E. A. Davidson u. W. M. Sams *905*
Tirschek, H., s. Pfleger, L. *910*
Tischendorf, W., s. Klostermann, G. F. *843*
Titone, s. Huger *854*
Tixier-Vidal, A. 1014, *1027*
Todaro, F. *613*
Töndury, G. 625, 637, 640, 673, *682*
Togashi, Y., s. Yoshida, Y. *915*
Tompkins, J., u. I. M. Weinstein *905*

Tomsa, W. 493, 497, 583, 586, 594, 597, 598, 599, 600, *612, 622, 623*
Tood and Bowman 493, 599, *612, 622, 623*
Tornabuoni, G. 896, *917*
Toro-Genkel, L. 809, *853*
Torres, E. A., J. C. Radicé, N. U. Villafane u. S. Vaccaro 873, *905*
Torsuev, N. A. 675, *682*
Tosti, A. 498, *612*, 873, *905*
— u. L. Fazzini 873, *905*
Touraine, A., u. P. Renault 838, *860*
Toussant *782*
Tovo u. de Bernardi 729
Toyama, I., u. T. Nagashima 824, *855*
Tranck, A., s. Darier, J. *616*
Tranzer, J. P., u. A. G. E. Pearse 102, 103, *140*
Traub, E. F. 816, *853*
Tremer, H. M., s. Sobin, S. S. *612*
Tretjakoff, D. 933, 934, 936, *1027*
Tright, H. van 996, *1027*
Trimble, M. E., s. Argyris, T. S. *1032*
Trotter, M. 699, *707*
— s. Duggins, O. H. *180*
Trotter, W. R., u. K. C. Eden 877, *908*
Trubowitz, S., u. Ch. F. Sims 824, *855*
Truffi, G. 354, 357, 569, *376*, 580, 581, 583, 584, 586, 594, 597, 598, 606, *622, 623*, 639, 640, *682*
Trujillo-Cenóz, O. 953, *1027*
Trump, B. F., s. Ericsson, J. L. E. *331, 332*
Trupke, I., s. Grassmann, W. *128*
Tryb, H. A. 875, 879, *908*
Trygstad 827, *857*
Tsou, K.-C., s. Rosa, C. G. *136*
— s. Seligman, A. M. *137*
Tsuchiya, K. 230, *266*, 664, *682*
Tuba, J., s. Shanks, J. A. *855*
Tunbridge, R. E., R. N. Tattersall, D. A. Hall, W. T. Astbury u. R. Reed 874, *905*
— s. Hall, D. A. *904*
Turiaf, J., u. F. Basset 117, *140, 910*
— s. Basset, F. *121, 908*
Turnbridge, R. E., R. N. Tattersall, D. A. Hall, W. T. Astbury u. R. Reed 449, *489*
— Hall, D. A. *485*

Turner, C. N., s. Althausen, T. L. *916*
Tusques, J. 978, *1027*
Twitty, V. C. 105, *140*

Uchida, T., s. Demura, K. *856*
Uden, N. van, s. Ferreira-Marques *904*
Ueda, M. 664, *682*
Ueda, Y., s. Kataoka, H. *904*
Ugo, A., s. Parvis-Preto, V. *614*
Uher, V. *784*
Ullrich, K. J., s. Schulz, I. *266*
Umbreit, Ch. 829, *857*
Umrath, K., s. Adrian, E. D. *423*
Underwood, G., s. Bellairs, A. d'A. *1016*
Underwood, L. J., s. Montgomery, H. *907*
Undeutsch, W., s. Hering, H. *847, 856, 858*
— u. H. Hering, s. Berner u. Heyde *855*
— u. H. Hernig, s. Cruse *857*
— s. Schneider, W. *852*
Ungar, H. 801, 802, *849*
— s. Katzenellenbogen, I. *904*
Unna 869
Unna, P. 583, 606, 607, *623*
Unna, P. G. 10, 11, 13, 14, 15, 17, 18, 19, 20, 21, 23, 29, 30, 50, 51, 75, 76, 81, *140, 141*, 791, *846*
— u. L. Golodetz 18, 20, 76, *141*
Unna jr., P. 494, *612, 622*
Unrau, S. A., s. Atkinson, S. *178*
Unshelm, E. 833, 834, 841, *860*
Urbach, E. 798, 814, 815, *849*, 853, *853*, 881, 885, *910*
— E. Epstein u. K. Lorenz *910*
— u. C. Wiethe 870, *905*
Urbach, F., s. Wood, M. G. *905*
Usher, B., u. I. M. Rabinowitsch 885, *910*
Ussing, H. H. 978, 981, *1027*
— s. Koefoed-Johnsen, V. *1021*
Usuku, G., u. J. Gross 986, *1027*
Utiger, R. D., Th. Lemarchand-Beraud u. A. Vannotti 877, *908*
Uttley, M., s. Ashmore, H. *178*

Vaccaro, S., s. Torres, E. A. *905*
Valentino, A. 826, *855*
Vanable, J. W. 986, *1027*

Vandekerckhove, M. 796, 800, 836, *849, 860*
Vandenbroucke, J., G. de Groote u. L. O. Standeert *337*
Vandendriessche, L., s. Ruyssen, R. *331*
Vannotti, A., s. Utiger, R. D. *908*
Varley, H., s. Huger *854*
— s. Jackson, S. H. *854*
Vassar, P. S., u. F. C. Culling 864, *903*
Vastarini-Cresi, G. 494, 513, 551, 553, *612, 615, 620*
Vater-Pacini 377
Vaupel-v. Harnack, M., s. Oksche, A. *1024*
Vazques, T. T., F. J. Dixon u. A. L. Neil 866, *903*
Veil, W. 285, *337*
Velde, van der 413, *428*
Vercander, E., s. Bellmann, S. B. *615*
Vernall, D. G. 148, *183*
Verne, J. 62, *141*
— u. V. Vilter 948, *1027*
Verne, J.-P., s. Sézary, A. *917*
Vero, F. 816, *853*
Versari, A. 494, *612*
Vesey, C. M. L., u. D. S. Wilkinson 796, 836, *849*, 860
Veslot, Duperrat, Browaes, Garnier u. Pley 882, *910*
Vester, G., s. Teller, H. 489, *707*
Vezekény, K. N., s. Szodoray, L. *852*
Vidal-Leloir 872, *905*
Viglioglia, P., s. Kaminsky, A. *848*
Vignolo-Lutati, C. 686, 695, 699, 700, *707*
Vilanova u. Gräflin 799, 800
— s. Woodburne *853*
Vilanova, X. *861*
— u. J. Piñol Aguadé 796, 800, 802, 803, *849, 861*
— — u. J. M. Moragas *849*, 879, *908*
Vilar, O., s. Mancini, R. E. *487*
Villafane, N. U., s. Torres, E. A. *905*
Villiger, W., s. Durrer, H. *1017*
Vilter, V. 950, 951, *1027*
— s. Verne, J. *1027*
Viragos-Kis, F., s. Fazekas, I. G. *784*
Virchow, R. 863, 875, *903, 908*
Visetti, M., s. Ormea, F. *619*
Viterbo, B., s. Montanari, G. D. *783*

Vitry, G., u. Y. Privat 435, 450, *489*
Vitry, M., s. Lortat, G. *856*
Voegt, H., s. Lossie, H. *858*
Völker, O. 1005, 1010, *1027*
Vogel, A. 31, 32, 33, *141*, 462, *489*
Vogell, W. 289, *337*
— s. Braun-Falco, O. 122, *123*
— s. Macher, E. *611*
— s. Petry, G. *135*
Vogt, A., u. H. G. Kochem 865, *903*
— s. Letterer, E. *902*
Vogt, D., s. Röckl, H. *910*
Vohwinkel, K. H. 272, *337*, 691, 704, *707*
Voit 745, *783*
Voit, K., s. Feulgen, R. *127*
Volk, R. 816, *853*
Volkmann, R. v. 61, *141*
Volland, W. 114, *141*
— u. W. Pribilla 896, *917*
Volterra, M. 536, *620*
Voss, H. 85, *141*, *843*
Voss, M. 471, *489*, *611*
Voute, C. L. 979, 982, 983, *1028*
Vrla, V., s. Kutscher, W. *909*

Wachstein, M., u. E. Meisel 437, *489*
— s. Bradshaw, M. 122, *615*
Wada 378
Wada, M. *784*
— u. T. Takagaki 224, *266*
Waelsch, L. 329, *336*, *337*
Wagner 707, 872, *905*
Wagner, B. M. 863, *903*
Wagner, Ch. E. *786*
Wagner, G. 683, 693, 700, *707*
Wagner, H. O., u. C. Müller 1012, *1028*
Wagner, H., s. Wetzstein, R. *337*
Wagner, H. J. 730, 765, *785*
Wagner, L., s. Rotter, W. 614, *681*
Wahlgren, F., s. Lofgren, S. *848*
Wail 831, *857*
Wainfeld, S., s. Pierini, L. E. 796, *861*
Wainger, C. K., u. W. F. Lever 794, *846*
Walcher, K. 724, 752, 759, 763, *782*, *783*, *784*
Walchshofer, E. 698, *707*
Waldeyer, W. 11, *141*
Wales, R. T., s. Martin, E. A. *222*
Walker, B. E., s. Leblond, C. P. *131*

Walker, S. M., u. G. R. Schrodt 55, *141*
Wall, P. D. *1031*
Wallace, W. S. 883, *910*
Waller, J. I. 823, 824, *855*
Wallin, O. 962, *1028*
Walls, E. W., u. T. J. Buchanan 497, 534, *612*, *620*
Walp, L., s. Hammett, F. S. *129*
Walser 751
Walsh jr., T. S. 570, *622*
Walter, C., s. Dannenberg, A. M. *484*
Walter, P. 383, 406, *428*, *1031*
Walters, V., s. Scholander, P. F. *1026*
Walther, D. 794, *846*, *853*
Walther, H. 798, 799, *850*
Walton, D. C., u. M. G. Witherspoon 779, *786*
Ward, W. H., u. H. P. Lundgren 17, *141*
— s. Lundgren, H. P. *131*
Ward-Hendrick, A. 820, *843*
Waring, H. 946, 947, 948, 950, 951, 965, 991, *1028*
Warren, C., s. Savill, A. *182*
Washburn jr., W. W., u. T. G. Blocker jr. 69, 77, *141*
Wassermann, F. 440, 451, 455, 456, 458, 461, 475, *489*, 640, *682*, 788, 819, 827, *845*, *857*
— u. T. F. McDonald 456, 460, 461, *489*, 490, 788, *845*
Wassermann, H. 788, *845*
Wassilev, W., s. Kadanoff, D. *425*
Wassner 817, 818
Watamuki, S., s. Takeuchi, T. *140*
Watanabe, H. 323, *337*
Watanabe, S. 563, *620*
Watson, E. M., u. R. H. Pearce 875, *908*
— s. Österreicher, D. L. *856*
— s. Pearce, R. H. *488*
Watson, G. G. 1014, *1028*
Watson, M. L. 40, *141*, 499, *612*
WaHiaux, R., s. Duve, C. de 97, *126*, *141*
— s. Duve, C. de, B. C. Pressman, R. Gianetto u. F. Appelmans *126*
Watzka, M. 326, *337*, 551, *620*
Way, St. C., u. A. Memmesheimer 275, 277, 329, *337*, 704, *707*
— s. Alderson, H. E. *846*
Weakley, D. R., s. Steigleder, G. K. *139*, *376*

Wearn, J. T. 530, *620*
Weber, G. 76, *141*, 794, *846*, 875, *908*, 989, *1028*
— u. G. Roth 805, *861*
— s. Braun-Falco, O. *123*, *135*
— s. Korting, G. W. *907*
Weber, R. 986, 987, *1028*
Weber-Christian, s. de Granciansky, P. *860*
Weck, A. de, s. Brun, R. *220*
Wecke, H., s. Oehlert, W. *848*, *859*
Weddel 357
Weddell, G. 377, 379, *428*, 564, 565, 566, *620*, 921, 956, *1028*, *1031*
— u. S. Miller *428*
— u. W. Pallie 565, 567, *620*
— — u. E. Palmer 411, *428*, *1031*
— u. E. Palmer *428*, 702, *707*
— — u. W. Pallie 376, *1032*
— s. Allenby, C. F. *423*
— s. Lele, P. P. *426*, *1022*
— s. Miller, S. *426*, *1031*
— s. Pawlowski *427*
Weerd, J. W. de, s. Best, E. W. *846*
Wegelius, O., s. Asboe-Hansen, G. *906*
Wegener, F. 811, *861*
Wegner, A. J. 893, *916*
Wehrmann, R., s. Herrmann, W. P. *847*
— s. Kimmig, J. *130*, *844*
— s. Wiskemann, A. *916*
Weibel, E. R., u. U. W. Schnyder 40, 41, 43, *141*
Weibel, J., s. Ericsson, J. L. E. *331*, *332*
Weichhardt, E., s. Schmitt-Rhode, J. M. *911*
Weiden, S., s. Althausen, T. L. *916*
Weidenreich, F. 15, 21, 23, 29, *141*, 387, *428*, *915*
Weidinger, A., s. Derksen, J. C. *125*
— s. Derksen, J. *375*
Weidman, F., s. Margolies, A. *222*
Weidman, F. D. 790, *843*
— u. W. Freeman 882, *910*
— u. L. W. Shaffer 887, *912*
Weigert 791, *846*
Weill, J. P., s. Woringer, Fr. 853, *860*
Weiner, G., s. Woringer, F. *850*
Weiner, J. S., u. K. Hellman 224, *266*
— u. K. Hellmann *1030*
Weinig, E., u. P. Zink 717, 760, *780*

Weinmann, J. P., s. Meyer, J. 133, 706
Weinmann, P., s. Potter, B. 905
Weinmann, W. 777, 786
Weinstein, A., H. C. Francis u. B. F. Sprofkin 882, 911
Weinstein, G. D. 69, 141
Weinstein, I. M., s. Tompkins, J. 905
Weinstock, A., s. Wilgram, G. E. 141, 142
Weiß 775
Weiß, E. 494, 612
— u. M. Hohanel 612
Weiß, F. 788, 845
Weiss, P. 453, 490, 642, 682
— u. W. Ferris 2, 3, 35, 37, 141, 364, 376, 970, 973, 974, 975, 1028
— s. Willer, B. 615
Weiß, R. S., s. Mook, W. H. 910
Weiß, S., u. W. R. Frazier 531, 533, 620
— u. B. Nickau 530, 620
Weissenfels, N. 915
— s. Danneel, R. 1017
Weismann, B., u. K. Meyer 875, 908
Weitkamp, A. W. 196, 223
Weitzel, G., s. Lennert, K. 131
Weitkamp, A. W., A. M. Smiljamic u. S. Rothman 196, 223
Wellings, S. R., u. G. R. Philp 326, 337
— u. V. Siegel 110, 113, 115, 141, 915
Wells 921
Wells, G. C. 92, 93, 95, 141, 877, 908
— s. Nicolaides, N. 222
Wells, G., s. Stoughton, R. 489
Wells, M., s. Muckle, T. J. 866
Welton, D. G., s. Belote, G. H. 908
Wende, s. Goi 746
Wenzel, H. G. 473, 490
Werkgartner, A. 735, 766, 767, 782, 784, 785
Werle, E., s. Schauer, A. 488
Werner, S., s. Hagen, E. 424
Wersäll, J., s. Engström, H. 424
— s. Flock, Å. 1018
— s. Frithiol, L. 127
— s. Lowenstein, O. M. 1022
Wertheimer, E., u. B. Shapiro 459, 460, 490
— s. Shapiro, B. 844
Wertheimer, H. E. 787, 788, 789, 844, 845
Wertheimer, M., s. Wertheimer, N. 612, 620

Wertheimer, N., u. M. Wertheimer 497, 530, 612, 620
Werthemann, A. 620
Wessells, N. K. 1032
— u. K. D. Roessner 1031
— s. Kallman, F. 1029
West, G. B., s. Riley, J. F. 488
Westfall, J. A., s. Eakin, R. M. 1017
Westling, H., s. Lindberg, S. 680
Wetzel, N. C., u. Y. Zottermann 491, 494, 496, 531, 533, 534, 595, 598, 604, 612, 620, 622, 623
Wetzstein, R., u. H. Wagner 271, 337
Wewalka, F. 917
Weyers, H. J., s. Brandsma, C. H. 850
Weyhbrecht, H. 867, 899, 903, 918
— u. G. W. Korting 871, 905
— s. Braun, W. 903
Weyrich, G. 735, 782
Whitear, M. 966, 968, 969, 984, 1028
Whitting, H. W., s. Miller, L. 1033
Widlan, S., s. Mishima, Y. 680, 914
Widmer, C., s. Hatefi, Y. 129
Wiedemann, E. 993, 1028
Wiedmann, A. 116, 141, 387, 428, 436, 490, 563, 620, 882, 911, 915
— s. Niebauer, G. 426, 487, 914
Wiener, A. 67, 141
Wiener, R., A. Jannaccone, J. Eisenberg, S. I. Griboff, A. W. Ludwig u. L. J. Soffer 877, 908
Wiethe, C. 870, 905
— s. Urbach, E. 905
Wifling, L., s. Beck, F. 903
Wigley, J. E. 900, 918
— u. C. D. Calnan 805, 830, 850, 857
Wilander, O., s. Jorpes, E. 486
Wilder, R. M., s. Butt, H. R. 916
Wildman, A. B. 511, 615
Wile, U. J., u. J. S. Snow 871, 905
Wilgram u. Caulfield 59
Wilgram, G. F. 25, 26, 40, 58, 59, 141
— J. B. Caulfield u. W. F. Lever 2, 3, 4, 21, 33, 36, 37, 38, 40, 141
— — u. E. B. Madgic 21, 31, 32, 35, 36, 37, 38, 40, 141

Wilgram, G. F., u. A. Weinstock 25, 26, 33, 35, 141, 142
— s. Caulfield, J. B. 124
Wilkinson, D. S., s. Vesey, C. M. R. 849, 860
Wilks, S. S., u. R. T. Clark 786
Willer, B., P. Weiß u. V. Hamburger 499, 500, 615
Williams 811
Williams jr., Ch. H., R. H. Gibbs u. H. Kamin 90, 142
Williams-Ashman, H. G., s. Ortiz, E. 1023
Williamson, J. R. 460, 461, 490, 788, 845
— u. P. E. Lacy 788, 827, 845, 857
Willis, R. A. 820, 823, 843
Wilson, D. M. 953, 1028
Wilson, H. T. H., s. Becker, J. F. 903
Wilson, J. W., s. Novy, F. G. 855
Wilson, R. B., u. C. A. McWhorter 665, 682
Wimpfheimer, C. 270, 337
Wimtrup, B. 524, 620
Winer, L. H. 815, 853, 867, 873, 887, 903, 905, 912
— S. M. Bierman u. Th. Sternberg 877, 908
Wingo, W. J., s. Foraker, A. G. 127
— s. Foraker, A. E. 180
Winigrad, A. J., s. Sheldon, H. 844
Winkelmann 411
Winkelmann, R. K. 354, 357, 367, 376, 428, 492, 495, 497, 507, 511, 520, 530, 547, 564, 594, 595, 596, 597, 598, 604, 612, 615, 620, 622, 674, 675, 682, 921, 1032
— u. J. V. Hultin 283, 337, 697, 707
— u. H. Montgomery 283, 309, 337
— u. T. T. Myers 1004, 1028
— u. L. S. Osment 413, 428
— S. R. Scheen jr., R. A. Pyka u. M. B. Coventry 354, 376, 604, 623, 1030
— s. Bourlond, A. 423
— s. Kim, R. 907
— s. Muller, S. A. 848, 852
— s. Perry, H. O. 861
— s. Rollins, T. G. 859
— s. Wolff, K. 142
— s. Wolff, K., u. K. Holubar 142

Winkelmann, R. K., s. Zollmann, P. E. *429*
Winkler, A., s. Konrad, J. *907*
Winter, G. D. *1033*
Winter, W., u. O. Braun-Falco 286, *338*
— s. Braun-Falco, O. *123, 331, 780, 781*
Winzler, R. J. 875, *908*
Wirth, H., s. Schenk, G. P. *916*
Wise, F. 816, *853*, 899, *918*
— u. Ch. R. Rein 871, *905*
Wiseman, A., s. Meirowsky, E., u. L. W. Freeman *132*
Wiskemann, A. 887, *912*
— u. R. Wehrmann 894, *916*
— u. K. Wulf 894, *916*
Wislocki, G. B. 85, *142*
— H. Bunting u. E. W. Dempsey 85, *142*, 437, 450, *490*, 526, *620*
— D. W. Fawcett u. E. W. Dempsey 23, 78, 79, 80, *142*
— s. Bunting, H. *264, 331, 483*
— s. Dempsey, E. W. *125*
Witherspoon, M. G., s. Walton, D. C. *786*
Witkowski, J., s. Hurley, H. J. *264, 265*
Witschi, E. 1015, *1028*
Witt, I., s. Hensel, H. *424*
Witterlin, s. Parrisius, W. *611*
Wittig, R. 272, *338*
— s. Nikolowski, W. *706*
Wittkowski, J. A., s. Hurley, H. J. *333*
Wittneben, W., s. Jaensch, W. *613*
Witzel, M., u. O. Braun-Falco 162, 163, *183*
Wodniansky, P. 875, 876, 877, 879, *908*
— s. Tappeiner, J. 852, *853, 908, 910, 912*
Wöhlisch, E., R. du Mesnil de Rochemont u. H. Gerschler 445, 447, *490*
Woellwarth, C. v. 969, *1028*
Wohlfahrt, T. A. 952, *1028*
Wohlfahrt-Bottermann 333, 378
Wohlfarth-Bottermann, K. E., s. Komnick, H. *1021*
Wohlwill, Fr., s. Hegler, C. *853*
Woito 746
Wolbach, S. B. 158, 160, *183*
Wolf, J. 80, *142*
Wolf, M. 802, *850*
Wolff, F., u. M. Laufer *785*
Wolff, J. 304, *338*

Wolff, K. 99, 101, 102, 115, 116, 117, 119, 120, *142*, 176, *183*, 527, 539, 550, 559, *620*, 885, 886, *911*
— u. F. G. Schnellander 560, 561, 562, *620*
— u. R. K. Winkelmann 117, *142*
— — u. K. Holubar 117, *142*
Wolman, M. 449, 457, *490*, 871, 882, 885, 905, *911*
— u. J. J. Bubis 863, *903*
Wolpers, C. 440, 443, 449, *490*
Wolstenhome, G. E., s. Lansing, A. J. *904*
Wong, R. L., s. Benditt *483*
Wood, C., s. Gross, S. *853*
Wood, M. G., K. Pranich u. H. Beerman 273, *338*
— F. Urbach u. H. Beerman 871, *905*
Wood, R. L. 31, *142*
Wood, W. J., s. Keech, M. K., u. R. Reed *486*
Woodburne 799
— Philpott, Vilanova u. Graflin *853*
Woodburne, A. R., s. Busman, G. J. *917*
Woodhouse-Price, L. R. 804, *850*
Woods, E. F., s. Gillespie, J. M. *128*
Woods, H. J., s. Astbury, W. T. *120*
— s. Jeffrey, G. M. *130*
Woods, M. W. 110, *142*
— s. Du Buy *125*
Wool, I. G., u. R. S. Harris, s. Lerner, A. B. *1022*
Woolf, D. L., s. Evans, M. J. *424*
Woollard, H. H. 272, 277, *338, 566, 620*
Woolley, P. 991, *1028*
Woolner, M. E., s. Hofmann, K., u. E. T. Schwartz *1020*
Woringer, F. 806, 808, 815, 830, 841, *850, 853*, 857, *860*
— u. J. P. Weill 815, 837, *853, 860*
— u. G. Weiner *850*
— s. Pautrier, L. M. *135, 848, 855*
— s. Roederer, J. 852, *910*
Wozniak, L., s. Ruszczak, Z. *903*
Wright, I. S., u. A. W. Durjee 530, *620*
Wright, M. R. 950, 951, 984, *1028*
— u. A. B. Lerner 950, 982, *1028*
Wright, P. A. *1028*

Wrigth, P. G., s. Luck, C. P. *1032*
Wulf, K., s. Wiskemann, A. *916*
Wunderer, H. 956, *1028*
Wyllie, L.-M.-A., s. Breathnach, A. S. *123, 678, 912, 913*
— s. Breathnach, A. S., u. D. Goodwin *123*
Wynkoop, E. M. 148, *183*, 699, *707*

Yada, S., M. Okane, Y. Sano u. Y. Fukumori 752, *783*
Yajima, H., s. Hofmann, K. *1020*
— s. Hofmann, K., N. Yanaihara, T. Liu u. J. Lande *1020*
— s. Raben, M. S. *1024*
Yamada, H. 297, *338*
— u. S. Miyake 398, *429*
Yamada, I., s. Higashi, H. *1020*
Yamada, K. 184, 185, *223*
— s. Okajima, K. *487*
Yamagata, S., s. Kataoka, H. *904*
Yamagishi, M., s. Kurosumi, K. *333*
Yamamoto, T., J. Ito, T. Ohno, T. Ohyama, H. Omoto u. S. Seino 414, *429*
Yamato, K., s. Sevastinos, E. *859*
Yamazaki 96
Yamazaki, K. *429*
Yamine 497
Yamomoto, T. *429*
Yanagisawa, N. 268, *338*, 663, *682*
Yanaihara, N., s. Hofmann, K. *1020*
— s. Hofmann, K., H. Yajima, T. Liu u. J. Lande *1020*
Yanazaki 387
Yang, S. H., s. Goodall, A. M. 610, *613*
Yoshida, Y., u. Y. Togashi *915*
Yoshino, S., s. Katsuki, Y. *1021*
Yasuda, K. 268, 279, 284, 312, 321, *338*
— T. Aoki u. W. Montagna *1029*
— R. A. Ellis u. W. Montagna 268, 287, 292, 293, 294, 297, 299, 300, *338*
— H. Furusawa u. N. Ogata 236, 242, 248, 260, *266*, 268, 312, *338*
— — u. O. Saeki 268, 305, *338*

Yasuda, K., u. H. Kagemoto 268, 277, 305, 306, *338*
— — u. K. Kobayashi 268, 305, *338*
— H. Machida u. T. Suzuki 268, 284, 312, *338*
— u. W. Montagna 176, *183*, 202, *223*, 236, 242, 248, 253, *266*, 268, 305, 321, *338*, 482, *490*
— T. Suzuki u. H. Machida 268, 321, *338*
— s. Montagna, W. *1029*
— s. Montagna, W., u. R. A. Ellis *265*
— s. Shimai, K. *335, 337*
Yasuda, T., s. Ohmura, H. *335*
Yasui, I. 270, 271, 277, 322, 323, *338*
— u. H. Kagemoto 271, 307, 309, 310, 311, *334, 338*, 665, *682*
— u. T. Suzuki 268, 306, *338*
Yasuma, A., u. T. Ichikawa 67, *142*
Yasunobu, K. T. 114, *142*
Yoshimura, F., u. M. Irie 299, *338*
Youatt, G., s. Rogers, G. E. *136*
Young, J. Z. 932, 933, *1028*
— u. C. W. Bellerby 933, *1028*
Yum, S. S., s. Montagna, W. *426*
Yun, J. S., s. Montagna, W. *133, 182, 222, 265, 334, 614, 618, 621, 1029*
Yuyama 240, 243

Zacks, M. A. 899, *918*
Zachariae, H. 638, *682*
Zaias, N. 342, 343, 344, 348, *376*, 669, 670, 671, 672, 673, *682*
Zak, F. G., s. Montagna, W. *133, 222*
— s. Montagna, W., u. R. Noback *334*
Zakon, S. J., s. Rony, H. R. *223*
Zander, R. 62, *142*, 342, 353, 364, *376*
Zastava, V. 627, *682*

Zaun, H. 163, *183*, 873, *905*
— s. Braun-Falco, O. *179*
— s. Heite, H. J. *705*
— s. Nödl, F. *902*
— s. Rassner, B. *182*
Zavarini, G. 803, 832, *850*, 860
Zeek, P., u. E. M. Madden 806, 807, 809, *850*
Zeiger *781*
Zeiger, K. 15, 17, *142*
Zeisler, E. P., u. M. R. Caro 885, *911*
Zeitlhofer, J. 804, *850*
Zelesnikow, I. G. 636, 639, 669, *682*
Zelickson, A. S. 31, 37, 38, 44, 56, 78, 87, 118, 119, *142*, 176, *183*, 258, 260, 261, 288, *338*, 495, 536, 541, 543, *612, 621*, 638, *682, 915*
— u. J. F. Hartmann 13, 14, 21, 31, 37, 38, 55, 56, 57, 58, 59, 60, 103, 104, 107, 108, 109, 110, 117, *142*, 891, *915*
— H. M. Hirsch u. J. F. Hartmann 110, 115, *142*, 891, *915*
— s. Hirsch, H. M. *913*
Zeligman, I., u. L. F. Hubener 188, *223*
Zeller u. Hetz 836, *861*
Zenin, B. A. 398, *429*
Zetterqvist, H., s. Sheldon, H. *138*
Zettner, A. 948, *1028*
Zeumer, G. 802, *850*
Zezschwitz, K. A. v. 879, *908*
Ziegler, D. M., s. Doeg, K. A. *125*
— s. Green, D. E. *128*
Ziegler-Günder, I. 931, 977, *1028*
Ziegler, H. 339, 346, *376*
Ziegler, I. 931, 965, *1028*
Zieler *850*
Zieler, C., u. L. Arzt, s. Brünauer, St. R. *845*
Zieler, K., s. Arzt, L. *681*
Ziemke *784*
Ziemke, E. *784*
Zierz 805, *850*
Zika, K., u. E. Kominkora *622*

Zillinsky, s. Collen, W. S. *847*
Zillner, E. 747, *783*
Zimmer, J. G., u. D. J. Demis 531, 533, *621*
Zimmerli, E., u. W. Lutz 900, *918*
Zimmermann, A. A. 105, *142*, 649, 676, *682*, 890, *915*
— u. S. W. Becker jr. 104, 105, *142*, 387, *429, 682*, 890, *912, 915*
— u. Th. Cornbleet 105, 106, 110, *142*, 387, *429*, 890, *915*
— s. Becker jr., S. W. *423, 677*
Zimmermann, K. W. 152, 154, *183*, 536, *621*
Zimmermann, S. B., u. H. C. Dalton 950, *1028*
Zink, P. 780, *784*
— s. Weinig, E. *780*
Ziswiler, V. 1006, *1028*
Zocchi, S. 833, *860*
— s. Baccaredda-Boy, A., G. Moretti u. F. Crovato *615*
Zöllner 881
Zöllner, N. 881, 882, 888, *911, 912*
Zollinger, H. U. 438, *490*, 720, *781*
Zollmann, P. E., u. R. K. Winkelmann *429*
Zoon, J. J. 899, *918*
— L. H. Jansen u. A. Hovenkamp 872, *905*
Zorzoli, G. 310, *338*, 663, *682*
Zottermann, Y., s. Wetzel, N. C. *612, 620, 622, 623*
Zuber, H., s. Schwyzer, R. *1026*
Zuelzer, G. 778, *786*
Zugibe, F. T. 525, *621*
Zuick, K. H. *784*
Zurhelle, E., s. Brocq *853*
— s. Hoffmann, E. *854*
Zweifach, B. W. 552, *621*
— M. M. Black u. E. Schorr 88, *142*
— s. Chambers, R. *610, 616, 622*
Zwijndregt, H. A. v., s. Carol, W. L. L. *846*
Zypen, E. van der 379, 382, 398, *429*

Sachverzeichnis

Abt-Letterer-Siwesche Erkrankung, Nosologie 882
Acantholyse, Beziehung von Fibrillen zu Desmosomen 40
—, „lamellated bodies" 59
—, Veränderungen der Haut der späten Leichenzeit 732
Acanthosis nigricans benigna, experimentelle Pathologie des Fettgewebes 826
— sebacea, Fettstarre der frühen Leichenzeit 724
Acetalphosphatide, Arteriolen der Haut, Histochemie 537
—. Histiocytose und Xanthogranulomatose 883
—, Kapillaren der Haut, Histochemie 537
—, Venolen der Haut, Histochemie 537
Acetylcholinesterase, arteriovenöse Anastomosen, Histochemie 556
— in Herbstschen Körperchen bei Vögeln 1005
—, Histochemie der Keratinocyten 92
—, — des Nagels 367
—, — der Talgdrüsen 196, 204
—, histochemischer Nachweis in apokrinen Schweißdrüsen 321
Acetylcholin, Innervation der Haut 418
Achsel s. auch Axilla
Achselgeruch, Beziehung zum Eisengehalt der apokrinen Schweißdrüsen 311
Achselhaare, Eisengehalt 310
Achseldrüsen, apokrine, Haarkomplexentwicklung 657
Achselhaut, Faserverlauf im Stratum papillare 468
—, Musculus cutis diagonalis 481
Acinus, glandulärer, Gefäßversorgung 581
Acranier, Corium 923
—, Epidermis 922
—, freie Nervenendigungen der Haut 925
—, Haut der, vergleichende Histologie 922

Acranier, Innervation des Integumentes 923, 925
—, mit Kapseln versehene Nervenendigungen der Haut 926
—, Lymphgefäße der Haut 923
—, Quatrefagessche Körperchen 925, 926
—, Sinneszellen im Epithel 926
—, Subcutis 923
Acrodermatitis chronica atrophicans Pick-Herxheimer, Fettgewebsatrophie der Haut 793
Acroreaktion, Kupfernachweis auf der Haut bei Elektrounfällen 775
Acrosyringium, ekkrines, fetale Haut, Glykogengehalt 632
—, —, — —, Phosphorylase-Aktivität 632
—, Elektronenmikroskopie 666
—, Embryonalentwicklung der ekkrinen Drüsen 664
—, Ultrastruktur der ekkrinen Drüsen 665
Acrotrichium, Haarkomplexentwicklung 654
ACTH, Einfluß auf Melanophorenpigmente bei Tieren 949
—, — auf die Reptilienhäutung 990
—, lipid mobilisierende Wirkung am menschlichen Fettgewebe 827
Acupunktur, Innervation der Haut 412
Adenosindiphosphatase, Kapillaren der Haut, Histochemie 537
— in Langerhans-Zellen 119
—, Venolen der Haut, Histochemie 537
Adenosinmonophosphatase, Arteriolen der Haut, Histochemie 527, 537
—, Kapillaren der Haut, Histochemie 537
—, Venolen der Haut, Histochemie 537, 550
Adenosintriphosphatase, Arteriolen der Haut, Histochemie 527, 537

Adenosintriphosphatase, Blutgefäßneubildung der Haut, Histochemie 560
—, Cytochemie, myoepitheliale Zellen 236
—, Epithelzellmembranen bei Amphibien 981
—, helle Zellen, Cytochemie 243
—, Histochemie der Gewebsmastzellen 437
—, Histotopochemie des Haarfollikels 176
—, Histochemie der Keratinocyten 99
—, histochemischer Nachweis in apokrinen Schweißdrüsen 324
—, Histiocyten der Haut 435
—, Kapillaren der Haut, Histochemie 537
—, Langerhans-Zellen 119, 120
—, Melanocyten 115
—, —, Lokalisation, Vergleich mit Dopa-oxydase-Reaktion 116
—, Venolen der Haut, Histochemie 537, 550
—, weiche Hornschicht bei Reptilien 989
ADH s. Hormon, antidiuretisches
Adiponecrosis subcutanea neonatorum, Ätiologie und Pathogenese 833
— —, autoallergische oder hyperergische Phänomene 835
— —, Bedeutung traumatogener Reize für die Reaktion des Gefäßnervensystems 835
— — —, dünnschichtchromatographische Untersuchungen 834
— — —, experimentelle Fettgewebsschädigung 830
— — —, Fettgewebsschädigung durch Injektionen 830
— — —, Fettgewebsveränderung durch Kälte 831
— — —, mikrochemische Untersuchungen 833
— — —, Patho-Histologie 806

Adiponeogenese, postmortale Fettphanerose 745
Adipositas, Beeinflussung der Fettspeicherung 459
Adipozire 741
—, Hydroxylstearinsäure 746
Adrenalektomie, Beeinflussung der Fettspeicherung 459
Adrenalin, Aktivierung der alkalischen Phosphatase in apokrinen Schweißdrüsen 323
—, Chalone-Wirkung 65
—, lipidmobilisierende Wirkung am menschlichen Fettgewebe 827
—, Wirkung auf die Mastzellen 438
—, Einfluß auf Melanophorenpigmente bei Tieren 950
—, — auf die Melanophoren bei Reptilien 991
—, — auf Mitoserate 64
Adventitia capillaris s. Pericyten
Affenfurche, Entwicklung bei intrauteriner Rubeolavirus-Infektion 636
— bei Mongolismus 636
Afterfedern bei Vögeln 1006
Agnoszierung 729
Akne vulgaris, buccale Talgdrüsen 217
Akrogerie, Fettgewebsatrophie der Haut 794
Albino, Melanocytenzahl 691
Alcianblau-Färbung bei aktinischer Elastose 874
—, Arteriolen der Haut 525
— der Bindegewebsgrundsubstanz 450
— bei Mucinosis follicularis 880
—, Mucopolysaccharide, Histochemie der Keratinocyten 79
Alcianblau-PAS-Färbung, Darstellung der Uratablagerungen in der Haut 889
Aldehydfuchsin-Färbung bei Mucinosen 879
—, Darstellung elastischer Fasern 448
Aldolase, Corium 474
—, histochemischer Nachweis in apokrinen Schweißdrüsen 310, 313
Algenrasen, postmortale Veränderungen der Haut 735
Algor, Haut der frühen Leichenzeit 708
—, Hautveränderungen an Leichen 708
Aliesterasen, Histochemie der Keratinocyten 92

Aliesterasen, histochemischer Nachweis in apokrinen Schweißdrüsen 322
Alkohol, postmortale, percutane Resorption 779
Alkoholintoxikation, Livores 711
Allergie, Fettgewebe als Schockorgan 840
Alloxan-Technik, Histochemie der Keratinocyten 67
Alopecia mucinosa, Klinik und Pathohistologie 880
— praematura, Haarfollikel 168
— senilis, Haarfollikel 168
Alopecie, androgenetische, Haarfollikel 168
Alpha-Cytomembran, Lipide, Histochemie der Keratinocyten 84
—, Melanocyten, Elektronenmikroskopie 110
—, —, Melaninsynthese 115
—, Morphologie der Keratinocyten 22, 57
—, Nomenklatur 58
Alpha-Helix, Keratinstruktur 50
Alpha-Keratin, Röntgendiffraktionsmethode, Schwefelgehalt 75
Alpha-naphthol-Esterasen, Histochemie der Keratinocyten 92
Altersamyloidose 866
Altersdimorphismus, Gefiedertypen bei Vögeln 1015
Altersnagel, Anatomie 342
—, Histologie 360
Alterspigmentierung der Haut 685
Altmann's Technik, Färbung der Mitochondrien 55
Amido-Schwarz, Darstellung des Stratum corneum 15
Aminosäuren, Einbau in die Haarwurzelzellen 175
—, Histochemie der apokrinen Schweißdrüsen 305
—, — der Keratinocyten 67
—, Histotopographie im Haarfollikel 172
—, freie, in Häutungszellen bei Reptilien 990
Aminopeptidasen, Arteriolen der Haut, Histochemie 527, 537
—, Basalzellen, Cytochemie 253
—, Blutgefäße der Haut, Histochemie 498
—, Blutgefäßneubildung der Haut, Histochemie 560
—, Haarbalg 474

Aminopeptidasen in Häutungszellen bei Reptilien 990
—, Histochemie von Brandwunden der Haut 772
—, — der Keratinocyten 101
—, — der Leichenhaut 721
—, Histotopochemie des Haarfollikels 176
—, Kapillaren der Haut, Histochemie 537
— in Langerhans-Zellen 119, 120
—, Nachweis in Fibrocyten des Coriums und der Subcutis 431
—, Pinocytose-Mechanismus der Histiocyten 435
—, Schweißdrüsen 474
—, Tropokollagenbildung 433
—, Venolen der Haut, Histochemie 537
Aminophosphorylase, epidermaler Schweißdrüsen-Ausführungsgang 260
amitotische Zellteilung, Epidermis 62
Ammoniaksaponifikation, Biochemischer Mechanismus 746
Amnionepithel, Embryologie der Epidermis 626
Amphibien, adulte, Corium der 982
—, —, Epidermis der 978
—, —, Haut der 978
—, —, Subcutis der 982
Amphibienhaut, Veränderungen während der Metamorphose 986
—, vergleichende Histologie 969
Amphibien, Larvenhaut der 970
Amphibienlarven, Epidermis der 970
—, Hautatmung der 976
—, Subcutis der 976
Ampulle, intradermaler Schweißdrüsen-Ausführungsgang 249
Amylase, experimentelle Fettzellnekrose 831
Amylo-1,6-Glukosidase, Histochemie, Talgdrüsen 196, 201
Amyloid, Ablagerungen im Fettgewebe bei Fettgewebsatrophie der Haut 794
Amyloidablagerungen, Histologie der 867
Amyloid, Bindung an Kongorot 863, 866
—, chemische Struktur 862, 864

Amyloid, Dichroismus 863
—, Differenzierung zwischen periretikulärem und perikollagenem Amyloid 866
—, Elektronenmikroskopie 863, 864
—, Färbung mit Thioflavin T 864
—, Fettabsorption 864
Amyloidfibrille, Unterschied zur Kollagenfibrille 865
—, Ultrastruktur 865
Amyloid, Gammaglobulinnachweis 866
—, histochemische Darstellung 863
—, intracelluläre Bildung 865
—, klassische Färbemethoden 864
—, Polarisationsmikroskopische Untersuchungen 865, 866
—, primäres, Einteilung nach Missmahl 866
—, —, Herkunft 865
Amyloidringe, Amyloidablagerung im Fettgewebe 868
Amyloid, Rot-Metachromasie 863
Amyloidschollen, Histologie der Amyloidablagerungen in der Haut 867
Amyloid, sekundäres, Antigen-Antikörper-Reaktion 865
—, —, Herkunft 865
—, Sezernierung vom RES 864
—, Sudanophilie 864
—, Tryptophantest 864
Amyloidose, Ablagerungs- und Speicherkrankheiten der Cutis 862
—, Ähnlichkeit mit Hyalinose 871
—, Diskussion der Immunopathie 866
—, Einteilung nach Missmahl 866
—, Einteilungsschema 865
—, experimentelle, Immunologie 865
— bei familiärem Mittelmeerfieber 866
— als Folge einer entsprechenden Grundkrankheit 866
— — des multiplen Myeloms 866
—, hereditäre 866
—, idiopathische 866
—, kardiopathische familiäre 866
—, neuropathische familiäre 866

Amyloidose, perikollagene 866
—, —, Polarisationsoptische Untersuchung 863, 866
—, periretikuläre 866
—, —, polarisationsoptische Untersuchung 863, 866
—, primäre, Einteilungsschema 865
—, sekundäre, Einteilungsschema 865
—, —, Hautbefall 865
—, typische, klassische, echte, Einteilungsschema 865
— mit Urticaria und Taubheit einhergehend 866
Amylophosphorylase, Cytochemie myoepithelialer Zellen 236
—, Histochemie der fetalen ekkrinen Drüsen 665
—, Histochemie des Nagels 367
Amylo-1,4 → 1,6-transglucosidase, Histochemie der Keratinocyten 77, 91
Anämie, idiopathische refraktäre, Hämochromatosesyndrom 895
—, Livores 711
—, sideroachrestische, Hämochromatosesyndrom 895
Anagen, Strukturveränderungen des Haarfollikels 158, 160, 162
Anagenhaare, dysplastische, Haarwurzelstatus 163
—, normale, Haarwurzelstatus 163
Analhaut, glatte Muskulatur 479
Anastomosen, arterio-venöse, Altersveränderungen der Fingerhaut 700
—, —, Embryonalentwicklung 640
—, —, Histogenese der 513
—, —, des Corium 599
—, —, der Haut, äußerer Durchmesser 553
—, —, —, Anzahl 552
—, —, —, arterielle Äste 553
—, —, —, Elektronenmikroskopie 557
—, —, —, Histochemie 556
—, —, —, innerer Durchmesser 553
—, —, —, Innervation 398, 401, 566
—, —, —, Kaliberschwankungen 552
—, —, —, regionäre Verteilung 552
—, —, —, Schaltstücke 553
—, —, —, Struktur 553

Anastomosen der Haut, äußerer Durchmesser, Thermoregulation 552
—, —, —, Typen 551
—, —, —, vergleichende Anatomie, Blutgefäße der Haut 500, 503, 507, 509, 511
— erster Ordnung, Gefäßnetz der Haut 569, 572
— zweiter Ordnung, Gefäßnetz der Haut 569
— der Gesichtshaut, Altersveränderungen 700
Anatomie, vergleichende, der Blutgefäße der Haut 499, 500
Androgene, Einfluß auf Mikoserate 64
—, — auf Trennung epithelialer Verwachsungen durch Verhornung 635
Anetodermia erythematosa maculosa Jadassohn, Fettgewebsatrophie der Haut 793
Aneurysmabildung bei Periarteriitis nodosa cutanea 810
Angiitis, allergische, granulomatöse, riesenzellhaltige (Churg-Strauss), Patho-Histologie 809, 811
—, senile, riesenzellige Angiitis Erbslöh 809
Angioblasten 499
Angiokeratoma corporis diffusum Fabry, Histochemie 884
— — —, Klinik und Histologie 884
— — —, Lipidablagerung in der Haut 881
— — —, Polarisationsmikroskopie 884
Angiolipom, Patho-Histologie 820
Angiome, kapilläre, bei Angiokeratoma corporis diffunum Fabry 884
Anilin, Färbung von Hyalin 869
Anisotropie, Talgdrüsen 201
„annulate lamellae", Ultrastruktur der apokrinen Schweißdrüsen 300
Anoxybiose, Autolyse der frühen Leichenzeit 719
Antephase, Mitose der Keratinocyten 65
Antikörper, Bildung in Plasmazellen 438, 439
Antimon, Nachweis im Pulverschmauch 766
Antimonvergiftung, Mumifikation 740

Antistreptolysintiter, Erhöhung bei Erythema nodosum 836
Anus, embryonale Entwicklung 635
Apophase, Mitose der Keratinocyten 65
„apopilose baceous unit", Ausführungsgang apokriner Schweißdrüsen 284
Apoplexie, neurogene Lipome 838
Arachidonsäure, Aufbau des Fettes in der Subcutis 789
Arginin, Histotopographie im Haarfollikel 172
argyrophile Faser s. Faser, argyrophile
Argyrophilie elastischer Fasern 445
Argyrose, Einteilung 898
—, experimentelle, Silberspeicherung im RES 899
—, lokale, gewerblich bedingte, Histologie 898
—, universelle, Klinik und Histologie 899
Arrectores plumarum in der Vogelhaut 1001
Arsenvergiftung, Mumifikation 740
Arteriae incubatoriae bei Vögeln 1001
Arteria intersegmentalis, Mesodermentwicklung 637
Arterien der Haut 517
— —, Altersveränderungen 702
— —, Histologie 523
— —, Innervation 565
— —, metamere Verteilung 518
— —, „mixed cutaneous arteries" 518
— —, Pharmakodynamik 566
— —, „pure cutaneous arteries" 518
— —, segmentale Verteilung 518, 521
— —, Übergang in Arteriolen 524
— —, Verteilung in Subcutis und Corium 567
Arteriitis, generalisierte (Berblinger), Patho-Histologie 809, 811
—, nekrotisierende (Müller-Hoppe), Patho-Histologie 809, 811
— temporalis Horton-Magath-Brown, Patho-Histologie 809, 811
Arteriolen der Hautanhangsgebilde 580
— der Haut 519

Arteriolen der Haut, Definition 524
— —, Durchmesser 523
— —, Elektronenmikroskopie 525, 527
— —, Gefäßarkaden 520, 522
— —, Histochemie 525, 537, 556
— —, Histologie 523
— —, Innervation 565
— —, mehr oberflächliche, Elektronenmikroskopie 529
— —, Pharmakodynamik 566
— —, tief subcutane, Elektronenmikroskopie 527
— —, Übergang von Arterien 524
— —, — zu Kapillaren 524
— —, Patho-Histologie gefäßbedingter Erkrankungen des subcutanen Fettgewebes 808
Arteriolitis allergica (Ruiter), Patho-Histologie 809
Arteriosklerose, Ätiologie der Lipome 839
— der Blutgefäße der Haut 700
—, Glykogenanreicherung im Gewebe 886
Arterio-venöse Anastomosen s. Anastomosen, arteriovenöse
Arthritis, Glykogenanreicherung im Rheumaknötchen 886
Arthus-Phänomen, hyperergische Reaktion bei Periateriitis nodosa cutanea 811
— bei Periarteriitis nodosa 837
Artiodactyla, vergleichende Anatomie, Blutgefäße der Haut 510
AS-Esterasen, Histochemie der Keratinocyten 92, 95
—, Kapillaren der Haut, Histochemie 537
—, Venolen der Haut, Histochemie 537
Astrablau-Färbung der Bindegewebsgrundsubstanz 450
— bei Mucinosis follicularis 880
Atherom, Identitätsfeststellung 730
Atmungsfermente in braunem Fettgewebe 819
ATPase s. Adenosintriphosphatase

Atrophia cutis senilis, Pathologie der Haut 789, 790
— striata neurotica, neurotrophische Atrophien der Haut 792
Atropin, Einfluß auf Pigmentablagerung in der Haut 898
Augenflecke bei Selachiern 947
Augenlid, Subcutiskonstruktion 477
Auriaris, Klinik und Histologie 900
Autolyse der Haut, chemische und histochemische Befunde 720
— —, Experimente 732
— — beim Fetus 721
— —, frühe Leichenzeit 718
— —, morphologische Befunde 720
Autolytische Aktivität, intradermaler Schweißdrüsen-Ausführungsgang 250
AVA s. Anastomosen, arteriovenöse
Axilla s. auch Achsel
Axillardrüsen, hormonelle Einflüsse auf apokrine Schweißdrüsen 329
Axillarhaut, Amyloidablagerung 868
—, physiologisches Hämosiderin-Vorkommen 897
Axillarorgan, Lokalisation apokriner Schweißdrüsen 272
Axone, Blutgefäße der Haut 564
—, Innervation der Haut 379, 391, 396, 419, 422
—, Mitochondriengehalt, Innervation der Haut 384, 408, 419
Axolemm, Innervation der Haut 379, 387
Azanfärbung, Basalmembran 462

Bakerscher Hämateintest, Fettsynthese 461
Bakersche Reaktion bei Histiocytose und Xanthogranulomatose 883
Ballendrüsen, historischer Überblick über apokrine Schweißdrüsen 268
Bariumcarbonat und Mennige, Injektionsmethoden 497
Bariumchloridfärbung, Darstellung kollagener Fasern 446

Barium, Nachweis im Pulverschmauch 766
Barnett-Reaktion, Kapillaren der Haut 536
—, Arteriolen der Haut 526
Basalfüßchen, Basalmembran 462, 465
Basaliom, ektopische apokrine Schweißdrüsen 273
Basalmembran, Altersveränderung des Coriums 693
— bei Amphibien 973
—, Bildung der 463
—, Bindegewebsgrundsubstanz, Stoffwechsel 451
—, Desmosomen der Keratinocyten 36
—, Elektronenmikroskopie 2, 3, 463
—, embryonale Entwicklung 639
—, Entstehung der, bei Amphibien 974
—, Epidermis, Innervation der Haut 379, 391, 398
—, fetale Haut, Glykogengehalt 632
—, — —, Phosphorylase-Aktivität 632
—, Fettspeicherung 460
—, Haarentwicklung, PAS-Reaktion 649
—, Histochemie 463
—, Kapillaren der Haut 534, 539, 541
—, — —, Histochemie 539
—, — —, Innervation der Haut 398
—, korio-epidermale Verknüpfung 2, 3
—, mikroskopische Anatomie der apokrinen Schweißdrüsen 280
—, — und submikroskopische Anatomie von Corium und Subcutis 461
—, morphologische Entwicklung des Haarbulbus 651
—, myoepitheliale Zellen 482
—, PAS-reaktive Substanzen 79
—, Regeneration der, bei Amphibien 975
—, schematische Darstellung 464
—, Ultrastruktur der apokrinen Schweißdrüsenzellen 288
—, univacuoläre Fettzelle 456
—, Veränderungen der Haut in der späten Leichenzeit 732
— der Vogelhaut 999
—, Vorkommen von Mucopolysacchariden im Nagel 363

Basalmembran, Weite des epidermalen Spaltes 3
Basalmembranzapfen 465
„basal membrane" s. Basalmembran
„basal plate" 35
Basalschicht, Embryologie der Epidermis 627
— der fetalen Epidermis, Ultrastruktur 631
Basalzellen, Basalmembran 250
—, Cytoplasma 250
—, Desmosomen 250
—, endoplasmatisches Reticulum 251
— -Epitheliom, Ultrastruktur der ekkrinen Drüsen 665
—, Epidermis, Durchmesser 10
—, fetale Epidermis, Glykogengehalt 631, 632
—, — —, Phosphorylase-Aktivität 631
—, Fibrocyten 250
—, Funktion 253
—, Glykogen 251, 253
—, intercelluläre Kanäle 251
—, intradermaler Schweißdrüsen-Ausführungsgang, Elektronenmikroskopie 250
—, intraepidermaler Schweißdrüsen-Ausführungsgang, Cytochemie 252
—, kollagene Fasern 250
—, marklose Nervenfasern 250
—, Melaningehalt bei Mucinose 879
—, Mikrovilli 250, 253
—, Mitochondrien 250, 253
— der Nagelmatrix, Ultrastruktur 374
—, Natriumrückresorption 253
—, Plasmamembran 250
—, Tonofilamente 254, 257
—, Ultrastruktur der ekkrinen Drüsen 665
„basement membrane", Nomenklatur 2, 3
Basophilie, Epidermis 58
Bauer-Feulgen-Reaktion, Darstellung des Glykogenvorkommens in der Haut 886
Baufett 458, 459
Becherzellen bei Knochenfischen 958
Benzin, postmortale percutane Resorption 779
Benzol, postmortale percutane Resorption 779

Benzpyren-Fluorescenzmethode, Lipiddarstellung bei Angiokeratoma corporis diffusum Fabry 884
Bernsteinsäuredehydrogenase, Histochemie des Coriums und des subcutanen Fettgewebes 641
—, — der fetalen ekkrinen Drüsen 668
—, — — Epidermis 633
—, — der Haarkomplexentwicklung 659
—, — der Leichenhaut 721
—, — der apokrinen Schweißdrüsen 310, 316
—, Histotopochemie des Haarfollikels 176
Berliner Blau, Injektionsmethoden 497
Berliner Blau-Reaktion bei Hämochromatose 896
Beryllium, Fremdkörpergranulom der Haut 900
Best-Carmin-Reaktion, Darstellung des Glykogenvorkommens in der Haut 886
Bichatscher Fettkörper, Atrophie bei Lues und Encephalitis 829
Bindegewebe, Aggregationsweise der Bauteile 453
—, embryonales, Histochemie 641
—, Fasern, normale Histologie von Haut und Subcutis 439
—, Fermentaktivität 474
—, Grundsubstanz, Altersveränderung des Coriums 693
—, —, Fermentaktivität 474
—, —, Herkunft 451
—, —, normale Histologie von Haut und Subcutis 450
—, —, schematische Darstellung der Aggregation 877
—, —, Stoffwechsel 451
—, —, Ultrastruktur 451
— der Haut, spezifische Differenzierung 642
—, Histologie der Fasern 439
—, — der zelligen Bestandteile 430
—, Hyalinisierung 869
—, retikuläre Entstehung 455
—, Subcutis 475
— als Verschiebeschicht bei Reptilien 992
—, zellige Bestandteile, normale Histologie von Corium und Subcutis 430
Bindegewebsscheide, arteriovenöse Anastomosen 555

Bizzozerosche Knötchen, embryonale Nagelentwicklung 364
Blasenbildung, subepidermale, bei Porphyria cutanea tarda 894
Blauer Naevus, dermale Melanocytenansammlung 891
Blausäurevergiftung, Livores 711
Blauzellen, Aufbau der Federfarben bei Vögeln 1011
Blei, Nachweis im Pulverschmauch 766
Blitzverbrennungen bei Atomexplosionen 772
„blocking arteries" s. Anastomosen, arteriovenöse, der Haut 551
„blocking veins" s. Anastomosen, arteriovenöse, der Haut 551
Blutbildung s. Hämatopoese
Blutgefäßerkrankungen, Ätiologie der Necrobiosis lipoidica 837
Blutgefäße der fetalen Haut, Glykogengehalt 632
— — —, Phosphorylase-Aktivität 632
— der Haut 491
— —, der Haut, „permanent blood networks of mammals", vergleichende Anatomie 501
— —, Abnahme der Anzahl im Alter 790
— —, altersabhängige Degeneration 563
— —, Altersabhängigkeit der Gefäßwanddicke zum Gefäßdurchmesser, Meßwerte 701
— —, Altersveränderungen 685, 700
— —, biologische Modifikationen 558
— —, Degenerationsphänomene 563
— —, Elastica-Veränderungen im Alter 702
— —, Embryologie 499, 511, 514
— —, embryonale Entwicklung 639
— —, Funktion 492
— —, Gefäßwandverdickung im Alter 700
— —, Granulierung der Lamina elastica interna 563
— —, histochemische Methoden 496, 498
— —, histologische Methoden 496, 498

Blutgefäße der Haut, historische Betrachtungen 493
— —, hyaline Degeneration 563, 700
— —, Hyperplasie der Lamina elastica interna 563
— —, Injektionsmethoden 496, 497
— —, Innervation 564
— —, kapillaroskopische Methoden 495, 496
— —, Meßwerte des Lumens, Altersabhängigkeit 700
— —, neugebildete, Elektronenmikroskopie 562
— —, Histochemie 559
— — des Neugeborenen 515, 517
— —, neurocutanes Geflecht 564
— —, perinatale Entwicklung 499, 511, 514
— —, periodische Regeneration 558
— —, permanent blood networks of mammals, vergleichende Anatomie 501
— —, permanente Regeneration 558
— —, physikalische Methoden 496, 498
— —, Regeneration 492
— —, senile Kopfhaut 563
— —, sklerotische Alterationen 563
— —, technische Betrachtungen 495
— —, Veränderungen bei Mucinosen 880
— —, vergleichende Anatomie 499, 500
— —, Verlaufsrichtung im Alter 700
— des Nagels, Altersveränderung 699
— des Stratum laxum bei Reptilien 993
—, Veränderungen bei Lipogranulomatosis subcutanea hypertonica Gottron 799
Blutgerinnung, postmortale 717
Blutinseln 499
Blut, pH-Wert, postmortal 719
Blutzirkulation, avaskuläre, der Epidermis 491
„bobbin" 35
Branchiostoma lanceolatum, Haut und Zentralnervensystem 921, 924
Brandblasen 496
—, Differenzierung zwischen vitaler und postmortaler Entstehung 768, 769

Brandblasen an der Leichenhaut, Differenzierung an Fäulnisblasen 769
Branderythem, Verbrennungen der Leichenhaut 768
Brandleiche 771
Bromphenolblau-Färbung, Histochemie der fetalen ekkrinen Drüsen 668
Brustdrüse, Altersveränderungen 698
—, männliche, Altersveränderungen 698
—, weibliche, Altersinvolution 698
Brutflecke, besondere Vascu-lierung bei Vögeln 1001
Bürstenzellen, neutrale Muco-polysaccharide 465
Bulbus s. Haarzwiebel
Bulbusbildung, Haarcyclus 160
Bulbuszapfen, morphologische Entwicklung des Haarkomplexes 649
Bursae synoviales subcutaneae, Konstruktion der Subcutis 477
Butyrylcholinesterase, arterio-venöse Anastomosen, Histochemie 557
—, Histochemie, Talgdrüsen 204

Calamus der Feder bei Vögeln 1005
Calcinose, Patho-Histologie 887
Calcium, Histochemie der Keratinocyten 66
— -Nachweis im Fibrin, Fibrinoid und Hyalin 871
Calciumphosphat in der Amphibienhaut 981
Capillaren s. Kapillaren
Carboanhydrase, helle Zellen, Cytochemie 241
—, Histochemie der Keratinocyten 102
Carbonyl-Anhydrase, Histochemie der Keratinocyten 66
Carbonylgruppen-Reaktion nach Ashbel und Seligman, Reaktion von Fibrin, Fibrinoid und Hyalin 871
Carnivora, vergleichende Anatomie, Blutgefäße der Haut 507
Carotinämie durch Ernährung 898
Carotin, chemische Konstitution 897

Carotinoide, Ablagerung und Speicherung in der Haut 897
—, Blutspiegel, regulierende Faktoren 897
—, histologischer Nachweis 898
Carotinose, Prädilektionsstellen 898
—, Bedeutung der Schweißdrüsen 898
Casella-Reaktion, Darstellung des Glykogenvorkommens in der Haut 886
„cell boundary" s. Plasmamembran
„cellular elongation region" 147
Centriole, Langerhans-Zelle 117
Ceruminaldrüsen, Altersveränderungen 697
—, Embryologie 663
—, Embryonalentwicklung der apokrinen Schweißdrüsen 270
Cetacea, vergleichende Anatomie, Blutgefäße der Haut 508
Chalone, Mitoserate in der Epidermis 65
China-Tinte, Injektionsmethoden 497
Chiroptera, vergleichende Anatomie, Blutgefäße der Haut 503
1-(4-chloromercuriphenylazo)-naphthol-2-Reagens, Histochemie der Keratinocyten 70
Cholera, postmortale Hyperthermie 709
Cholesterinase, ekkrine Schweißdrüsen 262
Cholesterin, braunes Fett 457
—, Darstellung bei extracellulärer Cholesterinose Kerl-Urbach 885
—, Definition 881
Cholesterinester, Histochemie, Talgdrüsen 196
Cholesterin, freies, Histochemie, Talgdrüsen 200
—, Histochemie der apokrinen Schweißdrüsen 307
—, — der Keratinocyten 81
—, — der Talgdrüsen 200
Cholesterinkristalle, Histologie des Xanthoms 881
Cholesterinose, extracelluläre, Kerl-Urbach 881
— Kerl-Urbach, Patho-Histologie 885

Cholinesteraseaktivität, Beziehung zur Phosphorylaseaktivität in apokrinen Schweißdrüsen 312
Cholinesterasen, arteriovenöse Anastomosen, Histochemie 556
—, Basalzellen, Cytochemie 253
—, Histochemie des Coriums und des subcutanen Fettgewebes 641
—, — der embryonalen Nerven 676
—, — der fetalen Haut 631
—, — der Keratinocyten 92, 96
—, — des Nagels 366
—, — der Talgdrüsen 203
—, — der Kapillaren der Haut 537
—, Langerhans-Zelle 119
—, Nervenentwicklung in der Haut 674
—, spezifische, Arteriolen der Haut, Histochemie 527, 537
—, unspezifische, histochemischer Nachweis in apokrinen Schweißdrüsen 321
—, Venolen der Haut, Histochemie 537
Chondrichthyes, Bau der Haut 941
—, Haut der, vergleichende Histologie 941
Chondroitinsulfat B, Histochemie der Keratinocyten 79
Chondroitinsulfat, Bausteine der Grundsubstanz 875
—, Bindegewebsgrundsubstanz 450
— der Bindegewebsgrundsubstanz, Altersveränderung 452
—, Färbung des Amyloid 863
—, Funktion des Papillarkörpers 469
Chondrosulphatase, histochemischer Nachweis in apokrinen Schweißdrüsen 325
Chorda dorsalis, Querschnitt Embryo 625
Chordata, Corium 922
—, Epidermis 921
—, Feinstruktur des Integuments 921
—, Subcutis 922
Chrom, Darstellung der Struktur der Kollagenfibrille 442
Chromatinkörperchen in Fibrocyten 693

Chromatophoren, Definition 104
— bei Knochenfischen 964
— bei Neunaugen 932
Chromhidrosis, Pigmentgranula in apokrinen Schweißdrüsen 278
—, saure Phosphatase in apokrinen Schweißdrüsen 323
—, Zusammenhang mit ektopischen apokrinen Schweißdrüsen 273
Chrysiasis cutis, Klinik und Histologie 900
Chymotrypsin, Histochemie der Keratinocyten 101
Ciliardrüse, Wachsmodell, makroskopisches Aussehen der apokrinen Schweißdrüsen 274
Cilien, Ultrastruktur der ekkrinen Drüsen 665
Citrullin, Histotopographie im Haarfollikel 172
„clear cells" s. auch helle Zellen
—, Melanocyten-Darstellung 106
—, Transformation der Lymphocyten 62
Coccidioidomykose, Erythema nodosum 836
Cölom, Querschnitt Embryo 625
Coenzym A, Fettsäuresynthese 789
Coenzym Q s. Ubiquinon
CO-Hämoglobin, Bestimmung zur Feststellung eines Schwelbrandes 768
—, Nachweis im Gewebe nach absolutem Nahschuß 767
—, Nachweis bei Schußverletzungen 765
Colcemid, Einfluß auf Mitoserate 64
Colloidmilium, Pseudomilium colloidale Pellizari 872
Colloidome miliaire, Pseudomilium colloidale Pellizari 872
Condyloma, Melaningranula 112, 113
Conjunctiva, postmortale Vertrocknung 725
Conjunctivom mit hyaliner Degeneration, Pseudomilium colloidale Pellizari 872
Contact burns 772
Corium, Altersveränderung 691
—, Bindegewebsfasern, Altersveränderung, Histologie 694

Corium, corio-epidermale Verknüpfung 2
—, Dicke, Altersabhängigkeit 691
—, —, Altersveränderung, Meßwerte verschiedener Körperregionen 692
—, — beim Fetus und beim Neugeborenen 639
—, Elastizitätsunterschiede 472, 473
—, Embryologie der Haut 625
—, embryonale Entwicklung 636
— -Epidermis-Interface, Histologie der normalen Haut 4
—, Fermentaktivität 474
—, fetales, Glykogengehalt 632
—, —, Phosphorylase-Aktivität 632
—, Gefäßeinbau 478
—, glatte Muskulatur 479
—, Hämatopoese im Embryonalleben 637
—, Histochemie 474
—, intrafibrilläre Kittsubstanz, Altersveränderung 693
—, Maceration 465
—, mikroskopische und submikroskopische Anatomie 461, 471
—, Musculi cutis diagonales 481
—, normale Histologie 430
—, pathologische Kalkablagerungen 887
—, Stratum papillare 465
—, Stratum reticulare 470
—, Veränderungen durch elektrischen Strom 777
—, Vorkommen von Mucopolysacchariden im Nagel 363
—, Wassergehalt 733
—, Zahl der Mastzellen 438
—, Zug und Reißfestigkeit 472
Cornea-Epithel, Keratohyalinbildung 56
„cortical preceratinization region" 147
Cortison, Abhängigkeit der Epidermisdifferenzierung bei Vögeln 998
—, Hypertrophie des braunen Fettgewebes 829
Corynebacterium acues, Talgfollikel 192
Cosmoidschuppen bei Knochenfischen 962

Craniota, Haut der, vergleichende Histologie 927
Cristae intermediae, Embryonalentwicklung ekkriner Drüsen 663
„Cristae limitantes", Nervenentwicklung in der Haut 674
Cruor, Livores 711
Ctenoidschuppen bei Knochenfischen 962
Cupula, Aufbau der Sinnesknospen bei Tieren 953, 955
— bei Knochenfischen 969
Cuticula, Haarkomplexentwicklung 655
—, Morphologie der apokrinen Schweißdrüsen 275
—, Struktur der inneren Wurzelscheide 150
Cuticulazellen, Elektronenmikroskopie des Haarfollikels 155
„cuticular border", epidermaler Schweißdrüsen-Ausführungsgang 258
—, Oberflächenzellen 254, 256
Cutis s. auch Haut
—, Amyloidablagerungen 867
—, Embryologie der Haut 625
—, epidermale Verknüpfung 2
— -Melanoblasten, Terminologie 891
—, Metachromasie in der Strangfurche 759
—, Verschieblichkeit 478
—, Verschmälerung in der Strangfurche 759
Cyanose, Differentialdiagnose Livores 714
Cyan-Wasserstoff, postmortale percutane Resorption 779
Cycloidschuppen bei Knochenfischen 962
Cystein, Biochemie der Keratinisation 73
— -Desulfhydrase, Histochemie der Keratinocyten 103
Cystin, Biochemie der Keratinisation 73
—, direkter Einbau in keratogene Zonen des Haarfollikels 175, 177
—, Gehalt in Epidermis, Haar und Nagel 74
Cytidin-H³, Autoradiographie in Keratinocyten 70
cytochrine Sekretion, Melaningranula 113

Cytochromoxydase, Arteriolen der Haut, Histochemie 526, 537
—, Basalzellen, Cytochemie 253
—, Cytochemie, myoepitheliale Zellen 235
—, dunkle Zellen, Cytochemie 248
—, helle Zellen, Cytochemie 241
—, Histochemie des Coriums und des subcutanen Fettgewebes 641
—, — der Haarkomplexentwicklung 659
—, — der fetalen ekkrinen Drüsen 668
—, — — Epidermis 633
—, — der Keratinocyten 85
—, — der Leichenhaut 721
—, — der Talgdrüsen 196, 202
—, histochemischer Nachweis in apokrinen Schweißdrüsen 310, 318
—, — in Fibrocyten von Corium und Subcutis 431
—, Histotopochemie des Haarfollikels 176
—, Histotopografie der Keratinocyten 78
—, Kapillaren der Haut, Histochemie 537
—, Oberflächenzellen, Cytochemie 256
—, Venolen der Haut, Histochemie 537
Cytopempsis, Fettverdauung 461
—, Innervation der Haut 419
Cytosiderose der Bantu-Neger, Hämochromatosesyndrom 895
Cytosome, Elektronenmikroskopie der Mucinosis follicularis 880

Daktyloskopie, Identitätsfeststellung bei Fäulnisleichen 751
—, — in der späten Leichenzeit 751
Deckplatte bei Amphibien 971
—, Neunaugen, vergleichende Histologie 927, 931
„D-cells", Mitose der Keratinocyten 66
Dedifferenzierungsphase, Haarcyclus 158
„deep network", verg leichnde Anatomie, Blutgefäßeeder Haut 501, 511

„Dégénérescence colloid du derme", Pseudomilium colloidale Pellizari 872
Dehydrogenasen, Histochemie der fetalen Epidermis 633
Dehydroliponsäure-Dehydrogenase, Arteriolen der Haut, Histochemie 526, 537
—, Kapillaren der Haut, Histochemie 537
—, Venolen der Haut, Histochemie 537
Denaturierung des Kollagens bei Knochenfischen 961
Dendriten der Langerhans-Zelle, Morphologie 117
— der Melanocyten, Funktion 114
Dendritenzellen, Darstellung, Verteilung und Häufigkeit 106
— der Haut, Melanocyten-Kontakt, Innervation der Haut 387
—, Melanocyten 891
—, normale Histologie der Haut 103
—, pigmentierte 106
—, Terminologie 104
—, Verwandtschaft oder Identität mit Keratinocyten 104
—, weiße 106
„dense melanosomes", Elektronenmikroskopie der Melanocyten 115
Dentin bei Selachiern 945
Depotfett 458, 459, 478
—, Anatomie des Fettgewebes 789
Depressoren in der Vogelhaut 1003
dermal autofluorescent cells, Histiocyten-ähnliche Zellen 436
„Dermalmembran", Nomenklatur Basalmembran 462
„dermal (subpapillary) network", vergleichende Anatomie, Blutgefäße der Haut 501, 506, 507, 508, 510
Dermatitis lichenoides purpurica pigmentosa Gougerot, sekundäre Hämosiderose der Haut 897
Dermatitis solaris subita recidivans, Fluorescenzmikroskopie 893
Dermatofibroma protuberans, Glykogenvorkommen in Endothelzellen und in der glatten Muskulatur 886
Dermatoglyphen 224

Dermatom, Embryologie der Haut 673
—, Mesodermentwicklung 637
—, Querschnitt Embryo 625
— bei Reptilien 996
—, trapezförmige, bei Vögeln 1004
Dermatomyositis, Fettgewebsatrophie der Haut 793
Dermatosis pigmentaria progressiva Schamberg, sekundäre Hämosiderose der Haut 897
Dermatrophia chronica idiopathica maculosa, Fettgewebsatrophie der Haut 793
Dermis, Embryologie der Haut 625
Desmosomen bei Amphibien 973, 979
— bei Amphibienlarven 973
—, „attachment plaque" 32, 33
—, Berührung mit epidermalen Fasern 40
—, „composite" 31
—, Elektronenmikroskopie der Basalmembran 4
—, epidermale Nerven 381
—, Froschhaut 31
—, junctionale, Keratinocyten 35
—, Keratinocyten 19, 31
—, —, Beziehung zu Fibrillen 36
—, „modified" 31
—, Morphologie der Keratinocyten 31
—, „regular" 31, 32
—, -SH-Gruppen und -S-S-Gruppen in Keratinocyten 74
—, „simple", Morphologie der Keratinocyten, Ultrastruktur 31, 34
—, Stratum spinosum 10
— -Tonofilamentkomplex der fetalen Epidermis, Schema 630
—, Ultrastruktur der ekkrinen Drüsen 665
— —, Epidermis der fetalen 628, 631
Desoxyribonuclease s. DNase
Desoxyribonucleinsäure s. DNS
Desulfhydrase, Histochemie der Keratinocyten 103
Diabetes mellitus, Ätiologie der Necrobiosis lipoidica 837
— —, Carotinämie 898
— —, Hämochromatose 895

Diabetes mellitus, Kombination mit Pfeifer-Weber-Christian-Syndrom und Pankreasschäden 836
—, Lipogenese in der Haut 528
—, neurotrophische Atrophie der Haut 792
Diaphorase, Nomenklatur 89
Diastase-resistente Polysaccharide, Histochemie der Keratinocyten 79
Diastase, Stratum corneum 15
—, Wirkung auf Basalmembran 463
Dichophase, Mitose der Keratinocyten 65
Diffusionstotenflecke, Druckanämie der Leichenhaut 756
—, Veränderungen der späten Leichenzeit 732
Digitonin, Histochemie, Talgdrüsen 200
Dihydroliponsäure-Dehydrogenase, histochemischer Nachweis in apokrinen Schweißdrüsen 310, 321
2,2′-dihydroxy-6,6′-dinaphthyl-disulfid-Reagens, Histochemie der Keratinocyten 70
Dimethylaminobenzaldehyd-Methode, Kapillaren der Haut 536
Diphosphopyridinnucleotid-Diaphorase, Blutgefäßneubildung der Haut, Histochemie 559
Disulfid-Gruppen s. -S-S-Gruppen
DNA s. DNS
DNase, Histochemie der Keratinocyten 100
—, Pinocytose-Mechanismus der Histiocyten 435
DNS, Abbau, Autolyse der Leichenhaut 721
—, Histochemie der Keratinocyten 68
—, — der Wundheilung 754
—, Histotopographie im Haarfollikel 174
—, Kapillaren der Haut, Histochemie 537
—, -Synthese, Autoradiographie Epidermis 63
—, Chalone-Wirkung 65
—, „mitosis operon" 65
—, Venolen der Haut, Histochemie 537
Dopachinon, Melaninstoffwechsel 890

Dopachrom, Melaninstoffwechsel 890
Dopa, Melaninsynthese 890
Dopa-oxydase-Reaktion, Vergleich der Lokalisation mit ATPase-Aktivität in Melanocyten 116
—, Melaninstoffwechsel 890
—, Melaninsynthese 890
Dopa-Reaktion, Darstellung der Melanocyten 114
— der Dendritenzellen und Keratinocyten 106
—, embryonale Entwicklung der Melanocyten 676
—, Färbung der weißen Dendritenzellen 106
„droplet secretions", Sekretionsmodus apokriner Schweißdrüsen 327
Druckanämie der Leichenhaut 755
Druckatrophie der Haut, Blutgefäßveränderungen 792
— —, Pathologie 781
Druckkammern, Subcutis 475
Drüsen, apokrine, Verwandtschaft mit ekkrinen Drüsen 664
—, ekkrine, Ausführungsgang 664
—, —, —, Histochemie 556
—, —, Basalmembran 664
—, —, Durchmesser des Ausführungsganges 669
—, —, Embryologie 663
—, —, embryonaler Ausführungsgang, Elektronenmikroskopie 667
—, —, Histochemie der Embryonalentwicklung 665
—, —, Histologie verschiedener Entwicklungsstadien 664
—, —, Maße der Zellkerngröße 669
—, —, Ultrastruktur 665
—, —, Verwandtschaft mit apokrinen Drüsen 664
—, —, Volumen in verschiedenen Stadien des Embryonallebens 668, 669
Drüsenleisten, epidermale, Embryonalentwicklung ekkriner Drüsen 663
—, Nervenentwicklung in der Haut 674
—, Ultrastruktur der ekkrinen Drüsen 665
Drüsenzellen, Aldolaseaktivität 310, 313
—, apokrine, atypische, Ultrastruktur der apokrinen Schweißdrüsen 300

Drüsenzellen, apokrine, Schweißdrüsen, Histochemie, PAS-reaktive Granula 308
—, —, Ultrastruktur 287
—, —, —, intercellulare Canaliculi 301
—, ekkrine, Vakuolisierung im Alter 696
—, Glycerinaldehyd-3-Phosphat-Dehydrogenase-Nachweis 310, 313
—, Histochemie der apokrinen Schweißdrüsen, Eisengehalt 309
— bei Knochenfischen 958
—, Morphologie der apokrinen Schweißdrüsen 275
—, Phosphorylaseaktivität 310, 312
—, seröse, bei Selachiern 942
—, Stofftransport durch myoepitheliale Zellen 482
—, Zellmembran 287
Duftdrüsen bei adulten Amphibien 983
—, myoepitheliale Zellen 482
Duftorgane, Lokalisation apokriner Schweißdrüsen 271
Durodentin bei Selachiern 946
Dyskeratose, Keratohyalin 43
Dyslipoidose, Pathologie des subcutanen Fettgewebes 795
Dysproteinämie bei Pseudomilium colloidale Pellizari 873

Eberthsche Figuren bei Amphibienlarven 971
Ehrlichsche Mastzellen, normale Histologie 436
Eimersches Organ, Innervation der Epidermis 383
Einschußwunde, Basophilie 765
Eisen, Ablagerung in der Haut 895
—, apokrine Schweißdrüsen, Beziehung zu Achselgeruch 311
—, Histochemie der apokrinen Schweißdrüsen 309
—, — der Talgdrüsen 196, 201
—, — der Keratinocyten 66
— in den Sekretzellen apokriner Schweißdrüsen, Altersveränderungen der Haut 697
—, Nachweis im Pulverschmauch 766
—, tägliche Aufnahme und Resorption 895
—, — Ausscheidung 895

Eisenhämatoxylin, Darstellung von Myofibrillen 482
Eisenpartikel, Ultrastruktur der apokrinen Schweißdrüsen 295
Eisen-Reaktion, kolloidale, Arteriolen der Haut 525
Eisentherapie, Hämochromatosesyndrom 895
Eisenthesaurismose, Terminologie 895
Ektoderm, Anusentwicklung 635
—, Darstellung der Mehrschichtigkeit durch Gewebekultur 627
—, Embryologie der Haut 624
—, Entwicklungsmechanik, Selbststeuerung 641
—, Haarentwicklung 644
—, primäres, Embryologie der Haut 624
—, sekundäres, Embryologie der Haut 624
—, symmetrische Verdickungen, topographische Unterschiede der embryonalen Epidermis 634
Elastase, Bindegewebsgrundsubstanz 450
—, Corium 474
—, Darstellung der Fibrillen der elastischen Fasern 449, 450
—, experimentelle Fettzellnekrose 451
—, Stoffwechsel des Bindegewebes 452
Elastica-Färbung, Darstellung kollagener Fasern 448
—, Gefäßdarstellung in Corium und Subcutis 478
—, Kalkablagerungen in der Haut 887
Elastica-Farbstoff, Darstellung elastischer Sehnen 479
Elastica interna, arteriovenöse Anastomosen 554
Elastin, Basalmembran, Histochemie 539
—, Degeneration bei Pseudomilium colloidale Pellizari 872
—, Elastase 450
—, Entstehung elastischer Fasern 447
—, Histochemie des Nagels 371
—, Nachweis bei aktinischer Elastose 873
—, Struktur der elastischen Faser 448
Elastinfibrille, Ultrastruktur der elastischen Faser 449
Elastoblast, Entstehung der elastischen Faser 447

Elastophilie, Argyrose 899
Elastose, aktinische 693
—, —, Pseudomilium colloidale Pellizari 873
—, senile, Porphyria cutanea tarda 894
—, Altersveränderung des Nagels 699
—, senile 693
Elastosis colloidalis conglomerata, Pseudomilium colloidale Pellizari 872
Elastosis senilis, aktinische Elastose 873
Eleidin, Glykogen 77
Elektrounfälle, Veränderung der Leichenhaut 774
Elementarfibrille s. Mikrofibrille
Elementargranula, Innervation der Epidermis 382
Embryologie, Blutgefäße der Haut 499, 511, 514
—, Entwicklungsbewegung 642
—, Formentwicklung 642
— der Haut 624
—, Lageentwicklung 642
—, Strukturentwicklung 642
—, Entwicklung der apokrinen Schweißdrüsen 268
Embryonalschild, Embryologie der Epidermis 626
Encephalitis, Fettgewebsatrophie 829
Endangitis obliterans, Morphologische Befunde der Autolyse der Haut 720
Endangiosis fibroblastica, Pathologie der gefäßbedingten Entzündungen des Fettgewebes 795
Endarteriitis obliterans bei Erythema induratum Bazin 798
— —, Patho-Histologie des subcutanen Fettgewebes 795
Endarteriitis productiva fibrosa, Ätiologie der Necrobiosis lipoidica 837
— — —, Patho-Histologie der Necrobiosis lipoidica 815
Endkolben, Hautinnervation bei Reptilien 996
β-endo-N-acetylhexosaminidase bei Amphibienlarven 986
Endophlebitis obliterans bei Erythema nodosum adiponecroticans 797
— — bei Erythema induratum Bazin 798
— —, Patho-Histologie des subcutanen Fettgewebes 795

Endothelien, arteriovenöse Anastomosen 554
—, Kapillaren der Haut 534, 539
Endothelzellen, argyrophile Faserbildung 443
Endopeptidasen, Histochemie der Keratinocyten 101
Endoplasmatisches Reticulum, Nomenklatur 58
Endovasculitis obliterans bei Erythema nodosum chronicum perilobulare 797
Entoderm, Anusentwicklung 635
Entwicklungsbewegung, Entwicklungsmechanik 642
Entzündung, forensische Pathologie 754
—, Schema des zeitlichen Ablaufes der morphologischen und histochemischen Veränderungen 754
Enzymaktivitäten, maximale, Arteriolen der Haut 527
Enzyme, helle Zellen, Cytochemie 241
—, hydrolytische, dunkle Zellen 248
—, mucolytische, Regulierung der Mucopolysaccharidmenge der Haut 877
—, proteolytische, Dekomposition der Haut in der späten Leichenzeit 733
—, —, Histochemie der Intermediärzone der Epidermis 18
—, —, — der Keratinocyten 101
—, —, — der Leichenhaut 721
„epidermal eccrine sweat duct unit" 664
epidermaler Schweißdrüsen-Ausführungsgang, Cytochemie 260
— —, Elektronenmikroskopie 258
— —, Embryonalhaut 260
— —, Hautoberfläche 258
„epidermal-Langerhans-cell-unit" 117
„epidermal sweat duct unit" s. epidermaler Schweißdrüsen-Ausführungsgang 258
Epidermicula, Struktur des Haarfollikels 149
Epidermin, Faserproteinstruktur 50
Epidermis, Altersveränderung 686
—, amitotische Zellteilung 62

Epidermis, Basalmembran 462
—, Basophilie durch Ribosomen 58
—, corio-epidermale Verknüpfung 2
—, Cytochromoxydaseaktivität 85
—, „dermo-epidermal interface" 4
—, Dicke 8
—, —, Altersveränderung, Meßwerte in verschiedenen Regionen 687
—, — bei Feten 636
—, — bei Neugeborenen 636
—, — an der unbedeckten Haut 685
—, Druckatrophie bei Amyloidablagerungen 867
—, Elektronenmikroskopie 9
—, Embryologie 625
—, —, regionäre Unterschiede 626
—, embryologische Determinierung 642
—, embryonale, Melanocytenanordnung 676
—, fetale, Histochemie 631
—, —, Ultrastruktur 628
—, —, Verhornung durch Gewebekultur 627
—, Frühentwicklung 625
—, Grad der Differenzierung 20
—, Histochemie 556
—, Histologie der normalen Haut 1
—, intercellulärer Spalt der Keratinocyten 23
—, Kohlenhydratstoffwechsel 76
—, Mitose-Index 62
—, Mitosezahlen 690
— des Neugeborenen 636
—, —, Mitoserate 636
—, nichtpigmentierte, Dendritenzellen 106
—, nichtverhornte, Plasmamembran der Keratinocyten 21
—, normale Histologie des Haut 8
—, pathologische Kalkablagerungen 887
—, Penetration von Gasen 778
—, Phasen der embryonalen Entwicklung 626
—, Pigmentierung, Altersabhängigkeit 691
—, postmortale Vertrocknung nach vitaler Verletzung 727
—, Regeneration 8
—, Regenerationsfähigkeit 690

Epidermis, Regenerationszeit 61
—, Schwefelgehalt 73
—, spezifische 642
—, unverhornte, Begriffsbestimmung 17
—, —, intercellulärer Spalt 24
—, Veränderungen durch elektrischen Strom 777
—, verhornte, Begriffsbestimmung 17
—, Verhornung 11
—, Verschmälerung, Altersveränderung 686
Epidermiszellen, Bildung der Basalmembran 463
—, Zellgrenze 20, 628
Epinephrin s. Adrenalin
Epithel der Haut, Embryologie, topographische Unterschiede 633
Epithelhörnchen der embryonalen Eichel, Embryologie der Epidermis 634
Epitheliale Verwachsungen, Trennung von 635
Epithelien, Modulationsfähigkeit 642
Epithelkeim, primärer, Haarentwicklung 644
Epithelmuskelzellen, Muskulatur der Haut 482
Epitheloidzellen, Fremdkörpergranulom 901
Epithel, Phosphorylase 474
Epithelpfröpfe, Embryologie der Epidermis 634
Eponychium, Anatomie des Nagels 342
—, fetale Haut, Glykogengehalt 632
—, —, Phosphorylase-Aktivität 632
—, Histologie 352
—, mikroskopische Untersuchung des embryonalen Nagels 346
Erektion der Mamille, Mechanismus 479, 480
Ergastoplasma, Ultrastruktur der apokrinen Schweißdrüsen 300
Erythema elevatum et diutinum, extracellulare Cholesterinose Kerl-Urbach 885
Erythema induratum Bazin, Ätiologie und Pathogenese 836
— —, Patho-Histologie 798
— — —, des subcutanen Fettgewebes 795
Erythema induratum, Disposition 837

Erythema induratum nodosum Patho-Histologie 799
Erythema nodosum adiponecroticans, Patho-Histologie 796
Erythema nodosum, Ätiologie und Pathogenese 836
— — nach Applikation von Jodkalium, Patho-Histologie 798
Erythema nodosum chronicum perilobulare, Patho-Histologie 796
Erythema nodosum lipogranulomatosum, Patho-Histologie 796
Erythema nodosum, medikamentöses 836
— —, Patho-Histologie des subcutanen Fettgewebes 795
— —, Realisationsfaktor 836
— — trichophyticum, Patho-Histologie 798
— — bei Tumormetastasen im subcutanen Fettgewebe 826
Erythrocyanose, Disposition zu Erythema induratum 837
Erythrocytenagglutination 534
Erythrophoren bei Knochenfischen 964
— der Reptilienhaut 991
— bei Selachiern 948
Esterase-Aktivität in Fettgewebsgranulomen 834
Esterasen, dunkle Zellen, Cytochemie 248
—, epidermaler Schweißdrüsen-Ausführungsgang 260
— in der Epidermis der Vogelhaut 998
—, Exoenzyme der Epidermis 93
— in Fettzellen 456
—, helle Zellen, Cytochemie 242
—, Haarbalg 474
—, Histochemie der apokrinen Schweißdrüsen 321
—, — des Coriums und des subcutanen Fettgewebes 641
—, — der fetalen ekkrinen Drüsen 668
—, — — Haut 633
—, — der Gewebsmastzellen 437
—, — der Intermediärzone der Epidermis 18
—, — der Keratinocyten 92
—, intercellulärer Spalt Stratum corneum 23
—, Nachweis in Fibrocyten von Corium und Subcutis 431

Esterasen, Oberflächenzellen, Cytochemie 256
—, Pinocytose-Mechanismus der Histiocyten 435
—, spezifische, Histochemie der Keratinocyten 92
—, unspezifische, Arteriolen der Haut, Histochemie 526
—, —, Histochemie der Haarkomplexentwicklung 659
—, —, — der Keratinocyten 92
—, —, — der Leichenhaut 721
—, —, — der Talgdrüsen 196, 202
—, —, — der Wundheilung 754
—, —, Histotopochemie des Haarfollikels 176
—, —, Kapillaren der Haut, Histochemie 538
—, —, in Langerhans-Zellen 119
—, —, Venolen der Haut, Histochemie 537, 550
—, weiche Hornschicht bei Reptilien 989
Excoriationen der Leichenhaut 755
—, Strangmarke 758
Exocytose, Sekretionsmodus der apokrinen Schweißdrüsen 326
Exoenzyme, Indoxylacetat-Esterase der Epidermis 95
Exopeptidasen, Histochemie der Keratinocyten 101
Exoplasmatheorie, Fibrillogenese 440
Expulsionsphase, Haarcyclus 158
Exsudat, entzündliches, Argyrophilie elastischer Fasern 445, 448
„external compound membrane", Keratinocyten, Ultrastruktur 34
Extremitätenhaut, Anatomie des Gefäßnetzes 570, 571, 578
Extremitätenknospen, Mesodermentwicklung 637

Fadenfedern bei Vögeln 1006
Fadenzellen bei Schleimaalen 938
Fäulnisblasen der Haut 731
Fäulnisemphysem der Haut, Veränderungen der späten Leichenzeit 732
Farben der Vogelfedern 1009
Farbwechsel, physiologischer, bei Amphibienlarven 977

Farbwechsel, physiologischer, bei Knochenfischen 965
—, —, bei Reptilien 991
—, —, bei Selachiern 946
Farbzellen bei adulten Amphibien 982
— bei Amphibienlarven 977
—, hormonale Beeinflussung der, bei Knochenfischen 965
— bei Knochenfischen 964
—, nervöse Beeinflussung der, bei Knochenfischen 965
— bei Reptilien 991
Fascia cruris, Gefäßeinbau 478
Fasern, argyrophile, Altersveränderung des Coriums 693
—, —, Basalmembran 462, 463, 464, 465
—, —, Darstellung 444
—, —, Elektronenmikroskopie 444
—, —, Faserentwicklung 443
—, —, Fremdkörpergranulom 901
—, —, der Haut, Embryologie 638
—, —, mechanische Eigenschaften 444
—, —, Mesodermentwicklung 637
—, —, myoepitheliale Zellen 482
—, —, normale Histologie von Corium und Subcutis 443
—, —, Stratum papillare 467
—, —, Subcutis 475
—, —, univacuoläre Fettzellen 456
—, Corium- und Fettgewebsentwicklung 638
—, Definition epidermaler Fibrillen 37
—, dermale, Basalmembran 3
—, elastische, Altersveränderung, PAS-Reaktion 693
—, —, bei Amyloidablagerung in der Haut 868
—, —, Argyrophilie 445
—, —, chemische Analyse 447, 448
—, —, Darstellung 448
—, —, Degeneration bei Pseudomilium colloidale Pellizari 872
—, —, degenerative Veränderung und Kalkablagerung 887
—, —, Elektronenmikroskopie 449
—, —, Embryologie 638
—, —, Entstehung 447
—, —, Fixierungsmethode 448

Fasern, elastische, Histochemie 449
—, —, Mesodermentwicklung 637
—, —, Musculus arrector pili, Haarkomplexentwicklung 656
—, —, Neubildung bei pathologischen Kalkablagerungen im Gewebe 888
—, —, normale Histologie von Corium und Subcutis 447
—, —, Papillarkörperatrophie 469
—, —, Silberimprägnierung bei der Argyrose 899
—, —, Stratum papillare 467
—, —, Stratum reticulare 471
—, —, Subcutis 474, 475
—, —, Textur 454
—, —, Veränderung bei Mucinosen 879
—, —, Verlauf in der Haut der Fingerbeere 468
—, epidermale, Anordnung 38
—, —, Berührung mit Desmosomen 39
—, —, Dichte 38
—, —, Durchmesser 38
—, —, Ultrastruktur 33
— der fetalen Haut, Glykogengehalt 632
— — —, Phosphorylase-Aktivität 632
—, interfilamentöse Substanzen 42
—, kollagene, Altersdegeneration 447
—, —, Altersveränderung des Coriums 693
—, —, an der Haut 685
—, —, bei Amyloidablagerung in der Haut 868
—, —, Basalmembran 3, 462, 463, 464
—, —, Degeneration, Papillarkörper 469
—, —, Elektronenmikroskopie der Basalmembran 4
—, —, Entstehung im Corium 473
—, —, aus Fibrillen 443
—, —, Fermentaktivität 474
—, —, des Fettgewebes, Veränderung bei neurotrophischer Atrophie 792
—, —, der Haut, negative Doppelbrechung durch Einwirkung von elektrischem Strom 778
—, —, Mesodermentwicklung 637
—, —, normale Histologie von Corium und Subcutis 445

Fasern, kollagene, Stratum papillare 467, 468, 469
—, —, Stratum reticulare 470
—, —, Subcutis 474, 475, 476
—, —, Textur 454
—, —, univacuoläre Fettzellen 456
—, —, Zugfestigkeit 447
—, —, Zug- und Reißfestigkeit des Coriums 472
— der Langerhans-Zelle, Elektronenmikroskopie 117
—, Melanocyten, Elektronenmikroskopie 108, 109
—, präkollagene, normale Histologie von Corium und Subcutis 443
Faserreticulum, arteriovenöse Anastomosen 554
Federbälge der Vogehaut 1001
Federfluren bei Vögeln 998
Federn, Hautderivat der Vögel 1005
—, Morphologie bei Vögeln 1005
— bei Vögeln 997
Federraine bei Vögeln 998
Federstrukturen, genetische Faktoren der, bei Vögeln 1009
Federwachstum der Vögel 1006
— —, Mutanten 1009
Ferntastsinn bei Chondrichthyes 951
Ferri-Ferricyanidreaktion, Melanindarstellung 890
Ferritin, Hämochromatose 896
—, Ultrastruktur der apokrinen Schweißdrüsen 295
Fersenpolster, Konstruktion der Druckpolster der Subcutis 475
Fett, Biosynthese im Fettgewebe 789
—, braunes 456
Fettcystenbildung bei Spontanpanniculitis Typ Rothmann-Makai 802
Fettentspeicherung 460
Fettgewebe, Allergisierung 840
—, allgemeine Pathologie 787
—, Altersatrophie 478
—, Anatomie 788
—, autoradiographische Untersuchungen 829
—, Bindegewebsfasern 788
—, Blutdurchströmung 788
—, braunes, Funktion 819
—, Stoffwechselbeeinflussung durch periphere Nerven 819, 829

Fettgewebe, braunes, Untersuchungen beim Früh- und Neugeborenen 640
—, Corium 468
—, embryonale Entwicklung 636
—, experimentelle Pathologie 826
—, Fettorgan 458
—, Fettsäuremuster bei Säuglingen und bei Erwachsenen 834
—, Glykolyse 789
—, Hämatopoese 788
— der Haut, Altersveränderungen 703
—, Mechanismus der Reaktionsprozesse 839
—, normale Histologie von Corium und Subcutis 455
—, plurivacuoläres 456
—, prospektive Potenz 819
—, Regeneration, experimentelle Pathologie 827
—, Respirationsmessungen normaler und pathologischer Zellen 827
—, Speicherung und Entspeicherung 459
—, subcutanes, Altersveränderungen 703
—, —, bindegewebige Sklerosierung bei Hautatrophie 795
—, —, Embryonalentwicklung 640
—, —, funktionelle Bedeutung 458
—, —, gefäßbedingte Erkrankungen, Patho-Histologie 808
—, —, Tumoren 818
—, Subcutis 474
—, Wasserretention 459
Fettgewebserkrankungen, Ätiologie und Pathogenese 832
Fettgewebsgranulom, Bildung durch hohen Gehalt an gesättigten Fettsäuren in der Nahrung 830
— nach Diathermie oder Starkstrom, Ätiologie und Pathogenese 833
—, spontan auftretendes, Patho-Histologie 803
Fettgewebsnekrosen, Ätiologie und Pathogenese 832
— der Brustdrüse, Patho-Histologie 803
—, spontan auftretende, Patho-Histologie 803
—, traumatogene, Patho-Histologie 803

Fettgewebstumoren, Ätiologie und Pathogenese 819, 838
Fettläppchen, Fettorgane in der Subcutis 475
Fettorgan, Fettgewebe 458
—, normale Histologie von Corium und Subcutis 455
— in der Subcutis 475
Fettphanerose, postmortale 745
Fettsäure-Ester, Arteriolen der Haut, Histochemie 526, 537
—, Kapillaren der Haut, Histochemie 537
—, Talg 196
—, Venolen der Haut, Histochemie 537
Fettsäuremobilisierung, Einfluß von Hormonen, experimentelle Pathologie 827
Fettsäuren, Arteriolen der Haut, Histochemie 526, 537
—, Fischlers Reagens 81, 82, 83
—, freie, Bestimmung im Serum bei normalen und adipösen Personen 828
—, —, Talg 197, 199, 203
—, Histochemie der apokrinen Schweißdrüsen 307
—, — der Kapillaren der Haut 537
—, — der Keratinocyten 83
— im Serum bei Adiponecrosis subcutanea neonatorum 833
—, Venolen der Haut, Histochemie 537
Fettsäuresynthese 789
Fettsclerem, Patho-Histologie der Adiponecrosis subcutanea neonatorum 806
Fettspeicherung 457, 460, 478
—, Stoffwechsel der Bindegewebsgrundsubstanz 452
Fettstarre, Haut der frühen Leichenzeit 724
Fettstoffwechsel, Einfluß der Temperatur 828
—, — des vegetativen Nervensystems 828
Fettstoffwechselhormon, experimentelle Pathologie des Fettgewebes 826
Fettsynthese 460
Fetttröpfchen, Elektronenmikroskopie, Talgdrüsen 213, 216
—, Histochemie der Keratinocyten 83
—, Morphologie der Keratinocyten 58

Fettvakuolen, Elektronenmikroskopie, Talgdrüsen 209
Fettverdauung, Cytopempsis 461
—, Fettspeicherung 461
—, Pinocytose 461
Fett, weißes, chemische Analyse 456, 457
—, —, Leichenhaut 724
—, —, Unterscheidung von braunem Fett 456
Fettzellen, Abstammung von Fibroblasten 827
—, Amyloidringe 868
—, argyrophile Faserbildung 443
—, einfache seröse Atrophie 791
—, elektronenmikroskopisches Bild der Speicherung 457
—, experimentelle mechanische Belastung 829
—, — Untersuchungen zur Differenzierung 827
—, fetale Haut, Glykogengehalt 632
—, —, Phosphorylase-Aktivität 632
—, Fettstoffwechsel der univacuolären Fettzelle 460
—, Größe der 828
—, normale Histologie von Corium und Subcutis 439
—, Pluripotenz 789
—, plurivacuoläre 455
—, Schwund bei Lipodystrophie 792
—, seröse 461
—, Subcutis 474, 475
—, Turgorverlust bei neurotrophischer Atrophie der Haut 792
—, — bei Werner-Syndrom 793
—, univacuoläre 455
—, Wucheratrophie 791
Fettzellschwund bei Atrophia cutis senilis 790
Feulgen-Reaktion, Arteriolen der Haut 526
—, Färbung von Hyalin 869
—, Feststellung eines Vitalschadens der Haut 768
„fibre", Definition 37
Fibrillen, Definition 37
—, Dicke im Corium 693
—, Elektronenmikroskopie 52, 53
—, — der Basalmembran 3
—, — des Haarfollikels 155
—, — des Stratum corneum 16
—, epidermale, Anastomosen 38

Fibrillen, epidermale, Anordnung 38
—, —, Desorganisation 40
—, —, Dichte 38
—, —, Elektronenmikroskopie 9, 51
—, —, Entwicklung zu Keratinfibrillen 42
—, —, Keratocyten 19
—, —, Morphologie der Keratinocyten 36
— in Hornzellen 17
— im Hyalin, Darstellung 869
—, Intercellularbrücken der Keratinocyten 20
— der Keratinocyten, Beziehung zu Desmosomen 40
—, „keratin-pattern" 51
—, kollagene, Aufbau 442
—, —, Bildung der 440
—, —, Bildungsmechanismus 440
—, —, embryonale Entwicklung der Basalmembran 639
—, — Faser 446
—, —, Fibroblasten von Corium und Subcutis 432
—, —, Unterschied zur Amyloidfibrille 865
—, -SH-Gruppen und -S-S-Gruppen in Keratinocyten 74
—, „speckled pattern" 42, 43
—, Ultrastruktur der T-Zellen 12
— der unbedeckten Haut, Altersveränderung, Elektronenmikroskopie 693
Fibrillogenese, Exoplasmatheorie 440
—, extracelluläre Genese 440
—, intracelluläre Genese 440
Fibrin, histochemische Reaktionen 870
—, Keratinisation 18
—, Leitstruktur im Bindegewebe 454
Fibrinoid, histochemische Reaktionen 870
Fibroblasten, Aggregation der Bauteile im Bindegewebe 453, 454
—, Amyloidsynthese 865
—, argyrophile Faserbildung 443
—, Aufbau der kollagenen Fibrille 442
—, Bildung der Basalmembran 463
—, Elektronenmikroskopie 432, 433

Fibroblasten, embryonale, Faserbildung in der Gewebekultur 638
—, Entstehung elastischer Fasern 447
—, fetale Haut, Glykogengehalt 632
—, — —, Phosphorylase-Aktivität 632
—, Herkunft der Bindegewebsgrundsubstanz 451
—, Kollagenese 440
—, Kollagensynthese, Elektronenmikroskopie 432
—, Leitstruktur im Bindegewebe 454
—, Mucopolysaccharidsynthese 441, 875
—, Mucoproteine in fetalen 641
—, normale Histologie von Corium und Subcutis 431
—, Plasmazellherkunft 439
—, Reticulin-Bildung 445
—, Stammzelle der Fettzellen 827
—, Stratum papillare 467
—, Stratum reticulare 470
—, Tropokollagen 441
Fibrocyten des Corium, Zahl der, Altersveränderung 693
— — und der Subcutis, elektronenmikroskopisches Bild 431
—, Glykogenablagerung bei Glykogenspeicherkrankheit 886
—, normale Histologie von Corium und Subcutis 431
—, Plasmalemmoberfläche 431, 432
—, Speicherfähigkeit 434
—, Umwandlung zu Histiocyten 434
—, — zu Pericyten 434
Fibrolipom, Entartung zu einem Fibrosarkom oder Liposarkom 824
—, Patho-Histologie 820
„filament", Definition 37
Filamente, Elektronenmikroskopie des Haarfollikels 154
„filament-matrix-complex", Röntgen-Diffraktionsmethode 75
Finger, Subcutiskonstruktion 477
Fingerbeere, Gefäßversorgung 356
—, Haut der, Verlauf elastischer Fasern 468
—, Histologie des Nagels 353

Fingerbeere, mikroskopische Untersuchung des embryonalen Nagels 347
—, Nervenentwicklung in der Haut 674
—, postmortale Vertrocknung 727
Fingerhaut, Bau der Subcutis 477
Fischlersche Reaktion, Histiocytose und Xanthogranulomatose 883
— —, Histochemie der Keratinocyten 81, 82, 83
Fischler-Färbung, Talgdrüsen 199
„flash burns" 772
Fleckfieber, idiomuskulärer Wulst 722
—, spontan auftretende Fettgewebsnekrosen und Fettgranulome 803
Fluorescenz, Darstellung des Stratum corneum 15
Flügelzellen, Struktur der inneren Wurzelscheide 151
Follikelatrophie, Altersveränderungen der Haut 703
Follikelhüllen, bindegewebige, Struktur des Haarfollikels 153
Folsäure, Wirkung auf die Proteinsynthese in Keratinocyten 70
—, — auf die RNA-Synthese in Keratinocyten 70
Fordyce spots, Talgdrüsen 217
Fremdkörper, Ablagerung und Speicherung in der Haut 900
— Historöntgenographie 901
—, Polarisationsmikroskopie 901
—, Röntgenabsorptionsspektrographie 901
Fremdkörpergranulom, Ähnlichkeit mit Lipogranulom 839
—, Klinik und Histologie 900
Fremdkörperzellen, Fremdkörpergranulom 901
Fruktose, Einfluß auf Mitoserate 64
Fusi, Struktur des Haarfollikels 146, 148
Fußleisten, embryonale Entwicklung 636
Fußsohle, Bau der Basalmembran 465

Gänsehaut, postmortale Fettstarre 724
—, Rigor 722

Gammaglobulin, Nachweis im Bereich von Amyloidablagerungen 866
Ganglienleiste, Embryologie der Haut 673
Ganoblasten bei Selachiern 944
Ganoidschuppen bei Knochenfischen 962
Gasemphysem bei Wasserleichen 744
Gefäße, Einbau in Corium und Subcutis 478
Gefäßeinheit s. ,,vascular unit"
Gefäßektasie, Altersveränderungen der Blutgefäße der Haut 700
Gefäßfibrinoid 869
Gefäßhyalin 869
Gefäßnerven, Innervation der Epidermis 378
—, — der Haut 398
—, sensible Endkörperchen der Haut 411
—, subepidermales Nervengeflecht 389
Gefäßnetz des Corium 519, 572
— —, regionäre Unterschiede 575
— eines glandulären Acinus 581
— der Haut, Aufbau des 567
— —, cutanes 519, 567
— —, —, regionale Unterschiede 568
— —, fasziales 519, 567
— —, —, regionale Unterschiede 568
— —, musculo-cutanes 570
— —, perifollikuläres, Anatomie 583
— —, —, horizontale Äste 583, 586
— —, —, longitudinale Äste 583
— —, —, permanenter Anteil 586
— —, —, Statik und Dynamik 583
— —, —, transitorischer Anteil 586
— —, —, vergleichende Anatomie 589
— —, periglanduläres 581
— —, —, Anatomie 581
— —, schematische Darstellung 605
— —, subepidermales 519, 575
— —, subpapilläres 519, 573
— —, venöses 595, 597
— des Nagels 579, 580
Gefäßplexus, subcutaner, bei Vögeln 1000, 1003

Gefäßreichtum des Stratum laxum bei Knochenfischen 966
Gefäßspasmus, Ätiologie der traumatogenen Fettgewebsnekrose 803
Gefäßverteilung, Haut 491
—, parenchymatöse Organe 491
Gehörgang, Subcutiskonstruktion 477
Genitalhaut, glatte Muskulatur 479
gerader Gang, Oberflächenzellen 256
Geriatrie, Altersveränderung der Haut 683
Geschlechtschromatin, Bestimmung in der Haut zur Identitätsfeststellung 729
— in der Epidermis des Frühgeborenen 636
— der Epidermiszellen, Altersabhängigkeit 690
— in Talgdrüsen, Altersveränderung 696
Geschlechtsdimorphismus, Gefiedertypen bei Vögeln 1015
Geschlechtshöcker, topographische Unterschiede der embryonalen Epidermis 635
Gesichtshaut, Anatomie des Gefäßnetzes 569, 575
Gewebe, periunguales, Anatomie des Nagels 342
—, —, Histochemie 361
—, —, Histologie 352
—, —, mikroskopische Untersuchung des embryonalen Nagels 346
Gewebslipasen, Ätiologie der Fettgewebserkrankungen 832
Gewebsmastzellen s. auch Mastzellen
—, Bildung der Mucopolysaccharide 875
—, Elektronenmikroskopie 437
— der Haut, normale Histologie 436
—, Hautstoffwechsel 473
—, Heparinbildung 437
—, Herkunft 438
—, Histaminbildung 437
—, Serotonin 437
Gewebswasserverschiebung, postmortale, Haut der frühen Leichenzeit 718
Gewichtsverlust, postmortaler 739
gewundener Gang, Oberflächenzellen 256

Gicht, neurotrophische Atrophie der Haut 792
Gichtanfall, Mechanismus 888
Giemsa-Färbung, Fetttröpfchen in Keratinocyten 83
Giftdrüsen bei adulten Amphibien 983
— bei Knochenfischen 959
Gitterfasern bei Amyloidablagerung in der Haut 868
— im Fettgewebe 788
—, glatte Muskulatur 479
—, normale Histologie von Corium und Subcutis 443
—, plurivacuoläres Fettgewebe 456
—, Subcutis 475
—, Vermehrung bei Mucinosen 879
Glandulae alae nasi, Heterotopie apokriner Schweißdrüsen 272
Glandulae ceruminales, myoepitheliale Zellen 482
Glandula vestibularis, Embryonalentwicklung der apokrinen Schweißdrüsen 268
Glashaut, Haarkomplexentwicklung 653
—, Struktur der bindegewebigen Haarfollikelhüllen 153
Glasmembran, Struktur der äußeren Wurzelscheide 152
Glatze, Blutgefäße der Haut 563
Glatzenbildung, Haarfollikel 168
— bei männlichen Vögeln 1014
Glomus cutaneum, arteriovenöse Anastomosen 554
Glomus digitale, arteriovenöse Anastomosen 554
Glomusorgan, Gefäßversorgung der Fingerbeere 356
Glomus subunguale, Entwicklung arterio-venöser Anastomosen 640
Glossy skin and fingers, neurotrophische Atrophien der Haut 792
Glucagon, lipid-mobilisierende Wirkung am menschlichen Fettgewebe 827
Glucose, Arteriolen der Haut, Histochemie 525, 537
—, Einfluß auf Mitoserate 64
—, Kapillaren der Haut, Histochemie 536, 537
Glucose-6-Phosphatase, Corium 474
—, Histotopochemie des Haarfollikels 176

Glucose-6-phosphat-Dehydrogenase, Histochemie der Keratinocyten 90
—, histochemischer Nachweis in apokrinen Schweißdrüsen 310, 315
—, Pinocytose-Mechanismus der Histiocyten 435
Glucose, Venolen der Haut, Histochemie 537, 550
α-Glucosidase, Pinocytose-Mechanismus der Histiocyten 435
β-Glucuronidasen, Arteriolen der Haut, Histochemie 527, 537
—, Basalzellen 253
—, Blutgefäßneubildung der Haut, Histochemie 559
—, dunkle Zellen, Cytochemie 248
— in Fettzellen 456
—, Haarbalg 474
—, helle Zellen, Cytochemie 242
—, Histochemie der Gewebsmastzellen 437
—, — der Intermediärzone der Epidermis 18
—, — der Keratinocyten 100
—, — des Musculus arrector pili 481
—, — der Talgdrüsen 196, 202
—, histochemischer Nachweis in apokrinen Schweißdrüsen 325
—, Histotopochemie des Haarfollikels 176
—, Kapillaren der Haut, Histochemie 537
—, Pinocytose-Mechanismus der Histiocyten 435
—, myoepitheliale Zellen 482
—, Nachweis in Fibrocyten von Corium und Subcutis 431
—, Tropokollagenbildung 433
—, Venolen der Haut, Histochemie 537
Glutamat-Dehydrogenase, Histochemie der Keratinocyten 90
—, histochemischer Nachweis in apokrinen Schweißdrüsen 310, 320
Glycerinaldehyd-3-Phosphat-Dehydrogenase, histochemischer Nachweis in apokrinen Schweißdrüsen 310, 313
Glycerin-1-Phosphat-Dehydrogenase, histochemischer Nachweis in apokrinen Schweißdrüsen 310, 314

Glycerin-1-Phosphat-Oxydase, histochemischer Nachweis in apokrinen Schweißdrüsen 310, 314
β-Glycerophosphatase, Arteriolen der Haut, Histochemie 527, 537
—, Kapillaren der Haut, Histochemie 537
—, Venolen der Haut, Histochemie 537, 550
α-Glycerophosphat-Dehydrogenase, Histochemie der Keratinocyten 90
Glycin, Autoradiographie der Epidermis 68
Glycolipoprotein, Histochemie der Keratinocyten 85
Glykogen, Ablagerung und Speicherung in der Cutis 885
—, Arteriolen der Haut, Histochemie 525, 537
—, arteriovenöse Anastomosen, Histochemie 556
—, Bedeutung bei der Zellteilung und Keratinbildung des Nagels 362
—, Cytochemie, myoepitheliale Zellen 236
—, dunkle Zellen, Cytochemie 247
— im embryonalen Bindegewebe 641
—, Fettsynthese 460
—, funktionelle Bedeutung im Cytoplasma 886
— im Haarkeim 648
—, Histochemie der apokrinen Schweißdrüsen 307
—, Histochemie der Basalmembran 463
—, — des embryonalen Nagels 673
—, — der fetalen ekkrinen Drüsen 665
—, — der Haarkomplexentwicklung 659
—, — der Keratinocyten 76
—, — des Nagels 361
—, — der Talgdrüsen 196, 201
—, histochemischer Nachweis von Amylo-Phosphorylase in glykogenhaltigen Zellen 367
—, Histotopographie im Haarfollikel 170
—, intradermaler Schweißdrüsen-Ausführungsgang 250
—, Kapillaren der Haut, Histochemie 536, 537
— im Lumen apokriner Drüsen des Haarfollikels 657
—, Mesodermentwicklung 637

Glykogen im Muskulus arrector pili, Haarkomplexentwicklung 656
—, Nachweis in Fettzellen 456
—, Oberflächenzellen, Cytochemie 257
—, Phosphorylase und Amylo-1,4 → 1,6-transglucosidase in der Epidermis 91
— der Schleimhautepithelien, Altersveränderung 690
—, Schweißdrüsen, ekkrine 227
—, Synthese in der Haut 474
—, Ultrastruktur der ekkrinen Drüsen 665
—, — der fetalen Epidermis 628, 629, 631
— im unteren Haarfollikelabschnitt, Haarkomplexentwicklung 653
—, Venolen der Haut, Histochemie 537
—, Verteilung in der fetalen Epidermis 631, 632
—, Vorkommen während der Embryonalentwicklung des Nagels 362
— in den Zellen des Infundibulums und des Haarkanals 654
Glykogenese, Keratinocyten 77
Glykogengehalt der Leichenhaut 721
— in Sekretzellen apokriner Schweißdrüsen 697
Glykogengranula, Elektronenmikroskopie, Talgdrüsen 208
Glykogenose, Abbauhemmung des Glykogens 886
Glykogenschwund bei Verbrennungen 768
Glykogenspeicherkrankheit, Glykogenvorkommen in der Haut 886
Glykolyse, Enzyme der, Histochemie der apokrinen Schweißdrüsen 312
— und Fettsynthese 789
Gold, Ablagerung und Speicherung in der Cutis 900
Gold-Färbung der weißen Dendritenzellen 106
Golgi-Apparat, Beziehung zur Zentriole in Keratinocyten 59
—, Elektronenmikroskopie 57
—, „lamellated bodies" 59
—, Langerhans-Zelle 117
—, Lipide, Histochemie der Keratinocyten 84

Golgi-Apparat der Melanocyten, Elektronenmikroskopie 109
—, —, Melaninsynthese 115
—, mikroskopische Anatomie der apokrinen Schweißdrüsen 278
—, Morphologie der Keratinocyten 57
—, Ort der Melanogenese 110, 111, 112
—, Phasenkontrastmikroskopie 57
—, Talgdrüsen 195, 200, 205, 209, 215, 216
—, Ultrastruktur der apokrinen Schweißdrüsen 299
Golgi-Elemente, Oberflächenzellen 256
Golgi-Mazzoni-Körperchen, Innervation der Haut 377
Gomori-Methode, Blutgefäße der Haut 498
—, Darstellung von Kalkablagerungen in der Haut 887
—, Kombination mit Toluidin-Färbung, Blutgefäße der Haut 498
— bei Mucinosen 879
Gram-Färbung, Darstellung des Stratum corneum 15
—, Fetttröpfchen in Keratinocyten 83
Gram-positive Substanzen, Histochemie der Keratinocyten 80
Grandy-Körperchen, Innervation der Haut 377
Granula, amorphe, Elektronenmikroskopie des Haarfollikels 155
—, dunkle, Ultrastruktur der apokrinen Schweißdrüsen 293
—, helle, Ultrastruktur der apokrinen Schweißdrüsen 292
—, Histochemie der apokrinen Schweißdrüsen, Eisengehalt 310
—, Übergangsformen zwischen hellen und dunklen, Ultrastruktur der apokrinen Schweißdrüsen 297
—, Ultrastruktur der Myoepithelzellen 303
„granular layer", Nomenklatur Stratum intermedium 11
Granulom, eosinophiles, Nosologie 882
—, lipophages 839
—, —, bei Spontanpanniculitis Typ Pfeifer-Weber-Christian 801

Granuloma anulare, Glykogenanreicherung im Hautbindegewebe 886
Granulomatose, Fettgewebsinfiltration 824
Granumolatosis disciformis, Glykogenanreicherung im Hautbindegewebe 886
— — chronica et progressiva Miescher, Ätiologie und Pathogenese 837
— — — —, Patho-Histologie 815
— — — —, — des Paraffinoms 805
— tuberculoides pseudosclerodermiformis chronica, Patho-Histologie 815
Gravidität, hormonelle Einflüsse auf apokrine Schweißdrüsen 329
Grenzflächenpräparate, epidermocutane 166
Grenzzone, Nomenklatur, Intermediärzone 17
Grubenorgane, kleine, bei Knochenfischen 969
Grundsubstanz, Definition 874
—, mesenchymale, Beziehung zu den Zellen des Bindegewebes und zum Blut 876
—, —, Regulierung der Mucinmenge 876
—, —, schematische Darstellung der Degradation 876
Guanophoren bei Knochenfischen 964
— der Reptilienhaut 991

Haar, Altersveränderungen 698
—, Durchmesser der Filamente 51
—, Elektronenmikroskopie der Filamente 52
—, Epidermicula 149
—, Epidermiculaschuppen 150
—, Fusi 148
—, Haarfarbe 148
—, Haarkomplexentwicklung 655
—, Haarmark 148
—, Haarrinde 148
—, „keratin pattern" 75
—, Keratinstruktur 50
—, keratogene Zone, fetale Haut, Glykogengehalt 632
—, — —, — —, Phosphorylase-Aktivität 632
—, Melaninaufnahme durch Keratinocyten, Elektronenmikroskopie 114

Haar, Melanogenese 110, 111, 112
—, Motivbild des Stratum papillare 467
—, Schaftbreite 147
—, sensible Nervenformationen 400
—, Terminalfasern, Nervenapparat des Haares 401
— des Tragus, Meßwerte 661
—, topographische Entwicklung der Haare 658
—, Wachstumsgeschwindigkeit 178
—, Wachstum, synchronisiertes 162
—, Zusammenhang mit Tween 60-Esterase 95
—, Wurzelscheide, Innervation der Haut 386, 401, 402
Haarbalg, Basalmembran 462
—, Fermentaktivität 474
—, glatte Muskulatur 479
—, Goldablagerung 900
—, Musculus arrector pili 481
—, Stratum reticulare 470
—, Struktur der bindegewebigen Haarfollikelhüllen 154
Haarbeet, morphologische Entwicklung des Haarkomplexes 649
Haarbildung, Induktionswirkung des Mesoderms 647
Haarbulbus der fetalen Haut, Glykogengehalt 632
— — — —, Phosphorylase-Aktivität 632
Haarcyklus, Blutgefäße der Haut 558
—, Funktion der dermalen Haarpapille 647
—, perifolliculäres Gefäßnetz 586
—, Stadien, Gefäßversorgung 502
—, Strukturveränderungen des Haarfollikels 157
Haare, dystrophische, Haarwurzelstatus 163
Haarentwicklung und hormonelle Einflüsse auf apokrine Schweißdrüsen 329
— nach STÖHR, schematische Darstellung 646, 648, 651
Haarfollikel, aktiver, fetale Haut, Glykogengehalt 632
—, —, —, Phosphorylase-Aktivität 632
—, —, Struktur 143
—, Altersabhängigkeit der Anzahl 704
—, Altersveränderungen 165, 698

Haarfollikel, Amyloidablagerung 868
—, Anlagen 227
—, apokrine Drüsen, Embryonalentwicklung 657
—, Autoradiographie 175
—, Bulbus 144
—, Bulbuszapfen, Melanocytenverteilung in der embryonalen Haut 677
—, dermale Papille 144
—, Ductus pilo-sebaceus 144
—, Ebene, kritische 177
—, embryonale Entwicklung der Melanocyten 676
—, Enzymaktivitäten 175, 176
—, fetale Gefäßentwicklung 513
—, Funktion 157
—, Glashaut 144
—, Haarbalg 144
—, Histochemie 143, 169
—, Histologie 143
—, Histotopographie anorganischer Substanzen 170
—, — von Kohlenhydraten 170
—, Harnpfropfbildung 699
— der Kopfhaut, Altersveränderungen an den Kapillaren 700
—, Musculus arrector pili 144
—, Nervenapparat des Haares 408
—, Penetration von Gasen 778
—, Struktur der Haarzwiebel 145
—, Strukturveränderungen 157
— des Tragus, Meßwerte 661
—, unterer Abschnitt, embryonale Haarkomplexentwicklung 652
—, Venen des 597
—, Wachstumsdynamik 143
—, Wurzelscheiden 144
—, Zusammenhang mit apokrinen Schweißdrüsen, historischer Überblick 268
Haarkanal, Haarkomplexentwicklung 653, 656
—, morphologische Entwicklung des Haarkomplexes 647, 649, 650, 653
—, Struktur der inneren Wurzelscheide 152
Haarkeim, Entwicklungsmechanik der Haut 644
— der fetalen Haut, Glykogengehalt 632
—, — —, Phosphorylase-Aktivität 632
—, Glykogengehalt der fetalen Epidermis 631

Haarkeim, Haarentwicklung 644
—, morphologische Entwicklung des Haarkomplexes 645, 647
Haarkeratin, Intermediärzone 18
Haarkomplex, Embryologie der Haut 644
—, fetaler, quantitative Daten 660
—, Meßwerte am Tragus Neugeborener 661
Haarkomplexentwicklung, Haarkanal 653, 656
—, Histochemie 659
—, Infundibulum 653, 656
—, Isthmus 653
—, Talgdrüse 653
—, Wulst 653
Haarmatrix, Histologie der Dendritenzellen der Haut 103
Haarmuskeln, Mesodermentwicklung 637
—, morphologische Entwicklung des Haarkomplexes 649, 650, 656
Haarpapille, dermale, Funktion beim Haarcyclus 647
— der fetalen Haut, Glykogengehalt 632
— — —, Phosphorylase-Aktivität 632
—, Goldablagerung 900
—, Melanocytenverteilung in der embryonalen Haut 676
—, Nervenapparat des Haares 402
Haarrinde, Haarkomplexentwicklung 655
Haarscheibe, Nervenapparat des Haares 407
—, subepidermales Nervengeflecht 384
Haarscheidenkegel, Haarkomplexentwicklung 655
Haarstengel, Strukturveränderungen des Haarfollikels 160
Haarstrich, Entwicklungsmechanik der Haut 643
—, epidermale Drüsenleisten 663
—, Haarbalgmuskel 481
—, Papillarkörper 467
—, topographische Entwicklung der Haare 658
Haarverteilungsmuster, Haarwurzelstatus 163
Haarvorkeim, Embryonalentwicklung ekkriner Drüsen 664
—, morphologische Entwicklung des Haarkomplexes 644

Haarwirbel, topographische Entwicklung der Haare 658
Haarwulst, Struktur der äußeren Wurzelscheide 152
Haarwurzelscheide, Goldablagerung 900
Haarwurzelstatus 163
Haarzapfen, fetale Haut, Glykogengehalt 632
—, — —, Phosphorylase-Aktivität 632
—, morphologische Entwicklung des Haarkomplexes 649
—, sensorische Nervenfasern, Entwicklung im Embryo 675
Haarzwiebel, Anisotropie 147
—, Fusi 146
—, Haarmatrix 145
—, kritische Ebene 145
—, Melanocyten 146
—, Struktur 145
Hämalaun-Eosin-Färbung, Hyalinosis cutis et mucosae 870
Hämangioblastom, Patho-Histologie 821
Haemangioma capillare, Patho-Histologie 821
Haemangioma cavernosum, Patho-Histologie 821
Hämangiopericytom, Glykogenvorkommen in Endothelzellen und in der glatten Muskulatur 886
Hämatopoese im embryonalen Corium 637
— in der embryonalen Haut 638
— im subcutanen Fettgewebe 788
Hämatoxylin-Eosin-Färbung bei aktinischer Elastose 873
—, Blutgefäße der Haut 498
—, Melanocyten 107
— von Gefäßhyalin und Gefäßfibrinoid 869
—, Pseudomilium colloidale Pellizari 872
Hämochromatose, Diagnose durch Leberbiopsie 896
—, histologischer Eisennachweis 895
—, Klassifikation 895
—, Patho-Histologie 896
—, Terminologie 895
Hämocytoblasten, Plasmazellherkunft 439
Hämolyse, Hämochromatosesyndrom 895
—, postmortale 731

hämorrhagische Diathese, sekundäre Hämosiderose der Haut 897
hämorrhagisches Mikrobid (STORCK), Patho-Histologie 809
Hämosiderin, Hämochromatose 896
—, physiologisches Vorkommen 896
Hämosiderinablagerung in der Haut 895
Hämosiderose, Eisenablagerung 895
—, Terminologie 895
Häutung der Amphibien 979
—, hormonale Steuerung bei Reptilien 990
— bei Reptilien 987, 989
Häutungsschicht bei Reptilien 988
Halbdesmosomen bei Amphibienlarven 973, 975
Hale-PAS-Reaktion, Veränderungen der Haut in der späten Leichenzeit 732
Hale-Reaktion, Altersveränderungen der Blutgefäße der Haut 702
—, Darstellung des Amyloid 863
—, embryonale Fasern 638
„half-desmosome" 35
Handleisten, embryonale Entwicklung 636
Handrücken, Bau der Basalmembran 465
Hand-Schüller-Christiansche Erkrankung, Nosologie 882
—, Patho-Histologie 882
Handteller, Bau der Basalmembran 465
Harnsäure, physiologischer Abbau der Purine 888
Harnsäurespiegel im Blut, Erhöhung und Uratablagerung in der Haut 888
Haut, Ablagerung und Speicherung 862
—, — von Hyalin 868
— der Acranier, vergleichende Histologie 922
Hautabschürfungen, Histologie an der Leiche 757
— an der Leiche 757
Haut, altersabhängige Elastizitätsunterschiede 472, 473
—, Altersbestimmung in der frühen Leichenzeit 729
—, — postmortaler Schnittwunden 762
—, Altersveränderung 683
—, — beim Astheniker 704

Haut, Altersveränderung, Geschlechtsunterschiede 703
—, —, Konstitutionsunterschiede 704
—, —, beim Pykniker 704
—, —, rassische Unterschiede 704
—, Atrophie der, Begriffsbestimmung 789
—, Autolyse in der frühen Leichenzeit 718
—, bedeckte, Altersveränderungen 684
—, behaarte, Innervation 377, 386, 400
—, Blutgefäße 491
—, Blutvolumen 492
—, Carotinoidablagerung und Speicherung in der Haut 897
—, Cysten und Atrophie der Haut 792
—, degenerative Altersatrophie 684
—, Dehnbarkeit, Faser-Textur 472
—, Dekomposition in der späten Leichenzeit 733
—, Dicke der, Altersabhängigkeit 686
—, einfache Altersatrophie 684
—, Eisen- und Hämosiderinablagerung 895
—, Elastizitätsmodul 472
—, Embryologie der 624
—, embryologische Determinierung 642
—, — Differenzierung 642
—, — Potenzbeschränkung 642
—, Entwicklungsmechanik 641
—, Faltenbildung 468
—, Fäulnisblase der späten Leichenzeit 731
—, Fäulnishinweis durch Grünverfärbung 731
—, Felderung und Papillarkörper 468
—, Fettwachspanzerung in der späten Leichenzeit 747
—, Fremdkörperablagerung und Speicherung 900
—, geschlechtsgebundene Elastizitätsunterschiede 473
—, Gewalteinwirkungen auf die Leichenhaut 752
—, glatte Muskulatur der 479
—, Goldablagerung und Speicherung 900
—, Glykogenablagerung und Speicherung 885
— der Hände, Berufsmerkmale 729

Haut, Hiebverletzungen 762
—, Identitätsfeststellung in der frühen Leichenzeit 729
—, Innervation 377
—, Kalkablagerung und Speicherung 887
—, Kohlenhydratstoffwechsel 76
—, Melaninablagerung und Speicherung 889
—, mikroskopische Veränderungen der späten Leichenzeit 732
—, mikroskopische und submikroskopische Anatomie der Muskulatur der 479
—, Morphologie der Altershaut 705
— der Neunaugen, vergleichende Histologie 927
—, normale Histologie 1
—, Penetration von Gasen 778
—, pH-Wert in der frühen Leichenzeit 718
—, Pigmentgehalt der bedeckten und unbedeckten Haut 685
—, Porphyrinablagerung und Speicherung 892
—, postmortale Hauttemperaturen 708
—, — Resorption von Gasen 778
—, — Veränderungen durch Fauna 734
—, — — durch Fliegen 734
—, — — durch Flora 735
—, — Vertrocknung nach Verletzung 727
—, Putrifikation 730
—, regionale Festigkeitsunterschiede 760
— der Rundmäuler, vergleichende Histologie 927
—, Saponifikation, Veränderungen in der späten Leichenzeit 741
—, Schnittverletzungen 761
—, Silberablagerung und Speicherung 898
—, Skeletmuskulatur, mikroskopische und submikroskopische Anatomie der 482
—, Stichverletzungen 761
—, Stoffwechsel 473
—, Tätowierungen 729
—, Tumoren und Atrophie der Haut 792
—, unbedeckte, Altersveränderungen 684
—, Uratablagerung und Speicherung 888

Haut, Veränderungen an Leichen 708
—, — in der späteren Leichenzeit 730
—, vergleichende Histologie der 920
—, Vergrößerung durch Papillarkörper 467
—, Vertrocknung nach agonaler Verletzung 727
—, — in der Agone 724
—, — in der frühen Leichenzeit 724
—, — nach Nekrophageneinwirkung 728
—, — nach postmortalen Verletzungen 728
—, — post mortem 725
—, Wassergehalt 724
Hautamyloidose, sekundäre 868
Hautanhangsgebilde, Arteriolen und Kapillaren 580
—, Venen der 595
—, — und Venolen 597
Hautatmung bei Amphibienlarven 976
— bei Knochenfischen 966
Hautatrophie nach allergischen Prozessen 793
—, entzündlich bedingte, umschriebene Atrophie des subcutanen Fettgewebes 794
—, entzündliche, Pathologie der Haut 789
— nach infektiösen Prozessen 793
—, mechanisch bedingte, Pathologie der Haut 790
—, neurotrophische, Pathologie der Haut 790
—, nichtentzündliche, Pathologie der Haut 789
—, primäre, physiologisch bedingte 789, 790
—, sekundär degenerative, Pathologie der Haut 790
—, — entzündliche, Pathologie der Haut 790, 793
— nach toxischen Prozessen 793
Hautbindegewebe, pathologische Glykogenanreicherung 886
Hautblutungen an der Leiche 755
—, postmortale 716
—, —, Abhängigkeit vom Lebensalter 716
—, — idiomuskulärer Wulst 716
—, Vortäuschung vitaler 717
Hautdrüsen bei adulten Amphibien 982
— bei Vögeln 998

Hautepitheliom, sekundäre Hautamyloidose 868
Hautfelderung und Spaltlinien 471
Hautinnervation bei Acraniern 923, 925
— bei Amphibien 978, 984
— bei Knochenfischen 968
— bei Neunaugen 933
— bei Schleimaalen 940
—, segmentale, bei Reptilien 995
—, —, bei Vögeln 1004
— bei Selachiern 956
Hautmuskulatur, Funktion der, bei Vögeln 1003
—, zentral-nervöse Kontrolle der, bei Vögeln 1003
Hautnerven, Blutgefäße 564
—, Gefäßversorgung 594, 598
Hautoberfläche, Esteraseaktivität 93, 94
—, proteolytische Aktivität 102
Hautrezeptoren, Innervation der Haut 383, 412
Hautsinnesknospen bei Neunaugen 934
Hautsinnesorgane bei Neunaugen 933
— bei Reptilien 995, 996
Hautspannung durch Fäulnisgasblähung 763
Hauttemperatur, Einfluß auf die Autolyse in der frühen Leichenzeit 719
Hauttransplantation, topographische Differenzierung des Bindegewebes 642
Hautturgor, Hyaluronsäure 452
—, Papillarkörperatrophie 469
Hautvenolen, regionäre Unterschiede 598
Hautwunden an der Leiche, Histochemie 754
—, vitale Differenzierung von agonalen oder postmortalen Verletzungen 753
—, — Reaktionen 753
Hautzirkulation, Mechanismus der, bei Reptilien 994
Heidenhain's Hämatoxylin, Färbung der Mitochondrien 55
Hemiatrophia faciei progressiva, neurotrophische Atrophien der Haut 792
„hemi-desmosome" 35
Henlesche Schicht, Haarkomplexentwicklung 655
— —, Struktur der inneren Wurzelscheide 150

Heparin, Beeinflussung des Bindegewebsstoffwechsels 875
—, Bildung in Gewebsmastzellen 437
Herbst'sche Körperchen, Acetylcholinesterasegehalt bei Vögeln 1005
— —, Aufbau, bei Vögeln 1004
— — als Druckreceptoren der Vögel 1005
Herzmassage, extrathorakale, Hautveränderungen 727
Hibernom, Patho-Histologie 821
—, Tumoren des subcutanen Fettgewebes 819
Hibernoma malignum, Patho-Histologie 824
Hidrocystom, schwarzes, Zusammenhang mit ektopischen apokrinen Schweißdrüsen 273
Histamin, Arteriolen der Haut, Histochemie 526, 537
—, Bildung in Gewebsmastzellen 437
—, Embryologie der Mastzellen 638
—, Freisetzung, postmortale 759
— in der Haut von vitalen und postmortalen Erhängungsfurchen 759
—, Kapillaren der Haut, Histochemie 537
—, Stoffwechselaktivität des Papillarkörpers 474
—, Venolen der Haut, Histochemie 537
Histidin, Einbau in Keratohyalin 47
—, Pauly-Reaktion in Keratinocyten 67
Histidindecarboxylase, Histochemie der Gewebsmastzellen 437
Histiocyten, DAF-Zellen 436
—, Elektronenmikroskopie 434
—, Entstehung aus Fibrocyten 434
—, epitheloidzellige Transformation bei Spontanpanniculitis Typ Pfeifer-Weber-Christian 801
—, fetale Haut, Glykogengehalt 632
—, —, Phosphorylase-Aktivität 632
— im Fettgewebe 788
— der Haut, Herkunft 436
—, Hautstoffwechsel 473
—, neurohormonale Zellen 436

Histiocyten, neurovegetative Zellen 436
—, normale Histologie von Corium und Subcutis 434
—, Speicherfähigkeit 434
—, Stratum papillare 467
—, Zellen mit chromaffinen Granula 436
Histiocytose, Elektronenmikroskopie 883
—, Histologie 882
—, Lipidablagerung in der Haut 881
Histiomonocyten, Ähnlichkeit mit Histiocyten der Haut 436
Histologie, vergleichende, der Haut 920
Histoplasmose, Erythema nodosum 836
Hodensack, post mortale Vertrocknung 726
Hormon, antidiuretisches, bei Amphibien 981
Hornalbumosen, Hornmembran der Keratinocyten 21
—, Stratum corneum, Biochemie 51
Hornhaut, Innervation 384
Hornmembran 30
—, Cystingehalt 76
—, Keratinocytenmorphologie 20
—, -SH- und -S-S-Gruppen 75
—, Stratum corneum, Biochemie 51
—, — intermedium 18
Hornschicht, harte, bei Reptilien 989
— der Haut, Wassergehalt 733
— s. auch Stratum corneum 15
—, weiche, bei Reptilien 989
„horny cell membrane" 30
„horny membrane" s. Hornmembran
Hornzellen, Anzahl der Fibrillen 54
—, Dicke der Plasmamembran 23
—, Durchmesser 17
—, Elektronenmikroskopie der Fibrillen 53
—, Fibrillenveränderung 40
—, Invagination 19, 20
—, Keratinocytenoberfläche 19
—, Keratohyalin 11
—, Lipide, Histochemie 84
—, Plasmamembran 22
—, Struktur 17
—, T-Zellen 12

Hornzellen, Transformation und Interzellularraum 25
—, Ultrastruktur, des Nagels 373
—, Zellhöhe 17
Hornzellmembran, Histochemie 30
—, Interzellularspalt 30
Hoyer-Grosser's Organe, arteriovenöse Anastomosen 554
Huxleysche Schicht, Haarkomplexentwicklung 655
— —, Struktur der inneren Wurzelscheide 150
Hyalin, Ablagerung und Speicherung in der Cutis 868
—, bindegewebiges 869
—, conjunctivales, Begriffsbestimmung 869
—, Darstellbarkeit 868
—, Definition 869
—, epitheliales, Begriffsbestimmung 869
—, Gefäßhyalin 869
—, histochemische Reaktionen 870
Hyalinbildung, bindegewebige 869
Hyalinisierung 869
Hyalinose, Ähnlichkeit mit Amyloidose und Paramyloidose 871
Hyalinosis cutis et mucosae, Ablagerung und Speicherung in der Haut 870
— — —, Pathogenese 871
Hyalodentin bei Knochenfischen 963
Hyalom, Pseudomilium colloidale Pellizari 872
Hyaluronidase, Bindegewebsgrundsubstanz 450
—, Corium 474
—, experimentelle Fettzellnekrose 831
—, Regulierung der Mucopolysaccharidmenge der Haut 877
—, Stoffwechsel des Bindegewebes 452
—, Unterscheidung verschiedener Mucopolysaccharide 453
—, Wirkung auf Basalmembran 463
—, Zusammensetzung der Grundsubstanz 874
Hyaluronsäure, Bausteine der Grundsubstanz 875
— der Bindegewebsgrundsubstanz, Altersveränderung 452
—, Bursae synoviales in der Subcutis 478

Hyaluronsäure, Funktion des Papillarkörpers 469
—, Stoffwechsel der Bindegewebsgrundsubstanz 452
—, Wasserbindung im Bindegewebe 452
Hydrolasen, Arteriolen der Haut, Histochemie 526
—, Kapillaren der Haut, Histochemie 538
Hydroxyapatit, Placoidschuppen bei Selachiern 946
β-Hydroxybuttersäure-Dehydrogenase, Histochemie der Keratinocyten 90
β-Hydroxy-Butyl-Dehydrogenase, Histotopochemie des Haarfollikels 176
Hydroxyprolin, Gehalt im Kollagenmolekül, bei Knochenfischen 962
—, Kollagenbestandteil bei Amphibien 975
—, Kollagenfibrille 865
Hydroxy-Steroid-Dehydrogenase, Histochemie, Talgdrüsen 196, 202
Hyperkeratose, Amyloidablagerungen in der Epidermis 867
— bei Angiokeratoma corporis diffusum Fabry 884
—, epidermolytische, „lamellated bodies" 59
—, Fetttröpfchen in Keratinocyten 83
—, Mitochondrien- und Fibrillenanzahl 56
—, Nexus der Keratinocyten 35
—, Psoriasis 11
—, Uratablagerungen in der Haut 889
Hypersensitivitätsangiitis (ZEEK), Patho-Histologie 809, 811
Hyperthermie, postmortale 709
Hyperthyreose, Mucinanreicherung beim prätibialen, lokalisierten Myxödem 877
—, Mucingehalt bei diffusem Myxödem 877
Hypertonie, Ätiologie der Lipome 839
—, Endarteriopathia chronica deformans, Patho-Histologie 817
—, Meßwerte über Gefäßwanddicke und Gefäßdurchmesser in Abhängigkeit vom Alter 701
Hypochlorämie, idiomuskulärer Wulst 722

„hypodermal (cutaneous) network", vergleichende Anatomie, Blutgefäße der Haut 501, 506, 507, 510
Hyponychium, Anatomie des Nagels 340, 342
—, Embryologie des Nagels 671
—, Histochemie 361
—, Histologie 351, 353
—, mikroskopische Untersuchung des embryonalen Nagels 346
—, Terminologie 340
Hypophyse, hormonelle Einflüsse auf apokrine Schweißdrüsen 330
Hypophysektomie, Beeinflussung der Fettspeicherung 459
—, Einfluß auf die Melanophoren bei Reptilien 991
Hypostase, Druckanämie der Leichenhaut 756
—, Hautblutungen der Leichenhaut 757
Hypothermie, agonale 709
—, postmortale 709
Hypotonie, Ätiologie der Necrobiosis lipoidica 837

Ichtyosis, „lamellated bodies" 59
Identitätsfeststellung, Haut der späten Leichenzeit 751
idiomuskulärer Wulst 722
— —, Hautblutungen 757
Imbibitions-Argyrose, lokale, Histologie 899
Immunoelektrophorese der Haut, Identitätsfeststellung 729
IMW s. idiomuskulärer Wulst
Inaktivitätsatrophie, Pathologie der Haut 790, 791
Inanitionsatrophie des Fettgewebes, Pathologie der Haut 790
Indolreaktion, Reaktion von Fibrin, Fibrinoid und Hyalin 871
Indoxylacetat-Esterase der Epidermis 95
—, Histochemie der Keratinocyten 92, 95
Indoxylesterase, Kapillaren der Haut, Histochemie 537
—, Venolen der Haut, Histochemie 537
Infundibulum, Haarkomplexentwicklung 653, 656
Injektionsverletzung, Differenzierung zwischen vitaler und postmortaler 761

Insulin, Einfluß auf Mitoserate 64
—, Fettsynthese 460
—, tierexperimentelle Befunde über Einfluß auf Muskelfasern und Fettzellen der Subcutis 833
Insulinlipodystrophie, Ätiologie und Pathogenese 832
— bei Alloxan-Diabetes-Ratten 831
—, Patho-Histologie 804
Insulinlipohypertrophie, Patho-Histologie 805
Insulinlipom, Ätiologie und Pathogenese 833, 839
—, Patho-Histologie 805
Insulinmast 459
Innervation, apokrine Schweißdrüsen 284
— der Haut 377
— der Sinnesknospen bei Chondrichthyes 953, 955
—, Ultrastruktur der Myoepithelzellen 304
„inosculation", Blutgefäße der Haut 559
Inosintriphosphatase in Langerhans Zellen 119
Interfilamentöse Substanz, Keratin 51
„interfilamentous substance", Definition 37
Intermediär-Drüsen, Altersveränderungen apokriner Schweißdrüsen 697
Intermediärzone, Bedeutung der Konzentration hydrolytischer Enzyme 96
—, Cytochromoxydaseaktivität 85
—, Esteraseaktivität 93
—, β-Glucuronidase-Aktivität 101
—, Histochemie 18
—, RNase-Aktivität 100
—, saure Phosphataseaktivität 98
„intermediate cells", Transformation der Lymphocyten 62
Intermedin, Einfluß auf Pigmentverteilung 948
Interzellularbrücken, Keratinocyten 20
—, Morphologie der Keratinocyten 31
Interzellularspalt, Biochemie des Stratum corneum 51
—, Keratinocyten, -SH- und -S-S-Gruppen 75
—, Polarisationsmethode 30
—, Röntgen-Diffraktionsmethode 30

intradermaler Schweißdrüsen-Ausführungsgang, Basalzellen 249
— —, Oberflächenzellen 254
— —, periphere Zellen 249
„Intrafibrillar matrix", Definition 37
„Intrafilamentous matrix", Definition 37
„intrinsic capacity" s. Kapillaren der Haut
Iodin-Test, Basalzellen 253
—, helle Zellen, Cytochemie 242
Ionenpumpe in der Amphibienepidermis 980, 981
Iridocyten bei Amphibienlarven 977
— bei Knochenfischen 964
— bei Neunaugen 933
Isocitrat-Dehydrogenase, Histochemie der Keratinocyten 90
—, NAD-abhängige, histochemischer Nachweis in apokrinen Schweißdrüsen 310, 316, 318
—, NADP-abhängige, histochemischer Nachweis in apokrinen Schweißdrüsen 310, 316, 318
Isthmus, Haarkomplexentwicklung 653

Janus-Grün, Färbung von Mitochondrien 55
„junctional complex", epidermaler Schweißdrüsen-Ausführungsgang 258
— —, Oberflächenzellen 256
„— desmosomes" 35
— —, Histologie der normalen Epidermis 4
„— granule" 35

Kachexie, idiomuskulärer Wulst 722
Kältereceptoren im Körperkern von Vögeln 1001
Kältezittern, reflektorisches, bei Vögeln 1001
Kalium, Histochemie der Keratinocyten 66
—, Nachweis im Fibrin, Fibrinoid und Hyalin 871
Kalkablagerungen im Gewebe, Elektronenmikroskopie 888
— und Speicherung in der Haut 887
Kandelaber-Arterien 572, 581
— der Haut 521, 523
Kandelaber-Venolen 546
Kantharidenpflaster, kapillaroskopische Methoden 496, 531

Kapillaren, embryonale, Darstellung durch Injektionsmethoden 639
— der Haut, allgemeine Charakteristica 529
— —, Altersabhängigkeit 530
— —, Altersveränderungen 700
— —, Basalmembran 534, 539, 541
— —, Belichtung der Hautareale 530
— —, Definitionen 524, 529
— —, Diät 531
— —, Elektronenmikroskopie 539
— —, Endothelien 534, 539
— —, Endothelschlauch 529
— —, eineiige Zwillinge 530
— —, Gitterfasern 535
— —, Grad der Gefäßdehnung 530
— —, Größe der Oberfläche 530
— —, Größe des Versorgungsgebietes 530
— —, Heredität 530
— —, histangiöse Zone 529
— —, Histochemie 536
— —, Innervation 566
— —, „intrinsic capacity" 546
— —, jahreszeitliche Abhängigkeit 531
— —, kapillaroskopische Bilder 530
— —, Klassifikation 539
— —, Konstitutionstypus 530
— —, Mesodermentwicklung 637
— —, metabolischer Austausch 546
— —, morphofunktionelle Lokalisation 530
— —, Neurastheniker 530
— —, papilläre, regionäres Verteilungsmuster 533
— —, Papillarschlingen 533
— —, Pericyten 534, 536, 539, 542
— —, Silbernitrat-Färbung nach GOMORI 535
— —, Struktur 534
— —, Thermoregulation 546
— —, Unterschiede der Gefäßlokalisation 530
— der Hautanhangsgebilde 580
—, Patho-Histologie gefäßbedingter Erkrankungen des subcutanen Fettgewebes 808

Kapillarendothelien, embryonale, Darstellung durch alkalische Phosphatase-Reaktion 640
kapillaroskopische Methoden, Nachteile 497
Kapillarvenen der Haut 548
Karyolyse der Haut, Morphologie der Autolyse 720
— —, Veränderungen in der späten Leichenzeit 732
Karyoplasma, Morphologie der Keratinocyten 60
Kaschin-Beck-Krankheit, Hämosiderosesyndrom 895
Katagen, Strukturveränderungen des Haarfollikels 158, 162
Katagenbewegung, Haarcyclus 158
Katagenhaare, Haarwurzelstatus 163
Katagenphasen, Dynamik der 159
Katecholamin-Granula, Innervation der Haut 384
Kathepsin bei Amphibienlarven 986
Keimschicht, intraepidermaler Schweißdrüsen-Ausführungsgang 258
Keratin, amorphes, Elektronenmikroskopie des Haarfollikels 156
—, anisotrope Fibrillen, Darstellung 30
—, Definition 37
—, faseriges, Elektronenmikroskopie des Haarfollikels 156
—, Histochemie des Nagels 371
—, histochemische Untersuchung des Nagels 369
—, — — —, Basophilie 370
—, Klassifikation 49
—, Röntgendiffraktionsuntersuchungen 49
—, Ultrastruktur des Nagels 374
Keratin A, Histochemie der Hornzellmembran 30
—, Hornmembran der Keratinocyten 20
—, Interzellularspalt des Stratum corneum 30
—, Stratum corneum, Biochemie 51
—, Stratum intermedium 18
Keratin B, Hornmembran der Keratinocyten 21
—, Stratum corneum, Biochemie 51

„keratin pattern" 44, 45
—, Keratinfibrillen 52
—, -SH- und -S-S-Gruppen in Keratinocyten 75
α-Keratin, Intermediärzone 18
—, Struktur 50
—, Synthese in der Federscheide bei Vögeln 1007
β-Keratin, Struktur 50
—, Synthese der Federzellen bei Vögeln 1007
Keratin-Fibrillen, Entwicklung 42
Keratinisation, DNase-Aktivität der Epidermis 100
—, Elektronenmikroskopie des Haarfollikels 154
—, Entwicklung der Keratinfibrillen 42
—, epidermaler Schweißdrüsen-Ausführungsgang 260
— der Epidermis bei Vögeln 999
—, β-Glucuronidaseaktivität 101
—, Intermediärzone 17
—, Mucopolysaccharidsynthese 80
—, RNase-Aktivität 100
—, Stratum intermedium 11, 18
—, Sulfhydrylgruppen 71
Keratinocyten, Alpha-Cytomembran 57
—, Desmosomen 31
—, Einfluß auf Melaninbildung 113
—, Elektronenmikroskopie 19
—, — der Basalmembran 4
—, — der Intermediärzone der Epidermis 18
—, Enzyme in 85
—, Fetttröpfchen 58
—, Fibrillenveränderung 41
—, funktionelle Beziehung zu Langerhans-Zellen 117
—, Golgi-Apparat 57
—, Histochemie 66
—, interzellulärer Spalt 23
—, „lamellated bodies" 58
—, Melaninaufnahme 114
—, Mitose-beeinflussende Faktoren 64
—, Mitosezahl 62
—, Morphologie 18
—, — der, Mitochondrien 55
—, Nexus 34
—, Nucleinsäuren, Histochemie 68
—, Nucleus 60
—, Plasmamembran 20
—, —, in der unverhornten Epidermis 21

Keratinocyten, Regeneration 61
—, Ribosomen 47, 57
—, Transformation zu Dentritenzellen 104
—, — aus Lymphocyten 62
—, T-Zellen 14
—, Zelloberfläche 18
—, —, -SH- und -S-S-Gruppen 75
—, Zellrelief 18
„Keratinosomes", Intercellularspalt der Keratinocyten 26
Keratin-Polysaccharid-Komplex, Altersveränderung des Nagels 699
Keratogenese, Wirkung der sauren Phosphatase 366
„keratogene Zone" 147
„keratogenous zone", Nomenklatur Intermediärzone 17
Keratohyalin, ATPase-Aktivität der Epidermis 99
—, Bildung 43
—, Dyskeratose 43
—, Elektronenmikroskopie der Epidermis 9
—, Embryologie der Epidermis, Periderm-Austausch 627
—, Embryologie des Nagels 671
—, Entwicklung der Keratinfibrillen 43
—, epidermale Fasern 39
—, Glykogen 76
—, Gram-positive Substanzen 80
—, Hale-PAS-positive Substanzen 81
—, Histochemie des embryonalen Nagels 673
—, Keratinisation 44
—, Keratinocyten 19
—, Nexus der Keratinocyten 35
—, RNA-Gehalt 69
—, pathologischer Mangel 11
—, Pauly-Reaktion 67
—, Psoriasis 43
—, saure Phosphataseaktivität der Epidermis 99
—, Stratum spinosum 11
— -Synthese 80
—, T-Zellen 14
—, Ultrastruktur der fetalen Epidermis 629, 631
—, — des Stratum intermedium 13
Keratohyalinbildung, Haarkomplexentwicklung 654
— durch Mitochondrien 56
Kerato-Hyalin-Granula, Altersveränderung der Epidermis 688

Kerato-Hyalin-Granula, epidermaler Schweißdrüsen-Ausführunsgang 260
—, Stratum intermedium 11
Keratohyalinkörner, Ultrastruktur der ekkrinen Drüsen 665
Keratose, senile, intraepidermaler Schweißdrüsen-Ausführungsgang 258
Kern s. auch Nucleus
Kernelongation, Fehlbeurteilung durch Artefakte 776
—, Histologie der Elektrounfälle 775
Kernmembran, Keratinocyten 22, 60
Kernpyknose, Morphologie der Autolyse der Haut 720
Kiemendarm, Mesodermentwicklung 637
Kinocilium, Aufbau der Sinnesknospen bei Tieren 953
Kirchhofsrosen, Haut der frühen Leichenzeit 710
Kittmasse, Basalmembran 464
Kloake, Anusentwicklung 635
Kloakenmembran, Anusentwicklung 635
Knäueldrüsen, Subcutis 474
Knochenfische, Corium der 960
—, Epidermis der 957
—, Haut der, vergleichende Histologie 956
—, Subcutis der 961
Knochengewebsbildung nach pathologischen Kalkablagerungen im Gewebe 888
Kohlenhydrate, Histochemie der apokrinen Schweißdrüsen 307
—, — der Keratinocyten 76
Kohlenmonoxyd, postmortale percutane Resorption 778
Kohlenmonoxydintoxikation, Livores 711
—, Mumifikation 740
Kohlensäure, postmortale percutane Resorption 778
Kohlensäureanhydratase, Histotopochemie des Haarfollikels 176
Kolbenhaar, Strukturveränderungen des Haarfollikels 157
Kolbenhaarbildung, präsumptive Phase, Haarcyclus 158
Kolbenzellen bei Knochenfischen 959
—, Neunaugen 930

Kollagen, Aminosäureanalyse 440
—, Bindegewebsgrundsubstanz 450
—, chemische Analyse 440
—, Degeneration bei der Atrophia cutis senilis 790
—, — bei Pseudomilium colloidale Pellizari 872
—, Entstehung 440
—, — elastischer Fasern 447
—, Schrumpfung, Altersverschmälerung des Coriums 691
—, Ultrastruktur 440
Kollagenase bei Amphibienlarven 986
—, Bindegewebsgrundsubstanz 450
—, Corium 474
—, Stoffwechsel des Bindegewebes 452
—, Wirkung auf Basalmembran 463
Kollagenfaserbildung über argyrophiles Zwischenstadium 443
Kollagenfibrillen s. auch Fibrillen, kollagene
— der Haut, Embryologie 638
Kollagensynthese, Elektronenmikroskopie des Fibrocyten 432
Kollazin, Entartung des Kollagen bei Atrophia cutis senilis 790
Kolloid, epitheliales Hyalin, Begriffsbestimmung 869
Kongorot, chemische und physikalische Bindung an Amyloid 863, 866
—, Reaktion von Fibrin, Fibrinoid und Hyalin 870
Kontaktmikroradioskopie, Blutgefäße der Haut 498
Konturfedern, große, bei Vögeln 1003, 1006
Kopfhaar, Stratum intermedium 12
Kopfhaut, Amyloidablagerung 868
—, Anatomie des Gefäßnetzes 569, 575
—, Gefäßveränderungen im Alter 700
—, Glykogengehalt 76
—, Stratum papillare 465
Körnerzellen, fetale Epidermis, Glykogengehalt 632
—, — —, Phosphorylase-Aktivität 632
— bei Knochenfischen 959
—, Neunaugen 929
Korbzellen, Muskulatur der Haut 482

Kossa-Färbung, Darstellung von Kalkablagerungen in der Haut 887
Kragen, Struktur der äußeren Wurzelscheide 152
Krausesche Endkolben, Altersveränderungen 702
— Körperchen, Histologie der Innervation des Nagels 358
— —, Innervation der Haut 377
Kraurosis penis, Fettgewebsatrophie der Haut 794
Kraurosis vulvae, Fettgewebsatrophie der Haut 794
Kreatinurie und idiomuskulärer Wulst 722
Kresylviolett, Färbung des Amyloid 863
Kupfer, Nachweis in der Haut nach Elektrounfällen 775

Labrocyten, normale Histologie der Gewebsmastzellen der Haut 436
Lactat, Einfluß auf Mitoserate 64
Lactat-Dehydrogenase, Histochemie der Gewebsmastzellen 437
—, — der Keratinocyten 90
—, — der apokrinen Schweißdrüsen 310, 314
Lactieren, glatte Muskulatur 479
Lagomorpha, vergleichende Anatomie, Blutgefäße der Haut 506
„lamellated bodies", Interzellularspalt der Keratinocyten 26
— —, lysosomale Funktion 59
— —, Morphologie der Keratinocyten 58
— —, Virusinfektion 59
Lamellenkörperchen s. auch Vater-Pacinisches Lamellenkörperchen
— am Federbalg bei Vögeln 1003
Lamina densa, Bildung durch Epidermiszellen 463
— —, Elektronenmikroskopie 464
— —, Nomenklatur Basalmembran 462
Langerhanssches Netz der Larvenhaut 971
Langerhanszell-Organellen, Elektronenmikroskopie der Histiocytose und Xanthogranulomatose 883

Langerhans-Zellen, Abstammung 116
—, ATPase-Aktivität 115
—, Elektronenmikroskopie 118
—, Embryologie der Haut, Nervenentwicklung 116
—, Enzymaktivität 119
—, Keratinocytenoberfläche 19
—, Melaningranula in 119
—, mesenchymale Herkunft 117
—, Morphologie 117
—, Nervenentwicklung in der Haut 676
—, neuroektodermale Herkunft 625
—, normale Histologie der Haut 116
—, Phagocytose 117
—, Pigmentbildung 117
—, Proteinsynthese 116
—, Schwannsche Zelle 116
—, Verwandtschaft mit Melanocyten 116
—, Zugehörigkeit zum neurovegetativen oder neurohormonalen System 116
Langhans-Zellen, Fremdkörpergranulom 901
Lanugo, Haarkomplexentwicklung 655
—, Nervenapparat des Haares 404
—, perifolliculäres Gefäßnetz 589
Lateralisnerven, Wurzeln der, bei Chondrichthyes 953
Laugenverätzung, Veränderung der Leichenhaut 774
Laurinsäure, Aufbau des Fettes in der Subcutis 789
Lebercirrhose, Hämochromatose 895
Lecithinase, experimentelle Fettzellnekrose 831
Lederhaut, Embryologie der Haut 625
—, Histologie des Nagels 354
—, mikroskopische Untersuchung des embryonalen Nagels 348
Leichenhaut, Carbonisierung 771
—, Differenzierung zwischen agonalen und vitalen Verletzungen 752
—, Einwirkung stumpfer Gewalt 755
—, Hautveränderungen 708
—, mikroskopische Befunde von Hautverletzungen 752
—, Schußverletzungen 764
—, spitze Hautverletzungen 760
—, Temperatur 708

Leichenwachs 741
Leichenwachsbildung 744
—, forensisch-kriminalistische Bedeutung 747
Leichenzehrer 734, 740
— und Mumifikation, forensisch-kriminalistische Bedeutung 741
—, Vortäuschung von Schrotschußverletzungen 764
— im Wasser 748
Leitungsgeschwindigkeit, Nervenapparat des Haares 408
—, Nerven der Subepidermis 389
Lemnocyten, Innervation der Haut 379
—, Mitochondrien, sensible Endkörperchen der Haut 422
Lentigo senilis 685
Lepra, Erythema nodosum 836
Leuchtbildmethode, Diagnostik der Argyrose 899
—, Diagnose der Auriasis 900
Leucin, Autoradiographie der Epidermis 68
Leucinaminopeptidase, Histochemie der apokrinen Schweißdrüsen 325
—, — von Corium und subcutanem Fettgewebe 641
—, — der fetalen ekkrinen Drüsen 668
—, — der Haarkomplexentwicklung 659
—, —, Kapillaren der Haut 539
—, — der Talgdrüsen 196, 202
—, — der Wundheilung 754
Leucylaminopeptidase, Histochemie der Gewebsmastzellen 437
l-Leucyl-4-methoxy-β-naphthylamid, Nachweis von proteolytischen Enzymen in der Haut 102
l-Leucyl-β-naphthylamid, Nachweis von proteolytischen Enzymen in der Haut 102
Leukämie, lymphatische, Erythema nodosum als Primärsymptom 836
—, —, Fettgewebsinfiltration 824
—, myeloische, Erythema nodosum als Primärsymptom 836
—, —, Fettgewebsinfiltration 824
—, Regenerationszeit der Epidermis 61

Leukoderma syphiliticum, Dendritenzellen der Haut 103
Leukophoren bei Selachiern 946
Leydig'sche Zellen der Larvenhaut 971
Lichen amyloidosus, Histologie der Amyloidablagerung in der Epidermis 867
Lichen myxoedematosus, Einteilung der Mucinosen 878
— —, Erhöhung der Blut-Mucopolysaccharide 876
— —, Histologie 879
Lichen ruber planus, Fettgewebsatrophie der Haut 793
— — — —, Fetttröpfchen in Keratinocyten 83
Lichen sclerosus et atrophicus, Fettgewebsatrophie der Haut 794
Lichtdermatose, Porphyrinablagerung in der Haut 894
Liebermann-Burchard-Reaktion, Histochemie, Talgdrüsen 200
Lillie's performic acid-Schiff-Reaktion, Histochemie der Keratinocyten 82, 83
Linolensäure, Aufbau des Fettes in der Subcutis 789
Lipase-Aktivität bei Tumormetastasen im subcutanen Fettgewebe 826
Lipasen, experimentelle Fettzellnekrose 831
— in Fettzellen 456
—, Funktion der Tela subcutanea 788
—, Histochemie der apokrinen Schweißdrüsen 322
—, — der Intermediärzone der Epidermis 18
—, — der Keratinocyten 92
—, — der Talgdrüsen 196, 203
Lipatrophia anularis, Ätiologie 813
— —, Patho-Histologie 813
Lipoatrophie, Begriffsbestimmung 805
„lipid droplets" s. Fetttröpfchen
Lipide, Ablagerung und Speicherung in der Cutis 880
—, arteriovenöse Anastomosen, Histochemie 556
— und Carotinoide im Blut 898
—, Cytochemie, myoepitheliale Zellen 236
—, Definition 880

Lipide, Histochemie der apokrinen Schweißdrüsen 306
—, — der Basalmembran 463
—, — der Intermediärzone der Epidermis 18
—, — der Keratinocyten 81
—, — der Talgdrüsen 196
—, interzellulärer Spalt, Stratum corneum 23
—, intradermaler Schweißdrüsen-Ausführungsgang 250
—, Plasmamembran der Keratinocyten 22
— in den Sekretzellen apokriner Schweißdrüsen, Altersveränderungen der Haut 697
Lipidgehalt in ekkrinen Schweißdrüsen, Altersabhängigkeit 696
Lipid-Synthese, Talgdrüsen 196, 204
Lipoblast, Fettspeicherung 460
Lipoblastom, Tumoren des subcutanen Fettgewebes 818
Lipoblastoma cutis, Patho-Histologie 820
Lipochondrien, Ultrastruktur der apokrinen Schweißdrüsen 297
Lipochrome 457
—, Aufbau der Federfarben bei Vögeln 1009
—, braunes Fett 458
—, echte, Carotinoide 897
Lipodystrophia progressiva Simons, Patho-Histologie 805
Lipodystrophie, Begriffsbestimmung 805
—, medikamentöse, Patho-Histologie 804
—, neurotrophische Atrophie der Haut 792
Lipofuscin, mikroskopische Anatomie der apokrinen Schweißdrüsen 278
—, saure Phosphatase in apokrinen Schweißdrüsen 323
—, Ultrastruktur der Myoepithelzellen 303
Lipofuscingranula, Ultrastruktur der apokrinen Schweißdrüsen 294
Lipogenese in der Haut von Diabetikern 828
— und Wachstumshormon 827
Lipoglykoprotein, Histochemie der Keratinocyten 83
Lipoglykoproteinose, Hyalinosis cutis et mucosae 870

Lipogranulom, Ähnlichkeit mit Fremdkörpergranulom 839
—, ätiologische Faktoren 840
—, — und Pathogenese 832
— nach Einwirkung thermischer Noxen, ionisierender Strahlen und Pankreasextrakten 831
—, Fermentaktivität und Riesenzellen 834
—, resorptive Entzündung 840
—, sklerosierendes, Patho-Histologie 805
—, Stoffwechselstörung der Fettzelle 891
Lipogranulomatose, Pathologie des subcutanen Fettgewebes 795
Lipogranulomatosis subcutanea hypertonica Gottron, Patho-Histologie 799, 816
Lipogranulomatosis subcutanea Rothmann-Makai, Ätiologie und Pathogenese 835, 840
— — —, Patho-Histologie 802
Lipogranulombildung nach Anwendung von Medikamenten 830
Lipohypertrophie, Begriffsbestimmung 805
Lipoide, Definition 880
—, Histotopographie im Haarfollikel 171
Lipoidose, Lipidablagerung in der Haut 881
Lipoidproteinose, Ablagerung und Speicherung in der Haut 870
— und erythropoetische Porphyrie 872
Lipoidspeicherkrankheit, systematisierte 881
Lipom, Ätiologie und Pathogenese 838
—, Entwicklung zu einem Liposarkom 823
— bei Panniculitis Rothmann-Makai 838
Lipomatosis cutis, Patho-Histologie 820
Liponekrose, Pathologie des subcutanen Fettgewebes 795
Lipophagen bei Spontanpanniculitis Typ Pfeifer-Weber-Christian 801
Lipophagie bei Spontanpanniculitis Typ Rothmann-Makai 802
Lipophanerose, Veränderungen der Haut in der späten Leichenzeit 742

Lipophoren bei Knochenfischen 965
— bei Neunaugen 933
Lipopigment, Ultrastruktur der apokrinen Schweißdrüsen 297
β-Lipoproteide, Carotinoidbindung im Blut 897
—, Lipidtransport 788
Lipoprotein, Histochemie der elastischen Faser 449
— -Membranen, Ubiquinon-Aktivität 102
Lipolyse, Funktion der Tela subcutanea 788
Liposarkom, Patho-Histologie 823
lipotropes Hormon s. Lipotropin
Lipotropin, experimentelle Pathologie des Fettgewebes 826
Lippenrot, embryonale Nervenentwicklung 676
Liquor, pH-Wert, postmortal 719
Livores, Differentialdiagnose Cyanose 714
—, Diffusionstotenflecke 710
—, Druckanämie der Leichenhaut 756
—, Haut der frühen Leichenzeit 710
—, hypostatische 710
—, Körperhaltung 711
—, mikroskopische und makroskopische Befunde in verschiedenen Zeiten nach dem Tode 712
—, percutane Permeation von Gasen 714
—, postmortale Reoxydation 714
—, Reoxydation des Hämoglobins durch percutane Resorption von Sauerstoff 778
Lobärpneumonie, Livores 711
Lokomotion, Histiocyten 434
„longitudinal connecting surface", Keratinocyten, Ultrastruktur 34
Lues, Erythema nodosum 836
—, Fettgewebsatrophie 829
Lugol'sche Lösung, Darstellung des Glykogenvorkommens in der Haut 886
luisches Exanthem, Fettgewebsatrophie der Haut 793
Lungenödem, postmortale Blutungen 716
Lunula, Anatomie des Nagels 340, 342

Lupus erythematodes, Fettgewebsatrophie der Haut 793
Lymphgefäße der Haut, Altersveränderungen 702
— —, embryologische Studien durch Injektionsmethode 640
— —, embryonale Entwicklung 639
Lymphknoten, braunes Fettgewebe 458
Lymphoblasten, Plasmazellherkunft 439
Lymphocyten, Transformation zu Keratinocyten 62
Lymphogranuloma inguinale, Erythema nodosum 836
Lymphogranulomatosis maligna Paltauf-Sternberg, Fettgewebsinfiltration 824
lymphoretikuläre Hyperplasie, Fettgewebsinfiltration 824
Lymphräume, Gefäßnerven der Haut 398, 400
— bei Schleimaalen 939
Lysosomen bei Amphibien 979
—, Cytochemie, myoepitheliale Zellen 236
—, epidermaler Schweißdrüsen-Ausführungsgang 260
—, Epidermis, β-Glucuronidaseaktivität 101
—, helle Zellen 242
—, Histiocyten 435
—, Langerhans-Zellen, Elektronenmikroskopie 118
—, mikroskopische Anatomie der apokrinen Schweißdrüsen 277
—, PAS-reaktive, Diastaseresistente Substanz, Histochemie apokriner Schweißdrüsen 309
—, saure Phosphataseaktivität 97, 98
—, — — in apokrinen Schweißdrüsen 323
—, Schweißdrüsen 227, 229

Maceration, abakterielle 721
—, Corium 465
„macula adhaerens", Desmosomen der Keratinocyten 31
„macula occludens" bei Amphibien 980
— —, Keratinocyten, Ultrastruktur 34
Magnesium, Histochemie der Keratinocyten 67
Makroglobulinämie Waldenström, Fettgewebsinfiltration 824

Makrophagen s. auch Histiocyten
—, Entstehung aus Fibrocyten 434
—, periglanduläre, Eisennachweis 311
Malat-Dehydrogenase, Histochemie der Gewebsmastzellen 437
—, — der Keratinocyten 90
—, histochemischer Nachweis in apokrinen Schweißdrüsen 310, 316
Malatenzym, histochemischer Nachweis in apokrinen Schweißdrüsen 310, 315
Malic Enzyme s. Malatenzym
Mallory-Azan-Technik, Blutgefäße der Haut 498
Mallory-Färbung, Fremdkörpergranulom 901
—, Hyalinosis cutis et mucosae 870
Mallory's Bindegewebsfärbung, Reaktion von Fibrin, Fibrinoid und Hyalin 870
Malpighizellen, Melanin-Phagocytose 891
Malteserkreuz, Histiocytose und Xanthogranulomatose 883
Mamma s. auch Brustdrüse
—, Fettgewebsnekrose, Patho-Histologie 803
—, Metachromasie der Bindegewebsgrundsubstanz 450
—, myoepitheliale Zellen 482
—, spezialisierte Drüsen der Haut, Embryologie 661
Mammacarcinom, Vorkommen von Myoepithelzellen 279
Mammadrüsen, Embryologie, Haarkomplex 661
Mamille, glatte Muskulatur 479
—, Vorkommen freier Talgdrüsen 661
Mantelzellen, Aufbau der Sinnesknospen bei Tieren 953
Marasmus febrilis, Inanitionsatrophie des Fettgewebes der Haut 790
Markscheide der Nerven der Haut, Begriffserklärung 379
— der Nervenfasern der Haut 377, 381, 383, 400, 405, 419
Markzellen, Elektronenmikroskopie des Haarfollikels 155
Masson-Färbung, Blutgefäße der Haut 498
Massonsche Silbermethode, embryonale Entwicklung der Melanocyten 676

Masson's Trichromfärbung, Reaktion von Fibrin, Fibrinoid und Hyalin 870
Mastzellen, Anzahl in der Haut des Neugeborenen 638
—, arteriovenöse Anastomosen 555
— und Bindegewebsstoffwechsel 875
—, Embryologie 638
—, fetale Haut, Glykogengehalt 632
—, — —, Phosphorylase-Aktivität 632
—, Funktion des Papillarkörpers 469
—, Geschlechtsunterschiede der Altersveränderungen 704
—, Gewebsmastzellen der Haut, normale Histologie 436
—, Herkunft der Bindegewebsgrundsubstanz 451
—, Histamingehalt im Embryonalleben 638
—, Mucopolysaccharidbildung 438
—, Stratum papillare 467
—, Transformation zu Melanocyten 105, 106
—, Turgorverlust der Haut 453
—, Vermehrung bei Amyloidablagerungen in der Epidermis 867
—, — bei Mucinosen 879
—, Zahl, Altersveränderung 694
—, Zellgehalt in der Haut 438
Mastzellgranula 437
—, Entstehung 438
—, histogenetische Verwandtschaft mit Melaningranula 105
Matrix, Anatomie des Nagels 340, 342
—, mikroskopische Untersuchung des embryonalen Nagels 345
—, morphologische Entwicklung des Haarbulbus 651
—, — — des Haarkomplexes 649, 650, 651
—, Terminologie des Nagels 340
Matrixzellen, Struktur des Haarfollikels 154
Mauser, beeinflussende Faktoren der, bei Vögeln 1011
—, hormonelle Steuerung, bei Vögeln 1011, 1014
Mauthner'sche Neurone bei Chondrichthyes 953

Mechanoreceptoren, Innervation der Haut 384
—, Nervenapparat des Haares 410
—, sensible Endkörperchen der Haut 414
MDH s. „melanin dispersing hormone"
Mediaabscesse bei Periarteriitis nodosa cutanea 810
Medullaranlage, Frühentwicklung der Epidermis 625
Medullarplatte, Embryologie der Epidermis 626
Meibom'sche Drüsen 218
— —, Entwicklungsmechanik der Haut 643
— —, Histochemie der Haarkomplexentwicklung 659
— —, spezialisierte Drüsen, Haarkomplexentwicklung 661
Meißnersche Tastkörperchen, Altersveränderungen 702
— —, Anlage, Nervenentwicklung in der Haut 675
— —, Bedeutung des Papillarkörpers 469
— —, Histologie der Innervation des Nagels 358
— —, Innervation der Haut 377, 385
— —, sensible Endkörperchen der Haut 412, 417
Melanin, Ablagerung und Speicherung in der Haut 889
—, Aufbau der Federfarben bei Vögeln 1009
— der Basalzellen bei Mucinose 879
—, Beziehung zu Esteraseaktivität in der Epidermis 93
—, cytochrine Sekretion 113
—, Differentialdiagnose durch Histochemie 890
—, Elektronenmikroskopie der Epidermis 9
—, histochemische Eigenschaften 890
— in Langerhans-Zellen 119
—, Struktur des proteingebundenen 890
„melanin dispersing hormone" bei Neunaugen 933
— — — bei Selachiern 948
Melaninablagerung bei Hämochromatosesyndrom 895
Melaningranula, Anzahl, rassische Unterschiede 107
—, „dense" 113
—, Elektronenmikroskopie 110
—, — des Stratum basale 56
—, Haarkomplexentwicklung 655

Melaningranula, histogenetische Verwandtschaft mit Mastzellen 105
—, „light" 113
—, Morphologie der Keratinocyten 59
—, Synthese 890
—, Umwandlungsvorgang 113
Melaninphagocytose, Theorien über den Mechanismus 892
„melanin stimulating hormone" bei Amphibienlarven 977
— — — bei Reptilien 991
Melaninstoffwechsel, biochemische und morphologische Grundlagen 889
Melaninsynthese, Lokalisation 115
Melanoblasten, Abstammung, experimentelle Embryologie 105
—, Definition 104
—, morphologische Entwicklung des Haarkomplexes 649
—, Terminologie 891
Melanocyten, Abstammung 103
—, —, experimentelle Embryologie 105
—, Altersabhängigkeit der Anzahl in der Haut 691
—, ATPase-Aktivität 115
—, Dendritenfunktion 114
—, dermale, Melaninsynthese 891
—, „dermal melanocytes" 105
—, Drüsenzelleigenschaften 891
—, ektodermale Herkunft 105
—, Elektronenmikroskopie 108, 891
—, Embryologie der Haut, Nervenentwicklung 674
—, Enzymaktivität 114
—, „epidermal melanin unit" 113
—, Fasern und Fibrillen, Elektronenmikroskopie 108
—, Fixierung in der Epidermis 107
—, Haarkomplexentwicklung 652, 655
— der Haut, neuroektodermale Herkunft 625
—, Innervation der Haut 387
—, Interzellularbrücken 104
—, Keratinocytenoberfläche 19
—, -Keratinocyten-Relation der Epidermis 113, 114
—, Kontakt mit Dendritenzellen der Epidermis 387

Melanocyten, Melaninbildung, Diskussion 103
— des menschlichen Haares, Morphologie 113
—, Morphologie 107
—, neoplastische, Nachweis der Melaninsynthese in Melanosomen durch Dopa-C^{14} 115
—, Nervenentwicklung in der Haut 676
—, normale Abstammung 890
—, — Histologie der Haut 103
—, Perikaryon 107
—, Plasmamembran 107
—, rassische Unterschiede 107
—, retinale, Desmosomen 107
—, Struktur der äußeren Wurzelscheide 153
—, Teilungsvorgang, Diskussion 103
—, Terminologie 891
—, Unterscheidung von Melanophagen durch saure Phosphatase-Reaktion 892
—, Verteilung in der embryonalen Epidermis 676
—, „wahre" 106
—, Zahl in der Haut 107
—, — bei Negern, Albinos und Vitiligoherden 691
Melanocytenoberfläche, Morphologie 107
„melanocyte-stimulating-hormone" bei Selachiern 948, 950
—, α- und β-Typ 948
Melanodendrocyt, Definition 104
Melanodermie, universelle, autochthone Melaninbildung 892
Melanogenese 110
—, Biochemie 114
—, rassische Unterschiede 106
„melanogenetische Ebene", Struktur der äußeren Wurzelscheide 153
Melanogenocyt, Definition 104
Melanom, malignes, Metastasierung in das subcutane Fettgewebe 825
— der Maus, Autoradiographie der Melaningranula 110
— —, Tyrosinaseaktivität in Melanocyten 115
—, universelle Melanodermie mit autochthoner Melaninbildung 892
Melanomzellen, Melanosomensynthese 891
—, PAS-Reaktion 890
Melanosomen, Elektronenmikroskopie verschiedener Stadien 112

Melanosomen, embryonale Entwicklung der Melanocyten 676
—, Lokalisation der Melaninsynthese 115
—, — der Tyrosinaseaktivität 890
—, Polymorphismus, Elektronenmikroskopie der Melanocyten 891
—, Synthese 890
Melanophagen, Melanin-Phagocytose 891
—, Terminologie 891
—, Unterscheidung von Melanocyten durch saure Phosphatase-Reaktion 892
Melanophagengranula, PAS-Reaktion 890
Melanophoren bei adulten Amphibien 982
—, Definition 104
—, doppelte Innervation der, bei Knochenfischen 966
— bei Knochenfischen 960, 964
— in nackten Hautregionen bei Vögeln 1005
— bei Neunaugen 932
— bei Reptilien 990
— bei Selachiern 942, 947
—, Terminologie 891
Melatonin bei Amphibienlarven 978
Melantonin, Einfluß auf die Melanophorenpigmente bei Tieren 949
Membran, adepidermale, bei Amphibien 973, 974
—, —, embryonale Entwicklung der Basalmembran 639
—, mucöse, „lamellated bodies" 59
Membrana reuniens, topographische Unterschiede fetaler Epithelien der Epidermis 634
„membrane-coating granules", Intercellularspalt der Keratinocyten 26
Menopause, Altersinvolution der Brustdrüse 698
Menstruationscyclus, hormonelle Einflüsse auf apokrine Schweißdrüsen 329
Merkel'sche Tastkörperchen bei Vögeln 1005
Merkelsche Tastscheiben, Histologie der Innervation das Nagels 358
— —, Innervation der Haut 377, 384
— —, Nervenapparat des Haares 406

Merkelsche Tastzellen, Nervenentwicklung in der Haut 674
— — bei Reptilien 996
Merkel'sche Zellen bei Amphibien 984
Mesaxon, Innervation der Haut 379
—, Nervenapparat des Haares 410
—, sensible Endkörperchen der Haut 421
—, subepidermales Nervengeflecht 389, 391, 392
Mesektoderm, Mesodermentwicklung 637
Mesenchym, Mesodermentwicklung 637
Mesenchymzellen, fetale Haut, Glykogengehalt 632
—, — —, Phosphorylase-Aktivität 632
—, ruhende, Ähnlichkeit mit Reticulumzelle 439
Mesoderm, Beschreibung beim menschlichen Embryo mit 4 Ursegmenten 636
—, Embryologie der Haut 624
—, Haarentwicklung 644
—, induktive Haarbildung 647
Metachromasie, Arteriolen der Haut, Histochemie 525
—, arteriovenöse Anastomosen, Histochemie 556
—, Darstellung von Schleimstoffen in der Haut 877
—, Differenzierung der vitalen von der postmortalen 757
—, dunkle Zellen 249
Metamerie, Embryologie der Haut 625
Metamorphose bei Amphibien 969, 981, 984
Met-Hämoglobin, Differentialdiagnose der Grünverfärbung der Leichenhaut 731
Methionin, Autoradiographie der Epidermis 68
—, Einbau in keratogene Zonen des Haarfollikels 177
Methylenblau-Färbung der weißen Dendritenzellen 106
Methylblau-Methode, Nervenentwicklung in der Haut 674
Methylthiouracil, Einfluß auf die Reptilienhäutung 990
Mieschersche Radiärknötchen s. Radiärknötchen
Mikrobid, leukoklastisches (MIESCHER-STORCK), Patho-Histologie 809

Mikrofibrille, Durchmesser 443
—, Entstehung der 443
—, kollagene, Ultrastruktur 446
—, —, — der Bindegewebsgrundsubstanz 451
—, Ultrastruktur der Basalmembran 463, 464
Mikroincineration, Histotopographie der Epidermis 66, 67
Mikroradiographie, Talgdrüsen-Zellen 194
Mikrosomen der Epidermis, β-Glucuronidase-Aktivität 101
— der Langerhans-Zelle 117
—, RNS-Gehalt in Drüsenzellen der apokrinen Schweißdrüsen 277
Mikrotubuli der Melanophoren bei Knochenfischen 964
Mikrovilli, Elektronenmikroskopie des Periderms 627, 628, 629
—, —, Talgdrüsen 205
—, epidermaler Schweißdrüsen-Ausführungsgang 258
—, Uktrastruktur der ekkrinen Drüsen 665
Milchdrüsen, Haaranlage, Embryonalentwicklung 661
—, Schweißdrüsen, Embryonalentwicklung 661
—, Talgdrüsen, Embryonalentwicklung 661
Milchgänge, Embryonalentwicklung 661
Milchleiste, embryonale Entwicklung spezialisierter Drüsen der Haut 661
—, topographische Unterschiede der embryonalen Epidermis 634, 635
Milchstreifen, Entwicklungsmechanik der Haut 644
—, topographische Unterschiede der embryonalen Epidermis 634, 635
Millon-Reaktion, Reaktion von Fibrin, Fibrinoid und Hyalin 871
Mineralsalze, Einlagerung von, bei Knochenfischen 963
Mitochondrien im Axon, Innervation der Haut 380
—, Cytochromoxydase-positive Granula in der Epidermis 86
— der ekkrinen Schweißdrüsen, Altersveränderungen 696

Mitochondrien der Epidermis, NADH- und NADPH-Tetrazolium-Reduktase-Aktivität 90
—, spezifische Coenzym-gebundene Dehydrogenasen 90
—, Ubiquinon-Aktivität 103
— der Keratinocyten, Anzahl in verschiedenen Epidermisschichten 55
—, ATPase-Aktivität 99
—, Elektronenmikroskopie 55
—, Succinyldehydrogenase 55
— der Langerhans-Zelle 117
— in Lemnocyten, sensible Endkörperchen der Haut 422
— der Meissnerschen Tastkörperchen, Zerfall 419
— der Melanocyten, Elektronenmikroskopie 109
—, Melanogenese 110
—, mikroskopische Anatomie der apokrinen Schweißdrüsen 277
— der Schwannschen Zelle, sensible Endkörperchen der Haut 422
—, subepidermales Nervengeflecht 392
— in den seniblen Endkörperchen der Haut 417
—, Ubiquinon-Aktivität in den Lipoprotein-Membranen 102
—, Ultrastruktur der apokrinen Schweißdrüsen 290, 291
—, — des Stratum basale 56
Mitochondrienmembran, Keratinocyten 22
Mitose, beeinflussende Faktoren 64
Mitose-Achse, Lage in der Epidermis 63
Mitose-Index, Epidermis 62
Mitosen, Autoradiographie 63
—, Haarentwicklung 645
—, Nagelwachstum 350
—, Papillarkörper 469
—, Vorkommen in apokrinen Schweißdrüsen 279
—, Zahl in der Epidermis 61, 62
—, —, Altersabhängigkeit 690
—, — und Lokalisation während Haarcyclus 161
Mitosenrate der Epidermis des Neugeborenen 636
—, Haarcyclus 161

„mitosis operon", Mitose der Keratinocyten 65
Mollsche Drüsen, Embryonalentwicklung der apokrinen Schweißdrüsen 268
— —, Histochemie der Haarkomplexentwicklung 659
Mongolenfleck, dermale Melanocytenansammlung 891
—, Entstehung 890
—, pathologische Melaninablagerung in der Haut 889
Mongolismus, Entwicklung der Affenfurche 636
Monoaminoxydase, Basalzellen, Cytochemie 253
—, Cytochemie, myoepitheliale Zellen 236
—, helle Zellen, Cytochemie 242
—, Histochemie des Coriums und des subcutanen Fettgewebes 641
—, — der fetalen ekkrinen Drüsen 668
—, — — Epidermis 633
—, — der Haarkomplexentwicklung 659
—, — der Keratinocyten 87
—, — der apokrinen Schweißdrüsen 321
—, — der Talgdrüsen 196, 202
—, Histotopochemie des Haarfollikels 176
—, Kapillaren der Haut, Histochemie 537
—, myoepitheliale Zellen 482
—, Nachweis in Fibrocyten von Corium und Subcutis 431
— in der unverhornten Epidermis 87
—, Venolen der Haut, Histochemie 537
Monocyten, Ähnlichkeit mit Histiocyten der Haut 436
—, Identifizierung durch Peroxydase-Reaktion 436
Monocytenleukämie, akute, Erythema nodosum als Primärsymptom 836
Montgomery-Drüsen 218
—, Embryonalentwicklung 661
—, Milchzuckernachweis 663
Moorleiche, Moormumifikation 749
Moormumienhaut, Konsistenz 750
—, Veränderungen der Haut in der späten Leichenzeit 749
Morbus Addison, idiomuskulärer Wulst 722

Morbus Besnier-Boeck-Schaumann, Erythema nodosum 836
— —, — —, Patho-Histologie 796
— —, Manifestation des Sarkoid Darier-Roussy 800
Morbus Fox-Fordyce, altersbedingte Veränderungen der mikroskopischen Anatomie der apokrinen Schweißdrüsen 283
— —, Gestagenwirkung auf 330
— —, histochemischer Glykogennachweis in apokrinen Schweißdrüsen 309
— —, hormonelle Einflüsse auf apokrine Schweißdrüsen 330
— —, Veränderung der apokrinen Schweißdrüsen 697
Morbus Raynaud, Glykogenanreicherung im Gewebe 886
Morbus Werlhof, Ätiologie der Lipome 839
„mosaic pattern", Haarcyclus 162
Motivbild nach HORSTMANN, Stratum papillare 467
MSH s. „melanocyte-stimulating-hormone"
Mucicarmin-Färbung, Darstellung der Schleimstoffe der Haut 878
— von Hyalin 869
Mucin, Ablagerung und Speicherung in der Haut 874
—, Anreicherung bei endokrinen Störungen 876
— der mesenchymalen Grundsubstanz, Regulierung der Mucinmenge 876
Mucinosen, Einteilung 878
—, histologische Veränderungen 878
—, Mastzellvermehrung 875
—, Vermehrung der sauren Mucopolysaccharide 875
—, Zusammensetzung des Mucins 875
Mucinosis follicularis, Elektronenmikroskopie 880
— —, Klinik und Patho-Histologie 880
— —, „lamellated bodies" 59
— —, Sensibilitätsstörungen 880
— —, Verminderung der Schweißsekretion 880
Mucophanerosis intrafollicularis et seboglandularis, Klinik und Pathohistologie 880

Mucopolysaccharidablagerung und Hypoxie 880
Mucopolysaccharide in der Amphibienhaut 979
—, Analyse der kollagenen Faser 440
—, argyrophile Faser 444
—, arteriovenöse Anastomosen, Histochemie 556
— in den Basalzellen der fetalen Epidermis 631
—, Bildung in Mastzellen 438
—, Bindegewebsgrundsubstanz 450
— der Bindegewebsgrundsubstanz, Altersveränderung 452
—, Bursae synoviales in der Subcutis 478
—, dunkle Zellen 247
—, Fibroblastentheorie 875
—, Funktion im Zellstoffwechsel des Nagels 364
—, Gram-positive Substanzen in Keratinocyten 80
— der Haut, enzymatische Regulierung 877
—, Hautmesenchymmatrix 637
—, Herkunft der Bindegewebsgrundsubstanz 451
—, Histochemie der Keratinocyten 78
—, — des Nagels 362
—, histochemischer Nachweis 877
—, — — in Phagosomen 435
—, interzellulärer Spalt der Epidermiszellen 23
—, Isthmus, Haarkomplexentwicklung 653
—, Kittmasse der Basalmembran 464
—, kollagene Faser 446
—, „lamellated bodies" 59
—, Matrix der Fibroblasten 432
—, Nachweis bei aktinischer Elastose 874
—, neutrale, Arteriolen der Haut, Histochemie 525, 537
—, —, Bedeutung für die Basalmembran 465
—, —, embryonale Entwicklung der Basalmembran 639
—, —, Histochemie der Basalmembran 463
—, —, Kapillaren der Haut, Histochemie 536, 537
—, saure, Abbau durch β-Glucuronidase im Intercellularspalt der Epidermis 101

Mucopolysaccharide, saure, Analyse der elastischen Faser 448
—, —, Arteriolen der Haut, Histochemie 525, 537
—, —, Bestandteil des Siderinpigmentes 896
—, —, Blutgefäßneubildung der Haut, Histochemie 559
—, —, Chemie des Amyloid 863
—, —, dunkle Zellen 249
—, —, Funktion des Papillarkörpers 469
—, —, Histochemie apokriner Schweißdrüsen 309
—, —, — der Basalmembran 463
—, —, — der Gewebsmastzellen 437
—, —, Histotopographie im Haarfollikel 171
—, —, Kapillaren der Haut, Histochemie 536, 537
—, —, Synthese durch Kapillarendothelien bei Permeabilitätsstörungen 864
—, —, Veränderungen der Haut in der späten Leichenzeit 732
—, —, Vermehrung im Blut bei Mucinose 875
—, —, — bei Mucinosen 875
—. Stoffwechsel in der Bindegewebsgrundsubstanz 451
—, Synthese 80
—, — bei Kollagenbildung 441
—, Übertragergewebe 452
—, Ultrastruktur der Bindegewebsgrundsubstanz 451
—, Unterscheidung verschiedener Typen durch Hyaluronidasen 453
—, Venolen der Haut, Histochemie 537, 550
—, Vorkommen in den Intercellularräumen der Epidermis 363
—, — im embryonalen Nagel 363
—, Wasserretention im Fettgewebe 459
—, Zugehörigkeit zu Stützgewebe des Nagels 364
—, Zusammensetzung der Grundsubstanz 874
Mucoproteide, Bausteine der Grundsubstanz 875
—, Depolymerisierung durch Schilddrüsenhormon 877
Mucoproteine, braunes Fett 457
—, Histochemie des embryonalen Bindegewebes 641

Mucus Malpighii, Nomenklatur Stratum spinosum 10
Mueller's Methode, Kapillaren der Haut, Histochemie 537
Mumienhaut, makroskopischer Befund 740
—, mikroskopischer Befund 740
Mumifikation, forensisch-kriminalistische Bedeutung 741
—, partielle 740
—, primäre, Vertrocknung der Leichenhaut 739
—, sekundäre, Fäulnis der Leichenhaut 739
—, totale 740
—, Veränderungen der Haut in der späten Leichenzeit 739
—, Zeitdauer 740
Mumifizierung, artifizielle 739
—, natürliche 739
Mundlippen, postmortale Vertrocknung 726
Mundschleimhaut, Epithel, Altersveränderung 690
—, —, Mitochondrien- und Fibrillenanzahl 56
Mund-zu-Mund-Beatmung, Hautveränderungen 728
Murexidprobe, Uratnachweis in den Tophi 889
Musculi cutis diagonales 481
Musculus arrector pili 481
— — —, Gefäßversorgung 594, 598
— — —, glatte Muskulatur 479
— — — des fetalen Haarkomplexes, Anzahl 660
— — —, fetale Haut, Glykogengehalt 632
— — —, — —, Phosphorylase-Aktivität 632
— — —, Histochemie 481
— — —, morphologische Entwicklung des Haarkomplexes 649, 650, 656
— — —, Rigor 722
— — —, subepidermales Nervengeflecht 394, 397, 398, 399
— — —, Veränderung bei Mucinosen 879
— — —, Volumen in verschiedenen Stadien des Embryonallebens 660
Musculus sexualis, glatte Muskulatur 480
Muskulatur, cutane, bei Reptilien 993
—, glatte, der Haut 479
—, —, —, Altersveränderung 695

Muskulatur, glatte, der Haut, Mesodermentwicklung 637
— der Haut, mikroskopische und submikroskopische Anatomie der 479
—, mimische, mikroskopische und submikroskopische Anatomie 482
—, postmortale Erregbarkeit 723
Muskelschicht, arteriovenöse Anastomosen 554
Muskeltraining, Einfluß auf Mitoserate 64
Mycosis fungoides, Fettgewebsinfiltration 824
Myelitis, neurotrophische Atrophie der Haut 792
—, segmentale, neurogene Lipome 838
Myelom, multiples, Amyloidose 866
Myoepithelzellen, Aldolaseaktivität 310, 313
— der ekkrinen Drüsen, Embryonalentwicklung 664
—, Glycerinaldehyd-3-Phosphat-Dehydrogenase-Nachweis 310, 313
—, Glycerin-1-Phosphat-Dehydrogenaseaktivität 310, 314
—, Glycerin-1-Phosphat-Oxydaseaktivität 310, 315
—, Histochemie, Glykogengehalt 309
—, Hypertrophie, hormonelle Einflüsse auf apokrine Schweißdrüsen 329
—, mikroskopische Anatomie der apokrinen Schweißdrüsen 279
—, Morphologie der apokrinen Schweißdrüsen 275
—, Phosphorylaseaktivität 310, 312
—, Ultrastruktur der apokrinen Schweißdrüsen 288, 301
—, —, Innervation 304
—, —, Mikrotubuli 303
—, —, Myofilamente 302
—, —, der Zellkerne 303
—, Vorkommen bei Mammacarcinom 279
Myofibrillen, glatte Muskulatur 479
—, myoepitheliale Zellen 482
Myofilamente, Ultrastruktur der Myoepithelzellen 302
Myosin, Keratinisation 18
Myristinsäure, Aufbau des Fettes in der Subcutis 789
Myxodermie, euthyreotische, Mucinosen 878

Myxödem, Carotinämie 898
—, prätibiales, Erhöhung der Blut-Mucopolysaccharide 876
Myxoedema circumscriptum praetibiale bei Hyperthyreose, Einteilung der Mucinosen 878
Myxoedema diffusum bei Hyperthyreose, Einteilung der Mucinosen 878

Nabelschnur, postmortale Vertrocknung 726
Nackenhaut, Anatomie des Gefäßnetzes 570
NADasen, Arteriolen der Haut, Histochemie 537
—, Kapillaren der Haut, Histochemie 537
—, Venolen der Haut, Histochemie 537
NADH-Tetrazolium-Reductase, helle Zellen, Cytochemie 241
—, Histochemie der Keratinocyten 89
—, histochemischer Nachweis in apokrinen Schweißdrüsen 310, 318
—, Histotopochemie des Haarfollikels 176
—, Histotopographie der Ubiquinon-reaktiven Formazan-Granula 103
— in Mitochondrien der Keratinocyten 56
Nadi-Reaktion, Histochemie der Keratinocyten 85
NADPasen, Arteriolen der Haut, Histochemie 537
—, Kapillaren der Haut, Histochemie 537
—, Venolen der Haut, Histochemie 537
NADPH-Tetrazolium-Reductase, helle Zellen, Cytochemie 241
—, Histochemie der Keratinocyten 89
—, histochemischer Nachweis in apokrinen Schweißdrüsen 310, 318
—, Histotopochemie des Haarfollikels 176
—, Histotopographie der Ubiquinon-reaktiven Formazan-Granula 103
— in Mitochondrien der Keratinocyten 56
NADP-Reductase, Arteriolen der Haut, Histochemie 526
—, Venolen der Haut, Histochemie 550

NAD-Reductase, Arteriolen der Haut, Histochemie 526
—, Blutgefäßneubildung der Haut, Histochemie 560
—, Venolen der Haut, Histochemie 550
Naevoxanthoendotheliom, Nosologie, Histiocytose 882
Naevus coeruleus, Melaninsynthese 892
— lipomatodes cutaneus superficialis Hoffmann-Zurhelle, Patho-Histologie 823
— ota, dermale Melanocytenansammlung 891
— papillomatosus, Syntopie mit apokrinen Schweißdrüsen 272
— sebaceus, heterotope apokrine Schweißdrüsen 272
— syringocystadenomatosus, Syntopie mit apokrinen Schweißdrüsen 272
— verruciformis, Syntopie mit apokrinen Schweißdrüsen 272
Naevuszellen, Melanosomensynthese 891
Nagel, Altersnagel, Anatomie des 342
—, Altersveränderung 699
—, Anatomie des 340
—, Basophilie des Keratins, Histochemie 370
—, distale Grenzfurche, Embryologie 670
—, — Leiste, Embryologie 670
—, dorsal plume, Embryologie 670
—, Elektronenmikroskopie 373
—, Embryologie des 342, 669
—, Entwicklung des 372
—, Gefäßversorgung, Histologie 354
—, fetale Haut, Glykogengehalt 632
—, — —, Phosphorylase-Aktivität 632
—, Histochemie 361
—, — des, Enzyme 365
—, — des, Mucopolysaccharide 362
—, — der Nagelentwicklung 673
—, — des, Ribonucleinsäure 364
—, histochemische Untersuchung der alkalischen Phosphatase 366
—, — — der Amylo-Phosphorylase 367

Nagel, histochemische Untersuchung der Cholinesterase 366
—, — — der PAS-positiven Substanzen im Nagelkeratin 369
—, — — der sauren Phosphatase 365
—, — — der Sulfohydrylgruppen im Keratin 370
—, Histologie des 349
—, Innervation, Histologie 357
—, Literatur über Histologie und Histochemie 374
—, mikroskopische Untersuchung des embryonalen Nagels 344
—, Nageleinheit 340
—, normale Histologie und Histochemie 339
—, Pigmentierung des 350
—, primäres Nagelfeld, Embryologie 670
—, proximale Matrix, Embryologie 670
—, proximaler Nagelwall, Embryologie 670
—, Rillenbildung im Alter 699
—, Struktur des embryonalen 673
—, terminale Matrix, Nomenklatur 671
—, Terminologie 340
—, Venen des 598
—, vergleichende Anatomie 339
Nagelanlage, Lokalisation, Embryologie 669
Nagelbett, s. auch Hyponychium
—, Anatomie des Nagels 340, 342
—, Embryologie des Nagels 671
—, fetale Haut, Glykogengehalt 632
—, — —, Phosphorylase-Aktivität 632
—, Terminologie 340
Nagelentwicklung, Elektronenmikroskopie 672
Nagelfeld, Embryologie des Nagels 343
Nagelfurche, Anatomie des Nagels 340, 342
Nagelhäutchen, Anatomie des Nagels 342
Nagelmatrix, Anatomie des Nagels 341
—, Basalzellen, Ultrastruktur 374
—, Histochemie 361
Nagelplatte, Anatomie des Nagels 341

Nagelplatte, Embryologie des Nagels 671
—, fetale Haut, Glykogengehalt 632
—, — —, Phosphorylase-Aktivität 632
Nageltasche, hintere, Embryologie des Nagels 671
Nagelwachstum 350
Nagelwall, Anatomie des Nagels 340, 342
„nail bed", Embryologie des Nagels 671
Naphthol-AS-Esterase, Histochemie der fetalen ekkrinen Drüsen 668
—, Methode, Histochemie der fetalen Haut 633
— -Reaktion, Histochemie der Haarkomplexentwicklung 659
α-Naphthol-Esterase, Histochemie der fetalen ekkrinen Drüsen 668
α-Naphthol-Reaktion nach Gomori, Histochemie der Haarkomplexentwicklung 659
α-Naphthylesterase, Kapillaren der Haut, Histochemie 537
—, Venolen der Haut, Histochemie 537
Narbenbildung 471
Nasenbluten, postmortales 715
Nasenrückenhaut, Stratum papillare 465
Natrium, Histochemie der Keratinocyten 67
Natriumlinolenat, Hemmung des O_2-Verbrauchs im subcutanen Fettgewebe 828
Natriumpumpe, ATP-ase-Aktivität in der Epidermis 100
Natriumrückresorption, Basalzellen 253
Natriumtransport, helle Zellen 244
Natternhemd 990
Necrobiosis lipoidica cum et sine diabete, Glykogenanreicherung im Hautbindegewebe 886
— — diabeticorum, Patho-Histologie 814
— —, Ätiologie und Pathogenese 837
— —, Lipidablagerung in der Haut 881
— —Patho-Histologie 884
— —, — der medikamentösen Lipodystrophie 804
— —, — des Paraffinoms 805

Necrobiosis maculosa, Ätiologie und Pathogenese 837
— —, Glykogenanreicherung im Hautbindegewebe 886
— —, Patho-Histologie 815
Necrosis progressiva subcutanea neonatorum, Patho-Histologie 808
Nekrophagen, Hautveränderungen der späten Leichenzeit 733
Nekrophagenzusammensetzung, Abhängigkeit von Milien 733
Nekrothermometrie 710
Neogenese, Blutgefäße der Haut 558
nephrotisches Syndrom, Carotinämie 898
Nervenapparat des Haares 377, 378, 386, 400
Nerven, arteriovenöse Anastomosen der Haut 566
—, cholinesterasepositive, in ekkrinen Drüsen der Haut 664
—, Darstellung durch Färbemethoden 378, 379, 387, 398
—, — durch Phasenkontrastmikroskopie 378
—, Embryologie der Haut 673
—, epidermale, Innervation der Haut 378—389
—, —, Wurzelscheiden 401
— der fetalen Haut, Glykogengehalt 632
— — —, Phosphorylase-Aktivität 632
—, Gefäßnerven der Haut 398—400
— der Haut, Altersveränderungen 702
— —, Neuroektodermale Herkunft 625
—, Innervation der Hautarterien 565
—, — der Hautarteriolen 565
—, — der Hautvenen 566
—, — der Hautvenolen 566
—, Leitungsgeschwindigkeit der Hautnerven 389, 408
—, Markscheiden der Hautnervenfasern 377, 381, 383, 400, 405, 419
—, Nervenapparat des Haares 400—410
—, perivasale, sensorische 564
—, vegetative 564
—, Regeneration 384
—, sensible Endkörperchen der Haut 411—423
—, sensorische, Ausbreitung während der embryonalen Entwicklung 675

Nerven, subepidermales Nervengeflecht 389—398
—, vegetative, Speicherungsmechanismus der Fettzellen 461
—, —, im univacuolären Fettzellgewebe 456
Nervenendapparate, Innervation der Haut 377, 378, 383, 384
—, Nervenapparat des Haares 401
—, sensible Endkörperchen der Haut 411
Nervenendigungen der Haut, Embryologie 674
Nervenfaserbündel, Blutgefäße der Haut 564
Nervenfasern, arteriovenöse Anastomosen 555
—, cerebrospinale, Innervation der Haut 379, 384, 386, 389, 406, 421
—, epidermale 378
—, —, der Kopfhaut 412
—, hederiforme Endigungen, Embryologie 674
—, intraepidermale, Zahl in der Embryonalentwicklung 675
—, markarme, Innervation der Haut 379, 381
—, —, sensible Endkörperchen der Haut 421
—, markreiche, Innervation der Haut 379
—, —, sensible Endkörperchen der Haut 421
—, perikapilläre, Hautkapillaren 566
—, perivaskuläre, ,,vegetative end formation'' 564
—, vegetative, Innervation der Haut 379, 384, 386
—, —, Nervenapparat des Haares 406, 407
—, —, sensible Endkörperchen der Haut 421
Nervennetz, subcutanes, bei Vögeln 1004
Nervenplexus, cutaner, bei Knochenfischen 968
—, subepidermaler 379, 380, 387, 389, 410
—, —, nach Röntgenbestrahlung 393, 396, 397
Nervensystem, Frühentwicklung 673
Nervus facialis, Innervation der Skeletmuskulatur der Haut 482
— spinalis, Embryologie der Haut 673
Neunaugen, Corium der 932
—, Deckplatte der 927, 931

Neunaugen, Epidermis der 927
—, Haut der, vergleichende Histologie 927
—, Innervation der Haut 933
—, Subcutis der 932
Neuralleiste, alkalische Phosphatase-Aktivität 633
—, Embryologie der Haut 624
—, Querschnitt Embryo 625
Neuralleistenabkömmlinge, Embryologie der Haut 673
Neuralleistenzellen bei Knochenfischen 964
Neuralrohr, Querschnitt Embryo 625
Neurocutanes Geflecht, Blutgefäße der Haut 564
Neuroeffectorgebiet, Innervation der Haut 379, 382, 387
Neuroektoderm, Embryologie der Haut 625
,,neuroepitheliale'' Verbindungen, Innervation der Haut 383
— —, Nervenapparat des Haares 410
Neurofibrillen, Blutgefäße der Haut 564
Neurofibrom, Syntopie mit apokrinen Schweißdrüsen 272
Neurofibromatosis generalisata, nervale Induktion lipomatöser Tumoren 838
Neurofilamente, Innervation der Haut 384
Neuromasten bei Knochenfischen 969
—, Seitenliniensystem bei Chondrichthyes 951, 954
Neurotubuli, Innervation der Haut 384
Neuralfett, Definition 880
—, Histochemie der apokrinen Schweißdrüsen 307
,,nexus'', Keratinocyten-Ultrastruktur 34
Niere, Hochdruckniere, Succinyldehydrogenaseaktivität 88
Nilblau-Färbung, Esteraseaktivität des Stratum corneum 95
Nilblausulfat-Färbung, Darstellung von Neutralfetten bei Adiponecrosis subcutanea neonatorum 808
—, Histochemie der Keratinocyten 81
— bei Histiocytose und Xanthogranulomatose 883
—, Talgdrüsen 197

Nilblau-Sulfat, Kapillaren der Haut 537
—, Reaktion von Fibrin, Fibrinoid und Hyalin 870
Ninhydrin-Schiff-Technik, Histochemie der Keratinocyten 67
Nitroprussid-Färbung, Histochemie der Keratinocyten 70
—, -SH- und -S-S-Gruppen in Keratinocyten 72
Nitroprussid-Methode, Kapillaren der Haut, Histochemie 536
Nodular-Vasculitis, Patho-Histologie 799
„nodule of Bizzozero" 31
„nodule of Ranvier" 31
Noradrenalin, Einfluß auf Melanophorenpigmente bei Tieren 950
Nuclease, Histochemie der Intermediärzone der Epidermis 18
—, — der Keratinocyten 100
Nucleinsäuren, Histochemie der apokrinen Schweißdrüsen 305
—, —, arteriovenöse Anastomosen 556
—, — der Keratinocyten 68
Nucleolus, Morphologie der Keratinocyten 60
Nucleoproteine, Arteriolen der Haut, Histochemie 526, 537
—, arteriovenöse Anastomosen, Histochemie 556
—, Kapillaren der Haut, Histochemie 536
—, Venolen der Haut, Histochemie 537, 550
5-Nucleotidasen, Histochemie, Arteriolen der Haut 527, 537
—, —, Blutgefäßneubildung der Haut 561
—, —, Kapillaren der Haut 537
—, —, Venolen der Haut 537
—, Histotopochemie des Haarfollikels 176
Nucleus, Elektronenmikroskopie, Talgdrüsen 205
—, Lipide, Histochemie der Keratinocyten 84
—, Morphologie der Keratinocyten 60

Oberflächenzellen, Absorption 257
—, Cytochemie 256
—, Desmosomen 255

Oberflächenzellen, Elektronenmikroskopie 254
—, endoplasmatisches Reticulum 256
—, Ergastoplasma 256
—, Ergastoplasma 256
—, Funktion 257
—, Glycogen 256
—, intradermaler Schweißdrüsen-Ausführungsgang 254
—, Mitochondrien 254
—, Mikrovilli 255
—, Mucopolysaccharide 258
—, Natriumtransport 257
—, Pinocytose 255, 257
—, Plasmamembran 255
—, Sekretion 255
—, Stützzellen 257
Oberhäutchen bei Reptilien 989
„Odland's bodies", β-Glucuronidaseaktivität 101
— —, Interzellularspalt der Keratinocyten 26
Odontoblasten bei Selachiern 944
Oedeme, postmortale Gewebswasserverschiebung 718
Ölcysten bei Atrophie des subcutanen Fettgewebes 794
Ölrot O, Reaktion von Fibrin, Fibrinoid und Hyalin 870
Ölsäure, Aufbau des Fettes in der Subcutis 789
Oestradiol, direkte Wirkung auf apokrine Schweißdrüsen 330
Oestrogene, Einfluß auf Mitoserate 64
—, medikamentöses Erythema nodosum 836
—, Wirkung auf Mastzellen 438
Ohrmuschel, Subcutiskonstruktion 477
Ohrschmalzdrüsen, Embryologie 663
Orcein, Darstellung argyrophiler Fasern 444
—, — elastischer Fasern 448
Orcein-Färbung bei aktinischer Elastose 873
— elastischer Fasern des Stratum reticulare 471
Orthokeratose bei Psoriasis, Fetttröpfchen in Keratinocyten 83
Osmidrosis, Vorkommen von Eisen im apokrinen Sekret 311
Osmium, Darstellung der Schichten des Stratum lucidum 13
—, — des Stratum corneum 15

Ovariektomie, hormonelle Einflüsse auf apokrine Schweißdrüsen 329
—, Lipogranulombildung 840
Palisadengeflecht, Nervenapparat des Haares 402
Palma, Stratum corneum 15
—, Stratum lucidum 14
Palmitinsäure, Aufbau des Fettes in der Subcutis 789
Palor, Haut der frühen Leichenzeit 710
Pankreascarcinom, Metastasierung in das subcutane Fettgewebe 825
Pankreaserkrankungen, Kombination mit Pfeifer-Weber-Christian-Syndrom und Diabetes mellitus 836
Panniculitis nach Anwendung von Medikamenten 830
—, artifizielle Ätiologie 840
— nach Einwirkung thermischer Noxen, ionisierender Strahlen und Pankreasextrakten 831
—, experimentelle Auslösung 829
—, Lipogranulom 830
— nodularis febrilis non suppurativa Pfeifer-Weber-Christian bei Tumormetastasen im subcutanen Fettgewebe 826
— — non suppurativa, Patho-Histologie 800
—, Pathologie des subcutanen Fettgewebes 795
— bei Poliomyelitis 799
— Rothmann-Makai, Lipome 838
— subacuta nodosa migrans Vilanova-Piñol-Aguadé, Patho-Histologie 803
— carnosus, Skeletmuskulatur der Haut 482
Papillarkörper, s. auch Stratum papillare
—, Altersatrophie 469
—, Basalmembran 462
—, Bedeutung des 469
—, Fermentaktivität 474
—, Funktion 468
—, Gefäßeinbau 478
—, Geschlechtsunterschiede 467
—, Hautoberflächenvergrößerung 467
—, Metachromasie der Bindegewebsgrundsubstanz 450
—, Rückbildung 466
—, Tastempfindung 469
Papillarleisten, Negativbild 466

Papillarmuster, embryonale Entwicklung 636
Papillarlinienmuster der Fingerbeere, Identitätsfeststellung 729
Papillarschlingen, Durchmesser 534
—, Erythrocytenagglutination 534
—, Länge 533
—, Morphologie 533
Papillen der Haut, Geschlechtsbestimmung zur Identitätsfeststellung 729
— —, Hautstruktur 4, 5, 6, 7
—, dermale, Struktur des Haarfollikels 153
—, morphologische Entwicklung des Haarkomplexes 649, 650
Papillenhaar, Strukturveränderungen des Haarfollikels 157
Papillenhals, morphologische Entwicklung des Haarbulbus 652
Papillenpolster, morphologische Entwicklung des Bulbus 651
—, — — des Haarkomplexes 649
Papillenrest, Strukturveränderungen des Haarfollikels 160
PAS-Granula, diastaseresistente, „lamellated bodies" 59
PAS-positiver Grenzstreifen, Veränderungen der Haut in der späten Leichenzeit 732
PAS-positive Substanzen, Histochemie der Keratinocyten 78
— —, histochemische Untersuchung des Nagelkeratins 369
— in Sekretzellen apokriner Schweißdrüsen, Altersveränderungen der Haut 697
PAS-Reaktion, aktinische Elastose 874
—, apokrine Drüsen, Haarkomplexentwicklung 657
—, Arteriolen der Haut, Histochemie 525
—, arteriovenöse Anastomosen 556
—, Basalmembran, Altersveränderung des Coriums 693
—, Basalmembran, Haarentwicklung 649
—, Bindegewebsgrundsubstanz 450
—, Darstellung des Amyloid 863

PAS-Reaktion, Darstellung des Glykogenvorkommens in der Haut 886
—, — von Schleimstoffen in der Haut 877
—, elastische Fasern 449
—, embryonale Fasern 638
—, fetale Epidermis 631
—, Fetttröpfchen in Keratinocyten 83
— am Gefrierschnitt, Reaktion von Fibrin, Fibrinoid und Hyalin 871
— im Haarkeim 648
—, Histochemie der Basalmembran 462
—, — der Intermediärzone der Epidermis 18
—, — der Keratinocyten 84
—, — —, Glykogen 77
— im Infundibulum, Haarkomplexentwicklung 654
—, Kapillaren der Haut, Histochemie 536
—, kollagene Faser 446
—, Lamina densa 464
— der Melaningranula 890
—, Musculus arrector pili 481
— am Paraffin-Schnitt, Reaktion von Fibrin, Fibrinoid und Hyalin 871
— bei Porphyria cutanea tarda 894
—, Stratum corneum 15
—, Ultrastruktur der Bindegewebsgrundsubstanz 451
PAS-reaktive Lipoproteide, Histochemie der apokrinen Schweißdrüsen 309
— Polysaccharide, Histochemie der Keratinocyten 78
— Substanz, Diastase-resistente, Nachweis in apokrinen Schweißdrüsen 307, 309
Pappenheim-Färbung, Fetttröpfchen in Keratinocyten 83
Papulose atrophiante maligne (Degos), Patho-Histologie 809
Paraffinom, experimentell erzeugte lipogranulomatöse Reaktion 830
—, Fremdkörpergranulome 901
—, Patho-Histologie 805
Parakeratose, Fetttröpfchen in Keratinocyten 83
—, Mitochondrien- und Fibrillenanzahl 56
—, Nexus der Keratinocyten 35
—, Protofilamente 54
—, Stratum intermedium 11

Parakeratotische Fetttröpfchen 83
Paramyloid, Darstellung 863
Paramyloidose, Ähnlichkeit mit Hyalinose 871
—, Einteilungsschema der Amyloidosen 865
Parasympathicus, Hemmwirkung auf den Fettstoffwechsel 829
Pathothesaurismosen, Fettgewebsatrophie der Haut 794
Pauly-Reaktion, Epidermis 67
Pektinase, Wirkung auf Basalmembran 463
Pellagra, neurotrophische Atrophie der Haut 792
Pelzdunen bei Vögeln 1005
Pemphigus, „tonofilament-desmosome complex" 40
Penis, Musculus sexualis 480
—, Subcutiskonstruktion 477
Periarteriitis nodosa, Ätiologie und Pathogenese 837
— — cutanea benigna 809
— — —, Patho-Histologie 809
—, Einteilung in allergische und nicht-allergische Formen 837
— —, Radiärknötchen, Patho-Histologie des Erythema nodosum 796
— —, Typ Kussmaul-Maier-Gruber, Patho-Histologie 813
— —, — —, Sonderformen 809
Pericardialplatte, Embryologie der Epidermis 625
Pericyten, argyrophile Faserbildung 443
—, Entstehung aus Fibrocyten 434
—, Kapillaren der Haut 534, 536, 539, 542
Periderm, Embryologie der Epidermis 627
—, embryonales, bei Vögeln 998
—, der fetalen Epidermis, Glykogengehalt 631
—, funktionelle Anpassung der fetalen Haut 627
Periderm-Hornschicht der fetalen Epidermis, Phosphorylase-Aktivität 632
—, Glykogengehalt 632
Peridermzellen, Elektronenmikroskopie, Mikrovilli 630, 631
— eines Fetus, Elektronenmikroskopie 627

Peridermzellen, Umwandlung zu Hornzellen 629
„perifollicular networks", vergleichende Anatomie, Blutgefäße der Haut 501, 508, 511
Perikaryon, Melanocyten 107
Perinatale Entwicklung, Blutgefäße der Haut 499, 511, 514
Periost, Subcutiskonstruktion der Ferse 476
Periphlebitis bei Erythema nodosum lipogranulomatosum Carol 797
Perissodactyla, vergleichende Anatomie, Blutgefäße der Haut 508
Peritonitis, Putrifikation in der späten Leichenzeit 730
Perjodat-Leukofuchsin-Methode, Darstellung der Grundsubstanz 874
Perjodsäure-Schiff-Reaktion s. PAS-Reaktion
—, Darstellung argyrophiler Fasern 444
Perjodsäure-Silbersalz-Methode, Darstellung der Ultrastruktur argyrophiler Fasern 444
Perl-Färbung, Talgdrüsen 201
Perlorgane bei Knochenfischen 957
Peroxydase, histochemischer Nachweis in Phagosomen 435
Pepsin, Wirkung auf Basalmembran 463
Perthesche Blutungen, Hautveränderungen der frühen Leichenzeit 717
Pertinax-Körperchen, Altersveränderungen des Nagels 699
Pfeifer-Weber-Christian-Syndrom, Ätiologie und Pathogenese 835
—, Kombination mit Pankreasschäden und Diabetes mellitus 836
—, Spontanpanniculitis, Patho-Histologie 800
Phagocytose, Histiocyten 434
Phagosomen, Fibrocyten von Corium und Subcutis 431
—, Pinocytose der Histiocyten 435
„phanerogenous zone", Histochemie der Keratinocyten 71
Pharmakodynamik, Arteriolen der Haut 566

Phenolase, melaninbildende, enzymhistochemischer Nachweis 890
— s. auch Phenoloxydase
Phenol-Oxydase, Histochemie der Melanocyten 114
Phenylalanin, Autoradiographie der Epidermis 68
Phosphamidase, Histochemie der Keratinocyten 100
Phosphatase, alkalische, Aktivität in Capillarendothelien des Coriums und der Subcutis 641
—, —, Arteriolen der Haut, Histochemie 526, 537
—, —, arteriovenöse Anastomosen, Histochemie 556
—, —, Basalzellen, Cytochemie 253
—, —, Blutgefäße der Haut 498, 505, 511
—, —, Blutgefäßneubildung der Haut, Histochemie 559, 561
—, —, Cytochemie, myoepitheliale Zellen 236
—, —, Darstellung von Capillarendothelien 639
—, —, dunkle Zellen, Cytochemie 248
—, —, in Fettzellen 456
—, —, Haarbalg 474
—, —, helle Zellen, Cytochemie 243
—, —, Histochemie von Brandwunden der Haut 772
—, —, — des embryonalen Nagels 673
—, —, — der fetalen ekkrinen Drüsen 665
—, —, — der fetalen Epidermis 633
—, —, — der Haarkomplexentwicklung 659
—, —, — der Keratinocyten 99
—, —, — der Leichenhaut 721
—, —, — des Musculus arrector pili 481
—, —, — des Nagels 366
—, —, — der Talgdrüsen 204
—, —, — der Wundheilung 754
—, —, histochemischer Nachweis in apokrinen Schweißdrüsen 323
—, —, Histologie, Altersabhängigkeit der Aktivität in den Kapillaren der Haut 701, 702
—, —, Histotopochemie des Haarfollikels 176

Phosphatase, alkalische, Kapillaren der Haut, Histochemie 537
—, —, Kombination mit Injektionsmethoden, Blutgefäße der Haut 498
—, —, myoepitheliale Zellen 482
—, —, Nachweis in Fibroblasten von Corium und Subcutis 431
—, —, Pinocytosemechanismus der Histiocyten 435
—, —, Venolen der Haut, Histochemie 537, 550
— in der Epidermis der Vogelhaut 998
— der Pulpazellen bei Vogelfedern 1008
—, saure, Arteriolen der Haut, Histochemie 526, 537
—, —, arteriovenöse Anastomosen, Histochemie 556
—, —, Corium 474
—, —, dunkle Zellen, Cytochemie 248
—, —, helle Zellen, Cytochemie 242
—, —, Histochemie von Brandwunden der Haut 772
—, —, — von Corium und subcutanem Fettgewebe 641
—, —, — der fetalen ekkrinen Drüsen 667
—, —, —, — Epidermis 633
—, —, — der Gewebsmastzellen 437
—, —, — der Haarkomplexentwicklung 659
—, —, — der Intermediärzone der Epidermis 18
—, —, — der Keratinocyten 96
—, —, — der Leichenhaut 721
—, —, — des Nagels 365
—, —, — der Talgdrüsen 196, 202
—, —, — der Wundheilung 754
—, —, histochemischer Nachweis in apokrinen Schweißdrüsen 322
—, —, Histotopochemie des Haarfollikels 176
—, —, intradermaler Schweißdrüsen-Ausführungsgang 250, 253
—, —, Kapillaren der Haut, Histochemie 537
—, —, Oberflächenzellen, Cytochemie 256
—, —, Pinocytose-Mechanismus der Histiocyten 435

Phosphatase, saure, im Rattenleberhomogenat 97
—, —, Unterscheidung von Melanophagen und Melanocyten 892
—, —, Ultrastruktur der apokrinen Schweißdrüsen 296
—, —, Venolen der Haut, Histochemie 537
—, weiche Hornschicht bei Reptilien 989
Phosphatase-Präparation, alkalische, Gefäßnetz des Corium 575, 578, 590
6-Phosphogluconat-Dehydrogenase, Histochemie der Keratinocyten 90
—, histochemischer Nachweis in apokrinen Schweißdrüsen 310, 315
Phospholipide, Arteriolen der Haut, Histochemie 526, 537
—, „Baker's acid hematein test" 81, 82
—, Basalzellen, Cytochemie 253
—, braunes Fett 457, 458
—, helle Zellen, Cytochemie 241
—, Fettsynthese 461
—, Histochemie der apokrinen Schweißdrüsen 306
—, — der Intermediärzone der Epidermis 18
—, — der Keratinocyten 81
—, — der Talgdrüsen 196, 198, 200
—, Kapillaren der Haut, Histochemie 537
—, „lamellated bodies" 59
Phospholipoide, Histotopographie im Haarfollikel 172
Phosphomonoesterasen, Histochemie der Keratinocyten 96
—, histochemischer Nachweis in apokrinen Schweißdrüsen 322
Phosphor, Histochemie der Keratinocyten 67
Phosphormolybdänsäure, Darstellung elastischer Fasern 449
Phosphorwolframsäure, Darstellung der Struktur der Kollagenfibrille 442
Phosphorylase, Basalzellen, Cytochemie 253
—, dunkle Zellen, Cytochemie 248
— in der fetalen Epidermis 632

Phosphorylase, Glykogensynthese in der Haut 474
—, Haarbalg 474
—, helle Zellen, Cytochemie 242
—, Histochemie der apokrinen Schweißdrüsen 310, 312
—, — des Coriums und des subcutanen Fettgewebes 641
—, — des embryonalen Nagels 673
—, — der fetalen ekkrinen Drüsen 665
—, — der fetalen Epidermis 633
—, — des Haarfollikels 176
—, — der Haarkomplexentwicklung 659
—, — der Keratinocyten 77, 91
—, —, Talgdrüsen 196, 201
—, Kapillaren der Haut, Histochemie 537
—, Venolen der Haut, Histochemie 537
Photoreceptoren bei Schleimaalen 940
pH-Wert der Haut der frühen Leichenzeit 718
Pickworth-Färbung, Blutgefäße der Haut, Histochemie 498
Pigmentanomalien, Identitätsfeststellung 730
Pigmente, Basalzellen 253
—, dermale, Abtransport 892
—, fluorescierende, Aufbau der Federfarben bei Vögeln 1009
—, intraepidermaler Schweißdrüsen-Ausführungsgang 258
—, photolabile, bei Neunaugen 930, 947
— in der Vogelhaut 1005
Pigmentgranula, mikroskopische Anatomie der apokrinen Schweißdrüsen 278
— in Sekretzellen apokriner Schweißdrüsen, Altersveränderungen der Haut 697
Pigmentierung, Alterspigmentierung 691
— der Haut, Altersabhängigkeit 691
Pigmentzellen, Nervenentwicklung in der Haut 676
— bei Selachiern 946
—, Stratum papillare 467
—, Terminologie 104, 105
Pikrinsäure, Gelbtönung von Haut, Haaren und Nägeln, Identitätsfeststellung 730
Pikrocarmin, Darstellung des Stratum corneum 15

Pilocarpin, Aktivierung der alkalischen Phosphatase in apokrinen Schweißdrüsen 323
—, Einfluß auf Pigmentablagerung in der Haut 898
Pingranliquose, Patho-Histologie 817
Pinocytose, Fettspeicherung 460
—, Fettverdauung 461
—, Fibrocyten 434
—, — von Corium und Subcutis 431
—, helle Zellen 243
—, Histiocyten 434, 435
—, Innervation der Haut 384, 385
—, Nervenapparat des Haares 409
—, neutrale Mucopolysaccharide 465
—, sensible Endkörperchen der Haut 421
Pinocytoseblasen bei Knochenfischen 966
Pinosomen, Pinocytose der Histiocyten 435
Pityriasis rubra pilaris, Fetttröpfchen in Keratinocyten 83
Pityrosporon ovale, Talgfollikel 192
PJS-Reaktion s. PAS-Reaktion
Placoidschuppen bei Selachiern 941, 943, 944
Plantarhaut, Dicke der Plasmamembran des Stratum corneum 23
—, Stratum corneum 15
—, Stratum lucidum 13
Plasmalemm, Innervation der Haut 379
Plasmalemmvesikulation, Histiocyten-Pinocytose 435
Plasmalogen, braunes Fett 457
—, Histochemie der Keratinocyten 84
Plasmalreaktion, Histiocytose und Xanthogranulomatose 883
—, Histochemie Musculus arrector pili 481
Plasmamembran, Alpha-Cytomembran der Keratinocyten 22
—, Intrazellularspalt des Stratum corneum 30
— der Keratinocyten, Dicke 22, 23
—, Kernmembran der Keratinocyten 22

Plasmamembran, Mitochondrienmembran der Keratinocyten 22
—, Morphologie der Keratinocyten 21
—, Zelloberfläche der Keratinocyten 20
Plasmaproteine, Bindegewebsgrundsubstanz 450
Plasmazellen, Antikörperbildung 439
—, Elektronenmikroskopie 438
—, Hautstoffwechsel 473
—, Herkunft 439
—, normale Histologie des Coriums und der Subcutis 438
Plasmocyt s. Plasmazellen
Plasmocytom, Fettgewebsinfiltration 824
Plattenepithel-Carcinom, Mitosezahl in der Epidermis 62
Platysma, mikroskopische und submikroskopische Anatomie 482
—, postmortale Kontraktionen 723
Platz-Quetschwunden an der Leichenhaut 755
„Plexus sousbasaux" 384
Plexus, vergleichende Anatomie, Blutgefäße der Haut 500
Polarisationsmethode, Interzellularspalt 30
Poliomyelitis, Panniculitis 799
Polyneuritis, neurogene Lipome 838
Polysaccharid, diastaseresistentes, Histochemie der fetalen ekkrinen Drüsen 665
—, —, Kohlenhydratstoffwechsel der Haut 76
—, Oberflächenzellen 257
Porenendothel, Gefäßnerven der Haut 398, 400
Porphyria congenita Günther, Patho-Histologie 893
— —, Photosensibilisierung 893
— cutanea tarda, Hautbiopsie, fluorescenzmikroskopischer Porphyrinnachweis 894
— —, Leberbiopsie, fluorescenzmikroskopischer Porphyrinnachweis 893
Porphyrie, erythropoetische, und Lipoidproteinose 872

Porphyrinablagerung in der Haut, fluorescenzmikroskopische Befunde 893
— und Speicherung in der Haut 892
Porphyrine, kupferhaltige, Aufbau der Federfarben bei Vögeln 1009
Praekeratin, Durchmesser 54
—, Keratinstruktur 50
Praemelanin, embryonale Entwicklung der Melanocyten 676
—, Melanogenese 110
Praemelanosomen, Elektronenmikroskopie 115
— in der embryonalen Epidermis 676
—, Lokalisation der Tyrosinaseaktivität 890
Praemitotische Erholungsphase, Adrenalinwirkung 65
Praeputium penis, Musculus sexualis 480
— —, Subcutiskonstruktion 477
„preelongation region" 147
presumptive keratin granules, Ultrastruktur der apokrinen Schweißdrüsen 294
„pre-terminal network", perivaskuläre Nervenfasern 564
Preußischblau-Färbung, Histochemie der Keratinocyten 70
—, Injektionsmethoden 497
—, Keratohyalin 71
—, -SH- und -S-S-Gruppen in Keratinocyten 72
„Primary fibrillar melanosomes", Histochemie der Melanocyten 115
Primaten, vergleichende Anatomie, Anhangsgebilde der Haut 506
—, — —, Blutgefäße der Haut 505
Primitivknoten, Embryologie der Epidermis 626
—, Entwicklungsmechanik der Haut 645
Probeexcisionen mit dem Elektrokauter, Artefakte 776
„progenitor cells", Mitose der Keratinocyten 66
Progerie, Fettgewebsatrophie der Haut 794
Prophase, Mitose der Keratinocyten 65
Protein, Bursae synoviales in der Subcutis 478
—, Depolymerisation durch elektrischen Strom 777

Protein, Histochemie der apokrinen Schweißdrüsen 305
—, — der Basalmembran 463
—, — der Keratinocyten 67
Proteinsynthese, Fibroblasten 433
—, Haarfollikel 177
—, Keratinocyten 47, 68
—, Langerhans-Zelle 116
—, „speckled pattern" der Epidermis-Fibrillen 49
Protofibrille s. auch Mikrofibrille
—, Elektronenmikroskopie der elastischen Faser 449
—, Struktur der elastischen Faser 448
„Protofilament", Definition 37
—, Elektronenmikroskopie des Haares 52
—, — des Haarfollikels 155
—, Parakeratose 54
—, Röntgen-Diffraktions-Methode 54
—, Struktur 54
Protoporphyrin, Photosensibilisierung 893
Protoporphyrinämische familiäre Lichturticaria, Fluorescenzmikroskopie 893
— Lichturticaria, Photosensibilisierung 893
Protozoen, neutrale Mucopolysaccharide 465
Protyrosinase, Melaninsynthese 890
Pseudoakanthosis nigricans, Talgdrüsen 201
Pseudocholinesterasen, Histochemie der Keratinocyten 92
—, — des Nagels 367
—, — der Talgdrüsen 203
Pseudomilium colloidale Pellizari 872
— — —, historöntgenographische (mikroradiographische) Untersuchungen 873
Pseudoxanthoma elasticum, Kalkablagerung in den elastischen Fasern 888
Psoriasis, Autoradiographie mit Histidin-H^3 68
—, Dicke der Plasmamenbran der Epidermiszellen 23
—, Fetttröpfchen in Keratinocyten 83
—, Fibrillenstruktur 49
—, Hyperkeratose 11
—, Keratinfibrillen, Entwicklung 42

Psoriasis, Keratinocyten-Verknüpfung 34
—, Keratohyalin 43
—, Keratohyalinmangel 11
—, „lamellated bodies" 59
—, Mitochondrien und Fibrillenanzahl 56
—, Mitosezahl in der Epidermis 62
—, Nexus der Keratinocyten 35
—, Parakeratose 11
—, RNA-Synthese 70
—, Stratum spinosum 10, 11
—, Sulfhydryl- und Disulfidgruppen in Keratinocyten 70
—, Ultrastruktur der T-Zellen 12
—, Zunahme der Zellschichten im Stratum basale 10
Pterinophoren bei adulten Amphibien 982
— bei Amphibienlarven 977
— bei Knochenfischen 964, 965
Pterylose, embryonale, bei Vögeln 998, 1001
Pubertas praecox, Embryonalentwicklung der apokrinen Schweißdrüsen 270
— —, hormonelle Beeinflussung der apokrinen Schweißdrüsen 328
Pulverschmauchniederschläge an der Schußhand, Differenzierung von Mord und Selbstmord 766
Purpura anularis teleangiectodes Majocchi, sekundäre Hämosiderose der Haut 897
—, rheumatica Schoenlein-Henoch, Patho-Histologie 809
—, vasculäre, Ätiologie der Necrobiosis lipoidica 837
Putrifikation der Haut, Hautveränderungen in der späteren Leichenzeit 730
Pyknose der Kerne, mikroskopische Veränderungen der Haut der späten Leichenzeit 732
Pyroninophilie, Autolyse der Leichenhaut 721
Pyruvat, Einfluß auf Mitoserate 64

Quatrefagessche Körperchen, Acranierhaut 925, 926
„quintuple-layered cell interconnection", Keratinocyten-Ultrastruktur 34

Radiärknötchen, Faserneubildung bei Periarteriitis nodosa cutanea 811
—, Patho-Histologie des Erythema nodosum 796
Radii der Feder bei Vögeln 1005
Radiographie, Kombination mit Injektionsmethoden 497
Radspeichenstruktur, Plasmazellen der Haut 438
Rami der Feder bei Vögeln 1005
Raphe perinei, Haut, Stratum papillare 466
Receptoren für Berührungsreize bei Amphibien 984
„recovery phase", Blutgefäßneubildung der Haut, Histochemie 560
Rectumbiopsie, Amyloidose 866
Regaud's Hämatoxylin, Färbung der Mitochondrien 55
Regeneration, Blutgefäße der Haut 558
„regression phase", Blutgefäßneubildung der Haut, Histochemie 560
„rejection phase", Blutgefäßneubildung der Haut, Histochemie 561
Reptilienhaut, Corium der 991
—, Epidermis der Schuppenoberseite 988
—, Subcutis der 995
—, vergleichende Histologie 987
RES, Amyloid-Sezernierung 864
—, Silberspeicherung bei der experimentellen Argyrose 899
Resorcin-Fuchsin, Darstellung argyrophiler Fasern 444
—, Darstellung elastischer Fasern 448
Resorcin-Fuchsin-Färbung, aktinische Elastose 873
Resorptive Mechanismen, intradermaler Schweißdrüsen-Ausführungsgang 250
Reteleisten, Altersveränderung der Epidermis 686
Rete Malpighii, Nomenklatur Stratum spinosum 10
Rete mucosum, Nomenklatur Stratum spinosum 10
Retezellen, Veränderung in den Strommarken 776
Reticuloendothel des Coriums 637
Reticuloendotheliales System s. RES

Reticulo-Endotheliose, Ätiologie, Inanitionsatrophie des Fettgewebes der Haut 791
reticulo-histiocytäres System, Pluripotenz, Fettgewebe-Reaktion 840
Reticulosarkomatose, Fettgewebsinfiltration 824
Reticulose, Abgrenzung von Reticulosarkomatose und Hodgkin-Sarkom durch Cytophotometrie 824
—, Fettgewebsinfiltration 824
Reticulum, Argyrophilie von Fasern 445
—, endoplasmatisches 232
—, —, Elektronenmikroskopie, Talgdrüsen 204, 208, 211, 216
—, —, Ultrastruktur der apokrinen Schweißdrüsen 300
—, terminales, perivasculäre Nerven 564
Reticulumzelle, argyrophile Faserbildung 443
—, Entwicklung der Fettorgane der Haut 455
—, Fettspeicherung 460
—, normale Histologie von Corium und Subcutis 439, 443
—, Speichertätigkeit 439
—, Umwandlung zu Makrophagen 439
Retikulinfasern, argyrophile, Histologie der Reticulumzelle 439
Retinacula cutis 474
Retraktoren der Vogelhaut 1001
Rheumaknötchen, Glykogenanreicherung 886
Rheumatismus, neurotrophische Atrophie der Haut 792
Rhexisblutung, Livores der frühen Leichenzeit 713
—, postmortale, Differentialdiagnose 715
—, —, durch postmortale Muskelkontraktionen 723
rhino-pharyngo-bronchiale Granulomatose Wegener, Patho-Histologie 809, 811
Ribonuclease s. RNase
Ribonucleinsäure s. RNA
Ribonucleoproteide, Basalzellen, Elektronenmikroskopie 251
Ribonucleoprotein, dunkle Zellen 245
—, Talgdrüsen 193
Ribosomen, Durchmesser 57
—, Keratinocyten 47, 49

Ribosomen, Kollagenbildung in Fibroblasten 433
— der Melanocyten, Syntheseort für Melanin 115
—, mikroskopische Anatomie der apokrinen Schweißdrüsen 277
—, Morphologie der Keratinocyten 57
—, Ultrastruktur der apokrinen Schweißdrüsen 300
—, — der Plasmazellen der Haut 438
Riesenzellen bei Atrophie des subcutanen Fettgewebes 794
—, Fremdkörpergranulom 901
Rigor, Haut der frühen Leichenzeit 722
Ringblutung, Schußverletzungen der Haut 765
Ringgeflecht, Nervenapparat des Haares 402
RNA-Abbau, Autolyse der Leichenhaut 721
—, Gehalt in der Verhornungszone bei Vogelfedern 1008
—, Histochemie der Keratinocyten 69
—, — des Nagels 364
—, — der Wundheilung 754
—, Histotopographie im Haarfollikel 174
—, Keratohyalin 47
—, mikroskopische Anatomie der apokrinen Schweißdrüsen 277
—, Proteinsynthese bei der Nagelentwicklung 364
RNase, Histochemie der Keratinocyten 100
—, Histotopochemie des Haarfollikels 176
—, Pinocytose-Mechanismus der Histiocyten 435
RNA-Synthese, Autoradiographie in Keratinocyten 70
— in Keratinocyten 69, 70
RNS s. RNA
Rodentia, vergleichende Anatomie, Blutgefäße der Haut 507
Röntgen-Diffraktionsmethode, Intercellularspalt 30
—, Keratinstruktur 75
Röntgenmikroskopie, Blutgefäße der Haut 499
—, Kombination mit Injektionsmethoden 497
Röntgenstrahlen, Durchlässigkeit des Stratum corneum 15

Rothmund-Syndrom, Fettgewebsatrophie der Haut 793, 794
Rouget's Zellen s. Pericyten
"rough cisternae", Nomenklatur der Ribosomen 58
Rubeolavirus, intrauterine Infektion, Entwicklung von Affenfurchen 636
Rückenhaut, Anatomie des Gefäßnetzes 570, 576
Ruffinische Körperchen, Histologie der Innervation des Nagels 358
— —, Innervation der Haut 377
Ruhr, idiomuskulärer Wulst 722
Rundmäuler, Haut der, vergleichende Histologie 927
Rundzell-Infiltrate in der Altershaut 695
Rußaspiration, Feststellung eines Schwelbrandes 768

Säugetierhaut, Literaturübersicht 1029
Säuglingsatrophie, Fettentspeicherungsmechanismus 461
Saftkanälchen der ekkrinen Drüsen, Embryonalentwicklung 664
Saisondimorphismus, Gefiedertypen bei Vögeln 1015
Salpetersäureverätzung, Veränderung der Leichenhaut 773
Salzsäureverätzung, Veränderungen der Leichenhaut 773
Sammelvenole, primäre, arteriovenöse Anastomosen 553
Saponifikation, biochemischer Mechanismus der 746
— der Haut, histologischer Befund 746
— —, makroskopisches Aussehen 746
— —, postmortal 741
Sarcoma idiopathicum Kaposi, Glykogenvorkommen in Endothelzellen und in der glatten Muskulatur 886
Sarkoid Darier-Roussy, Ätiologie und Pathogenese 836
— —, Patho-Histologie 800
— —, des subcutanen Fettgewebes 796
Satoshe Silbermethode, Nervenentwicklung in der Haut 675
Sauerstoff, postmortale percutane Resorption 778

Sauerstoffmangel, Einfluß auf Mitoserate 64
Schaltstücke, myoepitheloide, arteriovenöse Anastomosen 554
Schambergsche Dermatose, Eisenpigment in den Langhans-Zellen 896
Schaumzellen, Histologie der Hand-Schüller-Christianschen Erkrankung 883
Schimmelpilze, postmortale Veränderungen der Haut 737, 739
Schläfenhaut, Stratum papillare 465
Schlaf, Einfluß auf Mitoserate 64
Schlafmittelvergiftung, Verbrennungsreaktion auf der Haut 768
Schleimaale, Corium der 938
—, Epidermis der 936
—, Haut der, vergleichende Histologie 936
—, Innervation der Haut 940
—, Subcutis der 939
Schleimhaut, Cytochromoxydase-positive Granula 86
—, Vertrocknungen post mortem 725
Schleimhautepithelien, Altersveränderung 690
Schleimhautvertrocknungen in der Agone 724
Schleimdrüsen bei adulten Amphibien 983
—, alveoläre, bei Schleimaalen 936, 939
Schleimstoffe, histochemische Darstellung 877
Schleimzellen, kleine, bei Schleimaalen 937
— bei Selachiern 942
Schmerzempfindung, Innervation der Haut 379, 384
Schmorl-Reaktion, Melanindarstellung 890
Schreckmauser bei Vögeln 1014
Schreckstoffe bei Amphibienlarven 971
— bei Knochenfischen 959
Schürfsaum bei Ausschußverletzungen 767
— bei Schußverletzungen der Haut 765
Schultz'sche Färbung, Reaktion von Fibrin, Fibrinoid und Hyalin 870
Schuppen, Aufbau bei Reptilien 992
— bei Knochenfischen 956, 962

Schuppen, Regeneration der, bei Knochenfischen 963
Schuppenanlagen bei Reptilien 993
Schuppenreste bei adulten Amphibien 982
Schußverletzungen, absoluter Nahschuß 766
—, Ausschußverletzungen 767
— der Haut, Fernschuß 764
— —, Nahschuß 765
—, Histologie 765
— der Leichenhaut 764
Schwannsche Zelle, Embryologie der Haut 674
— —, Innervation der Haut 379, 391, 392, 393, 395, 408, 409, 418, 419, 420, 421
— —, Mitochondrien der, subepidermales Nervengeflecht 392
— —, Zahl, Nervenentwicklung in der Haut 675
Schwanzleiste, topographische Unterschiede der embryonalen Epidermis 635
Schwefel, geheilt in der Epidermis 72, 73
—, Histochemie der Keratinocyten 67
Schwefelsäureverätzung, Veränderungen der Leichenhaut 773
Schwefelwasserstoff, Grünfärbung der Leichenhaut 731
—, postmortale percutane Resorption 779
Schweiß, Eisengehalt 310
—, Enzym der Hautoberfläche 94
Schweißdrüsen, Aminopeptidase 474
—, Amyloidablagerung 868
—, apokrine 224, 226
—, —, altersbedingte Veränderungen der mikroskopischen Anatomie 282
—, —, Altersveränderungen 696
—, —, atypische 278
—, —, Basalmembran 280
—, —, cystische Erweiterung der Lumina 697
—, —, Ektopie 272
—, —, elektronenmikroskopische Anatomie 287
—, —, Embryonalentwicklung 268
—, —, Entwicklung bei Pubertas praecox 270
—, —, Epithelzellenatrophie 697
—, —, Gefäßversorgung 583

Schweißdrüsen, apokrine, Glycerin-1-Phosphat-Dehydrogenaseaktivität 310, 314
—, —, Glykogengehalt bei Morbus Fox-Fordyce 309
—, —, Heterotopie 272
—, —, Histochemie 305
—, —, —, Eisen 309
—, —, —, Enzyme des energieliefernden Stoffwechsels 311
—, —, —, Kohlenhydrate 307
—, —, —, Lipide 306
—, —, —, Phosphorylase 310, 312
—, —, histochemischer Nachweis von Acetylcholinesterase 321
—, —, — — von Adenosintriphosphatase 324
—, —, — — von Aliesterasen 322
—, —, — — von alkalischer Phosphatase 323
—, —, — — von Bernsteinsäure-Dehydrogenase 310, 316
—, —, — — von Chondrosulphatase 325
—, —, — — von Cytochromoxydase 310, 318
—, —, — — von Dihydroliponsäure-Dehydrogenase 310, 321
—, —, — — von Esterasen 321
—, —, — — der Glucose-6-Phosphat-Dehydrogenase 310, 315
—, —, — — von β-Glucuronidase 325
—, —, — — von Glutamatdehydrogenase 310, 320
—, —, — — von Glycerinaldehyd-3-Phosphat-Dehydrogenase 310, 313
—, —, — — von Glycerin-1-Phosphat-Oxydase 310, 314
—, —, — — von Leucinaminopeptidase 325
—, —, — — von Lipasen 322
—, —, — — von Malat-Dehydrogenase 310, 316
—, —, — — von Malatenzym 310, 315
—, —, — — der Monoaminoxydase 321
—, —, — — von NADH-Tetrazoliumsalzreductase 310, 318
—, —, — — von NAD-Isocitrat-Dehydrogenase 310, 316, 318

Schweißdrüsen, apokrine, histochemischer Nachweis von NADP-Isocitrat-Dehydrogenase 310, 316, 318
—, —, — — von NADPH-Tetrazoliumsalzreductase 310, 318
—, —, — — von 6-Phosphat-Gluconat-Dehydrogenase 310, 315
—, —, — — von sauren Phosphatasen 322
—, —, — — von Thiaminpyrophosphatase 324
—, —, — — von Ubichinon 310, 318, 320
—, —, Histologie des sekretorischen Abschnittes 280
—, —, historischer Überblick 267
—, —, hormonelle Beeinflussung 328
—, —, Innervation, mikroskopische Anatomie 284
—, —, „intermediäre" Drüsen 697
—, —, „kuppelförmige Sekretion" 277
—, —, Lactat-Dehydrogenase-Aktivität 310, 314
—, —, Lokalisation 271
—, —, Lumeninhalt, mikroskopische Anatomie 281
—, —, makroskopisches Aussehen 273
—, —, mikroskopische Anatomie 275
—, —, — des Ausführungsganges 284
—, —, — der Myoepithelzellen 279
—, —, — der Zellen des intermediären Abschnittes 279
—, —, Morbus-Fox-Fordyce 283
—, —, Morphologie des Drüsenepithels 275
—, —, im Kindesalter 270
—, — des sekretorischen Abschnittes 275
—, —, mukoide Metaplasie 697
—, —, PAS-Reaktivität des Cuticularsaumes 276
—, —, postmortale Veränderungen 285
—, —, Sekretionsmodus 325
—, —, sekretorische Ausbuchtungen der Drüsenzellen 276
—, —, Ultrastruktur des Ausführungsganges 304

Schweißdrüsen, apokrine, Ultrastruktur, irreguläre Korpuskeln mit kristalliner Innenstruktur 297
—, —, —, Mitochondrien 290, 291
—, —, — der Myoepithelzellen 301
—, —, —, Plasmalemm 289
—, —, —, Zellkern 289, 290
—, —, Volumen 271
—, —, Vorkommen von Mitosen 279
—, —, Zellkerne der Drüsenzellen 277
—, Argyrose der Basalmembran 899
—, Bedeutung bei der Carotinosis 898
—, Dermatoglyphen 224
—, ekkrine 224
—, —, Altersveränderung 696
—, —, Anatomie 224
—, —, Anlagen 225
—, —, Cholesterinase 226
—, —, Cytochemie 224
—, —, dunkle Zellen 237, 244
—, —, Elektronenmikroskopie 224
—, —, Entwicklung 225
—, —, epidermaler Schweißdrüsen-Ausführungsgang 258
—, —, Esterasen 228
—, —, Gefäßnetz, Altersabhängigkeit 696
—, —, Gefäßversorgung 261, 581
—, —, gerader Gang 230
—, —, Geschlechtsunterschied der Altersveränderungen 704
—, —, gewundener Gang 230, 249
—, —, Glycerin-1-Phosphat-Dehydrogenaseaktivität 314
—, —, Glykogen 227
—, —, Glykogengehalt in der frühen Leichenzeit 721
—, —, Handfläche 225
—, —, helle seröse Zellen 230
—, —, — Zellen 237
—, —, histochemischer Phosphorylasenachweis 312
—, —, hydrolytische Enzyme 228
—, —, Innervation 262
—, —, intradermaler Ausführungsgang 249, 253
—, —, intraepidermaler Gang 230
—, —, Lactat-Dehydrogenaseaktivität 314

Schweißdrüsen, ekkrine, Lipidgehalt, Altersabhängigkeit 669
—, —, Malatenzymaktivität 315
—, —, Lysosomen 227, 229
—, —, myoepitheliale Zellen 230
—, —, ——, Elektronenmikroskopie 231
—, —, Nervenversorgung 226
—, —, PAS-positive Substanzen, Altersabhängigkeit 696
—, —, Phosphatasen, saure 228
—, —, 6-Phosphat-Gluconat-Dehydrogenaseaktivität 315
—, —, Pigmentgehalt, Altersabhängigkeit 696
—, —, der Ratte 243
—, —, Schleimzellen 230
—, —, sekretorische Schlinge 230, 244
—, —, sekretorischer Tubulus 230
—, —, im Senium 241
—, —, Sohlen 225
—, —, Verteilung 224
—, —, Zahl 224
—, Embryonalentwicklung, quantitative Daten 668
—, foetale Gefäßentwicklung 513
—, Funktion 224
—, Glykogenablagerung bei Glykogenspeicherkrankheit 886
—, Goldablagerung 900
—, Histologie der Fingerbeere 353
—, Innervation 378, 395, 398, 409
—, merokrine 224
—, Monoaminoxydaseaktivität 87
—, Musculus arrector pili 481
—, myoepitheliale Zellen 482
—, Öffnungen 224
—, Venen der 598
Schweißdrüsenausführungsgang, epidermaler, Elektronenmikroskopie 227, 229
—, Motivbild 467
—, Penetration von Gasen 778
—, Stratum reticulare 470
—, Veränderungen durch elektrischen Strom 777
Schweißporen 224
Schweißrückresorption, Oberflächenzellen 257

Schweißsekretion, Oberflächenzellen 257
Schwitzen, helle Zellen 243
Sclerema adiposum, Patho-Histologie 805
— neonatorum, Ätiologie und Pathogenese 835
— — —, Patho-Histologie 805
Scorch burns 772
„scotch tape" 496, 531
Scrotalhaut, Stratum papillare 466
Scrotum, Glykogengehalt 76
—, Musculus sexualis 480
—, Subcutiskonstruktion 477
Sehnen, elastische, Elastica-Darstellung 479
—, —, Gefäßeinbau 479
—, —, Musculus arrector pili 481
—, —, Zugfestigkeit 447
Seitenlinien-Sinnesorgane bei Chondrichthyes 951, 954
Seitenlinien-System bei Amphibien 978, 984
— bei Knochenfischen 968
— bei Neunaugen 933
— bei Schleimaalen 940
— bei Selachiern 956
Sekret als Gift bei Selachiern 942
Sekretgranula, Innervation der Epidermis 382
—, mikroskopische Anatomie der apokrinen Schweißdrüsen 277
Sekretion, helle Zellen 243
Sekretionsgranula, Beziehung zu Lipopigmenten 307
—, dunkle Zellen 245
—, Sekretionsmodus der apokrinen Schweißdrüsen 326
—, Ultrastruktur der apokrinen Schweißdrüsen 292
Sekretionsmodus, apokrine Schweißdrüsen 325
Sekretkörnchen der ekkrinen Drüsen, Embryonalentwicklung 664
Sekundärhaare, topographische Entwicklung der Haare 658
Sempersches Trockenpräparat, Papillarleisten 466
Sengverbrennungen 772
sensible Endkörperchen, Innervation der Haut 411
Selachier, Corium der 943
—, Epidermis der 941
—, Haut der 941
—, Subcutis der 943
„Selby-Odland's bodies", Interzellularspalt der Keratinocyten 26

Seligman-Reaktion, Arteriolen der Haut 526
—, Histochemie der Keratinocyten 71
—, Kapillaren der Haut 536
Sepsis, Putrifikation in der späten Leichenzeit 730
Serotonin, Bildung in Gewebsmastzellen 437
Sexualhormone, Beeinflussung der apokrinen Schweißdrüsen 328
-SH-Gruppen, Arteriolen der Haut, Histochemie 526, 537
—, arteriovenöse Anastomosen, Histochemie 556
—, Cytochemie, myoepitheliale Zellen 236
—, Embryologie des Nagels 671
—, grampositive Substanzen 80
—, Histochemie des embryonalen Nagels 673
—, — der Intermediärzone der Epidermis 18
—, — der Keratinocyten 70
—, — der Talgdrüsen 196, 201
—, Histotopographie im Haarfollikel 173
—, — der Kopfhaut 73
—, Kapillaren der Haut, Histochemie 537
—, Keratinisationsvorgang 72
—, Keratinocyten, Rassenunterschiede 72
—, Keratohyalin 44
—, Oberflächenzellen, Cytochemie 257
—, Reaktion von Fibrin, Fibrinoid und Hyalin 871
—, Umwandlung zu -S-S-Gruppen bei der Keratinisation 75
—, Venolen der Haut, Histochemie 537
—, Vorkommen in Gemeinschaft mit Succinyldehydrogenase in der Epidermis 88
Shunt, Gefäßversorgung des Nagels 355
Shwartzmann-Sanarelli-Phänomen, experimentell erzeugte Panniculitis 830
Siderose, Terminologie 895
Silber, Ablagerung und Speicherung in der Cutis 898
Silberimprägnation, Nervenentwicklung in der Haut 674
Silberimprägnationsmethode nach Gomori, Darstellung der Tophi 889

Silicium, Histochemie der Keratinocyten 66
Silikongummi, Injektionsmethoden 497
Sinushaare, morphologische Entwicklung des Haarkomplexes 647
Sinnesknospen, Aufbau der, bei Tieren 953
—, s. auch Neuromasten
— der Seitenlinienorgane bei Amphibien 984
Sinneszellen bei Schleimaalen 940
Skelettmuskulatur der Haut, mikroskopische und submikroskopische Anatomie 482
Skleroblasten bei Knochenfischen 963
Skleroedema adultorum, Euthyreose, Einteilung der Mucinosen 878
— —, Metachromasie durch Hyaluronsäure 879
Skleromyxödem, Enteilung der Mucinosen 878
—, Erhöhung der Blut-Mucopolysaccharide 876
—, Glykogenanreicherung im Bindegewebe 886
—, Histologie 879
Skleroprotein, Histochemie des Nagels 371
—, Zusammensetzung der Grundsubstanz 874
Sklerotom, Querschnitt Embryo 625
Sohlenhorn, Anatomie des Nagels 340, 342
—, Embryologie des Nagels 671
—, Terminologie des Nagels 340
Somatopleura, Corium- und Subcutisentwicklung 637
—, Querschnitt Embryo 625
Spaltlinien, Corium 471, 472
—, Richtungswechsel während des Embryonallebens 638
Speicheldrüsen, myoepitheliale Zellen 482
Sperrarterien, Pathogenese der Mucinosen 880
Sphincter colli, Skeletmuskulatur der Haut 482
Sphincter, intradermaler Schweißdrüsen-Ausführungsgang 249
Sphingosin, Definition der Lipoide 881
Spinalnerven, Embryologie der Haut 673
Spinnenzellen bei Schleimaalen 937

„spinous layer", Nomenklatur Stratum spinosum 10
Spontanpanniculitis Typ Pfeifer-Weber-Christian, Patho-Histologie 800
— — Rothmann-Makai, Patho-Histologie 802
— — —, Pathogenese und Ätiologie 835
Squalen, Talg 196
Squamatenhaut, Häutungsvorgänge 987
-S-S-Gruppen, Cytochemie, myoepitheliale Zellen 236
—, Histochemie des embryonalen Nagels 673
—, — der Keratinocyten 70
—, Histotopographie im Haarfollikel 173
—, — der Kopfhaut 74
—, Kapillaren der Haut, Histochemie 537
—, Keratinisationsvorgang 72
—, Keratinocyten, Rassenunterschiede 72
—, Keratohyalin 44
—, Oberflächenzellen, Cytochemie 257
—, Umwandlung bei der Keratinisation 75
—, Venolen der Haut, Histochemie 537
Stachelzellen, fetale Epidermis, Glykogengehalt 632
—, — —, Phosphorylase-Aktivität 632
—, Keratocyten 19
—, Keratohyalin 11
—, Stratum spinosum 10
— in der Vogelhaut 999
Stachelzellschicht s. Stratum spinosum
Stearinsäure, Aufbau des Fettes in der Subcutis 789
Steatonekrose, Pathologie des subcutanen Fettgewebes 795
—, Spontanpanniculitis Typ Rothmann-Makai 802
Steroide, Einfluß auf Amphibienhäutung 979
Steroid-Metabolismus, Talgdrüsen 188, 202
Stirnhaut, Elastizität 473
—, Musculus cutis diagonalis 481
—, Stratum papillare 466
Strangfurchen, Hautläsionen an der Leiche 758
—, Histamingehalt der Haut 759
Strangmarke, Differenzierung zwischen vitaler und postmortaler 759

Strangmarke, Hautläsionen an der Leiche 758
Stratum acanthoticum, Nomenklatur Stratum spinosum 10
— anoxybioticum, Glykogenstoffwechsel 78
— basale, Alpha-Cytomembran 58
— —, Altersveränderung der Epidermis 686
— —, Amylo-1,4→1,6-transglucosidaseaktivität 91
— —, AS-Esteraseaktivität 95
— —, ATPase-Aktivität 99
— —, Basophilie 8
— —, Carboanhydraseaktivität 102
— —, Cholinesteraseaktivität 96
— —, Cytochromoxydasepositive Granula 86
— —, Elektronenmikroskopie der Epidermis 9
— —, Fibrillen, Elektronenmikroskopie 41
— —, Fibrillenveränderungen 40
— —, β-Glucuronidase-Aktivität 101
— —, Keratinocyten 4
— —, Keratohyalinsynthese 49
— —, Melanocytenverteilung in der embryonalen Haut 676
— —, Mitosen 62
— —, Monoaminoxydaseaktivität 87
— —, normale Histologie 8
— —, Phosphorylaseaktivität 91
— —, Planta und Palma, Esteraseaktivität 95
— —, proteolytische Aktivität 101
— —, Ribosomen 58
— —, spezifische Coenzymgebundene Dehydrogenasen 90
— —, Succinyldehydrogenaseaktivität 87
— —, „true melanocytes" 106
— —, Ubiquinon-Aktivität 102
— —, Übergangszellen 10
— —, Ultrastruktur, Desmosomen 33
— —, Unterscheidung von Stratum spinosum 8
— —, Zentriole 59
— compactum s. Stratum reticulare

Stratum corneum, alkalische Phosphataseaktivität 99
— —, Altersveränderung der Epidermis 688
— —, Amylo-1,4→1,6-transglucosidaseaktivität 92
— —, AS-Esteraseaktivität 95
— —, Carboanhydraseaktivität 102
— — compactum, Elektronenmikroskopie 14
— — —, Intermediärzone 17
— —, Cytochromoxydaseaktivität 85
— —, Dicke 14, 15
— —, — an der unbedeckten Haut 685
— —, —, Verhältnis zur Dicke des Stratum germinativum, Meßwerte 742
— —, DNAse-Aktivität 100
— —, Elektronenmikroskopie 16, 18, 24
— —, — der Epidermis 9
— —, — der Fibrillen 51
— —, Fetttröpfchen 83
— —, Fibrillen, Elektronenmikroskopie 41
— —, Histochemie Glykogen 77
— —, Keratinisation 11
— —, Keratinstruktur 51
— —, „keratin-pattern" 75
— —, Keratohyalinbildung 44
— —, Mikroradiographie 15
— —, normale Histologie der Epidermis 14
— —, Pauly-Reaktion 68
— —, Phosphamidaseaktivität 100
— —, Phosphorylaseaktivität 92
— —, proteolytische Aktivität 101
— —, Ribosomen 58
— —, RNase-Aktivität 100
— —, Röntgenstrahlendurchlässigkeit 15
— —, saure Phosphataseaktivität 96
— —, Schichten des 15
— —, spezifische Coenzymgebundene Dehydrogenasen 90
— —, Succinyldehydrogenaseaktivität 87
— —, Syncytiumbildung 15
— —, Talgdrüsen-Gang 192
— —, T-Zellen 12
— —, Ubiquinon-Aktivität 102
— —, Ultrastruktur 26, 27, 28, 29

Stratum corneum, Ultrastruktur, Desmosomen 33
— —, Veränderungen durch elektrischen Strom 777
— —, Zellmembrangehalt 30
— cylindricum, Nomenklatur Stratum basale 8
— disjunctum, Planta und Palma 15
— germinativum, Dicke, Verhältnis zur Dicke des Stratum corneum, Meßwerte 742
— —, Embryologie der Epidermis 627
— —, Mitosen 62
— —, morphologische Entwicklung des Haarkomplexes 645
— —, Veränderungen durch elektrischen Strom 777
— granulosum, Altersveränderungen der Epidermis 688
— —, Nomenklatur Stratum intermedium 11
— infrabasale, Schichten des Stratum lucidum 13
— intermedium, alkalische Phosphataseaktivität 99
— —, Alpha-Cytomembran 58
— —, Amylo-1,4→1,6-transglucosidaseaktivität 92
— —, AS-Esteraseaktivität 95
— —, ATPase-Aktivität 99
— —, Cholinesteraseaktivität 96
— —, Cytochromoxydaseaktivität 85
— —, Desulfhydrase-Aktivität 103
— —, Elektronenmikroskopie der Epidermis 9
— —, Embryologie der Epidermis 627
— —, fetale Epidermis, Glykogengehalt 631
— —, — —, Ultrastruktur 631
— —, Fibrillenveränderung 40
— —, β-Glucuronidaseaktivität 101
— —, Histochemie, Glykogen 76
— —, interzellulärer Spalt 23
— —, Invagination der Zelloberflächen 20
— —, Karyoplasma 60, 61
— —, Keratohyalinsynthese 47
— —, Kernmembran 60

Stratum intermedium, „lamellated bodies" 59
— —, Melanocytenverteilung in der embryonalen Haut 676
— —, Monoaminoxydaseaktivität 87
— —, NADH- und NADPH-Tetrazolium-Reduktase-Aktivität 90
— —, normale Histologie der Epidermis 11
— —, Phosphamidaseaktivität 100
— —, Phosphorylaseaktivität 92
— —, proteolytische Aktivität 101
— —, Ribonukleinsäuresynthese 47
— —, Ribosomen 58
— —, spezifische Coenzymgebundene Dehydrogenasen 90
— —, Succinyldehydrogenaseaktivität 87
— —, Ubiquinon-Aktivität 102
— —, Ultrastruktur 13
— lucidum, Aliesterasen 95
— —, Altersveränderung der Epidermis 688
— —, Amylo-1,4 → 1,6-transglucosidaseaktivität 92
— —, AS-Esteraseaktivität 95
— —, Cholinesteraseaktivität 96
— —, DNAase-Aktivität 100
— —, Histochemie Glykogen 77
— —, normale Histologie der Epidermis 13
— —, Palmarhaut 13
— —, Phosphorylaseaktivität 92
— —, Plantarhaut 13
— —, proteolytische Aktivität 101
— —, Ribosomen 58
— —, Schichten 13
— —, T-Zellen 12
— Malpighii, Nomenklatur Stratum spinosum 10
— oxybioticum, Glykogenstoffwechsel 78
— papillare, kollagene Fasern 467
— —, mikroskopische und submikroskopische Anatomie des Corium 465
— —, Motivbild 467
— —, normale Histologie des Stratum intermedium 12
— —, Papillarlinienmuster zur Daktyloskopie 752

Stratum papillare, Stoffwechselfunktion der Haut 473
— reticulare, Altersveränderung, Epidermis 691
— —, —, Mikroskopie 688, 689
— —, Faserverlaufsrichtung 471
— —, Fermentaktivität 474
— —, Gefäßeinbau 478
— —, mechanische Funktion 473
— —, mikroskopische und submikroskopische Anatomie des Coriums 470
— —, Musculus arrector pili 481
— —, Musculus sexualis 480
— —, Planta und Palma 15
— spinosum, Alpha-Cytomembran 58
— —, Altersveränderung der Epidermis 686
— —, —, Meßwerte der Zelldurchmesser in verschiedenen Regionen 689
— —, Amylo-1,4 → transglucosidaseaktivität 92
— —, AS-Esteraseaktivität 95
— —, ATPase-Aktivität 99
— —, Carboanhydraseaktivität 102
— —, Elektronenmikroskopie der Epidermis 42
— —, Epidermisdicke 10
— —, Fibrillenveränderung 40
— —, β-Glucuronidase-Aktivität 101
— —, Histochemie Glykogen 76
— —, interzellulärer Spalt 23
— —, — — in der unverhornten Epidermis 24
— —, Mitosen 12
— —, Monoaminoxydaseaktivität 87
— —, normale Histologie 10
— —, Phosphamidaseaktivität 100
— —, Phosphorylaseaktivität 92
— —, Planta und Palma, Esteraseaktivität 95
— —, proteolytische Aktivität 101
— —, Ribosomen 58
— —, spezifische Coenzymgebundene Dehydrogenasen 90
— —, Succinyldehydrogenaseaktivität 87
— —, Ubiquinon-Aktivität 102

Stratum reticulare, Übergangszellen 10
— —, Unterscheidung vom Stratum basale 8
— —, Zentriole 59
— subpapillare, Fasern 468
— —, Gefäßeinbau 478
— —, Musculus arrector pili 481
— —, Stratum papillare 465
— —, — reticulare 470
— vasculosum bei Vögeln 1000, 1003
Strommarke, Begriffsbestimmung 776
—, Differenzierung zwischen reaktiver und nichtreaktiver Region 777
—, — zwischen vitaler und postmortaler Entstehung 775
—, makroskopischer Befund 776
—, Metallisation 775
—, mikroskopischer Befund 777
—, Veränderung der Leichenhaut 774
„striated melanosomes", Histochemie der Melanocyten 115
Strukturfarbe bei Vogelfedern 1010
Subcutis, fetale, Glykogengehalt 632
—, —, Phosphorylase-Aktivität 632
—, Funktion 788
—, Gefäßeinbau 478
—, glatte Muskulatur 479
—, granulomatöse Reaktion auf unterschiedliche Schädigungen 839
—, Konstruktion 475
—, lamellärer Bautyp 477
—, mikroskopische und submikroskopische Anatomie 461, 474
—, mikroskopische Untersuchung des embryonalen Nagels 348
—, Musculi cutis diagonales 481
—, Musculus sexualis 480
—, normale Histologie 430
—, pathologische Kalkablagerungen 887
—, „Primitivorgan" 788
—, tuberculoide Entzündungen 799
subepidermales Nervengeflecht s. Nervenplexus, subepidermaler

„subepidermal network", vergleichende Anatomie, Blutgefäße der Haut 501, 506, 507, 508, 510
„subfascial network", vergleichende Anatomie, Blutgefäße der Haut 501, 506, 507, 511
Succinyldehydrogenase, altersabhängige Aktivität in der Epidermis 88
—, Arteriolen der Haut, Histochemie 526, 537
—, Basalzellen, Cytochemie 252
—, Blutgefäße der Haut, Histochemie 498
—, Blutgefäßneubildung der Haut, Histochemie 560
—, Cytochemie, myoepitheliale Zellen 235
—, dunkle Zellen, Cytochemie 248
— in der Epidermis, regionäre Unterschiede 88
— in Fettzellen 456
—, helle Zellen, Cytochemie 241
—, Histochemie der Keratinocyten 87
—, — des Musculus arrector pili 481
—, — der Talgdrüsen 196, 202
—, Histotopographie der Keratinocyten 78
—, Kapillaren der Haut, Histochemie 537
—, Lokalisation der Mitochondrien 87
— in Mitochondrien der Keratinocyten 56
—, Nachweis in Fibrocyten von Corium und Subcutis 431
—, Oberflächenzellen, Cytochemie 256
—, Sulfhydrylgruppen in Keratinocyten 72
—, Tropokollagenbildung 433
—, Venolen der Haut, Histochemie 537, 550
Sucquet-Hoyer's arterielles System, fetale Gefäßentwicklung 513
Sucquet-Hoyerscher Kanal, Histologie der Innervation des Nagels 360
Sudanfärbung, Histochemie der Keratinocyten 81
—, Talgdrüsen 197
Sudan III-Färbung, Darstellung von Kristalleinschlüssen in Fettzellen bei Adiponecrosis subcutanea neonatorum 808

Sudan III-Färbung, Differenzierung verschiedener Fettzelltypen 788
—, extracelluläre Cholesterinose Kerl-Urbach 885
—, Kapillaren der Haut 537
— bei Necrobiosis lipoidica 885
Sudan IV-Färbung, Arteriolen der Haut 526
Sudanophilie elastischer Fasern 449
Sudanschwarz-B-Färbung, Arteriolen der Haut 526
—, Esteraseaktivität des Stratum corneum 95
—, Histochemie der Keratinocyten 83
—, Reaktion von Fibrin, Fibrinoid und Hyalin 870
—, Zellmembranen der Intermediärzone 93
Sudanschwarz-Scharlachrot-Färbung bei Angiokeratoma corporis diffusum Fabry 884
Sulfathiazol, medikamentöses Erythema nodosum 836
Sulfat-Inkorporation, Amyloid, Autoradiographie 864
Sulf-Hämoglobin, Vorkommen in der Leiche 731
Sulfhydryl-Gruppen s. -SH-Gruppen
Sulfomucopolysaccharide, Bindegewebsgrundsubstanz, Metachromasie 450
„suprafascial network", vergleichende Anatomie, Blutgefäße der Haut 501, 506, 507, 511
Supronal, medikamentöses Erythema nodosum 836
Sympathicus, Hemmwirkung auf den Fettstoffwechsel 829
—, Schweißdrüsen, ekkrine 262
Synapsen, Innervation der Haut 379, 380, 382
—, sensible Endkörperchen der Haut 418
Synaptische Bläschen, Innervation der Haut 382
— —, Nervenapparat des Haares 410
— —, sensible Endkörperchen der Haut 418
„synaptic vesicles" s. synaptische Bläschen
Synovia, Subcutis 478
Syringomyelie, neurogene Lipome 838
—, neurotrophische Atrophie der Haut 792

Tabes dorsalis, neurotrophische Atrophie der Haut 792
Tätowierungen, Identitätsfeststellung in der frühen Leichenzeit 729
Talg, Enzyme der Hautoberfläche 94
—, RNase-Aktivität 100
Talgdrüsen, Acinus 192
—, —, Basalmembran 192
—, —, undifferenzierte Basalzellen 192
—, äußeres Genitale 218
—, Altersveränderung 695
—, Amyloidablagerung 868
—, Anatomie 184
—, apokrine, fetale Haut, Glykogengehalt 632
—, —, — —, Phosphorylase-Aktivität 632
—, Augenlid 218
—, ausdifferenzierte Zellen 216
—, Brustdrüse 218
—, cell turnover 220
—, Cervix 219
—, Degeneration bei Mucinosis follicularis 880
—, Dichte der Zellen 194
—, ekkrine, fetale Haut, Glykogengehalt 632
—, —, — —, Phosphorylase-Aktivität 632
—, ektopisches Vorkommen 216
—, Elektronenmikroskopie 184, 204
—, endokrine Kontrolle 187
—, Färbemethoden 197
—, foetale Gefäßentwicklung 513
—, freie, des fetalen Haarkomplexes, Anzahl 660
—, —, Volumen in verschiedenen Stadien des Embryonallebens 660
—, Geschlechtsunterschiede der Altersveränderungen 704
—, Goldablagerung 900
—, Golgi-Zonen 195, 200, 205, 209, 215, 216
—, Haarkomplexentwicklung 653
—, Histochemie 184, 195
—, — der Haarkomplexentwicklung 659
—, histochemischer Phosphorylasenachweis 312
—, Histologie 184, 192
—, Innervation 204, 378, 394, 398, 409
— der Kopfhaut, Altersveränderungen an den Arteriolen 700

Talgdrüsen, Langerhans'sche Zellen 195
—, Larynx 219
—, Lippe 217
—, makroskopisches Aussehen apokriner Schweißdrüsen 274
—, Melanocyten 195
—, Mitochondrien 195, 204, 207, 212, 216
—, Monoaminoxydaseaktivität 87
—, morphologische Entwicklung des Haarkomplexes 649, 650, 653
—, Mundschleimhaut 217
—, Musculus arrector pili 481
—, Oesophagus 219
—, perinatales Verhalten 187
—, periphere Zellen 205
—, Plattenepithel, geschichtetes 192, 219
—, Pluripotenz 219
—, Ribonucleoproteine 193
—, Schleimhaut 216
—, Sekretion, holokrine 192
—, Speicheldrüsen 218
—, Talgdrüsengang 192
—, —, Stratum corneum 192
—, teildifferenzierte Zellen 210
—, Tonofilamente 219
— des Tragus, Meßwerte 661
—, Venen der 597
—, Verteilung 184
—, Volumen 185
—, Wachstum und Proliferation 219
—, Zellen, Lipid-produzierende 192
Talgfollikel 192
—, Corynebacterium acnes 192
—, Pityrosporon ovale 192
Talgproduktion, Geschlechts- und Altersunterschiede 187
Tastballen, Embryologie des Nagels 670
Tastempfindung, Bedeutung des Papillarkörpers 469
Tastfasern, Nervenapparat des Haares 407
Tastkörperchen, Innervation der Haut 377, 384, 385, 406, 411, 412, 413, 414, 415, 417, 418, 419
Tastorgane, Feinbau in der Reptilienhaut 996, 997
Tela subcutanea s. Subcutis
Telogen, Strukturveränderungen des Haarfollikels 158, 160, 162
Telogenhaare, Haarwurzelstatus 163

Terminalfasern, gerade 401
—, zirkuläre 401
Terminalhaar, Innervation 400
Testosteron, direkte Wirkung auf apokrine Schweißdrüsen 330
—, Einfluß auf Glatzenbildung bei Vögeln 1014
Tetanus, postmortale Hyperthermie 709
Tetrachlorkohlenstoff, postmortale percutane Resorption 779
Thermoregulation, Anastomosen, arteriovenöse, der Haut 552
—, Beziehungen zum physiologischen Farbwechsel bei Reptilien 994
— der Haut, Mechanismus bei Vögeln 1000
— — bei Reptilien 994
—, zentral-nervöse Regulation bei Reptilien 995
Thesaurismosis lipoidica hereditaria, Klinik und Histologie 884
Thiaminpyrophosphatase, histochemischer Nachweis in apokrinen Schweißdrüsen 324
Thioaminosäuren, Einbau in die Haarwurzelzellen 175
Thioflavin T, Amyloid-Nachweis 864
Thionin-Weinsteinsäure-Einschlußfärbung bei Histiocytose und Xanthogranulomatose 883
Thiouracil, Einfluß auf die Reptilienhäutung 990
Thrombangiitis obliterans, Patho-Histologie der Periarteriitis nodosa cutanea 811
— —, Spontanpanniculitis Typ Pfeifer-Weber-Christian 802
Thyreoidektomie, Lipogranulombildung 840
Thyreotoxikose, Veränderungen des mesodermalen Gewebes beim Embryo 638
Tyrosin, Histotopographie im Haarfollikel 172, 177
—, L-Tyrosin, Melaninsynthese 889
Tyrosinase, Nachweis in weißen Dendritenzellen 106
—, s. auch Phenoloxydase
Tyrosinaseaktivität, Lokalisation 890

Tyrosinase-Reaktion, Darstellung der Melanocyten 114
—, Melaninsynthese 889, 890
Tyrosingehalt der Basalmembran bei Amphibien 975
Thyroxin, Einfluß auf Amphibienhäutung 979
—, — auf das Federwachstum bei Vögeln 1009
—, — auf die Reptilienhäutung 990
—, Wirkung auf die Mastzellen 438
Tierfraß, Veränderungen der Haut in der späten Leichenzeit 734, 736, 737
„tight junction", Keratinocyten, Ultrastruktur 34
„tissue operon", Mitose der Keratinocyten 65
Todesschweiß, Vertrocknungen der Haut 725
Todesursache, Livores 713
Todeszeitbestimmung durch Histologie von Hautverletzungen 758
— durch Livoresmessung 711
— durch Rigormessung 722
— durch Temperaturmessung 709
Toluidinblau-Färbung bei aktinischer Elastose 874
—, Amyloid 863
—, arteriovenöse Anastomosen, Histochemie 556
—, embryonale Fasern 638
—, Fetttröpfchen in Keratinocyten 83
— bei Mucinosen 879
— bei Mucinosis follicularis 880
Tonofibrillen, Keratinisation in der Intermediärzone 18
—, Morphologie der Keratinocyten 36
—, Nagelwachstum 350
—, Struktur der äußeren Wurzelscheide 153
—, Ultrastruktur der fetalen Epidermis 628, 631
—, Verlaufsrichtung 469
„tonofilament-desmosome complex" 40
Tonofilamente, Ultrastruktur der ekkrinen Drüsen 665
Tophi, lokale begünstigende Faktoren 888
—, Patho-Histologie 889
—, Uratnachweis 889
Totenflecke s. Livores
Toutonsche Riesenzellen, Histologie 883
— —, Xanthom 881

TPN-Reductase, Blutgefäße der Haut, Histochemie 498
Tragus des Neugeborenen, Meßwerte der Haarkomplexe 661
„transitional cells" s. Übergangszellen und T-Zellen
„transitional layers", Nomenklatur Intermediärzone 17
„transitional region", Nomenklatur Intermediärzone 17
„transitional zone", Nomenklatur Intermediärzone der Epidermis 17
Transitionsgrade, perifolliculäres Gefäßnetz 588
„transparent chamber technique", Blutgefäße der Haut 558
Transplantat, Blutgefäße der Haut 559
Triglyceride, Biosynthese im Fettgewebe 789
—, ungesättigte, Talgdrüsen 197
Trichohyalin, Elektronenmikroskopie des Haarfollikels 156
—, Haarkomplexentwicklung 655
—, Struktur der inneren Wurzelscheide 150, 151
Trichophytie, Erythema nodosum 836
Trisymptom Gougerot, Patho-Histologie 809
Tropokollagen, Aggregation der Moleküle 442
—, Bildung in Fibroblasten und Fibrocyten 432, 433
—, Kollagenese 441
—, Stoffwechsel in der Bindegewebsgrundsubstanz 451
—, Ultrastruktur der Bindegewebsgrundsubstanz 451
—, Verdickung der Mikrofibrille 443
Trypsin, experimentelle Fettzellnekrose 831
—, Histochemie der Gewebsmastzellen 437
—, Wirkung auf Basalmembran 463
Trypsinverdauung zur Darstellung des Hyalin 869
Tryptophan, Histotopographie im Haarfollikel 172
—, Kapillaren der Haut, Histochemie 537
— -Test 864
—, Venolen der Haut, Histochemie 537

TSH, lipid-mobilisierende Wirkung am menschlichen Fettgewebe 827
Tubarruptur, Livores 714
Tuberkulin-Reaktion, hyperergische Reaktion bei Periarteriitis nodosa cutanea 811
—, Periarteriitis nodosa 837
Tuberkulose, Ätiologie des Erythema nodosum 836
Tubulus, sekretorischer, Schweißdrüsen 230
Tumoren, epitheliale, pathologisches Glykogenvorkommen 886
—, maligne, idiomuskulärer Wulst 722
— des subcutanen Fettgewebes 818
Tunica dartos, Entwicklung des Musculus sexualis 480
— —, Gefäßeinbau 479
— —, Gefäßversorgung 594, 598
— — labialis, glatte Muskulatur 481
— —, postmortale Kontraktionen 723
Turnbullblau-Methode bei Hämochromatose 896
Tween-Esterasen, Kapillaren der Haut, Histochemie 537
—, Venolen der Haut, Histochemie 537, 550
Tween 60-Esterasen, Epidermis, Zusammenhang mit Haarwachstum 95
—, Histochemie der Keratinocyten 92, 95
Tysou's Drüsen 218
T-Zelle, Elektronenmikroskopie, Keratohyalin 48
—, Fibrillenveränderung 40
—, Intermediärzone der Epidermis 18
—, Invagination 19, 20
—, Karyoplasma 61
—, Keratinocytenoberfläche 19
—, Keratohyalin 43
—, Kernstruktur 60
—, Lipide, Histochemie 84
—, normale Histologie der Epidermis 12
—, Planta 14
—, Plasmamembran 22
—, Plasmamembrandicke 23
—, Ribosomen 58
—, Stratum infrabasale 14
—, Transformation und Interzellularraum 25
—, Typenunterscheidung 14
— s. auch Übergangszellen

Ubichinon, histochemischer Nachweis in apokrinen Schweißdrüsen 310, 318, 320
Ubiquinon, Histochemie der Keratinocyten 102
—, Kapillaren der Haut, Histochemie 537
—, Venolen der Haut, Histochemie 537, 550
„Übergangsepithelien", Nomenklatur Intermediärzone der Epidermis 17
Übergangsschichten, Nomenklatur Intermediärzone 17
Übergangszellen, Epidermis 10
— s. auch T-Zellen
Übertragergewebe, Mucopolysaccharide 452
Uhlenhuthsche Präcipitation der Haut, Identitätsfeststellung 729
Ulcus, hypostatisches, Glykogenanreicherung im Gewebe 886
Unna-Tanzer-Livini-Färbung, Blutgefäße der Haut 498
Untergrund-Effekt bei Amphibienlarven 979
— bei Knochenfischen 965
— bei Reptilien 991
— bei Selachiern 947, 950
Unterhautbindegewebe, Reliefbild bei Reptilien 988
Uran, Histochemie der Keratinocyten 66
Uranylacetat, Darstellung epidermaler Fibrillen 40, 51
—, — der Fibrillen 44, 45
—, — der Schichten des Stratum corneum 17
Urate, Ablagerung und Speicherung in der Haut 888
—, Nachweis in den Tophi 889
Uridine-H^3, RNA-Synthese in Keratinocyten 70
Urocanic acid 69
Urogenitalseptum, Anusentwicklung 635
Uroporphyrin, Photosensibilisierung 893
—, Vorkommen in der normalen menschlichen Haut 894
Ursegmente, Embryologie der Haut 673
—, Entwicklung von Corium und Subcutis 637
—, Frühentwicklung der Epidermis 625
Urwirbel, Embryologie der Haut 625, 673

Urwirbel, Mesodermentwicklung 637
UV-Mikrospektrographie, Proteindarstellung in Keratinocyten 67
—, RNA in den Keratinocyten 69
UV-Schiff-Reaktion, Histochemie der Keratinocyten 82, 83

Vacuolen, sekretorische, Ultrastruktur der apokrinen Schweißdrüsen 299
—, Ultrastruktur der apokrinen Schweißdrüsen 299
Vakat-Wucherung, Altersveränderungen des subcutanen Fettgewebes 703
van Gieson-Färbung bei aktinischer Elastose 873
—, Blutgefäße der Haut 498
—, Fremdkörpergranulom 901
—, Hyalinosis cutis et mucosae 870
Vasa vasorum, arteriovenöse Anastomosen 553
Vascular Allergy Harkavy, Patho-Histologie 809, 811
„vascular units" der Hautanhangsgebilde, Morphologie 590, 606
— — —, unterschiedliche Durchmesser 592
Vasculitis, Ätiologie des Erythema nodosum 796
— nodularis, Patho-Histologie 799
— —, —des subcutanen Fettgewebes 795
Vaselinom, Fremdkörpergranulome 901
Vasodilatation, perivaskuläre Nervenfasern 565
Vasokonstriktion, perivaskuläre Nervenfasern 565
Vater-Pacinische Körperchen, Anlage, Nervenentwicklung in der Haut 675
— —, Gefäßversorgung 594
— —, Innervation der Haut 377, 385, 400, 411, 415, 416, 418
Venen der Haut, Altersveränderungen 702
—, elastische Fasern 550
—, Gefäßwand 547
—, Innervation 566
—, Muskelfasern 550
—, Struktur 547, 550
—, Typen 546
—, Venenklappen 550
—, Verteilung in Subcutis und Corium 595
—, terminale 546

Venolen der Haut, Durchmesser 546
— —, elastische Fasern 548
— —, elastische Membran 548
— —, Elektronenmikroskopie 550
— —, Filamente 550
— —, Histochemie 537, 550
— —, Innervation 566
— —, Muskelfasern 548
— —, perivasculäre kollagene Fasern 550
— —, regionäre Unterschiede 598
— —, Struktur 547, 549
— —, Typen 546
— —, Venenklappen 549
Venolen, Patho-Histologie gefäßbedingter Erkrankungen des subcutanen Fettgewebes 808
Verätzungen der Leichenhaut 773
Verbindung, dermo-epidermale, Festigkeitsverlust bei Porphyria cutanea tarda 894
Verbrennung, Verletzungen der Leichenhaut 768
Verbrühung, Hautveränderung an der Leiche 772
Verdoglobin, Vorkommen in der Leiche 731
Vergiftung, postmortale Hyperthermie 709
Verhoeff-Färbung, Blutgefäße der Haut 498
Verhornung, Embryonalentwicklung des Nagels 364
— bei Reptilien 987
—, Struktur des Haarfollikels 154
—, Wachstum der Vogelfeder 1008
Vermoderung, Dekomposition der Haut in der späten Leichenzeit 733
Vernix caseosa, Epidermis des Neugeborenen 636
Versilberung, Basalmembran 462
Verruca seborrhoica, Keratohyalinbildung 49
— vulgaris, Fetttröpfchen in Keratinocyten 83
Verwesung, Dekomposition der Haut in der späten Leichenzeit 733
Vibices, postmortale Rhexisblutungen 715
Vibrationssinn bei Vögeln 1005

Vitamin A, Abhängigkeit der Epidermisdifferenzierung bei Vögeln 998
—, Carotinosis 898
— -Mangel, Keratohyalinbildung 56
Vitamin C, Wirkung auf die Proteinsynthese in Keratinocyten 70
—, — auf die RNA-Synthese in Keratinocyten 70
Vitamine, Einfluß auf Mucingehalt der Haut 877
Vitaminmangel und Inanitionsatrophie des Fettgewebes der Haut 791
Vitiligo, Langhans-Zelle 116
Vitiligoherde, Melanocytenzahl 691
Vögel, Haut der, vergleichende Histologie 997
Vogelhaut, Corium der 999
—, Epidermis der 998
—, Subcutis der 999, 1001

Wachstumshormon und Lipogenese 827
Wärmekontraktur an der Brandleiche 771
Wangenhaut, Musculus cutis diagonalis 481
Warburg-Ferment s. Cytochromoxydase 85
Waschhaut, zeitliche Verhältnisse der Entstehung 743
Waschhautbildung, Saponifikation der Leichenhaut 741
Wassermannsche Fettorgane, normale Histologie von Corium und Subcutis 455
— —, Subcutis 475
Wasserleiche, Abhängigkeit der Veränderungen von der Wassertemperatur 744
—, Hautveränderungen der späten Leichenzeit 741
—, Schätzung der Zeit des Wasseraufenthaltes nach Hautveränderungen 742
—, Treibverletzungen 747
Wasserretention im Fettgewebe 459
Weigert-Färbung, Blutgefäße der Haut 498
Weigertsche Resorcinfärbung bei Mucinosen 879
Werner-Syndrom, Fettgewebsatrophie der Haut 793
Wiederbelebungsversuche, Hautvertrocknung nach agonaler Verletzung 727
Wimperhaare, Entwicklungsmechanik der Haut 643

Wimpern, Fehlen von Haarbalgmuskeln 657
Wirbelbildungen bei Vogelfedern 1014
Wismuthvergiftung, Mumifikation 740
Wucheratrophie des subcutanen Fettgewebes 794
Wulst, elastische Fasern, Haarkomplexentwicklung 653
—, Haarkomplexentwicklung 653
Wundheilung, Blutgefäße der Haut 558
—, histochemische Veränderungen 754
—, intraepidermaler Schweißdrüsen-Ausführungsgang 258
—, Kollagenfaserbildung 443
—, Mastzellen und Bindegewebsgrundsubstanz 453
—, modulationsfähige Epithelien 642
Wundränder bei Ausschußverletzungen 767
— -Retraktion, vitale Reaktion 763
Wurzelfüßchen, korio-epidermale Verknüpfung 2
Wurzelscheide, äußere, embryonale Haarkomplexentwicklung 652
—, —, fetale Haut, Glykogengehalt 632
—, —, — —, Phosphorylase-Aktivität 632
—, —, Struktur des Haarfollikels 152
—, fibröse, Haarkomplexentwicklung 653
—, Haar, enzymatischer Abbau bei der Haarkomplexentwicklung 656
—, —, Innervation der Haut 386, 401, 402
—, Haarkomplexentwicklung 655
—, Haarwurzelstatus 163
—, innere, Haar der fetalen Haut, Glykogengehalt 632
—, —, — —, Phosphorylase-Aktivität 632
—, —, Struktur des Haarfollikels 150
—, mesodermale, morphologische Entwicklung des Haarkomplexes 649, 650, 653

Xanthogranulomatose, Histologie 882
—, Lipidablagerung in der Haut 881

Xanthom und Glykogenspeicherkrankheit 886
—, Histologie 881
—, Lipidablagerung in der Haut 881
Xanthomatose, normocholesterinämische, disseminierte 881
Xanthomzelle, Elektronenmikroskopie 882
—, Entstehung 881
—, Zerfallsprodukte 882
Xanthophoren bei Amphibienlarven 977
— bei Knochenfischen 964
— in nackten Hautregionen bei Vögeln 1005
— der Reptilienhaut 991
— bei Selachiern 946
Xanthophyll, chemische Konstitution 897
Xanthoproteinreaktion, Reaktion von Fibrin, Fibrinoid und Hyalin 871

Zehe, Subcutiskonstruktion 477
Zehenbeere, Nervenentwicklung in der Haut 674
Zeis-Drüsen 218
Zellen, dunkle, Cytochemie 247
—, —, ekkrine Schweißdrüsen 237, 244, 245
—, —, Elektronenmikroskopie 245
—, —, endoplasmatisches Reticulum 245
—, —, Ergastoplasma 245
—, —, Fluoreszenz 247
—, —, Funktion 248
—, —, Glucosamin 248
—, —, Glycoprotein 249
—, —, Golgi-Apparat 245
—, —, Interzellularspalt 245
—, —, „junctional complexes" 245
—, —, Lipide 247
—, —, Microtubuli 247
—, —, Mikrovilli 245
—, —, Mitochondrien 247
—, —, Mucin 248
—, —, Mucopolysaccharide 248
—, —, Natriumrückresorption 248
—, —, Nucleus 245
—, —, Pigment 247
—, —, Plasmamembran 247
—, —, Ribosomen 245
—, —, Schleimzellen 245
—, —, Sekretion 246
—, —, sekretorische Vakuolen 247, 249

Zellen, dunkle, Synthese 245, 248
—, —, Tonizität 248
—, —, Tonofilamente 247
—, —, Vakuolen 246
—, —, Zentriolen 247
—, helle, Anzahl 237
—, —, atrophische 243
—, —, Basalmembran 237
—, —, Cytochemie 241
—, —, Cytoplasma 239
—, —, ekkrine Schweißdrüsen 237
—, —, Elektronenmikroskopie 237
—, —, extrazelluläre Substanzen 237
—, —, Funktion 243
—, —, glattes endoplasmatisches Reticulum 240
—, —, Glykogen 239, 241
—, —, Golgi-Apparat 241
—, —, interstitielle Flüssigkeiten 243
—, —, Interzellularspalt 237
—, —, interzelluläre Kanälchen 237
—, —, intrazelluläre Kanälchen 237, 243
—, —, „junctional complexes" 237
—, —, Lipideinschlüsse 240
—, —, Lipofuscin 241
—, —, Melanocyten-Darstellung 106
—, —, Membranfluß 243
—, —, Mikrotubuli 241
—, —, Mikrovilli 237
—, —, Mitochondrien 238, 240
—, —, mitotische Aktivität 237
—, —, Nucleus 240
—, —, Plasmamembran 238
—, —, rauhes endoplasmatisches Reticulum 241
—, myoepitheliale, Abstammung 280
—, —, acidophile 235
—, —, anisotrope 235
—, —, Basalmembran 232
—, —, Cytochemie 235
—, —, Desmosomen 232
—, —, Elektronenmikroskopie 231
—, —, Esterasen, Cytochemie 236
—, —, Fibrocyten 232
—, —, Funktion 236
—, —, glattes endoplasmatisches Reticulum 232
—, —, Glykogengranula 232
—, —, Golgi-Apparat 233
—, —, Impulsübertragung 236

Zellen, myoepitheliale,
kollagene Fasern
232
—, —, Kontraktion 236
—, —, Lipide 233
—, —, Lipofuscin 233, 236
—, —, Lysosomen 234
—, —, marklose Nervenfasern
232
—, —, Mitochondrien 232
—, —, Muskulatur der Haut
482
—, —, Myofilamente 232, 234
—, —, Pigmente 233
—, —, Pinozytose-Aktivität
236
—, —, Plasmamembran 232
—, —, Proteinsynthese 236
—, —, rauhes endoplasmatisches Retikulum 233

Zellen, myoepitheliale,
Receptoren 236
—, —, Sekretion 236
—, —, Zellteilung 236
Zellgrenze der Epidermiszellen
20
— der fetalen Epidermis 628
—, Plasmamembran 22
Zellmembran der Keratinocyten, ATPase-Aktivität
99
—, Ultrastruktur apokriner
Drüsenzellen 287
Zell-Regeneration, Epidermis
61
Zelltod, Autolyse der Leichenhaut 721
Zementsubstanz, amorphe,
Elektronenmikroskopie des
Haarfollikels 155

Zentriole, Beziehung zum
Golgi-Apparat 59
—, Morphologie der Keratinocyten 59
Zifferblattmotiv, Embryonalentwicklung ekkriner Drüsen 663
Zink, Histochemie der Keratinocyten 66
Zirkonium, Fremdkörpergranulom der Haut
900
Zone, keratogene, Haarwurzelstatus 163
—, —, Strukturveränderungen
des Haarfollikels 158
,,zonula occludens", Keratinocyten, Ultrastruktur 34
Zungenepithel, Plasmamembran 22

SONDERDRUCK AUS
HANDBUCH DER HAUT- UND GESCHLECHTSKRANKHEITEN
J. JADASSOHN

ERGÄNZUNGSWERK

HERAUSGEGEBEN GEMEINSAM MIT
R. DOEPFMER · O. GANS · H. GÖTZ · H. A. GOTTRON · J. KIMMIG
A. LEINBROCK · G. MIESCHER† · TH. NASEMANN · H. RÖCKL · C. G. SCHIRREN
U. W. SCHNYDER · H. SCHUERMANN† · H. W. SPIER · G. K. STEIGLEDER
H. STORCK · A. WIEDMANN

VON

A. MARCHIONINI†

SCHRIFTLEITUNG

C. G. SCHIRREN

ERSTER BAND / ERSTER TEIL
NORMALE UND PATHOLOGISCHE ANATOMIE DER HAUT I
HERAUSGEGEBEN VON

O. GANS UND G. K. STEIGLEDER

SPRINGER-VERLAG / BERLIN · HEIDELBERG · NEW YORK
(PRINTED IN GERMANY)

THE EPIDERMIS

BY

ISSER BRODY

WITH 54 FIGURES

SONDERDRUCK AUS

HANDBUCH DER HAUT- UND GESCHLECHTSKRANKHEITEN

J. JADASSOHN

ERGÄNZUNGSWERK

HERAUSGEGEBEN GEMEINSAM MIT
R. DOEPFMER · O. GANS · H. GÖTZ · H. A. GOTTRON · J. KIMMIG
A. LEINBROCK · G. MIESCHER† · TH. NASEMANN · H. RÖCKL · C. G. SCHIRREN
U. W. SCHNYDER · H. SCHUERMANN† · H. W. SPIER · G. K. STEIGLEDER
H. STORCK · A. WIEDMANN

VON

A. MARCHIONINI †

SCHRIFTLEITUNG
C. G. SCHIRREN

ERSTER BAND / ERSTER TEIL

NORMALE UND PATHOLOGISCHE ANATOMIE DER HAUT I

HERAUSGEGEBEN VON
O. GANS UND G. K. STEIGLEDER

SPRINGER-VERLAG / BERLIN · HEIDELBERG · NEW YORK
(PRINTED IN GERMANY)

HISTOLOGIE, HISTOCHEMIE UND WACHSTUMSDYNAMIK DES HAARFOLLIKELS

VON

HANSOTTO ZAUN

MIT 20 ABBILDUNGEN, DAVON 2 FARBIGE

SONDERDRUCK AUS
HANDBUCH DER HAUT- UND GESCHLECHTSKRANKHEITEN
J. JADASSOHN

ERGÄNZUNGSWERK

HERAUSGEGEBEN GEMEINSAM MIT

R. DOEPFMER · O. GANS · H. GÖTZ · H. A. GOTTRON · J. KIMMIG
A. LEINBROCK · G. MIESCHER† · TH. NASEMANN · H. RÖCKL · C. G. SCHIRREN
U. W. SCHNYDER · H. SCHUERMANN† · H. W. SPIER · G. K. STEIGLEDER
H. STORCK · A. WIEDMANN

VON

A. MARCHIONINI †

SCHRIFTLEITUNG
C. G. SCHIRREN

ERSTER BAND / ERSTER TEIL
NORMALE UND PATHOLOGISCHE ANATOMIE DER HAUT I

HERAUSGEGEBEN VON
O. GANS UND G. K. STEIGLEDER

SPRINGER-VERLAG / BERLIN · HEIDELBERG · NEW YORK
(PRINTED IN GERMANY)

HISTOLOGY, HISTOCHEMISTRY AND ELECTRON MICROSCOPY OF SEBACEOUS GLANDS IN MAN

BY

J. S. STRAUSS and P. E. POCHI

WITH 22 FIGURES

SONDERDRUCK AUS
HANDBUCH DER HAUT- UND GESCHLECHTSKRANKHEITEN
J. JADASSOHN
ERGÄNZUNGSWERK

HERAUSGEGEBEN GEMEINSAM MIT
R. DOEPFMER · O. GANS · H. GÖTZ · H. A. GOTTRON · J. KIMMIG
A. LEINBROCK · G. MIESCHER† · TH. NASEMANN · H. RÖCKL · C. G. SCHIRREN
U. W. SCHNYDER · H. SCHUERMANN† · H. W. SPIER · G. K. STEIGLEDER
H. STORCK · A. WIEDMANN
VON
A. MARCHIONINI†

SCHRIFTLEITUNG
C. G. SCHIRREN

ERSTER BAND / ERSTER TEIL
NORMALE UND PATHOLOGISCHE ANATOMIE DER HAUT I
HERAUSGEGEBEN VON
O. GANS UND G. K. STEIGLEDER

SPRINGER-VERLAG / BERLIN · HEIDELBERG · NEW YORK
(PRINTED IN GERMANY)

ECCRINE SWEAT GLANDS: ELECTRON MICROSCOPY CYTOCHEMISTRY AND ANATOMY

BY

RICHARD A. ELLIS

WITH 23 FIGURES

SONDERDRUCK AUS
HANDBUCH DER HAUT- UND GESCHLECHTSKRANKHEITEN
J. JADASSOHN

ERGÄNZUNGSWERK

HERAUSGEGEBEN GEMEINSAM MIT
R. DOEPFMER · O. GANS · H. GÖTZ · H. A. GOTTRON · J. KIMMIG
A. LEINBROCK · G. MIESCHER† · TH. NASEMANN · H. RÖCKL · C. G. SCHIRREN
U. W. SCHNYDER · H. SCHUERMANN† · H. W. SPIER · G. K. STEIGLEDER
H. STORCK · A. WIEDMANN

VON

A. MARCHIONINI †

SCHRIFTLEITUNG

C. G. SCHIRREN

ERSTER BAND / ERSTER TEIL
NORMALE UND PATHOLOGISCHE ANATOMIE DER HAUT I
HERAUSGEGEBEN VON

O. GANS UND G. K. STEIGLEDER

SPRINGER-VERLAG / BERLIN · HEIDELBERG · NEW YORK
(PRINTED IN GERMANY)

APOKRINE SCHWEISSDRÜSEN

VON

OTTO BRAUN-FALCO

MIT 46 ABBILDUNGEN, DAVON 1 FARBIG

SONDERDRUCK AUS
HANDBUCH DER HAUT- UND GESCHLECHTSKRANKHEITEN
J. JADASSOHN

ERGÄNZUNGSWERK

HERAUSGEGEBEN GEMEINSAM MIT
R. DOEPFMER · O. GANS · H. GÖTZ · H. A. GOTTRON · J. KIMMIG
A. LEINBROCK · G. MIESCHER† · TH. NASEMANN · H. RÖCKL · C. G. SCHIRREN
U. W. SCHNYDER · H. SCHUERMANN† · H. W. SPIER · G. K. STEIGLEDER
H. STORCK · A. WIEDMANN

VON

A. MARCHIONINI†

SCHRIFTLEITUNG
C. G. SCHIRREN

ERSTER BAND / ERSTER TEIL
NORMALE UND PATHOLOGISCHE ANATOMIE DER HAUT I

HERAUSGEGEBEN VON
O. GANS UND G. K. STEIGLEDER

SPRINGER-VERLAG / BERLIN · HEIDELBERG · NEW YORK
(PRINTED IN GERMANY)

NORMALE HISTOLOGIE UND HISTOCHEMIE DES NAGELS

VON

GEORGES ACHTEN

MIT 34 ABBILDUNGEN

SONDERDRUCK AUS

HANDBUCH DER HAUT- UND GESCHLECHTSKRANKHEITEN

J. JADASSOHN

ERGÄNZUNGSWERK

HERAUSGEGEBEN GEMEINSAM MIT

R. DOEPFMER · O. GANS · H. GÖTZ · H. A. GOTTRON · J. KIMMIG
A. LEINBROCK · G. MIESCHER† · TH. NASEMANN · H. RÖCKL · C. G. SCHIRREN
U. W. SCHNYDER · H. SCHUERMANN† · H. W. SPIER · G. K. STEIGLEDER
H. STORCK · A. WIEDMANN

VON

A. MARCHIONINI†

SCHRIFTLEITUNG

C. G. SCHIRREN

ERSTER BAND / ERSTER TEIL

NORMALE UND PATHOLOGISCHE ANATOMIE DER HAUT I

HERAUSGEGEBEN VON

O. GANS UND G. K. STEIGLEDER

SPRINGER-VERLAG / BERLIN · HEIDELBERG · NEW YORK
(PRINTED IN GERMANY)

ZUR INNERVATION DER HAUT

VON

E. HAGEN

MIT 47 ABBILDUNGEN

SONDERDRUCK AUS
HANDBUCH DER HAUT- UND GESCHLECHTSKRANKHEITEN
J. JADASSOHN

ERGÄNZUNGSWERK

HERAUSGEGEBEN GEMEINSAM MIT
R. DOEPFMER · O. GANS · H. GÖTZ · H. A. GOTTRON · J. KIMMIG
A. LEINBROCK · G. MIESCHER† · TH. NASEMANN · H. RÖCKL · C. G. SCHIRREN
U. W. SCHNYDER · H. SCHUERMANN† · H. W. SPIER · G. K. STEIGLEDER
H. STORCK · A. WIEDMANN

VON

A. MARCHIONINI †

SCHRIFTLEITUNG
C. G. SCHIRREN

ERSTER BAND / ERSTER TEIL
NORMALE UND PATHOLOGISCHE ANATOMIE DER HAUT I

HERAUSGEGEBEN VON
O. GANS UND G. K. STEIGLEDER

SPRINGER-VERLAG / BERLIN · HEIDELBERG · NEW YORK
(PRINTED IN GERMANY)

DIE NORMALE HISTOLOGIE VON CORIUM UND SUBCUTIS

VON

WOLFGANG SCHMIDT

MIT 22 ABBILDUNGEN

SONDERDRUCK AUS
HANDBUCH DER HAUT- UND GESCHLECHTSKRANKHEITEN
J. JADASSOHN

ERGÄNZUNGSWERK

HERAUSGEGEBEN GEMEINSAM MIT
R. DOEPFMER · O. GANS · H. GÖTZ · H. A. GOTTRON · J. KIMMIG
A. LEINBROCK · G. MIESCHER† · TH. NASEMANN · H. RÖCKL · C. G. SCHIRREN
U. W. SCHNYDER · H. SCHUERMANN† · H. W. SPIER · G. K. STEIGLEDER
H. STORCK · A. WIEDMANN

VON

A. MARCHIONINI†

SCHRIFTLEITUNG
C. G. SCHIRREN

ERSTER BAND / ERSTER TEIL
NORMALE UND PATHOLOGISCHE ANATOMIE DER HAUT I

HERAUSGEGEBEN VON
O. GANS UND G. K. STEIGLEDER

SPRINGER-VERLAG / BERLIN · HEIDELBERG · NEW YORK
(PRINTED IN GERMANY)

THE BLOOD VESSELS OF THE SKIN

BY

GUISEPPE MORETTI

WITH 165 FIGURES. THEREOF 10 IN COLOUR

SONDERDRUCK AUS
HANDBUCH DER HAUT- UND GESCHLECHTSKRANKHEITEN
J. JADASSOHN
ERGÄNZUNGSWERK

HERAUSGEGEBEN GEMEINSAM MIT
R. DOEPFMER · O. GANS · H. GÖTZ · H. A. GOTTRON · J. KIMMIG
A. LEINBROCK · G. MIESCHER† · TH. NASEMANN · H. RÖCKL · C. G. SCHIRREN
U. W. SCHNYDER · H. SCHUERMANN† · H. W. SPIER · G. K. STEIGLEDER
H. STORCK · A. WIEDMANN
VON
A. MARCHIONINI †

SCHRIFTLEITUNG
C. G. SCHIRREN

ERSTER BAND / ERSTER TEIL
NORMALE UND PATHOLOGISCHE ANATOMIE DER HAUT I
HERAUSGEGEBEN VON
O. GANS UND G. K. STEIGLEDER
SPRINGER-VERLAG / BERLIN · HEIDELBERG · NEW YORK
(PRINTED IN GERMANY)

EMBRYOLOGIE DER HAUT

VON

HERMANN PINKUS u. **ANTOINETTE TANAY**

MIT 37 ABBILDUNGEN

SONDERDRUCK AUS
HANDBUCH DER HAUT- UND GESCHLECHTSKRANKHEITEN
J. JADASSOHN

ERGÄNZUNGSWERK

HERAUSGEGEBEN GEMEINSAM MIT

R. DOEPFMER · O. GANS · H. GÖTZ · H. A. GOTTRON · J. KIMMIG
A. LEINBROCK · G. MIESCHER† · TH. NASEMANN · H. RÖCKL · C. G. SCHIRREN
U. W. SCHNYDER · H. SCHUERMANN† · H. W. SPIER · G. K. STEIGLEDER
H. STORCK · A. WIEDMANN

VON

A. MARCHIONINI†

SCHRIFTLEITUNG

C. G. SCHIRREN

ERSTER BAND / ERSTER TEIL
NORMALE UND PATHOLOGISCHE ANATOMIE DER HAUT I
HERAUSGEGEBEN VON

O. GANS UND G. K. STEIGLEDER

SPRINGER-VERLAG / BERLIN · HEIDELBERG · NEW YORK
(PRINTED IN GERMANY)

DIE ALTERSVERÄNDERUNGEN DER HAUT

VON

H. J. CRAMER

MIT 7 ABBILDUNGEN

SONDERDRUCK AUS
HANDBUCH DER HAUT- UND GESCHLECHTSKRANKHEITEN
J. JADASSOHN

ERGÄNZUNGSWERK

HERAUSGEGEBEN GEMEINSAM MIT
R. DOEPFMER · O. GANS · H. GÖTZ · H. A. GOTTRON · J. KIMMIG
A. LEINBROCK · G. MIESCHER† · TH. NASEMANN · H. RÖCKL · C. G. SCHIRREN
U. W. SCHNYDER · H. SCHUERMANN† · H. W. SPIER · G. K. STEIGLEDER
H. STORCK · A. WIEDMANN

VON

A. MARCHIONINI †

SCHRIFTLEITUNG

C. G. SCHIRREN

ERSTER BAND / ERSTER TEIL
NORMALE UND PATHOLOGISCHE ANATOMIE DER HAUT I

HERAUSGEGEBEN VON

O. GANS UND G. K. STEIGLEDER

SPRINGER-VERLAG / BERLIN · HEIDELBERG · NEW YORK
(PRINTED IN GERMANY)

HAUTVERÄNDERUNGEN AN LEICHEN

VON

G. DOTZAUER u. L. TAMÁSKA

MIT 22 ABBILDUNGEN, DAVON 5 FARBIG

SONDERDRUCK AUS
HANDBUCH DER HAUT- UND GESCHLECHTSKRANKHEITEN
J. JADASSOHN

ERGÄNZUNGSWERK

HERAUSGEGEBEN GEMEINSAM MIT
R. DOEPFMER · O. GANS · H. GÖTZ · H. A. GOTTRON · J. KIMMIG
A. LEINBROCK · G. MIESCHER† · TH. NASEMANN · H. RÖCKL · C. G. SCHIRREN
U. W. SCHNYDER · H. SCHUERMANN† · H. W. SPIER · G. K. STEIGLEDER
H. STORCK · A. WIEDMANN

VON

A. MARCHIONINI †

SCHRIFTLEITUNG

C. G. SCHIRREN

ERSTER BAND / ERSTER TEIL
NORMALE UND PATHOLOGISCHE ANATOMIE DER HAUT I

HERAUSGEGEBEN VON

O. GANS UND G. K. STEIGLEDER

SPRINGER-VERLAG / BERLIN · HEIDELBERG · NEW YORK
(PRINTED IN GERMANY)

ALLGEMEINE PATHOLOGIE DES FETTGEWEBES

VON

GÜNTER EHLERS

MIT 15 ABBILDUNGEN

SONDERDRUCK AUS
HANDBUCH DER HAUT- UND GESCHLECHTSKRANKHEITEN
J. JADASSOHN

ERGÄNZUNGSWERK

HERAUSGEGEBEN GEMEINSAM MIT

R. DOEPFMER · O. GANS · H. GÖTZ · H. A. GOTTRON · J. KIMMIG
A. LEINBROCK · G. MIESCHER† · TH. NASEMANN · H. RÖCKL · C. G. SCHIRREN
U. W. SCHNYDER · H. SCHUERMANN† · H. W. SPIER · G. K. STEIGLEDER
H. STORCK · A. WIEDMANN

VON

A. MARCHIONINI †

SCHRIFTLEITUNG
C. G. SCHIRREN

ERSTER BAND / ERSTER TEIL
NORMALE UND PATHOLOGISCHE ANATOMIE DER HAUT I
HERAUSGEGEBEN VON
O. GANS UND G. K. STEIGLEDER

SPRINGER-VERLAG / BERLIN · HEIDELBERG · NEW YORK
(PRINTED IN GERMANY)

ABLAGERUNG UND SPEICHERUNG IN DER CUTIS

VON

CHRISTOPH EBERHARTINGER, HERWIG EBNER u. GUSTAV NIEBAUER

SONDERDRUCK AUS
HANDBUCH DER HAUT- UND GESCHLECHTSKRANKHEITEN
J. JADASSOHN

ERGÄNZUNGSWERK

HERAUSGEGEBEN GEMEINSAM MIT
R. DOEPFMER · O. GANS · H. GÖTZ · H. A. GOTTRON · J. KIMMIG
A. LEINBROCK · G. MIESCHER† · TH. NASEMANN · H. RÖCKL · C. G. SCHIRREN
U. W. SCHNYDER · H. SCHUERMANN† · H. W. SPIER · G. K. STEIGLEDER
H. STORCK · A. WIEDMANN

VON

A. MARCHIONINI †

SCHRIFTLEITUNG
C. G. SCHIRREN

ERSTER BAND / ERSTER TEIL
NORMALE UND PATHOLOGISCHE ANATOMIE DER HAUT I
HERAUSGEGEBEN VON
O. GANS UND G. K. STEIGLEDER

SPRINGER-VERLAG / BERLIN · HEIDELBERG · NEW YORK
(PRINTED IN GERMANY)

VERGLEICHENDE HISTOLOGIE DER HAUT

VON

H. U. KOECKE

MIT 21 ABBILDUNGEN